Canine *and* Feline Cytopathology

A COLOR ATLAS AND INTERPRETATION GUIDE

4th EDITION

Canine *and* Feline Cytopathology

A COLOR ATLAS AND INTERPRETATION GUIDE

Rose E. Raskin, DVM, PhD, DACVP, MRCVS
Professor Emerita of Veterinary Clinical Pathology
College of Veterinary Medicine
Purdue University
West Lafayette, Indiana

Denny J. Meyer, DVM, DACVP, DACVIM (SAIM)
Veterinary Clinical Pathologist and Small Animal Internist
Lauderdale-by-the-Sea, Florida

Katie M. Boes, DVM, MS, DACVP
Clinical Pathologist
Antech Diagnostics
Blacksburg, Virginia

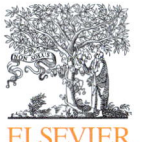
ELSEVIER

Elsevier
3251 Riverport Lane
St. Louis, Missouri 63043

CANINE AND FELINE CYTOPATHOLOGY: A COLOR ATLAS
AND INTERPRETATION GUIDE, FOURTH EDITION

ISBN: 978-0-323-68368-5

Copyright © 2023 by Elsevier, Inc. All rights reserved.

No part of this publication may be reproduced or transmitted in any form or by any means, electronic or mechanical, including photocopying, recording, or any information storage and retrieval system, without permission in writing from the publisher. Details on how to seek permission, further information about the Publisher's permissions policies and our arrangements with organizations such as the Copyright Clearance Center and the Copyright Licensing Agency, can be found at our website: www.elsevier.com/permissions.

This book and the individual contributions contained in it are protected under copyright by the Publisher (other than as may be noted herein).

Notice

Practitioners and researchers must always rely on their own experience and knowledge in evaluating and using any information, methods, compounds or experiments described herein. Because of rapid advances in the medical sciences, in particular, independent verification of diagnoses and drug dosages should be made. To the fullest extent of the law, no responsibility is assumed by Elsevier, authors, editors or contributors for any injury and/or damage to persons or property as a matter of products liability, negligence or otherwise, or from any use or operation of any methods, products, instructions, or ideas contained in the material herein.

Previous editions copyrighted © 2016, 2010, and 2001.

Library of Congress Control Number: 2021942956

Executive Content Strategist: Jennifer Catando
Senior Content Development Specialist: Mary Hegeler
Publishing Services Manager: Catherine Jackson
Senior Project Manager/Specialist: Carrie Stetz
Design Direction: Renee Duenow

Printed in India

Last digit is the print number: 9 8 7 6 5 4 3 2 1

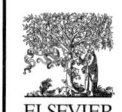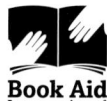

CONTRIBUTORS

Julie Allen, BVMS, MS, DACVIM, DACVP
Veterinary Information Network
Davis, California

Tara Arndt, DVM, Cert LAM, Dip LAS (Path), DACVP
Senior Clinical Pathologist
Labcorp Drug Development
Madison, Wisconsin

Anne M. Barger, DVM, MS, DACVP
Clinical Professor
Veterinary Clinical Medicine
University of Illinois
Urbana, Illinois

Katie M. Boes, DVM, MS, DACVP
Clinical Pathologist
Antech Diagnostics
Blacksburg, Virginia

Ul-Soo Choi, DVM, PhD
Professor
Veterinary Clinical Pathology
College of Veterinary Medicine, Chonbuk National University
Iksan si, Republic of Korea

Francisco O. Conrado, DVM, MSc, DACVP
Assistant Professor of Clinical Pathology
Biomedical Sciences
Cummings School of Veterinary Medicine at Tufts University
North Grafton, Massachusetts

Pierre Lucien Deshuillers, DVM, MS, PhD, DACVP
Associate Professor of Clinical Pathology
Départment des Sciences Biologiques et Pharmaceutiques
Ecole Nationale Vétérinaire d'Alfort
Maisons-Alfort, France

Kristin J. Fisher, DVM, MS
Veterinary Clinical Pathologist
Valley Central Veterinary Referral and Emergency Center
Whitehall, Pennsylvania

Bente Flatland, DVM, MS, DACVIM, DACVP
Professor and Clinical Pathology Laboratory Director
Biomedical and Diagnostic Sciences
College of Veterinary Medicine
University of Tennessee
Knoxville, Tennessee

Maria Elena Gelain, DVM, PhD, DECVCP
Professor
Dipartimento di Biomedicina Comparata e Alimentazione
University of Padua
Padua, Italy

Jessica Anne Hokamp, DVM, PhD, DACVP
Assistant Professor of Veterinary Biosciences
The Ohio State University
Columbus, Ohio

Shannon Jones Hostetter, DVM, PhD, DACVP
Associate Professor
University of Georgia
Athens, Georgia

Davide De Lorenzi, PhD, DECVCP, SCMPA
AniCura Veterinary Hospital "I Portoni Rossi"
Veterinary Laboratory
Cytopathology Unit
Zola Predosa, Italy

Carlo Masserdotti, DVM, DECVCP, Spec Bioch Clin
Consultant in Clinical Pathology
Laboratorio Veterinario San Marco
Padua, Italy

Denny J. Meyer, DVM, DACVP, DACVIM (SAIM)
Veterinary Clinical Pathologist and Small Animal Internist
Lauderdale-by-the-Sea, Florida

Laureen M. Peters, DVM, MVM, MRCVS, FHEA, DACVP
Lecturer in Veterinary Clinical Pathology
Department of Pathobiology and Population Sciences
The Royal Veterinary College
Hatfield, United Kingdom

Laura Pintore, DVM, PhD DECVCP
Specialist in Veterinary Clinical Pathology
Malpensa AniCura Veterinary Clinic
Samarate, Italy

José A. Ramos-Vara, DVM, PhD, DECVP
Professor of Comparative Pathobiology–ADDL
College of Veterinary Medicine
Purdue University
West Lafayette, Indiana

Rose E. Raskin, DVM, PhD, DACVP, MRCVS
Professor Emerita of Veterinary Clinical Pathology
College of Veterinary Medicine
Purdue University
West Lafayette, Indiana

Davis M. Seelig, DVM, PhD, DACVP
Associate Professor of Veterinary Clinical Sciences
College of Veterinary Medicine
University of Minnesota
St. Paul, Minnesota

Laura Snyder, DVM, DACVP
Clinical Pathologist
Companion Animal Group
IDEXX Laboratories
Westbrook, Maine

Laia Solano-Gallego, DVM, PhD, DECVCP
Professor
Department of Animal Medicine and Surgery
College of Veterinary Medicine
Autonomous University of Barcelona
Barcelona, Spain

From Rose:
I dedicate this fourth edition to my fellow cytopathologists and veterinary colleagues around the world who have shared comments and materials to further improve and expand each edition of this textbook over the 20 years of its existence. Thank you also for your friendship.

To my family and friends, who remain my source of emotional strength. To my girlfriend Sherill since childhood, who is like a sister to me; I am grateful for your friendship. Love to my daughter Hannah, brother Richard, and stepson James, who all give me a sense of life's purpose.

From Denny:
To my wife of 51 years, and to the Antonacci and Meyer families—Booyah! You are my life's symphony. Let the music continue.

From Katie:
To the two who gave me life and the three who give life meaning. I am forever grateful for the love, lessons, and support from my mom, dad, husband, and daughters. Mom, your discipline and work ethic still surpass my own. Dad, thank you for sharing your love of animals, nature, and science. Eddie, your genuine goodness, zeal, and creativity always inspire me.

To my mentors who endured my naivety. Rose, Craig, Joanne, John, Dennis, and Alan, I hope to faithfully convey your knowledge, patience, and enthusiasm to new generations of veterinarians.

To my colleagues with shared journeys toward enlightenment in the beautiful art of veterinary pathology.

From all Editors:
To all the veterinary students, residents, and practitioners who have touched our lives and made us feel that what we do is worthwhile: you give us purpose, and we thank you.

People Touch Our Lives—Bits and Pieces
People important to you, people unimportant to you,
cross our life, touch it with love and carelessness and move on.
There are people that leave you, and you breathe a sigh of relief,
and you wonder why you ever came in contact with them.
There are people who leave, and you breathe a sigh of remorse,
and wonder why they had to go and leave such a gaping hole.
People move in and out of each other's lives,
and each leaves a mark on the other.
You find you are made up of bits and pieces of all who have ever touched your life,
and you are more because of it, and would be less if they had not touched you.
Pray to always accept the bits and pieces in humility and wonder
and never question and never regret.
—*Adapted from the poem "People Touch Our Lives" by Lois A. Cheney*

PREFACE

The fourth edition has been completely revised with expanded content, 700 new images, two new chapters, new quick reference charts, enhanced procedural appendices, additional Key Point callouts, and a distinctive, differentiating title change. Cytopathology is a branch of pathology that studies and diagnoses diseases on the cellular level. The discipline was founded in 1928 by George Nicolas Papanicolaou, for whom the "Pap smear" was named. Dr. Victor (Vic) Perman, one of my (D.J.M.) influential mentors at the College of Veterinary Medicine at the University of Minnesota, published one of the first collages of veterinary cytopathology.[1] Time spent with him at the two-head microscope and encouragement for the expanded use Diff-Quik–stained specimens for diagnosis indelibly "stained" my career, which eventuated to partnering with Rose for the development of this Atlas. I am forever grateful to him and to Rose for her tenacious drive for perfection embodied in this benchmarking fourth edition.

Cytopathology is the use of samples of free cells or tissue fragments for diagnosis, in contrast to histopathology, which studies whole tissue structure. Cytopathology is commonly used to investigate diseases involving a wide range of body sites to aid in the diagnosis of neoplasia, infectious diseases, and immune-mediated and other noninfectious inflammatory conditions. The diagnostic application of cytopathology, a branch of pathology, is historically and less precisely referred to as "cytology," a term that means the study of cells. Cytology encompasses cell metabolism, cell communication, cell cycle, and cell composition. Since the diagnostic specimen is applied to a glass slide directly following aspiration biopsy, collected via exfoliation or following cytocentrifugation of a fluid for subsequent staining and microscopic examination, often using a "smear" technique, in this sense, it is referred to as a *cytologic preparation*. To encourage a better appreciation of the pathology discipline, the term *cytopathology* in this Atlas applies to the disease-related changes of cells, while *cytology* is reserved for the microscopic anatomy of normal cells from the body systems. This is akin to the tissue pathologist's reference to histopathology for diseased tissue sections and histology as a branch of microscopic anatomy.

As in the previous edition, figure legends indicate structure sizes either with internal bars or magnification noted relative to the original objective lens used during image capture. The notations for the objectives are **LP** (low power) for 4× or 10×, **IP** (intermediate power) for 20× or 40×, and **HP oil** (high power oil) for 50×, 60×, or 100× oil immersion.

Readers will appreciate that all photomicrographs in this edition were reviewed meticulously to correct previous chromatic concerns and to improve crispness and clarity, producing a truer representation as is observed microscopically.

We are excited to present the fourth edition and hope it becomes a well-used reference for those engaged in veterinary cytopathology.

Rose, Denny & Katie

---

[1] Perman V, Alsaker RD, Riis RC. *Cytology of the Dog and Cat.* Denver; American Animal Hospital Association; 1979:1–159.

ACKNOWLEDGMENTS

Teamwork = Cooperative effort by the members of a group or team to achieve a common goal.
Achievement = Something accomplished successfully, especially by means of exertion, skill, practice, or perseverance.
Exemplary = Of such high quality that it should serve as an example to be imitated.

—*American Heritage Dictionary, 4th edition*

An Atlas that successfully covers the broad scope of cytopathology could not be completed without the assistance of an editorial staff, many of whom are transparent to us. Thanks to Jennifer Catando, Senior Content Strategist, for suggesting and supporting a fourth edition as well as managing the communications to assist in signing on our 22 chapter authors for the new edition. Noteworthy recognition of folks at Elsevier is extended to Mary Hegeler, Senior Content Development Specialist, who exhibited remarkable patience as we pushed timelines and provided congenial encouragement to successfully meet the publication milestones, particularly during the home office workplace environment necessitated by the COVID-19 pandemic. We wish to acknowledge Elsevier staff for their critical support of efforts to improve chromatically many of the photomicrographs. Lastly, the worker bees of the editing staff in concert with the marketing and production specialists, Kristin Wilhelm and Carrie Stetz, worked adroitly with diligent attention to detail, a noteworthy challenge and accomplishment. Collectively, the team effort produced a significantly revised product of exceptional quality for which we, the editors, are all very excited, pleased, and proud.

Denny and I are thrilled to have worked with Katie Boes, who as a busy Associate Professor at Virginia Tech at the time and mothering a young family, joined our editorial team to review finished chapters and contributed several impactful chapters and a new reference chart of infectious agents. We thank her for bringing her creativity, experience, and diligence to this project.

We wish to express our sincere appreciation to the contributing authors of the fourth edition. They are represented both by the seasoned and the newer, most promising purveyors of cytopathology today. Their collective expertise and extraordinary scholarship have significantly expanded the wealth of information featured in this new edition. They made an exemplary commitment and altruistically added one more burden to their primary professional duties to share their cytopathologic expertise. Thank you for eagerly and successfully partnering with us. We hope you share in our pride with the final product: simply put, it is awesome! Booyah!

We would be remiss if we did not acknowledge the previous contributors whose text and photomicrographs formed the foundation on which many chapters were constructed. Our sincerest gratitude is extended to all the subject matter experts listed below; you're truly the best, thank you.

Rose, Denny & Katie

Acquisition and Management of Cytology Specimens
  Denny J. Meyer (1st–3rd)
  Sara L. Connolly (2nd)
  Hock Gan Heng (2nd)

General Categories of Cytologic Interpretation
  Rose E. Raskin (1st–3rd)

Skin and Subcutaneous Tissues
  Rose E. Raskin (1st–3rd)

Hemolymphatic System
  Rose E. Raskin (1st–3rd)

Respiratory Tract
  Mary Jo Burkhard (1st–3rd)
  Amy Valenciano (1st)
  Anne Barger (1st)
  Laurie M. Millward (2nd)

Body Cavity Fluids
  Sonjia M. Shelly (1st)
  Alan H. Rebar (2nd)
  Craig A. Thompson (2nd–3rd)

Oral Cavity, Gastrointestinal Tract, and Associated Structures
  Claire B. Andreasen (1st–3rd)
  Albert E. Jergens (1st–3rd)
  Denny J. Meyer (1st–2nd)
  Shannon Jones Hostetter (3rd)

Dry-Mount Fecal Cytology
  Heather L. Wamsley (2nd–3rd)
  Amy L. Weeden (3rd)

The Liver
  Denny J. Meyer (1st–3rd)

Urinary Tract
  Dori L. Borjesson (1st–3rd)
  Keith DeJong (2nd–3rd)

Microscopic Examination of the Urinary Sediment
  Denny J. Meyer (1st–3rd)

Reproductive System
  Kristin L. Henson (1st)
  Laia Solano-Gallego (2nd–3rd)
  Carlo Masserdotti (3rd)

Musculoskeletal System
  David J. Fisher (1st)
  Anne M. Barger (2nd–3rd)

Central Nervous System
  Kathleen P. Freeman (1st)
  Rose E. Raskin (1st)
  Davide De Lorenzi (2nd–3rd)
  Maria T. Mandara (2nd–3rd)

Eyes and Adnexa
  Rose E. Raskin (1st–3rd)

Endocrine/Neuroendocrine System
  A. Rick Alleman (1st–2nd)
  Ul Soo Choi (2nd–3rd)
  Tara Arndt (3rd)

Advanced Diagnostic Techniques
  Janice M. Andrews (1st)
  David E. Malarkey (1st)
  José A. Ramos-Vara (2nd–3rd)
  Anne C. Avery (2nd–3rd)
  Paul R. Avery (2nd–3rd)

APPENDICES
  Rose E. Raskin (3rd)

CONTENTS

1 **Acquisition and Management of Cytologic Specimens**, 1
Kristin J. Fisher and Denny J. Meyer
General Sampling Guidelines, 1
Diagnostic Imaging-Guided Sample Collection, 1
Managing the Cytologic Specimen, 3
Staining the Specimen, 10
Submitting Cytology Specimens to a Reference Laboratory, 13

2 **General Categories of Cytologic Interpretation**, 15
Rose E. Raskin
Normal Tissue, 15
Hyperplastic Tissue, 15
Cystic Mass, 15
Inflammation or Cellular Infiltrate, 15
Neoplasia, 22
Common Cell Relationships, 29

3 **Integumentary System**, 35
Rose E. Raskin and Francisco O. Conrado
Normal Histology, 35
Normal Skin Cytology and Artifacts, 35
Noninfectious Inflammatory Disorders, 35
Infectious Inflammatory Disorders, 45
Non-neoplastic Tumors, 61
Neoplastic Tumors, 64
Response to Tissue Injury, 117

4 **Hemolymphatic System**, 124
Rose E. Raskin
General Considerations for Lymphoid Tissues, 124
Lymph Nodes, 124
Spleen, 156
Thymus, 171

5 **Respiratory System**, 182
Katie M. Boes
Nasal Cavity, 182
Larynx, 199
Trachea, Bronchi, and Lungs, 204

6 **Body Cavity Fluids**, 242
Katie M. Boes
Sample Collection and Technique, 242
Fluid Sample Handling, 243
Normal Cytology and Artifacts, 245
Cellular and Fluid Responses to Injury, 247
Peritoneal Effusions, 250
Pleural Effusions, 264
Pericardial Effusions, 269
Neoplastic Effusions, 272
Bicavitary Effusions, 279
Effusion Ancillary Diagnostics, 279

7 **Oral Cavity, Gastrointestinal Tract, and Associated Structures**, 287
Shannon Jones Hostetter
Oral Cavity, 287
Salivary Gland, 292
Esophagus, 296
Gastrointestinal Cytopathology, 301
Stomach, 301
Intestine, 307
Colon, Cecum, and Rectum, 313

8 **Pancreas (Exocrine and Endocrine)**, 322
Julie Allen
Normal Anatomy and Histology, 322
Sample Collection, 322
Normal Cytology and Artifacts, 324
Pancreatic Cystic Lesions, 324
Tissue Injury (Necrosis, Mineralization), 324
Pancreatic Nodular Hyperplasia, 325
Noninfectious Inflammatory Disorders, 325
Infectious Inflammatory Disorders, 329
Miscellaneous Nonneoplastic Tumors, 331
Neoplastic Tumors, 331

9 **Hepatobiliary System**, 339
Laureen M. Peters and Denny J. Meyer
Sample Collection and Technique, 339
Normal Cytology and Artifacts, 340
Responses to Tissue Injury, 341
Inflammation and Infection, 357
Neoplasia, 362

10 **Fecal and Rectal Cytopathology**, 377
Francisco O. Conrado
Sample Collection and Processing, 377
Normal or Incidental Microscopic Findings, 379
Abnormal Microscopic Findings, 381
Fecal Leukocytes, 383
Other Cell Types, 386

11 **Urinary System**, 397
Laura Snyder and Davis Seelig
Kidneys, 397
Ureters, 406
Urinary Bladder and Urethra, 406

12 **Urine**, 414
Jessica Anne Hokamp and Denny J. Meyer
Complete Urinalysis, 414
Urine Collection, 414
Specimen Processing and Slide Preparation, 414
Microscopic Examination and Reporting, 416

13 **Reproductive System**, 440
Laia Solano-Gallego and Carlo Masserdotti
    Female Reproductive System, 440
    Male Reproductive System, 467

14 **Musculoskeletal System**, 485
Anne M. Barger
    Normal Joint Anatomy and Synovial Fluid Production, 485
    Synovial Fluid Evaluation, 485
    Skeletal Muscle, 498
    Bone, 499

15 **Nervous System**, 512
Davide De Lorenzi and Laura Pintore
    Cerebrospinal Fluid, 512
    Cytopathology of Nervous System Tissue, 538

16 **Eyes and Ears**, 558
Pierre L. Deshuillers and Rose E. Raskin
    Eye and Orbital Structures, 558
    Eyelids, 558
    Conjunctivae, 559
    Nictitating Membrane, 565
    Sclera, 567
    Cornea, 567
    Iris, Ciliary Body, and Aqueous Humor, 571
    Retina, 574
    Choroid and Vitreous Body, 575
    Orbital Cavity, 576
    Nasolacrimal Apparatus, 582
    Otic Cytopathology, 582
    External Ear and Pinna, 582
    Middle Ear, 590
    Inner Ear, 592

17 **Endocrine and Neuroendocrine Systems**, 596
Ul-Soo Choi and Tara Arndt
    Thyroid Gland, 596
    Parathyroid Glands, 604
    Extra-Adrenal Paragangliomas, 605
    Adrenal Gland, 607
    Carcinoids, 613
    Summary, 614

18 **Advanced Diagnostic Techniques**, 618
José A. Ramos-Vara and Maria Elena Gelain
    Immunodiagnosis, 618
    Electron Microscopy, 635
    Histochemical Stains, 639
    Flow Cytometry, 642
    Lymphocyte Clonality Testing, 655
    Detection of Translocations, Chromosomal Aberrations, and Gene Mutations, 659

Appendix
1 **Microscope and Telecytopathology Basics**, 665
2 **Selected Stains and Protocols**, 672
3 **Peculiar Findings and Polarizing Materials**, 675
4 **Mitotic Figures and Chromatin Patterns**, 685
5 **Advanced Collection and Preparation Techniques**, 689
6 **Composing Pathology Reports**, 691
7 **Specialized Diagnostic Testing Sites**, 696
8 **Quick Reference for Morphologic Features of Microorganisms**, 700
9 **Quality Management Recommendations for Veterinary Diagnostic Cytopathology Services**, 706

Index, 713

CHAPTER 1

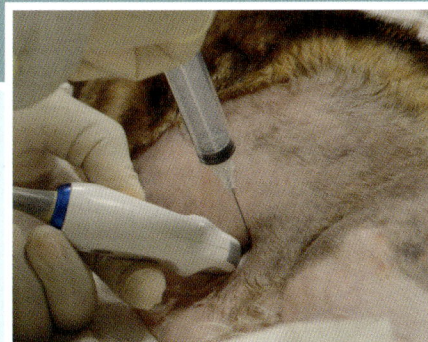

Acquisition and Management of Cytologic Specimens

Kristin J. Fisher and Denny J. Meyer

Management of cytologic specimens is a major factor affecting the accuracy of microscopic examination of tissue. Several successful steps are necessary for accurate results, including acquisition of a representative specimen, proper application to a glass slide, adequate staining, and examination with a high-quality microscope or digital microscopy. The objective of this chapter is to provide general recommendations for managing samples to ensure the most accurate diagnosis.

GENERAL SAMPLING GUIDELINES

Before executing any sampling procedure, a cytology kit should be prepared and dedicated for that purpose. Suggested contents are listed in Box 1.1. Six or more slides are placed on a firm, flat surface such as a surgical tray immediately before initiating the sampling procedure (Fig. 1.1). The surface of the glass slide should be routinely cleaned with a paper towel or laboratory tissue wipe to remove "invisible" glass particles that can interfere with the spreading procedure.

Table 1.1 lists biopsy techniques, example specimens, and suggested cytologic preparation techniques. The collection of specimens for cytologic evaluation from cutaneous and subcutaneous tissues and abdominal organs and masses in smaller animals is generally accomplished with a 22- or 25-gauge, 1- to 1½-inch needle firmly attached to a 6 or 12 mL syringe. Needle gauge is a contributing factor to fine-needle aspirate sample quality. However, it does not affect the overall ability to make a diagnosis. Samples obtained using 25-gauge needles resulted in less blood contamination yet increased cellular trauma compared with 22-gauge needle samples (Arai et al., 2019). For internal organs, especially in larger animals, a 2½- to 3½-inch spinal needle is used. The added length amplifies the area for cell collection and enhances the diagnostic yield—cores of hepatic tissue can be obtained with a longer needle. The stylet can be left in place as the cavity is entered to avoid contamination during the "searching" process of locating the tissue of sampling interest.

The general steps for obtaining a cytologic specimen are illustrated in Figure 1.2. After appropriate cleansing and disinfectant application, the tip of the needle is inserted into the tissue of interest, the plunger retracted slightly (0.5–1 mL of vacuum), the needle advanced and retracted in several different directions, the plunger released, the needle withdrawn, and the specimen placed on a glass slide or in an ethylenediaminetetraacetic acid (EDTA)-containing purple-top tube as appropriate. If fluid is obtained from a mass lesion, the site is completely drained, the needle withdrawn, the fluid placed in an EDTA tube, and the procedure repeated with a new needle directed at firm tissue. Both specimens are examined microscopically. To enhance operator flexibility in fluid collection, a butterfly needle can be used to attach the needle and syringe (Fig. 1.3). Positioning and redirection of the needle are easier and accommodate patient movement.

Suction is not a prerequisite for obtaining a cytologic specimen. A technique based on the principle of capillarity, referred to as *fine-needle capillary sampling,* can be performed by placing a needle into the lesion with or without a syringe attached (Mair et al., 1989). The technique has diagnostic sensitivity similar to that of aspiration with suction when used to sample many tissue types. Its major advantages are to reduce blood contamination from vascular tissues such as the liver, spleen, kidney, and thyroid and to reduce lysis of fragile cell populations. Cells are displaced into the cylinder of the needle by capillary action as the needle is incompletely retracted and redirected into the tissue three to six times. Personal preference is justified when deciding between suction and non-suction aspiration sampling for collection of the specimen. Through trial and error, the operator may determine that each has value for sampling different tissues.

> **KEY POINT** Acquisition of the cytology specimen is an art that can be honed only by practice. Selecting an appropriate mode of sampling enhances the probability of obtaining accurate diagnostic information.

> **KEY POINT** Dry wipe the surface of the glass slide to remove "invisible" glass particles that cause spreading deficiencies prior to sample collection. Never reuse washed glass slides.

DIAGNOSTIC IMAGING-GUIDED SAMPLE COLLECTION

Cytology sample collection can be performed under the guidance of fluoroscopy, ultrasound, and computed tomography. Ultrasound guidance is the preferred method because of its widespread availability and portability. In addition, ultrasound provides real-time monitoring of precise needle placement. The technique and indications are detailed elsewhere (Nyland et al., 2002a). Ultrasound-guided fine-needle aspiration biopsy (FNAB) is indicated for cytologic evaluation of nodules and masses detected on ultrasound and to evaluate organomegaly when a diffuse cellular infiltrate such as lymphoma and mast cell tumor is suspected. It is helpful in cases in which lesions are not easily

BOX 1.1 Contents of the Cytology Kit

Clippers
Cleansing and disinfectant wipes
Syringes: 6–12 mL, 20 mL if necessary
Needles: 1- and 1½-inch—20- to 25-gauge; 2½- or 3½-inch spinal needle with stylet
Bone marrow aspiration needles and core biopsy materials
Scalpel blades: #10 and #11
Culture swabs and cotton-tipped applicator sticks for slide preparation
Box of precleaned glass slides with frosted end
Tubes: EDTA (purple top) and serum (red top without separator or plain white tube)
Butterfly catheters 21- to 23-gauge and intravenous extension tubing
Pencil or solvent resistant slide-specific black marker
Hair dryer

EDTA, Ethylenediaminetetraacetic acid.

TABLE 1.1 Biopsy Techniques, Associated Specimens, and Cytologic Preparation Techniques

BIOPSY TECHNIQUE	SPECIMEN	PREPARATION TECHNIQUE
A. Sampling solid tissue		
1. Suction biopsy	Unknown mass	Spread, suspension cytospin
2. Non-suction biopsy	Vascular tissue	Direct smear, spread
B. Fluid aspiration biopsy		
1. Bloody fluid	Effusion (pericardial)	Buffy coat smear
2. Non-bloody fluid	Effusions, synovial fluid, cerebrospinal fluid, urine	Direct, sediment, cytospin
3. EDTA syringe	Bone marrow	Particle spread
C. Incisional biopsy	Soft tissue, bone marrow core	Imprint of cut section, tissue roll
D. Excisional biopsy	Masses, lymph node, eye, testicle	Imprint
E. Scraping biopsy	Firm tissue, skin, conjunctiva	Imprint, spread
F. Swab	Vaginal, fecal, oral, ocular	Imprint, roll
G. Washes	Prostate, urinary bladder, respiratory tract, peritoneal lavage	Sediment, cytospin

EDTA, Ethylenediaminetetraacetic acid.

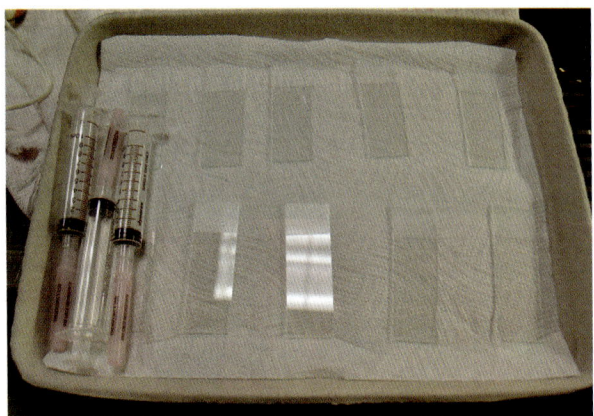

■ **FIGURE 1.1 Cytologic preparation.** Slide tray with needles, syringes, and clean glass slides. Having the proper setup before fine-needle aspiration biopsy facilitates appropriate management of the sample.

accessed for surgical biopsy (Cohen et al., 2003). If cytologic evaluation proves inconclusive, histologic evaluation is recommended. One of the main benefits to ultrasound-guided FNAB is that it can be performed in most patients without chemical restraint or local anesthesia. If chemical restraint is needed, agents that promote panting should be avoided because they lead to excessive movement and gas ingestion (Nyland et al., 2002a).

Biopsy Guidance

Ultrasound-guided FNAB is most frequently performed by the freehand technique. The freehand technique consists of holding the transducer in one hand and inserting the needle with the other at an oblique angle to the long axis of the transducer but still within the scan plane (see Fig. 1.2B–C). This technique requires more skill but allows for greater flexibility. If the needle cannot be seen initially during the procedure, slightly move the transducer into the path of the needle while gently probing with the needle. Enhanced visualization of the needle can be achieved by ensuring needle placement is within the focal zone of the transducer. Biopsy guides are available to help direct the course of the needle, but these are rarely used in clinical practice and limit transducer movement.

Equipment and Technique

Sterility is maintained during the procedure. Routine skin preparation should be performed before needle puncture through the skin (see Fig. 1.2A). The transducer can be sterilized with transducer-compatible disinfectant and sterilizing solutions (a list of which can be found in the user manual of the ultrasound machine). After the diagnostic ultrasound evaluation of the site of interest, the coupling gel is wiped off, and alcohol or sterile water is used as the coupling medium during the FNAB procedure. The use of a coupling gel is avoided because it can introduce potentially misleading artifacts into the cytologic specimen (Fig. 1.4).

The most commonly used needles are 20- to 25-gauge hypodermic and spinal needles. These are inexpensive and long enough to pass through the skin and body wall and still reach most lesions. Larger-bore needles are easier to visualize and generally increase the reliability of sample collection, but they increase the risk of hemorrhage. A larger-bore needle can be used when aspirating viscous fluids. When the needle is placed in the lesion, the stylet is removed, and the needle is moved up and down within the lesion until a small amount of fluid or blood is seen within the hub of the needle (Fagelman and Chess, 1990). This method generally produces a sample with less blood contamination. Alternatively, a syringe can be attached to the needle for better handling—a few milliliters of negative pressure can be applied while moving the needle up and down. The negative pressure should be released before removing the needle from the lesion. When possible, two or three samples should be obtained from each biopsy site; a new needle is used for each sample taken. A large lesion may have a necrotic center; therefore, samples should also be collected from the margins.

Complications

Complications associated with ultrasound-guided FNAB are uncommon and depend on the experience of the operator, size of needle, and type of lesion aspirated (Léveillé et al., 1993). Patients should be evaluated for bleeding disorders before FNAB, especially when highly vascular tissues and internal

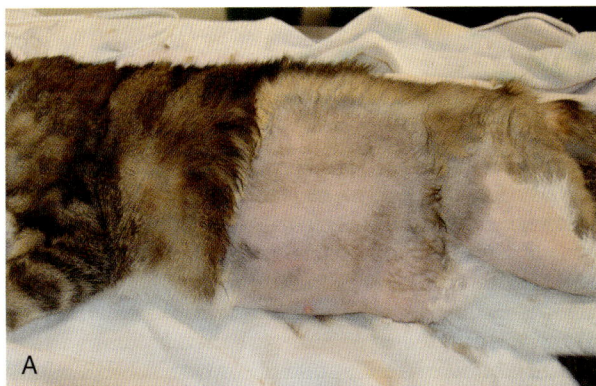
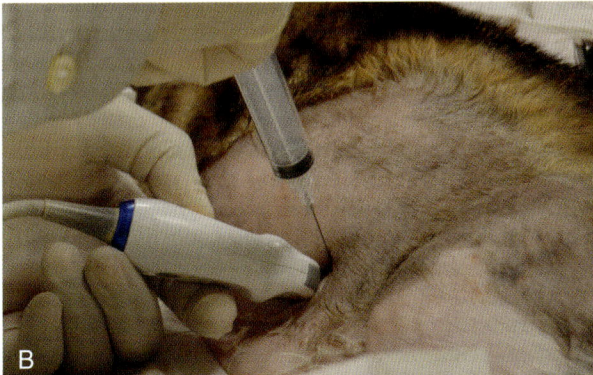
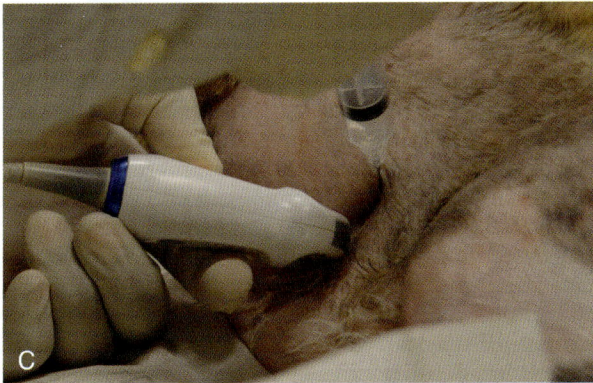

■ **FIGURE 1.2 Ultrasound-guided fine-needle aspiration biopsy.** **A,** The patient should be positioned for ease of access to the aspiration site and the area clipped, cleaned, and disinfected before the needle is inserted. **B,** The needle is inserted into the tissue and redirected three or four times using a non-suction aspiration technique. The same concept generally applies to the use of the technique for sampling sites within the thorax or abdomen. **C,** Freehand technique involving a small of amount of suction applied for aspiration biopsy.

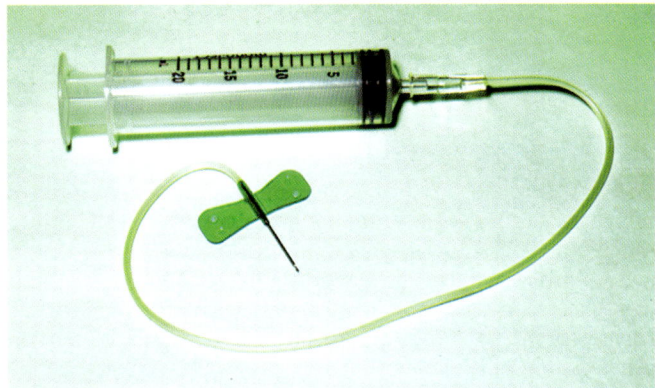

■ **FIGURE 1.3 Butterfly needle.** The use of a butterfly needle attached to the syringe allows more flexibility with fractious patients when removing fluid. A three-way stopcock can be placed between the butterfly tubing and syringe to facilitate the removal of large amounts of fluid.

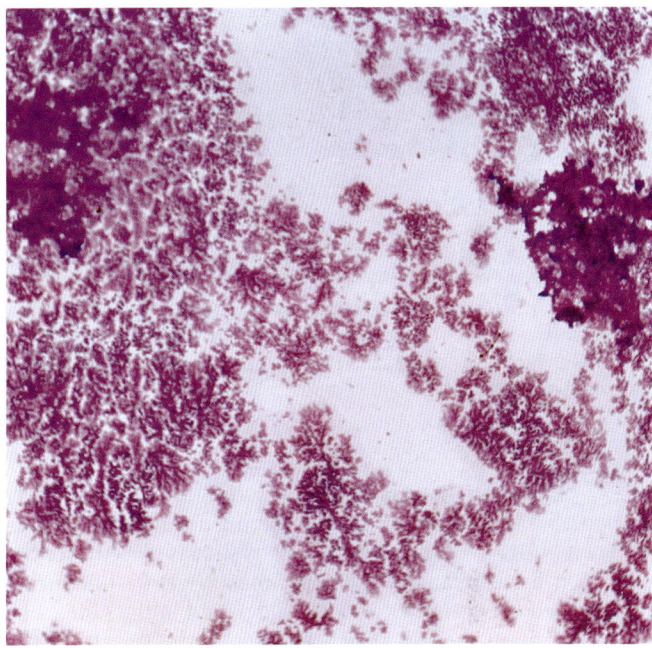

■ **FIGURE 1.4 Ultrasound gel.** It is important to remove any ultrasound gel on the patient and transducer before aspiration. The gel may enter the needle during placement and appear as bright pink or magenta amorphous material on the cytology slide that often obscures diagnostic features and potentially causes cytologic misinterpretation, such as a mucus-producing tumor or amyloid. (Wright; LP.)

organs are sampled. Occasional needle tract metastases are rare but have been reported in animals (Nyland et al., 2002b; Vignoli et al., 2007; Warren-Smith et al., 2011). They are most frequently reported in tumors of the urogenital tract (Klopfleisch et al., 2011). Because pneumothorax can develop after FNAB of the thoracic structures, the patient should frequently be observed for 12 to 24 hours after the procedure.

> **KEY POINT** Sample two to three areas of a lesion, when possible, to enhance the acquisition of a diagnostic specimen; this is especially prudent if necrotic tissue or a cyst is encountered.

MANAGING THE CYTOLOGIC SPECIMEN

The following section describes the more common preparation techniques used in veterinary medicine to obtain diagnostic specimens.

Spread (Compression) Preparation

The spread technique is one of most frequently used, adaptable techniques for the management of cytology specimens that are semisolid, mucus-like, or concentrated by centrifugation. Solid tissue does not generally compress and spread evenly for use of this method. A small amount of material is placed on a clean glass slide approximately ½ inch (1 cm) from the frosted end (Fig. 1.5A). A common mistake is the initial placement of

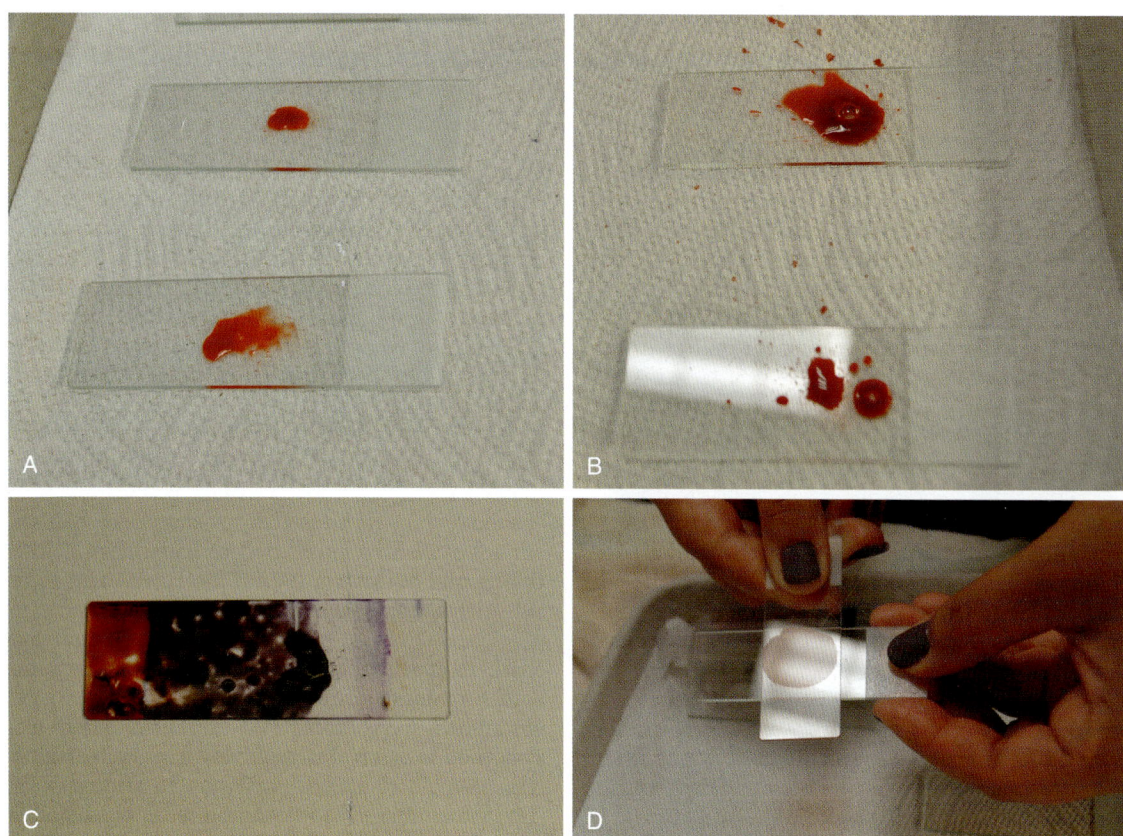

■ **FIGURE 1.5 Spread slide biopsy preparation. A,** The application of only a small drop or a portion of the specimen on the glass slide near the frosted end is an important initial step for making a quality cytologic preparation. **B** and **C,** Placing too much material on the slide results in a preparation that is too thick or spreads too close to the slide edges for diagnostic purposes. **D,** The specimen is gently but firmly compressed between the two glass slides held at 90 degrees.

excess sample on the glass slide, resulting in an excessively thick preparation that precludes obtaining diagnostic information (Fig. 1.5B–C). A second clean glass slide is placed over the specimen at right angles. The specimen is gently but firmly compressed between the two glass slides, and in the same continuous motion the top slide is slid across the surface of the bottom slide away from the frosted end while ensuring the flat surface of both slides remain evenly in contact (Fig. 1.5D). The objective is to redistribute the material such that there are monolayer, uniform stain penetration and microscopic examination of cell morphology. A properly prepared glass slide is characterized by a feather-shaped (oblong) area, with a monolayer end referred to as the "sweet spot" (Fig. 1.6). An alternate technique is to place the top slide parallel to the bottom slide (Fig. 1.7).

> **KEY POINT** Compression and spread of the specimen involve continuity; pauses can interfere with the spread of cellular material. Keep the flat surfaces of the two slides evenly in contact. A common mistake is to slightly angle the upper slide near the end of the gliding motion by allowing a slight counterclockwise rotation of the wrist (clockwise if left-handed) to occur, causing cell lysis or uneven spread of the specimen. A scraping sound of glass on glass can be heard when this occurs. Wiping each slide before the procedure helps ensure uniform spread of the cytologic specimen.

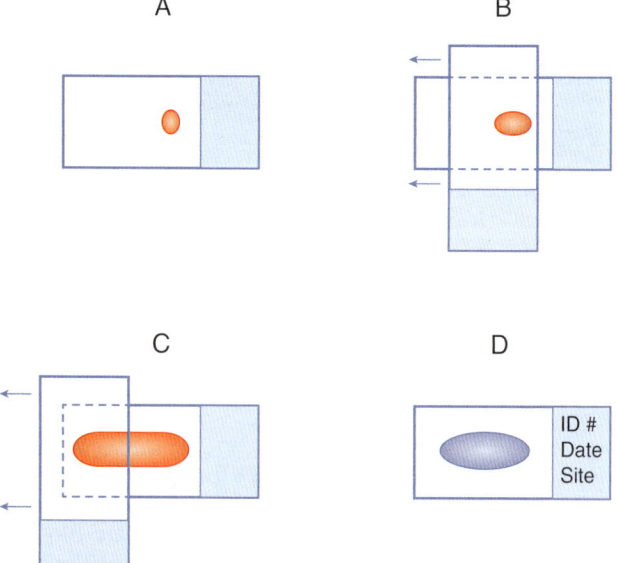

■ **FIGURE 1.6 Preparing the spread slide.** The small specimen (**A**) is gently compressed between the two glass slides (**B**), and in the same continuous motion (**C**) the top slide is glided along the surface of the slide with the material spread away from the frosted end, resulting in a feather-shaped specimen. The location of the "sweet spot" is demonstrated by a thin region of the oval area (**D**) on this appropriately labeled and stained preparation of a cytologic specimen.

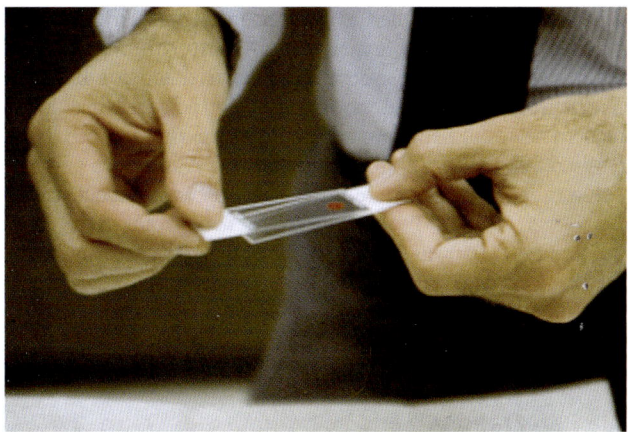

■ **FIGURE 1.7 Spread slide biopsy preparation.** An alternative method to spread the material is to hold the slides at 180 degrees, placing the top slide parallel to the bottom slide and gliding apart with an outward motion using even pressure.

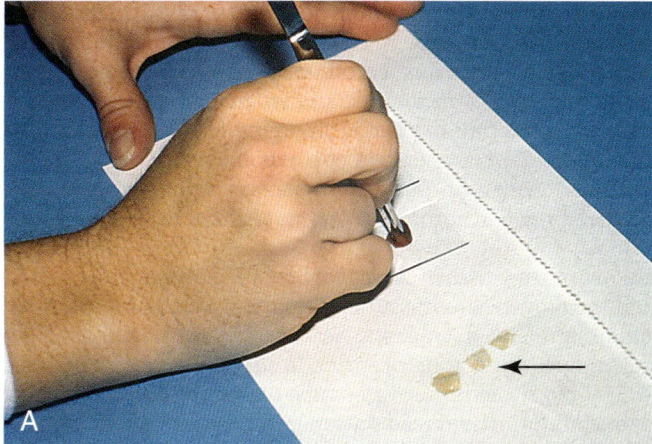

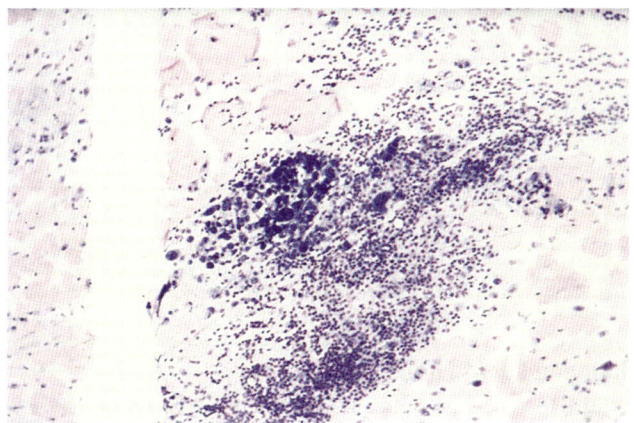

■ **FIGURE 1.8 Slide preparation.** The clear area to the left represents the guide track of the automated stainer that has partially scraped off the only cytologic material present on the slide because it was located too close to the slide's end. (Wright; LP.)

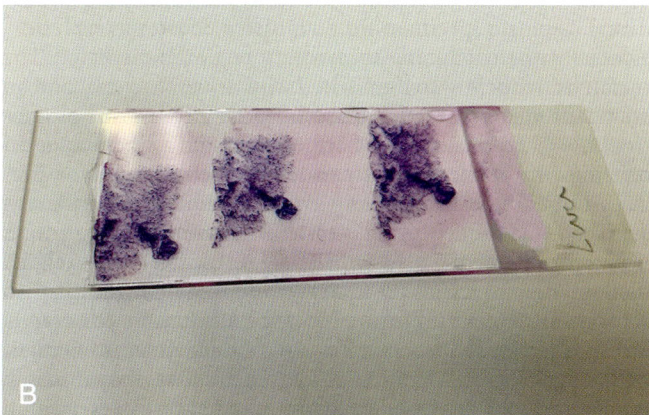

■ **FIGURE 1.9 A,** Impression smear biopsy. The touch imprint technique. The cut surface of the specimen is firmly blotted on a paper towel (note wet spots, *arrow*) until tacky and then firmly touched multiple times to the surface of a clean glass slide. **B,** A well-prepared and well-stained touch preparation.

> **KEY POINT** The *sweet spot* in a cytologic specimen refers to the thin monocellular location on a slide that facilitates successful microscopic examination. Note that the spread of the specimen close to the end or edges of the slide may not be adequately examined microscopically because of the inability of the 40× dry and 50× and 100× oil objectives to focus properly due to the slide's location on the stage. Furthermore, when slides go through an automated stainer, their guiding tracks can scrape off diagnostic material that is too close to the end of the slide (Fig. 1.8). Material placed too close to the end of the specimen will not adequately stain (see Fig. 1.5C).

> **KEY POINT** If the spread preparation appears too thick, it probably is. Make another one. If the cytology specimen appears to be too close to the end or edge of the slide, it probably is. Make another one. If you have doubts regarding the quality of the preparation, make additional preparations, especially if submitting to a referral laboratory; the price is the same generally whether submitting one or five spread preparations.

Touch Imprint (Impression Smear) and Scrape Biopsies

Cells often exfoliate from excised tissue when the cut surface is touched to a glass slide. This type of cytologic preparation permits immediate evaluation of a surgical biopsy before being placed in fixative and provides the pathologist with a second means of evaluating the tissue. The interpretation by the submitting practitioner can be then compared with the histopathologic findings. This technique is helpful during a surgical procedure to evaluate real time if (1) the histologic biopsy will be diagnostically adequate or if more tissue is needed and if (2) a definitive diagnosis may be obtained to facilitate immediate case management decisions. An example of this benefit is the accuracy observed with the intraoperative cytologic diagnosis of intracranial granular cell tumors (Levitin et al., 2019). The cut surface of the excised tissue is blotted on a paper towel or gauze to remove blood and tissue fluid. The specimen is considered adequately tacky for cells to exfoliate when the paper towel or gauze sticks to it. The tissue specimen is then touched firmly to the central area of a clean glass slide in several places (Fig. 1.9). Note that the surface of the slide with the cytologic specimen should be the same as the frosted surface of the slide or labeled if unfrosted slides are used to ensure proper staining and examination microscopically. Imprint areas that appear too thick can be finessed to a monolayer by the gentle use of the compression technique. Touch imprints should be made of each area of tissue specimen that appears grossly different. This technique is the preferred method for samples taken via endoscopy (Jergens et al., 2000).

Tissues with a fibrous texture, such as fibromas, fibrosarcomas, and reactive fibroplasia, may not exfoliate adequately with a touch imprint technique. The surface of these firm, often pale-appearing tissues needs to be abraded with a scalpel blade and then touched to the surface of a glass slide. If the specimen has been removed with an intact capsule, the capsule is incised before making the touch imprint. In addition, or alternatively, a scalpel blade can be used to scrape off a layer of cells to make a touch imprint or spread preparation (Fig. 1.10). The scraping or abrading biopsy technique is effective for obtaining a diagnostic cytologic specimen from an ulcerated cutaneous lesion, especially when neoplasia or mycotic infection is suspected. The surface is frequently contaminated with debris, bacteria, and an attendant mixed inflammatory cell reaction composed of neutrophils, macrophages, and fibroplasia that, if using only a direct imprint of the surface, can cause a misdiagnosis or preclude obtaining a diagnostic specimen. The ulcerated surface is aggressively debrided using moistened gauze or by aggressive, deep scraping of the area with a scalpel blade. The exfoliated material obtained with the scalpel blade is used to make touch imprints or spread preparations. If the lesion is large enough, an aspirate biopsy specimen may be obtained as a complementary diagnostic technique. For certain bullous skin diseases, touching a glass slide to a freshly ruptured bulla can be used to identify acantholytic epithelial cells along with nondegenerate neutrophils, referred to as a Tzanck preparation, which is supportive of a tentative diagnosis of an immune-mediated skin disorder (see Fig. 3.23).

Small tissue samples, such as those obtained with an endoscopic biopsy instrument, cutting biopsy needle, or bone marrow core biopsy needle, can be gently touched or rolled on a slide using another glass slide or displaced with a 22- or 25-gauge needle (Fig. 1.11). One may perform a compression preparation if there is extra tissue not needed for histologic examination.

Cotton Swab Biopsy Technique

Cotton-tipped swabs help exfoliate cells from mucosal surfaces and collect viscous or fluid discharges, particularly from the nose, ear, and external genitalia. The cotton tip of the applicator stick is used to swab the mucosal surface or the discharge directly, which is then used to roll along—not paint—the glass slide surface, generally forming two parallel rows for examination (Fig. 1.12).

Tape Preparations

The use of tape is most commonly used for initial, in-house evaluation of superficial skin lesions and is most helpful in identifying infectious agents such as *Malassezia* and *Demodex canis*. It is often well tolerated by patients. Clear tape is placed on the skin lesion, and the lesion can be compressed for increased exfoliation. A drop of blue stain, either the blue stain from the aqueous Romanowsky (AR) set or new methylene blue (NMB), is placed on a glass slide. The tape is removed from the skin and fixed upon the slide. This technique may be more beneficial than the scrape technique for identifying *Demodex canis* organisms (Hodges, 2013).

> **KEY POINT** Cytologic sample acquisition needs to be thoughtfully aligned with the type of lesion to be sampled, and cytologic sample preparation requires attention to detail; both are an art honed by experience.

Management of Fluids

A fluid specimen should be immediately placed in an EDTA tube to prevent clot formation. Excess fluids should be placed in either plain red-top tubes or other additives for possible

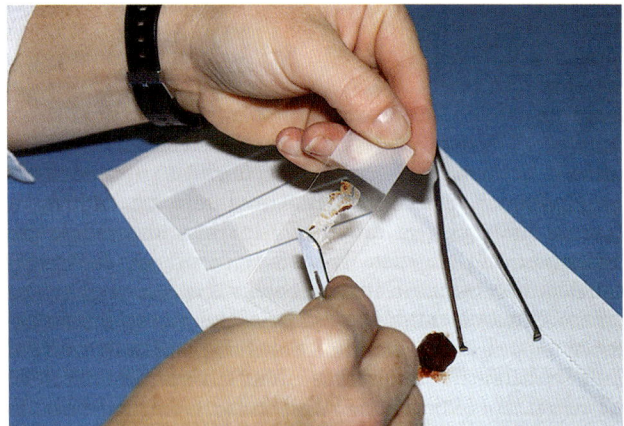

■ **FIGURE 1.10 Tissue scraping biopsy.** If the tissue does not adequately exfoliate, a scalpel blade is used to scrape or abrade the surface of the tissue. The tissue can be then touched to the glass surface. Another option is to place some of the specimen from the edge of the blade onto a glass slide and make a spread preparation. (From Meyer DJ. The management of cytology specimens. *Compend Contin Educ Pract Vet.* 1987;9:10-17.)

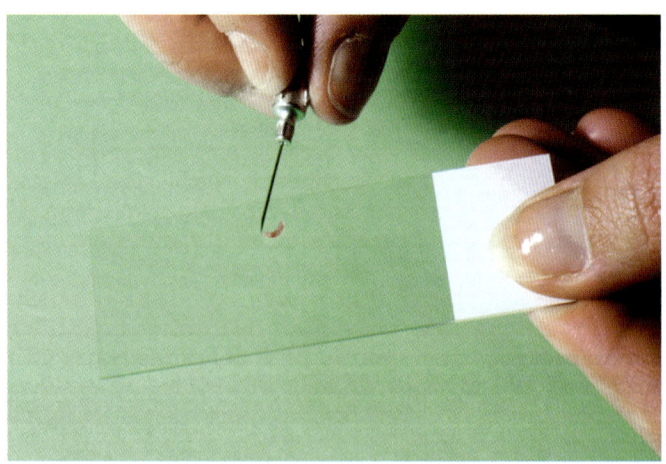

■ **FIGURE 1.11 Tissue rolling technique.** Small pieces of tissue that cannot be grasped with a forceps for imprinting can be gently rolled on a slide using a 25-gauge needle. This allows for exfoliation of a thin layer of cells. If the tissue is not friable, multiple slides may be made.

chemical analysis (see Chapter 6). Most fluids with a plasma-like consistency can be handled in a fashion similar to the preparation of a blood smear. A small drop of fluid is placed approximately one-half inch (1 cm) from the frosted end. The angled edge of a second glass slide, with the acute angle facing the operator, is backed into the specimen and drawn away from the frosted end as the fluid begins to spread along its edge (Fig. 1.13). The speed at which the slide is moved depends on the viscosity of the sample—the thinner the specimen, the faster the slide should be moved to distribute the specimen evenly and thinly. For a viscous fluid specimen such as synovial fluid, the spreader slide is moved with a slow

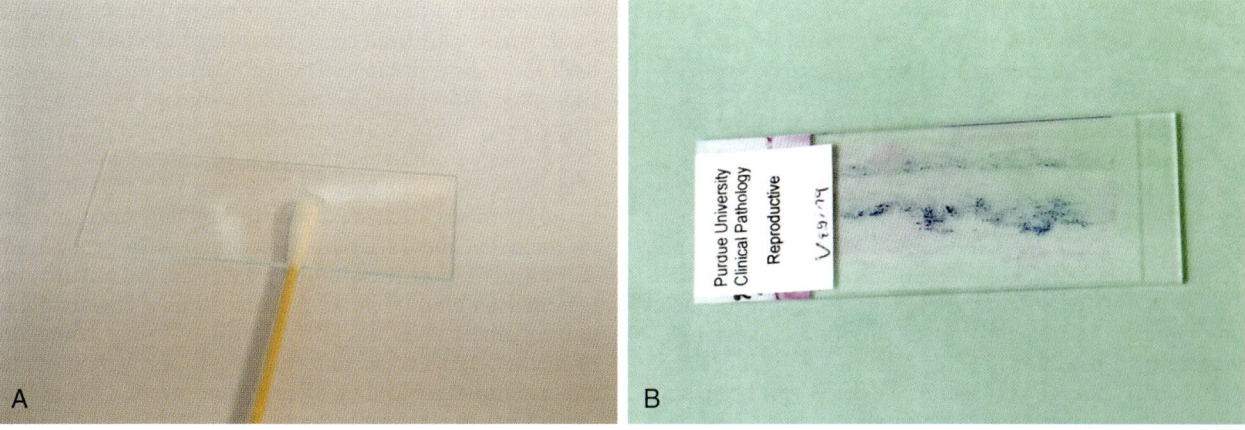

■ **FIGURE 1.12 Swab biopsy technique. A,** The swab smear preparation is made by rolling the cotton tip over the slide, forming two lines of cytologic specimen. **B,** A stained vaginal smear made using the swab technique.

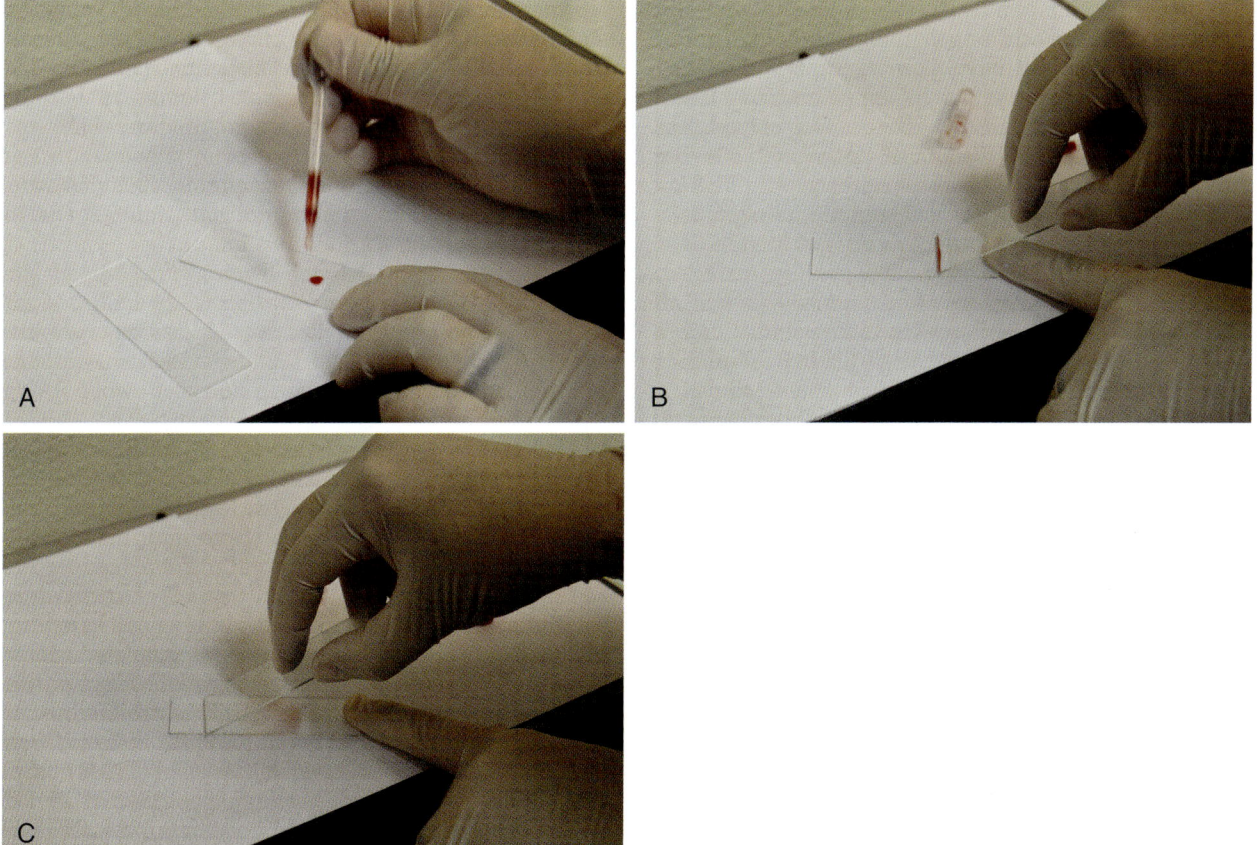

■ **FIGURE 1.13 Fluid material preparation. A,** The procedure for making a cytologic preparation from a fluid specimen. A small drop of the specimen is placed approximately one-half inch (1 cm) from the frosted end of the slide. **B,** The spreader slide is slowly backed into the drop. **C,** Just as the fluid begins to spread along its edge, the spreader slide is glided away from the frosted end.

and even movement. The spread technique can be used for high-viscosity samples. When in doubt regarding which approach is better suited for a viscous specimen, use both techniques.

All fluid initially applied to the slide must remain on the slide (Fig. 1.14). It is tempting to go off the end of the slide with excess fluid, referred to as the "edge of the cliff syndrome," but the result is the potential loss of diagnostic material, which is thrown into the garbage with the spreader slide. An ideal fluid preparation is shown in Figure 1.14B. The edge of the cliff syndrome poses a notable threat to pleural and peritoneal fluids that contain clumps of neoplastic cells. These cellular clumps often follow the spreader slide, finally sticking to the surface when the fluid dissipates (Fig. 1.15). To avoid this cytologic disaster when excess fluid remains, simply stop one-half inch from the end of the specimen slide, apply the spreader slide to another clean glass slide, and repeat the spreading procedure. When minimal excess fluid remains, the fluid can be permitted to slowly flow back on itself for a short distance. The thin part of the stained cytology slide preparation can be used to estimate cell numbers and the relatively thick, concentrated part (where the excess fluid is dried) can be evaluated for types of cells or infectious agents (Fig. 1.14C). Although not an optimal preparation, this "poor man's centrifuge" technique may be useful in emergency settings for the initial, rapid triage of a fluid specimen.

Sedimentation preparations can also be used to concentrate cells in bloody, cloudy, or wash fluids. The sample can be centrifuged in the same tube in which it was submitted *after*

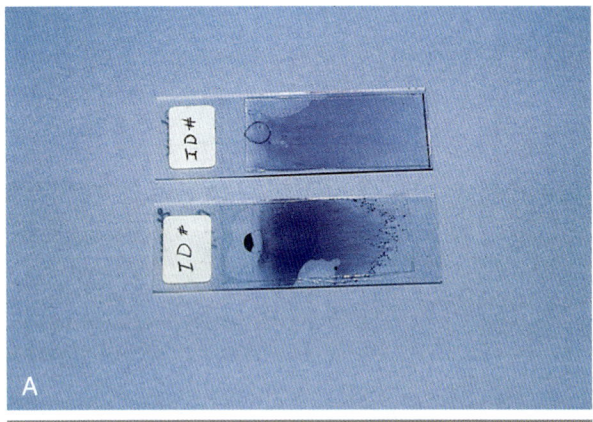
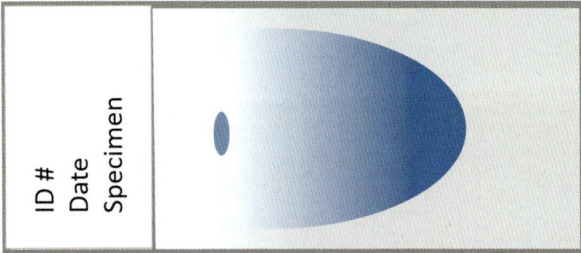
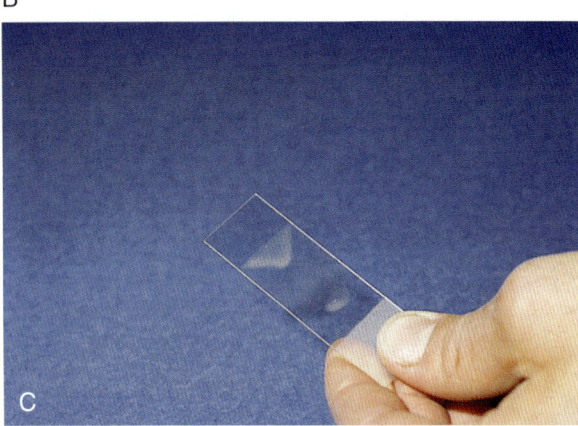

■ **FIGURE 1.14 Slides prepared from fluid. A,** All of the original fluid drop should remain on the slide; the temptation to go off the ends of the slide with excess fluid must be avoided. The upper slide demonstrates the "edge of the cliff syndrome" in which the excess fluid was drawn off both the sides and end of the slide. The lower slide illustrates retention of the feathered edge on the slide. **B,** Ideal slide preparation in which fluid does not extend to the sides or end of the slide and allows complete staining by an automatic stainer. Complete information is shown on label. **C,** Excess fluid that remains is allowed to partially flow back and is air dried as illustrated by the small opaque dried fluid triangle near the nonfrosted end of the slide. Alternatively, the edge of the spreader slide with the excess fluid adhering to it is transferred to another clean slide and another smear is made.

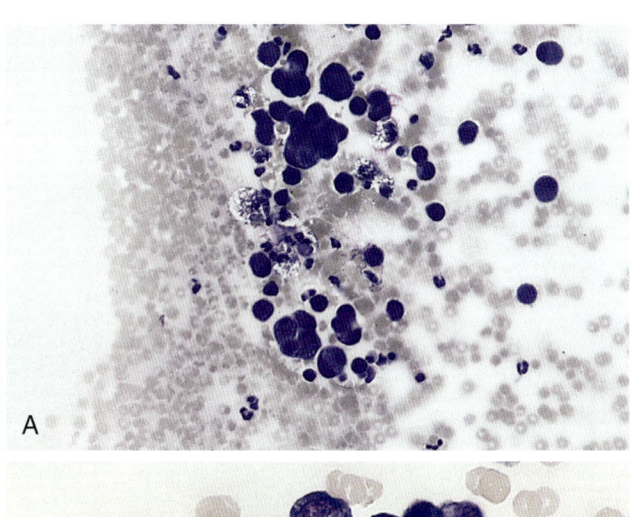
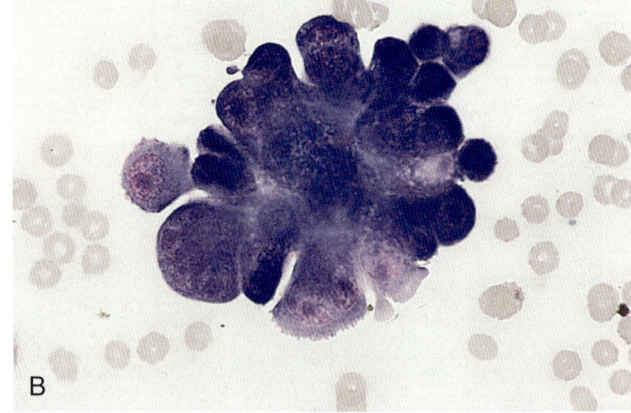

■ **FIGURE 1.15 Slide examination of feathered edge. A,** Examination of the feathered edge of the lower slide shown in Figure 1.14A demonstrates clumps of cells of diagnostic value located along the feathered edge emphasizing the need to leave the excess fluid on the slide. The thinner area to the right of the diagnostic cell clumps closer to the frosted end of the slide was composed of erythrocytes without diagnostic cell clumps. (Wright; IP.) **B,** A cytologic diagnosis of an adenocarcinoma was made by examining the cell clump structure and cell morphology. (Wright; HP oil.)

direct preparations have been made. After centrifugation, the majority of supernatant is removed with a pipette or carefully decanted with an applicator stick and the cell concentrate resuspended in the remaining fluid. A direct smear or spread preparation can be made from the concentrated cell specimen. It is important to remember that estimates of cell counts cannot be made on concentrated samples, only from the direct smear. After the cytologic preparation has been made, cell blocks can be made from the remaining cell concentrate for histopathologic or immunohistochemical evaluation. (Refer to Appendix 5 for more information.)

The diagnostic yield of a predominantly bloody fluid specimen may be enhanced with the buffy coat concentration technique. A microhematocrit tube is prepared as if to measure a hematocrit. The tube is broken just below the cellular concentrate (buffy coat) and gently expelled onto two or three slides (Fig. 1.16). A direct smear or spread technique is used to spread the specimen. The buffy coat technique is valuable for hemorrhagic pericardial, peritoneal, and pleural samples. It is also useful for the examination of peripheral blood for neoplastic cells and cell-associated infectious organisms.

Transudates and cerebrospinal fluid are low in protein and cell numbers. The use of a cytocentrifuge (cytospin) is recommended for the capture of all the cells (Fig. 1.17). For cerebrospinal fluid, a cytologic preparation should be made—ideally within 30 to 60 minutes because the low specific gravity predisposes to cellular lysis. When inflammatory cells, neoplastic cells, or infectious agents are present, the diagnostic integrity may be maintained for up several hours with immediate refrigeration (Meyer et al., 2004).

> **KEY POINT** For the management of fluid samples, routinely make direct, centrifuged (or buffy coat), and cytocentrifugation (if possible) preparations and assess each for the best diagnostic yield.

> **KEY POINT** Concentrated samples, such as sediment and cytocentrifuge preparations, cannot be used to estimate cell counts and should be used only to evaluate cell types present and their morphology.

> **KEY POINT** Cells may be washed off during the staining process of direct smear preparations made from low-protein fluids such as urinary sediments, cerebrospinal fluids, and transudates. Premade serum-coated slides facilitate the adhesion of the cells from these specimens. Several drops of the excess serum not used for clinical chemistries are applied to the entire non-frosted surface of a glass slide and air dried or dried with a no-heat hair dryer. From 10 to 20 of these slide preparations are made. When dry (not sticky to the touch), the slides are placed in a slide box and stored in the freezer to prevent bacterial growth. Before use, the slide is brought to room temperature. It is critical that no condensation develops on the surface because it causes cell lysis.

> **HELPFUL HINT** A hair dryer set on no heat or small personal fan facilitates rapid, even drying of fluid specimens. Heat fixation is not recommended for cytologic preparations.

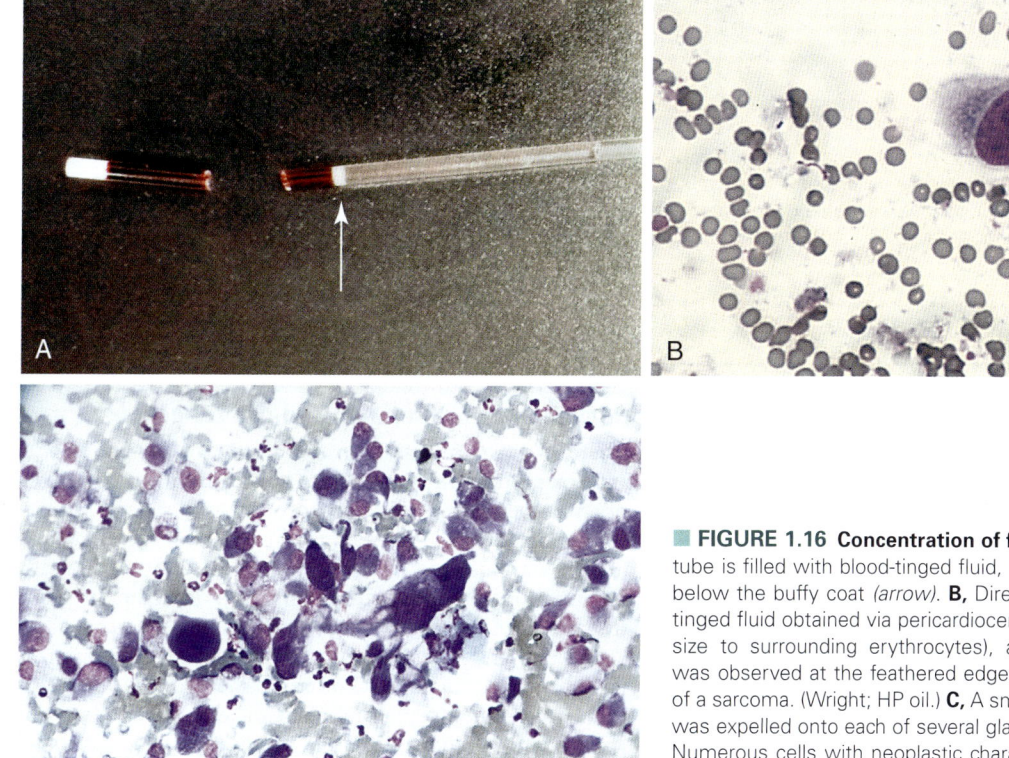

■ **FIGURE 1.16 Concentration of fluids. A,** A microhematocrit tube is filled with blood-tinged fluid, spun down, and broken just below the buffy coat *(arrow)*. **B,** Direct smear made from blood-tinged fluid obtained via pericardiocentesis. A rare large (contrast size to surrounding erythrocytes), atypical spindle-shaped cell was observed at the feathered edge microscopically, suggestive of a sarcoma. (Wright; HP oil.) **C,** A small amount of the buffy coat was expelled onto each of several glass slides and gently spread. Numerous cells with neoplastic characteristics of a sarcoma are observed microscopically at the feathered edge, affirming the cytologic diagnosis. (Wright; HP oil.)

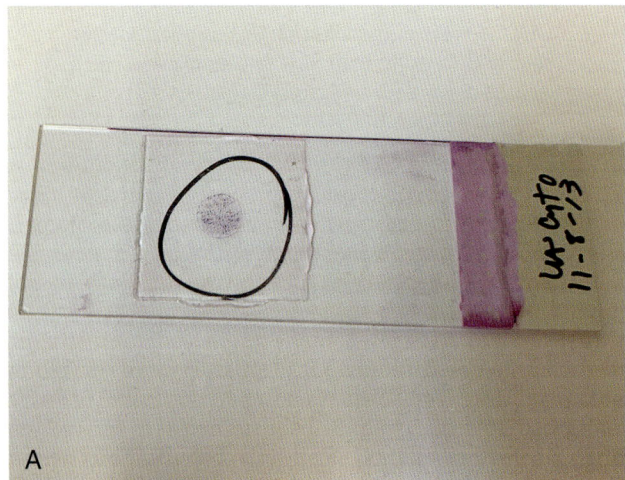

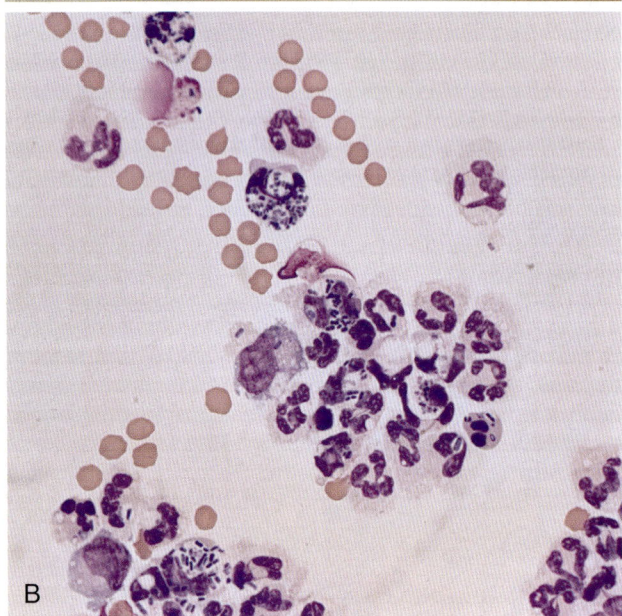

■ **FIGURE 1.17** Cytospin preparation. **A,** Cytospins are used to effectively concentrate cells in fluids with sparse nucleated cellularity. **B,** A cytospin preparation of a dilute urine sample illustrates the presence of segmented neutrophils with intracellular bacteria; these were not observed on the direct smear preparation.

STAINING THE SPECIMEN

Romanowsky and NMB stain are the two most commonly used stains in veterinary medicine for cytologic specimens. Air-dried slides are the preferred method of initial preparation. Rapid drying prevents cell shrinkage. One exception is the procedure of wet fixation before the slide dries for the Papanicolaou stain.

Papanicolaou Stain

The Papanicolaou (Pap) stain is used routinely in the human medical profession for selected cytologic specimens. The stain accentuates nuclear detail and is valuable in detecting early morphologic aberrations indicative of dysplasia and neoplasia. It is not commonly used in veterinary medicine because it offers no distinct diagnostic advantage for veterinary specimens. A rapid Pap staining procedure has been described in veterinary medicine for the reader to explore (Jorundsson et al., 1999).

New Methylene Blue Stain

NMB is a basic dye that stains nuclei, most infectious agents, platelets, and mast cell granules. In veterinary medicine, it is most commonly used in hematology to identify reticulocytes and Heinz bodies. Eosinophil granules do not stain, nor do erythrocytes, which appear microscopically as translucent circular areas. Because there is no alcohol fixation, adipocytes associated with lipomas and adipose tissue can be easily recognized. Cholesterol crystals often associated with follicular cysts are highlighted with NMB. The stain solution consists of 0.5 g of NMB dissolved in 100 mL of 0.9% saline. Full-strength formalin (1 mL) is added as a preservative. The stock solution is kept refrigerated. For clinical use, a small stoppered bottle is replenished from the stock solution; the stain is passed through filter paper first to remove all precipitate and contaminants (Fig. 1.18). A convenient filter alternative is the use of a syringe filter (0.45 μm), as shown in Figure 1.18B, which minimizes the waste from filtering large amounts of stain. Procedurally, a small drop of stain is applied directly to an air-dried cytology or hematology preparation. A dust-free coverslip (wiped with a paper towel or tissue paper) is placed on the drop of stain, which spreads by capillary movement. Larger coverslips, 20 × 40 mm or 20 × 50 mm, allow more of the specimen to be examined. The excess stain is removed by tilting and touching the glass slide onto filter paper or a paper towel. The specimen should be examined immediately because the water-based stain evaporates. An NMB-stained cytologic specimen is useful for the detection of nucleated cells, bacteria (both gram-positive and gram-negative bacteria stain dark blue), fungi, and adipose tissue. It is a valuable triage stain for blood and fluid specimens examined on an emergency basis. The NMB-stained slide can be preserved by removing the coverslip before it dries onto the slide and rinsing and fixing the slide with methanol followed by a permanent Romanowsky stain; however, the quality is variable. A better strategy is to make cytologic preparations for both the NMB stain and the Romanowsky stain.

HELPFUL HINT NMB is a diagnostically valuable, pragmatic, cost-effective stain for examining cytologic preparations, blood smears, and urine sediments in veterinary practice. The added responsibility of filtering the stock stain periodically to remove stain particulates, which mimic bacteria, is well worth the time invested.

Romanowsky Stain (Methanolic and Aqueous)

There are two formulations of Romanowsky stains used in veterinary medicine. AR stain is commonly used in general practice because of its ease of use and speed. Methanolic Romanowsky (MR) staining is often used in commercial laboratory settings and teaching hospitals. Both Romanowsky formulations involve methanol fixation of an air-dried slide as the first step.

Wright and Giemsa stains are types of methanol-based, polychromatic stains that contain basic dyes, azures, that stain DNA/RNA blue/purple, and an acidic dye, eosin, that stains alkaline cytoplasmic components pink/red. The polychromatic stain imparts the basophilic and eosinophilic tinctorial properties observed on blood films. Wright stain is used widely in

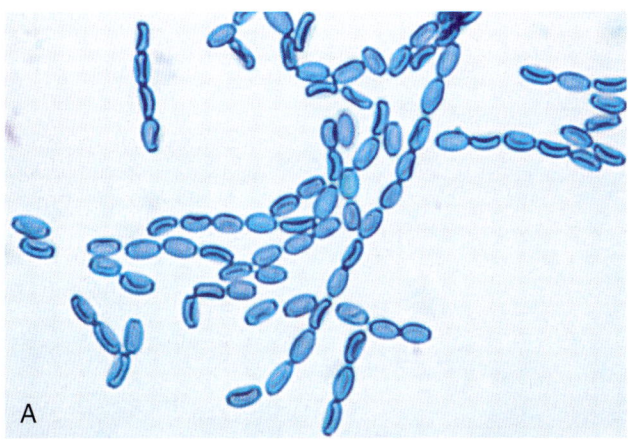
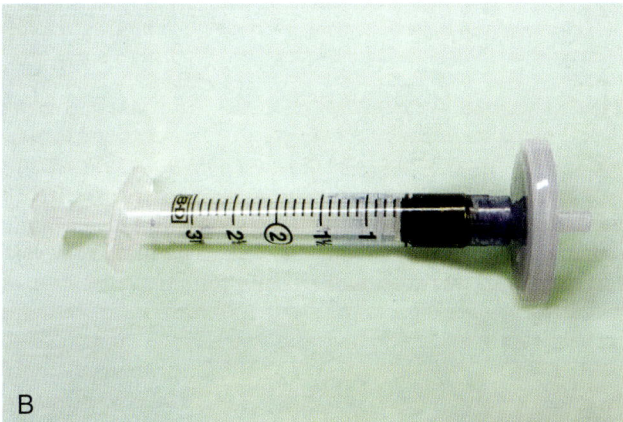
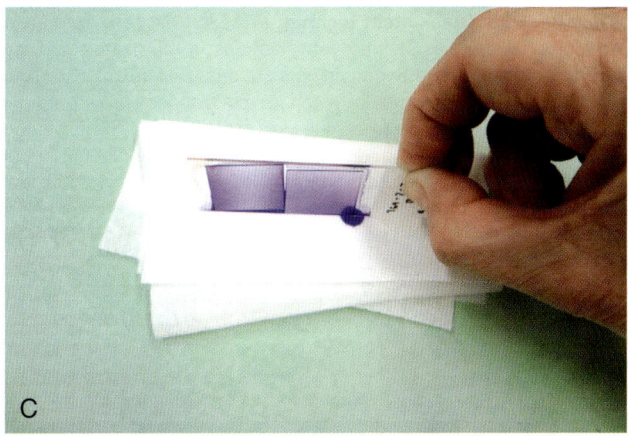

■ **FIGURE 1.18 New methylene blue. A,** This unfiltered stain contains chains of budding yeast as a contaminant. **B,** Contaminants may be removed using a 0.45 μm filter attached to a syringe filled with stain. Just before use, the stain is filtered as a simple drop that is directly applied to an air-dried slide. **C,** The coverslip is applied, and excess stain is removed by tilting the slide at right angles and blotting onto an absorbent sheet.

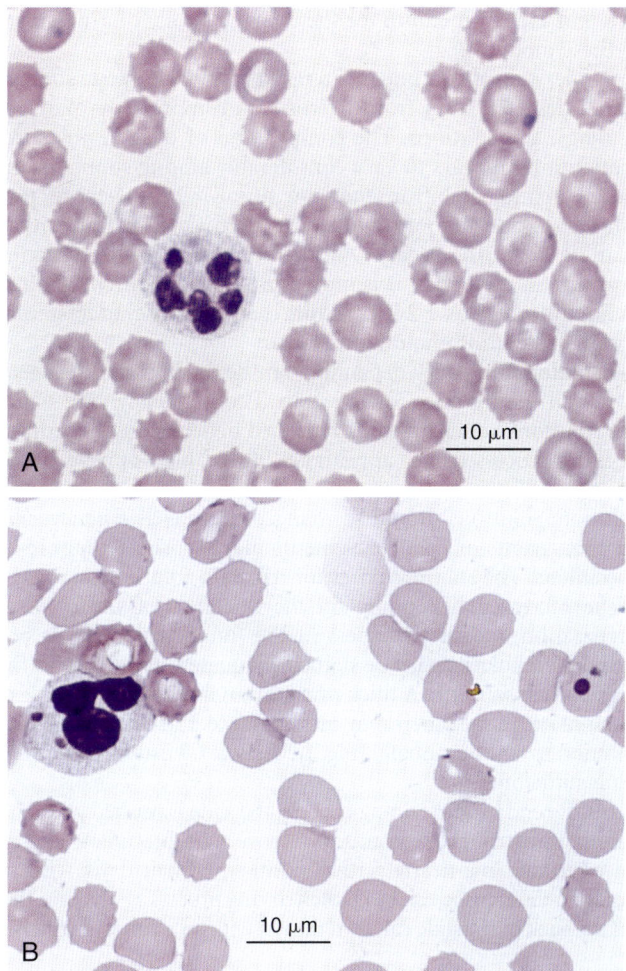

■ **FIGURE 1.19 Staining for distemper inclusion bodies. A,** The cytoplasmic viral inclusions within the neutrophil stain pale blue, as do the surrounding erythrocytes. (Methanolic Romanowsky; HP oil.) **B,** Canine distemper inclusion bodies stain dark purple, accentuating their identification. (Aqueous Romanowsky; HP oil.)

human medical and veterinary laboratories because it results in well-stained blood films. Other MR stains used alone or in various combinations include Leishman and May-Grünwald-Giemsa. Some MR stains are intended to be used as a stat stain. One example of a rapid Wright-Giemsa stain is Camco Quik Stain II (Fisher Scientific).

AR stains include quick-staining stains such as Diff-Quik (RAL Diagnostics) and Shandon Kwik-Diff Stain (Epredia).

These polychromatic stains are commonly used in veterinary practice because of their time-saving convenience. One advantage of AR over MR is the improved visibility of distemper viral inclusion bodies (Fig. 1.19). Mast cell granules, basophil granules, and cytotoxic lymphocyte granules do not stain reliably with AR (Allison and Velguth, 2010). Lengthening the fixation time does not improve the quality of granule staining in mast cell tumors (Jackson et al., 2013). For the diagnostic consideration of a mast cell tumor as differential consideration as a round cell tumor initially stained with AR, an MR stain or NMB-stained specimen is recommended for confirmation. Primary granules and toxic granulation may also stain weaker, according to a Wescor manual comparing automated AR (7120/7121) and MR (7150/7151) Aerospray instruments. With an AR stain, the granule contents are washed away in the water-diluted stain solution. In the MR stain, a precipitate initially forms primarily from a concentrated anhydrous azure B dye solution that stabilizes the granules prior to diluted staining. Although both AR and MR incorporate an initial methanol fixation, they differ in the azure dye type and concentration, pH, and solvent medium for the thiazine family of azures used in these methods.

Understained specimens can result from inadequate staining times, depleted stain from overuse, and improperly managed cytologic preparations. The composition of dyes in polychromatic stains appears to vary considerably among suppliers and from batch to batch from the same supplier. Furthermore, prolonged storage at room temperature (25°C; 77°F) can impair staining intensity because of the formation of degradation products in methanol. It is most convenient to purchase stains in liquid form. Box 1.2 lists factors that can cause understained specimens with Romanowsky stains.

Staining times vary depending on the thickness of the specimen and the freshness of the stain. The frequency with which the solutions are changed or refreshed depends on the number of slides processed. The appearance of dull-blue–appearing nuclei that lack sharp chromatin detail is one indication of a weak solution. Solutions should be changed completely whenever infectious agents or cellular elements inappropriately appear on specimens. The staining times for AR stain solutions may need to be increased depending on the thickness of the cytology preparation and the freshness of the stain. A pleural effusion with low cellularity may be stained adequately with three to five dips in each solution. A thick preparation from a lymph node or bone marrow specimen may require 60 to 120 seconds in each solution to stain optimally (Fig. 1.20). Box 1.3 lists basic staining time guidelines.

At the end of the staining process, the slide is washed with cold running water for 20 seconds to remove stain precipitate and allowed to dry in a nearly vertical position. (A hair dryer with no heat or a fan may be used to hasten drying process.) Any stain film on the back of the slide can be removed with an alcohol-moistened

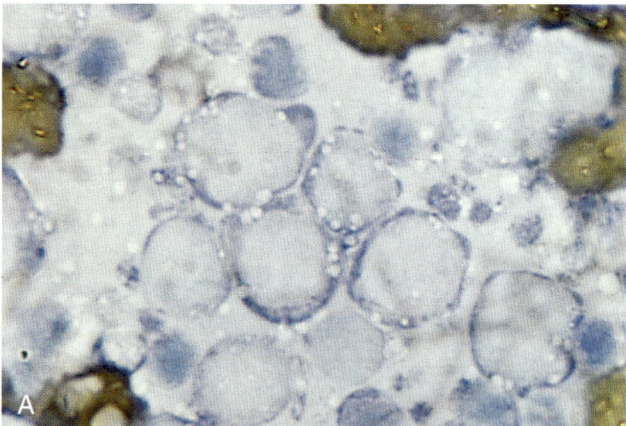
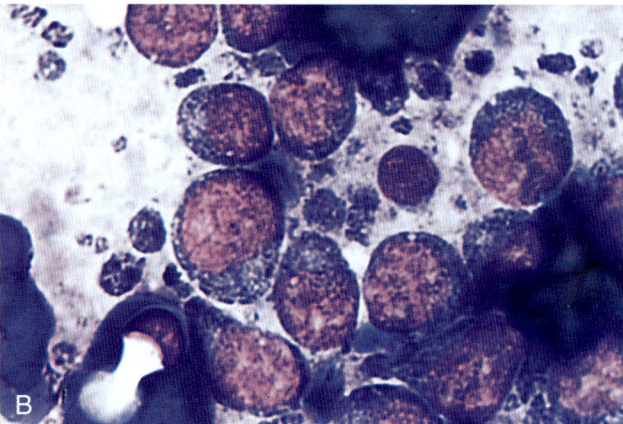

■ **FIGURE 1.20 Quick stain technique. A,** This aspirate from an enlarged lymph node was stained with five dips in the fixative and then five dips into each of the two staining solutions. Cell outlines are seen, but the detailed cytomorphology cannot be diagnostically discerned. (Diff-Quik; HP oil.) **B,** The same slide was replaced into the fixative for approximately 60 seconds and then into the staining solutions for approximately 60 seconds in each station while slowly moving the slide up and down for enhanced stain exposure. A cytologic diagnosis of lymphoma can now be made. A small lymphocyte near the center is a helpful size comparator. (Diff-Quik; HP oil.)

BOX 1.2 Causes of Abnormal Staining

Excessive Blue (Erythrocytes Appear Blue)
Prolonged contact time with the stain
Inadequate wash
Specimen too thick
Stain or diluent too alkaline—pH >7; check with pH paper
Exposure of specimen to formalin or its fumes (e.g., open formalin container)
Delayed fixation

Excessive Pink
Prolonged washing
Insufficient contact time with the stain
Stain or diluent too acidic—pH >7; erythrocytes can appear orange or bright red—formic acid can result from the oxidation of methanol with prolonged exposure to air; fresh methanol is recommended
Mounting the coverslip before the specimen is dry

Inadequately Stained Nucleated Cells and Erythrocytes
Insufficient contact time with one or more of the staining solutions
Surface of a second glass slide covers the specimen on the first slide (can occur when staining two slides back to back in Coplin jars)

Precipitate on the Stained Specimen
Inadequate washing of the slide at the end of the staining period
Inadequate filtration of the stain
Unclean slides

BOX 1.3 Suggested Procedure for Staining Cytologic Specimens Using Aqueous Romanowsky Solutions[a]

Fixative: 60–120 seconds
Solution 1: 30–60 seconds
Solution 2: 5–60 seconds[b]
Rinse under cold tap water: 15 seconds
Examine staining adequacy using low power; eosinophilia or basophilia can be enhanced by returning to solution 1 or solution 2, respectively, followed by a rinse.
Air dry and examine

[a]Suggested times are based on fresh stains; the stains weaken with time and use, and longer times will be required. Consistently understained specimens are an indication for replenishing with fresh stain.
[b]The shortest times are suggested for hypocellular fluids that are low in protein such as transudates, cerebrospinal fluid, and urine sediments.

gauze pad. The stained specimen is initially examined microscopically using the 10× or 20× objective for staining quality and uniformity. If acceptable, a coverslip is placed on the specimen if the 40× objective is to be used. A temporary mount is made by placing a small drop of immersion oil on the specimen followed by placement of a coverslip. A permanent mount is made with a commercially available coverslip xylene-based mounting medium (e.g., Eukitt; Sigma-Aldrich).

> **KEY POINT** A coverslip is always required for sharp focus when the 40× objective ("dry" objective) is used to examine the cytology specimen. A second drop of oil is placed on top of the coverslip when using the oil objective, but be careful not to then flip back to the "dry" objective because bathing it in oil can damage internal rubber rings if not quickly cleaned.

> **KEY POINT** Two staining stations are recommended. One is used for "clean" specimens such as blood films, effusions, and lymph node aspirates, and the other is used for "dirty" specimens such as skin scrapings, fecal and intestinal cytology, and suspected abscesses. The latter stain should be changed more frequently to avoid subsequent contamination and misdiagnosis.

SUBMITTING CYTOLOGY SPECIMENS TO A REFERENCE LABORATORY

The cytology specimen is frequently submitted to a commercial veterinary laboratory for examination. They have personnel specifically trained to process cytologic specimens, such as to make buffy coat and cytospin preparations of fluid specimens, as well as board-certified clinical pathologists to examine cytologic specimens. Their diagnostic expertise is most effective if the specimen is properly prepared with attendant clinical information provided (Christopher et al., 2008).

Fluid specimens should be placed immediately in EDTA tubes to prevent clot formation. If the fluid will be in transit longer than 24 hours, two or more direct slide preparations should be made to accompany the tube. Red-topped and purple-topped blood collection tubes should not be considered sterile; preexisting contaminant bacteria can cause cytologic misdiagnosis and erroneous culture results. Only use containers supplied by the laboratory dedicated for bacterial and fungal culture (contact the laboratory). See Appendix 7 for additional information about submitting specimens for specialized diagnostic testing.

As previously indicated, touch imprint biopsies can be helpful adjuncts to the histologic examination of formalin-fixed tissues. However, formalin vapors can drastically alter the staining characteristics of cytologic smears (Fig. 1.21). When touch imprints are sent along with formalin-fixed tissues to the laboratory, they must be placed in tightly sealed separate packages, never placed together in the same package. Breakage can occur when glass slides are submitted in cardboard containers. Rigid plastic containers offer more reliable protection. If there is a lack of familiarity with a particular sample submission procedure, the laboratory should always be contacted for advice.

Digital microscopy is becoming more readily available to general practitioners. Several devices are available for using cell phone cameras to capture images (see Appendix 1). After these images have been captured, they can be digitally sent to a clinical pathologist for review. A major limitation of this method is that the images may not be representative of the slide or lesion as a whole. In addition, clinical agreement between the digital image and the glass slide diagnosis was significantly higher when images were taken by an experienced cytologist compared with those taken by an inexperienced cytologist (Brooker et al., 2019). Other forms of digital microscopy are emerging, including whole-slide image (WSI) scanning and region of interest digital cytology. WSI scanning has been validated in veterinary medicine but is most commonly used in teaching hospitals, research institutions, and large commercial laboratories because the process is expensive and time consuming. The newer WSI scanners have a function that scans at different focal fields, allowing for the lack of uniformity observed

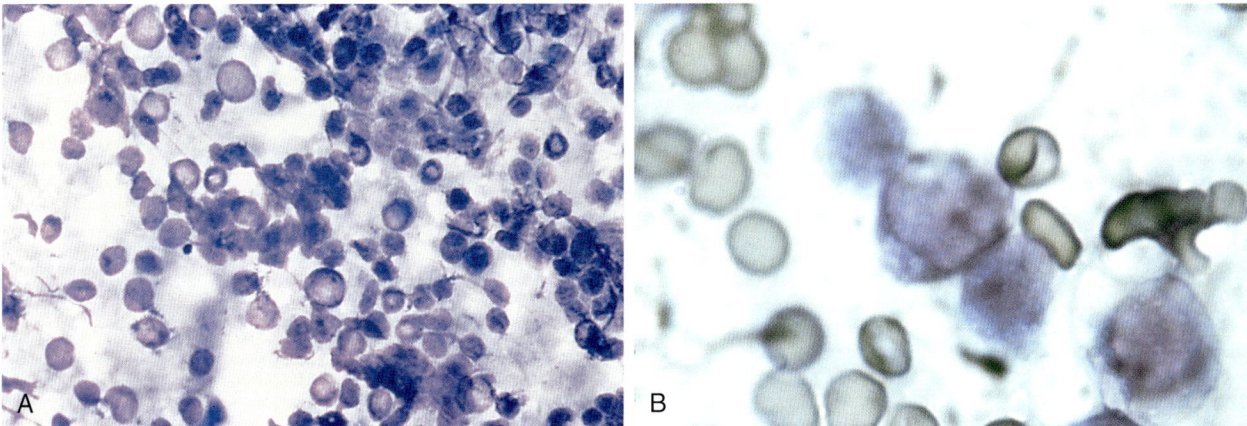

■ **FIGURE 1.21 Formalin effects. A,** This spread preparation from an aspirate biopsy of an enlarged lymph node was inadvertently exposed to formalin fumes before staining. The cells lack cytomorphologic features for accurate diagnostic discernment; therefore, this is a nondiagnostic sample. (Wright; HP oil.) A cytologic diagnosis of lymphoid hyperplasia was made from a second aspirate (not shown). **B,** This hematology slide was inadvertently exposed to formalin while managing the biopsy sample for histologic evaluation. Erythrocyte morphology lacks clarity and has a greenish or yellowish tint; several leukocytes present have indistinct morphology and are not identifiable. (Romanowsky; HP oil.)

of cytologic specimens (Bonsembiante et al., 2019). In these cases, the entire slide is scanned and reviewed by a clinical pathologist using a computer program. An alternate form of digital microscopy involves scanning only the region of interest. This process decreases the file storage space, time, and financial investment. After a slide has been stained and prepared, a trained technician is responsible for identifying and collecting images from the region of interest (Blanchet et al., 2019). These images are then sent digitally to a clinical pathologist for interpretation. As technology continues to advance, it is possible that computer screens will supplement microscopes as another means for the evaluation of the cytologic specimen.

> **KEY POINT** Formalin fumes are pervasive and rapidly penetrating, even through plastic. They alter the staining and morphology of hematology and cytopathology specimens. Keep open formalin containers away from these specimens even if opened only momentarily.

> **HELPFUL HINT** Each individual slide should be labelled with patient name, owner name, date submitted, and location of lesion to ensure proper processing. Clinical information should be included with the submission.

> **KEY POINT** Digital microscopy is becoming more readily available for examination of cytopathology specimens.

REFERENCES

Allison RW, Velguth KE. Appearance of granulated cells in blood films stained by automated aqueous versus methanolic Romanowsky methods. *Vet Clin Pathol.* 2010;39:99-104.

Arai S, Rist P, Clancey N, et al. Fine-needle aspiration of cutaneous, subcutaneous, and intracavitary masses in dogs and cats using 22- vs 25- gauge needles. *Vet Clin Pathol.* 2019;48:287-292.

Blanchet C, Fish E, Miller A, et al. Evaluation of region of interest digital cytology compared to light microscopy for veterinary medicine. *Vet Pathol.* 2019;56:725-731.

Bonsembiante F, Bonfanti U, Cian F, et al. Diagnostic validation of a whole-slide imaging scanner in cytological samples: diagnostic accuracy and comparison with light microscopy. *Vet Pathol.* 2019;56:429-434.

Brooker AJ, Krimer PM, Meichner K, et al. Impact of photographer experience and number of images on telecytology accuracy. *Vet Clin Pathol.* 2019;48:419-424.

Christopher MM, Hotz CS, Shelly SM, et al. Use of cytology as a diagnostic method in veterinary practice and assessment of communication between veterinary practitioners and veterinary clinical pathologist. *J Am Vet Med Assoc.* 2008;232:747-754.

Cohen M, Bohling M, Wright J, et al. Evaluation of sensitivity and specificity of cytologic examination: 269 cases (1999–2000). *J Am Vet Med Assoc.* 2003;222:964-967.

Fagelman D, Chess Q. Nonaspiration fine-needle cytology of the liver: a new technique for obtaining diagnostic samples. *Am J Roentgenol.* 1990;155:1217-1219.

Hodges J. Using cytology to increase small animal practice revenue. *Vet Clin North Am Small Anim Pract.* 2013;43(6):1385-1408.

Jackson DE, Selting KA, Spoor MS, et al. Evaluation of fixation time using Diff-Quik for staining of canine mast cell tumor aspirates. *Vet Clin Pathol.* 2013;42:99-102.

Jergens AE, Andreasen CB, Miles KG. Gastrointestinal endoscopic exfoliative cytology: techniques and clinical application. *Compend Contin Educ Pract Vet.* 2000;22(10):941-951.

Jorundsson E, Lumsden JH, Jacobs RM. Rapid staining techniques in cytopathology: a review and comparison of modified protocols for hematoxylin and eosin, Papanicolaou and Romanowsky stains. *Vet Clin Pathol.* 1999;28:100-108.

Klopfleisch R, Sperling C, Kershaw O, et al. Does the taking of biopsies affect the metastatic potential of tumours? A systematic review of reports on veterinary and human cases and animal models. *Vet J.* 2011;190:e31-e42.

Léveillé R, Partington BP, Biller DS, et al. Complications after ultrasound-guided biopsy of abdominal structures in dogs and cats: 246 cases (1984-1991). *J Am Vet Med Assoc.* 1993;203(3):413-415.

Levitin HA, Foss K, Hague D, et al. The utility of intraoperative impression smear cytology of intracranial granular cell tumors: three cases. *Vet Clin Pathol.* 2019;48:282-286.

Mair S, Dunbar F, Becker PJ, et al. Fine needle cytology—Is aspiration suction necessary? A study of 100 masses in various sites. *Acta Cytol.* 1989;33:809-813.

Meyer DJ, Harvey JW. Evaluation of fluids: effusions, synovial fluid, cerebrospinal fluid. In: Meyer DJ, Harvey JW, eds. *Veterinary Laboratory Medicine: Interpretation and Diagnosis.* Philadelphia: Saunders; 2004:245-259.

Nyland TG, Mattoon JS, Herrgesell EJ, et al. Ultrasound-guided biopsy. In: Nyland TG, Mattoon JS, eds. *Small Animal Diagnostic Ultrasound.* 2nd ed. Philadelphia: Saunders; 2002a:30-48.

Nyland TG, Wallack ST, Wisner ER. Needle-tract implantation following US-guided fine-needle aspiration biopsy of transitional cell carcinoma of the bladder, urethra and prostate. *Vet Radiol Ultrasound.* 2002b;43(1):50-53.

Vignoli M, Rossi F, Chierici C, et al. Needle track implantation after fine needle aspiration biopsy (FNAB) of transitional cell carcinoma of the urinary bladder and adenocarcinoma of the lung. *Schweiz Arch Tierheilkd.* 2007;149(7):314-318.

Warren-Smith CMR, Roe K, de la Puerta B, et al. Pulmonary adenocarcinoma seeding along a fine needle aspiration tract in a dog. *Vet Rec.* 2011;69:181-182.

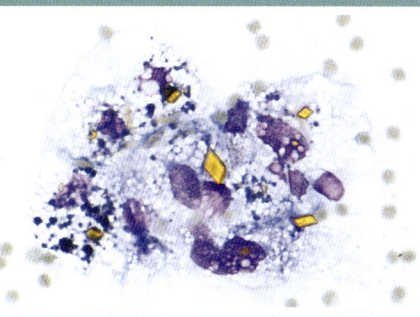

CHAPTER 2

General Categories of Cytologic Interpretation

Rose E. Raskin

Cytologic classifications assist in the diagnosis, prognosis, and management of a case. Interpretations can generally fit into one or more of five cytodiagnostic groups (Box 2.1). A sixth category can be used for nondiagnostic or artifact interpretations. Nondiagnostic samples usually result from insufficient cellular material, poor specimen distribution, or excessive blood contamination.

> **KEY POINT** Interpretation of cytologic material may include more than one category, such as inflammation along with a response to tissue injury or neoplasia with inflammation.

NORMAL TISSUE

Normal tissue is generally composed primarily of mature cell types, although some organs such as integumentary routinely contain immature basal epithelium. Normal cells display uniformity in cellular, nuclear and nucleolar size, and shape. Cytoplasmic volume is usually high relative to the nucleus (Figs. 2.1 and 2.2).

HYPERPLASTIC TISSUE

Hyperplasia is a non-neoplastic enlargement of tissue that can occur in response to hormonal disturbances or tissue injury. Hyperplastic tissue has a tendency to enlarge symmetrically in comparison with neoplasia. Cytologically, hyperplastic cells may appear similar to normal tissue but have a higher nuclear-to-cytoplasmic or nucleocytoplasmic ratio than normal mature cells. Examples of hyperplastic responses include nodular proliferations within the parenchyma of the prostate (Fig. 2.3) and pancreas (Fig. 2.4).

BOX 2.1   General Categories of Cytodiagnostic Interpretation

Normal or hyperplastic tissue
Cystic mass
Inflammation or cellular infiltrate
Response to tissue injury
Neoplasia
Nondiagnostic sample

CYSTIC MASS

Cystic lesions contain liquid or semisolid material. The low-protein liquid usually contains a small number of cells. These benign lesions may result from proliferation of lining cells or tissue injury. Examples include seroma (Fig. 2.5), salivary mucocele, apocrine sweat gland cyst, follicular or infundibular cyst (see Fig. 3.71), and cysts associated with noncutaneous glands such as the mammary gland or prostate (Fig. 2.6).

INFLAMMATION OR CELLULAR INFILTRATE

Inflammatory conditions are classified cytologically by the predominance of the cell type involved. Recognition of the inflammatory cell type often suggests an etiologic condition.

Purulent or suppurative lesions contain greater than 85% neutrophils; they are classified by the presence or absence of nuclear degeneration of the neutrophil. Nondegenerate neutrophils are morphologically normal with mature condensed chromatin and well-segmented purple lobes. These neutrophils predominate in relatively nontoxic environments such as immune-mediated diseases (Fig. 2.7A), neoplastic lesions, and sterile conditions caused by irritants such as urine and bile (Fig. 2.7B).

Degenerate neutrophils display early signs of oncotic necrosis with observable cellular and nuclear swelling with decreased nuclear stain intensity. In cytology, this early recognizable change is termed *karyolysis* (Fig. 2.8). Karyolysis results from decreased mitochondria function to produce adenosine triphosphate (ATP) that maintains transmembrane ion pumps. This function failure results in an influx of calcium, sodium, and water (hydropic degeneration), leading to damaged cell membranes and activated endonucleases that degrade RNA and DNA. This often indicates rapid cell death in a toxic or injurious environment. Degenerate neutrophils predominate in bacterial infections, particularly gram-negative types that produce endotoxins. Cytologically, under conditions of neutrophil degeneration, small infectious agents must be found intracellularly to confidently report it as septic neutrophilic inflammation (Fig. 2.9). *Karyolysis* as a histologic term describes cell death in the form of a ghost nucleus or nuclear remnants that precede eventual nuclear loss or dissolution.

In contrast to acute cell injury involving cellular and nuclear swelling, cell death may occur more slowly through a shrinkage phenomenon (apoptosis). Although apoptosis often occurs in isolated cells during normal physiologic cell aging (Fig. 2.10), it may be found alongside pathologic cell death characterized by

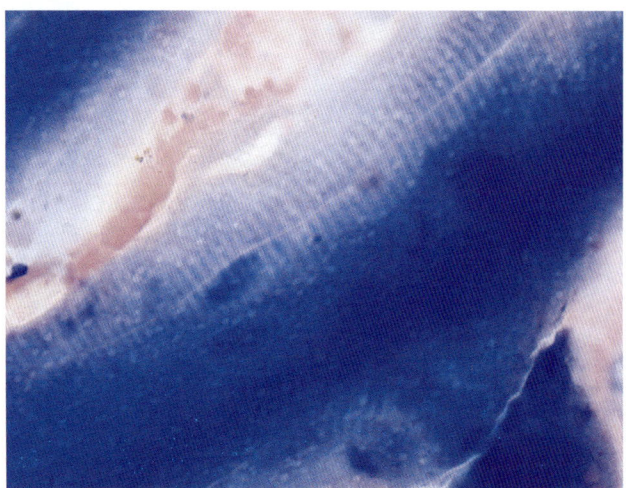

FIGURE 2.1 Normal skeletal muscle. Tissue aspirate. Dog. Numerous threadlike myofibrils compose each cell with small, condensed, and oval nucleus. Cross-striations, characteristic of skeletal muscle, are visible against the dark blue cytoplasm. (Modified Wright; HP oil.)

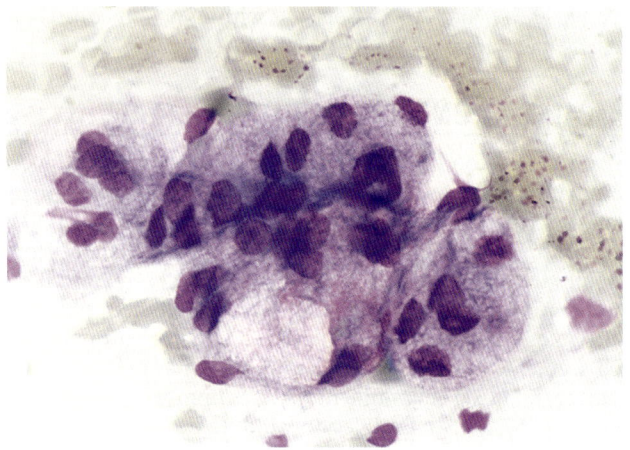

FIGURE 2.2 Normal salivary gland. Tissue aspirate. Dog. The gland has uniform features of nuclear size, nucleocytoplasmic ratio, and cytoplasmic content. (Wright-Giemsa; HP oil.)

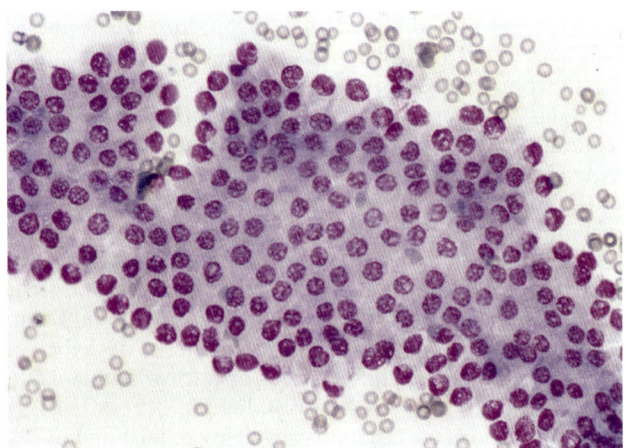

FIGURE 2.3 Canine prostatic hyperplasia. Tissue aspirate. Dog. The presenting clinical sign in this case involves blood dripping from the prepuce. Cytopathology reveals the nuclear size is uniform; however, the nucleocytoplasmic ratio is increased as indicated by the close proximity of nuclei to each other. (Wright-Giemsa; HP oil.)

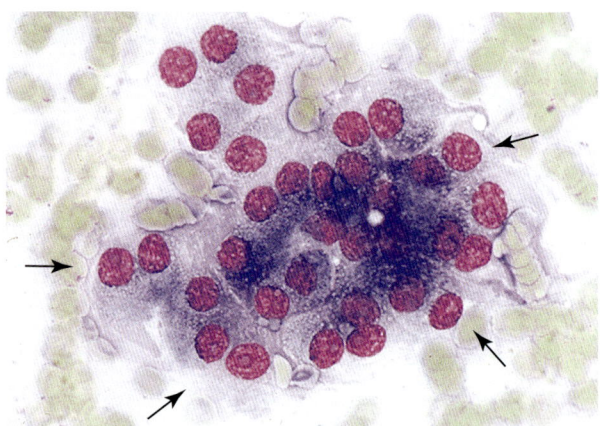

FIGURE 2.4 Nodular hyperplasia of the pancreas. Tissue aspirate. Dog. Ultrasound examination revealed a hypoechoic mass in the area of the pancreas. Hyperplastic parenchymal organs commonly display binucleation *(arrows)*. (Wright-Giemsa; HP oil.)

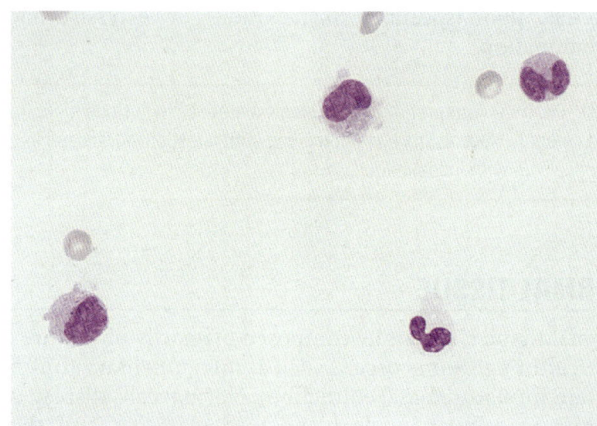

FIGURE 2.5 Seroma. Tissue aspirate. Dog. Blood-tinged fluid is removed from a swelling on the neck. There is low cellularity (3800/μL) and low protein content (2.5 g/dL). The direct smear contains a mixed cell population with large mononuclear cells having fine cytoplasmic granularity along with low numbers of erythrocytes. (Wright-Giemsa; HP oil.)

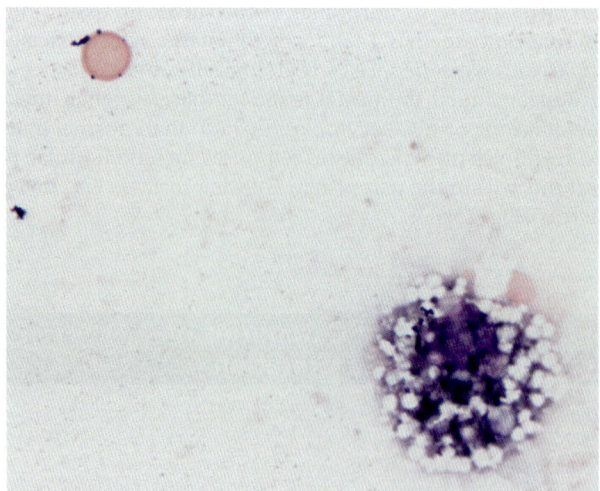

FIGURE 2.6 Prostatic cyst. Tissue aspirate. Dog. Low cellularity is apparent and a single mononuclear cell is shown, presumed to be a macrophage containing dark granular material, likely cystic debris. (Modified Wright; HP oil.)

CHAPTER 2 *General Categories of Cytologic Interpretation* 17

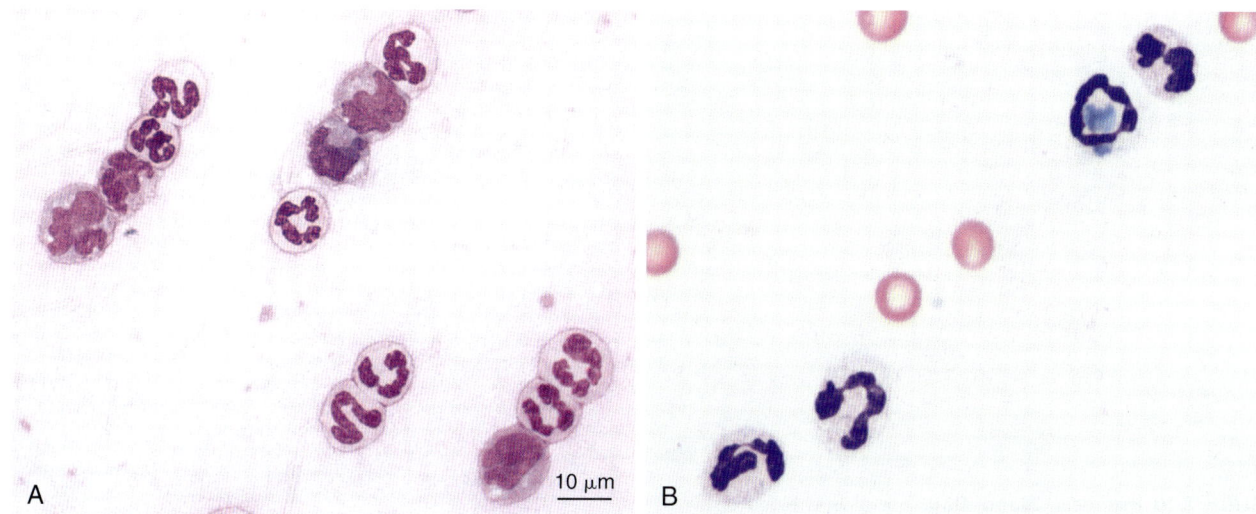

■ **FIGURE 2.7 A, Nondegenerate neutrophils. Synovial fluid. Dog.** This fluid is from a Doberman pinscher with an immune-mediated response to trimethoprim-sulfadiazine. There are eight neutrophils and five large mononuclear cells in windrowing or linear fashion. (Wright-Giemsa; HP oil.) **B, Nondegenerate neutrophils. Abdominal fluid. Dog.** Abdominal fluid following bile duct rupture with intact neutrophils, one of which has phagocytized green-gray mucus. (Modified Wright; HP oil).

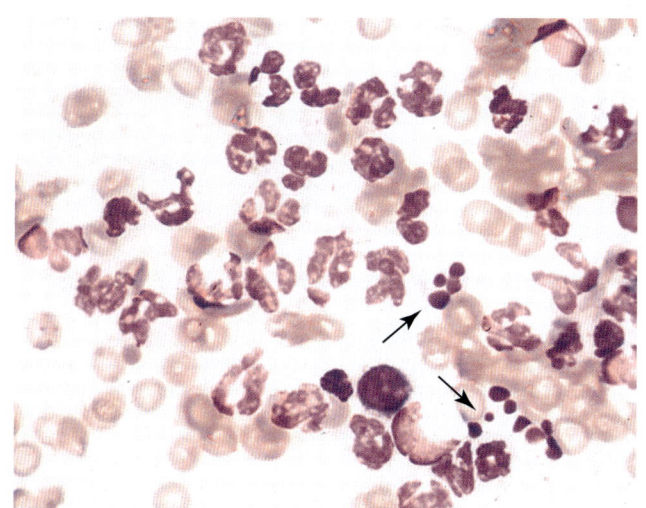

■ **FIGURE 2.8 Degenerate neutrophils, karyorrhexis. Tissue aspirate. Dog.** Mild to moderate karyolysis of neutrophils is evident by the decreased nuclear stain intensity and swollen nuclear lobes. Pyknosis of multiple nuclear segments appears as dark, dense, round structures, termed *karyorrhexis (arrows)*, in this case of bacterial dermatitis. (Wright-Giemsa; HP oil.)

■ **FIGURE 2.9 Bacterial sepsis. Tissue aspirate. Dog.** Markedly karyolytic neutrophils are present with intracellular coccoid bacteria. Karyolysis is so severe that the cells are barely recognizable as neutrophils. A fragmented erythrocyte is helpful for size comparison to demonstrate neutrophil swelling. (Modified Wright; HP oil.)

widespread nuclear destruction and necrosis. Increased nuclear staining (*hyperchromia*) with coalescence of the nucleus into a single or two dark basophilic round segments characterizes *pyknosis* (Fig. 2.11). If pyknosis is related to a slow, progressive change within a relatively nontoxic environment, an intact cell membrane may be present around the shrunken, more eosinophilic cell as occurs with normal cell aging. An end stage of nuclear breakdown termed *karyorrhexis* or *karyohexis* (Mastrorilli et al., 2013) may be seen as the result of pyknosis of hypersegmented nuclei (see Fig. 2.8) or fragmentation of chromatin of an individual dying cell (Fig. 2.12) as seen on both cytology and histology.

Histiocytic or *macrophagic* lesions contain a predominance of macrophages, suggesting chronic inflammation (Fig. 2.13). Foamy, often vacuolated, and phagocytic cells characterize this type of inflammation. In contrast, granulomatous lesions consisting of macrophages that morphologically resemble epithelial cells form in response to foreign material or persistent intracellular infectious agents and have a secretory rather than phagocytic activity. These cells are therefore termed *epithelioid macrophages* and are recognized by their abundant basophilic cytoplasm and large polygonal shape (Fig. 2.14). Epithelioid macrophages under the influence of cytokines and other inflammatory mediators undergo macrophage fusion to form

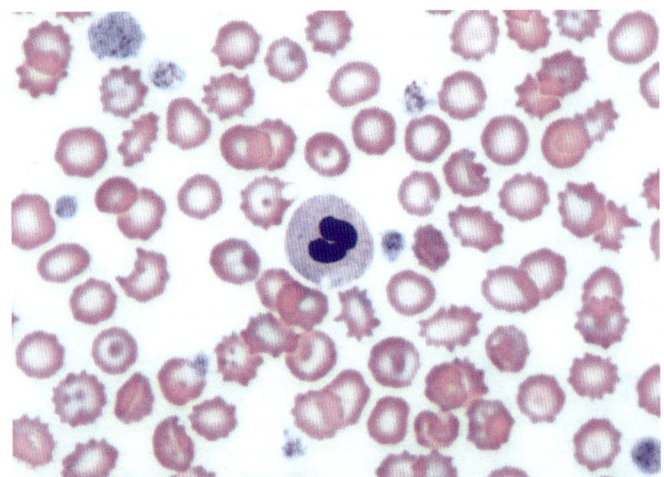

■ **FIGURE 2.10 Pyknosis. Blood. Dog.** Two-day-old blood displays cell aging and early pyknosis with rounded dense nuclear condensation and increased cytoplasmic eosinophilia. This change in the color of the cytoplasm is attributed to consolidation of cellular components or loss of ribosomal RNA, which is responsible for cytoplasmic basophilia. (Modified Wright; HP oil.)

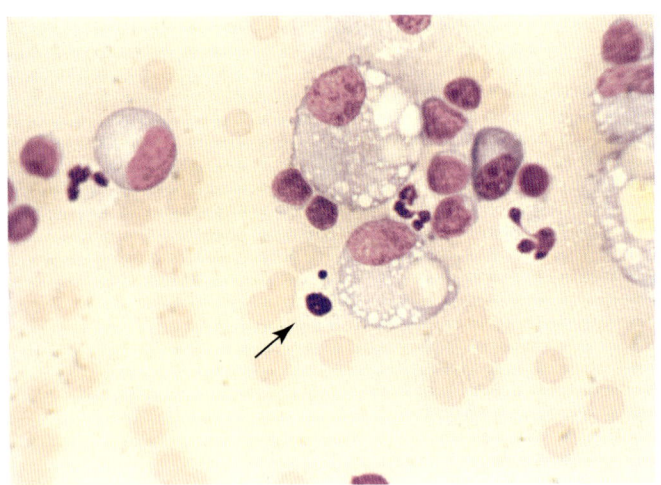

■ **FIGURE 2.11 Pyknosis. Chylous effusion. Dog.** Chronic inflammation of this fluid produces neutrophils with nuclei that have condensed into a large, often single, dark, round structure *(arrow)* related to the slow progression of cellular change in this nonseptic environment. The pyknotic cell *(arrow)* in this case also contains a second, smaller round nuclear fragment. (Wright; HP oil.)

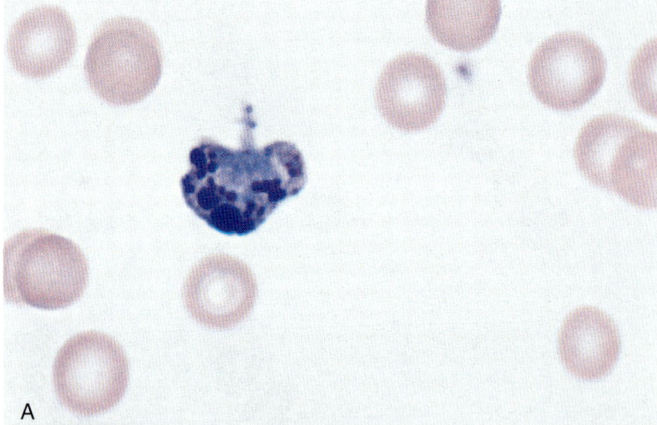

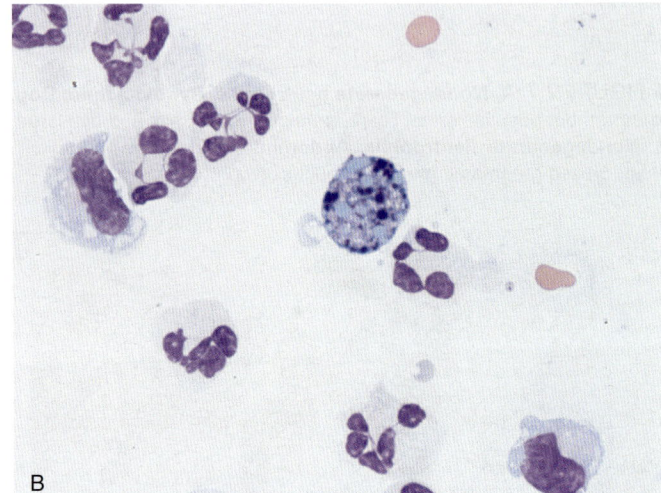

■ **FIGURE 2.12 A, Karyorrhexis. Bone marrow aspirate. Dog.** Fragmentation of the nucleus in this leukemic patient. (Modified Wright; HP oil). **B, Karyorrhexis. Abdominal fluid. Cat.** Nondegenerate neutrophils and two small mononuclear cells are present along with unknown cell that appears to contain blue and purple-black fragments. (Modified Wright; HP oil.)

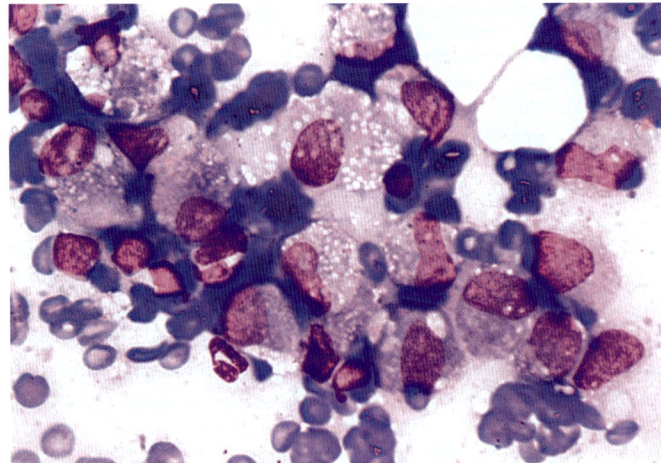

■ **FIGURE 2.13 Macrophagic inflammation. Tissue imprint. Dog.** Nodular lung disease with numerous large mononuclear cells having abundant foamy gray cytoplasm that also contains multiple colorless vacuoles. (Wright-Giemsa; HP oil.)

giant multinucleated forms (Fig. 2.15). Granulomas are often associated with foreign body reactions or fungi and appear cytologically by the presence of epithelioid macrophages or multinucleate cells.

Mixed cell inflammatory lesions contain a mixture of neutrophils and macrophages (Fig. 2.16) that also may include increased numbers of lymphocytes or plasma cells. This type of inflammation is often associated with foreign body reactions, fungal infections, mycobacterial infections, panniculitis, lick granulomas, and other chronic tissue injuries. The term *pyogranulomatous* should be reserved for a population of neutrophils and epithelioid macrophages with or without multinucleate giant cells (see Fig. 2.14).

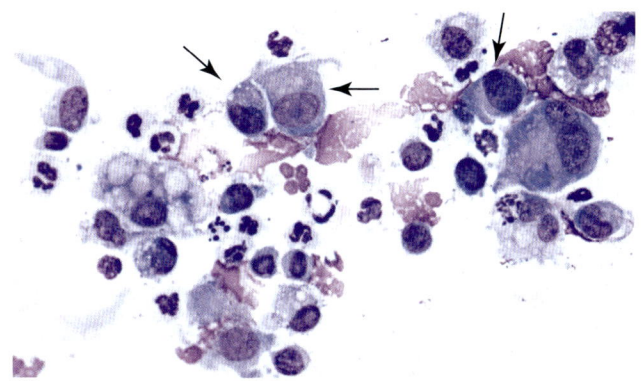

■ **FIGURE 2.14 Pyogranulomatous inflammation. Tissue aspirate. Dog.** Long-standing bacterial infection created a mixture of degenerate neutrophils, epithelioid macrophages *(arrows)*, binucleated giant cell, lymphocytes, and a vacuolated phagocytic macrophage. Note the presence of karyorrhexis *(near center)*. A plump fibroblast is seen in the upper left. (Modified Wright; HP oil.) (From Raskin RE. Tail mass in a dog. *NAVC Clinician's Brief*. 2006;Nov:13-15.)

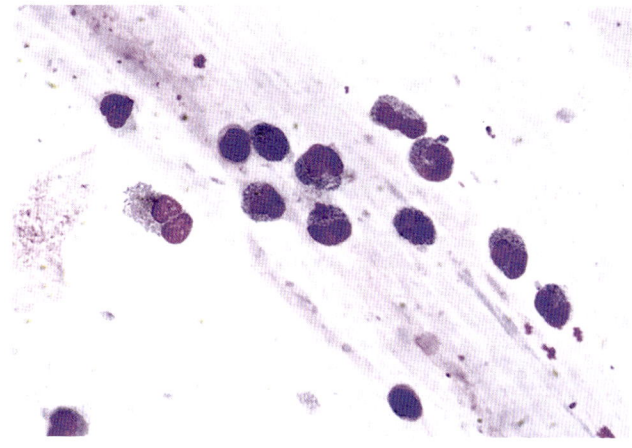

■ **FIGURE 2.17 Eosinophilic inflammation. Transtracheal wash. Cat.** Clinical presentation of a chronic cough in this cat with suspected pulmonary allergy. Fluid contains 95% eosinophils. Shown are several eosinophils that stain pink to orange and adhere to pink mucous material that prevents full stain penetration. (Wright-Giemsa; HP oil.)

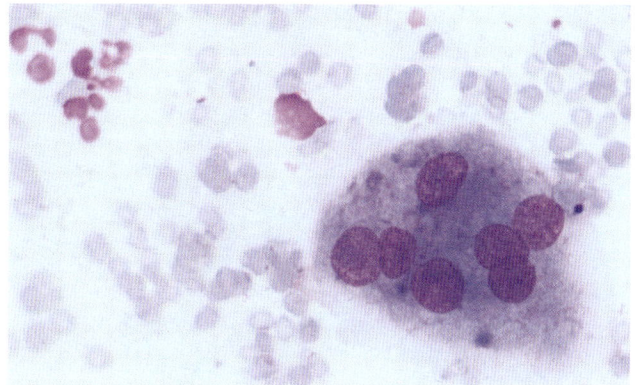

■ **FIGURE 2.15 Multinucleate giant cell. Tissue aspirate. Cat.** Skin lesion with pyogranulomatous inflammation, including many giant cells related to the presence of fungal hyphae (not shown). Shown is a cell with seven distinct nuclei and abundant blue-gray granular cytoplasm. (Wright-Giemsa; HP oil.)

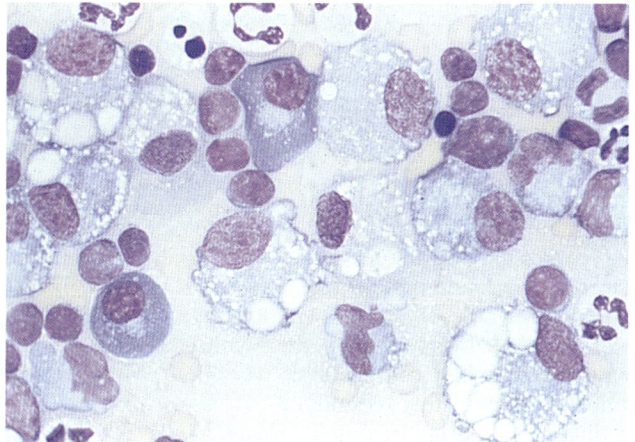

■ **FIGURE 2.16 Mixed cell inflammation. Chylous effusion. Dog.** Chronic chylous effusion contains a variety of cell types, including non-degenerate neutrophils, vacuolated macrophages, small to medium lymphocytes, and two mature plasma cells. (Wright; HP oil.)

Eosinophilic lesions contain greater than 10% eosinophils in addition to other inflammatory cell types (Fig. 2.17). These lesions may appear with or without mast cell involvement. It is common to see rust or brown granules in the cytoplasm of eosinophils on cytology in contrast to the pink-red cell color seen in blood. An eosinophilic inflammatory response is associated with eosinophilic granuloma, hypersensitivity or allergic conditions, parasitic migrations, fungal infections, mast cell tumors, and other neoplastic conditions that induce eosinophilopoiesis such as lymphoma. This combination of eosinophilic inflammatory conditions has been referred to as "worms, wheezes, and weird diseases."

Lymphocytic or *plasmacytic* infiltration is often associated with allergic or immune reactions, early viral infections, and chronic inflammation. The lymphoid population is heterogeneous, with small or intermediate-sized lymphocytes and plasma cells mixed with other inflammatory cells (see Fig. 2.16). In contrast, a monomorphic population of lymphoid cells without other inflammatory cells present may suggest lymphoid neoplasia.

Cytologic samples often contain evidence of tissue injury in addition to cyst formation, inflammation, or neoplasia. These changes include hemorrhage, proteinaceous debris, cholesterol or calcium crystals, necrosis, and fibrosis.

Pathologic *hemorrhage* should be distinguished from blood contamination encountered during the cytologic collection. Blood contamination is associated with the presence of numerous erythrocytes and platelets, whereas acute hemorrhage is associated with engulfment of erythrocytes by macrophages termed *erythrophagocytosis* (Fig. 2.18). Care must be taken to evaluate direct smears first before reporting the findings of processed materials. For example, the simple act of centrifugation to create a sediment smear from body fluids can activate macrophages to engulf nearby erythrocytes, an observation absent on the direct smear. Chronic hemorrhage is associated with foamy macrophages containing degraded blood pigment within their cytoplasm—for example, blue-green to black hemosiderin granules (Figs. 2.19 and 2.20) or yellow rhomboid

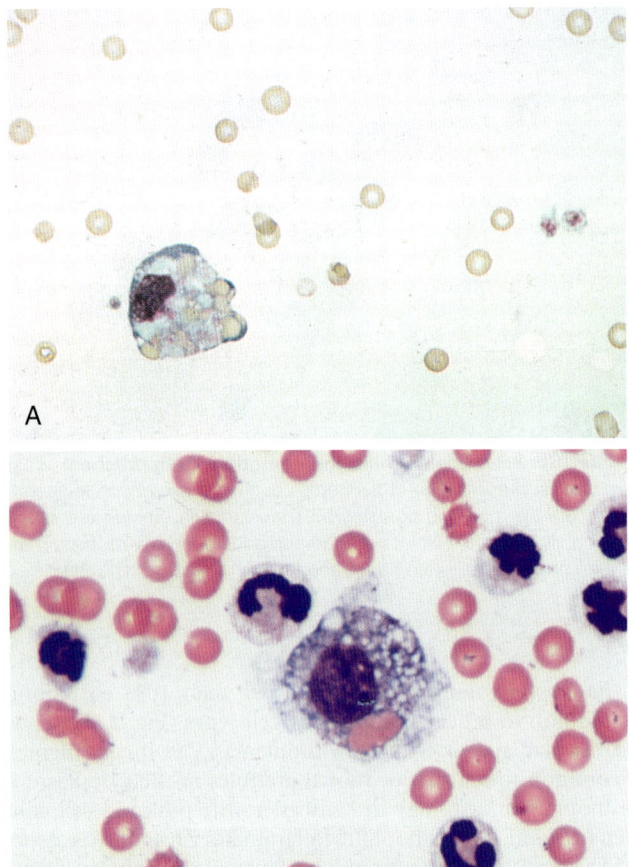

FIGURE 2.18 A, Erythrophagocytosis. Cerebrospinal fluid. Cat. Many erythrocytes are in the background of this direct smear along with one large macrophage that has engulfed numerous intact red cells. The cat had a confirmed infection (titer 1:1600) with feline coronavirus (feline infectious peritonitis). Erythrophagocytosis in this case supports the presence of acute hemorrhage. (Wright; HP oil.) **B, Erythrophagocytosis postcentrifugation artifact. Pleural fluid. Dog.** Sedimentation of the fluid induced macrophage engulfment of erythrocytes. Blood contamination, not acute hemorrhage, is present in this case. This was supported by frequent platelets and the absence of erythrophagocytosis in the direct smear. (Modified Wright; HP oil.)

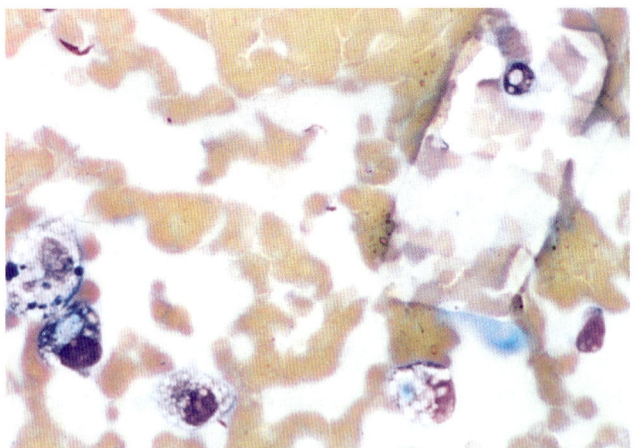

FIGURE 2.19 Chronic hemorrhage with hemosiderin. Tissue aspirate. Dog. Several foamy macrophages are present in this follicular cyst lesion. The macrophage directly below the cholesterol crystal contains blue-green granular material in the cytoplasm consistent with hemosiderin, a breakdown product of erythrocytes. On the *left edge* is a macrophage with large black granules suggestive of hemosiderin. (Wright; HP oil.)

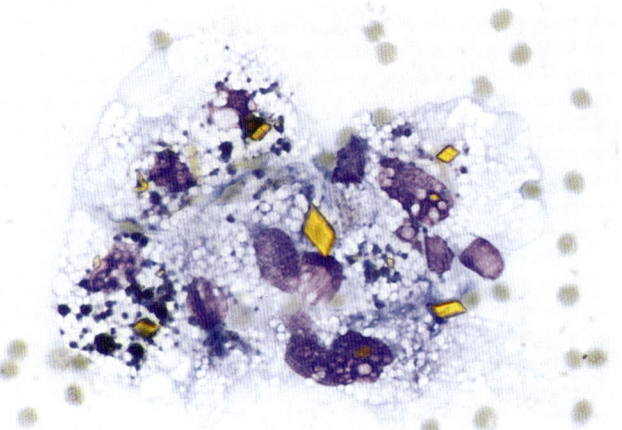

FIGURE 2.20 Chronic hemorrhage with hematoidin and hemosiderin. Pericardial fluid. Dog. Vacuolated macrophages with bright yellow rhomboid crystals (hematoidin) of variable size appear in this hemorrhagic fluid related to hemoglobin breakdown in an anaerobic environment. Several macrophages also contain black granular material consistent with hemosiderin. (Wright-Giemsa; HP oil.)

hematoidin crystals (see Fig. 2.20). Hemosiderin represents an excess aggregation of ferritin molecules or micelles. This form of iron storage becomes visible by light microscopy and stains blue with the Prussian blue reaction. Hematoidin crystals do not contain iron and are often formed during anaerobic breakdown of hemoglobin such as may occur within tissues or body cavities. Hematomas often contain phagocytized erythrocytes if the lesion is acute or hemosiderin-laden macrophages if the lesion is chronic.

Proteinaceous debris may be seen within the background of the preparation. Mucus stains lightly basophilic and appears amorphous (Fig. 2.21). Lymphoglandular bodies (Fig. 2.22) are cytoplasmic fragments from fragile cells, usually lymphocytes, which are discrete, round, lightly basophilic structures (Flanders et al., 1993). *Nuclear streaming* refers to linear pink to purple strands of nuclear remnants (Fig. 2.23) produced by excessive tissue handling of normal tissue during cytologic preparation or by compressing necrotic material on slides. Clear to light-pink amorphous strands representing collagen (Fig. 2.24) may be admixed with spindle cells and endothelium within a fibrovascular stroma. However, when these collagen fibers undergo damage (as in the collagenolysis associated with mast cell tumor), degranulating eosinophils release collagenase that produces dense, hyalinized pink collagen bands (Fig. 2.25). On histology, these necrotic collagen bands may form flame figures (Fig. 2.26), which may appear in several eosinophilic dermatopathic conditions. Amyloid is an uncommon pathologic protein found in tissues composed of several types between cells

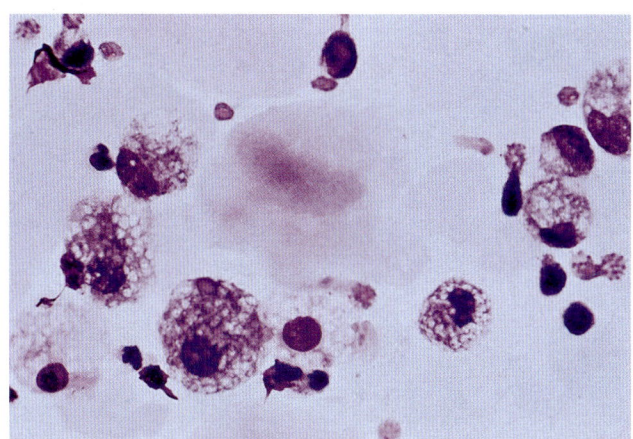

■ **FIGURE 2.21 Mucus. Salivary mucocele. Dog.** The background contains pale pink-blue amorphous material representative of mucus. Numerous foamy macrophages or mucinophages compose the predominant population. (Wright; HP oil.)

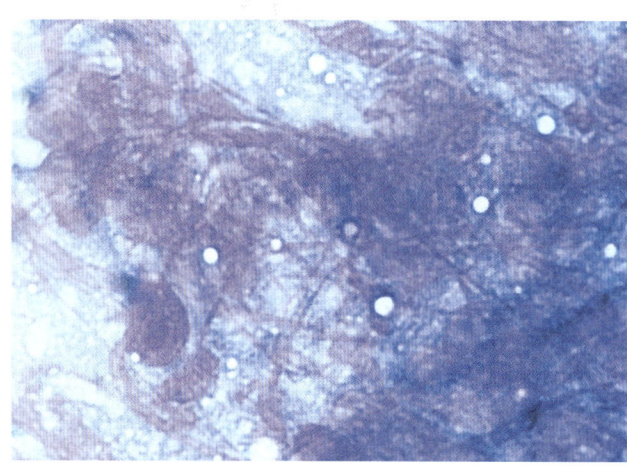

■ **FIGURE 2.23 Nuclear streaming. Tissue aspirate.** Purple strands of nuclear material are formed from ruptured cells either as an artifact of slide preparation or from fragile cells that are frequently neoplastic. (Wright-Giemsa; HP oil.) (Courtesy Denny Meyer, University of Florida.)

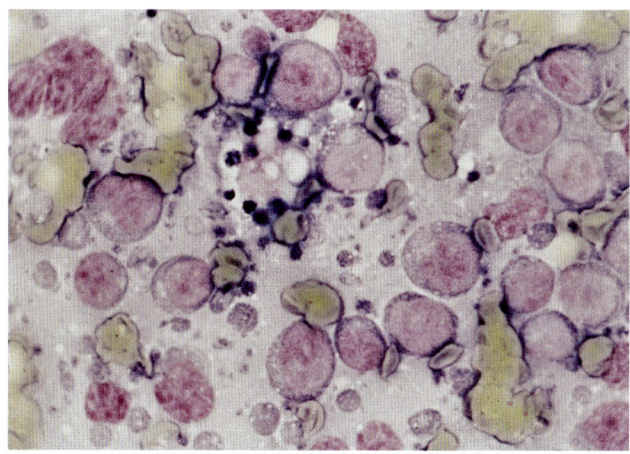

■ **FIGURE 2.22 Lymphoglandular bodies. Tissue aspirate. Dog.** The background of this lymph node preparation contains numerous small, blue-gray cytoplasmic fragments called *lymphoglandular bodies* that are related to the rupture of the fragile neoplastic lymphocytes. A large vacuolated macrophage has phagocytized cellular debris appearing as large blue-black particles. (Wright; HP oil.)

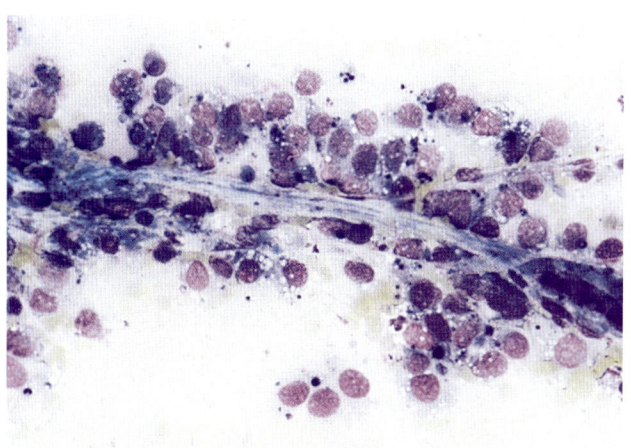

■ **FIGURE 2.24 Collagen fibers. Tissue aspirate. Dog.** Clear to light pink strands of intact strands of connective tissue may resemble fungal hyphae. Collagen fibers have poorly defined margins and a variable diameter, unlike hyphae, which have uniform width and distinct borders. Fibrin may appear similar but is often associated with evidence of bleeding. (Wright-Giemsa, HP oil.)

(Woldemeskel, 2012). It appears amorphous, eosinophilic, and hyaline and may be associated with chronic inflammation, plasma cell tumors (see Fig. 3-198A–B), or familial amyloidosis (Fig. 2.27). Cytoplasmic granules from neoplastic mast cells have been found within neutrophils from circulating blood and splenic cytology in both dogs (Conrado and Raskin, 2017) and cats (Fig. 2.28).

Cholesterol crystals represent evidence of cell membrane damage with lipid degeneration that appears in the background of some cytologic preparations. These crystals most often appear transparent, rectangular, and as stacked plates, particularly when background staining is enhanced, for example, with new methylene blue stain (Fig. 2.29). These crystals are most often associated with epidermal or follicular cysts. Other shape forms are possible for cholesterol as shown in Fig. A3.3C–D.

Necrosis and *fibrosis* may occur together or separately in some cytologic preparations. Dead or necrotic cells appear fuzzy or blurred with indistinct cell or nuclear outlines and lack recognition of cell origin (Fig. 2.30). A reparative response accompanying tissue injury involves increased fibroblastic activity. It is common to see very reactive fibrocytes (Fig. 2.31) along with severe inflammation. One must be careful not to overinterpret this reactivity as a neoplastic condition because fibroblasts display anaplastic features such as open and ropy chromatin, prominent nucleoli, and high nucleocytoplasmic ratios compared with mature fibrocytes. Abundant well-differentiated mast cells may be associated with fibroplasia, and care should be taken not to misdiagnose mast cell tumor in these situations.

Mitosis may be evident with increased cell turnover under normal physiologic and reparative influences in addition to a

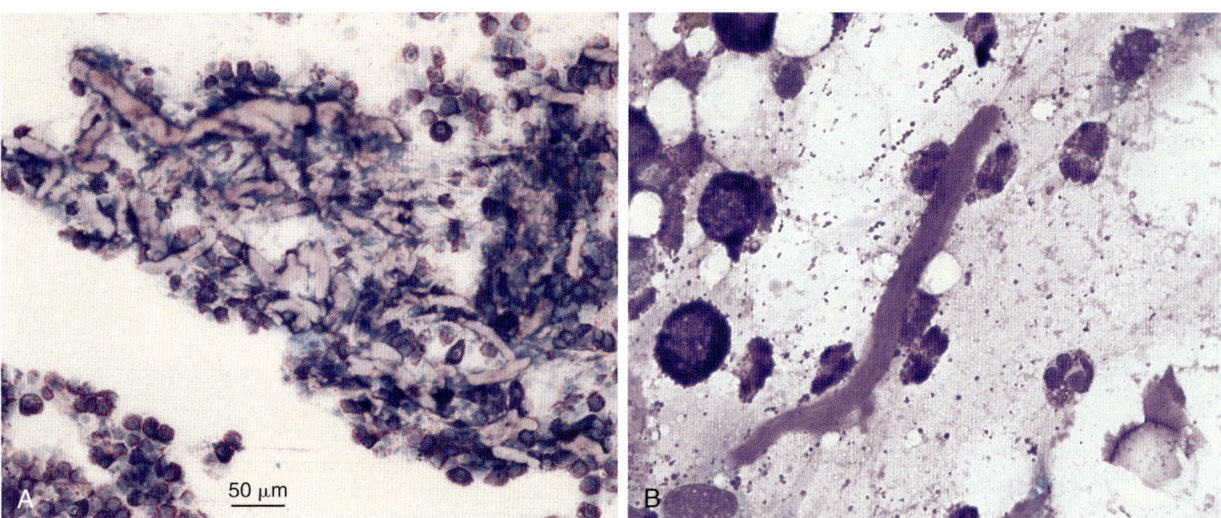

■ **FIGURE 2.25 Collagenolysis. Skin aspirate. Dog. A,** Haphazard bands of collagen appear bright pink and hyalinized owing to the breakdown of the fibers through release of collagenase by degranulating eosinophils. This type of connective tissue damage occurs commonly in canine mast cell tumors. Interspersed among tumor cells are eosinophils and their granules. (Wright; IP.) **B,** Hyalinized collagen surrounded by eosinophils with two mast cells nearby from a mast cell tumor. (Wright; HP oil.)

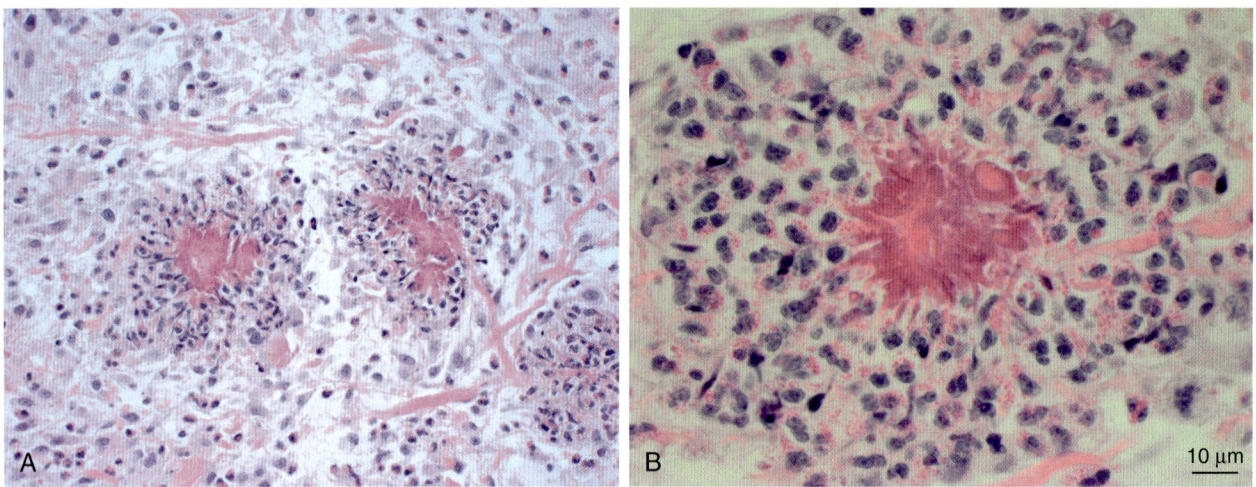

■ **FIGURE 2.26 Collagenolysis. Flame figures. Skin tissue section. Dog.** Same case in A and B. **A,** Two flame figures appear composed of aggregates of necrobiotic collagen with eosinophilic granules surrounded by dense dermal eosinophilic infiltrates. (H&E, IP.) **B,** One flame figure consists of necrobiotic collagen with eosinophilic granules surrounded by a monomorphic population of eosinophils from a case of eosinophilic dermatitis of unknown etiology. (H&E, IP.)

neoplastic proliferation (Fig. 2.32). Normal-appearing mitotic figures are common in hyperplastic lymph nodes and regenerative bone marrow. For examples, see Fig. A4.1A–I. Differences between normal and abnormal mitotic figures are discussed in more detail elsewhere (Tvedten, 2009).

NEOPLASIA

General Features

Neoplasia is initially considered when a monomorphic or monotypic cell population is present and significant inflammation is lacking. Further division into benign and malignant types involves cytomorphologic characteristics. *Benign cells* display uniformity in nuclear and cell size, nucleocytoplasmic ratio, and other nuclear features. *Malignant cells* often display three or more criteria of cellular immaturity or atypia, which are necessary to identify before making a diagnosis of malignancy (Table 2.1 and Figs. 2.32 to 2.38). Suggest performing histopathologic examination with cases having an equivocal diagnosis or severe inflammation that might mask neoplasia.

Cytomorphologic Categories

Neoplasms may be divided into four general categories to assist in making the cytologic interpretation and providing a list of differential diagnoses (Perman et al., 1979; Alleman and Bain, 2000). The categories listed in Table 2.2 are *not* based on cell origin or function but rather on their general cytomorphologic characteristics. The first two terms, *epithelial* and *mesenchymal*, are taken from embryologic histology (Noden and de Lahunta, 1985).

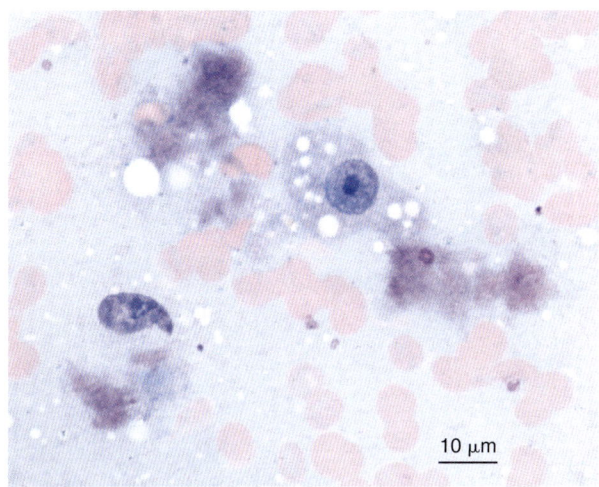

■ **FIGURE 2.27 Amyloid. Tissue aspirate. Dog.** Amorphous magenta material surrounds a hepatocyte from a Shar Pei with familial amyloidosis. (Modified Wright, HP oil.)

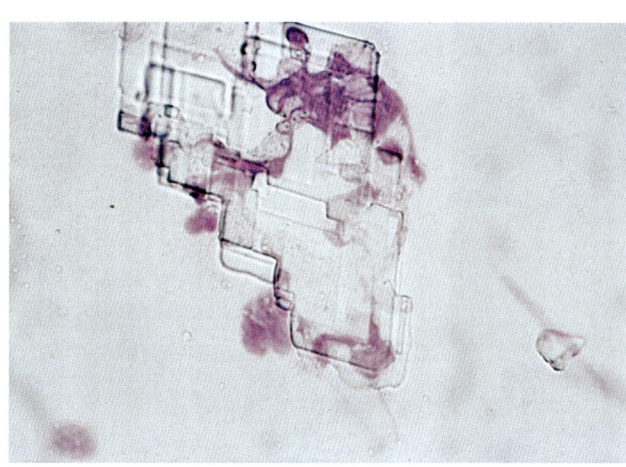

■ **FIGURE 2.29 Cholesterol crystal. Tissue aspirate.** Clear rectangular plates with notched corners are characteristic of cholesterol. This is often associated with degenerate squamous epithelium, as in follicular cysts. Crystals are highlighted against background cellular debris or by using an aqueous-based stain. (New methylene blue; HP oil.) (Courtesy Denny Meyer, University of Florida.)

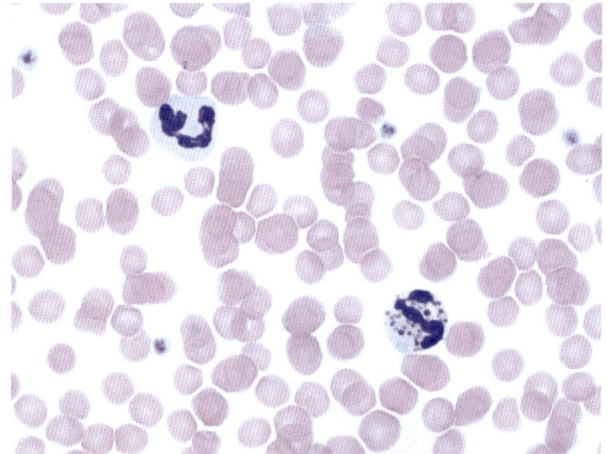

■ **FIGURE 2.28 Phagocytosis of mast cell granules. Blood smear. Cat.** Multiple and variably sized magenta to dark purple inclusions within a neutrophil *(right)* from a case of splenic and bone marrow mast cell tumor. (Modified Wright, HP oil.) (Courtesy Athema Etzioni and Rose Raskin, Purdue University. Presented at the 2005 ASVCP case review session.)

Epithelial Neoplasms

Epithelial neoplasms such as embryonal epithelium often associate with glandular or parenchymal tissue and lining surfaces. These neoplasms display a clustered cell arrangement with ball shapes or monolayer sheets. Examples of epithelial neoplasms include lung adenocarcinoma (Fig. 2.39), perianal adenoma (hepatoid tumor), trichoblastoma, sebaceous adenoma, urothelial cell carcinoma (Fig. 2.40), and mesothelioma. Specific cytologic features of epithelial neoplasms are listed in Box 2.2 such as tight cell junctions termed *desmosomes* (Fig. 2.41).

Mesenchymal Neoplasms

Neoplasms with a mesenchymal appearance resemble the embryonic connective tissue, mesenchyme. This tissue is loosely arranged with usually abundant extracellular matrix and individualized spindle, oval, or stellate cells (Bacha and Bacha, 2000).

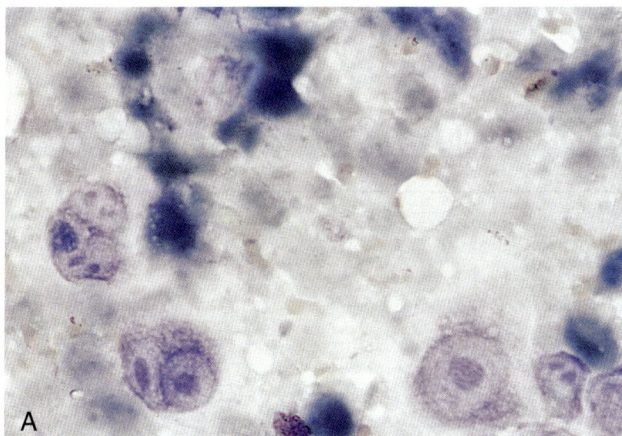
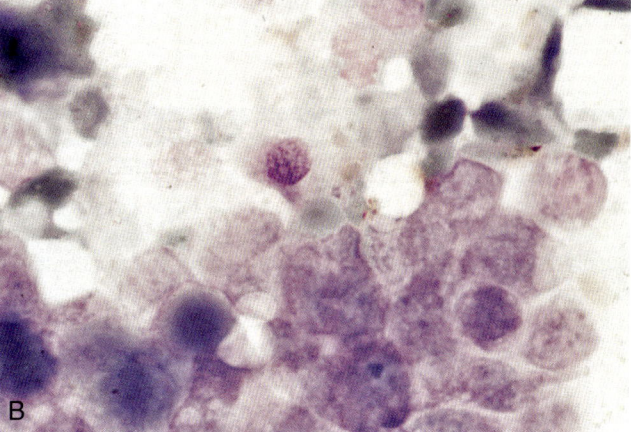

■ **FIGURE 2.30 Necrosis. Tissue aspirate. Dog.** Same case in A and B. **A,** Prominent nucleoli remain visible; other tissue has degenerated into dark blue-gray amorphous debris representative of necrotic material. The sample was from a case of prostatic carcinoma in which the necrotic site was focal. (Wright-Giemsa; HP oil.) **B,** Cell outlines remain visible; nuclear swelling is evident during this example of acute cell death. (Wright-Giemsa; HP oil.)

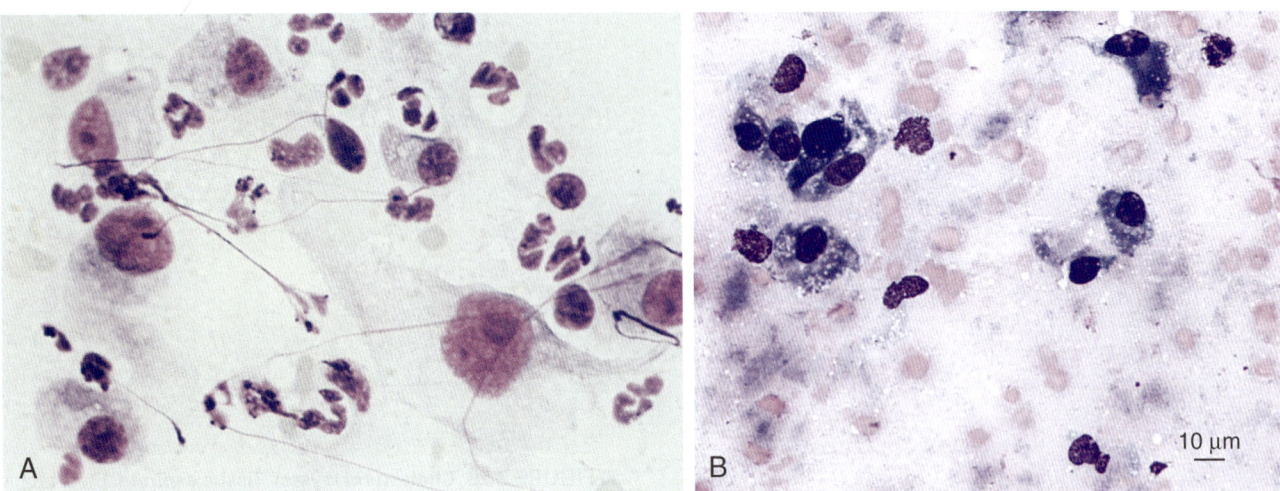

■ **FIGURE 2.31 A, Reactive fibroplasia. Tissue scraping. Cat.** Oral mass with associated septic inflammation. Pictured are several plump mesenchymal cells with a stellate to spindle appearance and prominent nucleoli along with suppurative inflammation. The severity of the inflammatory response warrants caution in suggesting a malignant mesenchymal mass or sarcoma. Note the nuclear streaming appears as purple strands. (Aqueous Romanowsky; HP oil.) **B, Postnecrosis fibroplasia. Tissue aspirate. Dog.** Facial swelling related to myositis. The background contains amorphous gray material supportive of necrosis. Several fibroblasts indicate a reparative process after tissue damage. (Modified Wright; HP oil.)

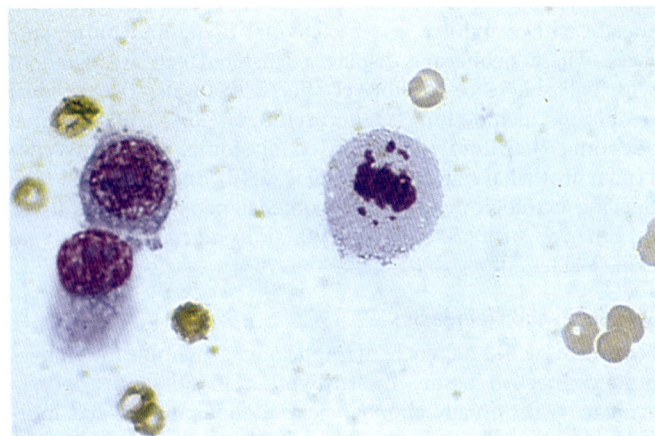

■ **FIGURE 2.32 Abnormal mitotic figure. Tissue aspirate. Dog.** Cell in metaphase with multiple lag chromatin outside the center. (Wright-Giemsa; HP oil.)

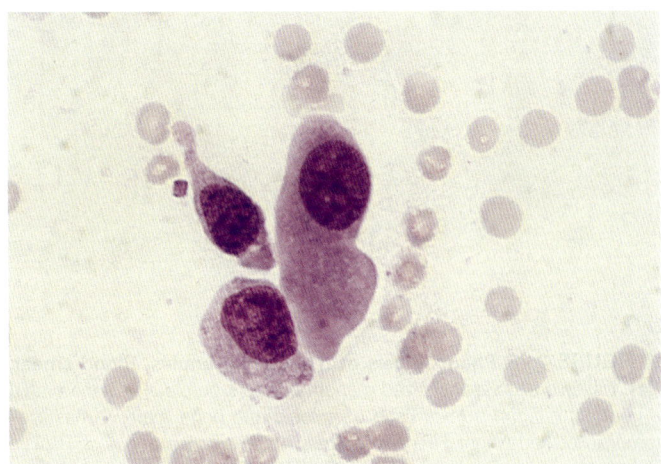

■ **FIGURE 2.33 Pleomorphism. Tissue aspirate. Dog.** Urothelial cell carcinoma cells display variability in size and shape supportive of malignancy. (Wright-Giemsa; HP oil.)

TABLE 2.1	Cytologic Criteria Used to Identify Malignant Cells
CRITERION	**MORPHOLOGIC FEATURES**
Abnormal mitotic figures	Abnormal chromosomal fragments may appear with uneven length of chromatin strands and as isolated or lag chromatin. Increased numbers may be suggestive but not definitive for malignancy (see Fig. 2.32).
Pleomorphism	Variation in the size, shape, or maturation state of cells and their nuclei (see Fig. 2.33).
Nucleocytoplasmic ratio	High or variable nuclear-to-cytoplasmic ratio between cells of similar origin (see Fig. 2.34).
Anisokaryosis	Variation in nuclear size between cells of similar origin (see Fig. 2.34).
Coarse chromatin	Ropy chromatin or clumping of nuclear chromatin is common in immature cells (see Fig. 2.35).
Nucleolar changes	Variation in nucleolar size (anisonucleosis), enlarged, multiple, or variably shaped nucleoli (see Fig. 2.36).
Nuclear molding	Abnormal nuclear shape related to the rapid growth of cells in which tight cell spacing occurs without normal crowd inhibition (see Fig. 2.37).
Multinucleation	Two or more nuclei occupy the same cell. Binucleation may be found in hyperplasia of some tissues (see Fig. 2.38).

CHAPTER 2 General Categories of Cytologic Interpretation

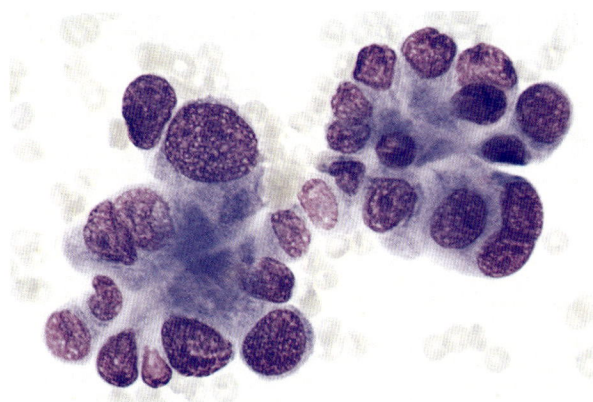

FIGURE 2.34 Anisocytosis, anisokaryosis. Tissue aspirate. Dog. Lung adenocarcinoma specimen has several features of malignancy. These features include high and variable nucleocytoplasmic ratio, anisokaryosis, binucleation, and coarse nuclear chromatin. (Wright-Giemsa; HP oil.)

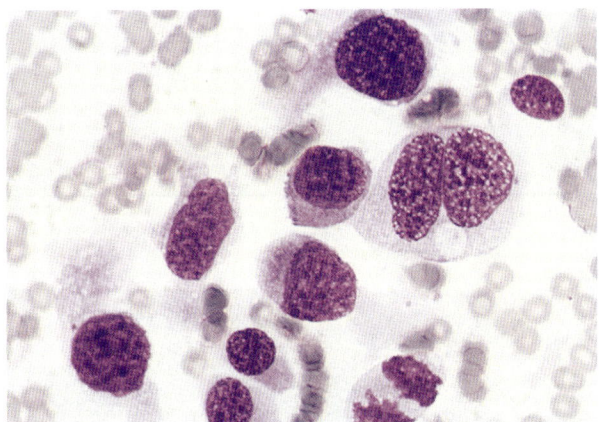

FIGURE 2.35 Coarse chromatin. Tissue aspirate. Dog. Same case as Figure 2.33. The ropy nuclear material is mottled with light and dark spaces and is described as coarsely stippled (see Fig. A4.4). This appearance is often associated with neoplastic urothelial epithelium but may be seen with other tissues. Binucleation is seen in one cell, and a mitotic figure is present on the bottom edge. (Wright-Giemsa; HP oil.)

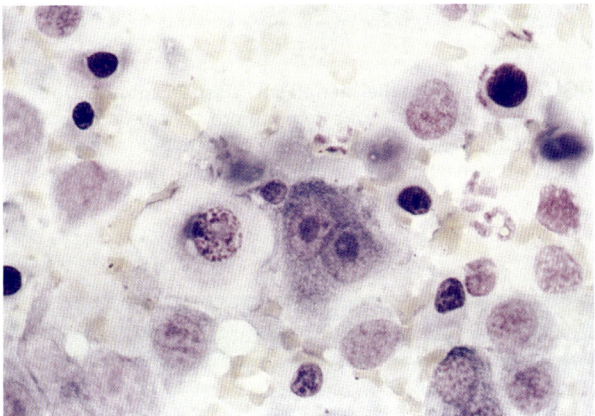

FIGURE 2.36 Prominent nucleoli. Tissue aspirate. Dog. Same case as Figure 2.30. A binucleate cell with very large single nucleoli in each nucleus is present. A prominent nucleolus is noted in the adjacent cell, which also displays coarse chromatin or chromatin clumping. (Wright-Giemsa; HP oil.)

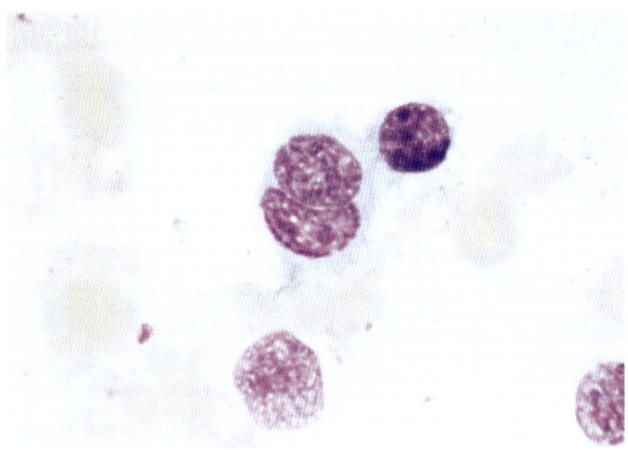

FIGURE 2.37 Nuclear molding. Tissue aspirate. Dog. Nasal chondrosarcoma pictured with a binucleate cell in which one nucleus is wrapped around the other within the same cell. This feature is present in malignant tissues and relates to the lack of normal inhibition of cell growth. (Wright-Giemsa; HP oil.)

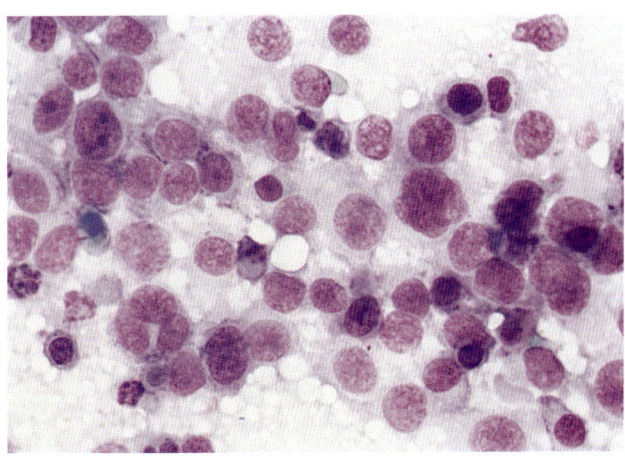

FIGURE 2.38 Multinucleation. Tissue imprint. Dog. Pheochromocytoma with two multinucleate cells, one in the lower *left side* with three nuclei and the other to *the right of center* with an irregularly shaped nuclear region. Multinucleation is also found in epithelial, mesenchymal, and round cell neoplasms. (Wright-Giemsa; HP oil.)

Benign and malignant mesenchymal neoplasms involve connective tissue elements, such as fibroblasts, osteoblasts, adipocytes, myocytes, and vascular lining cells. Examples of mesenchymal neoplasms include hemangiosarcoma (Fig. 2.42), osteosarcoma (Fig. 2.43), fibroma, and amelanotic melanoma (Fig. 2.44). Specific cytologic features of mesenchymal neoplasms are listed in Box 2.3.

Round Cell Neoplasms

Round cell neoplasms have discrete, round cellular shapes and involve hematopoietic cells. Therefore, their nuclear size is roughly two to four times the diameter of an erythrocyte. The five categories of round cell neoplasms include transmissible venereal tumor (Fig. 2.45), lymphoma (Fig. 2.46), mast cell tumor, plasmacytoma, and histiocytic tumors. Specific cytologic characteristics of round cell neoplasms are listed in Box 2.4.

TABLE 2.2 Four Cytomorphologic Categories of Neoplasia

CATEGORY	GENERAL FEATURES	IMAGE	EXAMPLES
Epithelial	Clustered, tight arrangement of cells		Urothelial cell carcinoma, lung tumors, sebaceous adenoma
Mesenchymal	Individualized, spindle to oval cells		Hemangiosarcoma, osteosarcoma, fibroma
Round cell	Individualized, round, discrete cells		Transmissible venereal tumor, lymphoma, mast cell tumor, plasmacytoma, histiocytic tumors
Naked nuclei	Loosely adherent cells with bare round nuclei		Thyroid tumors, Sertoli cell tumors, paragangliomas, neuronal cells, apocrine gland tumors

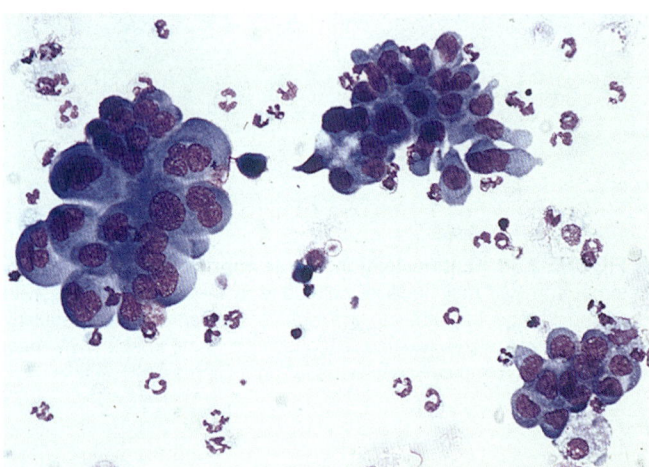

■ **FIGURE 2.39 Epithelial neoplasm. Lung lavage. Dog.** Large clusters of cohesive cells having distinct cell borders from a case of lung adenocarcinoma. (Wright-Giemsa; IP.) (Courtesy Robert King, Gainesville, FL.)

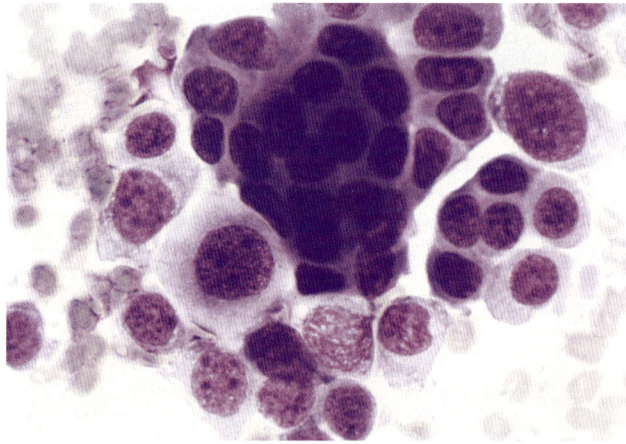

■ **FIGURE 2.40 Epithelial neoplasm. Tissue aspirate. Dog.** Same case as Figure 2.33. Cells are formed into tight balls or as sheets. Nuclei are round to oval, and cells are large, round to polygonal with distinct cytoplasmic borders. (Wright-Giemsa; HP oil.)

Naked Nuclei Neoplasms

Neoplasms with a naked nuclei cytomorphology have a loosely adherent cellular arrangement with free nuclei. This cytologic appearance is an artifact related to the fragile nature of these cells. These neoplasms are usually associated with endocrine, neuroendocrine, and neural tissues (Perman et al., 1979). In addition, anal sac adenocarcinoma frequently displays this

BOX 2.2 Specific Cytologic Features of Epithelial Neoplasms

- Cells exfoliate in tight clumps or sheets.
- Cells adhere to each other and may display distinct tight junctions, termed desmosomes (see Fig. 2.41).
- Cells are large and round to polygonal with distinct, intact cytoplasmic borders.
- Nuclei are round to oval.

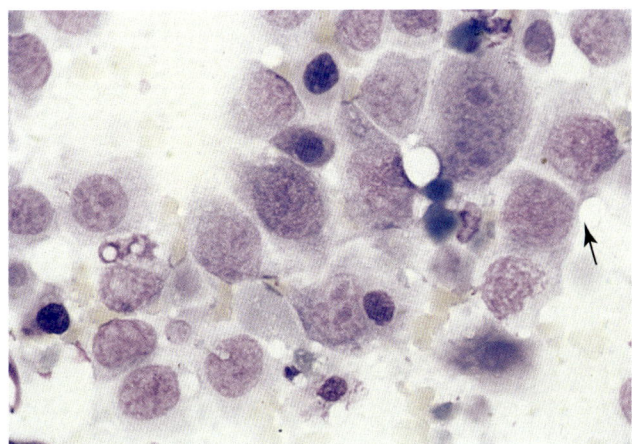

■ **FIGURE 2.41 Desmosomes. Tissue aspirate. Dog.** Same case as Figure 2.30. A sheet of carcinoma cells with prominent desmosomes. These clear lines *(arrow)* between adjacent cells represent tight junctions that are characteristic of epithelial cells. (Wright-Giemsa; HP oil.)

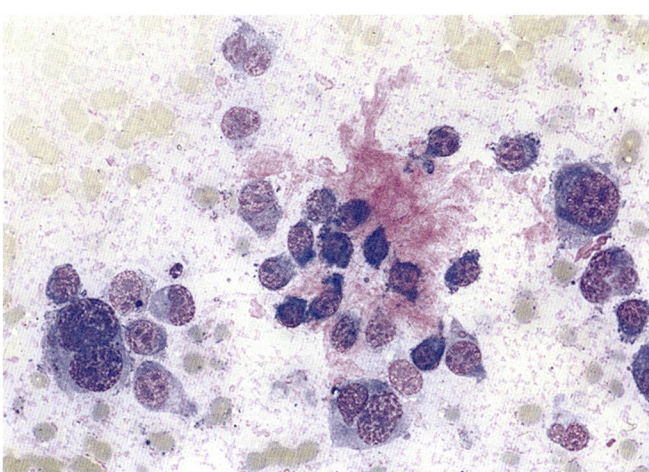

■ **FIGURE 2.43 Mesenchymal neoplasm. Tissue aspirate. Dog.** The finding of individualized pleomorphic cells with abundant extracellular eosinophilic osteoid material is consistent with osteosarcoma. Binucleate and multinucleate forms are common and seen in this sample. (Wright-Giemsa; HP oil.)

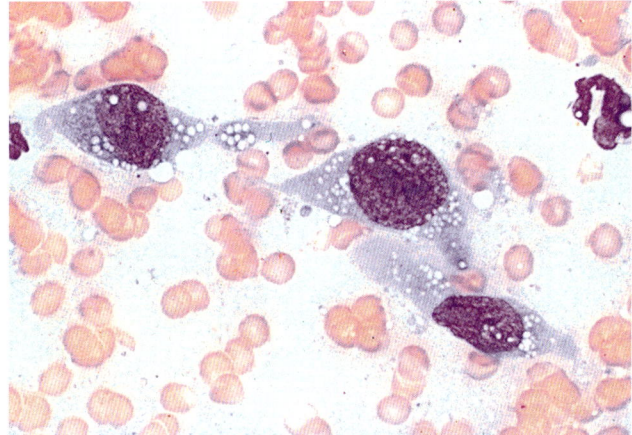

■ **FIGURE 2.42 Mesenchymal neoplasm. Tissue imprint. Dog.** Neoplastic cells exfoliate individually and appear oval, spindle, or fusiform. This bone lesion was confirmed as hemangiosarcoma on histopathologic examination. Characteristic of hemangiosarcoma cytology is a poorly cellular sample with large plump mesenchymal cells that contain numerous small punctate colorless cytoplasmic vacuoles. (Wright-Giemsa; HP oil.)

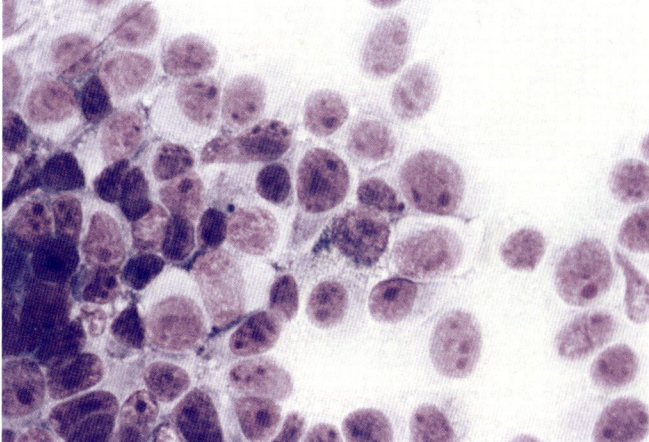

■ **FIGURE 2.44 Mesenchymal neoplasm. Tissue imprint. Dog.** Round to oval nuclei, anisokaryosis, high nucleocytoplasmic ratio, prominent and variably shaped nucleoli, and individualized cells with poorly distinct cytoplasmic borders suggest a malignant mesenchymal neoplasm. This lesion is from a gum mass with a confirmed histopathologic diagnosis of amelanotic melanoma. One cell in the center contains small amounts of melanin pigment granules. (Aqueous Romanowsky; HP oil.)

pattern when aspirated and should be considered when the naked nuclei cytomorphology is encountered (see Figs. 3.121 and 3.122). Typical examples include thyroid tumors (Fig. 2.47), islet cell tumors, paragangliomas (Fig. 2.48), and neuropil. Specific cytologic features of naked nuclei neoplasms include those listed in Box 2.5.

KEY POINT The use of the four cytomorphologic categories may help classify neoplastic lesions by their general cellular features and arrangement, thereby suggesting specific tumor types. Remember that these categories may not fit well for some neoplasms, especially for poorly differentiated tumors. It is recommended that biopsy specimens for histopathologic examination be taken to determine the specific tumor type and extent of the lesion under most circumstances.

BOX 2.3 Cytologic Features of Mesenchymal Neoplasms

- Cells usually exfoliate individually (however, aggregates of cells are seen occasionally bound by an extracellular matrix) (see Fig. 2.44).
- Cells are oval, stellate, or fusiform with often indistinct cytoplasmic borders.
- Samples are often poorly cellular.
- Cells are usually smaller than epithelial cells.
- Nuclei are round to elliptical.

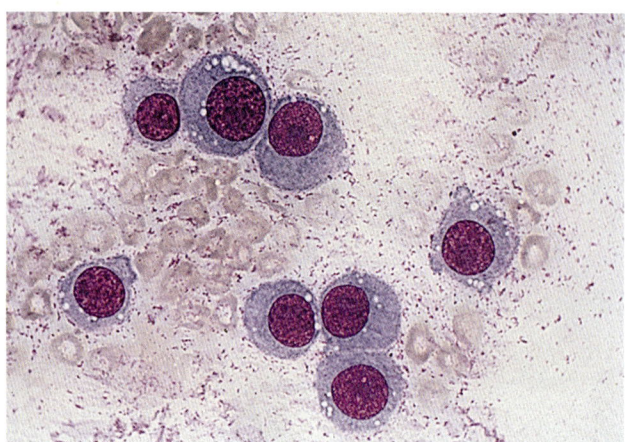

■ **FIGURE 2.45 Round cell neoplasm. Tissue aspirate. Dog.** This fleshy vulvar mass is composed of round cells bearing a single prominent nucleolus and moderately abundant cytoplasm with frequent punctate colorless cytoplasmic vacuolation. The cytologic diagnosis is transmissible venereal tumor. (Wright-Giemsa; HP oil.)

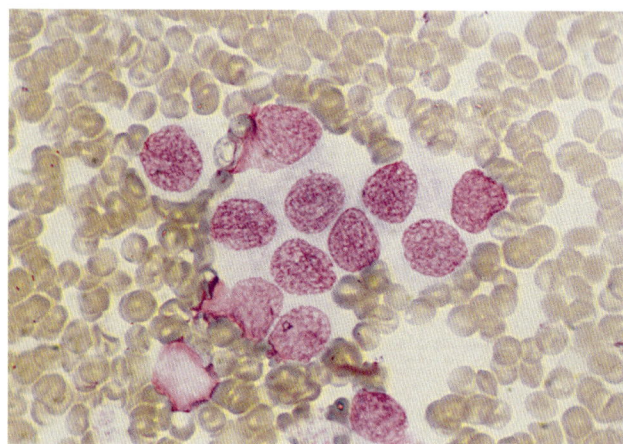

■ **FIGURE 2.47 Naked nuclei neoplasm. Tissue aspirate. Dog.** Cervical mass in the area of the thyroid from an animal with a honking cough. Cytologically, the sample presents as a syncytium of round nuclei with relatively uniform features. This is characteristic of an endocrine mass. Typically, the distinction between hyperplasia, adenoma, and carcinoma is difficult on cytopathology and sometimes histopathology. (Wright-Giemsa; HP oil.)

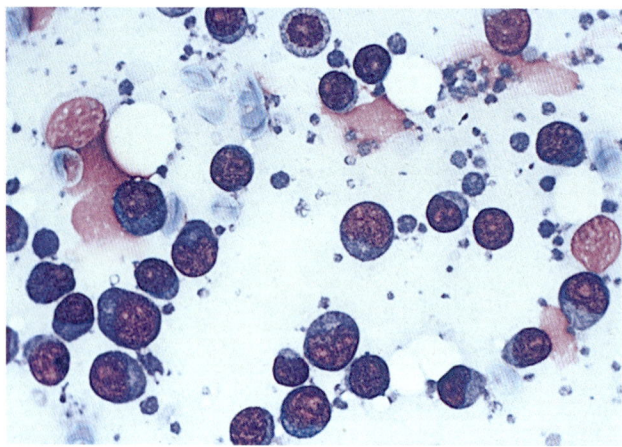

■ **FIGURE 2.46 Round cell neoplasm. Tissue aspirate. Dog.** Discrete cells with a round shape, distinct cytoplasmic borders, and a very high nucleocytoplasmic ratio are characteristic of lymphoid cells. This sample is taken from a lymph node effaced by lymphoma cells. (Wright-Giemsa; HP oil.)

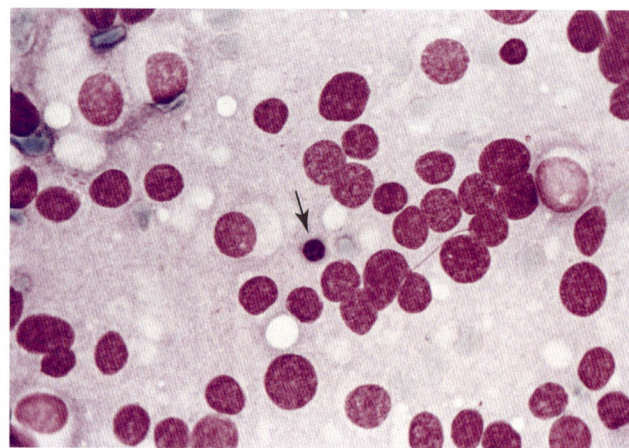

■ **FIGURE 2.48 Naked nuclei neoplasm. Tissue imprint. Dog.** Clinical signs include a head tilt and temporal muscle atrophy. Magnetic resonance imaging suggested a mass involving the osseous bulla. Surgery found a mass at the bifurcation of the common carotid artery. Cytologically, the preparation contains mostly loose or free round nuclei against a finely granular eosinophilic background. Although most nuclei are similarly sized, an occasional cell appears larger. Few intact cells remain with pale cytoplasm at the edges and center. Adjacent to the center intact cell is a nucleated red cell *(arrow)* suggestive of extramedullary hematopoiesis. The histopathologic diagnosis is paraganglioma, specifically a malignant chemodectoma in this case, because it metastasized and was thought to involve the chemoreceptor organ in that site. (Wright-Giemsa; HP oil.)

BOX 2.4 Specific Cytologic Characteristics of Round Cell Neoplasms

- Cells exfoliate individually, having distinct cytoplasmic borders.
- Cells are generally round.
- Samples are moderately cellular.
- Cells are usually smaller than epithelial cells.
- Nuclei are round to indented.

KEY POINT The five round cell neoplasms are easily remembered by the acronym T-LyMPH, which identifies **t**ransmissible venereal tumor, **ly**mphoma, **m**ast cell tumor, **p**lasmacytoma, and **h**istiocytic tumors, all of which are associated with the hematopoietic system (Table 2.3).

BOX 2.5 Specific Cytologic Features of Naked Nuclei Neoplasms

- Cells often exfoliate in loosely attached sheets with many free nuclei present and indistinct cytoplasmic borders.
- Occasional cell clusters may be present with distinct cell outlines.
- Cells are generally round to polygonal.
- Samples are highly cellular.
- Nuclei are round to indented, often with no to minimal anisokaryosis.

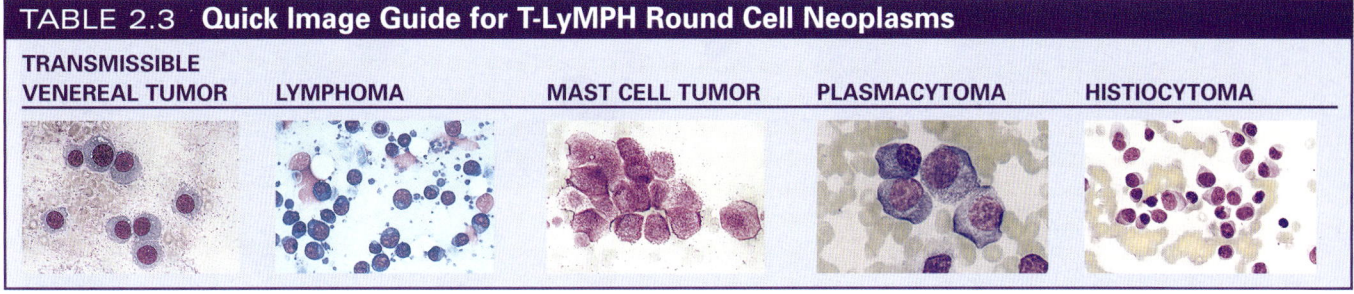

TABLE 2.3 Quick Image Guide for T-LyMPH Round Cell Neoplasms

TRANSMISSIBLE VENEREAL TUMOR	LYMPHOMA	MAST CELL TUMOR	PLASMACYTOMA	HISTIOCYTOMA

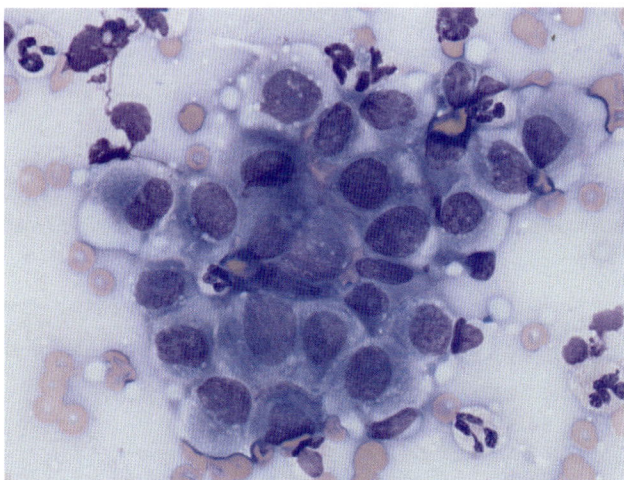

■ **FIGURE 2.49 Pavement pattern. Tissue aspirate. Dog.** Sheet of adherent epithelial cell from a nasal transitional cell carcinoma producing a cobblestone appearance. (Wright-Giemsa; HP oil.)

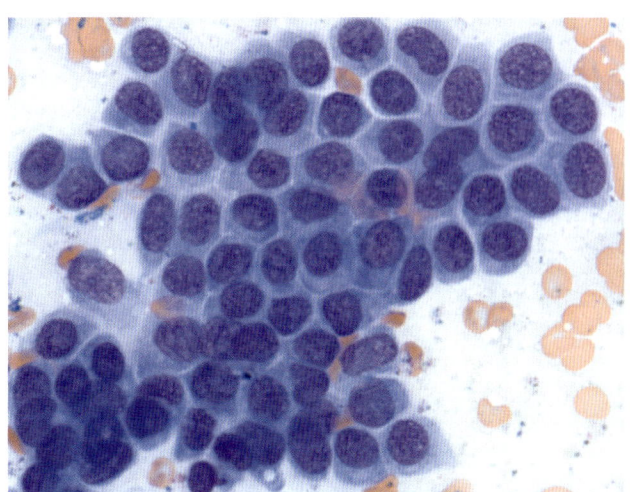

■ **FIGURE 2.50 Pavement pattern. Tissue aspirate. Dog.** Single layer of adherent mesothelium creates a mosaic pattern. (Wright-Giemsa; HP oil.)

COMMON CELL RELATIONSHIPS

Cell-to-Cell Relationships

Four types of cell-to-cell relationships were described earlier under the cytomorphologic categories of neoplasia, which assist in the identification of tissues involving neoplasia (see Table 2.2). Several architectural patterns are used to describe both cytologic and histologic biopsies involving normal or diseased tissues (Masserdotti, 2006). Most of the patterns relate to epithelial tissue, but *storiform* and *perivascular* apply to connective tissue and endocrine organs.

Pavement pattern (Figs. 2.49 and 2.50) involves layers of cells that exfoliate as flat sheets with an interlocking mosaic pattern, also termed *cobblestone*. Examples include squamous cells from keratinized and nonkeratinized surfaces, urothelial epithelium of the urinary bladder or nose, and mesothelium.

Honeycomb pattern (Figs. 2.51 and 2.52) is characteristic of cuboidal and columnar cells from multilayered or stratified epithelium that exfoliates as three-dimensional clusters. Examples include tissue from the gastrointestinal tract and prostate.

Acinar pattern (Figs. 2.53 and 2.54) describes the ring of cuboidal cells around a center filled often with secretory material from such organs as the pancreas, thyroid, salivary gland, and lung. Acini are similar in shape to *rosettes*, but the latter contains cell extensions within the center or may appear to have

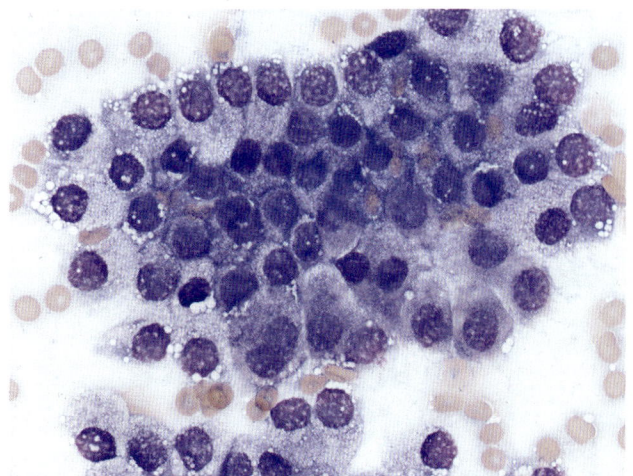

■ **FIGURE 2.51 Honeycomb pattern. Tissue aspirate. Dog.** Hyperplastic prostatic epithelium presents similar to the pavement pattern except these are cuboidal rather than flat cells, appearing more three dimensional. (Wright-Giemsa; HP oil.)

a lumen as with ependymomas. Pseudo-rosettes lack cells of the tumor in the center and may instead surround vascular tissue, mineral, or extracellular mucin. Both rosettes and pseudo-rosettes are common in the nervous system and pancreatic endocrine tumors (see Fig. 8.23A).

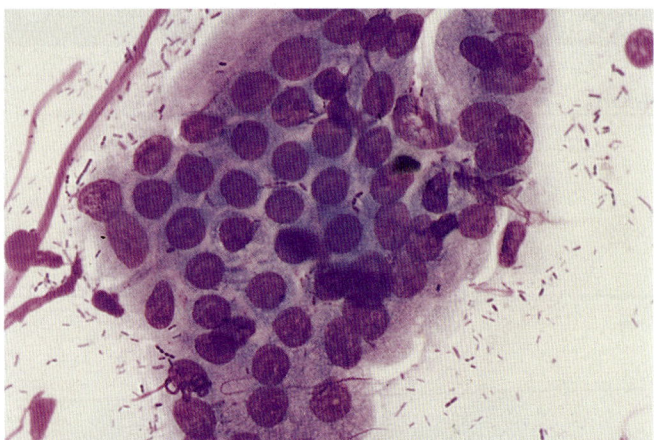

■ **FIGURE 2.52 Honeycomb pattern. Tissue imprint.** Cuboidal to columnar colonic epithelium produces a multidimensional appearance in lieu of a flat sheet of cells. (Wright; HP oil.)

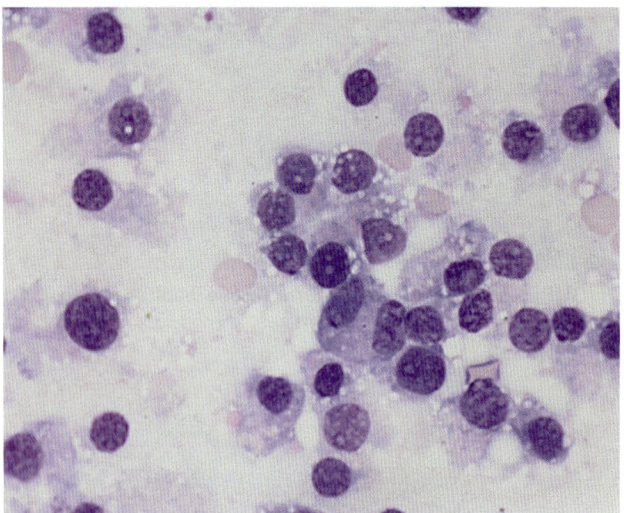

■ **FIGURE 2.53 Acinar pattern. Tissue aspirate. Dog.** A ring of nuclei encircles a pale center. This sample is from a thyroid adenocarcinoma. (Wright-Giemsa; HP oil.)

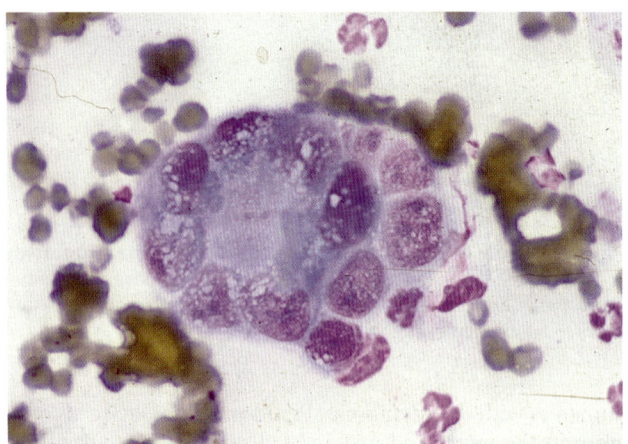

■ **FIGURE 2.54 Acinar pattern. Tissue aspirate. Cat.** A cluster of salivary gland epithelial cells is arranged in the shape of a ball from an adenocarcinoma. (Wright-Giemsa; HP oil.)

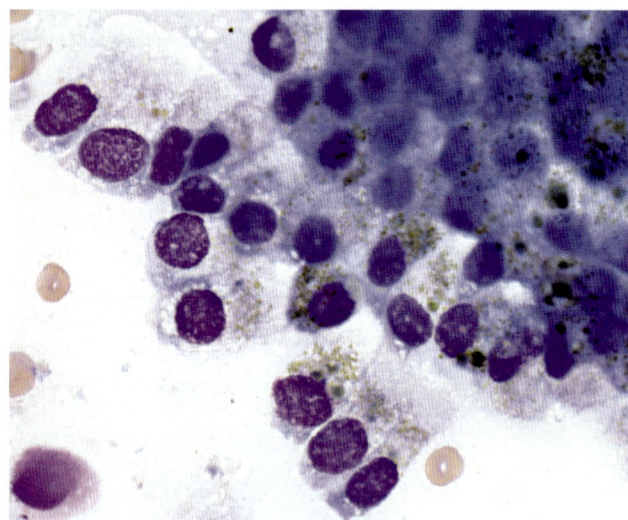

■ **FIGURE 2.55 Palisade pattern. Tissue imprint. Dog.** A single layer of cells forms a row with nuclei lining up to resemble a picket fence in this sample of benign prostatic hyperplasia. (Modified Wright; HP oil.)

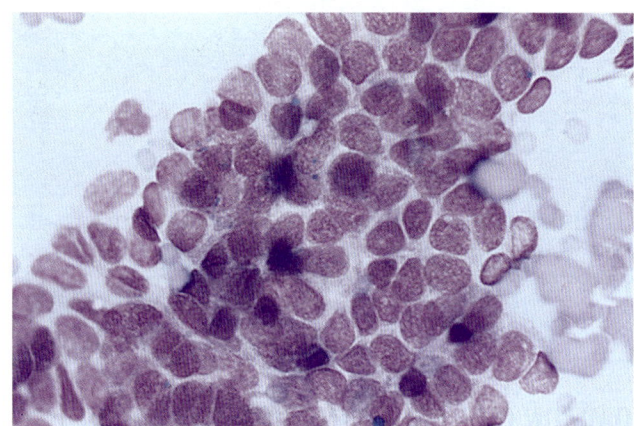

■ **FIGURE 2.56 Palisade pattern. Tissue aspirate. Cat.** In this mammary adenoma, there is a row of nuclei forming the edges of the specimen. (Wright-Giemsa; HP oil.)

Palisade pattern (Figs. 2.55 and 2.56) involves the linear arrangement of nuclei with a basilar orientation resembling a picket fence. Examples of this pattern include cells from the upper respiratory tract, gastrointestinal tract, or squamous basal epithelium as found in follicular tumors (e.g., trichoblastoma).

Papillary pattern (Figs. 2.57 and 2.58) is characterized by an extended area of growth having a central vascular stalk with an outer palisade layer of cells. It may resemble a ball of cells or morula. Examples involve mammary tissue, mesothelium, ovarian adenocarcinomas, and choroid plexus carcinoma.

Trabecular pattern (Figs. 2.59 and 2.60) denotes large cell clusters branching off in multidimensional cellular tracts. Examples of this pattern include hepatoid or perianal gland tumors, and hepatic, mammary, or gastrointestinal glandular tissue.

Storiform pattern (Figs. 2.61 and 2.62) relates to a swirling or haphazard streaming of mesenchymal cells within bundles of stroma. Examples include most soft tissue sarcomas such as myxosarcoma, fibrosarcoma, or other spindle cell tumors.

CHAPTER 2 *General Categories of Cytologic Interpretation* 31

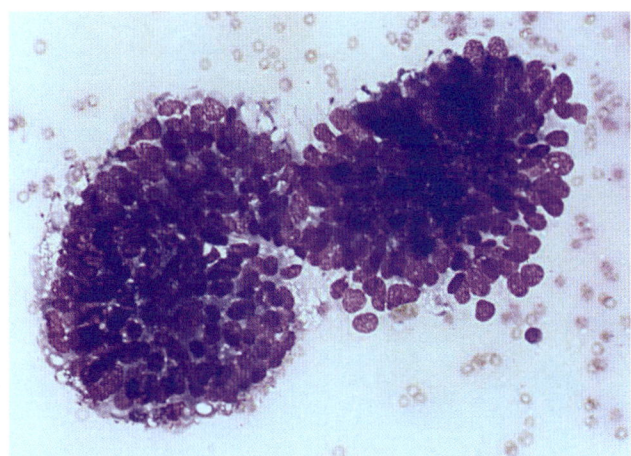

■ **FIGURE 2.57 Papillary pattern. Cytologic preparation. Dog.** A cluster of cohesive neoplastic epithelial cells from an ovary adenocarcinoma forms a ball of cells off an extended growth. (May-Grünwald-Giemsa; IP.)

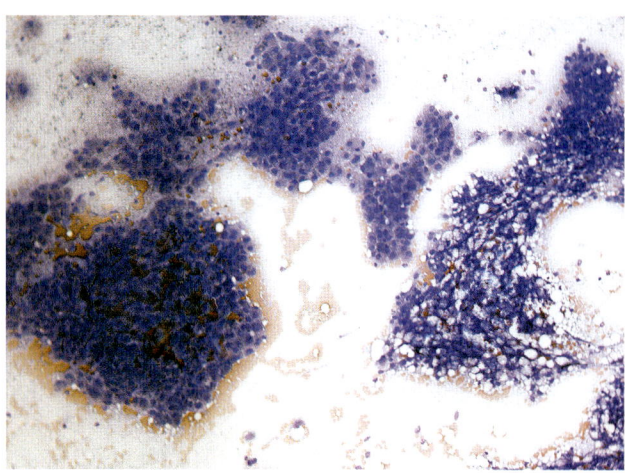

■ **FIGURE 2.60 Trabecular pattern. Tissue aspirate. Dog.** Dense branching and solid large collections of hepatocytes are sampled in this case of nodular hyperplasia with mild vacuolar change. (Modified Wright; LP.)

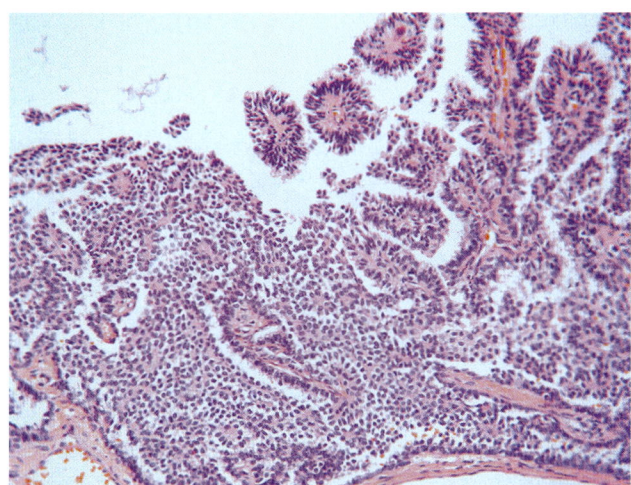

■ **FIGURE 2.58 Papillary pattern. Ovary tissue section. Dog.** There is dense proliferation of hyperchromic epithelial cells forming surface extensions off a central vascular stalk. (H&E; LP.)

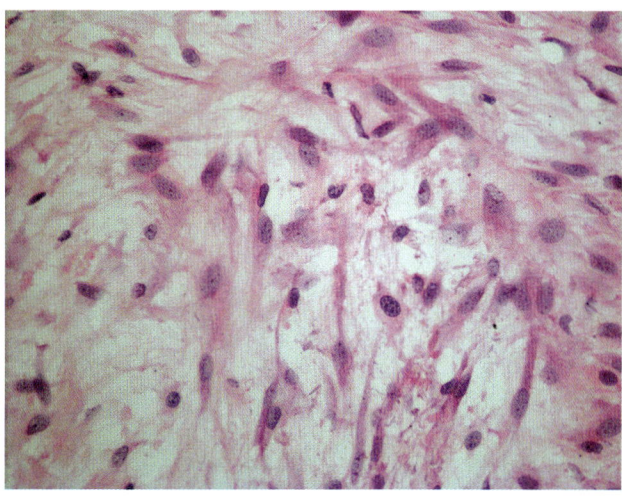

■ **FIGURE 2.61 Storiform pattern. Tissue aspirate. Dog.** Myxosarcoma with intersecting and haphazard orientation of mesenchymal cells in an extracellular matrix. (Modified Wright; IP.)

Perivascular pattern (Figs. 2.63 and 2.64) is characterized by orientation of cells around blood vessels or other vascular structures such as capillaries lined by endothelium and sometimes containing erythrocytes. Examples of this pattern can be seen in reproductive tissues such as ovarian granulosa cell tumor, interstitial testicular or Leydig cell tumor, and perivascular wall tumors.

Cell-in-Cell Relationships

Emperipolesis is a phenomenon distinct from phagocytosis in which live hematopoietic cells wander within host cells but are neither targeted nor actively destroyed and may remain viable for a time in the host cell after which the internalized cell may be disintegrated by the host cell via a lysosome-mediated mechanism or undergo apoptosis. This may be seen in normal physiologic conditions such as canine diestrus (Fig. 2.65) as well as in neoplasia.

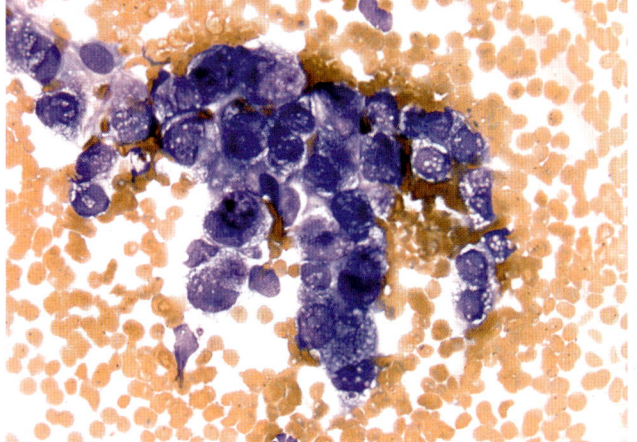

■ **FIGURE 2.59 Trabecular pattern. Tissue aspirate. Dog.** Gastric adenocarcinoma with large branches of proliferating cells. (Modified Wright; HP oil.)

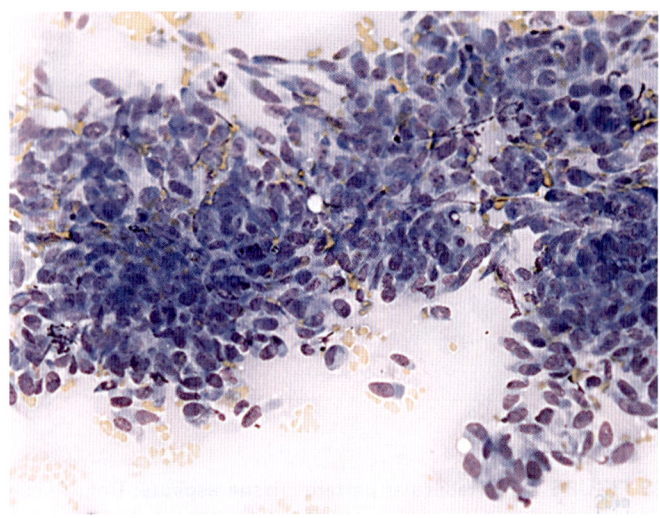

■ **FIGURE 2.62 Storiform pattern. Tissue aspirate. Dog.** Linear streaming of mesenchymal cells from a keloidal fibrosarcoma. (Modified Wright; IP.)

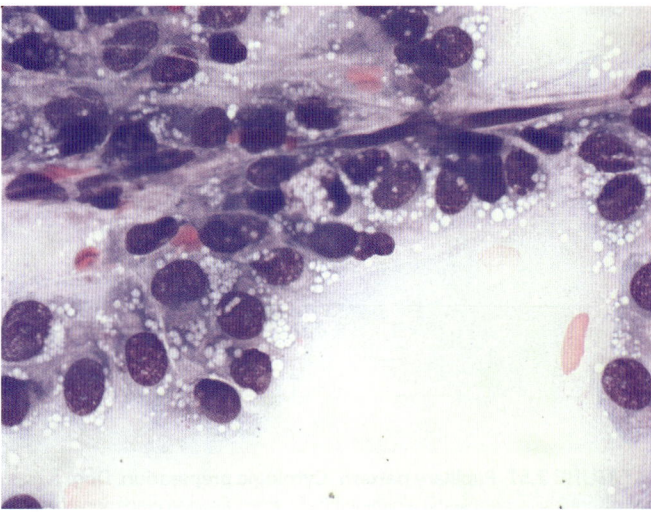

■ **FIGURE 2.64 Perivascular pattern. Tissue aspirate. Dog.** Neoplastic mesenchymal cells are attached to the capillary lining in this perivascular wall tumor of the skin. (Modified Wright; HP oil.)

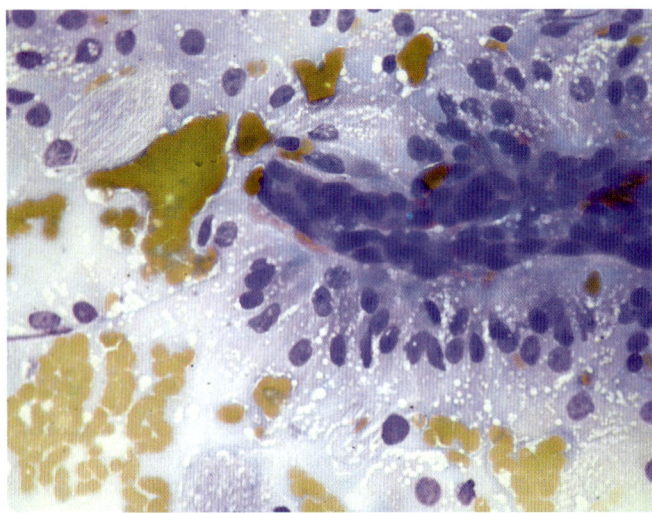

■ **FIGURE 2.63 Perivascular pattern. Tissue aspirate. Dog.** Prominent capillaries are lined by neoplastic ovary granulosa cells from a metastatic lesion to the pancreas. (Modified Wright; HP oil.)

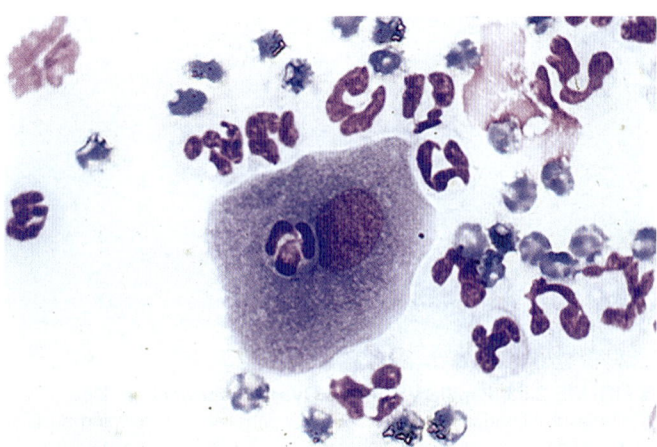

■ **FIGURE 2.65 Emperipolesis. Vaginal smear. Dog.** In this diestrus stage, a neutrophil appears inside an intermediate squamous epithelial cell. In this process, the neutrophil remains intact until degradation by the host cell or programmed apoptosis. (Wright-Giemsa; HP oil.)

Entosis appears similar to emperipolesis by containing a live cell, except in entosis, the target and host cells are of homotypic origin. The internalized cell may survive for a short time, divide within the host, or die by lysosome-mediated degradation and nonapoptotic cell death (Yang and Li, 2012). Unfortunately, cytology taken at one time period cannot confirm whether the target cell actively entered the host or if the host actively engulfed the target, especially when the target cell appears intact (Fig. 2.66A).

Cannibalism involves active engulfment of cellular material by nonprofessional phagocytes (Melendez-Lazo et al., 2015). Entosis and cannibalism differ as entosis involves only a homotypic live cell invasion, whereas cannibalism may engulf dead or living cells and involve homotypic or heterotypic cells. When a target cell lacks internal structure or appears degraded and not apoptotic within the host, it likely has been cannibalized (Fig. 2.66B). Erythrocytes cannibalized by tumor cells are an example of xenocannibalism such as occurs in hemangiosarcoma (Fig. 2.67) and T-cell or B-cell lymphoid neoplasia (Fig. 2.68B).

Phagocytosis is a term reserved for cell engulfment by professional phagocytes such as macrophages (see Fig. 2.18). Use of the term *cannibalism* is not appropriate under these circumstances.

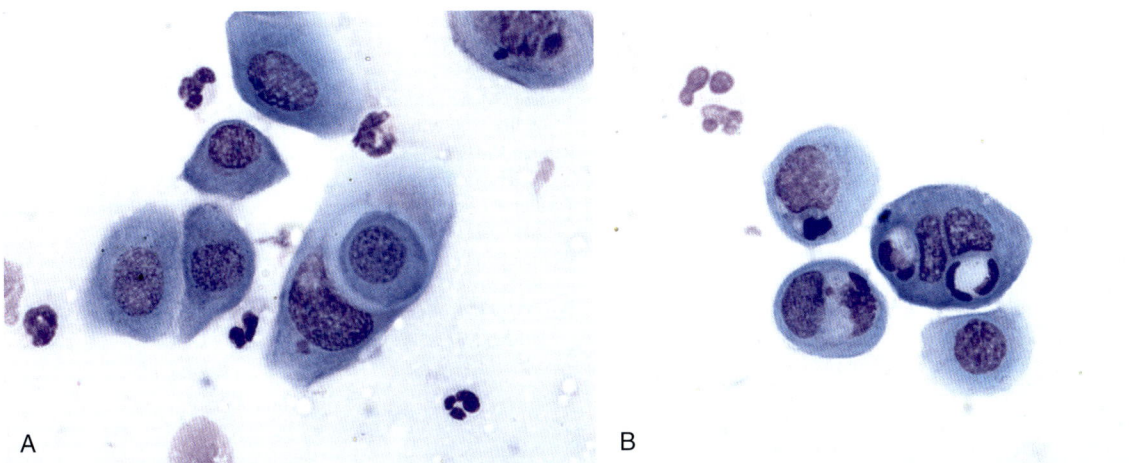

FIGURE 2.66 Cell-in-cell presentation. Corneal scraping. Dog. Same case in A and B. **A, Homotypic.** Clinical diagnosis is corneal ulcer and rare coccoid bacteria are present (not shown). One intact squamous cell is within a host squamous cell. This presentation is likely an example of entosis; however, homotypic cannibalism could be considered. **B, Heterotypic.** One squamous cell *(upper left)* contains a possible apoptotic remnant. The binucleated squamous cell *(upper right)* contains two neutrophils showing some nuclear degradation and condensation, while the host squamous cell *(lower left)* contains the early disintegrated nucleus of another possible squamous cell. Emperipolesis with apoptosis is possible for two cells, but cannibalism is likely occurring with the degraded squamous cell. (Wright-Giemsa; HP oil.)

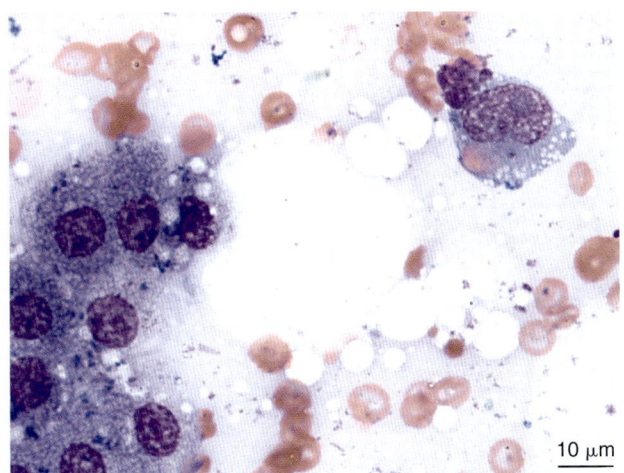

FIGURE 2.67 Erythrocyte engulfment. Tissue aspirate. Dog. A single neoplastic mesenchymal cell contains an erythrocyte with nearby hepatocyte onlookers. Hemangiosarcoma cells may exhibit xenocannibalism. (Wright-Giemsa; HP oil.)

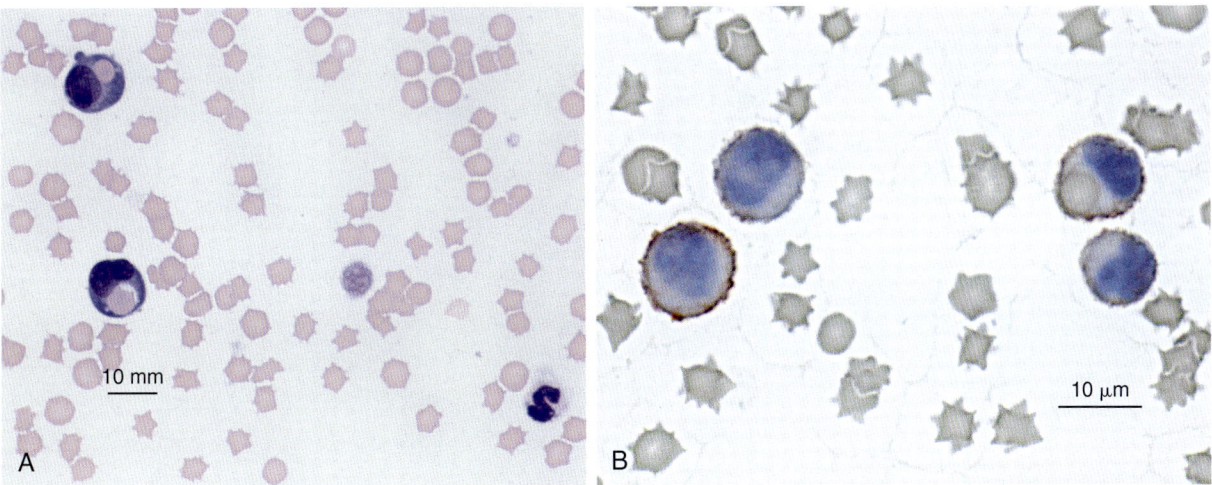

FIGURE 2.68 Erythrocyte engulfment. Blood smear. Cat. Same case in A and B. **A,** Frequent engulfment of erythrocytes by neoplastic lymphoid cells. This is an example of xenocannibalism. (Modified Wright; HP oil.) **B,** Immunocytochemistry demonstrates a positive membrane reaction and indicates a B-cell leukemia of lymphocytes with engulfed erythrocytes. (Anti-CD20/AEC; HP oil.)

REFERENCES

Alleman AR, Bain PJ. Diagnosing neoplasia: the cytologic criteria for malignancy. *Vet Med.* 2000;95:204-223.

Bacha WJ, Bacha LM. *Color Atlas of Veterinary Histology.* 2nd ed. Philadelphia: Lippincott Williams & Wilkins; 2000:13-15.

Conrado FO, Raskin RE. What is your diagnosis? Purple granules within neutrophils of a dog. *Vet Clin Pathol.* 2017;46:639-640.

Flanders E, Kornstein MJ, Wakely PE, et al. Lymphoglandular bodies in fine-needle aspiration cytology smears. *Am J Clin Pathol.* 1993;99:566-569.

Masserdotti C. Architectural patterns in cytology: correlation with histology. *Vet Clin Pathol.* 2006;35:388-396.

Mastrorilli C, Welles EG, Hux B, et al. Botryoid nuclei in the peripheral blood of a dog with heatstroke. *Vet Clin Pathol.* 2013;42:145-149.

Melendez-Lazo A, Cazzini P, Camus M, et al. Cell cannibalism by malignant neoplastic cells: three cases in dogs and a literature review. *Vet Clin Pathol.* 2015;44:287-294.

Noden DM, de Lahunta A. *The Embryology of Domestic Animals.* Baltimore: Williams & Wilkins; 1985:10-11.

Perman V, Alsaker RD, Riis RC. *Cytology of the Dog and Cat.* South Bend, IN: American Animal Hospital Association; 1979:4-7.

Tvedten H. Atypical mitoses: morphology and classification. *Vet Clin Pathol.* 2009;38:418-420.

Woldemeskel M. A concise review of amyloidosis in animals. *Vet Med Int.* 2012;2012:427296.

Yang YQ, Li JC. Progress of research in cell-in-cell phenomena. *Anat Rec.* 2012;295:372-377.

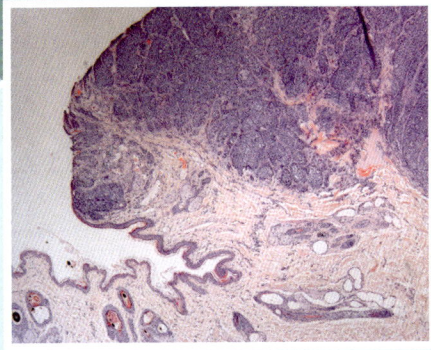

CHAPTER 3

Integumentary System

Rose E. Raskin and Francisco O. Conrado

NORMAL HISTOLOGY

There are regional differences in the histology of the skin of dogs and cats related to the thickness of the epidermis and dermis (Fig. 3.1). In general, the epidermis is composed of four layers of squamous epithelium, including a keratinized or corneal layer, a granular layer, a spinous layer, and a basal layer (Fig. 3.2). The adnexal structures of the epidermis include hair follicles, sweat glands, and sebaceous glands (Fig. 3.3). Sebaceous glands of dogs contain variably sized sebocytes and lipid droplets, whereas those of cats are small and uniform (Figs. 3.4 and 3.5).

The hair follicle is divided into three segments termed *infundibulum,* extending from the epidermis to the sebaceous duct; *isthmus,* from the sebaceous duct to insertion of the arrector pili muscles; and *inferior,* or *bulbar,* from the arrector pili muscles to the bulb (see Fig. 3.3). Surrounding the hair shaft are several layers, one of which is the external root sheath (ERS) that joins the epidermis in the infundibular region, appearing eosinophilic and extends into the deeper hair shaft regions, appearing very pale pink related to the glycogen-rich cytoplasm (Fig. 3.6). The internal root sheath lying between the ERS and the hair shaft is composed of eosinophilic cells with large trichohyalin granules (see Fig. 3.6) produced by the matrical cells of the bulb. The mitotically active cells of the bulbar segment have large basophilic nuclei with scant cytoplasm containing melanin (see Fig. 3.6A).

The dermis present below the epidermal layer contains the adnexal structures, smooth muscle bands, blood and lymphatic vessels, nerves, and variably sized collagen and elastic fibers. Beneath the dermis lies the subcutis, composed of loose adipose tissue and collagen bundles.

The nailbed region consists of the nail as dense compressed clear keratinocytes with a spinous layer and a columnar basal cell layer. The dermis abuts the periosteum of the third phalanx bone.

NORMAL SKIN CYTOLOGY AND ARTIFACTS

Normal cytology of the dermis and subcutis contains a mixture of epidermal squamous epithelium and well-differentiated glandular elements as well as mature adipose and collagen tissue. Basal epithelial cells are round and deeply basophilic with a high nucleocytoplasmic ratio. Cells of the other epidermal layers are known as *keratinocytes* because they contain keratin. Polygonal cells of the granular layer are evident cytologically by the presence of pink to magenta keratohyalin granules within an abundant lightly basophilic cytoplasm having a small, contracted nucleus. The most superficial keratinized layer consists of flattened, sharply demarcated, blue-green hyalinized squames that lack a nucleus. Elongated dark-blue to purple squames are termed *keratin bars,* which represent rolled or coiled cells. Melanocytes from neural crest origin are located within the basal layer of the epidermis or hair matrix. Their brownish-black to greenish-black fine granules may be seen in some keratinocytes. Also present may be a low number of mast cells from perivascular and perifollicular sites.

The anal sacs are two invaginations of epidermis that create a receptacle for a normally yellow-brown watery to slightly viscous material, which may contain small amounts of solid particles. Lining the anal sacs is a thin layer of keratinizing stratified squamous epithelium that is surrounded by skeletal muscle. Cytologically, low numbers of keratinocytes with few coccoid to rod bacteria are present without evidence of inflammation (Fig. 3.7).

Of the glandular elements of the skin, the sebaceous glands are the most recognizable cytopathologically related to their bubble-like cytoplasmic appearance (Fig. 3.8).

NONINFECTIOUS INFLAMMATORY DISORDERS

Acral Lick Dermatitis and Lick Granuloma

Acral lick dermatitis is a chronic inflammatory response to persistent licking or chewing of a limb, producing a thickened, firm, raised plaque lesion that often ulcerates (Fig. 3.9). Causes include infectious agents, hypersensitivity reactions, trauma, and psychogenesis. On cytopathology, there is a mixed population of mononuclear inflammatory cells, including plasma cells, along with intermediate squamous epithelium (Fig. 3.10) related to acanthosis (i.e., hyperplasia of the epidermal stratum spinosum layer). The healing response to surface erosion may produce fibroblastic cells, which appear in the cytopathologic specimens as plump, fusiform cells along with numerous erythrocytes related to increased vascularization. Lesions may also involve a secondary bacterial infection with suppuration. Treatment will be determined by the underlying cause and frequently involves control of the superficial pyoderma.

> **Cytopathologic differential diagnosis:** foreign body reaction, arthropod bite reaction.

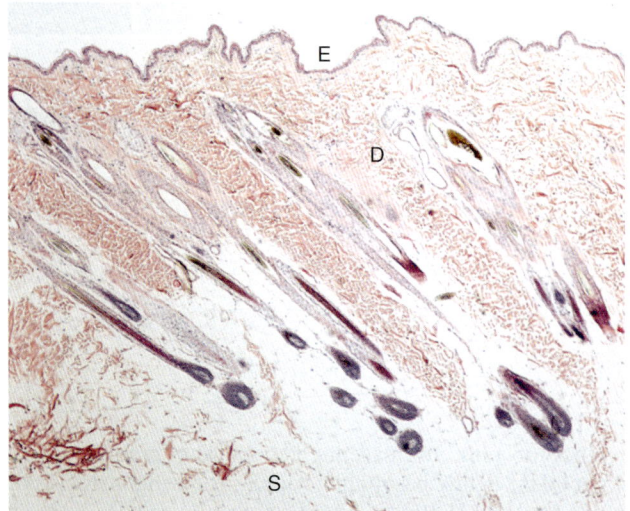

■ **FIGURE 3.1 Normal skin histology. Dog.** Section of haired skin from the hip area showing the epidermis (E), dermis (D), and subcutis (S). Note the compound hair follicles common in the dog and cat. (H&E; LP.)

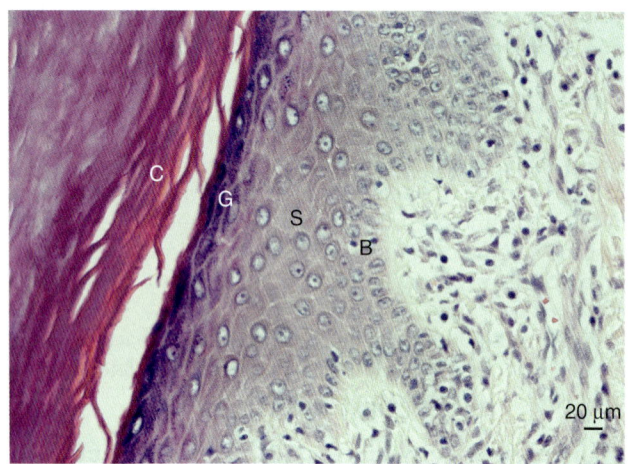

■ **FIGURE 3.2 Normal footpad skin histology. Cat.** Four squamous epithelial layers of skin: corneal (C), granular (G), spinous (S), and basal (B). (H&E; IP.)

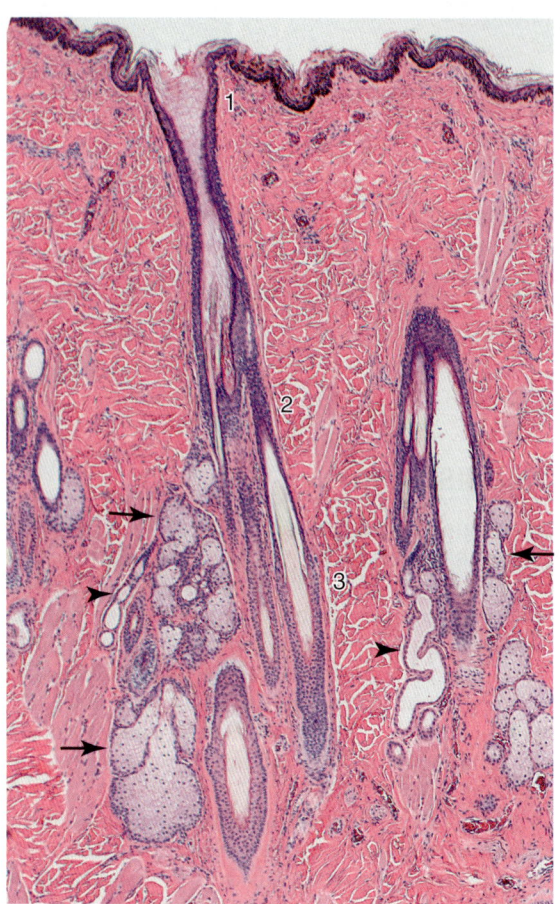

■ **FIGURE 3.3 Normal skin histology. Dog.** The adnexal structures of the epidermis include hair follicles *(1–3)*, sebaceous glands *(arrows)*, and sweat glands *(arrowheads)*. The hair follicle is divided into three segments termed infundibulum *(1)* extending from the epidermis to the sebaceous duct, isthmus *(2)* from the sebaceous duct to insertion of the arrector pili muscles, and inferior or bulbar *(3)* from the arrector pili muscles to the bulb. Dense collagen bundles fill much of remaining dermis. (H&E; LP.)

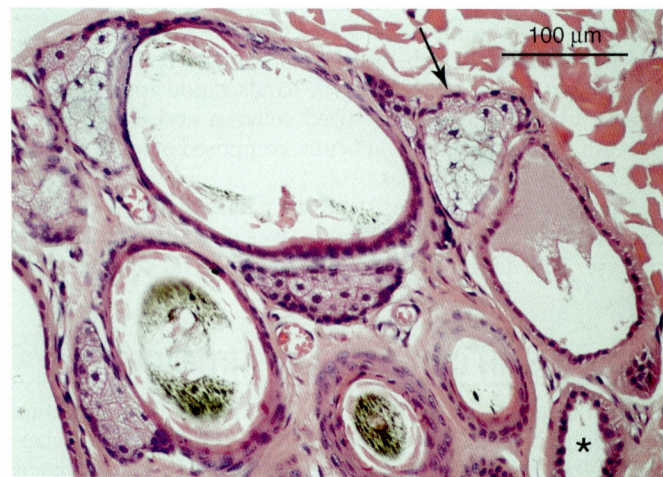

■ **FIGURE 3.4 Normal sebaceous gland histology. Dog.** The variably sized vacuoles within the sebocytes help to characterize canine sebaceous glands. The *asterisk* indicates the lumen of an apocrine gland. (H&E; IP.)

Foreign Body or Vaccine-Induced Reactions

Foreign body reactions are caused by penetration of plant, animal, or inorganic material into the skin, producing an erythematous wound that progresses to a nodular response that often drains fluid. On cytopathology, a mixed inflammatory response is present, composed mostly of macrophages and lymphocytes with smaller numbers of neutrophils and possibly eosinophils. Multinucleate giant cells are frequently present (Fig. 3.11). A fibroblastic response is common. A secondary bacterial infection may occur. Treatment includes surgical exploration or excision with histopathologic biopsy and culture if warranted.

Vaccine-induced inflammatory reactions may contain magenta or blue-gray stained globular material. Magenta material results from adjuvants composed of mucopolysaccharides as seen

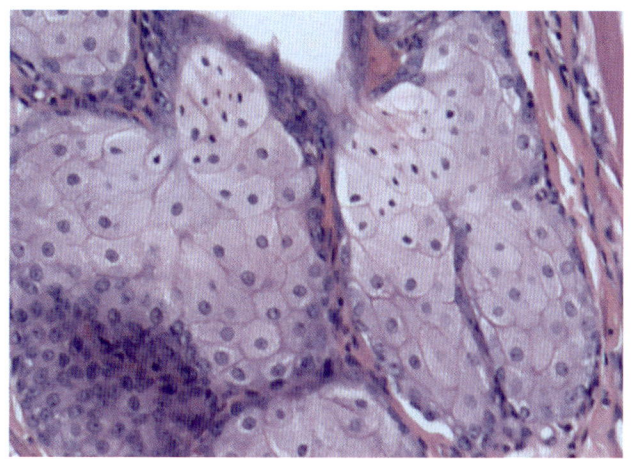

■ **FIGURE 3.5 Normal sebaceous glands histology. Cat.** The small and uniform-appearing lipid droplets within the sebocytes help to characterize feline sebaceous glands. (H&E; IP.) (Courtesy Mark Bennett, University of Bristol, UK.)

with Rabvac 1 and Fel-O-Vax Lv-K (Elanco) vaccines (Fig. 3.12). Blue-gray material reflects a metal-containing adjuvant as associated with Imrab 3 TF (Merial), a rabies vaccine, which reacts with Morin stain that detects aluminum (Fig. 3.13) (Scruggs and LeBlanc, 2015).

A recent report involved the presence of a mixed macrophagic and neutrophilic inflammation concurrent with nonstaining spherical structures, measuring approximately 120 to 180 μm in diameter and having multiple fine surface lines (Rigas and Latouche, 2021). History indicated subcutaneous injections of an extended-release suspension of moxidectin incorporated into sterile microspheres for the purpose of heartworm disease prevention (ProHeart). Subcutaneous swellings developed 2 to 3 weeks postinjection.

> *Cytopathologic differential diagnosis:* fungal, bacterial, noninfectious, or arthropod bite inflammatory lesions.

Arthropod Bite Reaction

Bites from insects, ticks, and spiders, for example, may induce a mild to severe reaction usually characterized by erythema and swelling with acute necrosis that appears as eosinophilic furunculosis or later as a granuloma on histopathology (Gross et al., 2005). Cytopathology reveals a mixed inflammatory infiltrate composed of neutrophils, macrophages, and usually increased numbers of eosinophils related to a hypersensitivity reaction (Figs. 3.14 and 3.15). These lesions often regress spontaneously, but some may require additional wound care.

> *Cytopathologic differential diagnosis:* bacterial, fungal, noninfectious, or foreign body reactions.

Nodular Panniculitis and Steatitis

Causes of noninfectious panniculitis include trauma, foreign bodies, vaccine-induced reactions, immune-mediated conditions, drug reactions, pancreatic conditions, nutritional deficiencies, and idiopathic. The condition appears in cats and

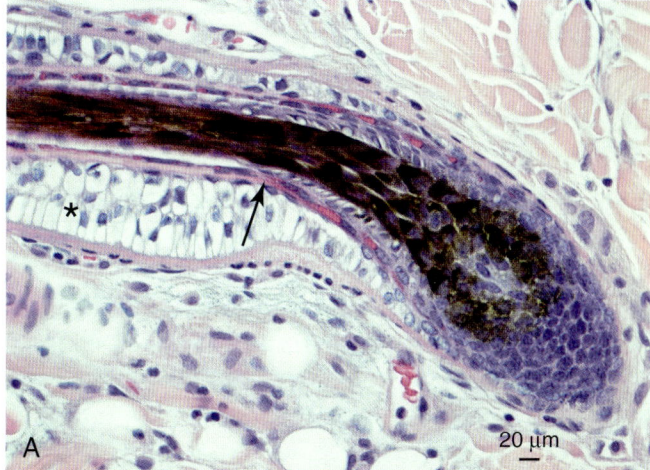
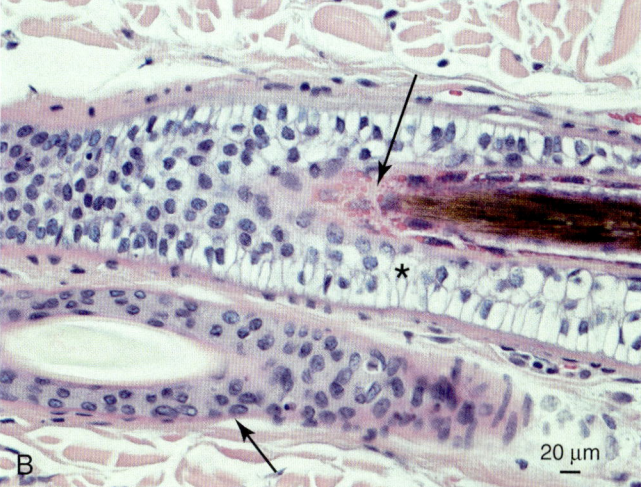

■ **FIGURE 3.6 Normal hair shaft histology. Dog.** Same case in A and B. **A, Inferior, matrical, or bulb region.** The bulbar segment consists of mitotically active cells appearing as large basophilic nuclei with scant cytoplasm. The external root sheath (*asterisk*) appears very pale related to the glycogen-rich cytoplasm. The internal root sheath (*arrow*) is composed of eosinophilic cells containing large trichohyalin granules. (H&E; IP.) **B, Isthmus region.** The internal root sheath contains large trichohyalin granules (*long arrow*). The external root sheath near the inferior region (*asterisk*) is pale staining, but in the isthmus it appears eosinophilic (*short arrow*) related to keratin aggregates. (H&E; IP.)

dogs as solitary or multiple, firm to fluctuant, raised, well-demarcated lesions. These may ooze an oily yellow-brown fluid (Fig. 3.16). Sites of prevalence include the dorsal trunk, neck, and proximal limbs. On cytopathology, nondegenerate neutrophils and macrophages predominate against a vacuolated background composed of adipose tissue (Figs. 3.17 and 3.18). Small lymphocytes and plasma cells may be numerous, especially in lesions induced by vaccination. Frequently, macrophages present with abundant foamy cytoplasm or as giant multinucleated forms. When chronic, evidence of fibrosis is indicated by the presence of plump fusiform cells with nuclear immaturity. The fibrosis may be so extensive as to suggest a mesenchymal neoplasm. The prognosis is usually best for solitary lesions, which respond to surgical excision. Histologically, sterile panniculitis may demonstrate inflammatory cells

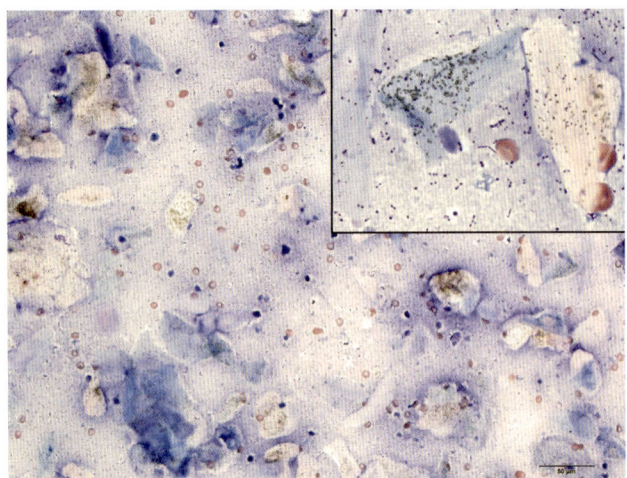

■ **FIGURE 3.7 Anal sac contents. Tissue aspirate. Dog.** Material was obtained during aspiration of an adjacent anal tumor. Against a granular basophilic background composed of a mixed bacterial population with small amount of blood are squamous epithelial cells and keratinized debris. *Inset:* Higher magnification showing keratinized squamous epithelial cells with associated melanin granules and an extracellular, mixed bacterial population. (Wright-Giemsa; IP.)

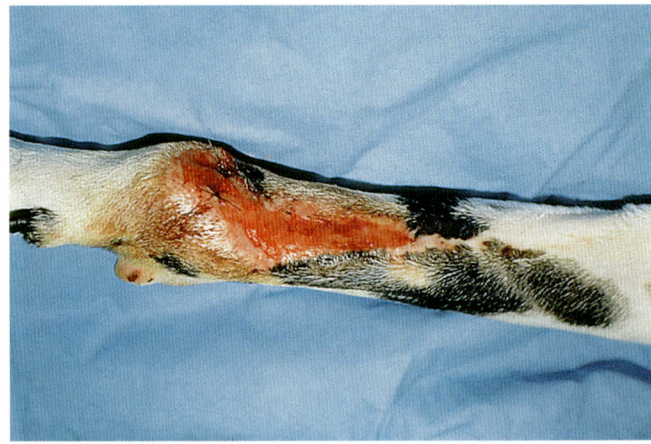

■ **FIGURE 3.9 Lick dermatitis. Macroscopic specimen. Dog.** Thickened, ulcerated, hairless lesion on the limb. (Courtesy Rosanna Marsella, University of Florida.)

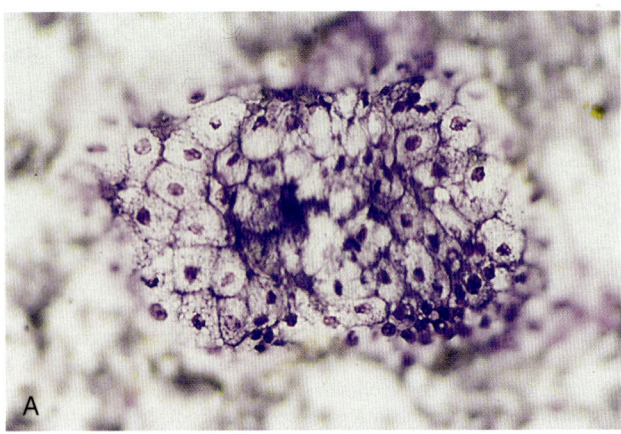

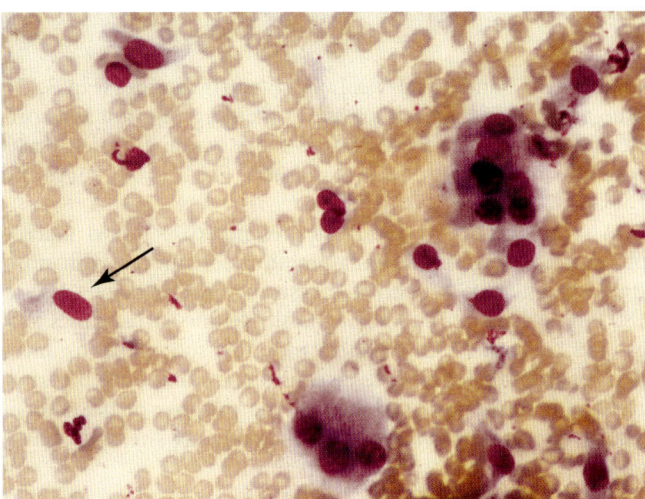

■ **FIGURE 3.10 Lick dermatitis. Tissue aspirate. Dog.** Sheets of intermediate squamous epithelium predominate related to the thickened epidermis found in these cases. Adjacent to the neutrophil in the lower left is a fibroblastic cell *(arrow)* present in response to stromal reaction. (Wright-Giemsa; HP oil.)

within the subcutis (Fig. 3.19) that extend into the dermis. Multiple lesions are often associated with systemic disease in young dogs, and treatment involves glucocorticoid administration. Dachshunds and poodles may be predisposed to this form of the disease. Culture and histopathologic examination are recommended to rule out infectious causes. Fungal stains should be applied to cytopathologic specimens.

Cytopathologic differential diagnosis: infectious panniculitis.

Eosinophilic Hypersensitivity Dermatitis

Eosinophilic hypersensitivity dermatitides occur rarely in dogs but are common in cats with most related to an underlying cause such as a hypersensitivity reaction to insects (fleas and mosquitoes), environmental allergens (atopic dermatitis), or

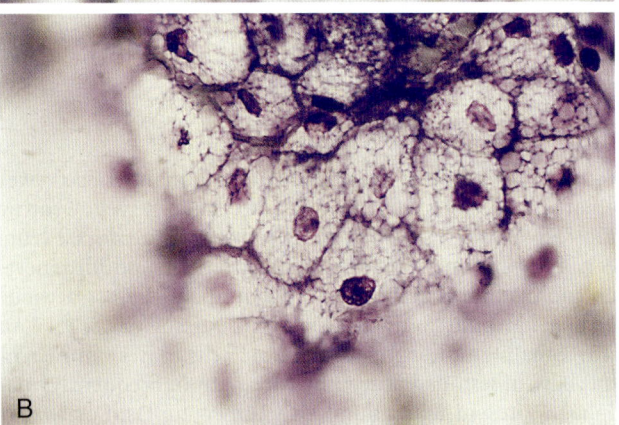

■ **FIGURE 3.8 Sebaceous gland aspirate. Dog.** Same case in A and B. **A,** The monomorphic population of vacuolated epithelial cells having a small, centrally placed nucleus is consistent with mature sebocytes. (Aqueous Romanowsky; HP oil.) **B,** Note the low nucleocytoplasmic ratio and the foamy cytoplasm with delicate streaks. (Aqueous Romanowsky; HP oil.)

foods (Bloom, 2006). In cats, this condition is referred to as *feline eosinophilic granuloma complex* (EGC). Included in EGC are three clinical presentations, namely eosinophilic plaque, eosinophilic granuloma, and indolent ulcer. Grossly, these lesions appear as focal, raised, alopecic, smooth or ulcerated, thickened areas of skin. Because the histopathologic findings are similar among all three presentations, tissue biopsy is only recommended to rule out other conditions such as neoplasia or fungal infections, which can appear similar.

Feline eosinophilic plaque presents initially as alopecic focal areas of intense pruritus that progress to ulceration with exudation. Sites commonly affected include the face, neck, ventral abdomen, perianal, and medial thigh regions (Fig. 3.20A). Lesions may become secondarily infected with bacteria and contain many neutrophils (Fig. 3.20B–D). On cytopathology, eosinophils and mast cells often predominate, with few lymphocytes. Treatment includes glucocorticoid administration and antibiotics if necessary.

Eosinophilic granuloma lesions may appear grossly as raised linear bands of yellow to erythematous tissue along the posterior legs or as papules and nodules on the nose, ears, chin, and feet. Ulceration may result from severe eosinophilic infiltration. Lesions have been seen in the oral cavity. On cytopathology, a mixed inflammatory response is seen, with macrophages, lymphocytes, plasma cells, neutrophils, and increased numbers of eosinophils and mast cells (Fig. 3.21). Rarely, multinucleate giant cells may be present. Collagen damage may occur owing to eosinophil granule release giving rise to the occasional appearance of amorphous basophilic material in the background. Eosinophil numbers are usually less than are seen in eosinophilic plaque. Surgical excision is recommended for solitary nodular lesions. For eosinophilic plaque and granuloma, the differential diagnosis includes cutaneous epitheliotropic T-cell lymphoma, mast cell tumor (MCT), squamous cell carcinoma or other neoplasms, or infectious granulomas (demodicosis, mycobacterial or fungal etiologies).

Indolent ulcer appears as an erosive to ulcerative lesion with slightly raised edges often on the midline of the upper lip, adjacent to the upper canine tooth, or hard palate. It is not painful or pruritic. The differential diagnosis for indolent ulcer includes squamous cell carcinoma and infectious agents such as

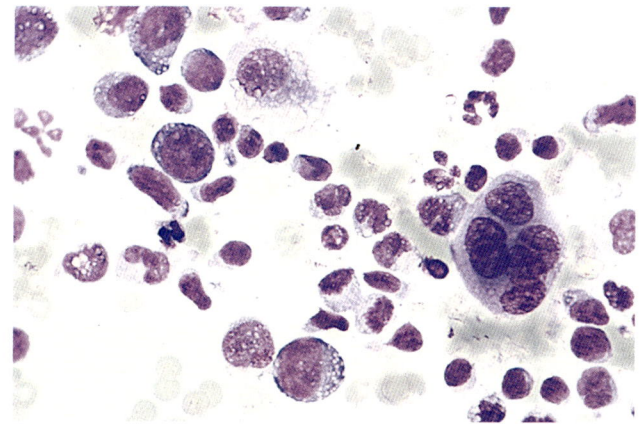

■ **FIGURE 3.11 Foreign body reaction. Tissue fluid sediment smear. Dog.** Small lymphocytes and macrophages predominate, with occasional neutrophils found. Note the giant cell, suggesting granulomatous inflammation. The inflammatory reaction was secondary to calcinosis circumscripta that was diagnosed on histopathology. (Aqueous Romanowsky; HP oil.)

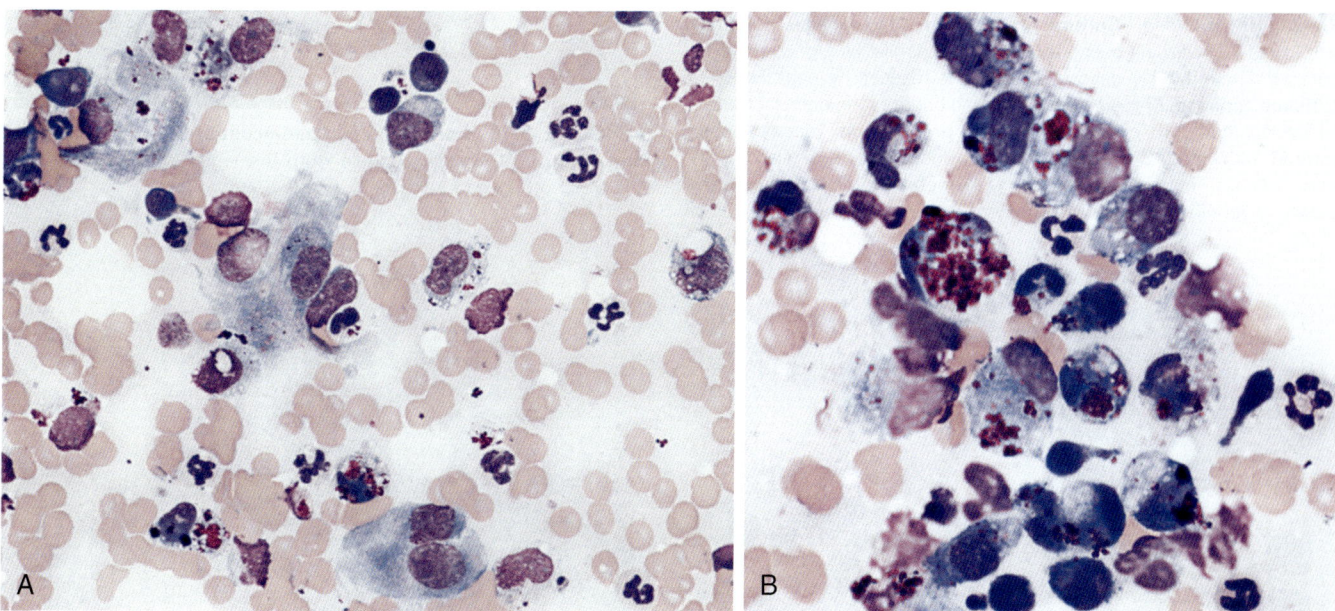

■ **FIGURE 3.12 Vaccine reaction. Mucopolysaccharide adjuvant. Tissue aspirate smear. Dog.** Same case in A and B. **A,** Firm subcutaneous swelling between the shoulder blades. A mixed inflammatory cell population composed of nondegenerate neutrophils, macrophages, fibroblasts, eosinophils (not shown), and occasional small and medium lymphocytes against a hemodiluted background. In some cases, a mixed population of lymphocytes may predominate (not shown). (Modified Wright; HP oil.) **B,** Many macrophages contain variably sized bright magenta globular material. Material that is occasionally present extracellularly (not shown) is consistent with the vaccine mucopolysaccharide adjuvant. (Modified Wright; HP oil.)

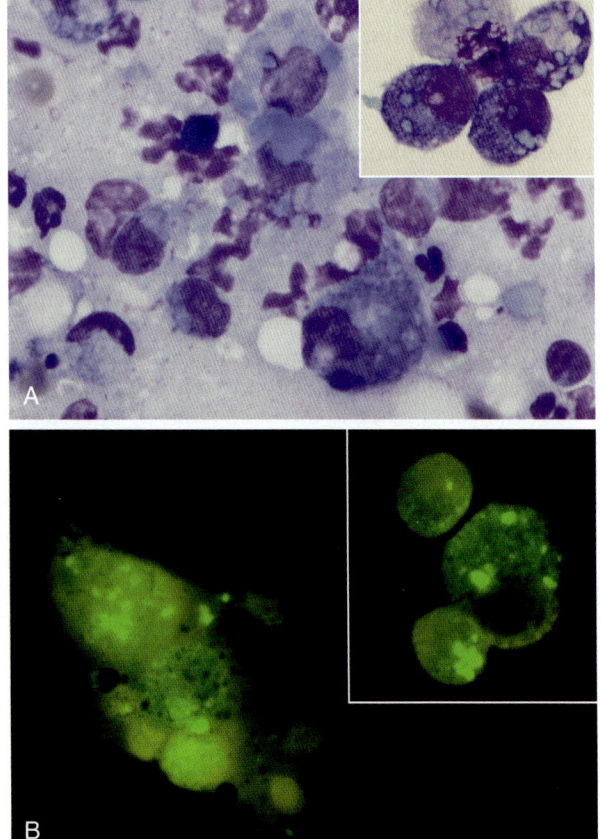

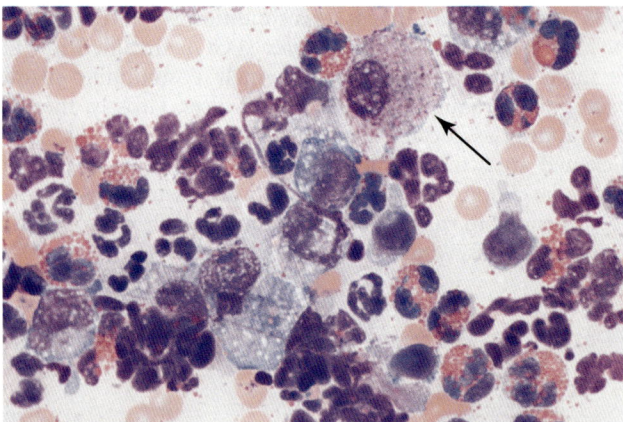

■ FIGURE 3.15 **Arthropod bite reaction. Tissue aspirate. Dog.** A small dermal mass on the muzzle displays a mixed inflammatory cell population with numerous eosinophils and one degranulated mast cell *(arrow)* in addition to many neutrophils, both degenerate and nondegenerate. (Modified Wright; HP oil.)

■ FIGURE 3.13 **Vaccine reaction. Metal adjuvant. Dog.** Same case in A and B. **A, Tissue aspirate.** Mixed neutrophilic and macrophagic inflammatory cells, many of which contain a blue-gray granular material. Extracellular material of the same color is present in the background. (Wright; HP oil.) *Inset:* **Culture preparation.** Macrophages cultured with Imrab 3 TF vaccine suspension display a similar blue-gray granular material as found in clinical cases of vaccine reaction. (Wright; HP oil.) **B, Tissue aspirate.** Macrophage containing bright green granular material (Morin stain; HP oil.) *Inset:* **Culture preparation.** Macrophages cultured with Imrab 3 TF vaccine suspension display a similar bright green granular material consistent with metal (aluminum) adjuvant. (Courtesy Jennifer Scruggs, University of Tennessee.)

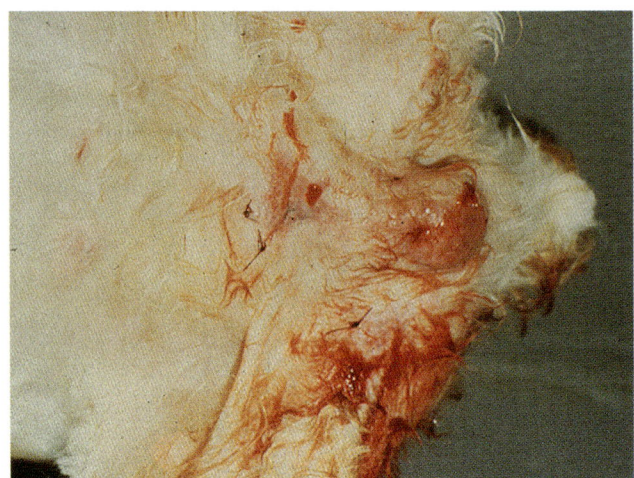

■ FIGURE 3.16 **Sterile nodular panniculitis. Macroscopic specimen. Dog.** Wet, draining nodule from the leg. (Courtesy Leslie Fox, University of Florida.)

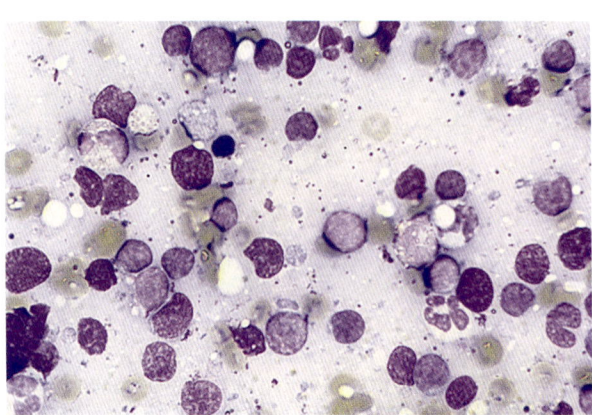

■ FIGURE 3.14 **Arthropod bite reaction. Tissue aspirate. Dog.** Small and intermediate-sized lymphocytes infiltrated this mass on the ventral neck in addition to low numbers of eosinophils and neutrophils. (Wright-Giemsa; HP oil.)

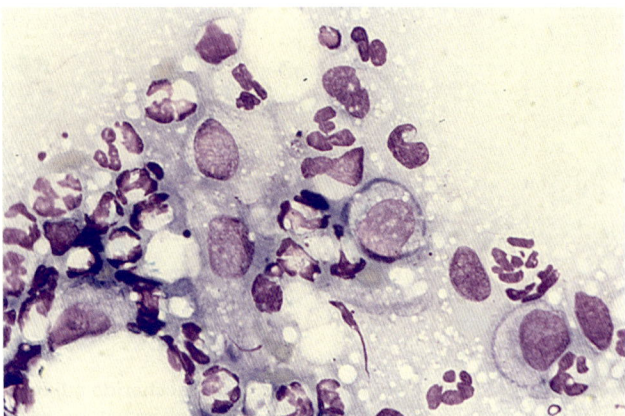

■ FIGURE 3.17 **Sterile nodular panniculitis. Tissue discharge. Dog.** Tracts drained in the lumbar region of this poodle for 1 year. Infectious agents were not found. Numerous degenerate neutrophils, several epithelioid macrophages, and occasional lymphocytes are present. (Wright-Giemsa; HP oil.)

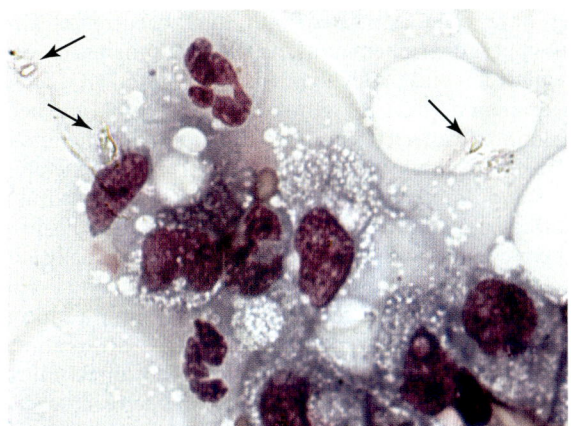

■ **FIGURE 3.18 Traumatic panniculitis. Tissue aspirate. Cat.** Subcutaneous mass on the ventral thorax (sternal) displays a background of free lipid and occasional yellow-green crystals, presumed to be mineral *(arrows)*. Shown are several macrophages with fine vacuolation and nondegenerate neutrophils. (Wright-Giemsa; HP oil.)

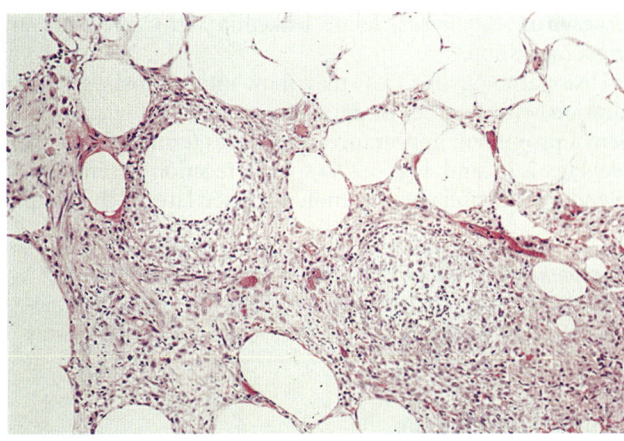

■ **FIGURE 3.19 Sterile nodular panniculitis. Tissue section. Dog.** Focal collections of neutrophils and macrophages appear within the subcutis of this animal, which was presented with multiple subcutaneous nodules. No evidence was found for an infectious agent. (H&E; LP.)

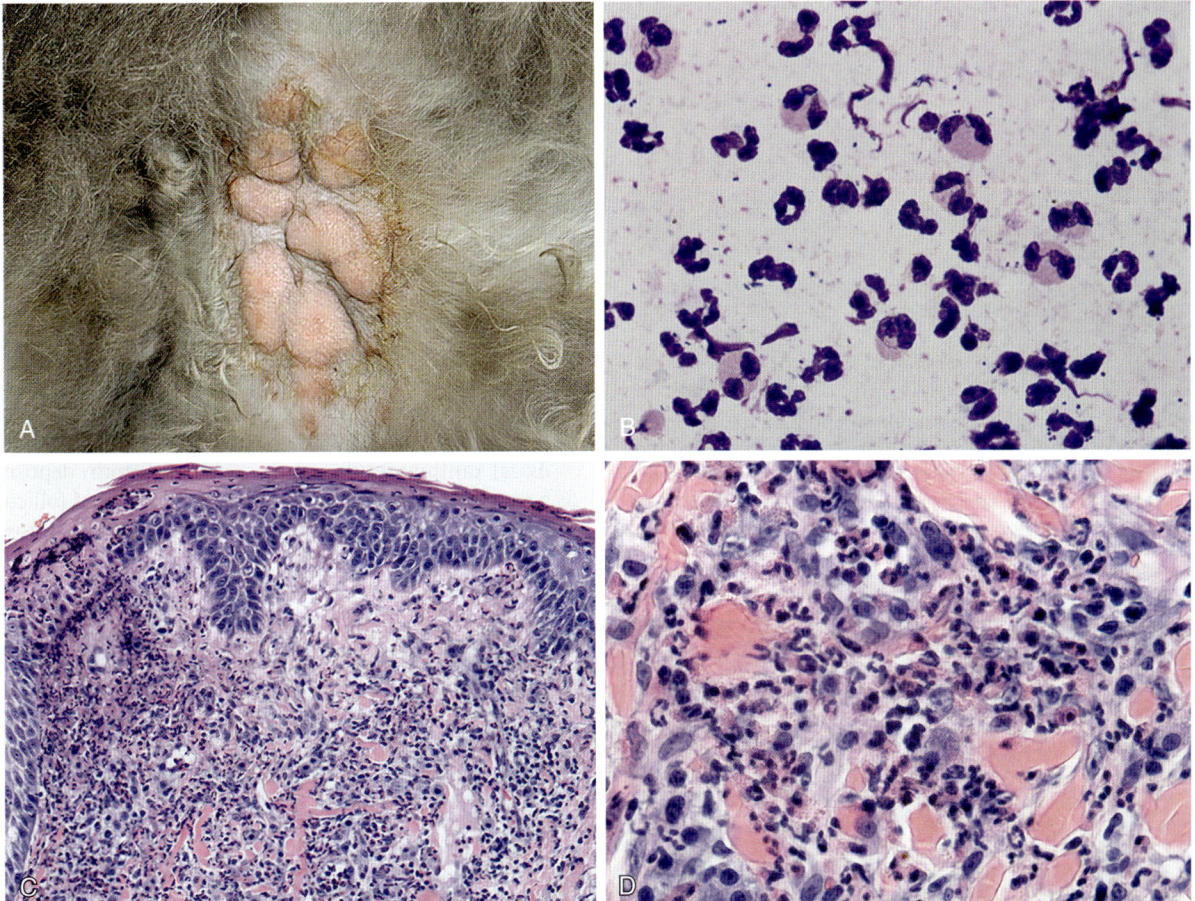

■ **FIGURE 3.20 Eosinophilic granuloma complex (eosinophilic plaque). Ventral abdomen. Cat.** Same case in A to D. **A, Gross lesion.** This 5-year-old domestic long-haired cat has coalescing skin nodules or plaques on the caudal abdomen (tail positioned to the right). The alopecic, erythematous lesions are pruritic as evidenced by wet-appearing fur and the cat's licking behavior reported in the history. **B, Plaque imprint.** A mixed population of inflammatory cells with two-thirds degenerate neutrophils and one-third eosinophils. Single and small clusters of coccoid bacteria appear within and neutrophils and extracellularly. (Aqueous Romanowsky; HP oil.) **C, Tissue punch biopsy.** Histopathology demonstrates a multifocal and expanded dermis infiltrated by large numbers of inflammatory cells. The overlying epidermis is mildly hyperplastic with parakeratotic hyperkeratosis and a cellular crust. There is focal erosion with near ulceration of the epidermis and basophilic foci within the epidermis is suggestive of bacterial colonies. (H&E; IP.) **D, Tissue punch biopsy.** Higher magnification to show the composition of the dermal cellular infiltrate. Eosinophils predominate with fewer neutrophils and mononuclear cells in decreasing magnitude. Hypereosinophilic hyalinized collagen bundles resembling flame figures owing to the release of eosinophil granules, are separated by the dense cell infiltrate. (H&E; HP oil.) (Courtesy Athema Etzioni, Tuskegee University.)

herpesvirus, calicivirus, feline leukemia virus infection, and *Cryptococcus* spp.

Histopathology for EGC may show intense eosinophilic infiltration with bundles of collagen separated by edema giving them a prominent appearance, sometimes termed *flame figures* (see Fig. 2.26 and Fig. 3.20D). This reaction resembles the Splendore-Hoeppli phenomenon discussed later in this chapter.

> ***Cytopathologic differential diagnosis:*** arthropod bite reaction, foreign body reaction, squamous cell carcinoma, mast cell tumor, cutaneous epitheliotropic T-cell lymphoma, bacterial and fungal agents.

Pemphigus Foliaceus

Pemphigus foliaceus is the most common autoimmune skin disease in dogs and cats. Drugs, chronic disease, and spontaneous causes have been associated with their occurrence. Grossly, lesions appear as erythematous macules that progress to white or yellow pustules and finally to crusts (see Fig. 16.74A). The head and feet are preferred sites, although the ears, trunk, and neck are also commonly affected in cats. Direct imprint of the underside of a crust or aspiration of a pustule reveals nondegenerate neutrophils and *acantholytic cells* appearing as round to oval individualized keratinocytes (Fig. 3.22; see Fig. 16.74B). Eosinophils may be present as well, but bacterial infection is usually lacking. Treatment includes antibiotics and immunotherapy. Excisional biopsy of early lesions is recommended that show a subcorneal vesicle with individualized or small clumps of keratinocytes (Fig. 3.23). Histologic examination along with direct immunofluorescent antibody tests or direct immunoperoxidase staining tests are necessary to distinguish the different pemphigus subtypes. Antinuclear antibody tests also may be helpful.

> ***Cytopathologic differential diagnosis:*** pyoderma.

Cutaneous Xanthoma and Xanthogranuloma

Xanthomatosis is an uncommon granulomatous inflammation in cats, dogs, birds, and amphibians; it is related to primary or secondary diabetes mellitus, high-fat diets, and hereditary hyperchylomicronemia (Gross et al., 2005; Banajee et al., 2011). The deposition of cholesterol and triglycerides in tissues results in lipid-laden macrophages. Grossly, the lesions are single or multiple, white to yellow plaques or nodules called *xanthomas* that may ulcerate or drain caseous material. Sites preferred are the face, trunk, and footpads. On cytopathology, aspirates contain numerous foamy macrophages (Fig. 3.24A) that stain positive with lipid stains (Fig. 3.24B). Histologically, cholesterol clefts and giant cells may be prominent (Fig. 3.24C). Larger vacuoles may be seen as well, as demonstrated in a case of idiopathic etiology (Fig. 3.25).

Focal xanthogranuloma may relate to keratin deposits acting as a source of lipids, such as seen with a variety of follicular conditions (Fig. 3.26A). Lymphocytes and occasional eosinophils

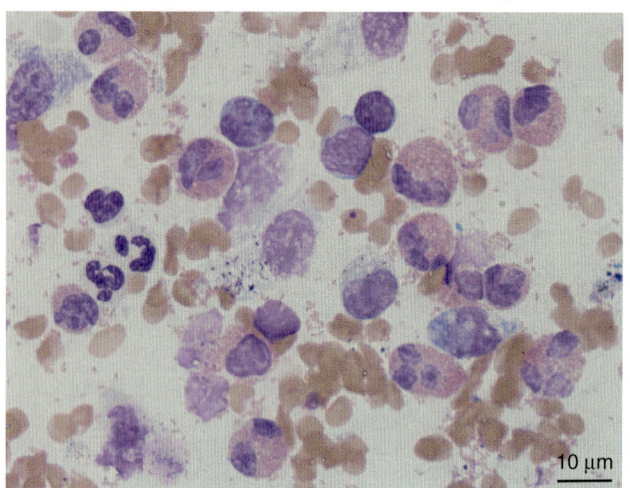

■ **FIGURE 3.21 Eosinophilic granuloma complex (eosinophilic granuloma). Lip mass. Tissue aspirate. Cat.** The lower lip is reported to be raised and firm and clinically most consistent with an eosinophilic granuloma. Admixed with eosinophils are nondegenerate neutrophils, small to medium lymphocytes, and fibroblasts. (Wright-Giemsa; HP oil.)

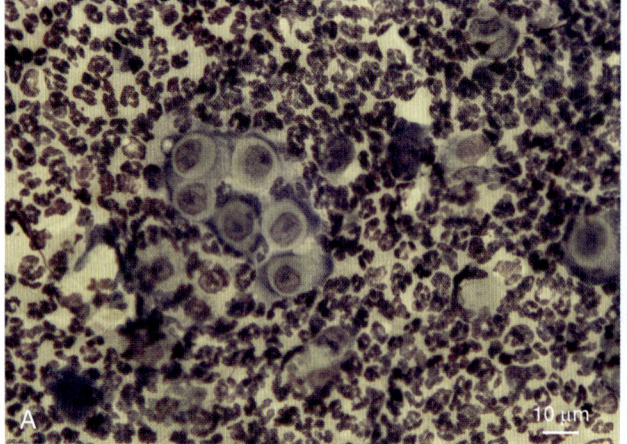
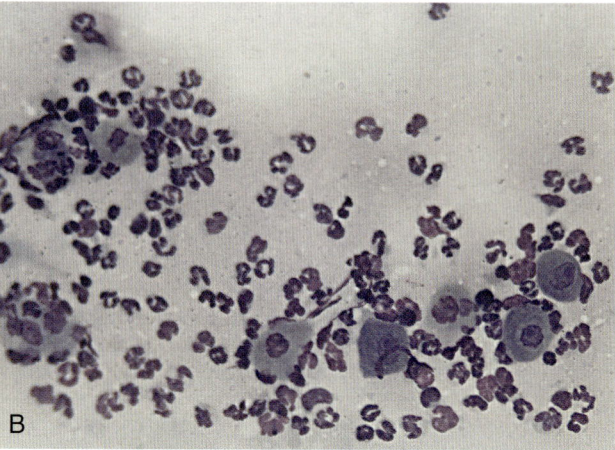

■ **FIGURE 3.22 Pemphigus foliaceus.** Same case in A and B. **A,** Surrounded by numerous nondegenerate neutrophils are a sheet of squamous epithelium that have a large round nucleus with prominent nucleolus surrounded by a clear halo. Cells appear rounded. (Modified Wright; HP oil.) **B,** In thinner areas, the rounded keratinocytes termed *acantholytic cells* can be seen clearly as individualized. (Modified Wright; HP oil.)

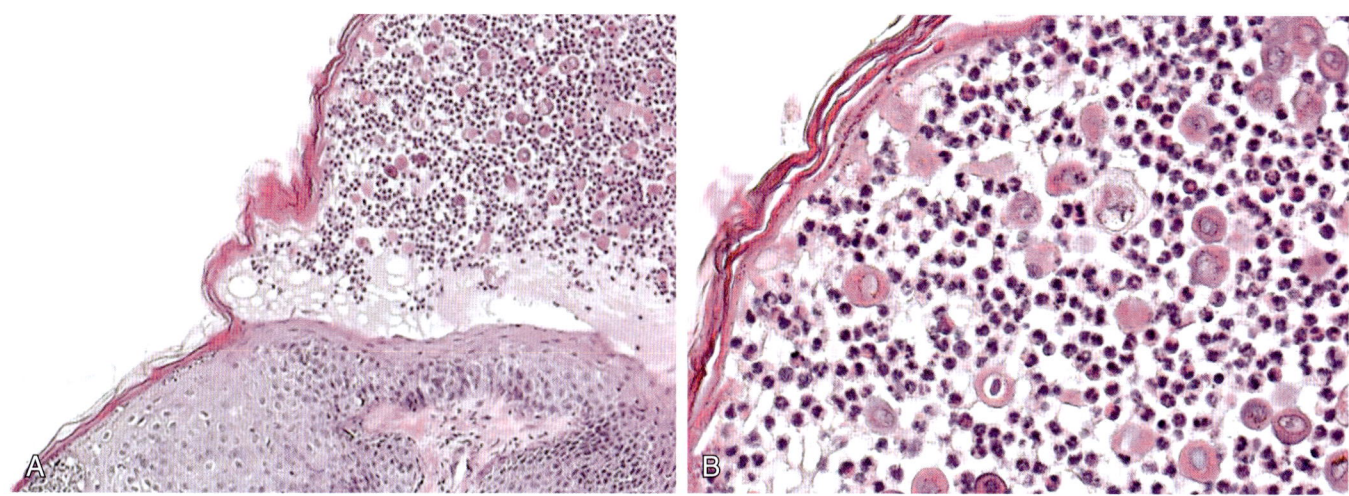

■ **FIGURE 3.23 Pemphigus foliaceus. Facial skin section. Cat.** Same case in A and B. **A,** Characteristic subcorneal pustule. **B,** Higher magnification of the pustule demonstrates the individualized acantholytic keratinocytes surrounded by numerous neutrophils. (H&E; HP oil.) (Courtesy Carlo Masserdotti, IDEXX, Italy. Presented at the 2018 ESVCP mystery case session.)

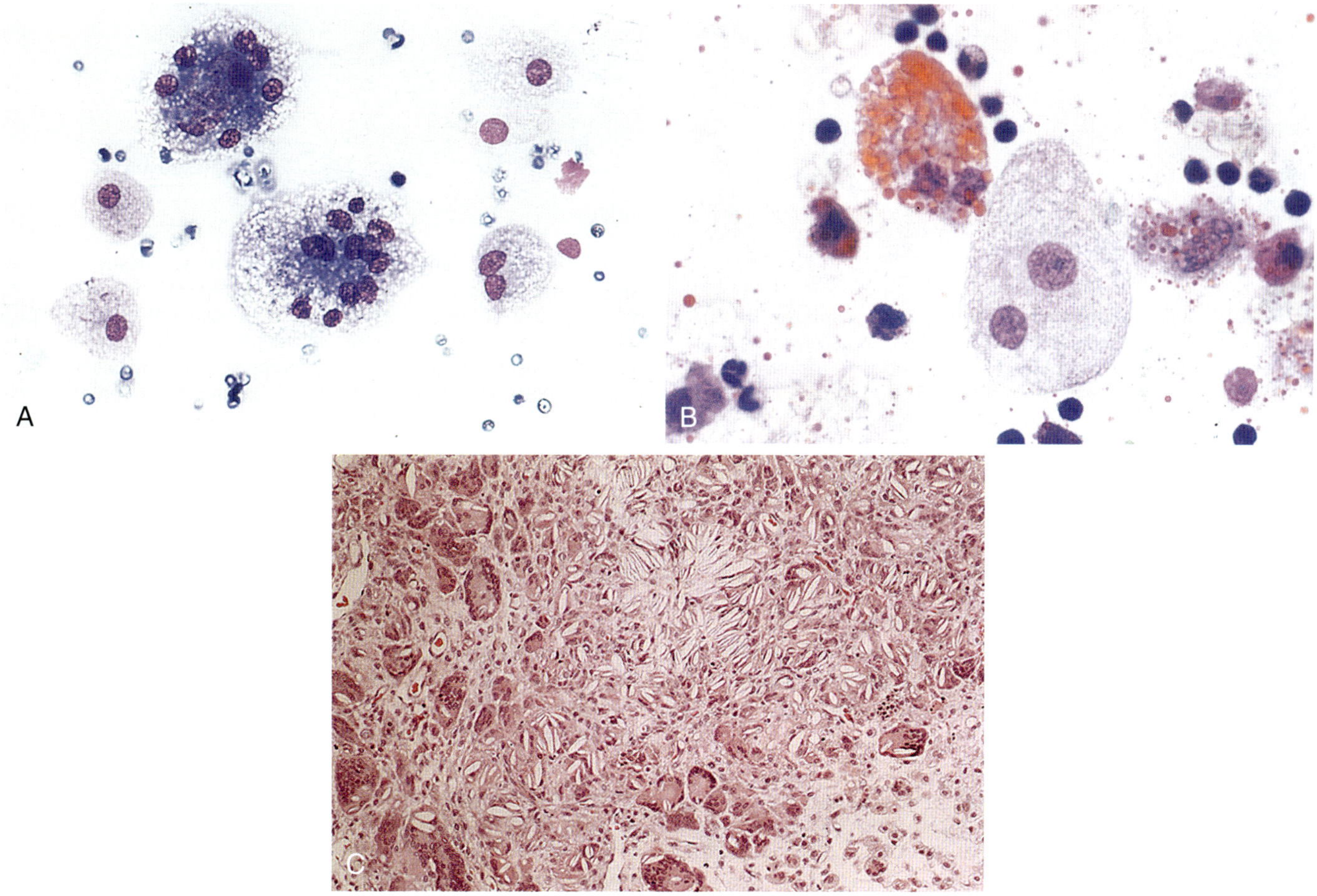

■ **FIGURE 3.24 Cutaneous xanthomatosis. Cat.** Same case in A to C. **A, Tissue aspirate.** Multinucleate giant cells and mononuclear foamy macrophages predominate in this specimen. This 1-year-old Siamese cat presented with multiple skin masses. (Wright-Giemsa; HP oil.) **B, Tissue aspirate.** This stain demonstrates the lipid content within the cytoplasm of variably sized macrophages. (Oil red O/new methylene blue; HP oil.). **C, Tissue section.** Aggregates of giant cells surround clusters of cholesterol clefts within the dermis. (H&E; IP.)

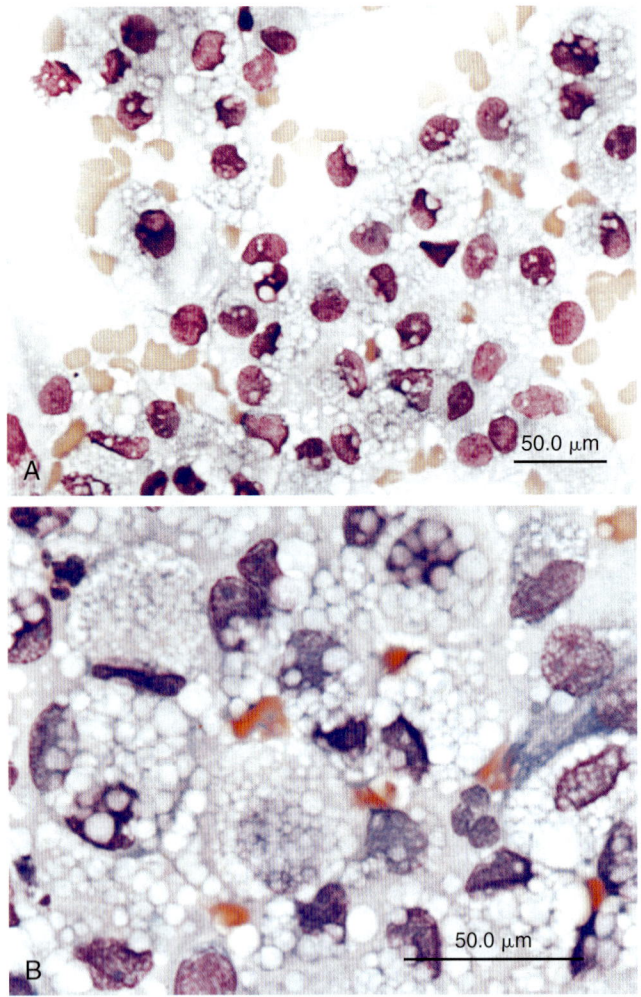

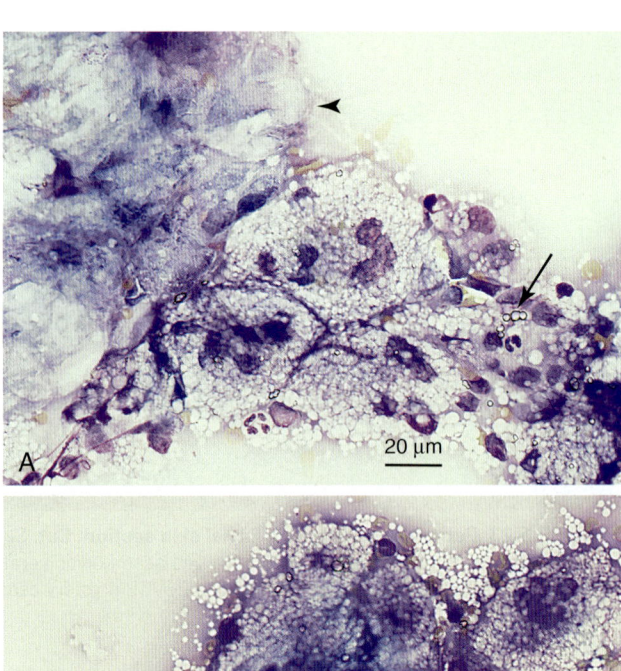

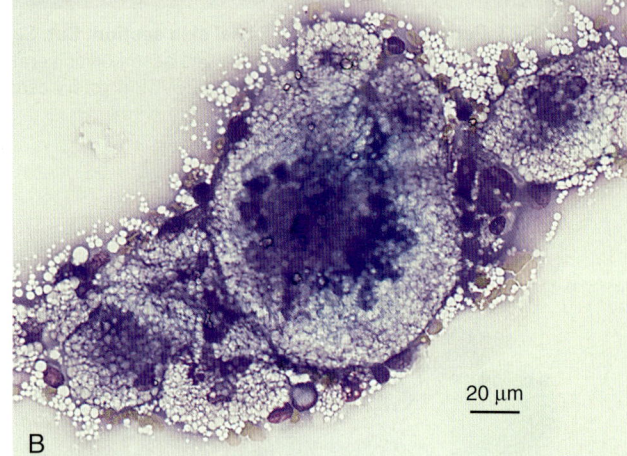

■ **FIGURE 3.25 Cutaneous xanthoma. Mass aspirate. Dog. A,** Cutaneous mass present on the ventral thorax. Nucleated cells are large round cells with large amounts of cytoplasm filled with many clear circular spaces, consistent with lipid. Nuclei have condensed chromatin and lack prominent nucleoli. Mild anisocytosis and anisokaryosis and occasional binucleation are noted. **B,** Higher magnification. (Wright-Giemsa; HP oil.) (From Banajee KH, Orandle MS, Ratterree W, et al. Idiopathic solitary cutaneous xanthoma in a dog, *Vet Clin Pathol.* 2011;40:95–98.)

■ **FIGURE 3.26 Xanthogranuloma. Foot mass. Tissue aspirate. Dog.** Same case in A and B. **A,** The dermal mass consists primarily of cell aggregates, characterized by abundant foamy cytoplasm with a single centrally located nucleus. Occasional lymphocytes and neutrophils are present as well as small amounts of mineral appearing as refractile round colorless granules *(arrow)*. Adjacent to the xanthomatous macrophages is a focus *(arrowhead)* of pale blue keratinized epithelium. Focal xanthogranuloma may relate to keratin deposits acting as a source of lipid. (Modified Wright; HP oil.) **B,** An aggregate of foamy macrophages is present, many of which are multinucleated. (Modified Wright; IP.) (Courtesy Tricia Bisby, Purdue University.)

or neutrophils are present as well as foamy macrophages, which may be multinucleated (Fig. 3.26B). These vacuolated xanthoma cells expressed CD18 to support macrophage origin. Treatment is aimed at identifying and controlling the underlying cause, if known.

> *Cytopathologic differential diagnosis:* sterile granuloma (e.g., foreign body reaction).

Sterile Granulomatous Dermatitis

Sterile granulomatous dermatitis and lymphadenitis have been referred to as *juvenile cellulitis* or *puppy strangles*. This is an infrequent lymphocutaneous disease seen in dogs ranging in age from a few weeks to 4 months for the juvenile form; it is less common in adults (Inga et al., 2020). Clinical signs involve lymphadenomegaly, fever, lethargy, and hyporexia. Skin lesions display papular nodules mostly on the face and ears but occasionally elsewhere. The disease appears most commonly in dachshunds, golden retrievers, Labrador retrievers, and Gordon setter breeds. Histopathology indicates nodular infiltrations of mostly macrophages with fewer neutrophils (pyogranulomas) around adnexal structures of the skin. Cytopathology reveals populations of mainly epithelioid macrophages with scattered nondegenerate neutrophils. The disease is considered idiopathic and may relate to immune dysfunction. Treatment is often successful with corticosteroids.

Feline Plasmacytic Pododermatitis

Cats rarely present with purple, spongy, soft, painless swellings of one or more footpads that are composed predominately of mature plasma cells and lesser numbers of neutrophils and small lymphocytes (Fig. 3.27). Despite looking for a variety of organisms, including *Mycobacterium* spp., *Bartonella* spp., *Ehrlichia* spp., *Anaplasma* spp., *Chlamydia felis*, *Mycoplasma* spp., *Toxoplasma gondii*, or feline herpesvirus type 1, none has been identified as a causative agent (Bettenay et al., 2007). Therefore, plasma cell pododermatitis is likely a purely immune-mediated condition. Immunohistochemical staining with kappa and lambda light chains show a mixed reaction indicating a non-neoplastic lesion (Dobromylskyi, 2015).

INFECTIOUS INFLAMMATORY DISORDERS

Viruses

Feline herpesvirus 1 (FeHV-1)-associated dermatitis occurs after upper respiratory disease. Ulcerative lesions around the eyes, nose, and muzzle relate to epidermal and follicular necrosis. Histopathology reveals a thick dermal infiltrate of eosinophils with occasional intranuclear inclusion bodies within keratinocytes (Sánchez et al., 2012). The presence of the virus may be confirmed with FeHV-1 immunohistochemistry. Imprints of the area when examined cytopathologically are blood contaminated numerous eosinophils and fewer neutrophils and macrophages; viral inclusions are not seen.

Bacteria

Acute Bacterial Abscess and Pyoderma

An abscess is a common subcutaneous lesion in cats and dogs, often related to bites or other penetrating wounds. This may be localized to the skin or associated with systemic signs. The area is firm to fluctuant, swollen, erythematous, warm, and painful. A creamy white exudate may be aspirated that is characterized on cytopathology by numerous degenerate neutrophils displaying karyolysis, karyorrhexis, and pyknosis (see Chapter 2). Bacteria may be found in association with the swollen, round nuclei. Case management includes culture and sensitivity tests, with treatment aimed at surgical incision and antibiotics.

Deep pyoderma manifests as a bacterial inflammation that extends into the dermis and hair follicles with subsequent damage to the follicle (furunculosis). The ruptured follicular wall releases fragments of the hair shaft as well as follicular keratin into the surrounding tissue that creates a foreign body reaction and pyogranulomatous inflammation with formation of a dermal nodule (Gross et al., 2005; Raskin, 2006b). *Staphylococcus intermedius* is typically the primary pathogen, but other bacteria and underlying conditions may occur to initiate the inflammation. Ulceration is common. Mixed inflammatory cells, including neutrophils and macrophages, are present (Fig. 3.28).

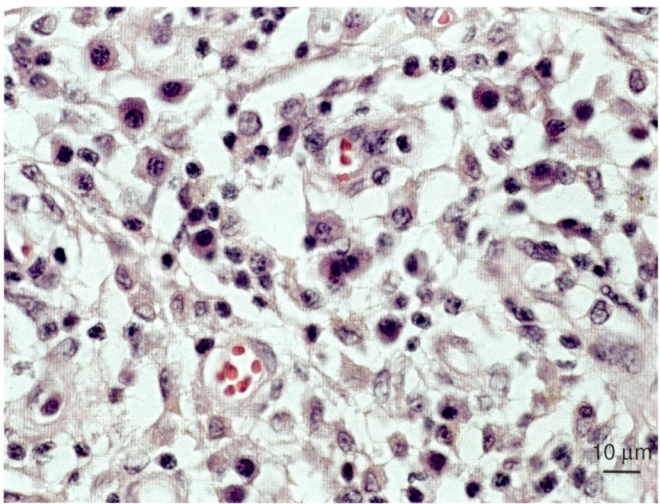

■ **FIGURE 3.27 Lymphoplasmacytic pododermatitis. Metacarpal food pad. Tissue section. Cat.** Multiple feet are affected in this animal, and the specimen is from a recurrent swelling. There is a densely cellular infiltrate composed of plasma cells, lymphocytes, and fewer macrophages. The condition is considered to be a purely immune-mediated condition, but evidence for infectious agents should be confirmed before immunosuppressant treatment is given. (H&E; HP oil.)

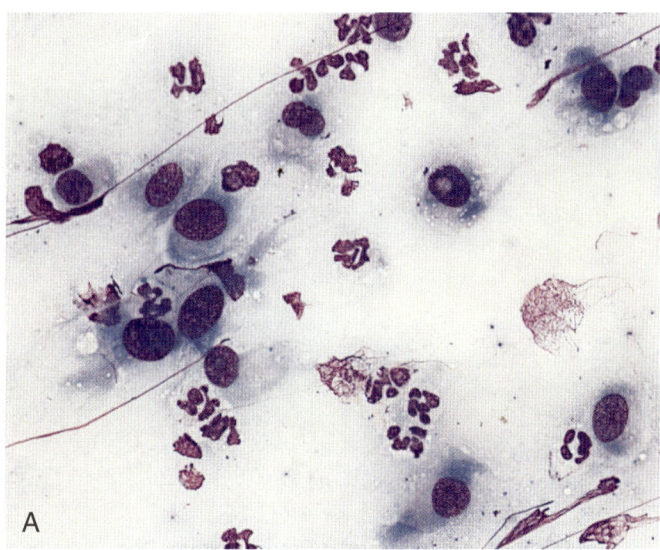 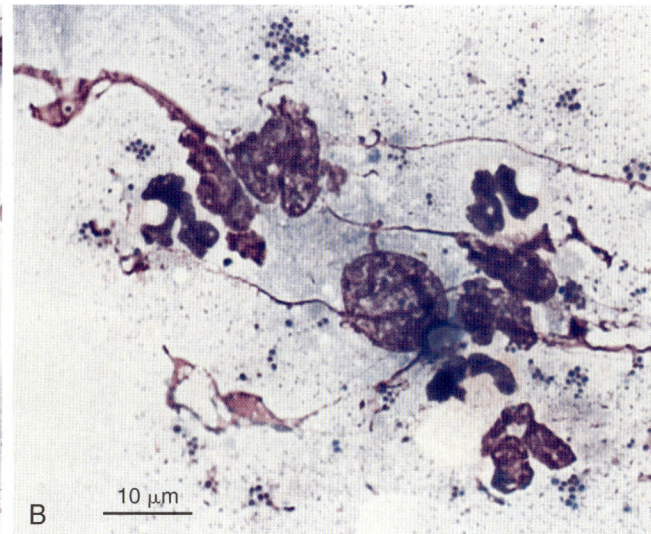

■ **FIGURE 3.28 Pyoderma. Tissue aspirate. Dog.** Same case in A and B. **A,** A persistent dermal mass on the tail consists of a mixed cell population of mostly degenerate neutrophils and plump stromal cells. (Modified Wright; HP oil.) **B,** Note the clusters of large cocci typical of *Staphylococcus* scattered in the background. (Modified Wright; HP oil.)

Suppurative inflammation may produce a proteinaceous mucinous discharge that displays a pattern like Curschmann's spirals from the respiratory tract (Fig. 3.29).

Clostridial Cellulitis

Clostridial infection is usually associated with penetrating wounds. The swollen skin may be crepitus with a serosanguineous wound exudate. Tissue aspirates may reveal large rods measuring 1 × 4 μm, some with a clear, oval, subterminal endospore, occurring singly or in short chains (Fig. 3.30A). *Clostridium* is an anaerobic gram-positive organism (Fig. 3.30B) but may stain variably as a result of a chronic infection or antibiotic therapy. The specimen background often contains cellular debris and lipid with few, if any, inflammatory cells. Neutrophils, when present, are often degenerate. Anaerobic culture is necessary for diagnosis. Treatment includes surgical management and appropriate antibiotic administration.

Rhodococcus equi Cellulitis

The presence of numerous neutrophils and macrophages, with the latter containing small rod to coccoid bacteria, should suggest infection from *Rhodococcus* spp. Case reports describe ulcerative swellings that often occur on extremities and involve adjacent lymph nodes (Patel, 2002). These are opportunistic bacteria that pose a higher risk to immunosuppressed animals.

Actinomycosis and Nocardiosis

The infection presents as subcutaneous swellings that progress to ulceration with exudation of red-brown fluid. The cause is often related to penetrating wounds. The infections may be associated with systemic signs that often include pyothorax. On cytopathology, degenerate neutrophils predominate, with macrophages and small lymphocytes also present. Bacteria may be intracellular or extracellular, the latter often found as dense clusters of organisms (Figs. 3.31 and 3.32). These

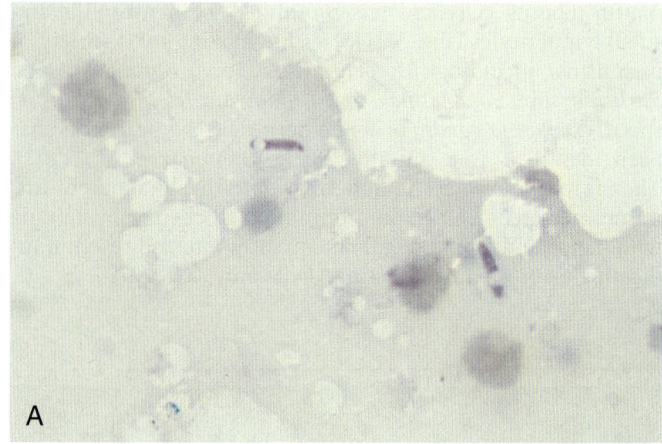
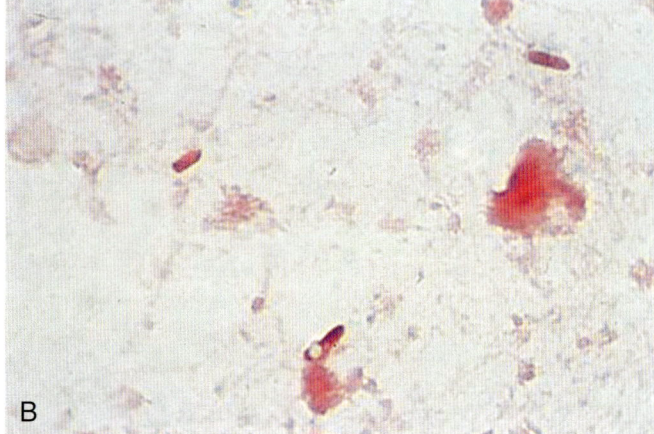

■ **FIGURE 3.30 Clostridial cellulitis. Tissue aspirate. Dog.** Same case in A and B. **A,** Bacilli with terminal spore formation in the subcutis of an animal with subcutaneous emphysema and adjacent bone lysis. (Wright-Giemsa; HP oil.) **B,** Gram-positive rods on aerobic culture were confirmed as *Clostridium* spp. (Gram; HP oil.)

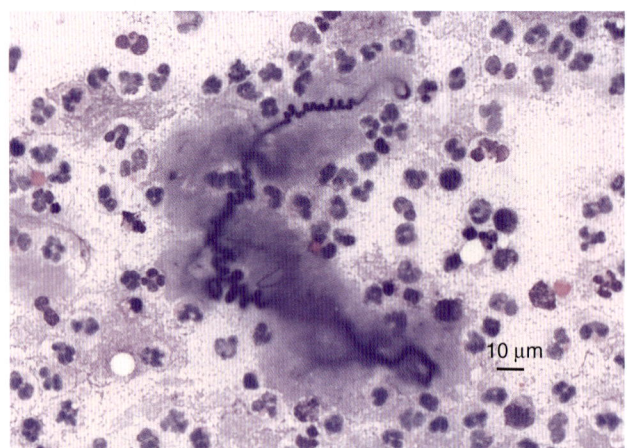

■ **FIGURE 3.29 Pyoderma with Curschmann's spirals. Fluid discharge smear. Dog.** Fluid discharge from a bite wound contains several mucoid strands resembling those more typically found in respiratory specimens. Marked suppurative inflammation noted in the background. (Modified Wright; IP.)

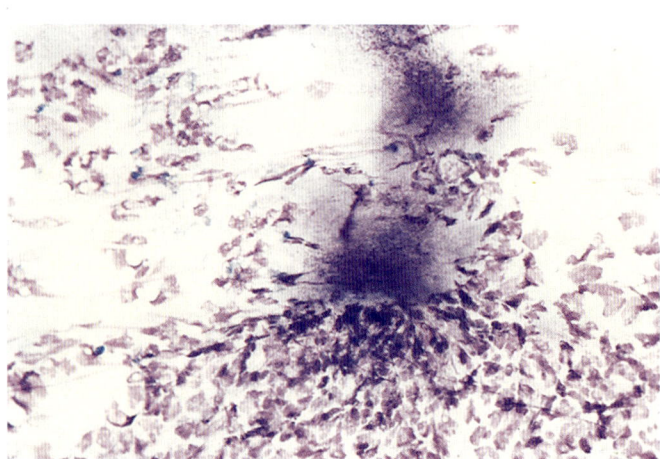

■ **FIGURE 3.31 Actinomycosis. Tissue aspirate. Dog.** Note the basophilic clusters of filamentous organisms that resemble amorphous debris. (Wright-Giemsa; HP oil.)

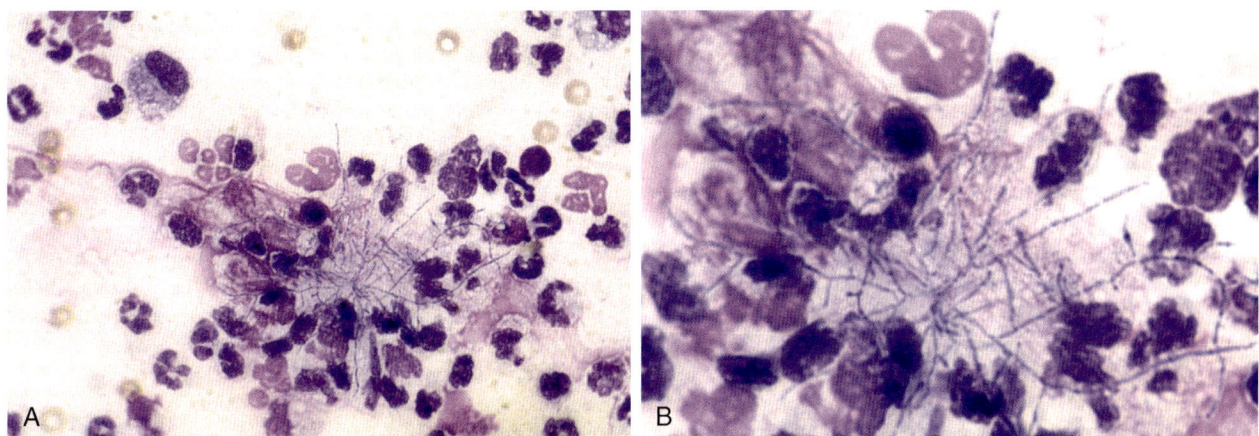

FIGURE 3.32 Nocardiosis. Tissue aspirate. Dog. Same case in A and B. **A,** Cluster of organisms surrounded by many degenerate neutrophils and few macrophages. Culture confirmed presence of *Nocardia* spp. (Wright-Giemsa; HP oil.) **B,** Branching, beaded, slender bacterial filaments are demonstrated in this fluid pocket from a dog with a swollen hind leg. (Wright-Giemsa; HP oil.)

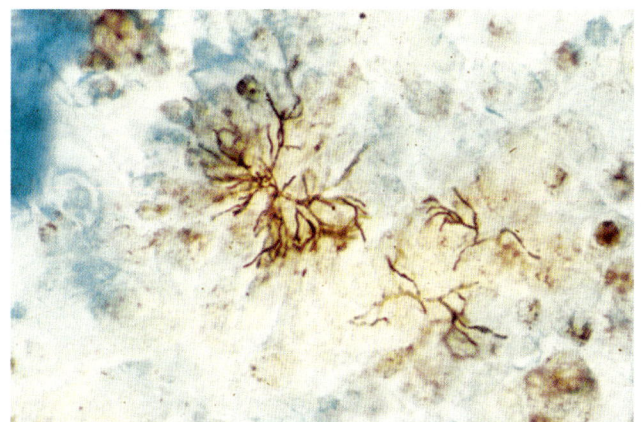

FIGURE 3.33 Actinomycosis. Tissue aspirate. Dog. Branching, beaded, slender bacterial filaments stain with a silver stain. (GMS; HP oil.)

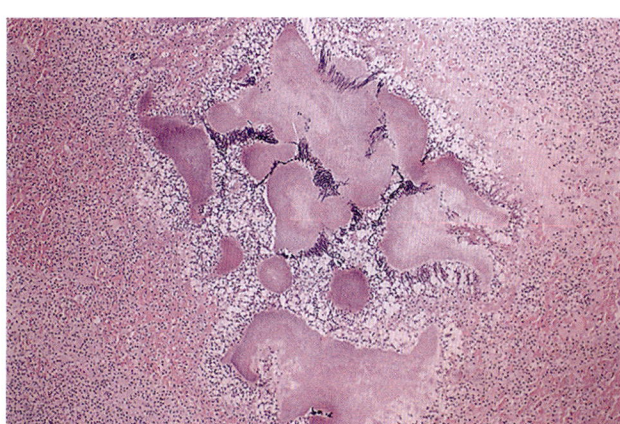

FIGURE 3.34 Actinomycosis. Tissue section. Pyogranulomatous cellulitis surrounding irregular islands of filamentous organisms that are gram positive but not acid fast. The periphery of these foci contain densely eosinophilic hyalinized material thought to represent antigen-antibody complexes. This reaction has been termed the *Splendore-Hoeppli phenomenon*. (H&E; LP.)

bacteria are slender, filamentous, branching, lightly basophilic rods with red spotted or beaded areas. They may be highlighted with a silver stain (Fig. 3.33). Histologically, inflammatory cells group around dense mats of organisms, forming dense eosinophilic hyalinized material (Fig. 3.34). *Actinomyces* spp. are gram positive but not acid fast, whereas *Nocardia* spp. are gram positive and variably acid fast. Culture is necessary for diagnosis of the specific type, and samples should be obtained anaerobically. Treatment includes surgical drainage and appropriate antibiotics.

Similar in morphology to *Actinomyces* spp. is *Actinomadura* spp. as noted in one recent case in a cat with a chronic nonhealing wound (Wells et al., 2018). Cytopathology reveals numerous multinucleate macrophages and gram-positive, acid-fast-negative, filamentous bacteria that polymerase chain reaction (PCR) and sequencing confirmed as *Actinomadura vinacea*.

> **KEY POINT** Look at the dense areas of the specimen for basophilic mats of bacteria.

Dermatophilosis

This is a rare infection that has been reported in cats and dogs, usually as the result of penetrating wounds contaminated with infected soil or water. The lesion presents as a firm, alopecic, subcutaneous draining mass. The thick gray exudate below the crusted surface is purulent, with numerous degenerate neutrophils but few eosinophils and macrophages. The organism appears as gram-positive branching filaments that segment horizontally and longitudinally into coccoid forms (Fig. 3.35). Diagnosis is made by morphologic identification of the organism on cytopathologic or histopathologic biopsy or through culture. Treatment involves appropriate antibiotics and appropriate wound management (Kaya et al., 2000).

Mycobacteriosis

Three clinical forms of mycobacteriosis in dogs and cats are recognized, which include internal tuberculous, localized cutaneous nodules (lepromatous), and spreading subcutaneous forms (Greene and Gunn-Moore, 2006). Diagnosis is best performed by tissue culture and histopathology. Definitive identification may be made by PCR of tissue specimens. Treatment may include surgical excision and appropriate antibiotics.

The tuberculous form is related to *Mycobacterium tuberculosis*, *Mycobacterium bovis*, or the opportunistic *Mycobacterium avium–intracellulare* complex. Contact with infected people, cattle, birds, or soil may be documented. The disease may also be associated with immunosuppressed animals. This form is characterized by a systemic disease with weight loss, fever, and lymphadenopathy. Although internal organs are most affected, skin nodules can appear on the head, neck, and legs of dogs and cats. These are slow-growing organisms that normally require 4 to 6 weeks to culture. Detection may be hastened to 2 weeks and may require PCR and other molecular techniques for identification. On cytopathologic specimens, macrophages contain few to many beaded bacilli, and some organisms may be extracellular (Fig. 3.36A). Acid-fast staining is helpful in the recognition of the organisms (Fig. 3.36B). Lymphocytes and neutrophils are more abundant than in lepromatous forms.

The lepromatous form in cats is caused by *Mycobacterium lepraemurium* and is common in wet, cooler climates with exposure to infected rodents. A novel, unnamed *Mycobacterium* spp. has been documented for dogs in Australia, New Zealand, and recently in the United States (Foley et al., 2002). In general, canine leproid granuloma cases involve immunocompetent, short-coated, large-breed dogs such as boxers and boxer mixed breeds being overrepresented. Nonpainful raised nodules are found on the head and distal limbs without systemic signs in cats. These nodules are soft to firm, fleshy, and often localized, with occasional ulceration and little exudation. Spontaneous remission has been reported in a cat (Roccabianca et al., 1996). Nodules in dogs are smooth to ulcerated, occurring frequently on the head, particularly the ears and muzzle. Cultivation of the organism is difficult. On cytopathology, macrophages containing numerous intracellular organisms predominate (Twomey et al., 2005) (Fig. 3.37). Other cells seen include lymphocytes, plasma cells, neutrophils, and occasional multinucleate giant cells.

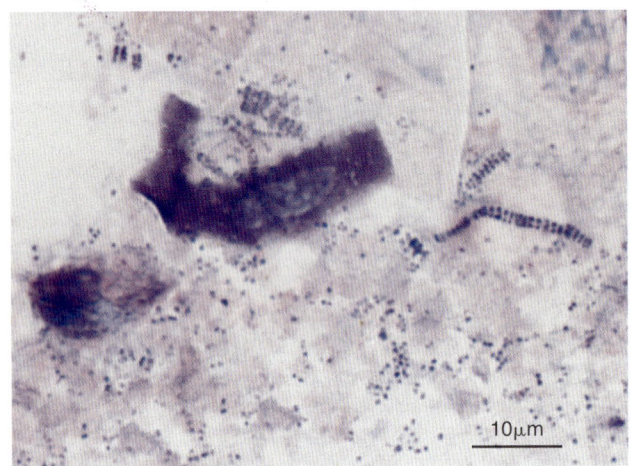

■ **FIGURE 3.35 Dermatophilosis. Tissue scraping. Horse.** *Dermatophilus congolensis* is seen as filamentous strands of paired coccoid bacteria. (Modified Wright; HP oil.)

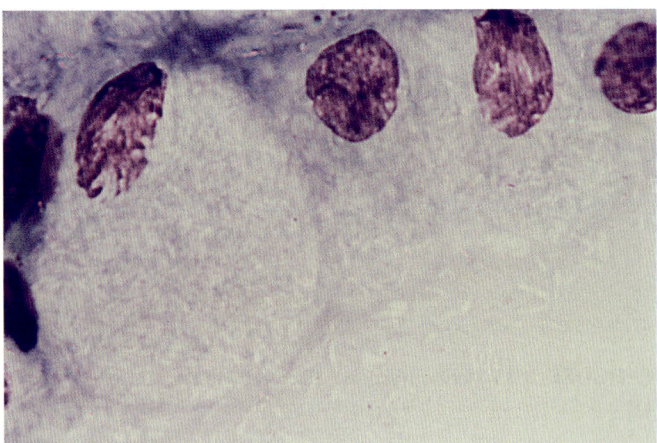

■ **FIGURE 3.37 Feline leprosy. Tissue imprint. Cat.** Negative-stained linear bacteria fill the cytoplasm and appear extracellular, visible against the proteinaceous background. (Giemsa; HP oil.) (Courtesy John Kramer, Washington State University. Presented at the 1988 ASVCP case review session.)

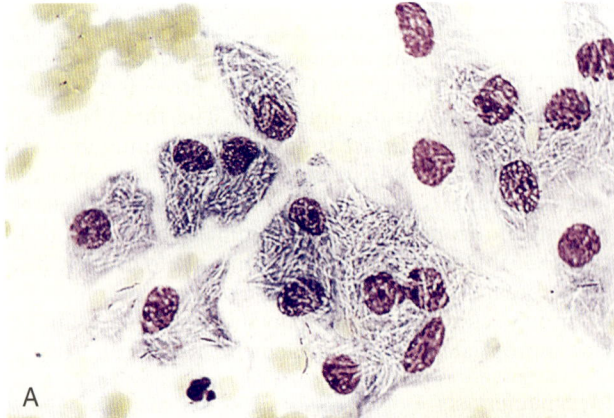
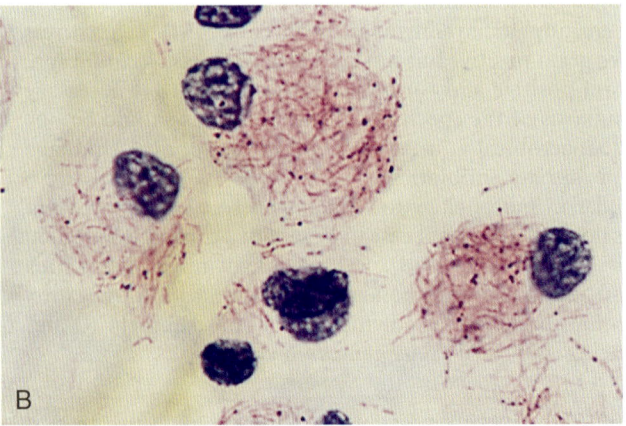

■ **FIGURE 3.36 Mycobacteriosis. Tissue aspirate. Cat.** Same case in A and B. **A,** A swollen area over the nose was confirmed positive for *Mycobacterium avium–intracellulare* complex. Note the abundance of negative-staining rods with the cytoplasm of macrophages. (Wright-Giemsa; HP oil.) **B,** Acid-fast stain is positive for the beaded linear bacteria. (Ziehl-Neelsen; HP oil.)

CHAPTER 3 Integumentary System

The more common presentation of cutaneous mycobacteriosis in dogs and cats involves fast-growing species having an atypical growth pattern or culture characteristic, such as *Mycobacterium fortuitum*, *Mycobacterium chelonei*, and *Mycobacterium smegmatis*. These are the result of inoculation with contaminated soil or standing water. Lesions are characterized by a spreading subcutaneous pyogranulomatous inflammation having frequent draining tracts. This form also lacks systemic signs. Bacterial culture of deep tissue sites is required, and growth may occur within 3 to 5 days. On cytopathologic specimens, a mixed population of neutrophils and macrophages predominates, with occasional lymphocytes, plasma cells, multinucleate giant cells, or reactive fibroblasts (Fig. 3.38A). Organisms are occasionally found on cytopathology with the aid of acid-fast staining (see Fig. 3.38). On histopathology, lesions appear diffuse, and organisms may be found within lipocysts surrounded by inflammatory cells. The prognosis for this form is guarded because response to antibiotics is often unrewarding.

> **KEY POINT** Mycobacterial organisms are gram positive and acid fast. They appear on cytopathology as nonstaining, long, thin rods because of the high lipid content of their cell walls.

Fungi
Localized Opportunistic Fungal Infections

Cutaneous or subcutaneous lesions occur as the result of penetrating wounds contaminated with infected soil or water, commonly in tropical or subtropical climates. Hyphae are narrow, septated with magenta granulation and acute angle formation. One common type is phaeohyphomycosis, caused by a group of dematiaceous (pigmented) fungi such as *Alternaria*, *Curvularia*, or *Bipolaris* spp. (Figs. 3.39 and 3.40). Although pigmentation is more likely detected on histopathology, slides may be stained with Fontana-Masson to enhance the staining. Hyphae produce bulbous or globose swellings. A second more rare type is hyalohyphomycosis, related to the hyaline hyphae, which are nonpigmented and appear pale. Specific fungi include *Paecilomyces* spp. (Figs. 3.41 and 3.42) as well as *Acremonium*, *Fusarium*, and *Pseudoallescheria* spp. Nodules develop slowly, usually on the extremities, later becoming ulcerated with draining tracts. On cytopathology, these fungi produce a pyogranulomatous inflammation with degenerate neutrophils, macrophages, multinucleate giant cells, lymphocytes, plasma cells, and mature fibroblasts. Yeast forms rarely occur. Bulbous swellings are less common in hyalohyphomycosis than phaeohyphomycosis. Diagnosis involves histopathologic

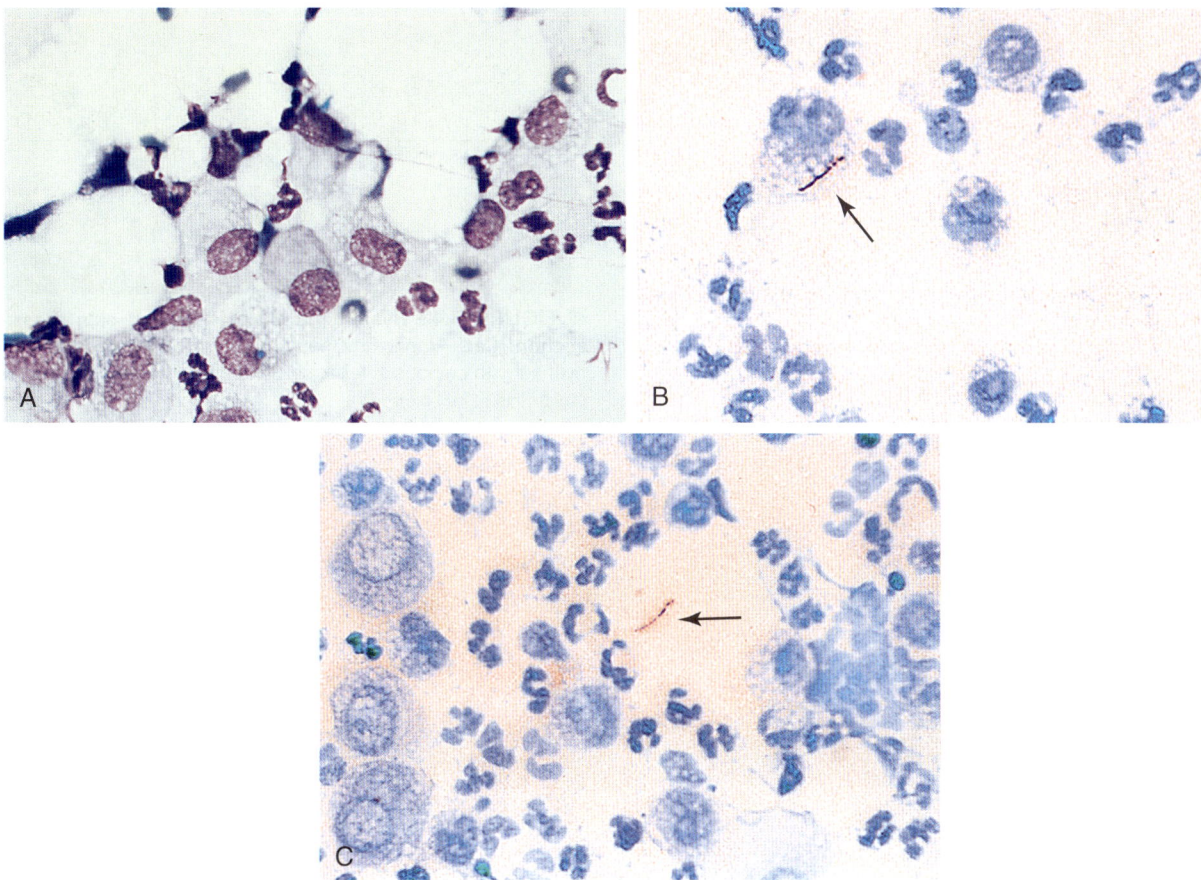

■ **FIGURE 3.38 Atypical mycobacteriosis. Tissue aspirate. Dog.** Same case in A to C. **A,** Frequent neutrophils and macrophages appear without obvious evidence of sepsis. Neutrophils are mildly degenerate in this 2 cm mass located on the back. (Wright-Giemsa; HP oil.) **B,** Single positive filamentous bacterium found within macrophage *(arrow)*. (Fite's acid-fast; HP oil.) **C,** Tissue aspirate. Single positive filamentous bacterium found within a lipocyst *(arrow)*. (Fite's acid-fast; HP oil.)

biopsy, tissue culture, PCR testing. Treatment involves surgical excision, but the prognosis is often poor to guarded.

Cutaneous Lesions From Systemic Fungal Infections

Cutaneous lesions from systemic fungal infections usually present as single or multiple nodules that ulcerate and drain a serosanguineous exudate. Regional lymphadenopathy is common along with affected organ systems. Examination of the exudate is diagnostic, but surgical excision with histopathologic biopsy is recommended. Serum titers, tissue culture, and PCR are helpful in difficult cases. In general, treatment is aimed at systemic antifungal therapy. Prognosis is guarded.

Blastomycosis. Blastomycosis is a pyogranulomatous or granulomatous inflammation of dogs and, rarely, cats that is related to yeast and rare hyphal forms of *Blastomyces dermatitidis* (Bulla and Thomas, 2009). The disease is endemic in areas around the Mississippi and Ohio River basins and in Canada. Lesions appear often on the extremities and nose. On cytopathologic specimens, degenerate neutrophils, macrophages, multinucleate giant cells,

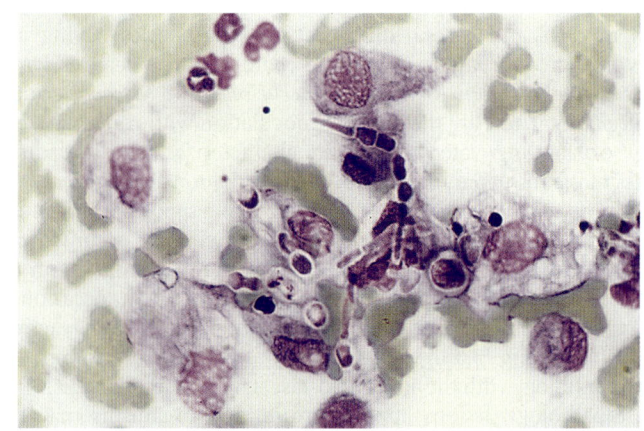

■ **FIGURE 3.41 Hyalohyphomycosis. Tissue aspirate. Cat.** This swollen digit contained hyphal structures with yeastlike swellings suspected to be caused by *Paecilomyces* spp. Numerous macrophages are noted along with few neutrophils. (Wright-Giemsa; HP oil.)

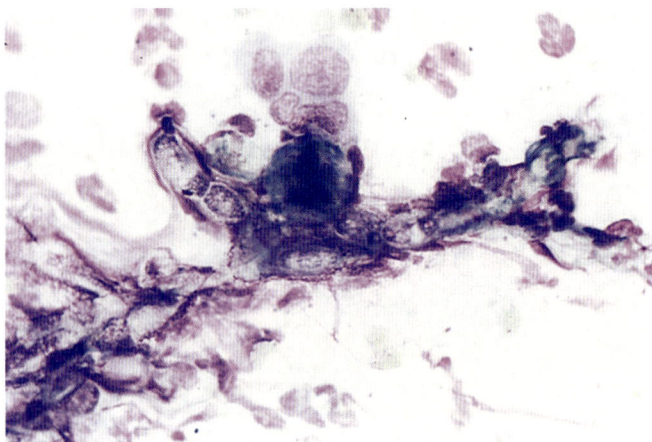

■ **FIGURE 3.39 Phaeohyphomycosis (pigmented fungi). Tissue aspirate. Dog.** Small mass on plantar surface of the foot was positive for *Curvularia* spp. on culture. Degenerate neutrophils and macrophages surround the fungal hyphae with yeastlike swellings. (Aqueous Romanowsky; HP oil.)

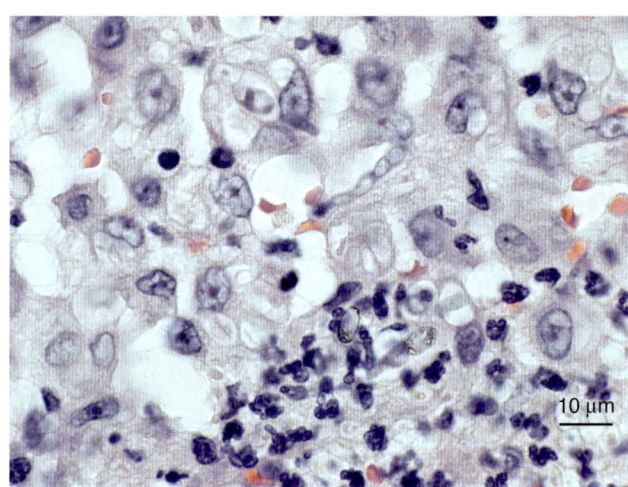

■ **FIGURE 3.42 Hyalohyphomycosis. Digital skin mass. Tissue section. Cat.** Among the neutrophils and macrophages are septate hyphae with bulbous swellings. Histopathologic diagnosis is paecilomycosis. (H&E; HP oil.)

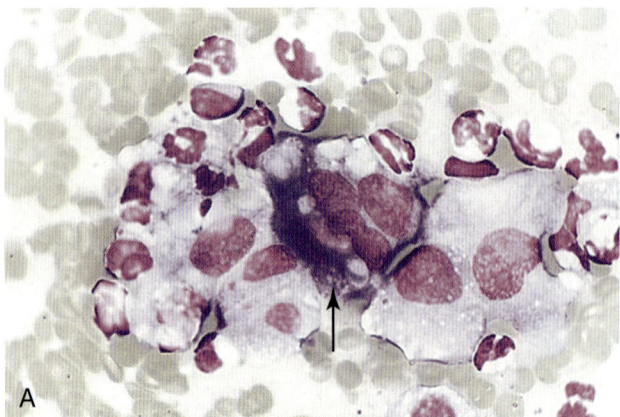

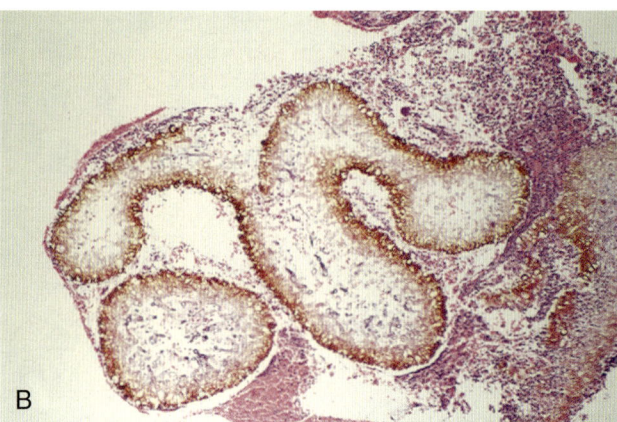

■ **FIGURE 3.40 Phaeohyphomycosis. Dog.** Same case in A and B. **A, Tissue aspirate.** Mixed inflammation with macrophages, degenerate neutrophils, and lymphocytes surround a hyphal structure *(arrow)* with yeast-like swellings. (Wright-Giemsa; HP oil.) **B, Tissue section.** Large colonies of brown fungi confirm the diagnosis of dematiaceous or pigmented fungi. (H&E; LP.)

and lymphocytes are present. Yeast forms measure 7 to 15 μm in diameter and have a refractile, deeply basophilic, thick cell wall (Figs. 3.43 and 3.44). Organisms may be phagocytized by macrophages or found extracellularly. Cell division occurs by budding that is broad based compared with the narrow-based budding of *Cryptococcus* spp. Structures stain positive with periodic acid–Schiff (PAS) (Fig. 3.45) and methenamine silver. Definitive diagnosis involves immunostaining of tissue sections and tissue culture. Serum tests involve agar gel immunodiffusion and enzyme-linked immunosorbent assay (ELISA) methods, but they have low sensitivity. A more sensitive quantitative antigen-based test for urine (93.5% sensitivity with some cross-reactivity to histoplasmosis) is available (see Appendix 7) that is more clinically useful (Spector et al., 2008). Confirmation of organisms found on cytopathologic biopsy may be performed by PCR with gene sequencing assays (Bulla and Thomas, 2009).

Coccidioidomycosis. Coccidioidomycosis, caused by *Coccidioides* spp., produces a pyogranulomatous response similar to that of blastomycosis in dogs and occasionally cats. It is endemic in the southwestern United States. The etiologic agents are *Coccidioides immitis*, most often seen in California or *Coccidioides posadasii*, seen in Arizona. On cytopathology, the organism appears as thick-walled spherules measuring 20 to 200 μm in diameter (Fig. 3.46). Within the basophilic spherule (Fig. 3.47) are uninucleate round endospores measuring 2 to 5 μm in diameter. The free endospores may be confused with yeast forms of *Histoplasma* or *Toxoplasma*. Empty small spherules resemble *Blastomyces*. Both cell wall and endospores stain positive with methenamine silver, whereas PAS stains the cell wall purple and the endospores red. Intact spherules are poorly chemotactic for neutrophils compared with free endospores, which attract many neutrophils. Serologic tests used include

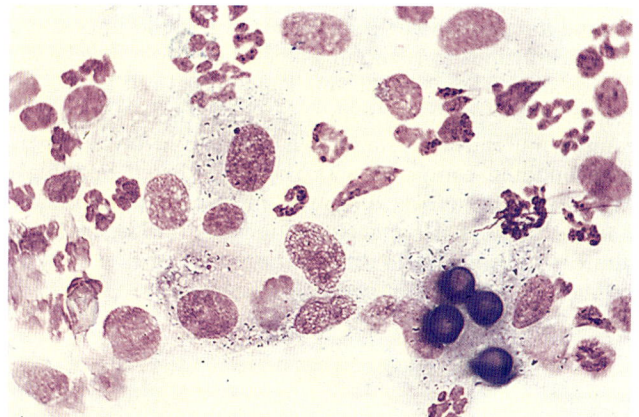

■ **FIGURE 3.43 Blastomycosis. Tissue imprint. Dog.** A mass on the digit revealed several deeply basophilic thick-walled budding yeast forms along with a mixture of macrophages and degenerate neutrophils. (Aqueous Romanowsky; HP oil.)

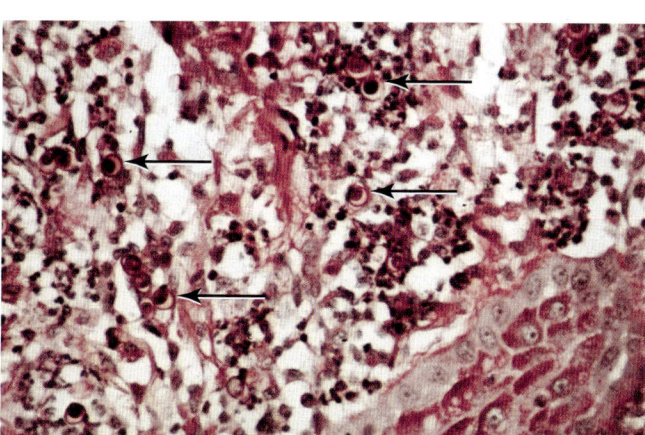

■ **FIGURE 3.45 Blastomycosis. Tissue section. Dog.** Dense accumulation of inflammatory cells surround densely stained yeast forms *(arrows)* whose thick cell wall collapses following fixation. (PAS; IP.)

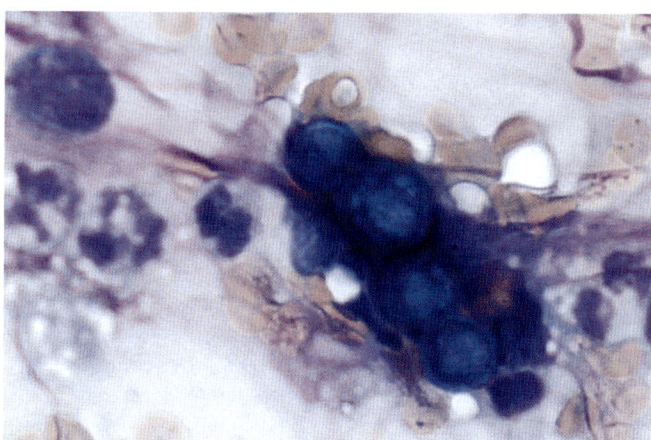

■ **FIGURE 3.44 Blastomycosis. Tissue imprint. Dog.** Four yeast forms are present that measure approximately the same size as the neutrophils in the field. The thick wall is visible on the deeply basophilic structures. (Modified-Wright; HP oil.)

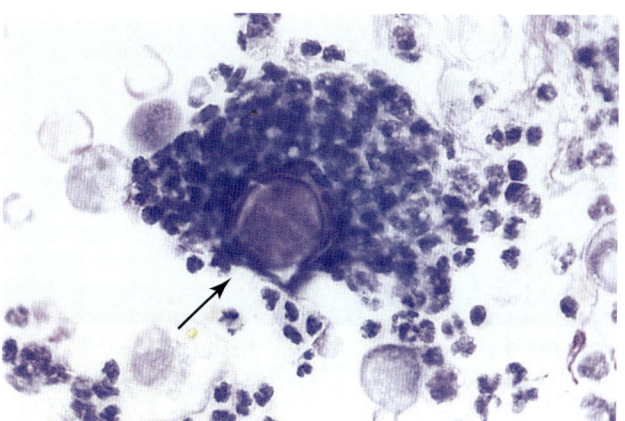

■ **FIGURE 3.46 Coccidioidomycosis. Tissue aspirate. Dog.** The animal presented with several semi-firm skin masses and no systemic signs. A purple, thick-walled spherule *(arrow)* measuring approximately 60 μm in diameter is surrounded by numerous degenerate neutrophils. (Modified Wright; HP oil.)

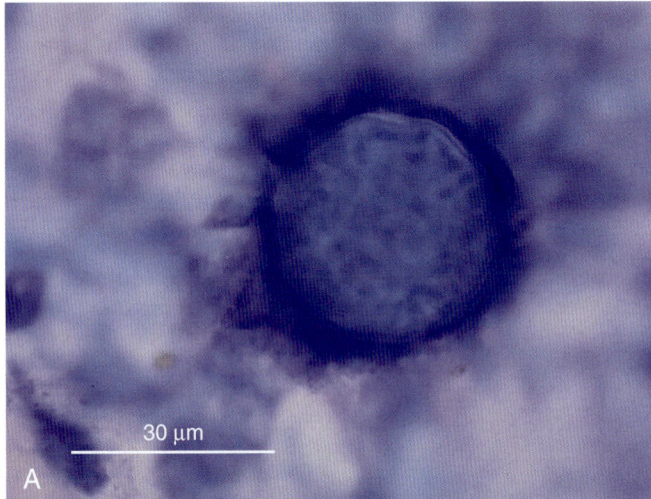

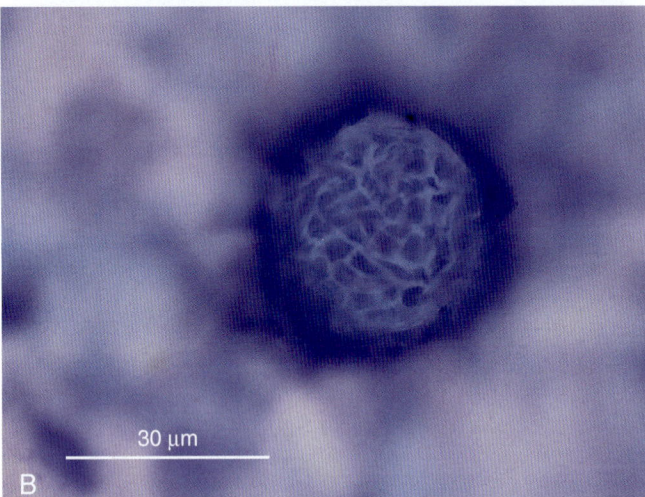

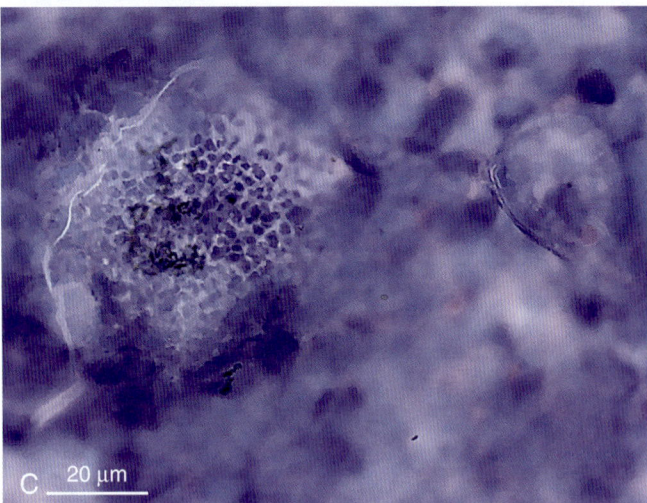

FIGURE 3.47 Coccidioidomycosis. Tissue aspirate. Dog. Same case in A to C. **A,** Within the scapular mass is a basophilic spherule. Focus is placed on the thick capsule wall. **B,** Refocusing demonstrates the developing endospores within the spherule. (Modified Wright; HP oil.) **C,** A small spherule *(right)* and a larger spherule *(left)* are seen; the latter appears ready to release numerous, small (2 μm), round endospores within the poorly defined mixed inflammatory response in the background. (Modified Wright; HP oil.)

tube precipitin (immunoglobulin M [IgM]), complement fixation (immunoglobulin G [IgG]), latex agglutination, and agar gel immunodiffusion (AGID). An enzyme immunoassay (EIA) for detection of IgG antibodies offers an alternative to AGID. Fluorescent antibody methods may be used on tissue biopsies. Combined antigen and antibody testing improves the sensitivity over antibody testing alone. Tissue culture is not recommended because of the public health risk. When results are equivocal, commercial testing using a DNA probe with a chemiluminescent label may be used (Beaudin et al., 2005).

Cryptococcosis. Cryptococcosis is found in several geographic areas but frequently in tropical or subtropical climates or with soil infected by pigeon droppings. Inhalation is considered the main route of entry with dissemination to the skin. Lesions in dogs and cats may present as crusts or erosions on the nose in addition to nodules. The cellular response is often granulomatous with macrophages predominating (Figs. 3.48 and 3.49). Other cells present include lymphocytes and multinucleate giant cells. There is minimal inflammation in immunocompromised patients and with organisms that retain their thick outer capsule. A causative agent, *Cryptococcus neoformans*, is found in cytopathologic specimens as a round to oval yeast form measuring 4 to 10 μm in diameter. Cell sizes may be variable, ranging from 2 to 20 μm. The internal cell body stains positive with methenamine silver and PAS, whereas the cell wall requires mucicarmine stain. Cell division involves narrow-based budding compared with the broad-based budding of *Blastomyces*. Definitive diagnosis involves immunostaining in tissue biopsies, latex agglutination test, ELISA, or fungal culture. Confirmation in difficult cases may involve PCR and detection of the *CAP59* gene. Another species, *Cryptococcus*

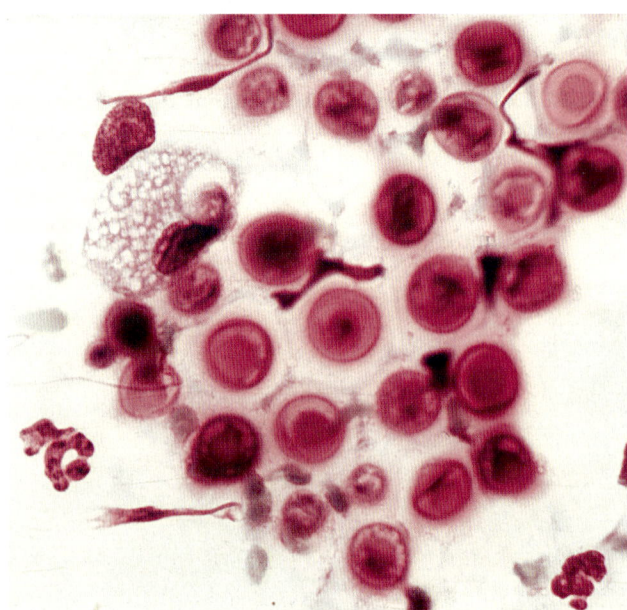

FIGURE 3.48 Cryptococcosis. Tissue aspirate. Cat. Subcutaneous mass in submandibular region contains clusters of yeast with mostly neutrophilic inflammation. Note the variable amount of clear lipid capsule surrounding the structures and the ingested yeast by the foamy macrophage. The scant capsule permits more antigenic stimulation and resulting inflammation to occur. A budding form is shown between the macrophage and a neutrophil. (Aqueous Romanowsky; HP oil.)

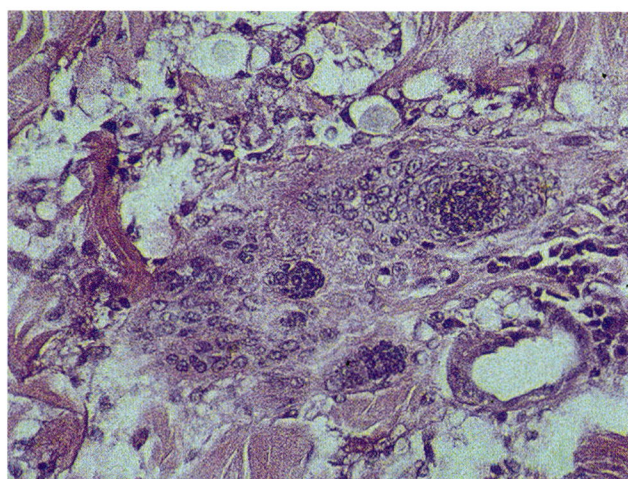

FIGURE 3.49 Cryptococcosis. Tissue section. Cat. Perifollicular inflammation related to the presence of numerous clear-walled yeast forms present in the upper left to center areas. (H&E; IP.)

gattii, is emerging into the northwest of the United States; it was previously thought to be restricted to tropical and subtropical regions in Australia, South America, Southeast Asia, and Africa. It may present with a small size similar to *Histoplasma* and with a narrow capsule (Lester et al., 2011). When present, the thick lipid capsule remains unstained with Romanowsky-type stains (Fig. 3.50A). As a result, the cytopathologic biopsy background appears vacuolated, often with many dense, round cell bodies. Stains such as new methylene blue and India ink are used to enhance the visibility of the capsule on unstained specimens (Fig. 3.50B).

Histoplasmosis. This disease produces a pyogranulomatous response by the agent *Histoplasma capsulatum* and is similar in geographic distribution to blastomycosis. Bird and bat droppings provide an ideal growth medium for the organisms. Cutaneous lesions (Fig. 3.51) are uncommon compared with those in gastrointestinal (GI) and hematopoietic organs. On cytopathology, macrophages predominate, but lymphocytes, plasma cells, and occasional multinucleate giant cells may be present. Numerous intracellular and extracellular oval yeast forms measuring 2 to 4 μm are frequently found in specimens (Fig. 3.52). They stain positive with PAS and methenamine silver. The yeast structures resemble the protozoan *Leishmania* except that *Histoplasma* has a clear halo due to cell shrinkage, and the cell body lacks a kinetoplast. Definitive diagnosis of histoplasmosis requires identification by cytopathology, immunostaining in tissue biopsy, or fungal culture. An enzyme quantitative antigen-based assay (MiraVista Diagnostics) similar to that for blastomycosis may be used to assist in the diagnosis. Molecular tests have been used on a limited basis.

Other systemic infections may involve *Aspergillus* spp., *Candida* spp., or *Paecilomyces* spp. These often occur in immunosuppressed patients.

Dermatophytosis

Dermatophytosis is a common infectious and often contagious disease to humans that frequently involves the superficial layers of the skin, hairs, and nails. *Microsporum* and *Trichophyton* spp. are the most common genera of dermatophytes associated with

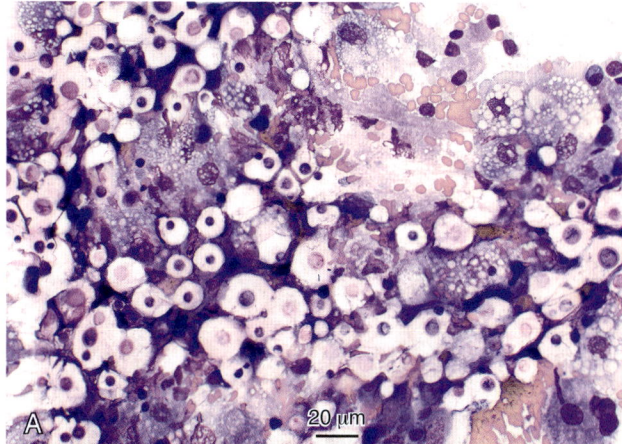
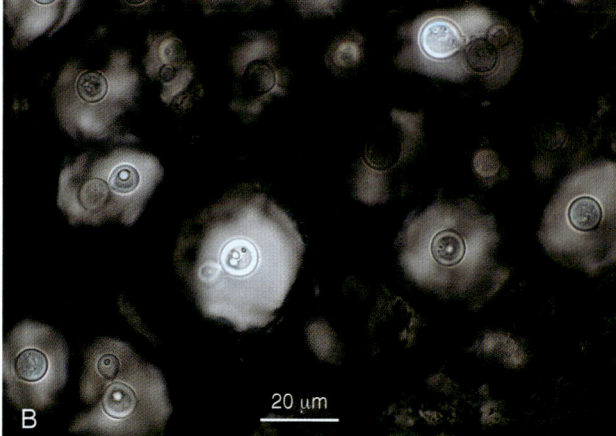

FIGURE 3.50 Cryptococcosis, *Cryptococcus gattii*. **Cat.** Same case in A and B. **A, Nasal tissue aspirate.** Numerous variably sized, round to ovoid yeasts are present, which have a thick, colorless to faint pink capsule and often a discernible thick wall around a pale to dark magenta center. Some of these yeasts exhibit narrow-based budding. This morphology is consistent with a *Cryptococcus* spp. Culture and molecular testing confirmed *C. gattii* infection. Several inflammatory cells present are predominantly highly vacuolated macrophages. (Wright-Giemsa; HP oil.) **B, Nasal flush.** (India ink; HP oil.)

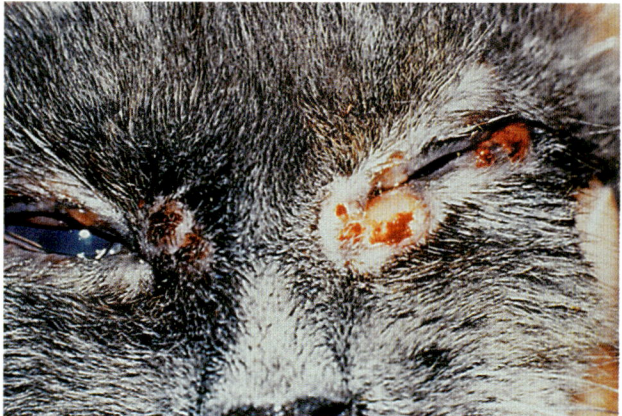

FIGURE 3.51 Histoplasmosis. Macroscopic specimen. Cat. Skin lesions and ocular lesions were present around the eyes in this cat. (Courtesy Heidi Ward, University of Florida.)

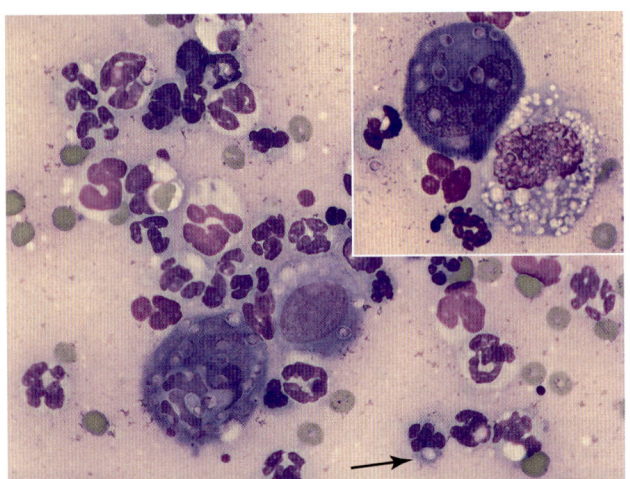

FIGURE 3.52 Histoplasmosis. Skin mass aspirate. Cat. Fluid material aspirated consists of an eosinophilic granular background with a mixed inflammatory cell population of nondegenerate neutrophils and macrophages. The macrophages have a foamy cytoplasm, and many contain one to multiple oval yeast (3 × 5 μm) structures *(arrows)* with a clear halo. (Modified Wright; HP oil.) *Inset:* In another field an extracellular yeast form is present *(left middle)*. (Modified Wright; HP oil.) (Courtesy Jennifer Bouschor, Kansas State University.)

dogs and cats. The lesions typically present with focal alopecia, broken hair shafts, crusts, scales, and erythema on the head, feet, and tail of dogs and cats (Caruso et al., 2002). Less commonly seen are raised or dermal nodules called kerions (Logan et al., 2006). A *kerion* forms when the infected hair follicle ruptures and both the fungus and keratin spill into the dermis, eliciting an intense inflammatory response (Fig. 3.53A) that may be painful. Cytopathologic specimens reveal a pyogranulomatous inflammation with degenerate neutrophils and large epithelioid macrophages. Arthrospores that measure 2 to 4 μm possess a thin, clear capsule (Fig. 3.53B) that is highlighted with PAS staining (Fig. 3.53C). The arthrospores and nonstaining hyphae are associated with hair shafts, which are best visualized using clearing agents with plucked hairs (Fig. 3.54). Additional staining using Grocott's methenamine silver (GMS) highlights the hyphae (Fig. 3.55). Fungal culture helps to diagnose the dermatophyte identity.

Compared with the more superficial kerion presentation, an uncommon presentation is termed a dermatophytic pseudomycetoma, usually seen in Persian cats, that is most often caused by *Microsporum canis* (Zimmerman et al., 2003). Clinically, the distinguishing features of mycetoma are formation of nodular inflammatory lesions with secondary fibrosis, formation of fistulae that often penetrate into deep tissue, and the presence of bacterial or fungal grains composed of dense aggregates of the organism. Pseudomycetoma is similar without the true fungal grains or pellets being formed. The lesion presents as a nodular granuloma with fistulous tracts deep into subcutaneous tissues, which can exist over long periods of time. On cytopathology, this involves macrophages with abundant foamy cytoplasm and numerous multinucleate giant cells (Fig. 3.56A). Arthrospores may be present along with fungal hyphae that have an irregular shape and size and may stain variably with Romanowsky-type stains (Fig. 3.56B). Positive staining occurs with PAS and methenamine silver to help reveal

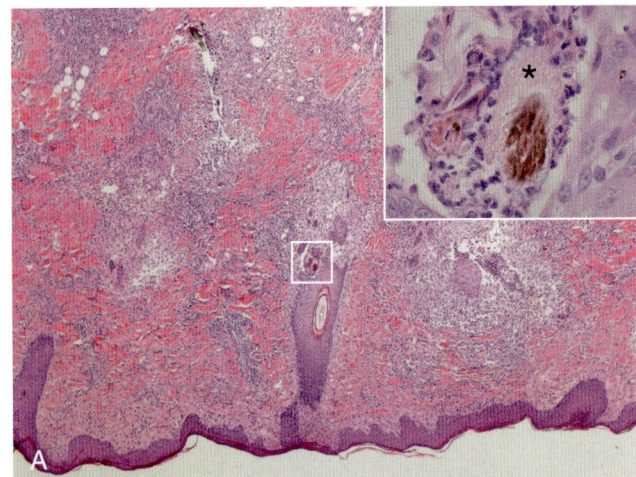
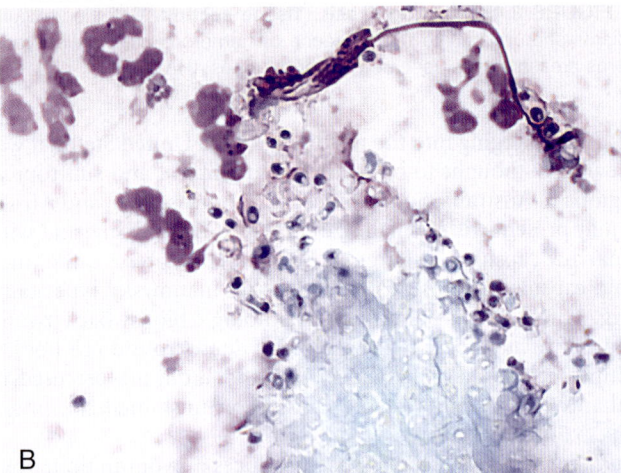
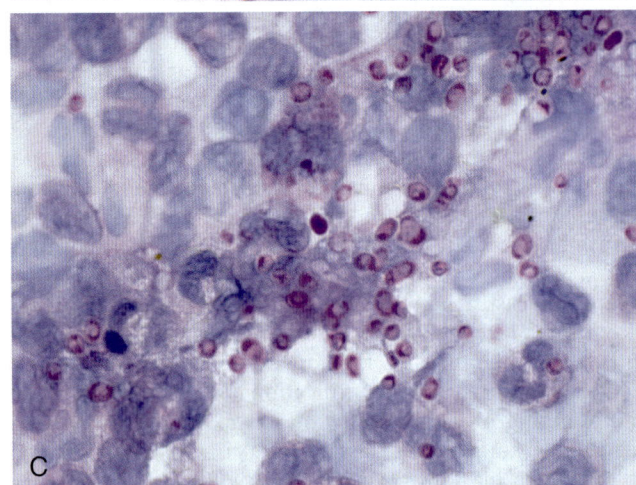

FIGURE 3.53 Dermatophytosis. *Microsporum canis*. Dog. Same case in A to C. **A, Tissue section.** This is from a firm raised erythematous nonulcerated alopecic nodule on the inner leg. The primary abnormality is folliculitis, furunculosis, and perifolliculitis as evidenced by the dense infiltrate around hair shafts. (H&E; LP.) *Inset:* High magnification demonstrates the dense collection of fungi *(asterisk)* around the pigmented hair. (H&E; HP oil.) **B, Tissue aspirate.** Degenerate neutrophils are present along with numerous ovoid arthroconidia that measure 3 to 4 μm long and have a thin cell wall. Pale blue keratin surrounds many of the yeasts. **C, Tissue aspirate.** Dermal nodule (kerion) with multiple pink oval arthroconidia within neutrophils and extracellularly. Culture results indicated *Microsporum canis* infection. (PAS; HP oil.) (Courtesy Michael Logan, Purdue University.)

CHAPTER 3 Integumentary System 55

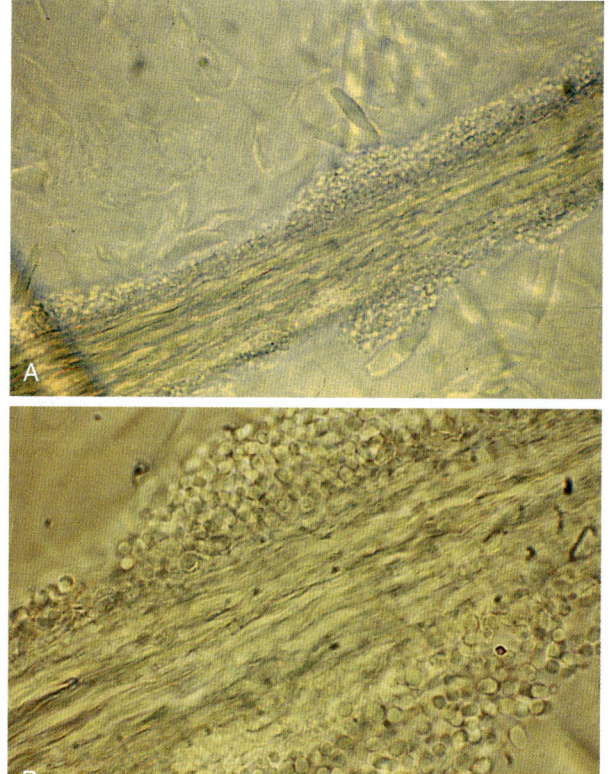

FIGURE 3.54 Dermatophytosis. Hair pluck. Same case in A and B. **A,** Low-magnification view of keratin-cleared hair shaft showing attached arthrospores. (Unstained; HP oil.) **B,** High-magnification view of keratin-cleared hair shaft, demonstrating arthrospores outside and fungal hyphae within the hair. (Unstained; HP oil.) (Courtesy University of Florida Dermatology Section.)

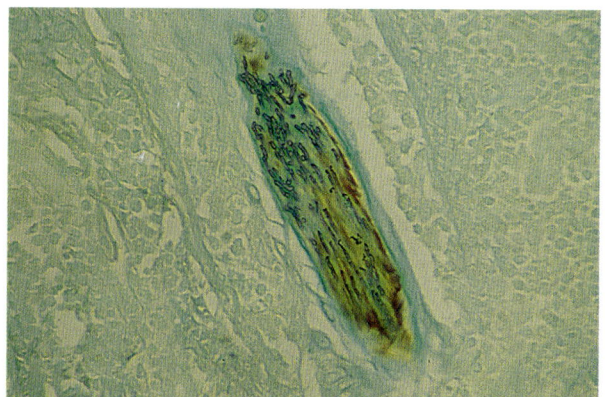

FIGURE 3.55 Dermatophytosis. Tissue section. Dog. Note the black-stained hyphae within the hair shaft from this tissue section of skin. Diagnosis confirmed as *Microsporum canis* by culture. (Gomori's methenamine silver; HP oil.)

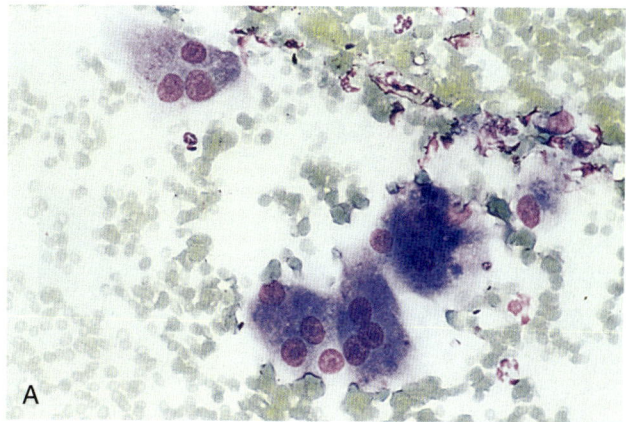

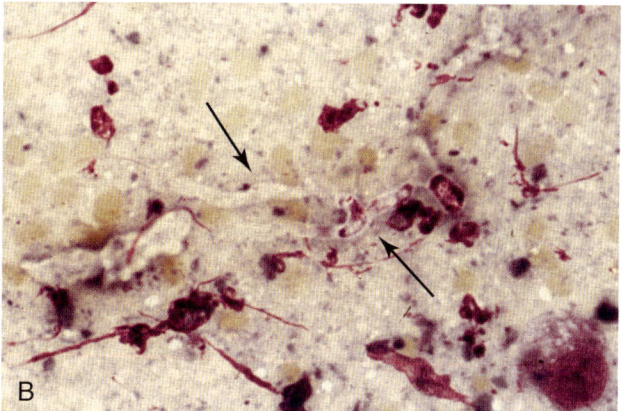

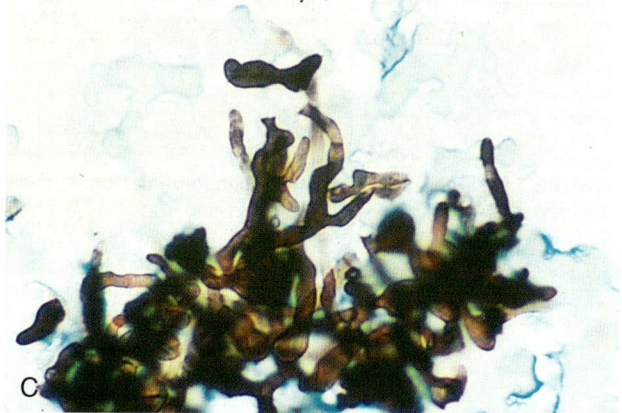

FIGURE 3.56 Dermatophytic pseudomycetoma. Tissue aspirate. Cat. Same case in A to C. **A,** Several multinucleate giant cells are present in this 3 cm superficial mass on the lateral abdomen of a Persian cat. (Wright-Giemsa; HP oil.) **B,** Fungal hyphae are variably visible with Romanowsky staining (*arrows*). Culture confirmed infection by *M. canis.* (Wright-Giemsa; HP oil.) **C,** Hyphal elements are clearly visible with silver staining. (Gomori's methenamine silver; HP oil.)

unstained hyphae (Fig. 3.56C). Treatment of the nodules involves surgical excision and antifungal drugs.

Malassezia

The causative agent, *Malassezia pachydermatis,* is an opportunistic invader of the skin and ear canal. It is associated with widespread seborrheic dermatitis and otitis externa in dogs. Organisms are found in surface scabs or crusts of exudative lesions (Fig. 3.57). Sites of predilection include the face, ventral neck, dorsum of paws, ventral abdomen, and caudal thighs. The skin infection involves primarily a mononuclear inflammation, with lymphocytes and macrophages, but secondary pyoderma may occur with the presence of focal neutrophils (Fig. 3.58). Romanowsky stains reveal purple, broad-based budding organisms characterized by a bottle or shoe shape. Treatment includes surface cleaning and appropriate antifungal agents.

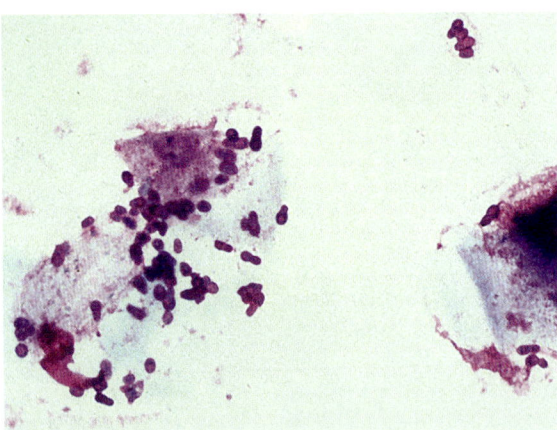

■ **FIGURE 3.57** *Malassezia* **otitis. Ear swab. Dog.** *Malassezia* spp. organisms adhere to keratinized squamous epithelium without evidence of inflammation. (Aqueous Romanowsky; HP oil.)

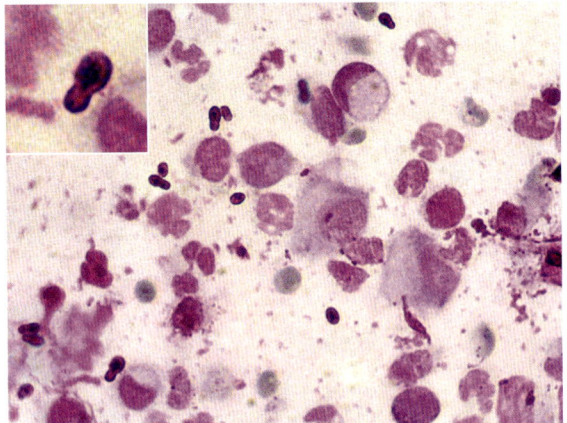

■ **FIGURE 3.58** *Malassezia* **dermatitis. Skin imprint. Dog.** Abundant budding yeast forms with a mixed-cell inflammatory response were noted in an animal with pustular dermatitis. Mildly degenerate neutrophils are present along with lymphocytes and macrophages. (Wright-Giemsa; HP oil.) *Inset:* Higher magnification of a single broad-based budding yeast with characteristic shoeprint morphology. (Wright-Giemsa; HP oil.)

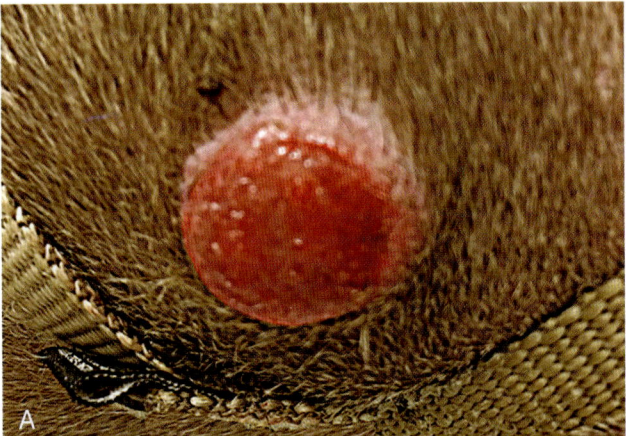

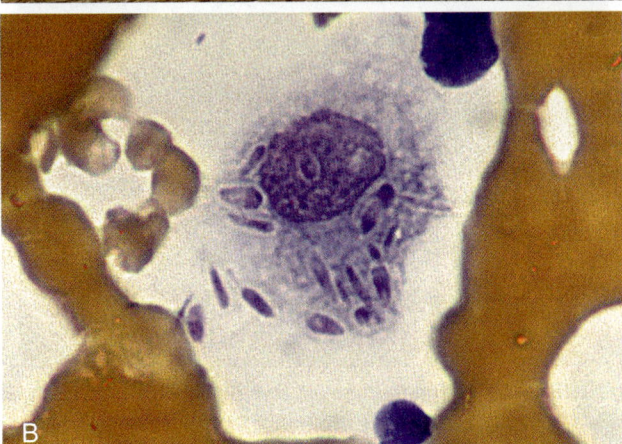

■ **FIGURE 3.59 Sporotrichosis. A, Muzzle nodule. Dog.** This 1.5-cm-diameter raised ulcerated lesion contained low numbers of yeast form. **B, Tissue imprint. Cat.** This 2 cm granulomatous lesion on one digit contains a macrophage with numerous oval to cigar-shaped yeast forms having a thin clear halo around the basophilic center. These structures measure 2×5 μm, approximately the width of an erythrocyte. (Wright; HP oil.)

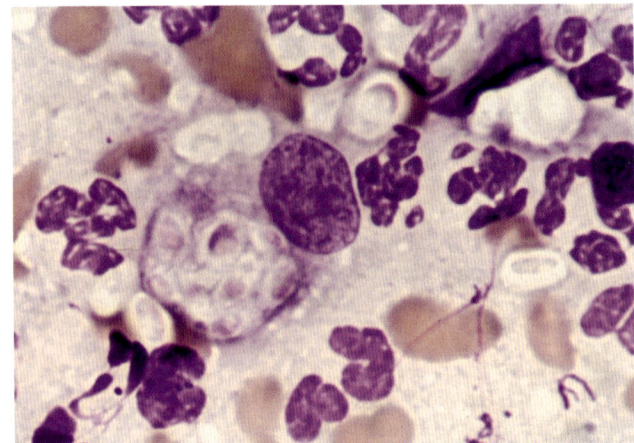

■ **FIGURE 3.60 Sporotrichosis. Cat. Tissue imprint.** Pyogranulomatous inflammation with engulfed yeast within a macrophage. These forms may have a round to oval shape, which is difficult to distinguish from *Histoplasma* spp. by morphology alone. Culture confirmed *Sporothrix* spp. (Romanowsky; HP oil.) (Courtesy Peter Fernandes, Texas A&M University.)

Sporotrichosis

Sporotrichosis is associated with immunosuppression, such as that occurring with glucocorticoid administration or concurrent disease. It presents in several clinical forms—cutaneous, respiratory, systemic, and the most frequent, cutaneous-lymphatic usually as the result of penetrating wounds (Welsh, 2003). Grossly, a dermal to subcutaneous nodule progresses into an ulcerated lesion that drains a serosanguineous exudate (Fig. 3.59A). In dogs, the skin of the trunk and extremities is preferred, whereas in cats, the large firm nodules appear on the limbs, feet, head, and tail base. The etiologic agent, *Sporothrix schenckii*, is a saprophytic fungus that appears classically as cigar-shaped yeast forms measuring 3 to 5 μm in diameter with a thin, clear halo around the pale-blue cytoplasm (Fig. 3.59B). The shape of the yeast is pleomorphic, with round to oval shapes (Fig. 3.60). A mycelial form occurs under cooler body temperatures as in nature (Fig. 3.61). On cytopathology, the yeast is located intracellularly or extracellularly, being abundant in cats and infrequent in dogs

(Bernstein et al., 2007). In dogs, pyogranulomatous inflammation with degenerative neutrophils is common, whereas macrophages and lymphocytes predominate in cats. The diagnosis is suggested from the characteristic cytopathologic appearance. The organism stains positive with both methenamine silver and PAS. Definitive diagnosis requires fungal culture of the exudate or tissue biopsy using immunofluorescence or immunoperoxidase techniques. Serologic testing is not definitive for current infection. A molecular test has been developed and used in a feline case (Kano et al., 2005). Surgical excision may be performed on single cutaneous lesions. Treatment of the systemic form involves a variety of antimicrobial drugs, which have been used with variable success. Prognosis is poor to guarded. Good response has been obtained with itraconazole (Bernstein et al., 2007).

> **KEY POINT** Organisms resemble those of histoplasmosis, which may be round or oval, but only sporotrichosis has cigar-shaped or slender yeast forms.

> **KEY POINT** The disease may spread to people, usually transmitted by cats.

Cytopathologic differential diagnosis: histoplasmosis, toxoplasmosis, cryptococcosis.

Oomycetes

Two agents, *Pythium insidiosum* and *Lagenidium* spp., are water molds of the oomycete class in the Stramenopila kingdom (Grooters et al., 2003). They differ from true fungi in producing motile flagellate zoospores, having cell walls without chitin, and having differences in nuclear division and cytoplasmic organelles. This disease is common in dogs and occasional in cats from tropical or subtropical climates, such as the southeastern United States. Animals are infected by standing in or drinking contaminated water. Systemic signs result from GI involvement and are more common than the cutaneous presentation. Dermal ulcerative nodules develop into draining tracts and serosanguineous exudation from sites that include the extremities, tail head, and perineum (Fig. 3.62A). Cytopathologic specimens consist of a pyogranulomatous inflammation with increased eosinophils and the presence of broad, poorly septate, and branching hyphal elements. Whereas *Pythium* hyphae are uniform, *Lagenidium* hyphae tend to have larger diameters and more bulbous shapes than *Pythium*. Methenamine silver stain is preferred over PAS stain to demonstrate the hyphae (Fig. 3.62B) because the organisms appear mostly colorless with Romanowsky stains (Fig. 3.62C). An ELISA serologic test for antibodies to oomycete antigens is helpful as a screening test. Culture of infected tissues followed by both morphologic and molecular identification of the pathogen is highly recommended. Immunohistochemistry uses a polyclonal antibody specific for *Pythium insidiosum*, not *Lagenidium*. However, distinction between the two oomycetes is best performed by rRNA gene sequencing or specific PCR amplification. Possible treatment involves wide surgical excision or amputation of affected limbs. Prognosis is guarded to poor.

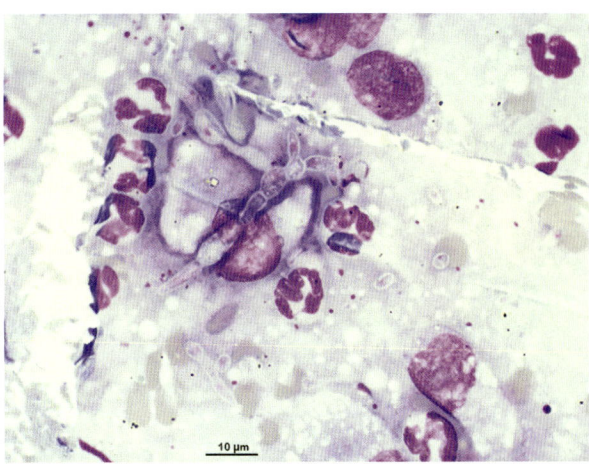

■ **FIGURE 3.61 Sporotrichosis. Cat. Nasal tissue imprint.** In addition to yeast forms, frequent mycelial forms measuring 3 to 5 μm in width appear with septation. Inflammatory cells involve neutrophils and macrophages. (Wright; HP oil.)

> **KEY POINT** Organisms stain poorly with Romanowsky stains and are best seen within dense clumps of inflammatory cells at low magnification. The presence of clear, uniformly sized, linear strands suggest hyphal elements, but these must be distinguished from collagen debris, which may also appear as unstained fibrin strands.

Algae
Protothecosis

Protothecosis is a rare disease in dogs and cats related to achloric algae, *Prototheca wickerhamii*, which is found in sewage-contaminated food and water. It is frequently associated with immunosuppression or concurrent disease. Cats usually develop a cutaneous disease, whereas dogs may develop both cutaneous and systemic forms. Systemic involvement primarily includes the GI tract, eye, and nervous system. Cutaneous lesions in dogs are chronic, nodular, exudative, and ulcerative, occurring on the trunk and extremities. Large, firm nodules on the limbs, feet, head, and tail base have been reported in cats. On cytopathologic specimens, the inflammation is granulomatous or pyogranulomatous. Epithelioid macrophages predominate, but lymphocytes, plasma cells, and occasional multinucleate giant cells may also be found. Organisms, present outside or within macrophages, measure 5 to 20 μm in diameter (Fig. 3.63A). They are round to oval with internal septation producing 2 to 20 endospores within the cell wall. The endospores are basophilic and granular with a single nucleus and have a clear halo around them. Both PAS and methenamine silver stains demonstrate the cell wall (Fig. 3.63B). Definitive diagnosis requires culture or tissue biopsy using immunofluorescence or immunoperoxidase techniques. Treatment involves surgical excision for cutaneous lesions. Antimicrobial drugs have been used with limited success in systemic forms. Prognosis is guarded to poor.

Protozoa
Leishmaniasis

This is an uncommon multisystemic disease with cutaneous presentation and regional lymphadenopathy. It is caused by the protozoan *Leishmania* spp., which is transmitted by sand

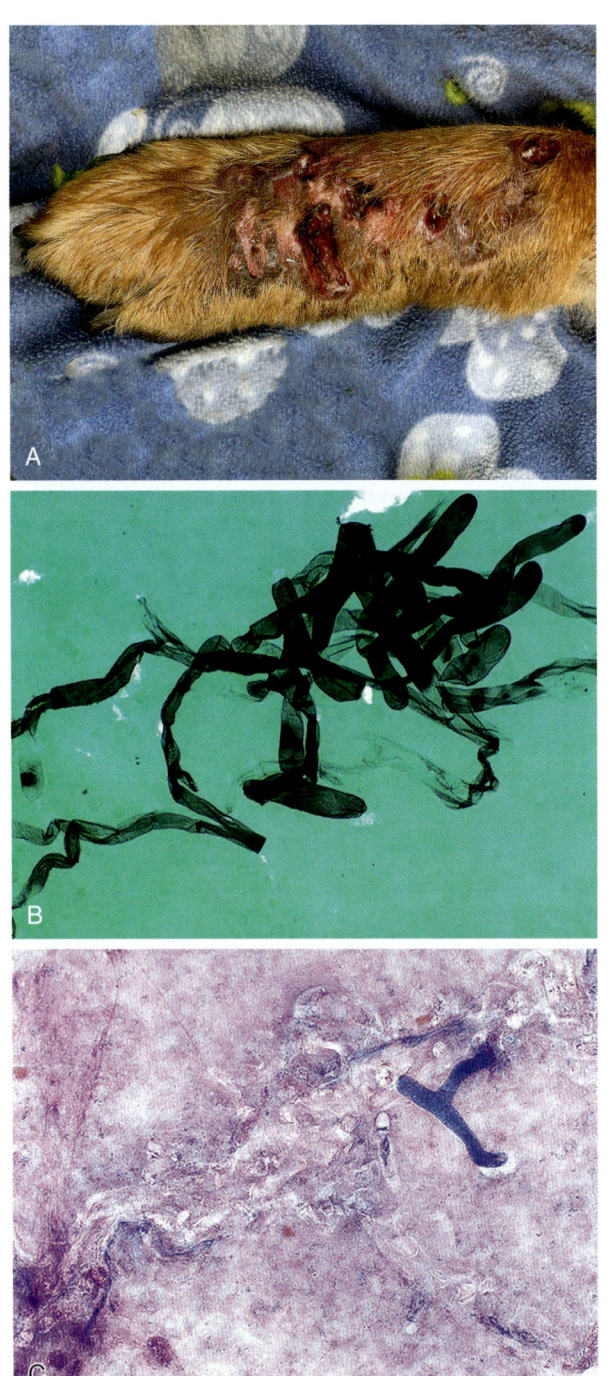

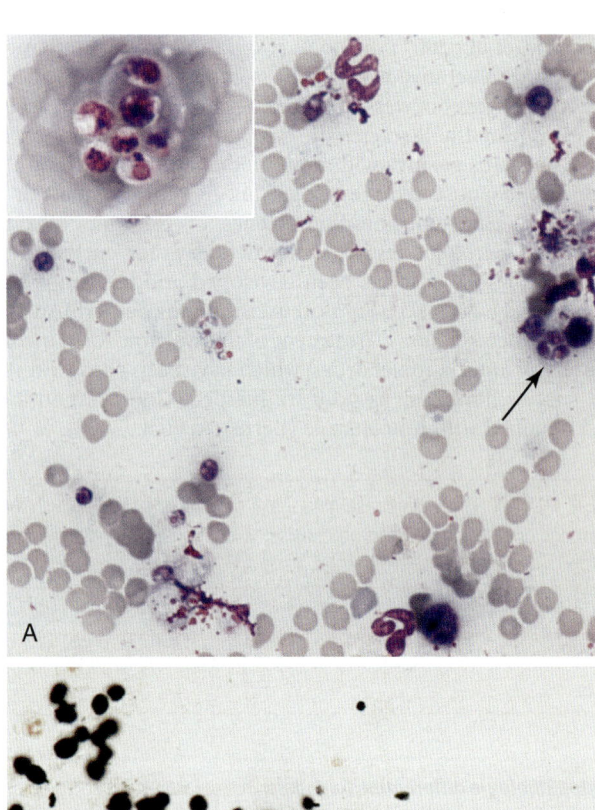

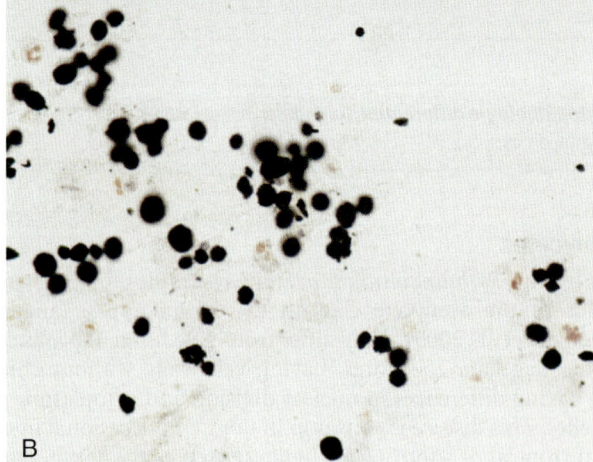

■ **FIGURE 3.62 Oomycetosis. Dog.** Same case A to C. **A, Macroscopic specimen.** This German shepherd dog had multiple lesions and draining tracts on the limb. **B, Tissue discharge.** A fluid pocket near the shoulder is aspirated and the specimen demonstrates the presence of non-septated hyphal structures. (GMS; HP oil.) **C,** Non-staining or poorly stained branching hyphal structures appear against a variably eosinophilic, proteinaceous background. *Pythium* serology was negative; however, an ELISA test revealed positive results to both *Pythium* and *Lagenidium*. PCR with direct sequencing confirmed *Lagenidium giganteum*. (Wright-Giemsa; HP oil.) (A, Courtesy Florian Wuillemin, Tufts University.)

■ **FIGURE 3.63 Protothecosis. Cat.** Same case and magnification in A and B. **A, Tissue aspirate.** This aspirate from a nasal skin nodule contains multiple basophilic round structures (endospores) occurring singly and in clusters *(arrow)* that measure approximately 3 to 12 μm in diameter. The cutaneous form of protothecosis is unique in cats. This animal had organisms that extended into the nasal cavity and to a draining mandibular lymph node. This cytopathology was initially considered to be of a nonencapsulated form of cryptococcosis; however, culture confirmed infection with *Prototheca wickerhamii*. Inset: Close-up view of sporulating organism with several endospores. (Wright-Giemsa; HP oil.). **B, Tissue swab.** Numerous silver positive round endospores of variable size are revealed in the nasal cavity swab of a cat with a cutaneous nodule. (GMS; HP oil.)

flies. One report found dog-to-dog transmission (McKenna et al., 2019). The disease is often associated with Mediterranean travel, although endemic areas such as Oklahoma and Ohio are found in the United States. It is more likely to occur in dogs than in cats. The condition may begin in the skin and then spread internally. Periorbital alopecia and scaling or ulcerative and erosive lesions of the nose are common signs that may progress to poorly demarcated cutaneous and mucocutaneous nodules. *Leishmania mexicana* has been associated with a nonsystemic, cutaneous form of the disease in cats from Texas and Mexico (Trainor et al., 2010). On cytopathology, macrophages predominate, but other cells present include lymphocytes, plasma cells, and occasional multinucleate giant cells. The intracellular organisms, termed *amastigotes*, measure 1.5 to 2.0×2.5 to 5 μm and possess a red nucleus and characteristic

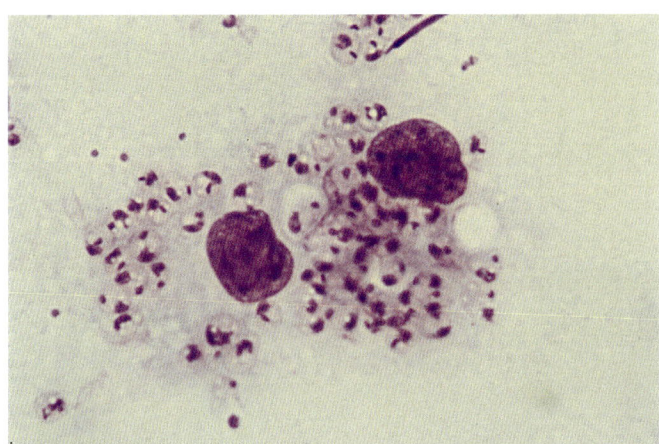

■ **FIGURE 3.64 Leishmaniasis. Tissue aspirate. Cat.** Ear nodule consists of macrophages with intracellular and extracellular organisms having a characteristic appearance of *Leishmania* spp. (Aqueous Romanowsky; HP oil.) (Courtesy Ruanna Gossett et al., Texas A & M University. Presented at the 1991 ASVCP case review session.)

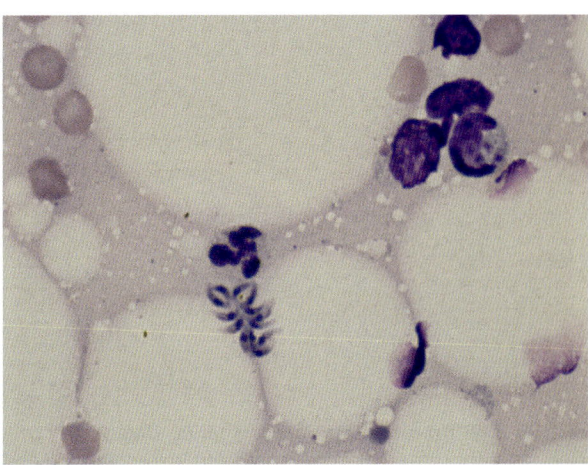

■ **FIGURE 3.65 Toxoplasmosis. *Toxoplasma gondii*. Ulcerated dermal mass. Tissue aspirate. Dog.** (Wright; HP oil.) Several banana-shaped tachyzoites are present in the background. PCR testing was used to confirm the diagnosis. (Courtesy Karen Dorsey, Oklahoma State University. Presented at the 2001 ASVCP case review session.)

bar-shaped kinetoplasts (Fig. 3.64). In addition to the skin, the bone marrow and lymphoid organs are common sites of involvement. Other laboratory abnormalities include polyclonal or monoclonal gammopathy and nonregenerative anemia. The characteristic cytopathology or culture is used to obtain a definitive diagnosis. Immunoperoxidase staining may also be performed on tissue biopsies. An indirect fluorescent antibody test is available for *Leishmania donovani*, but this only indicates previous exposure. Treatment involves pentavalent antimony compounds, itraconazole, or allopurinol for systemic disease and surgical excision for focal skin lesions. Prognosis is good to guarded; however, this is a zoonotic disease, and euthanasia may need to be considered.

Toxoplasmosis and Neosporosis

Cutaneous toxoplasmosis is uncommon but was reported in cats and dogs (Little et al., 2005; Park et al., 2007; Hoffmann et al., 2012). These conditions present as multiple and single nodules often after immunosuppressive therapy. The single nodule case (Park et al., 2007) displayed a necrotizing granulomatous panniculitis and vasculitis. Organisms were present within macrophages and other cells. They tested positive for *Toxoplasma gondii* and *Neospora caninum* antigens, and ultrastructural studies supported *T. gondii*. Furthermore, PCR and DNA sequence analysis was consistent with *T. gondii* infection. Reports of cutaneous neosporosis in dogs used immunohistochemistry for specific diagnosis of the tachyzoites (LaPerle et al., 2001; Gupta et al., 2011). Additional testing with PCR was specific for neosporosis and negative for *Sarcocystis* spp. and *T. gondii* (Gupta et al., 2011). Tachyzoites display a banana shape when intact (Fig. 3.65) but may lose this characteristic shape in necrotic areas. Treatment for both protozoal diseases involves long-term clindamycin administration.

Multicellular Parasites

Dracunculiasis is an uncommon parasitic condition in dogs and cats (Lucio-Forster et al., 2014) that causes pruritic, painful erythematous subcutaneous swellings that can be diagnosed by cytopathologic evaluation of aspirated tissue fluid or imprints from a lesion discharge. First-stage larvae from *Dracunculus insignis* measuring approximately 25 μm wide × 500 μm long appear pale blue when stained or granulated (Figs. 3.66 and A8.6F) and have a long, tapered tail. The life cycle involves ingestion of infected water fleas or frogs containing larvae that leave the digestive tract and migrate, usually to the limbs. Surgical excision is used to remove the adult nematode, which often measures 20 cm long (Beyer et al., 1999) but may reach lengths up to 120 cm. Anthelmintics appear ineffective in killing adults.

A common parasitic skin disease is demodicosis (Fig. 3.67). Neel et al. (2007) reported two different populations of demodectic mites present in skin scrapings from their case. Histologically, the mite is found within the hair shaft with a dense perifollicular inflammatory response (Fig. 3.68) consisting of neutrophils and macrophages.

Several recent reports of dirofilarial dermatitis note the presence of adult or larval parasites within the subcutaneous tissue of dogs and cats in Southern Europe, India, Russia, the Far East, and several African countries (Giori et al., 2010; Albanese et al., 2013; Sævik et al., 2014). Lesions are nodular with ulcerated or non-ulcerated surfaces (Fig. 3.69A). Adult males are 5 to 7 cm long, and females are 10 to 17 cm long. Microfilariae range from 260 to 360 μm in length. Aspirates may contain microfilaria and nematode fragments, including morula and embryonated eggs along with a mixed neutrophilic and eosinophilic inflammation (Fig. 3.69B–C). One type of dirofilariasis is caused by the mosquito-borne filarial nematode *Dirofilaria (Nochtiella) repens* and has been reported commonly in Italy and other parts of Southern Europe, in the Middle East, and rarely in Eastern and Northern Europe. In some cases, presence of the parasite is found in non-cutaneous sites (Paździor-Czapula et al., 2018). Diagnosis is by recognition of the adult nematode, microfilarial characteristics, and molecular confirmation. The character of the cephalic space is helpful to distinguish the microfilaria of *D. repens* from *D. immitis* (Liotta et al., 2013). Although lesions have minimal pathologic effects on animals, the main concern is its zoonotic significance to humans.

Other parasites causing incidental skin lesions include *Acanthocheilonema (Dipetalonema) reconditum*, *Dirofilaria immitis*, *Pelodera (Rhabditis) strongyloides*, and *Cuterebra* spp. (Fig. 3.70) (French and Blue, 1986; Bau-Gaudreault et al., 2018).

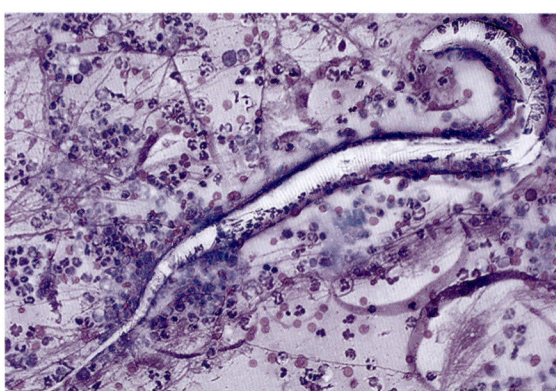

■ **FIGURE 3.66 Dracunculosis. Tissue imprint. Dog.** A 1–2 cm erythematous swelling with a 2 mm opening is noted on a hind limb. Nematode larvae are approximately 20–30 μm in diameter and up to approximately 400 μm in length, with long pointed tails and markedly striated cuticles. The inflammatory population consists primarily of non-degenerate to pyknotic and karyorrhectic neutrophils with lower numbers of mildly vacuolated macrophages. Morphology of this larva is consistent with *Dracunculus insignis*. (Modified Wright; IP.) (Courtesy Helen Michael et al., University of Minnesota. Presented at the 2011 ASVCP case review session.)

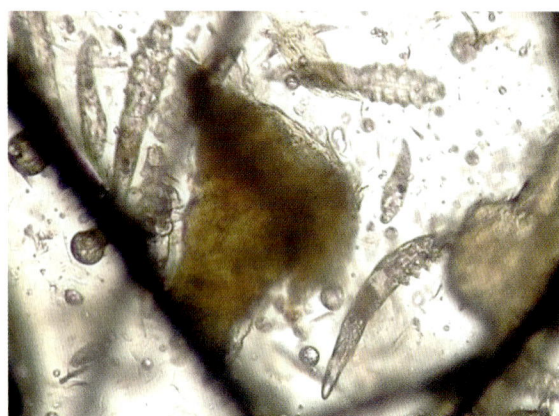

■ **FIGURE 3.67 Demodicosis. Skin scraping. Dog.** Multiple intact demodex mites among hair fragments (Unstained; IP.) (Courtesy Athema Etzioni, Tuskegee University.)

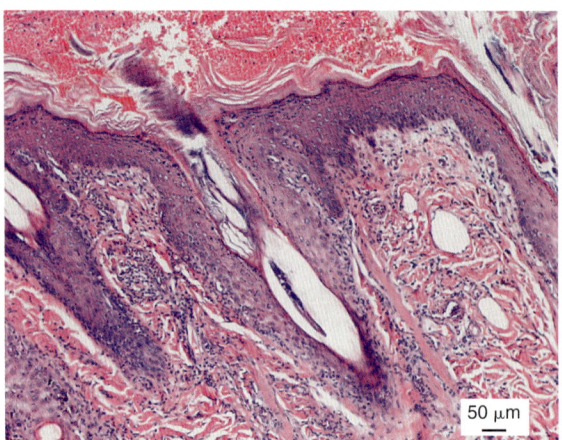

■ **FIGURE 3.68 Demodicosis. Tissue section. Dog.** Present within the shaft of the hair follicle is the mite with a mild mixed inflammatory cell population surrounding the follicle. (Courtesy Susan Ford, Vancouver, British Columbia, Canada.)

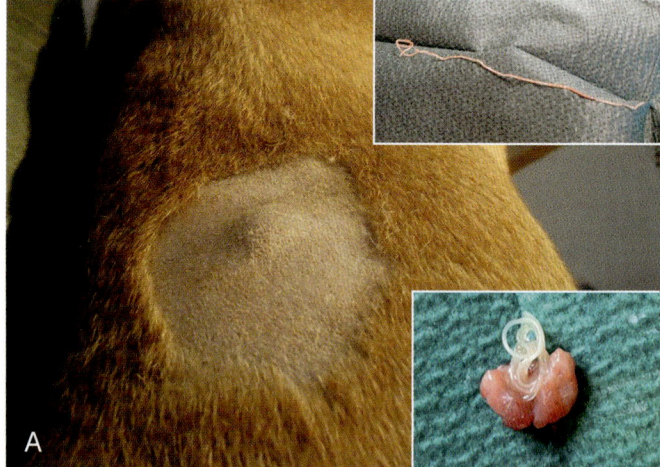

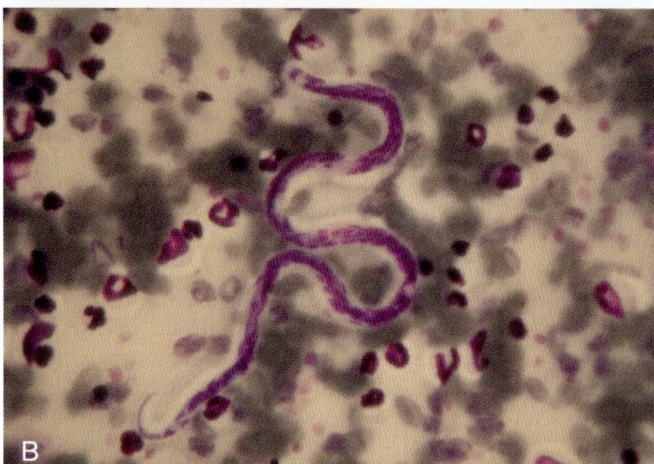

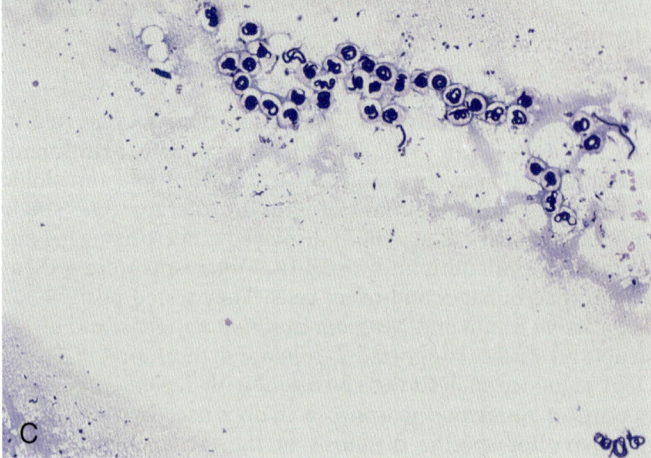

■ **FIGURE 3.69 Dirofilariasis. *Dirofilaria repens*. Dog. A, Macroscopic specimen.** Right lateral area is shaved demonstrating a smooth raised subcutaneous nodule. *Inset bottom:* Excised nodule shows the coiled nematode protruding from cut surface. *Inset top:* The extended worm measures approximately 17 cm in length. **B, Cytopathologic specimen.** Microfilaria is present along with many degenerate neutrophils. (Romanowsky; HP oil.) **C, Cytopathologic specimen.** Numerous embryonated eggs with coiled filarial worms (Romanowsky; LP.) (Courtesy Ernst Leidinger, Vienna, Austria.)

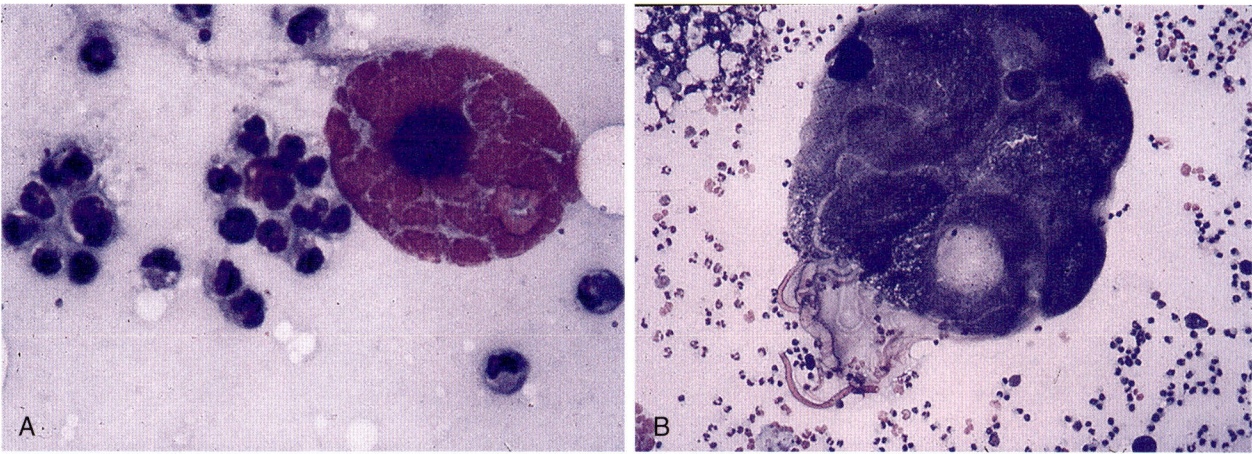

■ **FIGURE 3.70 Cuterebriasis. Abdominal wall subcutaneous mass. Tissue aspirate. Dog.** Same case in A and B. **A,** A raised, pink, nonpainful mass yielded numerous nondegenerate neutrophils along with a large cell estimated between 90 and 150 μm and containing a brightly staining eosinophilic granular material that resembles muscle tissue. (Romanowsky; HP oil.) **B,** In addition to the marked inflammatory reaction, there is large (between 300 and 500 μm) basophilic granular structure along with pink nonstaining tubular structures. (Romanowsky; IP.) (Courtesy Debbie Cunningham et al., Oklahoma State University. Presented at the 2002 ASVCP case review session.)

NON-NEOPLASTIC TUMORS

> **KEY POINT** The presence of only mature epithelium in a skin mass most often indicates a non-neoplastic condition.

Non-neoplastic noninflammatory tumorlike lesions account for approximately 10% of skin lesions removed from dogs and cats (Goldschmidt and Shofer, 1992). These include keratin-filled cysts, glandular hyperplasia, and increased collagen deposition.

Infundibular Cyst

Infundibular cysts, also termed *epidermal inclusion cysts* or *epidermoid cysts,* are found in one-third to one-half of the non-neoplastic noninflammatory tumor-like lesions removed in dogs and cats, respectively (Goldschmidt and Shofer, 1992). The peak incidence in dogs is between 4 and 8 years old (Goldschmidt and Goldschmidt, 2017). The cysts may be single or multiple, firm to fluctuant, with a smooth, round, well-circumscribed appearance. These are often located on the dorsum and extremities. The cyst lining arises from well-differentiated stratified squamous epithelium (Fig. 3.71). By definition, the lack of adnexal differentiation without a connection to the skin surface seen histologically is termed an *epidermal inclusion cyst.* The more common cyst is characterized by a distended hair follicle infundibulum that opens to the surface via a pore (see Fig. 3.71A). The distinction cannot be made by cytopathology. Keratin bars, squames, or keratinized superficial squamous cells predominate on cytopathologic specimens (Fig. 3.72). Degradation of cells within the cyst may lead to the formation of cholesterol crystals, which appear as negative-stained, irregularly notched, rectangular plates best seen against the amorphous basophilic cellular debris of the background (Fig. 3.73). They are thought to arise from frictional trauma leading to obstruction of follicular ostia when found on pressure points.

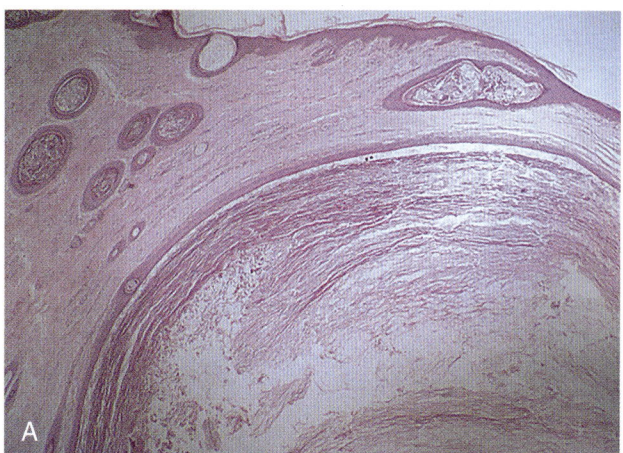
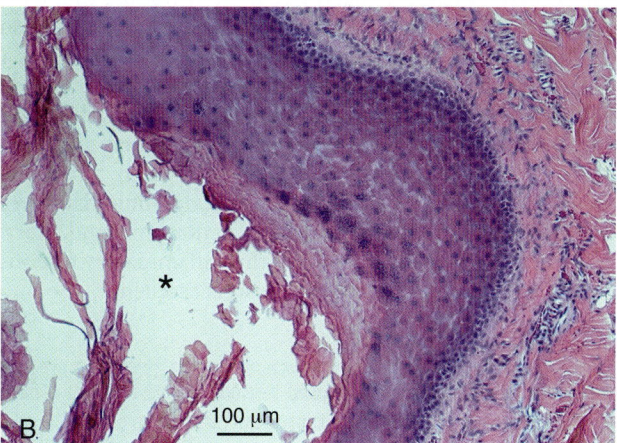

■ **FIGURE 3.71 Infundibular cyst. Tissue section. A, Dog.** The large cystic structure is composed of laminated keratin surrounded by a thin rim of stratified squamous epithelium. Note the nearby smaller cysts with pores that open to the surface, suggesting these are of follicular origin. (H&E; LP.) **B, Cat.** The lumen *(asterisk)* is lined by all four layers of epidermis indicating follicular origin. (H&E; LP.)

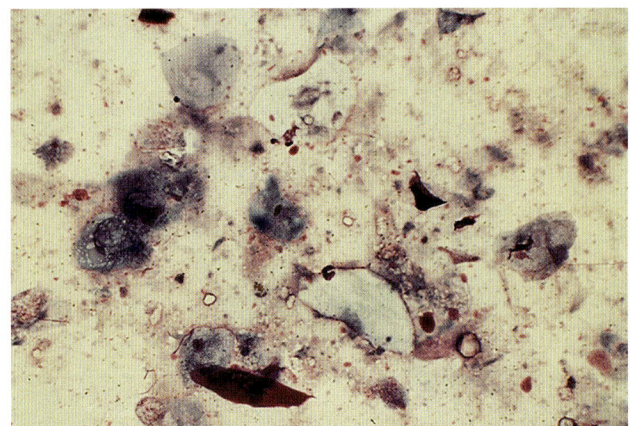

■ **FIGURE 3.72 Keratin-containing tumor. Tissue aspirate. Dog.** Amorphous cellular debris with anuclear squamous epithelium and keratin bars. (Wright; HP oil.)

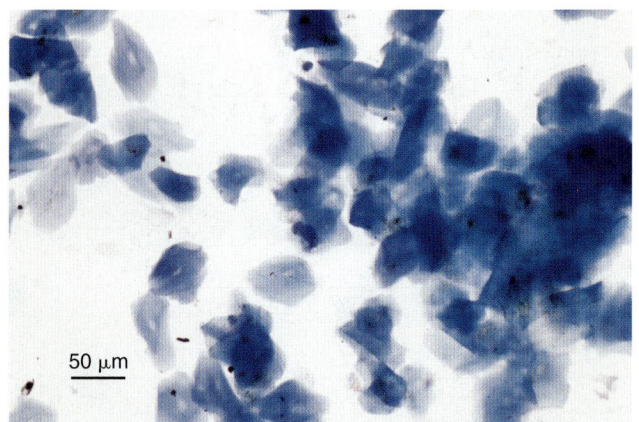

■ **FIGURE 3.74 Nailbed cyst. Tissue aspirate. Dog.** A dense collection of keratinized, sometimes pigmented, squamous epithelial cells is present as noted by their hyalinized turquoise color and angular shape. (Wright-Giemsa; IP.)

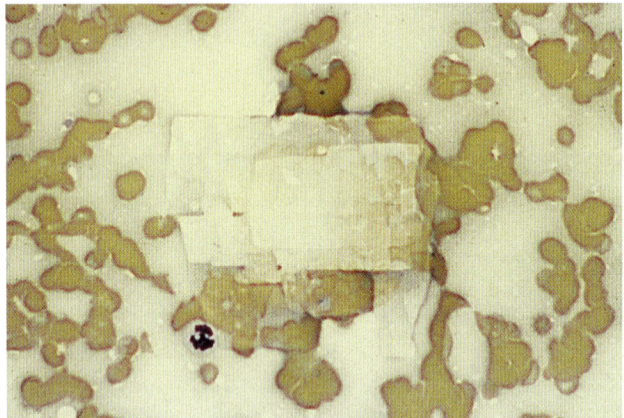

■ **FIGURE 3.73 Keratin-containing tumor. Tissue aspirate. Dog.** Cholesterol crystals appear as clear, rectangular plates visible against the proteinaceous background. (Wright; HP oil.)

Nailbed cysts (Fig. 3.74) likely occur from trauma that allows embedment of germ layer epidermis in underlying tissue, creating an epithelial inclusion cyst (Gross et al., 2005; Eu et al., 2017). In these cysts, pressure-induced lysis of the adjacent phalanx may result in periosteal proliferation and radiographic abnormalities suggestive of malignancy or osteomyelitis (Eu et al., 2017). The behavior of these masses is benign, but rupture of the cyst wall can induce a localized pyogranulomatous cellulitis (Fig. 3.75). When this occurs, neutrophils and macrophages may be frequent. To prevent this inflammatory response, surgery is suggested, and the prognosis is excellent.

> *Cytopathologic differential diagnosis:* keratoacanthoma, trichoepithelioma, dermoid cyst, melanoacanthoma, and other keratin-containing tumors.

Dermoid Cyst

Dermoid cyst occurs rarely in dogs and cats but resembles cysts of follicular origin in their cellular content. These cysts are associated with developmental abnormalities and may extend

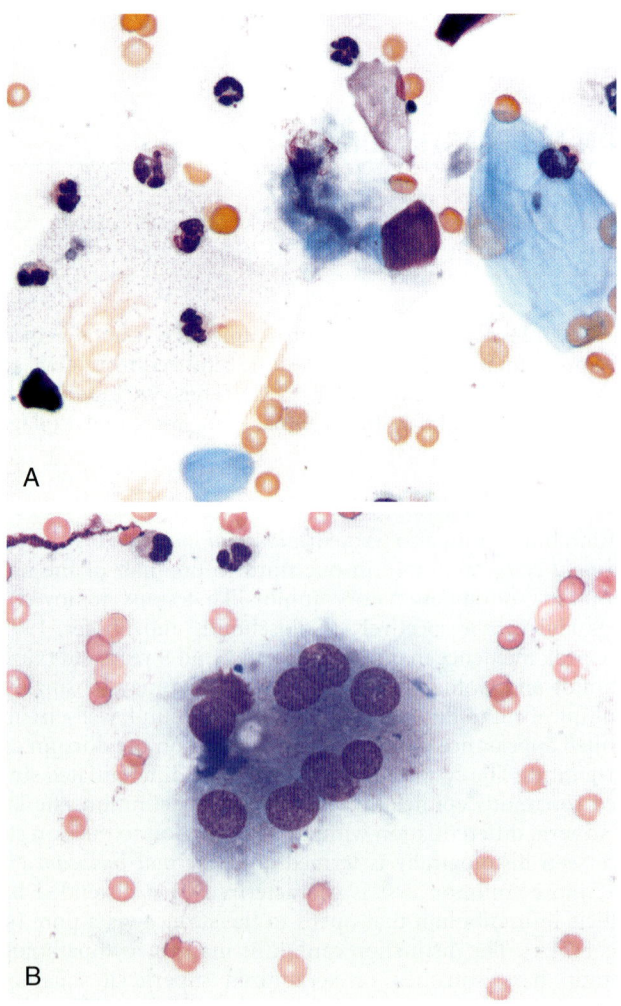

■ **FIGURE 3.75 Keratin inducing inflammation. Tissue aspirate. Dog.** Same case in A and B. **A,** Cholesterol crystal and squame remnants are present against a mildly hemodilute background. Nondegenerate and mildly karyolytic neutrophils react to the foreign material. (Modified Wright; HP oil.) **B,** Hemodilute background with the presence of a foreign body giant cell containing eight nuclei. The foreign material in this case is keratin and cholesterol. (Modified Wright; HP oil.)

deep to the spinal canal. Rhodesian ridgebacks, boxers, and Kerry blue terriers are reported to have a higher incidence. Histologically, the cyst is lined by squamous epithelium having small folliculosebaceous units radiating outward. The cyst is filled with abundant keratinized epithelium along with small hair follicles that are often pigmented as well as portions of other adnexal structures (Gross et al., 2005).

> **Cytopathologic differential diagnosis:** infundibular cyst, trichofolliculoma.

Apocrine Cyst

Apocrine cyst is a common lesion in dogs and cats that is formed from the occlusion of the apocrine or sweat gland duct. Grossly, it appears as a fluctuant swelling filled with light brown to colorless fluid that may become brown and gelatinous due to inspissation. On cytopathology, this fluid is usually acellular, having a clear background. Cuboidal to low columnar epithelium line these cysts (Fig. 3.76). Treatment involves surgical excision, and the prognosis is excellent.

> **Cytopathologic differential diagnosis:** apocrine gland hyperplasia, apocrine gland adenoma.

Ganglion Cyst

This is an uncommon condition in which patients present with a nonpainful, firm, raised mobile mass, generally near articular surfaces. Cysts are filled with pale-yellow mucinous fluid and may display internal shiny folds in the lining wall (Cho et al., 2000). The stained fluid smear has a magenta sheen consistent with mucopolysaccharide composition or synovial fluid. Microscopically, the background contains variably size eosinophilic amorphous deposits and there is a low to moderate mononuclear cellularity. The nucleated cells are round to oval, individualized with low nucleocytoplasmic ratio (Fig. 3.77). The round to oval

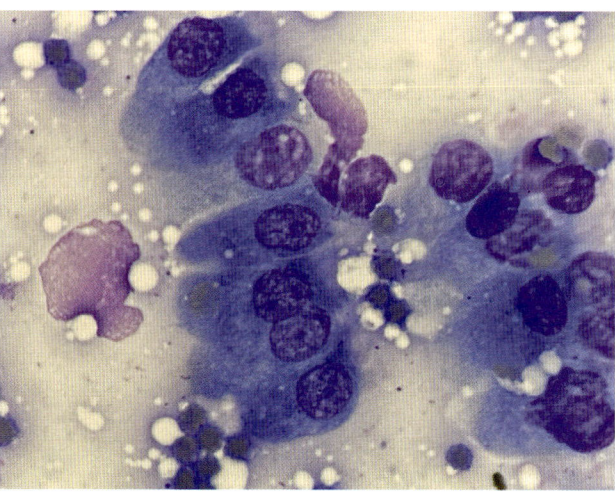

■ **FIGURE 3.76 Apocrine cyst. Digit mass. Tissue aspirate. Dog.** Cuboidal to low columnar cells with moderate amounts of basophilic cytoplasm line this non-neoplastic mass. The nuclei are round and basally located in palisading fashion with coarse chromatin and a single nucleolus. (Modified Wright; HP oil.) (Courtesy Linn Clarizio, Kansas State University.)

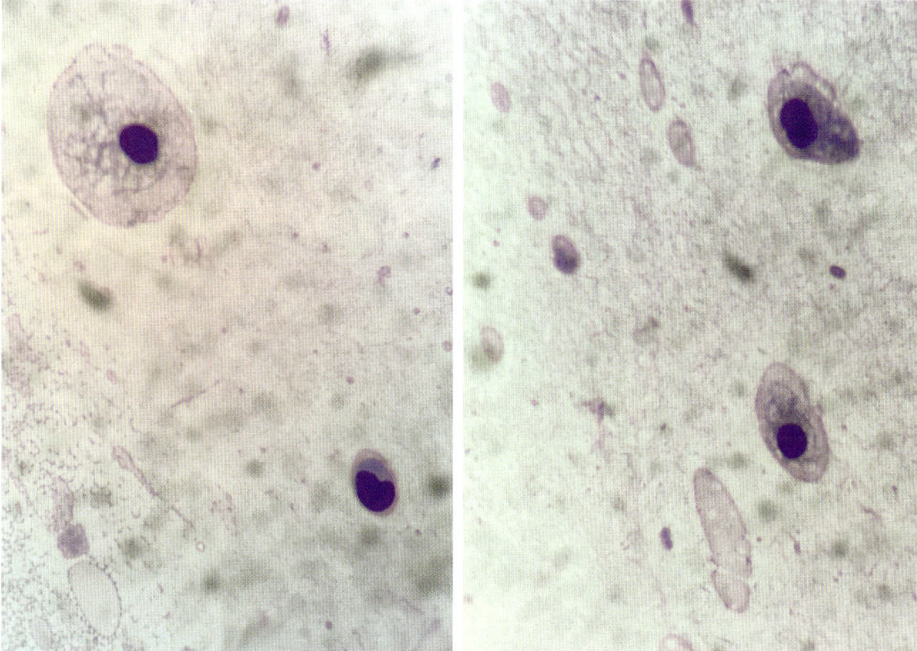

■ **FIGURE 3.77 Ganglion cyst. Carpal mass. Tissue aspirate. Dog.** The slide from this nonpainful mobile mass had a magenta shine consistent with mucopolysaccharide composition or synovial fluid. There is a low to moderate cellularity (estimated at 2000 cells/µL). *Left and right panels* are taken from different areas on the same slide. The background contains variably size eosinophilic amorphous deposits. The large nucleated cells are round to oval, individualized with low nucleocytoplasmic ratio. The round to oval nucleus is dense and displays mild anisokaryosis with occasional binucleation. The cytoplasm is pale eosinophilic to basophilic with mild foaminess. *Left panel* shows one lymphocyte along with a large mononuclear cell. (Modified Wright; HP oil.) (Courtesy TDDS/Synlab, Exeter, UK.)

nucleus is dense and display mild anisokaryosis with occasional binucleation. The cytoplasm is pale eosinophilic to basophilic with mild foaminess. These masses do not typically resolve on their own and require surgery to remove the cyst; otherwise, they often recur.

Nodular Sebaceous Hyperplasia

Sebaceous gland tumors are very common in dogs, and half of these tumors are nodular sebaceous hyperplasia. Grossly, nodular sebaceous hyperplasia presents as single to multiple masses and appear wartlike. Most are less than 1 cm in diameter. These tumors are very common in old dogs and less common in cats. Symmetrical proliferation of mature sebaceous lobules grouped around a keratinizing squamous-lined duct is the histopathologic basis used to classify the condition as hyperplasia (Fig. 3.78) (Gross et al., 2005). They are firm and elevated with a hairless, cauliflower or papilliferous surface (Fig. 3.79A). Mature sebaceous epithelial cells are seen on cytopathology, sometimes in clusters, or as individual pale, foamy cells with a small, dense, centrally placed nucleus, often mistaken for phagocytic macrophages. Distinction cannot be made cytopathologically and may even be difficult histologically when distinguishing between sebaceous hyperplasia and sebaceous adenoma (Fig. 3.79B–C). These benign proliferations have an excellent prognosis after surgical excision.

> *Cytopathologic differential diagnosis:* sebaceous adenoma, sebaceous hamartoma.

Hamartomas

These are nodular or plaque-like developmental abnormalities with mature tissue often hyperplastic for the site. *Sebaceous hamartoma* is a mid to deep dermal mass with normal to slightly hyperplastic sebaceous lobules and abundant surrounding collagenous tissue (Fig. 3.80). In contrast, *fibroadnexal hamartoma* or focal *adnexal dysplasia* is a non-neoplastic lesion composed of multiple adnexal structures such as hair follicles, sebaceous glands, and apocrine epithelium along with abundant surrounding collagenous tissue (Fig. 3.81). On cytopathology, the finding of dense collagen and hyperplastic sebaceous and/or follicular elements should suggest a possible hamartoma. Keratin released into the dermis from a ruptured hair follicle incites an acute inflammatory response that is often associated with fibroadnexal hamartomas. *Collagenous hamartoma* consists of dense dermal collagen and resembles fibroma on cytopathology (Fig. 3.82). Hamartomas are benign lesions that are best treated by surgery.

NEOPLASTIC TUMORS

One study (Villamil et al., 2011) indicated the common cutaneous neoplasms in dogs, which indicated lipoma, adenoma, and MCT as the top three. Refer to the report for further information about age and breed distribution.

Epithelial Cytomorphology
Viral Papilloma

Viral papillomas are usually solitary wartlike lesions, most often affecting older dogs and occasionally in cats that may lead to malignancy (Munday et al., 2017). They usually present as a raised growth with keratin-covered, finger-like projections (Fig. 3.83A) appearing on the head, limbs, or digits (Sprague and Thrall, 2001). On cytopathology, squamous epithelium in all stages of development is present, but mature forms with benign-appearing nuclei predominate, especially those with

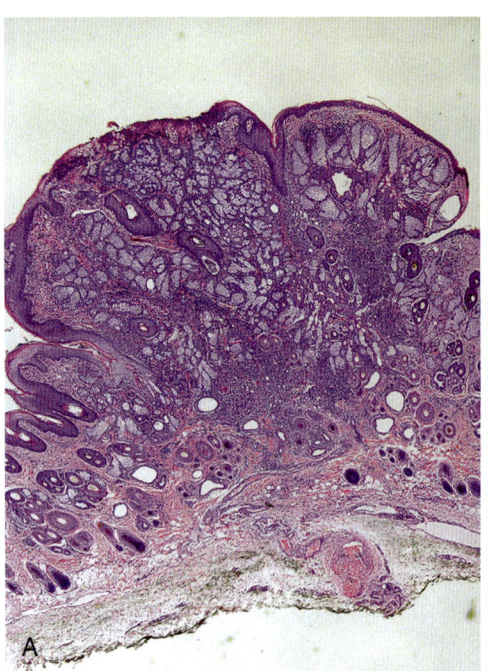
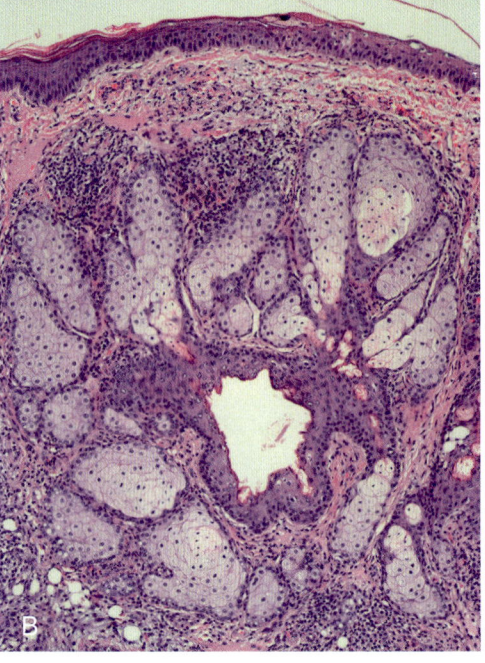

■ **FIGURE 3.78 Nodular sebaceous hyperplasia. Tissue section. Dog.** Same case in A and B. **A,** A raised papilliferous surface involves proliferation of sebaceous epithelium displacing hair follicles. (H&E; LP.) **B,** Characteristic histopathologic findings involve symmetrical proliferation of mature sebaceous lobules grouped around a keratinizing squamous-lined duct. (H&E; IP.)

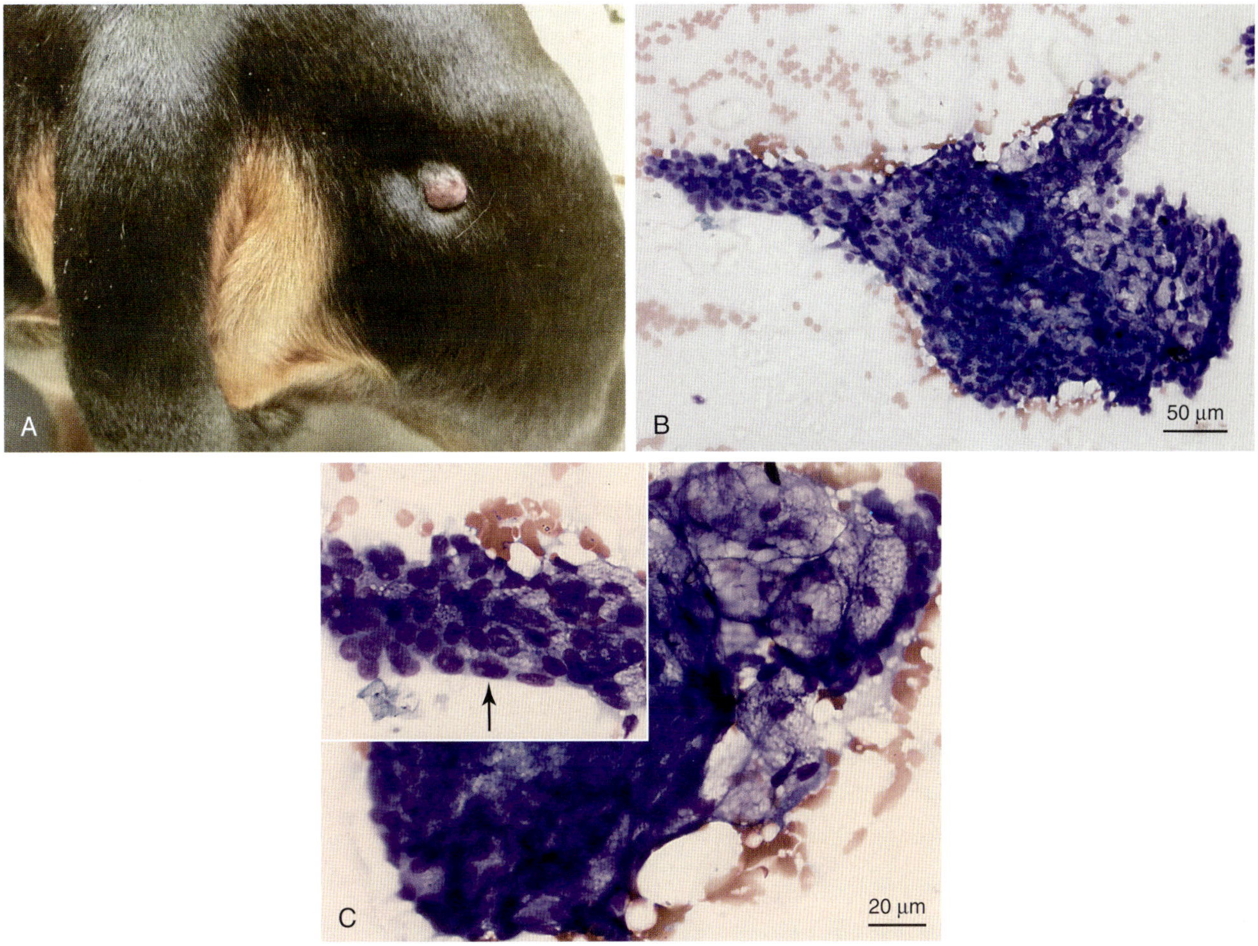

■ **FIGURE 3.79 Nodular sebaceous hyperplasia. Dog.** Same case in A to C. **A, Macroscopic specimen.** A 5 mm hairless raised dermal mass is present on the caudal thigh or rump area. **B, Tissue aspirate.** Nucleated cells primarily consist of mildly atypical sebaceous epithelial cells present in variably sized tightly cohesive clusters. (Wright-Giemsa; HP oil.) **C, Tissue aspirate.** These cells are polygonal or angular with distinct cytoplasmic borders and a moderate amount of pale basophilic cytoplasm with microvesicular vacuolization. *Inset:* Sebaceous glands are surrounded by reserve basal cells *(arrow)*. (Wright-Giemsa; HP oil.) (Courtesy Tracie Guy, University of Florida.)

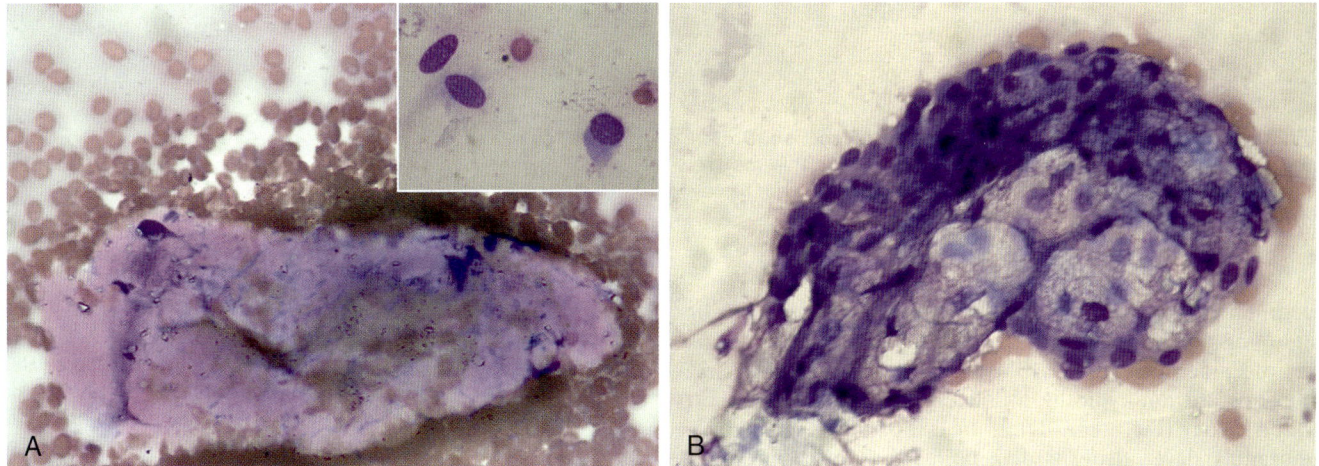

■ **FIGURE 3.80 Sebaceous hamartoma. Metatarsal mass. Tissue aspirate. Dog.** Same case in A and B. **A,** This 1 cm firm dermal mass is composed of two separate populations on different parts of the slide. Dense eosinophilic collagen was abundant. (Modified Wright; HP oil.) *Inset:* Three fibroblasts are shown indicating one nucleated cell population. **B,** Normal to hyperplastic sebaceous lobules are present as a second nucleated cell population. (Modified Wright; HP oil.) (Courtesy Eilidh Wilson, TDDS/Synlab, Exeter, UK.)

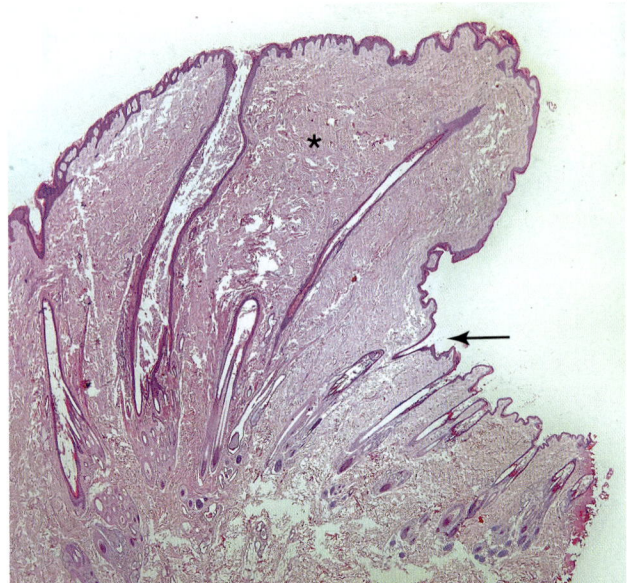

■ **FIGURE 3.81 Fibroadnexal hamartoma. Carpal mass. Tissue Section. Dog.** The dermis is expanded by a proliferation of collagen tissue *(asterisk)*. This fibrous nodule, about 5 mm in diameter, is demarcated by an *arrow*, where the collagen incorporates several dilated and skewed hair follicles. This lesion may also be termed *focal adnexal dysplasia*. (H&E; LP.) (Courtesy Margaret Miller, Purdue University.)

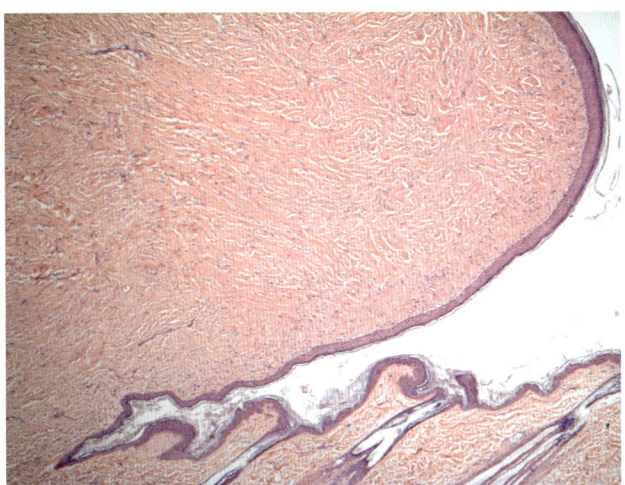

■ **FIGURE 3.82 Collagenous hamartoma. Tissue section. Dog.** A dense proliferation of normal collagen appears focally. This may resemble a fibroma on cytopathology. (H&E; LP.) (Courtesy Roger Easley, University of Florida.)

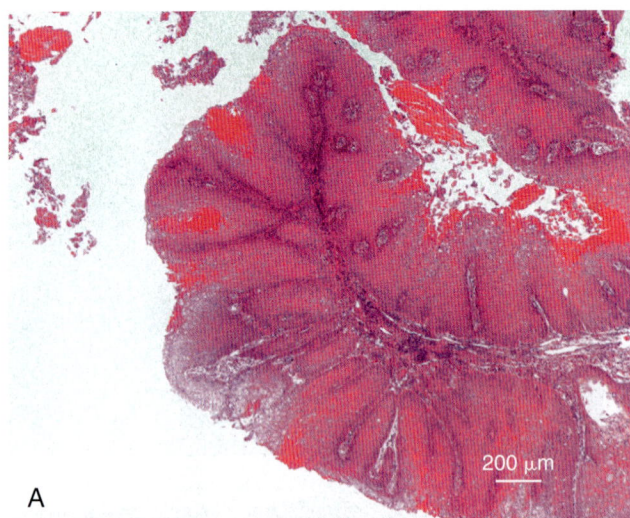

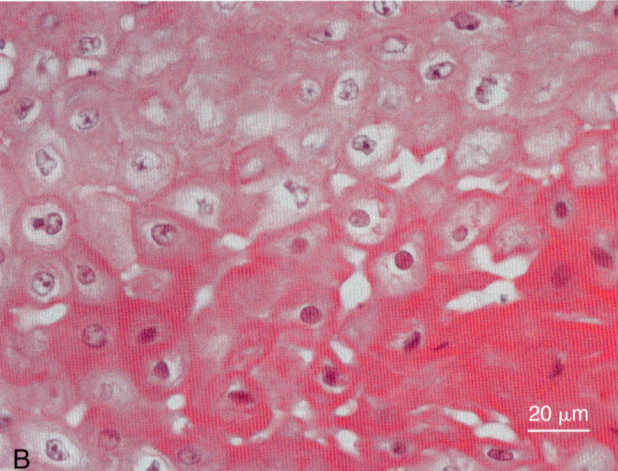

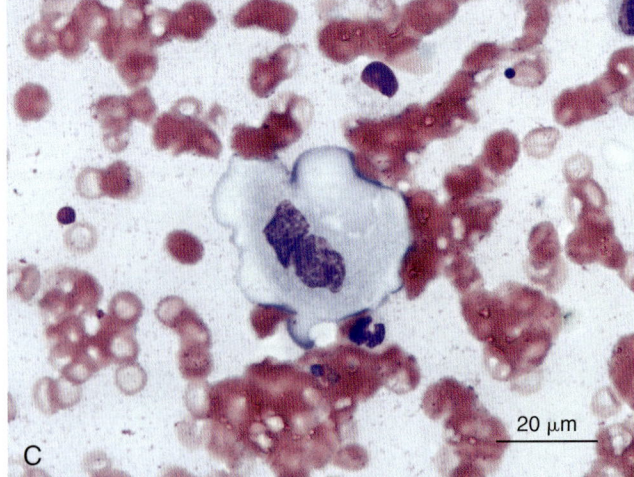

■ **FIGURE 3.83 Viral papilloma. Dog.** Same case in A to C. **A, Tissue section**. Papillary formation with a stalk-like exophytic structure. (H&E; LP.) **B, Tissue section.** Greater magnification of the thickened epidermis showing ballooning degeneration of keratinocytes with pale staining cytoplasm and open chromatin within round to irregular nuclear shapes. (H&E; HP oil.) **C, Tissue aspirate**. Presence of a single keratinized squamous epithelial cell with immature irregularly shaped nucleus and abundant pale staining cytoplasm. This degenerative change is consistent with papillomavirus infection; the individual cell is termed a *koilocyte*. (Wright-Giemsa; IP oil.)

pale bubbly or foamy cytoplasm consistent with *koilocytes* or ballooning degeneration of the squamous cells of the spinous layer of epidermis (Fig. 3.83B–C) (Moore et al., 2016). Viral inclusions are not typically found even when numerous on histopathology (Fig. 3.84A–D). If the cytopathic effect involves the granular layer, deposits of keratin may occur (Fig. 3.85) Keratin deposits are common. The viral papillomas usually regress within 2 months.

In contrast, squamous papillomas are not induced by papillomaviruses with normal epidermal differentiation and have no

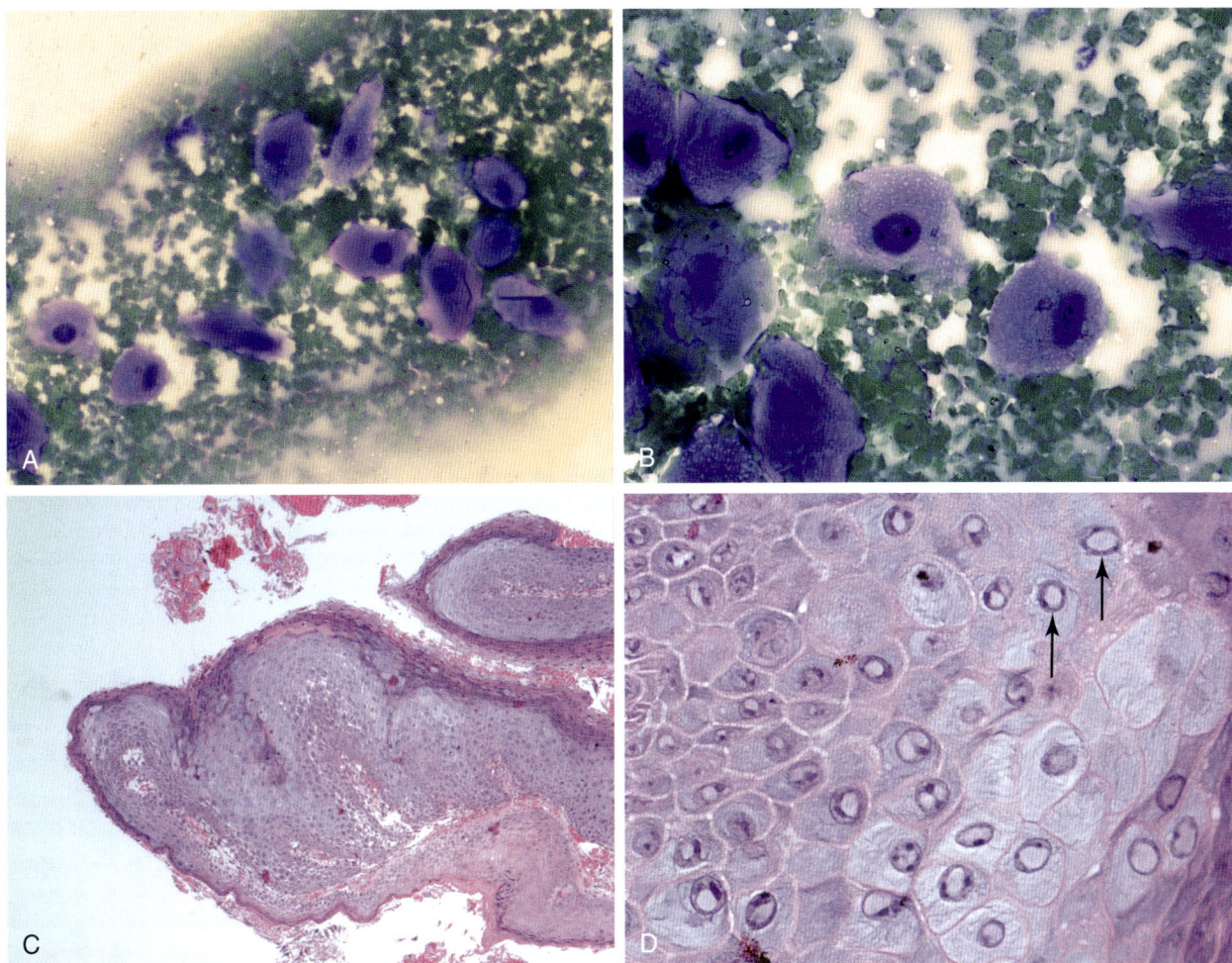

■ **FIGURE 3.84** **Viral papilloma. Digital mass. Dog.** Same case in A to D. **A, Tissue aspirate.** This 6 mm, circular, raised, and erythematous lesion displays moderate cellularity and marked hemodilution. Nucleated cells consist of individualized round to polygonal keratinized squamous epithelium. (May-Grünwald-Giemsa; HP oil.) **B,** Higher magnification demonstrates the nucleated keratinocytes with fine cytoplasmic vacuoles and blue-gray cytoplasmic deposits of keratin. The nucleus is round to elliptical with dense chromatin. These cells with ballooning degeneration and dysplasia are termed *koilocytes*. (May-Grünwald-Giemsa; HP oil.) **C, Tissue section.** The epidermis displays fingerlike projections. (H&E; L.P.) **D, Tissue section.** Several keratinocytes or koilocytes of the spinous layer contain glassy amphophilic nuclear inclusions *(arrows)* related to papillomavirus infection. (H&E; HP oil.) (Courtesy Chiara Piccinelli, University of Edinburgh, UK.)

presence of viral cytopathic effects such as koilocytes. They are not expected to resolve spontaneously compared with viral papillomas.

> ***Cytopathologic differential diagnosis:*** squamous cell carcinoma, keratoacanthoma, parakeratosis.

Squamous Cell Carcinoma

Squamous cell carcinoma is a common tumor in dogs and cats, occurring as solitary or multiple proliferative or ulcerative masses (Fig. 3.86). It accounts for 15% of skin tumors in cats but only 2% in dogs (Yager and Wilcock, 1994). For cats, the most common locations are the pinna, eyelids, face, and planum nasale. However, in dogs, this disease most frequently occurs on the head, abdomen, limbs, perineum, and digits (Goldschmidt and Goldschmidt, 2017). Tumors are usually locally invasive and may metastasize to regional lymph nodes. Those on the digit are considered to be highly malignant with a greater chance for metastasis. On cytopathology, purulent inflammation often accompanies immature or dysplastic squamous epithelium (Fig. 3.87A). The presence of one cell type within the cytoplasm of another, termed *emperipolesis*, may be noted in well-differentiated squamous cell carcinomas (Fig. 3.87B). Bacterial sepsis may occur if the surface has eroded. A tadpole shape with a tail-like projection and keratinized blue-green hyalinized cytoplasm may be a helpful criterion in determining the cell of origin (Garma-Avina, 1994). The neoplastic epithelium may appear as individual cells or as sheets of adherent cells. Squames and highly keratinized nucleated angular squamous epithelium with nuclear atypia predominate in well-differentiated tumors (Fig. 3.88). When these cells are concentrically arranged, they correspond to the keratin pearls seen histologically (Fig. 3.89). Moderately differentiated tumors have few angular cells and greater than 50% round or

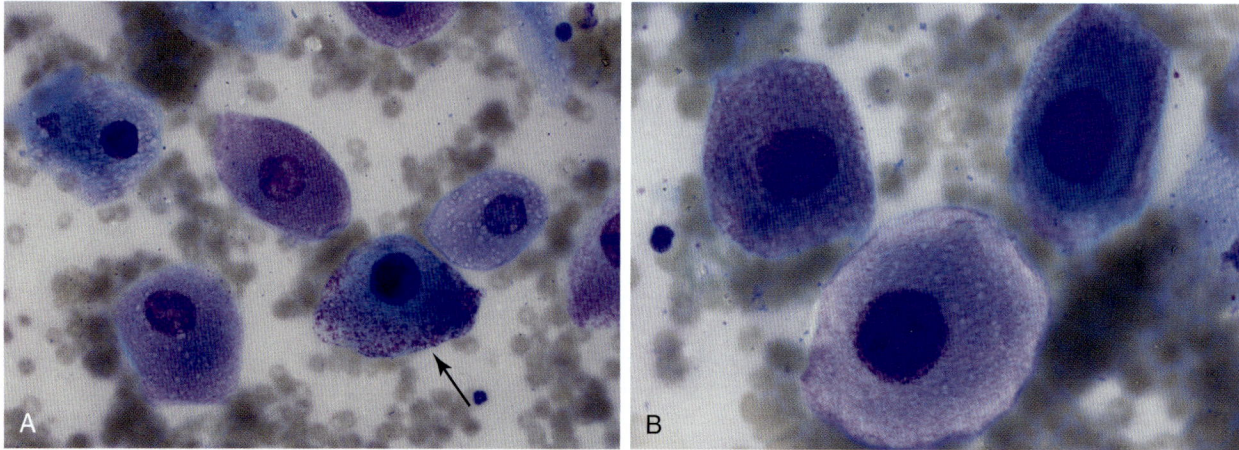

■ **FIGURE 3.85 Viral papilloma. Interdigital nodule. Tissue aspirate. Dog.** Same case in A and B. **A,** Individualized large squamous cells are present and appear oval to polygonal. These keratinized cells have an abundant aqua cytoplasm with eosinophilic stippling *(arrow)*. Anisocytosis is moderate and anisokaryosis is mild. The nucleocytoplasmic ratio is low. (Wright-Giemsa; HP oil.) **B,** The cytoplasm of these variegated cells is finely vacuolated, especially focally paranuclear. The round to oval nucleus measures two to four times the diameter of an erythrocyte with a coarsely clumped to condensed chromatin and no discernible nucleolus. (Wright-Giemsa; HP oil.) (Courtesy Jere Stern, University of Florida.)

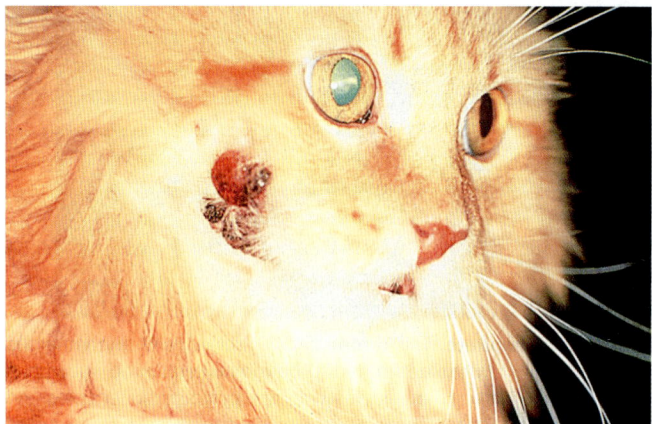

■ **FIGURE 3.86 Squamous cell carcinoma. Macroscopic specimen. Cat.** An ulcerative lesion on the face. (Courtesy Jamie Bellah, University of Florida.)

oval dysplastic cells (Fig. 3.90). Round, individualized cells having a high nucleocytoplasmic ratio predominate in the poorly differentiated tumors. Cellular and nuclear pleomorphism is marked in the poorly differentiated squamous cell carcinomas. Perinuclear vacuolation is thought to represent colorless keratohyalin granules and may be present most frequently in well and moderately differentiated tumor types (Fig. 3.91). Treatment considerations include surgical excision, cryosurgery, radiotherapy, intralesional chemotherapy, and photodynamic therapy. Prognosis is guarded because recurrence is common, especially in white-faced cats.

Multicentric in situ squamous cell carcinoma is common in cats, which may relate to papillomavirus and likely not related to sunlight exposure. It involves squamous epithelial cells with cytopathologic features of malignant transformation, but the histopathology does not show evidence of invasion through the basement membrane. Cells have moderately abundant pale basophilic cytoplasm, prominent nucleoli, and anisokaryosis. When hyperpigmented with the presence of dendritic melanocytes, they may be mistaken for malignant melanoma (Fig. 3.92).

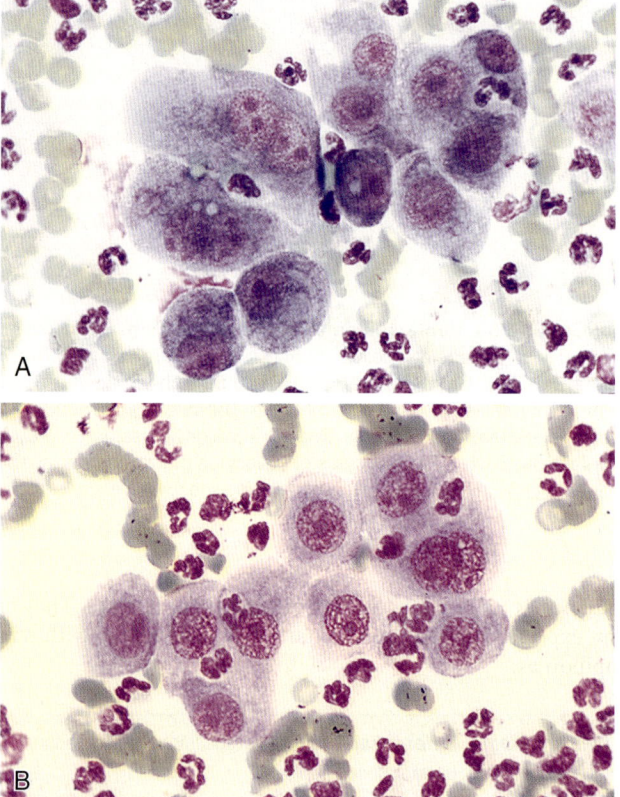

■ **FIGURE 3.87 Squamous cell carcinoma. Tissue aspirate. Dog.** Same case in A and B. **A,** Dysplastic epithelium with purulent inflammation from a mass on the nasal planum. (Wright-Giemsa; HP oil.) **B,** Emperipolesis noted by neutrophils migrating through epithelium. (Wright-Giemsa; HP oil.)

KEY POINT It is often difficult to determine if dysplastic changes are the result of the reaction to chronic inflammation or an indication of malignancy.

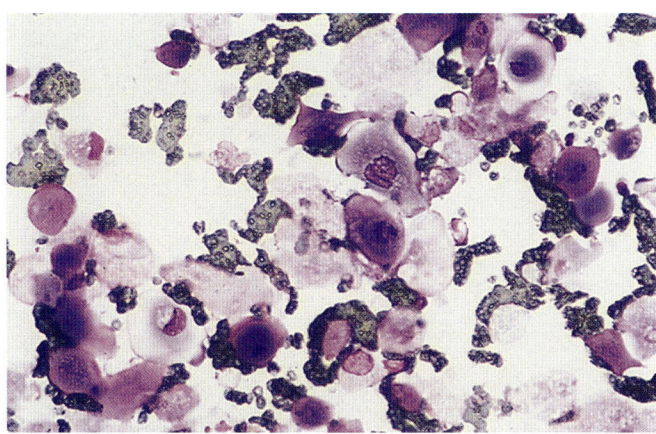

■ **FIGURE 3.88 Squamous cell carcinoma. Tissue aspirate. Cat.** Note the intermediate, superficial, and anucleated squame in this well-differentiated form of neoplasia found in a cheek mass. Many early stages of maturation have angular cell borders and keratinized cytoplasm suggesting dysplastic development. (Aqueous Romanowsky; HP oil.)

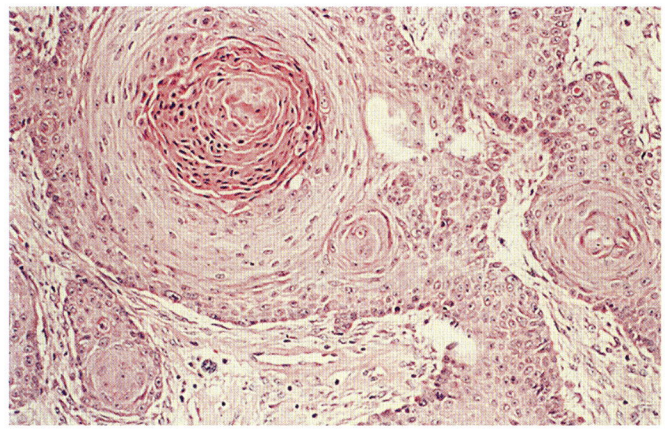

■ **FIGURE 3.89 Squamous cell carcinoma. Tissue section. Dog.** Keratin pearl in the center of a lobule of neoplastic squamous epithelium. (H&E; IP.)

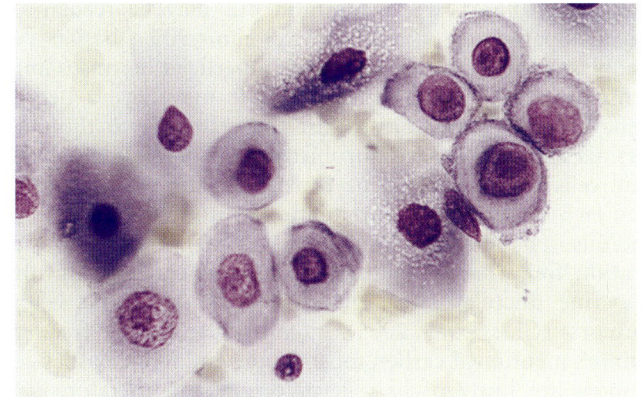

■ **FIGURE 3.90 Squamous cell carcinoma. Dysplastic squamous epithelium. Tissue aspirate. Dog.** Rounded cells and keratinized intermediate squamous epithelium similar to cells found in squamous cell carcinoma of a foot mass. (Aqueous Romanowsky; HP oil.)

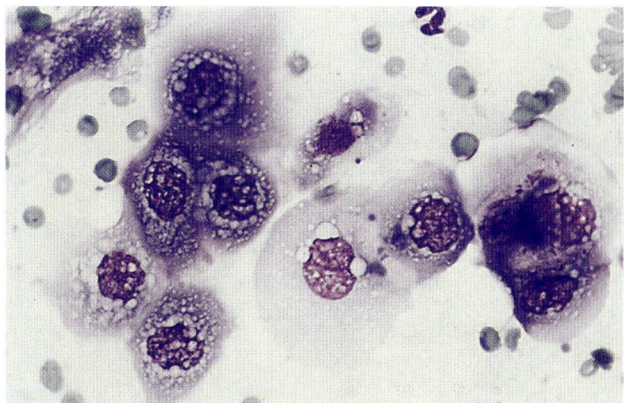

■ **FIGURE 3.91 Squamous cell carcinoma. Tissue aspirate. Cat.** Small sheets of epithelium with marked anisokaryosis and anisocytosis are present in this thigh mass. The keratinized cytoplasm displays prominent perinuclear vacuolation. (Aqueous Romanowsky; HP oil.)

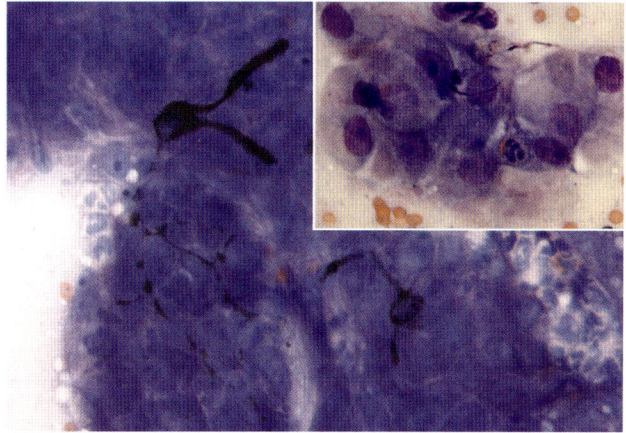

■ **FIGURE 3.92 Squamous cell carcinoma, in situ. Tissue aspirate. Cat.** A dense cluster of epithelial cells is infiltrated by dendritic melanocytes. Nondegenerate neutrophils are present in the background. These tumors when hyperpigmented with the presence of dendritic melanocytes may be mistaken for malignant melanoma. Histopathology is recommended. (Modified Wright; HP oil.) *Inset*: Squamous epithelial cells with cytopathologic features of malignancy. Cells have moderately abundant pale basophilic cytoplasm, prominent nucleoli, and anisokaryosis. (Modified Wright; HP oil.) (Courtesy Kathleen Tennant, University of Bristol, UK.)

Cytopathologic differential diagnosis: infundibular keratinizing acanthoma, squamous papilloma, basosquamous carcinoma.

Basosquamous Carcinoma

This uncommon neoplasm behaves as a low-grade malignancy and is composed primarily of basal cells with variably sized foci of squamous differentiation. It is generally found in adult dogs on the head, neck, and limbs. Cytopathology displays dense clusters of small basaloid cells with small amounts of basophilic cytoplasm (Fig. 3.93A). Evidence of keratinocytes with evidence of dyskeratosis may be found. Histopathologic specimens demonstrate a multilobulated localized mass within the dermis that may

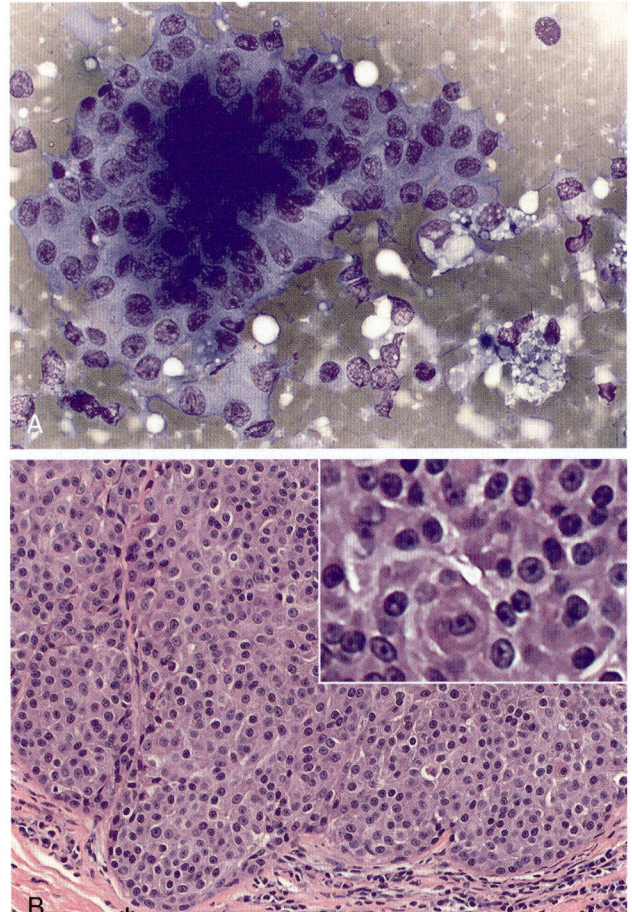

■ **FIGURE 3.93 Basosquamous carcinoma. Axillary mass. Tissue aspirate. Dog.** Same case in A and B. **A,** Moderately atypical epithelial cells predominate in this 3 cm dermal pedunculated mass. Cells are arranged in large cohesive clusters. These cells are round or oval, have variably distinct cytoplasmic borders, and a small to moderate amount of basophilic, finely stippled cytoplasm. The round or oval nucleus is central to paracentral, measures approximately 1.5 to 2.0 times the size of an erythrocyte, has coarse chromatin, and often contains one or more distinct nucleoli. The overall anisocytosis and anisokaryosis among this population are mild to moderate with a moderate nucleocytoplasmic ratio. (Wright-Giemsa; HP oil.) **B,** The multilobulated well-demarcated dermal mass appears to extend to the subcutis *(asterisk)*. The mass is composed of closely packed cells forming lobules supported by a thin fibrovascular stroma. The cells are medium and polygonal with variably distinct cellular borders and moderate amounts of granular, eosinophilic cytoplasm. The nuclei are central, oval, and medium with finely stippled chromatin and single, basophilic nucleoli. Anisokaryosis and mitotic activity are mild. (H&E; IP.) *Inset:* An area of abrupt differentiation into keratinized or dysplastic squamous cells is shown. (H&E; HP oil.)

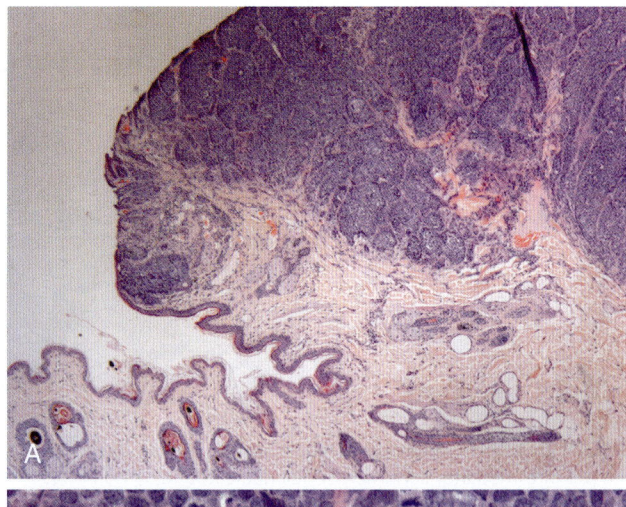
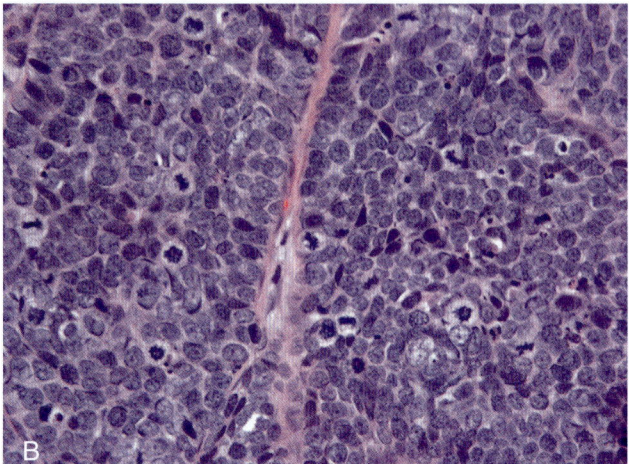

■ **FIGURE 3.94 Basal cell carcinoma. Neck mass. Tissue section. Cat.** Same case in A and B. **A,** This poorly demarcated dermal mass extends into the deep dermis and occasionally disperses as small cell clusters. (H&E; LP.) **B,** Small basaloid cells with high nucleocytoplasmic ratio are prominent without evidence of differentiation. Note the high frequency of mitotic figures. (H&E; IP.) (Courtesy Mark Bennett, University of Bristol, UK.)

extend to the subcutis (Fig. 3.93B). A central cyst with an abrupt differentiation of squamous cells may appear. Pleomorphism and mitotic activity are mild to moderate. Surgical excision is recommended but recurrence is possible if incompletely removed.

Germinal or Basilar Epithelial Neoplasms

Neoplasms that were formerly termed *basal cell tumor* are now mostly classified histologically by evidence supporting differentiation into epidermis, trichofollicular epithelium, or the adnexal structures of sweat and sebaceous glands. True basal cell tumors are uncommon but may be recognized on histopathology as a stromal circumscribed basilar cell neoplasm within the epidermis to superficial dermis (Goldschmidt et al., 2018). Although these may have a benign behavior, malignant forms exist that extend into the deep dermis and display pleomorphism (Fig. 3.94A). Small basaloid cells with high nucleocytoplasmic ratio are prominent and lack evidence of differentiation. Mitotic figures are numerous in basal cell carcinoma (Fig. 3.94B). Another consideration for a basilar epithelial tumor in cats may involve apocrine ductular sweat glands (see under Sweat Gland Tumors) (Gross et al., 2005). In contrast to the less frequent tumors mentioned earlier, most canine and feline basilar cell tumors are likely of hair germ origin and therefore best termed *trichoblastoma*.

Trichoblastomas are found commonly in dogs and cats and typically present as a benign single, firm, elevated, well-demarcated round intradermal mass that may be ulcerated

CHAPTER 3 *Integumentary System*

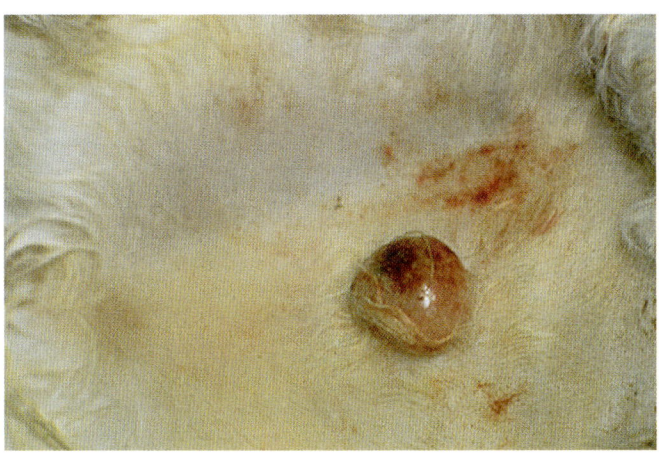

■ **FIGURE 3.95 Basilar epithelial neoplasm. Cat.** Note the single, firm, raised, alopecic, well-demarcated round intradermal mass. (Courtesy the University of Florida Dermatology Section.)

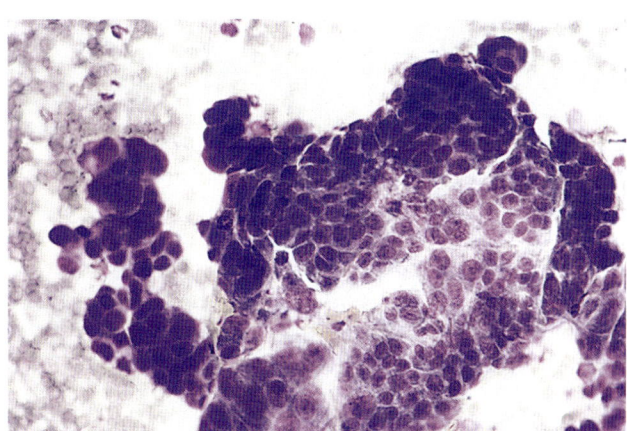

■ **FIGURE 3.97 Trichoblastoma. Tissue imprint. Dog.** Large clusters of tightly adherent uniform-appearing epithelial cells with intensely basophilic cytoplasm are present in this lip mass. Masses with this appearance are most likely termed *trichoblastoma* on histopathology. (Aqueous Romanowsky; HP oil.)

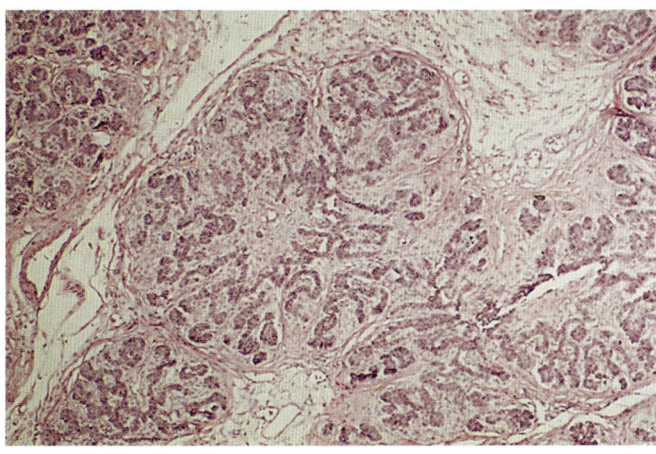

■ **FIGURE 3.96 Trichoblastoma. Tissue section. Dog.** Note the medusoid pattern with cords or ribbons of basal epithelium with palisading nuclei radiating out from the center. Between these cells is pink collagenous stroma. (H&E; LP.)

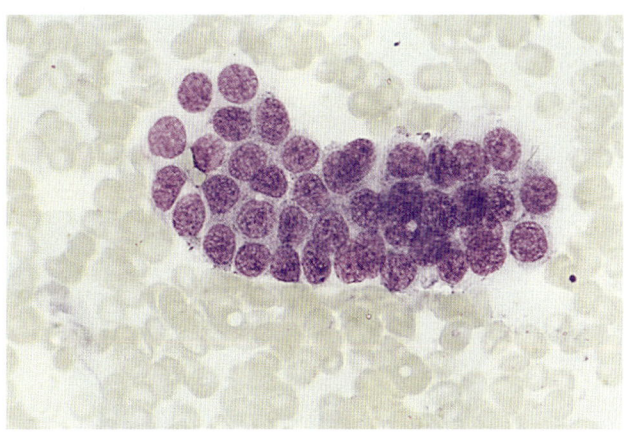

■ **FIGURE 3.98 Trichoblastoma. Tissue aspirate. Dog.** Tight cluster of uniform cells having a high nucleocytoplasmic ratio. The cytoplasm is scant and basophilic. This cytopathologic appearance of this mass is most consistent with a trichoblastoma seen on histopathology. (Wright-Giemsa; HP oil.)

or pigmented due to abundant melanin (Fig. 3.95). They are located mostly about the head with frequent occurrence on the neck. Histologically, they are arranged as solid, trabecular, or ribbons with palisading cells (Fig. 3.96). On cytopathologic specimens, basal epithelial cells are small cells characterized by high nucleocytoplasmic ratios, monomorphic nuclei, and deeply basophilic cytoplasm (Figs. 3.97 and 3.98). At times trichoblastomas may be pigmented and resemble melanocytic tumors (Figs. 3.99 and 3.100). A subtype termed *granular trichoblastoma* has been identified on cytopathology in which the cytoplasm of individualized cells appears abundant and finely granular (Fig. 3.101) (Asakawa et al., 2015). On cytopathology, a pink matrix (Fig. 3.102) along with spindle cells may be present with trichoblastomas and reflect the collagenous stroma (Adedeji et al., 2017). Classification of these basilar neoplasms is difficult on cytopathology, and histopathology is recommended to differentiate the different types (Bohn et al., 2006; Goldschmidt et al., 2018).

KEY POINT Because of their common origin, there is considerable overlap on cytopathology between basilar cell tumors and follicular or adnexal tumors.

Cytopathologic differential diagnosis: follicular tumors, sweat or apocrine gland tumors, sebaceous gland tumors.

Differentiated Follicular Neoplasms

Basal cells may predominate in these tumors, but foci of scattered keratinocytes (Fig. 3.103A) should suggest the presence of basal tumors with follicular differentiation (Fig. 3.103B). Hair follicle tumors are benign tumors that are usually solitary but may be multiple. They are usually found in older dogs. These are firm, raised, hairless, well-circumscribed masses that may ulcerate. Most often considered are trichoepithelioma and less

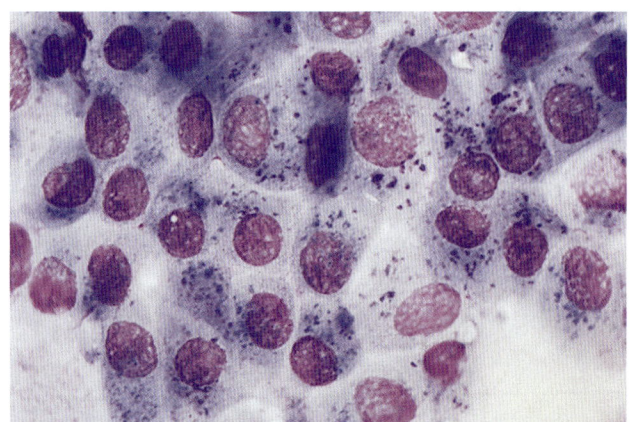

■ **FIGURE 3.99 Trichoblastoma. Neck mass aspirate. Dog.** Sheet of basal epithelium with prominent cytoplasmic granulation and pigmentation consistent with keratohyalin and melanin. (Wright-Giemsa; HP oil.)

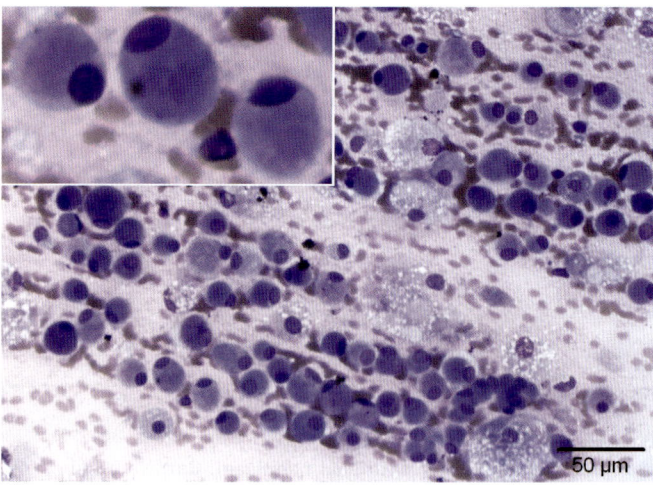

■ **FIGURE 3.101 Granular trichoblastoma. Cutaneous head mass, Tissue aspirate. Dog.** Cytopathologic specimens from a 2-cm-long, well-circumscribed, raised, alopecic mass are highly cellular and contain many monotypic individualized medium to large, round to polygonal cells arranged in linear arrays. Anisokaryosis is mild and anisocytosis is moderate. (Aqueous Romanowsky; IP.) *Inset:* Higher magnification of the same image to show cellular details. The cells have oval eccentric nuclei with smooth chromatin and a single indistinct nucleolus. The cytoplasm is abundant with distinct borders and moderate numbers of light purple granules. (Courtesy Midori Asakawa and Tracy Stokol, Cornell University.)

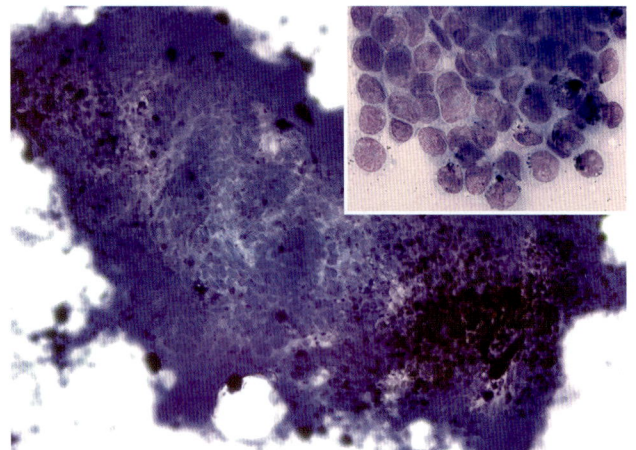

■ **FIGURE 3.100 Trichoblastoma. Pigmented cutaneous hock mass. Tissue aspirate. Dog.** A pleomorphic cell population is present in cohesive disorganized clusters, and many of the cells appear pigmented. (Wright-Giemsa; IP.) *Inset:* The predominant cell is a small to moderate basal cell that often contains numerous small melanin granules. Histopathology confirmed the diagnosis of trichoblastoma while melanoma was a consideration owing to the degree of pigmentation. (Wright-Giemsa; HP oil.) (Courtesy Roger Easley, University of Florida.)

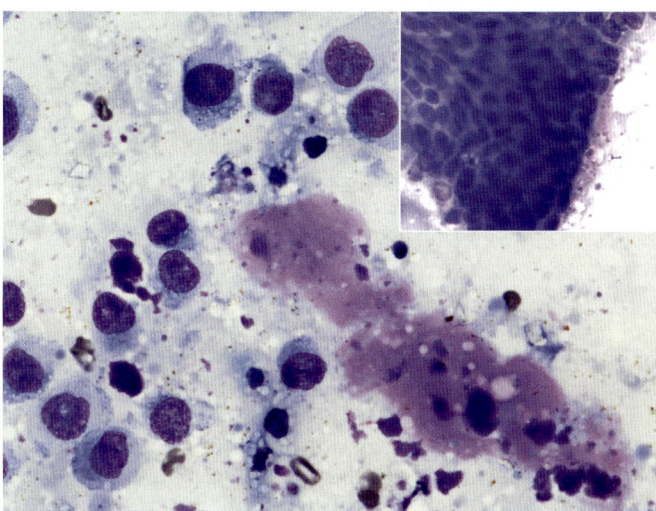

■ **FIGURE 3.102 Trichoblastoma. Thigh mass. Tissue aspirate. Cat.** This 0.5 cm cystic mass yielded a densely basophilic and granular background consistent with necrotic debris with rectangular colorless cholesterol crystals and occasional refractile mineralized material. Uniform basilar epithelial cells are present with a small amount of bright eosinophilic extracellular matrix, likely representing collagenous stroma. These cells are oval to polygonal and have variably distinct cytoplasmic borders and a scant amount of moderately basophilic cytoplasm. (Aqueous Romanowsky; HP oil.) *Inset:* Predominant in the specimen are large densely basophilic sheets of germinal epithelium. An eosinophilic matrix is shown to the right of the cell cluster. Histopathology confirmed a trichoblastoma with areas of cystic degeneration. (Aqueous Romanowsky; HP oil.)

commonly pilomatricoma or tricholemmoma. Trichoepithelioma and pilomatricoma are derived from hair matrix cells.

Trichoepitheliomas (Fig. 3.104) may have two cytopathologic presentations, which include mostly keratinizing anucleate to nucleated squamous cells or, to a lesser extent, basaloid cells undergoing keratinization along with keratin debris (Adedeji et al., 2017). Dense basophilic aggregates of keratinocytes and keratin may represent horn cysts. Histologically, the abrupt keratinization from the basal epithelium forming horn cysts helps to distinguish this tumor from basilar epithelial tumors with follicular differentiation. Treatment consists of surgical excision or cryosurgery. Prognosis is excellent, but they may metastasize with malignant variants (Jackson, 2010).

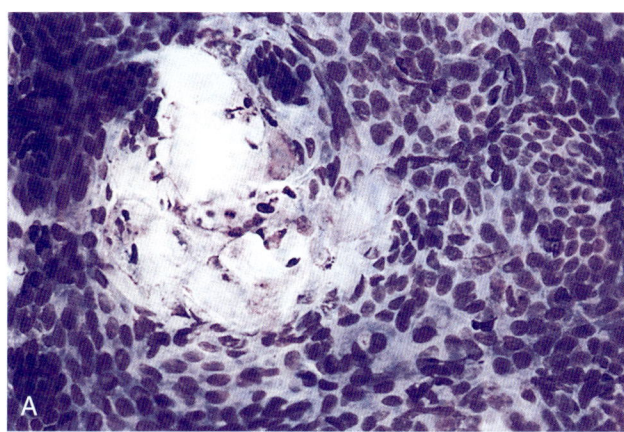
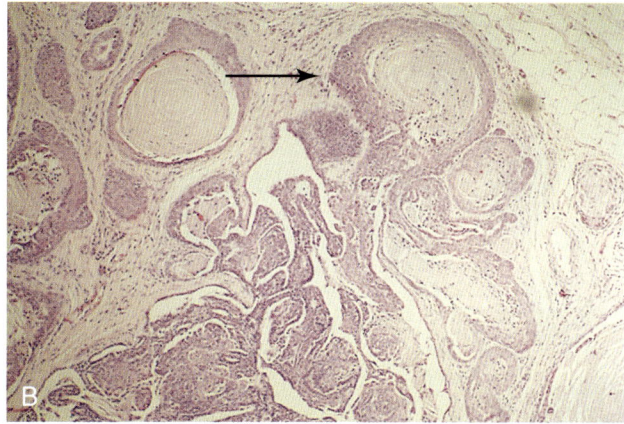

■ **FIGURE 3.103 Trichoblastoma with follicular differentiation. Shoulder mass. Dog.** Same case in A and B. **A,** Tissue aspirate. Dense clusters of basal epithelium compose the majority of cells. However, there is a small focus of keratinocytes suggesting follicular differentiation. (Aqueous Romanowsky; HP oil.) **B,** Tissue section. Note the gradual process of keratinization within the thickened basal epithelium (arrow). This tumor shows several areas of follicular differentiation; however, if basal epithelial cells were a minor component, the mass would be termed a *trichoepithelioma*. (H&E; LP.)

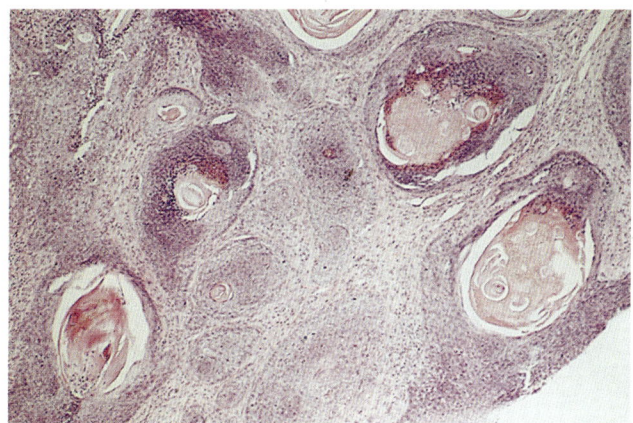

■ **FIGURE 3.104 Trichoepithelioma. Tissue section.** Note the keratinization in the center surrounded by a minor component of thickened basal epithelium, suggesting rudimentary hair formation. There is a gradual formation of keratin unlike the pilomatricoma. (H&E; LP.)

Pilomatricoma will show an abrupt change from germinal epithelium to keratinized epithelium with indistinct nuclear outlines in cells and occasional calcification (Figs. 3.105 and 3.106) (Masserdotti and Ubbiali, 2002). Unlike trichoepitheliomas, there is a lack of a granular layer. When keratin is released into the skin from a pilomatricoma, an intense inflammatory reaction occurs (Fig. 3.107). Occasionally encountered are keratin-filled masses that resemble a dermoid cyst but are melanized pilomatricomas containing pigmented ghost cells (Fig. 3.108).

Cytopathologic differential diagnosis: infundibular keratinizing acanthoma, infundibular cyst.

Keratoacanthoma

This is a benign neoplasm affecting the haired skin or nailbed. For the haired skin, infundibular keratinizing acanthoma represents a proliferation of the epithelium containing adnexal and follicular structures with a pore to the outside often with numerous horn cysts (Fig. 3.109). It may be predisposed in some breeds (Norwegian elkhounds, Keeshonds). Pore contents are similar to those of infundibular cyst. Keratinous debris, squames and superficial squamous cells, and cholesterol crystals characterize this tumor on cytopathologic specimens. Low numbers of basal cells are present. Treatment consists of surgical excision, cryosurgery, and retinoid, particularly for multiple tumor presentation. Prognosis is good.

A similar proliferation may occur in the nailbed and is termed *subungual keratoacanthoma*. The cytopathology, treatment, and prognosis are similar to that above for haired skin.

Cytopathologic differential diagnosis: infundibular cyst, trichoepithelioma.

Sebaceous Adenoma

Sebaceous adenoma appears as a single, smooth, raised, hairless cauliflower lesion or as an intradermal multilobulated mass that usually measures less than 1 cm in diameter similar to nodular sebaceous hyperplasia (Fig. 3.110). The overlying skin is alopecic and sometimes ulcerated. These are common in dogs, accounting for approximately 6% of all canine skin and subcutaneous tumors in one survey (Gross et al., 2005). Fifty percent of these tumors in older dogs occur on the head (Goldschmidt and Shofer, 1992). Multiple tumors occur infrequently. Although uncommon in cats, these tumors are most often found on the head and back. Cystic degeneration and lipogranulomatous inflammation may occur in the center of lobules. Compared with sebaceous hyperplasia, sebaceous adenomas do not retain normal orientation around hair follicles and may invade the panniculus. Mature sebocytes arranged in lobules or clusters predominate and are characterized on cytopathology by pale, foamy cytoplasm having a small, dense, centrally placed nucleus. A variable number of germinal epithelial cells having basophilic cytoplasm and a higher nucleocytoplasmic ratio may accompany the secretory cells.

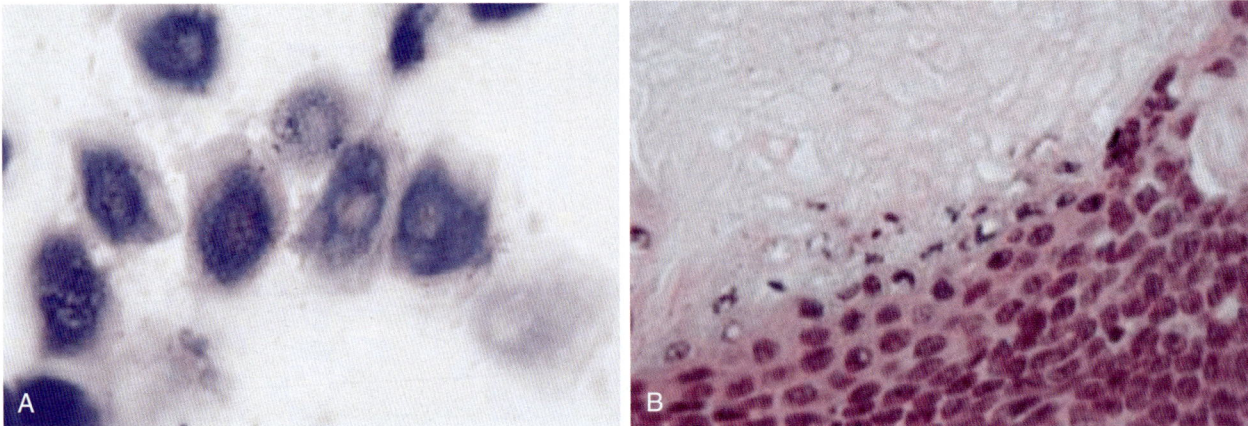

FIGURE 3.105 Pilomatricoma. Dog. Same case in A and B. **A, Tissue aspirate.** Ghost cells characterized by a central empty zone. (May-Grünwald-Giemsa; IP.) **B, Tissue section.** Histopathologic section showing the abrupt transformation of basaloid cells to ghost cells without evidence of the granular layer. (H&E; HP oil.) (From Masserdotti C, Ubbiali FA. Fine needle aspiration cytology of pilomatricoma in three dogs. *Vet Clin Pathol.* 2002;31:22–25.)

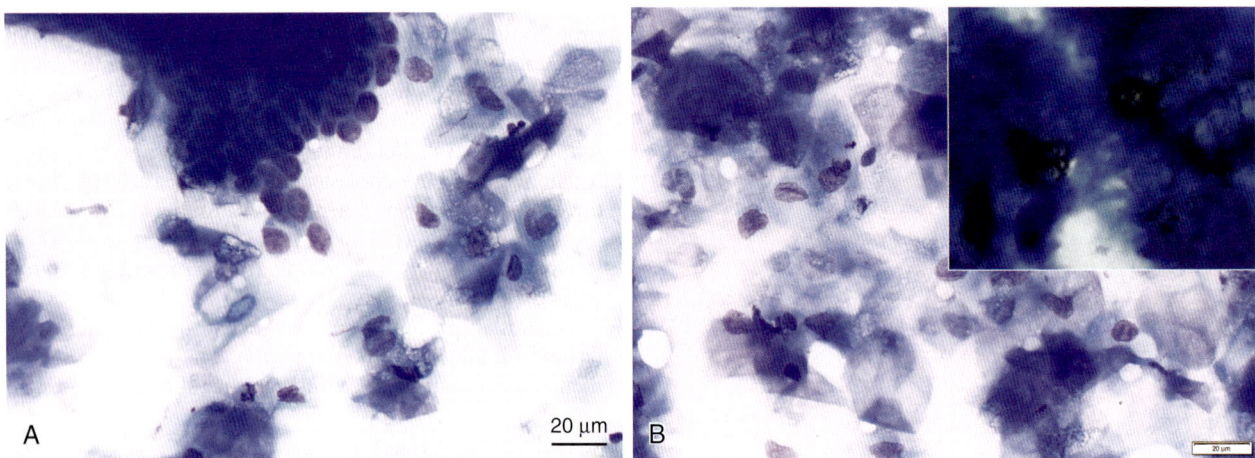

FIGURE 3.106 Pilomatricoma. Lateral neck mass. Tissue aspirate. Dog. Same case in A and B. **A,** Mildly atypical squamous epithelial cells are present as a large aggregate of basilar epithelium and as individualized keratinized cells without a transition phase. These individual cells have an abundant amount of aqua blue cytoplasm that contains several perinuclear vacuoles, consistent with keratinization. Some cells contain an ovoid to irregularly shaped nucleus. (Wright-Giemsa; HP oil.) **B,** The nucleus in this keratinized cell population is often missing, suggesting a ghost cell appearance. (Wright-Giemsa; HP oil.) *Inset:* Low amounts of refractile colorless granular mineral deposits are present. (Wright-Giemsa; HP oil.)

Necrotic centers containing amorphous basophilic debris with cells may be found related to cystic degeneration of sebocytes (Fig. 3.111). Treatment consists of surgical excision or cryosurgery. Prognosis is excellent.

> **KEY POINT** Histologic examination is necessary to distinguish between hyperplastic and adenomatous sebaceous tumors.

> ***Cytopathologic differential diagnosis:*** sebaceous hyperplasia, sebaceous hamartoma.

Sebaceous Epithelioma

Sebaceous epithelioma is similar in gross appearance to sebaceous adenoma. When present on the eyelid, it is termed *meibomian adenoma.* This is considered a low-grade malignant neoplasm. Histologically, germinal epithelium predominates, and small lobules of mature sebaceous epithelium are intermixed (Fig. 3.112A). On cytopathology, the tumor resembles a germinal cutaneous basilar neoplasm with small basophilic epithelial clusters along with scattered groups of mature sebocytes (Figs. 3.112B and 3.113). Occasional low numbers of individualized, well-differentiated squamous epithelial cells as keratinocytes appear related to sebaceous duct differentiation. Clinical behavior is benign, but the tumors may rarely recur locally. Prognosis is usually excellent after surgical excision.

> ***Cytopathologic differential diagnosis:*** sebaceous adenoma, cutaneous basilar epithelial neoplasm.

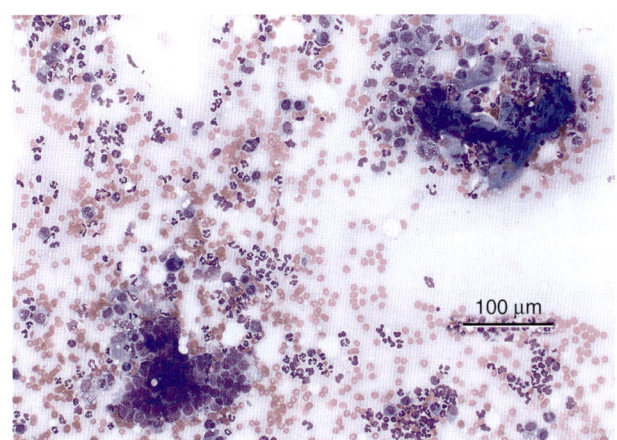

■ **FIGURE 3.107 Inflamed pilomatricoma. Tail mass aspirate. Dog.** This 3 cm mass yielded a background containing some amorphous bright blue material consistent with keratin *(upper right)*. Nucleated cells involve a mixture of inflammatory cells and epithelial cells with predominance of mature, nondegenerate neutrophils along with several mildly to moderately vacuolated macrophages. Mildly atypical basal epithelial cells are present in small tightly cohesive sheets *(lower left)*, and some appear partially lysed. Histopathology supported the diagnosis. (Wright-Giemsa; IP.)

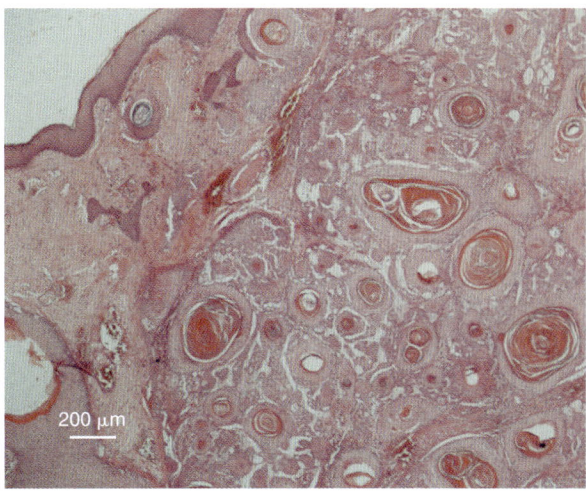

■ **FIGURE 3.109 Infundibular keratinizing acanthoma. Tissue section. Dog.** The proliferation of epithelium with follicular structures is shown. Not visible in this section is the pore to the outside demonstrating the epidermal inversion. (H&E; LP.)

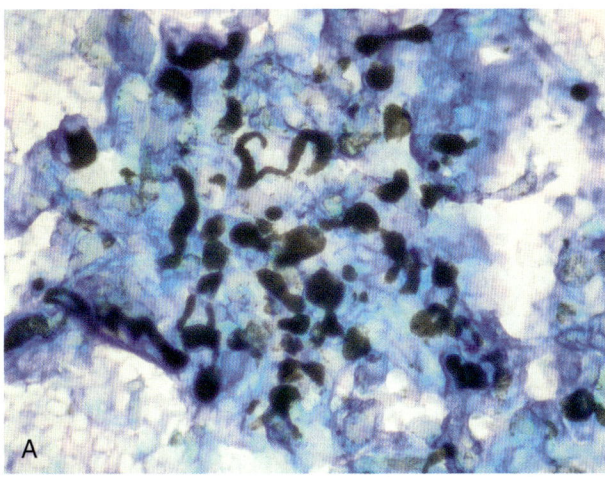

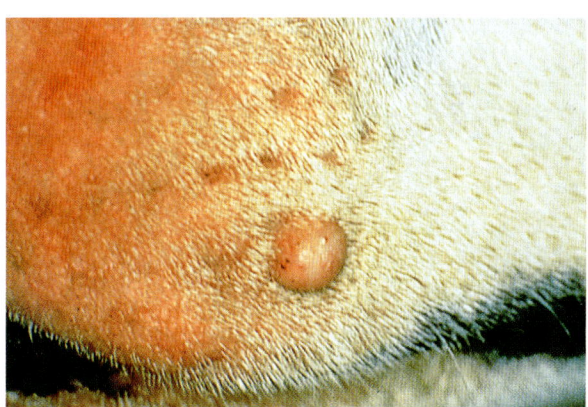

■ **FIGURE 3.110 Sebaceous adenoma. Macroscopic specimen. Dog.** Raised, alopecic, lobulated lesion present on the lip. (Courtesy University of Florida Dermatology Section.)

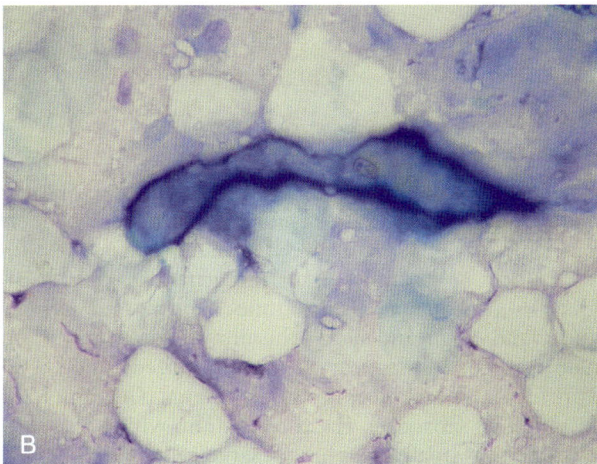

■ **FIGURE 3.108 Melanized pilomatricoma. Tissue aspirate. Dog.** Same case in A and B. **A,** Keratinized squamous epithelium admixed with pigmented keratinocytes. (Modified Wright; LP.) **B,** Higher magnification of a small nonpigmented keratin strand against the background of pale squamous epithelium. (Modified Wright; HP oil.)

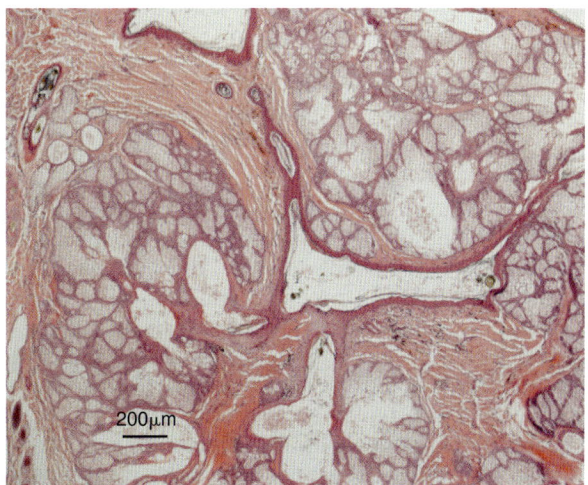

■ **FIGURE 3.111 Sebaceous adenoma. Tissue section.** A macroscopic polypoid skin mass consists of sebaceous lobules, dilated ducts, and areas of cystic degeneration of sebaceous cells. Lack of orientation of lobules around ducts supports the diagnosis of adenomatous growth rather than hyperplasia. (H&E; LP.)

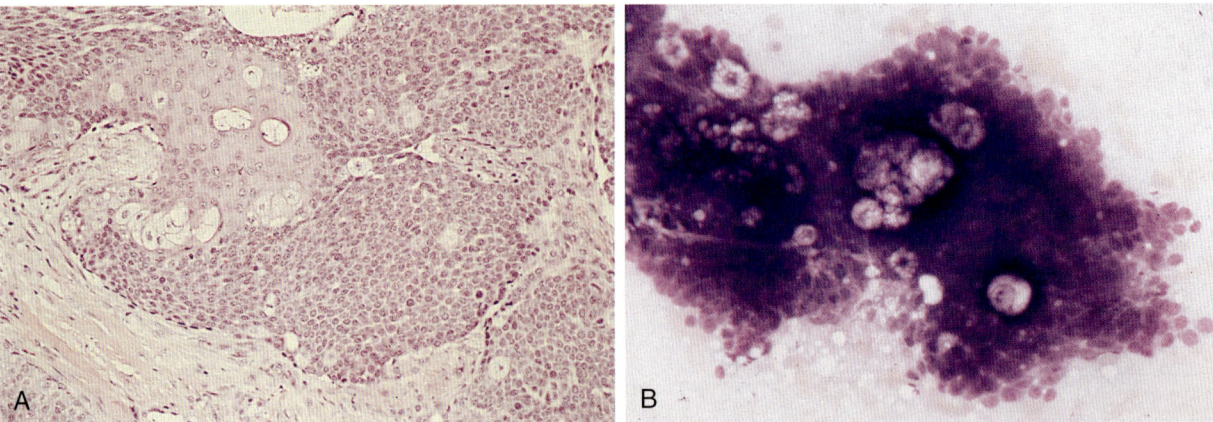

■ **FIGURE 3.112 Sebaceous epithelioma. Dog.** Same case in A and B. **A, Tissue section.** Dermal ear mass composed of lobules and islands of neoplastic basal epithelium with occasional foci of sebocytes and keratinocytes. (H&E; IP.) **B, Tissue aspirate.** Clusters of basal epithelium with scattered sebocytes are shown in this shoulder mass. Six months later, this mass was diagnosed as basal cell carcinoma because of progressive infiltration into subcutaneous tissues. (Wright-Giemsa; IP.)

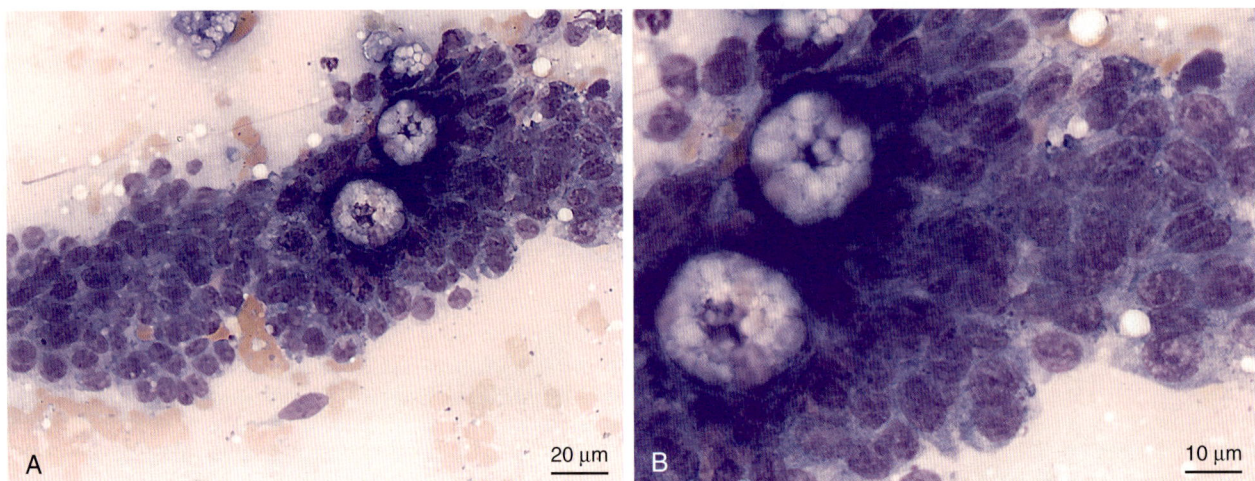

■ **FIGURE 3.113 Sebaceous epithelioma. Ear mass. Tissue aspirate. Dog.** Same case in A and B. **A,** This 1 cm pedunculated, lobulated mass on the inner pinna yielded a population of mildly atypical basilar epithelial cells present in large cell clusters. (Wright-Giemsa; HP oil.) **B,** High magnification shows the scattered mature sebocytes within the basilar epithelium. (Wright-Giemsa; HP oil.) (Courtesy Kellie Whipple, University of Florida.)

Sebaceous Carcinoma

Sebaceous carcinoma is an uncommon tumor found most frequently on the head of dogs. Cocker spaniels appear predisposed. It presents as a rapidly growing, large, ulcerated, poorly circumscribed mass. On cytopathologic specimens, pleomorphic glandular epithelial cells display malignant nuclear features such as anisokaryosis, prominent nucleoli, and frequent atypical mitotic figures. The finely vacuolated cytoplasm suggests sebaceous differentiation (Figs. 3.114 and 3.115). This malignant tumor is usually locally invasive but may occasionally metastasize to regional lymph nodes. Treatment consists of wide surgical excision. Prognosis is good.

Cytopathologic differential diagnosis: squamous cell carcinoma.

Perianal Gland Adenoma and Carcinoma

Perianal gland adenoma is a very common tumor mainly associated with intact male dogs, suggesting androgen dependency. Perianal gland tumors are rarely found in cats. The tumor may be single or multiple, occurring generally near the anus (Fig. 3.116), but it may also be found on the tail, perineum, prepuce, and thigh and along the dorsal or ventral midline. Initially, they grossly appear as smooth, raised round lesions that are lobulated and ulcerate as they enlarge. The tumor arises from modified sebaceous gland epithelium within the dermis that is lined by small basophilic reserve cells (Fig. 3.117). On cytopathology, sheets of mature, round hepatoid cells predominate characterized by abundant, finely granular, pinkish-blue cytoplasm (Fig. 3.118). Nuclei resemble those of normal hepatocytes, appearing round with an often single or multiple,

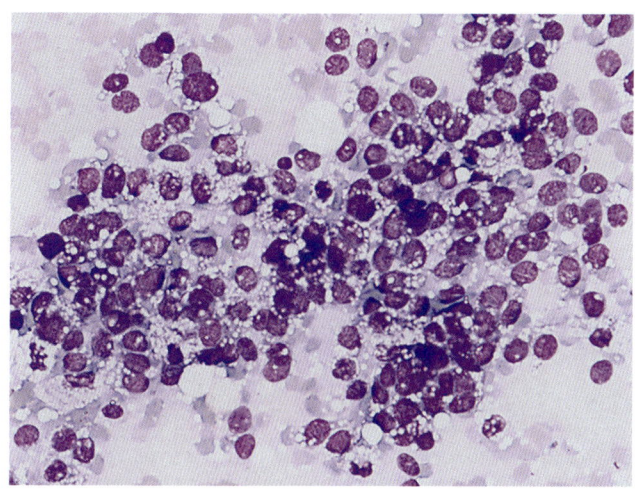

■ **FIGURE 3.114 Sebaceous carcinoma. Tissue aspirate. Dog.** A monomorphic population of cohesive cells in sheets and clumps noted in the shoulder mass. Malignant features include a high nucleocytoplasmic ratio, anisokaryosis, multinucleation, clumped chromatin, and prominent variable nucleoli. The cytoplasm is basophilic, with frequent clear, punctate vacuoles, suggestive of sebaceous differentiation. Histopathology confirmed the diagnosis. (Wright-Giemsa; HP oil.)

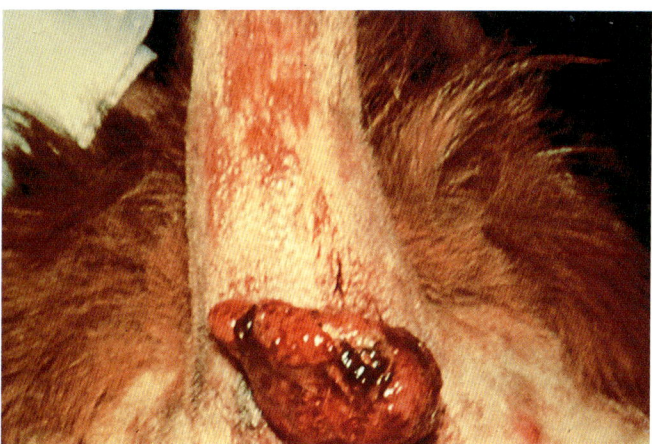

■ **FIGURE 3.116 Perianal gland tumor. Anal mass. Macroscopic specimen. Dog.** Large ulcerated mass present under the tail near the anus. (Courtesy Colin Burrows, University of Florida.)

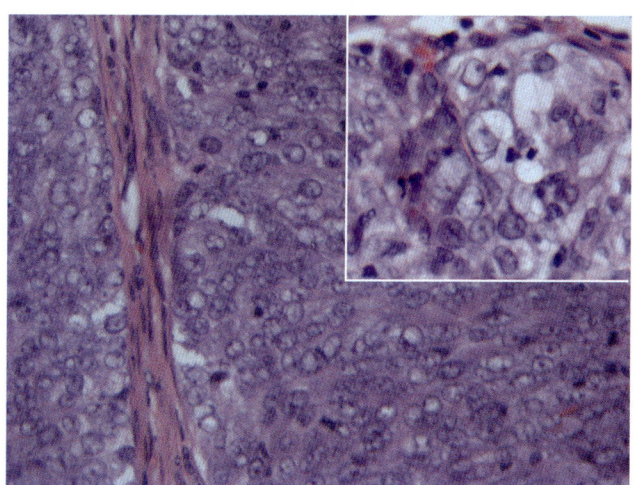

■ **FIGURE 3.115 Sebaceous carcinoma. Chin mass. Tissue section. Cat.** Fine fibrovascular stroma separate the malignant epithelial cell population into lobules. Numerous mitotic figures are scattered throughout, supporting malignancy. (H&E; IP.) *Inset:* Higher magnification of the same image demonstrates the focal vacuolated cytoplasm supportive of sebaceous origin. (Courtesy Mark Bennett, University of Bristol, UK.)

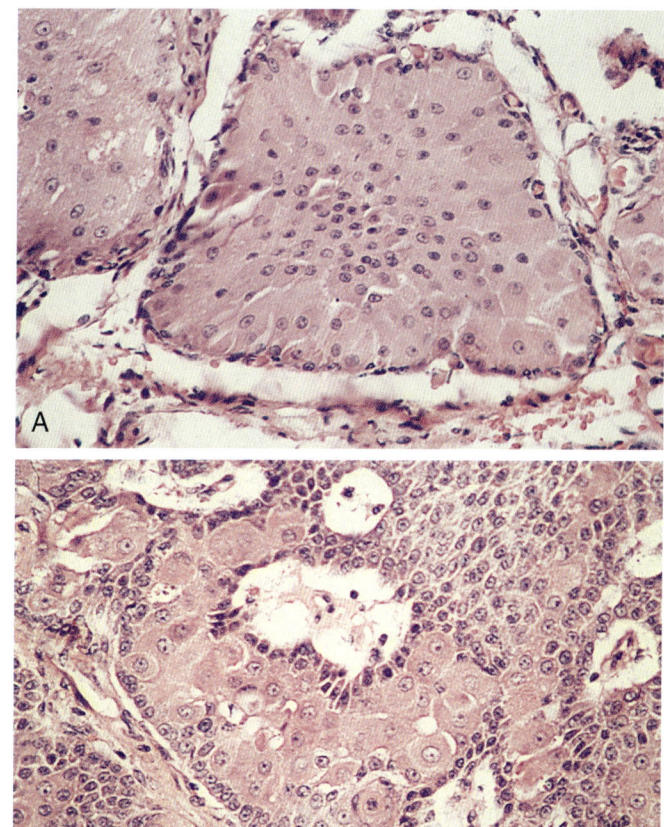

■ **FIGURE 3.117 Perianal gland tissue. Dog.** Same case in A and B. **A, Normal histology.** Within an unaffected area of tissue, the hepatoid cells, which are packets of modified sebaceous epithelium, display a uniform low nucleocytoplasmic ratio. Lining this glandular tissue are a low number of small basophilic reserve cells. (H&E; IP.) **B, Perianal gland adenoma. Tissue section.** In the affected region, there is a well-circumscribed lesion consisting of islands of polygonal hepatoid cells with mild to moderate anisocytosis with a dense proliferation of small basal reserve cells in the upper right area. (H&E; IP.)

prominent nucleolus. A low number of smaller basophilic reserve cells having a high nucleocytoplasmic ratio may also be present, but these lack features of cellular pleomorphism, Less commonly, a neoplasm of mixed hepatoid and basaloid or predominately reserve cells may occur (Fig. 3.119). Perianal gland adenomas are benign tumors that respond to surgical excision or cryosurgery, coupled with castration. Prognosis is good to excellent.

Perianal epithelioma is a low-grade malignancy that contains a preponderance of reserve cells (Fig. 3.120). Histologically,

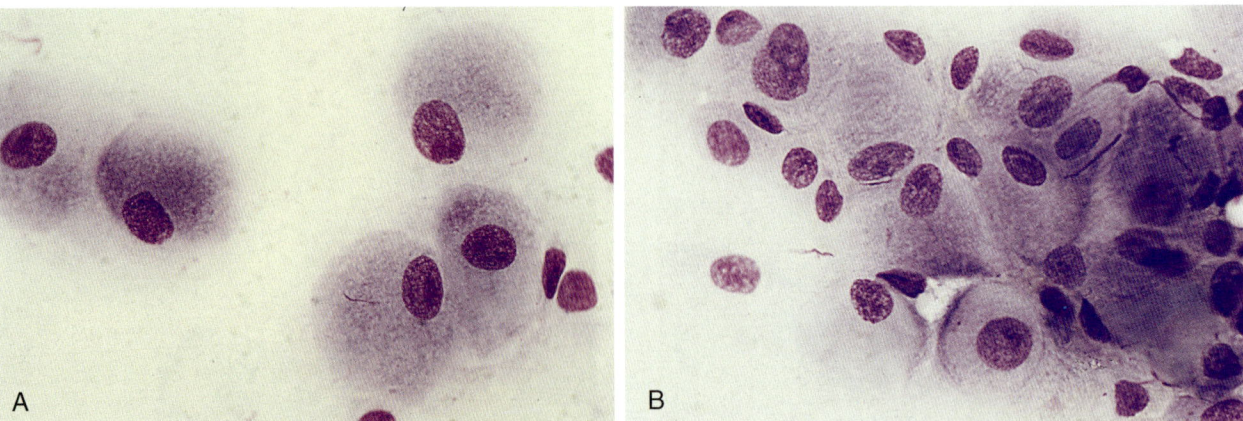

■ **FIGURE 3.118 Perianal gland adenoma. Tissue aspirate. Dog.** Same case in A and B. **A,** Individual hepatoid cells display a small, round nucleus and abundant pink-blue, finely granular cytoplasm. (Aqueous Romanowsky; HP oil.) **B,** Smaller basophilic reserve cells are interspersed between hepatoid cells. (Aqueous Romanowsky; HP oil.)

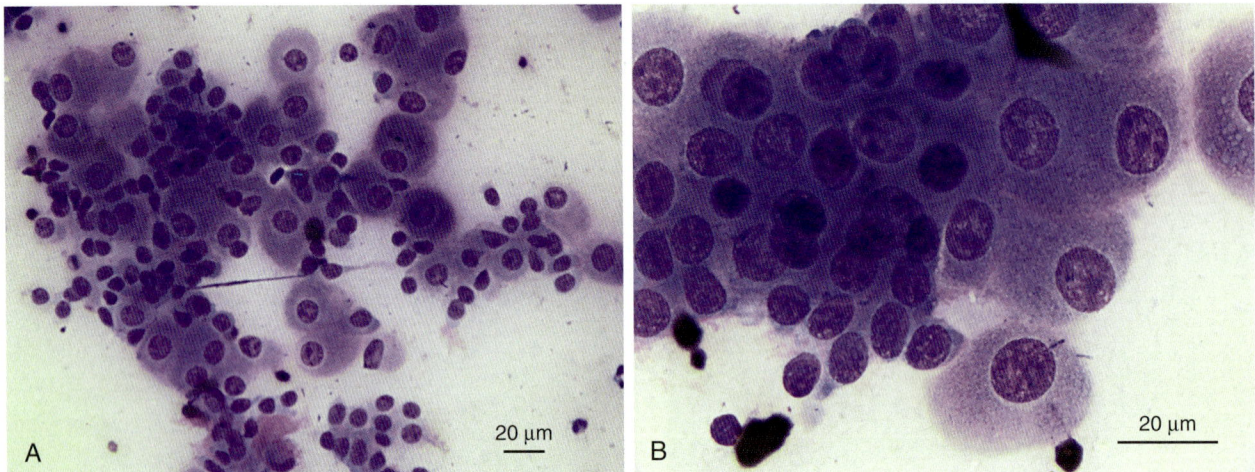

■ **FIGURE 3.119 Perianal gland adenoma. Cutaneous anal mass. Tissue aspirate. Dog.** Same case in A and B. **A,** There are two populations of cells in roughly equal proportions. One population consists of small (1.5 size of erythrocyte or 10 μm) round to oval nuclei with scant to moderate lightly basophilic cytoplasm that appear to form tight junctions. The nucleocytoplasmic ratio of these reserve cells is high, and only mild anisokaryosis is present. The second population consists of large hepatoid cells (30–35 μm in diameter) with round to oval nuclei (15 μm in diameter) having a single prominent central nucleolus along and abundant amphophilic (pink-blue) lightly granular cytoplasm. There is moderate anisokaryosis and occasional binucleation in this modified sebaceous gland epithelium. (Aqueous Romanowsky; IP.) **B,** Higher magnification shows cellular detail of the described cell populations. (Aqueous Romanowsky; HP oil.)

these appear unencapsulated and reserve cells display little nuclear atypia.

The malignant counterpart of this tumor may have a benign cytopathologic appearance, so histopathology is advised (McCourt et al., 2018). The percentage of reserve cells has no relevance in the determination of malignancy (Evans et al., 2018). In one cytopathologic study of perianal gland adenocarcinoma, nuclear pleomorphism was noted with anisokaryosis and coarse chromatin in reserve cells, and difficulty in distinguishing hepatoid from reserve cells helped determine perianal adenocarcinoma on cytopathology (Sabattini et al., 2019). The study also found in perianal adenocarcinoma that hepatoid cells were commonly vacuolated. The most common presenting signs are an ulcerated mass, perirectal pain or irritation, and tenesmus. Approximately 15% of malignancies show clinical evidence of metastasis at the time of diagnosis. The use of claudin-4 immunohistochemistry has been shown to be helpful in distinguishing between the positive expression of normal, hyperplastic, and neoplastic hepatoid cells and the negative expression by reserve cell-rich epitheliomas of the canine perianal gland (Jakab et al., 2009).

> ***Cytopathologic differential diagnosis:*** perianal gland hyperplasia, perianal gland epithelioma, well-differentiated perianal gland carcinoma.

Apocrine Gland Anal Sac Adenocarcinoma

There is an increased incidence of apocrine gland anal sac adenocarcinoma (AGASACA) in older, spayed female dogs, but a sex predilection has not been confirmed (Goldschmidt and

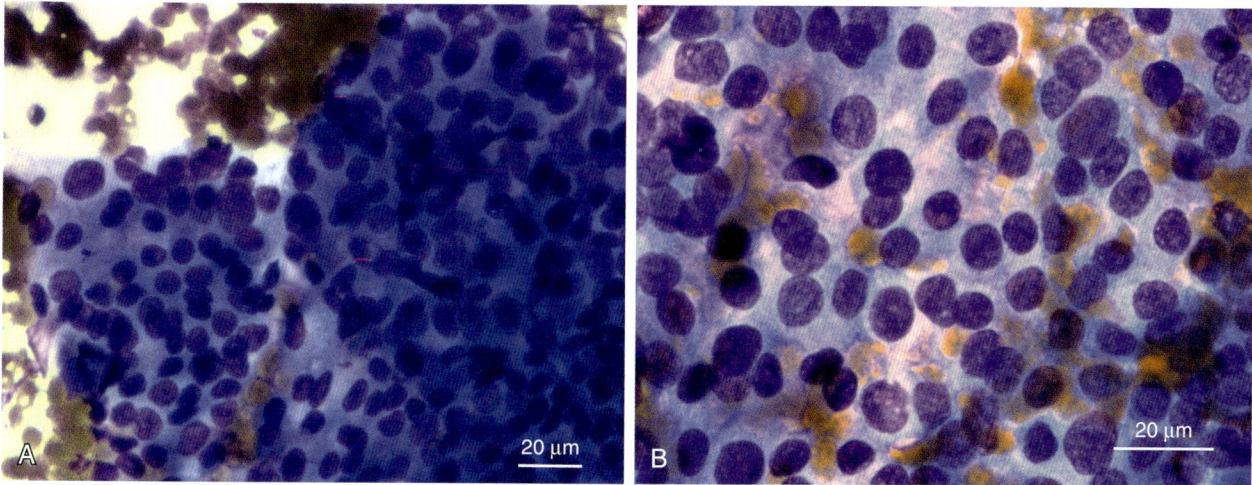

■ **FIGURE 3.120 Perianal gland epithelioma. Tissue aspirate. Dog.** Same case in A and B. **A,** Predominance of proliferative basal or reserve cells as a tight cell cluster. (Wright-Giemsa; HP oil.) **B,** Well-spread field composed entirely of reserve cells with small nucleoli and dense chromatin. (Wright-Giemsa; HP oil.)

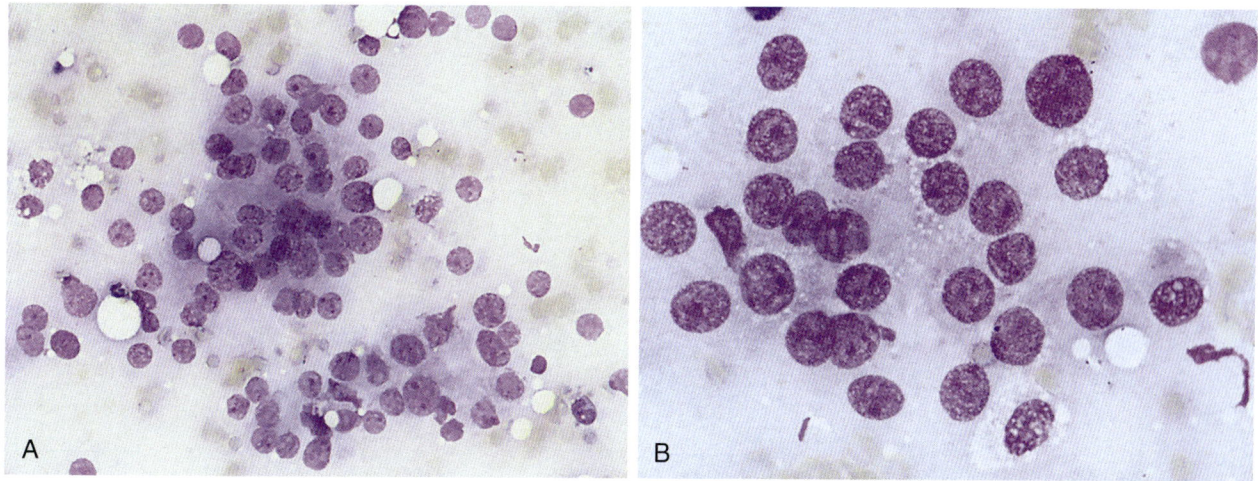

■ **FIGURE 3.121 Apocrine gland anal sac adenocarcinoma. Tissue aspirate. Dog.** Same case in A and B. **A,** Loosely cohesive cell clusters with indistinct cell borders resembling a naked nuclei appearance. (Wright-Giemsa; HP oil.) **B,** Malignant features include high and variable nucleocytoplasmic ratios, anisokaryosis, coarse chromatin, and prominent nucleoli. (Wright-Giemsa; HP oil.)

Shofer, 1992). The majority of cases involve dogs, but occasional cases have been reported in cats. Grossly, this is a subcutaneous mass firmly fixed around the anal sac that arises from the apocrine glands in the wall of these sacs. A paraneoplastic syndrome of hypercalcemia is associated with 50% to 90% of cases, which may result in renal disease (Ross et al., 1991).

Dense cell clusters with a papillary shape have poorly defined cell borders in the solid and anaplastic forms of AGASACA, often resembling a naked nuclei cytomorphology of neoplasia (Fig. 3.121A). Malignant characteristics are easily detected in glandular epithelium, which displays cellular and nuclear pleomorphism, a high nucleocytoplasmic ratio and, in some cases, multiple small cytoplasmic vacuoles (Fig. 3.121B). An acinar or rosette arrangement may be detected to aid in the diagnosis and distinguish it from perianal (hepatoid) carcinoma (Fig. 3.122). Recently, attention was given to a spindle cell form of AGASACA (Fig. 3.123), which may confound the diagnosis because its appearance is uncommon and suggests sarcoma. However, the spindle-shaped cells are not reactive to vimentin or desmin but are reactive to markers for epithelium and epithelial mucin or anal sac apocrine glandular material such as cytokeratin (clone CAM 5.2) and paradoxical concanavalin A (P-Con A) staining (Sakai et al., 2012). Treatment consists of wide surgical excision with postoperative radiation therapy. These malignant tumors commonly metastasize initially to regional lymph nodes. Prognosis is poor to fair.

Cytopathologic differential diagnosis: perianal gland carcinoma.

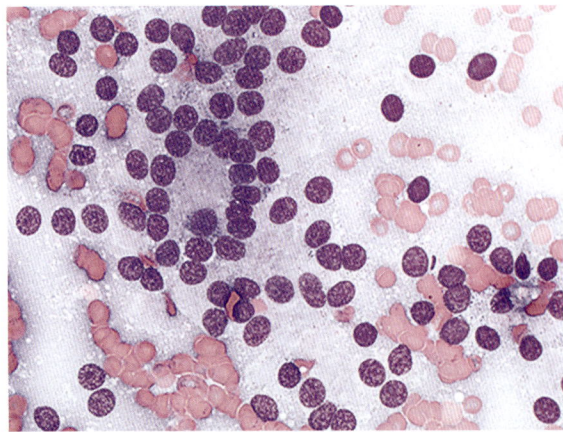

■ **FIGURE 3.122 Apocrine gland anal sac adenocarcinoma. Tissue aspirate. Dog.** An acinar arrangement with nuclei peripheralized within a loose sheet of cells helps diagnose this anal mass of glandular origin. Most cells embedded in pale basophilic cytoplasmic material appear lysed, as free nuclei that measure roughly one to two times the size of an erythrocyte with coarsely stippled chromatin and mild anisokaryosis. The diagnosis was confirmed by surgical excision and histopathologic evaluation. (Wright-Giemsa; HP oil.)

Sweat Gland Tumors

Of the benign sweat gland tumors found in dogs and cats, most commonly encountered are the apocrine cyst and apocrine ductular adenoma compared with the infrequent apocrine cystadenoma and apocrine secretory adenoma. Cyst cavities lined by cuboidal to columnar cells that contain granular secretory product may be seen with apocrine cystadenoma (Fig. 3.124). The use of immunohistochemistry may help distinguish glandular from ductular portions of apocrine glands (Kok et al., 2018).

Many apocrine ductular adenomas, especially those in cats, were previously classified as cystic basal cell tumors (Gross et al., 2005). These are noted by the solid basilar epithelium and cystic histologic appearances (Fig. 3.125). Necrotic cyst material may undergo dystrophic mineralization. Apocrine duct adenomas in dogs may contain abundant secretions with cholesterol crystals (Fig. 3.126A), which appear as clefts on histology (Fig. 3.126B). Although ductal epithelium may appear mildly anaplastic on cytopathology, these well-demarcated adenomas contain only occasional mitotic figures and are best confirmed by histopathology (Fig. 3.126C).

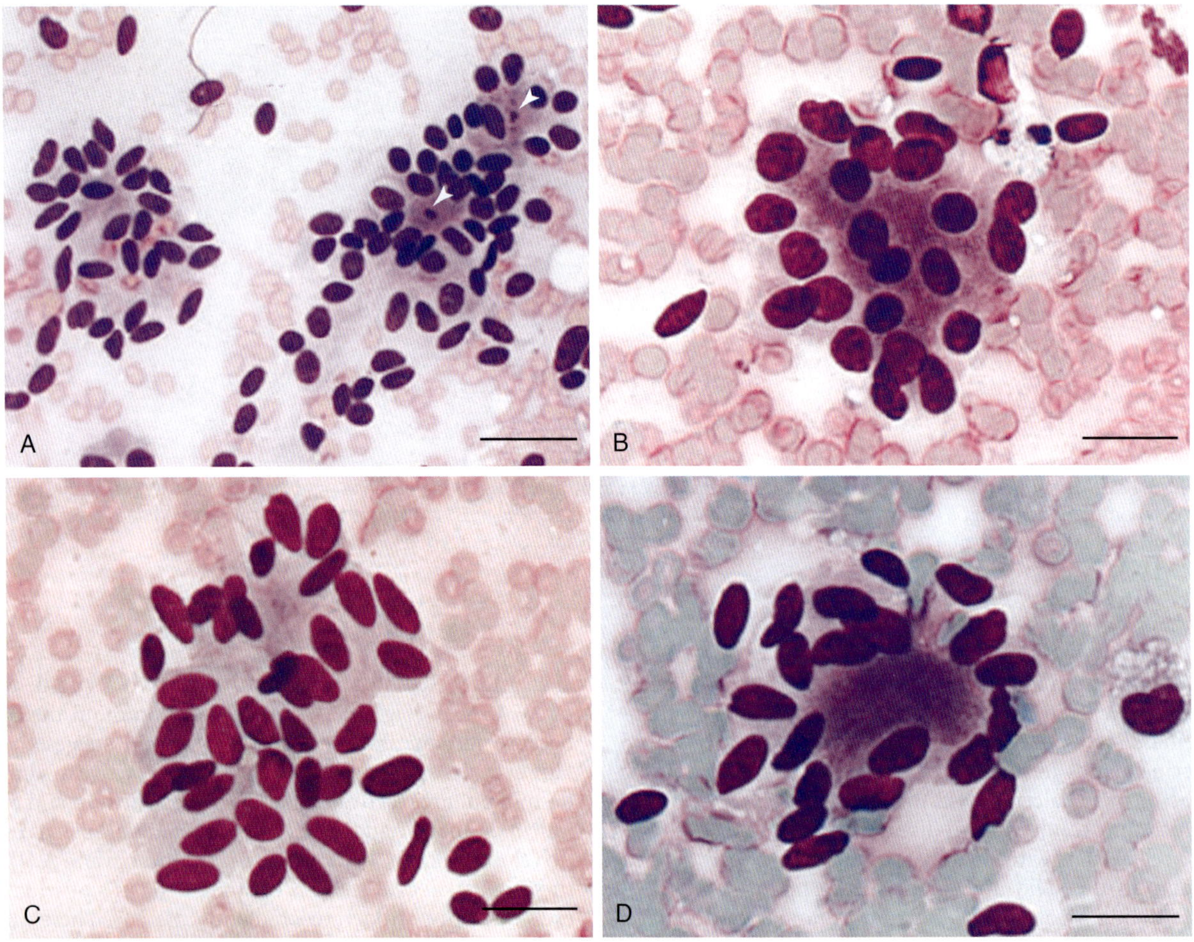

■ **FIGURE 3.123 Apocrine gland anal sac adenocarcinoma, spindle cell variant. Tissue imprint. Dog.** Impression smears of core biopsy samples of subcutaneous mass near the anus of an intact female dog. Hemacolor stain. **A,** Cells with elliptical nuclei are present in clusters. Some cells are radially arranged around small lumina that contain eosinophilic material *(arrowheads)*. Bar, 50 μm. **B,** Neoplastic cells with round nuclei and pale to basophilic cytoplasm with indistinct borders from a cluster. Bar, 20 μm. **C,** Spindle cells have pale cytoplasm with indistinct borders, fine homogenous chromatin, and a small indistinct nucleolus or no nucleolus. Mild anisokaryosis and anisocytosis are noted. Bar, 20 μm. **D,** Some spindle cells are radially arranged. Bar, 20 μm. (From Sakai H, Murakami M, Mishima H, et al. Cytologically atypical anal sac adenocarcinoma in a dog. *Vet Clin Pathol.* 2012;41:291–294.)

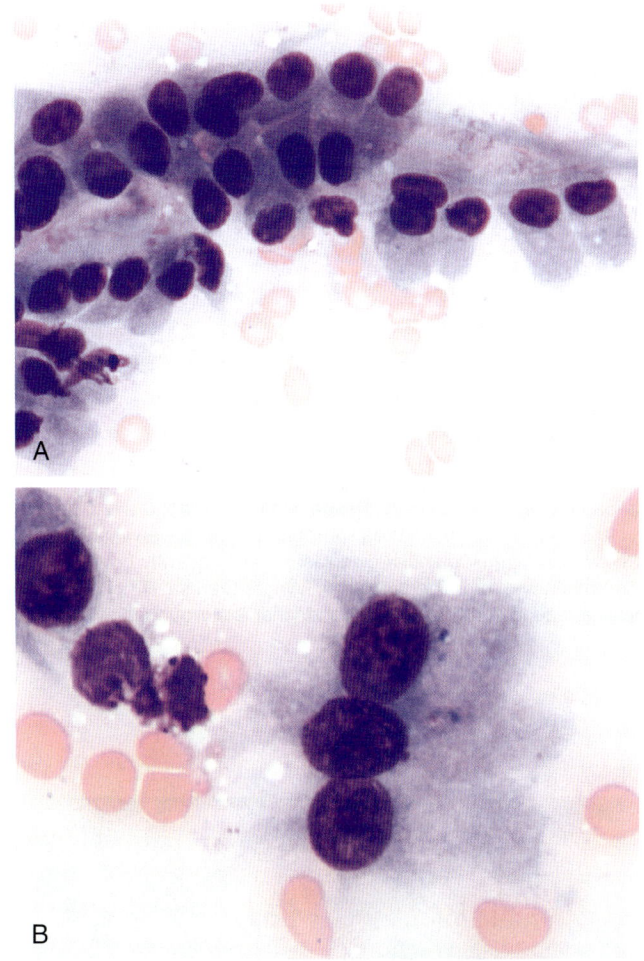

■ **FIGURE 3.124 Apocrine cystadenoma. Tissue aspirate. Dog.** Same case in A and B. **A,** Uniform population of cuboidal to low-columnar epithelium is present. Note the basilar location of the round nucleus. (Wright-Giemsa; HP oil.) **B,** The epithelial cells contain a dark, granular secretory material. (Wright-Giemsa; HP oil.)

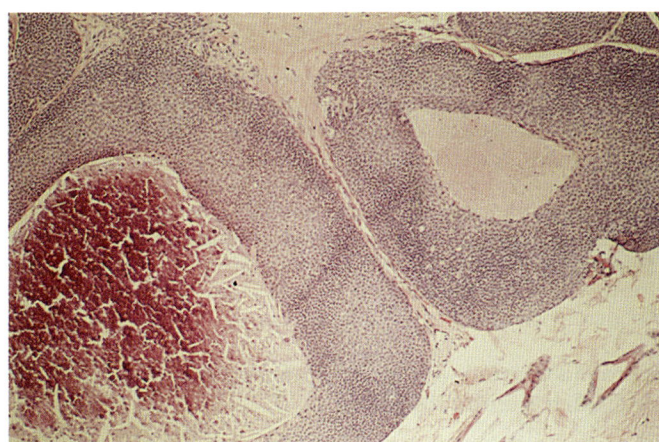

■ **FIGURE 3.125 Apocrine duct adenoma. Tissue section. Cat.** Head mass with basal epithelium proliferation surrounding centers containing cholesterol, calcium deposits, or liquefactive material. Masses of this nature were previously termed cystic basal cell tumor, which is no longer recognized as appropriate. (H&E; LP.)

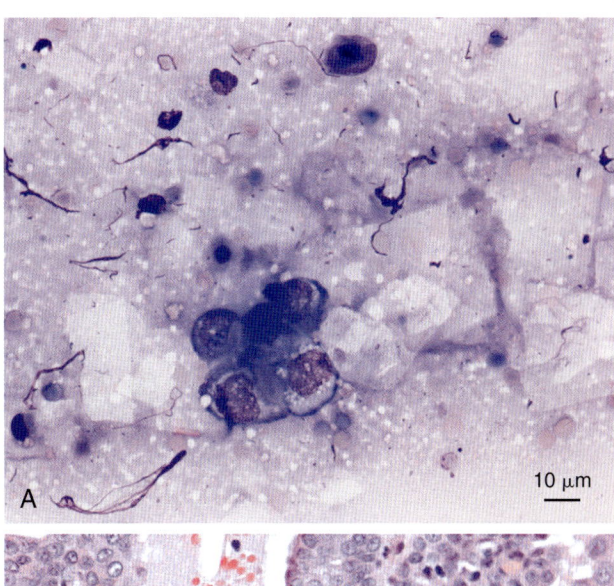
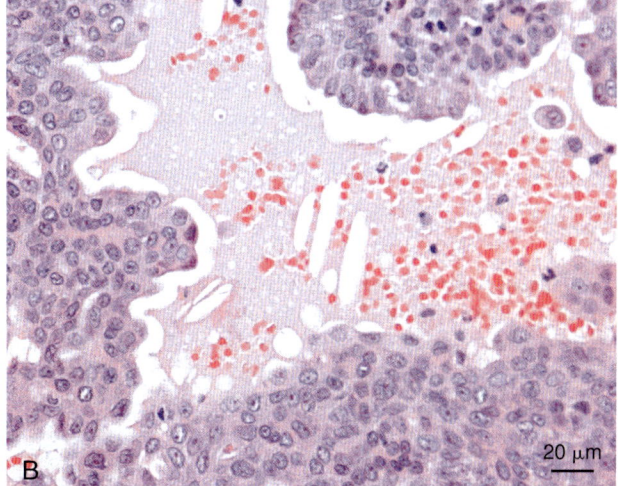
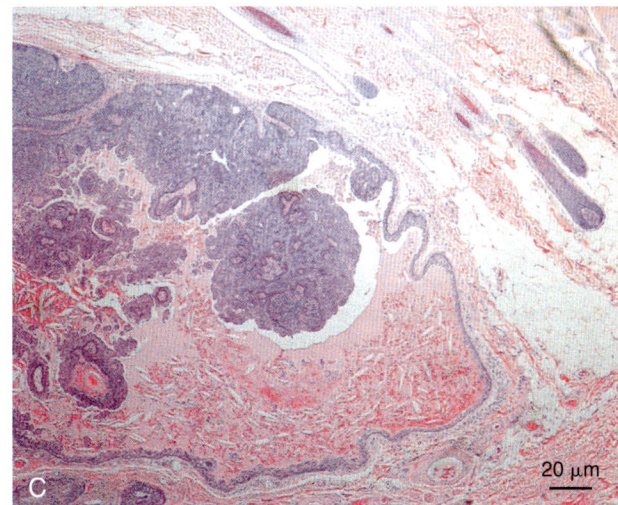

■ **FIGURE 3.126 Apocrine gland duct adenoma. Dog.** Same case in A to C. **A, Tissue aspirate.** Background consists of cholesterol crystals and granular basophilic material along with a cluster of duct epithelium. (Modified Wright; HP oil.) **B–C, Tissue section. B,** Higher magnification of ductular material showing cholesterol clefts (clear white angular structures) with blood and secretory granular substance. (H&E; IP.) **C,** Low-power magnification to demonstrate the single layer of ductular epithelium increasing in thickness and becoming adenomatous on the *upper left side*. (H&E; LP.)

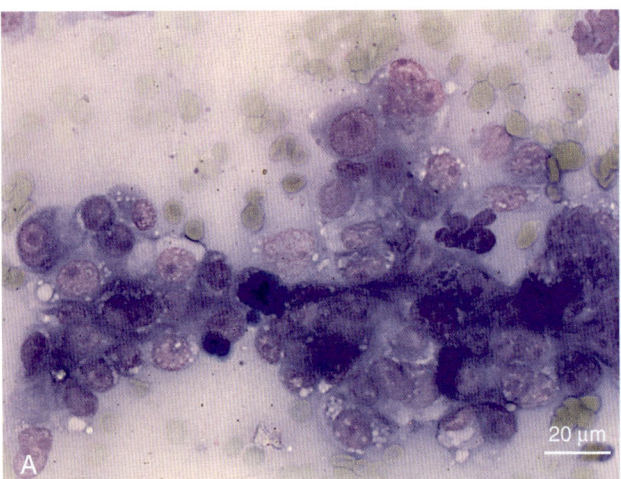
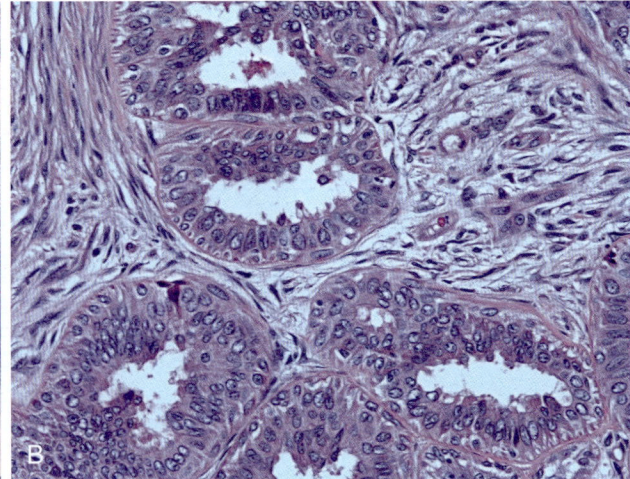

■ **FIGURE 3.127 Apocrine adenocarcinoma. Preputial dermal mass. Dog.** Same case in A and B. **A, Tissue aspirate.** The 2.0 × 2.0 cm firm, freely movable mass yielded a malignant epithelial cell population arranged in cohesive clusters. These cells are round or oval, have variably distinct cytoplasmic borders, and generally have a scant to moderate amount of basophilic and slightly granular cytoplasm that frequently contains small numerous punctate colorless vacuoles. One or more round nuclei have coarse chromatin with prominent nucleoli. (Wright-Giemsa; HP oil.) **B, Tissue section.** The multilobulated dermal mass is composed of malignant epithelial cells arranged around ductular glands that is surrounded by moderate to extensive desmoplasia (i.e., fibroplasia around carcinoma). (H&E; IP.)

Malignant sweat gland tumor is an uncommon apocrine secretory adenocarcinoma, accounting for up to 2% to 3% of skin tumors of dogs and cats, respectively (Gross et al., 2005). It is often located on the back, flanks, and feet of dogs and presents as a solitary, raised, well-circumscribed, and solid mass that often ulcerates. In older cats, most occur on the head and limbs, appearing as a solid, nodular mass. An alternate form observed in dogs and cats is an ulcerative, hemorrhagic, and frequently inflamed lesion that resembles acute dermatitis. Ductular epithelium is present as clusters of basophilic cells that display numerous criteria of malignancy in cytopathologic specimens (Fig. 3.127A). In some cases, significant fibroplasia occurs, so aspirates may yield fibroblasts along with epithelium (Fig. 3.127B). Treatment consists of wide surgical excision. Prognosis is fair to guarded because local recurrence and metastasis have been reported.

Cytopathologic differential diagnosis: mammary gland adenocarcinoma, anal sac adenocarcinoma, other adenocarcinomas, cutaneous basilar epithelial neoplasms.

Clear Cell Adnexal Carcinoma

This is an undifferentiated adnexal neoplasm that is slow growing and treated by surgical excision. Cells may resemble balloon cell malignant melanoma, so immunohistochemistry is necessary to confirm the diagnosis (Piviani et al., 2012). The cytopathologic appearance involves high cellularity, moderate to marked cellular pleomorphism, multinucleation, loose arrangement of individualized neoplastic cells, and a background containing ruptured cell cytoplasm that is blue-gray and granular (Fig. 3.128). Neoplastic cells are oval to polygonal to spindle shaped with wispy cytoplasmic borders. Criteria of malignancy are present, although the nucleocytoplasmic ratio is low. Nuclei are round to ovoid with coarse chromatin with prominent nucleoli often eccentrically placed.

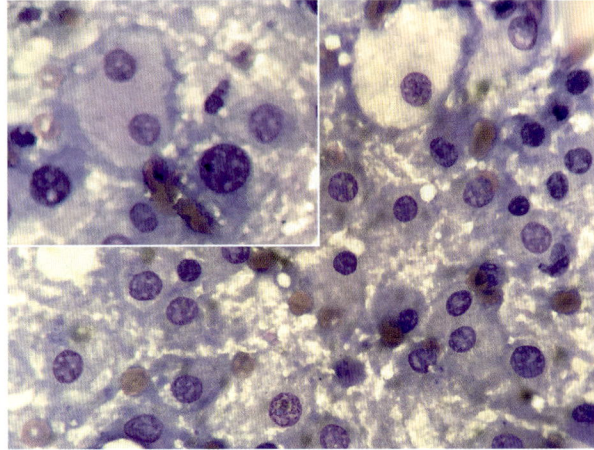

■ **FIGURE 3.128 Dog. Clear cell adnexal carcinoma. Thigh mass. Tissue aspirate. Dog.** There is high cellularity of moderately pleomorphic polygonal cells with a nucleus 1.5 to 2.5 × red blood cell diameter, multinucleation, coarse chromatin, small distinct nucleolus, and variably abundant blue-gray foamy cytoplasm. The neoplastic cells are arranged loosely against a background containing cellular debris and lipid droplets. This neoplasm is similar in morphology to balloon cell melanoma (Modified Wright; HP oil.) *Inset:* Higher magnification to demonstrate binucleation, moderate anisokaryosis, and wispy cytoplasmic borders. (Courtesy Robert Lukacs, TDDS/Synlab, Exeter, UK.)

Cutaneous Metastatic Carcinomas

Primary carcinomas that may metastasize to the skin via hematogenous or lymphatic routes include a duodenal adenocarcinoma (Juopperi et al., 2003), bronchogenic adenocarcinoma (Petterino et al., 2005), urothelial carcinoma from the bladder and prostate (Di Maria et al., 2020), and seminoma. Implantation

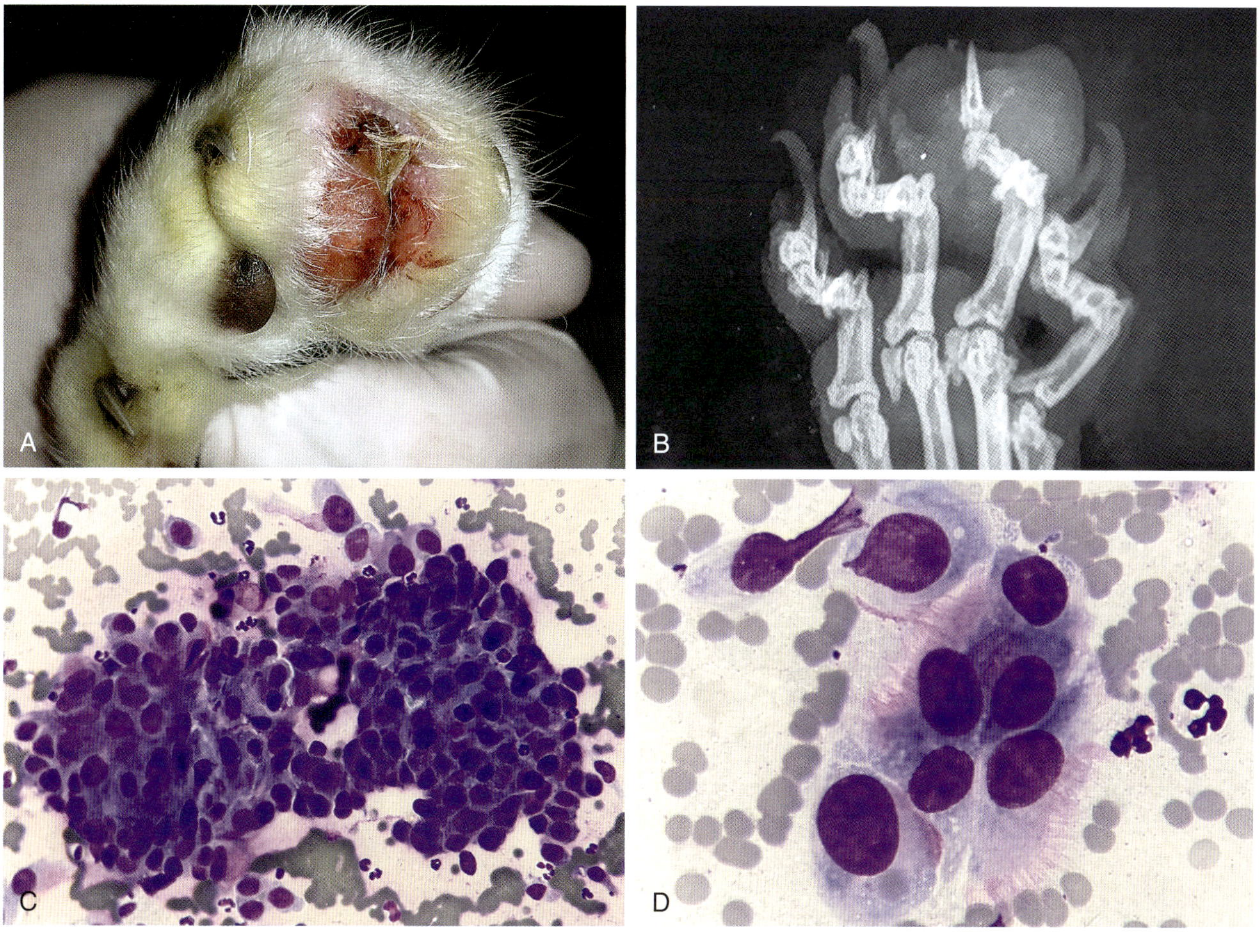

■ **FIGURE 3.129 MODAL (muscle, ocular, digit, aorta, lung) syndrome. Digit mass. Tissue aspirate. Cat.** Same case in A to D. **A,** Single ulcerated digit lesion. **B,** Mild osteolysis of the third phalanx and soft tissue swelling are evident on the radiograph of the digit. **C,** Moderately atypical epithelial cells are seen arranged in variably sized, cohesive sheets. (Aqueous Romanowsky; HP oil.) **D,** When individualized, a ciliated border is appreciated on the metastatic pulmonary epithelium. Further diagnostics should include thoracic evaluation to confirm suspected pulmonary neoplasia. (Aqueous Romanowsky; HP oil.) (Courtesy Santiago Kujman, Mar del Plata, Argentina.)

via biopsy procedures or surgery may also be responsible for metastasis. In cats only, there is a well-recognized association between pulmonary adenocarcinoma with phalangeal metastasis known as feline lung-digit syndrome (Fig. 3.129) (Gross et al., 2005; Vobornik et al., 2014). Based on a wider range of affected metastatic tissues, a new mnemonic for this condition was suggested namely, MODAL syndrome (for muscle, ocular, digit, aorta, and lung) (Thrift et al., 2017). Cytopathologic features resemble those of the primary site often with cilia but may appear more anaplastic (Figs. 3.129D and 3.130). The digits are considered to have high blood flow to this region, accounting for this metastatic location. There may be bony lysis in addition to dermal infiltration. Despite amputation, prognosis is poor.

Mesenchymal Cytomorphology
Fibroma
Fibroma is an uncommon tumor of adult dogs and cats, accounting for approximately 1% of cutaneous neoplasms in dogs (Yager and Wilcock, 1994). It presents as a solitary lesion on the extremities, head, flanks, and groin. Grossly, it is firm to soft, well circumscribed, hairless, and dome shaped or pedunculated. On cytopathology, variable numbers of spindle or fusiform cells with small, uniform, dense oval nuclei occur individually or

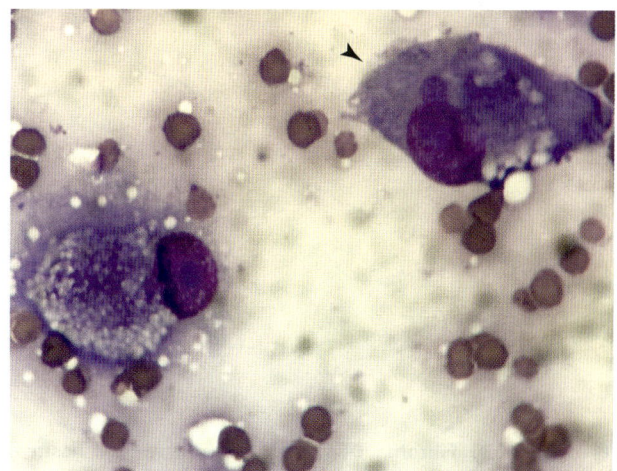

■ **FIGURE 3.130 MODAL (muscle, ocular, digit, aorta, lung) syndrome. Foreleg mass. Tissue aspirate. Cat.** Two atypical individualized columnar to ovoid epithelial cells are shown that have an abundant vacuolated to foamy basophilic cytoplasm. One cell displays cilia *(arrowhead)* on one edge of the cell. Because these are abnormal cells for this location, metastatic neoplasia should be considered. (Modified Wright; HP oil.) (Courtesy Matthew Harris, TDDS/Synlab, Exeter, UK.)

occasionally in small bundles. Generally, few cells exfoliate into cytopathologic preparations. Cytoplasm is lightly basophilic, and cell borders are poorly defined because they form cytoplasmic tails on opposite sides of the nucleus (Fig. 3.131A). Amorphous eosinophilic material representing intercellular collagen protein may be associated with the neoplastic cells. Histologically, spindle cells may be arranged loosely (Fig. 3.131B) or as dense collagen bundles that are found rarely on cytopathology (Fig. 3.131C). A subtype of fibroma termed *keloidal fibroma* contains abundant large hyalinized collagen fibers (Fig. 3.132). A rare subtype termed *fibromyxoma* has a mixture of both collagen and a mucinous matrix (Rosser et al., 2019). Fibromas are benign, and treatment consists of surgical excision. Prognosis is generally good except for occasional local recurrence after removal of large tumors.

> ***Cytopathologic differential diagnosis:*** myxoma, well-differentiated fibrosarcoma, neural sheath tumors, collagenous hamartoma, nodular dermatofibrosis.

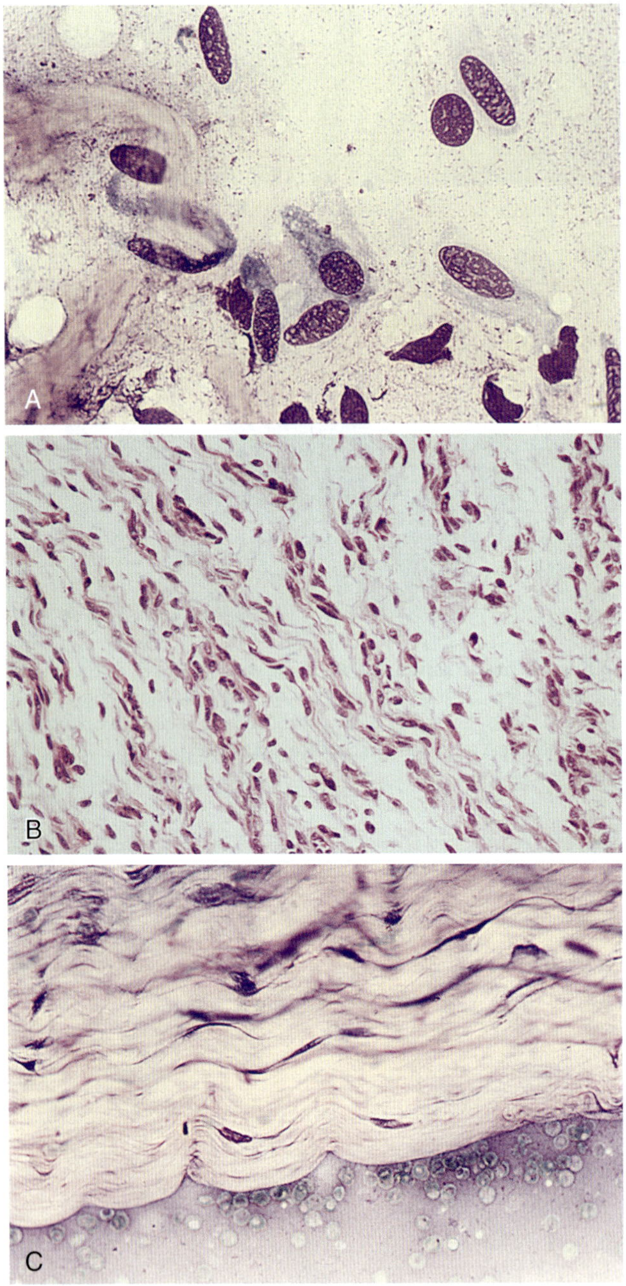

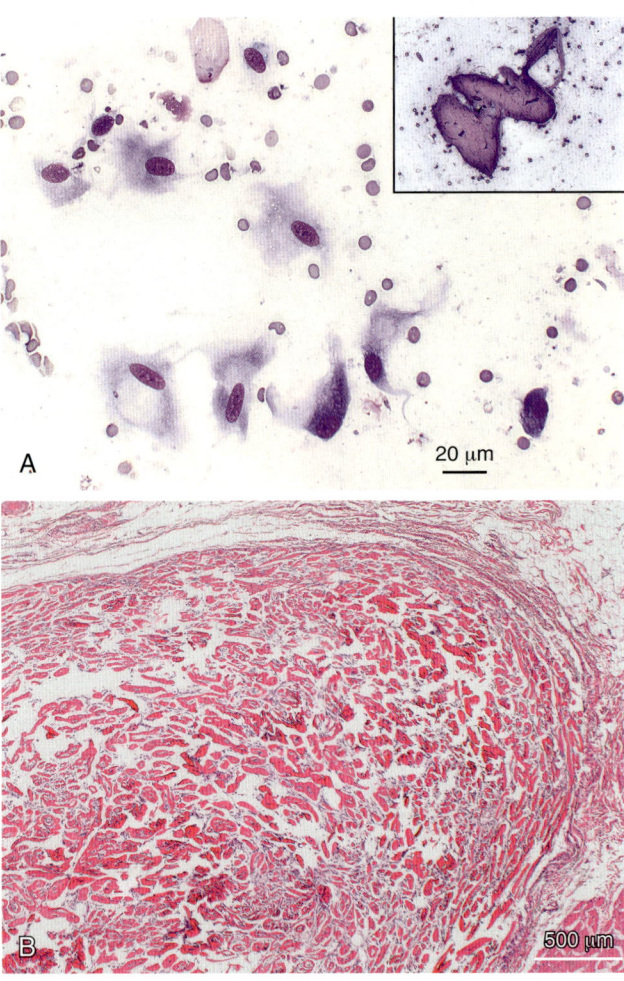

■ **FIGURE 3.131 Fibroma. Dog.** Same case in A to C. **A, Tissue imprint.** Spindle cells are present, with indistinct, lightly basophilic cytoplasm that extends from both ends of the oval nucleus. Note the amorphous eosinophilic material interspersed between cells from this metatarsal mass. (Aqueous Romanowsky; HP oil.) **B, Tissue section.** Loose proliferation of benign fibrocytes into wavy strands of collagen. (H&E; IP.) **C, Tissue imprint.** Dense bundles of collagen stained lightly pink, with basophilic oval nuclei enmeshed in the connective tissue. (Aqueous Romanowsky; HP oil.)

■ **FIGURE 3.132 Keloidal fibroma. Thoracic wall skin. Tissue aspirate. Dog.** Same case in A and B. **A,** The 1.0 cm subcutaneous nodule yielded a uniform mildly atypical mesenchymal cell population. The cells are mostly individualized, large, stellate to fusiform with indistinct cytoplasmic borders that frequently forms wispy projections. The oval or elongated nucleus measures 2 to 2.5 times the size of an erythrocyte, has coarsely stippled chromatin, and contains one or more, discernible nucleoli. The overall anisocytosis and anisokaryosis among this population are mild. (Wright-Giemsa; HP oil.) *Inset:* Focal dense aggregates and ribbons of hyalinized eosinophilic collagenous material are found on scanning. (Wright-Giemsa; IP.) **B, Tissue section.** The subcutaneous adipose tissue is expanded by a well-circumscribed, unencapsulated mass composed of mature fibrocytes surrounding abundant collagen fibers, some of which are broad, bright eosinophilic and hyalinized, and shiny. Mitotic figures are not noted. (H&E; LP.)

Fibrosarcoma

Fibrosarcoma is a common malignant tumor of dogs and cats; it is the fourth most common skin tumor in cats (Goldschmidt and Shofer, 1992), accounting for 15% to 17% of skin neoplasms. In young cats, it may be caused by the feline sarcoma virus and may be multiple. In older dogs and cats, fibrosarcomas are solitary with a predilection for the limbs, trunk, and head. They are poorly circumscribed and sometimes ulcerated (Fig. 3.133). They are invasive, and approximately 25% metastasize via hematogenous routes. Vaccine-induced fibrosarcomas, possibly related to subcutaneous-administered killed vaccines in cats, are locally invasive and aggressive (Gross et al., 2005).

On cytopathology, fibrosarcomas consist of abundant large, plump cells (Fig. 3.134) that occur individually or in aggregates often associated with pink, collagenous material. Multinucleate giant cells may be present occasionally. Nuclear pleomorphism may be marked compared with the benign counterpart. Cells are less uniform and generally have high nucleocytoplasmic ratios. Histopathology of conventional fibrosarcoma reveals intersecting bundles of spindle cells in herringbone fashion with minimal amounts of collagen (Fig. 3.135). In some cases, due to the amount of pink granular matrix and viscous nature of the material, these fibrosarcomas may resemble myxoid fibrosarcomas or myxosarcomas (Fig. 3.136).

An uncommon variant is the keloidal fibrosarcoma (Little and Goldschmidt, 2007; Evans et al., 2018). The characteristic feature is the abundance of dense hyalinized collagen bands seen on both histopathology and cytopathology associated with plump fibroblasts primarily with minimal inflammation (Figs. 3.137 to 3.139). These collagen bands closely resemble those fibers undergoing collagenolysis (termed *flame figures* on histology) in lesions associated with mast cells and eosinophilic inflammation, such as seen in MCTs (Fig. 3.140). However, the dense collagen in MCTs appears less eosinophilic and more

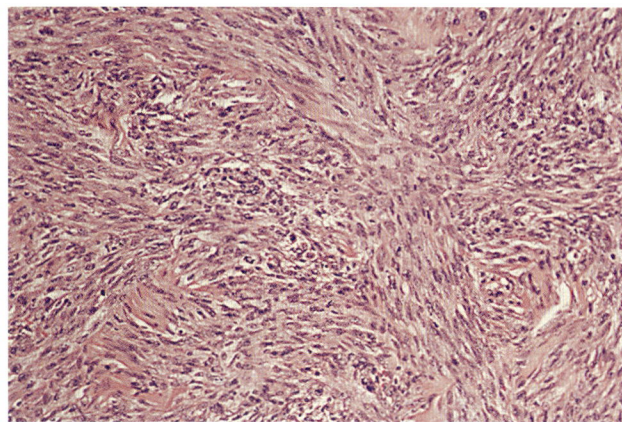

■ **FIGURE 3.135 Fibrosarcoma. Tissue section. Dog.** Broad interlacing bundles of spindle cells with malignant features are present. (H&E; IP.)

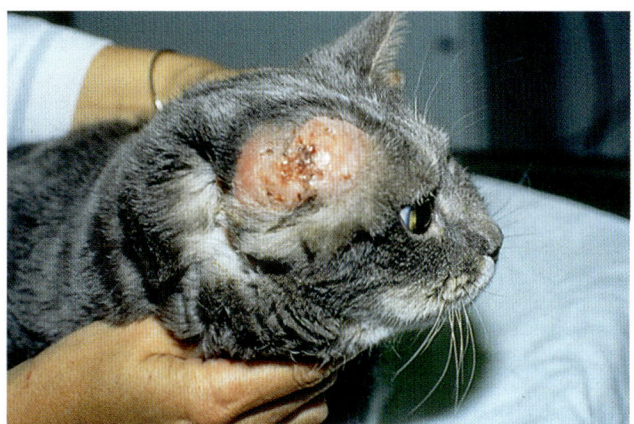

■ **FIGURE 3.133 Fibrosarcoma. Macroscopic specimen. Cat.** Recurrence of tumor in the site of previous surgery to remove the ear and surrounding tissue. (Courtesy Jamie Bellah, University of Florida.)

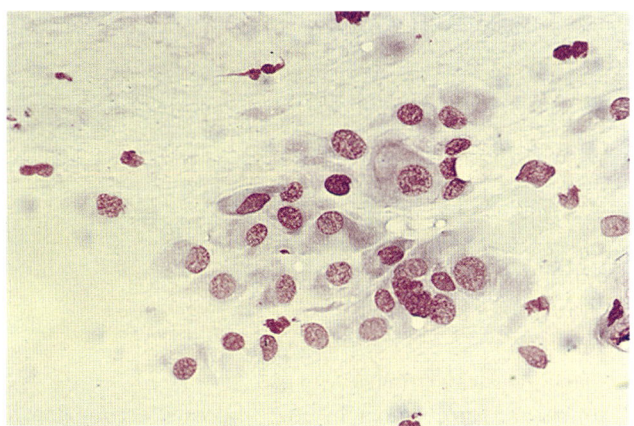

■ **FIGURE 3.134 Fibrosarcoma. Tissue aspirate. Cat.** Individualized plump oval cells with wispy cytoplasmic tails from a leg mass. Rare multinucleated cell noted as shown at *lower right*. (Aqueous Romanowsky; HP oil.)

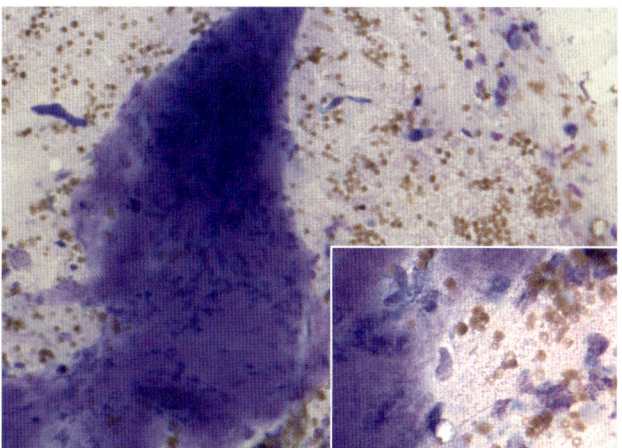

■ **FIGURE 3.136 Fibrosarcoma. Abdominal wall mass. Tissue aspirate. Cat.** This firm 8.0 × 3.0 cm subcutaneous mass yielded a mildly to moderately atypical mesenchymal cell population present in dense aggregates admixed with a moderate amount of bright eosinophilic extracellular matrix or as individual cells. These cells are oval to stellate to spindle shaped with a small to moderate amount of basophilic cytoplasm that frequently forms a wispy projection. (Wright-Giemsa; IP.) *Inset:* Higher magnification demonstrates the abundance of the eosinophilic granular matrix within the background. Myxosarcoma was a diagnostic differential. Histopathology supported the diagnosis of fibrosarcoma. (Wright-Giemsa; HP oil.)

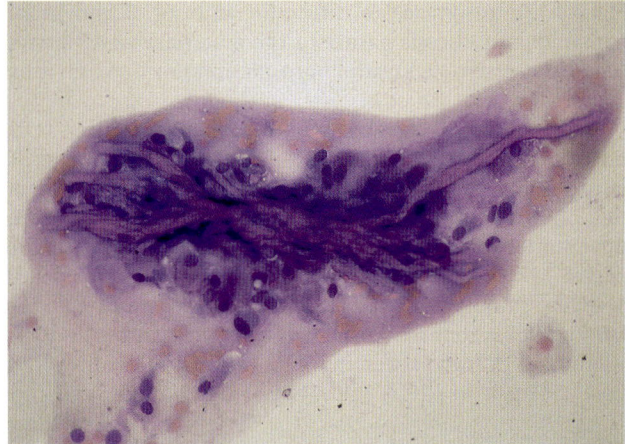

■ **FIGURE 3.137 Keloidal fibrosarcoma. Digital mass. Tissue aspirate. Dog.** This 2 × 2 cm subcutaneous nodule yielded a large number of pleomorphic fusiform and polygonal mesenchymal cells. These show moderate anisocytosis and anisokaryosis. Admixed with the cells are thick ribbons of hyalinized eosinophilic collagen. (Modified Wright; IP.) (Courtesy Oliver Coldrick, TDDS/Synlab, Exeter, UK.)

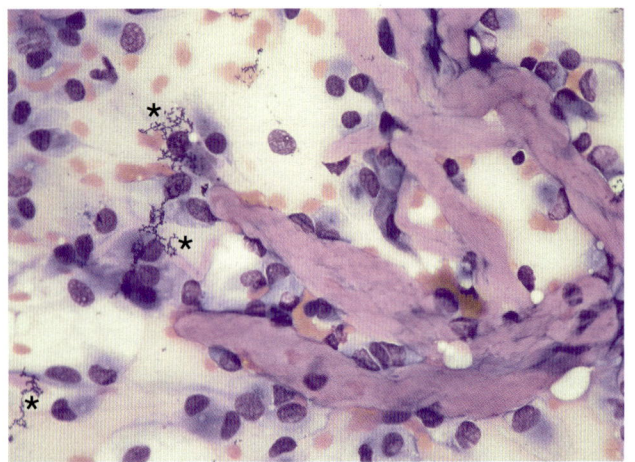

■ **FIGURE 3.138 Keloidal fibrosarcoma. Flank mass. Tissue aspirate. Dog.** This 1.5 cm soft subcutaneous mass adheres to deeper structures and yields numerous plump fibroblasts with round to oval nuclei. These cells have an oval to fusiform shape with wispy basophilic cytoplasmic borders. The characteristic feature is the abundance of dense hyalinized collagen bands without evidence of inflammation. Within the background are granular aggregates of stain precipitate *(asterisks)*, which should not be mistaken for bacteria. (Modified Wright; HP oil.) (Courtesy Clare Pitchford, TDDS/Synlab, Exeter, UK.)

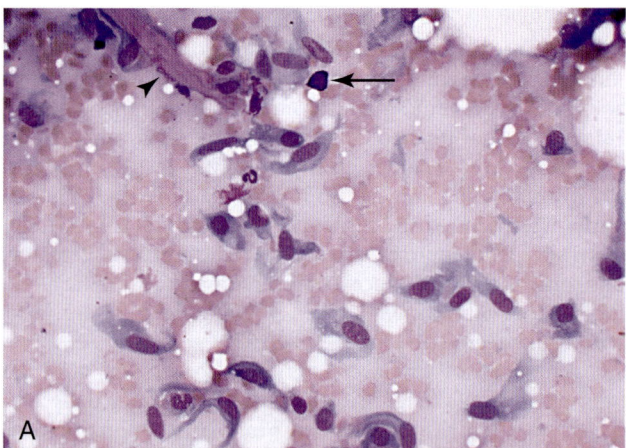

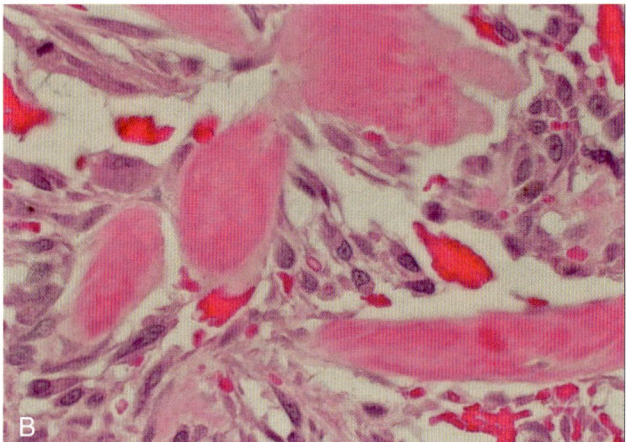

■ **FIGURE 3.139 Keloidal fibrosarcoma. Flank mass. Dog. A, Tissue aspirate.** A single 4 mm, nodular, firm, haired subcutaneous mass is evaluated. One dense linear band of hyalinized collagen *(arrowhead)* is shown closely associated with plump spindle cells. An occasional mast cell *(arrow)* is noted. (Wright-Giemsa; IP.) **B, Tissue section.** Among the dense collagen bands are immature fibroblasts, which have irregularly shaped nuclei with open chromatin and generally one prominent nucleolus. (H&E; IP.) (Courtesy Liz Little, University of Pennsylvania.)

fibrillar than the hyalinized collagen of the keloidal fibrosarcoma, which is bright magenta, glassy, and without distinct fibrillar appearance.

Treatment for fibrosarcoma consists of wide surgical excision, amputation, or both. Recurrence occurs in 30% of canine cases. Alternately, radiotherapy with or without hyperthermia may be helpful after surgery. Immunostimulants in combination with surgery and radiotherapy have also shown promising results. Chemotherapy alone has not proven effective in the treatment of fibrosarcoma but may be helpful when used with other modalities. Prognosis is good to poor depending on the site and degree of anaplasia.

> **KEY POINT** Histologic examination is necessary to distinguish between fibrosarcoma and other spindle cell mesenchymal malignancies or granulation tissue. Immunohistochemistry may be similarly useful in distinguishing tissue origin.

> *Cytopathologic differential diagnosis:* granulation tissue, neural sheath tumors, undifferentiated pleomorphic sarcoma, perivascular wall tumors, myxosarcoma.

Myxoma and Myxosarcoma

Myxomas are rare tumors in dogs and cats, accounting for fewer than 1% of skin tumors (Goldschmidt and Shofer, 1992). Myxomas are infiltrative growths with a soft, fluctuant feel that present as slightly raised masses. Common sites in

CHAPTER 3 Integumentary System

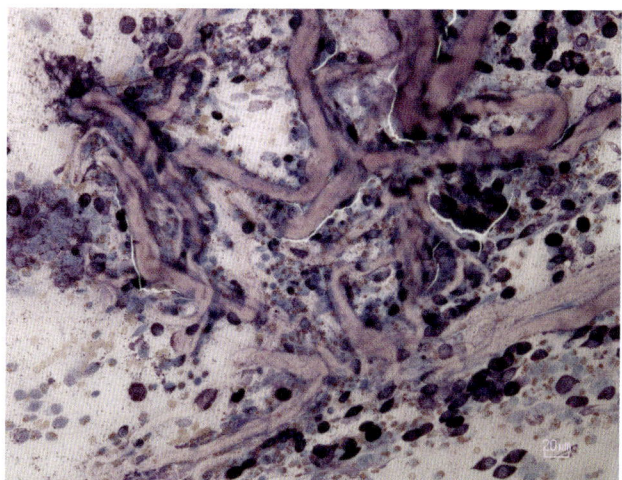

■ **FIGURE 3.140 Mast cell tumor. Collagen bundles.** Dense collagen in mast cell tumors appears less eosinophilic and more fibrillar than the hyalinized collagen of the keloidal fibrosarcoma, which is bright magenta, glassy, and without distinct fibrillar appearance. (Modified Wright; HP oil.) (Courtesy Yvonne Wikander, Kansas State University.)

Cutaneous Metastatic Sarcomas

Previously mentioned under hemangiosarcoma was the recognition of primary visceral hemangiosarcoma to metastasize to the skin. Other sarcomas include appendicular osteosarcoma (Gorman et al., 2006) and alveolar rhabdomyosarcoma (Otrocka-Domagala et al., 2015).

Nerve Sheath Tumors

This group encompasses subtypes such as neurofibroma, Schwannoma, and malignant neural sheath tumors, among others. Histopathology is necessary to confirm suspicions of these tumors because cytopathology reveals fusiform cells, similar to other spindle cell tumors (Fig. 3.143). These cells are large, oval, stellate or fusiform with variably indistinct cytoplasmic borders and a moderate amount of medium basophilic and finely stippled cytoplasm that frequently forms wispy projections. They may contain a few variably sized, variably distinct, colorless vacuoles. The round or oval nucleus is variably located, measures roughly 1.5 to 2.5 × red blood cell and has coarsely stippled chromatin, often containing one to three round or oval discernible variably sized nucleoli. The overall anisocytosis and anisokaryosis among this population are moderate, the nucleocytoplasmic ratio is generally moderate, and bi- or multinucleation are occasionally observed. Malignant neural sheath tumors may display pleomorphism with a plasmacytoid to fusiform appearance, multinucleation, and increased mitotic activity as reported in a cat (Tremblay et al., 2005) and demonstrated in a dog (Fig. 3.144). Because these neural origin tumors may be variable in cytomorphology, definitive diagnosis is best accomplished via immunohistochemistry from an excisional biopsy specimen (Figs. 3.145 and 3.146). Additional information and examples may be found in Chapter 15.

Perivascular Wall Tumors (Canine Hemangiopericytoma and Myopericytoma)

Perivascular wall tumors are common in dogs. They may be present in 7% of skin neoplasms (Goldschmidt and Shofer, 1992). The neoplastic cells are derived from the pericytes (hemangiopericytoma) and myopericytes (myopericytoma); both cells are located in the wall of blood vessels, adjacent to

dogs and cats include the limbs, thorax, and abdomen. Intercellular matrix is often present in the background as granular eosinophilic amorphous material in cytopathologic specimens (Fig. 3.141A). Alcian blue staining of the ground substance for mucin is diagnostic (Fig. 3.141B). Well-differentiated fusiform and stellate cells are found in low numbers in the benign lesion, which increase based on the degree of cellular and nuclear pleomorphism with the malignant form (Fig. 3.142A–D). Multinucleated cells are occasionally present in myxosarcomas. Treatment consists of surgical excision. Prognosis is good to fair because recurrence is common, but it rarely metastasizes.

> *Cytopathologic differential diagnosis:* fibroma, fibrosarcoma, neural sheath tumors, perivascular wall tumors.

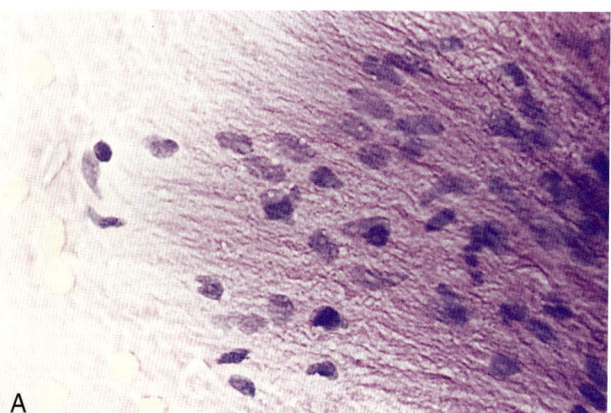 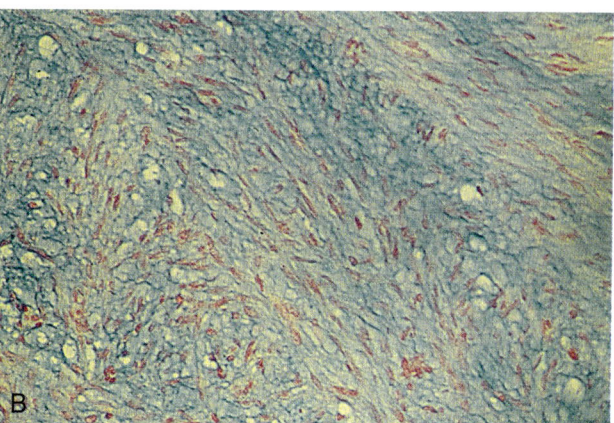

■ **FIGURE 3.141 Myxoma. Dog.** Same case in A and B. **A, Tissue aspirate.** Dense, granular eosinophilic intercellular matrix is present with small, dense nuclei suggesting a benign proliferation for this carpal mass. (Aqueous Romanowsky; HP oil.) **B, Myxoma. Tissue section.** The ground substance stains blue or positive for mucin shown between nuclei staining red. (Alcian blue; IP.)

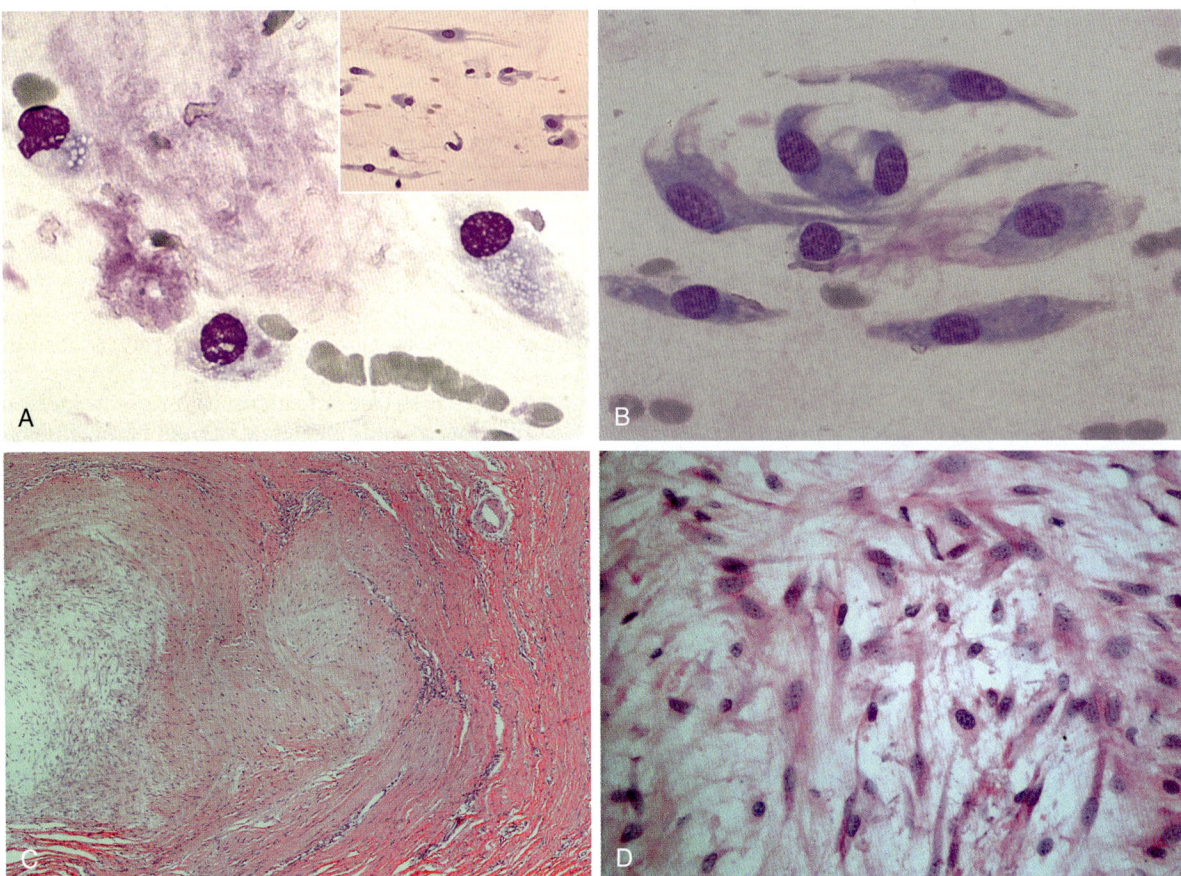

■ **FIGURE 3.142 Myxosarcoma. Metacarpophalangeal mass. Dog.** Same case in A to D. **A, Tissue aspirate.** A firm 3 × 2 × 2 cm subcutaneous mass is evaluated. An intracellular and extracellular granular brightly eosinophilic matrix is shown with plump individualized mesenchymal cells from a metacarpal mass. Note the windrowing of erythrocytes (Aqueous Romanowsky; HP oil.) *Inset:* Pleomorphic spindle cells with vesicular oval nuclei characterize the malignant form of myxomatous tumor. (Aqueous Romanowsky; HP oil.) **B, Tissue aspirate.** Cells appear stellate to fusiform with basophilic cytoplasm having wispy cell borders. Nuclei are oval with stippled chromatin and small distinct nucleoli. Between cells is a small amount of eosinophilic matrix. (Aqueous Romanowsky; HP oil.) **C, Tissue section.** A poorly demarcated, unencapsulated, sparsely cellular mass of neoplastic loosely packed cells mesenchymal cells streaming within a mucinous background (Alcian blue positive; not shown). (H&E; LP.) **D, Tissue section.** Individual cells are stellate to fusiform with eosinophilic cytoplasm having indistinct cell borders. Nuclei are oval with stippled chromatin and a small nucleolus. (H&E; IP.)

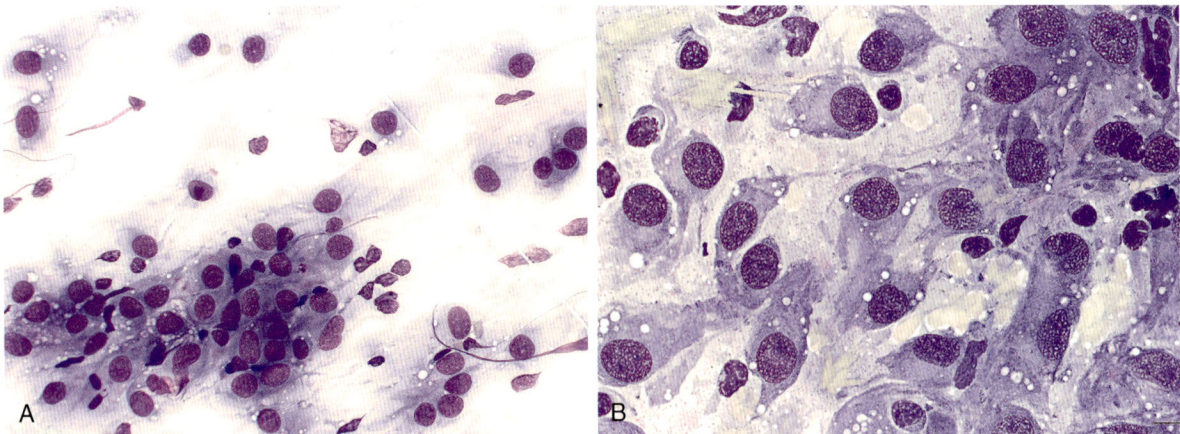

■ **FIGURE 3.143 Nerve sheath tumor. Subcutaneous flank mass. Tissue aspirate. Dog.** Same case in A and B. **A,** A 6.0 cm, asymmetric, variably firm, subcutaneous mass attached to the body wall. A moderately atypical mesenchymal population predominates, and cells are individualized or arranged in variably sized, variably cohesive aggregates. These cells are large, oval, stellate or fusiform, have variably indistinct cytoplasmic borders, and have a moderate amount of medium basophilic, finely stippled cytoplasm that frequently forms wispy projections and/or contains a few variably sized, variably distinct, colorless vacuoles. (Wright-Giemsa; HP oil.) **B,** The round or oval nucleus measures roughly 1 to 2.5 times the size of an erythrocyte and has coarsely stippled chromatin with one to three discernible nucleoli. The overall anisocytosis and anisokaryosis among this population are moderate. Histopathology confirmed the diagnosis of nerve sheath tumor. (Wright-Giemsa; HP oil.)

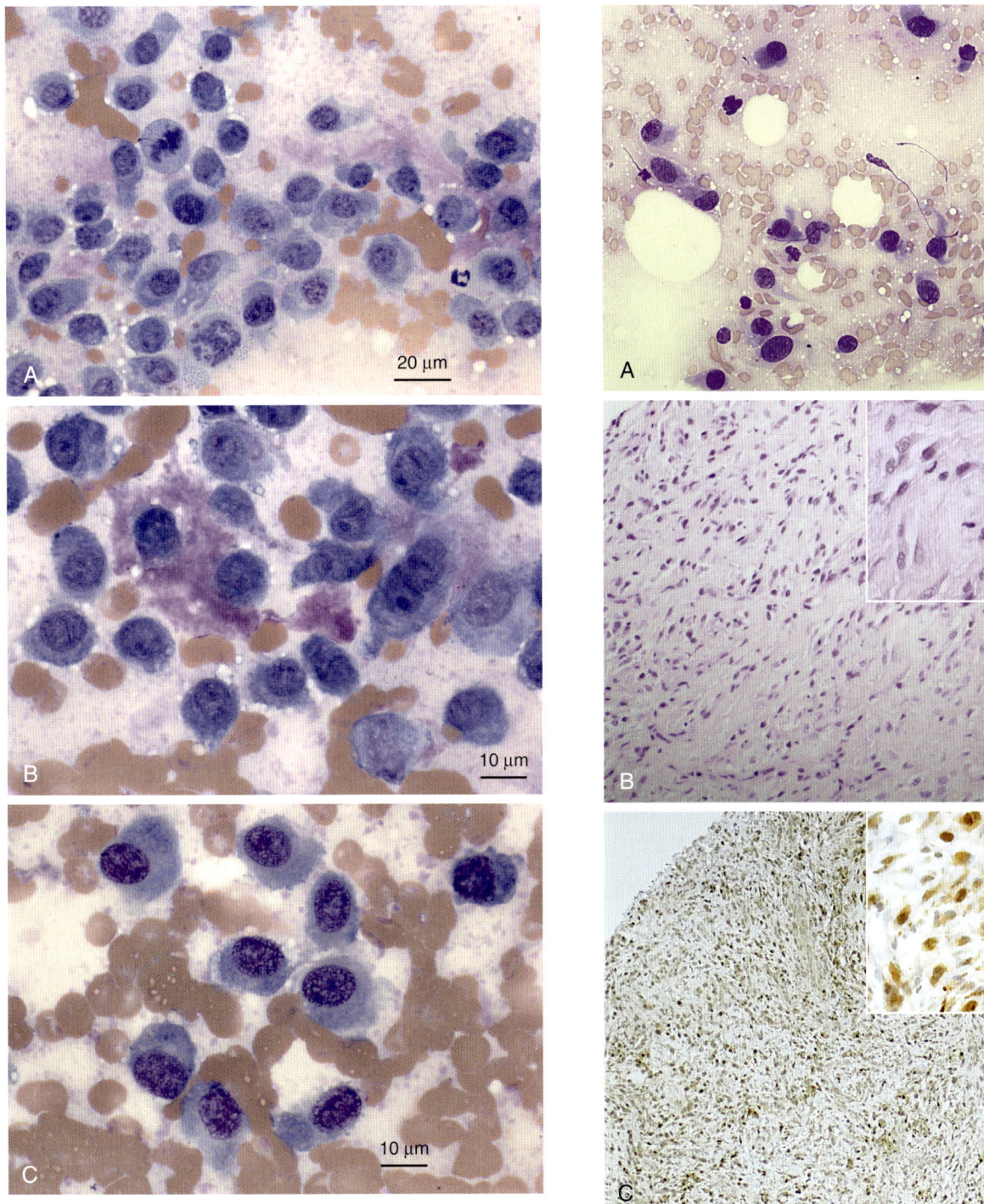

■ **FIGURE 3.144 Nerve sheath tumor. Perianal area mass. Cytopathologic specimen. Dog.** Same case in A to C. **A,** A firm 8.2 × 9.6 × 8.8 cm mass is evaluated. An individualized cell population with plasmacytoid features displays two mitotic figures. (Modified Wright; HP oil.) **B,** An eosinophilic extracellular matrix is present along with cells containing similar staining eosinophilic cytoplasmic globules. In these pleomorphic cells, nuclei that are occasionally multinucleated appear irregularly shaped with coarse chromatin and prominent multiple nucleoli. (Modified Wright; HP oil.) **C,** The plasmacytoid cells have an ovoid nucleus with coarse chromatin stippling and distinct nucleoli. Histopathology initially diagnosed the mass as soft tissue sarcoma. Further diagnostics with immunohistochemical support neural origin related to positive immunoreactivity to Olig-2 and CNPase. (Modified Wright; HP oil.)

■ **FIGURE 3.145 Nerve sheath tumor. C6 spinal nerve mass. Dog.** Same case in A to C. **A, Tissue imprint.** Individualized pleomorphic mesenchymal cells have several features of malignancy, including anisokaryosis, high nucleocytoplasmic ratio, nuclear and cellular pleomorphism, and prominent nucleoli. Cells are oval to stellate to fusiform. (Modified Wright; IP.). **B, Tissue section.** The neoplasm displays dense collagenous connective tissue with high cellular infiltration by proliferating mesenchymal cells. (H&E; IP.) *Inset:* The neoplastic cells have large, irregularly ovoid nuclei with a variable chromatin pattern and prominent nucleoli. (H&E; IP.) **C, Tissue section.** There is a strong diffuse positive immunoreactivity to the nerve sheath tumor marker. (S100/DAB; LP.) *Inset:* Nuclear and cytoplasmic reactivity support a positive response to this marker. (S100/DAB; IP.)

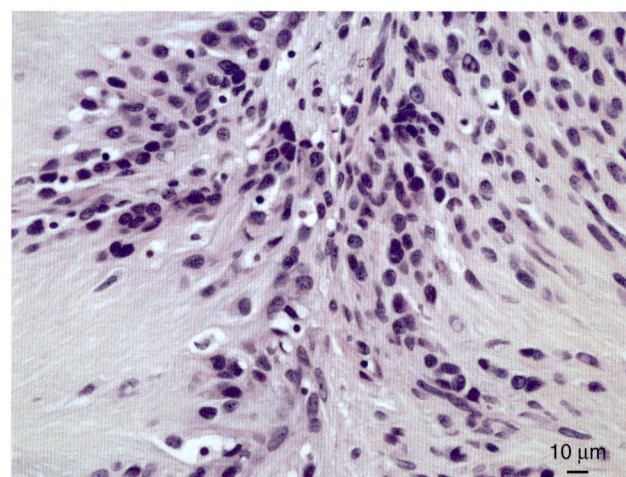

■ **FIGURE 3.146 Schwannoma. Flank mass. Tissue section. Cat.** A firm, spherical subcutaneous mass measuring 1.2 × 1.2 × 1.0 cm is evaluated. Most prominent are radially arranged variably sized cells with fine fibrillar and collagenous matrix. Oval and palisading nuclei composed the majority of nucleated cells. Ultrastructural studies support the presence of rudimentary myelin structures. Immunohistochemistry is positive for S-100 and vimentin. (H&E; IP.)

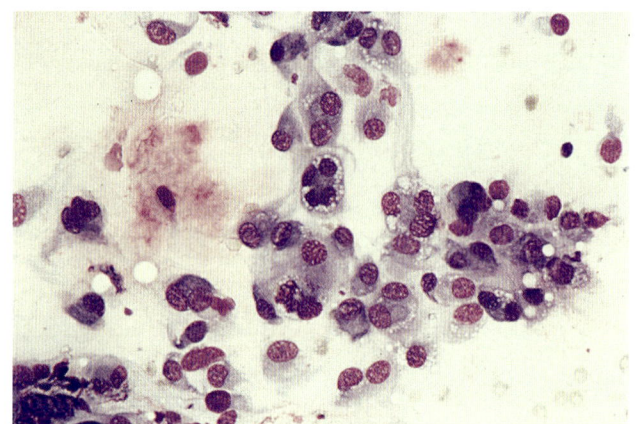

■ **FIGURE 3.147 Perivascular wall tumor. Tissue aspirate. Dog.** Slide preparation from a sternal subcutaneous mass is highly cellular, with aggregates of plump mononuclear or multinucleated mesenchymal cells. (Wright-Giemsa; HP oil.)

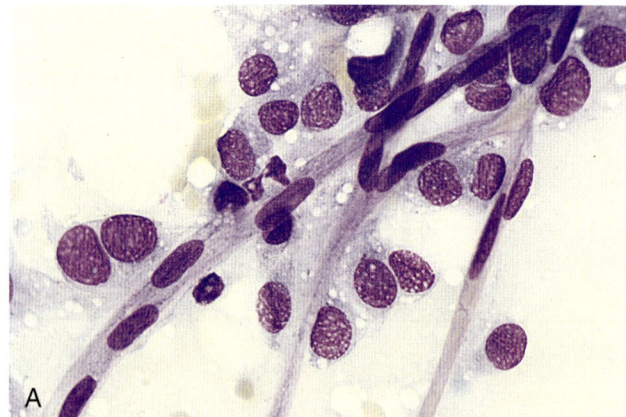

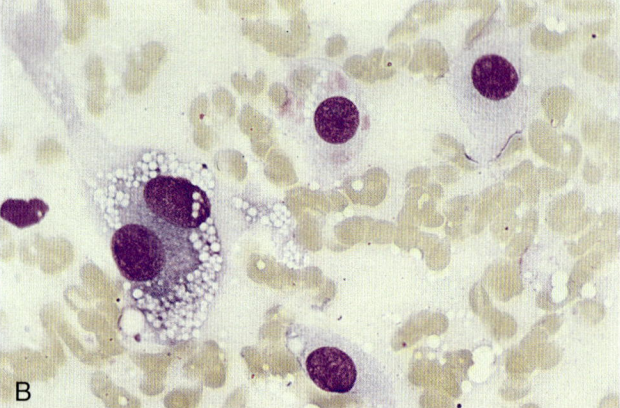

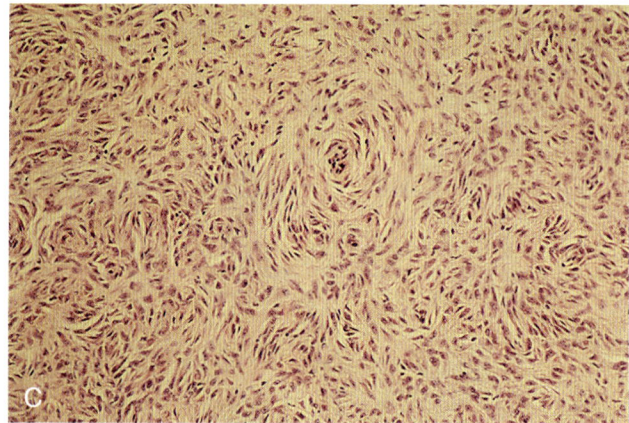

■ **FIGURE 3.148 Myopericytoma. Thigh mass. Dog.** Same case in A to C. **A, Tissue aspirate.** Plump spindle cells are shown adherent to the surface of capillaries. (Aqueous Romanowsky; HP oil.) **B,** The cytoplasm is basophilic with numerous small discrete vacuoles, and one cell contains eosinophilic globules. (Aqueous Romanowsky; HP oil.) **C, Tissue section.** Classic fingerprint whorls of plump spindle cells around blood vessels. This histologic pattern of perivascular wall tumor suggests myopericytoma related to the whorling. (H&E; IP.)

endothelium. A third cell type of perivascular tumor is derived from the glomus cell, which is discussed later in the chapter. The perivascular wall tumors are often solitary with a predilection for limb joints but are commonly found on the thorax and abdomen. They are firm to soft, multilobulated, and often well circumscribed. Cytopathologic preparations are moderately to highly cellular (Fig. 3.147). Plump spindle cells may be individualized or arranged in bundles and are sometimes adherent to the surface of capillaries (Fig. 3.148A). Associated cells may be a pink amorphous collagenous stroma. The cytoplasm is basophilic, often with numerous small, discrete vacuoles and occasional eosinophilic globules (Fig. 3.148B). Nuclei are ovoid, with one or more prominent central nucleoli. Histologically, they belong to a broad group of spindle cell tumors with the classic appearance of fingerprint whorls of plump spindle cells and a low mitotic index (Avallone et al., 2007) (Fig. 3.148C). Whereas staghorn vascular patterns are most associated with hemangiopericytoma, whirling and placentoid patterns are best associated with myopericytoma. Multinucleated cells termed *crown cells* (Figs. 3.149 and 3.150) are commonly seen (Caniatti et al., 2001). Lymphoid cells have been found in approximately 10% of cases. Treatment should vary as per the specific diagnosis, with wide surgical excision or amputation and radiotherapy with or without hyperthermia for the aggressive and recurrent disease termed *hemangiopericytoma*. Prognosis is fair because 20% to 60% recur locally, especially with conservative excision. Metastasis is rare. Myopericytoma is best distinguished using immunomarkers such as desmin, pan-actin, or calponin (Avallone et al., 2007). Prognosis is good because myopericytomas respond to surgical excision. A retrospective study of canine cutaneous perivascular wall tumors demonstrated local recurrence and rare metastasis in 12 of 55 cases reviewed (Stefanello et al., 2011). Good prognosis was associated with young age and tumor size smaller than 5 cm.

> ***Cytopathologic differential diagnosis:*** neural sheath tumors, well-differentiated fibrosarcoma, myxomatous tumors, undifferentiated pleomorphic sarcoma.

Undifferentiated Pleomorphic Sarcoma (Anaplastic Sarcoma With Giant Cells)

This form of sarcoma refers to a diverse group of soft tissue tumors formerly known as malignant fibrous histiocytoma that comprises a wide range of cell types and biological behaviors. It is occasionally found in dogs but is most common in cats (de Cecco et al., 2021). It is a pleomorphic spindle cell tumor (Fig. 3.151A),

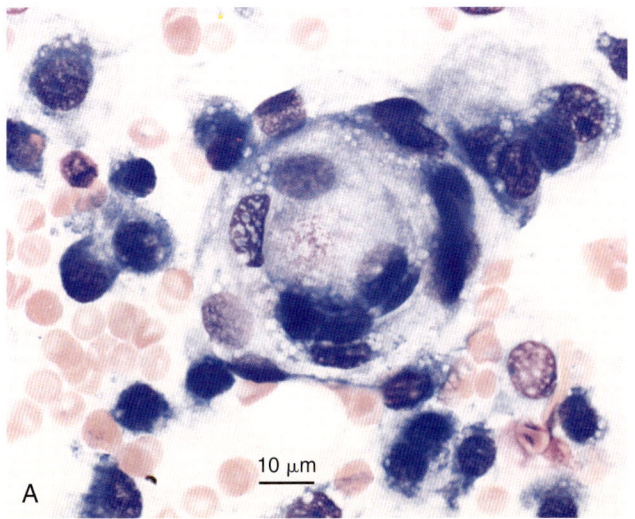
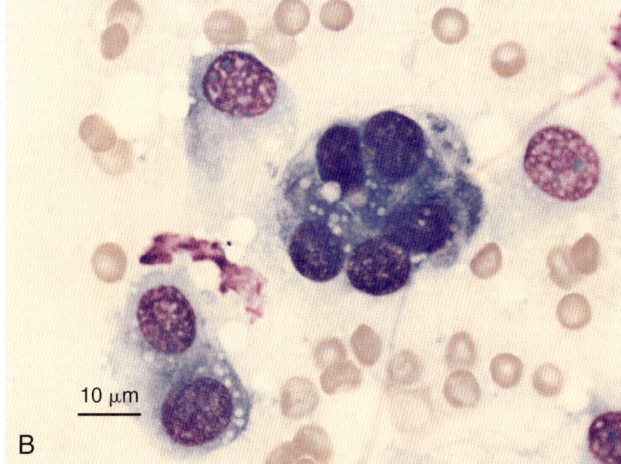

■ **FIGURE 3.149 Perivascular wall tumor. Tissue aspirate. Dog.** Same case in A and B. **A,** Characteristic circle of cells form the fingerprint whorl seen on histopathology. (Modified Wright; HP oil.) **B,** Crown cell presentation with a circle of cells having an unfilled center. (Modified Wright; HP oil.)

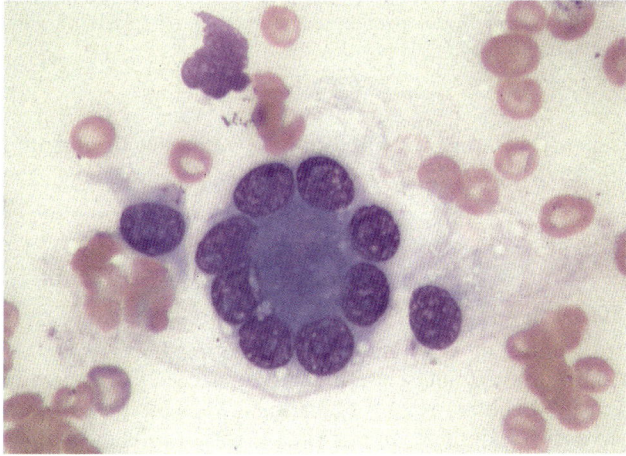

■ **FIGURE 3.150 Perivascular wall tumor. Tissue aspirate. Dog.** A circle formation of plump spindle cells having coarsely clumped chromatin and a single prominent nucleolus form a characteristic "crown" of cells. (Modified Wright; HP oil.) (Courtesy Andrew Torrance, TDDS/Synlab, Exeter, UK.)

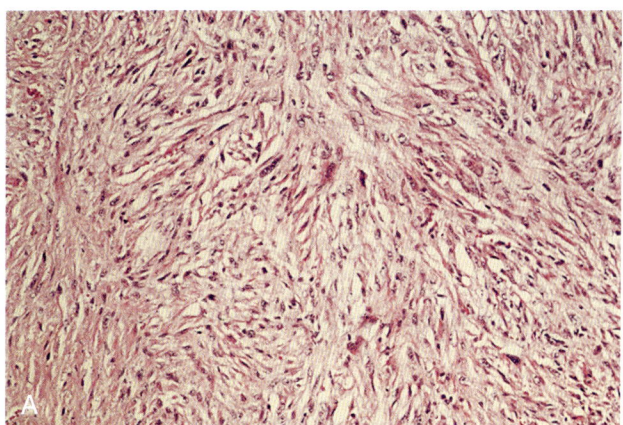
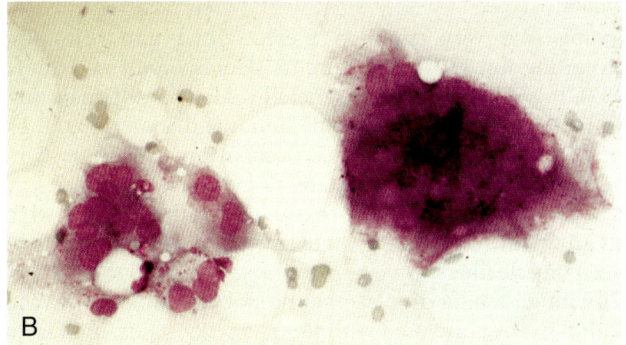

■ **FIGURE 3.151 Undifferentiated pleomorphic sarcoma. Thoracic skin mass. Cat.** Same case in A and B. **A, Tissue section.** Pleomorphic spindle cells form tightly swirling or interlacing (storiform) bundles. Note frequent multinucleated cells scattered throughout. This tumor recurred 3 months after previous surgical excision. (H&E; IP.) **B, Tissue aspirate.** Several variably sized giant cells are present. The cytoplasm contains fine eosinophilic granulation. (Wright-Giemsa; HP oil.)

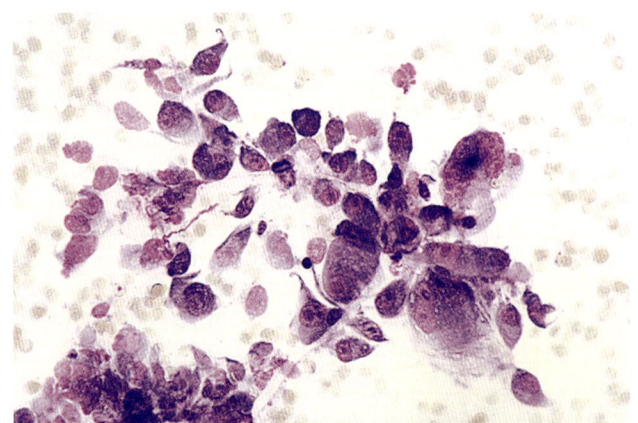

■ **FIGURE 3.152 Undifferentiated pleomorphic sarcoma. Flank mass aspirate. Dog.** A mixed population of plump spindle cells is present, with multiple criteria for malignancy, including increased and variable nucleocytoplasmic ratios, prominent nucleoli, anisokaryosis, and multinucleation. (Wright-Giemsa; IP.)

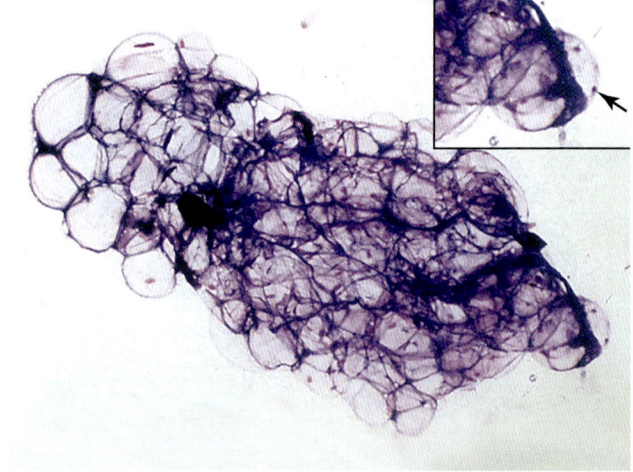

■ **FIGURE 3.153 Lipoma. Tissue mass aspirate. Dog.** Large aggregate of adipocytes. *Inset:* Higher magnification demonstrates the small dense nucleus displaced to the side of the cell *(arrow)* by the abundant clear staining lipid. (Romanowsky; LP.)

the origin of which likely involves a primitive dermal pluripotent precursor cell (myofibroblast) with accompanying inflammatory cells and multinucleate giant cells that are immunoreactive to the macrophage antibody (Iba1) (de Cecco et al., 2021). These tumors may be solitary or multiple, occurring mainly on the limbs of older dogs and cats, but they may occur in abdominal organs, lungs, and lymph nodes. They are firm and poorly circumscribed. A mixed population of multinucleated cells and plump spindle cells is seen on cytopathologic specimens (Figs. 3.151B and 3.152). Mononuclear inflammatory cells such as lymphocytes, plasma cells, and histiocytes may be present. Treatment involves radical excisional surgery and chemotherapy with or without radiotherapy. Prognosis is guarded because these tumors are locally invasive with frequent recurrence and may rarely metastasize, especially in cases containing higher percentages of giant cells.

Cytopathologic differential diagnosis: fibrosarcoma, sarcoma of other origins, granulation tissue, histiocytic sarcoma, nerve sheath tumors.

Lipoma

Lipoma is a very common mesenchymal tumor in dogs, accounting for 8% of skin tumors (Goldschmidt and Shofer, 1992). It is benign, affecting generally older, obese female dogs. It is present in 6% of cats (Goldschmidt and Shofer, 1992). The tumor may be single or multiple, occurring mainly on the trunk and proximal limbs. These are dome-shaped, well-circumscribed, soft, freely moveable masses within the subcutis, which can grow slowly, becoming quite large. Some may infiltrate between muscle fibers. On cytopathology, unstained slides appear wet with glistening droplets that do not dry completely. When alcohol fixatives are used with Romanowsky stains, lipid is dissolved, leaving slides often devoid of cells. When present, intact lipocytes have abundant clear cytoplasm with a small, compressed nucleus to one side of the cell (Fig. 3.153). Lipid may be best demonstrated with a water-soluble stain such as new methylene blue (Fig. 3.154) or the fat stain oil red O. An alternate form of lipoma consists of variable amounts of fibrous tissue and is termed *fibrolipoma*. Slides consist of fibroblasts and adipocytes without evidence of inflammation. Prognosis is

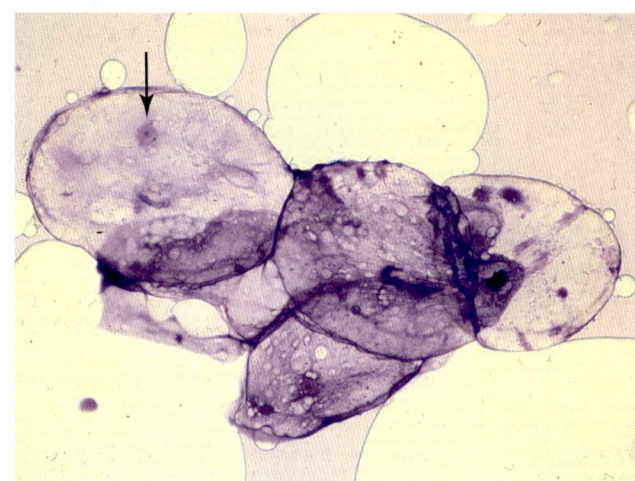

■ **FIGURE 3.154 Lipoma.** Adipocytes do not dissolve in the unfixed water-soluble stain making them more visible. Note the pyknotic basophilic nucleus *(arrow)* in relation to the massive cytoplasmic volume. (New methylene blue; HP oil.)

excellent; however, some infiltrative lipomas may be difficult to completely excise. Treatment involves surgical excision.

Cytopathologic differential diagnosis: normal subcutaneous fat.

Liposarcoma

Rare tumors of dogs and cats comprising fewer than 0.5% of skin tumors (Goldschmidt and Shofer, 1992), liposarcomas are usually solitary masses occurring anywhere, most often on the ventral abdomen. An association with a foreign body was documented in one report (McCarthy et al., 1996). They are firm, poorly circumscribed, and adherent to underlying tissues (Fig. 3.155A). Ulceration of the epidermis may occur. Dense aggregates of mesenchymal cells contain variable amounts of lipid vacuoles on cytopathology (Fig. 3.155B). Cells appear plump, spindle-shaped with large vesicular nuclei and prominent

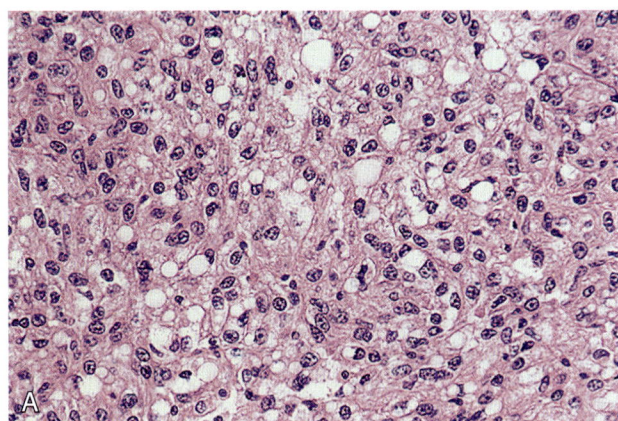

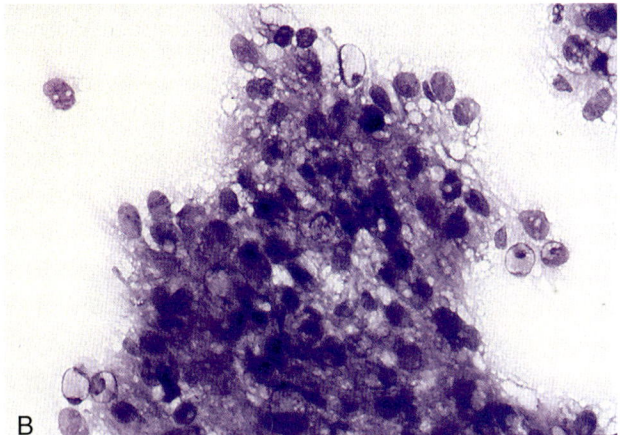

■ FIGURE 3.155 **Liposarcoma. Dog.** Same case in A and B. **A, Tissue section.** Lipid vacuoles are scattered between dense sheets of mesenchymal cells with vesicular nuclei. (H&E; IP.) **B, Tissue aspirate.** Large aggregates of mesenchymal cells with scattered lipid vacuoles that appear shrunken and well defined in this leg mass sample. (Aqueous Romanowsky; HP oil.)

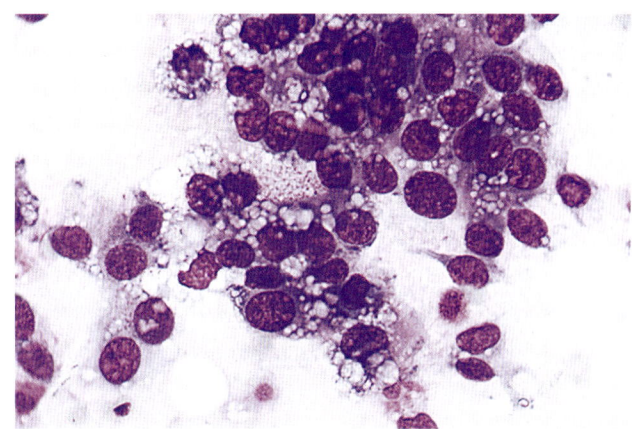

■ FIGURE 3.156 **Liposarcoma. Tissue aspirate. Dog.** Cells appear plump and spindle shaped, with large vesicular nuclei and prominent nucleoli with variably sized intracytoplasmic fat vacuoles. (Aqueous Romanowsky; HP oil.) (Courtesy of Peter Fernandes, Texas A&M University.)

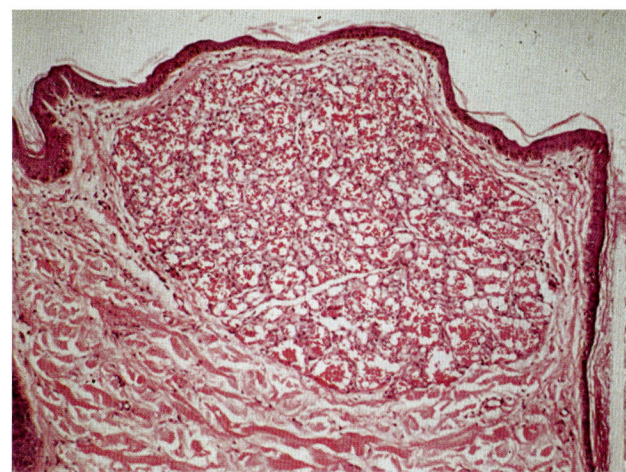

■ FIGURE 3.157 **Hemangioma. Tissue section. Dog.** Well-defined dermal nodule with endothelial proliferation and cavernous spaces filled with blood cells. (H&E; LP.)

nucleoli and may contain variably sized intracytoplasmic fat vacuoles (Fig. 3.156). A recent report of a liposarcoma demonstrated variable cytomorphology patterns, including naked nuclei and epithelial besides mesenchymal (McAloney et al., 2020). Multinucleated cells may be present. A myxoid variant may be associated with abundant Alcian blue staining, but cytoplasmic vacuoles should still be found within some cells to be considered lipoblasts (Boyd et al., 2005). This malignant tumor has moderate metastatic potential. Treatment involves wide surgical excision but may be coupled with radiation and hyperthermia to control recurrence. Prognosis is guarded because they are likely to recur and may metastasize.

Cytopathologic differential diagnosis: fibrosarcoma, undifferentiated pleomorphic sarcoma.

Hemangioma
Hemangiomas are benign tumors that are common in dogs and less common in cats, representing about 5% and 2% of skin masses, respectively (Goldschmidt and Shofer, 1992). They may be solitary or multiple. They present as discrete nodules present on the head, trunk, or limbs that appear dark red to purple and may feel spongy (Fig. 3.157). Aspirate biopsies appear bloody, resembling blood contamination. Small basophilic endothelial cells are infrequent. Evidence for acute or chronic hemorrhage is often noted, resulting in erythrophagocytosis or hemosiderin-laden macrophages. Platelets are not commonly seen. Treatment involves surgical excision or cryosurgery. Prognosis is excellent.

Cytopathologic differential diagnosis: hematoma, blood contamination.

Hemangiosarcoma (Angiosarcoma)
Hemangiosarcoma is a malignant infiltrative mass of the dermis or subcutis. It is an infrequent tumor of older dogs and cats, occurring in about 1% and 3% of skin tumors, respectively (Goldschmidt and Shofer, 1992). Studies show an association between dermal vascular tumors and solar radiation. Tumors are found more frequently in thin-haired areas such as the ventral abdomen of dogs and the ear pinnae of cats and may metastasize to the skin from primary visceral locations. Lesions are raised, poorly circumscribed, ulcerated, and hemorrhagic. Cytopathologic preparations often have low cellularity with

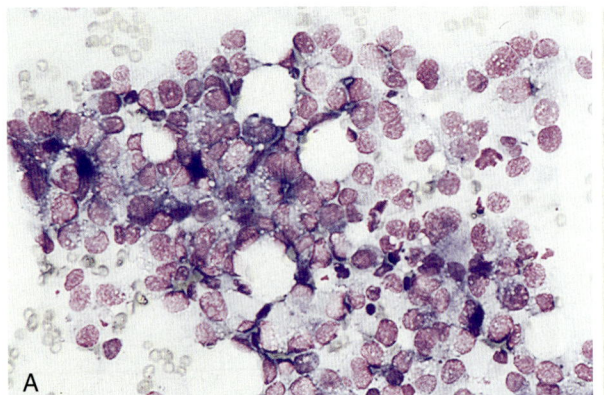
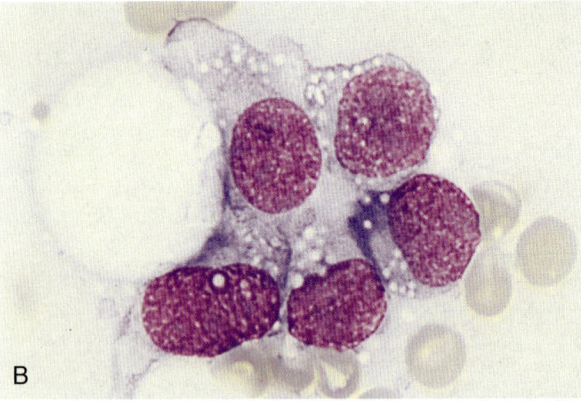

■ **FIGURE 3.158 Hemangiosarcoma. Tissue aspirate. Dog.** Same case in A and B. **A,** Large, dense aggregates of markedly pleomorphic mesenchymal cells from a skin mass. (Wright-Giemsa; HP oil.) **B,** Cells have high nucleocytoplasmic ratios, oval nuclei with coarse chromatin, and prominent multiple nucleoli. Note the punctate vacuoles in the cytoplasm seen commonly in this tumor. (Wright-Giemsa; HP oil.)

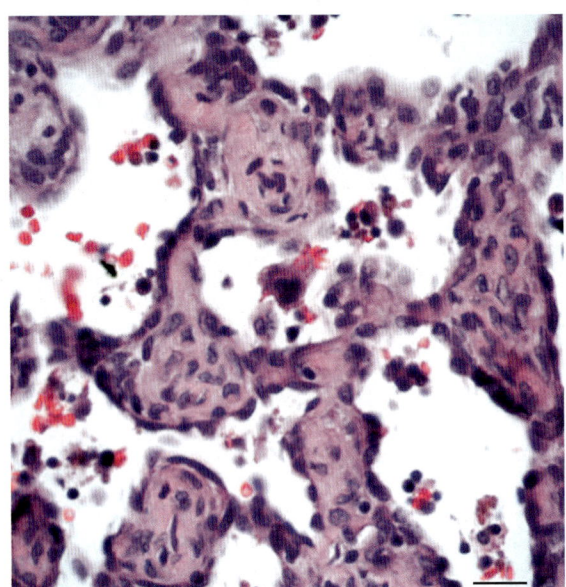

■ **FIGURE 3.159 Hemangiosarcoma. Tissue section. Dog.** Histologic section of a subcutaneous nodule overlying the left epaxial musculature of a dog. Vascular channels contain erythroid precursors and megakaryocytes. The diagnosis was hemangiosarcoma. (H&E.) Bar, 20 μm. (From Dunbar MD, Conway JA. What is your diagnosis? Cytologic findings from a subcutaneous nodule over the left epaxial musculature in a dog. *Vet Clin Pathol.* 2012;41:295–296.)

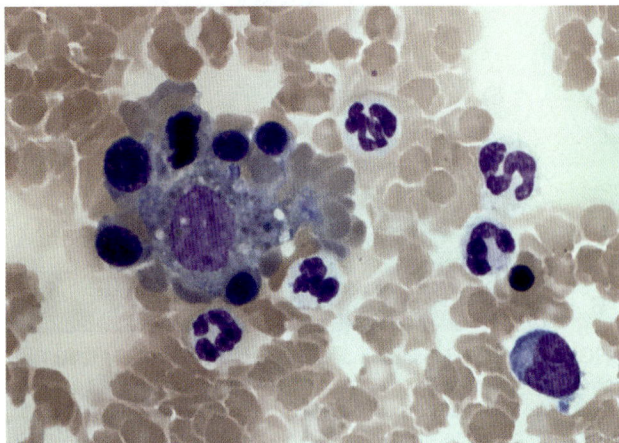

■ **FIGURE 3.160 Hemangiosarcoma. Inguinal mass. Tissue aspirate. Cat.** A lobulated mass measuring approximately 10 × 5 cm is evaluated. A single macrophage with developing erythroid precursors, termed an *erythroid island*, is present in the highly hemodilute and low cellular specimen. Rare poorly preserved atypical spindle cells and a megakaryocyte are also seen (not shown). There is a strong suspicion for hemangiosarcoma, which requires further diagnostic testing. (Wright-Giemsa; HP oil.) (Courtesy Jacqueline Dolan, University of Florida.)

numerous blood cells within the background as well as increased neutrophils. Solid, anaplastic cases of hemangiosarcoma may contain large dense aggregates of markedly pleomorphic mesenchymal cells (Fig. 3.158A). Neoplastic cells are pleomorphic, ranging from large spindle to stellate to epithelioid (Wilkerson et al., 2002). Cytoplasm is basophilic, having indistinct cell borders and frequent punctate colorless vacuoles. Cells have high nucleocytoplasmic ratios, oval nuclei with coarse chromatin, and prominent multiple nucleoli (Fig. 3.158B). Evidence of chronic hemorrhage with hemosiderin-laden macrophages, acute erythrophagia (Bertazzolo et al., 2005; Barger et al., 2012), and occasionally extramedullary hematopoiesis (Bertazzolo et al., 2005; Dunbar and Conway, 2012) may be associated with hemangiosarcoma (Figs. 3.159 and 3.160). Diagnosis may be assisted through immunohistochemistry using von Willebrand factor (factor VIII–related antigen), CD31, and vimentin (Bertazzolo et al., 2005). CD34 was shown to be too broad in reactivity in feline nonvascular tumors, so it cannot be recommended (Jennings et al., 2012). The epithelioid angiosarcomas were negative for cytokeratins. Treatment consists of radical surgical excision and, in the case of possible metastatic lesions, combination chemotherapy. Prognosis is guarded because of regional invasion and local recurrence. Metastasis is uncommon but is more likely to spread from those occurring within the subcutis.

Another malignant neoplasm of endothelium is that of lymphatic vessels, termed *lymphangiosarcoma*. These uncommon tumors of dogs and cats appear as a soft fluctuant mass on the cervical, trunk, or limb regions in generally adult animals, although dogs as young as 1 year old may be affected. Because bruising with erythema is common, it may appear as a weepy cellulitis. For cases in which cytopathology was performed, samples are consistent with mild neutrophilic inflammation with a high percentage of small mature lymphocytes (Curran et al., 2016). Histologically, the primitive clefts are empty and lack erythrocytes. PROX-1 activity is expressed by lymphatic vessels and is used as a specific marker.

> *Cytopathologic differential diagnosis:* fibrosarcoma, undifferentiated sarcoma, perivascular wall tumors, lymphangiosarcoma.

Rhabdomyosarcoma

The variable appearance of a subdermal neoplastic population appearing as round cells or mesenchymal cells in a juvenile animal, especially around the head, suggests the possibility of a skeletal muscle neoplasm. Subtypes include alveolar (Fig. 3.161), embryonal, and pleomorphic. Cell types involve myotubular cells, also termed *strap cells*, which are multinucleated and formed from fusion of small round rhabdomyoblasts (15–20 μm diameter). For further information and examples, see Chapter 14.

Melanocytic Tumors

Benign melanocytoma and malignant melanoma are common, accounting for 5% of canine skin tumors and 3% of feline skin tumors (Yager and Wilcock, 1994). Older animals are usually affected, as are those with dark skin pigmentation. Resident melanocytes may display a dendritic shape that is intertwined among the basal epithelial cells (Fig. 3.162). Gross features differ for benign and malignant forms. About 70% of the melanocytic dermal tumors are benign, appearing as mostly dark-brown to black, circumscribed, raised, dome-shaped masses covered by smooth, hairless skin (Fig. 3.163). Melanocytomas often consist of highly pigmented intraepidermal to dermal masses (Fig. 3.164A) composed of spindle to round cells containing abundant uniformly shaped and sized black-brown or green granules (Figs. 3.164B–C and 3.165). Nuclei in benign forms are small and uniform.

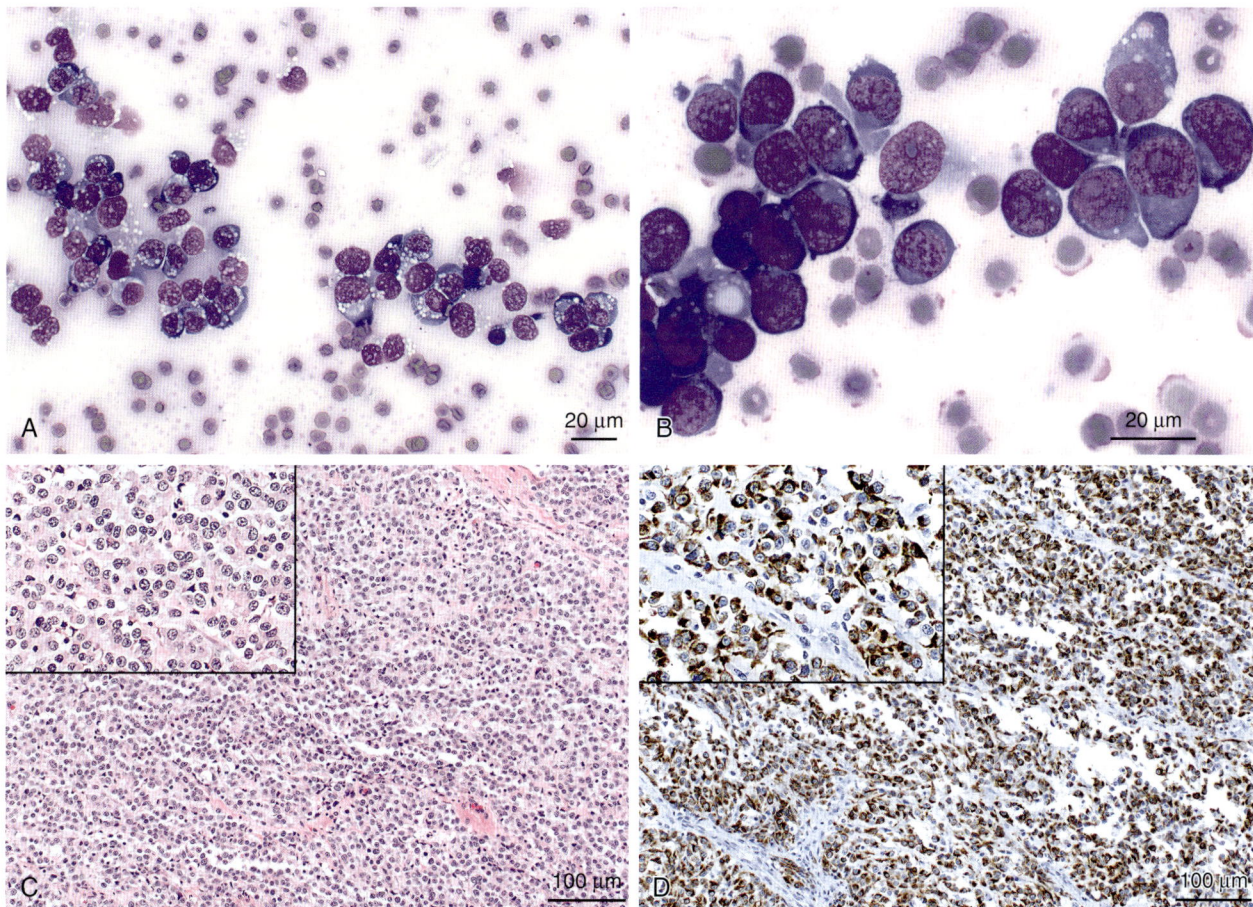

■ **FIGURE 3.161 Rhabdomyosarcoma. Orbital swelling. Dog.** Same case in A to D. **A, Tissue aspirate.** A cutaneous and subcutaneous mass in a juvenile dog yields an atypical population of mononuclear cells. Cells are typically seen arranged in variably sized, variably cohesive aggregates, as well as individualized that are scattered throughout the preparation. (Wright-Giemsa; HP oil.) **B, Tissue aspirate.** These cells are round or oval, have variably distinct to discrete cytoplasmic borders, and a small to moderate amount of medium to deeply basophilic cytoplasm that occasionally contains a small paranuclear clear zone, contains several small, variably distinct, colorless vacuoles, and/or forms small, bleblike projections. The round, oval, indented, or convoluted nucleus is paracentral to eccentric, measures roughly 1.5 to 3.0 times the size of an erythrocyte, and has coarsely stippled chromatin. Nuclei often contain one or more prominent nucleoli with anisonucleoliosis. The overall anisocytosis and anisokaryosis among this population are moderate. (Wright-Giemsa; HP oil.) **C, Tissue section.** Diffuse sheets of round cells. (H&E; IP.) *Inset:* Cells have round to ovoid open chromatin and distinct nucleoli. (H&E; IP.) **D, Tissue section.** Cells are immunoreactive to the muscle marker and negative to fibrous connective tissue bands. (Desmin/DAB; IP.) *Inset:* The cytoplasm is strongly positive to the immunomarker confirming the diagnosis of rhabdomyosarcoma. (Desmin/DAB; IP.)

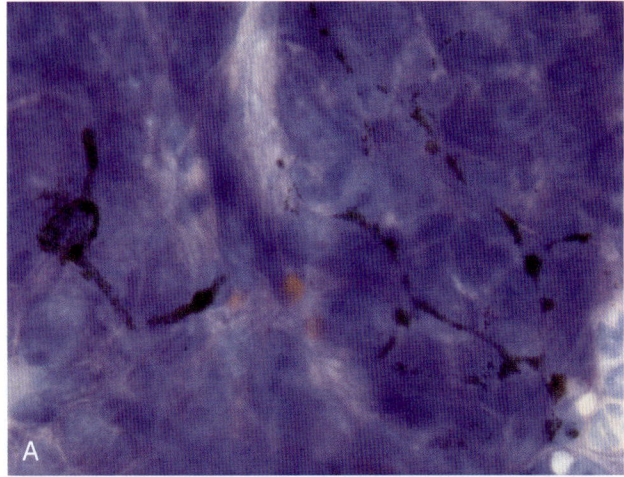
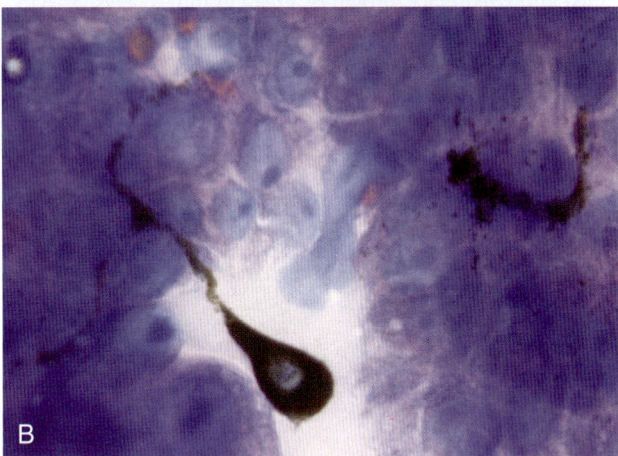

■ **FIGURE 3.162 Dendritic melanocytes. Dorsum mass. Tissue aspirate. Cat.** Same case in A and B. **A,** Interspersed between basal epithelial cells are resident melanocytes that display a dendritic shape. (Modified Wright; HP oil.) **B,** A pear-shaped cell with prominent nucleus is shown with dendrite-like cytoplasmic extensions. These cells likely represent a normal cell population and should not be mistaken for a melanocytic tumor. (Modified Wright; HP oil.) (Courtesy Kathleen Tennant, University of Bristol, UK.)

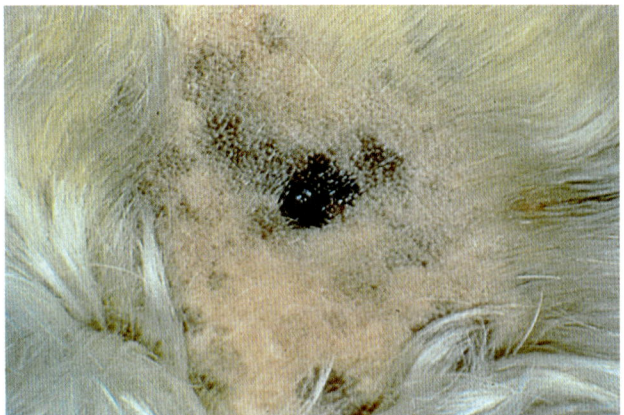

■ **FIGURE 3.163 Melanocytoma. Skin mass. Macroscopic specimen. Dog.** Note the dark-brown to black, circumscribed, raised, dome-shaped mass typical of most well-differentiated melanocytic tumors. (Courtesy Leslie Fox, University of Florida.)

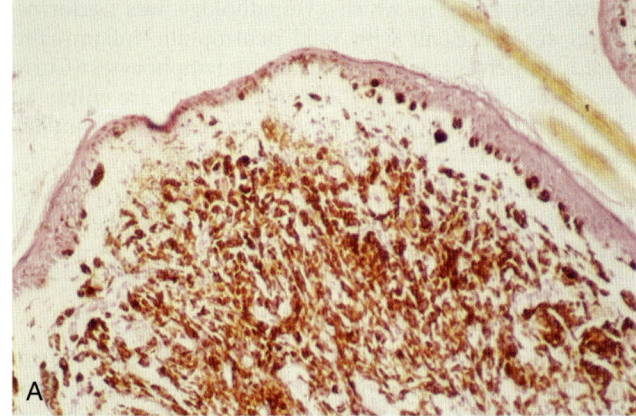
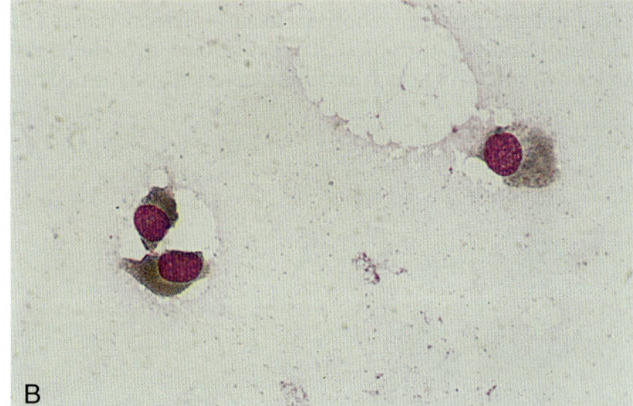
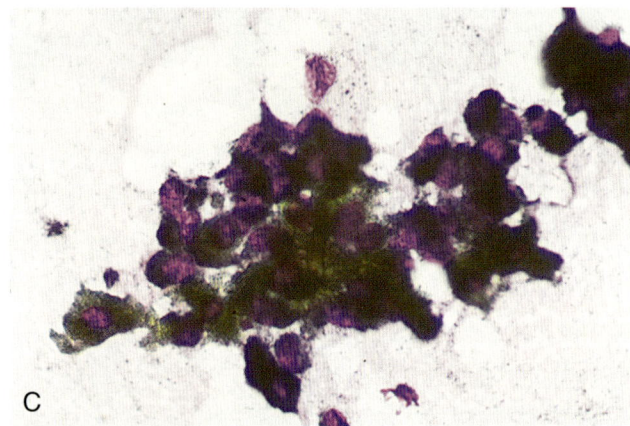

■ **FIGURE 3.164 Melanocytoma. Dog.** Same case in A to C. **A, Tissue section.** Melanocytes are present in the basal layer of the epidermis and within the superficial dermis arranged in clusters and diffusely. Cells are heavily pigmented in this mass on the back. (H&E; IP.) **B, Tissue imprint.** Individual fusiform cells with abundant melanin pigment. (Aqueous Romanowsky; HP oil.) **C, Tissue imprint.** Large aggregates of darkly pigmented cells are found that mask nuclear details. (Aqueous Romanowsky; HP oil.)

Malignant melanomas are variably pigmented, infiltrative, frequently ulcerated, and inflamed. On cytopathology, cells range from round to epithelial to mesenchymal cytomorphology patterns (Fig. 3.166A–C). They may mimic cutaneous plasmacytoma with an eccentric nucleus (see Fig. 3.166B). Nuclei are round to ovoid with malignant criteria of anisocytosis, anisokaryosis, coarse chromatin, and prominent nucleoli seen in the malignant

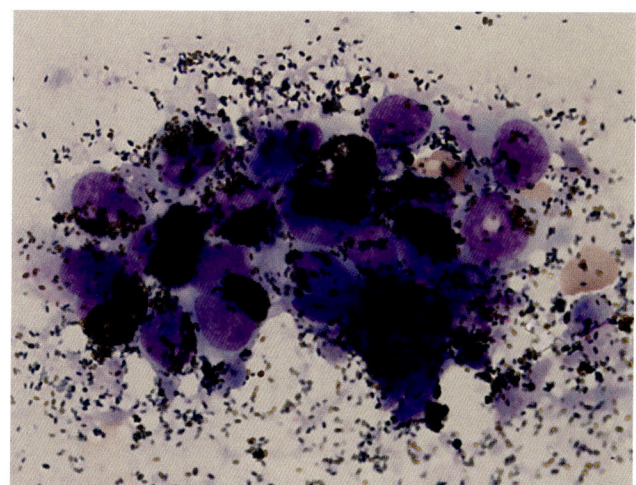

■ **FIGURE 3.165 Melanocytoma. Dog.** Nucleated cells consist primarily of mildly atypical mononuclear cells present as a dense aggregate. The oval or rounded cells (~20 μm in diameter) have a small to moderate amount of medium basophilic cytoplasm often containing few to many rod-shaped brown-black melanin granules. The round or oval nucleus is approximately twice the size of an erythrocyte with finely stippled chromatin and one or more small, round or oval distinct nucleoli. Anisocytosis and anisokaryosis are mild. (Wright-Giemsa; HP oil.) (Courtesy Tracie Guy, University of Florida.)

melanomas (see Fig. 3.166C). Poorly differentiated tumors may contain few or no cytoplasmic granules (see Fig. 3.166A–C); however, a gray, dust-like appearance in a few cells may help determine that the tumor is melanocytic (Fig. 3.167). When the diagnosis is in doubt, additional diagnostic stains are recommended.

The number of melanin granules will vary within a tumor, with deeper regions composed of fusiform cells having fewer granules compared with superficial areas composed of epithelioid cells. Special stains such as the Fontana-Masson stain is used on cytopathologic preparations to detect poorly visible melanin granules, especially useful for amelanotic melanomas. Prussian blue stain helps identify hemosiderin granules, which appear dark green and may resemble melanin granules. Additionally, the immunochemical stains Melan-A (Figs. 3.168 and 3.169), S-100, and PNL2 may help identify amelanotic melanoma and distinguish it from plasmacytoma with negative expression of CD18 and CD45 (Ramos-Vara et al., 2002).

An infrequent variant of amelanotic melanoma is balloon cell melanoma, which is difficult to distinguish from sebaceous carcinoma, liposarcoma, or clear cell adnexal carcinoma without melanocytic markers or ultrastructural evidence of melanosomes (Fig. 3.170) (Wilkerson et al., 2003). Cytopathology reveals large vacuolated to pale eosinophilic cytoplasm with low nucleocytoplasmic ratio, mild to moderate anisokaryosis, and low mitotic activity. These neoplasms may metastasize (Wilkerson et al., 2003).

On histopathology, an amelanotic round cell variant in dogs and cats may show a signet ring morphology having the nucleus pressed to the cell periphery by an abundance of eosinophilic cytoplasm causing the cell to appear plasmacytoid. On cytopathology, these amelanotic cells most resemble plasma cells or histiocytes with abundant dense basophilic cytoplasm and an eccentric nucleus containing prominent nucleoli (Albanese, 2017).

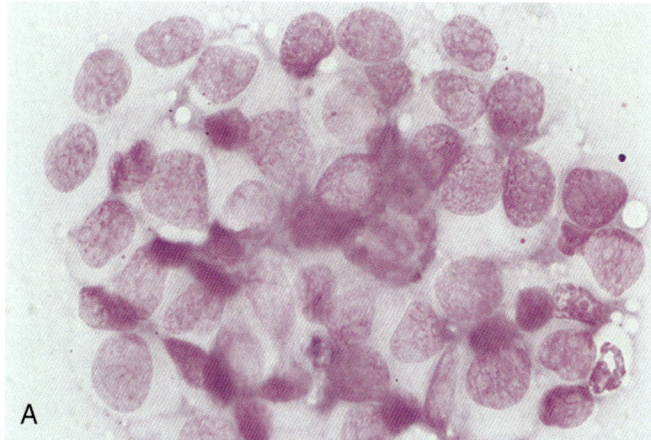

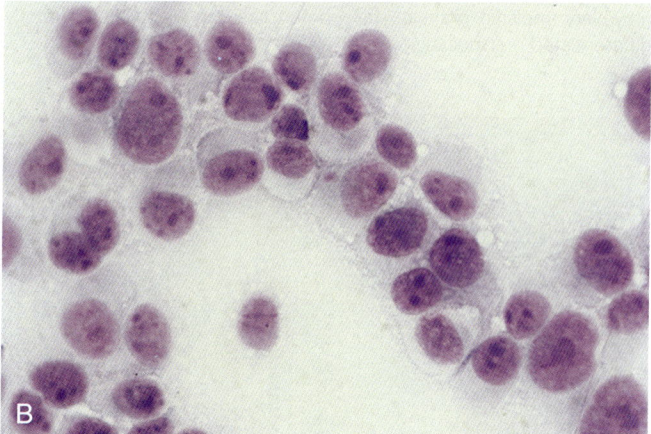

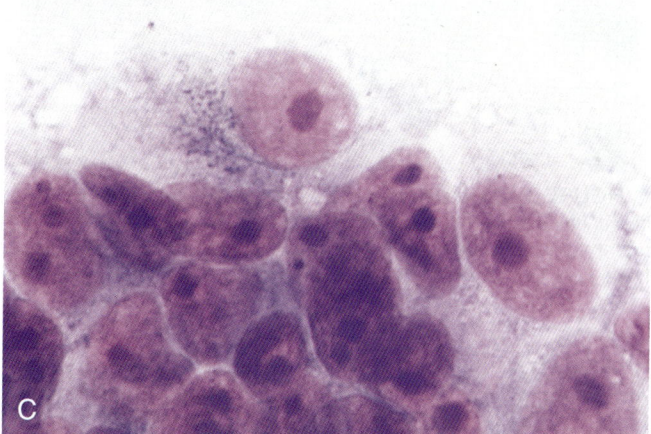

■ **FIGURE 3.166 Amelanotic melanoma. Oral mass. Dog.** Same case in A to C. **A, Tissue imprint.** Cells lacking pigment are clustered, giving a cohesive epithelial appearance. Abundant clear cytoplasm is present in the poorly differentiated type of melanoma. This gum lesion is associated with a poor prognosis. (Wright-Giemsa; HP oil.) **B, Tissue imprint.** In other parts of the slide, individualized cells with a plasmacytoid appearance are evident. Note the prominent and multiple nucleoli, anisokaryosis, coarse chromatin, and oval to round nuclei in the poorly differentiated melanoma. (Aqueous Romanowsky; HP oil.) **C, Tissue imprint. Dog.** Malignant features seen include large and multiple nucleoli, anisokaryosis, coarse chromatin, and variable nucleocytoplasmic ratios. Note the cell with a few dust-like, dark granules. (Aqueous Romanowsky; HP oil.)

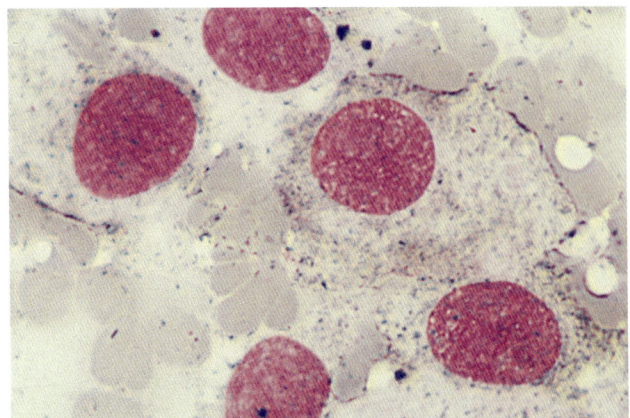

■ **FIGURE 3.167 Melanoma. Tissue aspirate. Dog.** The uniform fine, gray-black melanin granules help determine the diagnosis in poorly differentiated melanocytic tumors. (Wright-Giemsa; HP oil.)

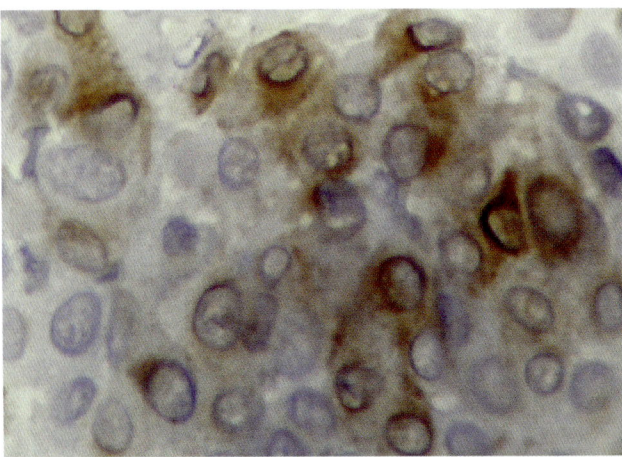

■ **FIGURE 3.169 Amelanotic melanoma. Cytopathologic specimen with previous Romanowsky staining. Tissue aspirate. Dog.** This slide was initially examined using a modified Wright stain, but the cell of origin was difficult to determine. After a heat-induced unmasking procedure, antibody was applied producing a positive reaction that identified the malignancy as melanoma. (Melan A/DAB; HP oil.) (Courtesy Julie Vickers, TDDS/Synlab, Exeter, UK.)

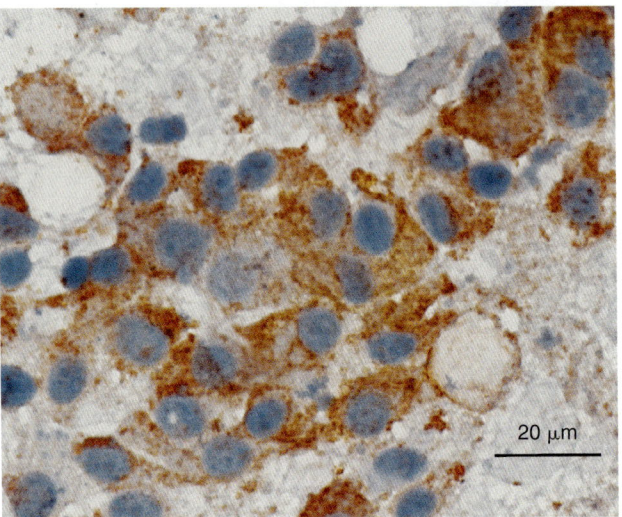

■ **FIGURE 3.168 Melanoma. Skin mass aspirate. Dog.** Prominent immunocytochemical staining in the cytoplasm of cells from a multicentric amelanotic melanoma. (Melan-A/AEC; HP oil.) (Courtesy Michael Logan, Purdue University.)

> ***Cytopathologic differential diagnosis for malignant melanoma:*** plasmacytoma, clear cell adnexal carcinoma, fibrosarcoma, other cutaneous spindle cell tumors.

Cutaneous Extraskeletal and Metastatic Osteosarcoma

Osteosarcomas within the subcutis can occur as a metastasis from a primary bone tumor (Fig. 3.171) or unrelated to bone, likely related to prior vaccination, trauma, or inflammation. Osteosarcoma may appear in several forms, including chondroblastic, fibroblastic, osteoblastic, and giant cell types. Cytopathology reveals an individualized oval cell with abundant cytoplasm that is basophilic and possibly granular with an eosinophilic osteoid or chondroid matrix. Use of alkaline phosphatase is recommended to help identify osteoblasts. See Chapter 14 for more information.

Round Cell Cytomorphology
Canine Histiocytoma

Canine histiocytoma is a very common benign, rapidly growing tumor of mainly young dogs, composing about 12% to 14% of skin masses (Goldschmidt and Shofer, 1992; Yager and Wilcock, 1994). Its origin is the Langerhans cell of the epidermis. It appears as a small, solitary, well-circumscribed, dome-shaped, red ulcerated, hairless mass, the so-called *button tumor*. It occurs commonly on the head, especially the ear pinnae, as well as on the hind limbs, feet, and trunk. Histologically, a nonencapsulated dense "top-heavy" dermal infiltrate of round cells is closely associated with hyperplastic epithelium (Fig. 3.172A). Mitotic figures are frequently found (Fig. 3.172B). On cytopathology, cells have variably distinct cytoplasmic borders (Fig. 3.173A). Nuclei are round, oval, or indented with fine chromatin and indistinct nucleoli (Fig. 3.173B). A variable number of small, well-differentiated lymphocytes, likely cytotoxic T cells, are common in regressing lesions and can sometimes appear to be the predominant cell type (Fig. 3.174). Cells exhibit

A rare type of a benign mixed melanocytic tumor is termed *melanoacanthoma*. It is composed of a melanocytoma and neoplastic follicular epithelium. Cytopathology in this type contains keratinocytes, cellular debris, and melanocytes (Goldschmidt and Goldschmidt, 2017).

Treatment for melanocytic tumors usually involves wide surgical excision. Prognosis depends on tumor site of origin and histologic characteristics that include mitotic activity and nuclear pleomorphism. Melanocytomas have a low mitotic rate and frequently have a good prognosis. Malignant melanomas may arise more often from the nail bed, lip, and other oral mucocutaneous junctions in dogs and cats. These forms appear to carry a guarded or poor prognosis related to frequent recurrence and metastasis.

> ***Cytopathologic differential diagnosis for melanocytoma:*** Normal skin melanocytes, normal pigmented basal cells, melanophages, hemosiderin-laden macrophages.

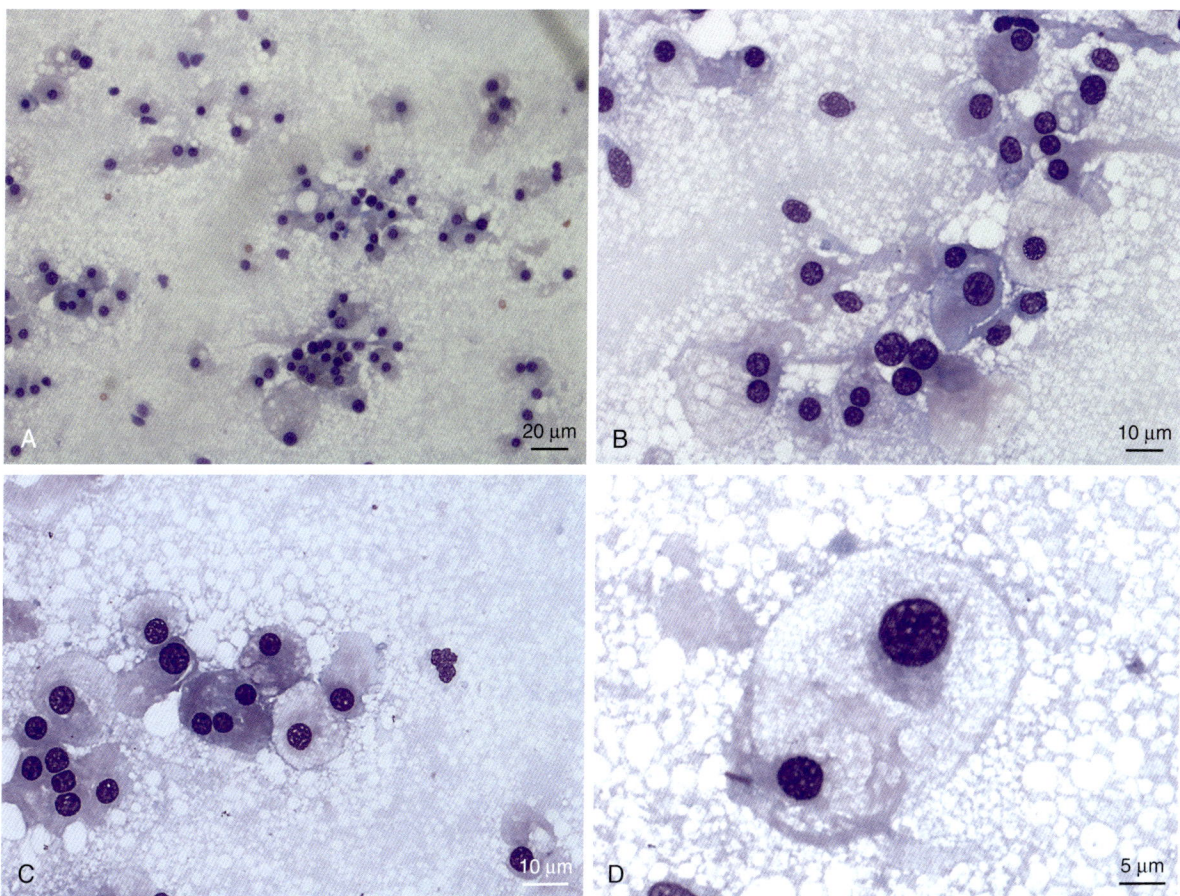

■ **FIGURE 3.170 Balloon cell melanoma. Cutaneous mass below eye. Tissue aspirate. Dog.** Same case in A to D. **A,** This 3 mm mass yielded a highly cellular specimen composed of atypical cells on a stippled, proteinaceous, basophilic background with many bare nuclei. The intact cells are pleomorphic, polygonal to oval in shape with variably distinct cellular borders and variable amounts of amphophilic cytoplasm, which sometimes includes clear vacuoles. (Wright-Giemsa; IP.) **B,** Moderate numbers of individual cells have markedly expanded cytoplasm. The nucleus is round, eccentrically located with coarse chromatin, and measures one to four times the diameter of an erythrocyte. (Wright-Giemsa; HP oil.) **C,** Multinucleation is observed with up to four nuclei seen. (Wright-Giemsa; HP oil.) **D,** Large vacuolated to pale eosinophilic cytoplasm with low nucleocytoplasmic ratio. Anisocytosis and anisokaryosis are marked. Histopathology supported the diagnosis. (Wright-Giemsa; HP oil.) (Courtesy Jacqueline Dolan, University of Florida.)

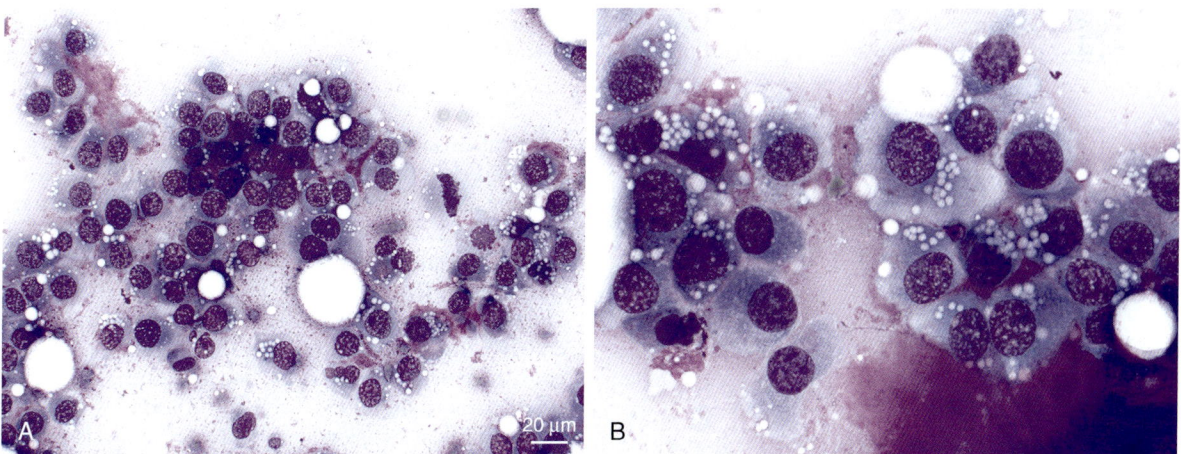

■ **FIGURE 3.171 Chondroblastic osteosarcoma. Lateral thoracic mass. Tissue aspirate. Dog.** Same case in A and B. **A,** This large (>10 cm) firm subcutaneous mass yielded a highly cellular population of moderately atypical mesenchymal cells. The cells are individualized as well, arranged in aggregates that are often admixed with an amorphous, bright eosinophilic (pink), extracellular matrix. (Wright-Giemsa; HP oil.) **B,** These cells are ovoid to fusiform, have indistinct cytoplasmic borders, and have a moderate to abundant amount of basophilic cytoplasm that contains distinct, colorless vacuoles. The round nucleus measures roughly 1.5 times the size of an erythrocyte and has coarsely stippled chromatin with one or more prominent nucleoli. Anisocytosis and anisokaryosis are moderate. This lesion is considered metastatic from a lesion on the radius 2 years prior that was histologically confirmed. (Wright-Giemsa; HP oil.)

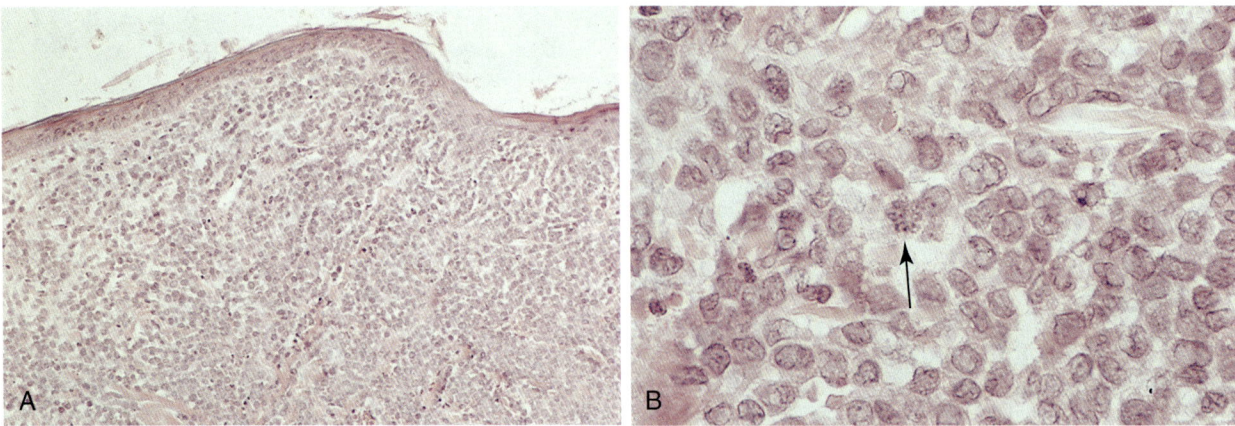

■ **FIGURE 3.172 Histiocytoma. Tissue section. Dog.** Same case in A and B. **A,** The dermis contains a diffuse nodular and dense infiltrate of round cells that is closely associated with hyperplastic epithelium. (H&E; IP.) **B,** Mitotic figures are frequently found among the pleomorphic histiocytic cells. One mitotic figure is shown in the center *(arrow).* (H&E; HP oil.)

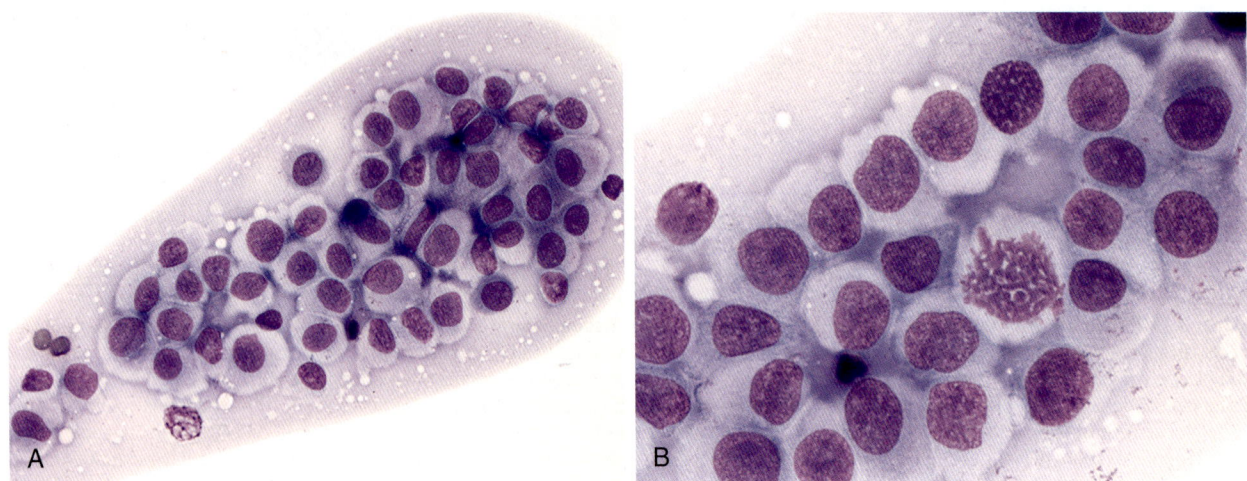

■ **FIGURE 3.173 Histiocytoma. Tissue aspirate. Dog.** Same case in A and B. **A,** Cells have variably distinct cytoplasmic borders in this mass from the tail. Few small dense lymphocytes are present between the larger histiocytic cells. Note the two erythrocytes for size comparison. (Wright-Giemsa; HP oil.) **B,** Nuclei are round, oval, or indented with fine chromatin and indistinct nucleoli. Anisocytosis and anisokaryosis are mild. A mitotic figure is present in the *center* as well as one small lymphocyte. (Wright-Giemsa; HP oil.)

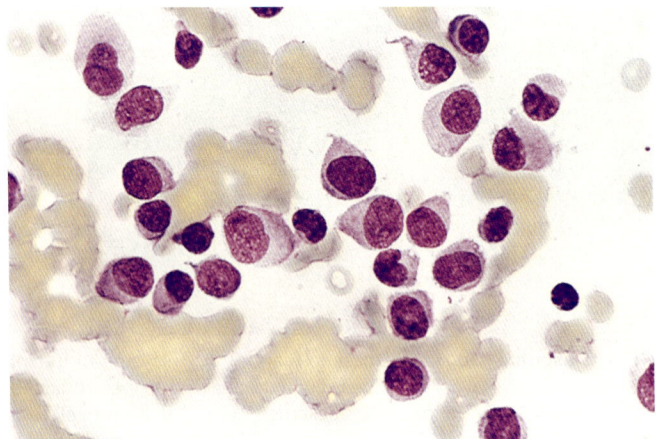

■ **FIGURE 3.174 Histiocytoma. Tissue aspirate. Dog.** Several lymphocytes are present, suggesting regression of the lesion in this elbow mass. (Aqueous Romanowsky; HP oil.)

minimal anisocytosis and anisokaryosis. The cytoplasm is abundant and clear to lightly basophilic (Fig. 3.175A). Cytochemical staining and immunostaining of these tumor cells may be positive for histiocytic markers (Fig. 3.175B), including nonspecific esterases, lysozyme, E-cadherin, Iba1, CD1a, CD11c, CD18, CD45, MHC II, and MUM1 (Pierezan et al., 2014; Moore, 2014; Stillwell and Rissi, 2018). MUM1 immunoreactivity was moderately strong in the nucleus but weak in the cytoplasm, contrasted with the marked nuclear and moderately strong cytoplasmic staining (Stillwell and Rissi, 2018). Treatment involves surgical excision if necessary. Prognosis is excellent to good because the tumor frequently regresses spontaneously within 3 months, and recurrence is rare.

> ***Cytopathologic differential diagnosis:*** lymphoma, plasmacytoma, benign cutaneous histiocytosis, systemic histiocytosis, Langerhans cell histiocytosis, nodular granulomatous dermatitis.

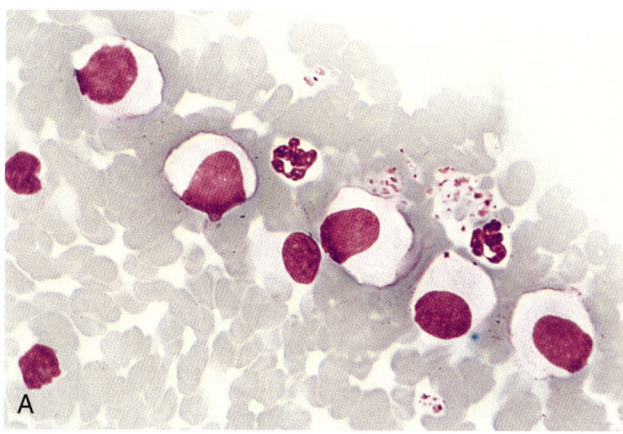 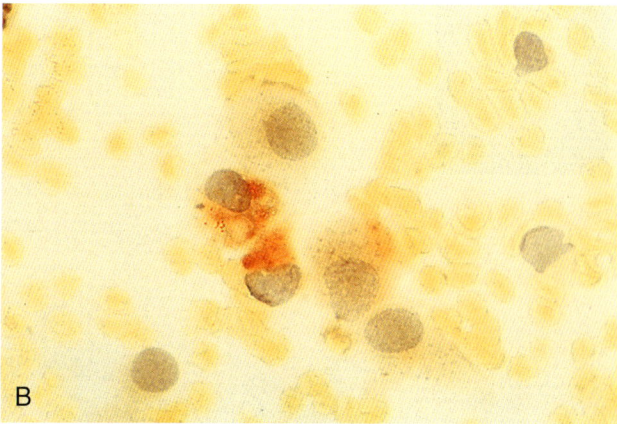

FIGURE 3.175 Histiocytoma. Tissue aspirate. Dog. Same case in A and B. **A,** The cytoplasm is abundant and clear to lightly basophilic and cells appear discrete in this lip mass. (Wright-Giemsa; HP oil.) **B,** Red cytoplasmic staining indicates positive reaction to this histiocytic cytochemical marker. (Alpha-naphthyl butyrate esterase; HP oil.)

Canine Cutaneous Langerhans Cell Histiocytosis

This rare dermal disease resembles histiocytoma except instead of a solitary lesion, there are multiple variably sized erythematous nodules. These lesions may fail to regress and become more aggressive, spreading to lymph nodes and visceral organs. Histiocytes may display more anisokaryosis and multinucleated cells than is typical for solitary histiocytoma with numerous mitotic figures. They display reniform, folded, or lobulated nuclei (Son et al., 2019). The immunophenotype is identical to canine histiocytoma as CD1a+, CD11c/CD18+, E-cadherin+, CD204−, and Iba1+ (Moore, 2014).

Feline Progressive Histiocytosis

Few cases of progressive histiocytosis have been identified in cats, presenting as single skin nodules usually around the head, neck, or lower extremities (Fig.3.176A) (Affolter and Moore, 2006). These may change into multiple intradermal masses that later ulcerate (Pinto da Cunha et al., 2014). Single or multinucleated histiocytic cells, which can resemble plasma cells, predominate (Fig. 3.176B–C). Cells express CD1a, CD1c, CD11b, CD18, Iba1, and MHC II and variably express E-cadherin (Fig. 3.176D). There may be CD3+ reactive lymphocytes intermixed between histiocytic cells. The disease slowly evolves into a fatal condition with invasion into regional lymph nodes and internal organs by neoplastic dendritic cells. Chemotherapy or immunosuppressive and immunomodulatory drugs have not been successful. Animals die or are euthanized from 1 month to 3 years (average, 13 months). The etiology is not known but appears to involve either interstitial dendritic cells or Langerhans cells depending on the environment (Hirabayashi et al., 2020). Cytopathologic specimens or fresh-frozen tissue specimens are necessary to diagnose the CD1 expression because formalin-fixation damages these cell surface molecules.

> **Cytopathologic differential diagnosis:** lymphoma, plasmacytoma, histiocytic sarcoma, granulomatous dermatitis.

Histiocytic Sarcoma

Histiocytic sarcoma, a tumor of neoplastic interstitial dendritic cells, occurs in dogs and cats as a localized or disseminated condition (Moore, 2014). A review of the clinical aspects of this disease is available (Kennedy et al., 2016). Localized histiocytic sarcomas are common in dogs and uncommon in cats. These are firm, often subcutaneous, masses located on the extremities and in periarticular sites. In contrast to histiocytomas and Langerhans cell histiocytosis, both of which originate in the dermis and are E-cadherin positive, histiocytic sarcomas originate within the subcutis from dermal dendritic cells that can extend into the dermis. Mass lesions are also observed in spleen, lung, lymph node, and other primary tissue sites.

Histiocytes are pleomorphic, mononuclear, as well as multinucleate giant cells with marked cytological atypia (Fig. 3.177A). The presence of multinucleate giant cells is similar to those seen in undifferentiated pleomorphic sarcoma. Low numbers of small lymphocytes may infiltrate these lesions (Fig. 3.177B). On cytopathology, these can have both a round cell and mesenchymal or spindle cell appearance. Individualized round cells contain abundant basophilic cytoplasm that may display vacuolation. Nuclei are vesiculated, round to indented, with one or more nucleoli. Marked anisokaryosis and anisocytosis are often observed (Figs. 3.177B and 3.178A).

The neoplastic cells are immunoreactive to CD1a, CD11c/CD18, CD45, and MHC II in the dog and cat (Fig. 3.178B). Recent studies indicate Iba1 and CD204 are useful in the diagnosis of histiocytic sarcoma using immunochemistry in both tissue sections and cytopathologic specimens (Pierezan et al., 2014; Kato et al., 2014). Preliminary studies (Hans et al., 2008) support expression by BLA.36, a marker often used for B cells, as an indicator of histiocytic disorders when other B-cell markers are nonreactive. Tumor cells lack E-cadherin expression, indicating these are likely not Langerhans cells. Histiocytic sarcomas are locally invasive with metastasis to draining lymph nodes. Prognosis is favorable in localized histiocytic sarcoma with early wide surgical excision or amputation of the limb followed by chemotherapy. Prognosis is poor with the disseminated form of the disease.

> **Cytopathologic differential diagnosis:** Langerhans cell histiocytosis, poorly granulated mast cell tumors, amelanotic melanoma, undifferentiated pleomorphic sarcoma, other sarcomas, reactive histiocytosis.

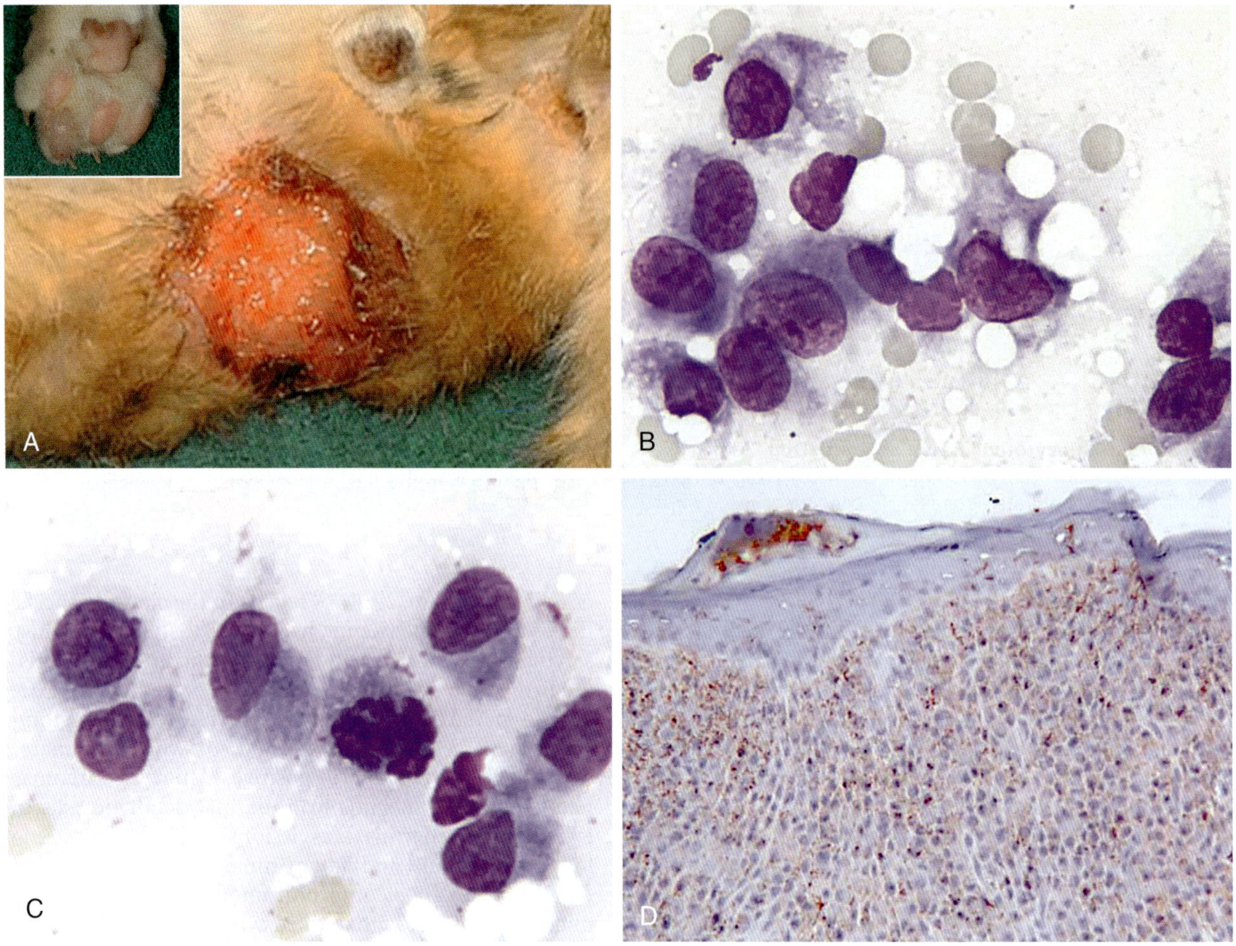

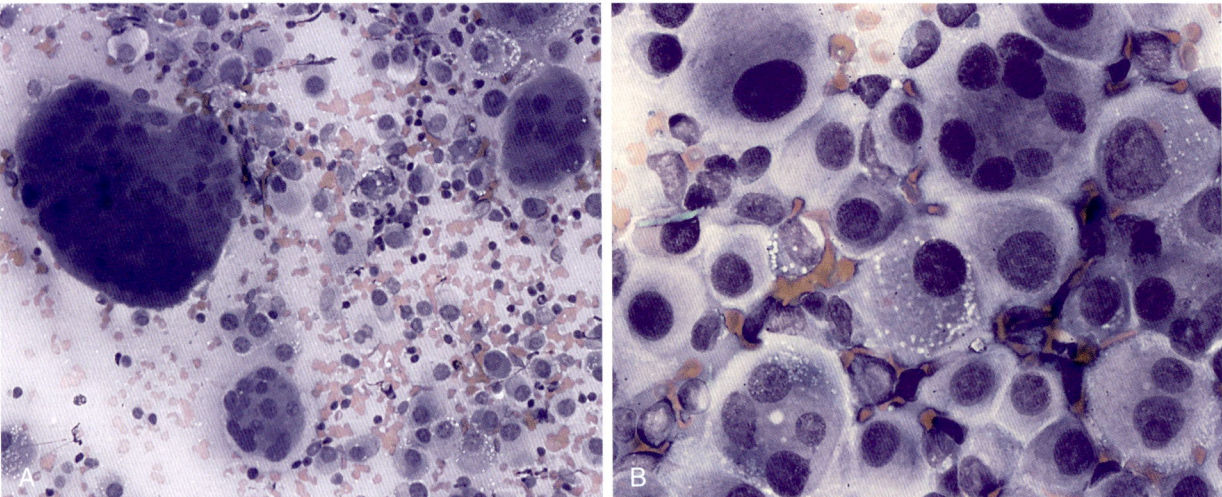

■ **FIGURE 3.176 Feline progressive histiocytosis. Cat.** Same case in A to D. **A, Macroscopic specimen.** Multiple skin nodules are present over the body, some of which are ulcerated as seen on the flank. *Inset:* Underside of the paw showing an alopecic interdigital nodular lesion. **B, Skin nodule imprint.** The predominant cell is mononuclear with moderate amounts of basophilic cytoplasm with variably distinct cell borders. (Wright-Giemsa; HP oil.) **C, Skin nodule imprint.** The nucleus is round to oval to irregular with finely stippled chromatin and a prominent nucleolus. A mitotic figure is shown in the center of the field. (Wright-Giemsa; HP oil.) **D, Tissue section.** Immunohistochemistry supports histiocytic origin with anti-CD1a positive reactivity. (CD1a/AEC; IP.) (Courtesy Janelle Renschler, North Carolina State University.)

■ **FIGURE 3.177 Histiocytic sarcoma. Cutaneous masses. Tissue aspirate. Dog.** Same case in A and B. **A,** Lateral thorax. A raised spherule mass that measures 0.5 inches yields a highly pleomorphic round cell population. Several multinucleate giant cells are present, some containing up to 30 nuclei. (Modified Wright; IP.) **B,** Dorsum. A raised spherule mass at mid spine that measures 0.5 inches yields a similar cell population as in A. Higher magnification of this population reveals the marked anisocytosis and anisokaryosis as well as several multinucleate giant cells. (Modified Wright; HP oil.) (Courtesy Michigan State University.)

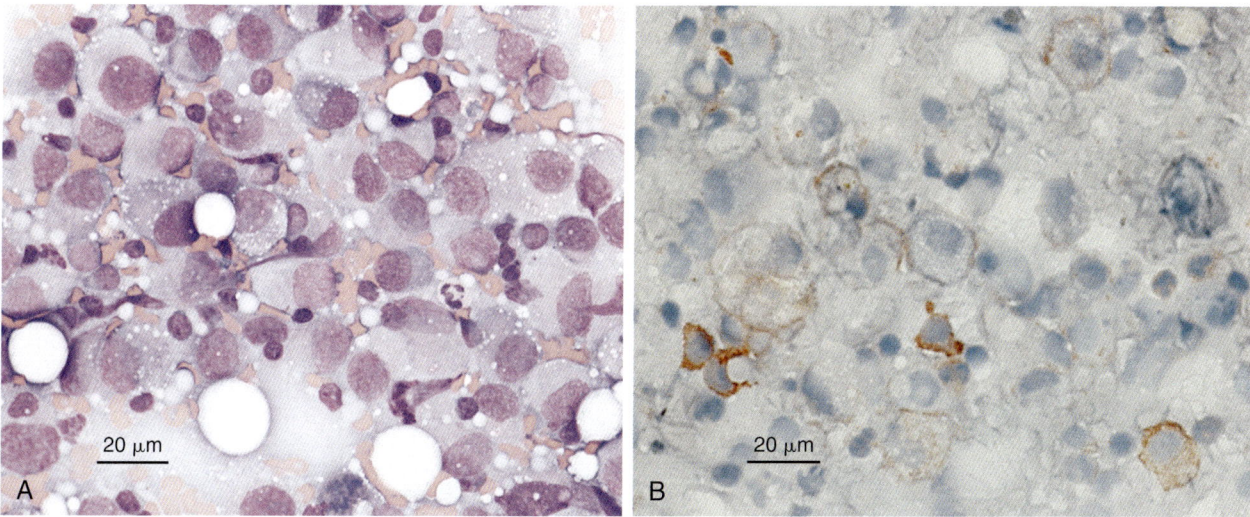

■ **FIGURE 3.178 Histiocytic sarcoma. Tissue aspirate. Dog.** Same case in A and B. **A,** Skin mass on the flank that 1 month later progressed to a similar proliferation of cells found around the head of the femur. Sample is highly cellular with large (20–30 μm) round cells as the predominant population. These cells have round to indented nuclei that are finely granulated with multiple small nucleoli. The grey cytoplasm is generally abundant with occasional small punctate vacuoles. The background contains free lipid and a mixture of lymphocytes and plasma cells. Anisocytosis, anisokaryosis, and variable nucleocytoplasmic ratios characterize the population. (Modified Wright; HP oil.) **B,** There is variable red granular membrane staining with immunocytochemistry to the anti-CD1a antigen, indicating the cell population is mostly composed of dendritic cells. Another consideration for the histiocytic appearance would be macrophagic origin, but this would be expected to be negative for CD1. (CD1a/AEC; HP oil.)

Reactive Histiocytosis (Cutaneous and Systemic)

In contrast to the neoplastic histiocytic diseases, a group of inflammatory conditions in dogs may mimic the cytopathologic appearance of histiocytic sarcoma. These reactive histiocytic diseases, such as systemic histiocytosis and cutaneous histiocytosis, have lesions dominated by activated interstitial dendritic cells and lymphocytes, which invade vessel walls, producing vasocentric infiltrates in skin, lymph nodes, and internal organs (only in systemic histiocytosis) (Moore, 2014). The "bottom-heavy" lesions of cutaneous histiocytosis appear as multiple cutaneous and subcutaneous firm nonpruritic nodules up to 4 cm in diameter composed of a mixed population of lymphoid and histiocytic cells (Fig. 3.179A–C). Histiocytes lack cytologic atypia, and multinucleate giant cells are rare. Common sites include the face, nose, neck, trunk, extremities, perineum, and scrotum.

Reactive histiocytes express dendritic cell markers such as CD1a, C11c, CD18, and MHC class II and, unlike those in histiocytic sarcoma, these dendritic cells express CD4, which indicates cell activation, and CD90 (Thy-1), which is expressed by normal interstitial dermal interstitial cells (Fig. 3.179D). Treatment may be attempted with immunosuppressive or immunomodulatory drugs to control the T-cell activation of these dendritic cells. It is worth noting that CD4 and CD11c cannot be evaluated in formalin-fixed tissue sections, whereas CD1a, CD90, CD18, MHC class II, and E-cadherin are possible. Therefore, cytopathologic specimens are extremely helpful in making a definitive diagnosis.

> *Cytopathologic differential diagnosis (cutaneous):* lymphoma, histiocytic sarcoma, plasmacytoma, multiple cutaneous histiocytoma, canine cutaneous Langerhans cell histiocytosis.

Mast Cell Tumor

Mast cell tumors accounts for about 20% of skin tumors in dogs, with higher prevalence in certain breeds such as boxers, Labrador and golden retrievers, Chinese Shar-Peis, bulldogs, Boston terriers, pit bull terriers, fox terriers, weimaraners, cocker spaniels, dachshunds, Australian cattle dogs, beagles, schnauzers, and pugs (Kiupel and Camus, 2019). The mean age in dogs is 9 years, but the disease may occasionally occur in puppies. In dogs, subcutaneous MCT should be differentiated from cutaneous MCT by histopathology because the former tends to have a less aggressive biologic behavior (Gill et al., 2020). Most commonly, MCT appears as solitary nonencapsulated nodules in the skin and less common in the subcutis. The gross appearance of MCT include hairless, raised, erythematous masses to nodular rashes or diffuse swellings. In dogs, MCTs are most common on the trunk and limbs and are generally solitary, nonencapsulated, and highly infiltrative into dermis or subcutis (Fig. 3.180). Tumors occurring on the perineum, scrotum, prepuce, and digits in dogs appear to be more aggressive (Gross et al., 2005).

If the tumor is located within the epidermis or outer dermis it is considered a cutaneous MCT (Fig. 3.181) but it is called subcutaneous if the majority of the mass is within the subcutis surrounded by adipose tissue. With observer variability and prognosis in mind, researchers have proposed a histologic two-tier scheme grading system for canine cutaneous MCT (Kiupel et al., 2011). This involves a low and high grade, the latter reflecting greater cellular and nuclear atypia, frequent mitotic figures, multinucleation, and karyomegaly.

Cytopathologic evaluation as a screening tool can easily make a diagnosis of MCT especially when methanolic Romanowsky stains such as Wright stain are applied (Fig. 3.182A). The presence of numerous cells densely packed with visible purple granules within the cytoplasm supports the diagnosis

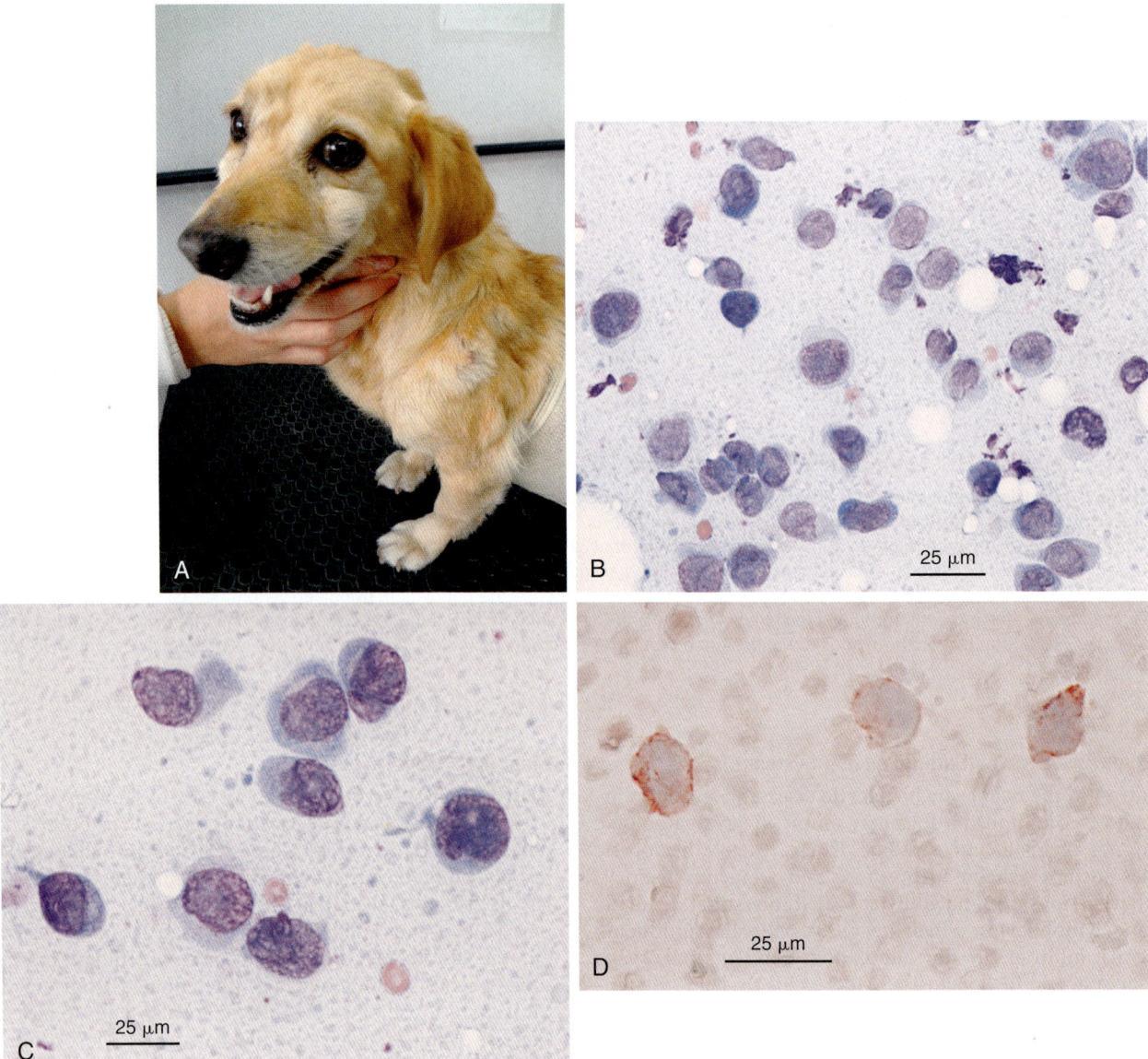

■ **FIGURE 3.179 Cutaneous histiocytosis. Dog.** Same case in A to D. **A,** Multiple variably sized nodules over the head, limb, and body and bilaterally on the muzzle below the eye. **B, Tissue aspirate.** Individualized cells with variable amounts of scant to moderate basophilic cytoplasm and pleomorphic irregularly round, indented, and reniform nuclei. (Modified Wright; HP oil.) **C, Tissue aspirate.** Higher magnification demonstrates presence of small Golgi zone and irregularly shaped nuclei. (Modified Wright; HP oil.) **D, Tissue aspirate.** Strong positive immunoreactivity with anti-CD90 (Thy1) indicating the presence of dermal interstitial dendritic cells, the presence of which supports a reactive histiocytosis. (CD90/AEC; HP oil.) (Courtesy Stella F. Valle, Porto Alegre, Brazil.)

of well-differentiated MCT, which often suggests a good prognosis. However, the use of aqueous Romanowsky quick stains minimizes the formation of a stain precipitate leaving a colorless or faintly granular cytoplasm even with a well-differentiated MCT (Fig. 3.182B–C). The presence of cytoplasmic granules may hide the high-grade features so destaining slides or using other stains that only reveal nuclear morphology such as hematoxylin and eosin or Papanicolaou are helpful (Ressel and Finotello, 2016) (Figs. 3.183 and 3.184).

Several researchers have attempted to use some aspects of the cutaneous mast cell histologic scheme for the grading of cytopathologic specimens (Barbosa et al., 2014; Scarpa et al., 2016) but found the criteria may need adjustment to better align with the less cellular samples. In one study, MCT was classified as high grade if on cytopathology, the cells were poorly granulated or had at least two of four findings: mitotic figures, binucleated or multinucleated cells, nuclear pleomorphism, or anisokaryosis (nuclei >1.5 times a typical mast cell nucleus) (Camus et al., 2016). This grading scheme had 88% sensitivity and 94% specificity relative to histopathologic grading. Even though cytopathology indicated more high-grade MCT than histopathology, the scheme proved to be an excellent screening test. Nuclear pleomorphism involving nuclear shapes that were neither round nor ovoid was found to be the least useful cytopathologic feature for survival prediction. An example of a canine high-grade MCT with the above cytopathologic findings

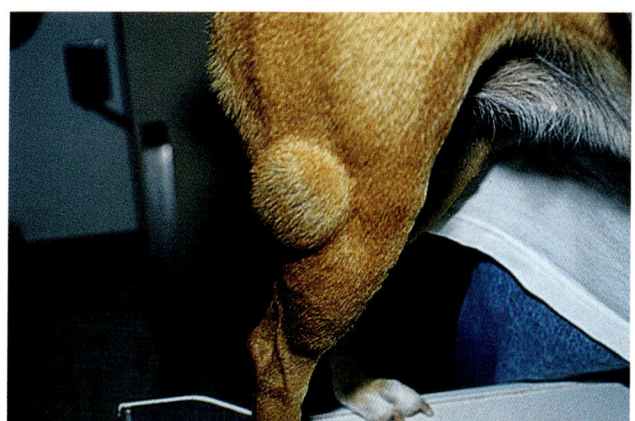

■ **FIGURE 3.180 Mast cell tumor. Leg mass. Macroscopic specimen. Dog.** Note the large, raised, haired nodule on the lateral stifle area that resembles grossly a lipoma.

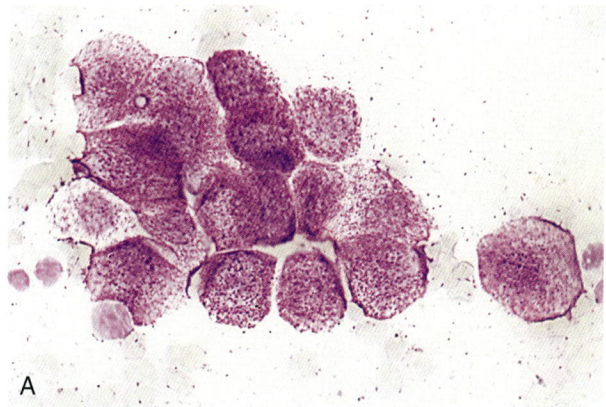

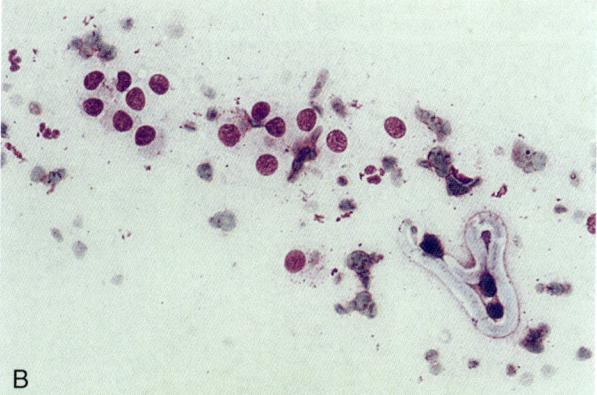

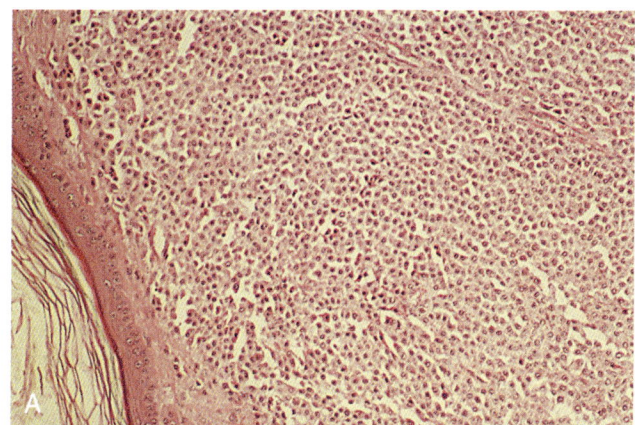

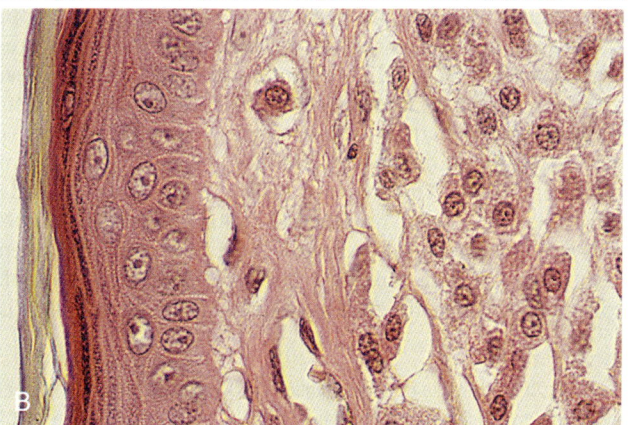

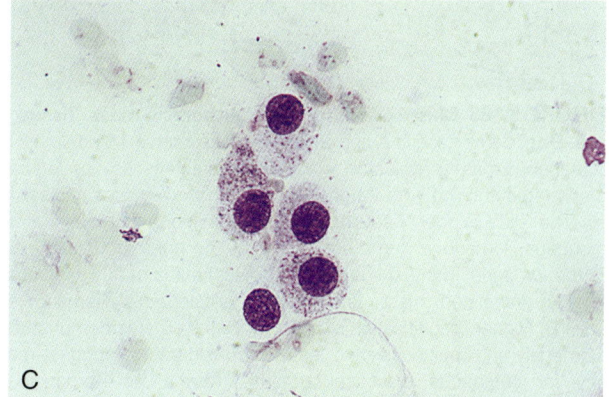

■ **FIGURE 3.181 Mast cell tumor. Tissue section. Cat.** Same case in A and B. **A,** Diffuse dense dermal infiltration of round cells. (H&E; IP.) **B,** Some granulation is present within the round cells. Nuclear size is uniform in this well-differentiated tumor. (H&E; HP oil.)

■ **FIGURE 3.182 Mast cell tumor. Tissue aspirate. Dog.** Same case in A to C. **A,** Variable staining of granules and anisokaryosis suggest a moderately differentiated tumor for this mammary area mass. (Wright-Giemsa; HP oil.) **B,** The water-soluble stain washes out the granular contents so that the mass appears to be poorly differentiated with cytopathology. Note the *Dirofilaria immitis* microfilaria in the *lower right* area among the poorly granulated mast cells. (Aqueous Romanowsky; HP oil.) **C,** Higher magnification of B. Note the light dusting of granulation in these cells related to the use of a water-soluble stain. Compare these cells with those in A that retain the granular contents using a methanolic Romanowsky stain. (Aqueous Romanowsky; HP oil.)

may also show variable intensity to different stains (Fig. 3.185A–D). Identification of mast cells by cytochemistry or immunochemistry involves Giemsa and toluidine blue staining for metachromatic granules (see Fig. 3.185D), in addition to chloroacetate esterase, omega-exonuclease, and antibodies for tryptase and KIT (Fernandez et al., 2005).

Eosinophils are more numerous in canine tumors than feline tumors. The background is usually filled with granules from ruptured mast cells and eosinophils. Degranulation may be associated with hemorrhage, vascular necrosis, edema, and collagenolysis. Collagen breakdown occurs through matrix metalloproteinases present in the neoplastic cells as well as

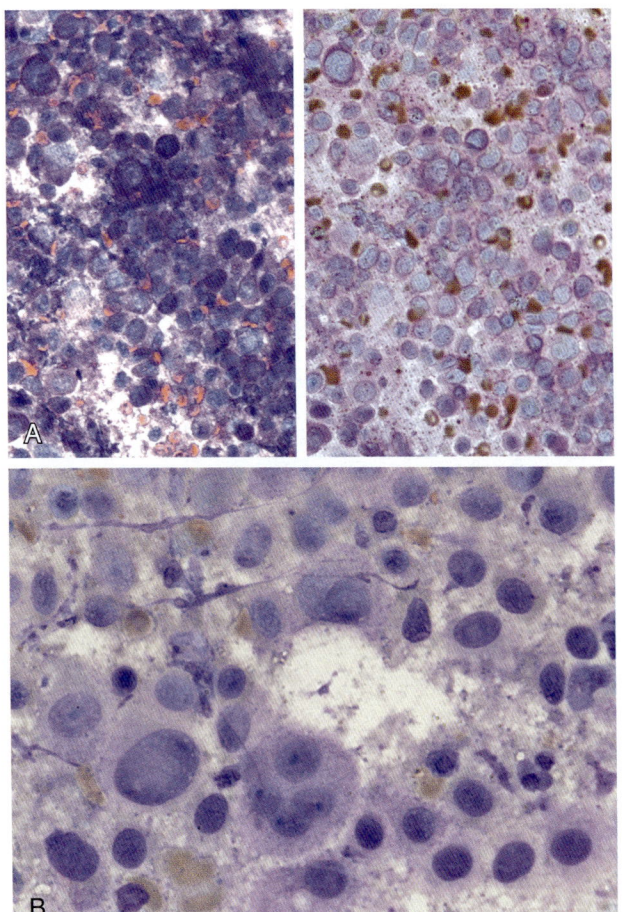

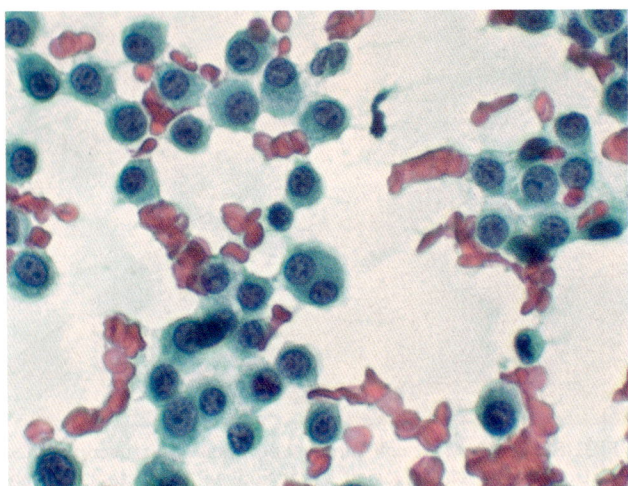

■ FIGURE 3.184 Mast cell tumor, poorly differentiated. Fine needle, non-aspiration. Dog. Mast cells exhibit a high degree of pleomorphism with prominent nucleoli as demonstrated with a stain that highlights nuclear and not cytoplasmic features. Note binucleated cell in center. (Papanicolaou stain; HP oil.) (Courtesy Noeme Sousa Rocha, FMVZ-UNESP Botucatu, Brazil.)

■ FIGURE 3.183 Mast cell tumor. Lateral thoracic mass. Tissue aspirate. Dog. Same case in A and B. **A,** One slide from a 1.5 cm × 1.5 cm subcutaneous mass is evaluated for staining characteristics. The *left panel* demonstrates staining with Wright-Giemsa, which disguises nuclear features. The slide is then destained using methanol and restained with an aqueous Romanowsky method shown in the *right panel*, same field as in the *left panel*. The result is improved visualization of nuclear features in highly granulated mast cells. (Methanolic/aqueous Romanowsky; HP oil.) **B,** Higher magnification of a similarly stained area demonstrating karyomegaly and multinucleation features considered to suggest malignancy for cutaneous mast cell tumors. (Methanolic Romanowsky-destained-restained aqueous Romanowsky; HP oil.)

inflammatory cells to enhance tissue invasion (Fig. 3.186). Fibroplasia may accompany MCT, and dense collagen bands often react to polarization (Figs. 3.187 to 3.189).

Treatment involves wide surgical excision, cryosurgery, radiotherapy, and chemotherapy. Prognostic tools in dogs involves the frequency of argyrophilic nucleolar organizer regions and Ki67 as indicators for cellular proliferation, both of which when increased were associated with decreased survival, as is also the case with KIT protein localization (Kiupel et al., 2004; Webster et al., 2007). Use of KIT protein evaluation along with proliferation markers and the two-tier approach has been shown to be most predictive of metastatic and recurrence potential for cytopathologic specimens (Sailasuta et al., 2014).

Mast cell tumors in cats represent the second most common skin tumor type, accounting for 12% to 20% of skin tumors (Goldschmidt and Shofer, 1992). These are usually solitary, well-circumscribed, dermal masses that occur on the head, neck, and limbs. Multiple masses are common in young Siamese cats (Gross et al., 2005). Small, well-differentiated lymphocytes may be associated with the feline tumors, but few or no eosinophils are expected. Tumor cells that resemble poorly granulated histiocytes are associated with the multiple form of MCT (Figs. 3.190 and 3.191). A significant number of young cats with multiple masses respond with spontaneous regression within months. For cats, the solitary form of the disease is generally considered benign with some exceptions of recurrence and invasion (Johnson et al., 2002). The cytopathologic and histopathologic correlation of a solitary feline case is demonstrated (Fig. 3.192). Mitotic index, KIT immunoreactivity score, and Ki67 index were significantly higher in mastocytic pleomorphic than in mastocytic well-differentiated or atypical/poorly granulated MCT histologic subtypes (Sabattini and Bettini, 2010). Most recently, feline MCTs were classified as high grade if there were more than 5 mitotic figures in 10 (40×) fields and at least two of the following criteria: tumor diameter larger than 1.5 cm, irregular nuclear shape, and nucleolar prominence/chromatin clusters (Sabattini and Bettini, 2019).

KEY POINT Giemsa or toluidine blue staining should be used to reveal cytoplasmic granules in poorly differentiated forms. It should be noted that aqueous Romanowsky stains often show a lack of granulation, especially in less differentiated forms of mast cell tumor. This is related to the water-soluble nature of the granule contents and an inability to form a stable precipitate. The use of wet fixation stains such as Papanicolaou helps to evaluate nuclear and nucleolar features because the granules are not visible with this stain.

Cytopathologic differential diagnosis: normal mast cells, chronic allergic dermatitis, lymphoma, balloon cell melanoma, histiocytoma, plasmacytoma.

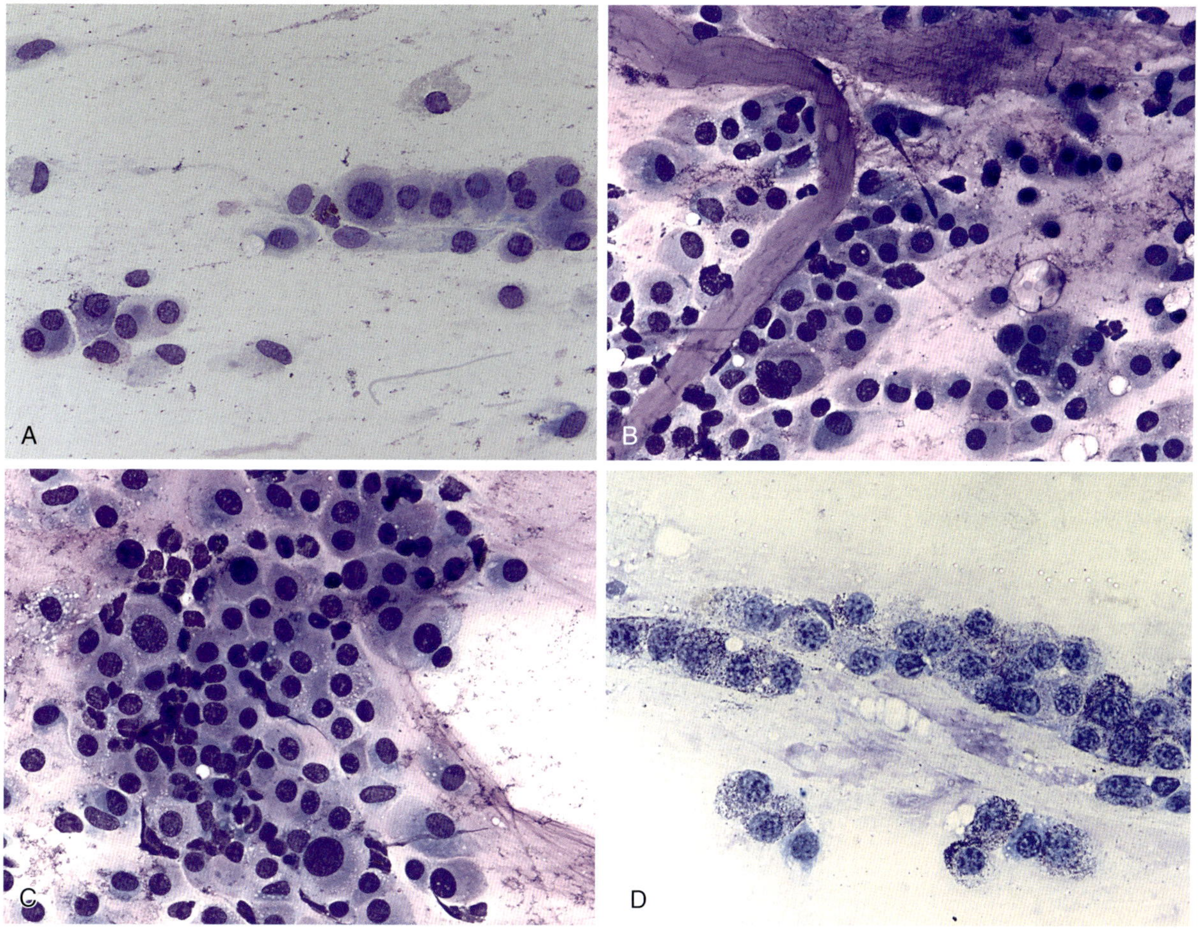

■ **FIGURE 3.185 Mast cell tumor, high grade. Caudal thigh mass. Tissue aspirate. Dog.** Same case in A to D. **A,** History involves recurrent mast cell tumor. Cells demonstrate moderate anisocytosis and mild to moderate anisokaryosis. Several binucleated cell are shown. The cytoplasm is poorly granulated with few fine magenta granules. (Wright-Giemsa; HP oil.) **B,** Collagen strands with associated mast cells. A multinucleated cell is readily visible. (Aqueous Romanowsky; HP oil.) **C,** Higher magnification demonstrates marked karyomegaly, a malignant feature. The cytoplasm of several cells contains numerous colorless punctate vacuoles. (Aqueous Romanowsky; HP oil.) **D,** A greater degree of cytoplasmic granulation is demonstrated with this stain compared with methanolic and aqueous Romanowsky staining. (Toluidine blue; HP oil.) (Courtesy Mary White, The Ohio State University.)

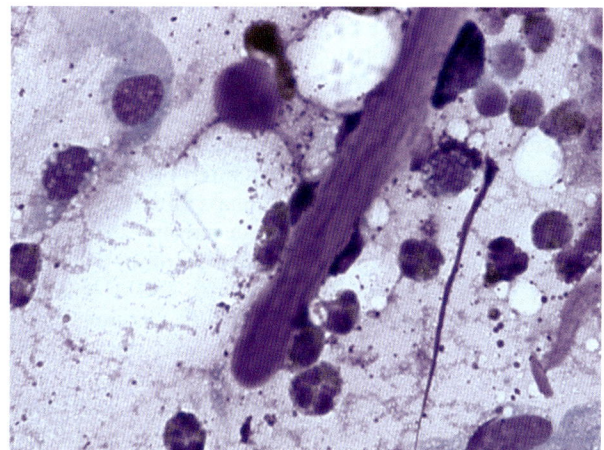

■ **FIGURE 3.186 Mast cell tumor, collagenolysis. Flank mass. Tissue aspirate. Dog.** Numerous eosinophils attach and surround a collagen strand, which appears fibrillar with linear streaks and more dense than normal, suggestive of degeneration. Several fibroblasts are present consistent with reactive fibroplasia that may accompany mast cell tumors. (Modified Wright; HP oil.) (Courtesy Jennifer Bouschor, Kansas State University.)

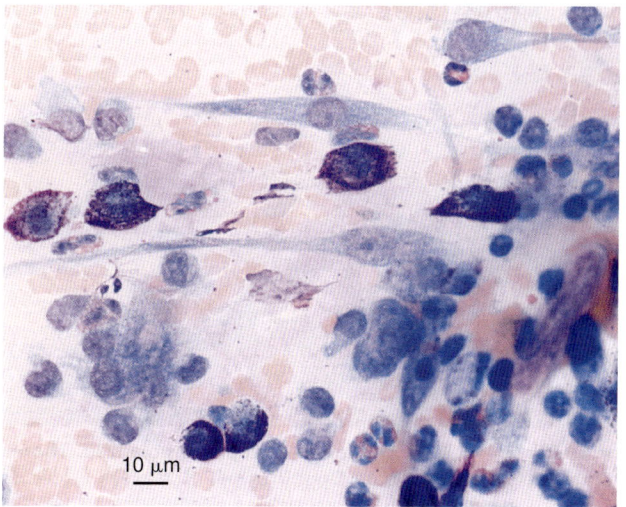

■ **FIGURE 3.187 Mast cell tumor, fibroplasia. Tissue aspirate. Dog.** Fibroplasia is frequent in this mast cell tumor as evidenced by the fibroblasts scattered among many eosinophils and mast cells. (Modified Wright; HP oil.)

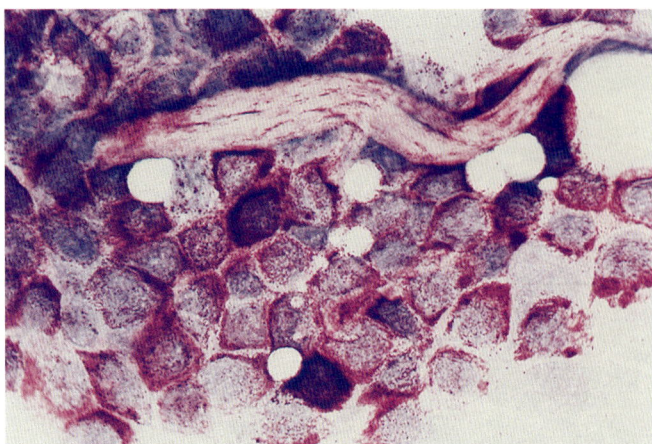

■ **FIGURE 3.188 Mast cell tumor, fibroplasia. Thoracic skin mass aspirate. Dog.** This moderately differentiated tumor contains pale-pink collagen strand. (Wright-Giemsa; HP oil.)

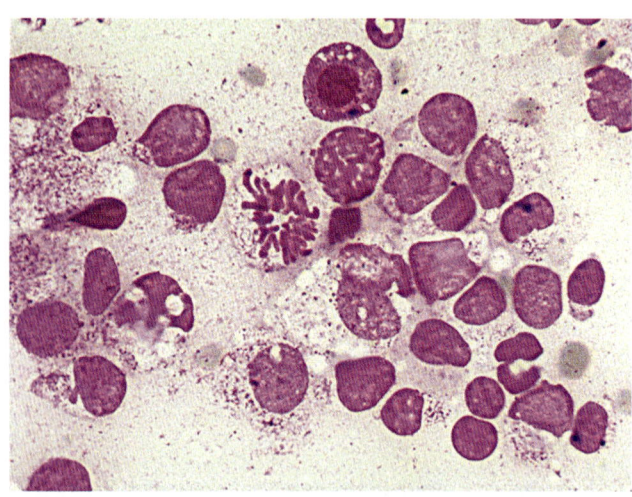

■ **FIGURE 3.190 Mast cell tumor. Digit mass imprint. Cat.** Note the granular background from released cytoplasmic granules. Cells are pleomorphic with a "histiocytic" appearance and contain a variable number of cytoplasmic granules. This 8-year-old cat had multiple digits on two feet affected by the same tumor. (Wright-Giemsa; HP oil.)

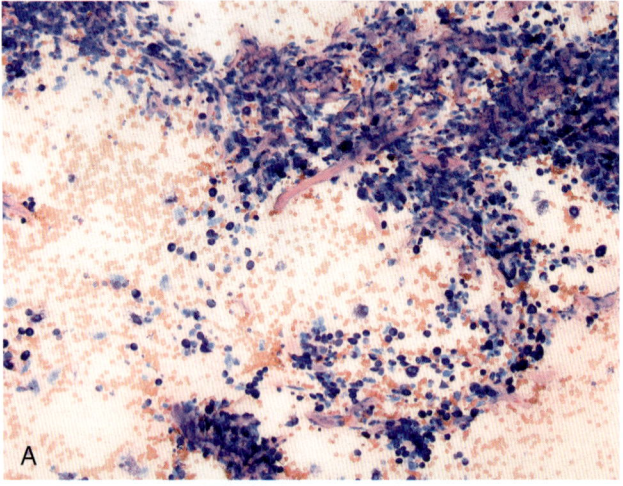

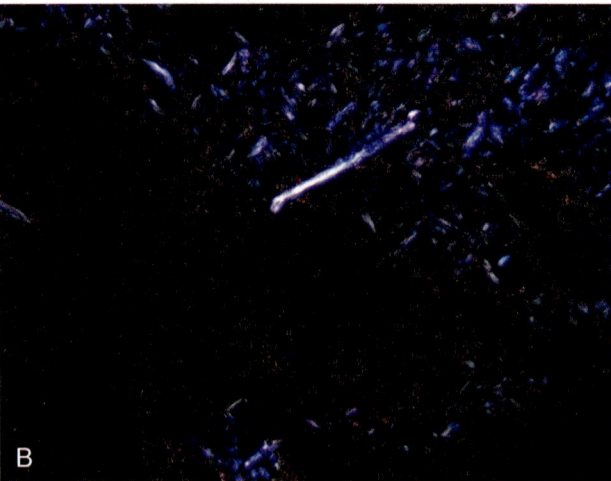

■ **FIGURE 3.189 Mast cell tumor, fibroplasia polarized. Thoracic dermal mass. Tissue aspirate. Dog.** This 2 × 2.3 cm mass yielded high cellularity with numerous highly granulated well-differentiated mast cells intertwined around many bright pink hyalinized collagen strands. (Wright-Giemsa; LP.) **B,** The same field when subjected to polarization demonstrates the birefringent nature of collagen. (Wright-Giemsa/Polarized; LP.) (Courtesy Jacqueline Dolan, University of Florida.)

Plasmacytoma

Plasmacytomas constitute about 2% of canine skin tumors and are rare in cats (Yager and Wilcock, 1994). They present as mostly solitary, well-circumscribed masses often on the digits, ears, and mouth. Aspirates are moderately to markedly cellular. Individual cells have variable amounts of basophilic cytoplasm in which borders are discrete (Fig. 3.193). Occasionally one may see cells with a pink periphery suggestive of a flame cell (Fig. 3.194) or a Mott cell (Fig. 3.195), supporting immunoglobulin production. Anisocytosis and anisokaryosis are prominent features. Nuclei are round to oval with fine to moderately coarse chromatin and indistinct nucleoli. The nuclei are often eccentrically placed and frequently binucleated. Multinucleated cells may be present (Figs. 3.196 and 3.197A). Amorphous eosinophilic material, representative of amyloid, is seen in fewer than 10% of plasmacytomas (Figs. 3.197B and 3.198). Amyloid may also appear as eosinophilic fibrillar material inside and surrounding neoplastic plasma cells as well as within histiocytes (Fig. 3.199) (Santos et al., 2017). Treatment involves wide surgical excision. Prognosis is generally good, but local recurrences are possible. Transition from extramedullary plasmacytoma to myeloma has been documented rarely in dogs and cats, the latter case after 5 months (Radhakrishnan et al., 2004). Identification of plasmacytomas can involve cytochemistry (RNA stains magenta with methyl green pyronin) or immunochemistry (CD45, CD79a, lambda chain, MUM1) (Majzoub et al., 2003; Ramos-Vara et al., 2007). MUM1 immunoreactivity was necessary to confirm the diagnosis in a rare occurrence of cytoplasmic granularity resembling a melanocytic tumor (Quiroz-Rocha et al., 2017). Recently, MUM1 was reported to be positive in both plasmacytomas and canine cutaneous histiocytomas but not histiocytic sarcomas; however, plasmacytomas were Iba1 negative unlike histiocytoma and histiocytic sarcoma (Stillwell and Rissi, 2018). The cytopathologic appearance of a peripheral neural sheath tumor in a cat displayed a morphologic resemblance to plasma cells, which suggests histopathology is best for these cases (Tremblay et al., 2005).

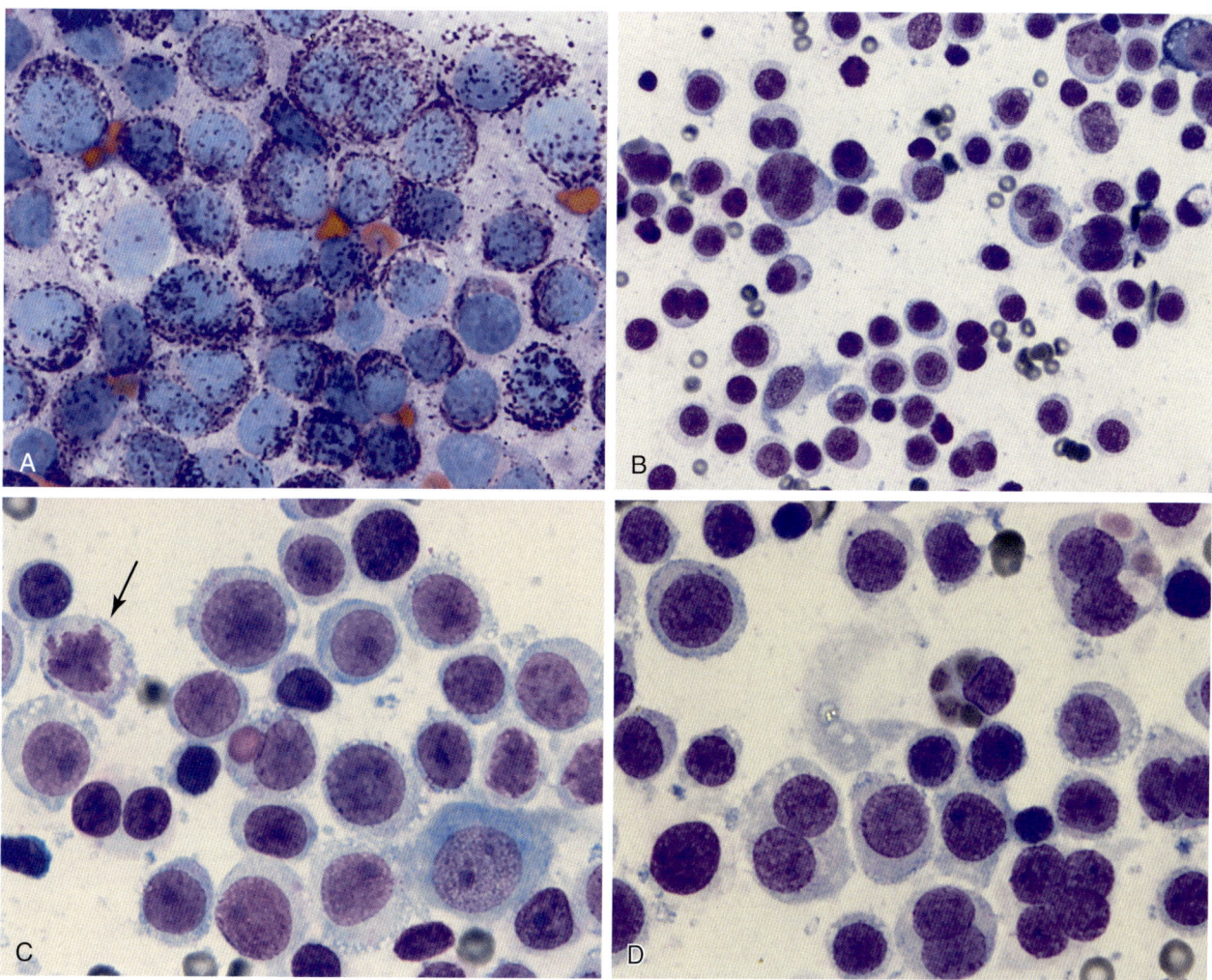

■ **FIGURE 3.191 Mast cell tumor. Inguinal area mass. Tissue aspirate. Cat. A,** This large (3 × 3 inch) round, firm, subcutaneous mass yielded a large population of moderately granulated mast cells. Two cells in the field display binucleation. (Modified Wright; HP oil.) **B,** A pleomorphic cell population is evident with this stain. Several binucleated and one multinucleated cells are shown. Cells have a high nucleocytoplasmic ratio and display moderate anisocytosis and anisokaryosis. (Aqueous Romanowsky; HP oil.) **C,** One mitotic figure *(arrow)* is present along with a mast cell with an intracytoplasmic erythrocyte. A single nucleolus is prominent in most of the cells including a plump fibroblast *(lower right)* (Aqueous Romanowsky; HP oil.) **D,** Two mast cells contain several erythrocytes, termed *xenocannibalism*. The erythrocytes appear to be phagocytized as they are found within vacuoles and partially degraded *(upper right)*. (Aqueous Romanowsky; HP oil.) (Courtesy Erica Corda, Michigan State University.)

> ***Cytopathologic differential diagnosis:*** lymphoma, histiocytoma, amelanotic melanoma, neuroendocrine (Merkel cell) tumor, peripheral nerve sheath tumor.

Cutaneous Lymphoma

Cutaneous lymphoma may occur as a primary disease of the skin or rarely as a manifestation of generalized lymphoma. It is more common in older dogs and cats, although its presence in juvenile dogs has been reported (Choi et al., 2004). Histologically, cutaneous lymphoma is divided into epitheliotropic and nonepitheliotropic types.

Prevalence of epitheliotropic lymphoma is 1% of skin tumors in dogs, and both types represent 2.8% of all feline skin tumors. Epitheliotropic lymphoma is more common in dogs than in cats (Gross et al., 2005). Lesions are solitary to multiple in the form of nodules, plaques, ulcers, erythroderma, or exfoliative dermatitis in the form of excessive scaling (Figs. 3.200 and 3.201). Pruritus may be common. B-cell lymphoma of the skin is extremely rare (Gross et al., 2005). Epitheliotropic lymphoma having neoplastic lymphocyte infiltrates of the epidermis and adnexa is termed *mycosis fungoides* (Fig. 3.202A). Sometimes focal collections of the neoplastic lymphocytes, termed *Pautrier microaggregates*, are formed within the epidermis. The cell of origin is usually a T lymphocyte with 80% expressing CD8 while the remaining 20% is double negative for CD4 and CD8 (Moore et al., 1994; Gross et al., 2005). When these neoplastic T lymphocytes are present both in the epidermis and peripheral blood, it is referred to as *Sézary syndrome* based on a similar presentation in humans. Canine pagetoid reticulosis is a form of CD3+ T-cell lymphoma in which TCRγδ (T-cell receptor gamma delta)-positive cells proliferate within the epidermis. In dogs and cats, lymphocytes are variable in appearance, with most being small to medium with round, indented, or convoluted nuclei (Fontaine et al., 2010, 2011) (Fig. 3.202B and C). Cytoplasm is scant to moderate and

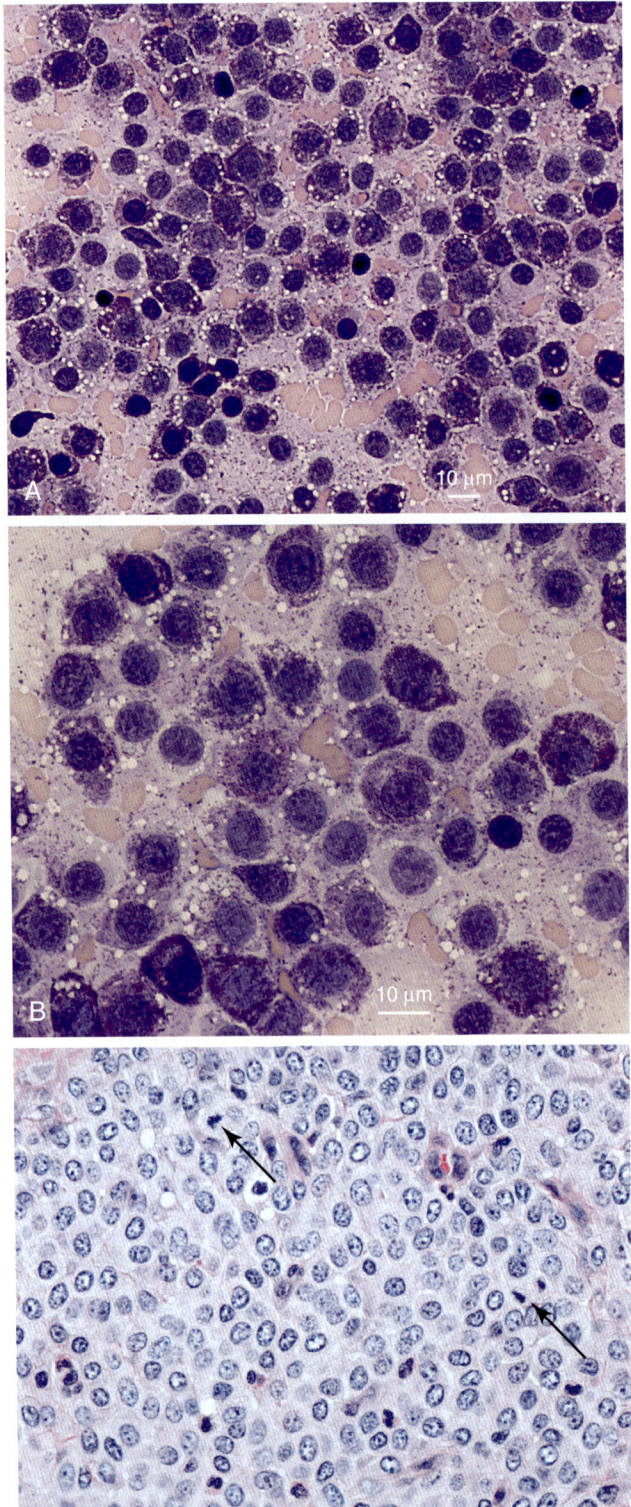

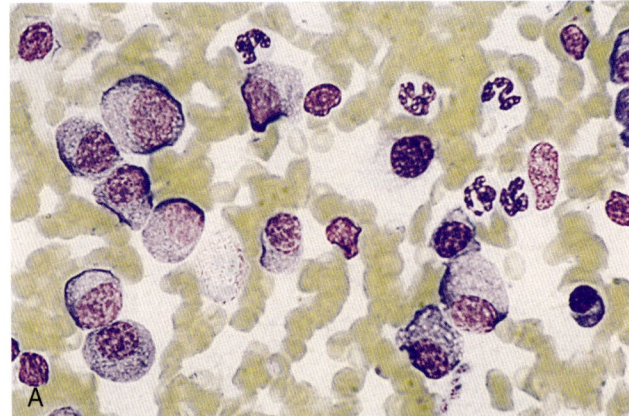

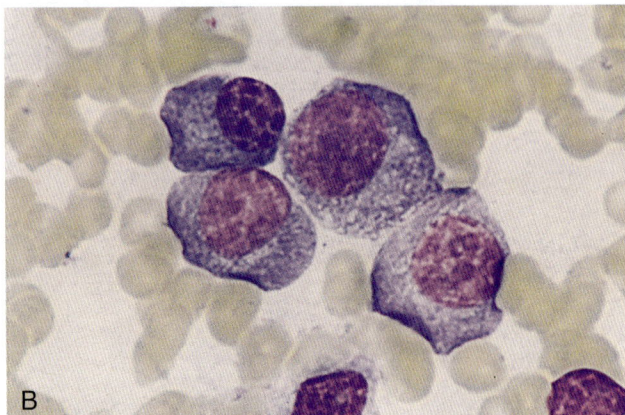

■ **FIGURE 3.193 Plasmacytoma. Tissue aspirate. Cat.** Same case in A and B. **A,** Cellular specimen with cells that have variable amounts of basophilic cytoplasm in which borders are discrete. Sample taken from a nasal planum mass. (Wright-Giemsa; HP oil.) **B,** Higher magnification of A. Note the plasmacytoid appearance with eccentrically placed nuclei and variably coarse chromatin. This case had a monoclonal production of gamma globulins. (Wright-Giemsa; HP oil.)

■ **FIGURE 3.192 Mast cell tumor. Solitary dermal neck mass. Cat.** Same case in A to C. **A, Tissue aspirate.** Variably granular mast cells with mild anisokaryosis. (Modified Wright; HP oil.) **B, Tissue aspirate.** Higher magnification shows many cells with numerous punctate vacuoles and variable granulation. (Modified Wright; HP oil.) **C, Tissue section.** Histologic section showing variably abundant cytoplasm and immature chromatin pattern with small nucleoli and occasional mitotic figures (arrows). (H&E; HP oil.)

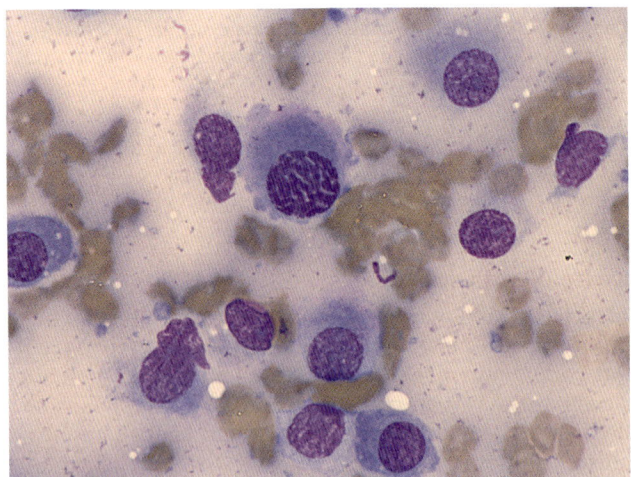

■ **FIGURE 3.194 Plasmacytoma. Hindlimb skin mass. Tissue aspirate. Dog.** This firm mass 5 × 5 cm yielded a pleomorphic population of neoplastic plasma cells. The cell at the *top center* has an eosinophilic corona to the periphery of the cytoplasm, termed a *flame cell*. This flame cell is in prophase as evidenced by the aggregated chromatin. (Modified Wright; HP oil.) (Courtesy Kansas State University.)

lightly basophilic. However, other cases of epitheliotropic lymphoma may show mostly medium lymphocytes with moderate amounts of lightly basophilic cytoplasm and frequent mitotic figures (Fig. 3.203). Nucleoli are usually indistinct but occasionally prominent. Uniformity of the lymphoid population without significant inflammation or plasma cell infiltration is suggestive of neoplastic lymphocytes. In general, treatment involving chemotherapy, radiotherapy, and immunotherapy has been unsuccessful in achieving long-term remission. Surgical excision may be helpful for solitary lesions (Choi et al., 2004). Prognosis is poor with median survival period of 6 months related to rapid progression, necessitating euthanasia. Nodal involvement, when present, usually occurs late in both types. Laboratory abnormalities such as monoclonal gammopathy, serum hyperviscosity, and hypercalcemia have been associated with cutaneous lymphoma.

Nonepitheliotropic lymphomas are more frequent in cats and uncommon in dogs. Of the nonepitheliotropic cutaneous lymphomas, some involve vaccine injection sites in cats (Roccabianca et al., 2016). In this study, lymphomas were classified mostly as a large B-cell with fewer anaplastic large T-cell, peripheral T-cell, and natural killer cell–like subtypes. On histopathology, features included necrosis, angiocentric lesions, and lymphoid aggregates. These lymphomas appear to develop within an environment of subacute to chronic inflammation.

In dogs, a form of nonepitheliotropic T-cell lymphoma termed *subcutaneous panniculitis-like T-cell lymphoma* is found that spares the dermis but involves the subcutis. Clinically, they appear as solitary or multiple raised erythematous variably sized (1–45 cm) masses. Histologically, cases are characterized by infiltration by small to medium or large CD3-positive T cells in a lace-like pattern that frequently rims adipocytes (Noland et al., 2018). Cytopathologic appearance demonstrates a mostly large-cell population of histiocyte-like cells having an oval to convoluted nuclear shape, frequent mitotic figures, and stippled chromatin with prominent nucleoli. The cytoplasm is basophilic, moderately abundant with small punctate clear vacuoles (Fig. 3.204). Behavior has been difficult to determine related to

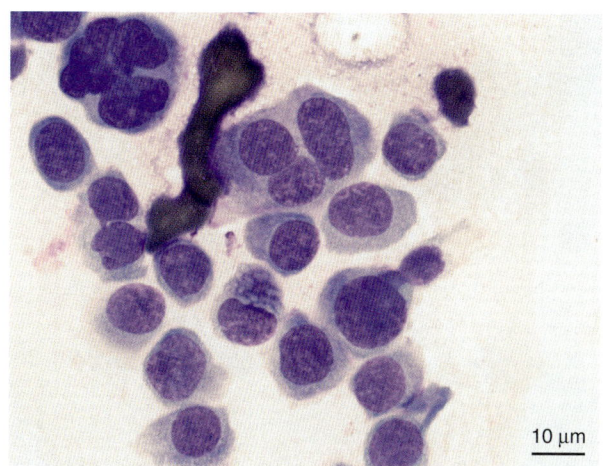

■ **FIGURE 3.195 Plasmacytoma. Carpal mass. Tissue aspirate. Dog.** A 1.0 cm firm raised dermal mass consists of a pleomorphic population of neoplastic plasma cells. One cell is shown with intracytoplasmic Russell bodies and is term a *Mott cell*. (Aqueous Romanowsky; HP oil.)

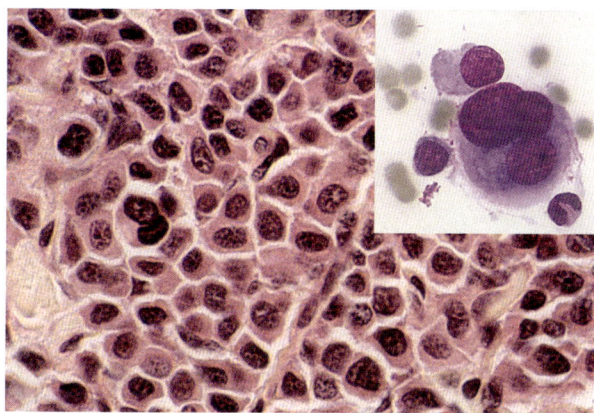

■ **FIGURE 3.196 Plasmacytoma. Digit mass. Tissue section. Dog.** There is dense dermal infiltration with pleomorphic round cells. Note the multinucleated cells to the *left of center,* which are a frequent finding in this tumor. (H&E; HP oil.) *Inset:* Tissue imprint. Multinucleated cell. (Wright-Giemsa; HP oil.)

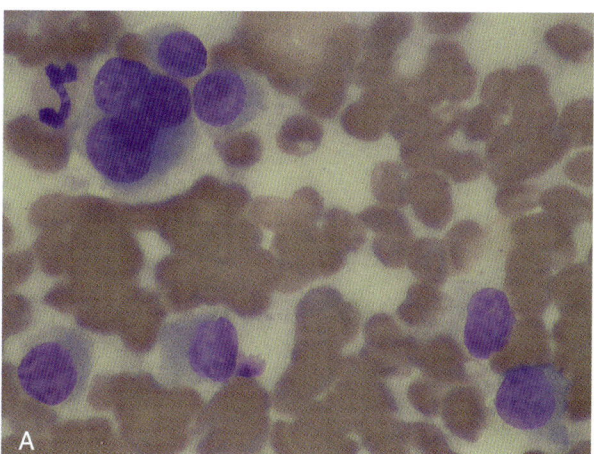
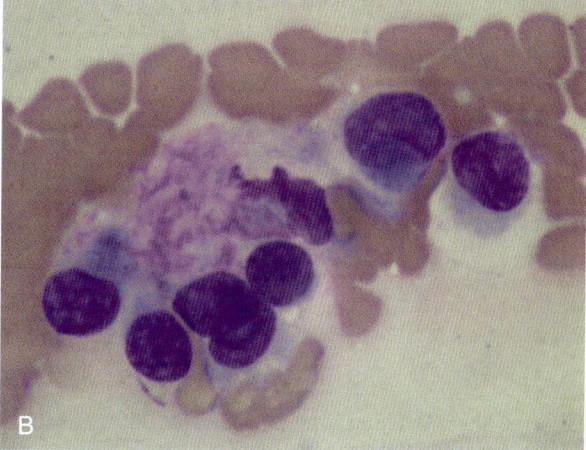

■ **FIGURE 3.197 Plasmacytoma with multinucleation and amyloid. Digital mass. Tissue aspirate. Dog.** Same case in A and B. **A,** There is mild anisocytosis and anisokaryosis in this population of neoplastic plasma cells. Multinucleation was frequent and shown is one multinucleated cell. (Modified Wright; HP oil.) **B,** Extracellular pink matrix consistent with amyloid is present in this specimen. (Modified Wright; HP oil.) (Courtesy Robert Lukacs, TDDS/Synlab, Exeter, UK.)

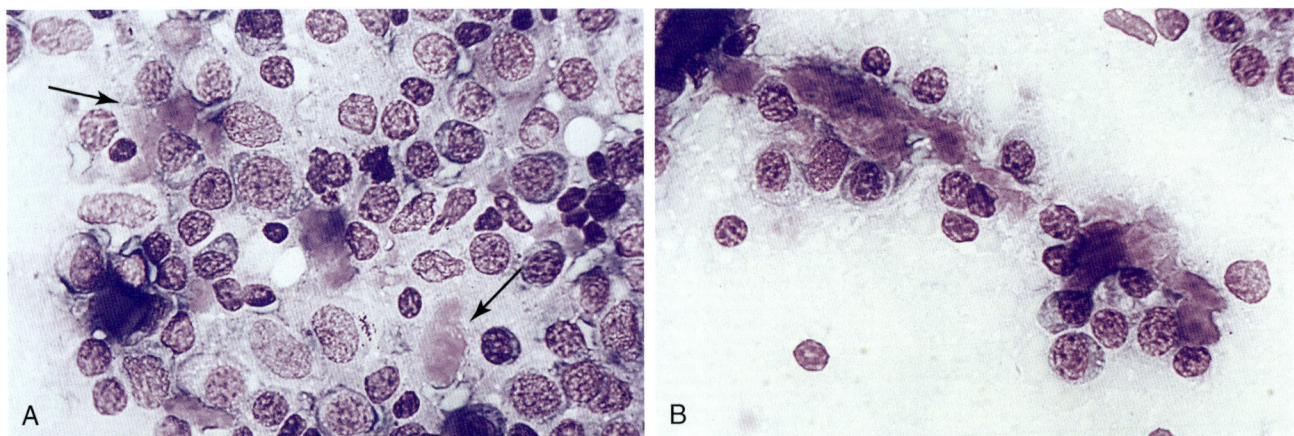

■ **FIGURE 3.198 Plasmacytoma with amyloid. Tissue imprint. Cat.** Same case in A and B. **A,** The specimen from a hock mass is densely cellular with marked anisocytosis and anisokaryosis. Several cells have a plasmacytoid appearance, whereas others appear histiocytic with abundant pale cytoplasm. Small amount of amyloid is present between cells *(arrows).* (Wright; HP oil.) **B,** Note the abundant pink amorphous material associated with plasmacytoid cells. (Wright; HP oil.) (Courtesy Gail Walter et al., Michigan State University. Presented at the 1992 ASVCP case review session.)

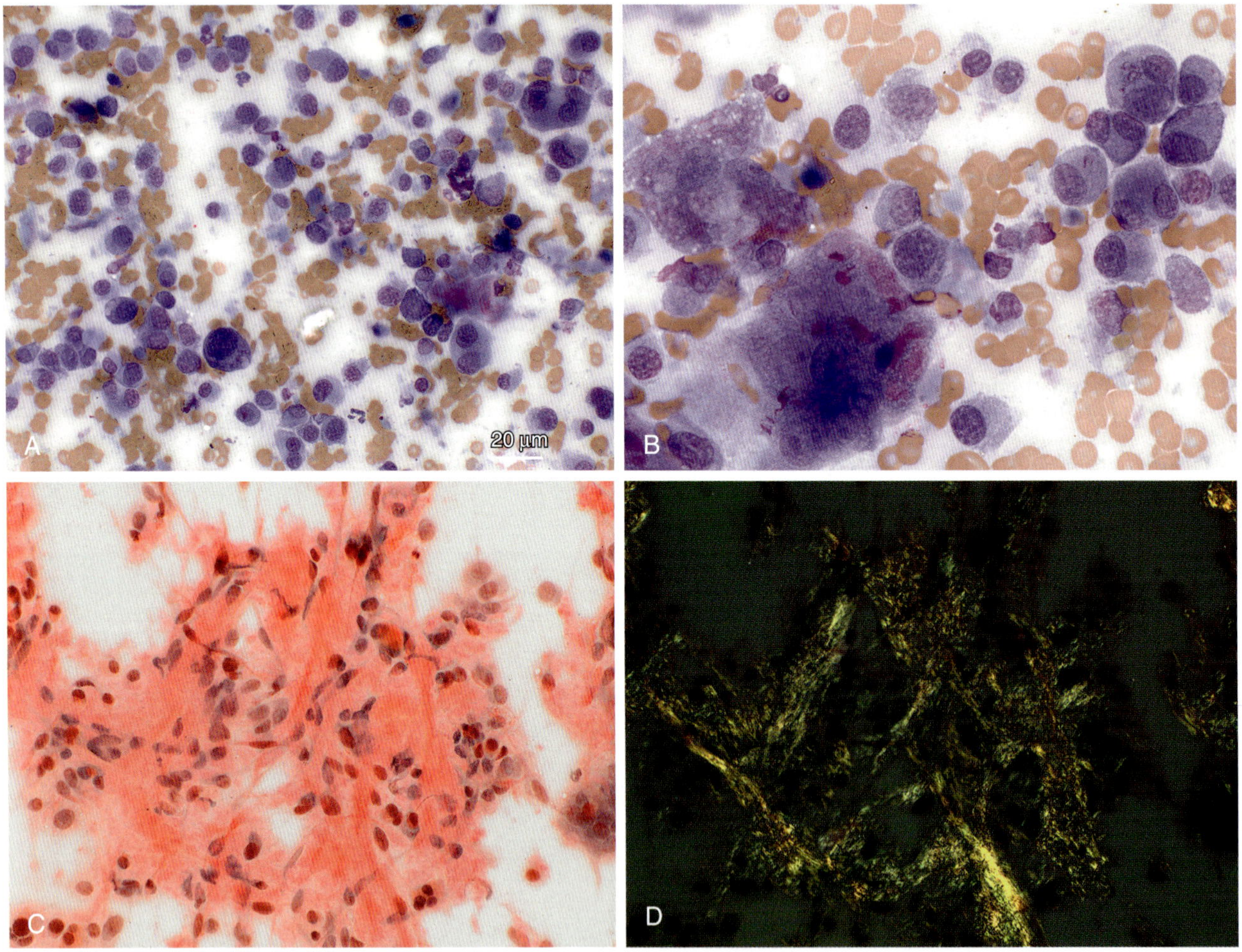

■ **FIGURE 3.199 Plasmacytoma with polarized amyloid. Tarsal mass. Tissue aspirate. Dog.** Same case in A to D. **A,** A 1.2 × 1.6 cm raised nodule on the plantar surface yielded a pleomorphic population of neoplastic plasma cells admixed with a moderate amount of amorphous to fibrillar bright eosinophilic extracellular and intracellular amyloid. (Wright-Giemsa; HP oil.) **B,** Higher magnification demonstrates intracellular fibrillar amyloid. (Wright-Giemsa; HP oil.) **C,** There are nodular aggregates of round cells that form dense sheets and cords separated by a fine fibrovascular stroma and moderate amounts of amyloid deposits. The red-orange stain highlights amyloid deposits. (Congo red; IP.) **D,** Polarization demonstrates the birefringent nature of amyloid that was highlighted by the Congo red stain. (Congo red/Polarized; IP.)

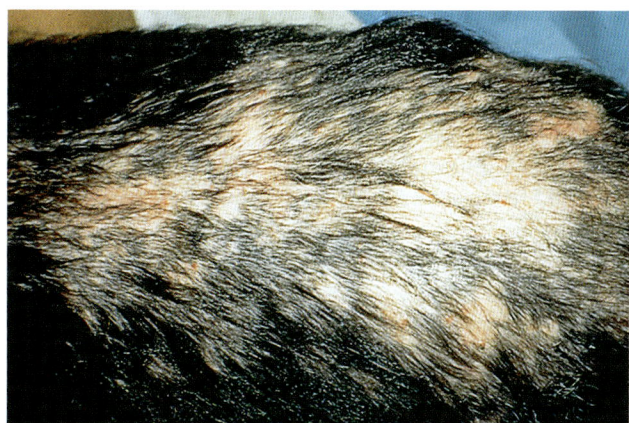

FIGURE 3.200 Mycosis fungoides. Dog. Plaques and nodules are present over the back. (Courtesy Janet Wojciechowski, University of Florida.)

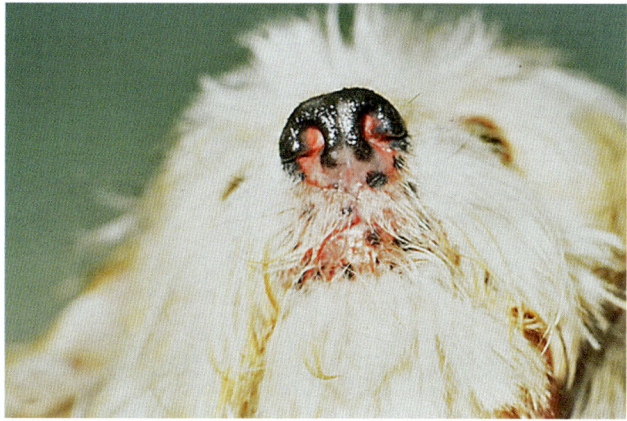

FIGURE 3.201 Mycosis fungoides. Dog. Depigmentation and crusting are noted around the nose and mouth. (Courtesy Janet Wojciechowski, University of Florida.)

the low frequency of this neoplasm, although cases examined survived 0.5 to 7 months (Noland et al., 2018).

> *Cytopathologic differential diagnosis:* chronic inflammatory dermatitis, histiocytoma.

Canine Transmissible Venereal Tumor

Canine transmissible venereal tumor is a tumor of dogs, most often in free-roaming sexually active animals living in temperate climates, related to transplantation of intact cells. Immunochemistry supports vimentin and CD45 and CD45RA immunoreactivity, indicating leukocyte origin with positive lysozyme and alpha-1-antitrypsin expression, supportive of histiocytic origin (Gross et al., 2005; Park et al., 2006). However, the cells do not appear to be of canine origin, having an abnormal karyotype with 59 chromosomes compared with a normal karyotype of 78 in dogs. PCR and molecular techniques to analyze the sequence of the long interspersed nuclear element may be used to identify tumor cells (Park et al., 2006). The tumor mostly appears on the skin of the external genitalia as well as the mucous membranes associated with sexual contact (Fig. 3.205); however, cutaneous lesions have been reported. A

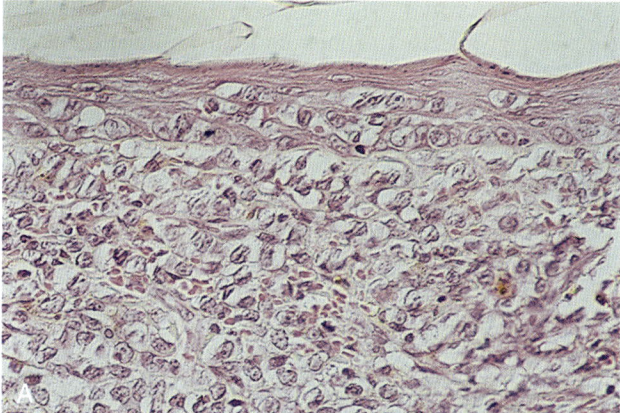
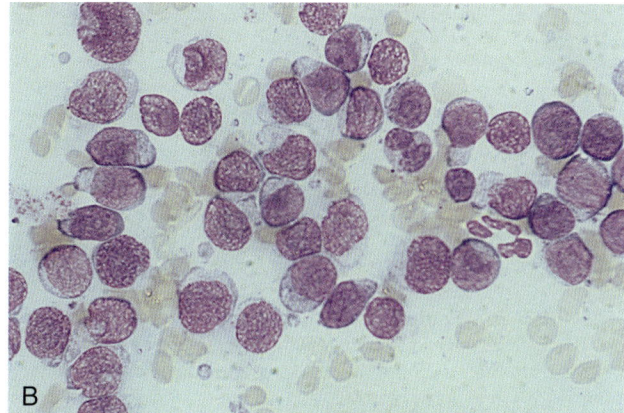
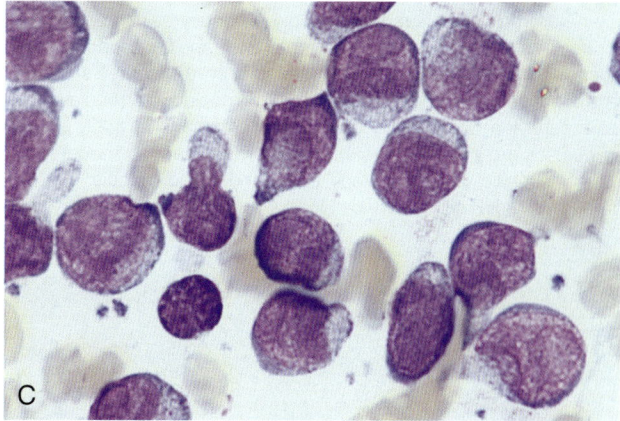

FIGURE 3.202 Mycosis fungoides. Dog. Same case in A to C. **A, Tissue section.** Neoplastic lymphocyte infiltrates involve the epidermis and dermis of the skin on the chest. Small focal collections of neoplastic cells, termed *Pautrier microaggregates,* are present within the epidermis. (H&E; HP oil.) **B, Tissue aspirate.** Lymphocytes are variable, ranging from small to large, with round, indented, or convoluted nuclei. Cytoplasm is scant to moderate and lightly basophilic. (Wright-Giemsa; HP oil.) **C, Tissue aspirate.** Higher magnification of B. Nuclear folds are common. Nucleoli are usually indistinct but occasionally prominent. Note the small lymphocyte at *bottom left* for comparison of cell size. (Wright-Giemsa; HP oil.)

case of a prepubertal female dog with skin lesions and no mucosal involvement has been reported (Marcos et al., 2006a). Grossly, the tumor is pink to red, poorly circumscribed, multinodular, raised to pedunculated, soft, friable, ulcerated, and hemorrhagic, with frequent necrosis and superficial bacterial infection (Fig. 3.206). The mass exfoliates easily by tissue impression, giving rise to a monomorphic population of large round cells with a round nucleus, coarse chromatin, and one or two prominent nucleoli. Mitotic figures may be seen. The cytoplasm is abundant and lightly basophilic and frequently contains multiple punctate vacuoles (see Fig. 3.206C). Associated with the tumor are small lymphoid cells and inflammatory cells, often with evidence of bacterial sepsis. Treatment involves chemotherapy, particularly with vincristine, radiotherapy, and surgical excision. Prognosis is good with chemotherapy. The tumors may regress spontaneously, presumably related to lymphocyte infiltration. Metastasis may occur (Park et al., 2006), and recurrence is high with surgical intervention.

> **Cytopathologic differential diagnosis:** other round cell tumors, amelanotic melanoma.

Naked Nuclei Cytomorphology
Thyroid Gland

Subcutaneous masses located adjacent to the trachea may be confirmed as thyroid glands by fine-needle aspiration. Classically, they consist of small sheets of closely or loosely attached cells, some of which contain black, granular intracytoplasmic

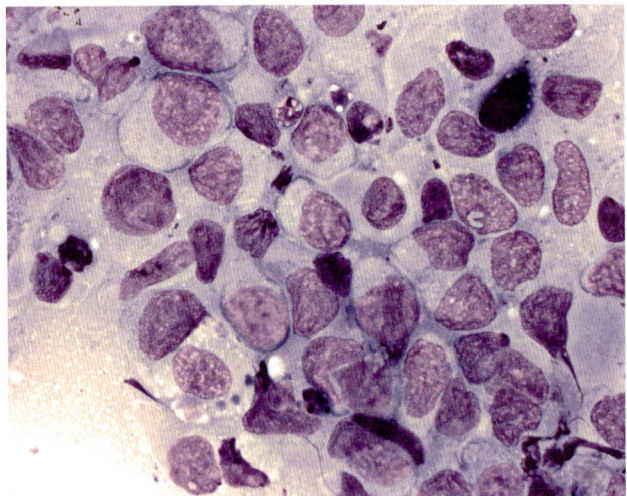

■ **FIGURE 3.203 Epitheliotropic lymphoma. Erosive skin imprint. Dog.** This animal has had a chronic skin condition originally attributed to an allergic dermatitis. Currently, the presentation involves multifocal erythematous and scaly patches and plaques, depigmentation, and erosive lesions. In addition, to surface neutrophilic inflammation (not shown), a large population of monotypic lymphocytes is present. These lymphocytes are moderately pleomorphic with mild to moderate anisocytosis and anisokaryosis. Nuclei measure 11 to 14 μm, suggesting these are medium to large lymphocytes. The nucleus is irregularly round to elongate and occasionally clefted. The chromatin is finely stippled, and nucleoli are not discernible. Cytoplasm is scant to moderate and lightly basophilic. Histopathology confirmed the diagnosis. (Aqueous Romanowsky; HP oil.) (Courtesy North Carolina State University.)

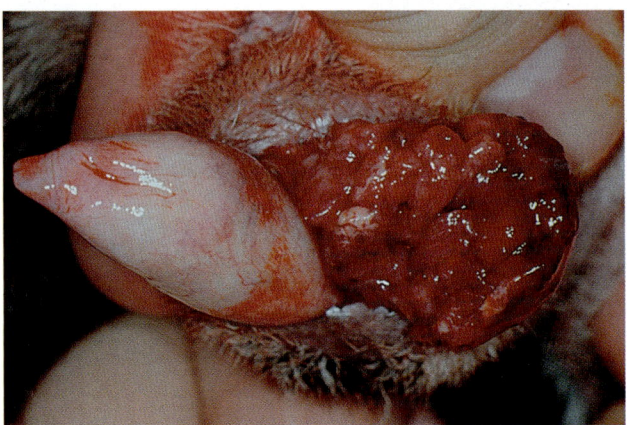

■ **FIGURE 3.205 Transmissible venereal tumor. Preputial mucocutaneous mass. Macroscopic specimen. Dog.** The tumor is soft, friable, and hemorrhagic.

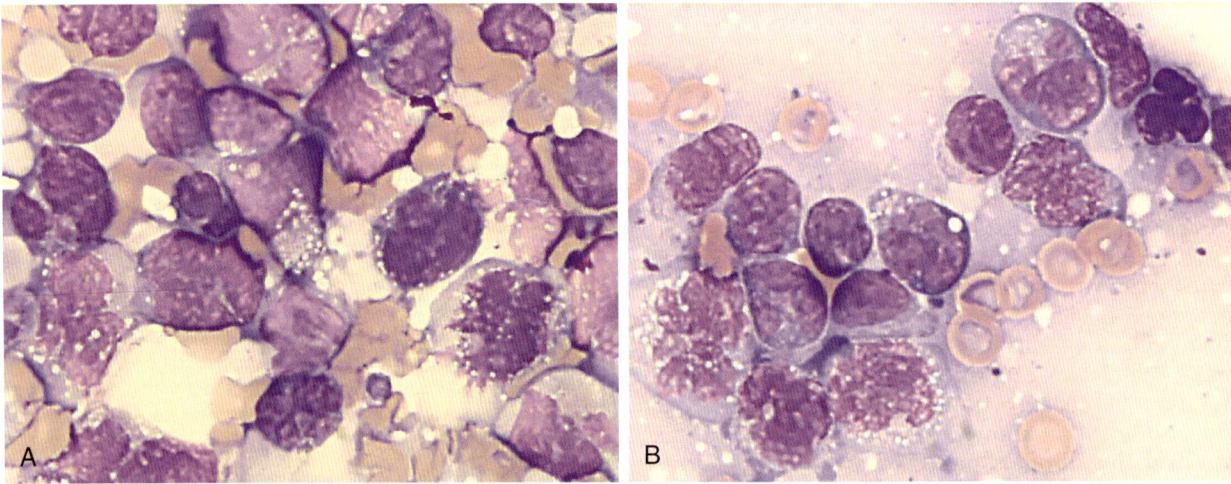

■ **FIGURE 3.204 Subcutaneous panniculitis-like T-cell lymphoma, gamma-delta subtype. Thoracic skin aspirate. Dog.** Same case in A and B. **A,** Large numbers of discrete cells are present and have a high nucleocytoplasmic ratio. The cytoplasm frequently contains variable numbers of small discrete, colorless vacuoles. The nuclei are round to cloverleaf to cleaved with smooth to finely stippled chromatin. Mitotic figures are seen frequently (one shown). (Wright-Giemsa; HP oil.) **B,** Compared with surrounding erythrocytes, the lymphocytes are medium to large. Histopathology noted a dense infiltration and effacement of subcutaneous tissue. There was positive immunoreactivity to CD3 and T-cell antigen receptor gamma-delta for the neoplastic population. (Wright-Giemsa; HP oil.) (Courtesy University of Florida.)

material (Fig. 3.207). The cytoplasmic border may or may not be apparent with the appearance of free nuclei. Occasionally, the cervical masses may present with no clinical signs other than a subcutaneous paratracheal mass on the neck as demonstrated by a recent report of a C-cell or medullary thyroid carcinoma (Bertazzolo et al., 2003). See Chapter 17 for further information about thyroid tumors.

Merkel Cell Tumor (Neuroendocrine Carcinoma)

Merkel cells are neuroendocrine cells widely dispersed throughout the skin and mucous membranes. They are a normal part of the epidermis (Fig. 3.208) and follicular epithelium, present at the bulge of the follicular isthmus near the attachment of the arrector pili muscle. Their function is believed to be associated with sensory mechanoreceptors (touch). Merkel cell tumors are rarely found in adult dogs and cats, in which the masses present as firm, intradermal, flesh-colored or red nodules or plaques up to 1.5 cm diameter. Cells are components of the amine precursor uptake

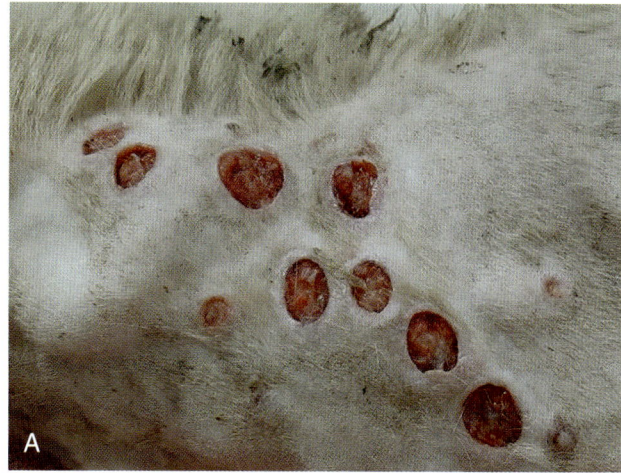
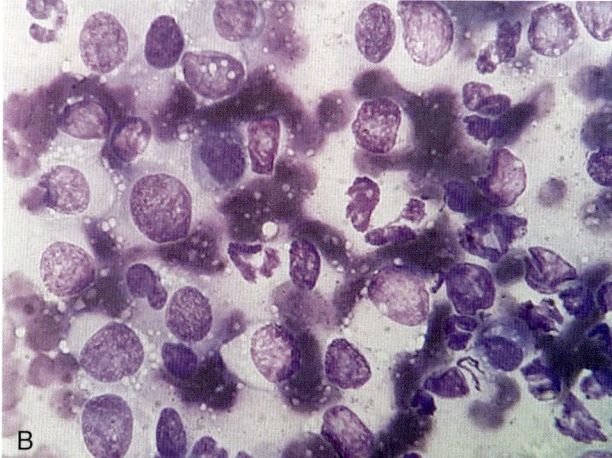
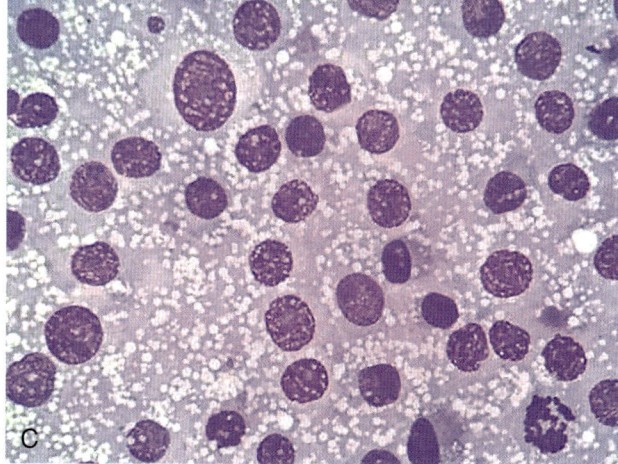

■ **FIGURE 3.206 Cutaneous transmissible venereal tumor. Dog.** Same case in A to C. **A, Macroscopic specimen.** Left lateral skin showing multiple circular ulcerated areas. **B, Tissue imprint.** Ulcerated surface consists of degenerate neutrophils and a uniform population of round cells. (Romanowsky; HP oil.) **C, Tissue aspirate.** Sample taken from a non-ulcerated area shows only the monomorphic population of round cells. Against a background of lysed cells and lipid droplets, variably sized round cells have moderate amounts of lightly basophilic cytoplasm containing frequent small punctate colorless vacuoles. The round nucleus displays mild anisokaryosis and an occasionally prominent nucleolus. A single mitotic figure is shown *(lower right)*. There was no evidence of a genital lesion in this adult stray animal. (Romanowsky; HP oil.) (Courtesy Perina Sumaco, Bali, Indonesia.)

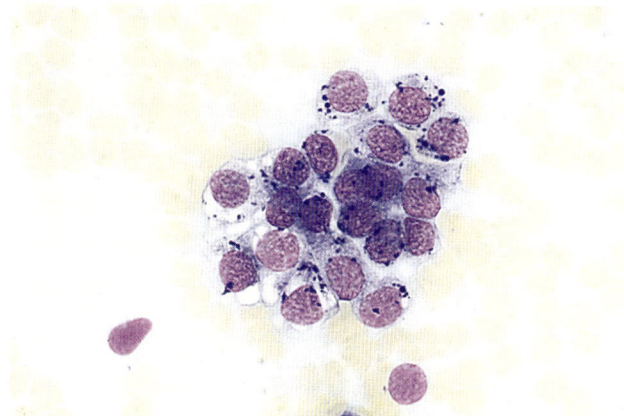

■ **FIGURE 3.207 Thyroid tissue. Tissue aspirate. Dog.** Subcutaneous masses located adjacent to the trachea may be confirmed as thyroid glands by fine-needle aspiration. Note the cohesive sheet of cells, many of which contain black, granular intracytoplasmic material thought to be tyrosine. (Wright-Giemsa; HP oil.)

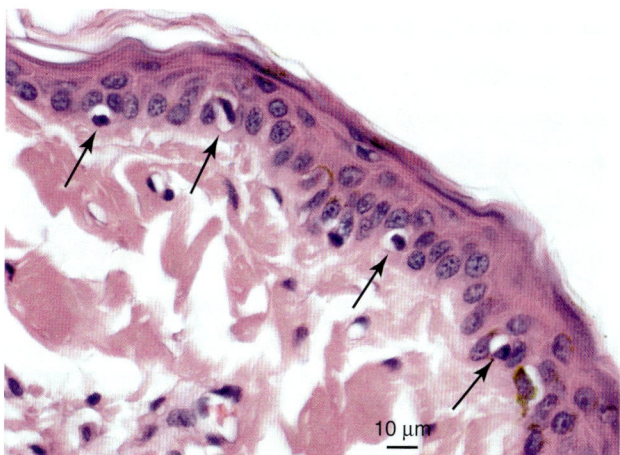

■ **FIGURE 3.208 Normal Merkel cells. Histology. Dog.** In the basal epithelial layer or at the epidermal-dermal junction lies the neuroendocrine cells, called Merkel cells *(arrows)*, which are associated with touch receptors. The nucleus is dense and round to oval. (H&E; HP oil.)

and decarboxylation (APUD) system. Ultrastructurally, the cells contain dense-core neurosecretory granules within the cytoplasm. The cells express neuron-specific enolase, chromogranin A, synaptophysin, and CK20 (Ramírez et al., 2014; Dohata et al., 2015). Histopathologic examination indicates the dermal mass is composed of closely packed cells separated by fine fibrovascular stroma (Fig. 3.209). Cytopathology describes the tumors as a monomorphic population of neoplastic round to polygonal cells mixed with many bare nuclei from lysed cells against a heavy background of proteinaceous material (Fig. 3.210). There is moderate anisocytosis and anisokaryosis. The cells have round to oval, central, or eccentric nuclei with coarse chromatin, prominent round nucleoli, small to moderate amounts of pale basophilic cytoplasm, and variably distinct cytoplasmic margins. A moderate number of binucleated cells are seen, and mitotic figures are rare (Joiner et al., 2010; Dohata et al., 2015). The neoplasm may resemble round cell neoplasms on cytopathologic examination. Canine cutaneous neuroendocrine tumors are typically benign but may metastasize as multiple masses develop as is more common in cats that have a high rate of recurrence and metastasis.

Glomus Tumor

This is an uncommon benign tumor arising from specialized smooth muscle cells surrounding small vessels called glomus bodies, which affect thermoregulation. This tumor appears as a firm dermal mass of a limb or digit in the dog and cat (Reed et al., 2018; Uchida et al., 2002). Cytopathology involves a sheetlike proliferation of epithelioid tumor cells with naked nuclei appearance enmeshed with capillaries (Fig. 3.211). Cells

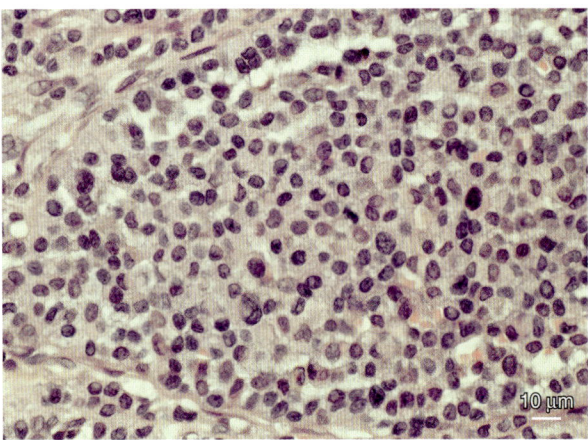

■ **FIGURE 3.209 Merkel cell carcinoma. Lip mass. Tissue section. Dog.** Neoplastic cells are arranged in a sheet of closely packed epithelial cells. A fine fibrovascular stroma separates the cells into lobular regions. The neoplastic cells have indistinct pale basophilic cytoplasm with round to ovoid to irregularly shaped nuclei with fine chromatin. There are mild anisokaryosis and occasional mitotic figures, one shown in the *center* of the field. (H&E; HP oil.)

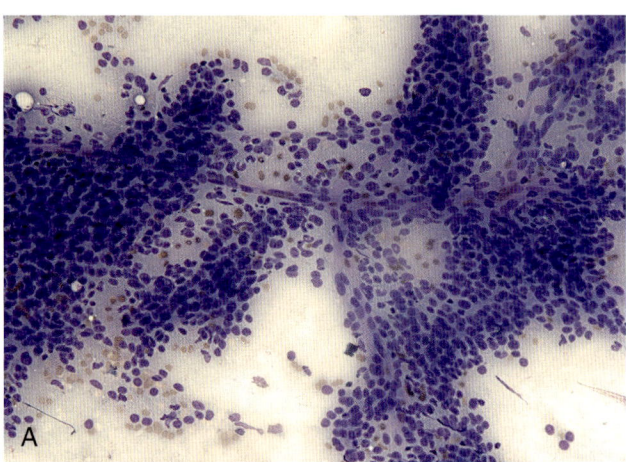

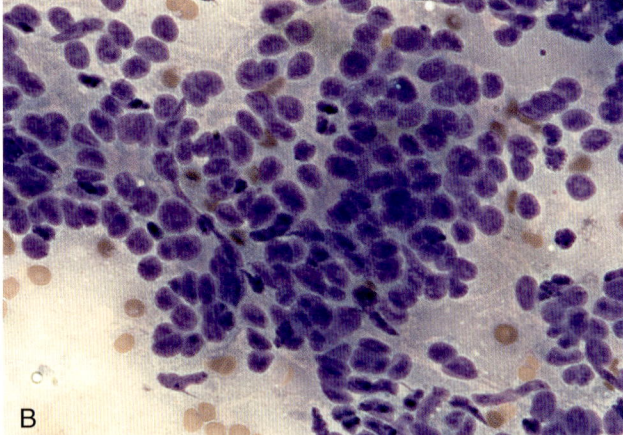

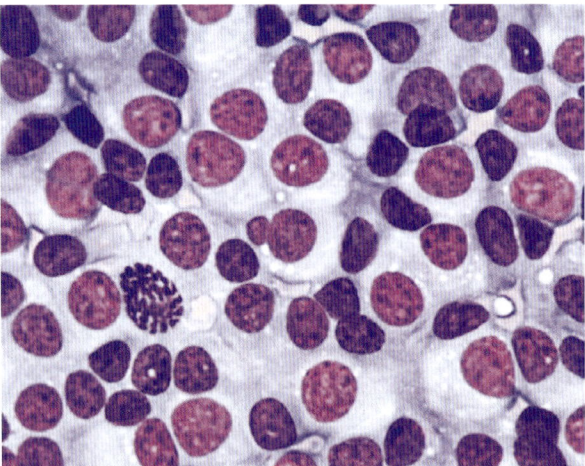

■ **FIGURE 3.210 Merkel cell carcinoma (neuroendocrine carcinoma). Cutaneous mass. Tissue aspirate. Dog.** Dense aggregates of neoplastic round to polyhedral cells against a proteinaceous background. The cells have moderate amounts of fine granular basophilic cytoplasm and central-to-eccentric nuclei with coarse chromatin. A single mitotic figure is present. (Modified Wright; HP oil.) (From Joiner KS, Smith AN, Henderson RA, et al. Multicentric cutaneous neuroendocrine (Merkel cell) carcinoma in a dog. *Vet Pathol.* 2010;47:1090–1094.)

■ **FIGURE 3.211 Glomus tumor. Intradermal mass on dorsum. Tissue aspirate. Dog.** Same case in A and B. **A,** The highly cellular specimen consists of free nuclei, scattered individual cells, and loose clusters of cells with poorly defined borders. Neoplastic cells are closely associated with capillaries that appear intertwined with the cells. (Aqueous Romanowsky; IP.) **B,** Higher magnification displays a naked nuclei cytomorphology with round to ovoid nuclei in a palisading arrangement. The nucleocytoplasmic ratio is high and cytoplasmic borders are indistinct. Cells exhibit mild anisocytosis and anisokaryosis. Histopathology with immunochemistry is performed and the neoplastic cells are immunoreactive to vimentin and smooth muscle actin supporting the final diagnosis. (Aqueous Romanowsky; HP oil.) (Courtesy Matthew Reed, Joint Pathology Center, Bethesda, MD.)

exhibit mild anisocytosis and anisokaryosis, small amounts of basophilic cytoplasm, round to ovoid nuclei with granular chromatin, and one to three small nucleoli. Tissue sections reveal a well-delineated circular lesion of epithelioid cells involving capillaries that are immunoreactive to vimentin and smooth muscle actin. Unlike perivascular wall tumors and smooth muscle tumors, spindle cells are not a feature of glomus tumor. Treatment is surgical excision.

RESPONSE TO TISSUE INJURY

Calcinosis Cutis and Calcinosis Circumscripta

Calcinosis cutis is an uncommon condition of calcium apatite deposition in the dermis, epidermis, or subcutis. It is associated with glucocorticoid use or hyperadrenocorticism and iatrogenic administration of calcium products for hypoparathyroid treatment in dogs (Gross et al., 2005). Paw calcification in cats has been documented in patients with chronic renal disease and hyperthyroidism (Bertazzolo et al., 2003; Declercq and Bhatti, 2005). In these diseases, metastatic calcification is related to hypercalcemia or hyperphosphatemia (or both) from hyperparathyroidism depositing into tissues likely susceptible to trauma. It other cases, there may be normal serum concentrations with dystrophic calcification of collagen or elastin via metaplasia into fibrocartilaginous tissue (Fig. 3.212). Sites of predilection include the dorsal neck, inguinal area, and axillary region. Grossly, erythematous papules or firm gritty whitish plaques develop and often ulcerate. On cytopathology, the white, gritty material (Bettini et al., 2005) appears densely granular in the background and a mixed inflammatory response occurs, including macrophages, giant multinucleated cells, neutrophils, lymphocytes, and plasma cells. Prognosis is good because these benign lesions resolve untreated over several months.

A clinical subgroup of calcinosis cutis is calcinosis circumscripta, which is uncommon in dogs and rare in cats. This is a well-circumscribed solitary lesion within the deep dermis and subcutis formed by dystrophic mineralization. It is mainly associated with young German shepherd dogs. The lesions often occur over joint areas or pressure points, at sites of previous trauma, or under the tongue (Gross et al., 2005; Marcos et al., 2006b). Mass texture is firm and gritty (Fig. 3.213). Histologically, the lesion is characterized by large lakes of mineralized deposits surrounded by dense fibrous connective tissue and foreign body giant cells (Fig. 3.214A). On cytopathology, it is similar to calcinosis cutis except fibroblasts are more frequently observed. Mineral deposits often present as refractile yellow-green granules of irregular size and shape that are best observed with a lowered microscope condenser (Fig. 3.214B). Purple fine granular material present in the background likely represents necrotic tissue, which may be prominent. Demonstration of calcium may be enhanced by use of cytochemical stains such as von Kossa and Alizarin red S (Marcos et al., 2006b; Raskin, 2006a). These focal benign lesions may be treated by surgical excision.

Responsive Fibroplasia

Firm subcutaneous swellings may arise from an exuberant fibroblastic response to tissue injury. Histologically, *granulation tissue* mass is composed of horizontally arranged proliferating fibroblasts transected by vertically proliferating endothelium from small blood vessels (Fig. 3.215). Mitoses and macrophages are commonly found. The plump, reactive fibroblasts seen on cytopathology have an ovoid vesicular nucleus and may resemble the fusiform cells seen in fibrosarcoma. Histopathology is recommended to distinguish the two conditions.

Scar tissue after surgery also involves the presence of a low to moderate number of plump mesenchymal cells on cytopathology (Fig. 3.216). Within MCT, it is common to find frequent fibroblasts with resulting dense collagen bands (Fig. 3.217).

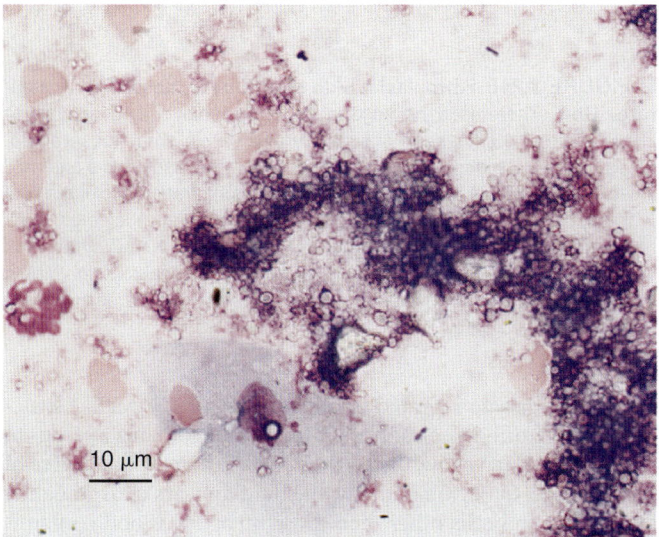

■ **FIGURE 3.212 Calcinosis cutis. Lip mass. Tissue aspirate. Dog.** The patient has hyperadrenocorticism. A squamous epithelium and a degenerate neutrophil are against a background of variably sized round to irregularly shaped refractile crystals, consistent with dystrophic mineralization. Occasional oral bacterial flora can be seen. (Modified Wright; HP oil.)

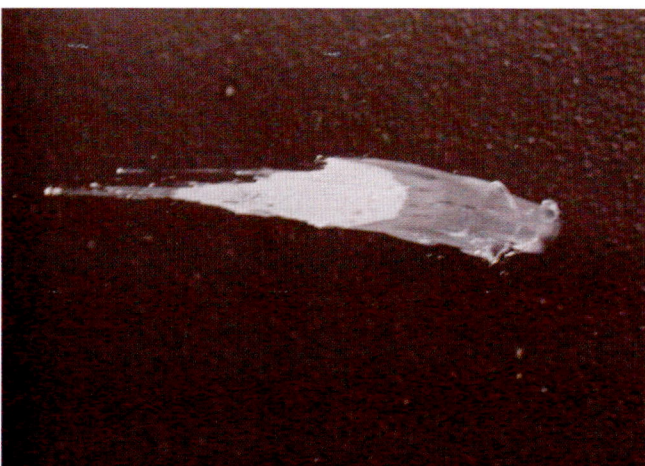

■ **FIGURE 3.213 Calcinosis circumscripta. Elbow mass. Macroscopic specimen. Dog.** An aspirate of the mass yielded a chalk-like white gritty material. Mineralization was thought to be related to constant trauma. (Unstained.)

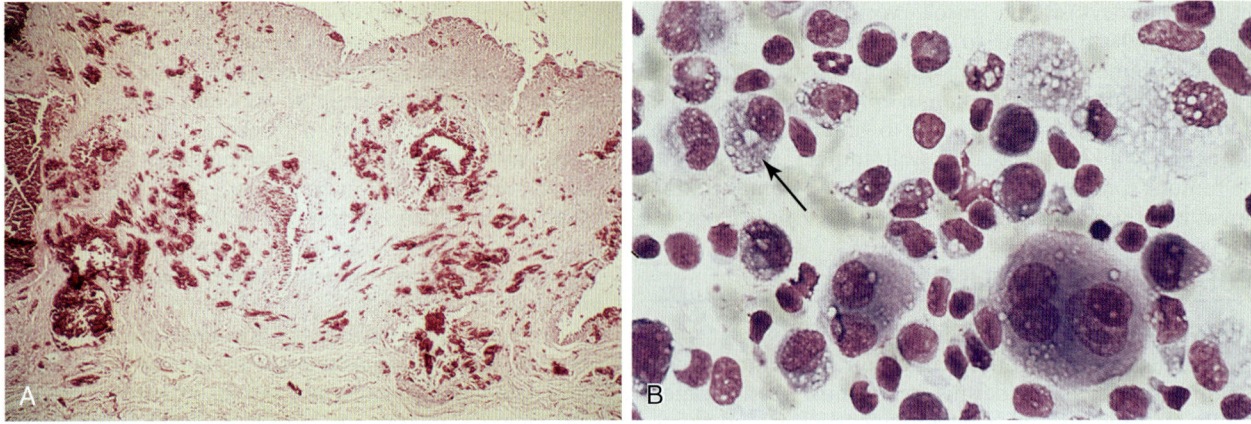

■ **FIGURE 3.214 Calcinosis circumscripta. Dog.** Same case in A and B. **A, Tissue section.** This multinodular dermal and subcutaneous mass is composed of central areas of mineralization that stain intensely red. These areas are surrounded by macrophages, giant cells, and dense, fibrous connective tissue. (H&E; LP.) **B, Tuber coxae mass aspirate.** Fluid from elbows and hip areas contained similar fluid, which was aspirated, sedimented, and smeared onto a slide. Highly cellular sample contained macrophages, giant cells, and lymphocytes. Within the background and phagocytic cells *(arrow)* are numerous clear refractile structures consistent with calcium crystals. (Aqueous Romanowsky; HP oil.)

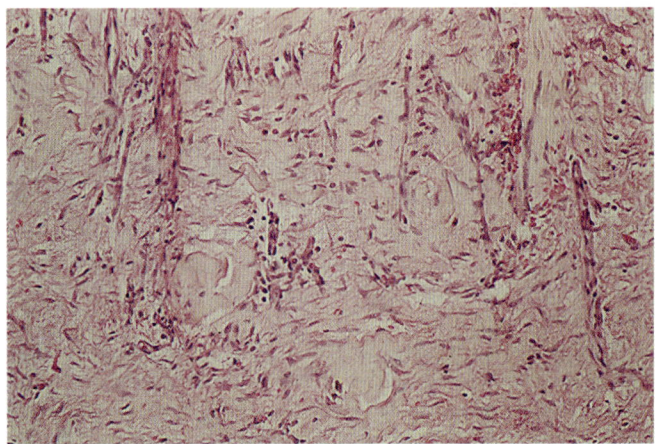

■ **FIGURE 3.215 Granulation tissue. Tissue section. Dog.** A mass on the dorsum contains dense, fibrous connective tissue layered horizontally with capillaries coursing through the tissue vertically. The reaction was secondary to noninfectious panniculitis. (H&E; IP.)

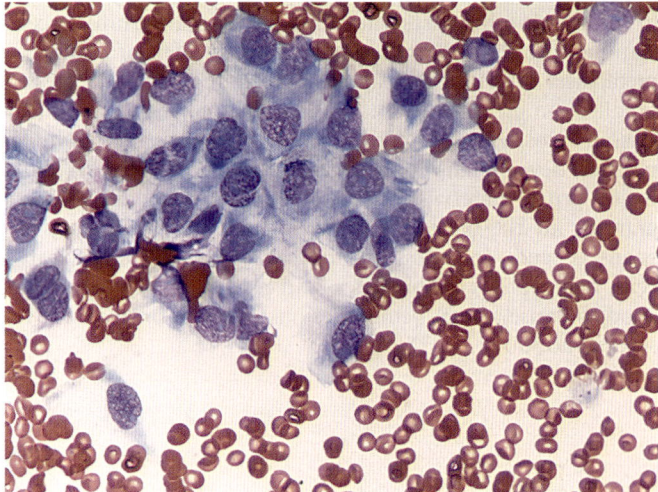

■ **FIGURE 3.216 Fibroplasia. Skin scar. Elbow mass. Tissue aspirate. Dog.** There is a homogeneous intermediate-sized spindle to irregularly round cells seen individually and within small loose aggregates. These cells demonstrate mild to moderate anisocytosis and mild anisokaryosis with a moderate nucleocytoplasmic ratio. Nuclei are oval with stippled chromatin and a single, round prominent nucleolus. Cells have moderate amounts of moderately basophilic wispy cytoplasm. With the location of this mass under a previous surgical excision site, it is most compatible with reactive fibroplasia. (Wright-Giemsa; HP oil.) (Courtesy Mary White, The Ohio State University.)

Hematoma

Grossly, the blood-filled mass of a hematoma can resemble neoplastic conditions such as hemangioma or hemangiosarcoma. Initially, when formed, a hematoma contains fluid identical in cell content to blood except that it lacks platelets. Shortly thereafter, macrophages engulfing erythrocytes (erythrophagocytosis) are common. Over time, the hemoglobin material breaks down, appearing as blue-green to black hemosiderin granules within the macrophage cytoplasm or remains extracellular as needle-like bilirubin crystals (Fig. 3.218). On occasion, *hematoidin crystals* appear as rhomboid golden crystals (see Fig. 2.20) produced from iron-poor hemoglobin pigment. As the healing continues, plump fibroblasts appear that can mimic a neoplastic mesenchymal cell population.

Hygroma

Hygroma is a swelling within the subcutaneous tissues that forms over bony prominences, commonly the elbow of large-breed dogs, secondary to repeated trauma or pressure. A cystlike structure forms from dense connective tissue that contains a serous to mucinous, clear, yellow, or red fluid, depending on the degree of hemorrhage. On cytopathology, the fluid appears clear to lightly basophilic, and cells other than those involving blood contamination include macrophages (Fig. 3.219) and reactive fibrocytes. Pathophysiology is similar to seroma formation.

Mucocele or Sialocele

Duct rupture related to trauma or infection leads to an accumulation of saliva within the subcutaneous tissues. The presence of

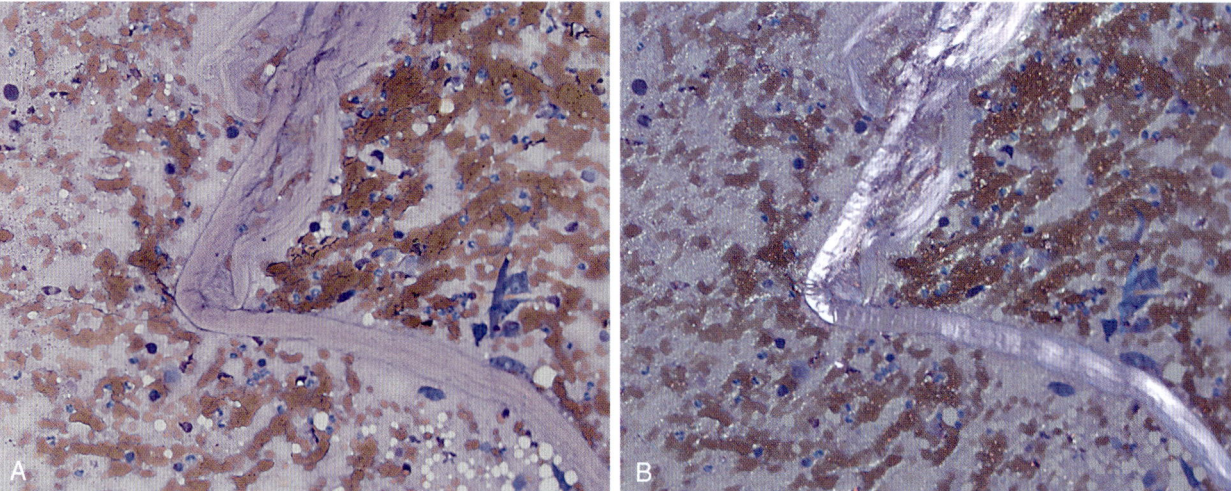

■ **FIGURE 3.217 Fibroplasia. Mast cell tumor. Tissue aspirate. Dog.** Same case in A and B. **A,** Against a hemodiluted background are a low number of well-differentiated mast cells along with thick collagen strands. (Wright-Giemsa; IP.) **B,** When the same field is subjected to polarization, the birefringent nature of collagen is apparent. (Wright-Giemsa/Polarized; IP.)

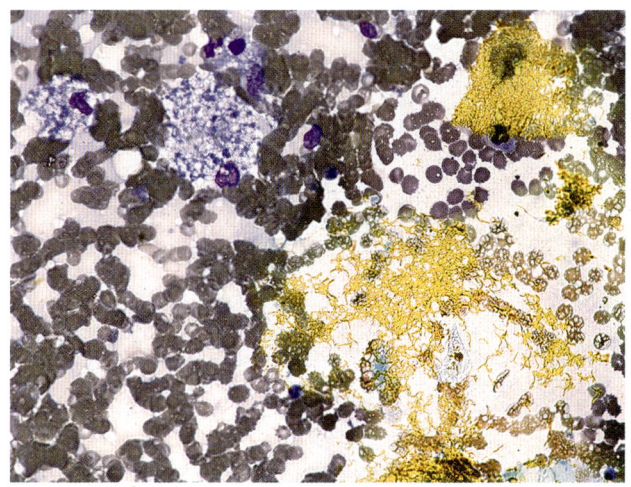

■ **FIGURE 3.218 Hematoma. Bilirubin/hematoidin crystals. Hip mass. Dog.** In addition to the macrophages containing blue-black hemosiderin granules, there is a cell-free deposition of bilirubin/hematoidin in the form of fine needle-like crystals. The bilirubin crystals are not expected to positively react with Prussian blue staining for iron. (Wright-Giemsa; IP.)

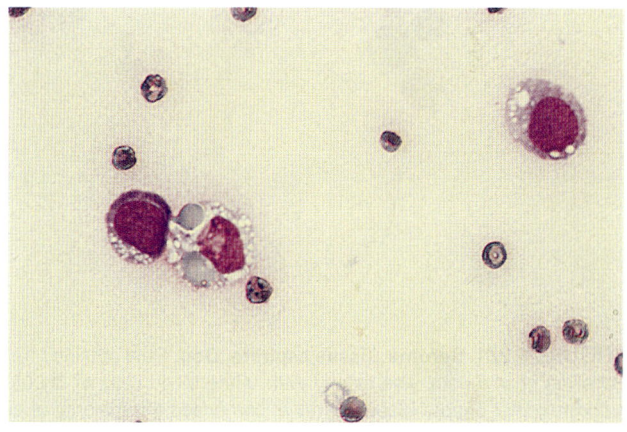

■ **FIGURE 3.219 Hygroma. Elbow swelling. Tissue aspirate. Dog.** The fluid obtained was orange and hazy with white blood cells <400/μL and protein of 3.3 g/dL. The background is lightly granular related to increased protein content. Cells were mononuclear phagocytes and exhibited erythrophagia as shown. (Wright-Giemsa; HP oil.)

a fluctuant mass containing clear to bloody fluid with stringlike features grossly suggests a salivary gland duct rupture. The cytopathologic specimen often stains uniformly purple from the high protein content. The background may contain scattered, pale basophilic, amorphous material, consistent with saliva. The fluid is often bloody with evidence of both acute and chronic hemorrhage. Erythrophagocytosis is common, and *hematoidin crystals* may be seen that are associated with chronic hemorrhage (Fig. 3.220A). The nucleated cells are predominately highly vacuolated macrophages that display active phagocytosis (Fig. 3.220B). Distinction between these cells and secretory glandular tissue may be difficult, especially when cells are individualized and nonphagocytic. Nondegenerate neutrophils are common, becoming degenerate when bacterial infection occurs.

Seroma

Injury may lead to a seroma, which is composed of clear to slightly blood-tinged fluid. The leaked plasma originates from immature capillaries created during granulation tissue formation. The fluid is poorly cellular and may require sedimentation before examination. Phagocytic macrophages predominate among a mixture of inflammatory cells (Fig. 3.221).

Mucinosis

Cutaneous mucinosis relates to an excess accumulation of mucin within the dermis. It may be hereditary in the Chinese Shar-Pei or in other breeds secondary to allergy and other inflammatory diseases or MCTs. The lesions appear as focal nodular, multifocal, or diffuse papular with variably sized

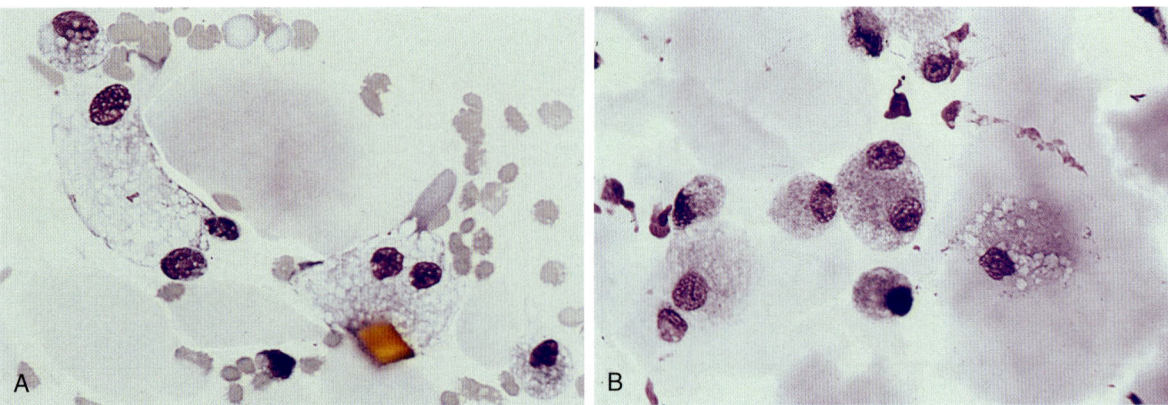

■ **FIGURE 3.220 Sialocele. Cervical mass aspirate. Dog.** Same case in A and B. **A,** Chronic hemorrhage is noted by the presence of a large yellow rhomboid crystal, termed *hematoidin*. The background contains pale-pink material, and vacuolated mononuclear cells are abundant. (Wright; HP oil.) **B,** The nucleated cells are predominately highly vacuolated mononuclear cells that are not easily identified as salivary gland epithelium or macrophages. Amorphous material in the background is consistent with mucus. (Aqueous Romanowsky; HP oil.)

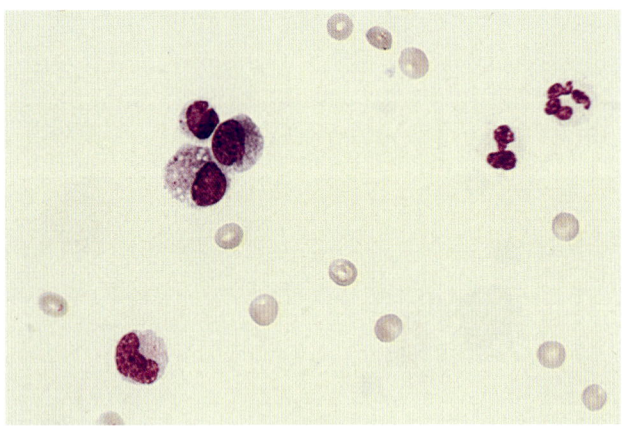

■ **FIGURE 3.221 Seroma. Tissue aspirate. Dog.** Fluid obtained from a swelling on the neck was bloody with white blood cells of 3800/µL and protein of 2.5 g/dL. Blood elements comprised the majority of cell types found. Mononuclear phagocytes as shown accounted for 24% of the cell population. (Wright-Giemsa; HP oil.)

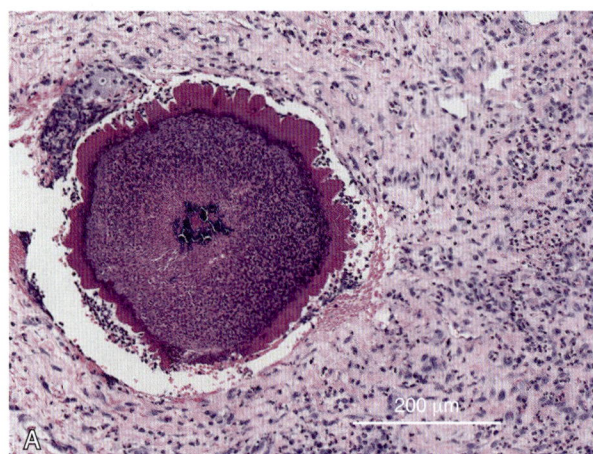
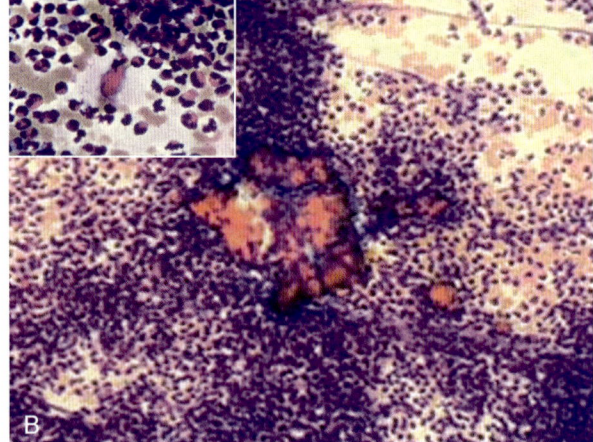

■ **FIGURE 3.222 Splendore-Hoeppli phenomenon. Pararectal mass. Dog.** Same case in A and B. **A, Tissue section.** A dense eosinophilic circular structure composed of radiating antigen-antibody complex material, inflammatory cells, tissue debris, and fibrin is present within the submucosa tissues along with reactive fibroblasts and collagenous stroma. (H&E; IP.) **B, Tissue aspirate.** Eosinophilic amorphous granular material is surrounded by an intense cellular infiltrate. This granular material correlates with the Splendore-Hoeppli immune complex material shown in A. (Romanowsky; IP.) *Inset:* High magnification reveals the cells are mostly eosinophils. A small piece of the eosinophilic immune complex granular material is also visible in the field. Culture revealed a *Staphylococcus aureus* infection. (Romanowsky; HP oil) (Courtesy Laura Snyder, Marshfield Labs.)

vesicles producing a bubbly appearance. If severe, the epidermis may slough, leading to an inflammatory response. Cytopathology demonstrates low cellularity against a light eosinophilic mucinous background with windrowing of cells and possibly collagen fibrils (Whipple et al., 2020). The cell population consists of few spindle mesenchymal cells with a variable number of mast cells and possibly other inflammatory cells such as eosinophils and neutrophils. The background is positive for Alcian blue stain (pH, 2.5) (Lawson, 2021). Nodular lesions may be surgically excised and severe cases treated with corticosteroids or immunosuppressants; however, most lesions regress over time.

Splendore-Hoeppli Reaction

This reaction may occur in cutaneous and mucocutaneous regions and involve a localized immunological response to an antigen–antibody precipitate related to fungi, parasites, bacteria, or biologically inert materials. The characteristic formation of the peribacterial or perifungal Splendore-Hoeppli reaction may be a protective mechanism to prevent phagocytosis and intracellular killing of the offending agent. The reaction is most commonly noted on histopathology but may be appreciated by cytopathology (see Figs. 3.34 and 3.222). Inflammatory cells may range from macrophages to eosinophils and neutrophils along with a lymphoplasmacytic population.

REFERENCES

Adedeji AO, Affolter VK, Christopher MM. Cytologic features of cutaneous follicular tumors and cysts in dogs. *Vet Clin Pathol.* 2017;46(1):143–150.

Affolter VK, Moore PF. Feline progressive histiocytosis. *Vet Pathol.* 2006;43:646–655.

Albanese F. Cytology of skin tumours. In: *Canine and Feline Skin Cytology.* Cham, Switzerland: Springer International Publishing; 2017:291–490.

Albanese F, Abramo F, Braglia C, et al. Nodular lesions due to infestation by *Dirofilaria repens* in dogs from Italy. *Vet Dermatol.* 2013;24:255–259.

Angus JC. Otic cytology in health and disease. *Vet Clin North Am Small Anim Pract.* 2004;34:411–424.

Asakawa MG, Lewis SM, Buckles EL, et al. What is your diagnosis? Cutaneous mass in a dog. *Vet Clin Pathol.* 2015;44(4):607–608.

Avallone G, Helmbold P, Caniatti M, et al. The spectrum of canine cutaneous perivascular wall tumors: morphologic, phenotypic and clinical characterization. *Vet Pathol.* 2007;44:607–620.

Banajee KH, Orandle MS, Ratterree W, et al. Idiopathic solitary cutaneous xanthoma in a dog. *Vet Clin Pathol.* 2011;40:95–98.

Barbosa DL, Paraventi MD, Strefezzi RF. Reproducibility of nuclear morphometry parameters from cytologic smears of canine cutaneous mast cell tumors—intra- and interobserver variability. *Vet Clin Pathol.* 2014;43: 469–472.

Barger AM, Skowronski MC, MacNeill AL. Cytologic identification of erythrophagocytic neoplasms in dogs. *Vet Clin Pathol.* 2012;41:587–589.

Bau-Gaudreault L, Overvelde S, Martin D. What is your diagnosis? Subcutaneous temporal mass from a cat. *Vet Clin Pathol.* 2018;47(2):324–325.

Beaudin S, Rich LJ, Meinkoth JH, et al. Draining skin lesion from a desert poodle. *Vet Clin Pathol.* 2005;34:65–68.

Bernstein JA, Cook HE, Gill AF, et al. Cytologic diagnosis of generalized cutaneous sporotrichosis in a hunting hound. *Vet Clin Pathol.* 2007;36:94–96.

Bertazzolo W, Dell'Orco M, Bonfanti U, et al. Canine angiosarcoma: cytologic, histologic, and immunohistochemical correlations. *Vet Clin Pathol.* 2005;34:28–34.

Bertazzolo W, Giudice C, Dell'Orco M, et al. Paratracheal cervical mass in a dog. *Vet Clin Pathol.* 2003;32:209–212.

Bertazzolo W, Toscani L, Calcaterra S, et al. Clinicopathological findings in five cats with paw calcification. *J Feline Med Surg.* 2003;5:11–17.

Bettenay SV, Lappin MR, Mueller RS. An immunohistochemical and polymerase chain reaction evaluation of feline plasmacytic pododermatitis. *Vet Pathol.* 2007;44(1):80–83.

Bettini G, Morini M, Campagna F, et al. True grit: the tale of a subcutaneous mass in a dog. *Vet Clin Pathol.* 2005;34:73–75.

Beyer TA, Pinckney RD, Cooley AC. Massive *Dracunculus insignis* infection in a dog. *J Am Vet Med Assoc.* 1999;214:366–368.

Bloom PB. Canine and feline eosinophilic skin diseases. *Vet Clin Small Anim.* 2006;36:141–160.

Bohn AA, Wills T, Caplazi P. Basal cell tumor or cutaneous basilar epithelial neoplasm? Rethinking the cytologic diagnosis of basal cell tumors. *Vet Clin Pathol.* 2006;35:449–453.

Boyd SP, Taugner FM, Serrano S, et al. Matrix "blues": clue to a cranial thoracic mass in a dog. *Vet Clin Pathol.* 2005;34:271–274.

Bulla C, Thomas JS. What is your diagnosis? Subcutaneous mass fluid from a febrile dog. *Vet Clin Pathol.* 2009;38:403–405.

Camus MS, Priest HL, Koehler JW, et al. Development of cytologic criteria for mast cell tumor grading with clinical outcome evaluation. *Vet Pathol.* 2016;53(6):1117–1123.

Caniatti M, Ghisleni G, Ceruti R, et al. Cytological features of canine haemangiopericytoma in fine needle aspiration biopsy. *Vet Rec.* 2001;149:242–244.

Caruso KJ, Cowell RL, Cowell AK, et al. Skin scraping from a cat. *Vet Clin Pathol.* 2002;31:13–15.

Cho KO, Park NY, Kang MI, et al. Ganglion cysts in a juvenile dog. *Vet Pathol.* 2000;37(4):340–343.

Choi US, Jeong SM, Kang MS, et al. Cutaneous lymphoma in a juvenile dog. *Vet Clin Pathol.* 2004;33:47–49.

Curran KM, Halsey CHC, Worley DR. Lymphangiosarcoma in 12 dogs: a case series (1998–2013). *Vet Comp Oncol.* 2016;14(2):181–190.

de Cecco BS, Argenta FF, Bianchi RM, et al. Feline giant-cell pleomorphic sarcoma: cytologic, histologic and immunohistochemical characterization. *J Feline Med Surg.* 2021;23(8):738–744.

Declercq J, Bhatti S. Calcinosis involving multiple paws in a cat with chronic renal failure and in a cat with hyperthyroidism. *Vet Dermatol.* 2005;16(1): 74–78.

Di Maria FM, Annoni M, Roccabianca P, et al. Cutaneous metastases of prostatic adenocarcinoma in two dogs. *Vet Clin Pathol.* 2020;49(3):459–464.

Dobromylskyi M. Feline plasma cell pododermatitis—a pathologist's eye view. *Control and Therapy Series.* 2015;279:41–45.

Dohata A, Chambers JK, Uchida K, et al. Clinical and pathologic study of feline Merkel cell carcinoma with immunohistochemical characterization of normal and neoplastic Merkel cells. *Vet Pathol.* 2015;52(6):1012–1018.

Dunbar MD, Conway JA. What is your diagnosis? Cytologic findings from a subcutaneous nodule over the left epaxial musculature in a dog. *Vet Clin Pathol.* 2012;41:295–296.

Eu WW, Pool R, Kelso N, et al. What is your diagnosis? Aspirate from a digit of a dog. *Vet Clin Pathol.* 2017;46(4):637–638.

Evans SJM, Connolly SL, Schaffer PA, et al. Basal cell enumeration does not predict malignancy in canine perianal gland tumor cytology. *Vet Clin Pathol.* 2018;47:634–637.

Evans SJ, Frank CB, Avery PR, et al. What is your diagnosis? Subcutaneous mass on a dog. *Vet Clin Pathol.* 2018;47(1):160–161.

Fernandez NJ, West KH, Jackson ML, et al. Immunohistochemical and histochemical stains for differentiating canine cutaneous round cell tumors. *Vet Pathol.* 2005;42:437–445.

Foley JE, Borjesson D, Gross TL. Clinical, microscopic, and molecular aspects of canine leproid granuloma in the United States. *Vet Pathol.* 2002;39: 234–239.

Fontaine J, Heimann M, Day MJ. Canine cutaneous epitheliotropic T-cell lymphoma: a review of 30 cases. *Vet Dermatol.* 2010;21(3):267–275.

Fontaine J, Heimann M, Day MJ. Cutaneous epitheliotropic T-cell lymphoma in the cat: a review of the literature and five new cases. *Vet Dermatol.* 2011;22(5):454–461.

French TW, Blue JT. What is your diagnosis? (Cuterebra). *Vet Clin Pathol.* 1986; 15:18–19.

Garma-Avina A. The cytology of squamous cell carcinomas in domestic animals. *J Vet Diagn Invest.* 1994;6:238–246.

Gill V, Leibman N, Monette S, et al. Prognostic indicators and clinical outcome in dogs with subcutaneous mast cell tumors treated with surgery alone: 43 cases. *J Am Anim Hosp Assoc.* 2020;56(4):215–225.

Giori L, Garbagnoli V, Venco L, et al. What is your diagnosis? Fine-needle aspirate from a subcutaneous mass in a dog. *Vet Clin Pathol.* 2010;39:255–256.

Goldschmidt MH, Goldschmidt KH. Epithelial and melanocytic tumors of the skin. In: Meuten DJ, ed. *Tumors in Domestic Animals.* 5th ed. Ames, IA: John Wiley & Sons; 2017:88–141.

Goldschmidt MH, Munday JS, Scruggs JL, et al. In: Kiupel M, ed. *Surgical Pathology of Tumors of Domestic Animals Vol 1: Epithelial Tumors of the Skin.* 3rd ed. Gurnee, IL: Davis-Thompson Foundation; 2018:74–81.

Goldschmidt MH, Shofer FS. *Skin Tumors of the Dog and Cat.* Oxford, UK: Pergamon Press; 1992:1–3, 50–65, 103–108, 271–283.

Gorman E, Barger AM, Wypij JM, et al. Cutaneous metastasis of primary appendicular osteosarcoma in a dog. *Vet Clin Pathol.* 2006;35(3):358–361.

Greene CE, Gunn-Moore DA. Mycobacterial infections. In: Greene CE, ed. *Infectious Diseases of the Dog and Cat.* 3rd ed. Philadelphia: Elsevier; 2006:462–488.

Grooters AM, Hodgin EC, Bauer RW, et al. Clinicopathologic findings associated with *Lagenidium* sp. infection in 6 dogs: initial description of an emerging oomycosis. *J Vet Intern Med.* 2003;17:637–646.

Gross TL, Ihrke PJ, Walder EJ, et al. *Skin Diseases of the Dog and Cat. Clinical and Histopathologic Diagnosis.* 2nd ed. Ames, IA: Blackwell Science; 2005.

Gupta A, Stroup S, Dedeaux A, et al. What is your diagnosis? Fine-needle aspirate of ulcerative skin lesions in a dog. *Vet Clin Pathol.* 2011;40:401–402.

Hans E, Raskin R, Bisby TM. Statistical evaluation of BLA.36 antigen antibody for hematopoietic tumors in dogs and cats [abstract]. In: *Proceedings of the ACVP/ASVCP Conference*. 2008:27.

Hirabayashi M, Chambers JK, Sumi A, et al. Immunophenotyping of nonneoplastic and neoplastic histiocytes in cats and characterization of a novel cell line derived from feline progressive histiocytosis. *Vet Pathol*. 2020;57(6):758–773.

Hoffmann AR, Cadieu J, Kiupel M, et al. Cutaneous toxoplasmosis in two dogs. *J Vet Diagn Invest*. 2012;24(3):636–640.

Inga A, Griffeth GC, Drobatz KJ, et al. Sterile granulomatous dermatitis and lymphadenitis (juvenile cellulitis) in adult dogs: a retrospective analysis of 90 cases (2004–2018). *Vet Dermatol*. 2020;31(3):219-e47.

Jackson K, Boger L, Goldschmidt M, et al. Malignant pilomatricoma in a soft-coated Wheaten terrier. *Vet Clin Pathol*. 2010;39:236–240.

Jakab C, Rusvai M, Szabo Z, et al. Expression of the claudin-4 molecule in benign and malignant canine hepatoid gland tumours. *Acta Vet Hung*. 2009;557:463–475.

Jennings RN, Miller MA, Ramos-Vara JA. Comparison of CD34, CD31, and factor VIII–related antigen immunohistochemical expression in feline vascular neoplasms and CD34 expression in feline nonvascular neoplasms. *Vet Pathol*. 2012;49(3):532–537.

Johnson TO, Schulman FY, Lipscomb TP, et al. Histopathology and biologic behavior of pleomorphic cutaneous mast cell tumors in fifteen cats. *Vet Pathol*. 2002;39:452–457.

Joiner KS, Smith AN, Henderson RA, et al. Multicentric cutaneous neuroendocrine (Merkel cell) carcinoma in a dog. *Vet Pathol*. 2010;47:1090–1094.

Juopperi TA, Cesta M, Tomlinson L, et al. Extensive cutaneous metastases in a dog with duodenal adenocarcinoma. *Vet Clin Pathol*. 2003;32:88–91.

Kano R, Watanabe K, Murakami M, et al. Molecular diagnosis of feline sporotrichosis. *Vet Rec*. 2005;156:484–485.

Kato Y, Funato R, Hirata A, et al. Immunocytochemical detection of the class A macrophage scavenger receptor CD 204 using air-dried cytologic smears of canine histiocytic sarcoma. *Vet Clin Pathol*. 2014;43(4):589–593.

Kaya O, Kirkan S, Unal B. Isolation of *Dermatophilus congolensis* from a cat. *J Vet Med B Infect Dis Vet Public Health*. 2000;47:155–157.

Kennedy K, Thomas R, Breen M. Canine histiocytic malignancies—challenges and opportunities. *Vet Sci*. 2016;3(1):2.

Kiupel M, Camus M. Diagnosis and prognosis of canine cutaneous mast cell tumors. *Vet Clin North Am Small Anim Pract*. 2019;49(5):819–836.

Kiupel M, Webster JD, Bailey KL, et al. Proposal of a 2-tier histologic grading system for canine cutaneous mast cell tumors to more accurately predict biological behavior. *Vet Pathol*.2011;48:147–155.

Kiupel M, Webster JD, Kaneene JB, et al. The use of KIT and tryptase expression patterns as prognostic tools for canine cutaneous mast cell tumors. *Vet Pathol*. 2004;41:371–377.

Kok MK, Chambers JK, Ong SM, et al. Hierarchical cluster analysis of cytokeratins and stem cell expression profiles of canine cutaneous epithelial tumors. *Vet Pathol*. 2018;55(6):821–837.

La Perle KM, Del Piero F, Carr RF, et al. Cutaneous neosporosis in two adult dogs on chronic immunosuppressive therapy. *J Vet Diagn Invest*. 2001;13(3):252–255.

Lawson CA. What is your diagnosis? Aspirate from a Chinese Shar-Pei with multiple skin nodules. *Vet Clin Pathol*. 2021;50(1):92–94.

Lester SJ, Malik R, Bartlett KH, et al. Cryptococcosis: update and emergence of *Cryptococcus gattii*. *Vet Clin Pathol*. 2011;40(1):4–17.

Liotta JL, Sandhu GK, Rishniw M, et al. Differentiation of the microfilariae of *Dirofilaria immitis* and *Dirofilaria repens* in stained blood films. *J Parasitol*. 2013;99(3):421–425.

Little LK, Goldschmidt M. Cytologic appearance of a keloidal fibrosarcoma in a dog. *Vet Clin Pathol*. 2007;36:364–367.

Little L, Shokek A, Dubey JP, et al. *Toxoplasma gondii*-like organisms in skin aspirates from a cat with disseminated protozoal infection. *Vet Clin Pathol*. 2005;34:156–160.

Logan MR, Raskin RE, Thompson S. "Carry-on" dermal baggage: a nodule from a dog. *Vet Clin Pathol*. 2006;35:329–331.

Lucio-Forster A, Eberhard ML, Cama VA, et al. First report of *Dracunculus insignis* in two naturally infected cats from the northeastern USA. *J Feline Med Surg*. 2014;16:194–197.

Majzoub M, Breuer W, Platz SJ, et al. Histopathologic and immunophenotypic characterization of extramedullary plasmacytomas in nine cats. *Vet Pathol*. 2003;40:249–253.

Marcos R, Santos M, Marrinhas C, et al. Cutaneous transmissible venereal tumor without genital involvement in a prepubertal female dog. *Vet Clin Pathol*. 2006a;35:106–109.

Marcos R, Santos M, Oliveira J, et al. Cytochemical detection of calcium in a case of calcinosis circumscripta in a dog. *Vet Clin Pathol*. 2006b;35:239–242.

Masserdotti C, Ubbiali FA. Fine needle aspiration cytology of pilomatricoma in three dogs. *Vet Clin Pathol*. 2002;31:22–25.

McAloney CA, Brown ME, Martinez MP, et al. What is your diagnosis? Subcutaneous mass in a dog. *Vet Clin Pathol*. 2020;49:161–163.

McCarthy PE, Hedlund CS, Veazy RS, et al. Liposarcoma associated with a glass foreign body in a dog. *J Am Vet Med Assoc*. 1996;209:612–614.

McCourt MR, Levine GM, Breshears MA, et al. Metastatic disease in a dog with a well-differentiated perianal gland tumor. *Vet Clin Pathol*. 2018;47(4):649–653.

McKenna M, Attipa C, Tasker S, et al. Leishmaniosis in a dog with no travel history outside of the UK. *Vet Rec*. 2019;184(14):441.

Moore AR, Libby AL, Khanal S, et al. Is this cell hollow? *Vet Clin Pathol*. 2016;45(1):8–9.

Moore PF. A review of histiocytic diseases of dogs and cats. *Vet Pathol*. 2014;51:167–184.

Moore PF, Olivry T, Naydan D. Canine cutaneous epitheliotropic lymphoma (mycosis fungoides) is a proliferative disorder of CD8+ T cells. *Am J Pathol*. 1994;144:421–429.

Munday JS, Thomson NA, Luff JA. Papillomaviruses in dogs and cats. *Vet J*. 2017;225:23–31.

Neel JA, Tarigo J, Tater KC, et al. Deep and superficial skin scrapings from a feline immunodeficiency virus-positive cat. *Vet Clin Pathol*. 2007;36:101–104.

Noland EL, Keller SM, Kiupel M. Subcutaneous panniculitis-like T-cell lymphoma in dogs: morphologic and immunohistochemical classification. *Vet Pathol*. 2018;55(6):802–808.

Otrocka-Domagała I, Paździor-Czapula K, Gesek M, et al. Aggressive, solid variant of alveolar rhabdomyosarcoma with cutaneous involvement in a juvenile Labrador retriever. *J Comp Pathol*. 2015;152(2–3):177–181.

Park CH, Ikadai H, Yoshida E, et al. Cutaneous toxoplasmosis in a female Japanese cat. *Vet Pathol*. 2007;44:683–687.

Park MS, Kim Y, Kan MS, et al. Disseminated transmissible venereal tumor in a dog. *J Vet Diagn Invest*. 2006;18:130–133.

Patel A. Pyogranulomatous skin disease and cellulitis in a cat caused by *Rhodococcus equi*. *J Sm Anim Pract*. 2002;43:129–132.

Paździor-Czapula K, Otrocka-Domagała I, Myrdek P, et al. *Dirofilaria repens*: an etiological factor or an incidental finding in cytologic and histopathologic biopsies from dogs. *Vet Clin Pathol*. 2018;47(2):307–311.

Petterino C, Guazzi P, Ferro S, et al. Bronchogenic adenocarcinoma in a cat: an unusual case of metastasis to the skin. *Vet Clin Pathol*. 2005;34:401–404.

Pierezan F, Mansell J, Ambrus A, et al. Immunohistochemical expression of ionized calcium binding adapter molecule 1 in cutaneous histiocytic proliferative, neoplastic and inflammatory disorders of dogs and cats. *J Comp Pathol*. 2014;151(4):347–351.

Pinto da Cunha N, Ghisleni G, Scarampella F, et al. Cytologic and immunocytochemical characterization of feline progressive histiocytosis. *Vet Clin Pathol*. 2014;43:428–436.

Piviani M, Sánchez MD, Patel RT. Cytologic features of clear cell adnexal carcinoma in 3 dogs. *Vet Clin Pathol*. 2012;41(3):405–411.

Quiroz-Rocha GF, Deravi N, Knight B, et al. What is your diagnosis? A pigmented round cell tumor. *Vet Clin Pathol*. 2017;46(3):538–539.

Radhakrishnan A, Risbon RE, Patel RT, et al. Progression of a solitary, malignant cutaneous plasma-cell tumour to multiple myeloma in a cat. *Vet Comp Oncol*. 2004;2:36–42.

Ramírez GA, Rodríguez F, Herráez P, et al. Morphologic and immunohistochemical features of Merkel cells in the dog. *Res Vet Sci*. 2014;97(3):475–480.

Ramos-Vara JA, Miller MA, Johnson GC, et al. Melan A and S100 protein immunohistochemistry in feline melanomas: 48 cases. *Vet Pathol*. 2002;39:127–132.

Ramos-Vara JA, Miller MA, Valli VEO. Immunohistochemical detection of multiple myeloma 1/interferon regulatory factor 4 (MUM1/IRF-4) in canine plasmacytoma: comparison with CD79a and CD20. *Vet Pathol.* 2007;44:875–884.

Raskin RE. Applied cytology: canine elbow mass. *NAVC Clinician's Brief.* 2006a;4:65–67.

Raskin RE. Applied cytology: tail mass in a dog. *NAVC Clinician's Brief.* 2006b;4:13–15.

Ressel L, Finotello R. Cytological grading of canine cutaneous mast cell tumours: is haematoxylin and eosin staining better than May-Grünwald-Giemsa? *Vet Comp Oncol.* 2016;15(3):667–668.

Rigas JD, Latouche JS. Spherule splendor. *Vet Clin Pathol.* 2021;50:7–8.

Roccabianca P, Avallone G, Rodriguez A, et al. Cutaneous lymphoma at injection sites: pathological, immunophenotypical, and molecular characterization in 17 cats. *Vet Pathol.* 2016;53(4):823–832.

Roccabianca P, Caniatti M, Scanziani E, et al. Feline leprosy: spontaneous remission in a cat. *J Am Anim Hosp Assoc.* 1996;32:189–193.

Ross JT, Scavelli TD, Matthiesen DT, et al. Adenocarcinoma of the apocrine glands of the anal sac in dogs: a review of 32 cases. *J Am Anim Hosp Assoc.* 1991;27:349–355.

Rosser MF, Wycislo KL, Duffy DJ, et al. What is your diagnosis? A ventral cervical mass in a dog. *Vet Clin Pathol.* 2019;48(1):125–127.

Sabattini S, Bettini G. Prognostic value of histologic and immunohistochemical features in feline cutaneous mast cell tumors. *Vet Pathol.* 2010;47:643–653.

Sabattini S, Bettini G. Grading cutaneous mast cell tumors in cats. *Vet Pathol.* 2019;56(1):43–49.

Sabattini S, Renzi A, Rigillo A, et al. Cytological differentiation between benign and malignant perianal gland proliferative lesions in dogs: a preliminary study. *J Small Anim Pract.* 2019;60(10):616–622.

Sævik BK, Jörundsson E, Stachurska-Hagen T, et al. *Dirofilaria repens* infection in a dog imported to Norway. *Acta Vet Scand.* 2014;56(1):1–6.

Sailasuta A, Ketpun D, Piyaviriyakul P, et al. The relevance of CD117-immunocytochemistry staining patterns to mutational exon-11 in c-kit detected by PCR from fine-needle aspirated canine mast cell tumor cells. *Vet Med Int.* 2014;2014:787498.

Sakai H, Murakami M, Mishima H, et al. Cytologically atypical anal sac adenocarcinoma in a dog. *Vet Clin Pathol.* 2012;41:291–294.

Sánchez MD, Goldschmidt MH, Mauldin EA. Herpesvirus dermatitis in two cats without facial lesions. *Vet Dermatol.* 2012;23(2):171–173.

Santos M, Canadas A, Puente-Payo P, et al. What is your diagnosis? Cutaneous ulcerated nodule in a geriatric dog. *Vet Clin Pathol.* 2017;46(3):535–537.

Scarpa F, Sabattini S, Bettini G. Cytological grading of canine cutaneous mast cell tumours. *Vet Comp Oncol.* 2016;14(3):245–251.

Scruggs JL, LeBlanc CJ. Identification of blue staining vaccine-derived material in inflammatory lesions using cultured canine macrophages. *Vet Clin Pathol.* 2015;44(1):152–156.

Son NV, Uchida K, Thongtharb A, et al. Establishment of cell line and in vivo mouse model of canine Langerhans cell histiocytosis. *Vet Comp Oncol.* 2019;17:345–353.

Spector D, Legendre AM, Wheat J, et al. Antigen and antibody testing for the diagnosis of blastomycosis in dogs. *J Vet Intern Med.* 2008;22:839–843.

Sprague W, Thrall MA. Recurrent skin mass from the digit of a dog. *Vet Clin Pathol.* 2001;30:189–192.

Stefanello D, Avallone G, Ferrari R, et al. Canine cutaneous perivascular wall tumors at first presentation: clinical behavior and prognostic factors in 55 cases. *J Vet Intern Med.* 2011;25:1398–1405.

Stilwell JM, Rissi DR. Immunohistochemical labeling of multiple myeloma oncogene 1/interferon regulatory factor 4 (MUM1/IRF-4) in canine cutaneous histiocytoma. *Vet Pathol.* 2018;55(4):517–520.

Thrift E, Greenwell C, Turner AL, et al. Metastatic pulmonary carcinomas in cats ('feline lung-digit syndrome'): further variations on a theme. *JFMS Open Rep.* 2017;3(1):1–8.

Trainor KE, Porter BF, Logan KS, et al. Eight cases of feline cutaneous leishmaniasis in Texas. *Vet Pathol.* 2010;47:1076–1081.

Tremblay N, Lanevschi A, Doré M, et al. Of all the nerve! A subcutaneous forelimb mass on a cat. *Vet Clin Pathol.* 2005;34:417–420.

Twomey LN, Wuerz JA, Alleman AR. A "down under" lesion on the muzzle of a dog. *Vet Clin Pathol.* 2005;34:161–133.

Uchida K, Yamaguchi R, Tateyama S. Glomus tumor in the digit of a cat. *Vet Pathol.* 2002;39(5):590–592.

Villamil JA, Henry CJ, Bryan JN, et al. Identification of the most common cutaneous neoplasms in dogs and evaluation of breed and age distributions for selected neoplasms. *J Am Vet Med Assoc.* 2011;239:960–965.

Vobornik S, Johnson M, Diesel A, et al. What is your diagnosis? Aspirate from a digit in a cat. *Vet Clin Pathol.* 2014;43(2):291–292.

Webster JD, Yuzbasiyan-Gurkan V, Miller RA, et al. Cellular proliferation in canine cutaneous mast cell tumors: associations with *c-KIT* and its role in prognostication. *Vet Pathol.* 2007;44:298–308.

Welsh RD. Sporotrichosis. *J Am Vet Med Assoc.* 2003;223:1123–1126.

Wells B, Burnum AL, Armstrong J, et al. *Actinomadura vinacea* isolated from a nonhealing cutaneous wound in a cat. *Vet Clin Pathol.* 2018;47:638–642.

Whipple KM, Kieran EA, Dark MJ, et al. What is your diagnosis? Cutaneous mass from a Shar-Pei dog. *Vet Clin Pathol.* 2020;49(2):365–366.

Wilkerson MJ, Chard-Bergstrom C, Andrews G, et al. Subcutaneous mass aspirate from a dog [epithelioid hemangiosarcoma]. *Vet Clin Pathol.* 2002;31:65–68.

Wilkerson MJ, Dolce K, DeBey BM, et al. Metastatic balloon cell melanoma in a dog. *Vet Clin Pathol.* 2003;32:31–36.

Yager JA, Wilcock BP. *Color Atlas and Text of Surgical Pathology of the Dog and Cat: Dermatopathology and Skin Tumors.* London: CV Mosby; 1994:243–244, 245–248, 257–271, 273–286.

Zimmerman K, Feldman B, Robertson J, et al. Dermal mass aspirate from a Persian cat. *Vet Clin Pathol.* 2003;32:213–217.

4 CHAPTER

Hemolymphatic System

Rose E. Raskin

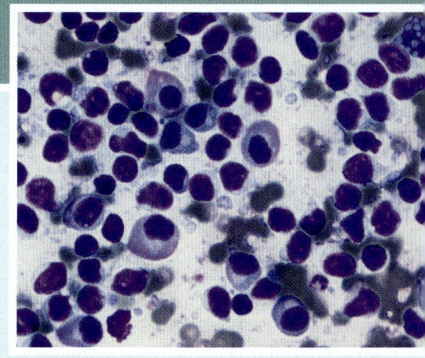

GENERAL CONSIDERATIONS FOR LYMPHOID TISSUES

The lymphoid organs commonly examined by cytopathology include the peripheral and internal lymph nodes, spleen, and occasionally the thymus. As a result of their similar cell populations, the following cytodiagnostic categories are used. It should be noted that more than one presentation might occur in a specimen at a time.

Cytodiagnostic Groups for Lymphoid Organ Cytopathology

- Normal tissue
- Reactive/hyperplastic tissue
- Inflammation
- Metastatic disease
- Primary neoplasia
- Extramedullary hematopoiesis

Cytopathologic Biopsy Considerations

The lymphosomes or lymphatic territories of the superficial lymphatic system in dogs were mapped, showing drainage into 10 regions (Fig. 4.1) (Suami et al., 2013). Mandibular lymph nodes are frequently enlarged and reactive because of their constant exposure to antigens but are a poor choice for biopsy with generalized lymphadenopathy.

In a study of cytopathologic and histopathologic correlation in dogs and cats, cytopathology of lymph nodes had a sensitivity of 67%, specificity of 92%, and accuracy of 77% for neoplasia (Ku et al., 2017). However, cytopathology was poorly sensitive for detecting mesenteric T-cell lymphoma, especially in cats, in which mature cell types predominated, and for metastatic sarcomas, in which distribution was often focal. Similarly, for the spleen, cytopathology correlated to histopathology in 61% of cases with problems occurring where tissue architecture was required to distinguish between reactive and neoplastic conditions (Ballegeer et al., 2007).

> **KEY POINT** Popliteal and superficial cervical (prescapular) lymph nodes are the preferred biopsy sites for generalized lymphadenopathy.

LYMPH NODES

Normal Lymph Node Anatomy and Histology

The canine or feline lymph node consists of a thin connective tissue capsule that surrounds cortical and medullary lymphoid tissue and extends inward as trabeculae. The outer cortex contains variably sized lymphatic nodules (Fig. 4.2A) composed primarily of B lymphocytes surrounded by a thin rim of small T lymphocytes. The diffuse lymphoid tissue between the nodules, composed primarily of T lymphocytes, extends deep into the paracortex, where macrophages and dendritic reticular cells act as antigen-presenting cells. The diffuse lymphoid tissue extends inward to form medullary cords (Fig. 4.2B), which contain B lymphocytes, plasma cells, macrophages, and other leukocytes. Between the cords are endothelial-lined sinuses in contact with dendritic reticular cells and reticular fibers. Lymph enters the afferent vessels that penetrate the capsule, through the subcapsular and cortical sinuses of the cortex, into the medullary sinuses and exits through efferent vessels at the hilus. Blood flow enters the hilus through arterioles that branch into the cortex to perfuse the lymphatic nodules. In this region, vessels enlarge to form postcapillary or *high endothelial venules* of the paracortex (Fig. 4.2C). These venules are important sites for the travel of lymphocytes from blood into the lymph node parenchyma that is related to the selective binding of the lymphocyte with the receptors on the endothelial cells. The venules drain into larger veins that exit via the hilus region.

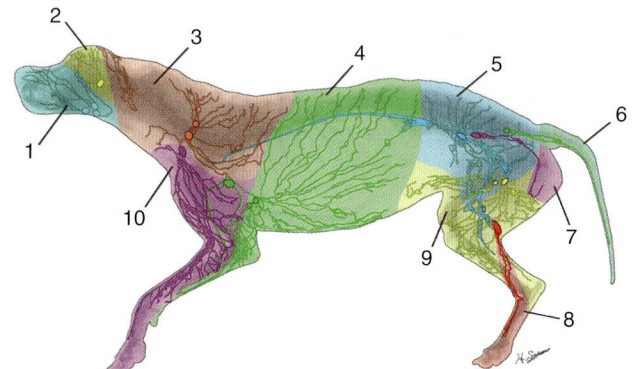

■ **FIGURE 4.1 Lymphosomes. Diagram. Dog.** Color-coded diagram of the lymphatic territories (lymphosomes) with lymphatic vessels shown distally from their corresponding lymph nodes: *1*, mandibular; *2*, parotid; *3*, dorsal superficial cervical; *4*, axillary; *5*, medial iliac; *6*, lateral sacral; *7*, internal iliac; *8*, popliteal; *9*, superficial inguinal; *10*, ventral superficial cervical. (From Suami H, Yamashita S, Soto-Miranda MA, et al. Lymphatic territories (lymphosomes) in a canine: an animal model for investigation of postoperative lymphatic alterations. *PLoS One.* 2013;8(7):e69222.)

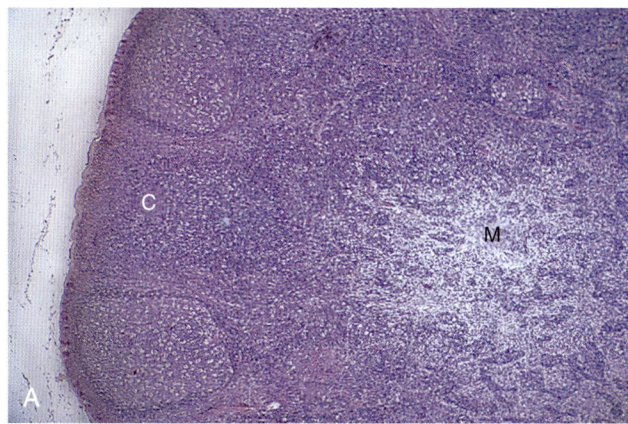
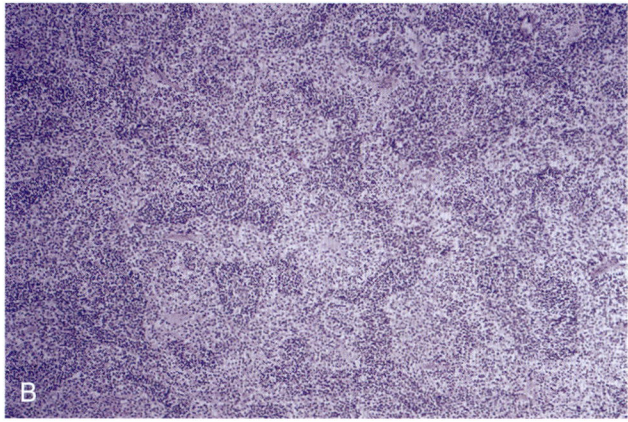
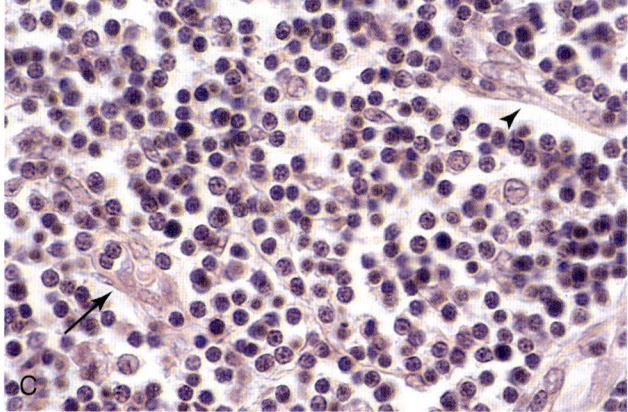

■ **FIGURE 4.2 Normal lymph node. Histology. Dog.** Same case in A to C. **A,** The cortex (C) contains variably sized lymphoid follicles, and the medullary (M) area contains cords of cells along endothelial-lined sinuses. (H&E; LP.) **B,** Medullary cords appearing as dark bands are composed of lymphocytes, plasma cells, and macrophages and lie adjacent to pale-stained sinus spaces. (H&E; LP.) **C,** The deep cortex contains high endothelial venules shown in the cross section *(arrow)* and longitudinal section *(arrowhead)*. Lymphocytes selectively adhere to receptors on the endothelium to leave the circulation and enter the lymph node. (H&E; HP oil.)

Indications for Lymph Node Biopsy

- *Lymphadenomegaly,* or enlargement of one or multiple lymph nodes, is detected by palpation, radiography, or ultrasonography and was the most common reason for cytopathology in one study (Amores-Fuster et al., 2015).
- *Evaluation of metastatic disease* involves evaluation of the lymph node(s) draining the primary lesion (Table 4.1). The sensitivity of cytopathology was 67% for sarcomas, 100% for carcinomas, 63% for melanomas, 75% for mast cell tumors, and 100% for other round cell tumors. The specificity varied between 83% and 96% (Fournier et al., 2018).
- *Classification of lymphoma* may be enhanced by cytopathologic specimens stained with Romanowsky stains, or by cytochemical and immunocytochemical stains (see Chapter 18 and Appendix 2) to distinguish B- and T-cell subtypes; the latter stains may be performed at specialized laboratories.

Lymph Node Collection and Specimen Preparation

The size of the lymph node should be considered. Very large nodes may yield misleading information because they frequently contain necrotic or hemorrhagic tissue. A mildly enlarged lymph node is preferred, and a sample from more than one location is desirable. If a large lymph node must be aspirated, the needle should be aimed tangentially to avoid hitting the direct center.

In performing aspirate smears, a 22-gauge needle is used alone or together with a 6 or 12 mL syringe. The needle is inserted into the node in several directions. With the syringe attached to the needle or butterfly catheter, quick and multiple withdrawal motions of the plunger are made to create negative pressure. The pressure on the plunger is released *before* removing the needle to avoid splattering the material within the syringe. An air-filled syringe is reattached, and the needle contents are expelled onto the approximate center of a glass slide. The aspirate appears creamy white and watery to viscous, indicating the presence of many leukocytes. The material is *gently* squashed with a second slide, sliding them apart horizontally. Smears are dried rapidly with a fan or hair dryer to avoid crenation effects.

An alternative method to aspiration biopsy uses the needle only, without suction. In this method, cells are drawn into the needle by capillary action (Fig. 4.3). This technique is preferred for lymphoid organs to prevent excess blood contamination.

When preparing impression smears from an excisional biopsy, it is important to blot excessive tissue fluids on a paper towel before touch preparations are made to increase the cellular yield. After the cut surface of the excised lymph node is blotted, the surface is then touched gently to a glass slide.

An alternative slide preparation technique using lymphoid tissue aspirates involves placing aspirate material, often multiple aspirations required, into 1 to 2 mL of physiologic 0.9% saline until solution becomes cloudy or turbid from sufficient cell numbers. Preparations should be made immediately by cytocentrifugation or by a fluid sedimentation method. A drop of sediment can be spread directly or as a squash prep, the latter of which is preferred. The squash technique allows structural elements to remain intact usually in the center. If transported to a laboratory, albumin or the patient's serum to approximately 10% of the solution is added to aid in maintenance of cell integrity during transit.

Preparing cell blocks of lymphoid tissue and processing them as histopathology with immunochemistry increased sensitivity for leishmaniasis (Guerra et al., 2019), but insufficiently cellular cell blocks could impair diagnosis (Heinrich et al., 2019). See more discussion about cell blocks in Appendix 5.

To avoid the formalin artifact, cytopathologic and histopathologic samples must be mailed separately when submitted to a referral laboratory.

TABLE 4.1	Commonly Sampled Lymph Nodes in Dogs (See Fig. 4.1)	
LYMPH NODE	LOCATION	DRAINAGE FEATURES
Mandibular (submandibular)	Group of two to four nodes located ventral to the angle of the jaw	Includes most of the head, including the rostral oral cavity
Superficial cervical (prescapular)	Group of two or three nodes located in front of the supraspinatus muscle	Includes the caudal part of the head (pharynx, pinna), most of the thoracic limb, and part of the thoracic wall
Axillary	One or two nodes located caudal and medial to the shoulder joint	Includes most of the thoracic wall, deep structures of the thoracic limb and neck, and the thoracic and cranial abdominal mammary glands
Superficial inguinal	Two nodes located in the furrow between the abdominal wall and the medial thigh	Includes the caudal abdominal and inguinal mammary glands, ventral half of the abdominal wall, penis, prepuce, scrotal skin, tail, ventral pelvis, and medial part of the thigh and stifle
Popliteal	One node located behind the stifle	Includes areas distal to the stifle
Medial iliac	One to two nodes near the caudal vena cava and aorta	Includes the skin of the pelvic area, pelvic limb, distal intestinal, and urogenital system

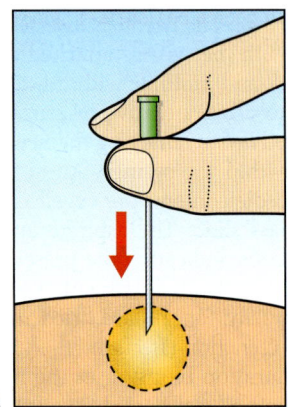 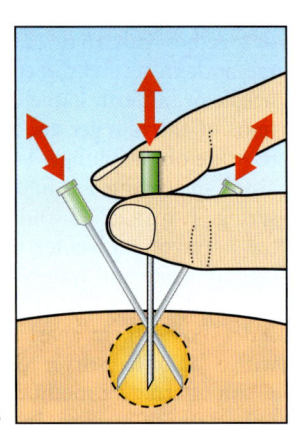 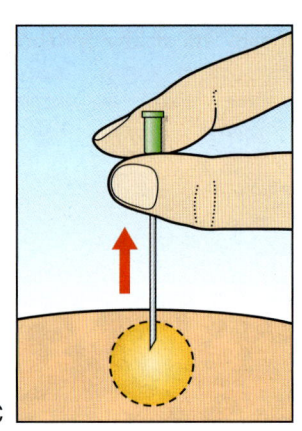 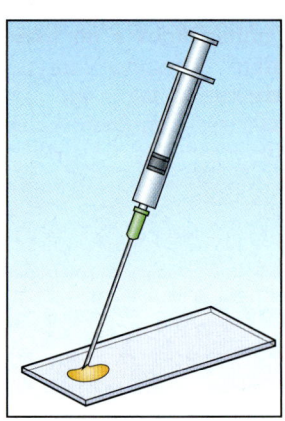

A B C D

■ **FIGURE 4.3 Fine-needle biopsy without suction.** Stepwise illustration of the biopsy procedure. **A,** The needle is inserted into the target tissue. **B,** The needle is moved back and forth inside target, varying the angle. **C,** The needle is withdrawn. **D,** The needle is attached to the syringe, and the sample is blown onto the microscopy slide. (From Orell SR, Sterrett GF, Whitaker D. *Fine needle aspiration cytology*, ed 4. Edinburgh: Churchill Livingstone; 1995.)

> **KEY POINT** The center of a very large lymph node should be avoided during aspiration.

> **KEY POINT** Aspirate smears must be spread gently because immature lymphoid cells are often quite fragile.

> **KEY POINT** The nonsuction method of collection is best to minimize blood contamination from lymphoid organ collection.

> **KEY POINT** Keep cytopathologic preparations away from formalin fumes to avoid premature fixation, which would result in poor staining and cellular detail.

Normal Lymph Node Cytology and Artifacts

Small, well-differentiated lymphocytes that measure 1 to 1.5 times the diameter of an erythrocyte in dogs and cats compose approximately 90% of the population (Fig. 4.4). The chromatin of

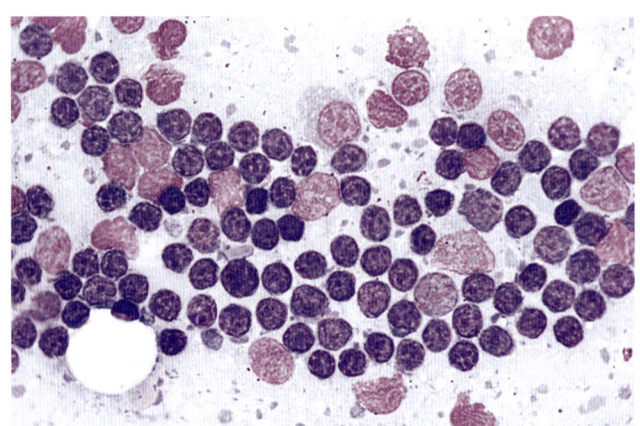

■ **FIGURE 4.4 Normal lymph node. Tissue aspirate. Dog.** This superficial cervical (prescapular) lymph node contains a majority of small lymphocytes. Low numbers of medium-sized lymphocytes are present as well as several lysed cells that appear light pink and lack cytoplasmic borders. (Wright-Giemsa; HP oil.)

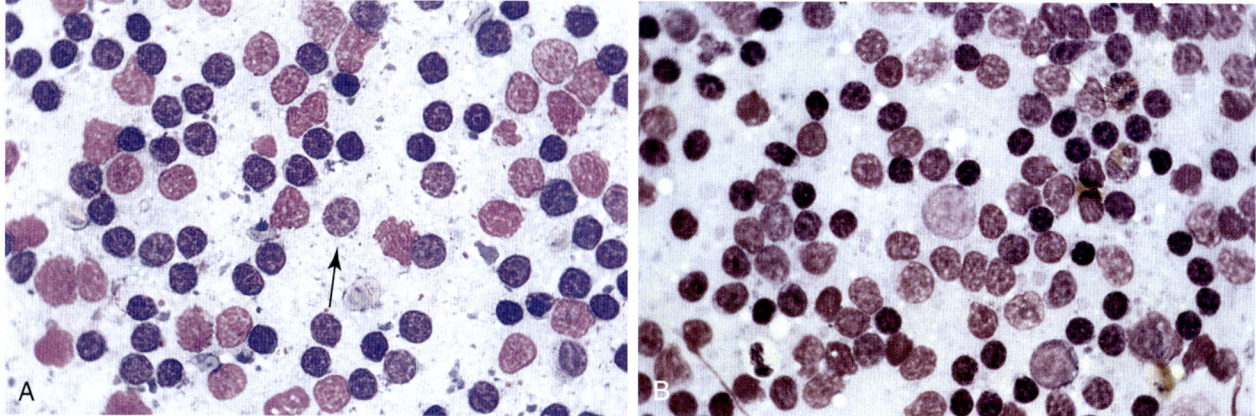

FIGURE 4.5 **Normal lymph node. Tissue aspirate. Dog.** Same case in A and B. **A,** This popliteal lymph node contains a majority of small lymphocytes. Note the medium-sized lymphocyte *(arrow)*. (Wright-Giemsa; HP oil.) **B,** A mixed cell population. Note the large lymphocyte in the center and occasional granulocytes. (Wright-Giemsa; HP oil.)

these cells is densely clumped with no visible nucleoli. Cytoplasm is scant. These cells are the darkest staining of all the lymphocytes. The medium (2–2.5 times) and large lymphocytes (>3 times) whose nuclei are measured relative to the erythrocyte diameter may be present in low numbers (<5%–10%) (Fig. 4.5). Their nuclei have a fine, diffuse, and light chromatin pattern. Nucleoli may be prominent. The cytoplasm is more abundant and often basophilic. Mature plasma cells represent a small portion of the cells found. Their chromatin is densely clumped, and often the nucleus is eccentrically placed within the abundant, deeply basophilic cytoplasm. A pale area or halo is seen adjacent to the nucleus, which indicates the Golgi zone. Occasional macrophages (histiocytes) appear as large mononuclear cells with abundant light cytoplasm, often containing cellular debris. Nuclear chromatin is finely stippled, and nucleoli may be found in activated macrophages. Mast cells and neutrophils also may be present in low numbers (Bookbinder et al., 1992). Arterial fragments with smooth muscle cells are rarely encountered (Fig. 4.6).

A flow cytometric study of normal canine lymph nodes indicated approximately equal numbers of T cells and B cells (Rütgen et al., 2015). More specific results for this study were CD3+ 55%, CD3ε+ 57%, CD5+ 52%, CD21+ 34%, CD79a+ 47%, and CD14+ 6%. There were 59% CD4+ and 21% CD8+ of CD3+ cells.

In attempting to aspirate the mandibular lymph node, it is quite common to sample salivary gland tissue (Fig. 4.7A–B). The mandibular lymph node is found directly ventral to the prominent part of the zygomatic arch, which is behind and below the eye, midway between the eye and ear. The mandibular salivary gland is located within the bifurcation of the external jugular vein and is posterior and dorsal to the lymph node (Fig. 4.7C).

Reactive or Hyperplastic Lymph Node

Enlargement of a lymph node under this condition is due to any local or generalized antigenic response, which may include infection, inflammation, immune-mediated disease, or neoplasia from an area that drains into the lymph node. Histologically, lymphoid nodules within the cortex form prominent germinal centers that develop after antigen stimulation (Fig. 4.8). Light and dark zones compose the germinal center. In addition to small

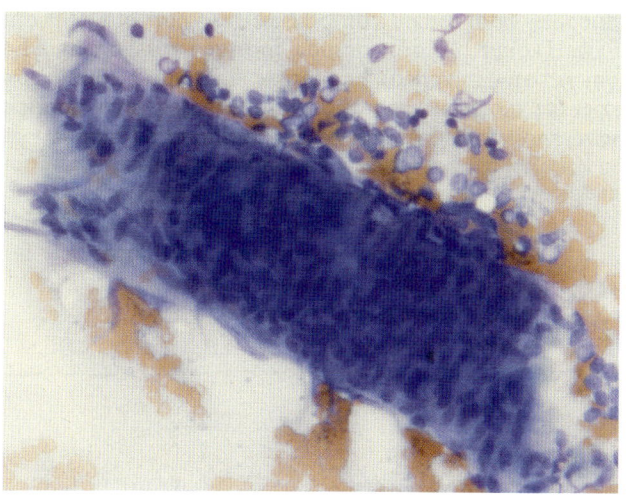

FIGURE 4.6 **Artery. Hyperplastic mandibular lymph node. Tissue aspirate. Dog.** Dense collection of uniform-appearing mesenchymal cells arranged in a linear array composed of smooth muscle tissue. Cells are fusiform with indistinct cytoplasmic borders and a scant to small amount of moderately basophilic cytoplasm. The elongated to cigar-shaped nucleus is central with finely stippled chromatin and no discernible nucleoli. Anisocytosis and anisokaryosis are mild.

lymphocytes, the center light zone contains reticular dendritic follicular cells, macrophages, and larger lymphoid cells (Fig. 4.9). In benign hyperplasia, the dark zone or mantle cell cuff expands from proliferation of small B lymphocytes that surround the pale portion of the germinal center with the thickest portion of the cuff at the apical end (see Fig. 4.9). The hyperplastic germinal centers often demonstrate polarity (Fig. 4.10) directed toward the antigen source, so that a dark mantle cell cuff is at one end (cortical) and a paler group of large lymphocytes appears at the other end (medullary). The presence of follicular polarity helps distinguish follicular hyperplasia from follicular lymphoma. In contrast to the heterogeneity of the germinal centers, the nodules in follicular lymphoma contain a monomorphic population of neoplastic lymphocytes. The expanded follicles may press against the capsule, producing a thin mantle zone, but there is no destruction of the subcapsular sinus as occurs with lymphoma.

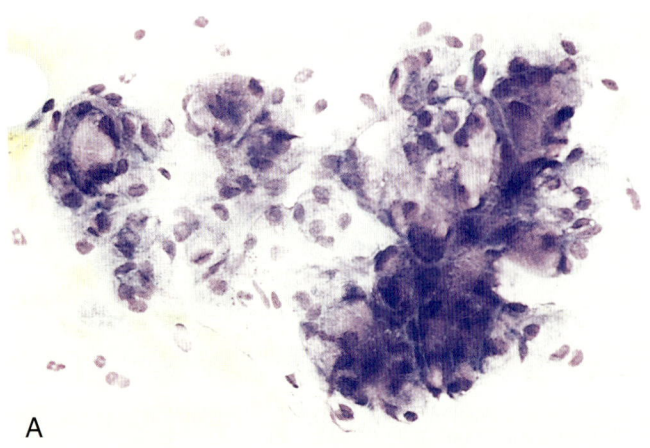

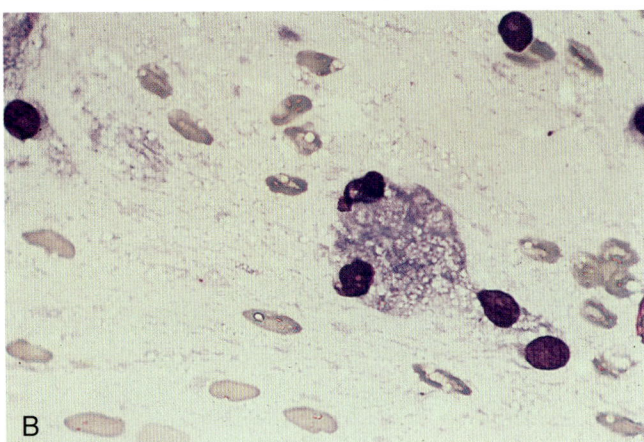

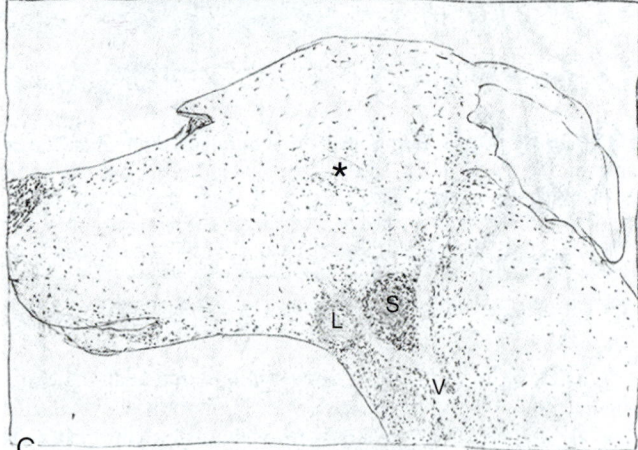

■ **FIGURE 4.7 Normal salivary gland. Tissue aspirate. Dog.** Same case in A and B. **A,** Attempted aspirate of the mandibular lymph node resulted in the collection of epithelial clusters. (Wright-Giemsa; HP oil.) **B,** Individual salivary gland cell with abundant foamy basophilic cytoplasm. Free nuclei in the background are easily mistaken for small lymphocytes. Note the basophilic granular background consistent with mucin and the manner erythrocytes appear within mucus as a string of cells. (Wright-Giemsa; HP oil.) **C,** Diagram showing the location of the mandibular salivary gland and mandibular lymph node. Dog. The *asterisk* indicates the bony prominence of the zygomatic arch. The mandibular lymph node (L) is directly ventral or perpendicular to the arch. Note the more posterior and dorsal location of the mandibular salivary gland (S) located within the bifurcation of the external jugular vein (V).

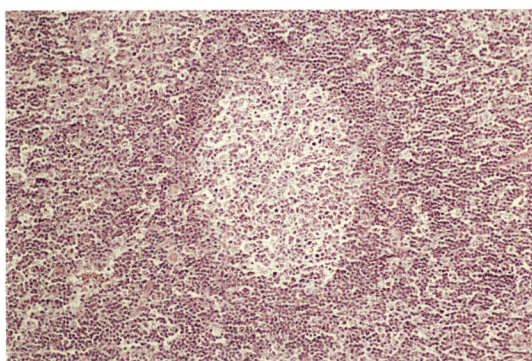

■ **FIGURE 4.8 Hyperplastic lymph node. Tissue section. Dog.** Prominent germinal center is composed of two zones, a dark zone with a thin rim of small, dense lymphocytes (mantle cells) and a light middle zone composed of larger lymphocytes, dendritic cells, and macrophages. (H&E; IP.)

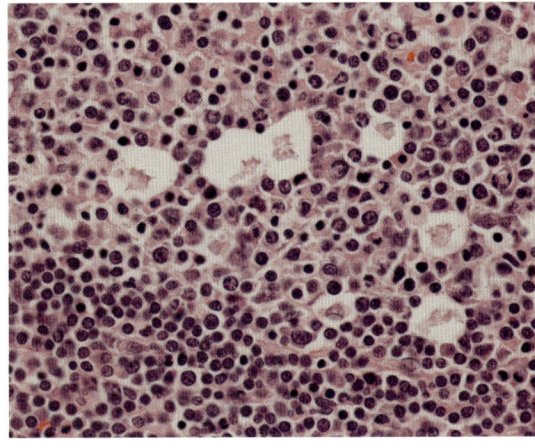

■ **FIGURE 4.9 Hyperplastic lymph node. Tissue section. Dog.** Light zone of a germinal center is shown; the dark mantle cell layer is in the *lower left*. The light zone is composed of large lymphocytes, dendritic cells, and macrophages; the latter cells appear as large, clear spaces with shrunken cellular material. The mantle cells are small, round to irregularly round cells with scant cytoplasm and a dense chromatin pattern. (H&E; HP oil.)

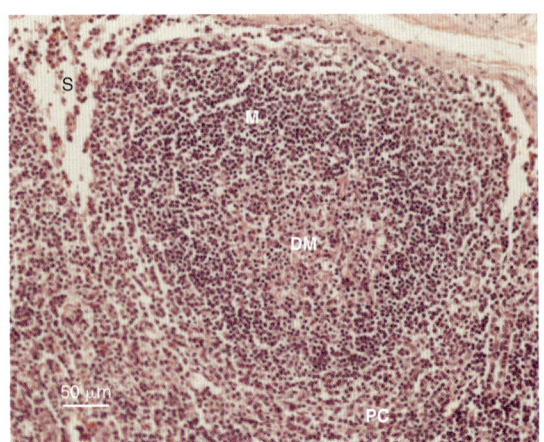

■ **FIGURE 4.10 Reactive lymph node, cortex. Tissue section. Dog.** Germinal center demonstrating polarity with subcapsular sinus (S) as the source of antigenic stimulation, cuff (M) of small mantle B lymphocytes, middle area (DM) of dendritic cells and lymphophagocytic macrophages or tingible bodies, and an area containing plasma cells (PC) below the germinal center. (H&E; IP.)

With expanded hyperplasia, marginal zone cells that surround the mantle cell cuff may increase in number, producing a heterogeneous population that expands into the paracortical region and mixes with resident T lymphocytes (Fig. 4.11A). Sampling these areas by cytopathology displays cell size variability without a marked increase in plasma cells.

The marginal zone cells have a medium cell size (nucleus approximately 2–2.5 times the erythrocyte diameter) and abundant cytoplasm contributing to the lighter color on histopathology. Marginal zone cells may be transformed to have marginated chromatin and contain a single large, centrally located nucleolus, but mitotic activity is low despite the immature appearance of these cells (Fig. 4.11B). Specialized paracortical blood vessels termed *high endothelial venules* in view of their cuboidal cell shape or rounded nucleus increase in prominence and number. The T lymphocytes from circulating blood enter the paracortex transmurally through these venules. Retention of these venules between follicles helps distinguish histologically paracortical hyperplasia from lymphoma in which they may be incorporated within the nodular or follicle-like neoplasia. In response to antigenic stimulation, plasma cells move from the paracortex and accumulate within the medullary cords (Fig. 4.12), where they produce antibodies.

On cytopathologic specimens, small lymphocytes predominate in reactive or hyperplastic lymph nodes, but there is an increase (>15%) in medium and/or large cell types of the total cell population (Fig. 4.13). Plasma cells are mildly to markedly increased in number and may be shifted toward

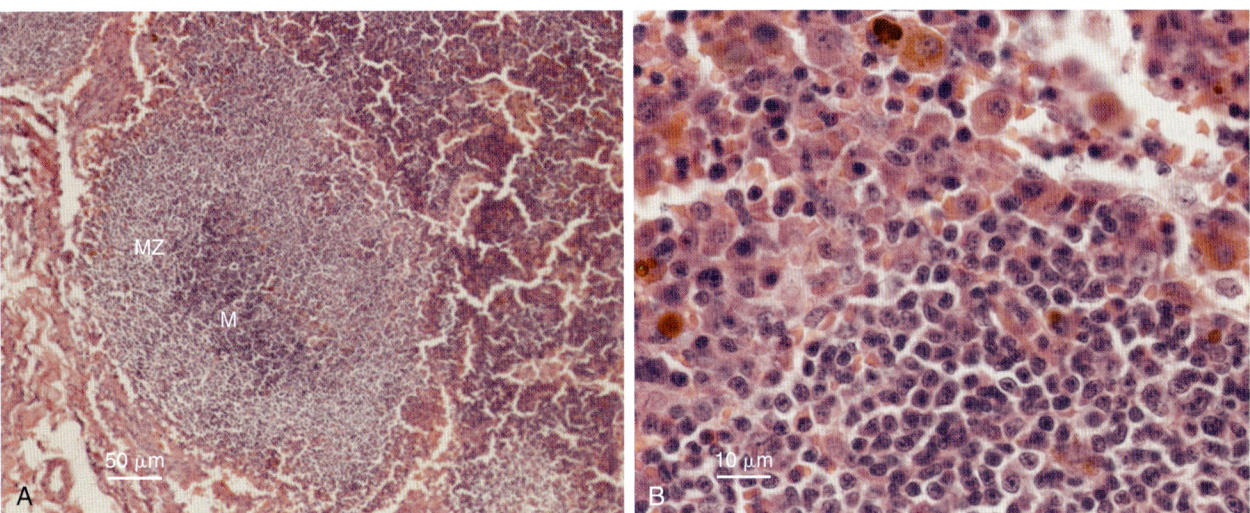

■ **FIGURE 4.11 Hyperplastic lymph node. Tissue section. Dog.** Same case in A and B. **A,** Prominent light-colored marginal zone cuff (MZ) surrounds the fading germinal center with residual mantle cells (M) recognized by their dark, small cell appearance. (H&E; LP.) **B,** Expanded marginal zone cells at the bottom frequently have vesicular chromatin and a single large, centrally located nucleolus. Note the lack of mitotic activity in this region. At the top is the medullary region filled with abundant macrophages, many of which contain a dark yellow pigment, presumed to be hemosiderin. (H&E; HP oil.)

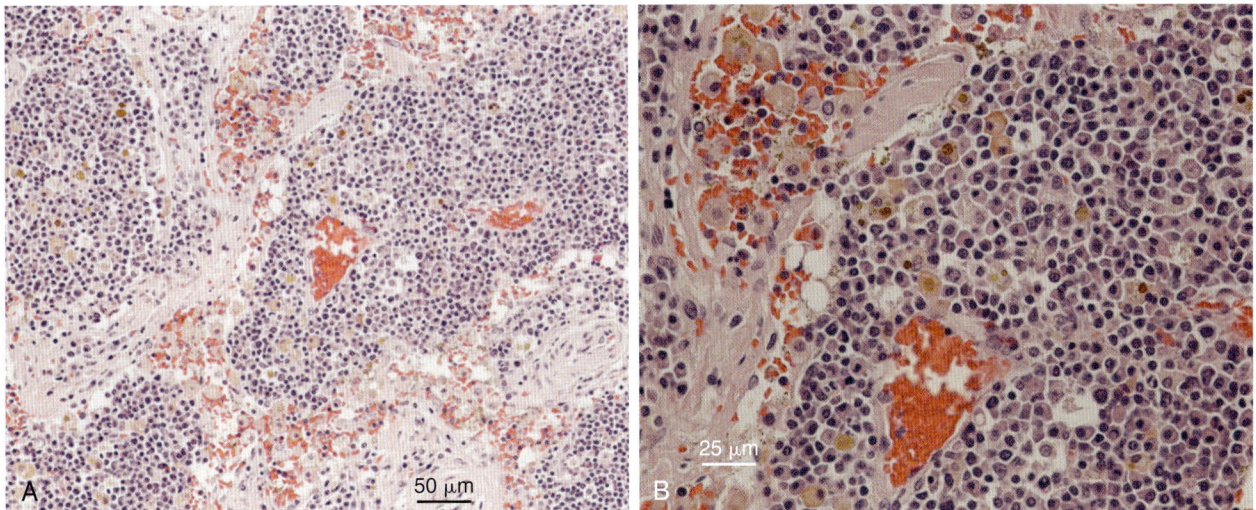

■ **FIGURE 4.12 Reactive lymph node. Tissue section. Dog.** Same case in A and B. **A,** Medullary cords filled with plasma cells and hemosiderin-laden macrophages are expanded and compressing the blood-filled sinuses between the cords. (H&E; IP.) **B,** Higher magnification of A. Medullary cords are filled with plasma cells readily identified by their eccentrically placed nucleus. (H&E; IP.)

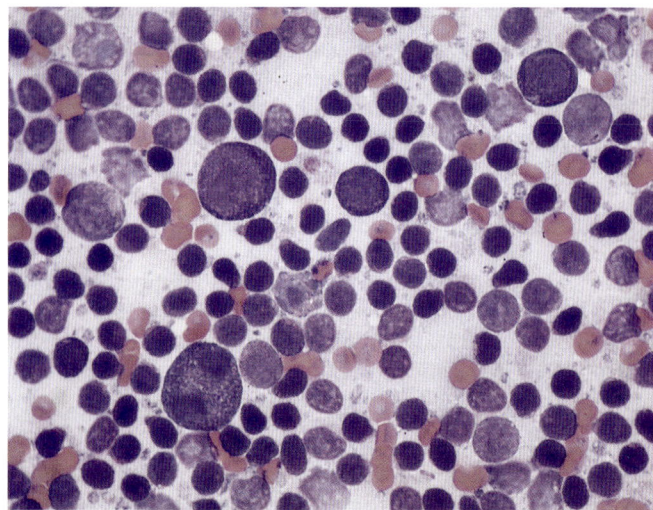

■ **FIGURE 4.13 Hyperplastic jejunal lymph node. Tissue aspirate. Cat.** There is an expansion of medium and large lymphoid cells along with a predominance of small lymphocytes. Clinical signs were related to the gastrointestinal system, and lymphadenomegaly was attributed to general immune stimulation. (Modified Wright; HP oil.) (Courtesy Clare Pitchford, TDDS, Synlab, Exeter, UK.)

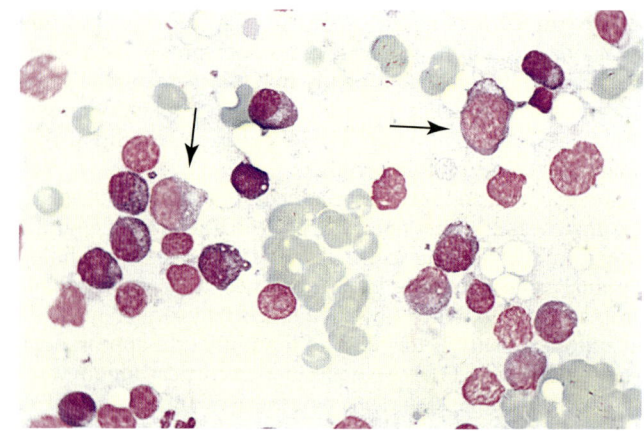

■ **FIGURE 4.15 Reactive lymph node. Tissue aspirate. Dog.** Plasma cells are moderately increased in number, and two appear shifted toward immaturity *(arrows)*. (Wright-Giemsa; HP oil.)

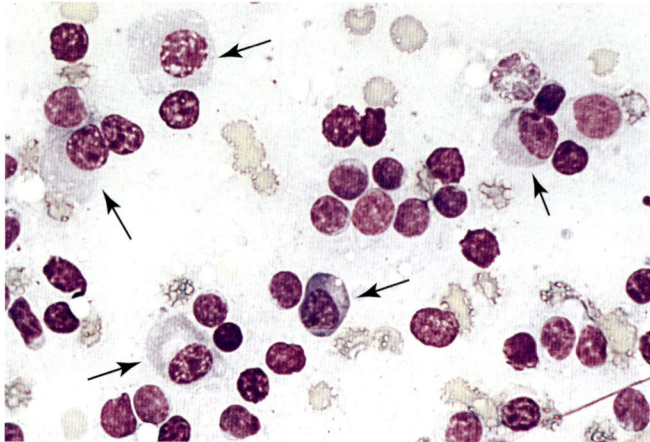

■ **FIGURE 4.14 Reactive lymph node. Tissue aspirate. Dog.** Many small lymphocytes are present along with several well-differentiated plasma cells *(arrows)*. Higher numbers of medium-sized lymphocytes than expected in normal lymph nodes are noted in the center. (Wright; HP oil.)

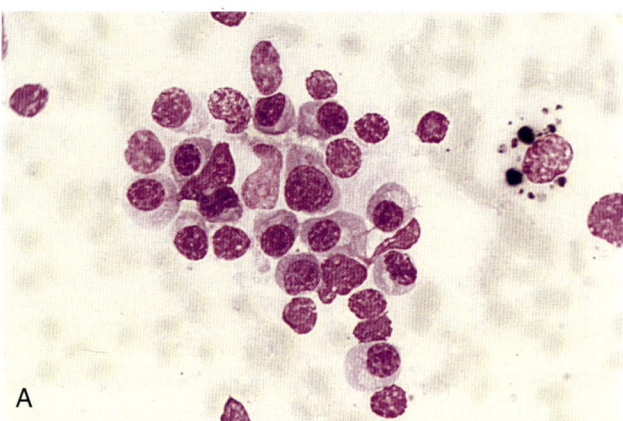

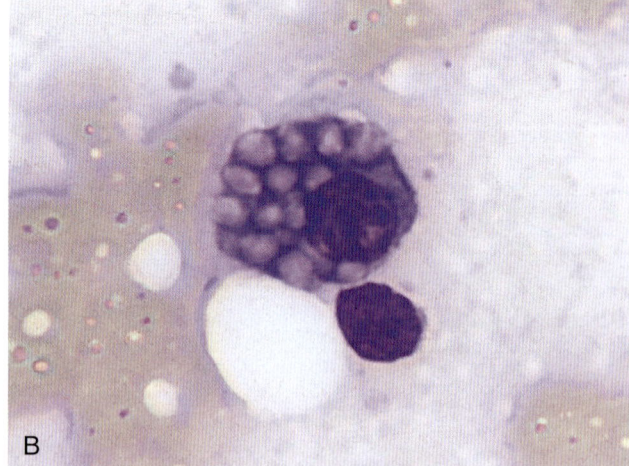

■ **FIGURE 4.16 Reactive lymph node. Tissue imprint. Dog.** Same case in A and B. **A,** Note the marked increase in plasma cell numbers composed of various degrees of differentiation. A hemosiderin-laden macrophage is present to the right of the field. (Aqueous Romanowsky; HP oil.) **B, Mott cell. Tissue imprint. Dog.** This plasma cell from a reactive lymph node is highly activated with an abundant basophilic cytoplasm that contains multiple large, pale vacuoles. The vacuoles, known as *Russell bodies*, represent packets of immunoglobulin secretions. (Aqueous Romanowsky; HP oil.)

immaturity (Figs. 4.14 to 4.16A). Some highly activated plasma cells, termed *Mott cells*, are characterized by abundant cytoplasm filled with multiple large, spherical, pale vacuoles that represent immunoglobulin secretions known as *Russell bodies* (Fig. 4.16B). The immunoglobulins within the cytoplasm may have an eosinophilic hue, giving rise to the term "flame cell" (Fig. 4.17). Occasionally, inclusions associated with the nucleus have been termed *Dutcher bodies*, which are intracytoplasmic inclusions that have invaginated into or overlay the nucleus resulting from the accumulation of immunoglobulin in the paranuclear cisterna (Fig. 4.18). Both Russell bodies and Dutcher bodies are periodic acid–Schiff (PAS) positive. Macrophages, neutrophils, eosinophils, and mast cells may also mildly increase in response

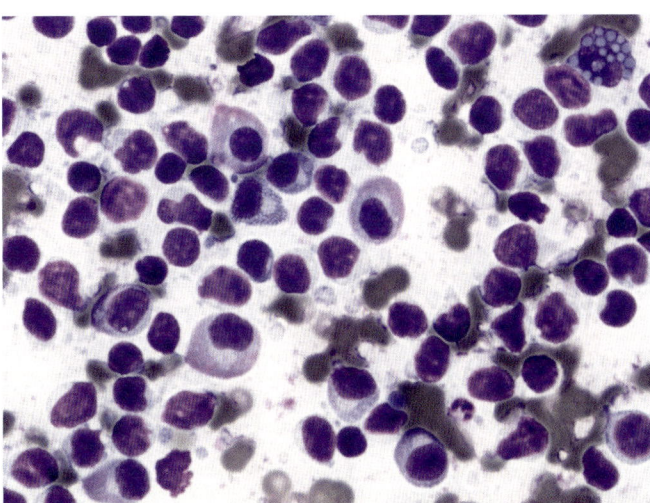

■ **FIGURE 4.17 Reactive mandibular lymph node. Tissue aspirate. Dog.** Marked increase in numbers of plasma cells, some of which display peripheral eosinophilic cytoplasm consistent with "flame cells" that contain immunoglobulin inclusions. Flame cells have been associated with immunoglobulin A and M. Note the Mott cell in the upper right corner. (Aqueous Romanowsky; HP oil.) (Courtesy Larissa Kipa, Michigan State University.)

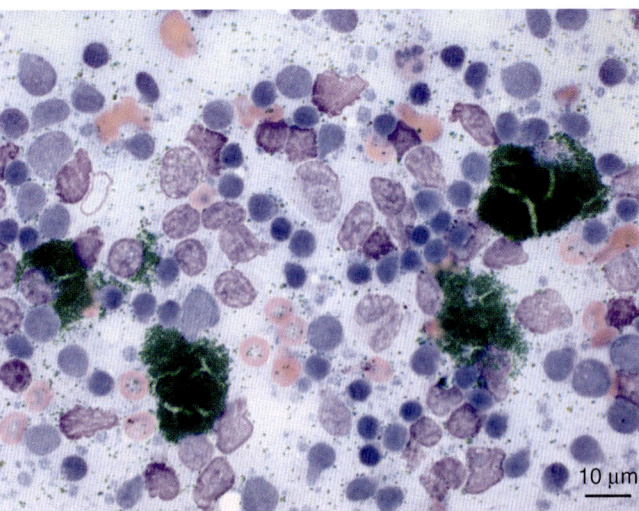

■ **FIGURE 4.19 Melanophages. Mandibular lymph node. Cytopathologic specimen. Dog.** Several pigment-laden macrophages are present, and granules are dispersed throughout the background. This may relate to injury to adjacent pigmented skin, but concern for melanoma should also be considered. (Wright-Giemsa; HP oil.) (Courtesy Rose Raskin, North Carolina State University.)

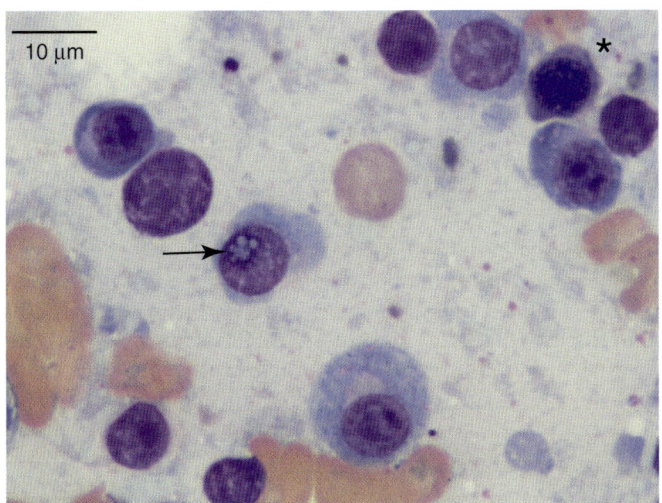

■ **FIGURE 4.18 Dutcher bodies. Reactive lymphoid tissue aspirate. Dog.** This specimen taken from the spleen demonstrates immunoglobulin inclusions within the nucleus *(arrow)* called *Dutcher bodies*. Although they appear within the nucleus, they are actually outside the nucleus and within invaginations of the nuclear membrane. Note the nucleated erythroid precursor *(asterisk)*. This patient presented with hyperglobulinemia. (Modified Wright; HP oil.) (Courtesy Natalia Strandberg, Purdue University.)

to antigen stimulation; however, these cells occur in lower numbers than expected for lymphadenitis. Melanin-containing cells (Fig. 4.19), such as melanophages, may be present in non-neoplastic conditions owing to damage pigmented tissues as well as from granules released from melanomas. In dogs in which oral pigmentation is common, melanophages in the mandibular lymph nodes are likely from gingivitis or stomatitis. The presence of green granules resembles hemosiderin, so Prussian blue staining may be necessary to verify the presence of melanin granules, which do not stain. Lymphoid hyperplasia was the most common cytopathologic diagnosis of lymph nodes in cats in one study (Amores-Fuster et al., 2015).

During early antigenic stimulation before germinal centers have developed, the paracortex responds with expansion and crowding of the cortex (Fig. 4.20A). Paracortical hyperplasia may precede plasma cell proliferation, and 2 weeks may pass before the appearance of prominent germinal centers. During this time, aspirate smears may contain a variably sized lymphoid population without significant numbers of plasma cells (Figs. 4.20B to 4.22).

A benign condition in young cats has been reported (Moore et al., 1986; Mooney et al., 1987) in which peripheral lymph nodes show marked enlargement that histologically resembles lymphoma (see Fig. 4.20A). Cells may be primarily medium and large lymphocytes with low numbers of small lymphocytes and plasma cells (see Fig. 4.20B). High endothelial venules are prominent in the paracortex in this condition. These cases generally regress spontaneously in 1 to 17 weeks (Mooney et al., 1987). In one study, the majority of cats were feline leukemia virus positive, and 1 of 14 cats progressed to lymphoma (Moore et al., 1986). Generalized lymphadenopathy is known to occur in cats infected with feline immunodeficiency virus (FIV) and *Bartonella* spp. (Kordick et al., 1999). In both dogs and cats, phenobarbital administration has been associated with lymph node hyperplasia resembling lymphoma that resolves with discontinuation of the drug (Lampe et al., 2017; Lieser and Schwedes, 2018).

Immunostaining of reactive lymph nodes demonstrates the paracortical expansion of T lymphocytes (Fig. 4.23A) and the development of the germinal centers (Fig. 4.23B–C).

Lymphadenitis

The predominant inflammatory cell population categorizes the type of inflammation in a lymph node.

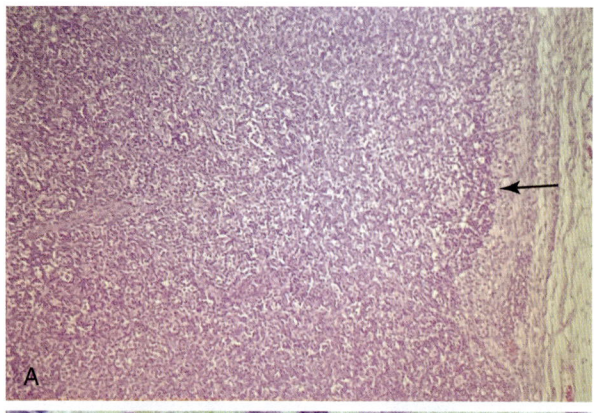

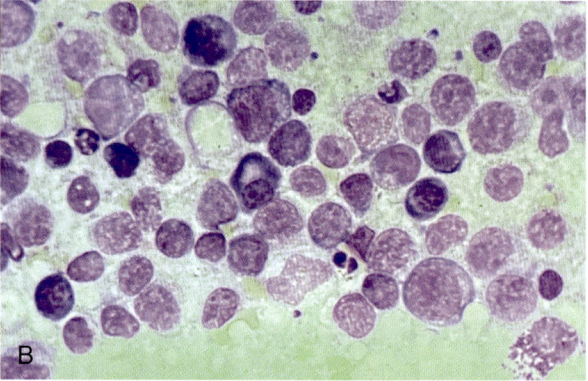

■ **FIGURE 4.20 Hyperplastic lymph node. Cat.** Same case in A and B. **A, Tissue section.** Peripheral node lymphadenopathy in this case is characterized by a paracortical expansion displacing normal lymphoid nodules and creating a homogenous appearance resembling lymphoma. At *right,* a thin band of small, dark lymphocytes *(arrow)* remains from the normal nodule. (H&E; LP.) **B, Reactive and hyperplastic lymph node. Tissue imprint.** This sample of superficial cervical lymph node contains a mixed population of small, medium, and large lymphocytes; plasma cells; and a mast cell *(lower right).* The majority of the lymphocytes are medium-sized with moderately coarse chromatin and indistinct nucleoli. (Aqueous Romanowsky; HP oil.)

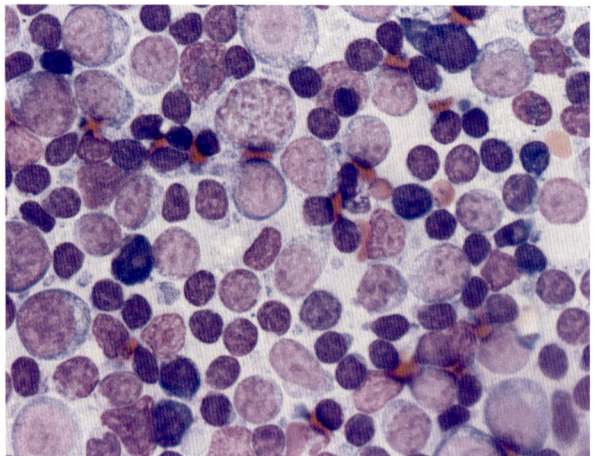

■ **FIGURE 4.21 Hyperplastic popliteal lymph node. Tissue aspirate. Cat.** There is an increased number of medium and large lymphoid cells. Note the cell in prophase (upper center). The patient presented with generalized hair loss, skin ulceration, and bent ears. There is generalized peripheral lymphadenomegaly. The clinical diagnosis is feline relapsing polychondritis, an immune-mediated condition of cartilage and connective tissue. (Wright-Giemsa; HP oil.) (Courtesy Jacqueline Dolan, University of Florida.)

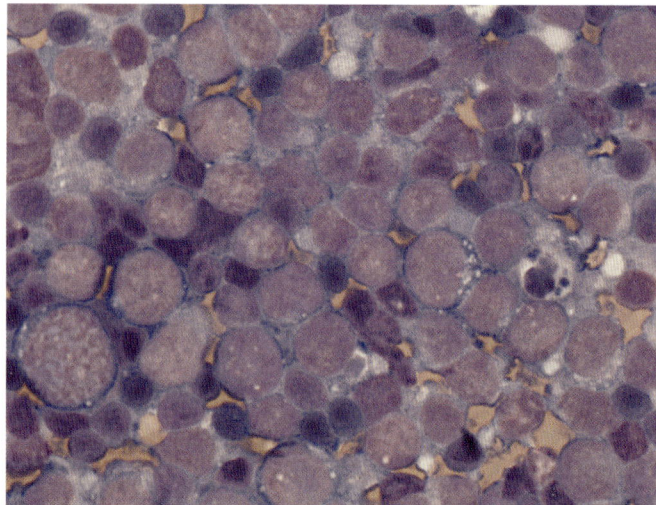

■ **FIGURE 4.22 Atypical lymphoid hyperplasia, lymph node. Tissue aspirate. Cat.** Aspirates from both mandibular lymph nodes were similar. This 10-year-old cat had been recently treated for hyperthyroidism and presented with ulcerative stomatitis. The cat was otherwise clinically normal and tested negative for feline leukemia virus and feline immunodeficiency virus. The specimen contained a predominant population of medium and large lymphocytes with occasional plasma cells (not shown). It is presumed that this is a paracortical hyperplastic response related to the oral lesion. (Wright; HP oil.)

Neutrophilic Lymphadenitis

Purulent or suppurative (Fig. 4.24) lymphadenitis involves greater than 5% neutrophils and may be associated with bacterial (Figs. 4.25 and 4.26), neoplastic, or immune-mediated conditions.

Eosinophilic Lymphadenitis

Greater than 3% eosinophils of the nucleated cell population are often related to fleabite hypersensitivity, feline eosinophilic skin disease (Fig. 4.27), hypereosinophilic syndrome, gastrointestinal eosinophilic sclerosing fibroplasia (Fig. 4.28), lagenidiosis (Fig. 4.29), and paraneoplastic syndrome for mast cell tumor (Fig. 4.30), as well as certain lymphomas (Thorn and Aubert, 1999) and carcinomas (Fig. 4.31).

Histiocytic or Mixed Cell Lymphadenitis

Inflammation of the lymph nodes may involve increased numbers of macrophages, which may be termed *histiocytic lymphadenitis* (Fig. 4.32) or mixed cell lymphadenitis (Fig. 4.33). The presence of neutrophils and epithelioid macrophages may be referred to as *pyogranulomatous lymphadenitis* (Fig. 4.34), even though a granuloma is best appreciated on histologic sections. Some cases of mixed cell inflammation have been associated with lymphoid neoplasia in nearby tissues (Fig. 4.35). Sinus histiocytosis may be appreciated by numerous histiocytes, which histopathologically depicts these macrophages fill the lymph node medullary sinuses to react with pathogens or during chronic inflammatory conditions.

Conditions associated with inflammatory responses include systemic fungal infections, opportunistic fungal infections (Tomlinson et al., 2011; Whipple et al., 2019) (Fig. 4.36; see also Fig. 4.34), mycobacteriosis (Fig. 4.37), leishmaniasis (Guerra et al., 2019), salmon fluke poisoning disease (Fig. 4.38),

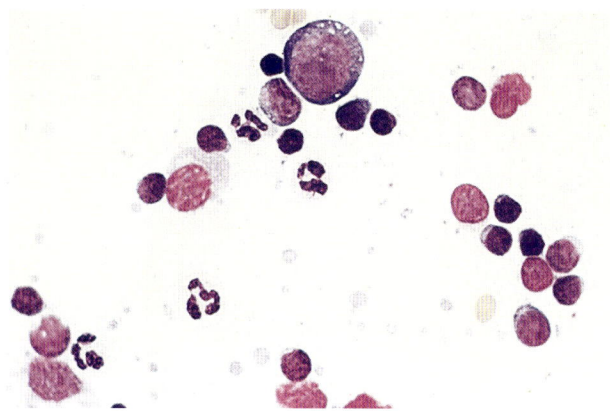

■ **FIGURE 4.24 Neutrophilic lymphadenitis. Tissue aspirate. Cat.** Four nondegenerate neutrophils are present along with small and medium lymphocytes. One large lymphocyte is also noted. (Wright; HP oil.)

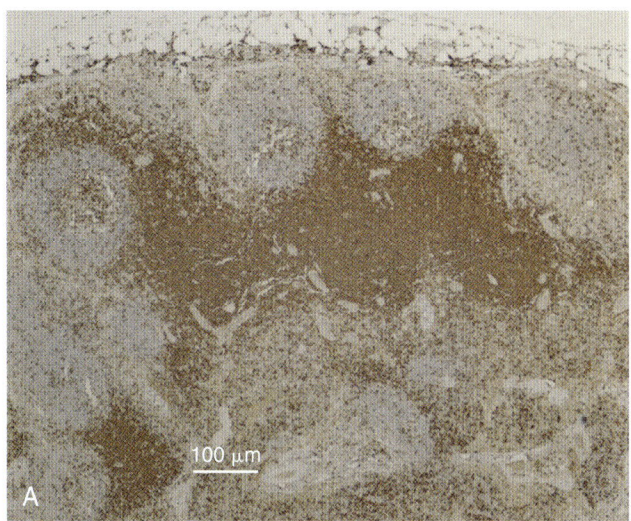

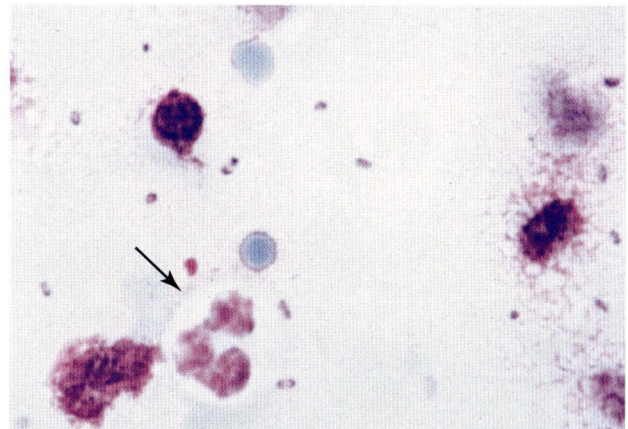

■ **FIGURE 4.25 Septic suppurative lymphadenitis. Tissue aspirate. Cat.** Bipolar coccobacillus bacteria confirmed as *Yersinia pestis* are present extracellularly adjacent to a degenerate neutrophil *(arrow)*. (Wright-Giemsa; HP oil.) (Courtesy Kyra Royals et al., Colorado State University. Presented at the 1996 ASVCP case review session.)

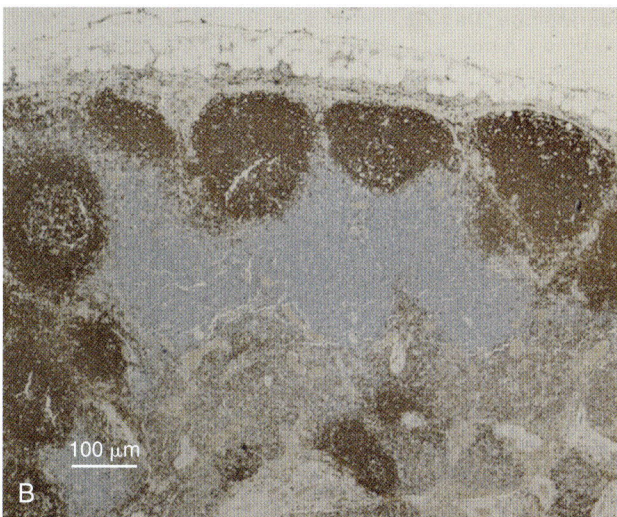

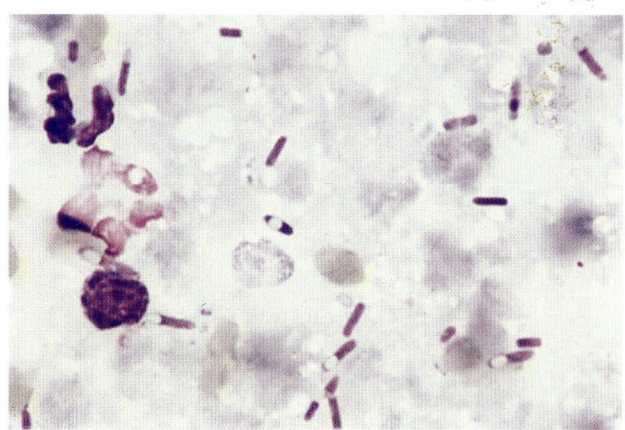

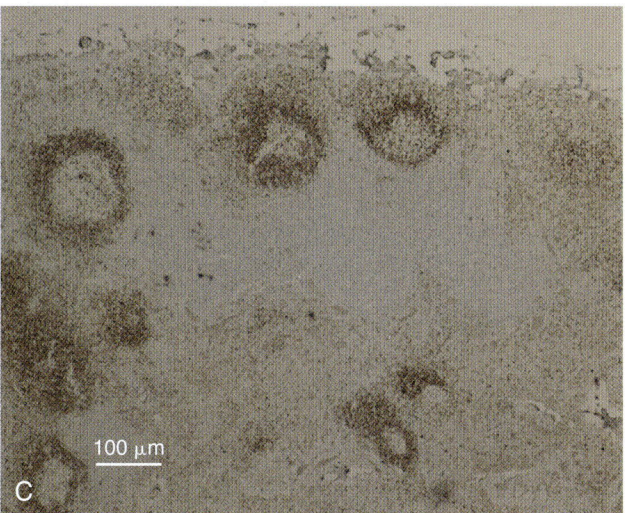

■ **FIGURE 4.23 Reactive lymph node. Tissue section. Immunohistochemistry. Dog.** Same case in A to C. **A,** Note the strong staining of T lymphocytes within the paracortex and scattered involvement within the medullary region (CD3/diaminobenzidine [DAB]; LP.) **B,** Strong staining of B lymphocytes within the germinal centers is demonstrated by the anti-CD20 reaction and negative staining within the paracortical areas. (CD20/DAB; LP.) **C,** Strong staining of mantle cell B lymphocytes is evident with weak, scattered staining within the cortex and medullary cords. (CD79a/DAB; LP.)

■ **FIGURE 4.26 Septic suppurative lymphadenitis. Tissue imprint. Dog.** The history included a dogfight 2 months before the present lymphadenomegaly. Most of the lymphoid cells are necrotic and appear as amorphous basophilic material. Note two intact degenerate neutrophils and one small lymphocyte. Large bacilli with subterminal and terminal swellings are numerous in the background, which culture confirmed as *Clostridium* spp. (Wright-Giemsa; HP oil.)

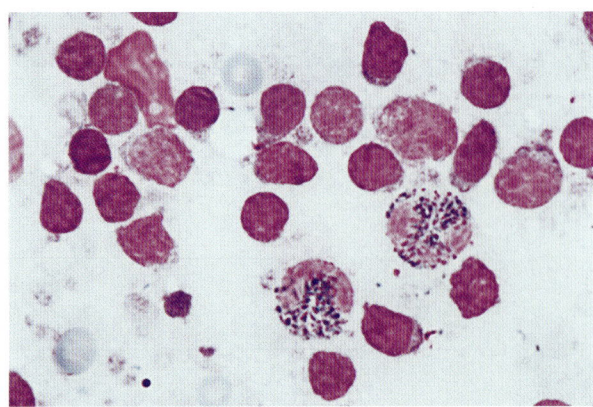

■ **FIGURE 4.27 Eosinophilic lymphadenitis. Tissue aspirate. Cat.** Two eosinophils are shown within a population of small lymphocytes from an animal with a rodent ulcer of the mouth. (Wright-Giemsa; HP oil.)

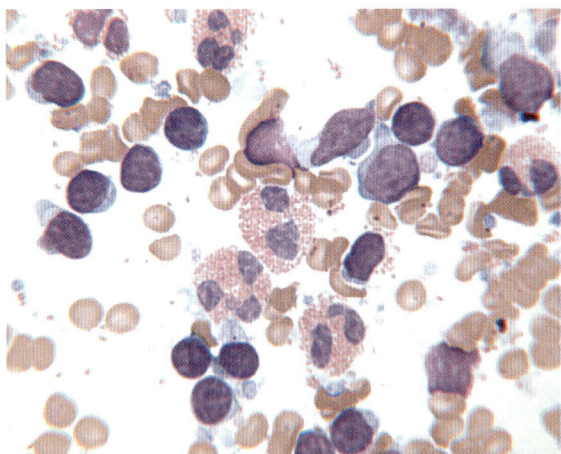

■ **FIGURE 4.28 Eosinophilic lymphadenitis. Mesenteric lymph node aspirate. Cat.** Five eosinophils are shown in this case of suspected gastrointestinal eosinophilic sclerosing fibroplasia. (Wright-Giemsa; HP oil.)

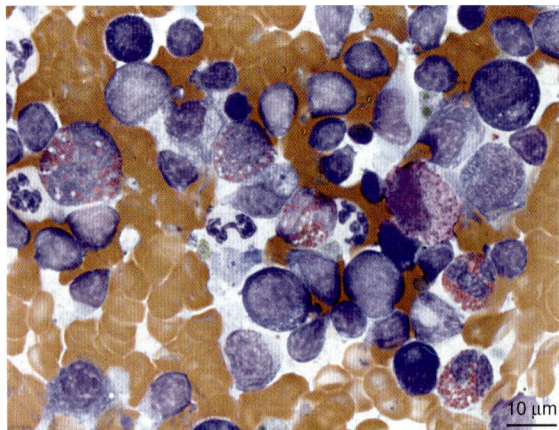

■ **FIGURE 4.29 Mixed cell lymphadenitis. Medial iliac lymph node aspirate. Dog.** Many eosinophils with fewer macrophages and neutrophils are present with a reactive lymphoid cell population in the area adjacent to skin lesions. Histopathology diagnosed cutaneous pyogranulomatous dermatitis and panniculitis with fungal hyphae. Confirmation of lagenidiosis was determined by culture. (Wright-Giemsa; HP oil.) (Courtesy Kellie Whipple, University of Florida.)

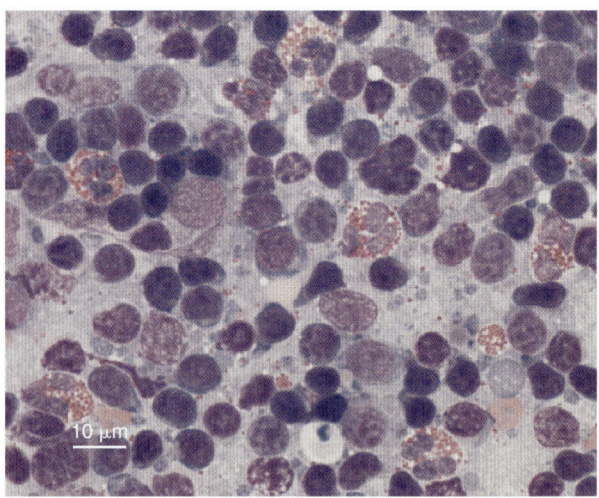

■ **FIGURE 4.30 Eosinophilic lymphadenitis. Mandibular lymph node aspirate. Dog.** The lymph node is examined for evidence of spread from a mast cell tumor on the nose. The lymphoid population is predominately small with low numbers of medium lymphocytes. Frequent eosinophils are present, but no evidence of metastatic tumor is found. (Wright; HP oil.)

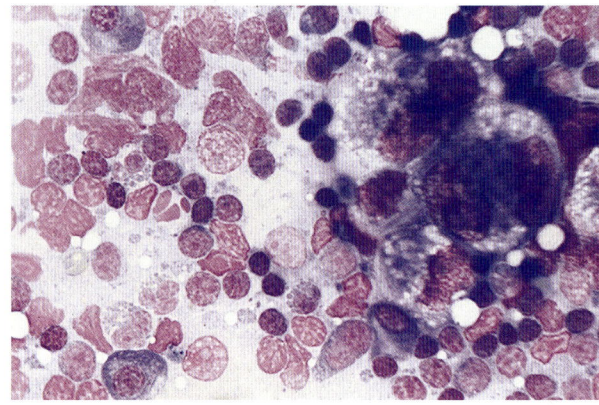

■ **FIGURE 4.31 Eosinophilic lymphadenitis. Tissue imprint. Dog.** Small lymphocytes predominate along with increased numbers of medium lymphocytes and eosinophils. At *right* is a cluster of pleomorphic epithelium from an animal with metastatic urothelial (transitional cell) carcinoma found within the sublumbar lymph node. (Wright-Giemsa; HP oil.)

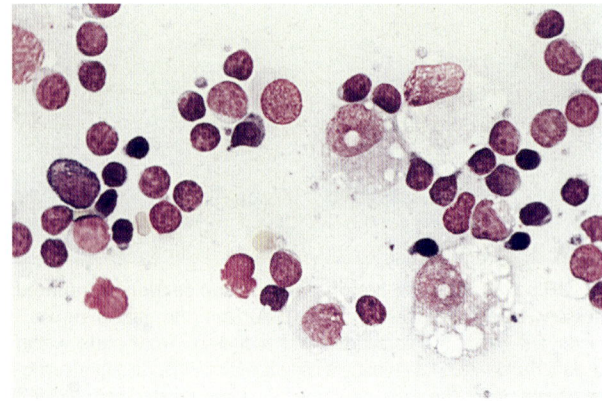

■ **FIGURE 4.32 Histiocytic lymphadenitis. Tissue aspirate. Cat.** Several macrophages are present along with small and medium-sized lymphocytes. (Wright; HP oil.)

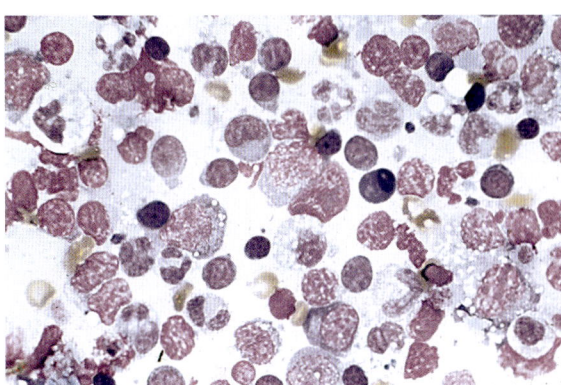

■ **FIGURE 4.33 Histiocytic and neutrophilic lymphadenitis. Tissue aspirate. Dog.** Numerous vacuolated macrophages and several degenerate neutrophils appear among a mixed population of lymphocytes. (Wright-Giemsa; HP oil.)

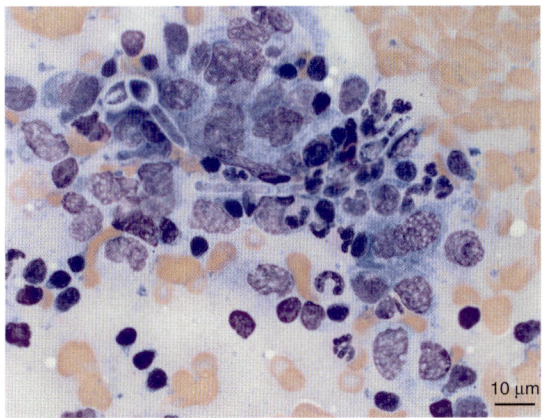

■ **FIGURE 4.34 Pyogranulomatous lymphadenitis with intralesional fungal hyphae. Popliteal lymph node aspirate. Dog.** A mixed cell population of epithelioid macrophages and neutrophils surrounds hyphal structures measuring 4 to 5 μm in width with bulbous swellings and septations. Final identification was *Curvularia* spp. (Wright-Giemsa; HP oil.) (Courtesy Amy DiDomenico, North Carolina State University.)

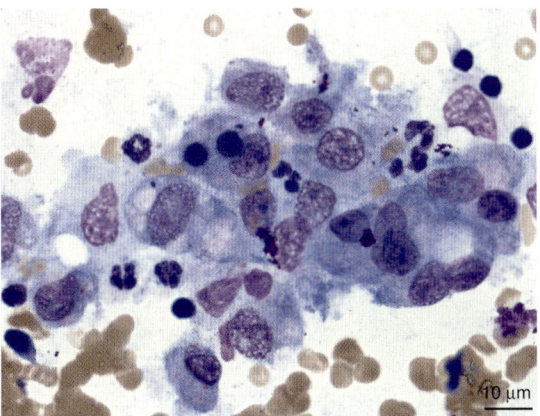

■ **FIGURE 4.35 Histiocytic lymphadenitis. Mesenteric lymph node aspirate. Cat.** A markedly enlarged and hypoechoic lymph node in a patient with renal lymphoma revealed a phagocytic histiocytic population along with moderate numbers of nondegenerate neutrophils. These histiocytes phagocytized red blood cells, amorphous basophilic debris, and leukocytes. Note the two apparent phagocytized lymphocytes off-center. (Wright-Giemsa; HP oil.) (Courtesy Francisco Conrado, University of Florida.)

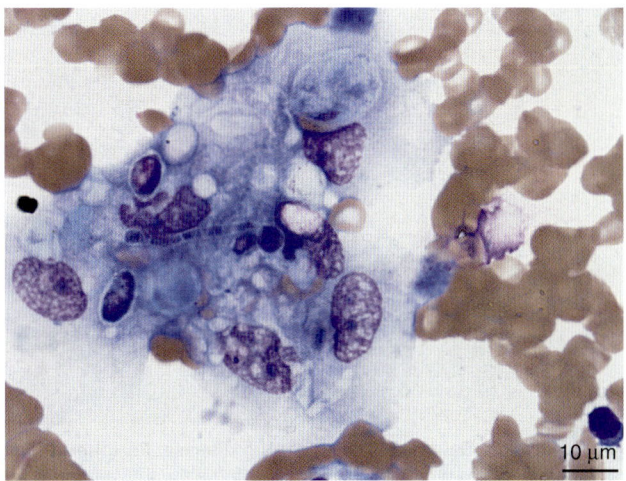

■ **FIGURE 4.36 Granulomatous lymphadenitis with intralesional fungal hyphae. Medial iliac lymph node aspirate. Dog.** A large aggregate of epithelioid and phagocytic macrophages is present. The septate fungal hyphae are approximately 3 μm in diameter with nonstaining, nonparallel walls and infrequent branching basophilic structures. Many oval to spherical yeast-like structures approximately 4 to 10 μm in diameter are present. Culture identified the fungus as *Talaromyces helicus*. (Wright-Giemsa; HP oil.) (Courtesy Tracie Guy, University of Florida.)

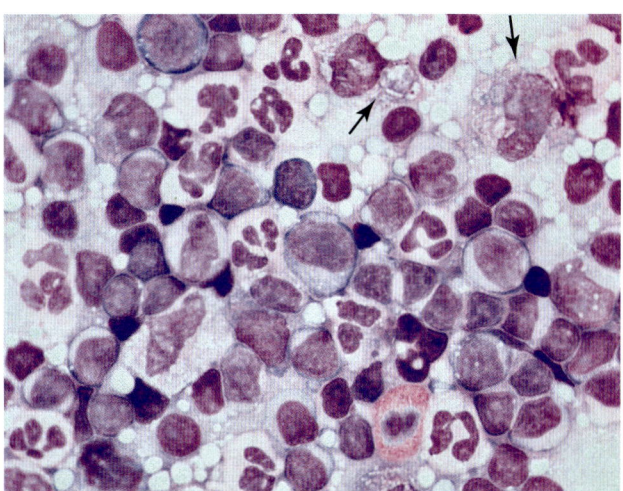

■ **FIGURE 4.37 Mixed neutrophilic-histiocytic lymphadenitis. Tissue aspirate. Cat.** Low numbers of negative staining rod bacteria *(arrows)* from an infection of *Mycobacterium avium*. (Romanowsky; HP oil.)

protothecosis (Whipple et al., 2020) (Fig. 4.39), and pythiosis. The systemic fungal diseases include blastomycosis (Fig. 4.40), cryptococcosis (Gerontiti et al., 2017) (Fig. 4.41), histoplasmosis (Fig. 4.42), and coccidioidomycosis. Feline infectious peritonitis may induce pyogranulomatous or mixed cell inflammation (Fig. 4.43).

In the United Kingdom, a condition common for English springer spaniels presents as a sterile idiopathic pyogranulomatous lymphadenitis along with pyrexia, lymphadenomegaly, and dermatologic or other system abnormalities (Dor et al., 2019; Ribas Latre et al., 2019). Other inflammatory reactions include a primary neutrophilic, macrophagic, or necrotizing response. Despite extensive investigations for etiologic agents, none was found. Treatment in the form of corticosteroids provided good

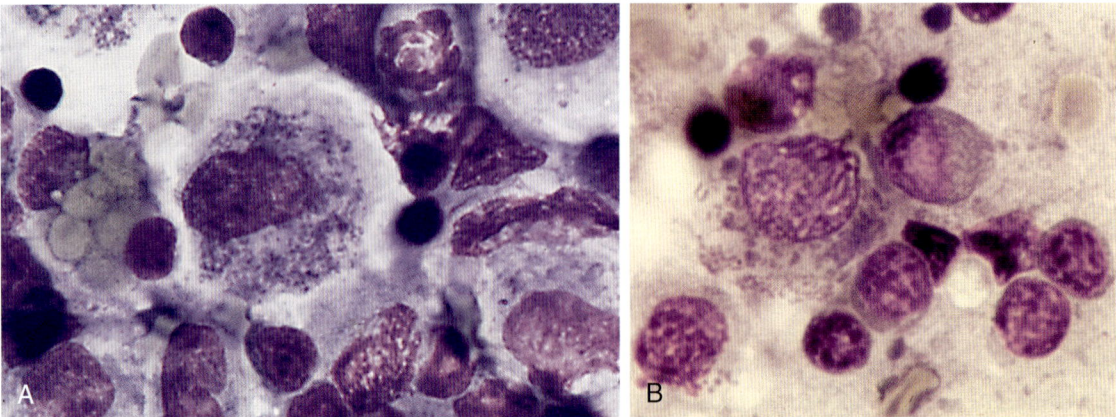

■ **FIGURE 4.38 Salmon fluke poisoning disease. Peripheral lymph node aspirate. Dog.** Same case in A and B. **A,** Numerous small basophilic granules are shown within a macrophage infected with *Neorickettsia helminthoeca*. (Romanowsky; HP oil.) **B, Lymph node aspirate.** Lymph nodes display increased numbers of medium lymphocytes and plasma cells in addition to the inflammatory response. Note the rickettsial organism within the macrophage. (Romanowsky; HP oil.) (Courtesy Jocelyn Johnsrude, IDEXX.)

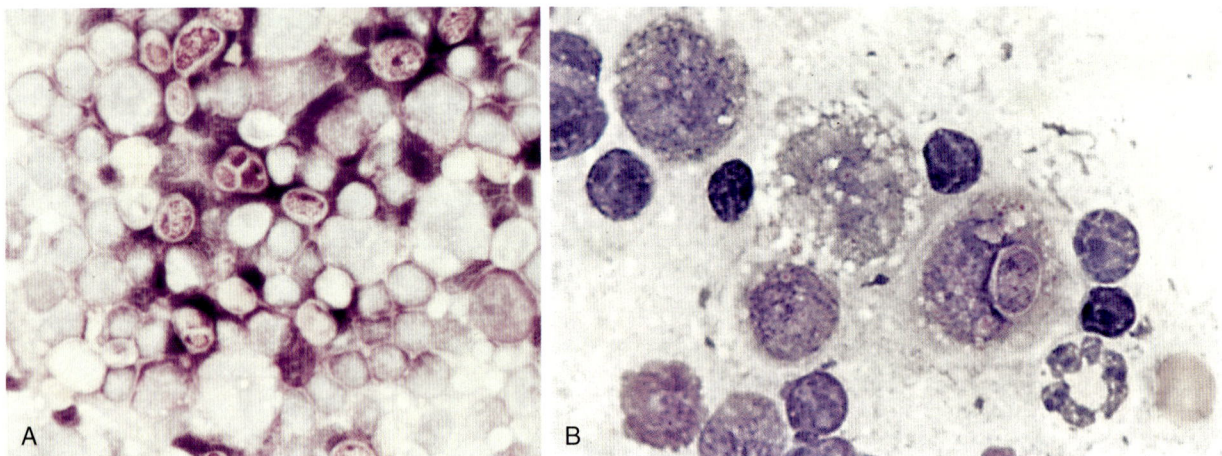

■ **FIGURE 4.39 Protothecosis. Dog. A, Colonic lymph node imprint.** Several round to oval structures are present that measure approximately 6 to 10 μm in length. These sporangiospores have a basophilic granular cytoplasm and thin, clear cell wall. Note the sporulated forms (sporangia) with multiple endospores (sporangiospores). (Aqueous Romanowsky; HP oil.) **B, Lymph node imprint.** Note the single endospore engulfed by a macrophage. (Aqueous Romanowsky; HP oil.) (A, Courtesy Karyn Bird et al., Texas A&M University. Presented at the 1988 ASVCP case review session. B, Courtesy Peter Fernandes, Texas A&M University.)

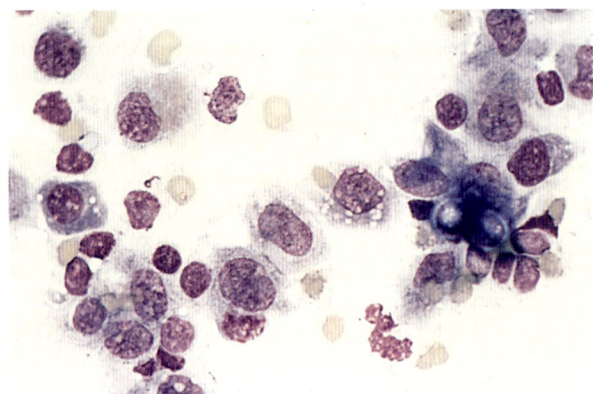

■ **FIGURE 4.40 Pyogranulomatous lymphadenitis with blastomycosis. Tissue aspirate. Dog.** Two round basophilic yeast structures are surrounded by a mixed inflammatory response, including epithelioid macrophages, degenerate neutrophils, small and medium lymphocytes, and plasma cells. (Wright; HP oil.)

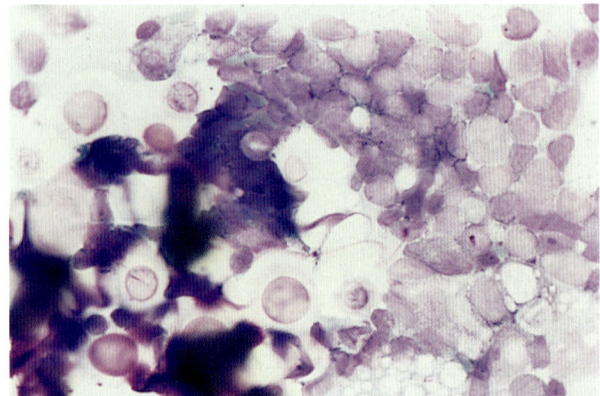

■ **FIGURE 4.41 Histiocytic lymphadenitis with cryptococcosis. Lymph node aspirate. Cat.** A subcutaneous mass behind the ear is present in this animal. A periauricular lymph node demonstrates numerous encapsulated yeast forms, consistent with *Cryptococcus* spp. Note the lymphocytes in the background with few inflammatory cells present. (Wright-Giemsa; HP oil.)

CHAPTER 4 Hemolymphatic System

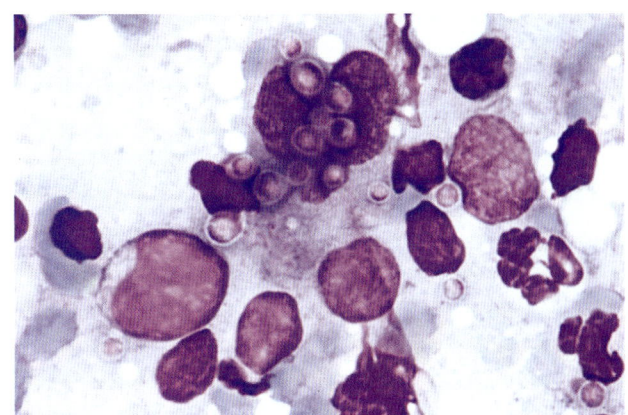

FIGURE 4.42 Pyogranulomatous lymphadenitis in histoplasmosis. Lymph node aspirate. Cat. Several intracellular small, oval yeast forms are present within a macrophage. Extracellular yeast structures are also found, including a mixed population of lymphoid cells and degenerate neutrophils. (Aqueous Romanowsky; HP oil.)

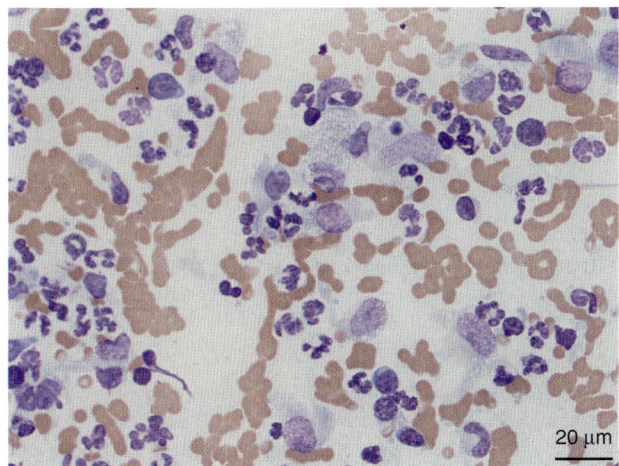

FIGURE 4.43 Neutrophilic and macrophagic lymphadenitis. Mesenteric lymph node aspirate. Cat. A 7-month-old kitten presented with a large (6 cm) hypoechoic abdominal lymph node. Nondegenerate and degenerative neutrophils are abundant along with phagocytic and epithelioid macrophages. The lymphoid population was mixed with evidence of reactivity. Feline infectious peritonitis was suspected. (Aqueous Romanowsky; HP oil.) (Courtesy Kellie Whipple, University of Florida.)

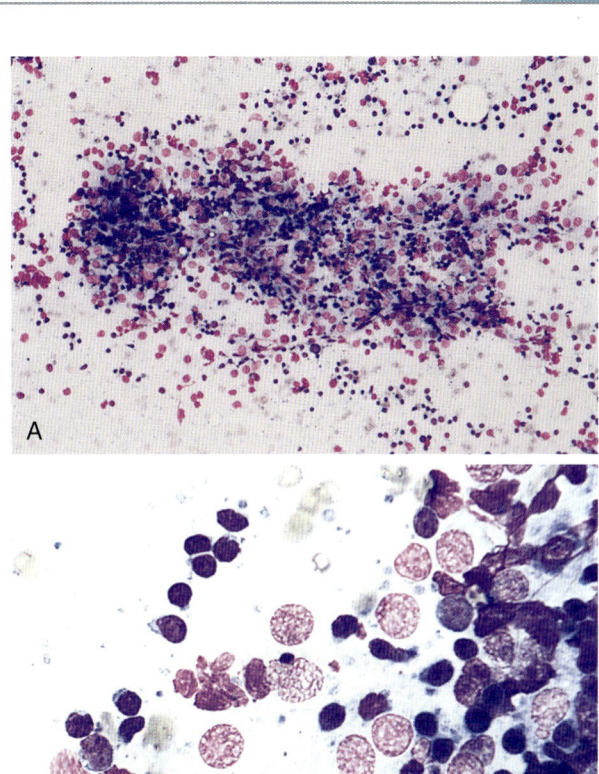

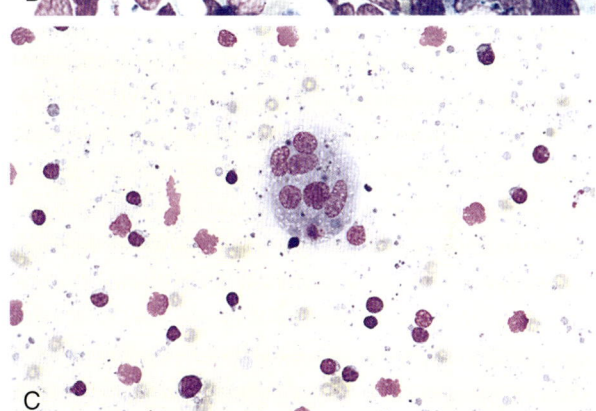

FIGURE 4.44 Histiocytic lymphadenitis with prominent vascular elements. Submandibular lymph node aspirate. Dog. Same case in A to C. **A,** Several aggregates of reticular (fibrohistiocytic) stroma surrounding blood vessels are noted in this lymph node draining an inflamed skin mass. Histopathology supported the clinical diagnosis of an immune-mediated disease by finding lymphoplasmacytic and suppurative vasculitis in several subcutaneous tissues. (Wright-Giemsa; IP.) **B,** Higher magnification displays a cohesive mass of large mononuclear cells having abundant clear cytoplasm. Small lymphocytes are present in the background. (Wright-Giemsa; HP oil.) **C,** Multinucleated giant cells were present in low numbers in this generalized histiocytic proliferation within the lymph node. Mixed lymphoid cell population is noted in the background. (Wright-Giemsa; HP oil.)

to excellent response, supporting an underlying immune-mediated etiology. Similar etiology is associated with canine juvenile cellulitis and vasculitis (Fig. 4.44).

Other noninfectious conditions include chronic drainage of injured tissues in addition to hemorrhage with hemosiderosis (Fig. 4.45) (see Fig. 4.11B) and Gamna-Gandy bodies (Attipa et al., 2017; Moore et al., 2017) (Fig. 4.46). See further discussion about the Gamna-Gandy bodies under Splenitis later in this chapter.

Lymphoma

Lymphoma is a very common spontaneous neoplasm in dogs and cats. One study found an incidence of 103 cases within a pet population of 130,684 insured dogs in the United Kingdom (Edwards et al., 2003). Within this population, boxers had significantly higher relative risks than did other breeds. The other breeds with increased relative risk included basset hound, St. Bernard, Scottish terrier, Airedale terrier, bulldog, Labrador retriever, Bouvier des Flandres, and Rottweiler (Edwards et al., 2003). Others with observed increased risk include golden retrievers and bullmastiffs. In

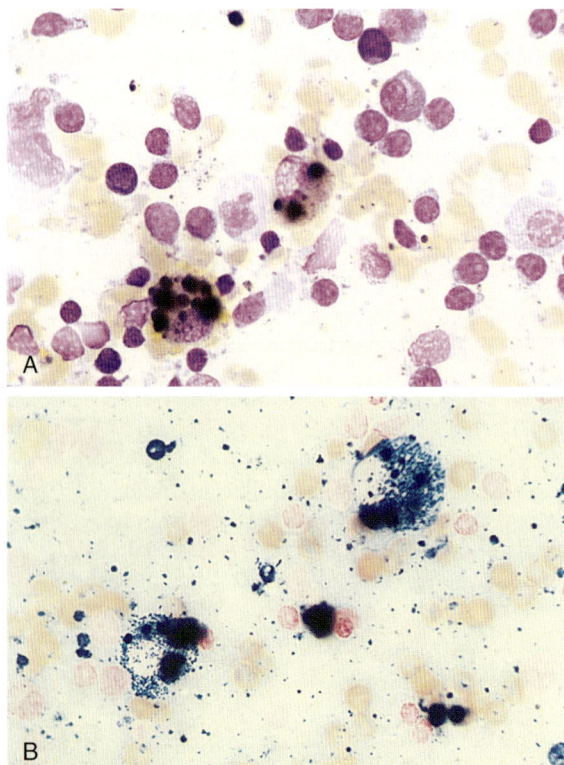

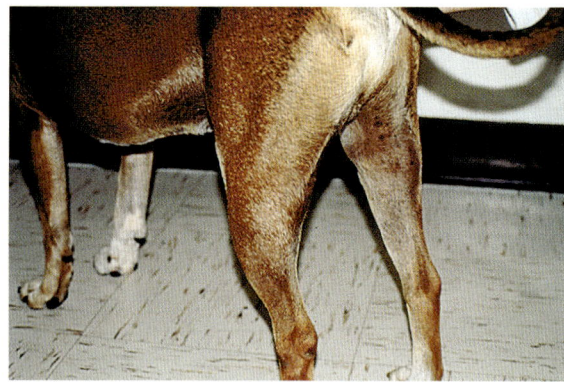

■ **FIGURE 4.47 Lymphoma. Dog.** Popliteal lymph node enlargement is shown. (Courtesy Leslie Fox, University of Florida.)

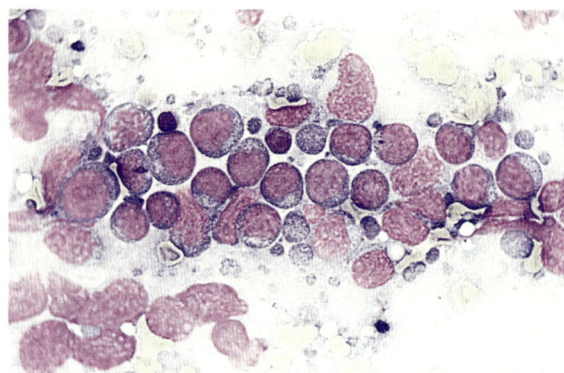

■ **FIGURE 4.45 Histiocytic lymphadenitis with hemosiderosis. Lymph node aspirate. Dog.** Same case in A and B. **A,** Numerous hemosiderin-laden macrophages are shown, characterized by large, coarse, black granules. The background contains several small dark granules consistent with hemosiderin. The lymphoid cell population is mixed, which is consistent with immune stimulation. A malignant neoplasm was previously diagnosed in the area drained by this submandibular lymph node. (Aqueous Romanowsky; HP oil.) **B, Hemosiderosis. Cytochemistry.** Iron stain demonstrates a large amount of coarse, blue-black, granular material both intra- and extracellularly. Note the small positively stained granules in the background. (Prussian blue; HP oil.)

■ **FIGURE 4.48 Lymph node aspirate. Dog.** Medium and large lymphocytes comprise 60% to 90% of the total cells in this lymph node, which are of B-cell origin. (Wright-Giemsa; HP oil.)

dogs, lymphoma was the most common diagnosis of lymph node cytopathology (Amores-Fuster et al., 2015). The boxer breed has a statistically higher frequency of T-cell lymphomas than Rottweilers or golden retrievers (Lurie et al., 2004; Comazzi et al., 2018). There appears to be geographic differences as noted in a European study where golden retrievers were not predisposed to T-zone lymphoma in non-UK European countries (Comazzi et al., 2018).

The term termed *lymphoma* is preferred over *lymphosarcoma*. It is clinically recognized as lymphadenomegaly (Fig. 4.47). The predominant neoplastic cell in dogs and cats is usually a medium or large lymphocyte; however, cats may display a small cell lymphoma within the alimentary tract (Twomey and Alleman, 2005). Medium-sized or large lymphocytes often comprise greater than 50% of the total cells in lymphoma (Fig. 4.48). An exception is the subtype of a B-cell lymphoma having a predominant population of macrophages or T cells, termed, respectively, *histiocytic-rich* or *T-cell–rich B-cell lymphoma*.

A micrometer such as an erythrocyte is best used to determine the size of the lymphocytes because neutrophils are more variable in size and less frequent in specimens (Fig. 4.49). The nucleus of a small, medium, and large canine lymphocyte is 1 to 1.5, 2 to 2.5, and more than 3 times a red blood cell (RBC) diameter, respectively (Box 4.1).

Terminology Concerns

A *lymphoblast* is defined as an enlarged (medium or large) lymphocyte that has been activated to divide. It is recognized

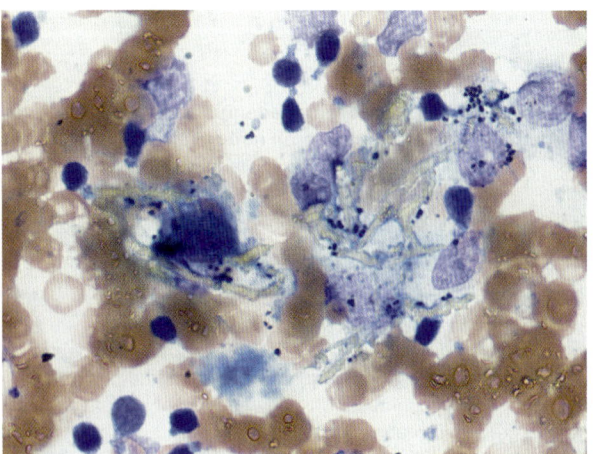

■ **FIGURE 4.46 Gamna-Gandy bodies. Histiocytic lymphadenitis. Medial iliac lymph node aspirate. Dog.** Against the background of small lymphocytes are histiocytes, some containing dark granular material presumed to be hemosiderin. Within the cell aggregates are light yellow linear structures (siderocalcific plaques) that represent evidence of prior hemorrhage. (Wright-Giemsa; HP oil.) (Courtesy Francisco Conrado, University of Florida.)

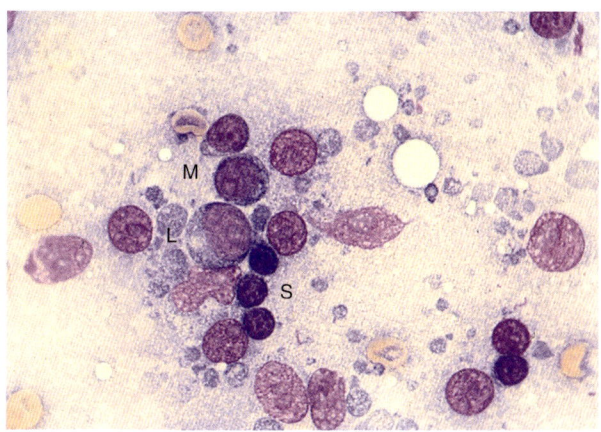

■ **FIGURE 4.49 Lymph node aspirate.** A micrometer such as the erythrocyte at the top of the field is used to determine the size of the lymphocytes present. Note the three dark-staining, small (S) lymphocytes in the center along with two intact medium (M) and one intact large (L) lymphocyte. Basophilic cytoplasmic fragments termed *lymphoglandular bodies* and pink remnants of lysed nuclei surround the intact cells. (Wright-Giemsa; HP oil.)

BOX 4.1 Cytopathologic Protocol and Terms Used to Evaluate Lymphoma Cases

Determine the cell size based on comparison of the nucleus to the size of an erythrocyte.
- Small: 1–1.5 × RBC diameter
- Medium: 2–2.5 × RBC diameter
- Large: ≥3 × RBC diameter

Determine the shape of the nucleus and its placement within the cytoplasm.
- Round: circular with no indentations
- Irregularly round: few indentations or convolutions
- Convoluted: several deep indentations
- Clefted: single deep indentation
- Central vs. eccentric placement

Determine the number, size, visibility, and location of nucleoli within the neoplastic lymphocytes.
- Single vs. multiple
- Large vs. small
- Indistinct: not visible or barely perceivable
- Prominent: easily visible
- Central vs. marginal or peripheral placement

Describe the cytoplasm by amount and color. Be sure to note presence of paranuclear Golgi zone or granulation.
- Scant: small rim around nucleus
- Moderate size: amount intermediate between scant and abundant
- Abundant: nearly twice the size of the nucleus
- Pale: light in color or clear
- Moderate basophilia: color intermediate between pale and dark blue
- Deep basophilia: royal blue or darker

Count the total number of mitotic figures in 10 highly cellular fields under 40× objective. (If using 50× objective, count 15 fields)
- Low mitotic count: 0–2 mitotic figures
- Moderate mitotic count: 3–5 mitotic figures
- High mitotic count: >6 mitotic figures

Tumor grade is morphologically based on cell size and mitotic count.
- Low grade: Low mitotic count and small cell size
- High grade: Moderate or high mitotic count and medium or large cell size

RBC, Red blood cell.

TABLE 4.2 Recognized Subtypes of Canine and Feline Lymphoid Malignancies Using Current WHO Classification

	B CELL	T CELL/NK CELL
Precursor (bone marrow)	Lymphoblastic leukemia or lymphoma[a]	Lymphoblastic leukemia or lymphoma[a]
Mature (peripheral)	Small lymphocytic lymphoma/CLL[a,b]	Granular lymphocytic leukemia or lymphoma[a]
	Prolymphocytic leukemia	Prolymphocytic leukemia
	Mantle cell lymphoma	Adult T-cell leukemia/lymphoma
	Marginal zone lymphoma (nodal, spleen,[a,b] MALT)	Hepatosplenic γδ T-cell lymphoma[a]
	Follicular lymphoma	Subcutaneous panniculitis-like lymphoma[a]
	Lymphoplasmacytic lymphoma[a] (including Waldenström macroglobulinemia[b])	Mycosis fungoides/Sézary syndrome[a]
		Peripheral T-cell lymphoma[a]
	Plasma cell neoplasms[a]: myeloma,[b] plasmacytoma	T-zone lymphoma[a]
	Diffuse large B-cell lymphoma[a] (including TCRBCL)	Enteropathy-type T-cell lymphoma[a]
		Angioimmunoblastic T-cell lymphoma
	Mediastinal (thymic) lymphoma[a]	Angiocentric T-cell lymphoma
	Primary effusion lymphoma	Anaplastic large cell lymphoma
		Aggressive NK cell leukemia/lymphoma

[a]Common lymphoid condition.
[b]Monoclonal gammopathy may occur.
CLL, Chronic lymphocytic leukemia; *MALT*, mucosa-associated lymphoid tissue; *NK*, natural killer; *TCRBCL*, T-cell–rich B-cell lymphoma; *WHO*, World Health Organization.

morphologically by an immature nucleus having fine granular chromatin with or without prominent nucleoli.

Lymphoblastic leukemia/lymphoma is a specific disease entity of lymphoid neoplasia according to the World Health Organization (WHO) classification, whose neoplastic cell arises from precursor lymphoid cells within the bone marrow (Table 4.2). *Lymphoblastic lymphoma* is applied to lymphoid tissue when there is less than 25% lymphoblasts in the bone marrow (Bain et al., 2010). *Acute lymphoblastic leukemia* is used when lymphoblasts involve greater than 25% of the bone marrow; this condition is usually characterized by the presence of stem cell marker CD34 on cell surfaces.

Mature B- and T-cell lymphomas arise from post–stem cell lymphocytes. *Chronic lymphocytic leukemia* arises from mature lymphocytes that proliferate within the bone marrow or accumulate within circulation. A subtype of lymphoid leukemia arises from the proliferation of granular lymphocytes within the red pulp region of the spleen that then circulate within the blood but do not originate from the bone marrow.

General Morphologic Considerations

Within the background of the preparation are *lymphoglandular bodies* (Fig. 4.50; see also Fig. 4.49) that result from the rupture

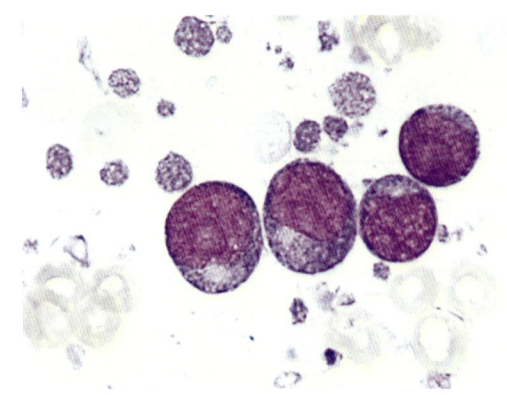

■ **FIGURE 4.50 Lymphoglandular bodies. Lymph node aspirate. Dog.** Prominent basophilic round structures of variable size indicate fragmentation of the cytoplasm. This appearance is often associated with lymphoma but is found in other conditions with fragile cells. (Wright-Giemsa; HP oil.)

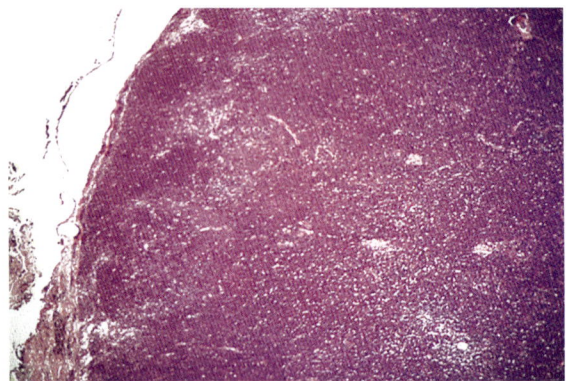

■ **FIGURE 4.51 Lymphoma. Lymph node. Tissue section. Dog.** A dense infiltration of neoplastic lymphocytes effaces the normal architecture, leaving no discernible cortex and medulla. (H&E; LP.)

for prognostic value (Ponce et al., 2004). In the past, the updated Kiel classification scheme was helpful to define high and low grade by size and mitotic activity. Currently, this has been largely replaced by use of the WHO classification to characterize disease entities for prognostic purposes (see Table 4.2) (Valli et al., 2011). However, the common nodal lymphoma subtypes seen on cytopathology can be distinguished by cell size, as shown later in this chapter. Histopathologic evaluation of lymphoma relies on cell size as well as architectural features to classify subtypes.

Diagnostic Considerations

Immunophenotyping the lymphoma into B- and T-cell types has been shown to assist in prognosis of canine lymphomas by determining clinical disease types (Raskin and Fox, 2003; Seelig et al., 2014). Antibodies against antigens (e.g., CD20, CD21, CD79a, Pax5, BLA.36) may be used to determine B-cell origin (Figs. 4.52 and 4.53) (Jubala et al., 2005), whereas those against CD3, CD4, CD5, and CD8 are useful for T-cell neoplasms (Fig. 4.54). Chapter 18 expands on the methodology and application of

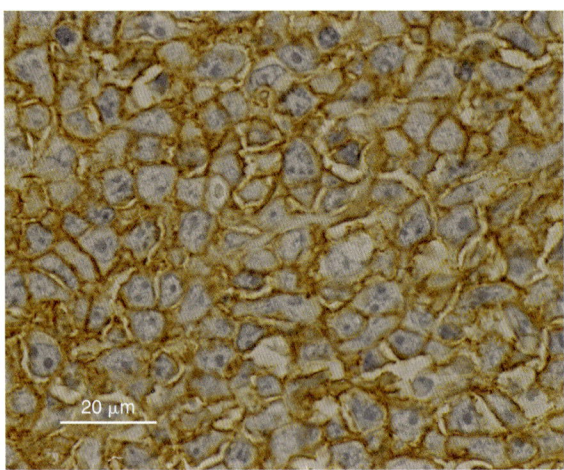

■ **FIGURE 4.52 Immunohistochemistry.** Note the uniform cell surface expression of CD20 indicating a B-cell origin using an immunoperoxidase technique. (CD20/DAB; HP oil.)

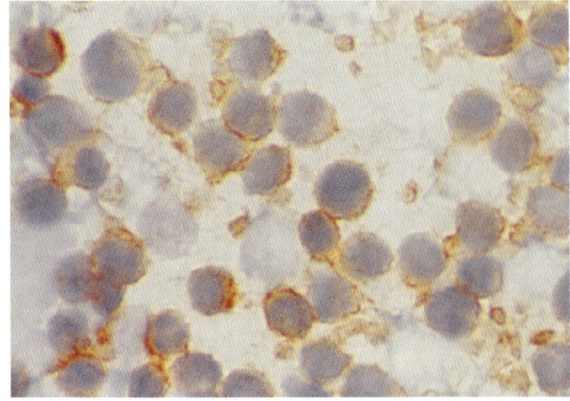

■ **FIGURE 4.53 Lymphoma. Lymph node aspirate as cytocentrifuged specimen. Immunocytochemistry. Dog.** Cell surface expression of CD21 indicates B-cell origin using aminoethylcarbazole as the chromogen. (CD21/AEC; HP oil.)

of lymphocytes and appear as small platelet-sized basophilic cytoplasmic fragments. Although these bodies may be seen in benign lymph node conditions, a higher frequency is expected in lymphoma because of the immaturity and fragility of these cells. Lysed nuclei may appear as lacy, amorphous eosinophilic material (see Figs. 4.48 and 4.49).

The population is often homogeneous (Fig. 4.51; see also Fig. 4.50), although early in the disease, there may be incomplete effacement of the lymph node. When cell populations are mixed, including different cell sizes present such as small and large lymphocytes, the diagnosis of lymphoma may require additional procedures such as histopathologic assessment, immunophenotyping, and polymerase chain reaction for antigen receptor rearrangement (PARR) (see Chapter 18). Surgical removal and histopathologic examination of the lymph node is recommended in all equivocal cases to help make a definitive diagnosis and classify the disease subtype (see Table 4.2) of lymphoma for treatment and prognostic purposes. Clinical staging, particularly stage V that involves blood, bone marrow, or miscellaneous sites and clinical substage, has prognostic importance for lymphoma as well as clinical substage (Jagielski et al., 2002).

Morphologic appearance of the neoplastic cells has been used along with immunophenotype to further classify the lymphomas

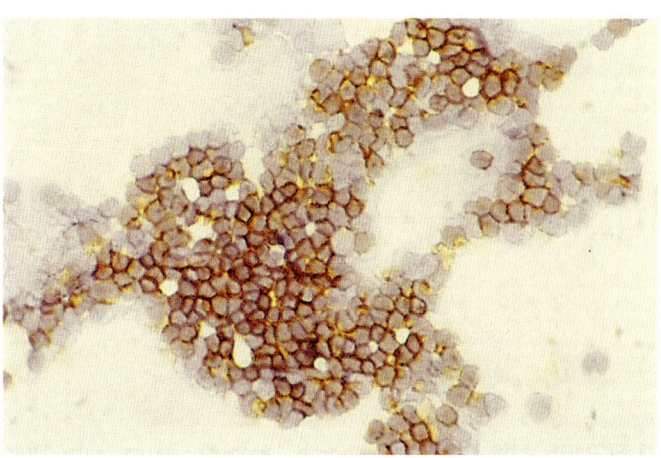

FIGURE 4.54 Peripheral T-cell lymphoma. Lymph node aspirate as cytocentrifuged specimen. Immunocytochemistry. Dog. A strong positive reaction is indicated by the brown cytoplasmic stain. (CD3/DAB; HP oil.)

leukocyte immunophenotyping. Studies have demonstrated that although the T-cell phenotype was often associated with a poor prognosis, significant prognostic differences were evident within the B- and the T-cell subtypes of canine lymphoma (Chiulli et al., 2003; Ponce et al., 2004). Therefore, B-cell types are not always "best," and T-cell types are not always "terrible." These studies support the use of a clinicomorphologic characterization of the disease in dogs, similar to the current hematopoietic neoplasm classification scheme for humans, which is based on clinical presentation, immunophenotype, anatomic site, morphology, cytogenetics, and clinical aggressiveness (Swerdlow et al., 2008). Description of some of the veterinary WHO subtypes shown in Table 4.2 may be found in the literature (Fry et al., 2003; Cienava et al., 2004; Valli et al., 2006; Valli et al., 2011).

Immunophenotyping is necessary initially to characterize the type of lymphoma and may be accomplished through a variety of techniques. Canine and feline lymphoid neoplasia may be immunophenotyped by flow cytometry of aspirate material (Dean et al., 1995; Grindem et al., 1998; Gibson et al., 2004), immunostaining of tissue sections (Fournel-Fleury et al., 1997; Vail et al., 1998; Kiupel et al., 1999; Fournel-Fleury et al., 2002), or direct immunostaining of aspirate cytopathologic preparations (Fisher et al., 1995; Caniatti et al., 1996; Chiulli et al., 2003). Fisher et al. (1995) demonstrated an excellent correlation of immunophenotype between immunostained canine cytopathologic and histopathologic samples. Studies support B-cell lymphomas account for approximately 60% of the cases, with the remainder being T-cell and null cell types (Teske and van Heerde, 1996; Fournel-Fleury et al., 1997; Ponce et al., 2004; Valli et al., 2013). Neoplasms of natural killer cell origin are occasionally encountered in veterinary medicine and are often suggested by the presence of CD3ε and granzyme immunoreactivity.

PARR is not indicated for phenotyping lymphoid neoplasms but rather is helpful in supporting the presence of clonality of a lymphoid cell population (high specificity), but a negative result does not rule out the possibility of clonality (low sensitivity). See Chapter 18 for further information on methodology and application of this molecular test in dogs and cats.

Another prognostic indicator involves use of cell proliferation markers in histopathologic and cytopathologic specimens to evaluate active cell turnover. The most commonly used proliferation markers are mitotic count, percent positivity of Ki-67 antigen, percent positivity of proliferation cell nuclear antigen (PCNA), and argyrophilic nucleolar organizing regions (AgNORs) quantitation (Vail et al., 1997; Kiupel et al., 1998; Kiupel et al., 1999; Dank et al., 2002; Hipple et al., 2003; Vajdovich et al., 2004; Whitten and Raskin, 2004; Bauer et al., 2007). Ki-67 recognizes an antigen expressed in all cell cycle phases except the resting stage (G0). PCNA increases during G1, becomes maximal at DNA synthesis (S), and decreases during G2, mitosis (M), and G0. Mitotic count reflects only the M phase. See Appendix 4 for recognition of mitotic phases. The most comprehensive marker appears to be AgNOR, which indicates proteins associated with loops of DNA involved in ribosomal RNA transcription. The quantity of AgNOR not only reflects the percentage of cells cycling but also increases when the cell cycle is faster. AgNOR counts correlated well with tumor grade (Kiupel et al., 1998). Studies on AgNOR frequency and area parameters demonstrated significant predictive potential for remission and survival time in treated and untreated cases of canine lymphoma (Kiupel et al., 1998; Kiupel et al., 1999). A later study found that use of nucleolar AgNOR counts may be more reliable prognostically than mean AgNOR or percent proliferative AgNOR counts for certain forms of canine lymphoid neoplasia (Whitten and Raskin, 2004).

Small Cell (1–1.5 × RBC Diameter) Lymphoma

T-zone lymphoma. T-zone lymphoma is a type of indolent lymphoma recognized morphologically and immunophenotypically as unique with a small cell or occasionally medium size and pale or clear cytoplasm, presence of "hand mirror" cells, loss of CD45 antigen (Seelig et al., 2014), and often the presence of CD21 antigen (Martini et al., 2015). It is a common subtype comprising 62% of all canine indolent lymphomas in one study (Flood-Knapik et al., 2013). Histopathologically, T-zone lymphoma shows neoplastic cells expanding the paracortex and medullary cords between fading germinal follicles without effacing the nodal architecture. Cytopathologically, there is a homogeneous population of CD3+ small lymphocytes that have sharp, shallow nuclear indentations, indistinct nucleoli, and a moderate volume of pale or clear cytoplasm. A hand mirror or single cytoplasmic extension called a *uropod* may be observed with T-zone lymphocytes (Yeuroukis et al., 2017) (Figs. 4.55 to 4.57). This type of lymphoma is indolent, with median survival of 637 to 760 days (Seelig et al., 2014; Martini et al., 2016). Golden retrievers and Shih Tzus are often associated with T-zone lymphoma, with demodicosis present in 10% to 50% of cases studied in the United States and Japan (Flood-Knapik et al., 2013; Mizutani et al., 2016).

Lymphoplasmacytic lymphoma. A mature B-cell neoplasm with an indolent course is *lymphoplasmacytic lymphoma* (Fig. 4.58). Cytopathologically, cells are a mixture of small and medium lymphocytes that often have a plasmacytoid appearance. Needle-like stacks, thick splinters of immunoglobulin (Fig. 4.58B), or round (Fig. 4.59) cytoplasmic inclusions have been recognized in a low percentage of these lymphoma cases. A monoclonal gammopathy may be present in these cases.

Small lymphocytic lymphoma. Small cell predominance may arise from solid tissues as small lymphocytic lymphoma (Fig. 4.60) or circulate in blood as chronic lymphocytic leukemia (Fig. 4.61). They arise from the same peripheral B cell and present with an indolent course. Cells are uniform, being small with scant cytoplasm. Nuclei are round with moderately

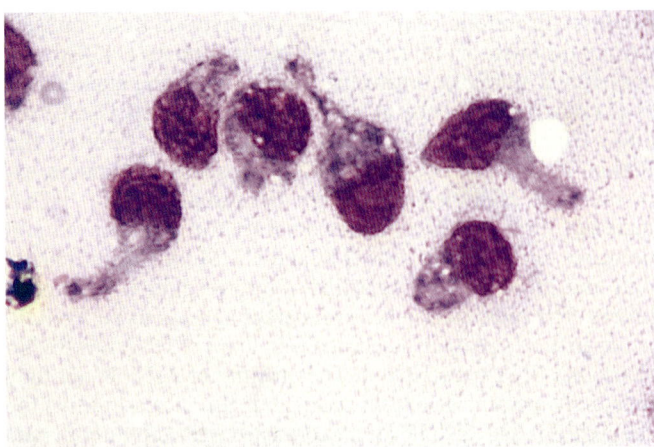

■ **FIGURE 4.55 T-zone lymphoma. Lymph node aspirate. Dog.** This animal also had cutaneous nodules, which appear similar on cytopathology and histopathology with these lymphocytes infiltrating the epidermis. Cells display a hand-mirror shape with cytoplasmic pseudopods that extend in different directions. (Wright-Giemsa; HP oil.)

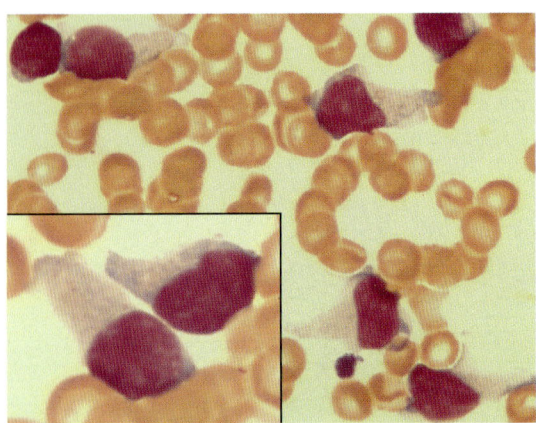

■ **FIGURE 4.56 T-zone lymphoma. Lymph node aspirate. Dog.** Uropod formation is frequent in this sample, with individual cells extended in different directions. Uropods are thought to help in binding the T cells to other cells and permit release of cytoplasmic contents. *Inset:* The pale cytoplasm in this case demonstrates the presence of few fine granules. (Romanowsky; HP oil.) (Courtesy Harold Tvedten, Swedish University of Agricultural Sciences.)

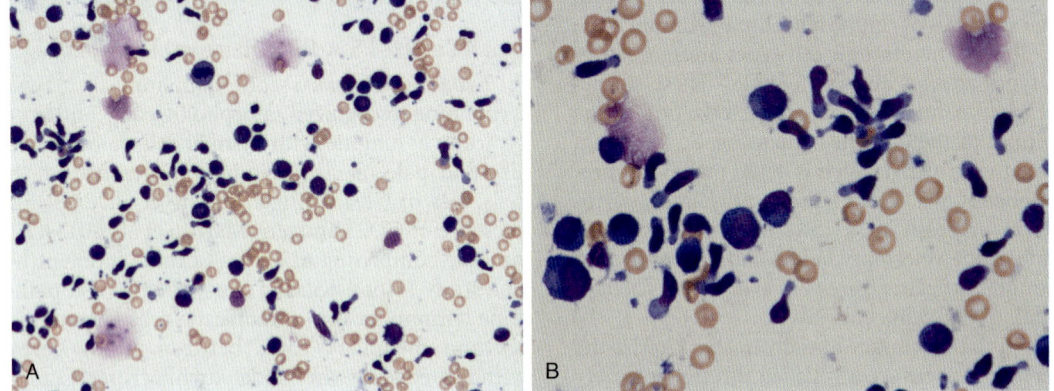

■ **FIGURE 4.57 T-zone lymphoma. Superficial cervical lymph node aspirate. Dog.** Same case in A and B. **A,** Mostly small cells are round or oval with distinct borders and have a small amount of deeply basophilic cytoplasm that often exhibits a cytoplasmic projection (uropod). Occasional mitotic figures are noted. **B,** Higher magnification of lymph node cells. Patient was treated for B-cell lymphoma, which was in remission before developing generalized demodicosis. There is a chronic lymphocytosis and flow cytometry of the blood revealed predominance of CD21+ cells, which were also in the lymph node. (Wright-Giemsa; HP oil.) (Courtesy Laura Black, University of Florida.)

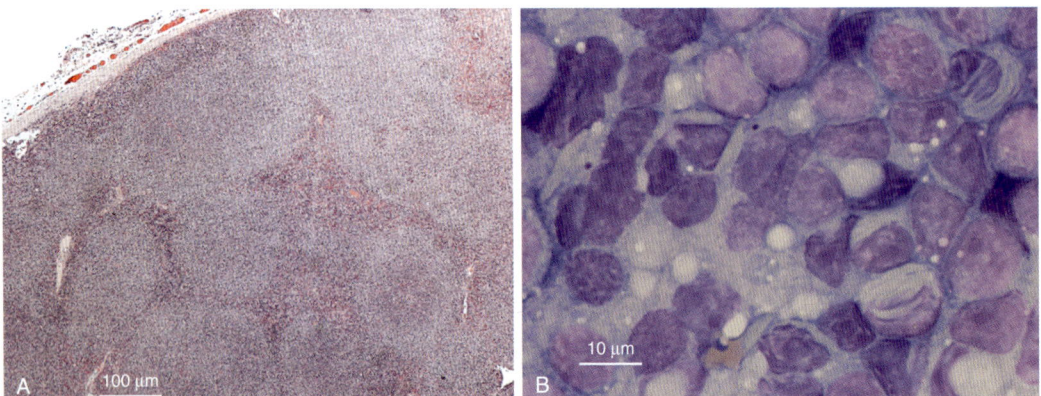

■ **FIGURE 4.58 Lymphoplasmacytic lymphoma. Inguinal lymph node. Dog.** Same case in A and B. **A, Tissue section.** Loss of normal lymph node architecture is indicated by expansive follicular areas having a uniform pale-staining appearance. This animal was clinically staged as IVa and had an indolent course of disease with more than 2 years survival despite the presence of a clonal proliferation that was verified by PARR. (H&E, LP.) **B, Tissue imprint.** A mixture of small and medium lymphocytes is present. Frequently observed within the cytoplasm are threadlike needle and splinter crystals, consistent with an atypical form of Russell bodies. Immunostaining was positive for CD21, CD45RA, and CD79a. (Wright-Giemsa; HP oil.)

dense clumped chromatin (see Fig. 4.61A). Monoclonal gammopathy may be associated with this leukemia in a low percentage of patients (see Fig. 4.61B). In humans, these CD5-positive cells are thought to arise from follicular mantle cells or circulating naïve cells (Swerdlow et al., 2008).

Follicular lymphoma. Follicular lymphomas arise from the germinal cells and expand the follicle, compressing surrounding paracortical tissue. Whereas normal germinal center possess tingible body macrophages filled with apoptotic debris, follicular lymphomas lack these macrophages. Callanan et al. (1996) evaluated eight natural and experimental cases of FIV-associated lymphomas in cats, finding a high prevalence of B-cell types with a similar follicular morphology. Follicular lymphoma is an uncommon form of lymphoma in dogs and cats and when present has an indolent course. Diagnosis require histopathology to evaluate the architectural involvement.

Medium Cell (2–2.5 × RBC Diameter) Lymphoma

Marginal zone lymphoma. A common but sometimes difficult subtype to recognize by cytopathology arises from the marginal zone layer surrounding the germinal center. This

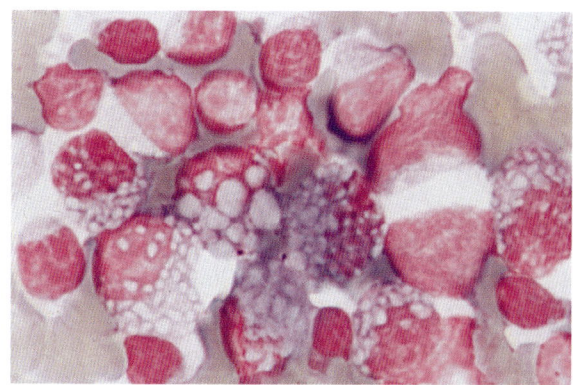

■ **FIGURE 4.59 Lymphoplasmacytic lymphoma. Prescapular lymph node aspirate. Dog.** A mixture of small and medium lymphocytes is present, some of which appear plasmacytoid. Frequently observed within the cytoplasm are variably sized, coarse, pebble-like inclusions, consistent with an atypical form of Russell bodies. The animal was clinically staged as Vb and had an aggressive course of disease with survival of 49 days. These cells were present in other sites, such as the kidney and rectum, suggesting a widely disseminated lymphoma. (Wright; HP oil.)

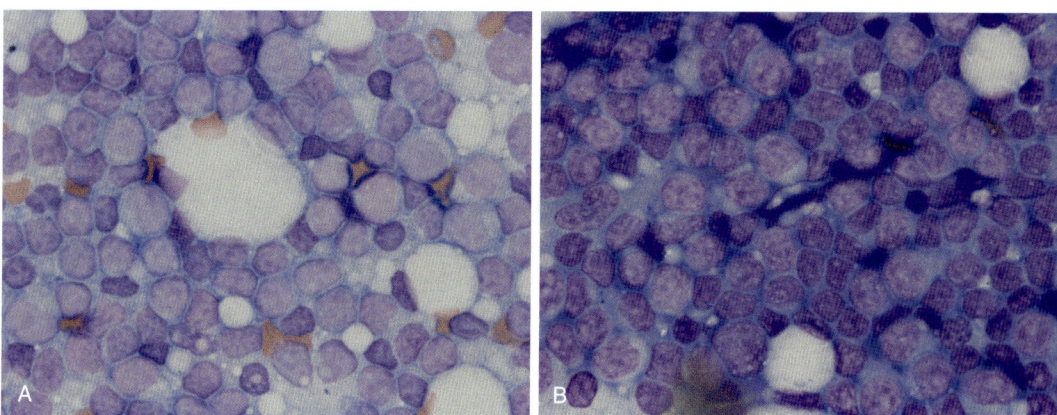

■ **FIGURE 4.60 Small B-lymphocytic lymphoma. Superficial cervical lymph node aspirate.** Same case in A and B. The patient presented 11 months earlier with splenic nodule diagnosed by flow cytometry as CD21+ population and positive PARR clonality for immunoglobulin gene. Histopathology of the spleen supported small B-lymphocytic lymphoma. **A,** The lymphoid population is composed mostly of small well-differentiated lymphocytes with a mildly expanded population of medium lymphocytes and rare large lymphoid cells. (Wright-Giemsa; HP oil.) **B,** Similar cytopathology as in A but with different stain to show a lack of cell immaturity. (Aqueous Romanowsky; HP oil.) (Courtesy Jacqueline Dolan, University of Florida.)

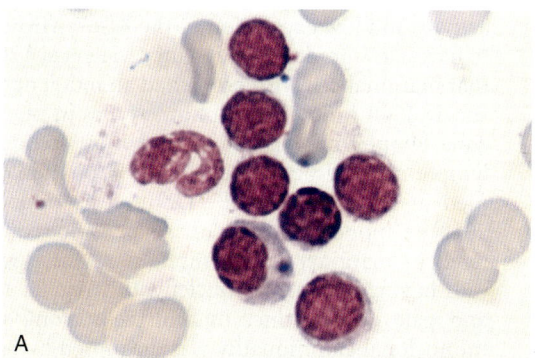
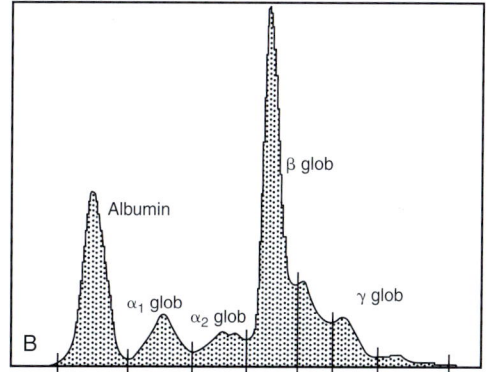

■ **FIGURE 4.61 B-cell chronic lymphocytic leukemia/small lymphocytic lymphoma. Dog.** Same case in A and B. **A, Bone marrow aspirate.** Both the bone marrow and spleen were involved in this case of a 13-year-old mixed breed dog with clinical stage Va. The neoplastic cells were uniformly round with generally scant cytoplasm and a low mitotic index. Cells expressed CD79a, CD21, and sIg. This disease had an indolent course with a survival of 160 days. (Wright-Giemsa; HP oil.) **B, Paraproteinemia. Serum protein electrophoretogram.** The densitometer scan indicates a monoclonal spike in the beta region indicative of immunoglobulin A or M. Immunoelectrophoresis confirmed immunoglobulin A production in the M-component.

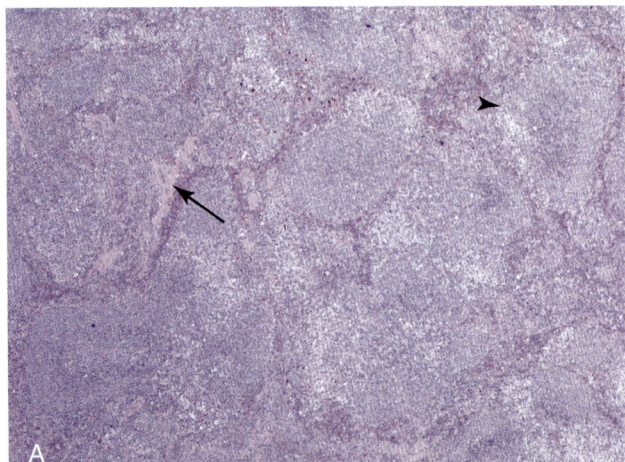
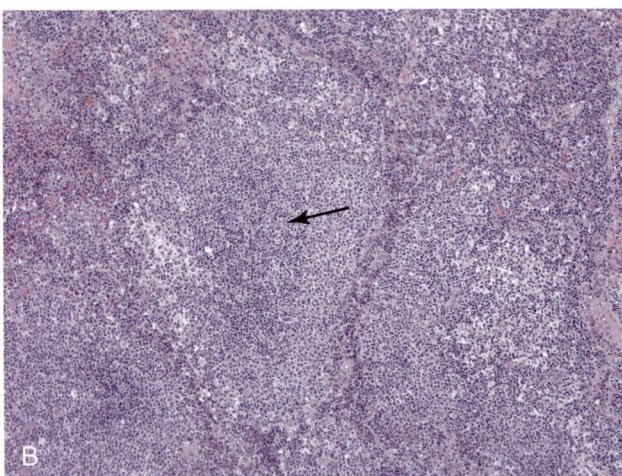

FIGURE 4.62 Marginal zone lymphoma. Mesenteric lymph node histologic section. Dog. Same case in A and B. **A,** Multiple follicles are expanded with a loss of normal architecture. Note the follicle *(arrowhead)* with reverse staining with lighter outside and dark inside. Hyalinosis of the fading follicle *(arrow)* with pink staining is shown. (H&E; LP.) **B,** Higher magnification of the follicle showing remnant small, dense-staining mantle cells *(arrow)* within the center of a pale proliferation of larger lymphoid cells. Note the poorly demarcated follicular margin with the expansion of malignant cells into the surrounding interfollicular areas compared with well-defined follicle with marginal zone expansion in Figure 4.11A. (H&E; LP.)

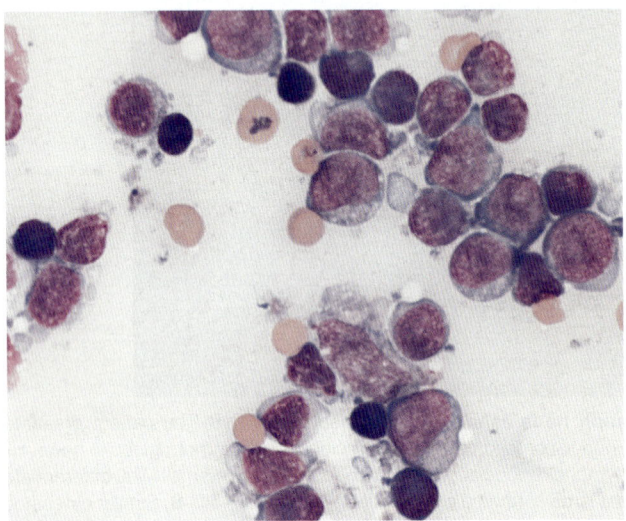

FIGURE 4.63 Marginal zone lymphoma. Mesenteric lymph node imprint. Dog. This field contains an increased number of medium-sized lymphocytes, most of which contain a single large, prominent nucleolus and moderate amounts of basophilic cytoplasm consistent with the marginal zone cell. The remaining nucleated cells are small and medium-sized lymphocytes having scant cytoplasm and in some fields (not shown) predominated. (Wright-Giemsa; HP oil.)

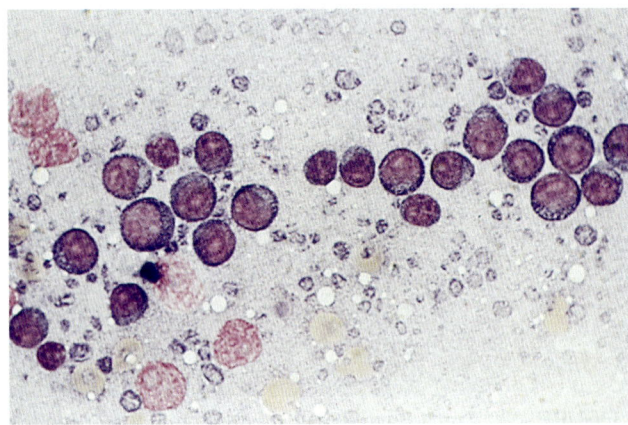

FIGURE 4.64 Marginal zone lymphoma. Lymph node aspirate. Medium-sized lymphoid cells exceed 30% of the cell population. Immunostaining was positive for CD21 and CD79. Note the large number of lymphoglandular bodies in the background, suggesting high fragility. (Wright-Giemsa; HP oil.)

indolent form of lymphoma is best diagnosed by histopathology (Fig. 4.62). There is a residual of small dark follicular cells with fading germinal centers and pink hyalinosis surrounded by medium-sized pale marginal zone cells. Cases can involve both lymph nodes and the spleen. On cytopathologic specimens, a mixture of small and medium lymphocytes is found with an increased percentage of immature, medium-sized lymphocytes, many with a single prominent nucleolus (Fig. 4.63). This unique-appearing cell type present in dogs contains only one large centrally placed nucleolus instead of multiple nucleoli (Figs. 4.64 and 4.65). This cell, termed *macronucleated medium-sized cell* (MMC) by Fournel-Fleury et al (1997), suggests its origin is the marginal perifollicular zone. Based on low mitotic activity and low expression of the Ki-67, MMC was considered to have a low grade of malignancy. Valli et al. (2006) determined that marginal cell lymphoma had an indolent course with long survival. Of indolent lymphoma types in one study, marginal zone lymphoma was the second most frequent after T-zone lymphoma and accounted for 25% of indolent cases with a median survival time of 21.2 months (Flood-Knapik et al., 2013). A monocytoid nuclear shape is not commonly encountered in marginal zone lymphoma. A case with monocytoid cells having convoluted nuclei with irregular nuclear contours and pale or indistinct nucleoli cells along with concurrent monoclonal gammopathy was diagnosed by histopathology of an extracted lymph node (Burgess et al., 2020). A similar example appears under marginal zone lymphoma of the spleen (see Fig. 4.136).

B-lymphoblastic leukemia/lymphoma. Neoplastic B-lymphoid cells arising from precursor cells within the bone marrow, which are medium cells that may quickly spread to lymph nodes and

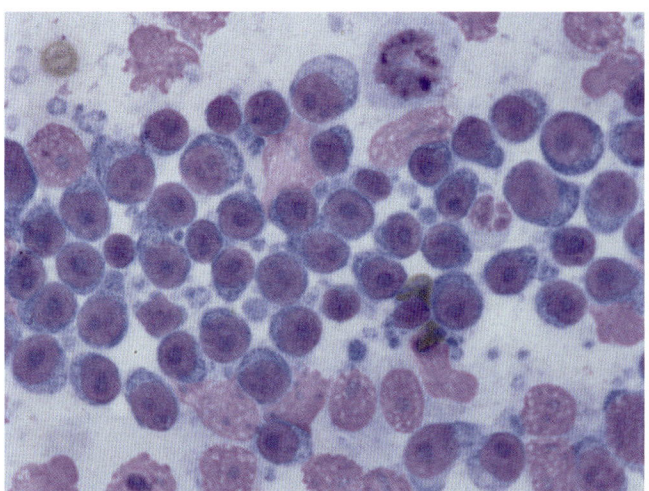

FIGURE 4.65 Marginal zone lymphoma. Popliteal lymph node aspirate. Dog. Nucleated cells consist of a monomorphic population of medium-sized lymphocytes (nuclei ~2 × RBC diameter). Nuclei are irregularly round and eccentrically located with a finely granular chromatin pattern and generally one prominent, ovoid centrally placed nucleoli. These medium lymphocytes have a moderate volume of blue cytoplasm with a paranuclear clearing (Golgi apparatus). Note the mitotic figure in the upper center field. (Aqueous Romanowsky; HP oil.) (Courtesy Brandy Kastl, Kansas State University.)

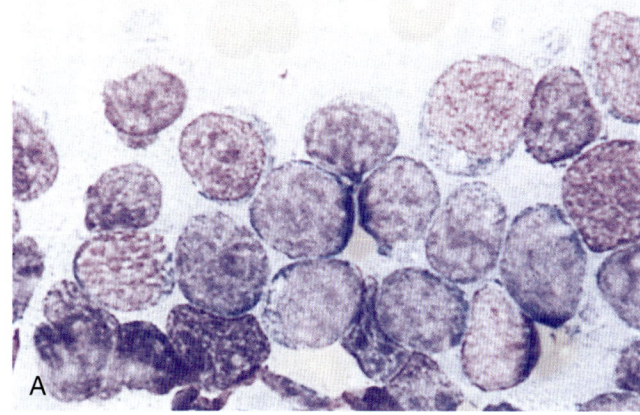
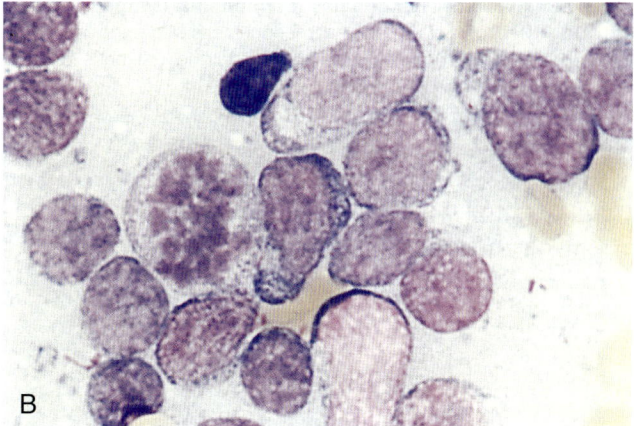

FIGURE 4.66 B-Lymphoblastic lymphoma. Lymph node aspirate. Dog. Same case in A and B. **A,** Precursor cells are medium-sized with round nuclei measuring 2 to 2.5 times RBC diameter. Nucleoli are generally indistinct. The cytoplasm is scant and moderately basophilic. Immunostaining was positive for CD21 and CD79a. These cells were present in the bone marrow and spleen as well in the 7-year-old cocker spaniel who survived only 29 days after diagnosis. (Wright-Giemsa; HP oil.) **B,** Mitotic activity is high for the lymphoblastic category. Note the small, dark-staining lymphocyte for size comparison. Most cells are medium sized with indistinct nucleoli and scant cytoplasm. (Wright-Giemsa; HP oil.)

present as lymphoblastic lymphoma when evaluated in solid tissues (Fig. 4.66). Cases of B-lymphoblastic leukemia/lymphoma had a highly aggressive course with a median of 48 days survival despite treatment (Raskin and Fox, 2003).

T-lymphoblastic leukemia/lymphoma. Similar to B cells, neoplasia may involve the precursor T cell, resulting in acute lymphoblastic leukemia or lymphoblastic lymphoma (Figs. 4.67 to 4.70). The lymphoblastic type was associated with a mediastinal mass in 8 of 13 cases and a paraneoplastic syndrome of hypercalcemia with 4 of 13 cases (Ponce et al., 2003). The morphologic features of the lymphoblast involve a medium-sized cell with nuclei measuring 2 to 2.5 times RBC diameter. The nucleus may be round or irregular, and the nucleoli are often small and indistinct, best appreciated with a new methylene blue wet mount (see Fig. 4.68). The cytoplasm is often scant. Mitotic activity is high (Box 4.1). Another diagnostic tool is cytochemical staining that is distinctive with a focal or dot appearance with alpha naphthyl acetate esterase, alpha naphthyl butyrate esterase, or acid phosphatase (see Fig. 4.69) (Raskin and Nipper, 1992). Prognosis for this morphologic type is poor owing to renal failure, which results from the hypercalcemia or from the diffuse and expansive infiltration of the bone marrow (see Fig. 4.70).

Other medium-sized lymphomas. For further discussion, see descriptions under small-sized T-zone lymphoma and large-sized peripheral T-cell lymphoma. Shown is an example of a predominant medium-sized lymphoma with occasional fine intracytoplasmic granules associated with an intestinal mass, likely enteropathy-associated T-cell lymphoma (Fig. 4.71)

Large Cell (≥3 × RBC Diameter) Lymphoma

Diffuse large B-cell lymphoma. Lymphoma of B-cell origin often arises from the follicular region of the cortex becoming diffusely infiltrative, hence the name *diffuse large B-cell lymphoma* (DLBCL). Follicular cells have a round nucleus, fine

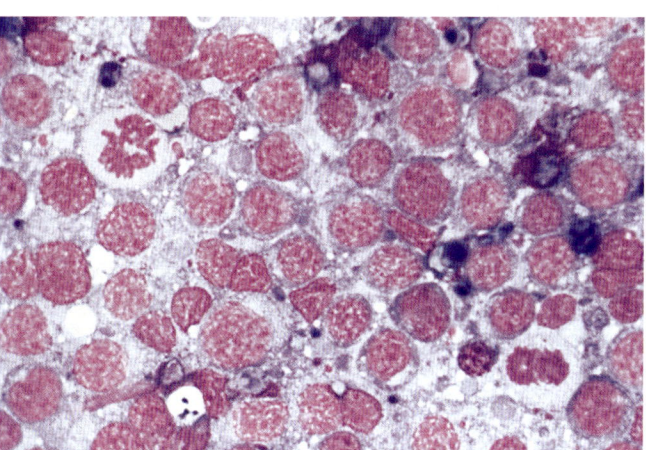

FIGURE 4.67 T-cell lymphoblastic lymphoma. Lymph node aspirate. Dog. The number of mitotic figures often exceeds 6 per 10 fields at 40× or 50× objectives. Cells have scant cytoplasm and nucleoli that are indistinct. (Wright-Giemsa; HP oil.)

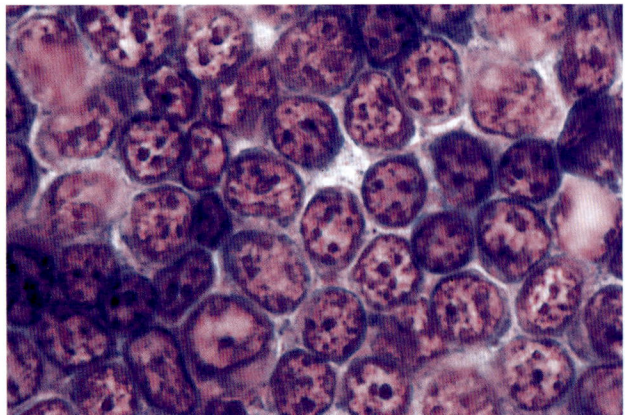

■ **FIGURE 4.68 T-cell lymphoblastic lymphoma. Lymph node aspirate. Dog.** Use of a wet mount procedure easily demonstrates the round or irregularly round nuclear shape and the presence of small multiple nucleoli. (New methylene blue; HP oil.)

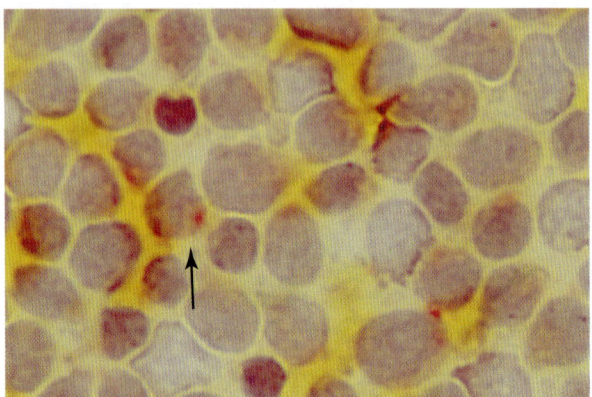

■ **FIGURE 4.69 T-cell lymphoblastic lymphoma. Lymph node aspirate. Dog. Cytochemistry.** Note the prominent focal staining of some lymphocytes *(arrow)*. Most of the other lymphocytes have weak focal staining. (Acid phosphatase; HP oil.)

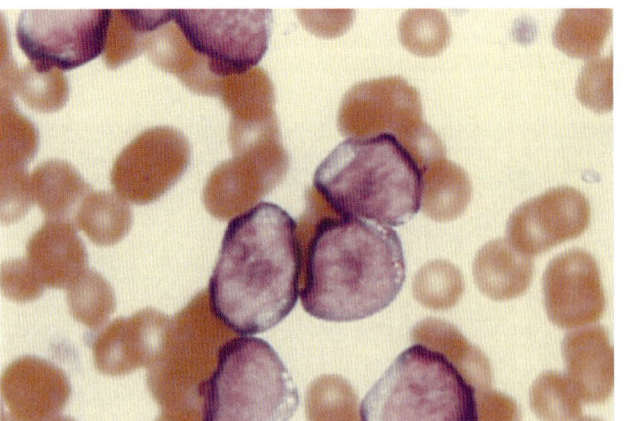

■ **FIGURE 4.70 T-cell lymphoblastic leukemia. Peripheral blood smear. Dog.** This 6-month-old English bulldog presented with anemia, thrombocytopenia, and marked leukocytosis (298,000/μL) of which most were immature lymphoid cells with irregularly round nuclei. Note the small, prominent nucleoli and fine chromatin within the nucleus. Besides the blood, involvement included the bone marrow and several peripheral lymph nodes. Clinical staging was Vb, and the disease was highly aggressive with survival of 17 days after initial diagnosis. (Wright-Giemsa; HP oil.)

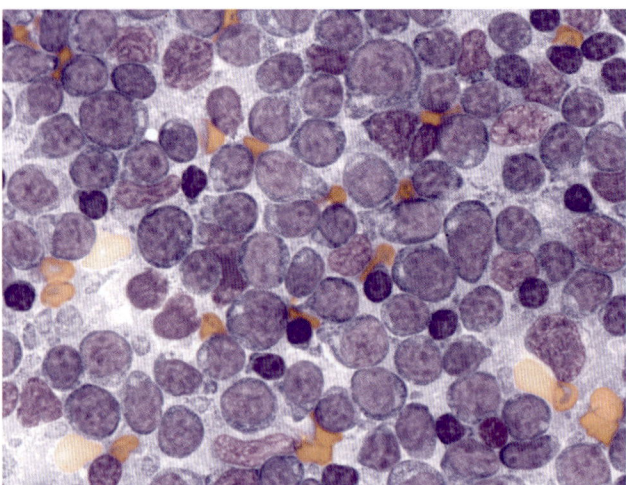

■ **FIGURE 4.71 Enteropathy-associated T-cell lymphoma. Mesenteric lymph node aspirate. Dog.** Clinically, the dog presented with evidence of intestinal thickening. A marked expansion of medium-sized lymphocytes within focal areas comprises approximately 60% to 65% of the lymphoid population. They have distinct cytoplasmic borders and a small amount of medium or deeply basophilic cytoplasm that in a few cells contains poorly visible fine eosinophilic granules. The round, oval, or convoluted eccentric nucleus is approximately 2 to 2.5 times RBC diameter with clumped chromatin and rarely one or two, round or oval, faintly distinct nucleoli. Few small and large lymphocytes are found. (Wright-Giemsa; HP oil.) (Courtesy Tracie Guy, University of Florida.)

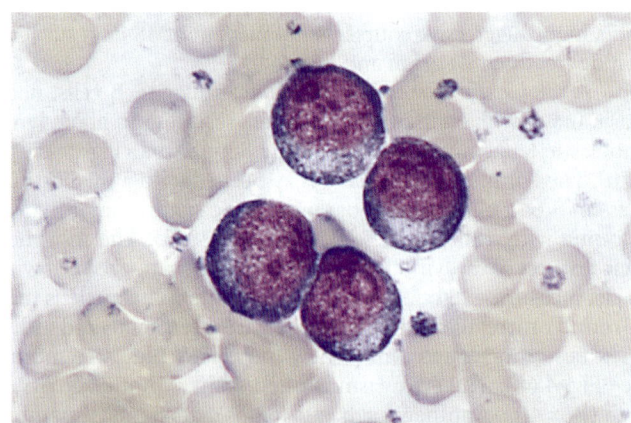

■ **FIGURE 4.72 Diffuse large B-cell lymphoma, monomorphic. Lymph node aspirate. Dog.** These medium to large cells have a round nucleus, fine chromatin pattern, and two to four small prominent and generally marginally placed nucleoli. The cytoplasm is scant and deeply basophilic. Immunostaining was positive for CD21, CD79a, and IgG. (Wright-Giemsa; HP oil.)

chromatin pattern, and prominent nucleoli and immunophenotyping supports B-cell origin (Figs. 4.72 to 4.76). The cytoplasm is scant to moderate and deeply basophilic with often a pale paranuclear area (Golgi zone). Cells may range in size to mostly large with occasional medium-sized cells. There may be one large, centrally placed nucleolus, but the large nuclear size differentiates this from marginal zone cells (see Figs. 4.75A and 4.76A), and mitotic counts are often high (see Fig. 4.76A). It is common to see frequent macrophages and lymphoglandular bodies from the fragile cells with high turnover (see Fig. 4.76).

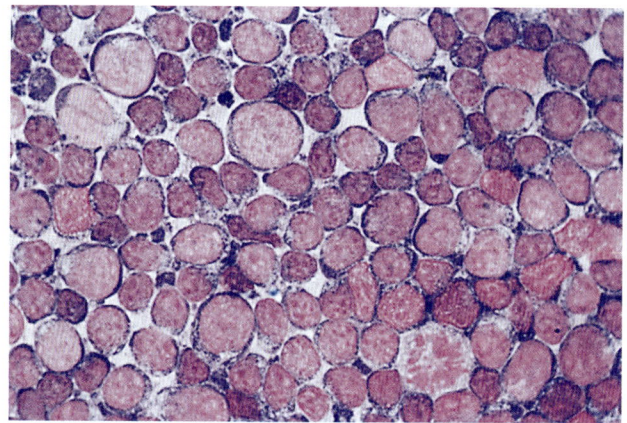

■ **FIGURE 4.73 Diffuse large B-cell lymphoma, polymorphic. Lymph node aspirate. Dog.** The lymphoid cell population contains an increased number of large blasts. Note the mitotic figure at the bottom of the field. Mitotic activity was high in this case. Immunostaining was positive for CD79a and IgG. (Wright-Giemsa; HP oil.)

The presence of the highly active macrophages within the densely cellular and basophilic cytoplasm gives rise to the expression of "starry sky" (see Fig. 4.76B).

In a canine study (Raskin and Fox, 2003), 30 of 62 lymphomas with these morphologies were diagnosed as DLBCL using the WHO classification. In this study, prognosis of DLBCL defined as survival after diagnosis differed within this group based on clinical substaging. Those dogs without signs of illness (substage a) had an indolent course with a median survival of 314 days compared with those displaying signs of illness (substage b), having a highly aggressive course and a median survival of only 24 days. Subtypes of DLBCL include T-cell rich or histiocytic rich forms.

Peripheral T-cell lymphoma. Peripheral T-cell lymphoma is a common morphology and accounted for nearly 40% of all T-cell lymphoma cases evaluated in one study (Fournel-Fleury et al., 2002). Twelve of 30 cases with peripheral T-cell lymphoma in this study presented with hypercalcemia, a common paraneoplastic condition with lymphomas of T-cell origin. This tumor

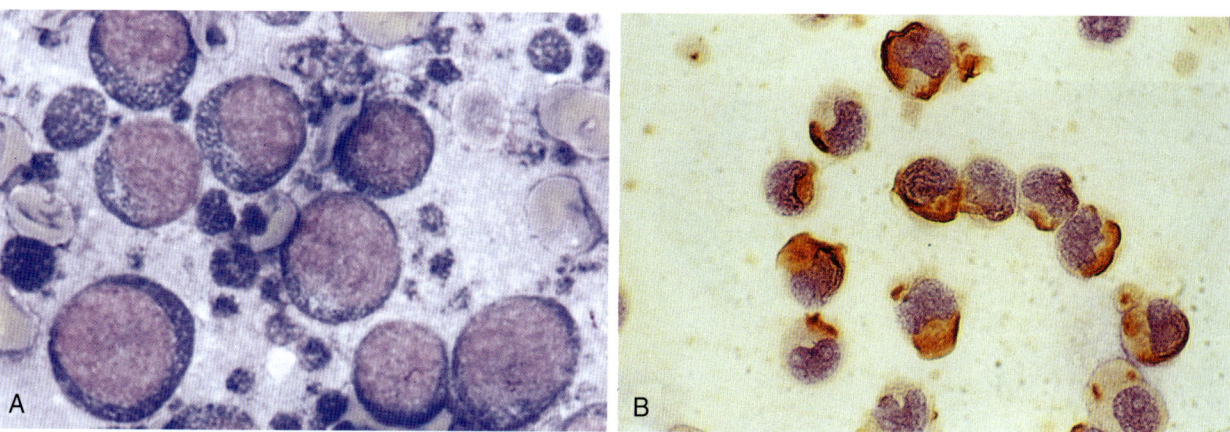

■ **FIGURE 4.74 Diffuse large B-cell lymphoma, polymorphic. Lymph node aspirate. Dog.** Same case in A and B. **A,** Prominent nucleoli can be seen in several cells. Numerous lymphoglandular bodies are present in the background. Immunostaining was positive for CD21, CD79a, and IgG. (Wright-Giemsa; HP oil.) **B, Lymph node aspirate cytocentrifuge specimen. Immunocytochemistry.** Positive immunoreactivity is indicated by dark-brown granular staining of the cytoplasm. (IgG/DAB; HP oil.)

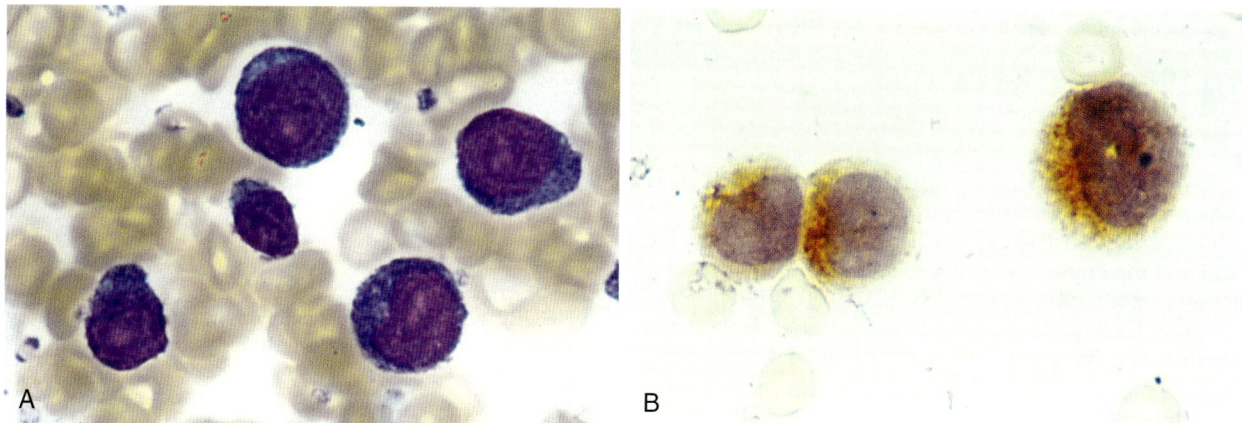

■ **FIGURE 4.75 Diffuse large B-cell lymphoma, polymorphic. Lymph node aspirate. Dog.** Same case in A and B. **A, Lymph node aspirate.** Several medium to large lymphoid cells are present, each containing one large centrally placed nucleolus. Immunostaining was positive for CD79a. (Wright-Giemsa; HP oil.) **B, Lymph node aspirate cytocentrifuge specimen. Immunocytochemistry.** Positive immunoreactivity is indicated by diffuse brown granular staining of the cytoplasm. (CD79a/DAB; HP oil.)

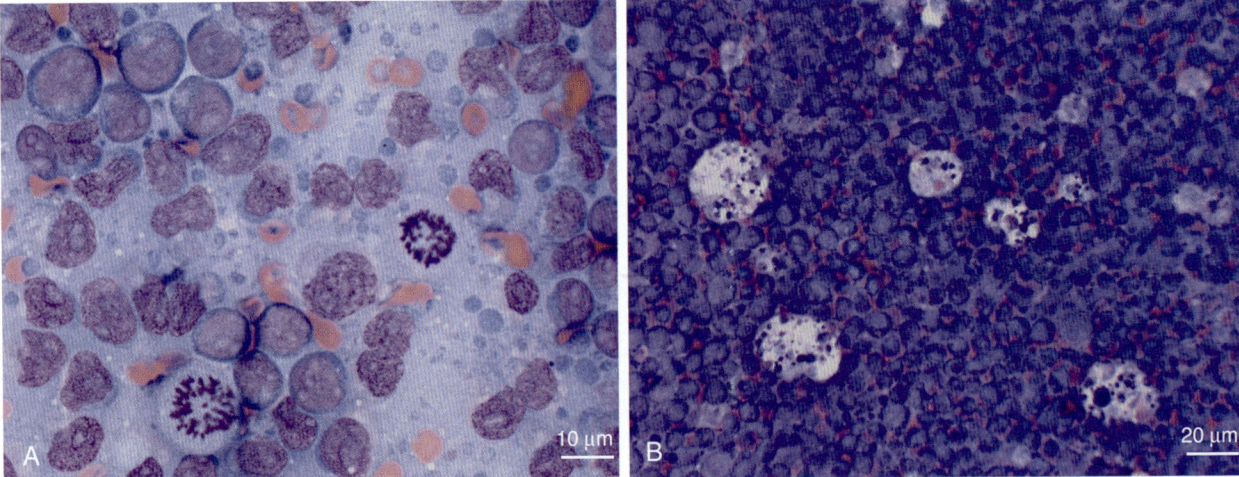

FIGURE 4.76 Diffuse large B-cell lymphoma. Mandibular lymph node aspirate. Dog. Same case in A and B. **A,** Among the lysed cells in the background are a uniform population of large (3 × RBC diameter) lymphocytes that display moderate anisocytosis and anisokaryosis. Cells have a round to oval nucleus with one to three prominent nucleoli and stippled chromatin with deeply basophilic cytoplasm. Frequent mitotic figures are seen. (Wright-Giemsa; HP oil.) **B,** Against the densely cellular neoplastic lymphoid cell population are several clear or lighter staining macrophages containing cellular debris, termed "starry sky." (Wright-Giemsa; HP oil.) (Courtesy Hiroyuki Mochizuki, North Carolina State University.)

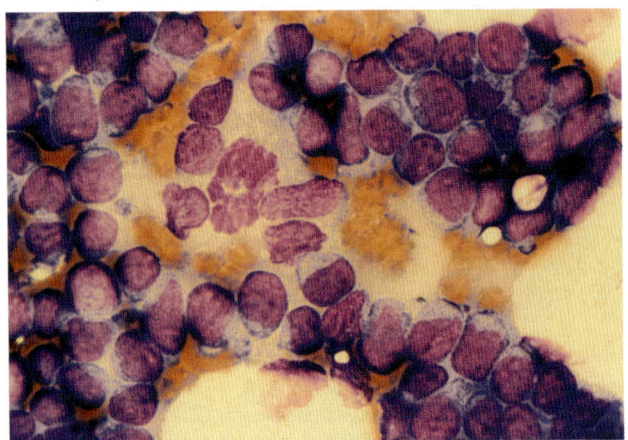

FIGURE 4.77 Peripheral T-cell lymphoma. Lymph node aspirate. Dog. Medium-sized lymphocytes predominate, displaying nuclear pleomorphism. Note the irregular nuclear shape, often with multiple indentations or serrations on one side. Chromatin is finely granular, and nucleoli are prominent in the large lymphocytes. The cytoplasm is moderately abundant and lightly basophilic. Immunostaining was positive for CD3 antigen. (Wright-Giemsa; HP oil.)

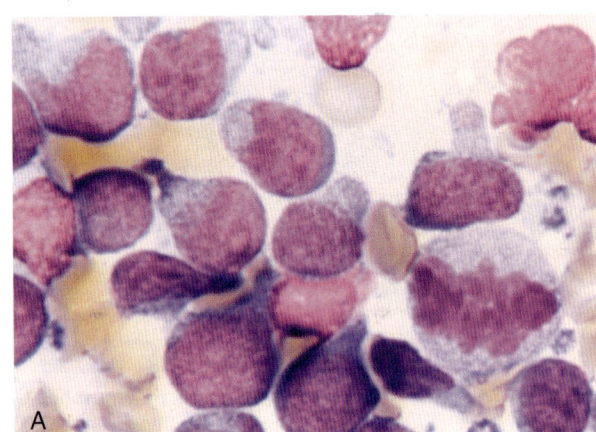

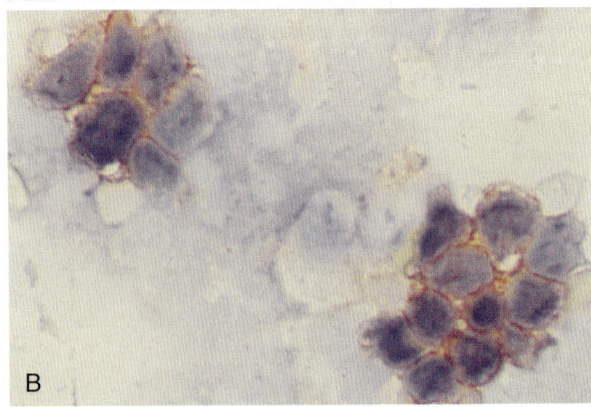

FIGURE 4.78 Peripheral T-cell lymphoma. Lymph node cytopathologic specimen. Dog. Same case in A and B. **A,** Notice the frequent serrated margins of the nuclei. This convoluted appearance of the nucleus is a distinctive morphologic feature of some T cells. Nucleoli are also prominent in this case. (Wright-Giemsa; HP oil.) **B, Lymph node cytocentrifuge preparation. Immunocytochemistry.** The cell surface CD3 is expressed using aminoethylcarbazole reaction. These cells also expressed CD45RA, an isoform of CD45 found on some B cells and nodal T-cell lymphomas. (CD3/AEC; HP oil.)

is composed of medium, large, or mixed medium and large cells that display considerable nuclear pleomorphism (Figs. 4.77 and 4.78). Often the nucleus is convex and smooth on one side, whereas the opposite side is concave with many irregular indentations or serrations and may be described as cerebriform (Figs. 4.79 and 4.80). Nucleoli are large and of variable shape and number. The cytoplasm is moderately abundant and moderately basophilic. Acid phosphatase focal staining can be observed in peripheral T-cell lymphoma in animals (Fig. 4.81). Eosinophilia may be associated with this subtype in people. In the human WHO classification, most forms of nodal T-cell lymphomas fall into the peripheral T-cell lymphoma, not otherwise specified category. In addition to CD3 immunoreactivity

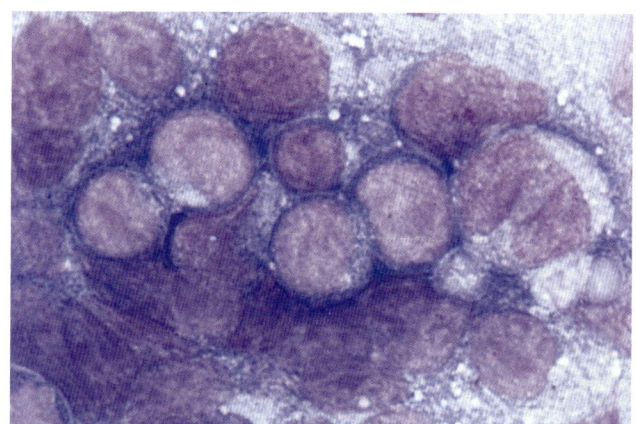

■ **FIGURE 4.79 Peripheral T-cell lymphoma. Lymph node aspirate. Dog.** The predominant cell population is medium sized with multiple convolutions of the nucleus. Nucleoli are indistinct. Immunostaining was positive for CD3 and CD8. (Wright-Giemsa; HP oil.)

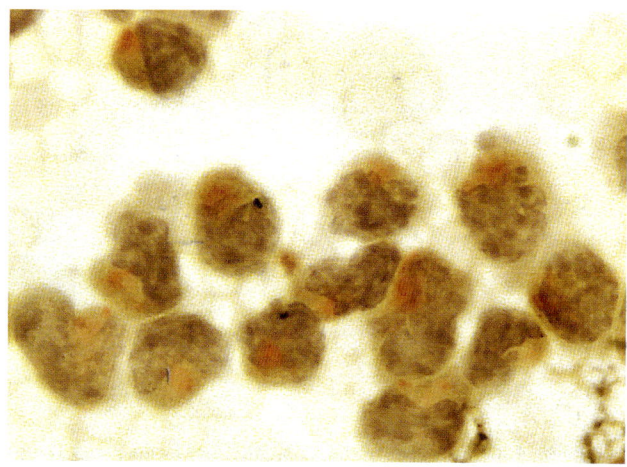

■ **FIGURE 4.81 Peripheral T-cell lymphoma. Cytopathologic specimen. Cytochemistry. Dog.** Focal red staining indicates a strong positive reaction associated with T cells. (Acid phosphatase; HP oil.)

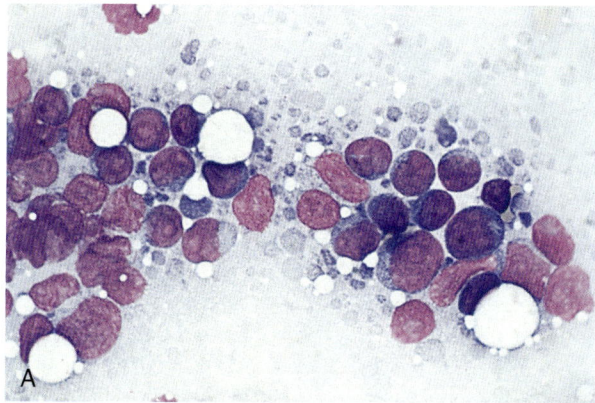

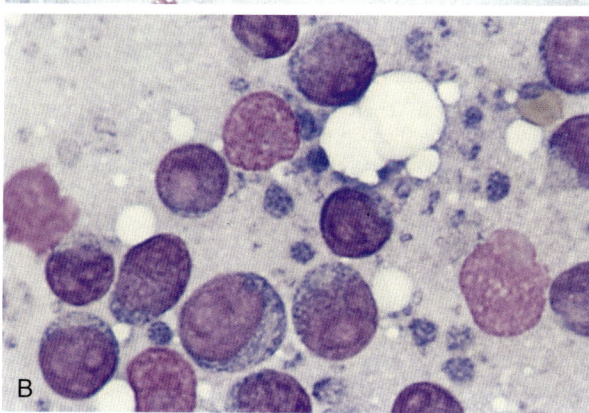

■ **FIGURE 4.80 Peripheral T-cell lymphoma. Lymph node aspirate.** Same case in A and B. **A,** Several large cells are present, with a single large, centrally placed nucleolus. Immunostaining was positive for CD3. (Wright-Giemsa; HP oil.) **B,** Higher magnification demonstrates the irregularly round nuclear shape and prominent nucleolus. The cytoplasm is moderately abundant and basophilic. (Wright-Giemsa; HP oil.)

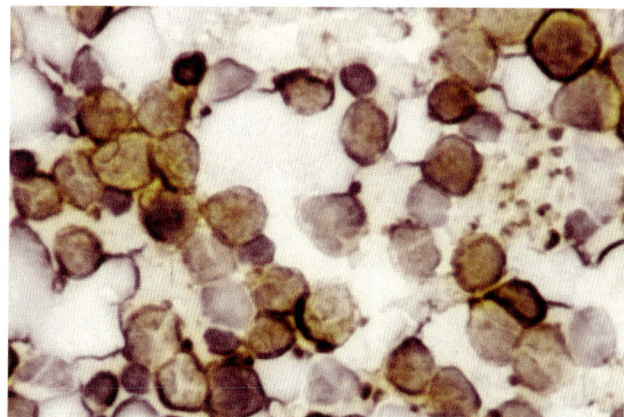

■ **FIGURE 4.82 Peripheral T-cell lymphoma. Lymph node cytopathologic specimen. Immunocytochemistry. Dog.** A strong positive reaction for expression of CD45RA is indicated by the brown cytoplasmic stain. This 8-year-old Shetland sheepdog was clinically staged as Vb and had an aggressive course of disease with a survival of 56 days. There was disease involvement of the spleen and bone marrow in addition to the lymph nodes. (CD45RA/DAB; HP oil.)

(see Fig. 4.78B), immunocytochemistry for the CD45RA isoform is often positive in nodal lymphomas (Fig. 4.82), whereas T-cell lymphomas in the skin or mucosal sites are generally negative.

Mediastinal B-cell lymphoma. Mediastinal B-cell lymphoma is an uncommon form of lymphoma thought to arise from thymic B cells from the medulla of the thymus. These masses are composed of large anaplastic cells (Fig. 4.83) having a histiocytic appearance and high mitotic activity, but they can have long survival with chemotherapy.

Hodgkin-like lymphoma. An uncommon presentation in cats and rarely in dogs is termed Hodgkin-like lymphoma. These cases usually involve a single lymph node around the head and neck or mediastinum (Walton and Hendrick, 2001; Steinberg and Keating, 2008). A distinguishing feature is the pleomorphic appearance of the cell population, especially the presence of a large single (Hodgkin) cell or multinucleated (Reed-Sternberg) lacunar cells, which are immunoreactive to CD79a, Pax5, and BLA36 (Newton et al., 2014) (Figs. 4.84 and 4.85).

> **KEY POINT** Lymphoma cells vary in size, shape, chromatin density, nucleolar features, and cytoplasmic characteristics. In addition to cellular morphology, attention should be given to immunophenotype, clonality, sites involved, and histology, especially when populations are heterogeneous, to best define the clinical behavior and therefore prognosis.

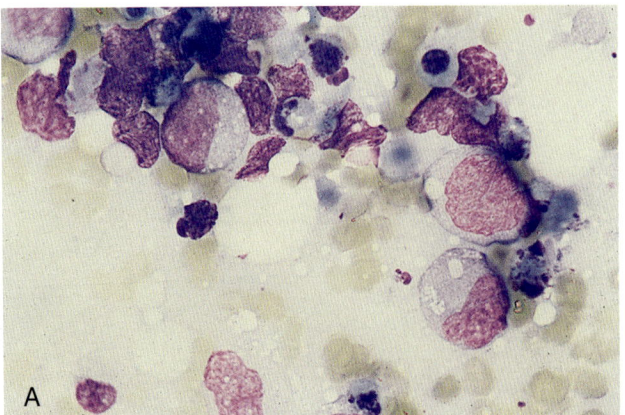
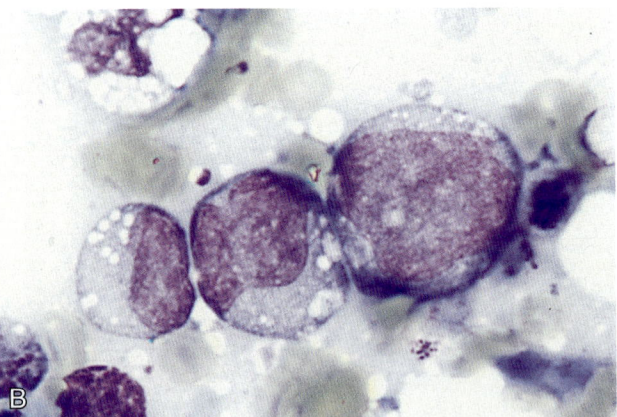

■ **FIGURE 4.83 Primary mediastinal (thymic) large B-cell lymphoma. Tissue aspirate. Dog.** Same case in A and B. **A,** Among the necrotic debris, several large intact cells are found that have histiocytic features based on their morphology with vacuolation. This 3-year-old Bassett hound was found to have a mediastinal mass with pleural fluid as well as lung and peripheral node involvement. Immunostaining was positive for IgG. (Wright-Giemsa; HP oil.) **B,** Note the large, variably sized anaplastic appearing cells with cytoplasmic vacuolation. Mitotic index was high (not shown). (Wright-Giemsa; HP oil.)

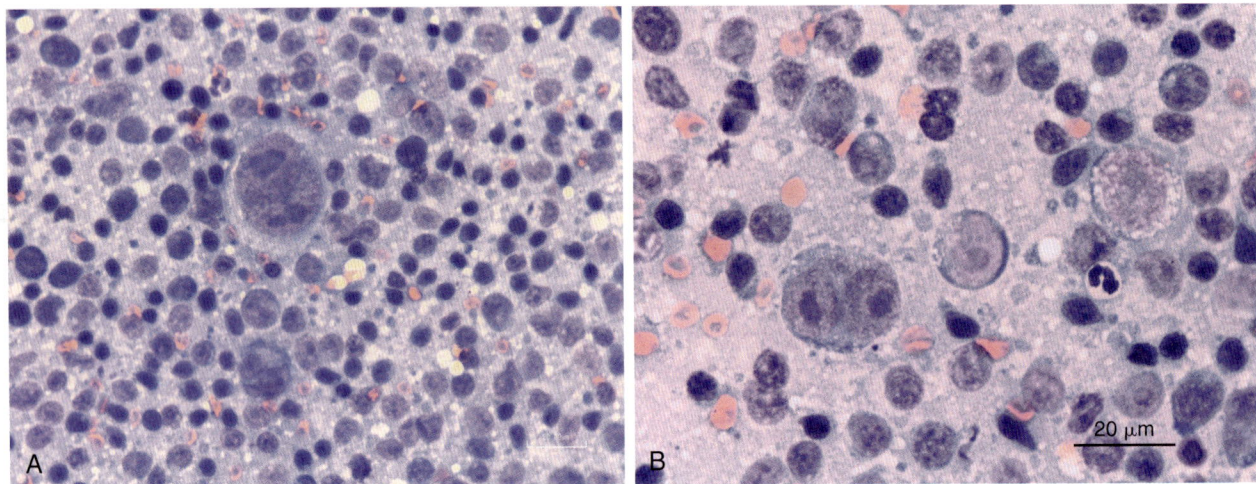

■ **FIGURE 4.84 Hodgkin-like lymphoma. Mediastinal lymph node aspirate. Cat.** Same case in A and B. **A,** Mixed cell population with increased numbers of medium and large lymphoid cells. Note the extremely large binucleated Reed-Sternberg cell in the center and a multinucleate cell just below it. (Romanowsky; HP oil.) **B,** Another field showing the mixed cells with the "owl-eyed" nuclei of a Reed-Sternberg cell. The cat had localized enlargement of one mandibular lymph node and a mediastinal lymph node. (Romanowsky; HP oil.)

Other Primary Neoplasia of Lymph Nodes

Rarely, vascular tumors arising from the lymph node have been reported. HogenEsch and Hahn (1998) described eight hemangiomas and one lymphangioma, mostly in the popliteal lymph node of aged dogs from a research colony, found as incidental lesions at postmortem. Stromal cell neoplasms may be considered, although they are very uncommon.

Metastasis to the Lymph Node

Metastasis is suggested by the presence of a cell population not normally expected in a lymph node, which for epithelial cells is relatively easier to detect because of their large cell size and clustered appearance (Figs. 4.86 and 4.87). These foreign cells often appear larger than surrounding lymphocytes and abnormal, displaying several cytopathologic features of malignancy (Fig. 4.86B). Histologically, metastasis to the lymph node may occur at the peripheral sinus or medullary sinuses related to lymphatic spread (Fig. 4.88).

Mesenchymal-appearing neoplasms are most difficult to recognize because of their individualized cell presentation. The presence of anaplastic round to spindle-shaped cells in a lymph node aspirate can support a diagnosis of malignancy (Fig. 4.89) (Desnoyers and St-Germain, 1994). Tumors such as melanoma may be easily confused with hemosiderin-laden macrophages (Grindem, 1994) (see Fig. 4.45A) related to the presence dark blue-black granules. Hemosiderin granules tend to be variable in size, large, and coarse compared with melanin granules that are small and finely granular (Fig. 4.90). Cytochemical staining, such as Fontana stain for melanin and Prussian blue for iron (Fig. 4.91), may be necessary to distinguish the two. Furthermore, immunochemistry may be helpful in amelanotic cases that lack visible granules (Fig. 4.92A) using markers such as S-100, Melan-A (Fig. 4.92B), PNL2, and others

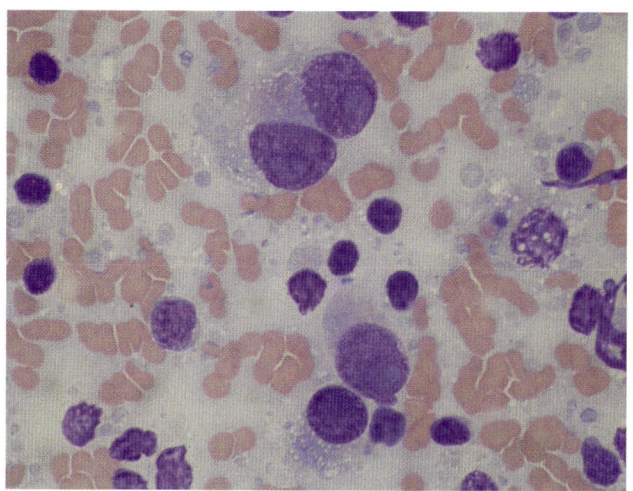

■ **FIGURE 4.85** **Hodgkin-like lymphoma. Cervical lymph node aspirate. Cat.** There is a mixed lymphocyte population composed of mostly small with lesser numbers of medium lymphocytes. Low to moderate numbers of atypical large to irregularly shaped cells measuring approximately 5 times RBC diameter are noted. Nuclei are round or oval with coarse chromatin; multinucleate variants of these cells is shown. These cells frequently contain one prominent round nucleolus. Histopathology supported the diagnosis. PARR test did not support clonality. (Modified Wright; HP oil.) (Courtesy David Buckeridge, TDDS, Synlab, Exeter, UK.)

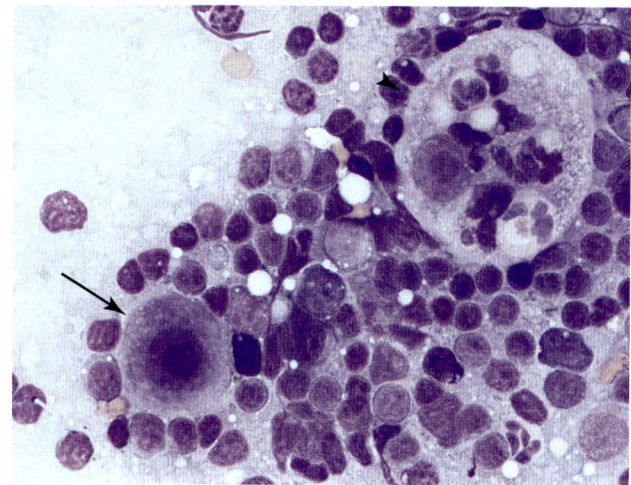

■ **FIGURE 4.87** **Metastatic squamous cell carcinoma. Mandibular lymph node aspirate. Dog.** Two large neoplastic squamous epithelial cells *(arrow and arrowhead)* stand out among the mixed lymphocytes (reactive lymphoid hyperplasia). These cells exhibit anisocytosis, have an increased and variable nucleocytoplasmic ratio, and have macronucleoli *(arrow)*. Emperipolesis was observed in a neoplastic squamous epithelial cell *(arrowhead)*. Emperipolesis is the presence of an intact cell within the cytoplasm of another cell. The engulfed cell (neutrophil) remains viable within the other and can exit at any time without causing structural or functional abnormalities in either cell. The biological process is not understood and has no known diagnostic importance. (Wright; HP oil.) (Courtesy Shannon Hostetter, Iowa State University.)

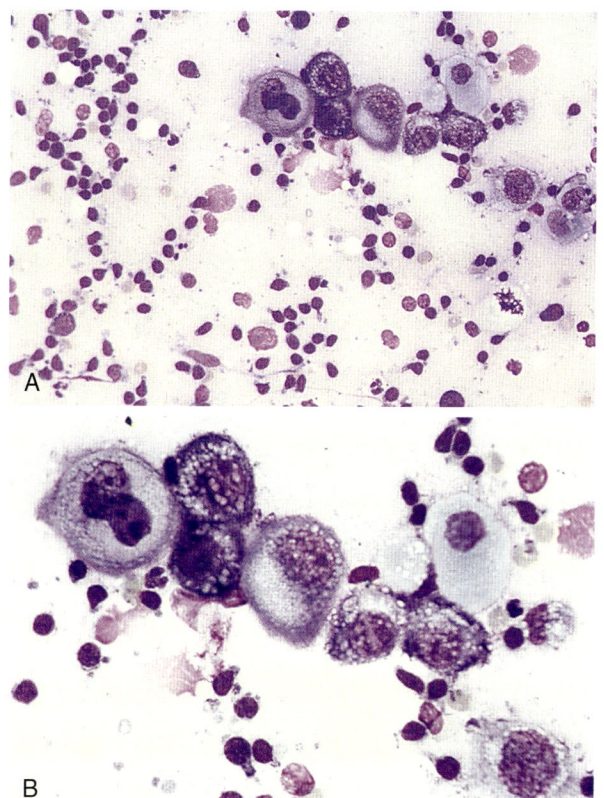

■ **FIGURE 4.86** **Metastatic squamous cell carcinoma. Lymph node aspirate. Dog.** Same case in A and B. **A,** A sheet of neoplastic squamous epithelium is surrounded by numerous small lymphocytes. (Wright-Giemsa; HP oil.) **B,** Higher magnification demonstrates the marked pleomorphism of the nuclei, coarse chromatin staining, and multiple, prominent, variably sized nucleoli. (Wright-Giemsa; HP oil.)

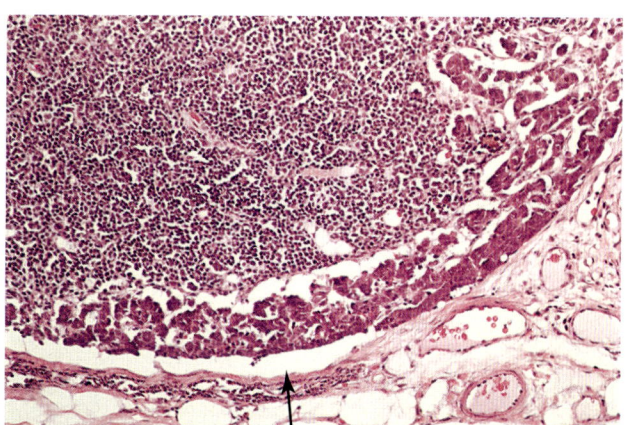

■ **FIGURE 4.88** **Metastatic carcinoma. Lymph node. Tissue section. Dog.** Neoplastic population has infiltrated the cortex beginning at the subcapsular sinus region *(arrow)*. (H&E; IP.)

(see Chapter 18). Use of Iba1 or lysozyme helps to distinguish melanophages from melanocytes when melanin in both of these cells is immunoreactive for Melan-A and PNL2 (Grossi et al., 2015). Agreement between cytopathologic and histopathologic assessment for lymph node metastasis for canine melanomas is overall poor and metastasis did not appear to correlate with survival in one study (Grimes et al., 2017).

Metastases from sarcomas are often difficult to discern among the normal reticular stromal elements. However, angiosarcomas have distinctive, large, individualized cells that may be prominent against the small lymphocytes (Fig. 4.93). Another

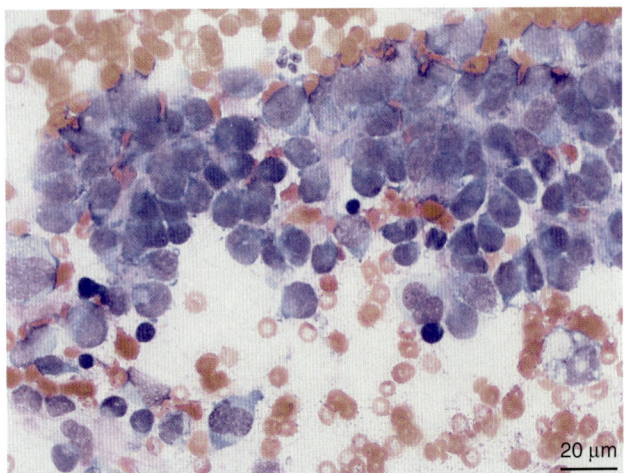

■ **FIGURE 4.89 Metastatic fibrosarcoma. Mandibular lymph node aspirate. Dog.** The dog had a previous diagnosis of fibrosarcoma. A moderately atypical mesenchymal cell population predominates arranged both in variably sized aggregates and individually throughout the preparation. The mesenchymal cells are stellate, fusiform, or irregularly oval; have variably indistinct cytoplasmic borders; and have a small to moderate amount of pale to moderately basophilic cytoplasm that frequently forms wispy projections. The round or oval nucleus is variably placed, measures roughly 1.5 to 3 times RBC diameter, and has stippled to coarse chromatin with usually one to three, round to oval, discernible nucleoli that vary in size. The overall anisocytosis and anisokaryosis among this population are mild to moderate; the nucleocytoplasmic ratio is moderate to high. A heterogeneous lymphoid population is also present composed of mostly small lymphocytes. (Wright-Giemsa; HP oil.) (Courtesy Kellie Whipple, University of Florida.)

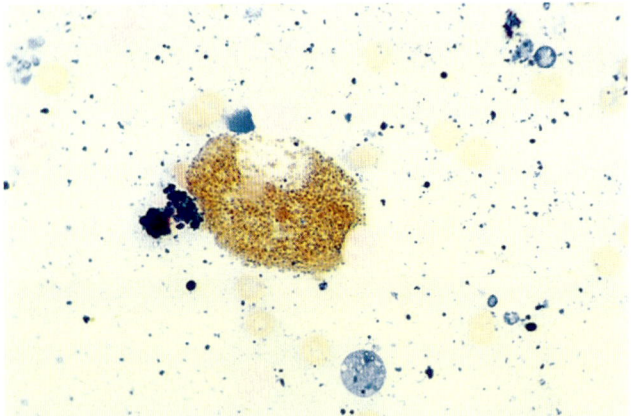

■ **FIGURE 4.91 Metastatic melanoma. Lymph node aspirate. Cytochemistry. Dog.** An iron stain helps to distinguish positive-staining background hemosiderin from a nonstaining cell containing melanin granules. Hemorrhage is often present in metastatic lesions. (Prussian blue; HP oil.)

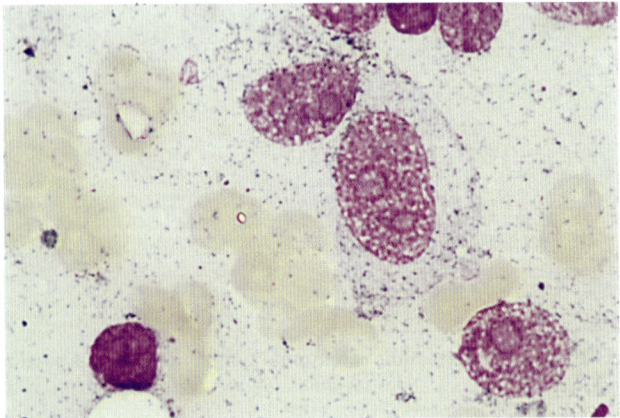

■ **FIGURE 4.90 Metastatic melanoma. Lymph node aspirate. Dog.** Fine black granules define the cell of origin. Prominent multiple nucleoli are also noted. Small lymphocytes are present in the background. (Aqueous Romanowsky; HP oil.)

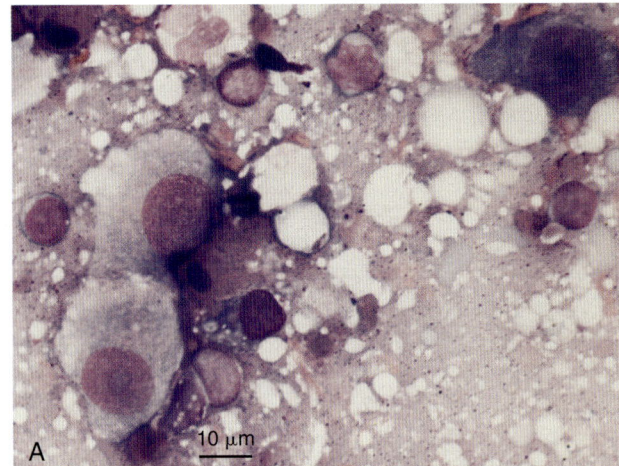

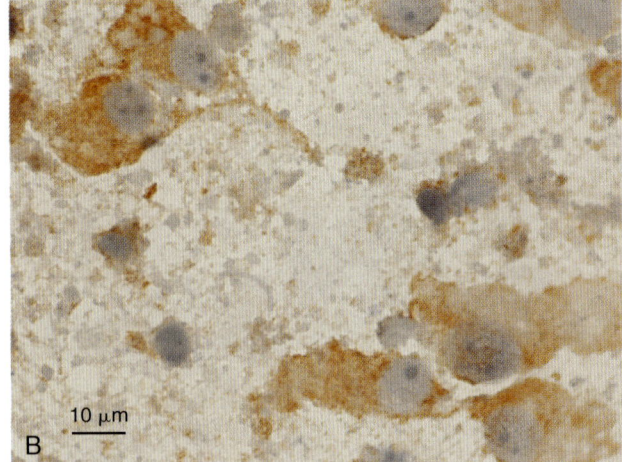

■ **FIGURE 4.92 Metastatic amelanotic melanoma. Lymph node aspirate. Cat.** Same case in A and B. **A,** Multiple masses on the leg and back with metastasis to regional lymph nodes. Shown are three large, poorly differentiated melanoma cells with prominent nucleoli against a background of small and medium lymphocytes. (Wright; HP oil.) **B, Immunocytochemistry.** The cytoplasm of several large neoplastic cells with prominent nucleoli is positive for Melan-A, a sensitive marker for melanin. A few small lymphocytes are unstained. (Melan-A/AEC; HP oil.)

sarcoma that is distinctive even when it has metastasized is the rhabdomyosarcoma. With multiple nuclei in a row, the *strap cell* is quite visible (Fig. 4.94). Demonstration of the presence of metastatic osteosarcoma in a regional lymph node can be assisted by the use of alkaline phosphatase staining as individual cells are then readily seen (see Appendix 2).

Metastatic hematopoietic neoplasms such as granulocytic leukemia cause mild to moderate lymphadenomegaly. The cell

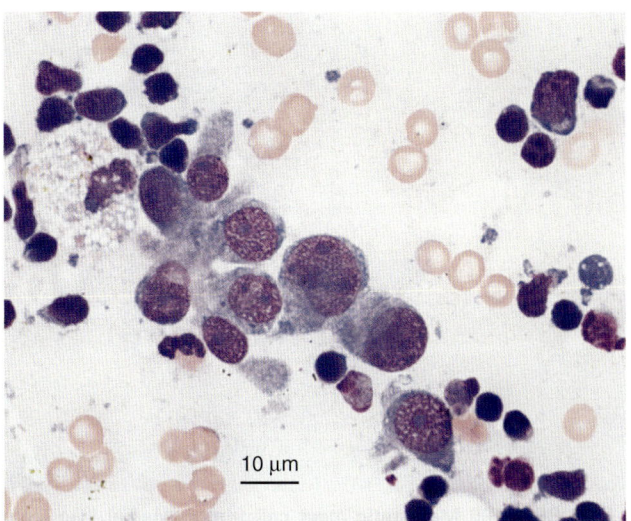

■ **FIGURE 4.93 Metastatic angiosarcoma. Popliteal lymph node aspirate. Dog.** Several large, individualized pleomorphic cells are surrounded by small lymphocytes. The original hock mass was removed 9 months earlier, but the leg presented as swollen with evidence of metastasis to the draining lymph node. (Wright; HP oil.)

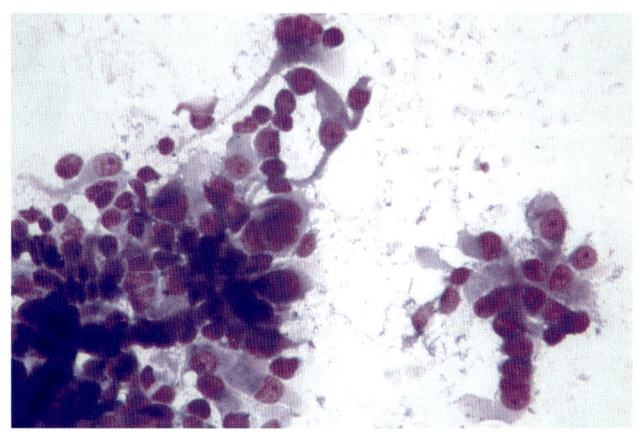

■ **FIGURE 4.94 Metastatic rhabdomyosarcoma. Lymph node aspirate. Dog.** Anaplastic mesenchymal cells in mononuclear and multinuclear forms. Note the characteristic cluster of nuclei in a linear fashion at the lower right side. (Aqueous Romanowsky; HP oil.)

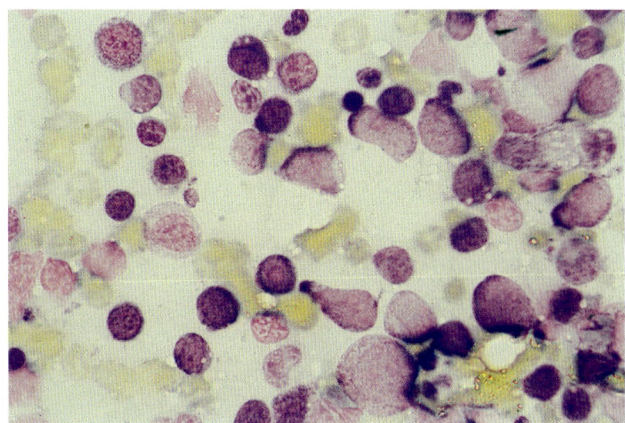

■ **FIGURE 4.95 Granulocytic leukemia. Lymph node aspirate. Dog.** Mixed cell population is present, with many large irregularly shaped myeloid precursor cells. (Wright-Giemsa; HP oil.)

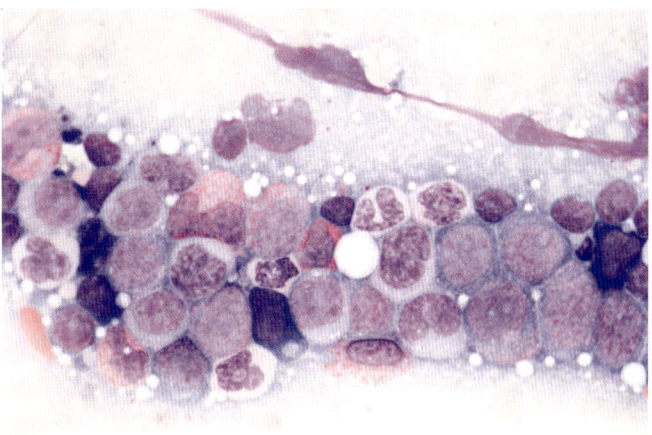

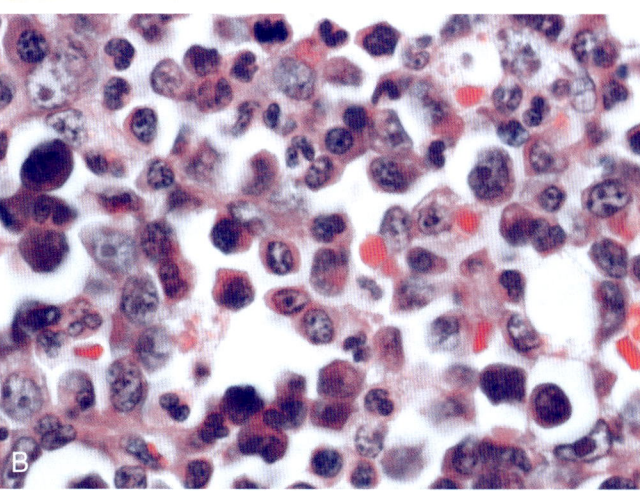

■ **FIGURE 4.96 Granulocytic leukemia. Lymph node aspirate. Dog.** Same case in A and B. **A,** Numerous large granulocytic precursors are present with evidence of maturation. (Wright-Giemsa; HP oil.) **B, Granulocytic leukemia. Lymph node. Tissue section.** Frequent presence of irregularly shaped blast cells with open chromatin and large prominent nuclei suggests myeloid origin along with segmented granulocytes. (H&E; HP oil.)

population appears mixed (Fig. 4.95), and dysplastic cells or granulated precursors may be present. In some cases, myoblasts may be indistinguishable from lymphoid precursors (Fig. 4.96A), and the histologic section often shows an increase in granulocytic precursors in various stages of maturation (Fig. 4.96B). Cytochemical staining for granulocytic origin may be indicated in poorly differentiated cases (Fig. 4.97).

Well-granulated mast cells may appear in low numbers, up to six per slide in clinically healthy dogs (Bookbinder et al., 1992), but increased cell numbers and the appearance of poorly granulated mast cells suggest metastasis (Figs. 4.98 to 4.100). The presence of eosinophils, especially in dogs, suggests degranulation and release of histamine.

Inflammation may accompany metastasis to lymphoid tissue, with eosinophils most commonly present as a paraneoplastic syndrome in canine mast cell tumors (Fig. 4.101) or some

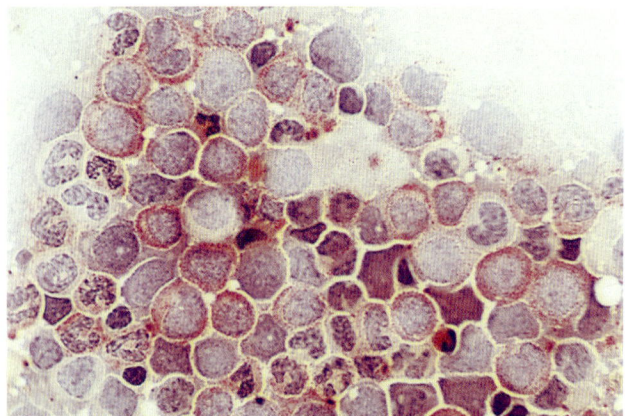

■ **FIGURE 4.97 Granulocytic leukemia. Lymph node aspirate. Cytochemistry. Dog.** Cytochemical staining is positive for this granulocytic marker. (Chloroacetate esterase; HP oil.)

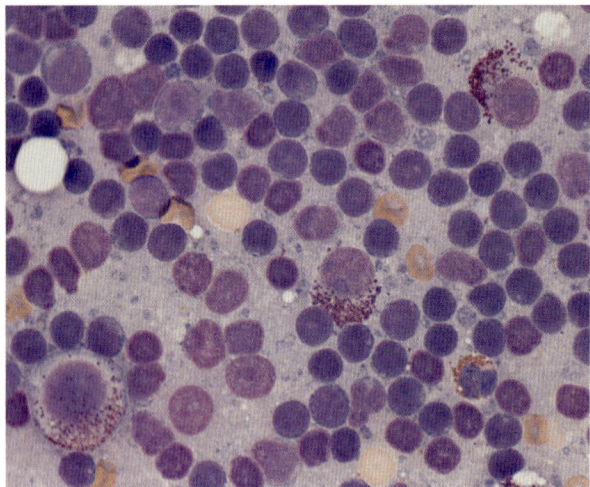

■ **FIGURE 4.98 Metastatic mast cell tumor. Lymph node aspirate. Dog.** Three mast cells and one eosinophil are shown in this submandibular lymph node draining an ulcerated mast cell tumor on the muzzle. These mast cells are moderately differentiated having prominent nucleoli and minimal granulation. The surrounding lymphoid cells are predominately small lymphocytes. (Wright; HP oil.)

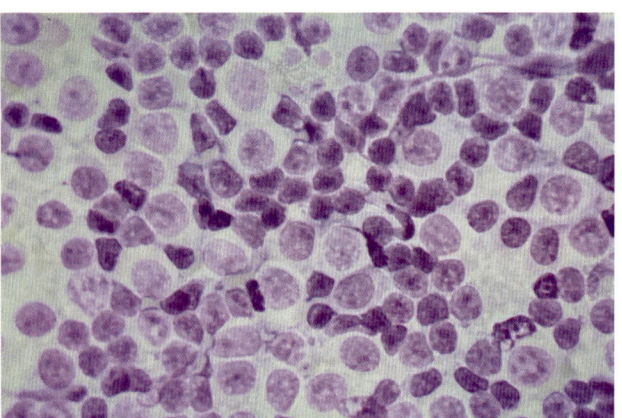

■ **FIGURE 4.99 Metastatic mast cell tumor. Lymph node aspirate. Cat.** Note the poorly granulated, round cells among the small lymphocytes, suggesting a poorly differentiated mast cell tumor. (Aqueous Romanowsky; HP oil.)

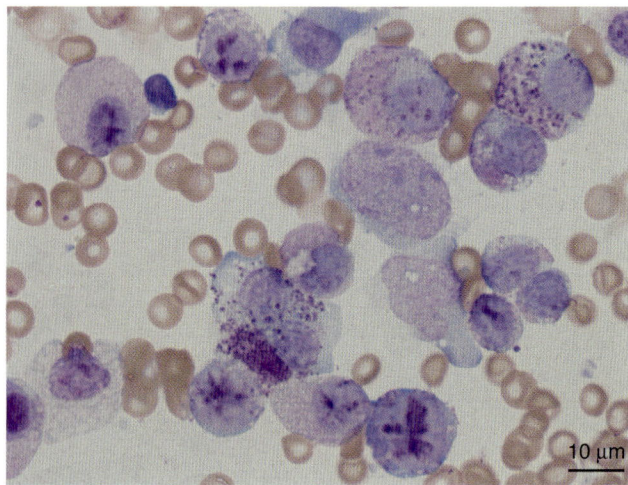

■ **FIGURE 4.100 Metastatic mast cell tumor. Medial iliac lymph node aspirate. Dog.** On ultrasound, the lymph node was enlarged, irregular, and heterogeneous. The preparation is composed of markedly atypical individual mast cells. These cells have a moderate amount of pale basophilic, highly vacuolated cytoplasm that contains a variable and few magenta granules. The round, eccentric nucleus measures 1.5 to 2.5 × RBC diameter, with clumped chromatin and no discernible nucleolus. Some of these round cells have a small amount of deeply basophilic cytoplasm that contains a fine dusting of magenta granules and a moderate number of clear, punctate vacuoles. The malignant population displays mild to moderate anisokaryosis, multinucleation, and variable nucleocytoplasmic ratios. A heterogeneous lymphoid population is present in lesser number, predominated by small lymphocytes. (Wright-Giemsa; HP oil.) (Courtesy Jere Stern, University of Florida.)

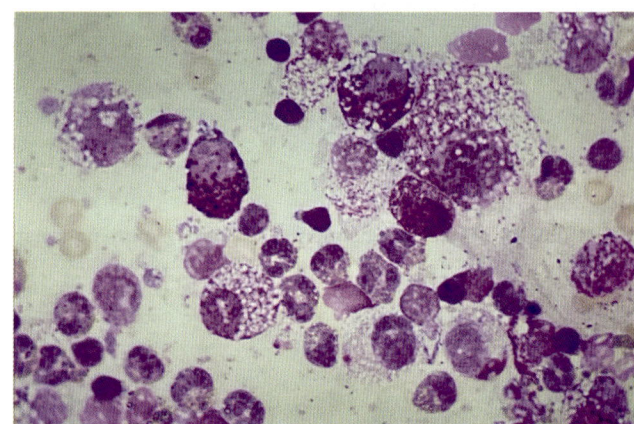

■ **FIGURE 4.101 Eosinophilic lymphadenitis. Tissue aspirate. Dog.** Numerous eosinophils are present along with several mast cells displaying variable degrees of degranulation and pleomorphism in an animal with a mast cell tumor. (Aqueous Romanowsky; HP oil.)

carcinomas (see Fig. 4.31). Neutrophils commonly occur with squamous cell carcinoma and may involve bacterial sepsis. The remaining lymphoid population in metastatic lymph nodes often appears immune stimulated, with cell types present as described under Reactive or Hyperplastic Lymph Node. Histiocytes may be part of the inflammatory reaction, especially to phagocytize cell debris and iron, but large numbers that form masses and encroach upon the cortical tissue should be considered neoplastic (Fig. 4.102).

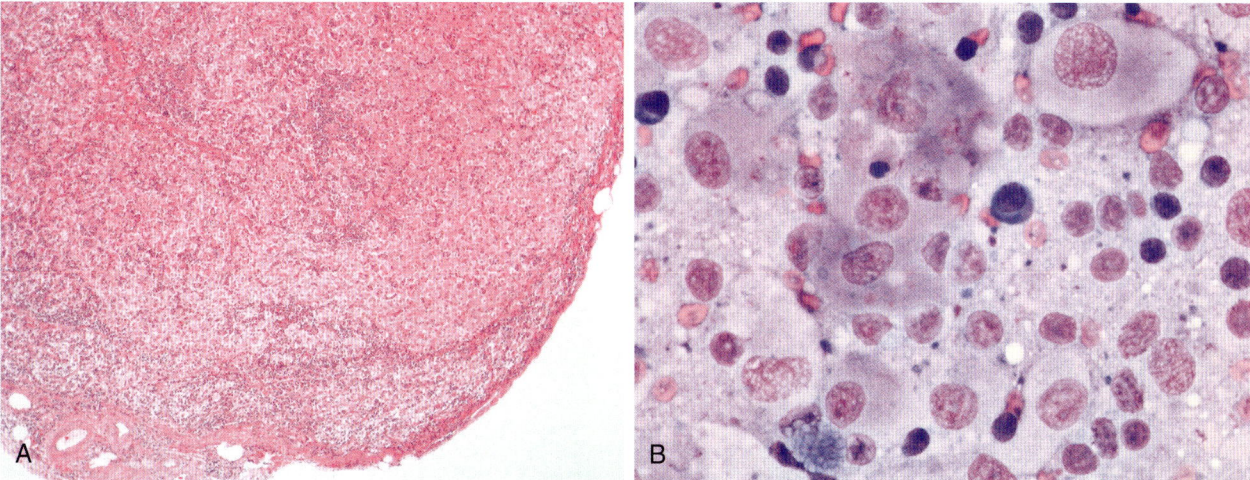

FIGURE 4.102 Metastatic histiocytic sarcoma from the colon. Mesenteric lymph node. Cat. Same case in A and B. **A, Tissue section.** There is a small remnant of remaining lymph node at the edge of the cortex. The lighter larger area is composed of malignant histiocytes. (H&E; IP.) **B, Tissue aspirate.** Numerous nonphagocytic histiocytes showing anisokaryosis displace most of the lymphocytes. (Wright-Giemsa; HP oil.)

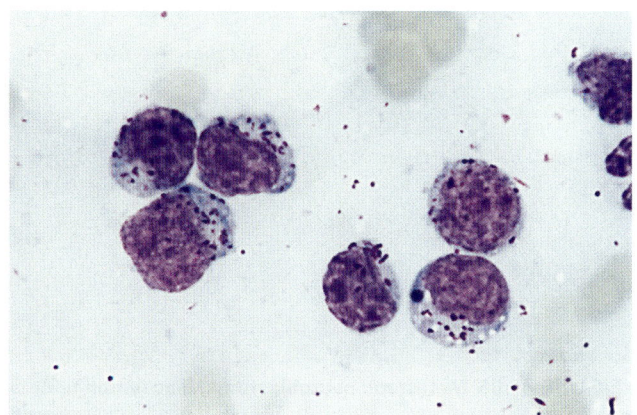

FIGURE 4.103 Metastatic large granular lymphoma. Intestinal lymph node aspirate. Cat. Nearly all cells present in this lymph node are medium sized, with moderately basophilic cytoplasm containing prominent purple granules. (Wright-Giemsa; HP oil.)

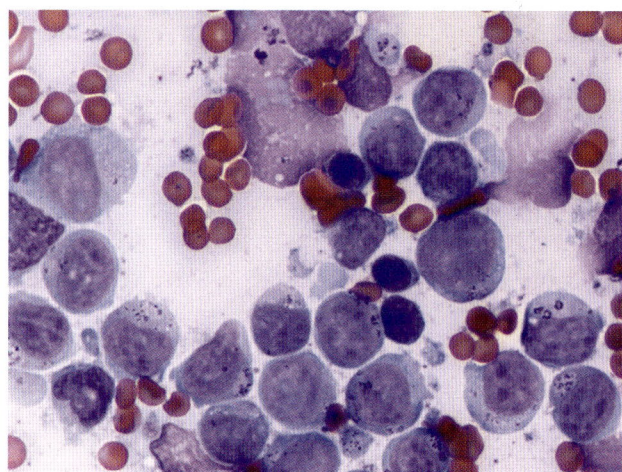

FIGURE 4.104 Metastatic large granular lymphoma. Jejunal lymph node aspirate. Cat. Patient found to have mild to moderate thickened intestines, irregular bowel loops, and enlarged and hypoechoic mesenteric lymph nodes. The majority of the nucleated cells (>80%) are a uniform population of medium to large lymphocytes that demonstrate moderate anisocytosis and anisokaryosis with a variable nucleocytoplasmic ratio. Nuclei are round to indented to irregular in shape, 2 to 4 × RBC diameter with finely to coarsely stippled chromatin and one to five variably sized and prominent nucleoli. Cells have mostly scant basophilic cytoplasm that often focally contains variable numbers of small fine to large coarse purple granules. (Modified Wright; HP oil.) (Courtesy Mary White, The Ohio State University.)

Lymphoid malignancies originating from the bone marrow or solid tissue sites such as the spleen or gastrointestinal tract may be easily recognized in lymph nodes when cells are coarsely granulated (Fig. 4.103) (Goldman and Grindem, 1997). The immunophenotypic features of feline large granular lymphocytes (LGLs) are similar to the small intestinal intraepithelial lymphocytes and hence may be the site of origin of this lymphoma in cats. These are medium to large cells with focal variably sized eosinophilic cytoplasmic granules (Fig. 4.104). The prognosis is poor for cats with LGL lymphoma, having a median survival in treated animals of 57 days (Krick et al., 2008). In dogs, by contrast, the red pulp of the spleen is the site of origin for these granular lymphocytes (Roccabianca et al., 2006). More discussion of lymphoma of canine granular lymphocytes is found under Splenic Lymphoma.

Early in the disease process, metastatic lesions will usually involve a small proportion of the entire cell population, usually less than 50%. In some cases, often late in the disease, the metastatic neoplasm may replace the lymph node parenchyma completely and interfere with the cytopathologic recognition of the tissue as lymph node (Figs. 4.105 and 4.106).

Extramedullary Hematopoiesis

Infrequently, evidence for extramedullary hematopoiesis of the erythroid, granulocytic, and/or megakaryocytic lines is found in the lymph node (Fig. 4.107). It is more likely to occur in animals having severe bone marrow disease such as myelophthisis (Santos et al., 2017).

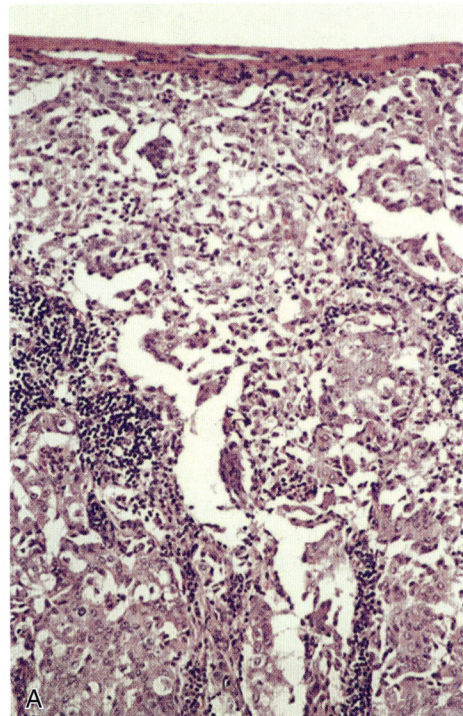

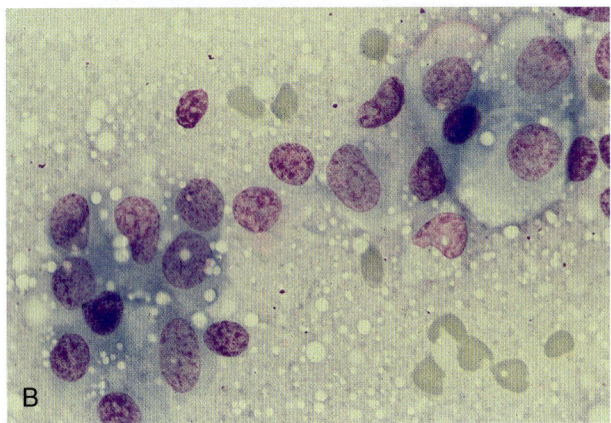

■ **FIGURE 4.105 Metastatic islet cell tumor. Gastric lymph node. Dog.** Same case in A and B. **A, Tissue section.** There is nearly complete effacement of the lymph node by an expansion of neoplastic cells. Note the remaining small, dark-staining lymphocytes at left center. (H&E; IP.) **B, Tissue imprint.** Clusters of intact cells are occasionally found, with most cells present resembling those on the left side, having naked nuclei with indistinct cell borders, typical of endocrine tissue. (Wright-Giemsa; HP oil.) (Courtesy Robin Allison et al., Colorado State University. Presented at the 1998 ASVCP case review session.)

SPLEEN

Normal Splenic Anatomy and Histology

The spleen is enclosed by a thick, smooth muscle capsule that extends inward as trabeculae (Fig. 4.108). The splenic parenchyma is divided into white pulp and red pulp. The white pulp consists of dense, periarterial lymphatic sheaths and lymphatic nodules, and the red pulp consists of erythrocytes contained within a reticular meshwork, within endothelial lined sinuses or blood vessels (Fig. 4.109A). The splenic artery enters the hilus of the spleen and branches into arteries that become the central

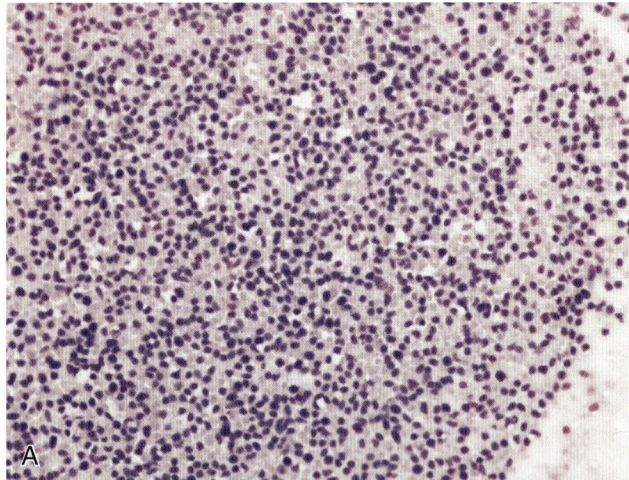

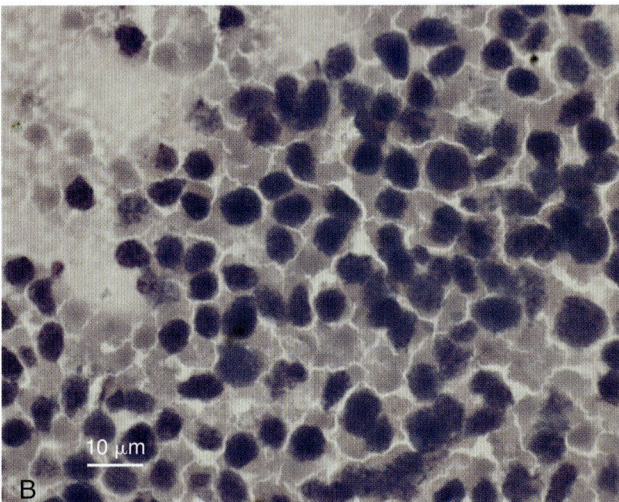

■ **FIGURE 4.106 Metastatic neuroblastoma. Iliac lymph node aspirate. Dog.** Same case in A and B. **A,** Low magnification reveals a highly cellular preparation with many individualized cells suggestive of lymphoid cells. (Wright; IP.) **B,** Higher magnification indicates that the cells appear to have more abundant pink cytoplasm than expected for lymphocytes, and there is moderate anisokaryosis. The loss of crisp nuclear features is related to necrosis occurring within this lymph node. The lack of cytoplasmic borders supports a naked nuclei appearance to the metastatic neoplasm. The primary neoplasm was found during an abdominal exploratory in which a large mass located beneath the lumbar spine incorporated the vena cava, kidney, and part of the pancreas. The mass was diagnosed as neuroblastoma in this 1.5-year-old boxer. (Wright; HP oil.)

arteries of the lymphatic sheaths. These vessels branch into pulp capillaries that are surrounded by concentric layers of macrophages within a reticular meshwork. The pericapillary macrophage sheaths, termed *ellipsoids*, are abundant in the marginal zone surrounding periarterial lymphatic sheaths adjacent to the red pulp (Fig. 4.109B).

Indications for Splenic Biopsy

- *Splenomegaly* may be detected by palpation, radiography, or ultrasonography.
- *Abnormal imaging features* such as increased nodule size (1–2 cm in diameter) and multiple number of splenic nodules, as well as presence of peritoneal fluid, suggest a higher

CHAPTER 4 Hemolymphatic System

suspicion for the presence of malignant neoplasia or inflammation (Yankin et al., 2020).
- *Evaluation of hematopoiesis* may be indicated when bone marrow disease is present.
- *Staging for disseminated neoplasia* provides prognostic tool for canine cutaneous mast cell tumor (Stefanello et al., 2009).

Splenic Aspirate Biopsy Collection

Aspiration may be performed in cases of thrombocytopenia, but body movements should be minimized by manual restraint or sedation. The needle and syringe may be coated with sterile 4% disodium ethylenediaminetetraacetic acid (EDTA) before aspiration to reduce the clotting potential of the specimen. A 1- to 1.5-inch, 21- or 22-gauge needle is used alone or attached to a hand-held 12 mL syringe or aspiration gun. In some cases, it may be preferable to use a 2.5- to 3.5-inch spinal needle. The animal is placed in right lateral or dorsal recumbency, and the area over the site is prepared surgically. The site is carefully determined by palpation or ultrasonography.

> **KEY POINT** The nonsuction method of cellular collection is preferred in vascular sites such as the spleen to reduce blood contamination and increase cellularity (LeBlanc et al., 2008).

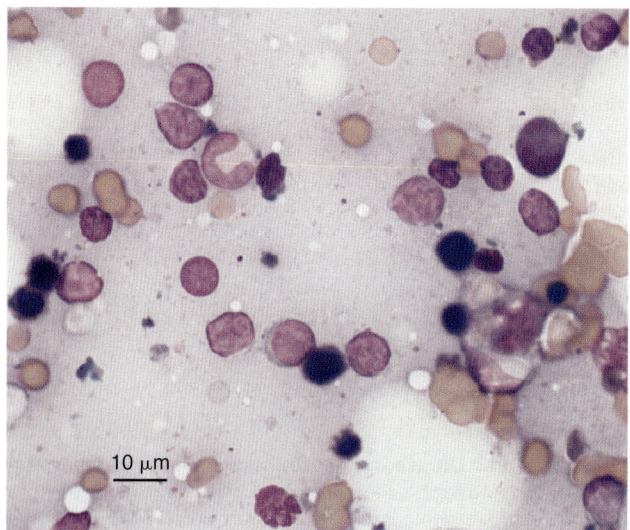

■ **FIGURE 4.107 Extramedullary hematopoiesis. Lymph node aspirate. Cat.** Among the small and medium-sized lymphocytes are variably sized, dense-staining erythroid precursors, some of which are closely associated with a macrophage displaying erythrophagocytosis. Complete blood count indicated pancytopenia with a hematocrit of 20% and lack of regeneration (i.e., polychromasia) in the blood smear. (Wright; HP oil.)

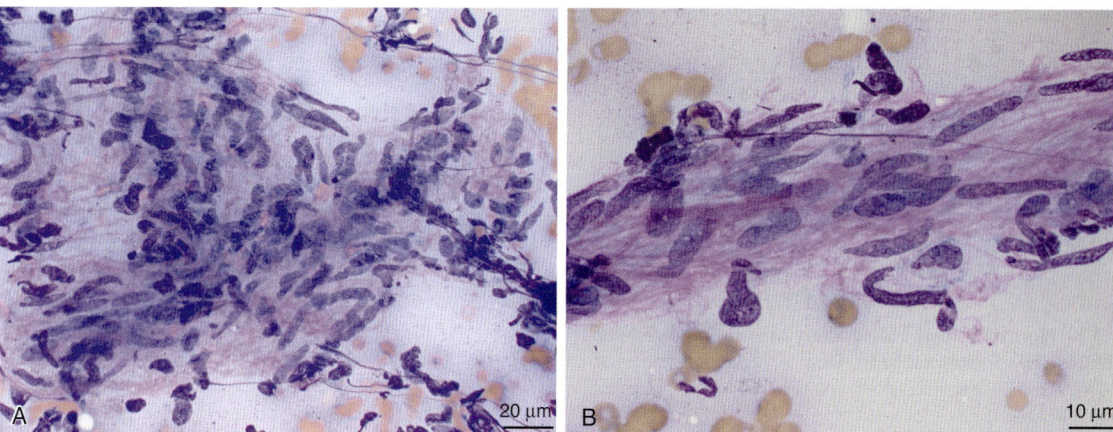

■ **FIGURE 4.108 Normal spleen. Tissue aspirate. Dog.** Same case in A and B. **A,** A uniform aggregate of mesenchymal cells is present, which likely represents splenic trabeculae composed of smooth muscle cells. (Wright-Giemsa; HP oil.) **B,** Higher magnification demonstrates the elliptical cigar-shaped nuclei within indistinct borders of pink fibrillar cytoplasm. (Wright-Giemsa; HP oil.) (Courtesy Allison Rowland, North Carolina State University.)

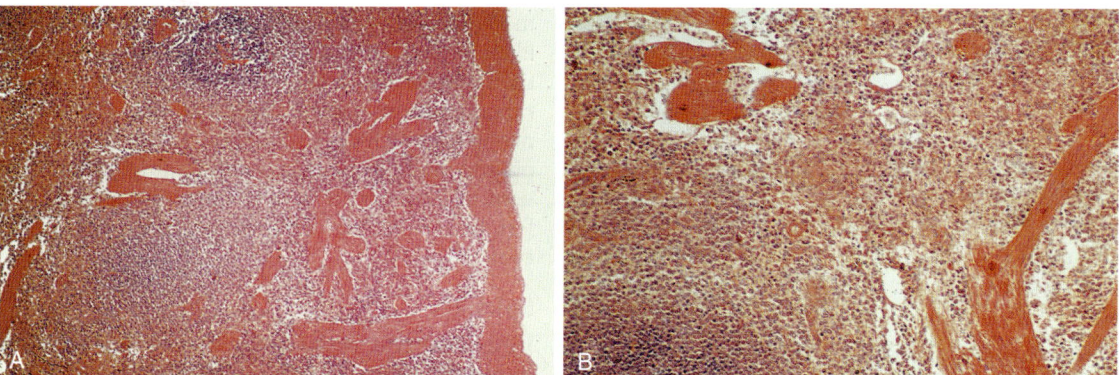

■ **FIGURE 4.109 Normal spleen. Tissue section. Cat.** Same case in A and B. **A,** A thick, smooth muscle capsule extends inward as trabeculae enclose the spleen. Note the dense, periarterial lymphatic sheath at top center of the field. (H&E; LP.) **B,** An ellipsoid, located in the center, is a capillary surrounded by concentric layers of macrophages within a reticular meshwork. (H&E; IP.)

Normal Splenic Cytology and Artifacts

Aspirate biopsy preparations contain large amounts of blood contamination, as evidenced by many intact erythrocytes and platelet clumps. Lymphoid cells present are similar to those of the normal lymph node (see Fig. 4.5A). Small lymphocytes predominate with occasional medium and large lymphocytes present. A few macrophages and plasma cells may be seen along with rare neutrophils and mast cells. Macrophages may contain small amounts of blue-green to black granular debris, compatible with hemosiderin. Occasional groups of macrophages within the red pulp may be admixed with the *reticular stroma* representing the ellipsoids or pericapillary histiocytic and reticular cell sheaths (Fig. 4.110). Circulating microfilaria (*Dirofilaria immitis*) may be present in splenic specimens owing to the high degree of blood contamination (Fig. 4.111).

Samples collected with the assistance of ultrasound often produce magenta debris in the background. This granular material represents ultrasound gel particles (Fig. 4.112) and can mimic necrotic tissue when mixed with blood. The material also may cause lysis or cellular swelling and therefore may

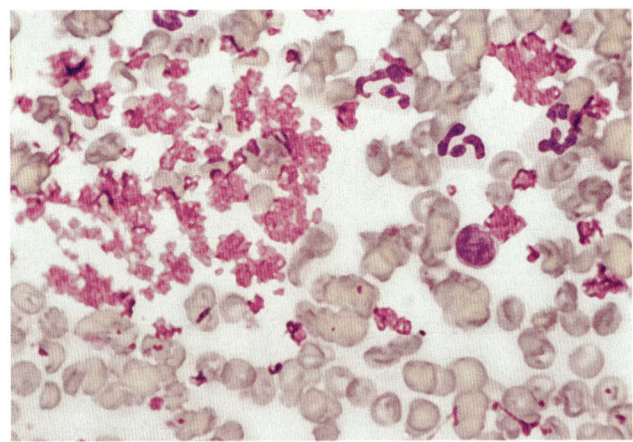

■ **FIGURE 4.112 Ultrasound gel. Transabdominal needle aspirate. Dog.** An attempt to sample the spleen produced a cytopathologic artifact. Note the pink to magenta, coarse, granular material in the background. (Wright; HP oil.) (Courtesy Kurt Henkel et al., Michigan State University. Presented at the 1996 ASVCP case review session.)

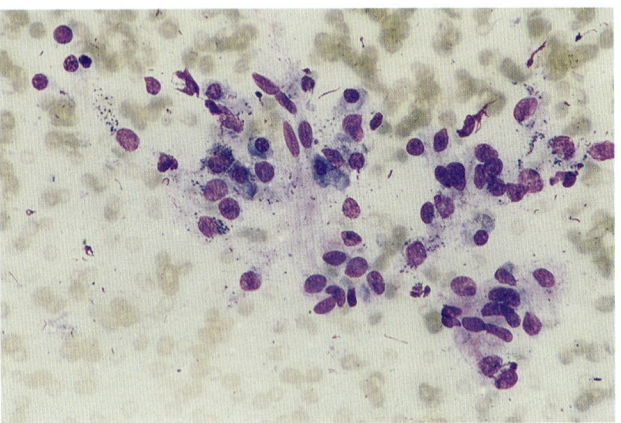

■ **FIGURE 4.110 Normal spleen. Pericapillary macrophage-reticular cell sheath (ellipsoid). Tissue aspirate. Dog.** A collection of macrophages is shown mixed with a reticular stroma representing an ellipsoid. (Wright-Giemsa; HP oil.)

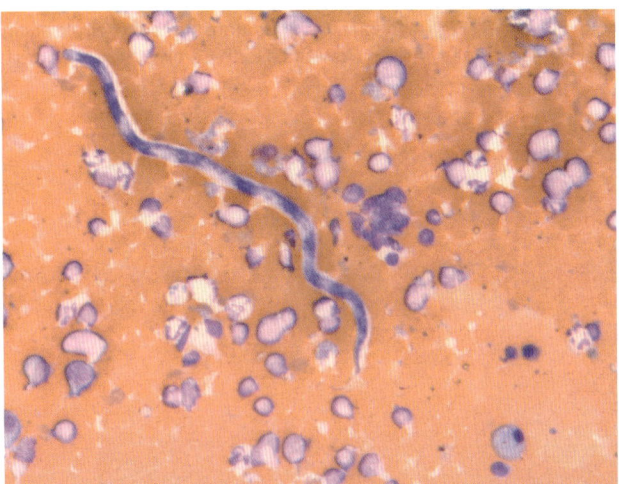

■ **FIGURE 4.111 Dirofilariasis. Spleen aspirate. Dog.** A microfilaria of *Dirofilaria immitis* is found within the hemodiluted background of a splenic preparation. (Wright-Giemsa; HP oil.) (Courtesy University of Florida.)

create unsuitable preparations for cytopathologic examination. See Chapter 1 for more information about imaging concerns.

Care should be taken when an incisional biopsy is taken of the spleen and impression smears are made. When the capsular surface is mistakenly imprinted instead of the parenchyma, uniform sheets of loosely attached mesothelium are seen (Fig. 4.113).

Reactive or Hyperplastic Spleen

Grossly, the reactive or hyperplastic spleen may present with nodular or diffuse enlargement. Lymphoid hyperplasia may result from antigenic reaction to infectious agents or the presence of blood parasites. Small lymphocytes still predominate, but there is an increase in medium-sized and large lymphocytes. Macrophages and plasma cells are often observed (Fig. 4.114). Frequent large collections of reticular stroma with increased numbers of mast cells are found at low magnification (Fig. 4.115). Hemosiderosis may be present with large amounts of coarse, dark granules (Fig. 4.116A). Capillaries may be more commonly observed with increased endothelial elements in the spleen (Fig. 4.116B).

A nodular presentation with lymphoid hyperplasia in the canine spleen had been termed *fibrohistiocytic nodule*. Within the firm, raised nodules are focal proliferations of spindle cells, macrophages, lymphocytes, and plasma cells (Fig. 4.117) that likely represent a response to another condition. It is now thought that this term can be applied to a mixture of conditions ranging from reactive lymphoid hyperplasia to malignant neoplasms, including histiocytic sarcoma, marginal zone lymphoma, and stromal sarcomas. Immunochemistry should be used to differentiate between them because the prognosis differs between these conditions (Moore et al., 2012; Sabattini et al., 2018).

Splenitis

Inflammatory cells increase in number with other noninfectious or infectious causes of disease. Noninfectious causes such as malignancy or immune reaction can incite neutrophilic or eosinophilic infiltration (Thorn and Aubert, 1999) (Figs. 4.118 to 4.120). The diagnosis of splenitis must be made cautiously if circulating

CHAPTER 4 *Hemolymphatic System*

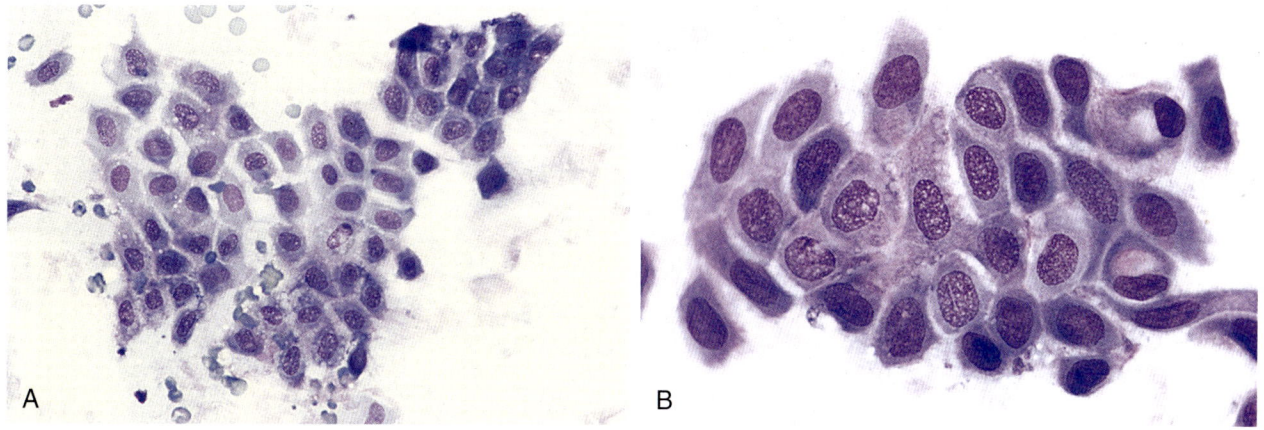

■ **FIGURE 4.113 Mesothelium. Splenic imprint. Dog.** Same case in A and B. **A,** Splenomegaly from suspected hypersplenism necessitated removal of the spleen. The outside surface was inadvertently imprinted onto the slide. Note a large sheet of interlocking cells. (Aqueous Romanowsky; HP oil.) **B,** Higher magnification demonstrates a uniform population of adherent cells with abundant basophilic cytoplasm. Clear spaces between cells represent cytoplasmic junctions. This benign sheet of cells is typical for mesothelial lining. The capsule on this spleen was prominently thickened grossly and on histopathology. (Aqueous Romanowsky; HP oil.)

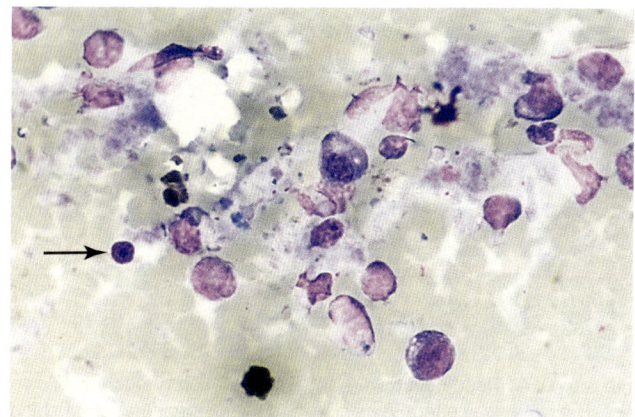

■ **FIGURE 4.114 Reactive spleen. Tissue aspirate. Dog.** An increase in medium-sized lymphocytes is present in comparison to the small lymphocyte indicated *(arrow)*. In addition, several plasma cells are noted along with a macrophage. (Wright-Giemsa; HP oil.)

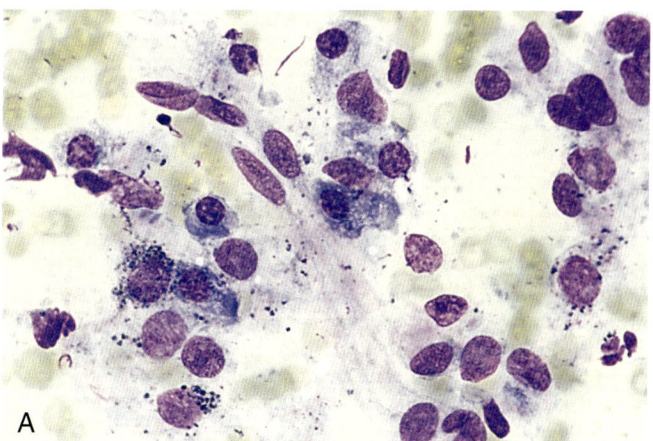

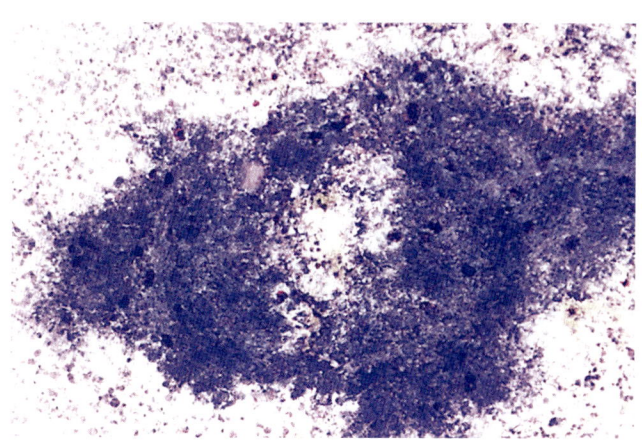

■ **FIGURE 4.115 Hyperplastic spleen. Tissue aspirate. Dog.** This animal was receiving chemotherapy for lymphoma. A very large aggregate of reticular stroma is shown infiltrated by an increased number of mast cells that appear as dark-purple cells sprinkled throughout. (Wright-Giemsa; IP.)

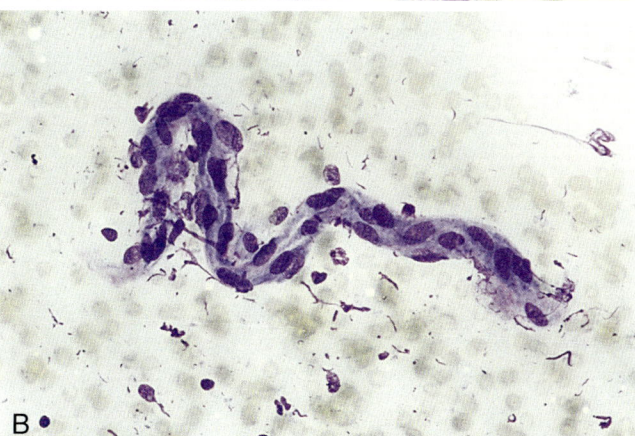

■ **FIGURE 4.116 Hyperplastic spleen. Tissue aspirate. Dog.** Same case in A and B. **A,** Hemosiderosis is recognized by the presence of hemosiderin-laden macrophages containing large amounts of coarse dark granules. (Wright-Giemsa; HP oil.) **B,** An endothelial-lined capillary is noted owing to endothelial hyperplasia. (Wright-Giemsa; HP oil.)

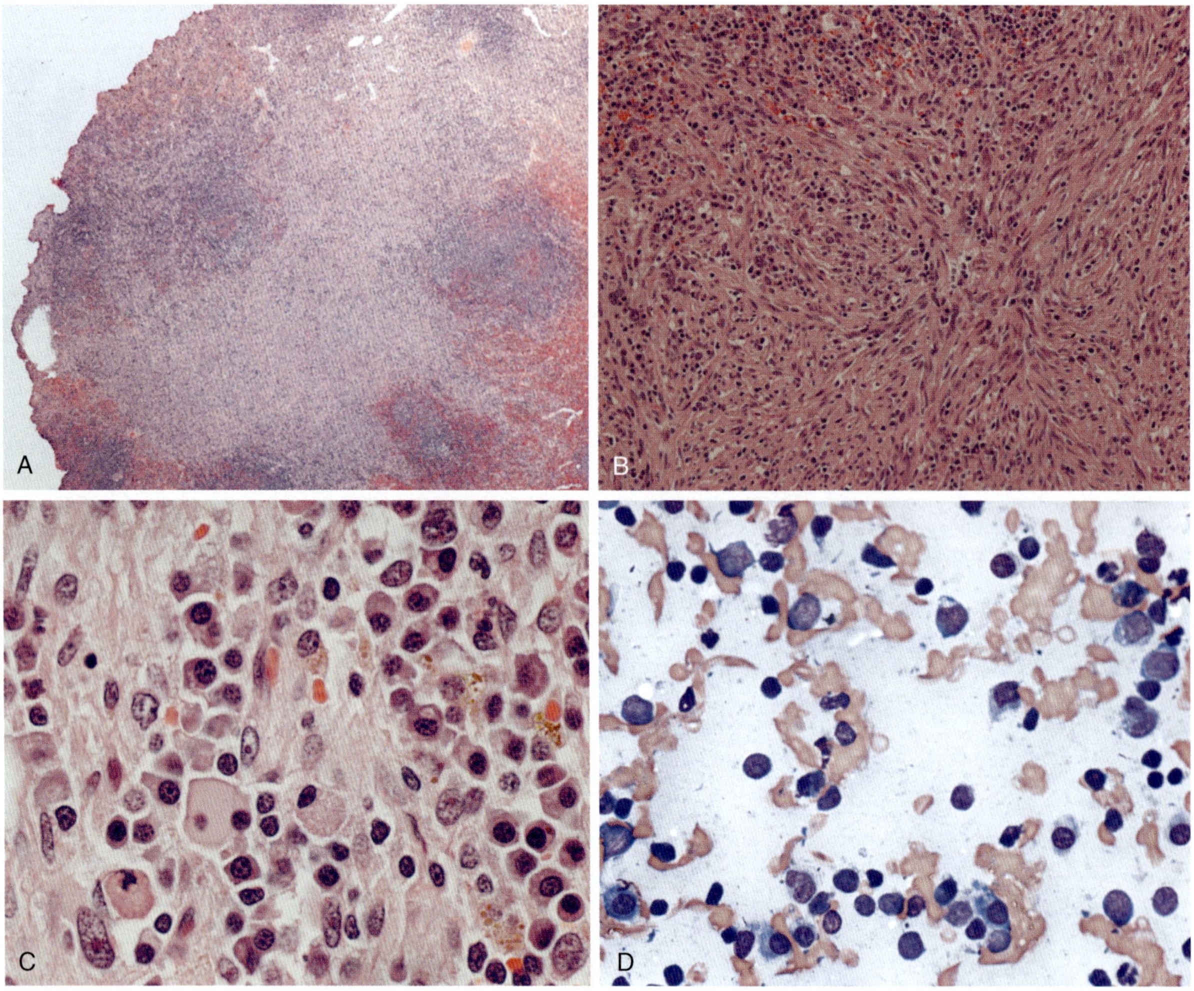

■ **FIGURE 4.117 Spleen. Lymphoid nodular hyperplasia. Dog.** Same case in A to D. **A, Tissue section.** A focal proliferation of eosinophilic connective tissue is shown placed between the multiple basophilic lymphoid follicles. The normal architecture is distorted by this proliferation of spindle cells. (H&E; L.P.) **B, Tissue section.** There are intersecting dense bands of plump spindle cells and connective tissue with scattered basophilic lymphoid cells. (H&E; I.P.) **C, Tissue section.** A higher magnification of the basophilic cellular areas indicate they are composed primarily of numerous plasma cells, small lymphocytes, and a few hemosiderin-laden macrophages. The background is composed of eosinophilic stroma. (H&E; HP oil.) **D, Tissue imprint.** The sample is cellular, composed of mostly small and medium lymphocytes with increased numbers of plasma cells against a hemodiluted background. Scattered plump mononuclear cells are present, a few of which have indistinct cytoplasmic borders that resemble the spindle cells in the tissue sections. (Modified Wright; HP oil.)

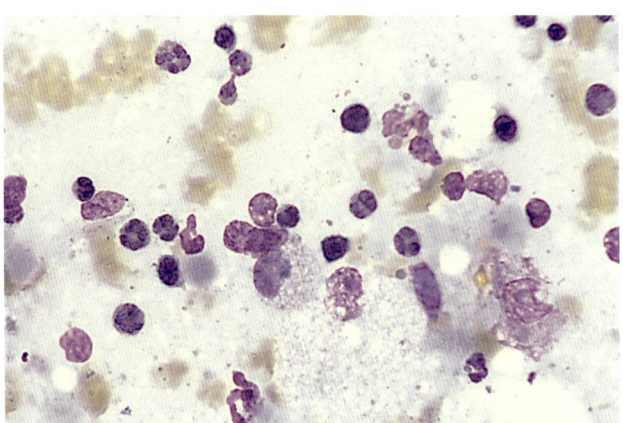

■ **FIGURE 4.118 Splenitis. Tissue aspirate. Dog.** Neutrophils, eosinophils, and foamy macrophages compose the severe inflammatory response in this animal with a necrotizing splenitis. (Wright-Giemsa; HP oil.)

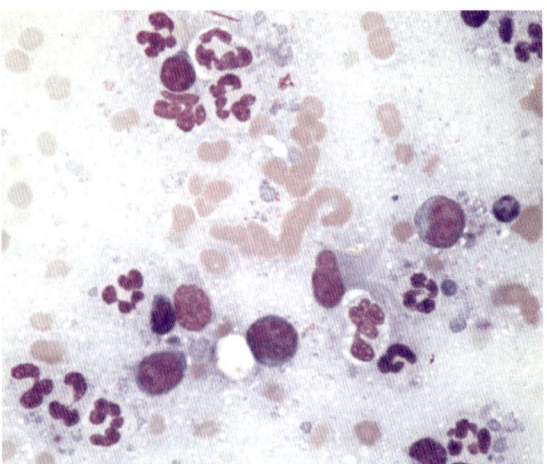

■ **FIGURE 4.119 Neutrophilic splenitis. Tissue aspirate. Cat.** Comparison with peripheral blood is helpful to rule out blood contamination. (Wright-Giemsa; HP oil.)

CHAPTER 4 Hemolymphatic System

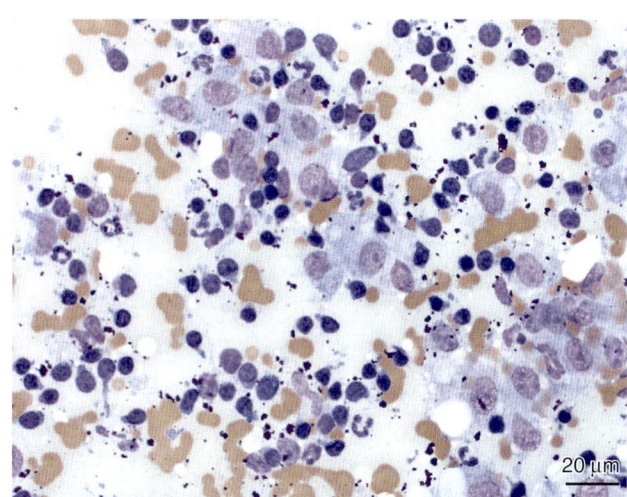

■ **FIGURE 4.120 Mixed macrophagic and neutrophilic splenitis. Splenic nodule aspirate. Cat.** Numerous hypoechoic splenic nodules are found on ultrasound in a patient diagnosed with renal lymphoma. The background contains amorphous to globular, pink-magenta ultrasound coupling gel. The lymphoid population is composed primarily of small lymphocytes, many of which have cytoplasmic extensions or uropods. An increase in medium lymphocytes is also noted. Significantly increased numbers of neutrophils and macrophages are present likely related to tissue damage from the neoplasia. (Wright-Giemsa; HP oil.) (Courtesy Francisco Conrado, University of Florida.)

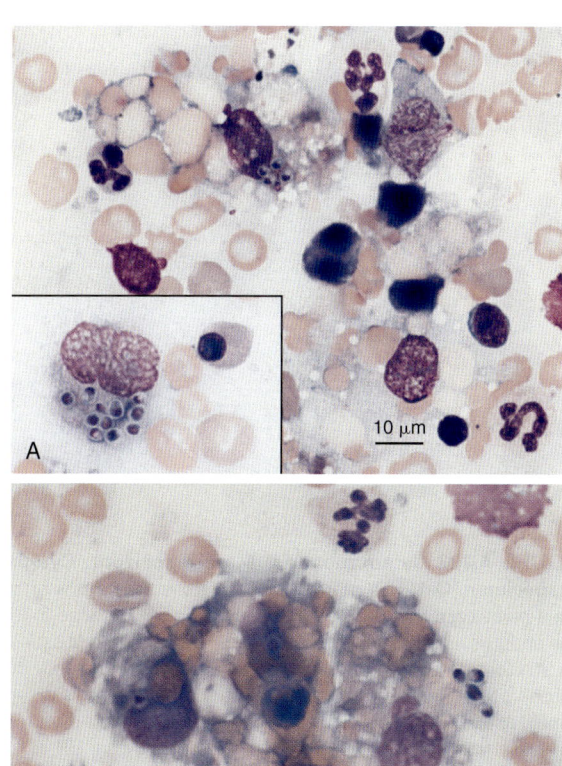

neutrophilia or eosinophilia is present. Macrophagic or histiocytic inflammation often occurs with the presence of systemic fungal infections such as histoplasmosis (Fig. 4.121), aspergillosis (Allen et al., 2018) or protozoal infections such as cytauxzoonosis (Figs. 4.122 and 4.123) and leishmaniasis in which amastigotes develop within parasitophorous vacuoles of the macrophages (Fig. 4.124). Mild to moderate histiocytic hyperplasia may be associated with immune-mediated hemolytic anemia and immune-mediated thrombocytopenia, as well as with other etiologies for hemolytic anemia (Figs. 4.125 and 4.126).

Sinus histiocytosis may be appreciated by the appearance of rosettes of lymphocytes around histiocytes or emperipolesis (lymphophagocytosis) of histiocytes having abundant pale blue vacuolated cytoplasm (Figs. 4.127 to 4.129). Histopathologically, these macrophages expand within the lymph node medullary sinuses and splenic red pulp to react with pathogens especially during chronic inflammatory conditions or with B-cell lymphoma (Fig. 4.129B).

In aged dogs, it is common to aspirate sidereocalcific plaques, also called siderotic plaques, fibrosiderotic nodules, or Gamna-Gandy bodies that lie along the splenic margins within or just under the fibrous capsule (Fig. 4.130) (Ryseff et al., 2014). These firm, sometimes calcified, masses mostly contain a form of blood pigment either as hemosiderin (blue-black) or hematoidin (golden yellow) that may be found within the associated macrophages or extracellularly along connective tissue fibers (Figs. 4.131 to 4.133A). They can result from previous hemorrhage as well as represent a senile change in dogs. Prussian blue stains positive in the presence of hemosiderin, whereas hematoidin that lacks iron is negative. Both Alizarin red S and Prussian blue can be used to stain these structures on previously stained preparations (see Figs. 4.130B and 4.133B–C) (Moore et al., 2017).

■ **FIGURE 4.121 Macrophagic splenitis. Histoplasmosis. Tissue aspirate. Dog.** Same case in A and B. **A,** A macrophage at the top contains yeast forms, but a concurrent extramedullary erythropoiesis is present. Note the many rubricytes and metarubricytes along with polychromatophils. (Wright; HP oil.) *Inset:* Multiple oval yeast forms measuring approximately 3 × 2 μm are present within a macrophage next to a metarubricyte. (Wright; HP oil.) **B,** The frequent erythrophagocytosis supports the presence of a hemophagic syndrome in light of the marked red cell destruction. This may occur with infection, such as in this case. The hematocrit decreased to 12.5% during this period of infection. (Wright; HP oil.)

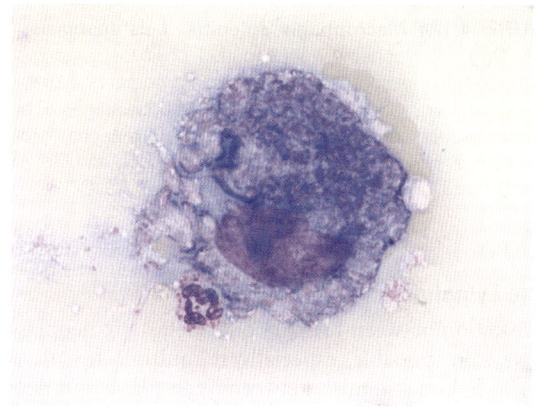

■ **FIGURE 4.122 Cytauxzoonosis. Immature schizont. Blood smear. Cat.** A parasitized macrophage with sporozoites is undergoing schizogony and expanding the cytoplasm with developing organisms. Note the prominent dark nucleolus, which is half the size of the adjacent granulocyte. The nucleus of the macrophage is markedly enlarged from normal. (Modified Wright; HP oil.) (Courtesy Kansas State University.)

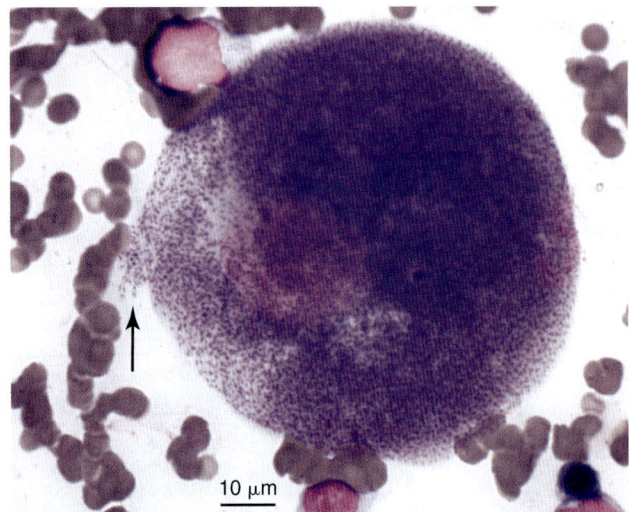

FIGURE 4.123 Cytauxzoonosis. Mature schizont. Cytopathologic specimen. Cat. This mature schizont from the bone marrow involves a parasitized mononuclear phagocyte similar to those found lining the endothelium of splenic vessels. Imprints of affected tissues may reveal schizonts that have blocked blood vessels and represent the tissue phase of the infection. Along the edge the mature schizont shown are small, about 1 μm, merozoites *(arrow)* that will infect erythrocytes after release from the ruptured schizont. (Wright-Giemsa; HP oil.)

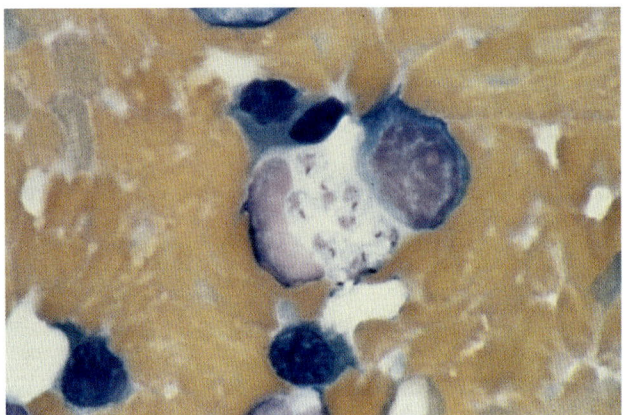

FIGURE 4.124 Macrophagic splenitis. Leishmaniasis. Tissue imprint. Dog. Macrophage with engulfed protozoal organisms confirmed as *Leishmania* spp. Note the organism contains a small, round nucleus and a short, rod-shaped kinetoplast. Various stages of erythroid precursors support a diagnosis of extramedullary hematopoiesis. (Wright-Giemsa; HP oil.) (Courtesy Cheryl Swenson and Gary Kociba, The Ohio State University. Presented at the 1987 ASVCP case review session.)

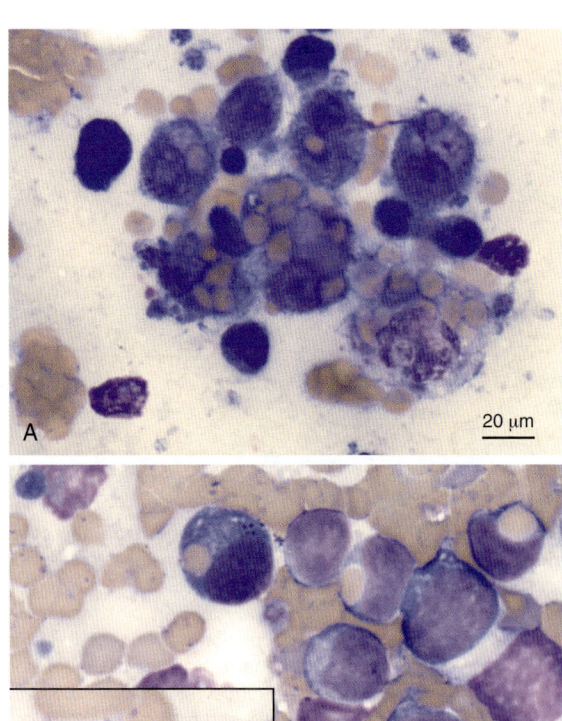

FIGURE 4.125 Hemophagocytosis. *Mycoplasma haemofelis* infection. Splenic aspirate. Cat. Same case in A and B. **A,** Macrophages have engulfed numerous parasitized erythrocytes. (Modified Wright; HP oil.) **B,** Individual erythrocytes are shown phagocytized by splenic macrophages. *Inset*: Note several ring and coccoid forms of hemotropic mycoplasma adhered to erythrocytes in the aspirate background. (Modified Wright; HP oil.) (Courtesy Joanne Messick, Purdue University.)

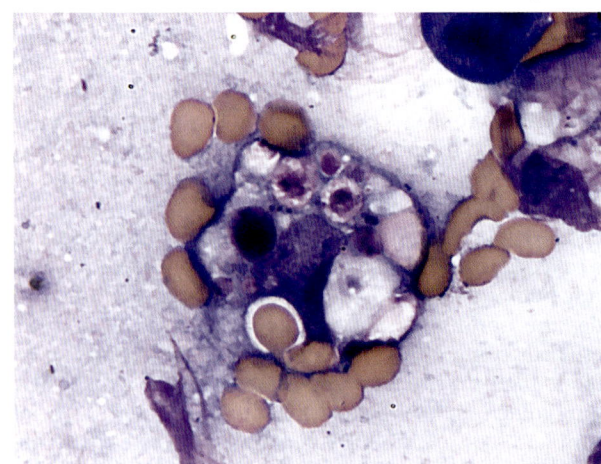

FIGURE 4.126 Rubriphagocytosis. Precursor-targeted immune-mediated hemolytic anemia (PIMA). Splenic imprint. Cat. The cat had a 3-year history of PIMA managed with prednisone and cyclosporine. The cat had a recent 1-month history of hemolytic anemia and severe splenomegaly. Mycoplasma was negative on PCR. Histopathology did not find evidence for a hemophagocytic neoplasm and supported cytopathology findings, which show prominent erythrophagocytosis and rubriphagocytosis. (Modified Wright; HP oil.) (Courtesy Erica Corda, Michigan State University.)

Splenic Lymphoma

Differentiation between primary and metastatic neoplasia may not always be possible, especially if multiple organs are involved. To help distinguish between hyperplasia and neoplasia, a blast cell count above 40% is often indicative of splenic lymphoma as demonstrated by PARR for verification (Williams et al., 2006). Lymphomas appear morphologically similar to the subtypes described in lymph nodes (Fig. 4.134). An uncommon presentation of splenic lymphoid neoplasia includes an anaplastic variant of diffuse large B-cell lymphoma. These cells are highly pleomorphic with variable nuclear shapes that may be

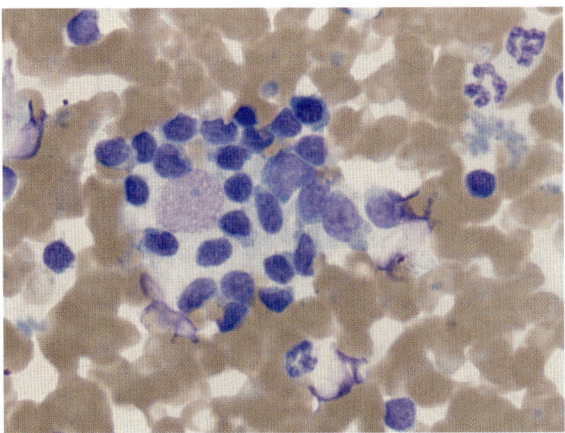

■ **FIGURE 4.127 Sinus histiocytosis. Splenic nodule aspirate. Dog.** Ultrasound identified a 1-cm-diameter, hypoechoic with hyperechoic center nodule on the spleen. Shown is a macrophage surrounded by small and occasional medium lymphocytes. Note the erythroid precursor with moderately basophilic cytoplasm at the 2 o'clock position outside the cuff of cells. (Wright-Giemsa; HP oil.) (Courtesy Jere Stern, University of Florida.)

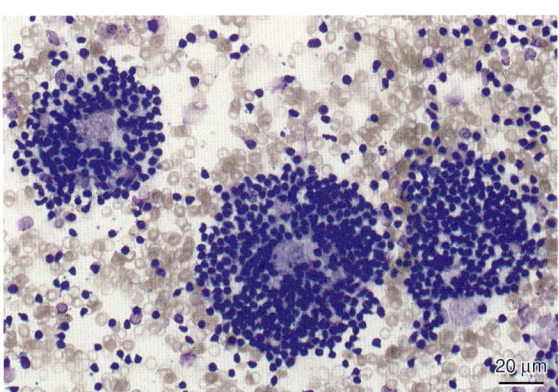

■ **FIGURE 4.128 Sinus histiocytosis. Unknown lymphoid tissue. Tissue aspirate. Dog.** A diagnosis of diffuse large B-cell lymphoma was determined at splenectomy 2 years earlier. Ultrasound identified a well-defined, ovoid, mildly heterogeneous, hypoechoic nodule in the region of the splenectomy site, while lymphoma has relapsed after treatment. Three of the numerous histiocytes are massively expanded by a cuff of small lymphocytes, which are generally intact. (Wright-Giemsa; HP oil.) (Courtesy Francisco Conrado, University of Florida.)

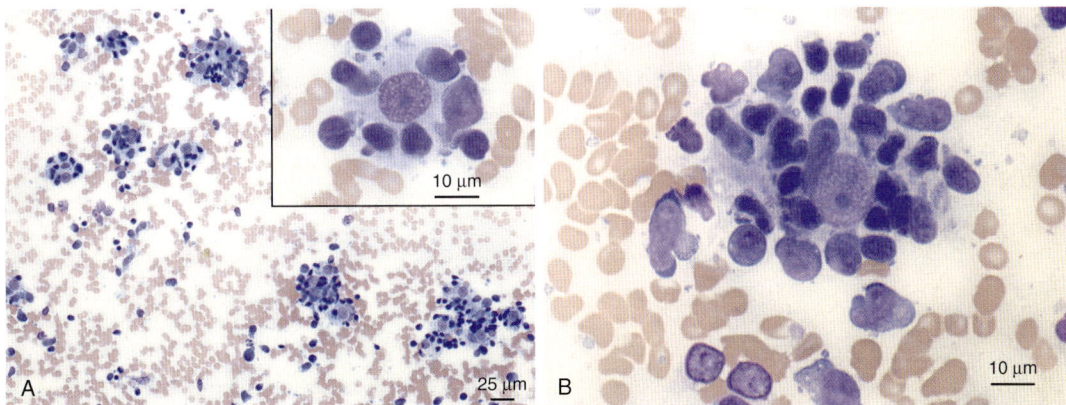

■ **FIGURE 4.129 Sinus histiocytosis with B-cell lymphoma. Splenic aspirate. Dog.** Same case in A and B. Upon staging and treatment for an oral melanoma, splenomegaly and peripheral lymphadenomegaly were found, and determined by PARR to have the same B-cell clonality in both sites. **A,** Numerous histiocyte aggregates. (Modified Wright; IP.) *Inset:* One aggregate appears to have internalized lymphocytes; however, the cells appear intact and may be present by emperipolesis or cytopolasmic invaginations. (Modified Wright; HP oil.) **B,** Another histiocyte aggregate shows cellular deterioration of internalized lymphocytes suggesting possible lymphophagocytosis. In addition, several medium lymphoid cells with a single prominent nucleolus (marginal zone cells) surround the histiocyte. (Modified Wright; HP oil.)

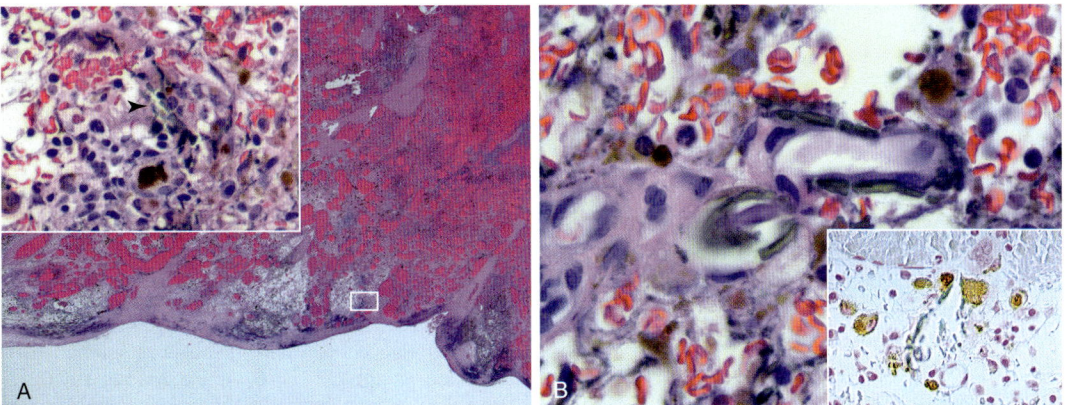

■ **FIGURE 4.130 Gamna-Gandy bodies. Spleen. Tissue section. Dog.** Same case in A and B. **A,** The subcapsular area of the spleen is pigmented and edematous. The rectangular area shown is magnified in the *inset*. (H&E; LP.) *Inset: Arrowhead* indicates a linear mineralized region. (H&E; IP.) **B,** Another region showing the yellow-green linear Gamna-Gandy bodies or siderocalcific plaques (H&E; HP oil.) *Inset:* Hemosiderin is contained within the Gamna-Gandy body as indicated by the blue-green reaction. (Prussian blue; HP oil.) (Courtesy University of Florida.)

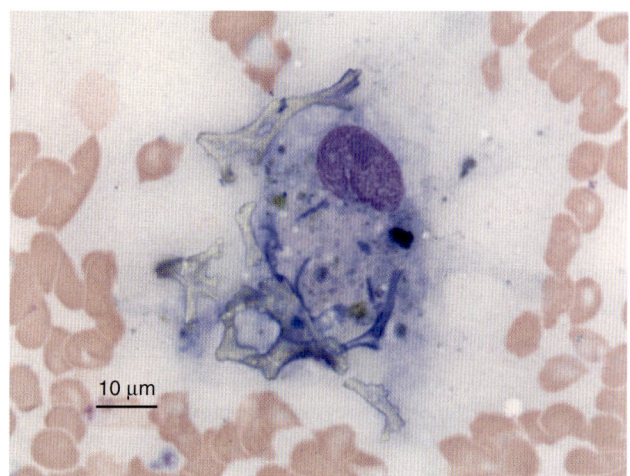

■ **FIGURE 4.131 Gamna-Gandy bodies. Splenic aspirate. Dog.** The dog has been receiving chemotherapy for lymphoma. Several pale-yellow linear structures are present within a macrophage and may be confused for fungal hyphae. (Modified Wright; HP oil.) (Courtesy Andrea Pires dos Santos, Purdue University.)

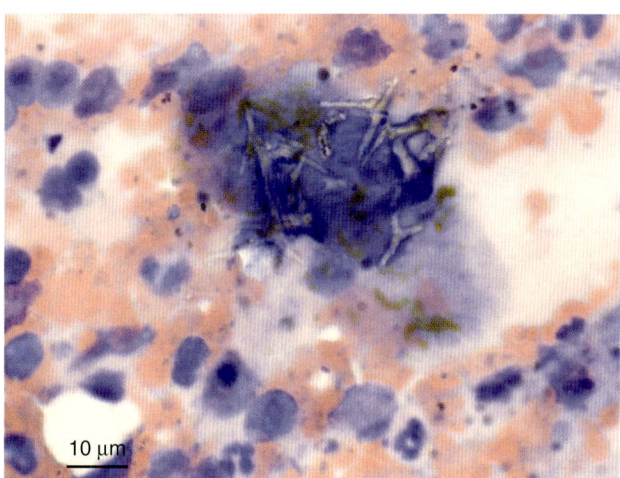

■ **FIGURE 4.132 Gamna-Gandy bodies. Spleen aspirate. Dog.** Patient presented for metastasis check for fibrosarcoma of the leg. Several clear linear structures are associated with an aggregate of histiocytes. Adjacent to these structures are yellow hematoidin, indicating chronic hemorrhage. (Modified Wright; HP oil.) (Courtesy Mara Varvil, Purdue University.)

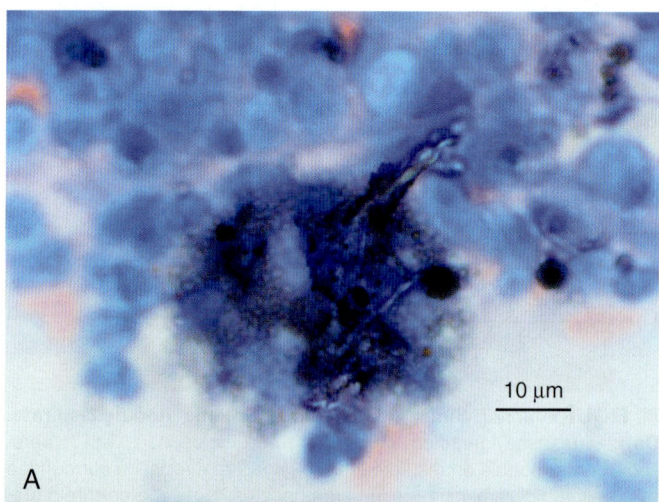

A

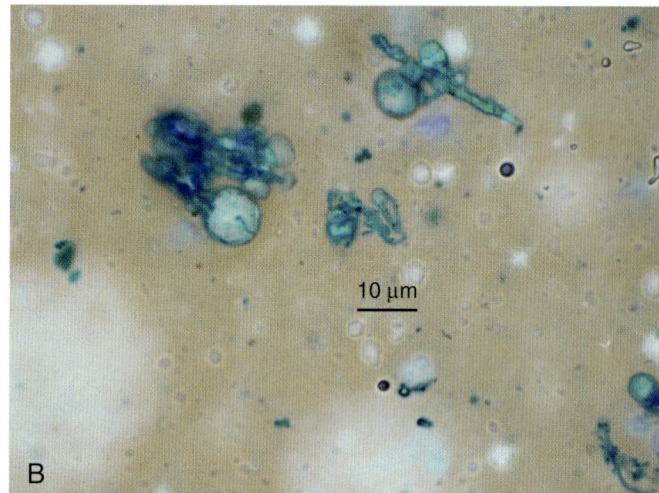

B

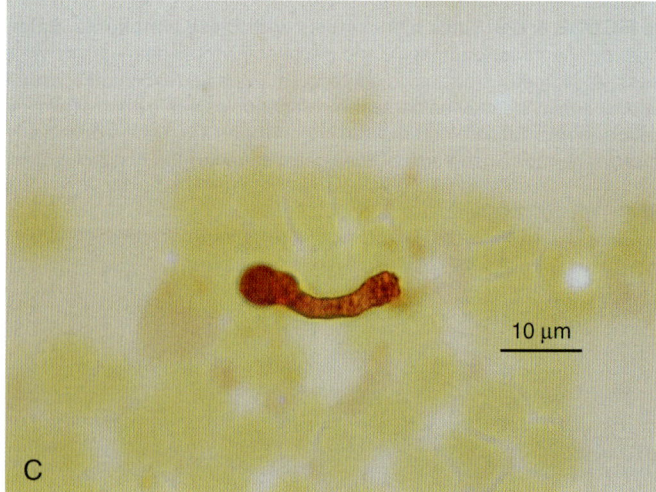

C

■ **FIGURE 4.133 Gamna-Gandy bodies. Splenic aspirate. Dog.** Same case in A to C. **A,** In addition to clear linear structures, the macrophages also contain dark granules, presumed to be hemosiderin. (Modified Wright; HP oil.) **B,** Ample positive staining linear and round crystalline material indicates the presence of iron. (Prussian blue; HP oil.) **C,** One positive stained crystalline structure is shown indicating the presence of calcium. (Alizarin red S; HP oil.) (Courtesy Natalia Strandberg, Purdue University.)

mistaken for histiocytic neoplasia (Fig. 4.135A–B). The presence of CD79a expression supports the diagnosis of B-cell origin (Fig. 4.135C).

Marginal zone lymphoma. Marginal zone lymphoma may be recognized in the spleen with the appearance of a mixed cell population (Fig. 4.136A), including those with a monocytoid appearance. In rare cases PAS-positive round cytoplasmic inclusions (Fig. 4.136B) may be seen in cases of marginal zone lymphoma as well as other forms of B-cell lymphoma. More often, an increase or predominance of medium-sized lymphocytes with a single, large, centrally located nucleolus is found (Fig. 4.137). One study found splenectomy with or without systemic chemotherapy beneficial in the treatment of canine splenic marginal zone lymphoma (Stefanello et al., 2011).

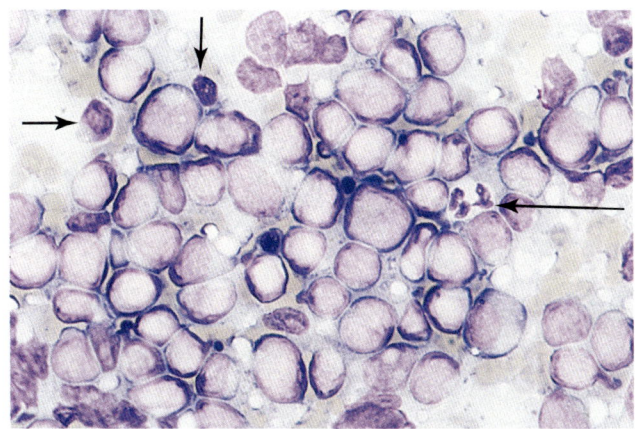

■ **FIGURE 4.134 Lymphoma. Splenic aspirate. Dog.** Same case as in Figures 9.24A and 9.72A. A population of neoplastic lymphocytes was aspirated from an enlarged spleen. The neutrophil *(long arrow)* and small lymphocyte *(short arrows)* are useful cell micrometers. (Wright; HP oil.)

Granular lymphocytic leukemia/lymphoma. Canine granular lymphocytes are thought to originate from the red pulp region of the spleen (McDonough and Moore, 2000; Workman and Vernau, 2003). The patient with granular lymphocytic leukemia often presents with marked granular lymphocytosis in circulation that is present also within the spleen (Fig. 4.138A–B). The bone marrow is usually not infiltrated by the neoplastic population (Lau et al., 1999). Clinical signs are variable, and progression of the neoplastic disease may be slow. Granules may be very small and difficult to see with use of aqueous Romanowsky stains (Fig. 4.138C–D). Immunophenotyping of these neoplastic granular lymphocytes usually indicates reactivity to CD3, CD8α, and CD11d antigens (Fig. 4.138E–F). Non-neoplastic conditions may produce a reactive granular lymphocytosis, which should first be ruled out.

Plasma cell neoplasia. Plasma cell tumor of the spleen may occur as a solitary extramedullary plasmacytoma (Fig. 4.139) or secondary to plasma cell myeloma. Splenic involvement of plasma cell myeloma with paraproteinemia was common in a study of 16 cats (Patel et al., 2005). An example of a cat with suspected myeloma and splenic involvement along with a monoclonal gammopathy displays both typical plasma cells as well as binucleation and karyomegaly in the spleen (Fig. 4.140). Use of immunocytochemistry with B-cell markers and MUM1 helps to identify a plasmacytoma when cells appear large and multilobulated like histiocytic cells (Fig. 4.141). Rare cytopathologic evidence of a collision tumor in a dog spleen involved a secretory plasmacytoma and a mast cell tumor (Pallatto and Bechtold, 2018).

Mantle cell lymphoma. Mantle cell lymphoma (MCL) arises from small B cells from the inner zone of cortical follicles in lymph nodes or near small arterioles in the spleen, bone marrow, or intestine. In dogs, MCL only appears as a solitary indolent splenic mass, but it is infrequent, accounting for only 0.5% to 1% of indolent lymphomas in dogs (Valli et al., 2006; Flood-Knapik et al., 2013). A mantle cell expansion is often associated with nodular lymphoid follicular hyperplasia in dogs, so molecular clonality testing is helpful to diagnose lymphoma. On histopathology, MCL appears as irregular and coalescing follicular structures composed predominantly of small cells with a scant amount of cytoplasm with irregular or indented deeply stained nuclei lacking obvious nucleoli. Cytopathologically, the

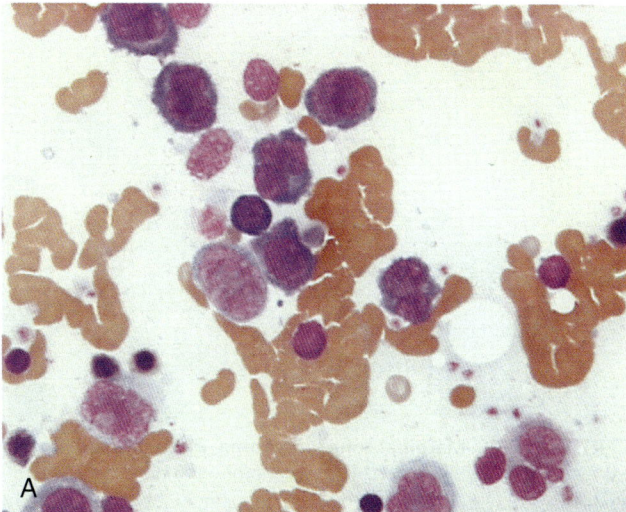
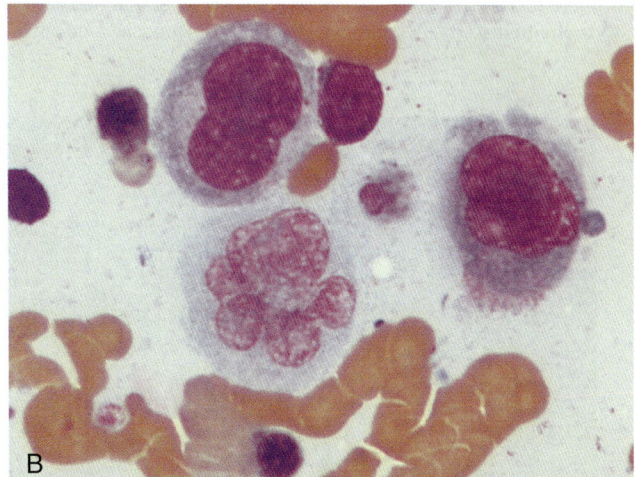
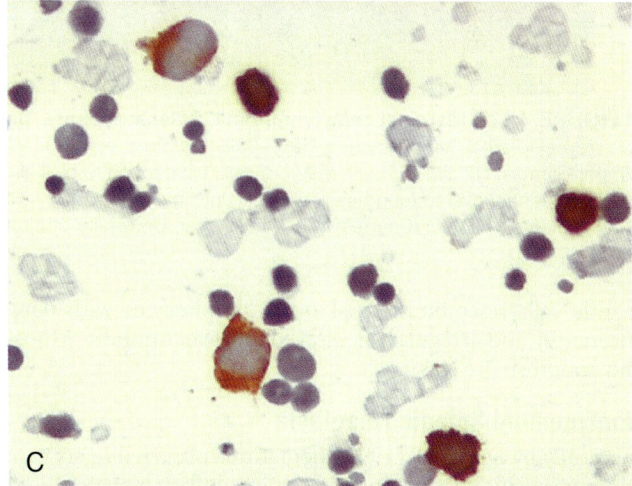

■ **FIGURE 4.135 Diffuse large B-cell lymphoma, anaplastic variant. Cytopathologic specimen. Cat.** Same case in A to C. **A,** This animal had bizarre and pleomorphic neoplastic cells in the spleen, liver, bone marrow, and abdominal fluid. Shown are several large cells measuring approximately 25 to 20 μm in diameter. Nuclei are highly lobulated, and cells resemble histiocytic cells. (Wright-Giemsa; HP oil.) **B,** Notice the uneven lobulation. (Wright-Giemsa; HP oil.) **C, Immunocytochemistry.** Many of large, pleomorphic, neoplastic cells stain diffusely red express CD79a antigen, a marker for the B-cell receptor. (CD79a/AEC; HP oil.)

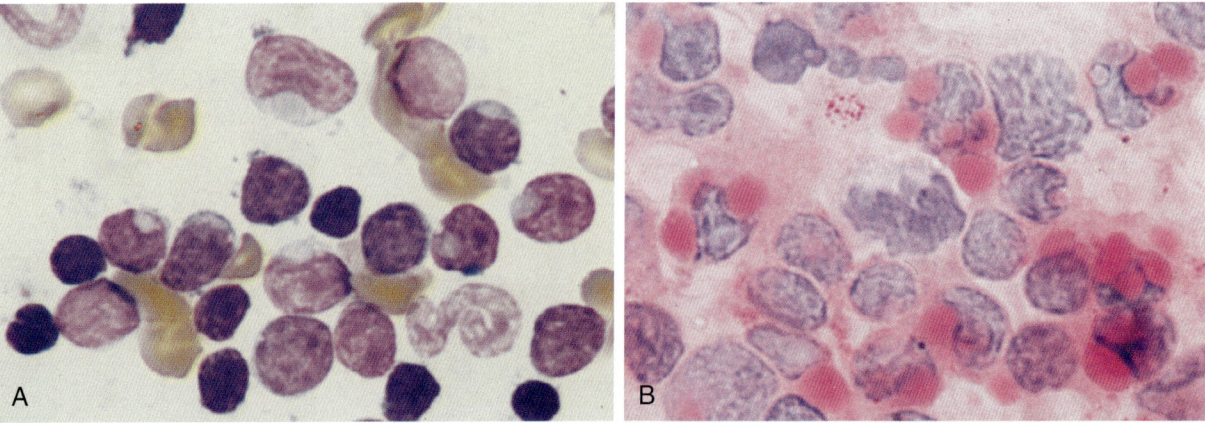

■ **FIGURE 4.136 Marginal zone lymphoma, disseminated. Bone marrow aspirate. Dog.** Same case in A and B. **A,** This 5-year-old pit bull terrier presented with a late form of this lymphoma with dissemination to the spleen, liver, lymph nodes, blood, and bone marrow. Lymphoid cells are variable in size, some of which display monocytoid features. Several medium-sized lymphocytes have a pale blue-gray inclusion that appears to indent the nucleus. This dog was clinically staged as Vb but had an indolent course of disease with a survival of 162 days. (Wright-Giemsa; HP oil.) **B, Cytochemistry.** The cytoplasmic inclusions stain positive consistent with immunoglobulin deposition. (PAS; HP oil.)

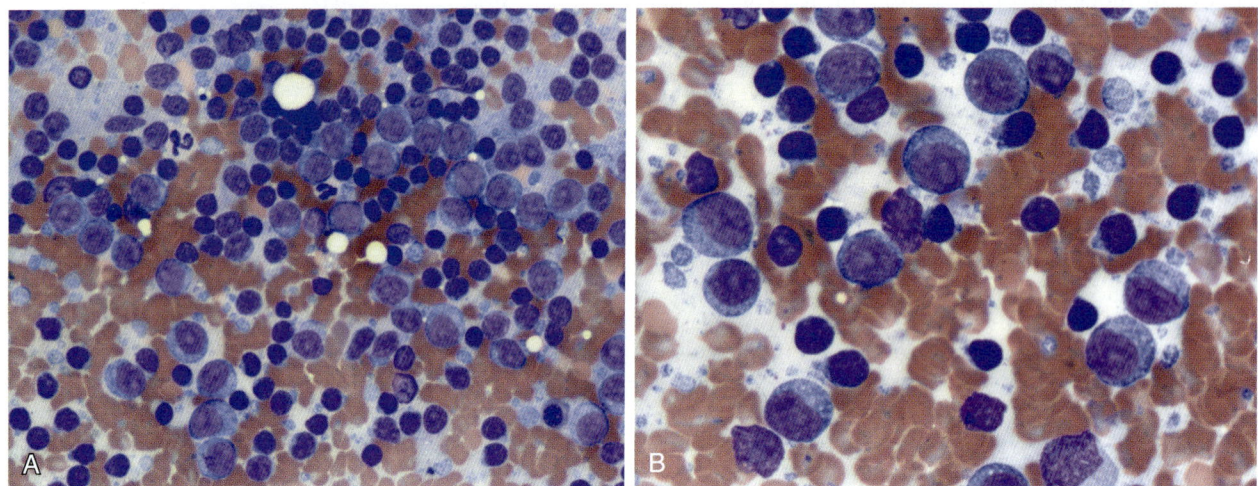

■ **FIGURE 4.137 Marginal zone lymphoma. Splenic aspirate. Dog.** Same case in A and B. **A,** Focal large sheets and aggregates of lymphoid cells revealed small lymphocytes (~50%–60%) admixed with a moderately expanded monomorphic medium lymphoid population (~40%–50%). (Wright-Giemsa; HP oil.) **B,** These medium cells have round to oval eccentric nuclei approximately 1.5 to 2 × RBC diameter with stippled chromatin, one large central oval to round nucleolus occupying one-third to two-thirds of the nucleus and small amounts of moderately basophilic cytoplasm. (Wright-Giemsa; HP oil.) (Courtesy Mary Leissinger, University of Florida.)

mantle cells resemble normal small lymphocytes with dense chromatin and irregular or cleaved nuclear outlines. Mitosis and apoptosis are lacking.

Nonlymphoid Splenic Neoplasia

In a study by Day et al. (1995), hematoma occurred in six cases and nonspecific changes such as extramedullary hematopoiesis, congestion, and hemosiderosis occurred in 16 of 87 canine biopsies. Hemangiosarcoma was the most commonly diagnosed splenic neoplasm (Day et al., 1995), involving 17 of 87 canine splenic biopsies. Hemangiosarcoma cells are similar to those in other sites. Scattered large, mesenchymal-appearing cells may be found scanning on low magnification (Fig. 4.142A). Extramedullary hematopoiesis, chronic hemorrhage, and lymphoid reactivity may accompany the tumor. Neoplastic cells are large with abundant cytoplasm having wispy, indistinct borders and frequently multiple punctate vacuoles (Figs. 4.142B–C and 4.143A). The nucleus is round with coarse chromatin and multiple prominent nucleoli. Use of immunostaining with anti-CD31 and von Willebrand factor (Fig. 4.143B–C) helps determine the cell of origin in mesenchymal neoplasia.

Other mesenchymal-appearing tumors in the canine spleen involve primarily fibrosarcoma, undifferentiated sarcoma, leiomyosarcoma, histiocytic sarcoma, osteosarcoma, chondrosarcoma (Kawabata et al., 2017), liposarcoma (Fig. 4.144A–C), myxosarcoma, mesenchymoma, and pleomorphic or anaplastic sarcoma with giant cells, formerly termed *malignant fibrous histiocytoma* (Hendrick et al., 1992; Spangler et al., 1994).

In cats, the most important cause of splenomegaly is mastocytoma, accounting for 15% of the total pathologic conditions submitted for diagnosis (Spangler and Culbertson, 1992). Diffuse enlargement of the spleen is detected on palpation or diagnostic

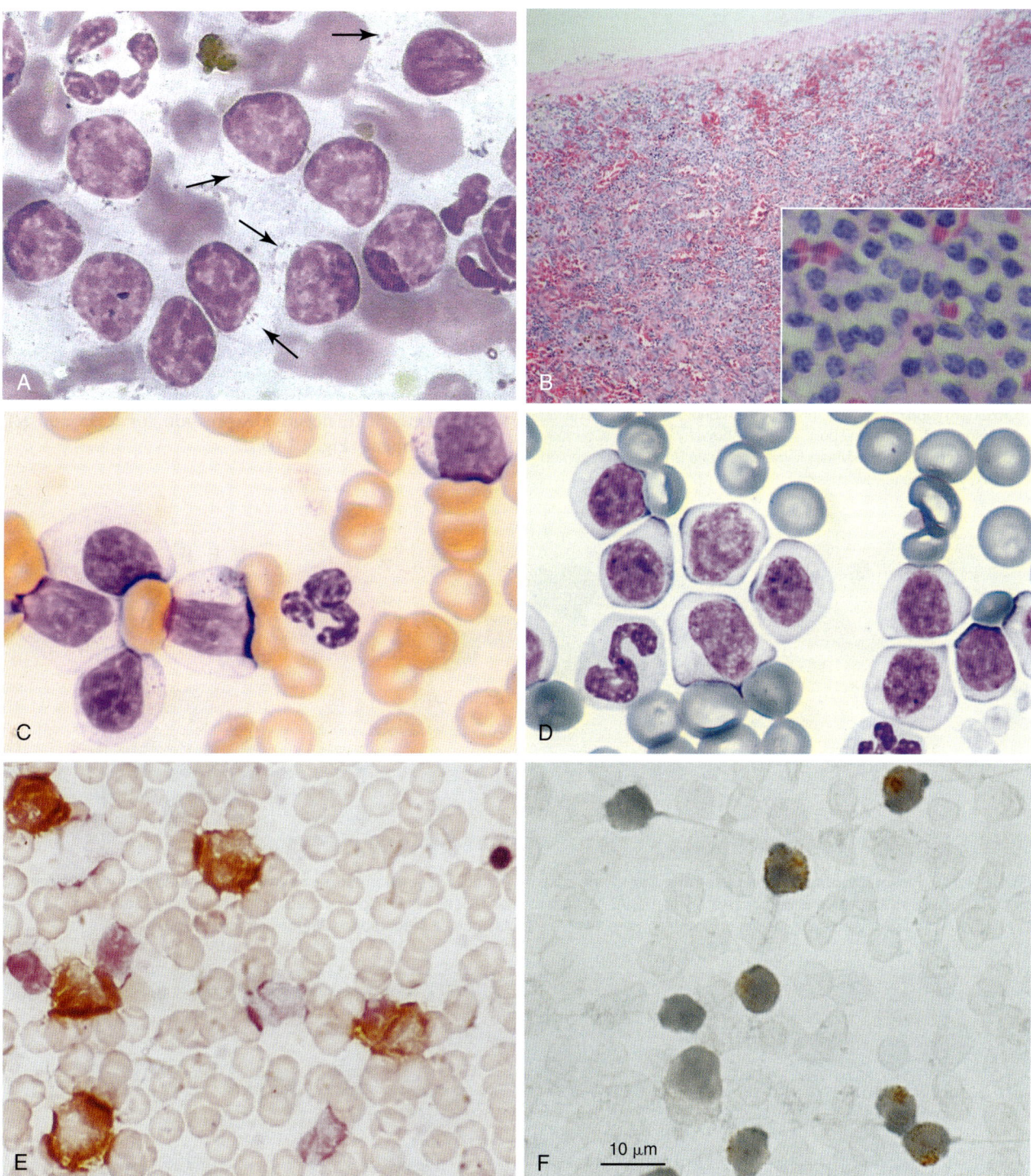

■ **FIGURE 4.138 Granular lymphocyte lymphoma/leukemia. Dog.** Same case in A to F. **A, Splenic imprint.** Several medium-sized lymphocytes with clumped chromatin and moderately abundant clear cytoplasm. Some of the cells visibly contain several fine azurophilic granules *(arrows)*. The spleen is the primary organ of involvement and was immunoreactive with CD3 antibody, a T-cell marker (not shown). (Wright-Giemsa; HP oil.) **B, Splenic section.** There is a loss of nodular structures with a dense infiltrate from the red pulp of pale lymphoid cells shown in the inset. (H&E; LP.) *Inset:* A dense uniform sheet of medium cells compared with erythrocytes. Cells are irregularly round with stippled chromatin and no discernible nucleoli. (H&E; HP oil.) **C, Blood smear.** The history involved 2 months of persistent lymphocytosis of counts exceeding 20,000/μL. Rickettsial infections were ruled out by titer tests. Note the typical abundant clear cytoplasm with small red granules arranged in a focal paranuclear manner. This cell population did not infiltrate the bone marrow. (Wright-Giemsa; HP oil.) **D, Blood smear.** Use of an aqueous-based stain did not demonstrate the cytoplasmic granules; therefore, methanolic Romanowsky stains are highly recommended. (Aqueous Romanowsky; HP oil.) **E, Immunocytochemistry.** Several lymphoid cells stain diffusely positive for the cell surface antigen. (CD8α/DAB; HP oil.) **F, Immunocytochemistry.** Several lymphoid cells react positive in a focal to diffuse manner for leukocyte integrin CD11d (formerly called alpha D). These positive cells arise from the red pulp region of the spleen. (CD11d/AEC; HP oil.)

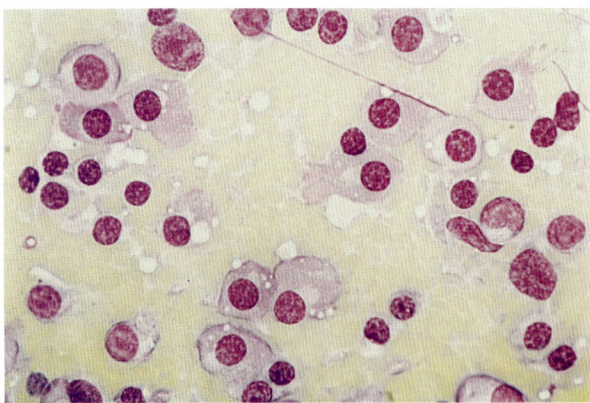

FIGURE 4.139 Plasmacytoma. Splenic imprint. Dog. Plasma cells composed the majority of cells present. Note the abundant eosinophilic cytoplasm typical for a "flame cell." Serum protein electrophoresis indicated a monoclonal gammopathy, which immunoelectrophoresis confirmed as an abnormal amount of immunoglobulin A. (Romanowsky; HP oil.) (Courtesy Christine Swardson and Joanne Messick, The Ohio State University. Presented at the 1989 ASVCP case reivew session.)

imaging (Fig. 4.145). Often a nearly pure population of highly granulated mast cells is present, several of which may display erythrophagocytosis (Fig. 4.146).

Other discrete cell tumors found in the spleen include myeloid leukemia and histiocytic sarcoma (Fig. 4.147). Histiocytic sarcoma may be localized to the spleen or disseminated (Affolter and Moore, 2002). This tumor arises from dendritic cells that are CD1+, CD4−, CD11c+, CD11d−, MHC II+, and ICAM-1+ in comparison to the hemophagocytic histiocytic sarcoma, which arises from macrophages and is associated with a rapid decline in health (Moore, 2014). Cats also display histiocytic neoplasms that possess similar characteristics (Friedrichs and Young, 2008). Marked erythrophagocytosis by Iba1+ or CD11d+ macrophages usually occurs in the spleen and bone marrow (Sills and Howerth, 2018) (Fig. 4.148A–B). BLA.36 appears to be a useful immunochemical marker for neoplastic histiocytic cells when positive concurrently with negative expression for CD3 and CD79a surface antigens (Fig. 4.148C).

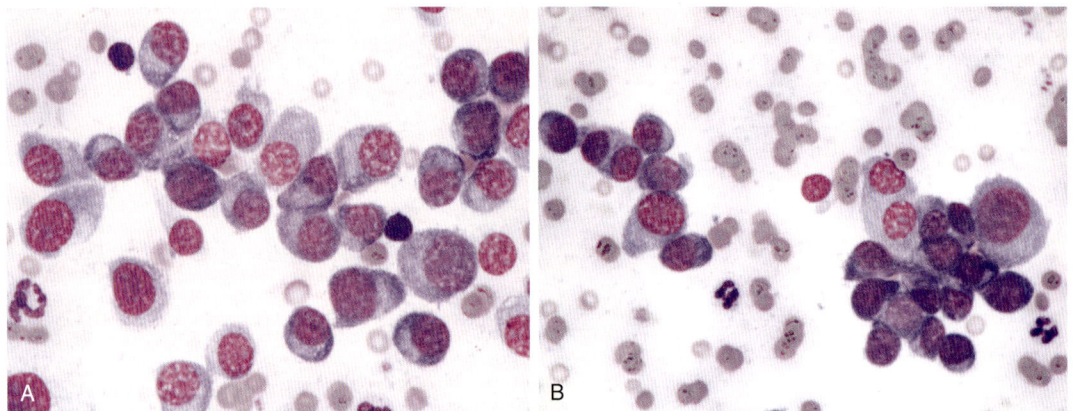

FIGURE 4.140 Plasmacytoma. Splenic aspirate. Cat. Same case in A and B. This patient presented with a fractured femur and a monoclonal gammopathy. It was suspected this began as a myeloma. **A,** Numerous plasma cells that appear mostly mature are present. (Wright-Giemsa; HP oil.) **B,** Another field demonstrates binucleation and pleomorphism of the plasma cell precursors. (Wright-Giemsa; HP oil.)

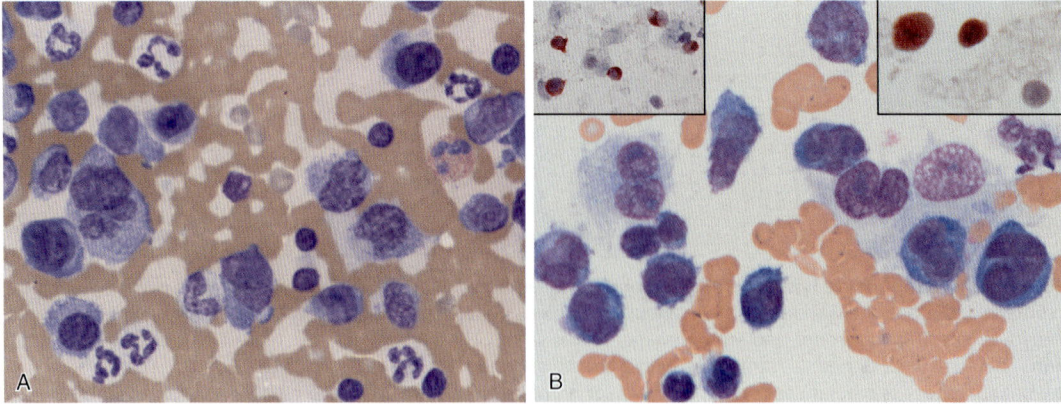

FIGURE 4.141 Plasmacytoma. Splenic aspirate. Cat. Same case in A and B. **A,** The nucleated cell population is heterogeneous with atypical round cells predominating. These cells have distinct cytoplasmic borders and a small to moderate amount of medium to deeply basophilic cytoplasm that may contain a prominent paranuclear clear zone and a few clear punctate vacuoles. The nucleus of these cells is often eccentric and highly pleomorphic ranging from oval to flower shaped, lobulated or ring form. The nucleus ranges from 2 to 4 × RBC diameter, with finely stippled to coarse chromatin and often contains one or two, round or oval, variably prominent nucleoli. (Wright-Giemsa; HP oil.) **B,** Occasional binucleation are observed. Among this population, there is marked anisocytosis and anisokaryosis with many mitotic figures (not shown). Lower numbers of small lymphocytes and well-differentiated plasma cells are found. (Wright-Giemsa; HP oil.) *Inset left:* Immunocytochemistry supports B-cell origin. (CD79a/AEC; HP oil.) *Inset right:* Immunocytochemistry supports plasma cell lineage. (MUM1/AEC; HP oil.) (Courtesy Mary Leissinger, University of Florida.)

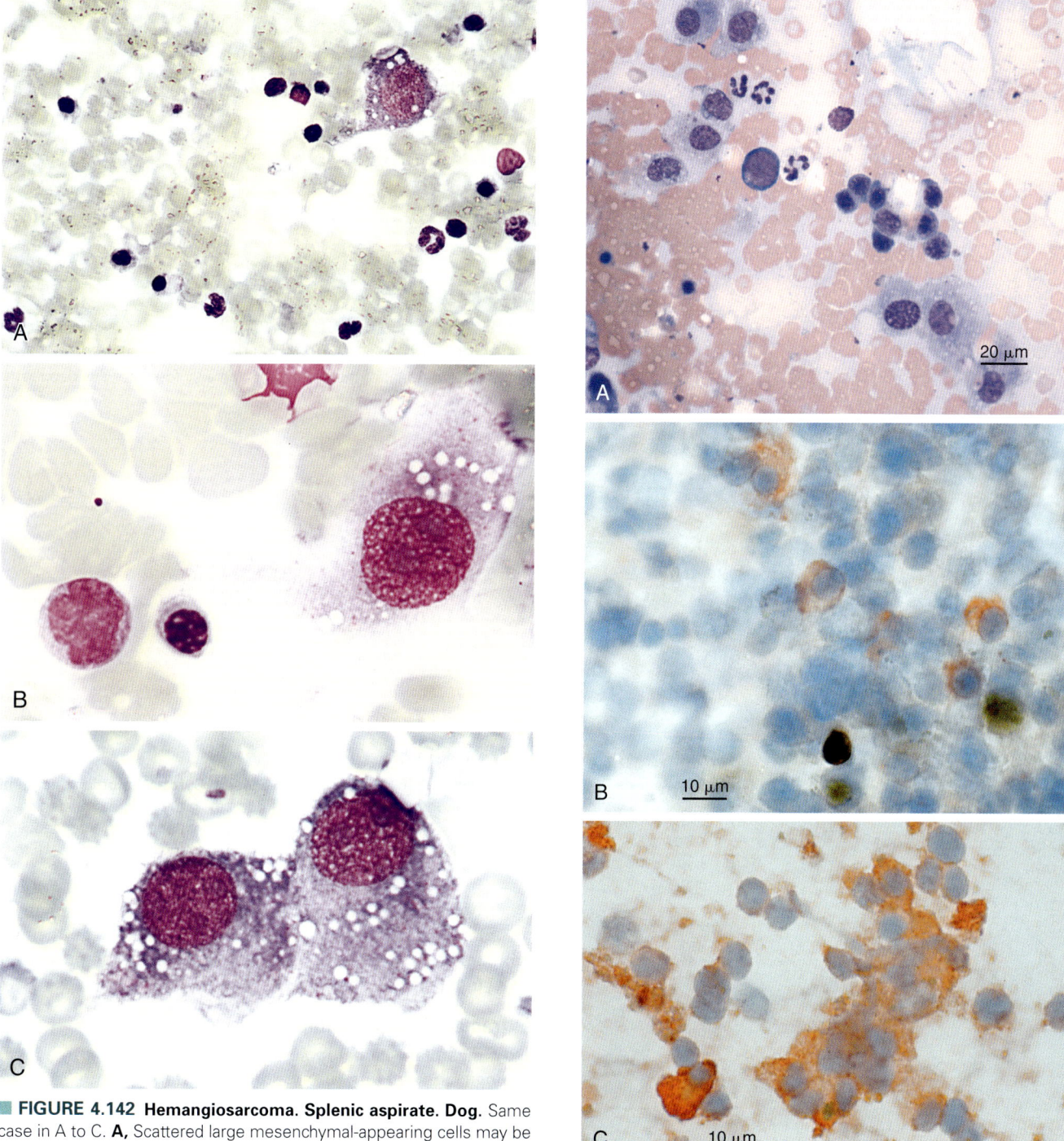

■ **FIGURE 4.142 Hemangiosarcoma. Splenic aspirate. Dog.** Same case in A to C. **A,** Scattered large mesenchymal-appearing cells may be found scanning on low magnification such as the one shown. (Wright-Giemsa; HP oil.) **B,** Medium lymphocyte, rubricyte, and large malignant cell. Note the round nucleus with coarse chromatin, multiple large nucleoli, and vacuolated cytoplasm with indistinct cell borders. Extramedullary hematopoiesis and lymphoid reactivity are commonly found in this condition. (Wright-Giemsa; HP oil.) **C,** Multiple punctate vacuoles are commonly found in the stellate cells of this neoplasm. (Wright-Giemsa; HP oil.)

■ **FIGURE 4.143 Hemangiosarcoma. Splenic aspirate. Dog.** Same case in A to C. **A,** Numerous neoplastic cells are present in aggregates. In the center is a group of erythroid precursors (extramedullary hematopoiesis). (Modified Wright; HP oil.) **B, Immunocytochemistry.** Cell surface reactivity present to endothelial antigen. (CD31/AEC; HP oil.) **C, Immunocytochemistry.** Strong reactivity with anti–von Willebrand factor also supports endothelial cell origin. (vWF/AEC; HP oil.)

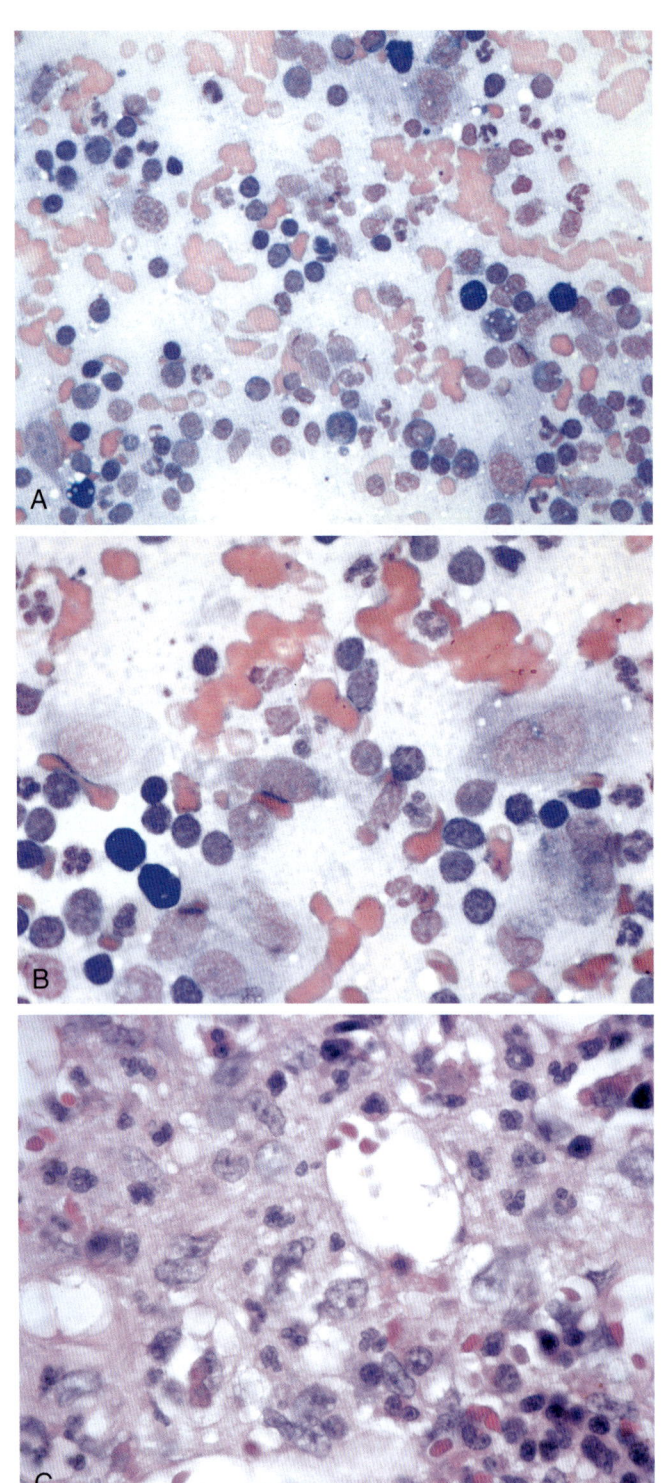

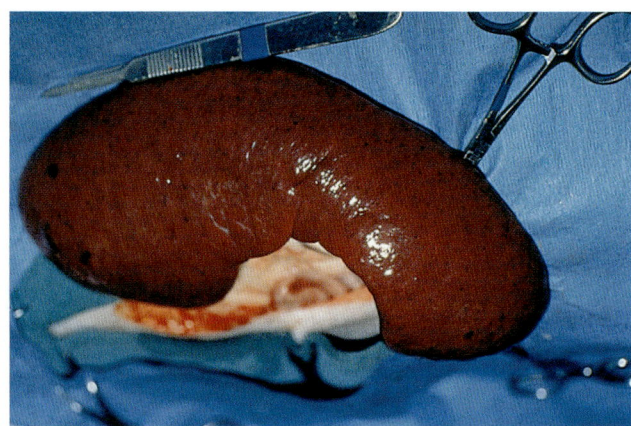

■ **FIGURE 4.145 Mastocytoma. Spleen. Macroscopic specimen. Cat.** Diffuse enlargement of the spleen is commonly found for this neoplasm.

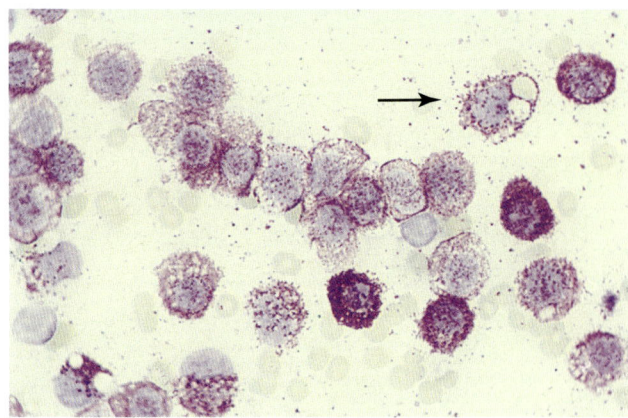

■ **FIGURE 4.146 Mastocytoma. Spleen. Cytopathologic specimen. Cat.** A monomorphic population of moderately to highly granulated mast cells is present. Note the cell *(arrow)* demonstrating erythrophagocytosis, a feature common for splenic mastocytoma. (Wright-Giemsa; HP oil.)

■ **FIGURE 4.144 Liposarcoma. Dog.** Same case in A to C. **A, Splenic imprint.** Four mesenchymal cells are present having wispy cell borders, round to oval nuclei, coarse chromatin, anisokaryosis, and prominent nucleoli. One cell is binucleated. (Wright-Giemsa; HP oil.) **B, Splenic imprint.** Some of the cells have small punctate vacuoles, which is similar to the primary liposarcoma discovered on the leg. (Wright-Giemsa; HP oil.) **C, Tissue section.** Neoplastic mesenchymal cells have foamy to vacuolated eosinophilic cytoplasm with indistinct cell borders. Nuclei are round to oval with vesicular chromatin with one or more prominent nucleoli. Low numbers of erythroid precursors and small lymphocytes are also seen. (H&E; HP oil.)

Occasionally, highly disseminated epithelial malignancies are found in the spleen. An example of secretory epithelium with anaplastic features (Fig. 4.149) and metastatic pheochromocytoma (Fig. 4.150) is shown.

Extramedullary Hematopoiesis

Extramedullary hematopoiesis was the most common cytopathologic abnormality in one study, accounting for 24% of the patients (O'Keefe and Couto, 1987). Although precursors from all three cell lines may be observed, erythroid cells are the most common, with metarubricytes, rubricytes, and prorubricytes present (Figs. 4.151 and 4.152). Care must be taken because erythroid precursors and lymphoid precursors appear very similar, and occasional late-stage erythroid precursors may be encountered commonly on splenic cytopathology. The finding of erythrblastic islands (Fig. 4.153) with developing rubricytes in contact with a macrophage for exchange of iron is strong evidence for extramedullary erythropoiesis. Mature megakaryocytes are easily observed during scanning at low magnification related to their large size. Conditions associated with extramedullary hematopoiesis include chronic hemorrhage, hemolytic anemia, chronic respiratory conditions, myeloproliferative disorders, and lymphoproliferative disorders.

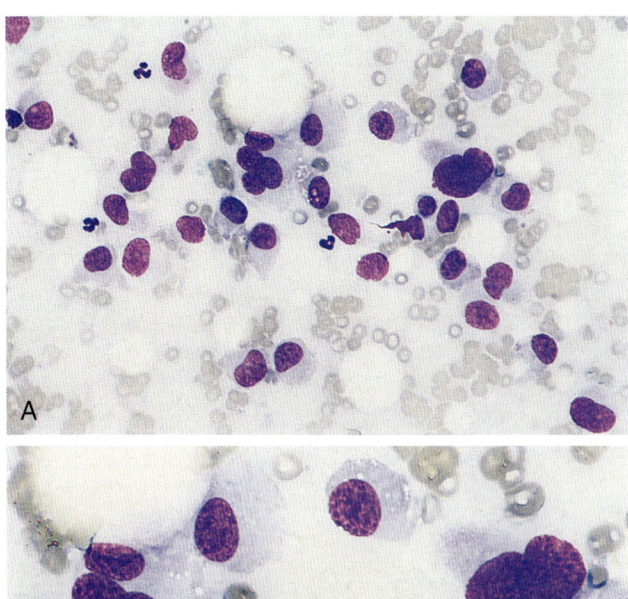

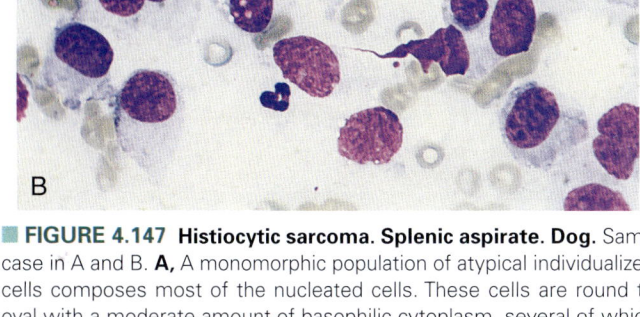

■ **FIGURE 4.147** **Histiocytic sarcoma. Splenic aspirate. Dog.** Same case in A and B. **A,** A monomorphic population of atypical individualized cells composes most of the nucleated cells. These cells are round to oval with a moderate amount of basophilic cytoplasm, several of which contain few punctate vacuoles. (Wright-Giemsa; HP oil.) **B,** Higher magnification demonstrates a lobulated cell *(right)* and a multinucleated cell *(left).* (Wright-Giemsa; HP oil.)

Appearing similar to extramedullary hematopoiesis is myelolipoma, an uncommon tumor in both dogs and cats, occurring in the liver or spleen. The presence of hematopoietic precursors with large amounts of lipid vacuoles in the background is strongly suggestive of this benign neoplasm (Fig. 4.154). It is often found unassociated with hematologic abnormalities. Ultrasound examination may demonstrate a small focal hyperechoic mass in the spleen or rarely a large mass (Al-Rukibat and Bani Ismail, 2006).

THYMUS

Normal Thymic Anatomy and Histology

Before puberty, the thymus has a prominent parenchyma divided into cortical and medullary regions (Fig. 4.155A). The outermost cortex is composed of small, densely packed lymphocytes without formation of lymphoid nodules. The central medulla is continuous between lobules that are formed by the inward extension of the thin connective tissue capsule. The medulla contains fewer and larger vesicular lymphocytes. The thymus is supported by a reticular network of stellate epithelial cells, which form loose cuffs around small vessels,

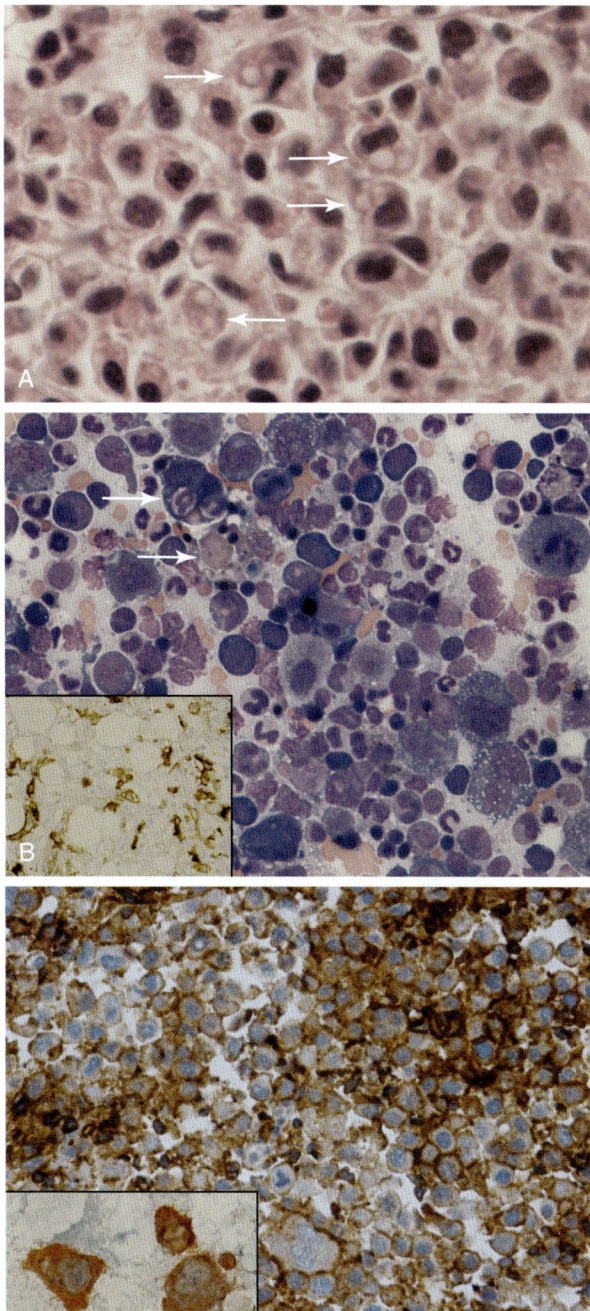

■ **FIGURE 4.148** **Hemophagocytic histiocytic sarcoma, disseminated. Dog.** Same case in A to C. **A, Splenic tissue section**. The spleen was replaced by a neoplastic population of histiocytic cells, several of which are shown displaying erythrophagocytosis *(arrows).* This 10-year-old Rottweiler presented with marked anemia and thrombocytopenia, along with clinical signs of lethargy and anorexia. (H&E; HP oil.) **B, Bone marrow aspirate**. Shown are large histiocytic cells, some of which display leukocytophagia and erythrophagia *(arrows).* (Wright; HP oil.). *Inset:* **Bone marrow core section**. Note the frequent expression of CD11d (brown reaction), a marker of splenic and bone marrow macrophages. (CD11d/DAB; IP.) **C, Spleen tissue section. Immunohistochemistry.** Nearly all cells in the spleen express BLA.36 on their cell surface in this tissue section but no immunoreactivity to CD3 and CD79a antigens supporting histiocytic origin. (BLA.36/DAB; IP.) *Inset:* **Bone marrow aspirate. Immunocytochemistry.** Three large bone marrow cells strongly express BLA.36 in this aspirate sample (BLA.36/AEC; HP oil.) (Courtesy Tricia Bisby, Purdue University.)

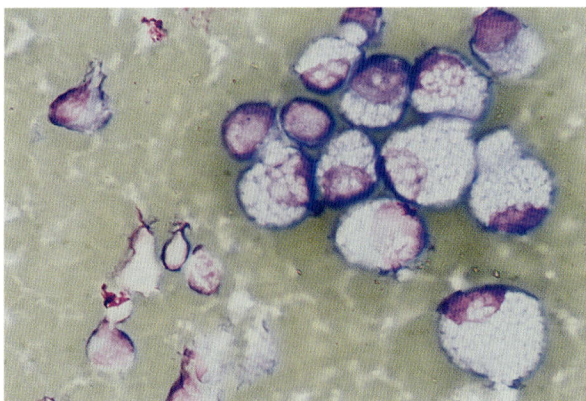

■ **FIGURE 4.149 Metastatic prostatic carcinoma. Splenic aspirate. Dog.** Cluster of individualized epithelial cells with marked anisokaryosis. Secretory nature of the tumor cells is suggested from the presence of abundant vacuoles in the cytoplasm. A carcinoma with similar-appearing cells was found in the prostate and was considered as the primary site. (Wright-Giemsa; HP oil.)

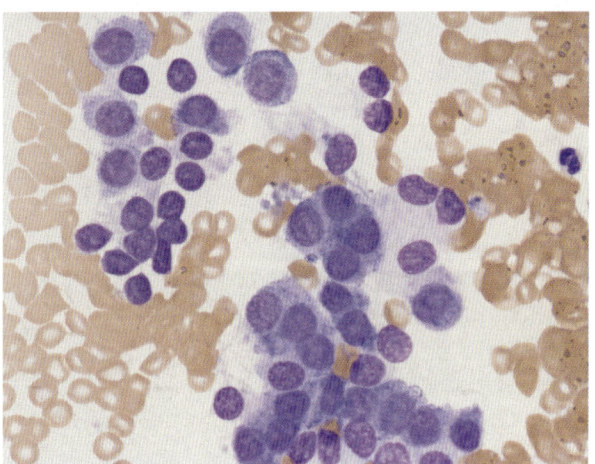

■ **FIGURE 4.150 Metastatic pheochromocytoma. Splenic nodule aspirate. Dog.** Nucleated cells consist predominately of epithelial cells with indistinct cell borders present in small clusters. When borders are visible, the cells appear round to polygonal with a centrally placed round or oval nucleus measuring 1 to 1.5 × RBC diameter with stippled to clumped chromatin that sometimes contains one to few small faint nucleoli. The cells have small to moderate amounts of lightly to moderately basophilic, often finely granular, cytoplasm. Anisocytosis and anisokaryosis is mostly mild, and the nucleocytoplasmic ratio is high. History includes a histopathologic diagnosis of malignant pheochromocytoma in one adrenal gland 7 months earlier to this presentation. (Wright-Giemsa; HP oil.) (Courtesy Mary Leissinger, University of Florida.)

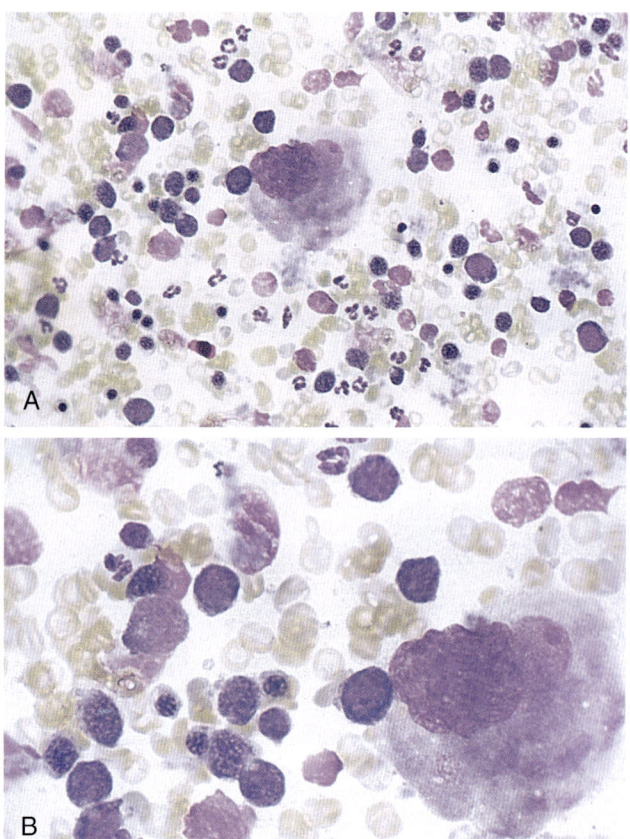

■ **FIGURE 4.151 Extramedullary hematopoiesis. Splenic aspirate. Dog.** Same case in A and B. **A,** A megakaryocyte and numerous erythroid precursors are detected in this sample from an animal that received chemotherapy 2 weeks earlier for lymphoma. (Wright-Giemsa; HP oil.) **B,** Higher magnification demonstrates low numbers of medium-sized lymphocytes with many rubricytes in addition to the mature megakaryocyte. (Wright-Giemsa; HP oil.)

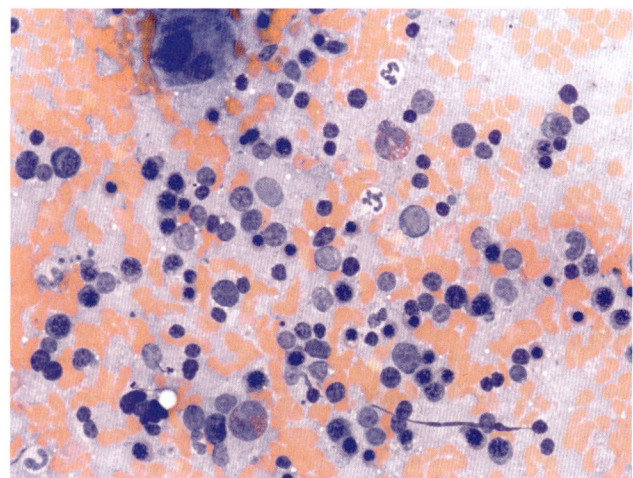

■ **FIGURE 4.152 Extramedullary hematopoiesis with reactive lymphoid hyperplasia. Splenic aspirate. Dog.** Hematopoietic precursors predominate comprised primarily of erythroid and megakaryocytic precursors with fewer myeloid precursors. A heterogeneous lymphoid population is also present. This response is likely secondary to this patient's reported immune-mediated thrombocytopenia. (Wright-Giemsa; HP oil.) (Courtesy Tracie Guy, University of Florida.)

termed *Hassall's corpuscles*. These concentric whorls of flattened reticular cells may become keratinized or calcified (see Fig. 4.155A–B). The reticular epithelium also gives rise to a ductal system within the medulla that may become cystic and lined by ciliated epithelium. After puberty, the thymic parenchyma begins to atrophy, becoming replaced by adipose tissue.

Indications for Thymic Biopsy
- *Enlargement*—detected by radiography and ultrasonography, often producing signs of dyspnea, pleural effusions, and dysphagia (swallowing difficulties)

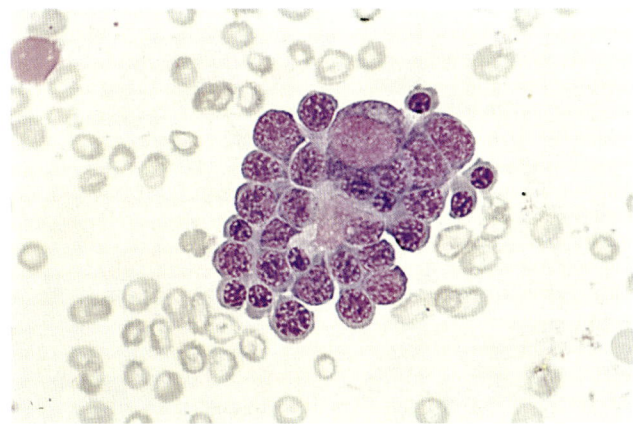

■ **FIGURE 4.153** **Extramedullary hematopoiesis. Splenic aspirate. Dog.** A nurse cell or a macrophage surrounded by various stages of erythroid development may be found in areas of increased erythropoiesis. (Wright-Giemsa; HP oil.)

- *Abnormal imaging features*—suggest the presence of hyperplasia or infiltrative processes

Normal Thymus Cytology and Artifacts

The thymus contains two different cell populations, lymphocytes and reticular epithelium. Cytologically, the cell population of the cortex is similar to that of the lymph node with the predominance of small, dense-staining lymphocytes (Fig. 4.156). Occasional mast cells are present. Large stellate cells with round vesicular nuclei representing the thymic epithelium are found scattered between the lymphocytes or in tight balls (Fig. 4.157), the latter arrangement become Hassall's corpuscles. These dense collections of epithelium appear similar to epithelioid macrophages having abundant pale-blue cytoplasm with cellular attachment to each other. If keratinized, the Hassall's corpuscles will be hyalinized and dark blue with Romanowsky staining and may be confused with mesothelium (Fig. 4.158).

Non-neoplastic Thymic Tumors

Branchial cysts or clefts of the thymus and are considered to be of common embryonic origin and are present as vestigial structures in the cranial mediastinum in dogs and rarely in cats (Zekas and Adams, 2002). Other cystic structures in the mediastinum include parathyroid, thyroglossal duct and pleural origins. The main clinical sign is dyspnea along with variable amounts of pleural fluid; however, they may be found incidentally. Aspiration of the cyst may reveal few or no cells with low protein. Alternatively, an aspirate may contain mucin only or ciliated epithelium (Fig. 4.159) related to their respiratory origins. Recently, transformation into carcinoma has been reported (Levien et al., 2010). Prognosis is variable depending on the severity of the clinical condition.

Thymic Lymphoma

Neoplasia of the lymphoid cells of the thymus is termed *thymic lymphoma*, having the appearance of lymphoma in other lymphoid organs as in the lymph node. Immunocytochemistry is a helpful adjunct to diagnosis (Fig. 4.160). In one canine study of mediastinal masses with immunophenotyping by flow cytometry along with PARR clonality assessment, there were six of

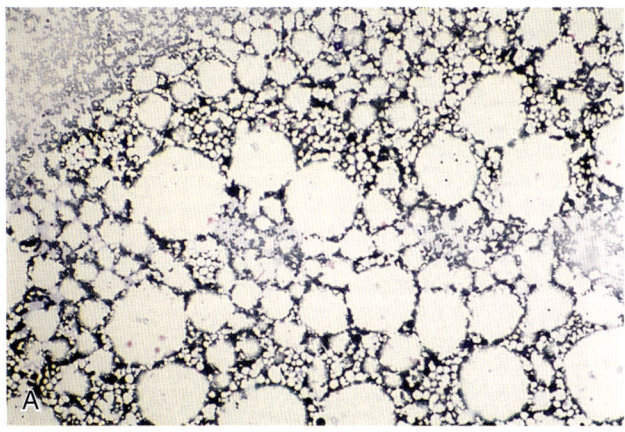

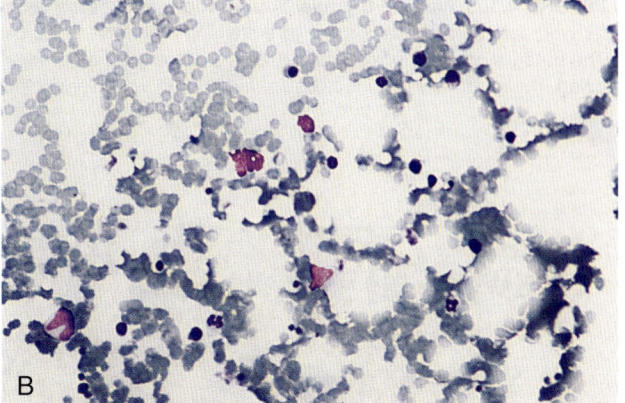

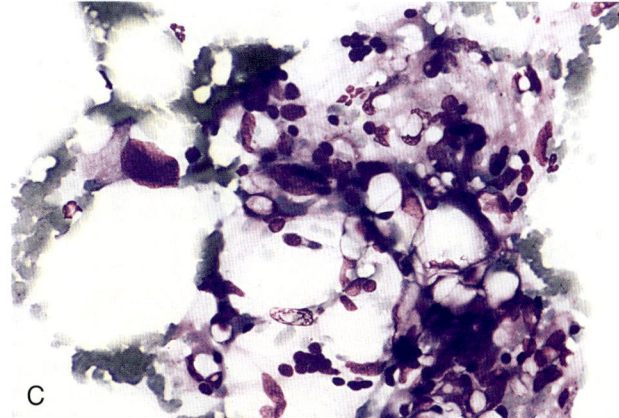

■ **FIGURE 4.154** **Myelolipoma. Splenic aspirate. Cat.** Same case in A to C. **A,** Low magnification demonstrates the massive amounts of variably sized clear vacuoles, consistent with lipid. (Wright-Giemsa; LP.) **B,** Dark-staining erythroid precursors are associated with the lipid material. (Wright-Giemsa; HP oil.) **C,** A megakaryocyte and collections of reticular stroma are present within the small discrete nodule on the splenic tail. (Wright-Giemsa; HP oil.)

T-cell origin and one of B-cell origin (Lana et al., 2006). One case had CD34+ phenotype with precursor lymphoblasts, but most thymic lymphoma tumors had a CD4+ phenotype, which is often associated with hypercalcemia.

Thymoma

Neoplasia of the thymic epithelial cells is termed *thymoma*. Clinical signs generally refer to swallowing, breathing, and general

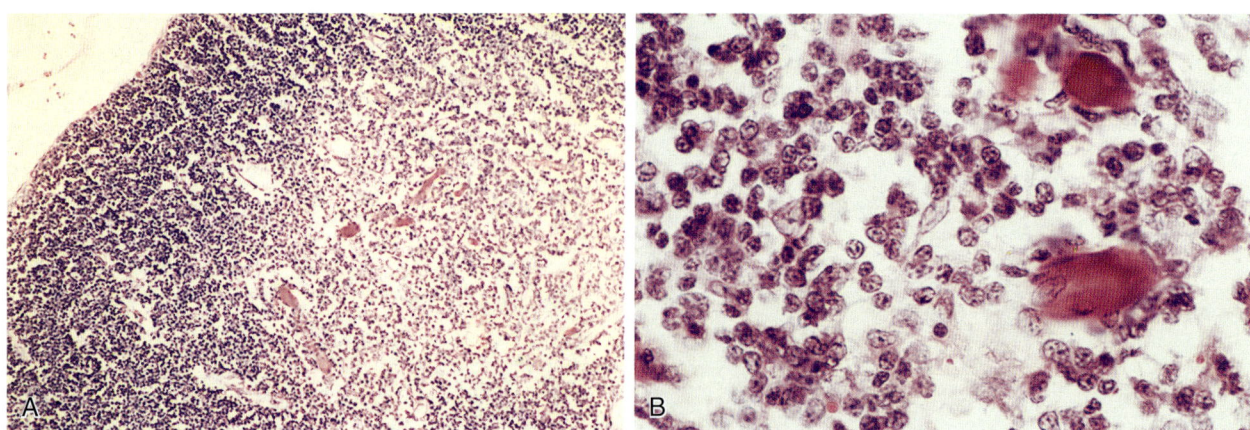

FIGURE 4.155 Normal thymus. Young dog. Same tissue section in A and B. **A,** The dense cortical area is composed of packed lymphocytes *(left)*, whereas the medulla is more pale staining *(right)*. Note the dark eosinophilic structures in the medulla called *Hassall's corpuscles*. (H&E; IP) **B,** The medulla contains eosinophilic Hassall's corpuscles that represent perivascular cuffs of flattened reticular stroma that become keratinized or calcified. The medullary lymphocytes are larger with vesicular nucleus. (H&E; HP oil.)

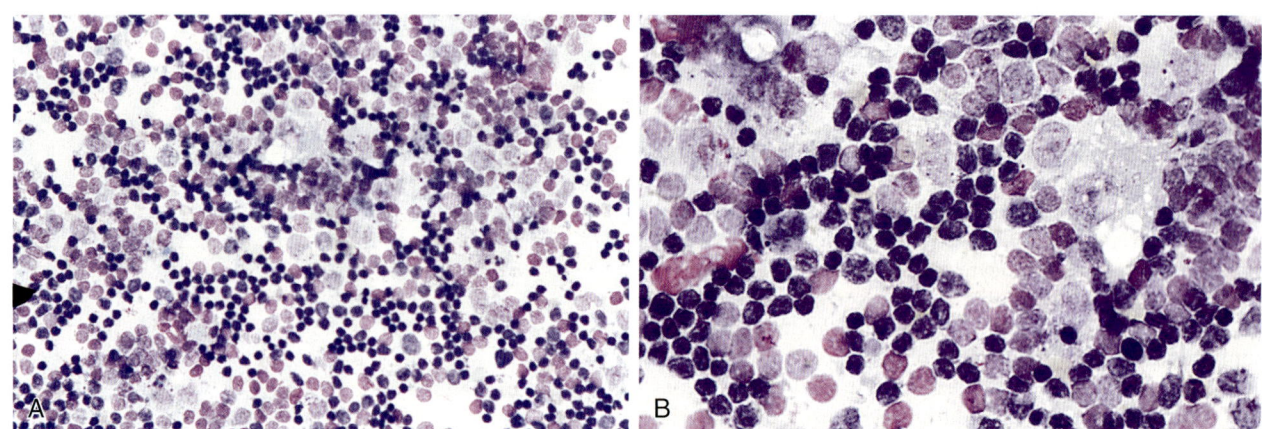

FIGURE 4.156 Normal thymus. Young dog. Same tissue aspirate in A and B. **A,** Many small, dark-staining lymphocytes are the predominant population, with fewer medium lymphocytes. Note the two large epithelial cells in the *top center* of the field. (Wright-Giemsa; HP oil.) **B,** Higher magnification demonstrates the large stellate reticular epithelium with vesicular nuclei. (Wright-Giemsa; HP oil.)

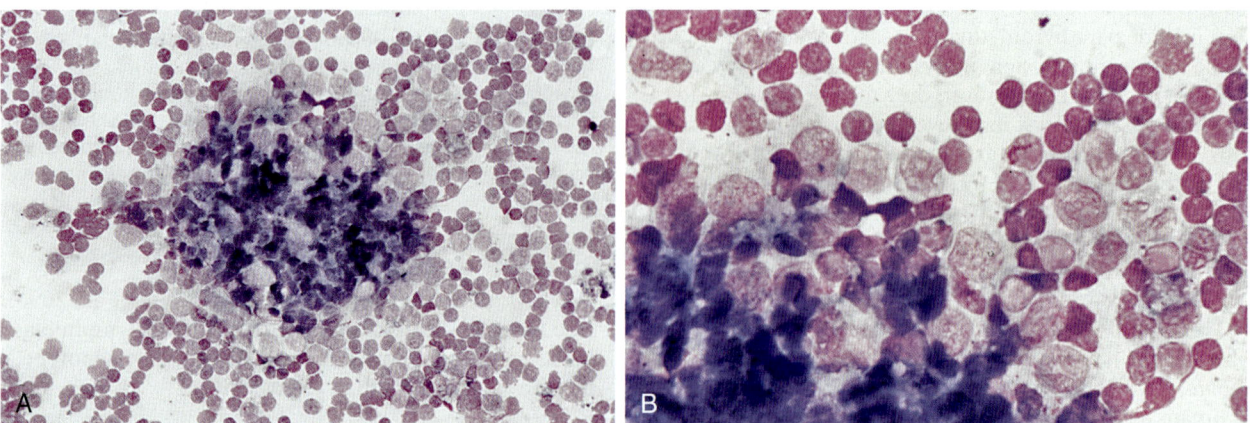

FIGURE 4.157 Normal thymus. Young dog. Same tissue aspirate in A and B. **A,** Thymic epithelium may be found in tight balls, possibly representing perivascular cuffs. (Wright-Giemsa; HP oil.) **B,** Higher magnification to demonstrate the small lymphocytes and thymic epithelium. (Wright-Giemsa; HP oil.)

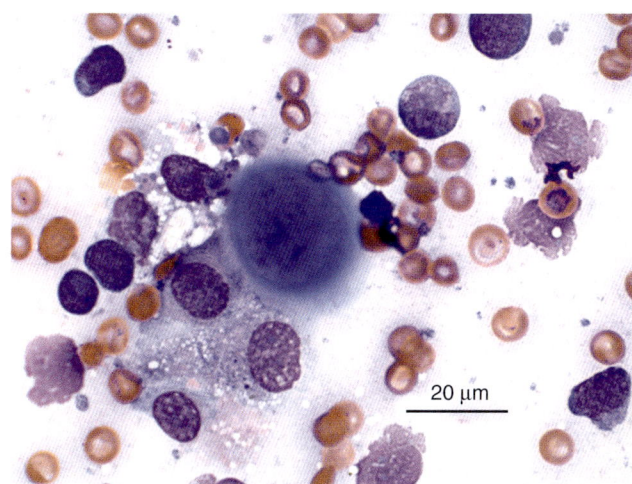

■ **FIGURE 4.158 Thymic lymphoma with mesothelial cell. Mediastinal mass aspirate. Dog.** A single mesothelial cell is found among several medium and occasional small lymphocytes. (Modified Wright; HP oil.) (Courtesy Andrea Pires dos Santos, Purdue University.)

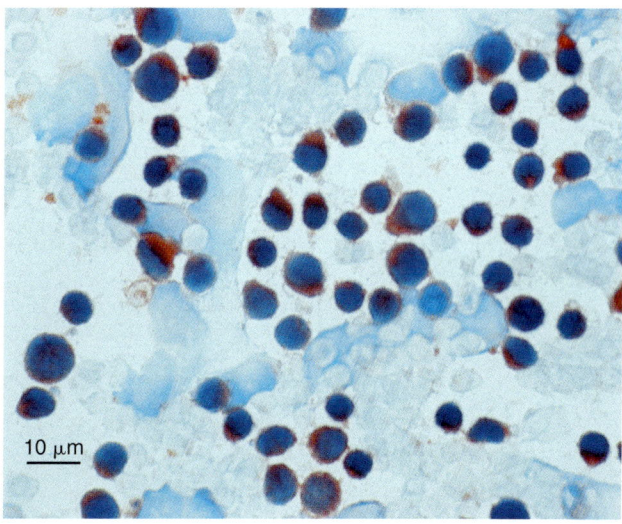

■ **FIGURE 4.160 Thymic T-cell lymphoma. Tissue aspirate. Immunocytochemistry. Cat.** Strong reactivity of both surface and cytoplasm to anti-CD3ε supporting T-cell origin. (CD3ε/AEC; HP oil.)

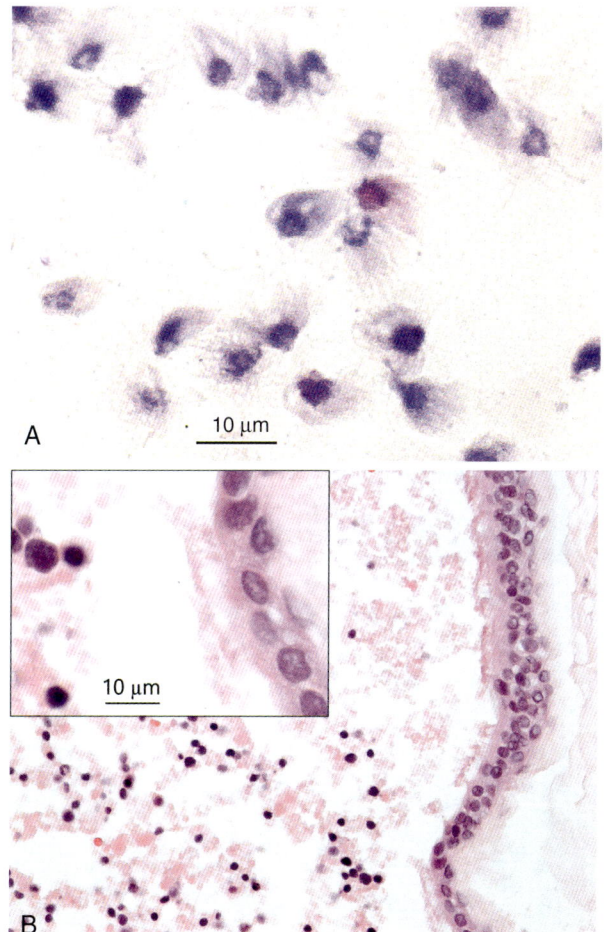

■ **FIGURE 4.159 Thymic cyst (branchial cleft). Dog.** Same case in A and B. **A, Tissue aspirate.** Cystic fluid was aspirated from a paraesophageal neck mass that contained ciliated cuboidal epithelium. The ciliated end supports the respiratory origin of these cells. (Modified Wright; HP oil.) **B, Tissue section.** Cells line a cyst filled with pyknotic cells, debris, and proteinaceous fluid. (H&E; IP). *Inset:* Closer view of cells demonstrates their ciliated surface. (H&E; HP oil.)

weakness with a mass seen radiographically in the cranial mediastinum (Fig. 4.161A). It usually takes one of three forms in dogs and cats such as epithelial thymoma (Fig. 4.161B), mixed lymphoepithelial thymoma, or lymphocyte-predominant thymoma based on the relative numbers of these two cell types. In the epithelial thymoma, the reticular epithelium predominates, with low numbers of mostly small lymphocytes remaining. The epithelial cells often appear as large cohesive, pale, mononuclear cells that resemble epithelioid macrophages (Fig. 4.162) or less commonly resemble spindle cells similar to fibroblasts. In the mixed cell thymoma, variably sized clusters of neoplastic epithelium appear with many small lymphocytes and fewer medium or large lymphocytes (Figs. 4.163 and 4.164). A lymphocyte-predominant thymoma contains many small lymphocytes and only scattered thymic epithelium with a loss of normal architecture (Fig. 4.165). Histopathologic subtypes are based on a WHO classification applied to animals, which relates to the cell morphology of the neoplastic epithelial cells, relative proportion of lymphocytes, mitotic count, and tissue invasion (Burgess et al., 2016).

Large numbers of well-differentiated mast cells are commonly found within thymomas and may give the false impression of a mast cell tumor or metastatic mast cells into a lymph node (Fig. 4.166; see also Fig. 4.163A). Eosinophilic material may be associated with cells in a thymoma (Andreasen et al., 1991), which closely resembles the colloid found in a thyroid tumor and may present a diagnostic dilemma. Thymic epithelium can be difficult to recognize, varying from indistinct cytoplasmic borders (Fig. 4.167; see also Figs. 4.162 and 4.163B) to well-defined cell borders (Fig. 4.168; see Fig. 4.164B). Immunohistochemistry can help determine thymic cells using anti-CD3 for T lymphocytes (see Fig. 4.165D) and cytokeratin markers for the thymic epithelium.

Clinically, increased survival has been demonstrated for dogs older than 8 years of age, dogs with the histologic subtype lymphocyte-predominant, and dogs without concurrent megaesophagus (Atwater et al., 1994). Myasthenia gravis and pure red cell aplasia are paraneoplastic syndromes associated with thymoma in addition to hypercalcemia. Elevated serum antibodies against acetylcholine receptor were demonstrated in dogs with

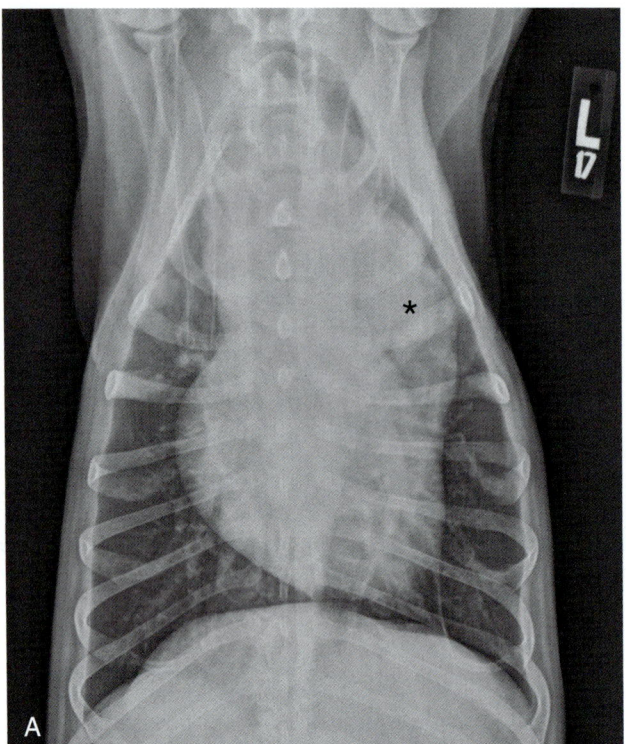

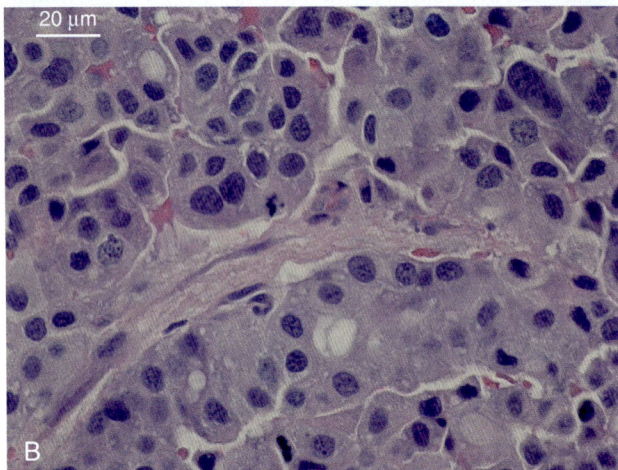

■ **FIGURE 4.161 Thymoma. Dog.** Same case in A and B. History involved an 8-month duration of ptyalism, lethargy, facial nerve paralysis, and weight loss. A high antibody titer against acetylcholine receptor supported the diagnosis of myasthenia gravis. **A, Radiograph.** The large cranial mediastinal mass *(asterisk)* extends caudally as determined by computed tomography. The mass surrounds the tracheal and esophagus, causing excessive drooling. **B, Tissue section.** The normal architecture is lost, and the most prominent cell type is an epithelial cell with moderate amount of pale eosinophilic cytoplasm and large round nucleus with dispersed chromatin with small or indistinct nucleoli. Occasional mitotic figures are found. There are low numbers of small lymphocytes with hyperchromatic nucleus and lack of nucleoli. (H&E; HP oil.) (A, Courtesy Carrie Fulkerson, Purdue University.)

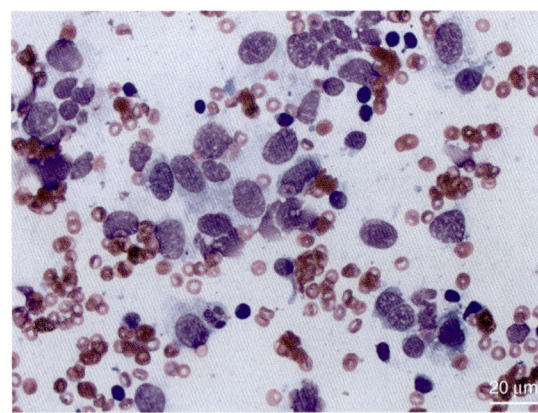

■ **FIGURE 4.162 Thymoma. Thoracic mass aspirate. Dog.** The majority of nucleated cells are moderately atypical epithelial cells present individually and rarely in small cohesive clusters. These cells are polygonal, angular, or oval with variably distinct cytoplasmic borders and a moderate amount of basophilic cytoplasm containing a few clear punctate vacuoles. The paracentral nucleus is approximately 1.5 to 2 × RBC diameter with coarse chromatin and one to few, round or oval, prominent nucleoli that vary in size. Among this population, anisocytosis and anisokaryosis are mild to moderate. Small lymphocytes are present in low numbers admixed with the epithelial cell population. History involved a previously excised thymoma 6 months earlier, suggesting local recurrence. (Wright-Giemsa; HP oil.) (Courtesy Tracie Guy, University of Florida.)

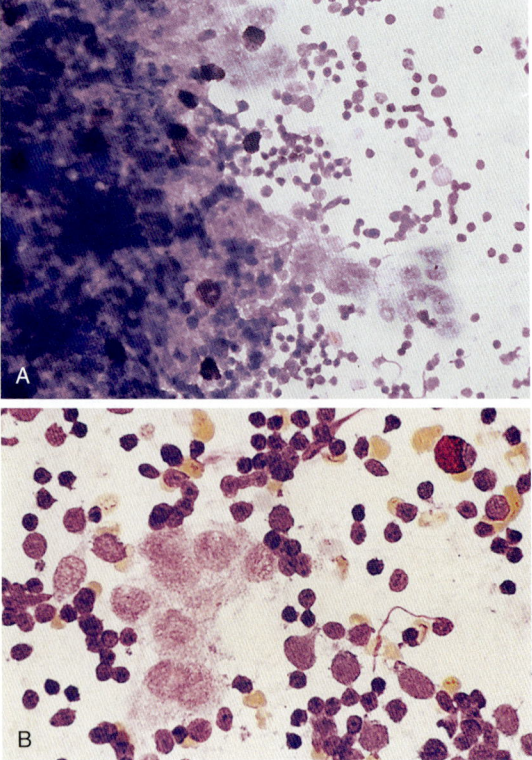

■ **FIGURE 4.163 Thymoma. Tissue aspirate. Dog.** Same case in A and B. **A,** Mixture of small lymphocytes and clusters of thymic epithelium suggests the lymphoepithelial histologic type. Note the scattered mast cells throughout the stroma at the left side seen as dark cells. (Wright-Giemsa; HP oil.) **B,** This animal presented with no clinical signs except radiographic evidence of a cranial mediastinal mass during screening for elective surgery. Note the small cluster of reticular epithelium that resembles spindle cells. A well-differentiated mast cell is shown in the *upper right corner*. (Wright-Giemsa; HP oil.)

megaesophagus and in about one-third of dogs with epithelial thymomas (Burgess et al., 2016). Owing to the close association between megaesophagus and myasthenia gravis, it is recommended that all dogs with megaesophagus and thymoma be tested for myasthenia gravis (Scott-Moncrieff et al., 1990). Cats

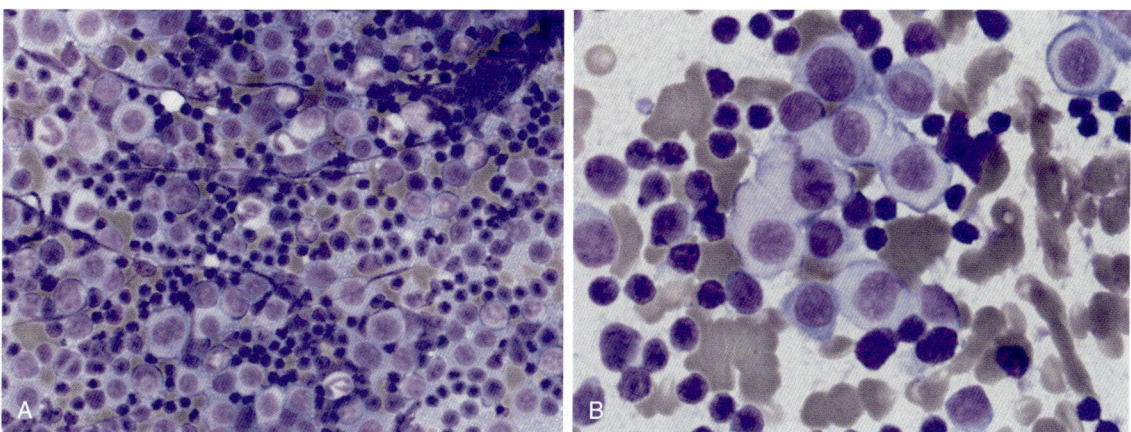

FIGURE 4.164 Mixed epithelial-lymphocytic thymoma. Mediastinal mass aspirate. Dog. Same case in A and B. **A,** There is a heterogeneous population of neoplastic epithelial cells and a mixed lymphoid population. The neoplastic epithelial cells are both individual and in small clusters. Anisocytosis and anisokaryosis are moderate with occasional binucleation observed. Occasional nondegenerate neutrophils are found. Low numbers of mast cells and mitotic figures are present but not shown. (Aqueous Romanowsky; HP oil.) **B,** Neoplastic cells are round with variably distinct cellular borders and a moderate amount of pale blue cytoplasm. The nucleus is oval to round, centrally located with stippled chromatin, and measures 1.5 to 3 × RBC diameter. One to four small nucleoli are observed. Of the lymphoid cell population, small lymphocytes predominate with fewer medium forms. (Aqueous Romanowsky; HP oil.) (Courtesy Jacqueline Dolan, University of Florida.)

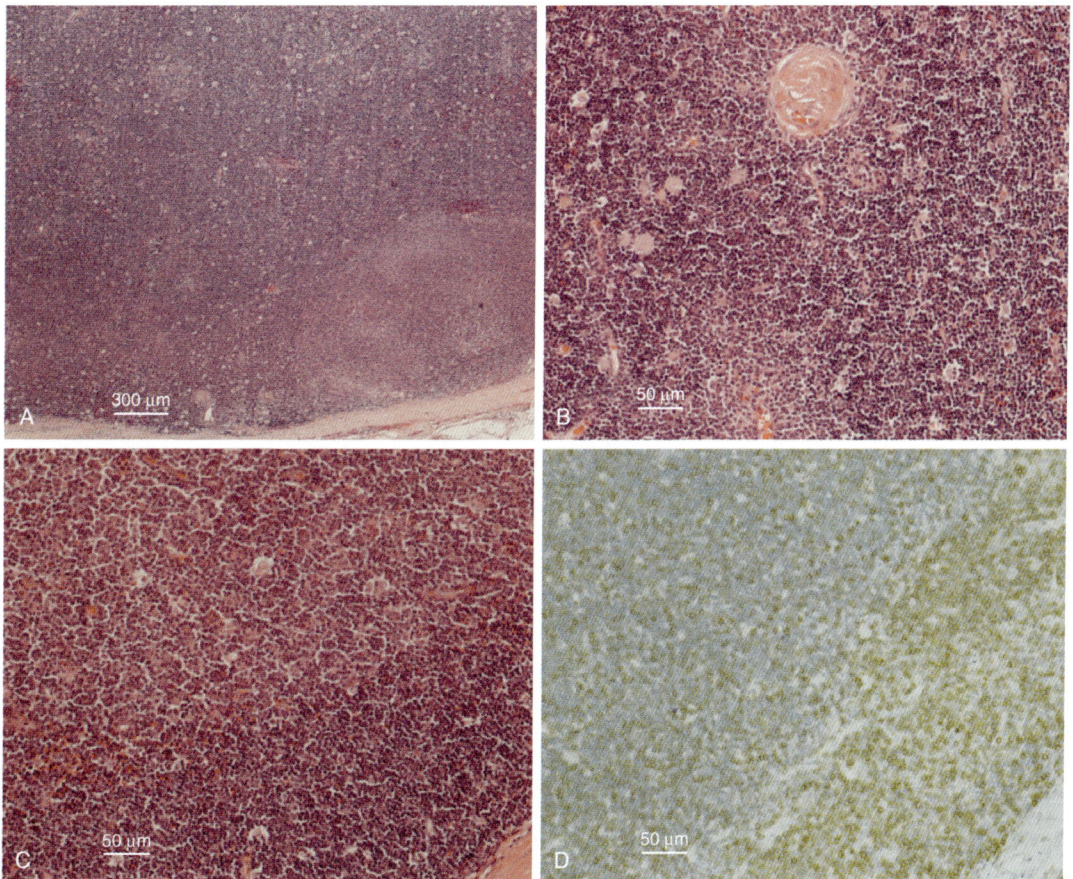

FIGURE 4.165 Thymoma, lymphocyte predominant. Tissue section. Dog. Same case in A to D. **A, Cortex.** The normal thymic architecture is lost in this mediastinal mass from a 3-year-old mixed-breed dog. There is disruption of the normal cortex by a focal proliferation of pale pink cells just under the thick, fibrous capsule. The majority of the cell population appears basophilic and diffuse. (H&E; LP.) **B, Hassall's corpuscle.** This is a higher magnification of the dense basophilic and cellular area from the case shown in A. Notice the circular pink area, called *Hassall's corpuscles,* which are composed of keratinized stromal cells that surround a blood vessel. (H&E; IP.) **C, Mixed cell population.** Notice the dense lymphocyte-rich cortical area adjacent to the capsule *(lower right).* Deep to the cortex is a well-defined mixed lymphocyte and epithelial region that stains paler than the cortex. This image complements the immunostaining shown in D. (H&E; IP.) **D, Immunohistochemistry.** This is the same magnification and area taken in C. The lymphocyte population is of T-cell origin based on the strong antibody expression in the cortex. The large area of thymic epithelial cells involves the paler areas. Thymic epithelium are best appreciated by immunoreactivity to cytokeratin (not shown). (CD3/DAB; IP.)

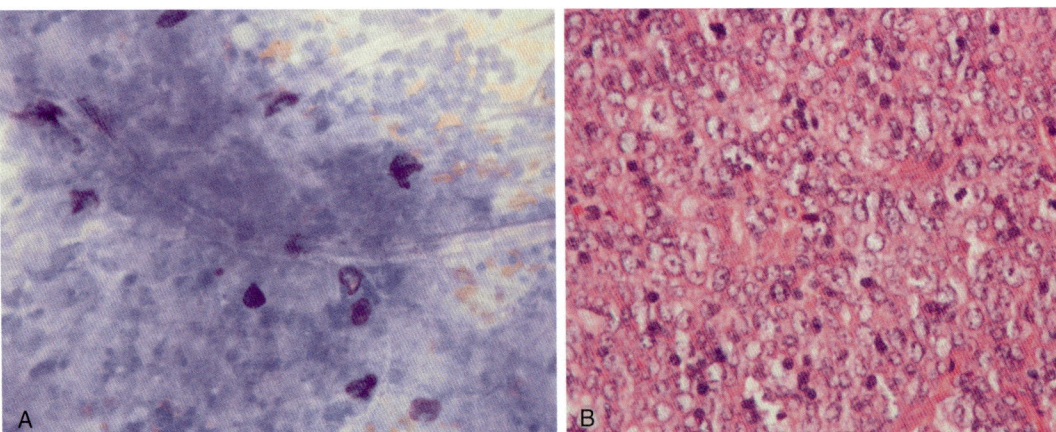

■ **FIGURE 4.166 Thymoma. Thymic mass. Dog.** Same case in A and B. **A, Tissue aspirate.** Low magnification of epithelial cluster with numerous scattered mast cells. (Wright-Giemsa; LP.) **B, Tissue section.** Numerous cells bearing light chromatin with prominent one or more nucleoli. Mast cells are not apparent without Giemsa staining. (H&E; HP oil.)

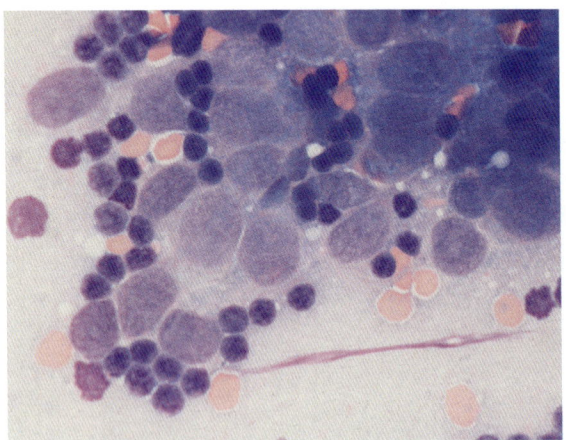

■ **FIGURE 4.167 Thymoma. Mixed epithelial-lymphocytic. Cytopathologic specimen. Dog.** Epithelial thymic cells have indistinct cell borders and have finely stippled chromatin with distinct nuclear outlines and high nucleocytoplasmic ratio. (Modified Wright; HP oil.) (Courtesy TDDS, Exeter, UK.)

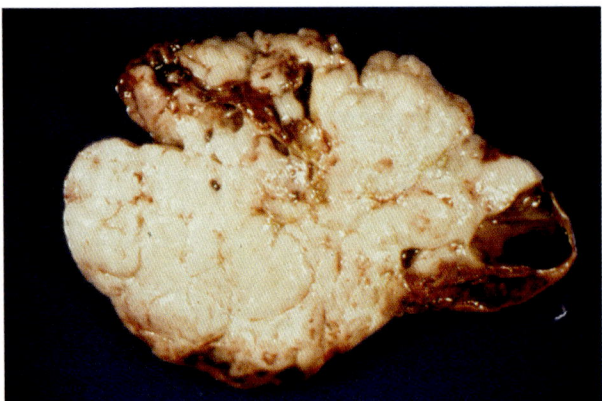

■ **FIGURE 4.169 Thymoma. Macroscopic specimen. German shepherd dog.** This large cranial mediastinal mass measured 12 × 10 × 8 cm. It was partially encapsulated, slightly firm, and tan with occasional mucus-containing cysts. (Courtesy Lois Roth, Angell Memorial Hospital. Presented at the 1997 ASVCP case review session.)

with thymoma were reported to have exfoliative skin lesions (Day, 1997; Scott et al., 1995). A case in a cat was present in an ectopic location and diagnosis involved histopathology with immunochemistry of the mass and flow cytometry of the lymphocyte population. Lymphocytes were double positive for CD4 and CD8, supporting the diagnosis of thymoma (Lara-Garcia et al., 2008). Thymoma masses are often large (Fig. 4.169), but because of their localized and often encapsulated appearance, surgical excision is recommended. Chylous effusion has also been associated with thymoma related to the infiltration of the tumor into the lymphatics. Another paraneoplastic condition associated with a dog with thymoma is T-cell lymphocytosis, which has a mixed cell type and is not similar to the double-positive lymphocytes of the thymic mass (Batlivala et al., 2010).

Recurrence of a thymoma with anaplastic features are concerning for malignancy (see Fig. 4.162). However, metastasis to the local lymph nodes or invasion into adjacent tissues supports thymic carcinoma (Fig. 4.170). Metastasis to the lung and liver is uncommon but has been reported in three of eight malignant canine cases in one study (Bellah et al., 1983). Reports of an uncommon occurrence of cystic thymomas in cats demonstrated metastasis in several of the cases (Patnaik et al., 2003).

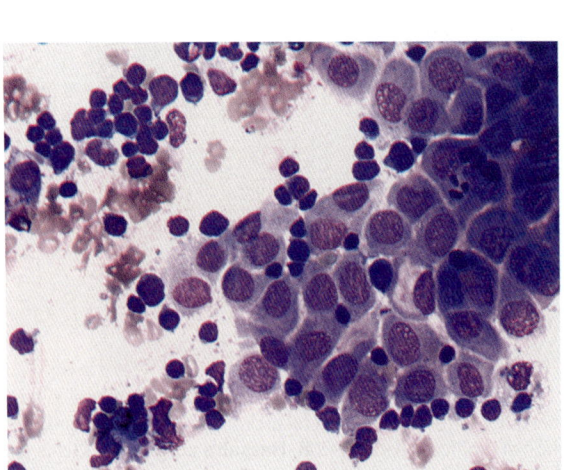

■ **FIGURE 4.168 Thymoma. Mixed epithelial and lymphocytic. Cytopathologic specimen. Dog.** Epithelial thymic cells from a case with distinct cytoplasmic borders, moderately coarse chromatin, and a moderate nucleocytoplasmic ratio. (Wright-Giemsa; HP oil.) (Courtesy Francesco Cian, Animal Health Trust, UK.)

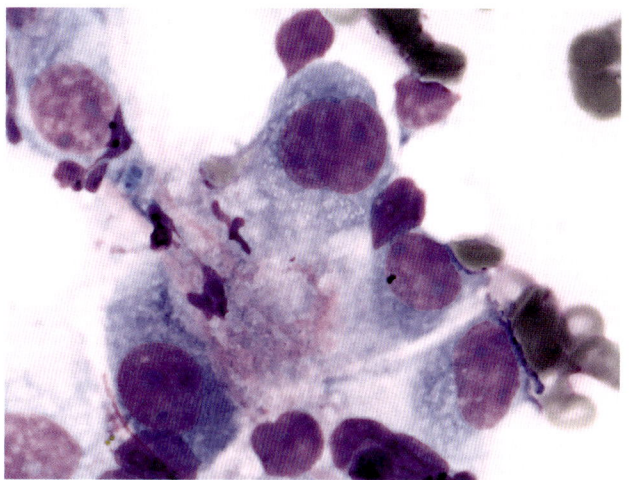

■ **FIGURE 4.170 Thymic carcinoma. Mediastinal mass aspirate. Dog.** The patient had a history of thoracic mass, dyspnea, and pleural effusion. The nucleated cells were composed primarily of large, cohesive sheets of polygonal cells, occasionally admixed with low amounts of pink fibrillar matrix. Cells have a round to oval nucleus, approximately 10 to 15 μm in diameter, with finely clumped chromatin, one to four small, prominent nucleoli, and moderate amounts of basophilic cytoplasm with indistinct borders and occasionally small vacuoles. Low to moderate numbers of small lymphocytes are also present in the background. Occasional well-granulated mast cells were noted along with erythrophagia, siderophagia, and phagocytized hematoidin (not shown). (Aqueous Romanowsky; HP oil.) (Courtesy Laureen Peters, The Royal Veterinary College, London.)

REFERENCES

Affolter VK, Moore PF. Localized and disseminated histiocytic sarcoma of dendritic cell origin in dogs. *Vet Pathol.* 2002;39:74-83.

Allen J, Hartley AN, Neel JA. What is your diagnosis? Splenic aspirate from a dog. *Vet Clin Pathol.* 2018;47(4):674-675.

Al-Rukibat RK, Bani Ismail ZA. Unusual presentation of splenic myelolipoma in a dog. *Can Vet J.* 2006;47(11):1112-1114.

Amores-Fuster I, Cripps P, Graham P, et al. The diagnostic utility of lymph node cytology samples in dogs and cats. *J Small Anim Pract.* 2015;56(2): 125-129.

Andreasen CB, Mahaffey EA, Latimer KS. What is your diagnosis? *Vet Clin Pathol.* 1991;20:15-16.

Attipa C, Brooks F, Wilson A, et al. What is your diagnosis? Lymph node aspirates from a dog with prominent lymphadenomegaly. *Vet Clin Pathol.* 2017;46(4):641-642.

Atwater SW, Powers BE, Park RD, et al. Thymoma in dogs: 23 cases (1980-1991). *J Am Vet Med Assoc.* 1994;205:1007-1013.

Bain BJ, Clark DM, Wilkins BS. Lymphoproliferative disorders. In: *Bone Marrow Pathology*. West Sussex, UK: Wiley-Blackwell; 2010:205.

Ballegeer EA, Forrest LJ, Dickinson RM, et al. Correlation of ultrasonographic appearance of lesions and cytologic and histologic diagnoses in splenic aspirates from dogs and cats: 32 cases (2002–2005). *J Am Vet Med Assoc.* 2007; 230(5):690-696.

Batlivala TP, Bacon NJ, Avery AC, et al. Paraneoplastic T cell lymphocytosis associated with a thymoma in a dog. *J Small Anim Pract.* 2010;51(9):491-494.

Bauer NB, Zervos D, Moritz A. Argyrophilic nucleolar organizing regions and Ki67 equally reflect proliferation in fine needle aspirates of normal, hyperplastic, inflamed, and neoplastic canine lymph nodes (n=101). *J Vet Intern Med.* 2007; 21:928-935.

Bellah JR, Stiff ME, Russell RG. Thymoma in the dog: two case reports and review of 20 additional cases. *J Am Vet Med Assoc.* 1983;183:306-311.

Bookbinder PF, Butt MT, Harvey HJ. Determination of the number of mast cells in lymph node, bone marrow, and buffy coat cytologic specimens from dogs. *J Am Vet Med Assoc.* 1992;11:1648-1650.

Burgess KE, DeRegis CJ, Brown FS, et al. Histologic and immunohistochemical characterization of thymic epithelial tumours in the dog. *Vet Comp Oncol.* 2016;14(2):113-121.

Burgess HJ, MacDonald Dickinson V, Kerr M, et al. Marginal zone lymphoma in a dog. *Vet Clin Pathol.* 2020;49:312-318.

Callanan JJ, Jones BA, Irvine J, et al. Histologic classification and immunophenotype of lymphosarcomas in cats with naturally and experimentally acquired feline immunodeficiency virus infections. *Vet Pathol.* 1996;33: 264-272.

Caniatti M, Roccabianca P, Scanziani E, et al. Canine lymphoma: immunocytochemical analysis of fine-needle aspiration biopsy. *Vet Pathol.* 1996;33: 204-212.

Chiulli FM, Raskin RE, Fox LE, et al. The clinical and pathological characteristics influencing the prognosis of 50 canine patients with lymphoid malignancies [abstract]. *Vet Pathol.* 2003;40:619.

Cienava EA, Barnhart KF, Brown R, et al. Morphologic, immunohistochemical, and molecular characterization of hepatosplenic T-cell lymphoma in a dog. *Vet Clin Pathol.* 2004;33:105-110.

Comazzi S, Marelli S, Cozzi M, et al. Breed-associated risks for developing canine lymphoma differ among countries: an European canine lymphoma network study. *BMC Vet Res.* 2018;14:232.

Dank G, Lucroy MD, Griffey SM, et al. bcl-2 and MIB-1 labeling indexes in cats with lymphoma. *J Vet Intern Med.* 2002;16:720-725.

Day MJ. Review of thymic pathology in 30 cats and 36 dogs. *J Small Anim Pract.* 1997;38:393-403.

Day MJ, Lucke VM, Pearson H. A review of pathological diagnoses made from 87 canine splenic biopsies. *J Small Anim Pract.* 1995;36:426-433.

Dean GA, Groshek PM, Jain NC, et al. Immunophenotypic analysis of feline haemolymphatic neoplasia using flow cytometry. *Comp Haematol Int.* 1995;5:84-92.

Desnoyers M, St-Germain L. What is your diagnosis? *Vet Clin Pathol.* 1994; 23:89.

Dor C, Gajanayake I, Kortum A, et al. Characterisation and outcome of idiopathic pyogranulomatous lymphadenitis in 64 English springer spaniel dogs. *J Small Anim Pract.* 2019;60(9):551-558.

Edwards DS, Henley WE, Harding EF, et al. Breed incidence of lymphoma in a UK population of insured dogs. *Vet Comp Oncol.* 2003;1:200-206.

Fisher DJ, Naydan D, Werner LL, et al. Immunophenotyping lymphomas in dogs: a comparison of results from fine needle aspirate and needle biopsy samples. *Vet Clin Pathol.* 1995;24:118-123.

Flood-Knapik KE, Durham AC, Gregor TP, et al. Clinical, histopathological and immunohistochemical characterization of canine indolent lymphoma. *Vet Comp Oncol.* 2013;11(4):272-286.

Fournel-Fleury C, Magnol JP, Bricaire P, et al. Cytohistological and immunological classification of canine malignant lymphomas: comparison with human non-Hodgkin's lymphomas. *J Comp Pathol.* 1997;117:35-59.

Fournel-Fleury C, Ponce F, Felman P, et al. Canine T-cell lymphomas: a morphological, immunological, and clinical study of 46 new cases. *Vet Pathol.* 2002;39:92-109.

Fournier Q, Cazzini P, Bavcar S, et al. Investigation of the utility of lymph node fine-needle aspiration cytology for the staging of malignant solid tumors in dogs. *Vet Clin Pathol.* 2018;47(3):489-500.

Friedrichs KR, Young KM. Histiocytic sarcoma of macrophage origin in a cat: case report with a literature review of feline histiocytic malignancies and comparison with canine hemophagocytic histiocytic sarcoma. *Vet Clin Pathol.* 2008;37:121-128.

Fry MM, Vernau W, Pesavento PA, et al. Hepatosplenic lymphoma in a dog. *Vet Pathol.* 2003;40:556-562.

Gerontiti S, Oikonomidis IL, Kalogianni L, et al. First report of canine systemic cryptococcosis owing to *Cryptococcus gattii* in Europe. *J Small Anim Pract.* 2017;58:58-59.

Gibson D, Aubert I, Woods JP, et al. Flow cytometric immunophenotype of canine lymph node aspirates. *J Vet Intern Med.* 2004;18:710-717.

Goldman EE, Grindem CB. What is your diagnosis? Seven-year-old dog with progressive lethargy and inappetence. *Vet Clin Pathol.* 1997;26(187):195-197.

Grimes JA, Matz BM, Christopherson PW, et al. Agreement between cytology and histopathology for regional lymph node metastasis in dogs with melanocytic neoplasms. *Vet Pathol.* 2017;54(4):579-587.

Grindem CB. What is your diagnosis? *Vet Clin Pathol.* 1994;23(72):77.

Grindem CB, Page RL, Ammerman BE, et al. Immunophenotypic comparison of blood and lymph node from dogs with lymphoma. *Vet Clin Pathol.* 1998;27:16-20.

Grossi AB, Hyttel P, Jensen HE, et al. Porcine melanotic cutaneous lesions and lymph nodes: immunohistochemical differentiation of melanocytes and melanophages. *Vet Pathol.* 2015;52(1):83-91.

Guerra JM, Fernandes NC, Réssio RA, et al. Evaluation of cytopathological techniques for the diagnosis of canine visceral leishmaniosis with lymph node samples. *J Comp Pathol.* 2019;172:62-71.

Heinrich DA, Avery AC, Henson MS, et al. Cytology and the cell block method in diagnostic characterization of canine lymphadenopathy and in the immunophenotyping of nodal lymphoma. *Vet Comp Oncol.* 2019;17(3):365-375.

Hendrick MJ, Brooks JJ, Bruce EH. Six cases of malignant fibrous histiocytoma of the canine spleen. *Vet Pathol.* 1992;29:351-354.

Hipple AK, Colitz CMH, Mauldin GH, et al. Telomerase activity and related properties of normal canine lymph node and canine lymphoma. *Vet Comp Oncol.* 2003;1:140-151.

HogenEsch H, Hahn FF. Primary vascular neoplasms of lymph nodes in the dog. *Vet Pathol.* 1998;35:74-76.

Jagielski D, Lechowski R, Hoffmann-Jagielska M, et al. A retrospective study of the incidence and prognostic factors of multicentric lymphoma in dogs (1998–2000). *J Vet Med A.* 2002;49(8):419-424.

Jubala CM, Wojcieszyn JW, Valli VEO, et al. CD 20 expression in normal canine B cells and in canine non-Hodgkin lymphoma. *Vet Pathol.* 2005;42:468-476.

Kawabata A, Husnik R, Donne VL, et al. Pathology in practice. *J Am Vet Med Assoc.* 2017;250(10):1113-1116.

Kiupel M, Bostock D, Bergmann V. The prognostic significance of AgNOR counts and PCNA-positive cell counts in canine malignant lymphomas. *J Comp Pathol.* 1998;119:407-418.

Kiupel M, Teske E, Bostock D. Prognostic factors for treated canine malignant lymphoma. *Vet Pathol.* 1999;36:292-300.

Kordick DL, Brown TT, Shin K, et al. Clinical and pathologic evaluation of chronic *Bartonella henselae* or *Bartonella clarridgeiae* infection in cats. *J Clin Microbiol.* 1999;37:1536-1547.

Krick EL, Little L, Patel R, et al. Description of clinical and pathological findings, treatment and outcome of feline large granular lymphocyte lymphoma (1996-2004). *Vet Comp Oncol.* 2008;6:102-110.

Ku CK, Kass PH, Christopher MM. Cytologic-histologic concordance in the diagnosis of neoplasia in canine and feline lymph nodes: a retrospective study of 367 cases. *Vet Comp Oncol.* 2017;15(4):1206-1217.

Lampe R, Manens J, Sharp N. Suspected phenobarbital-induced pseudolymphoma in a dog. *J Vet Intern Med.* 2017;31:1858-1859.

Lana S, Plaza S, Hampe K, et al. Diagnosis of mediastinal masses in dogs by flow cytometry. *J Vet Intern Med.* 2006;20:1161-1165.

Lara-Garcia A, Wellman M, Burkhard MJ, et al. Cervical thymoma originating in ectopic thymic tissue in a cat. *Vet Clin Pathol.* 2008;37:397-402.

Lau KWM, Kruth SA, Thorn CE, et al. Large granular lymphocytic leukemia in a mixed breed dog. *Can Vet J.* 1999;40:725-728.

LeBlanc CJ, Head L, Fry MM. Comparison of aspiration and non-aspiration techniques for obtaining cytology samples from the canine spleen [abstract]. *Vet Pathol.* 2008;45:735.

Levien AS, Summers BA, Szladovits B, et al. Transformation of a thymic branchial cyst to a carcinoma with pulmonary metastasis in a dog. *J Small Anim Pract.* 2010;51:604-608.

Lieser J, Schwedes CS. Pseudolymphoma in a cat on phenobarbital treatment. *J Small Anim Pract.* 2018;51:444-447.

Lurie DM, Lucroy MD, Griffey SM, et al. T-cell-derived malignant lymphoma in the boxer breed. *Vet Comp Oncol.* 2004;2:171-175.

Martini V, Marconato L, Poggi A, et al. Canine small clear cell/T-zone lymphoma: clinical presentation and outcome in a retrospective case series. *Vet Comp Oncol.* 2016;14(suppl 1):117-126.

Martini V, Poggi A, Riondato F, et al. Flow-cytometric detection of phenotypic aberrancies in canine small clear cell lymphoma. *Vet Comp Oncol.* 2015;13(3):281-287.

McDonough SP, Moore PF. Clinical, hematologic, and immunophenotypic characterization of canine large granular lymphocytosis. *Vet Pathol.* 2000;37:637-646.

Mizutani N, Goto-Koshino Y, Takahashi M, et al. Clinical and histopathological evaluation of 16 dogs with T-zone lymphoma. *J Vet Med Sci.* 2016;78:1237-1244.

Mooney SC, Patnaik AK, Hayes AA, et al. Generalized lymphadenopathy resembling lymphoma in cats: six cases (1972-1976). *J Am Vet Med Assoc.* 1987;190:897-899.

Moore AR, Leavell SE, Conrado FO, et al. Cytologic features and staining characteristics of Gamna-Gandy bodies from seven canine fine-needle aspirate preparations. *J Vet Diagn Invest.* 2017;29(6):920-925.

Moore AS, Frimberger AE, Sullivan N, et al. Histologic and immunohistochemical review of splenic fibrohistiocytic nodules in dogs. *J Vet Intern Med.* 2012;26:1164-1168.

Moore FM, Emerson WE, Cotter SM, et al. Distinctive peripheral lymph node hyperplasia of young cats. *Vet Pathol.* 1986;23:386-391.

Moore PF. A review of histiocytic diseases of dogs and cats. *Vet Pathol.* 2014;51(1):167-184.

Newton JA, de Vicente F, Haugland SP, et al. Extra-nodal subcutaneous Hodgkin's-like lymphoma and subsequent regression in a cat. *J Feline Med Surg.* 2014;17(6):543-547.

O'Keefe DA, Couto CG. Fine-needle aspiration of the spleen as an aid in the diagnosis of splenomegaly. *J Vet Int Med.* 1987;1:102-109.

Pallatto VA, Bechtold MA. Mast cell and plasma cell collision tumor in the spleen of a dog. *Vet Clin Pathol.* 2018;47:303-306.

Patel RT, Caceres A, French AF, et al. Multiple myeloma in 16 cats: a retrospective study. *Vet Clin Pathol.* 2005;34:341-352.

Patnaik AK, Lieberman PH, Erlandson RA, et al. Feline cystic thymoma: a clinicopathologic, immunohistologic, and electron microscopic study of 14 cases. *J Feline Med Surg.* 2003;5:27-35.

Ponce F, Magnol JP, Blavier A, et al. Clinical, morphological and immunological study of 13 cases of canine lymphoblastic lymphoma: comparison with the human entity. *Comp Clin Path.* 2003;12:75-83.

Ponce F, Magnol JP, Ledieu D, et al. Prognostic significance of morphological subtypes in canine malignant lymphomas during chemotherapy. *Vet J.* 2004;167:158-166.

Raskin RE, Nipper MN. Cytochemical staining characteristics of lymph nodes from normal and lymphoma-affected dogs. *Vet Clin Pathol.* 1992;21:62-67.

Raskin RE, Fox LE. Clinical relevance of the World Health Organization classification of lymphoid neoplasms in dogs [abstract]. *Vet Clin Pathol.* 2003;32:151.

Ribas Latre A, McPartland A, Cain D, et al. Canine sterile steroid responsive lymphadenitis in 49 dogs. *J Small Anim Pract.* 2019;60:280-290.

Roccabianca P, Vernau W, Caniatti M, et al. Feline large granular lymphocyte (LGL) lymphoma with secondary leukemia: primary intestinal origin with predominance of a CD3/CD8aa phenotype. *Vet Pathol.* 2006;43:15-28.

Rütgen BC, König R, Hammer SE, et al. Composition of lymphocyte subpopulations in normal canine lymph nodes. *Vet Clin Pathol.* 2015;44(1):58-69.

Ryseff JK, Duncan C, Sfiligoi G, et al. Gamna-Gandy bodies: a case of mistaken identity in the spleen of a cat. *Vet Clin Pathol.* 2014;43:94-100.

Sabattini S, Lopparelli RM, Rigillo A, et al. Canine splenic nodular lymphoid lesions: immunophenotyping, proliferative activity, and clonality assessment. *Vet Pathol.* 2018;55(5):645-653.

Santos M, Marcos R, Roccabianca P. The blood cell family on a lymph node road. *Vet Clin Pathol.* 2017;46:209-210.

Scott DW, Yager JA, Johnston KM. Exfoliative dermatitis in association with thymoma in three cats. *Feline Pract.* 1995;23:8-13.

Scott-Moncrieff JC, Cook JR, Lantz GC. Acquired myasthenia gravis in a cat with thymoma. *J Am Vet Med Assoc.* 1990;196:1291-1293.

Seelig DM, Avery P, Webb T, et al. Canine T-zone lymphoma: unique immunophenotypic features, outcome, and population characteristics. *J Vet Intern Med.* 2014;28(3):878-886.

Sills WS, Howerth EW. Pathology in practice. *J Am Vet Med Assoc.* 2018;252(9):1063-1066.

Spangler WL, Culbertson MR. Prevalence and type of splenic diseases in cats: 455 cases (1985-1991). *J Am Vet Med Assoc.* 1992;201:773-776.

Spangler WL, Culbertson MR, Kass PH. Primary mesenchymal (nonangiomatous/nonlymphomatous) neoplasms occurring in the canine spleen: anatomic classification, immunohistochemistry, and mitotic activity correlated with patient survival. *Vet Pathol.* 1994;31:37-47.

Stefanello D, Valenti P, Faverzani S, et al. Ultrasound-guided cytology of spleen and liver: a prognostic tool in canine cutaneous mast cell tumor. *J Vet Intern Med.* 2009;23(5):1051-1057.

Stefanello D, Valenti P, Zini E, et al. Splenic marginal zone lymphoma in 5 dogs (2001–2008). *J Vet Intern Med.* 2011;25:90-93.

Steinberg JD, Keating JH. What is your diagnosis? Cervical mass in a cat. *Vet Clin Pathol.* 2008;37(3):323-327.

Suami H, Yamashita S, Soto-Miranda MA, et al. Lymphatic territories (lymphosomes) in a canine: an animal model for investigation of postoperative lymphatic alterations. *PLoS One.* 2013;8(7):e69222.

Swerdlow SH, Campo E, Harris NL, et al. *WHO Classification of Tumours of Haematopoietic and Lymphoid Tissues.* 4th ed. Lyon, France: IARC Press; 2008.

Teske E, van Heerde P. Diagnostic value and reproducibility of fine-needle aspiration cytology in canine malignant lymphoma. *Vet Q.* 1996;18:112-115.

Thorn CE, Aubert I. Abdominal mass aspirate from a cat with eosinophilia and basophilia. *Vet Clin Pathol.* 1999;28:139-141.

Tomlinson JK, Cooley AJ, Zhang S, et al. Granulomatous lymphadenitis caused by *Talaromyces helicus* in a Labrador retriever. *Vet Clin Pathol.* 2011;40(4):553-557.

Twomey LN, Alleman AR. Cytodiagnosis of feline lymphoma. *Compend Contin Educ Pract Vet.* 2005;27:17-31.

Vail DM, Kravis LD, Kisseberth WC, et al. Application of rapid CD3 immunophenotype analysis and argyrophilic nucleolar organizer region (AgNOR) frequency to fine needle aspirate specimens from dogs with lymphoma. *Vet Clin Pathol.* 1997;26:66-69.

Vail DM, Moore AS, Ogilvie GK, et al. Feline lymphoma (145 cases): proliferation indices, cluster of differentiation 3 immunoreactivity, and their association with prognosis in 90 cats. *J Vet Intern Med.* 1998;12:349-354.

Vajdovich P, Psader R, Toth ZA, et al. Use of the argyrophilic nucleolar region method for cytologic and histologic examination of the lymph nodes in dogs. *Vet Pathol.* 2004;41:338-345.

Valli VE, San Myint M, Barthel A, et al. Classification of canine malignant lymphomas according to the World Health Organization criteria. *Vet Pathol.* 2011;48:198-211.

Valli VE, Vernau W, DeLorimier LP, et al. Canine indolent nodular lymphoma. *Vet Pathol.* 2006;43:241-256.

Walton RM, Hendrick MJ. Feline Hodgkin's-like lymphomas: 20 cases (1992-1999). *Vet Pathol.* 2001;38:504-511.

Whipple KM, Shmalberg JW, Joyce AC, et al. Cytologic identification of fungal arthritis in a Labrador retriever with disseminated *Talaromyces helicus* infection. *Vet Clin Pathol.* 2019;48(3):449-454.

Whipple KM, Wellehan JF, Jeon AB, et al. Cytologic, histologic, microbiologic, and electron microscopic characterization of a canine *Prototheca wickerhamii* infection. *Vet Clin Pathol.* 2020;49(2):326-332.

Whitten BA, Raskin RE. Evaluation of argyrophilic nucleolar organizer regions (AGNORS) as a prognostic indicator for canine lymphoproliferative diseases [abstract]. *Vet Pathol.* 2004;41:552.

Williams M, Avery A, Olver CS. Diagnosing lymphoid hyperplasia vs lymphoma in canine splenic aspirates. *Vet Pathol.* 2006;43:809.

Workman HC, Vernau W. Chronic lymphocytic leukemia in dogs and cats: the veterinary perspective. *Vet Clin North Am Small Anim Pract.* 2003;33:1379-1399.

Yankin I, Nemanic S, Funes S, et al. Clinical relevance of splenic nodules or heterogeneous splenic parenchyma assessed by cytologic evaluation of fine-needle samples in 125 dogs (2011-2015). *J Vet Intern Med.* 2020;34(1):125-131.

Yeuroukis CK, Thiman JM, Avery AC, et al. What is your diagnosis? Inguinal lymph node aspirate from a dog. *Vet Clin Pathol.* 2017;46(2):365-366.

Zekas LJ, Adams WM. Cranial mediastinal cysts in nine cats. *Vet Radiol Ultrasound.* 2002;43(5):413-418.

CHAPTER 5

Respiratory System

Katie M. Boes

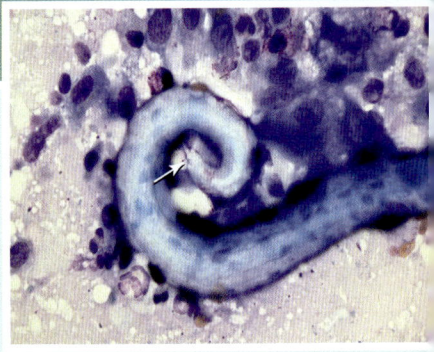

Cytopathologic evaluation of the respiratory tract provides invaluable diagnostic information that, when correlated with the history, clinical data, and imaging results, directly influences patient management. Cytopathologic features seen in the respiratory tract after injury, disease, and primary or metastatic neoplasia depend largely on the normal underlying structure and function of the cellular elements. Thorough examination of a high-quality sample is critical for obtaining meaningful cytopathology results. This chapter describes appropriate sampling techniques and cytologic interpretation of samples from the respiratory tract, including the nasal cavity, larynx, airways, and lung parenchyma.

NASAL CAVITY

Normal Anatomy and Histology

Beginning at the nares, the nasal cavity is divided by the nasal septum and terminates caudally as the osseous ethmoid plate. The passages that traverse through bony and cartilaginous sinuses are lined by a mucous membrane. The entrance to the nasal cavity, or vestibule, encompasses the nares and a narrow section of the anterior nasal cavity. The posterior portion, or nasal cavity proper, consists of extensive, delicate mucous membrane–lined turbinates. The nasolacrimal duct opens through the ventral lateral wall of the vestibule, allowing serous secretions from the conjunctival sac to flow into the rostral nasal cavity. At least in dogs, the nasolacrimal duct appears similar in both structure and function to that seen in humans (Hirt et al., 2012). Communicating with the nasal cavity are several paired, air-filled, mucosa-lined paranasal sinuses.

The vestibule is contiguous with the external skin and is lined by keratinized squamous epithelium at the nares that briefly transitions into a nonkeratinized squamous epithelium in the front of the nasal cavity. In dogs, this transitional nonciliated nasal epithelium consists of round to cuboidal cells that layer on each other and are thought to play a role in metabolizing inhaled and circulating xenobiotics related to their endowment with cytochrome P450 monooxygenase enzymes. The nasal cavity proper, nasal septum, and paranasal sinuses are lined by a ciliated, pseudostratified, columnar epithelium. Serous, mucous, and mixed tubuloalveolar glands are present in the rostral nasal cavity, whereas olfactory glands, albeit in low numbers in carnivores, are found in the caudal nasal cavity. In animals with a keen olfactory sense (macrosmatic) such as dogs and cats, olfactory receptor neurons are distributed throughout an olfactory recess near the rear of the nasal cavity. And, at least in dogs, this pattern of neuron distribution correlates well with the pattern of odorant deposition (Lawson et al., 2012). Nasal-associated lymphoid tissue (NALT) and lymphoid follicles are found in the submucosa of the caudal nasal cavity and are especially numerous in the nasopharynx.

The vomeronasal organ is bilaterally symmetric and located along the base of the nasal septum in the rostral part of the nasal cavity. The organ is composed of various components, including epithelium, ducts, glands, and connective tissue (Salazar et al., 1996) and, at least in dogs, is also rich in tissue of neuronal origin (Dennis et al., 2003). In addition to neuron cell bodies and axon fascicles, the sensory epithelium also expresses neuronal markers.

Sample Collection and Preparation

When history and clinical signs suggest a disease of the nasal cavity, the first diagnostic step is a thorough inspection of the external and internal nasal cavity; pharynx; hard and soft palates; and oral cavity, including examination of the gingiva and upper dental arcade, for oronasal fistulation and periodontal disease. Additionally, palpation for enlarged regional lymph nodes and subsequent aspirate biopsy and/or surgical biopsy may provide a valuable indirect means of achieving a diagnosis if disseminated or metastatic disease is present. Overall, persistent nasal disease can be a diagnostic challenge with failure to identify a definitive diagnosis in up to one third of canine patients despite a thorough and systematic diagnostic approach (Meler et al., 2008). Magnetic resonance imaging (MRI) and computed tomography (CT) provide additional data regarding the extent of the lesion, airway involvement, and three-dimensional localization (e.g., of foreign bodies). However, in most cases, radiographs remain a reliable tool to localize mass lesions for diagnostic sampling (Petite and Dennis, 2006; Jones and Ober, 2007), although they are less sensitive for differentiating inflammatory and neoplastic rhinitis (Kuehn, 2006). Adequate visual inspection of the nasal cavity endoscopically and localization of lesions via radiographs or other imaging techniques enable the appropriate collection techniques to be used. However, it should be noted that rhinoscopic assessment does not uniformly predict the presence or absence of inflammatory disease; thus, obtaining a sample for microscopic evaluation is critical (Johnson et al., 2004; Windsor et al., 2004). Examination by flexible endoscope is preferred because approximately 50% to 80% of the nasal cavity cannot be visualized through examinations by either a rigid endoscope or an otoscope (Elie and Sabo, 2006). In addition to visual inspection of the nasal cavity, flexible endoscopy permits diagnostic sampling of suspicious findings and removal of foreign bodies discovered serendipitously. If an endoscope is unavailable, an otoscope may be used to examine the rostral nasal cavity, and with aid of a dental mirror and light, a portion of the nasopharynx can also be visualized. Radiography and rhinoscopy should be performed before sampling because hemorrhage may hinder radiographic interpretation and obscure visualization during endoscopy.

A complete blood count (CBC) and coagulation profile should be performed before sampling because the majority of collection techniques result in hemorrhage owing to the rich venous plexuses underlying the nasal mucosa. Appropriate anesthetic restraint is tantamount for safe and successful procurement of tissue samples. General anesthesia allows appropriate restraint, placement of a properly inflated endotracheal tube, packing of the oropharynx with gauze, and tilting the patient's nose downward to protect against aspiration during sample collection.

Nasal Swabs

The presence of an acute or chronic nasal discharge indicates upper respiratory disease but is nonspecific and associated with inflammatory, infectious, or neoplastic disorders. Nasal discharge may be unilateral or bilateral and range from serous, suppurative, and mucoid to serosanguineous. Superficial and deep nasal swabs are easy to obtain and relatively nontraumatic but often do not provide much information beyond identifying superficial inflammation, secondary bacterial infection, hemorrhage, necrosis, and mucus, while the underlying disease process remains obscure. As a general rule, invasive techniques allowing collection of tissue deep to the nasal mucosa increase diagnostic potential. For example, successful detection of aspergillosis increases from positive detection of 13% to 20% of samples examined by a direct smear or blind swab to 93% to 100% positive detection in samples obtained by brush cytologic biopsy or incisional biopsy (De Lorenzi et al., 2006a). However, occasionally, the simplest technique can be rewarding, such as the diagnosis of cryptococcosis infection in cats using cytologic examination of a nasal swab.

> **KEY POINT** Cytopathologic examination of nasal exudate should be performed initially in any nasal disease. Although the diagnostic sensitivity is low, the technical ease and low cost of the procedure warrant evaluation.

Nasal Flush

Nasal flushing methods have been reviewed elsewhere (Smallwood and Zenoble, 1993). In general, invasive and aggressive techniques are more likely to yield diagnostic material. Nontraumatic nasal flushes only produce material for a definitive diagnosis in approximately 50% of the cases. A 6 to 10 Fr polypropylene or soft red rubber urinary catheter is inserted into the external nares to flush sterile, nonbacteriostatic, physiologic saline or lactated Ringer's solution through the nasal cavity (Fig. 5.1A). A traumatic nasal flush can be accomplished by beveling or nicking the tubing or catheter, creating a rough surface to aid in dislodging tissue. As with any instrument placed into the nasal cavity, penetration through the cribriform plate into the cranial vault can be avoided by measuring the distance from the external nares to the medial canthus of the eye and cutting the tubing or catheter to the appropriate length or marking the instrument with tape.

Small aliquots (5–10 mL) of fluid are introduced into the nasal cavity via a 20 to 35 mL syringe with alternating positive and negative pressure. As the fluid enters the cavity, the tubing or catheter is aggressively moved back and forth against the nasal turbinates in an attempt to free tissue fragments that can be collected on gauze sponges held below the external nares or reaspirated into the collection syringe. An alternative method involves directing a Foley catheter into the oral cavity and retroflexing around the soft palate into the nasopharynx, inflating the bulb, and lavaging the saline so that the fluid passes through the nasal cavity and out the external nares for collection (Fig. 5.1B).

The fluid and particulate matter retrieved should be placed into an ethylenediaminetetraacetic acid (EDTA)-anticoagulated tube. If the fluid is turbid, direct smears can be prepared for cytologic evaluation by placing a drop of the fluid on a clean glass slide and placing a second slide on top. After the fluid has spread between the slides, the two slides are pulled apart in a

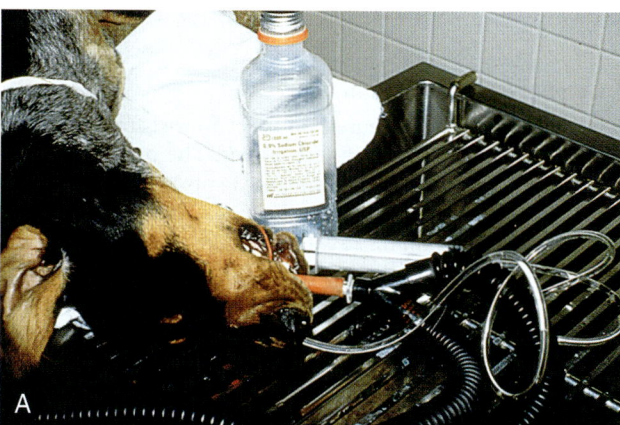
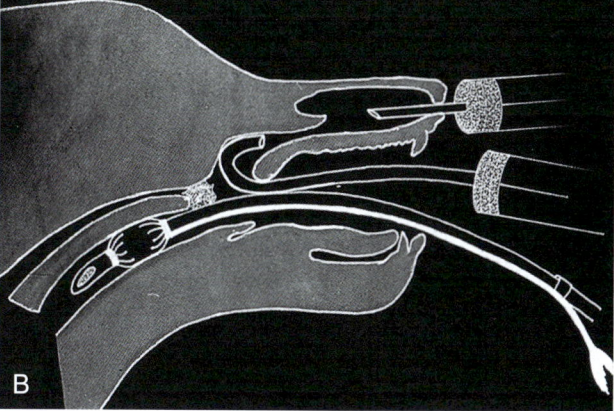

■ **FIGURE 5.1 Nasal flush procedure. A,** Placement of a flexible tube within the nasal cavity of an anesthetized dog and use of sodium chloride irrigation fluid. **B,** Diagram of an alternate technique demonstrating placement of a flexible tube retroflexed below and around the soft palate with collection of fluid from the external nares. (A, Courtesy Robert King, University of Florida. B, From Meyer DJ. The management of cytology specimens. *Compend Contin Educ Pract Vet.* 1987;9:10–16.)

horizontal fashion, with a slight amount of vertical pressure applied if small tissue fragments are present. If the fluid is relatively clear, the sample can be concentrated by centrifugation, and smears prepared from the sedimented material resuspended in a small volume of remaining supernatant similar to urine sediment preparation. Further concentration of the sample may be achieved via cytocentrifugation, if available. If large tissue chunks are retrieved, touch preparations may be prepared for cytologic evaluation. These techniques are detailed in Chapter 1. A small aliquot of fluid can be placed in a tube without any additives for culture and sensitivity, or the fluid may be applied to a culturette.

Fine-Needle Aspiration

Fine-needle aspiration (FNA) biopsy is most rewarding when mass lesions are present. If a visible external nasal mass is present, direct aspiration may be performed. To sample masses within the nasal cavity, the location is best identified by imaging techniques before aspiration. For FNA, a 1- to 1½-inch 22- to 23-gauge needle is attached to a 3 to 12 mL syringe. The needle is introduced into the mass while strong negative pressure is applied and released several times. The needle should be redirected and the procedure repeated; negative pressure is released before withdrawing the needle from the mass. Frequently, only minimal material is collected into the needle hub. Collected material should be expelled onto slides for cytologic preparation and evaluation. The technique is detailed in Chapter 1.

Imprint and Brush Cytology

Alligator biopsy forceps are used to obtain a pinch sample for impression (touch imprint) cytopathology and histopathology, whereas an endoscopic brush is used to collect tissue to roll on a glass slide for cytopathology. Both sampling techniques are typically performed with endoscopic guidance. Touch imprint cytology can also be performed on core biopsy samples obtained using a Tru-Cut biopsy needle. Similarly, the polypropylene portion of an indwelling catheter with the needle removed or a polypropylene urinary catheter with the end cut at 45 degrees can also be used to obtain tissue specimens. The catheter is pushed into the mass and rotated while applying negative pressure. Tissue can then be rolled on a glass slide or used to make touch imprints for cytologic evaluation before placing in 10% neutral buffered formalin. Brush cytologic biopsy often misses the deeper inflammatory cells and may not correlate well with histologic results (Michiels et al., 2003). Therefore deeper, more invasive samples are preferred wherever possible. In one study of 54 dogs with nasal tumors, brush and imprint cytopathology correctly identified neoplasia of epithelial origin in 88% and 90% of the cases, respectively (Clercx et al., 1996). However, in the same study, the ability to diagnose mesenchymal tumors was significantly lower because histologic diagnosis correlated with only 50% of imprint cytopathology impressions and 20% of those made by brush cytopathology. The diagnostic accuracy of brush cytopathology was evaluated in dogs with chronic nasal disease in which the gold standard used involved histologic diagnosis and/or clinical follow-up (Caniatti et al., 2012). In this study the brush technique had 71% sensitivity and 99% specificity, concluding good diagnostic accuracy for the technique in chronic lesions.

If the above procedures do not yield diagnostic samples or cannot be performed because of the nature of the lesion or small patient size, exploratory rhinotomy may be necessary to obtain an excisional biopsy from which impression smears for cytopathology can be prepared before the remainder of the tissue is preserved for histopathologic examination.

Normal Cytology and Oropharyngeal Contamination
Normal Cytology

Nasal swabs and flushes of healthy animals contain few cells, small amounts of mucus, and low numbers of a mixed population of extracellular bacteria (normal flora) found colonizing the surface of epithelial cells. Ciliated columnar respiratory epithelial cells from the posterior nasal cavity typically predominate; however, small numbers of squamous epithelial cells originating from the anterior nasal cavity may also be present. Respiratory epithelial cells can be seen singly or in small clusters, are columnar, and contain a round, basally located nucleus. Cilia, if present, are located opposite the nucleus and can be seen as an eosinophilic brush border (Fig. 5.2A). Goblet cells are also columnar with a basally located nucleus, but lack cilia, are plumper, and contain a moderate amount of cytoplasm with numerous prominent, round, purple-staining cytoplasmic mucin granules (Fig. 5.2B). Occasionally, basal epithelial cells may be seen. These cells are round to cuboidal with scant, deeply basophilic cytoplasm and round, centrally placed nuclei. On cytologic specimens, mucus appears as an eosinophilic amorphous extracellular material that often entraps cells. The canine and feline nasal cavity contains NALT and lymphoid follicles, particularly in the nasopharynx (Fig. 5.3). These islands of lymphocytes can respond similarly to other organized lymphoid tissue such as lymph nodes. The degree of hemorrhage observed is contingent on the collection procedure. Erythrocytes with platelet clumps and white blood cells in numbers and proportions consistent with blood (approximately one white cell per 500 to 1000 red cells) indicate iatrogenic contamination of the sample or peracute hemorrhage. The nasal cavity of normal dogs and cats harbors a mixed population of bacteria, including *Streptococcus* spp., *Staphylococcus* spp., *Escherichia coli*, *Pseudomonas* spp., *Proteus* spp., *Pasteurella* spp., *Mycoplasma* spp., *Corynebacterium* spp., and *Bordetella bronchiseptica*. Therefore, routine bacterial culture of nasal exudates is not diagnostically rewarding or cost-effective.

Oropharyngeal Contamination

Oropharyngeal contamination is seen most frequently in samples collected by flushing techniques. The presence of *Conchiformibius* spp. (formerly *Simonsiella* spp.) is a hallmark of oropharyngeal contamination (Euzéby, 2005; Xie and Yokota, 2005). *Conchiformibius steedae* and *Conchiformibius kuhniae* are the species found in dogs and cats, respectively. *Conchiformibius* spp. are large, rod-shaped, gram-negative bacteria that align in a palisade after division, resulting in a distinctive pattern that resembles stacked coins (Fig. 5.4A). Oropharyngeal contamination is also characterized by the presence of a mixed population of bacteria found extracellularly that colonize the surface of keratinized squamous epithelial cells. If oropharyngeal inflammation is present (e.g., periodontal disease), inflammatory cells may be seen associated with the oropharyngeal contamination (Fig. 5.4B).

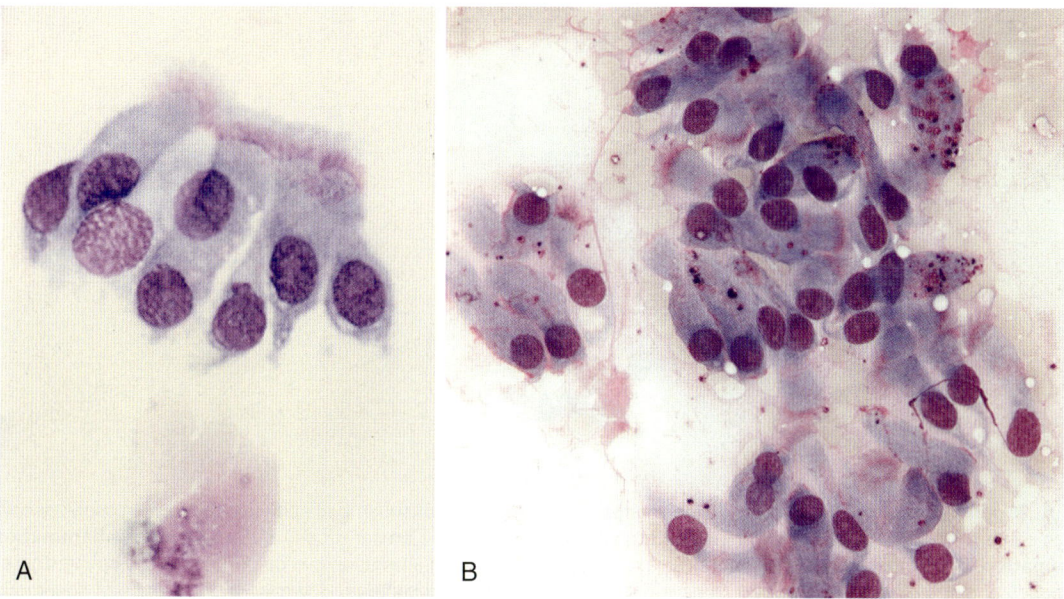

■ **FIGURE 5.2 Normal nasal epithelium. Tissue aspirate. A,** Ciliated columnar epithelium having basally located nuclei is found normally in the upper respiratory tract. (Wright-Giemsa; HP oil.) **B,** Goblet cells containing large, globular magenta granules admixed in with ciliated columnar epithelial cells. (Wright-Giemsa; HP oil.)

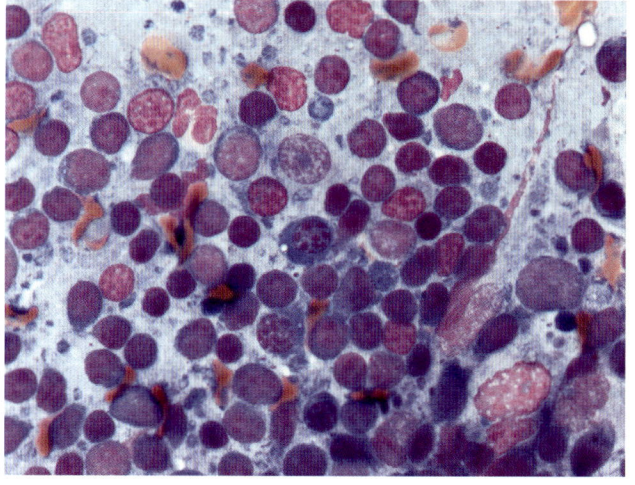

■ **FIGURE 5.3 Nasal-associated lymphoid tissue. Tissue aspirate. Dog.** This aspirate contains a heterogeneous mixture of small and medium lymphocytes, large lymphoid cells, and increased numbers of plasma cells, indicating mild reactive lymphoid hyperplasia. (Wright-Giemsa; HP oil.)

Cellular Responses to Injury
Hyperplasia and Dysplasia

Chronic inflammation secondary to various infectious and noninfectious etiologies (e.g., trauma, chronic irritation, or neoplasia) is common in the nasal cavity and can have a profound effect on the integrity and function of normal cellular constituents. Several adaptive mechanisms are employed by cells to survive amid the inflammatory stimulus. Increased numbers of cells, or *hyperplasia,* is one such mechanism and is often accompanied by dysplasia (Fig. 5.5A). Dysplasia is readily identified histologically as a loss of architectural organization but is more difficult to identify in cytopathologic preparations, which typically lack structural features. Samples from an inflamed nasal cavity with epithelial hyperplasia and dysplasia are likely to contain numerous clusters and sheets of epithelial cells with an increased nucleocytoplasmic ratio, mild to moderate anisocytosis, and increased cytoplasmic basophilia (Fig. 5.5B). Mitotic figures, although normal in appearance, may be increased in frequency as well. Epithelial hyperplasia and dysplasia are reversible but may represent early neoplastic changes and can be difficult to differentiate cytopathologically from a well-differentiated carcinoma. Goblet cell hyperplasia may be a feature of allergic rhinitis, especially when chronic.

In addition to hyperplasia of the epithelium, hyperplasia of the bony or cartilaginous portions of the nasal cavity has been reported, although it is uncommon (Rutherford et al., 2011).

Metaplasia

Another adaptive response to chronic irritation or inflammation is metaplasia. Metaplasia involves a change in cellular differentiation such that a susceptible specialized normal cell type is transformed to one that is better able to endure the environmental stress while losing specialized function. In the respiratory system, metaplasia is often characterized by the transformation of columnar respiratory epithelial cells to a more squamous phenotype, resulting in a loss of the ability to produce and secrete protective mucus. Cytopathologically, squamous metaplasia is detected by the presence of squamous epithelial cells either as the primary cell type or admixed with more normal respiratory epithelial cells (French, 1987). Cells may be present in sheets or individually depending on the degree of keratinization. Basilar cells tend to remain in clusters, whereas more keratinized squamous cells often appear individually and have angular borders; abundant hyalinized, basophilic cytoplasm; and small, and occasionally pyknotic or karyorrhectic, nuclei. As with hyperplasia, neoplastic transformation of the squamous cells may occur.

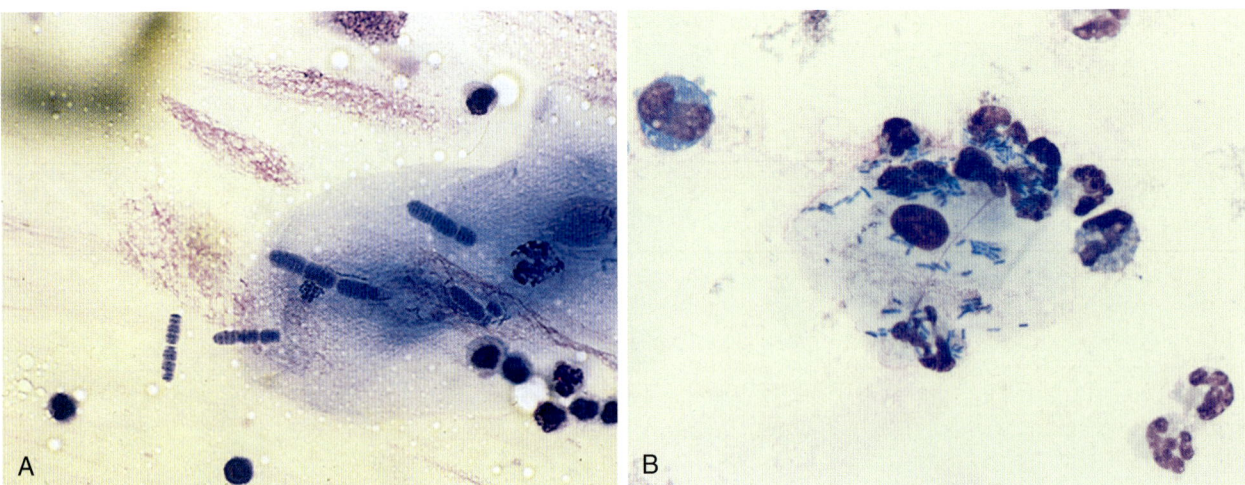

■ **FIGURE 5.4 A, Oropharyngeal contamination. Transtracheal wash.** Presence of squamous epithelial cells with closely associated *Simonsiella* bacteria suggests contamination by normal microflora or an oronasal fistula. (Wright-Giemsa; HP oil.) **B, Suppurative inflammation with oropharyngeal contamination. Bronchoalveolar lavage.** In this case the source of the inflammation can be difficult to determine. There is obvious suppurative inflammation and some neutrophils appear to have phagocytized several rod bacteria. However, the presence of squamous epithelial cells with adherent rod bacteria indicates oropharyngeal contamination which suggests that the inflammation and infection may be localized to the oral cavity. (Wright-Giemsa; HP oil.)

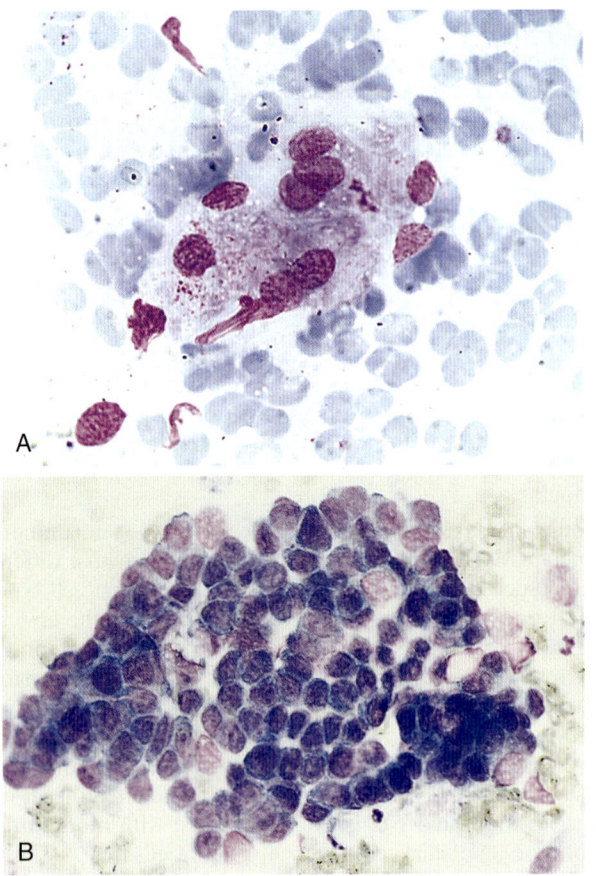

■ **FIGURE 5.5 A, Serous mucous glands of frontal sinus. Tissue imprint. Dog.** Clusters of hyperplastic glandular epithelium have an abundant, pale-blue to gray, foamy cytoplasm. (Wright-Giemsa; HP oil.) **B, Epithelial dysplasia/hyperplasia. Tissue aspirate.** This cluster of cells is characterized by increased cytoplasmic basophilia and moderate anisocytosis and anisokaryosis. (Wright-Giemsa; HP oil.) (A, Courtesy Rose Raskin, University of Florida.)

Nasal melanosis has also been suggested as a metaplastic transformation of the nasal respiratory mucosa and has been reported rarely in dogs with odontopathic (tooth- or socket-related infection) rhinitis (De Lorenzi et al., 2006b).

Noninfectious Inflammatory Disorders
Foreign Bodies
Nasal foreign bodies occur most commonly in dogs but have been reported in cats that often originate from plants such as plant awns, foxtails, or twigs (Henderson et al., 2004). Foreign bodies may be directly inhaled into the nasal cavity, or they may enter the cavity traumatically (e.g., buckshot) through the nares, through the nasal planum, or via the oral cavity by penetrating the palate. Cytopathologically, specimens are characterized by marked inflammatory reactions ranging from suppurative to pyogranulomatous often with significant hemorrhage and foreign material such as plant material or fibers. Secondary bacterial infection is common.

Allergic Rhinitis
Hypersensitivity may occur in the nasal cavity alone or concurrent with involvement of the lower airways. The inflammatory infiltrate associated with an allergic rhinitis is characterized predominantly by eosinophils, with lesser numbers of neutrophils, occasional mast cells, and occasional plasma cells (Fig. 5.6). Increased numbers of goblet cells and abundant mucus may also be seen along with rafts of hyperplastic respiratory epithelial cells. Other differentials for eosinophilic inflammation include parasitic and fungal infection. Mast cell tumors should also be considered when the mast cells are the predominant cell type. Typically, mast cells comprise only a small, scattered proportion of the inflammatory infiltrate in allergic rhinitis.

Lymphoplasmacytic Rhinitis
Until recently only occasional cases of idiopathic lymphoplasmacytic rhinitis had been described in dogs (Burgener et al.,

1987; Tasker et al., 1999b) and thought to be immune mediated (endogenous) rather than allergic (exogenous) in origin. However, a more recent study indicates that it may be more common than previously suspected (Windsor et al., 2004) and may be associated with and/or contribute to chronic nasal disease in dogs, resulting in turbinate remodeling and even bony destruction. Despite histologic evidence of bilateral disease in most dogs, a unilateral discharge was seen in some of the cases, indicating the need to examine both sides of the nasal cavity even in cases that appear localized in origin. Lack of response to glucocorticoid therapy (Windsor et al., 2004) suggests mechanisms other than immune-mediated disease. Other proposed etiopathogeneses include immune dysregulation, allergies, disruption of the normal microbial flora, and occult aspergillosis. The latter is associated with a lymphoplasmacytic rhinitis. However, analysis of cytokine profiles and toll-like and nucleotide oligomerization domain–like receptors (TLR and NOD, respectively) expression from nasal surgical biopsies from dogs with aspergillosis and idiopathic lymphoplasmacytic rhinitis indicates that the immunologic pattern of these diseases is quite different. Aspergillosis is associated with increased expression of TLRs 1, 4, 6–10, and NOD2 and induces a predominantly T-helper type 1 (Th1) response, whereas a partial Th2 response was detected in cases of idiopathic lymphoplasmacytic rhinitis (Peeters et al., 2007; Mercier et al., 2012). This type 2 response is in contrast to the type 1 cytokine profile reported in cats with chronic inflammation of the nasal cavity (Johnson et al., 2005), which suggests different pathogeneses between these species.

Chronic Sinusitis

Recurrent clinical signs of sneezing and nasal congestion may be related to infectious agents, parasites, allergies, foreign bodies, or neoplasia. A definitive cause may not be determined with cytology or histology in some of these cases. Cytopathologically, respiratory epithelium appears reactive as evidenced by hyperplasia, dysplasia, or metaplasia. Inflammatory infiltrates often consist of mixed mononuclear cells, including small to medium-sized lymphocytes, plasma cells, and macrophages (Fig. 5.7).

Infectious Inflammatory Disorders
Viruses

Viral infection of the upper airways often manifests as an acute and transient inflammatory process unless a secondary bacterial infection develops. Chronic rhinitis may develop if the viral infection results in turbinate damage and/or epithelial and glandular hyperplasia. Canine distemper virus (CDV), adenovirus types 1 and 2, and parainfluenza are the most common etiologies of canine viral rhinitis. Rarely disease may result from infection with herpes virus and reovirus. In cats, feline rhinotracheitis virus (feline herpesvirus I) and feline calicivirus tend to induce moderate to severe upper respiratory signs, whereas reovirus is more often associated with milder signs. Severe and recurrent rhinitis is common in cats infected with feline leukemia virus (FeLV) and feline immunodeficiency virus (FIV). Diagnosis of viral rhinitis is based on patient signalment, history (lack of appropriate vaccination, contact with other animals), clinical signs (mucopurulent nasal discharge, oral ulcers,

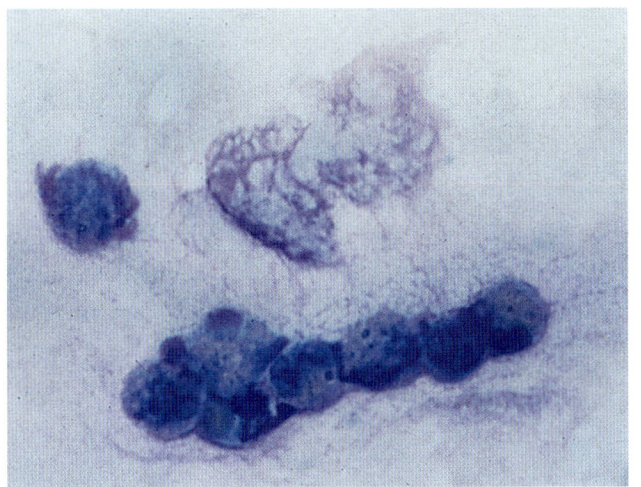

■ **FIGURE 5.6 Allergic rhinitis. Nasal flush. Dog.** Several eosinophils are enveloped in basophilic mucus, which affects the stain quality of the cells. (Wright-Giemsa; HP oil.)

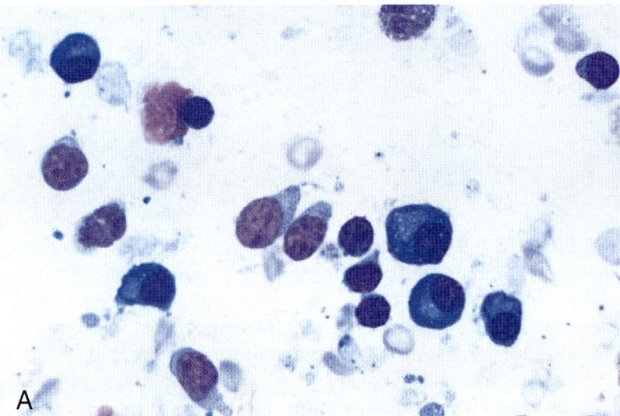
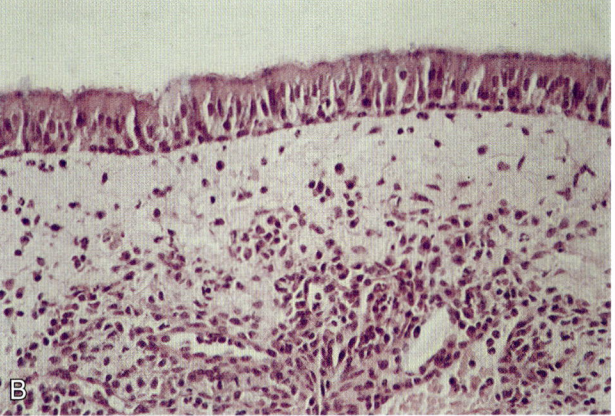

■ **FIGURE 5.7 A, Chronic inflammation. Tissue aspirate.** This mononuclear cell population is composed of small and medium-sized lymphocytes and well-differentiated plasma cells. (Wright-Giemsa; HP oil.) **B, Chronic rhinitis. Nasal mucosa. Cat.** Tissue section demonstrating intact respiratory epithelium with mild to moderate infiltration of mononuclear cells into the lamina propria below the layer of mucosal epithelium. (H&E; IP.) (B, Courtesy Rose Raskin, University of Florida.)

conjunctivitis, fever), direct fluorescent antibody testing of cells obtained from conjunctival scrapings, virus isolation, and/or serology. Cytopathologic findings associated with viral rhinitis are typically nonspecific with variable numbers and types of inflammatory cells. In addition, the cytopathology of viral rhinitis is often confounded by the effects of secondary bacterial infection. Viral inclusions are very rarely observed within the epithelial cells.

Bacteria

With the exception of *B. bronchiseptica* and *Pasteurella multocida,* which may cause acute rhinitis in dogs, primary bacterial rhinitis is rare. However, secondary bacterial infection is common and may accompany nasal neoplasia, viral infection, fungal infection, parasitic infection, trauma, foreign bodies, dental disease, or oronasal fistulation (Fig. 5.8). Infection with *Mycoplasma* spp. and *Chlamydophila* spp. (previously *Chlamydia* spp.) in cats may cause mild upper respiratory signs concurrently with conjunctivitis.

In recent years *Streptococcus equi* subspecies *zooepidemicus* has emerged as a cause of hemorrhagic pneumonia in both dogs and cats (Byun et al., 2009; Blum et al., 2010; Priestnall and Erles, 2011). It has also been recognized as a cause of rhinitis in both dogs (Piva et al., 2010) and in cats (Britton and Davies, 2010). In cats, the rhinitis has been associated with meningitis (Britton and Davies, 2010). The underlying mechanisms for the emergence of *S. zooepidemicus* as a pathogen of high virulence in dogs and cats remain unclear. In addition, although there is evidence for exposure to an equine reservoir in some cases, the source of infection for others is unknown (Priestnall and Erles, 2011).

Bacterial infection of the nasal cavity is identified cytopathologically by finding large numbers of a primarily monomorphic bacteria accompanied by a marked suppurative inflammatory response with numerous phagocytized bacteria (Fig. 5.9A). Mucus may be abundant and can obscure identification of bacteria in some cases (Fig. 5.9B–C). Culture of the nasal exudate reveals heavy growth of one type of organism, but a uniform population of organisms can also be detected with secondary or

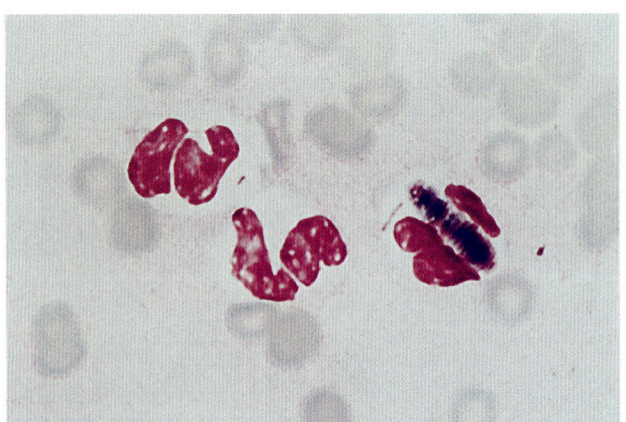

■ **FIGURE 5.8 Septic suppurative rhinitis. Nasal swab. Cat.** Three karyolytic neutrophils are present, one of which has phagocytized *Conchiformibius* spp. bacteria. An active bacterial infection was present in this animal with chronic sneezing and nasal discharge. (Wright-Giemsa; HP oil.) (Courtesy Rose Raskin, University of Florida.)

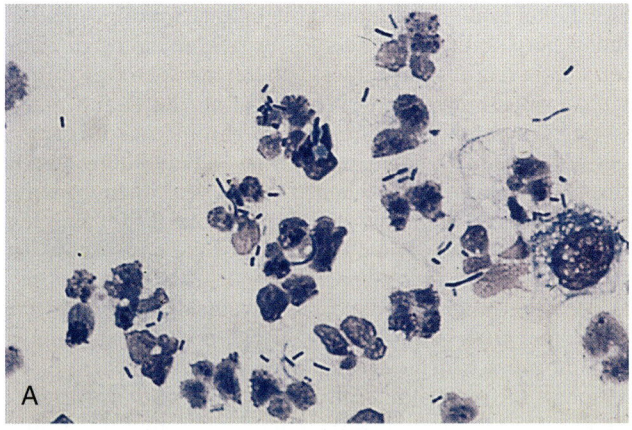

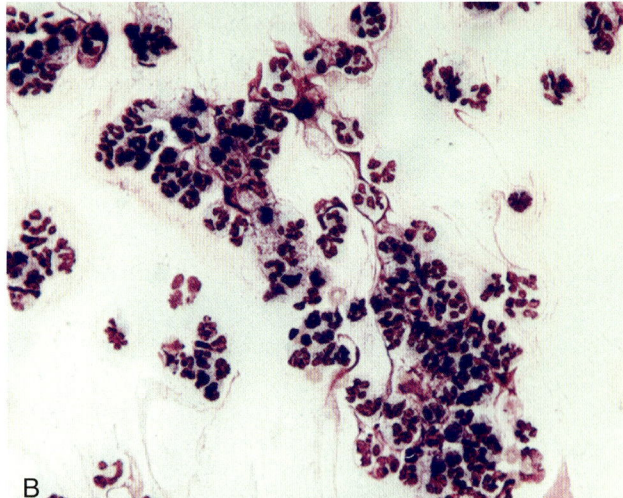

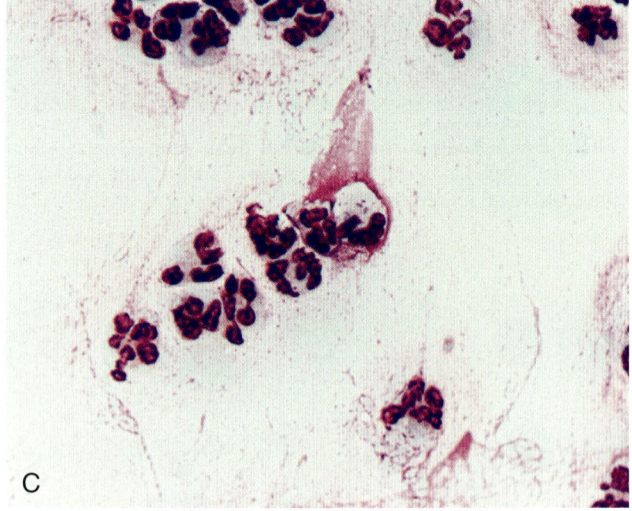

■ **FIGURE 5.9 A, Bacterial rhinitis. Nasal flush.** Large numbers of degenerate neutrophils and a monomorphic population of intracellular and extracellular rod bacteria, consistent with septic suppurative inflammation. (Wright-Giemsa; HP oil.) **B, Mucopurulent inflammation. Nasal flush.** Degenerate and nondegenerate neutrophils admixed with streams of mucus and nuclear debris. (Wright-Giemsa; HP oil.) **C, Septic mucopurulent inflammation. Nasal flush.** Closer view of B reveals the presence of intracellular short rod to cocci bacteria that can be difficult to differentiate from the extracellular mucus and cellular debris. (Wright-Giemsa; HP oil.)

opportunistic pathogens. Because primary bacterial rhinitis is uncommon, significant effort should be made to identify any possible underlying causes. The polymerase chain reaction (PCR) may also be useful to detect certain organisms, such as *Mycoplasma* spp. Identification of the bacteria as bacilli or cocci may aid in the initial institution of antimicrobial therapy as cocci are typically gram-positive and bacilli are typically gram negative. The presence of filamentous organisms forming mats of colonies suggests *Actinomyces* and *Nocardia* spp. Regardless, culture and sensitivity are necessary for proper identification of microorganisms and antimicrobial sensitivity.

Fungi

The diagnosis of fungal rhinitis can be complicated because fungal infection can be a primary or secondary, opportunistic disease. In addition, fungi such as *Aspergillus* spp., *Penicillium* spp., and *Cryptococcus* spp. can occasionally be cultured from the nasal cavity of clinically normal dogs and cats (Duncan et al., 2005). *Aspergillus* spp. and *Penicillium* spp. are the most common fungal agents in mycotic rhinitis in dogs, whereas *Cryptococcus* spp. occurs most frequently in cats. Upper respiratory involvement with *Histoplasma capsulatum* and *Blastomyces dermatitidis* has also been reported, but it is rare (Table 5.1).

Aspergillosis and penicilliosis can occur as focal or disseminated respiratory infections in dogs and cats. Both fungi are morphologically similar, necessitating culture for differentiation. Because these two fungi are frequent contaminants of the respiratory tract, diagnosis should be supported by a combination of culture, cytologic, or histologic identification of the organism and the presence of an inflammatory reaction. German shepherd dogs are predisposed to systemic aspergillosis.

Infection with *Aspergillus* spp. can be associated with purulent, granulomatous, or pyogranulomatous inflammation. Infection and inflammation may be present in the nasal cavity, frontal sinus, or both (Johnson et al., 2006). Cytopathologically, fungal hyphae are branching, septate, 5 to 7 μm wide, with straight, parallel walls and globose terminal ends. Hyphae can stain either intensely basophilic with a thin, clear outer cell wall

TABLE 5.1 Mycotic and Protozoal Organisms Commonly Seen in the Respiratory Tract of Dogs and Cats

ORGANISM	COMMON LOCATIONS	FORMS SEEN	SIZE (μm)	TYPICAL CELLULAR LOCATION	TYPICAL INFLAMMATION	CYTOPATHOLOGIC FEATURES
Fungi						
Aspergillus spp.	Nasal cavity, Lung	Hyphae	5–7	Extracellular	Granulomatous Pyogranulomatous	Septate, branching hyphae
Blastomyces dermatitidis	Airways, Lung	Yeast	5–20	Extracellular	Granulomatous Pyogranulomatous	Broad-based budding
Coccidioides spp.	Lung	Spherules Endospores	10–100 2–5	Extracellular	Granulomatous Pyogranulomatous	Spherules often seen
Cryptococcus spp.	Nasal cavity, Lung	Encapsulated yeast	8–40	Extracellular	Variable	Narrow-based budding
		Unencapsulated yeast	4–8	Intracellular (rare)		Mucoid capsule
Histoplasma capsulatum	Nasal cavity, Airways, Lung	Yeast	1–4	Intracellular or extracellular	Granulomatous Pyogranulomatous	Oval-shaped organisms
Penicillium spp.	Nasal cavity	Hyphae	5–7	Extracellular	Granulomatous Pyogranulomatous	Cytologically similar to *Aspergillus*
Pneumocystis spp.	Lung	Cysts	5–10	Intracellular or extracellular	Granulomatous	Free trophozoites difficult to identify
		Trophozoites	1–2		Pyogranulomatous	
Sporothrix schenckii	Airways, Lung	Yeast	2–7	Intracellular or extracellular	Granulomatous Pyogranulomatous	Oval- and cigar-shaped organisms
Protozoa						
Neospora caninum	Lung	Tachyzoites	1–7	Intracellular or extracellular	Mixed	Cytologically similar to *Toxoplasma* Suppurative
Toxoplasma gondii	Airways, Lung	Tachyzoites	1–4	Intracellular or extracellular	Mixed	Banana-shaped forms, single or clustered Suppurative
Mesomycetozoa						
Rhinosporidium seeberi	Nasal cavity	Endospores Sporangia	5–15 30–300	Extracellular	Mixed	Sporangia rare

or appear as negatively staining images against a cellular background (Fig. 5.10A–B). Hyphae may be difficult to identify when found in low numbers or in dense mats admixed with mucus, inflammatory cells, and cellular debris. Occasionally, round to ovoid blue-green fungal conidia may also be observed (Fig. 5.10C–D). Periodic acid–Schiff (PAS) or silver stains (GMS) facilitate detection of fungal structures. Fungal identification is most reliable by fungal culture, but differentiating *Aspergillus* spp. from *Penicillium* spp. may be achieved if fruiting bodies, which develop from *Aspergillus* spp. mycelia, are observed on cytopathologic examination. If direct examination is not feasible or unrewarding, detection of serum *Aspergillus*-specific antibodies provides good sensitivity and excellent specificity for the diagnosis of canine sinonasal aspergillosis. However, measurement of serum galactomannan antigen (a component of the cell wall of *Aspergillus* spp.) appears to be less useful (Billen et al., 2009). Similar to bacterial rhinitis, the presence of fungal elements does not rule out underlying neoplasia.

Cryptococcus spp. is a common cause of chronic upper respiratory disease in cats and is commonly detected in the nasal cavity of dogs (Trivedi et al., 2011). *Cryptococcus gattii* is been more commonly detected in cats, whereas *Cryptococcus neoformans* is more commonly detected in dogs; however, either can be seen in dogs or cats (Trivedi et al., 2011). Both *Cryptococcus neoformans* and *Cryptococcus gattii* have been reported in the nasal passages of dogs and cats in the absence of local or systemic infection (Duncan et al., 2005), suggesting that subclinical infection or asymptomatic carriage needs to be considered when the organism is serendipitously detected in healthy animals. In addition, other *Cryptococcus* species have been implicated in infection of dogs and cats (Poth et al., 2010; Kano et al., 2012). Inhalation is the suspected route of infection. Concurrent ocular, cutaneous, or neurologic disease may also be seen in animals with cryptococcal rhinitis. Immunity is speculated to play a role in the development of infections as well as in dissemination of infection throughout the body. Corticosteroid therapy during infection worsens the symptoms as well as the disease progression (Sykes and Malik, 2012). However, underlying diseases, especially immunosuppressive (e.g., FeLV, FIV), have not been proven to be predisposing factors to infection (Flatland et al., 1996). Organisms are readily identified in swabs of nasal exudates or imprints or aspirates from nasal masses (Fig. 5.11A–B). Positive identification of the organism via cytopathology is diagnostic; however, antigen detection serology and fungal culture are useful adjuncts. New methylene blue (Fig. 5.11C) and India ink can be used to demonstrate the negative staining capsule; however, care must be taken not to mistake air bubbles and fat droplets for organisms. *Cryptococcus*

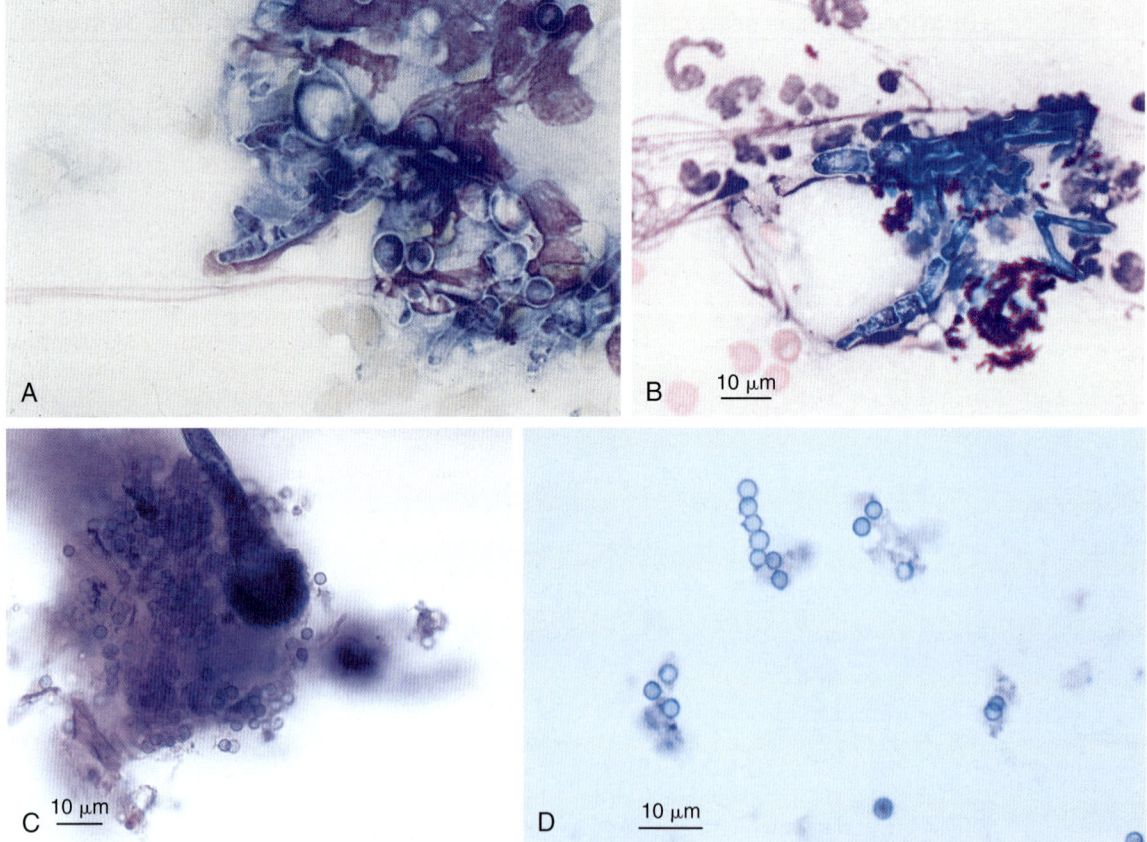

■ **FIGURE 5.10 Fungal rhinitis. A, Tissue aspirate.** Mat of branching fungal hyphae stains intensely basophilic with prominent septations and globose terminal ends. (Wright-Giemsa; HP oil.) **B, Nasal flush. Dog.** *Aspergillus fumigatus* hyphae shown with degenerate neutrophils are cultured from a secondary infection following treatment for cryptococcosis. (Wright; HP oil.) Same case in C and D. **Nasal swab. Dog. C,** Culture identified *Aspergillus fumigatus* in this patient having a unilateral serosanguineous discharge. An uncommon presentation shows one microphone-shaped conidiophore with attached cap or phialides from which the conidia extend. (NMB; HP oil.) **D,** Closer magnification of conidia at 3 μm in diameter. (NMB; HP oil.) (B–D, Courtesy Rose Raskin, Purdue University.)

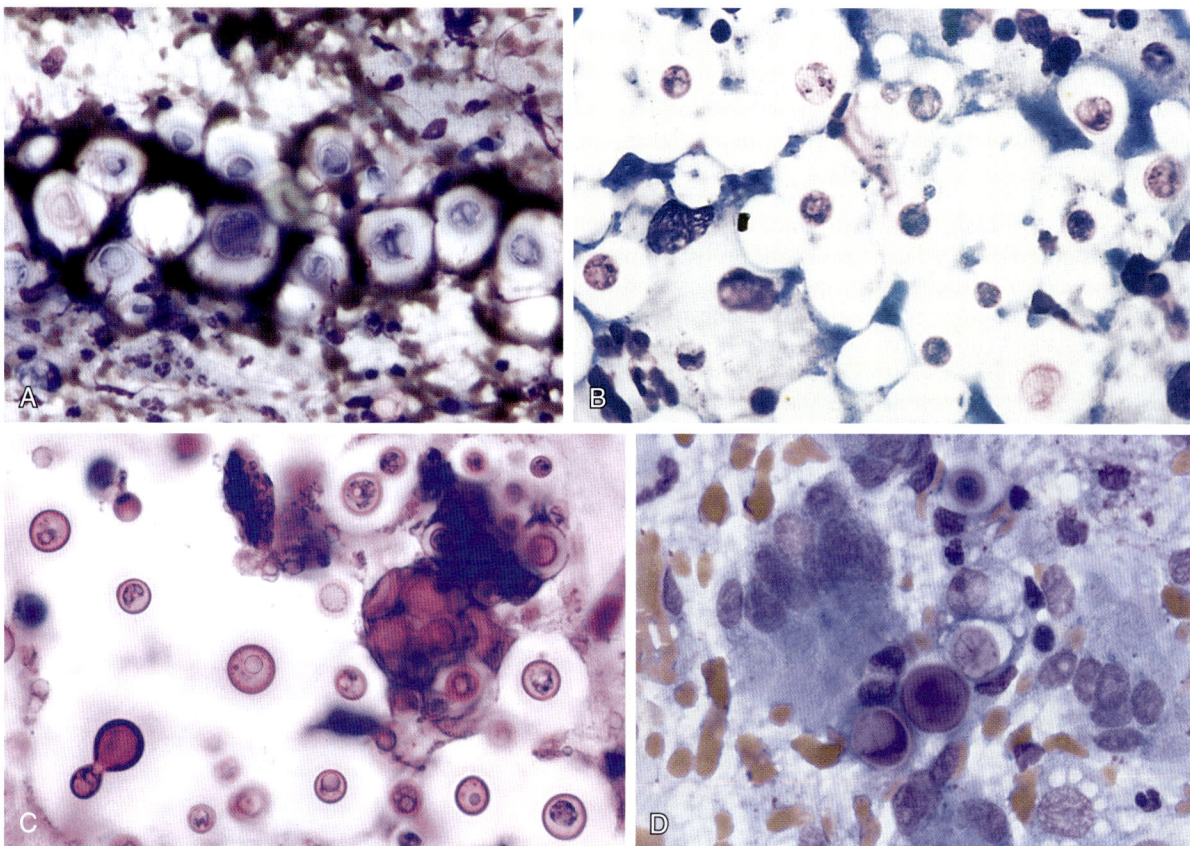

■ **FIGURE 5.11 Cryptococcal rhinitis. A, Nasal swab.** Numerous yeast forms with distinctive nonstaining, variably thick, mucoid capsules surrounding granular internal structures. The presence of concomitant inflammatory cells may be variable. (Wright-Giemsa; HP oil.) **B, Nasal swab.** Narrow-based budding is a feature of *Cryptococcus*. (Wright-Giemsa; HP oil.) **C, Nasal discharge. Cat.** Prominent budding and internal structure along with the capsule are highlighted by a water-soluble stain. (NMB; HP oil.) **D, Nasal surgical biopsy imprint. Cat.** Three yeast are present surrounded by respiratory columnar epithelium. Serology was positive for *Cryptococcus neoformans/gattii* antigen by the Remel latex agglutination test. (Wright-Giemsa; HP oil.) (C–D, Courtesy Rose Raskin, University of Florida.)

spp. are round to oval yeast that ranges 8 to 40 μm in diameter (including the capsule) (Fig. 5.11D). The organism has a granular internal structure that stains eosinophilic to purple and is surrounded by a thick, nonstaining, mucoid capsule. The capsule material can give the sample a mucinous texture. Occasionally, narrow-based budding may be seen. Unencapsulated or rough forms are 4 to 8 μm in size and are difficult to distinguish from *H. capsulatum*. Fungal culture and serology are useful in this case. The presence and type of inflammation range from the observation of a few to no inflammatory cells to robust pyogranulomatous inflammation to eosinophilic inflammation. The degree and type of inflammation may be related to characteristics of the capsule. Identification of the cryptococcal species by cytopathology is not possible (Lester et al., 2011).

Sporotrichosis has been rarely identified in samples from the nasal cavity of dogs (Cafarchia et al., 2007; Whittemore and Webb, 2007). The paucity of organisms and cytopathologic appearance is similar to that reported for *Sporothrix schenckii* from other canine samples. *Sporothrix schenckii* has also been isolated in the nasal cavity of cats with sporotrichosis and is more commonly detected in those with cutaneous lesions (Leme et al., 2007). One report involving various mammals found only a few to no fungal organisms in approximately one third of cases that cultured positive (Crothers et al., 2009). In feline patients in which both cytopathology and fungal culture were performed, sporothrix organisms were seen in 79% of the cases that were culture positive, making cytologic examination a relatively sensitive, low-cost initial diagnostic approach (Pereira et al., 2011).

Nasal mycosis caused by infection of cats by *Alternaria* spp., one of the dematiaceous fungi that induce phaeohyphomycosis, has been rarely reported in cats (McKay et al., 2001; Tennant et al., 2004). Cytopathologic findings include the presence of neutrophils, macrophages, lymphocytes, and plasma cells. Fungal organisms are pale staining and oval to round, with septate hyphae of approximately 7 to 14 μm having a narrow peripheral clear area and finely stippled eosinophilic internal material.

Algae

Prototheca spp. may produce a nasal mass in cats near the nares resulting from a cutaneous infection. Cytopathologically, aspirate or swab preparations reveal a mixture of inflammatory cells, mostly degenerate neutrophils and macrophages along with numerous sporulated and nonsporulated endospores. The endospores present as variably sized spheres having a thin, clear rim and a granular, dense center (see Chapter 3, Fig. 3.63).

Mesomycetozoa

Rhinosporidium seeberi occasionally infects the nasal cavity of dogs and, less commonly, cats, resulting in single to multiple polyps in which numerous small, miliary sporangia can be observed on the surface. Contact with flowing or standing water and trauma to the nasal mucous membranes are predisposing pathogenetic factors. Recent molecular analysis suggests that host-specific strains of *R. seeberi* may exist (Silva et al., 2005). Rhinosporidium is now considered to be an aquatic protist from the class *Mesomycetozoea* at the animal-fungal boundary and not a true fungus. Cytopathologic preparations contain variable numbers of sporangia and endospores (sporangiospores) (Gori and Scasso, 1994). Sporangia are variably sized, often very large (30–300 μm) (Fig. 5.12A–B), well-defined, globoid structures that undergo endosporulation to contain numerous small, round endospores (Fig. 5.12B–D). Sporangia are not commonly observed in stained smears because the wall of the sporangia are slightly refractile and do not stain. Sporangia can be observed in unstained direct preparations (Caniatti et al., 1998). Endospores within the sporangia are brown when observed microscopically before staining and appear as three different basophilic forms or stages of maturation with Romanowsky stains (Meier et al., 2006). Immature endospores are approximately 2 to 4 μm in diameter with lightly basophilic cytoplasm and a pink-purple nucleus encompassing one-third to one-half of the endospore and one to two smaller round magenta structures. Intermediate endospores are rarely described but appear to be spherical, granular, and basophilic structures approximately 5 to 8 μm in diameter with eosinophilic to globular internal structures and a variably sized, clear halo (see Fig. 5.12D). Mature endospores tend to predominate in cytologic preparations (see Fig. 5.12B–D). These structures are 8 to 15 μm in diameter, with a thick, hyalinized cell wall and a pale, magenta to nonstaining halo. The internal structure can be difficult to visualize in thick areas of the prep, but when endospores are spread out, numerous small spherical eosinophilic globular internal structures can be seen. PAS staining enhances the chance of finding the spores in cytologic and histologic specimens. Rhinosporidiosis incites a mixed inflammatory response consisting of neutrophils, plasma cells, and lymphocytes. Macrophages, mast cells, and eosinophils are

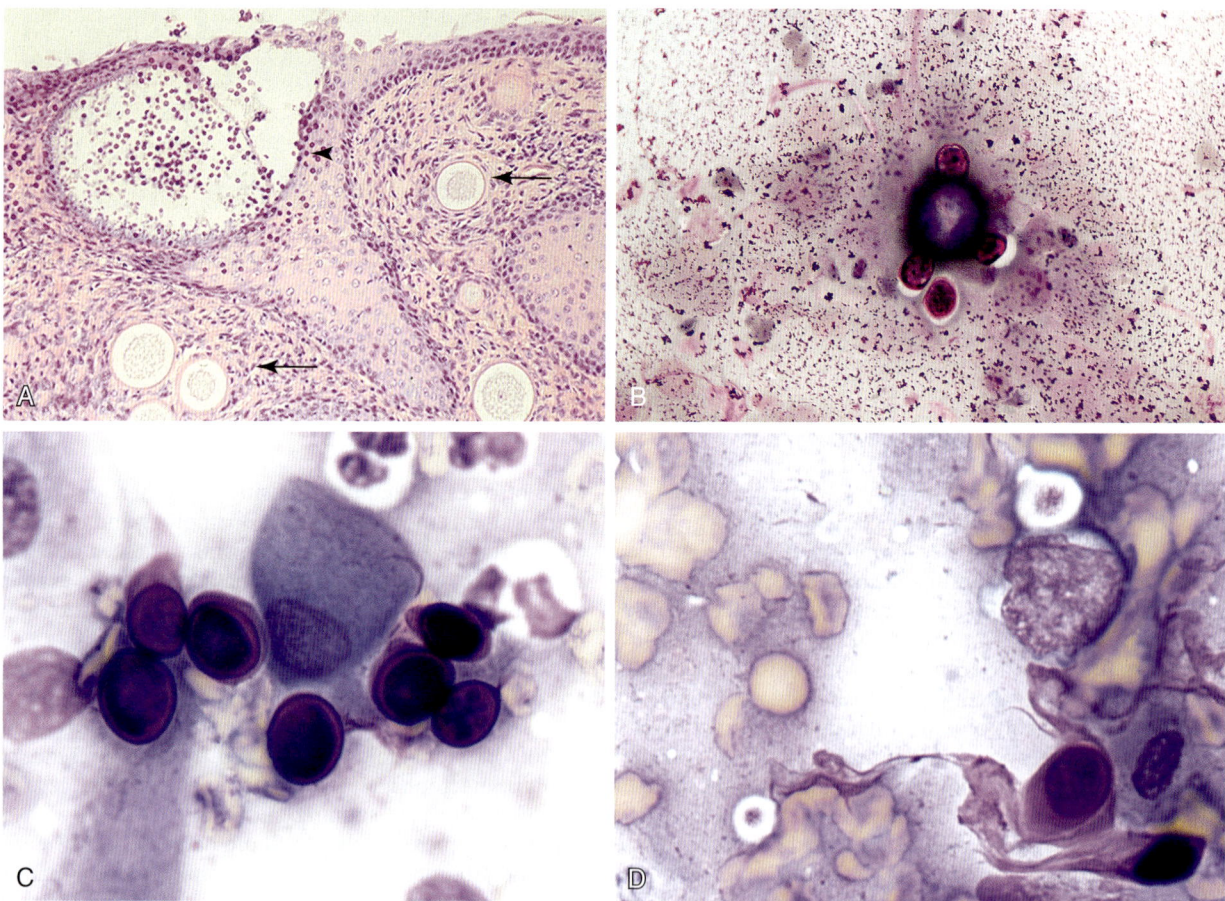

■ **FIGURE 5.12** Rhinosporidiosis. Nasal mass. Dog. **A, Sporangia and endospores. Histopathology.** Large mature sporangium with numerous endospores expels its contents to the surface *(arrowhead)*. Smaller, variably sized sporangia *(arrows)* are present within the lamina propria. (H&E; IP.) **B, Sporangium and endospores. Tissue imprint.** A small, immature sporangium is surrounded by four round, eosinophilic, mature endospores of *Rhinosporidium seeberi*. The sporangium is out of focus because of its larger thickness compared with the endospores. (Aqueous Romanowsky; HP oil.) Same case in C and D. **C, Endospores. Tissue imprint.** The capsule outlines and internal structures of seven mature endospores are visible along with an associated hyperplastic columnar respiratory epithelial cell. (Methanolic Romanowsky; HP oil.) **D, Endospores. Tissue imprint.** Two intermediate endospores and one mature endospore is shown. (Methanolic Romanowsky; HP oil.) (A, Courtesy John Bentinck-Smith et al., Mississippi State University. Presented at the 1984 ASVCP case review session. C–D, Courtesy Sara Hill et al., University of Minnesota. Presented at the 2008 ASVCP case review session.)

less commonly observed. Rosetting of inflammatory cells, particularly neutrophils, around the spores has been observed and is considered a useful feature in finding the spores during cytopathologic examination under low magnification.

Protozoa
Leishmania spp. may induce masses in the nasal cavity of dogs. Amastigotes can be identified in aspirate or surgical biopsies from dogs with leishmaniasis (Llanos-Cuentas et al., 1999).

Multicellular Parasites
Parasitic rhinitis is uncommon in dogs and cats and may or may not be associated with clinical signs (King et al., 1990). Infection with *Eucoleus boehmi* (formerly *Capillaria boehmi*) is diagnosed by finding the long, thin adult nematodes that measure 22 to 43 mm $\times$ 0.08 to 0.15 mm and embed within the mucosa of nasal passages and sinuses of dogs, red foxes, and wolves. Cases have been reported in Europe, North America, and South America. Clinical signs, when present, consist of a chronic nasal discharge, gagging, and sneezing. Diagnosis involves finding the ova by fecal flotation or rarely in nasal secretions along with fragments of adult worms (Piperisova et al., 2010). The ova are large (54–60 $\times$ 30–35 μm), ovoid, with two asymmetrical terminal plugs (opercula). Mixed or suppurative inflammation often containing eosinophils is present.

The nasal cavity and frontal sinuses of dogs may be inhabited by several forms of the arthropod parasite *Linguatula serrata*. Because the ova are infrequently seen in nasal exudates, this parasite is most readily diagnosed by direct visualization via rhinoscopy. The ova measure 90 $\times$ 70 μm; larvae, up to 500 μm; and nymphs, 4 to 6 mm. Infection with this parasite most commonly elicits mild signs such as sneezing and nasal discharge, but occasionally, severe clinical signs occur.

The nasal mite *Pneumonyssoides caninum*, which causes a mild, transient rhinitis, is best diagnosed by direct rhinoscopic visualization of the off-white, 1 to 2 mm adult mites inhabiting the nasal cavity and paranasal sinuses of dogs.

Non-neoplastic Tumors
Nasopharyngeal Polyps
Nasopharyngeal polyps are occasionally reported in dogs but occur most commonly in cats; they are characterized by hyperplasia of the mucous membranes or exuberant proliferation of fibrous connective tissue (White et al., 2021). Polyps originate within the nasopharyngeal region from the eustachian tube, middle ear, or nasopharynx. The majority of affected cats are young, often less than 1 year old (Moore and Ogilvie, 2001), whereas dogs are more often middle aged to older (Holt and Goldschmidt, 2011). The cause of nasal polyps remains unclear in most cases. Inflammatory nasopharyngeal polyps have the same epithelial and/or connective tissue hyperplasia but also contain a prominent inflammatory infiltrate. Polyps appear grossly as small, smooth, well-circumscribed, pedunculated masses arising from the mucosal surface of the nasal cavity. However, polyps may extend into the surrounding soft and bony tissues and cause turbinate destruction and bony lysis. Clinical signs are usually apparent when the polyp enlarges enough to occlude the nasopharynx. Cytopathologic findings include mature lymphocytes and plasma cells often admixed with rafts of epithelial cells and streams of matrix (Fig. 5.13). Small numbers of neutrophils and macrophages may also be present. Squamous metaplasia and/or dysplasia are frequently seen and, when present, can make the differentiation from epithelial neoplasia problematic.

Mesenchymal Nasal Hamartoma
A rare benign sinonasal tumor in cats younger than 2 years was diagnosed by squash preparations of endoscopic pinch biopsies in histologically confirmed cases of mesenchymal nasal hamartoma (Bottero et al., 2018). This study found the combined presence of cells appearing as osteoblasts and osteoclasts in addition to ciliated respiratory epithelium. All cells lacked atypia or malignant features. A receiver operating characteristic curve cut-off of three osteoblasts and two osteoclasts per 500 cells was diagnostic for this condition. The cytopathology is similar to osteosarcoma, but atypia is expected in the malignancy and not in this benign condition. Affected cats may present clinically with sneezing, stertorous breathing, and epistaxis.

Neoplastic Tumors
Although neoplasia of the nasal cavity and paranasal sinuses is uncommon in dogs and cats, a diagnosis of upper respiratory neoplasia usually carries a poor prognosis because the majority of nasal tumors are malignant. Carcinomas predominate in both dogs and cats. Neoplasia is more commonly diagnosed in older animals (lymphoma and transmissible venereal tumor [TVT] are notable exceptions). Although no sex predilection has been observed in dogs, male cats are more often affected than females.

Tumors can arise from any of the numerous tissue types found in the nasal cavity and paranasal sinuses with four distinct cytomorphologies (Table 5.2). Identification of the site of origin can be difficult because most malignant tumors are locally invasive and destructive and have extended into surrounding tissues by the time of diagnosis. The majority of tumors involve the caudal two-thirds of the nasal cavity near or adjacent to the cribriform plate. Less commonly, tumors may be located in the paranasal sinuses. Malignant neoplasia often involves the nasal turbinates and septum and can extend through the maxilla into the oral cavity. Extension into the orbit and cranial vault via erosion through the cribriform plate is less common but does occur. Metastasis to regional lymph nodes tends to occur late in the disease and is most often associated with epithelial tumors.

Cytopathologic and histopathologic diagnosis of malignant neoplasia depends on obtaining high-quality diagnostic samples. Emphasis should be placed on evaluation of samples obtained from deep tissues because secondary necrosis, inflammation, and hemorrhage are often prominent features of tumors involving the upper airways, which can confound the diagnosis.

Epithelial Neoplasia (Epithelial Cytomorphology)
Malignant epithelial tumors of the nasal cavity occur more frequently than their benign counterparts. The most common epithelial tumors of the nasal cavity include adenocarcinomas, squamous cell carcinomas (SCCs), and anaplastic or undifferentiated carcinomas. Adenocarcinomas are common in dogs and cats, whereas SCCs are more common in cats (Carswell and Williams, 2007). Cytopathologic samples from carcinomas tend to be moderately cellular. Neoplastic epithelial cells are present in small aggregates to larger sheets (Figs. 5.14 and 5.15). Adenocarcinomas can be identified by the presence of ring or rosette acinar arrangements that are best visualized at low magnification (e.g., 10$\times$ objective) (Fig. 5.16;

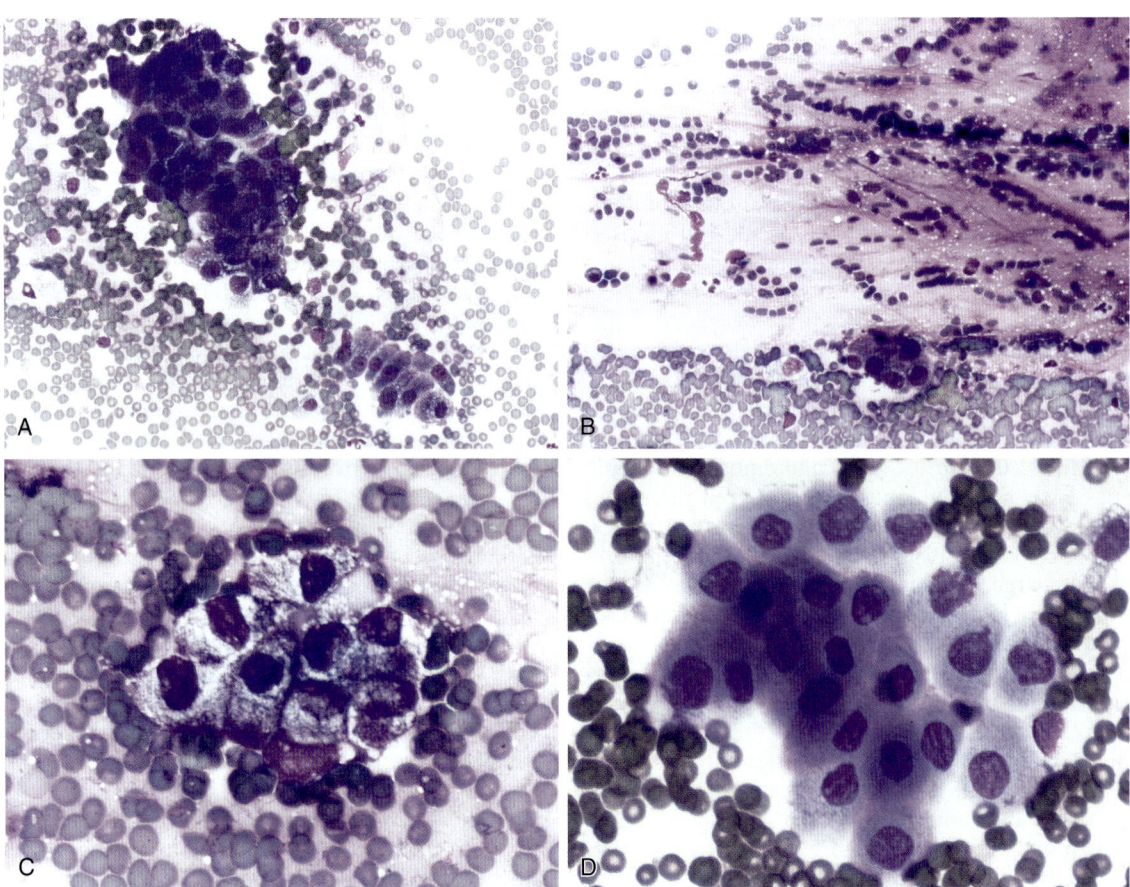

■ **FIGURE 5.13 Inflammatory nasopharyngeal polyp. Tissue imprint. Cat. A,** A cluster of hyperplastic respiratory epithelial cells (*top* and *left* of midline) and a row of columnar ciliated respiratory epithelial cells (*bottom* and *right* of midline) and a few scattered macrophages, plasma cells, and neutrophils. (Aqueous Romanowsky; IP.) **B,** Erythrocytes, neutrophils, macrophages, and plasma cells are windrowed within a thick, magenta matrix. A cluster of five cuboidal to columnar respiratory epithelial cells is present toward the bottom of the image. (Aqueous Romanowsky; IP.) **C,** Honeycomb-like sheet of vacuolated, hyperplastic respiratory epithelial cells without cilia. (Aqueous Romanowsky; HP oil.) **D,** Pavement pattern of squamous epithelial cells lined part of the polyp. (Aqueous Romanowsky; HP oil.)

TABLE 5.2 Neoplasia of the Nasal Cavity

CYTOMORPHOLOGY	BENIGN NEOPLASIA	MALIGNANT NEOPLASIA
Epithelial	Adenoma	Adenocarcinoma[a]
	Papilloma	Squamous cell carcinoma[a]
		Transitional carcinoma[a]
		Adenosquamous carcinoma
Mesenchymal	Fibroma	Fibrosarcoma[a]
	Chondroma	Chondrosarcoma[a]
	Osteoma	Osteosarcoma
	Leiomyoma	Leiomyosarcoma
		Undifferentiated sarcoma[a]
		Fibrous histiocytoma
		Hemangiosarcoma
		Liposarcoma
		Melanoma
Round cell		Lymphoma[a]
		Transmissible venereal tumor[a]
		Mast cell tumor[a]
		Plasmacytoma
Naked nuclei		Carcinoids
		Olfactory neuroblastoma

[a]Most common tumor types.

see Fig. 5.14B). Malignant epithelial cells are round to polygonal and typically display numerous criteria of malignancy. Such features include macrocytosis, moderate to marked anisocytosis, anisokaryosis, an increased nucleocytoplasmic ratio, and deeply basophilic cytoplasm that may contain numerous discrete, clear cytoplasmic vacuoles or one large, clear vacuole (signet ring form), suggestive of secretory product. Nucleolar criteria of malignancy should also be assessed, evaluating for the number of nucleoli per nucleus and any size or shape variations. Anaplastic cells may individualize and appear similar to lymphoid cells, but large cell size and periodic sheet formation are helpful in distinguishing the two types of neoplasms, although histopathologic examination without immunochemistry has difficulties. One study reviewed 232 histopathologic specimens of cats involving these two neoplasms and found a disputed diagnosis in 15 cases. Immunohistochemical staining of these disputed cases indicated that the original diagnoses were incorrect in 67% (10 of 15) and correct in 20% (3 of 15) (Nagata et al., 2014). Extracellular secretory material such as mucus may also be identified as eosinophilic, amorphous to fibrillar material. Some histologically classified carcinomas of the nasal and paranasal cavities were shown to react with neuroendocrine markers.

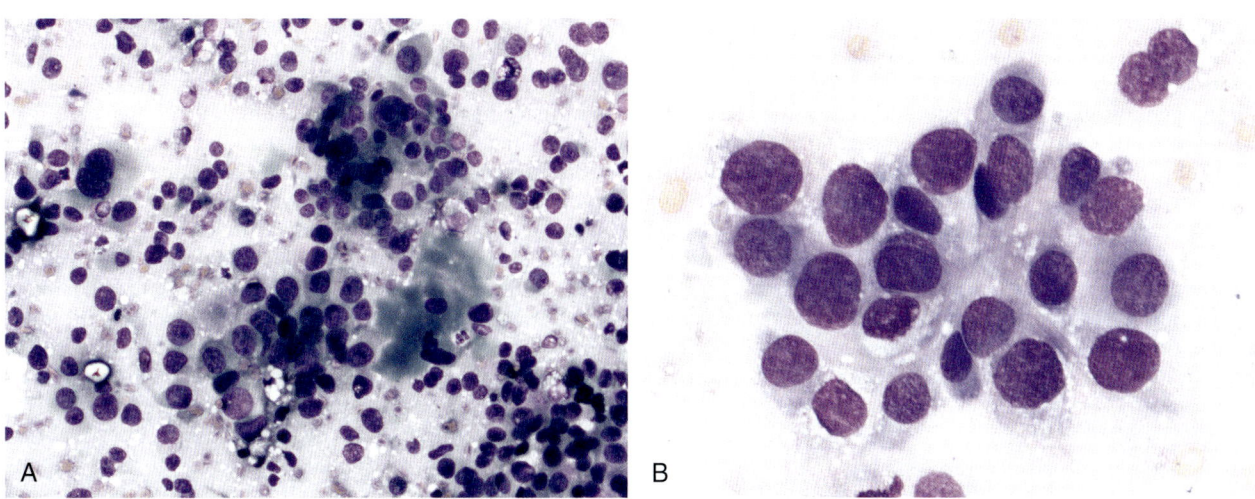

■ **FIGURE 5.14 Nasal adenocarcinoma. Tissue imprint. Dog.** Same case in A and B. **A,** Variably cohesive sheets and rows of pleomorphic polygonal to round cells with light basophilic cytoplasm and indistinct cell borders. The background contains lysed, round nuclei and an amorphous green-blue material (presumed mucus). (Wright-Giemsa; IP.) **B,** Glandular origin may be identified by the presence of acinar arrangements. (Wright-Giemsa; HP oil.)

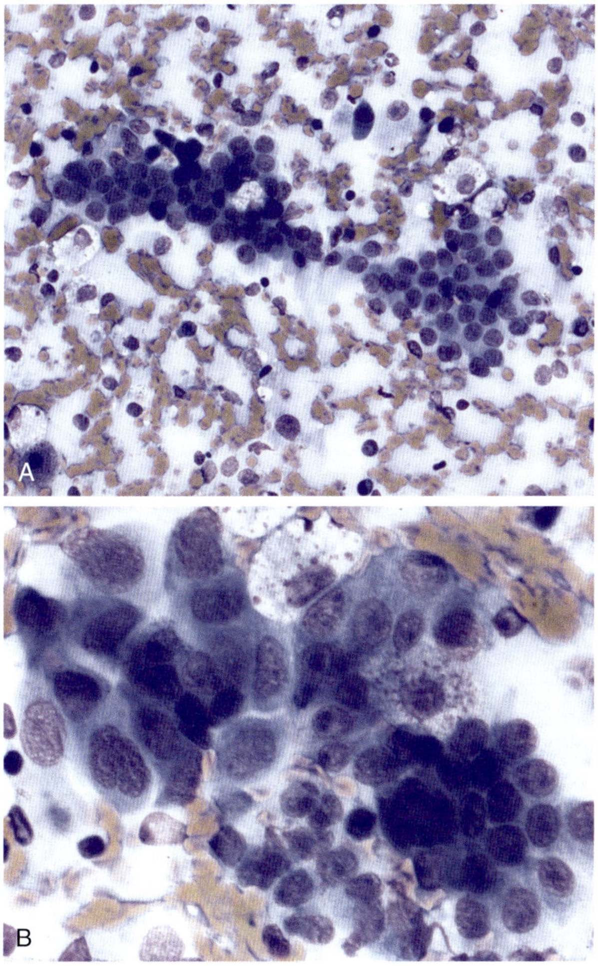

■ **FIGURE 5.15 Nasal adenocarcinoma, well-differentiated. Tissue imprint. Dog.** Same case in A and B. **A,** Honeycomb pattern of polygonal epithelial cells with scant to moderate cytoplasm and indistinct cell borders. (Wright-Giemsa; IP.) **B,** A transition from well-differentiated epithelial cells *(bottom right)* to more atypical epithelial cells *(top left)*. (Wright-Giemsa, HP oil.)

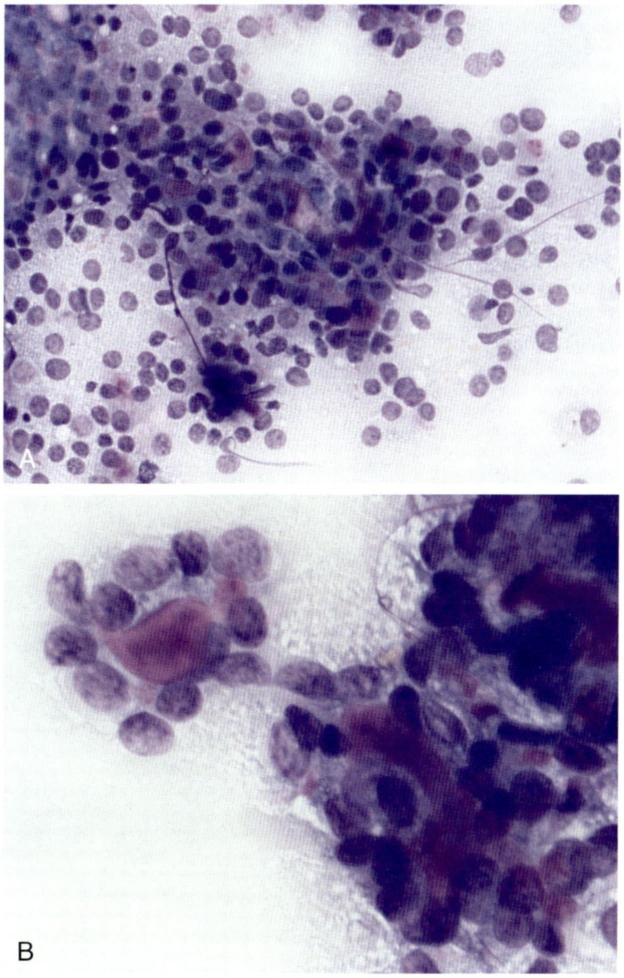

■ **FIGURE 5.16 Nasal adenocarcinoma, anaplastic. Tissue imprint. Dog.** Same case in A and B. **A,** Many lysed, round nuclei and fewer intact round cells surrounding and emanating from an eosinophilic matrical core. (Wright-Giemsa; IP.) **B,** The round nuclei show acinar formations with an eosinophilic central material. (Wright-Giemsa; HP oil.)

Squamous cell carcinoma can originate from the nasal cavity or the frontal sinus (de Vos et al., 2012). SCCs are distinguished by the presence of cells with angular borders containing abundant, homogenous, glassy cytoplasm and centrally placed nuclei. The neoplastic cells display a wide range in maturation—ranging from immature, small, cuboidal, nucleated, epithelial cells with deeply basophilic cytoplasm to more mature cells, identified as anucleate, fully keratinized cells containing abundant, pale, basophilic cytoplasm and sharply angulated borders. Evidence of asynchronous development may be present, such as the identification of fully keratinized cells with retained large nuclei (Fig. 5.17). Prominent anisokaryosis and variable chromatin patterns ranging from smooth (immature) to clumped (mature) may be seen. A few neoplastic squamous cells may also show a perinuclear clearing (perinuclear "halo") or even a few, small, clear, punctate, perinuclear vacuoles. Abundant keratinaceous debris represented as amorphous, basophilic extracellular material is often scattered about the slides. A common characteristic of SCC is the presence of a moderate to marked accompanying neutrophilic inflammatory response.

Similar in cytopathologic appearance to SCC is a neoplasm termed *transitional carcinoma*. This neoplasm arises from nonciliated nasal respiratory epithelium (Carswell and Williams, 2007). It may display a moderately abundant cytoplasm with numerous punctate vacuoles. Malignant features often involve anisokaryosis, multinucleation, coarse chromatin clumping, prominent nucleolus, and variable nucleocytoplasmic ratios (Fig. 5.18).

Careful documentation of the discussed characteristics with abundant criteria of malignancy is critical to a diagnosis of neoplasia of the nasal cavity. If criteria of malignancy are not readily apparent, diagnosticians should be cautious because cytopathologic differentiation of a well-differentiated carcinoma from benign epithelial neoplasia, epithelial hyperplasia, or squamous metaplasia may be impossible, particularly in the presence of inflammation.

Mesenchymal Neoplasia (Mesenchymal Cytomorphology)

Mesenchymal neoplasia of the nasal cavity is uncommon. Osteosarcoma, fibrosarcoma, and chondrosarcoma occur most commonly (Fig. 5.19). Chondrosarcomas are more likely to occur in young dogs with a possible increased risk in medium to large breeds (Lana and Withrow, 2001). Cytopathologic samples are typically of low cellularity, consisting of individualized and occasionally small, loose aggregates of oval, plump, or spindle-shaped cells (Fig. 5.20). Cytoplasmic borders are typically ill defined, and neoplastic cells may contain few to moderate numbers of fine eosinophilic to purple cytoplasmic granules. Matrix may be observed as streaming, brightly eosinophilic, fibrillar material, often intimately laced among the neoplastic cells. However, it is easily confused with mucus,

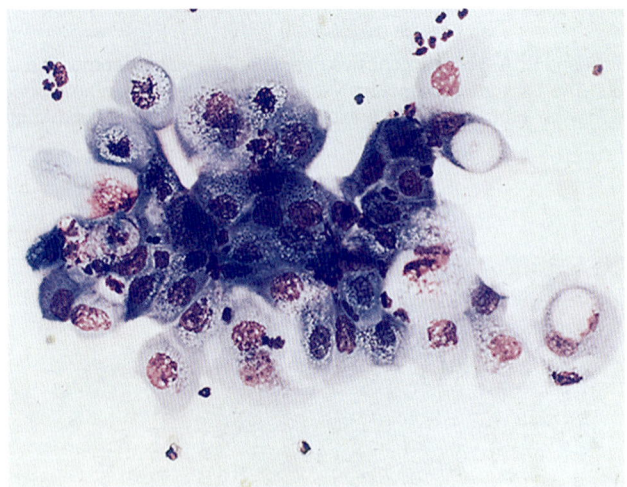

■ **FIGURE 5.17 Squamous cell carcinoma. Nasal flush.** Asynchronous keratinization, moderate pleomorphism, and perinuclear vacuolation are typical features of squamous cell carcinoma. The associated suppurative inflammation is commonly seen with this type of tumor. (Wright-Giemsa; HP oil.)

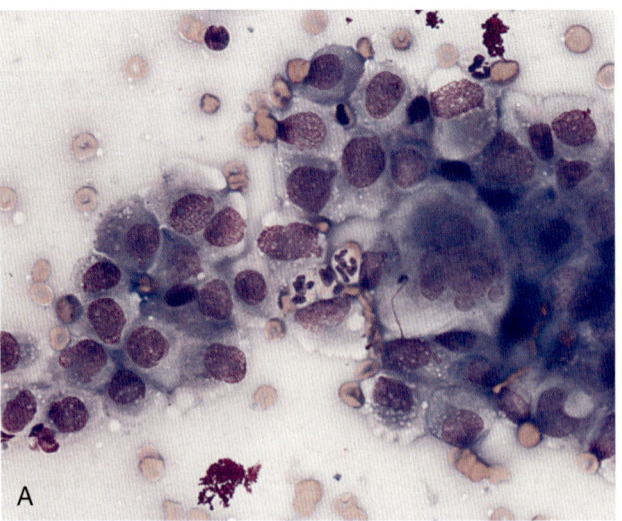 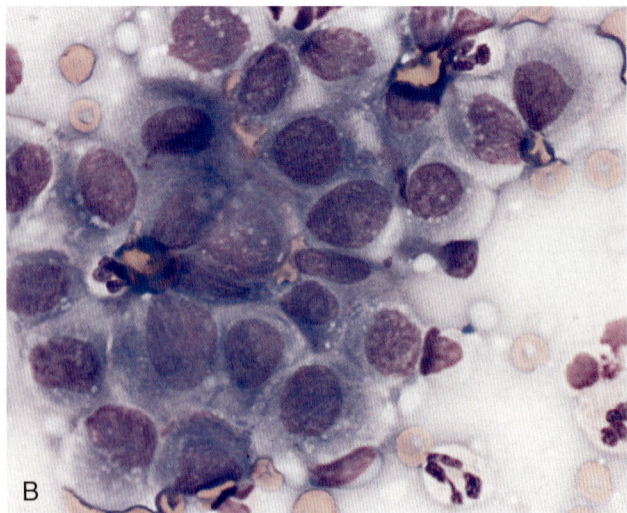

■ **FIGURE 5.18 Transitional carcinoma. Nasal mass imprint. Dog.** Same case in A and B. **A,** This appearance is similar to squamous cell carcinoma. Shown is a multinucleate cell with mild neutrophilic inflammation. Notice the pleomorphism of the transitional or nonciliated respiratory epithelium. The embedded neutrophils are a useful ruler for sizing the neoplastic cells. (Wright-Giemsa; HP oil.) **B,** Notice the moderately abundant cytoplasm with numerous punctate vacuoles. Malignant features involve anisokaryosis, coarse chromatin clumping, prominent nucleoli, and variable nucleocytoplasmic ratios (Wright-Giemsa; HP oil.) (Courtesy Rose Raskin, Purdue University.)

and the presence or absence of streaming eosinophilic material on a cytologic preparation should not be used to characterize the type of neoplasia.

A cytopathologic diagnosis of mesenchymal neoplasia is complicated by several factors. Mesenchymal neoplasia often exfoliates poorly, resulting in a hemodiluted sample that contains only a few pleomorphic spindle-shaped cells for evaluation. Also, significant inflammation can induce reactive fibroplasia that can be difficult to distinguish from fibrosarcoma. In this case, cytologic evaluation coupled with physical examination and historical and radiographic information raises the index of suspicion for mesenchymal neoplasia, warranting biopsy with histopathologic examination for definitive diagnosis. Additionally, histopathology is often necessary for classification of mesenchymal neoplasia because the more commonly seen mesenchymal tumors often lack distinguishing cytopathologic features.

Other types of mesenchymal tumors involving the upper airways (see Table 5.2) are uncommon but have cytopathologic features resembling soft tissue sarcomas in more common sites. Intranasal and sinus melanoma has been reported in both dogs (Hicks and Fidel, 2006) and cats (Mukaratirwa et al., 2001). Benign proliferations such as angiofibroma have been histologically described in the nasal cavity (Burgess et al., 2011).

Hemolymphatic Neoplasia (Round Cell Cytomorphology)

Hemolymphatic tumors such as lymphoma, plasmacytomas, mast cell tumors, TVTs, and histiocytic neoplasia can occur in the nasal cavity. These tumors yield highly cellular preparations composed of individualized, neoplastic, and discrete, round cells with distinct cytoplasmic borders. The morphology resembles that seen in other sites.

Lymphoma. Lymphoma is the most common round cell tumor reported in the nasal cavity of dogs and cats. In cats, the majority of nasal lymphomas are of B-cell origin, although T-cell lymphoma of the nasal cavity has also been reported (Mukaratirwa et al., 2001; Day et al., 2004; Santagostino et al., 2015). Lymphoma of the nasal cavity tends to be characterized by a monomorphic population of medium-sized or large, immature lymphoid cells with scant, deeply basophilic cytoplasm; large round nuclei; finely granular chromatin; and single to multiple nucleoli (Fig. 5.21A). Upper respiratory tract lymphomas in cats were aggressive, with survival varying from 0 to 301 days (mean, 53 days) (Santagostino et al., 2015). Anaplastic nasal carcinomas can individualize and resemble lymphoma, but the presence of very large cells and occasional sheet formation assist in making the proper diagnosis. Care should be taken to distinguish lymphoma from lymphoid hyperplasia or an inflammatory polyp. In lymphoid hyperplasia, a heterogeneous population of lymphocytes and plasma cells are present, with a predominance of small, mature lymphocytes and fewer intermediate and large lymphoid cells. In some cases, lymphoma is characterized by a predominance of intermediate-sized lymphocytes with an increased amount of cytoplasm and smooth chromatin lacking nucleoli. Even more problematic are cases in which the neoplastic population consists of small, well-differentiated lymphocytes (Fig. 5.21B). In such questionable cases, histopathology is imperative for definitive diagnosis of

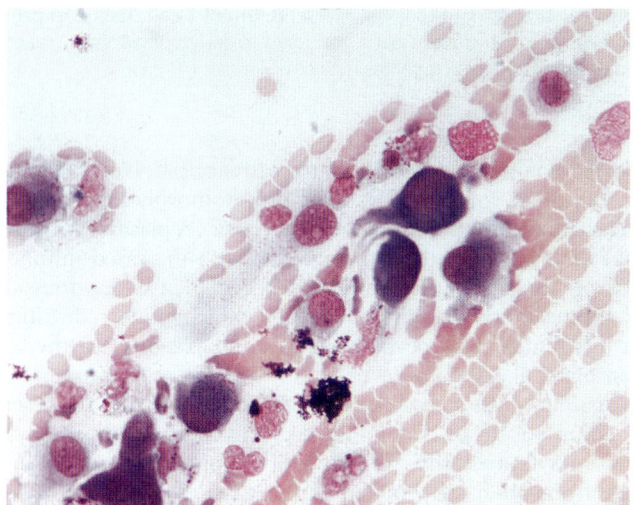

FIGURE 5.19 Frontal sinus sarcoma. Aspirate. Dog. Several individualized oval to spindle-shaped pleomorphic cells are present in a background of erythrocytes. Several cells contain a faint dusting of azurophilic granules, which may be observed in mesenchymal neoplasias. The suspected sarcoma was confirmed with histopathology. (Wright-Giemsa; HP oil.)

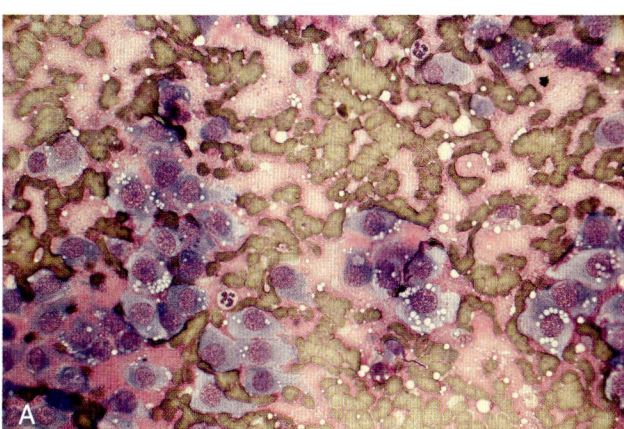 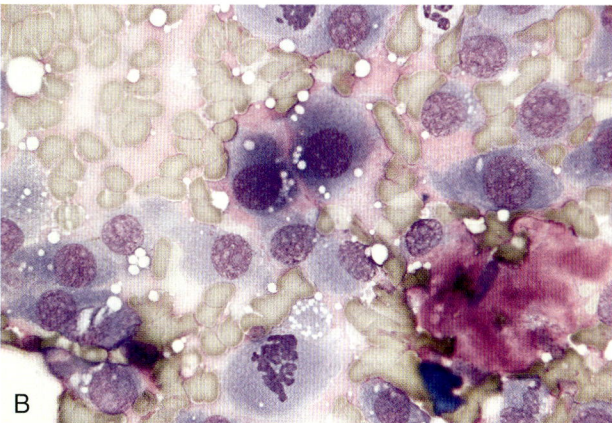

FIGURE 5.20 Nasal chondrosarcoma. Tissue imprint. Dog. A, Irregularly spindle-shaped to round cells enmeshed within bright, magenta, thick stroma. (Wright-Giemsa; HP oil.) **B,** The neoplastic cells contain round nuclei, multiple and prominent nucleoli, and mitotic figures. These cells are associated with a bright magenta, cartilaginous matrix *(bottom right).* (Wright-Giemsa; HP oil.)

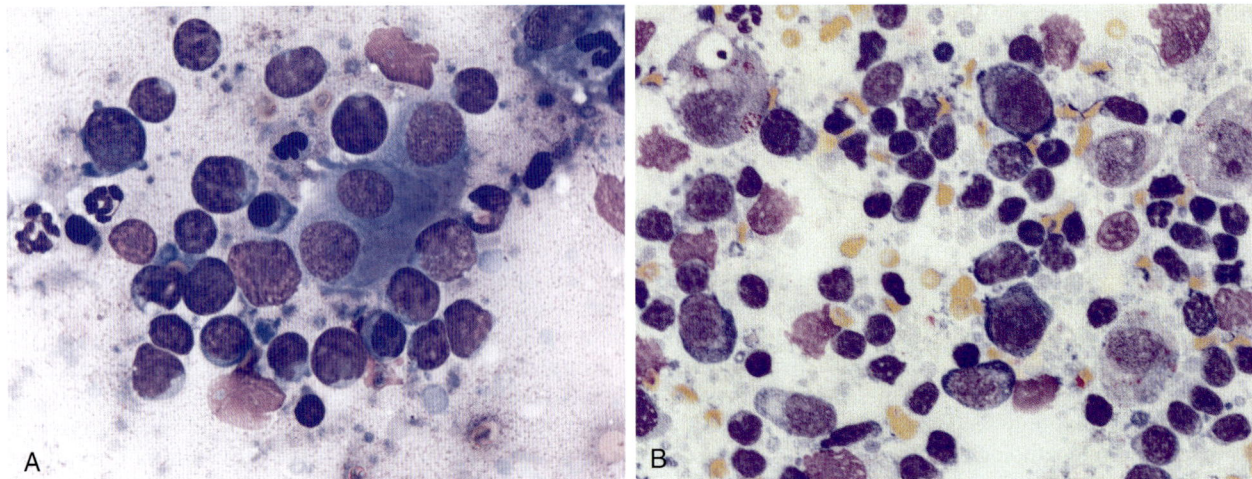

■ **FIGURE 5.21 Nasal lymphoma. A, Intermediate lymphoid cell.** Three reactive respiratory epithelial cells are present in the center surrounded by intermediate lymphoid cells with irregular nuclei (neutrophils for size comparison at *left*). (Wright-Giemsa; HP oil.) **B, Small T cell. Tissue imprint. Cat.** Many scattered small neoplastic lymphocytes with fewer interspersed, reactive inflammatory cells, including large lymphoid cells, macrophages, and neutrophils. Histopathology and immunohistochemistry were required for definitive diagnosis. (Wright-Giemsa; HP oil.)

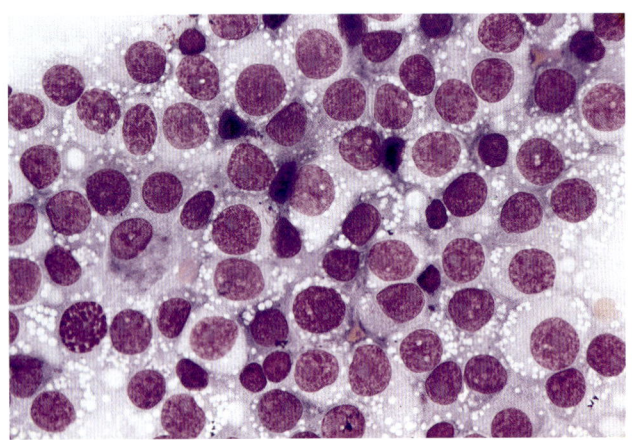

■ **FIGURE 5.22 Transmissible venereal tumor. Nasal mass imprint. Dog.** Highly cellular, moderately pleomorphic population of discrete cells with abundant pale cytoplasm, ropy chromatin, and distinct nucleoli. Note the presence of small dense lymphocytes intermixed in the specimen. Compare to Figs. 3.206 and 13.51. (Wright-Giemsa; HP oil.)

lymphoma. In one study in cats using comparison with histopathology, a diagnosis of lymphoma was attained by cytopathology in 12 of 25 (48%) cases, but a false-negative diagnosis of lymphoplasmacytic rhinitis was obtained in 11 cases (44%) (Santagostino et al., 2015).

Canine transmissible venereal tumor. Canine TVT is a contagious neoplasm involving the external genitalia of both sexes with a low occurrence of metastasis. Spread to the nasal cavity is thought to occur secondary to implantation from a primary genital tumor; however, there are several reports of primary intranasal TVT (Papazoglou et al., 2001). Cytologic preparations reveal large numbers of a monomorphic population of large, round cells with abundant, light to moderately basophilic cytoplasm containing numerous, distinct, small vacuoles. Nuclei are round with coarse to ropy chromatin with one or two large, prominent nucleoli. Mitoses are frequently observed (Fig. 5.22).

Cytopathologic classification into plasmacytoid, lymphocytoid, or mixed subtypes of TVT based on cytomorphologic appearance has been proposed (Flórez et al., 2012). A plasmacytic cytomorphology has also been associated with increased numbers of DNA breaks (Flórez et al., 2012) and increased expression of permeability glycoprotein (P-gp), which might contribute to differential subtype pathogenesis and response to therapy (Gaspar et al., 2010).

Histiocytic sarcoma. Canine histiocytic neoplasia can present as either a local or disseminated process. Localized histiocytic sarcomas tend to arise from the subcutis but occasionally originate from other sites, including the nasal cavity (Affolter and Moore, 2002). The morphology of cells in this report varied from site to site, as well as within different nodules of the same tumor; however, it was similar in phenotype and variation to those previously described.

Neuroendocrine and Neuroepithelial Neoplasia (Naked Nuclei Cytomorphology)

Neuroendocrine carcinomas or carcinoids have been rarely described in the nasal cavity of dogs (Patnaik et al., 2002; Sako et al., 2005), with a single report of metastasis (Koehler et al., 2012). Histologically, their features appear to be similar to those described elsewhere in the body (see Chapter 17). Cytopathologic characteristics have not been reported. Detection of neuroendocrine markers has been reported in several nasal and paranasal adenocarcinomas by histochemistry (argyrophilic stains) and immunohistochemistry (synaptophysin and chromogranin A) (Ninomiya et al., 2008).

The olfactory neuroblastoma or esthesioneuroblastoma is a rare neoplasm reported in dogs and cats that arises from the olfactory neuroepithelium (Brosinski et al., 2012). It can be difficult to differentiate from poorly differentiated sinonasal and neuroendocrine carcinomas, particularly by cytopathology (Cazzini et al., 2019). Histologically, it is composed of uniform small cells often organized in nests or lobules separated by a fibrovascular stroma. The cells consistently label with neuronal immunohistochemical stains such as neuron-specific enolase (NSE)

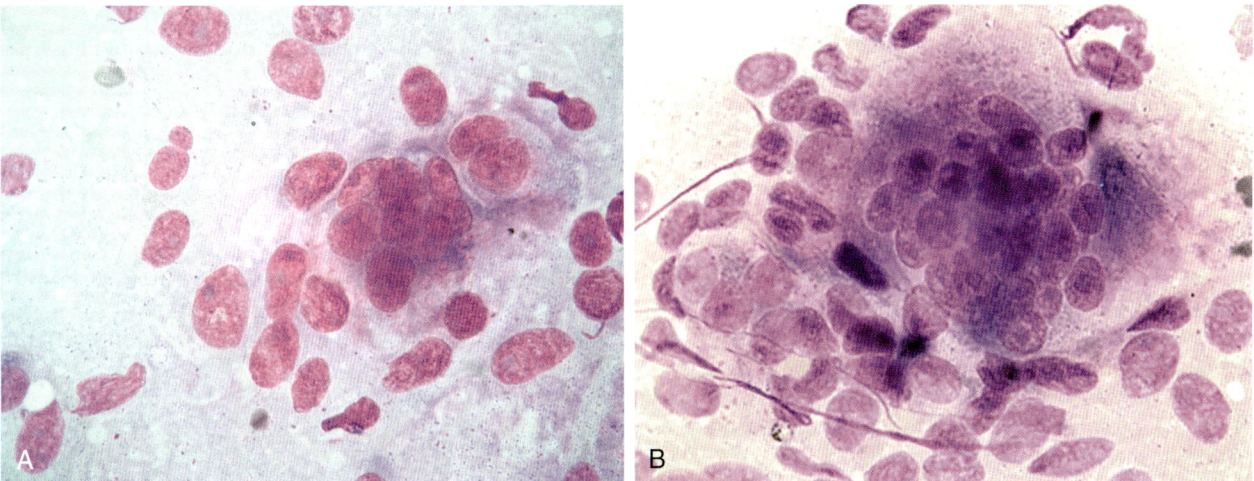

■ **FIGURE 5.23 Giant cell tumor of nasal bone. Nasal cavity mass scraping. Cat.** Same case in A and B. **A,** Monomorphic population of pleomorphic spindle-shaped cells with minimal faint-staining cytoplasm and a multinucleate cell with plump immature nuclei. Clinical signs for this 13-year-old cat involved bilateral epistaxis and serous ocular discharge from the affected side. (Aqueous Romanowsky; HP oil.) **B,** Large multinucleated cell with approximately 20 nuclei, surrounded by pleomorphic spindle-shaped cells, mimics a granulomatous inflammation; however there are no attendant inflammatory cells. Numerous multinucleate cells were present cytopathologically. Diagnosis confirmed by histopathology that noted bone involvement. (Aqueous Romanowsky; HP oil.) (Courtesy Dita Novakova, Czech Republic.)

and microtubule-associated protein-2 (MAP-2) (Brosinski et al., 2012).

Miscellaneous Neoplasia
Oncocytoma of the nasal cavity has been rarely reported in dogs and cats (Doughty et al., 2006) (see section on Laryngeal Oncocytoma later in this chapter for discussion of cytopathologic features). Giant cell tumor of bone (Fig. 5.23) of the sinonasal cavity is uncommon but has been noted in the cat (Jelínek et al., 2008) and should not be mistaken for granulomatous inflammation.

LARYNX

Normal Anatomy and Histology
The larynx is a musculocartilaginous portion of the upper respiratory tract that encompasses the vocal folds, arytenoid cartilage, and glottis. The larynx is composed of an elastic cartilage that is lined by a stratified squamous epithelium with collections of lymphoid tissue scattered throughout the lamina propria.

Sample Collection and Preparation
Respiratory stridor, dyspnea, and changes in or loss of vocal tone suggest laryngeal disease. Cytopathologic evaluation of the larynx is most useful for the characterization of mass lesions, infiltrative processes, or inflammatory disease and depends on obtaining adequate, representative samples. Laryngeal masses, although uncommon, may be detected and stabilized for sampling by palpation. Radiographs may help detect and localize mass lesions but may be difficult to interpret due to breed variations and superimposition of soft tissues. Ultrasonographic evaluation affords superior visualization of laryngeal masses and guidance for FNA. Ultrasound-guided aspiration through the ventral laryngeal cartilage has not been associated with significant complications, even in cats (Rudorf and Brown, 1998).

Laryngoscopy allows direct visualization and sampling of laryngeal masses but requires anesthesia. Lidocaine spray may be necessary for complete examination and sampling because of laryngospasm, especially in cats. Masses observed during laryngoscopy can be sampled directly by FNA biopsy or brush cytology, or alligator biopsy forceps may be used to obtain pinch samples for cytologic touch imprints. Intraluminal sampling may be associated with significant hemorrhage and edema, particularly in cats, which can result in laryngeal obstruction.

Normal Cytology and Oropharyngeal Contamination
Normal Cytology
Samples from the normal larynx typically are sparsely cellular with only scattered nonkeratinized squamous epithelial cells observed. Occasional aspirates or brush samples may demonstrate small aggregates of well-differentiated lymphocytes in addition to the epithelial cells.

Oropharyngeal Contamination
The cytopathologic findings of oropharyngeal contamination are similar to those described in the discussion of normal cytology and artifacts of the nasal cavity.

Cellular Responses to Injury
The laryngeal mucosa and vocal folds are reddened, thickened, and frequently edematous without evidence of mass lesions. Clinical signs of laryngeal dysfunction, such as coughing, gagging, and change in phonation, may be apparent. Suppurative inflammation is commonly present, although observation of etiologic agents is rare. Hemorrhage is identified by the presence of erythrophagocytic macrophages, whereas edema is characterized by a basophilic granular proteinaceous fluid background. In chronic inflammation, fibrosis or ossification of the larynx often occurs, resulting in sparsely cellular aspirates containing rare spindle-shaped cells.

Epithelial Hyperplasia and Dysplasia

Similar to squamous epithelial cells of other locations, the non-keratinized squamous epithelial cells of the larynx may become hyperplastic and dysplastic in response to chronic injury. These features may include increased cytoplasmic basophilia, increased nucleocytoplasmic ratios, nucleocytoplasmic maturation asynchrony, and keratinization.

Reactive Lymphoid Hyperplasia

Reactive lymphoid hyperplasia may occur secondary to infectious, inflammatory, or neoplastic disorders of the larynx. Reactive hyperplasia is differentiated from lymphoma by the heterogeneity of the lymphocyte population, orderly progression from lymphoblasts to small lymphocytes that predominate, and the presence of plasma cells or other inflammatory cells such as neutrophils, macrophages, and eosinophils.

Noninfectious Inflammatory Disorders
Local Irritation

Local irritation of the larynx may occur with inhaled irritants, intubation, chronic cough, or gastrointestinal reflux.

Granulomatous Laryngitis

Granulomatous laryngitis is a distinct but uncommon syndrome seen in dogs and cats that may mimic the appearance of neoplasia both grossly and cytopathologically (Oakes and McCarthy, 1994; Tasker et al., 1999a). Mass lesions can be large and may obstruct the laryngeal lumen. The cytopathologic appearance is similar to other granulomatous lesions and is characterized by the presence of large numbers of epithelioid macrophages. Lymphocytes may also be present. In chronic lesions, fibroplasia is prominent, and aspiration reveals increased numbers of plump, moderately pleomorphic, spindle-shaped cells easily confused with mesenchymal neoplasia. Etiologic agents are not observed, and the underlying cause of granulomatous laryngitis is unknown.

Infectious Inflammatory Disorders

The most common causes of laryngitis are infectious and include infectious tracheobronchitis (kennel cough) in dogs and viral rhinotracheitis and calicivirus in cats. Laryngeal abscesses are rare but may be caused by a penetrating foreign body.

Non-neoplastic Tumors
Laryngeal Cysts and Mucoceles

Laryngeal cysts and salivary mucoceles are uncommon findings in the laryngopharynx. Fluid aspirated from the cyst is typically of low cellularity and ranges from clear to milky in appearance. Mucoceles contain macrophages, nondegenerate neutrophils, and perhaps vacuolated salivary epithelial cells. In a case report of a laryngeal mucocele, variably sized basophilic amorphous, anuclear structures were present and were thought to represent inspissated saliva (Wiedmeyer et al., 2003). Mucoceles arising from the wall of the pharynx, although still uncommon, may induce marked upper airway obstruction, but they are difficult to diagnose without a thorough examination of the laryngopharynx (Benjamino et al., 2012).

Neoplastic Tumors

Primary laryngeal tumors have been identified in both dogs and cats. These tumors can arise from the epithelial or musculocartilaginous components of the larynx or from the lymphoid nodules. Lymphoma is the most commonly reported laryngeal tumor in cats followed by SCC. In dogs, carcinomas and SCC predominate.

Epithelial Neoplasia

Squamous cell carcinoma. The larynx is lined by squamous epithelial cells, so it is necessary to ensure that a deep sample is obtained because swabs, scrapings, or shallow aspiration result in exfoliation of the surface squamous lining. Aspirates from SCC tend to be of moderate cellularity. Individual cell morphology ranges from basal to fully keratinized squamous epithelial cells (Fig. 5.24). Basal cells are immature, cuboidal to

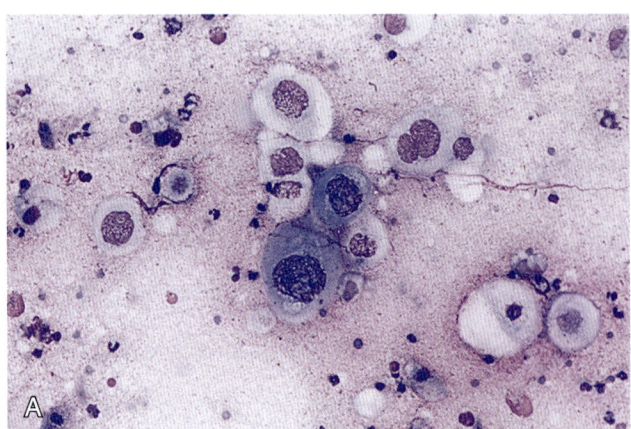

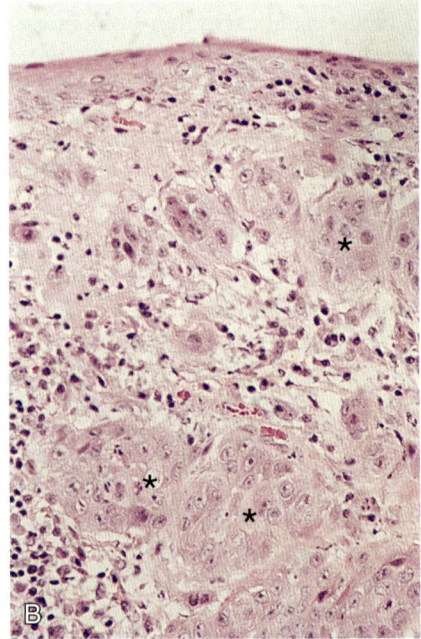

■ **FIGURE 5.24 Squamous cell carcinoma. A, Tissue aspirate.** Pleomorphic squamous epithelium with clear to basophilic cytoplasm embedded in a granular proteinaceous background and surrounded by a sprinkling of neutrophils and lymphocytes, which can be used to denote the size of the larger neoplastic squamous cells. (Wright-Giemsa; HP oil.) **B, Laryngeal mass. Cat.** Clinical signs included brief duration of dyspnea. Tissue section demonstrates islands of neoplastic squamous cells *(asterisks)* that extend into the deeper tissues. Lymphocytes, plasma cells, and neutrophils appear as small dense nuclei surrounding these islands indicating chronic active inflammation. (H&E; IP.) (B, Courtesy Rose Raskin, University of Florida.)

round, epithelial cells with deeply basophilic cytoplasm, large central nuclei, coarse chromatin, and prominent nucleoli. Mature squamous cells are large with angular borders and contain abundant homogenous cytoplasm and pyknotic or karyorrhectic nuclei. The presence of mature squamous cells alone in a laryngeal sample should not be interpreted as SCC. Multiple stages of epithelial cell development, cellular pleomorphism, and the presence of asynchronous cytoplasmic and nuclear maturation are necessary for a cytopathologic diagnosis of SCC. Suppurative inflammation is commonly associated with SCC and can confound the diagnosis because inflammation can induce squamous dysplasia.

Laryngeal Carcinoma

Carcinoma of the larynx is more prevalent in dogs than in cats. Aspirates are moderately cellular and contain small clusters or sheets of cohesive epithelial cells with round, centrally located nuclei, coarsely clumped chromatin, and basophilic cytoplasm. Well-differentiated carcinomas are characterized by a relatively uniform population of epithelial cells with only mild to moderate anisocytosis and anisokaryosis and single or indistinct nucleoli. Poorly differentiated carcinomas show moderate to marked pleomorphism between clumps of cells as well as within cells of the same cluster. Laryngeal adenocarcinomas are rare; however, they demonstrate acinar formation or ductular structures. These acini may secrete mucin that appears as blue-gray material within cuboidal to columnar epithelium that is best identified with mucicarmine histochemical staining (Fig. 5.25).

In addition to tumors arising from the larynx, perilaryngeal thyroid carcinomas (see Chapter 17) can invade the larynx and should be considered as a differential.

Mesenchymal Neoplasia

Tumors arising from the musculocartilaginous component are rare but include leiomyoma, leiomyosarcoma, fibrosarcoma (Fig. 5.26), chondrosarcoma, osteosarcoma, rhabdomyosarcoma, and rhabdomyoma (Figs. 5.27 and 5.28). Malignant melanoma and granular cell tumors may also arise from the

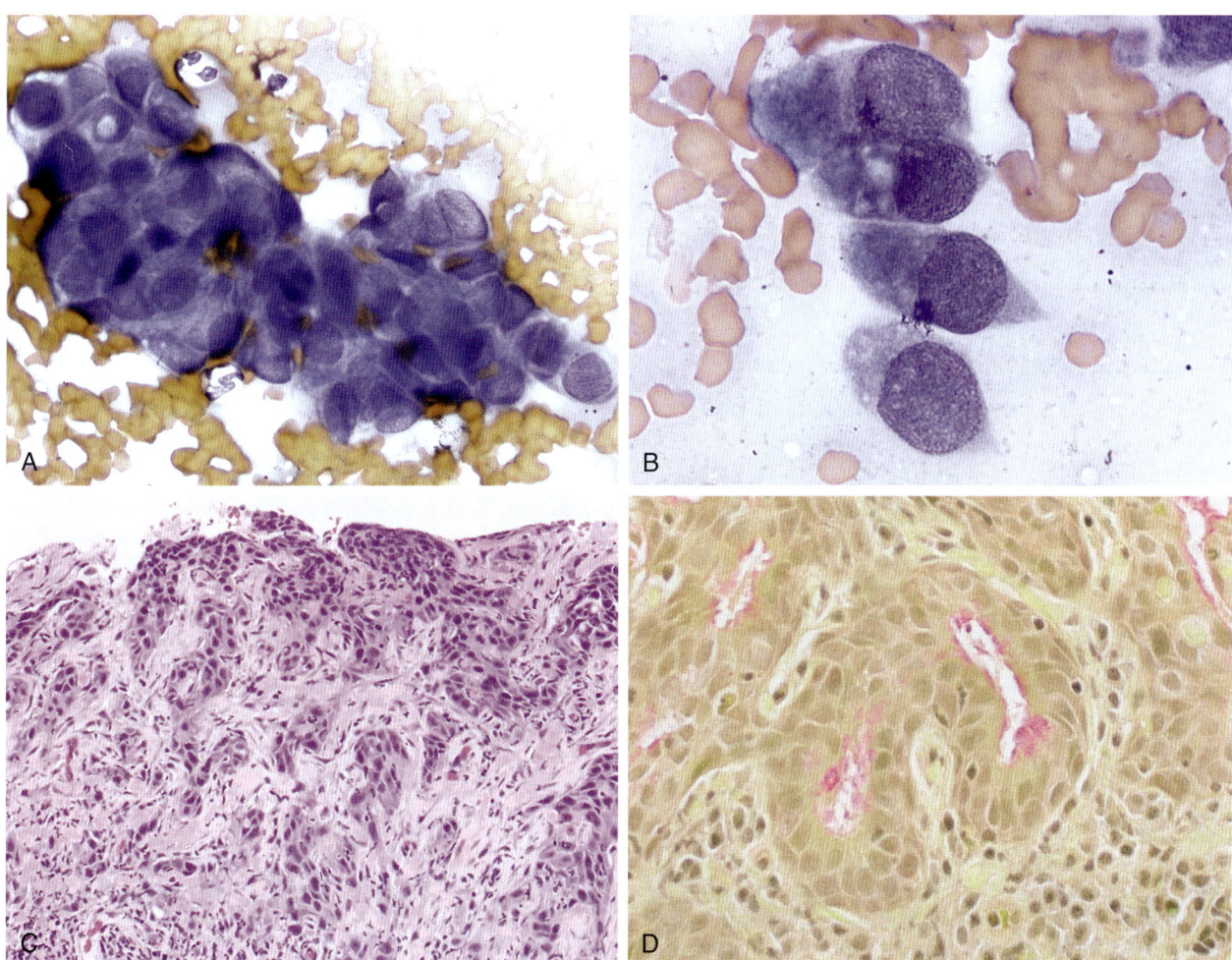

■ **FIGURE 5.25 Laryngeal adenocarcinoma. Cat.** Same case in A to D. **A, Tissue imprint.** The patient presented dyspneic with increased inspiratory respiratory effort from a laryngeal mass that occluded the airway. Epithelial cells have high nucleocytoplasmic ratio and form dense cords and tubular structures. (Wright; HP oil.) **B, Tissue imprint.** Close view of four cuboidal to columnar cells having a basal nucleus with the apical cytoplasm containing blue-gray mucoid material. (Wright; HP oil.) **C, Tissue section**. The surface is partially ulcerated with a subepithelial stroma expanded by a nonencapsulated, infiltrative proliferation of neoplastic epithelial cells that is arranged in nests and anastomosing trabeculae. (H&E; IP.) **D, Tissue section.** Histochemical staining indicates the presence of mucin particularly within acinar and tubular structures to identify the glandular function of the mass. (Mucicarmine; IP.) (A–B, Courtesy Rose Raskin. C–D, Courtesy Tuddow Thaiwong, Michigan State University.)

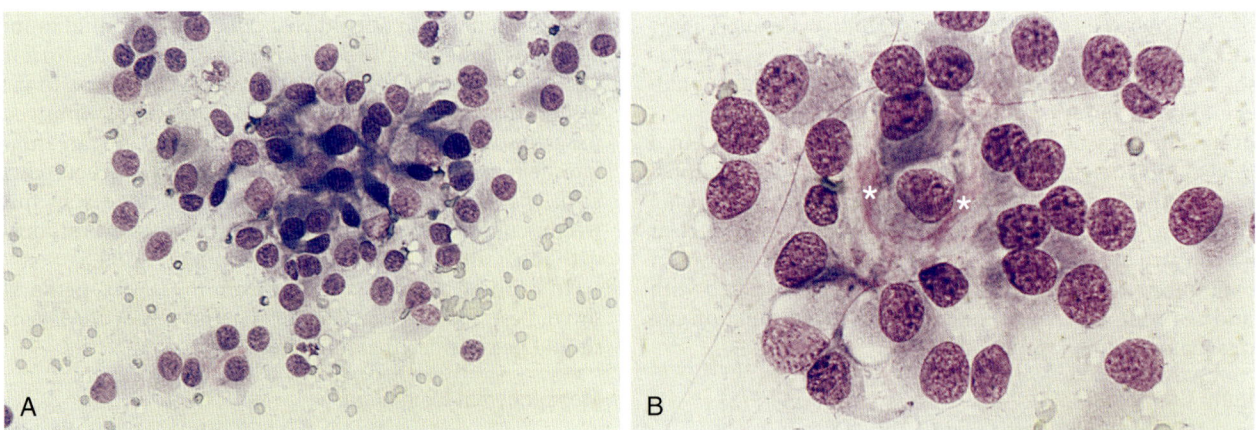

■ **FIGURE 5.26 Laryngeal fibrosarcoma. Mass imprint. Cat.** Same case in A and B. **A,** Aggregate of pleomorphic spindle-shaped cells with minimal faint-staining to dark basophilic cytoplasm in an animal with a month-long dysphonia and recent dyspnea. The erythrocytes can be used to denote the relatively large size of the neoplastic sarcoma cells. (Aqueous Romanowsky; HP oil.) **B,** A minimal amount of wispy eosinophilic intercellular matrix *(asterisk)* is associated with the neoplastic cells. Nuclei are oval to round with granular chromatin and indistinct small dark purple nucleoli. Cytoplasmic borders are wispy and indistinct. Immunohistochemistry was negative for muscle markers. (Aqueous Romanowsky; HP oil.) (Courtesy Rose Raskin, University of Florida.)

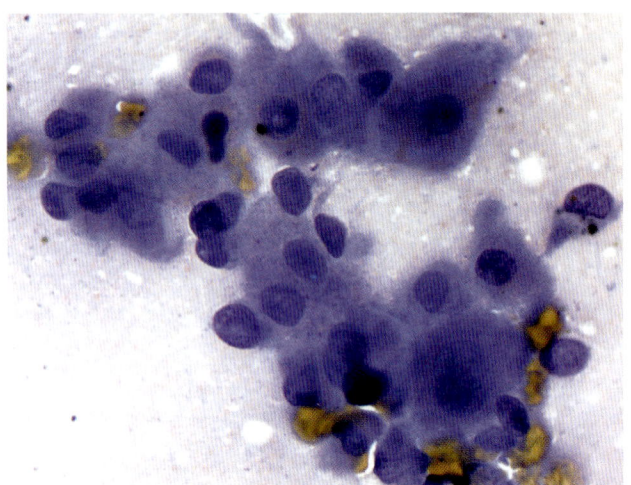

■ **FIGURE 5.27 Laryngeal rhabdomyoma. Mass imprint. Dog.** Variably sized, cuboidal to polygonal cells with moderate amounts of amphophilic, foamy to granular cytoplasm. Oncocytoma and rhabdomyoma are differentials for this cytopathologic appearance, and additional diagnostic tests are necessary to differentiate the two neoplasms. Electron microscopy and immunohistochemistry indicated that this mass was of muscle origin. (Methanolic Romanowsky; HP oil.) (Courtesy Shawn P. Clark et al., Purdue University. Presented at the 2002 ASVCP case review session.)

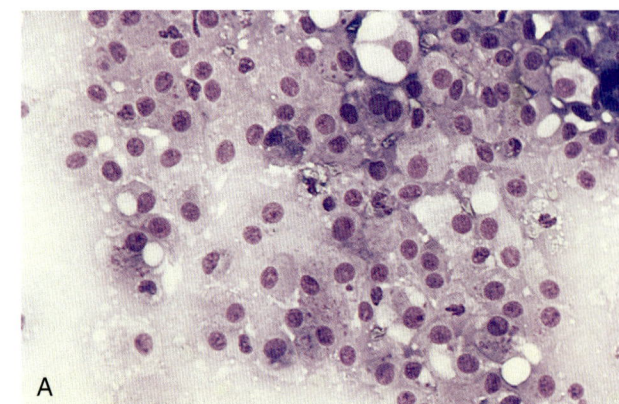

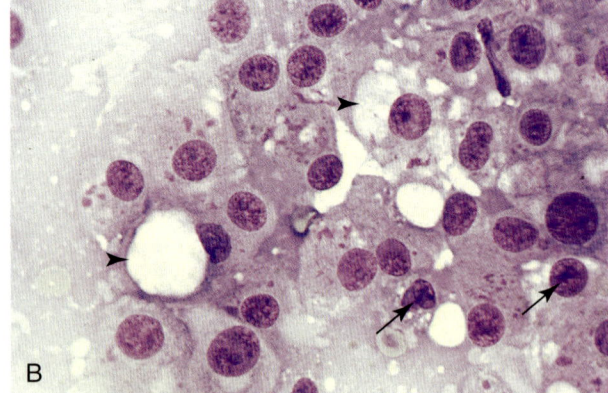

■ **FIGURE 5.28 Laryngeal rhabdomyoma. Cytopathology.** Same case in A and B. **A,** Highly cellular sample with a monomorphic population of large epithelioid-appearing cells having abundant eosinophilic cytoplasm. Large, distinct, clear vacuoles are present within the cytoplasm of several cells. (Aqueous Romanowsky; HP oil.) **B,** Nuclei are generally round with coarse chromatin and punctate, dark purple single or multiple nucleoli *(arrows)*. The cytoplasm of a few cells contain large vacuoles *(arrowheads)* or a dusting of pink granules. Vacuoles were negative for lipid or glycogen. The neoplastic cells were positive for sarcomeric actin, confirming its muscle origin. (Aqueous Romanowsky; HP oil.) (Courtesy Rose Raskin, University of Florida.)

laryngeal region in dogs. In general, these tumors resemble their counterparts arising in more common sites, although oncocytomas and rhabdomyomas may be difficult to differentiate without the use of additional diagnostics such as electron microscopy or immunohistochemical staining for desmin, myoglobin, or actin (Table 5.3). Laryngeal rhabdomyomas (see Figs. 5.27 and 5.28) have plump, large cells with abundant granular or foamy to vacuolated cytoplasm. Nuclei are large, round to oval, and centrally located with finely clumped chromatin and typically contain a single, indistinct nucleolus. Anisocytosis and anisokaryosis are common. The tumor frequently contains large areas of hemorrhage, which may result

TABLE 5.3 Comparative Diagnostic Features of Cytopathologically Similar Laryngeal Tumors

CHARACTERISTICS	RHABDOMYOMA	ONCOCYTOMA	GRANULAR CELL TUMOR
Cell of origin	Muscle	Oncocyte's speculate origin from transformed duct or glandular epithelium	Unknown; speculate neural tissue, possibly Schwann cells or meningeal cells
Behavior	Benign	Benign	Unclear
Signalment	Younger, middle aged	Younger, middle aged	Dogs > cats
Clinical presentation	Solitary, fleshy, well-circumscribed mass; originates from submucosa; projects into laryngeal lumen	Solitary, fleshy, well-circumscribed mass; originates from submucosa; projects into laryngeal lumen	Oral cavity is predominant site, but cutaneous and CNS forms also reported
Cytopathology	Large cells with abundant granular or foamy cytoplasm with large, central to eccentric nuclei with finely clumped chromatin and a single, indistinct nucleolus; multinucleate cells may be seen	Large, pale-staining epithelial cells with abundant foamy cytoplasm, large, centrally located, round nuclei with finely clumped chromatin and single, indistinct nucleolus	Variably sized round to polygonal cells with small, eccentric nucleus and abundant granular eosinophilic cytoplasm
Pleomorphism	Moderate	Moderate	Slight to moderate
Histology	Large polygonal cells with abundant eosinophilic granular cytoplasm arranged in sheets, cords, and acinar structures with fine fibrovascular stroma; striations may be seen	Large polygonal cells with abundant eosinophilic granular cytoplasm arranged in sheets, cords, and acinar structures with fine fibrovascular stroma; nuclei may be basally oriented	Variably sized oval to polygonal cells with abundant, pale, eosinophilic cytoplasm, distinct intracytoplasmic granules, distinct cell margins, and small nuclei
EM	Abundant mitochondria, myofibrils, Z-bands	Abundant mitochondria	Large numbers of membrane-bound lysosomal vacuoles
Diagnostic markers	Desmin[a] Myoglobin Actin PTAH	Cytokeratin[a] PTAH	All variably reported; no marker is consistent PAS (diastase resistant)[a] S-100 NSE Vimentin

[a]Most reliable.
CNS, Central nervous system; EM, electron microscopy; NSE, neuron-specific enolase; PAS, periodic acid–Schiff; PTAH, phosphotungstic acid hematoxylin.

in hemodiluted specimens with few neoplastic cells. Rhabdomyomas are similar cytopathologically to oncocytomas in other sites. Ultrastructurally, oncocytomas and rhabdomyomas or rhabdomyosarcomas contain numerous mitochondria and may be distinguished by finding myofibrils and Z-bands as evidence of muscle origin (Tang et al., 1994). Definitive diagnosis of muscle origin tumors is best accomplished with immunohistochemical staining for desmin, myoglobin, or actin (Meuten et al., 1985; Barnhart and Lewis, 2000).

Hemolymphatic Neoplasia

Lymphoma and plasmacytoma. Lymphoma of the larynx has the same diversity of appearance as lymphoma in other sites. Typically, a uniform population of immature lymphoid cells is observed (Fig. 5.29). Cytopathologic diagnosis of intermediate or small cell lymphoma is difficult because of the uniform, well-differentiated appearance of the lymphocytes. In these cases, a biopsy with histologic examination is necessary for diagnosis. Extramedullary plasmacytoma of the larynx has also been reported (Witham et al., 2012).

Miscellaneous Neoplasia

Laryngeal oncocytoma. Oncocytoma is a rare tumor of the larynx in small animals, especially younger dogs. A laryngeal oncocytoma typically presents as a well-circumscribed mass projecting from the laryngeal ventricle. Early reports of laryngeal oncocytomas in dogs were later reviewed (Meuten et al.,

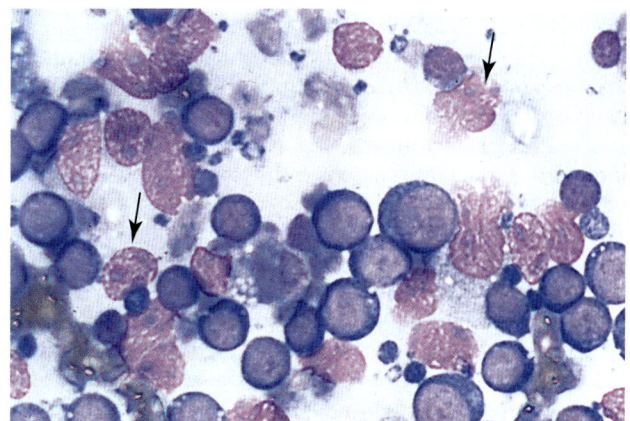

FIGURE 5.29 Laryngeal lymphoma. Tissue aspirate. Large pleomorphic lymphoid cells composed of round to oval nuclei with smooth chromatin and prominent nucleoli that are indistinct in the photomicrograph and have a variable amount of deeply basophilic cytoplasm. Pink-staining reticulated nuclei from ruptured neoplastic cells *(arrows)* helps reveal the nucleoli. (Wright-Giemsa; HP oil.)

1985) and found to be of muscle origin. Oncocytomas are benign tumors arising from oncocytes (oxyphil cells) that appear to be neuroendocrine in origin, although the exact genesis of these cells remains unclear. Others propose that these cells originate from transformation of ductular or seromucous gland epithelial cells (Doughty et al., 2006). Cytopathologically, the tumor is composed of moderately pleomorphic, large, pale-staining, loosely adhesive epithelial cells with abundant foamy to vacuolated cytoplasm. Nuclei are large, round to oval, and centrally located with finely clumped chromatin and typically contain a single, indistinct nucleolus. Anisocytosis and anisokaryosis are common. The tumor frequently contains large areas of hemorrhage that may result in hemodiluted specimens with few neoplastic cells. Rhabdomyomas and granular cell tumors can also originate from the larynx and may require examination by electron microscopy for definitive diagnosis (Tang et al., 1994). Oncocytomas possess abundant numbers of mitochondria in the cytoplasm and express cytokeratin (Doughty et al., 2006), whereas granular cell tumors stain positive for vimentin, S-100, and NSE (Patnaik, 1993). See Table 5.3 for a list of distinguishing features between several similar laryngeal neoplasms.

TRACHEA, BRONCHI, AND LUNGS

Normal Anatomy and Histology

The anatomic components of the remaining air passages include the trachea, bronchi, bronchioli, and alveoli. The trachea extends from the base of the larynx to the carina and is composed of incomplete cartilaginous rings supported by connective tissue and smooth muscle lined by ciliated, pseudostratified epithelium. The transition to pseudostratified epithelium begins as the larynx merges with the trachea and extends to the bronchi. Goblet cells are commonly found within the tracheal epithelium. Bronchi are similar in structure to the trachea; however, bronchial cartilaginous rings are complete rather than C-shaped. Smaller airways, or bronchioles, have no cartilaginous support, are composed of smooth muscle, and are lined by ciliated and nonciliated cuboidal epithelium. Terminal bronchioles branch into respiratory bronchioles that further divide into alveolar ducts, alveolar sacs, and alveoli. Alveoli are lined by flattened epithelium (type I pneumocytes) with lesser numbers of more cuboidal epithelial cells (type II pneumocytes). Type I pneumocytes typically cover more than 90% of the alveolar surface. Type II pneumocytes are responsible for synthesizing pulmonary surfactant. There is a support network of connective tissue underlying the epithelium consisting of fine reticular, collagenous, and elastic fibers with occasional fibroblasts. Intermingling between the alveoli is a large number of capillaries. The lung has a resident population of macrophages that exist primarily in the alveoli. When activated, alveolar macrophages become large, highly vacuolated, and highly phagocytic. Airways contain foci of bronchus-associated lymphoid tissue (BALT) as well as serous and mucus-secreting submucosal glands located in the submucosa and lamina propria. These may be sampled during evaluation of the respiratory tract if the overlying epithelium is damaged.

Sample Collection and Preparation

Tracheal wash (TW) and bronchoalveolar lavage (BAL) are relatively straightforward, inexpensive procedures with high diagnostic potential. The samples can be used for cytopathologic examination of airway disease as well as for culture and sensitivity. In animals with respiratory disease, it is important to obtain a cytologic sample in a manner that will yield a large number of well-preserved cells. Indications for sampling the airways are clinical or radiographic evidence of respiratory disease. TWs are helpful for examining the larger airways, whereas BAL focuses on the smaller airways and alveoli. It is important to note that studies have shown that 68% of cases have different cytopathologic characteristics in the TW fluid versus BAL fluid (Hawkins et al., 1995). In addition, even within a single technique such as BAL, slides prepared by cytospin have been shown to have a greater proportion of neutrophils than do slides prepared by smearing of pelleted cells (Dehard et al., 2008). Therefore, it is essential to interpret results based on the technique that is used. These techniques allow identification of inflammatory processes in the lungs without the risk of lung surgical biopsy. Although complications are minimal, appropriate sample handling, transport, and preparation are essential for an accurate and complete diagnosis. There are multiple techniques for collection from the tracheobronchial tract, several of which will be reviewed.

Tracheal Wash

The purpose of a TW is to collect fluid and/or cells from the trachea in a sterile fashion. Airway sampling can be achieved by direct penetration through the tracheal wall, termed transtracheal wash (TTW), or orally via an endotracheal tube, termed endotracheal wash (ETW). The former technique is usually reserved for larger dogs, and the latter is performed in smaller dogs and cats.

Direct aspiration of the tracheal lumen can be performed by entering through the cricothyroid ligament or between tracheal rings (Box 5.1; Fig. 5.30). General anesthesia impairs the cough reflex necessary to retrieve an adequate sample and is typically not used for TW procedures. Sterility should be maintained; therefore, the area of the cricothyroid ligament should be clipped and surgically prepared, and sterile gloves should be worn during the procedure. Generally, a 16-gauge catheter is recommended for dogs weighing more than 50 lb, an 18- or 19-gauge catheter is used in dogs weighing 20 to 50 lb, and a

---

BOX 5.1 Transtracheal Wash Procedure by Direct Tracheal Penetration

1. Place the animal in sternal recumbency for either technique.
2. Provide sedation if necessary depending on the demeanor of the patient.
3. Clip and surgically prepare the area of the cricothyroid ligament.
4. Palpate the cricothyroid ligament as an indentation between the thyroid and cricoid cartilage of the larynx.
5. Inject lidocaine into the skin and underlying subcutaneous tissue.
6. Use an appropriately sized jugular catheter (16- to 19-gauge) for the wash.
7. Insert the needle of the catheter bevel down through the lidocaine-injected area of skin.
8. Pass the needle through the ligament at a downward angle to avoid laceration of the larynx and to decrease risk of oropharyngeal contamination.
9. Pass the catheter over the needle, approximately to the level of the carina (fourth intercostal space).
10. Remove the needle, leaving the catheter in place.
11. Of the approximate 0.1–0.2 mL/kg of warm, sterile, nonbacteriostatic saline used for the wash, inject half of the volume rapidly to induce coughing (see Fig. 5.30).
12. Disconnect the syringe and replace with an empty syringe for aspiration.
13. Repeat aspiration until no more fluid is obtained.
14. Repeat the procedure with the remainder of the saline.

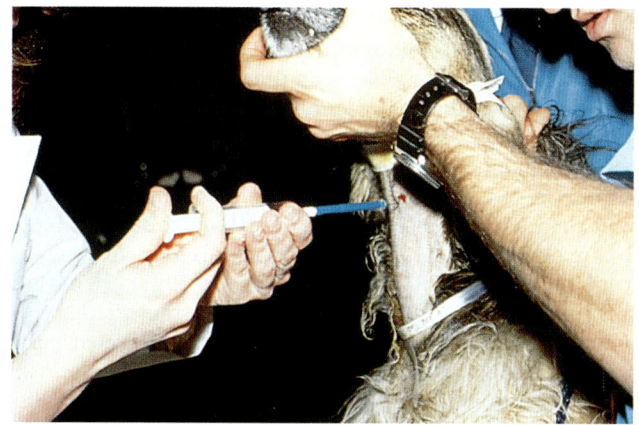

FIGURE 5.30 Transtracheal wash procedure. Injection of saline fluid after proper placement of catheter through the cricoid ligament in a dog. (Courtesy Robert King, University of Florida.)

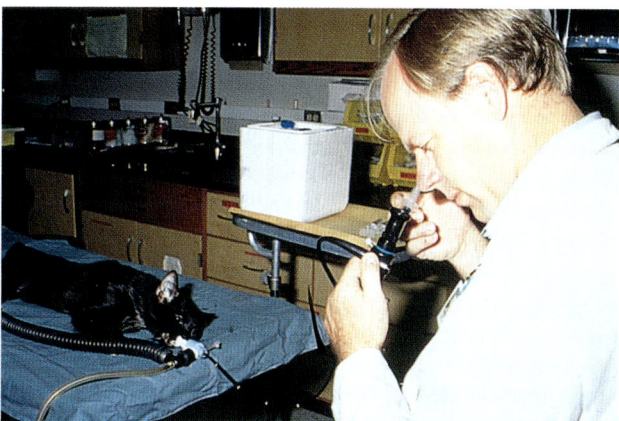

FIGURE 5.31 Bronchoalveolar lavage procedure. Placement of the fiberoptic scope through the endotracheal tube followed by injection of a saline fluid. (Courtesy Robert King, University of Florida.)

19-gauge catheter is recommended for cats and dogs weighing less than 20 lb. This method has the advantage that general anesthesia is not required. Also, the chance of oropharyngeal contamination is low, although still possible if the catheter goes cranially and through the vocal folds of the larynx. Complications with this technique are uncommon but may include subcutaneous emphysema, tracheal laceration, hemorrhage, hemoptysis, pneumomediastinum, and pneumothorax.

An alternative method is to perform the TW by way of an endotracheal tube. General anesthesia is required for this procedure because an endotracheal tube must be placed. Care must be taken not to contaminate the tip of the endotracheal tube in the oropharynx. After intubation, the cuff is inflated, and the animal is placed in lateral recumbency. A jugular catheter or sterile polypropylene urinary catheter is then inserted into the endotracheal tube and extended to the carina. A red rubber feeding tube should not be used because they easily collapse during aspiration of viscous material such as mucus (Smallwood and Zenoble, 1993). After the catheter is placed, saline is instilled and collected as described in Box 5.1.

Bronchoalveolar Lavage

Bronchoalveolar lavage is used to sample the smaller airways and alveoli and is therefore more effective than TW at sampling the lower respiratory tract. As for TWs, there are multiple techniques for BAL, each with variable advantages. All techniques yield highly diagnostic samples. The two techniques described here are bronchoscopy and BAL via an endotracheal tube.

Bronchoscopy is an excellent method for obtaining a BAL sample. Specific equipment is necessary to use this method, and the animal must be of adequate size to allow placement of the bronchoscope beyond the mainstem bronchus. The use of flexible endoscopes that are less than 5 mm in outer diameter for bronchoscopy in cats has been reported to yield highly diagnostic BAL samples with minimal complications (Johnson and Drazenovich, 2007). The animal must be maintained under general anesthesia. After placement of the endotracheal tube, the fiberoptic bronchoscope is passed through the endotracheal tube to allow visualization of the trachea and mainstem bronchi (Fig. 5.31). If radiographs have been taken before bronchoscopy, specific lobes of the lung may be selected based on localization or severity of the lesion. Warmed, sterile saline is injected through the biopsy channel in a volume equaling 5 mL/kg and can be aspirated in the same syringe by applying gentle suction (Hawkins et al., 1995). Saline can be injected as one large bolus or in two to three aliquots. Multiple lung lobes should be lavaged to increase the opportunity of identifying etiologic agents or cells with criteria of malignancy. It is advisable to keep animals on supplemental oxygen after the procedure, if not during, to decrease the risk of hypoxia. Advantages of this technique include the ability to visualize the airway, choose the lobe to be lavaged, and sample masses, if observed (McCauley et al., 1998).

Samples from multiple areas of the lung are often pooled and can increase the sensitivity of detection of neoplastic cells or infectious agents with diffuse disease. However, for animals with focal or segmental disease, the cytopathologic appearance, including total cell counts and cell differentials, are often very different depending on the site. Therefore, it may be more clinically relevant to process and evaluate samples from different lung segments or sites separately to maximize the identification of the underlying pathogenesis (Ybarra et al., 2012).

If a bronchoscope is unavailable or the patient is too small for the scope to pass through the endotracheal tube or beyond the main stem bronchus, a BAL may be performed via an endotracheal tube (Hawkins et al., 1994). The procedure has been well described in cats but may also be performed in dogs. Again, general anesthesia is required. After intubation, the animal should be placed in lateral recumbency, with the most severely affected side down. After inflation of the endotracheal tube cuff, a syringe adapter is attached to the end of the tube. Three separate aliquots of fluid (warm, sterile saline) should be used totaling 5 mL/kg. The first aliquot should be injected rapidly and followed immediately by application of suction using the same syringe until no more fluid is obtained. This procedure is repeated for the second and third aliquots. The rear of the animal may be elevated to assist with fluid retrieval.

Bronchoalveolar lavage results in localized edema, alveolar distention, mild to moderate congestion, and alveolar collapse. The primary complication of BAL techniques is a transient hypoxia that is associated with decreased compliance and ventilation/perfusion mismatch (Hawkins et al., 1995). The patient should be supplemented with oxygen for 5 to 20 minutes after the BAL and monitored with a pulse oximeter if available.

The sample should immediately be placed on ice and cytocentrifuged within 30 to 60 minutes of collection for optimal results (Hawkins et al., 1990). It is advisable to divide the samples from a BAL into two portions: one portion being placed into an EDTA tube to preserve cellular morphology and the other portion being placed into a sterile container that does not have anticoagulant for possible microbiologic culture. On cytopathologic evaluation, neutrophils and macrophages may phagocytize red blood cells, extracellular bacteria, and other debris if the sample is not prepared within the recommended time period, thus leading to erroneous interpretation of the sample. If the sample without anticoagulant is not immediately plated for bacterial culture, storage at 4°C (39°F) is advised to inhibit overgrowth of potential bacterial contaminants, such as *Escherichia coli* or *B. bronchiseptica* (Curran et al., 2020).

Cell counts can be performed on a standard hemacytometer or by an automated cell counter. The accuracy of these counts may be questionable because of increased mucus and lack of standardization of techniques; however, cell counts are crucial after BAL to establish adequacy of the sample (Hawkins and DeNicola, 1989). If less than 250 cells/μL are observed, the procedure should be repeated. Recent studies have suggested the use of urea dilution to standardize the cellular and noncellular components of BAL fluid samples for more adequate analysis of nucleated cell counts in epithelial lining fluid (Mills and Litster, 2006). A standardized procedure for sampling needs to be implemented in the hospital to ensure accurate interpretation of all BAL samples. Reproducibility for the enumeration of each cell type is increased with larger cell counts; this is particularly true for lymphocytes and bronchial epithelial cells. Thus, a standard procedure that includes a 500-cell differential has been recommended (De Lorenzi et al., 2009).

The sample should be examined grossly, and if large mucus plugs are observed, squash preparations should be made because cells and organisms are frequently embedded within mucus. The cellular component of the fluid should be concentrated. Cytocentrifugation is the preferred technique, if available. Alternatively, the sample may be centrifuged at 400 *g* (800 RPM) for 5 minutes and the supernatant removed, reserving 50 to 100 μL to resuspend the cell pellet. A concentrated direct smear can be made from this sample.

Bronchial Brushing

Bronchial brushings are obtained by use of bronchoscopy. Cytopathologic findings may be similar to those seen for BAL; however, in dogs with chronic coughs, bronchial brushings are more sensitive for detecting the presence of neutrophils and suppurative inflammation (Hawkins et al., 2006). Therefore, obtaining both lavage and brushing samples may be useful in certain cases.

Transthoracic Fine-Needle Aspiration

Transthoracic FNA is an excellent diagnostic method for obtaining material from the lung parenchyma for cytopathologic evaluation. This technique is most useful when diffuse parenchymal disease or discrete mass or masses are identified via imaging techniques, with discrete lesions yielding higher-quality specimens than those with diffuse interstitial involvement. Although a specific diagnosis may not be established in all cases, FNA is useful to categorize the lesion as inflammatory or neoplastic (Wood et al., 1998). When coupled with ultrasound for guided tissue sampling, FNA is an important and valuable tool for the diagnosis of thoracic lesions (Reichle and Wisner, 2000).

Although aspiration of the lung parenchyma is not without the potential for complications, especially in moribund patients or those in severe respiratory distress, these complications are fewer than with thoracotomy or transthoracic surgical biopsy and are typically minimal if a mass lesion is located closely adjacent to the thoracic wall (Teske et al., 1991). Hemostasis screening should be performed before transthoracic FNA, including a platelet count, prothrombin time, activated partial thromboplastin time, and, in predisposed breeds, von Willebrand factor antigen assay (vWF:Ag). Patients with abnormal hemostasis have a significantly increased risk of severe hemorrhage after FNA of the lung.

The patient may be placed in sternal recumbency or allowed to stand; however, proper restraint is critical. If the patient is distressed or struggling, sedation may be necessary to minimize risks. Local anesthetic may be injected into the anterior edge of the intercostal space because the intercostal vessels and nerves are located just posterior to each rib. Visualizing the mass or site to be aspirated by ultrasound is ideal because imaging guidance allows direct placement of the needle into the lesion, enhancing the likelihood that a diagnostic sample is obtained. Echoendoscopy is a useful technique when traditional ultrasound usage is not possible because of the presence of intervening bone or when an area to be scanned is beyond normal penetration depths. The echoendoscope is unique in that it has an ultrasound transducer at the end of a traditional endoscope. FNA samples of lung masses can be obtained using this technique (Gaschen et al., 2003). If ultrasound is not available, careful localization of the lesion using at least two radiographic views is essential. The right caudal lung lobe is typically sampled with diffuse disease; the standard sampling site is the seventh to ninth intercostal space, one third the distance from the spinal column to the costochondral junction. The most common mistake is to enter the chest too far caudally and aspirate the liver.

If the lesion to be sampled is close to the body wall, a 22- to 25-gauge, 2-inch needle attached to a 3 mL syringe can be used. If the lesion is deeper, a 22-gauge human spinal needle may be required to reach the site. In either case, the needle is introduced through the skin and intercostal muscles at a 90-degree angle to the chest wall in one controlled thrust. After the chest cavity has been entered, negative pressure is applied to the syringe by pulling back on the plunger slightly. The needle tip is advanced to the appropriate depth as estimated by examination of radiographs or by ultrasonographic visualization. The needle should be advanced, withdrawn slightly, and readvanced through the lesion while maintaining negative pressure. Advancing at slightly different angles will enhance the likelihood of obtaining a representative and diagnostic sample; however, it also increases the potential for complications. After sampling the lesion, the syringe is withdrawn, releasing the negative pressure in the syringe just before the needle leaves the chest cavity. Aspiration should be performed quickly, but in a controlled manner. Because the risk of complications increases with the length of time the needle is in the chest cavity, it is usually safer to perform multiple aspirations than to aspirate continuously from a single needle placement.

Typically, only a small amount of material is aspirated into the needle with little or no material seen in the hub of the needle. The syringe is detached from the needle, filled with air, and then reattached to the needle. The air is used to expel the aspirated material within the needle hub onto slides for preparation and staining. If fluid is aspirated, it should be transferred into an EDTA-anticoagulated tube for fluid analysis, including protein concentration and cell counts, as well as cytopathologic evaluation. If blood or hemorrhagic fluid is aspirated, the procedure should be halted and reattempted at another site. Aspiration of air alone may occur in cases of significant small airway disease. In this instance, aspiration should be repeated with caution because there is an increased risk of pneumothorax.

The patient should be checked frequently for the first few hours after aspiration to assess respiratory and cardiac function. A chest radiograph should be examined 1 hour after lung aspiration or at any time after aspiration if the patient's respiration worsens, to evaluate for the presence of pneumothorax, particularly tension pneumothorax.

Normal Cytology and Artifacts
Normal Cytology of the Tracheobronchial Tract

The trachea and bronchi are lined by pseudostratified, ciliated epithelial cells that are customarily observed in fluid from TW but not BAL samples (Box 5.2). These cells are elongate with a round, prominent nucleus and basophilic cytoplasm with cilia at the apical surface (Fig. 5.32). Cilia often detach from these cells if sample preparation is delayed and are visualized free in the background. It is therefore important to not confuse these cilia with bacterial rods (Andreasen, 2003). Cuboidal epithelium lines the bronchioles; therefore, these cells may be seen in both TW and BAL samples. Bronchiolar epithelium appears individually or in sheets. These cells are round to cuboidal, have moderate amounts of basophilic cytoplasm, and contain a round, centrally placed nucleus.

Bronchoalveolar lavage and TW samples from normal cats and dogs are of low cellularity. TW samples tend to be hypocellular when compared with BAL samples (Hawkins et al., 1995). Alveolar macrophages are the primary cell type observed in normal TW and BAL samples (Table 5.4). These cells often appear reactive and contain numerous small, discrete vacuoles in the cytoplasm filled with phagocytized debris (Fig. 5.33). Other leukocytes may be seen less frequently. Neutrophils typically represent less than 5% to 10% of the nucleated cell population (Hawkins and DeNicola, 1990; Vail et al., 1995); however, neutrophil populations greater than 20% have been reported (Padrid et al., 1991; Lecuyer et al., 1995). Other cell types observed in lesser numbers include lymphocytes (5% to 14%), eosinophils in species other than cats (<5%), and mast cells (<2%) (Hawkins and DeNicola, 1990; Padrid et al., 1991; Lecuyer et al.,

> **BOX 5.2 Comparison of Normal and Inflammatory Airway Cytology**
>
> **Normal Cytology of the Airway**
> - Ciliated columnar epithelial cells
> - Cuboidal epithelial cells
> - Macrophages, often activated
> - Mucus
> - Rare goblet cells
>
> **Common Changes With Inflammation**
> - Deeply basophilic, hyperplastic epithelial cells, frequently in sheets
> - Goblet cell hyperplasia
> - Inflammatory cells (e.g., neutrophils, macrophages)
> - Increased mucus and Curschmann's spirals

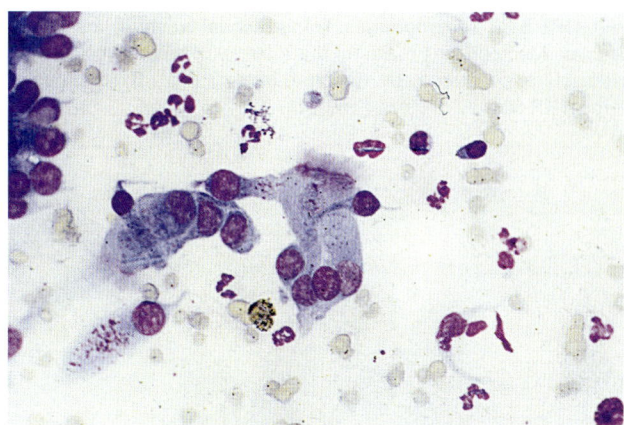

FIGURE 5.32 Normal epithelium. Transtracheal wash. Several oblong columnar epithelial cells with magnetic-staining cytoplasmic granules and eosinophilic cilia at the apical surface are present. Several smaller oval epithelial cells are attached. Scattered neutrophils can be used to denote relative size. (Wright-Giemsa; HP oil.)

1995; Vail et al., 1995). Rare goblet cells may be observed and are not considered an abnormal finding unless numbers are markedly increased. Goblet cells are approximately the size of macrophages but contain abundant cytoplasm filled with distinctive, deeply basophilic, uniform granules (Fig. 5.34). Immunophenotypic studies of canine lymphocytes found in BAL fluid determined the lymphocyte subpopulations were primarily T cells with a greater proportion of CD8 cells than blood, resulting in a CD4/CD8 ratio closer to 1:1 (Dirscherl et al., 1995; Vail et al., 1995).

Eosinophil numbers vary markedly between dogs and cats. Less than 5% is typical for samples from dogs, whereas 5% to

TABLE 5.4 Expected Total Cell Count and Percent Range for Cell Types Seen in Bronchoalveolar Lavage Samples From Clinically Healthy Dogs and Cats[a]

	TOTAL CELLS/ML	MACROPHAGE (%)	LYMPHOCYTE (%)	EOSINOPHIL (%)	NEUTROPHIL (%)	MAST CELL (%)
Dogs	<500	70–80	6–14	<5	<5	1–2
Cats	<400	70–80	<5	≤25	<6	<2

[a]Actual values may differ between techniques. These counts were compiled from the mean values of several references to be used as a general guide.

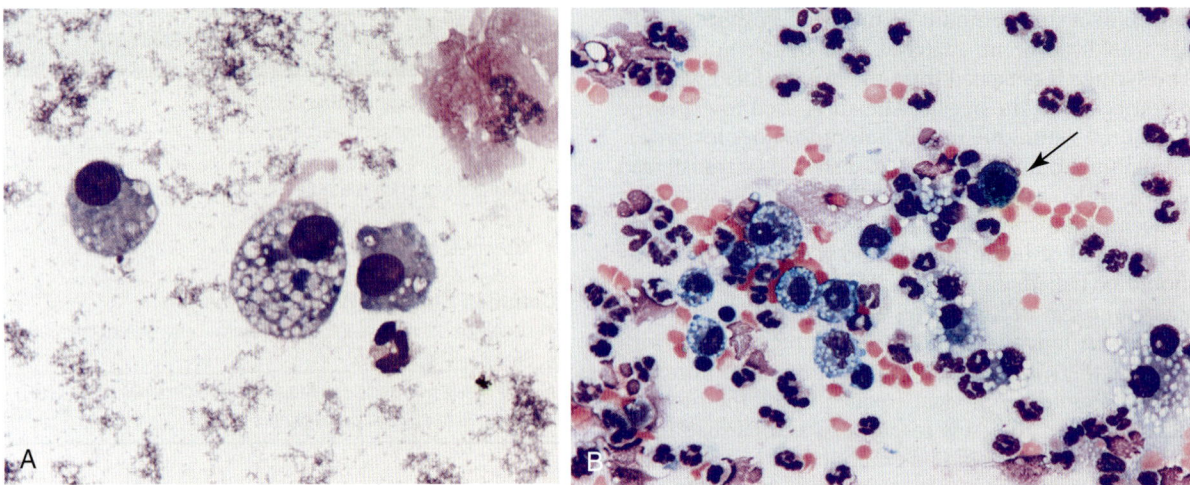

■ **FIGURE 5.33 Macrophages. Transtracheal wash. A,** Variably sized macrophages are characterized by abundant cytoplasm with small, discrete vacuoles. Macrophages make up the majority of cells in the tracheal and bronchiolar washes. The amorphous pinkish staining material is nuclear material form a ruptured cell. (Wright-Giemsa; HP oil.) **B,** Numerous macrophages are present with neutrophils and erythrocytes admixed. (Wright-Giemsa; HP oil.)

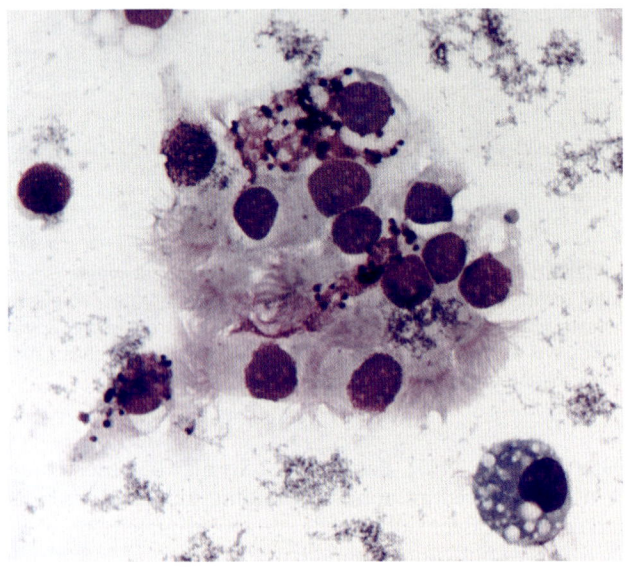

■ **FIGURE 5.34 Goblet cells. Bronchoalveolar lavage.** Goblet cells are simple columnar epithelial cells that secrete mucins. The variably sized mucin-laden cytoplasmic granules are denoted by dark magenta staining. They are admixed with ciliated columnar epithelial cells. One macrophage is present. (Wright-Giemsa; HP oil.)

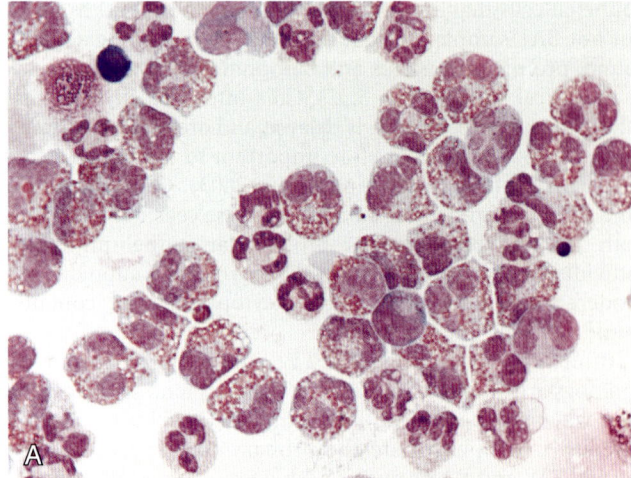

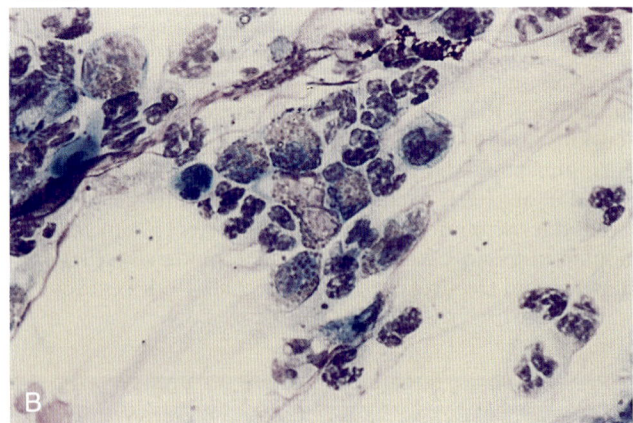

■ **FIGURE 5.35 Eosinophils. Transtracheal wash. A,** Abundant canine eosinophils from a tracheal wash. Note that some eosinophils have bean-shaped or oval nuclei. Neutrophils and one small lymphocyte are admixed. (Wright-Giemsa; HP oil.) **B,** When eosinophils are embedded in mucus, their granules may not stain pink but look bluish-gray because of the proteinaceous coating. Note dark granules of these canine eosinophils compared with A. (Wright-Giemsa; HP oil.)

28% eosinophils may be seen in BAL samples from healthy cats (Padrid et al., 1991; Hawkins et al., 1994; Lecuyer et al., 1995; Dye et al., 1996). The percentages of eosinophils in the airways of apparently healthy cats are extremely variable and thus should be interpreted carefully and in correlation with clinical signs and other diagnostic results. Eosinophils are often overlooked in samples because they can appear different than the typical eosinophil observed in blood. Eosinophils frequently become entrapped in aggregates of mucus and are unable to completely flatten, resulting in dark-red to brown-staining granules rather than the expected bright-pink to red granules (Fig. 5.35). In samples that have dried slowly (these are usually the samples with thick clumps of mucus), the granules also darken. It is common for the nucleus to be nonsegmented in cells, resembling eosinophils (Baldwin and Becker, 1993). These rare round cells with prominent pink to violet granules are consistent with globule leukocytes (Fig. 5.36). These cells are controversial in their origin, with some support that these cells may represent a form of mast cell or granular lymphocyte (Spoor et al., 2011). The cells are common within lining mucosa of the respiratory and gastrointestinal tract.

Normal Cytology of the Lung

Samples from healthy pulmonary tissue are sparsely cellular and contain primarily respiratory epithelial cells. Respiratory epithelial cells are lightly basophilic, columnar to cuboidal, and contain oval nuclei with granular chromatin situated towards the basilar aspect (Fig. 5.37). Cilia are commonly seen on the apical surface. Goblet cells may contain pink to purple granules. A small number of alveolar macrophages, erythrocytes, and white blood cells may also be seen. Mucus is often present in respiratory samples as ribbons of eosinophilic material but is typically sparse in aspirates from normal lung tissue. Obtaining a sample that is cytologically "normal" does not preclude the possibility of pulmonary disease but instead suggests that the lesion was not sampled. Reaspiration should be considered.

Oropharyngeal Contamination

Oropharyngeal contamination is a complication associated with several procedures for sampling the airways. Cytopathologically, this is observed as the presence of mature, keratinized, squamous epithelial cells, often coated with a mixed population of bacteria, including colonies of *Conchiformibius* spp., which are considered normal flora of the oropharyngeal cavity (see Fig. 5.4). Neutrophils are a common inhabitant of the oral cavity, particularly associated with dental disease. Airway samples with evidence of oropharyngeal contamination cannot be properly interpreted because it is impossible to determine the source of the inflammation. Rarely, a sample that appears to contain oropharyngeal contamination may represent a true biologic process, such as in the case of recurrent aspiration of pharyngeal material or a bronchoesophageal fistula (Burton et al., 1992). To differentiate these processes, the procedure should be repeated with increased effort to minimize the potential for oropharyngeal contamination.

Nonrespiratory System Aspirate

Occasionally, samples are obtained that are not consistent with the lung parenchyma. The two most common nonrespiratory cells seen with lung aspirates are mesothelial cells and hepatocytes. It is important to recognize these cells so as not to mistake them for a neoplastic population. Sheets of mesothelial cells are seen if the lung surface is scraped during the aspiration process. The sheets are composed of bland, monomorphic cells with angular, cohesive borders resembling fish scales, pale cytoplasm, and small, round central nuclei (Fig. 5.38). As the cells begin to

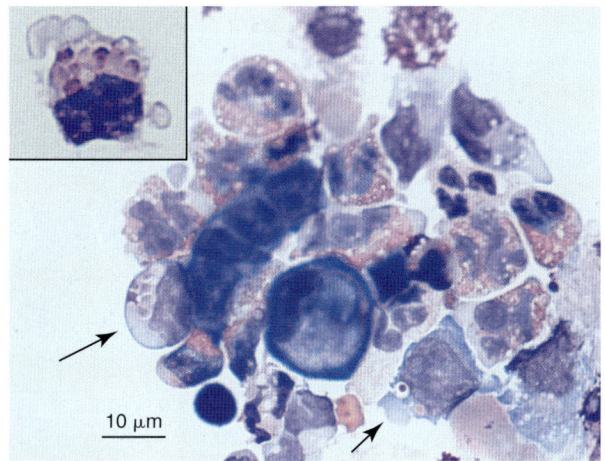

■ **FIGURE 5.36 Mixed cell inflammation with globule leukocytes. Endotracheal wash cytospin prep. Dog.** Numerous eosinophils are noted along with fewer neutrophils, lymphocytes, and globule leukocytes (*inset* and *arrows*). The patient presented with persistent sneezing and a productive cough. (Modified Wright; HP oil.) (Courtesy Sara Connolly, Purdue University.)

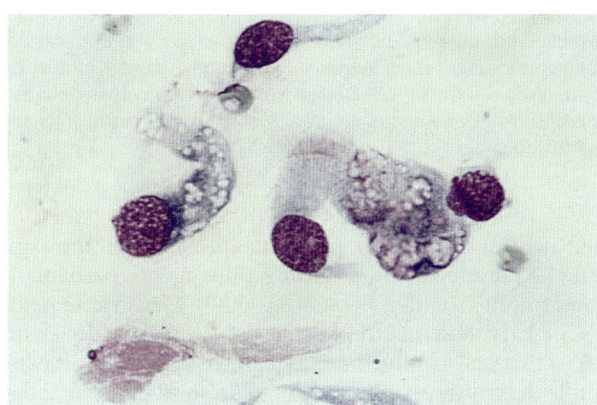

■ **FIGURE 5.37 Upper airway epithelium.** Ciliated columnar epithelium and goblet cells shown here are representative of those found in the trachea, bronchi, or large bronchioles. Epithelium becomes cuboidal in the small bronchioles. Two mucus-secreting cells with gray-blue foamy cytoplasm are shown. (Wright-Giemsa; HP oil.)

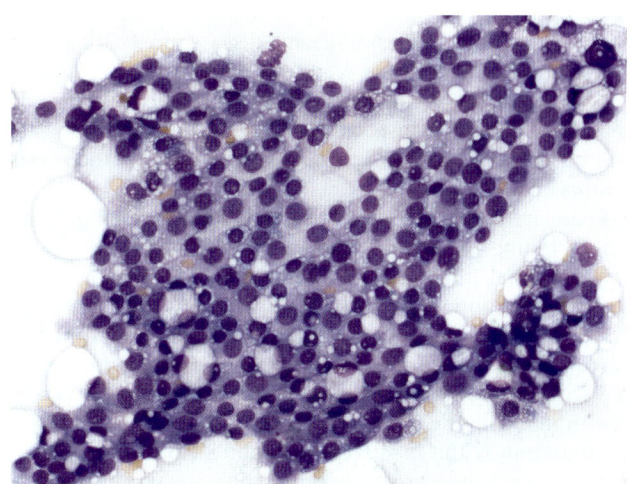

■ **FIGURE 5.38 Mesothelial cells. Lung aspirate.** A sheet of mildly pleomorphic mesothelial cells. Presence of mesothelial cells from an attempted lung aspirate biopsy indicates sampling of the surface lining only (pulmonary pleurae) and not a diagnostic specimen. (Wright-Giemsa; IP.)

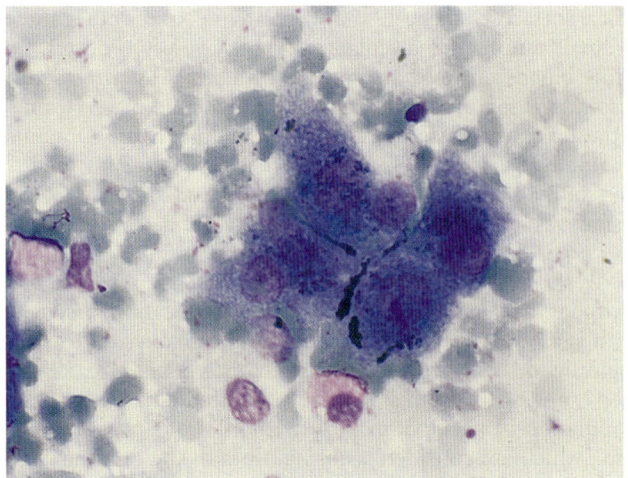

■ **FIGURE 5.39 Accidental liver aspirate.** Presence of hepatocytes with prominent canaliculi containing bile, consistent with cholestasis. The liver may be aspirated if the needle is placed too far caudally when attempting to sample the lung. (Wright-Giemsa; HP oil.)

exfoliate from the sheets, they round up, become more basophilic, and begin to demonstrate the glycocalyx halo (eosinophilic fringe) associated with more classical mesothelial cells seen commonly in thoracic and abdominal fluids. Aspiration of the liver occurs when the chest is entered too far caudally (Fig. 5.39).

Inflammation

Inflammation can be classified as acute neutrophilic, chronic active (mixed), chronic, eosinophilic, hemorrhagic, or neoplastic inflammation (Hawkins and DeNicola, 1990). Inflammatory cell populations change dramatically depending on the inciting cause of the inflammation. Neutrophils and eosinophils are observed in more acute processes, whereas increasing numbers of macrophages and lymphocytes, in addition to the neutrophils or eosinophils, are more consistent with chronic inflammation. Inflammation of the lung parenchyma consists predominantly of neutrophils, eosinophils, alveolar macrophages, epithelioid macrophages, or mixed cell population. The type of inflammation may suggest a specific disease process (e.g., large numbers of eosinophils are seen with allergic disease) or cause (e.g., granulomatous inflammation with fungal infection). Increased mucus is a nonspecific finding and may be associated with many pathologic processes of both infectious and noninfectious etiologies.

There are multiple causes of chronic bronchitis in dogs and cats, including congenital abnormality in structure of the airway, abnormal function of cilia, parasitic infestation, viral or bacterial infection, and inhalation of noxious substances such as smoke (Padrid and Amis, 1992). In chronic inflammation, macrophages become activated and may be bi- or multinucleated with highly vacuolated cytoplasm. Inflammation is commensurate with the underlying cause; however, suppurative inflammation is the most typical finding. Additional changes are consistent with chronic inflammation such as hyperplastic epithelial cells, goblet cell hyperplasia, and increased mucus.

Suppurative Inflammation

Neutrophils are the primary cell seen as part of a suppurative inflammatory process, both in acute and chronic inflammation.

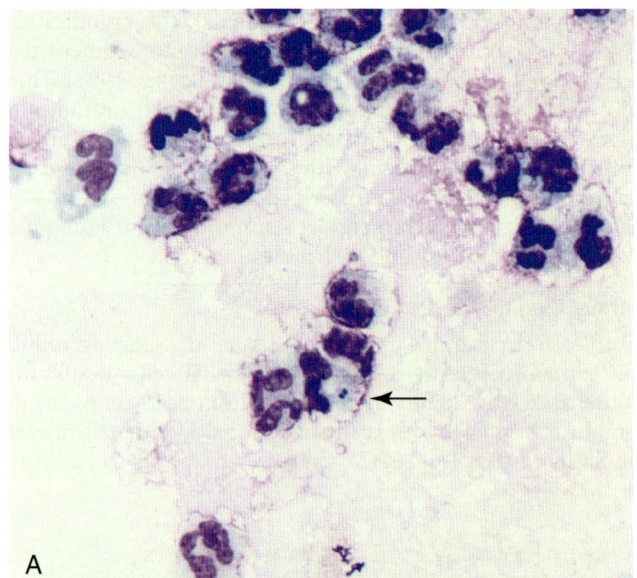

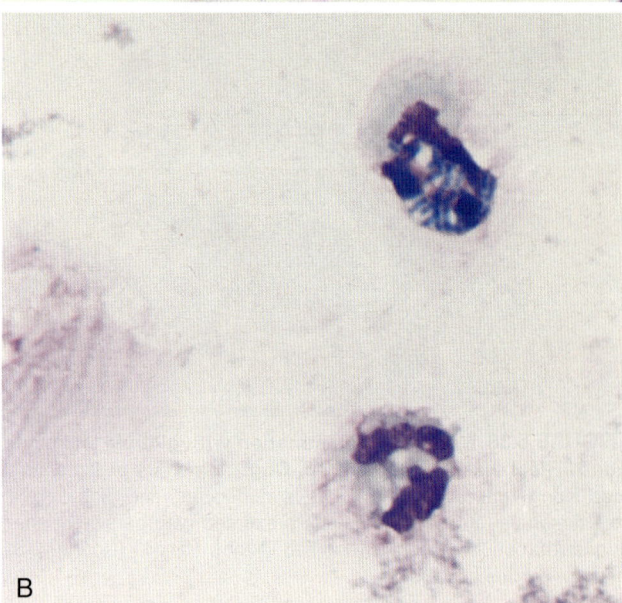

■ **FIGURE 5.40 Suppurative inflammation. Bronchoalveolar lavage. Dog. A,** The patient had infectious tracheobronchitis. Numerous well-preserved, primarily nondegenerate neutrophils that occasionally contain intracellular cocci *(arrow)*. Pinkish-gray mucus in the background. (Wright-Giemsa; LP.) **B,** Sample from a dog with infectious tracheobronchitis. Degenerate neutrophil contains intracellular bacteria. (Wright-Giemsa; LP.)

When neutrophils are the predominant cell type, the sample should be examined closely for infectious agents, particularly if the neutrophils are degenerate (Fig. 5.40). Degenerate neutrophils, or karyolytic neutrophils, have a swollen, paler-staining nucleus that has lost the discrete segmentation of healthy neutrophils. Karyolysis is induced by toxic substances or internal enzyme release. If a sample is not processed immediately, neutrophils can begin to degenerate due to enzyme release caused by cell degeneration. These neutrophils appear karyolytic even in the absence of bacteria. However, it is still recommended to culture any sample that contains karyolytic neutrophils.

Increased neutrophils may also be observed with noninfectious causes. Examples include neoplasia or aspiration of foreign substances (Colledge et al., 2013). Increased numbers of neutrophils are present in the first aliquot from BAL. This is thought to be caused by the relative adhesiveness of cells to the epithelial lining (Hawkins et al., 1994). The absolute and relative numbers of neutrophils increase with subsequent BAL or TW procedures.

Macrophagic and Mixed Inflammation
Alveolar macrophages are often seen in either acute or chronic forms of inflammation and may be the predominant cell type (Fig. 5.41). These cells are large, have abundant blue-gray foamy cytoplasm, and are frequently vacuolated and contain phagocytized material. A key feature to aid in the identification of alveolar macrophages is the eccentric position of the nucleus, which is usually round to oval. In chronic disease, binucleate and multinucleate forms may be seen. A mixed inflammatory response composed of nondegenerate neutrophils and macrophages is frequently seen in noninfectious pulmonary disease such as inhalation pneumonia, lung lobe torsion, or necrosis secondary to a neoplastic lesion.

Granulomatous Inflammation
Granulomatous inflammation is characterized cytopathologically by the presence of epithelioid macrophages and multinucleate giant cells. Epithelioid macrophages are blue-gray to pale pink with plump, round, well-defined cytoplasmic borders (Fig. 5.42A). Cells are frequently seen in small aggregates and are therefore termed *epithelioid*. Neutrophils may also be present (pyogranulomatous inflammation) as well as lesser numbers of plasma cells, lymphocytes, and eosinophils. Granulomatous or pyogranulomatous inflammation is seen in fungal infections such as blastomycosis (Fig. 5.42B), coccidioidomycosis, and aspergillosis. A foreign body or foreign material within the pulmonary parenchyma may provoke the same reaction.

Eosinophilic Inflammation
Clinical signs of allergic bronchitis and asthma include coughing, increased tracheal sensitivity, and crackles and wheezes on auscultation of the lung. Cytopathologically, this syndrome is characterized by increased mucus, Curschmann spirals, and increased numbers of eosinophils with varying numbers of macrophages, neutrophils, and mast cells in TTW and BAL fluids (Fig. 5.43). Other causes of increased eosinophils in BAL or TW include eosinophilic granulomas, aspergillosis, neoplasia, and rarely, bacterial pneumonia (Johnson and Vernau, 2011).

Eosinophils are typically sparse in lung samples (<5%). When eosinophils represent more than 10% of the nucleated cells, one should consider a hypersensitivity, parasitic, or infiltrative process. Eosinophilia in the lung may be seen with or without blood eosinophilia. Other inflammatory cell types may be seen, including small numbers of mast cells, lymphocytes, and plasma cells. Tumor-associated tissue eosinophilia is occasionally seen in dogs and cats, most reports of which are associated with malignant neoplasia.

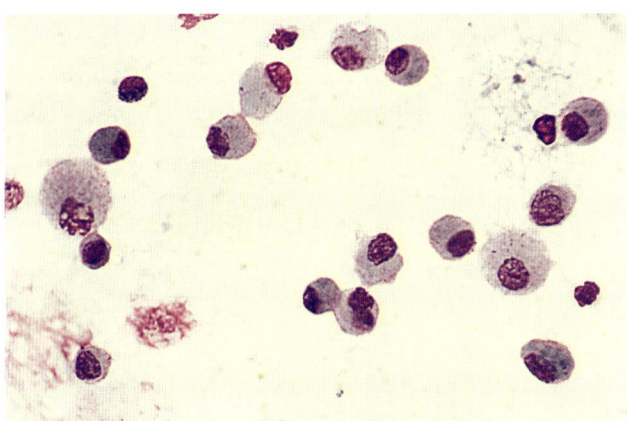

■ **FIGURE 5.41 Macrophagic inflammation. Bronchoalveolar lavage. Cat.** This diagnostic procedure was performed to rule out an active inflammatory condition in the lungs. The cell population consists primarily of alveolar macrophages distinguished by their eccentrically placed nuclei. The cytoplasm is blue-gray with distinct granules noted in some cells. These were later identified as Prussian blue positive for iron and consistent for chronic hemorrhage (see Fig. 5.48). (Wright-Giemsa; HP oil.) (Courtesy Rose Raskin, University of Florida.)

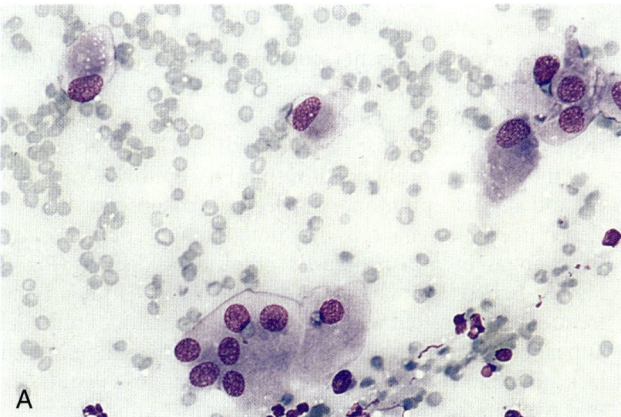
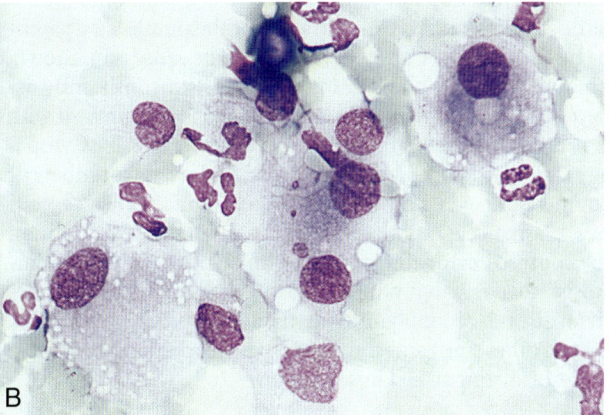

■ **FIGURE 5.42 Granulomatous inflammation. Lung aspirate. Dog.** Same case in A and B. **A,** A giant cell with many individualized nuclei is present along with several epithelioid macrophages that have abundant blue-gray cytoplasm and a distinct cytoplasmic outline. (Wright-Giemsa; HP oil.) **B,** Tissue aspirate contains epithelioid macrophages, neutrophils, and a thick-capsuled extracellular yeast consistent with *Blastomyces* (dark basophilic oval structure). Neutrophils can be used to guesstimate relative size. (Wright-Giemsa; HP oil.) (Courtesy Rose Raskin, University of Florida.)

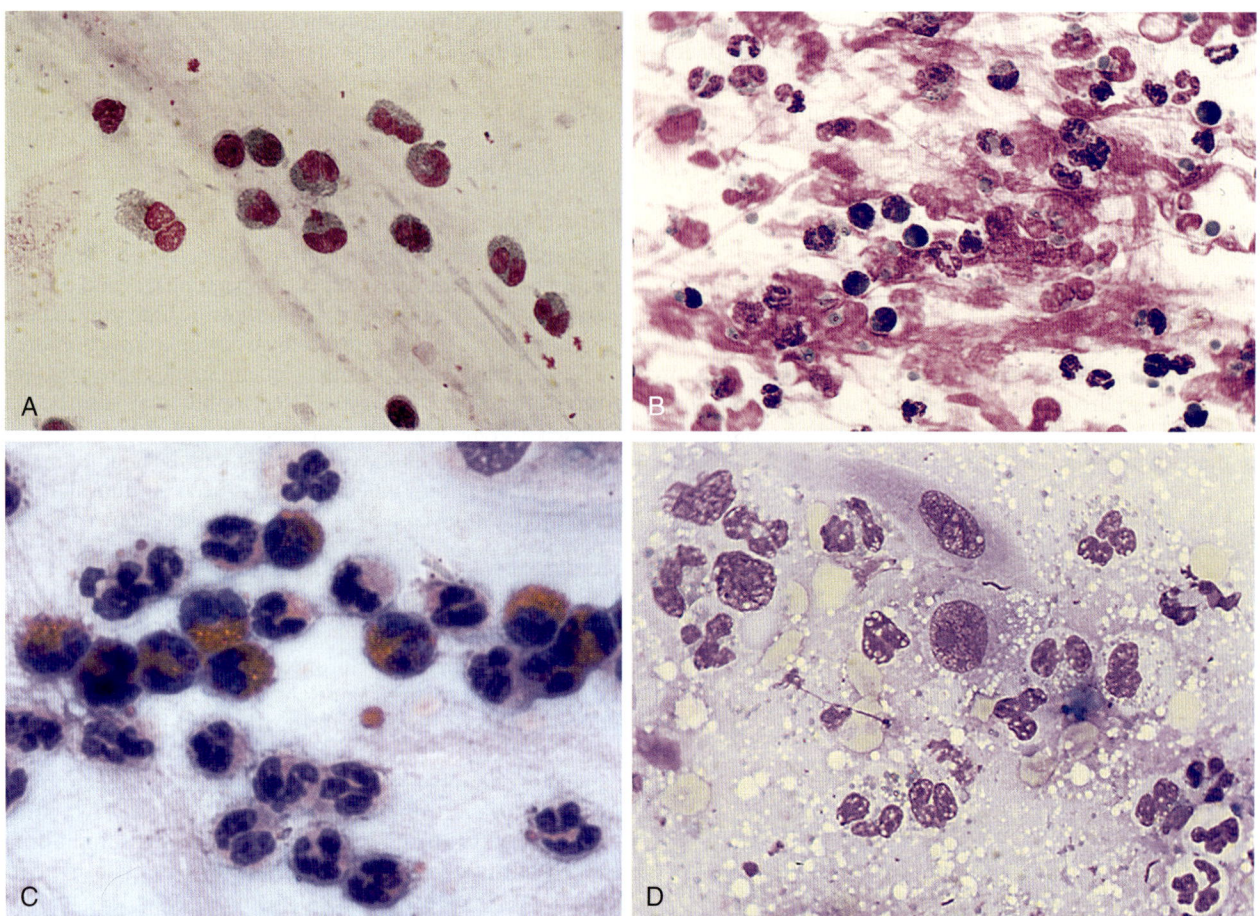

■ **FIGURE 5.43** Eosinophilic inflammation. **A, Bronchoalveolar lavage. Cat.** Numerous eosinophils (95% of the total nucleated cell population) were observed in this animal with a chronic cough suspected to have been caused by a hypersensitivity reaction. Most of the eosinophil granules stain bluish-gray. (Wright-Giemsa; HP oil.) **B, Sputum smear. Dog.** Numerous eosinophils are enmeshed in streams of pink-staining mucus from an animal with heartworm disease that exhibited frequent coughing. (Wright-Giemsa; HP oil.) **C, Endotracheal wash. Dog.** Many nondegenerate neutrophils and eosinophils in tracheal wash fluid from a dog with a chronic cough. The diagnosis was chronic bronchitis and immunosuppressive therapy was initiated. (Wright-Giemsa; HP oil.) **D, Eosinophilic granulomatosis. Bronchus exudate smear. Dog.** Mixed inflammatory cell population consisting of numerous eosinophils and low numbers of neutrophils and macrophages cells is shown along with a fibroblast *(top center)*. Histopathology of the pulmonary mass confirmed the diagnosis. (Aqueous Romanowsky; HP oil.) (A–B, Courtesy Rose Raskin, University of Florida. D, Courtesy Ruanna Gossett and Jennifer Thomas, Texas A&M University. Presented at the 1992 ASVCP case review session.)

Pulmonary eosinophilic granulomatosis is a syndrome identified in dogs characterized by infiltration of the pulmonary parenchyma by eosinophils (Calvert et al., 1988). The cause is unknown, but pulmonary eosinophilic granulomatosis is inconsistently associated with *Dirofilaria immitis* infection. Dogs may present with either a diffuse interstitial infiltrate or discrete masses. Cytopathology is similar in both instances and includes large numbers of eosinophils admixed with variable numbers of macrophages, neutrophils, plasma cells, and basophils (Fig. 5.43D). This condition may be confused cytopathologically with "lymphomatoid granulomatosis" that is a lymphoma causing angiocentric, angiodestructive disease of nonlymphoid tissues (typically lung, skin, kidney and other sites) and composed of a pleocellular population that must be distinguished histologically.

Response to Tissue Injury

Hyperplasia and Dysplasia of the Tracheobronchial Tract

Epithelial hyperplasia is a nonspecific change associated with inflammation that results in variably sized, deeply basophilic epithelial cells. Goblet cell hyperplasia may also be seen in inflammatory disease of the respiratory tract. Increased mucus is common and may present cytopathologically as inspissated mucus in a tight spiral coil, also known as a Curschmann spiral, which resembles a bottle washer brush (Fig. 5.44). These are designative of small airway disease (see Box 5.2) (Rebar et al., 1992).

Finding large numbers of respiratory epithelial cells is atypical and suggests pulmonary atelectasis, collapse, or hyperplasia. Respiratory epithelial cells may undergo hyperplastic or dysplastic changes in non-neoplastic pulmonary disease (Fig. 5.45). Hyperplasia of bronchiolar and alveolar type II pneumocytes is frequently associated with chronic inflammation. Epithelial cells appear atypical and share some features with malignant cells but lack sufficient criteria of malignancy to diagnose neoplasia. Normal columnar epithelial cells become more cuboidal and, when seen individually, may appear round. Nuclei assume a central instead of basilar form, are larger, and contain clumped nuclear chromatin and prominent nucleoli. The cytoplasm is more basophilic and may contain punctate vacuoles.

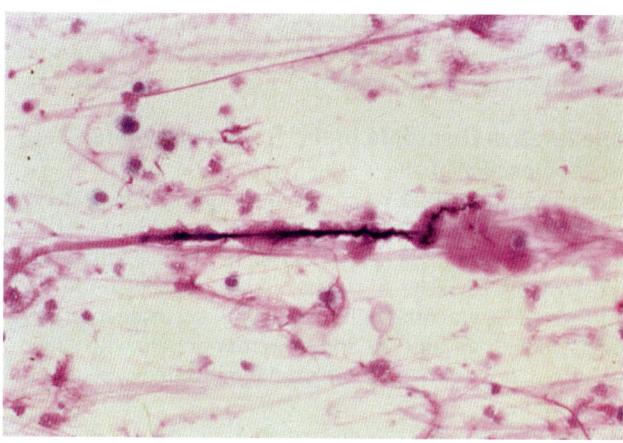

■ **FIGURE 5.44 Curschmann's spiral. Transtracheal wash.** Magenta-staining spiral-shape mucus plug considered to come from subepithelial mucous gland ducts of diseased bronchi such as chronic bronchitis. (Wright-Giemsa; HP oil.)

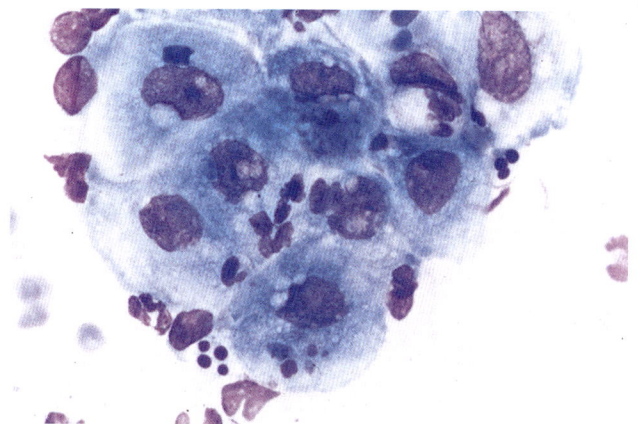

■ **FIGURE 5.46 Squamous metaplasia.** Squamous cells are ovoid with increased basophilia and increased hyalinization of the cytoplasm because of metaplastic transformation (conversion of one tissue type into another) secondary to chronic inflammation. A few neutrophil nuclei are present. (Wright-Giemsa; HP oil.)

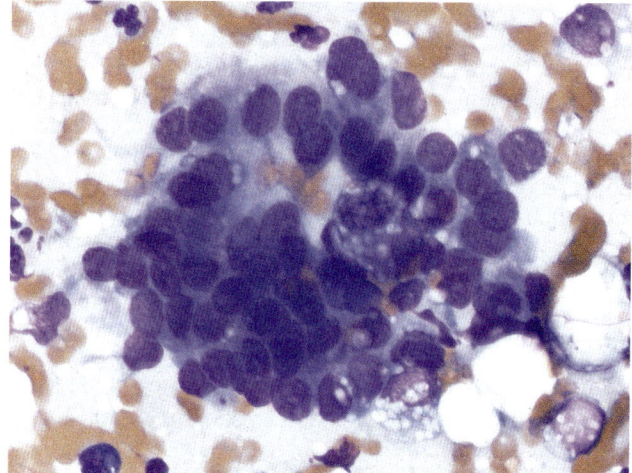

■ **FIGURE 5.45 Respiratory epithelial cell hyperplasia. Lung aspirate. Dog.** Rows and tight clusters of cuboidal to low columnar, respiratory epithelial cells with rare interspersed foamy macrophages, neutrophils, and plasma cells. The patient was diagnosed with pyogranulomatous pneumonia due to blastomycosis (not shown). (Wright-Giemsa; HP oil.)

Increased cell proliferation *(hyperplasia)* or asynchronous cytoplasmic and nuclear maturation *(dysplasia)* may occur secondary to chronic inflammation or tissue necrosis. These conditions can be difficult to differentiate cytologically from neoplasia. As a further complication, these cytopathologic changes may also be seen with preneoplastic changes that can progress to overt neoplasia. Reaspiration at a site more or less affected may be warranted to help characterize the degree of involvement or identify an underlying cause. If insufficient criteria of malignancy are present cytopathologically, a lung surgical biopsy is indicated.

Metaplasia of the Tracheobronchial Tract

Squamous metaplasia of the tracheobronchial tree has been described in dogs with chronic, experimental exposure to inhaled tobacco products and air pollutants (Roy et al., 1976; Hyde et al., 1978).

Metaplasia of the Lung

Metaplasia is the replacement of normal cells with a secondary but non-neoplastic population. Metaplasia can occur in response to hormonal or growth factor alterations or as part of an adaptive response to protect against chronic irritation. Aspirates from areas of squamous metaplasia are moderately cellular, yielding large, round to polygonal squamous epithelial cells that may be seen in sheets or individually (Fig. 5.46). Nuclei are relatively small in comparison to the cell size (low nucleocytoplasmic ratio). Occasional cells may contain pyknotic nuclei as part of the keratinization process. Lightly basophilic cytoplasm is abundant and may become folded or angular as the cells become keratinized. Anuclear superficial cells and keratin flakes may also be seen depending on the degree of keratinization. Squamous metaplasia can be difficult to differentiate from squamous neoplasia. In addition, SCC of the lung typically originates from areas of squamous metaplasia.

Necrosis

Necrotic material is frequently aspirated from lungs affected by either inflammatory or neoplastic changes. Necrosis is characterized cytopathologically by abundant amounts of basophilic granular to amorphous background material. Usually inflammatory or neoplastic cells are admixed within the necrotic debris; however, acellular aspirates or those with only remnant cell membranes or "ghost cells" may occasionally be obtained. In these cases, reaspiration is indicated, and particular care should be taken to obtain samples from the periphery of the lesion while avoiding the necrotic center.

Hemorrhage

Hemorrhage is characterized cytopathologically by one or more of several criteria, including erythrophagocytosis, hemosiderin-laden macrophages, and hematoidin crystals (Figs. 5.47 and 5.48A). Hemorrhage is a complication of many of the methods used to sample the respiratory tree, so the presence of erythrophagia, preferably with hemosiderin, is important to distinguish pathologic from iatrogenic hemorrhage or blood contamination. Hemorrhage is a common sequela to FNA of the pulmonary

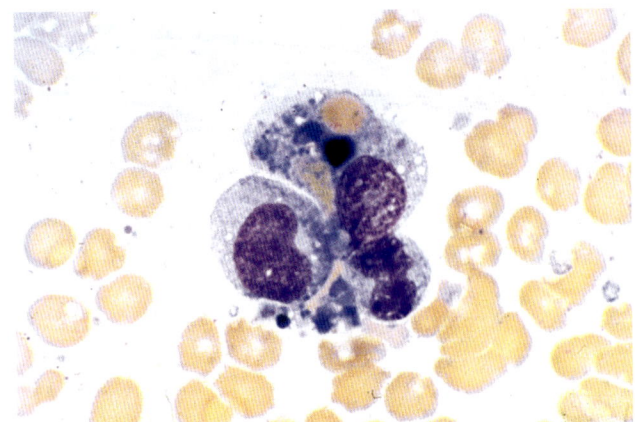

■ **FIGURE 5.47 Hemorrhage.** Macrophage has phagocytized erythrocytes and formed hemosiderin within its cytoplasm (variably sized dark blue structures). Erythrophagia and hemosiderin-laden macrophages are indicative of acute and chronic hemorrhage, respectively. (Wright-Giemsa; HP oil.)

parenchyma. Increased red blood cells in TW or BAL are observed with congestive heart failure, neoplasia, heartworm emboli, and coagulopathy. A high percentage of cats with respiratory inflammatory disease such as rhinitis and asthma had mild to moderate numbers of hemosiderophages in TW fluid (DeHeer and McManus, 2005). Prussian blue stain can be used to distinguish hemosiderophages (Fig. 5.48B).

Pulmonary Alveolar Proteinosis

This is an uncommon condition with prominent cytologic findings in lung aspirates or BAL (Silverstein et al., 2000; Camus and Ferris, 2020). Dogs and cats present with a chronic history of exercise intolerance, coughing, or prominent pulmonary interstitial pattern. After a couple of hours, a clear separation of milky sediment may be apparent grossly. Cytopathology often reveals abundant amounts of PAS-positive pale blue homogenous intracellular globules, suggestive of inspissated mucus or degenerate cells (Szatmári et al., 2015). This fluid may contain bronchial epithelial cells, cholesterol clefts, and low numbers of inflammatory cells. Pulmonary lavage may be therapeutic to reduce this excess accumulation of surfactant proteins.

Degenerative Disorders of the Tracheobronchial Tract
Tracheobronchomalacia

Tracheobronchomalacia results from the breakdown or degradation of the cartilaginous rings of the trachea and bronchial walls. In dogs, both acquired changes caused by chronic inflammation and heritable cartilage disorders appear to contribute to the pathogenesis. Cytopathologically, there is no distinctive pattern associated with this disease, and cases may present with suppurative, mixed, or lymphocytic inflammation (Singh et al., 2012).

Noninfectious Inflammatory Disorders of the Tracheobronchial Tract and Lungs
Hypersensitivity Airway Disorders

Canine allergic airway disorders include eosinophilic bronchitis, eosinophilic granuloma, and eosinophilic bronchopneumopathy, which are diagnosed based on a combination of clinical, radiographic, endoscopic, and cytologic findings (Johnson et al., 2019). All of these disorders are characterized by eosinophilic and neutrophilic inflammation in BAL fluid, but samples from dogs with eosinophilic bronchitis tend to have lower total nucleated cell counts and eosinophil percentages relative to the two other disorders (Johnson et al., 2019). Peripheral eosinophilia is more likely to occur with eosinophilic granuloma and eosinophilic bronchopneumopathy (Johnson et al., 2019).

Cats with feline asthma are often young at the onset of clinical signs and may be presented for cough, abnormal respiratory sounds, and dyspnea. BAL fluid cytopathology is expected to show increased eosinophil and neutrophil percentages with or without respiratory epithelial cell and goblet cell hyperplasia and dysplasia (Reinero et al., 2019; Grotheer et al., 2020). Cats with asthma may have positive bacterial cultures or PCR results for infectious agents, but the role of these organisms in disease pathogenesis is unclear (Reinero et al., 2019; Grotheer et al., 2020).

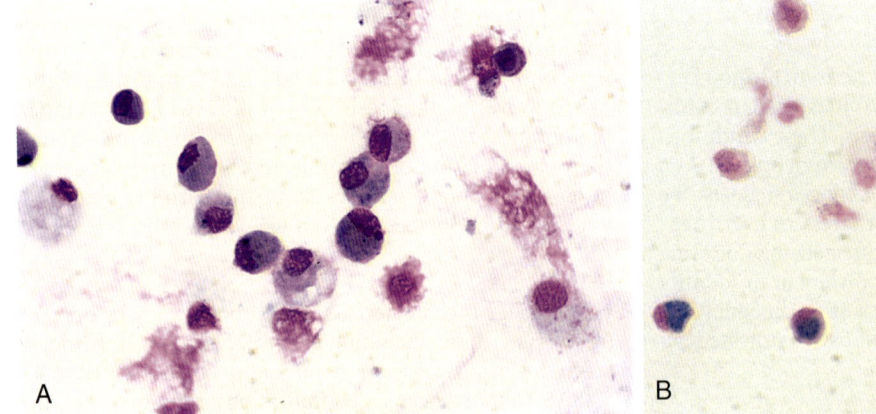
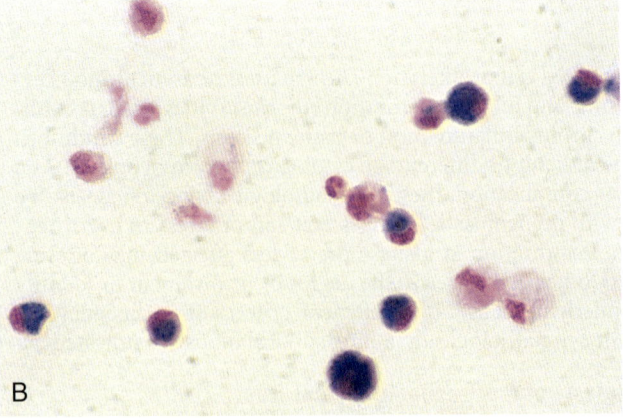

■ **FIGURE 5.48 Chronic Hemorrhage. Bronchoalveolar lavage.** Same case in A and B. **A,** Same case as in Figure 5.41. Alveolar macrophages stain blue-gray and finely granular owing to the presence of hemosiderin, verified in B. (Wright-Giemsa; HP oil.) **B,** Dense blue-black accumulations of iron within the cytoplasm of alveolar macrophages. Nuclear counterstain is red. (Prussian blue; HP oil) (Courtesy Rose Raskin, University of Florida.)

Feline Chronic Bronchitis

Feline chronic bronchitis is an idiopathic inflammatory respiratory condition in which cats are presented with similar clinical symptoms as cats with feline asthma (Reinero et al., 2019; Grotheer et al., 2020). BAL fluid cytopathology shows an increased neutrophil percentage without an increased eosinophil percentage and without infectious agents (Reinero et al., 2019; Grotheer et al., 2020). Bacterial culture results are negative (Reinero et al., 2019; Grotheer et al., 2020).

Lipid Pneumonia

Lipid pneumonia is a rarely reported disease in dogs and cats. This disease is classified as either exogenous lipid pneumonia caused by inhalation of fat or oil or as endogenous lipid pneumonia that is not associated with inhalation of external material (Lopez, 2000). Endogenous lipid pneumonia has been reported, albeit rarely, in both cats (Jerram et al., 1998; Jones et al., 2000) and dogs (Raya et al., 2006; Camus et al., 2013). Clinical signs of endogenous lipid pneumonia include dyspnea, cough, and mucus expectoration, but patients may be asymptomatic as well (Raya et al., 2006). Diagnosis of this disease is facilitated by radiography, sputum examination, lung aspiration, CT, and/or BAL. Cytopathology reveals variably sized, colorless, round structures (lipid droplets) and discrete, colorless, cytoplasmic vacuoles (phagocytized lipid) within macrophages (Fig. 5.49). Sudan IV stain or oil red O will create intense staining of the abundant lipid-rich vacuoles present in the macrophages. Histology of the lungs reveals multifocal interstitial pneumonia, characterized by interstitial fibrosis, accumulation of macrophages, lymphocytes, and small numbers of neutrophils in alveolar spaces, presence of multinucleated giant cells, and proliferation of type II pneumocytes (Raya et al., 2006). The exact etiology of this disease is uncertain; however, it is suspected to be related to diseases that incite airway obstruction. Chronic bronchitis, laryngeal paralysis, bronchogenic carcinoma, and *D. immitis* have been coexistent with endogenous lipid pneumonia in dogs and cats (Jerram et al., 1998; Jones et al., 2000; Raya et al., 2006; Camus et al., 2013).

Infectious Inflammatory Disorders of the Tracheobronchial Tract and Lungs

Neutrophils typically predominate in bacterial, protozoal, viral, and many fungal infections. In addition, macrophages, lymphocytes, and plasma cells may also be present.

Viruses

Viral tracheitis and bronchitis. Viral causes of canine infectious tracheobronchitis (kennel cough) include canine parainfluenza virus, canine adenovirus 2 (CAV-2), and CDV, and viral causes of feline respiratory disease complex include feline viral rhinotracheitis (feline herpesvirus 1) and feline calicivirus. Cytopathologic findings in acute viral infections tend to identify neutrophilic inflammation with or without a secondary bacterial infection. Viral inclusions are rarely observed on cytopathology with adenoviral or distemper viral infections.

Viral pneumonia. Viral infections are accompanied by neutrophilic inflammation. Although this is often caused by secondary bacterial infection, viral infections alone may induce an increase in absolute and relative neutrophil counts. Cats with FIV infection have significantly higher total cell counts and higher relative neutrophil numbers in BAL fluid (Hawkins et al., 1996). Canine distemper and adenovirus are the most common viral pathogens in dogs. Samples from suspected cases should be examined closely for viral inclusions. When seen, viral inclusions are found in respiratory epithelial cells coincident with clinical signs. Distemper inclusions are eosinophilic with aqueous Romanowsky staining, basophilic with methanolic Romanowsky staining, vary in size, and can be intranuclear or intracytoplasmic (Fig. 5.50). Inclusions may be observed in multiple cell types, including macrophages, lymphocytes, red blood cells, and epithelial cells. They can persist in lung tissue for more than 6 weeks. Infection with CAV-2 results in the presence of large, amphophilic or basophilic intranuclear inclusions that are most commonly seen in bronchiolar epithelial cells. Acidophilic intranuclear viral inclusions in lung tissue may be seen during the acute infection period in dogs infected with canine herpesvirus;

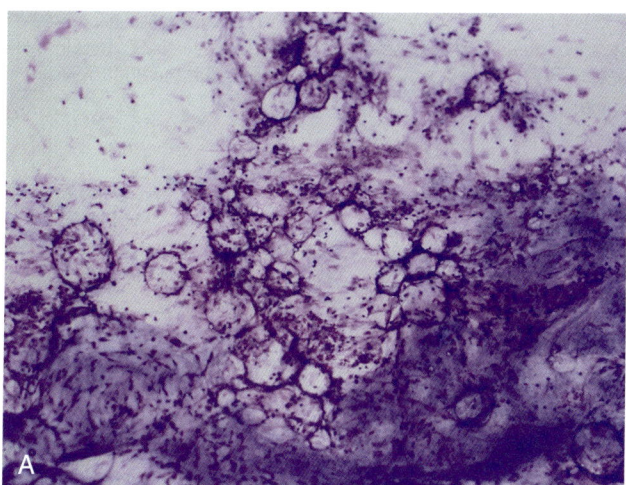 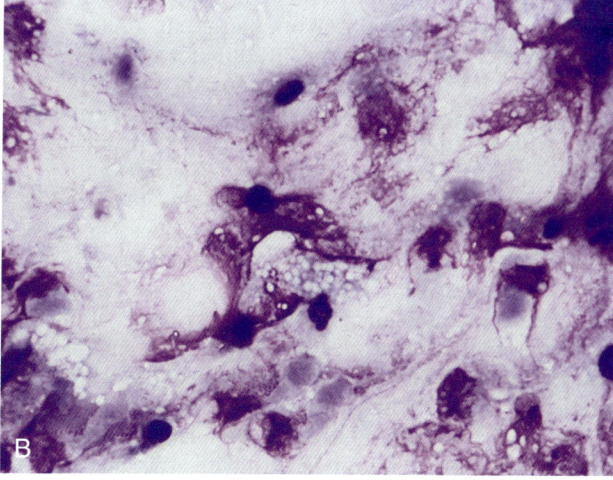

FIGURE 5.49 Lipid pneumonia. Endotracheal wash. Dog. A, Many variably sized lipid droplets admixed with abundant mucus and many inflammatory cells. (Modified Wright, IP.) **B,** Inflammatory cells are neutrophils and lipid-laden macrophages. (Modified Wright, HP oil.) (Courtesy Melinda Camus, University of Georgia.)

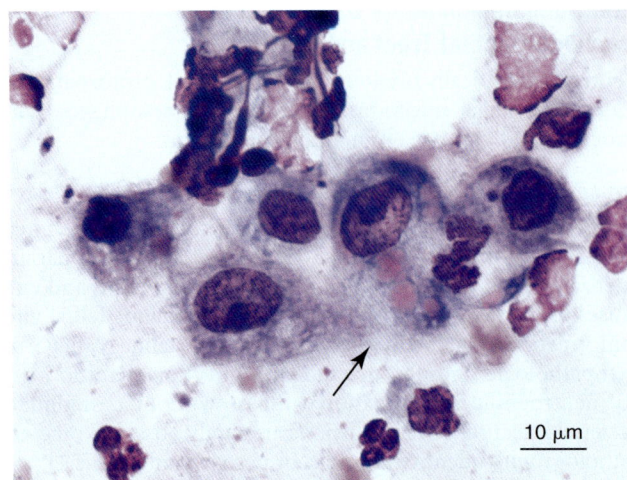

■ **FIGURE 5.50 Distemper inclusions. Lung imprint. Dog.** Pink-staining viral inclusions compatible with canine distemper are present in the macrophage *(arrow)*. (Romanowsky stain; HP oil.) (Courtesy Ron Tyler and Rick Cowell, Oklahoma State University. Presented at the 1982 ASVCP case review session.)

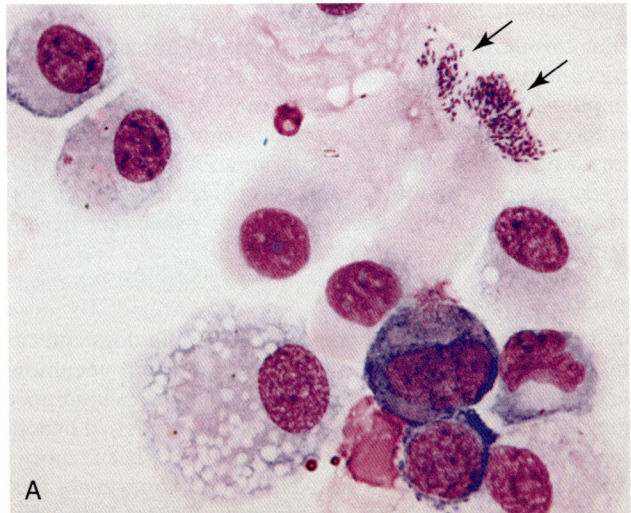

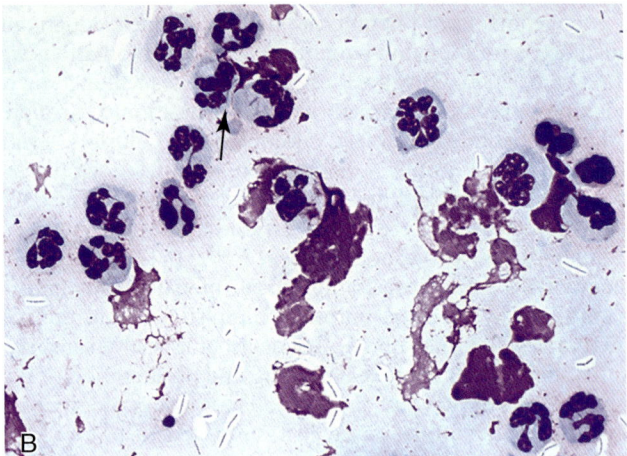

■ **FIGURE 5.51 Bacterial infection. A, Canine infectious tracheobronchitis. *Bordetella*. Bronchoalveolar lavage. Dog.** Columnar epithelium with a colony of tiny magenta-staining bacterial rods of *Bordetella bronchiseptica (arrows)* tightly adhered to cilia. Variably sized macrophages are present. (Wright; HP oil.) **B, Suppurative bronchitis. *Capnocytophaga*. Sputum. Dog.** Neutrophilic inflammation accompanies this infection from *Capnocytophaga cynodegmi* identified by culture and polymerase chain reaction testing. Note the thick clear-staining cell wall and short filamentous shape. Both intracellular *(arrow)* and extracellular bacteria are seen. (A, Courtesy Michael Scott, Michigan State University. B, Courtesy Heather Workman, University of California. Presented at the 2003 ASVCP case review session.)

however, these are more commonly demonstrated in nasal respiratory epithelium.

Experimental and natural infection with strains of the influenza virus has been reported in both dogs and cats (Kuiken et al., 2004; Crawford et al., 2005); however, there is substantial heterogeneity of the disease pathogenesis because of differences in viral strains, reservoirs, and host factors (Harder and Vahlenkamp, 2010).

Bacteria

Bacterial tracheitis and bronchitis. B. bronchiseptica is a bacterial agent of canine infectious tracheobronchitis (kennel cough). TW fluid cytopathologic findings are inflammation with bacterial bacilli adhered to the cilia of columnar respiratory epithelial cells (Fig. 5.51A). *Capnocytophaga cynodegmi*, a commensal organism of the canine and feline oral cavity, is reported in a dog having a severe bronchitis infection concurrent to a plant awn aspiration (Workman et al., 2008). This infection characterized by a prominent suppurative inflammation involves culture and PCR identification of this fastidious aerobic, capnophilic, gram-negative bacillus that is about 2 to 4 μm long with a thin, straight or slightly curved, filamentous shape having a thick clear-staining cell wall (Fig. 5.51B).

Bacterial pneumonia. Degenerate neutrophils are the most common cell type observed with bacterial pneumonia (Fig. 5.52). Mucus and numbers of macrophages are also frequently increased. The presence of intracellular bacteria, in the absence of oropharyngeal contamination, is diagnostic for bacterial pneumonia. Extracellular bacteria are also observed with pneumonia but may also be present because of contamination; therefore, identification of intracellular bacteria is necessary to confirm the diagnosis. Usually, a uniform bacterial population is present; however, a mixed population can be seen with aspiration pneumonia. Bacterial pneumonia may be accompanied by viral co-infections, such as parainfluenza viruses and respiratory coronaviruses (Viitanen, 2015).

Aspiration pneumonia may result from dysphagia, laryngeal dysfunction or paralysis, foreign body aspiration, esophageal dysfunction or stricture, seizures, oral gavage, or anesthesia. Typical respiratory fluid cytopathologic findings are neutrophilic inflammation with mixed bacteria within the background and phagocytized by neutrophils. Oropharyngeal squamous epithelial cells and bacterial flora, such as *Conchiformibius* spp., may represent aspiration and not oropharyngeal contamination. Foreign material may also be present and surrounded by or phagocytized by neutrophils and macrophages. Barium (Fig. 5.53), sucralfate (Fig. 5.54), or activated charcoal (see Fig. 6.54) may be observed if aspiration occurred during or after oral gavage of these substances (Colledge et al., 2013; Caudill et al., 2019).

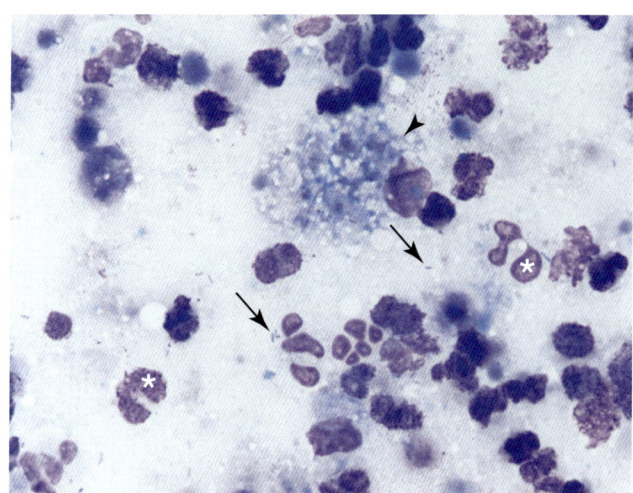

■ **FIGURE 5.52 Bacterial pneumonia. Lung aspirate.** Suppurative inflammation consists of large numbers of degenerate neutrophils *(asterisks)* with intra- and extracellular, short, rod-shaped bacteria *(arrows)* in a granular, necrotic background. A degenerate macrophage with phagocytized debris is also present *(arrowhead)*. (Wright-Giemsa; HP oil.)

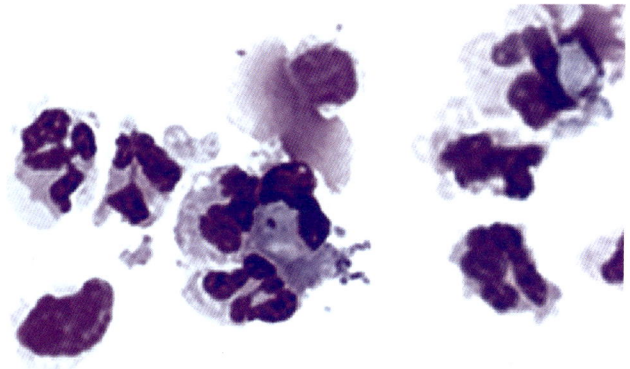

■ **FIGURE 5.54 Sucralfate aspiration. Tracheal wash. Dog.** Two neutrophils, *center* and *upper right*, contain relatively large bluish-gray oval to angular refractile structures after aspiration of administered sucralfate tablet suspension for the management of gastric ulcers. In addition to the sucralfate-aluminum complex, the tablets contain microcrystalline cellulose and starch. (Modified Wright; HP oil.) (Courtesy Sarah Johnson, Purdue University.)

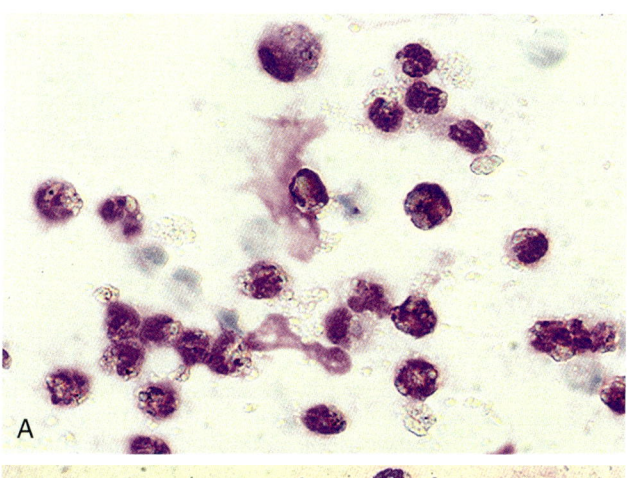

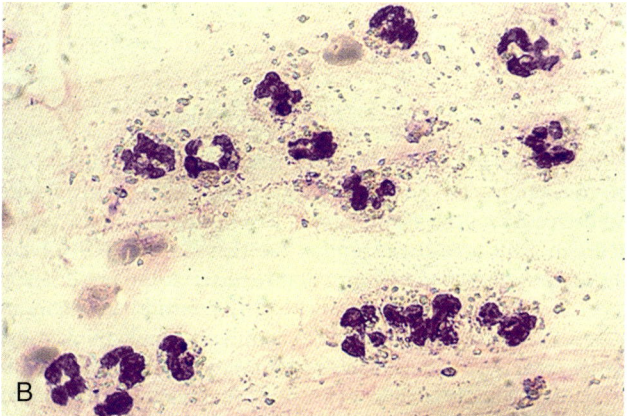

■ **FIGURE 5.53 Barium contrast media aspiration. Sputum smear. Dog. A,** Aspiration pneumonia occurred following the administration of barium contrast media for a diagnostic study of the digestive tract. Degenerate neutrophils contain yellow-green refractile crystals as well as extracellularly. (Wright-Giemsa; HP oil.) **B,** Degenerate neutrophils contain many tiny crystals, consistent with barium contrast media that appear yellow-green in this preparation. (Wright-Giemsa; HP oil.) (Courtesy Rose Raskin, University of Florida.)

Diatom algae (Fig. 5.55) were described in TW fluid from a dog that aspirated water in a drainage ditch (Benson et al., 2013). Dogs living in areas with environmental contaminants such as asbestos fibers have higher counts of ferruginous bodies in BAL fluids compared with control animals in Mexico and Italy (Vanda et al., 1998; Masserdotti and De Lorenzi, 2000). These particles are thin stick-shape or long needles with swollen ends that may be partially engulfed by macrophages. As the fiber or microdroplet is inhaled lodging in the alveoli, these golden particles become coated with ferritin material and react positive with Prussian blue staining for iron.

If *mycobacterial pneumonia* is suspected, macrophages should be examined closely for thin, negative-staining, filamentous bacteria (Fig. 5.56). Although most bacterial pneumonias are associated with suppurative inflammation, mycobacteriosis is typically associated with granulomatous or pyogranulomatous inflammation. In addition to neutrophils, Langhans multinucleate giant cells and large epithelioid macrophages with ill-defined cytoplasmic borders are seen along with variable numbers of neutrophils. *Mycobacteria* spp. do not stain with routine cytologic stains and can be difficult to visualize. However, careful examination of the cells and background material reveals the presence of distinctive negatively stained thin rods present both intra- and extracellularly. The organisms can be confirmed by acid-fast staining. Siamese cats appear to have increased susceptibility to mycobacteriosis (Jordan et al., 1994). One report of *Mycobacterium bovis* infection in a dog describes the presence of calcospherite-like bodies and caseous necrotic debris in tracheal mucus from this patient (Bauer et al., 2004). These findings are similar to what is seen in human patients with tuberculosis and are described as globular, lipidlike material and round, concentrically laminated crystalline structures, which take up the von Kossa stain for calcium and may be intermixed with proteinaceous mucus. A similar finding of microlithiasis in a cat was reported that was related to a chronic bronchopneumonia of unknown etiology (Brummer et al., 1989). The concentrically laminated crystals (Fig. 5.57) in this case were PAS positive as well composed of calcium carbonate.

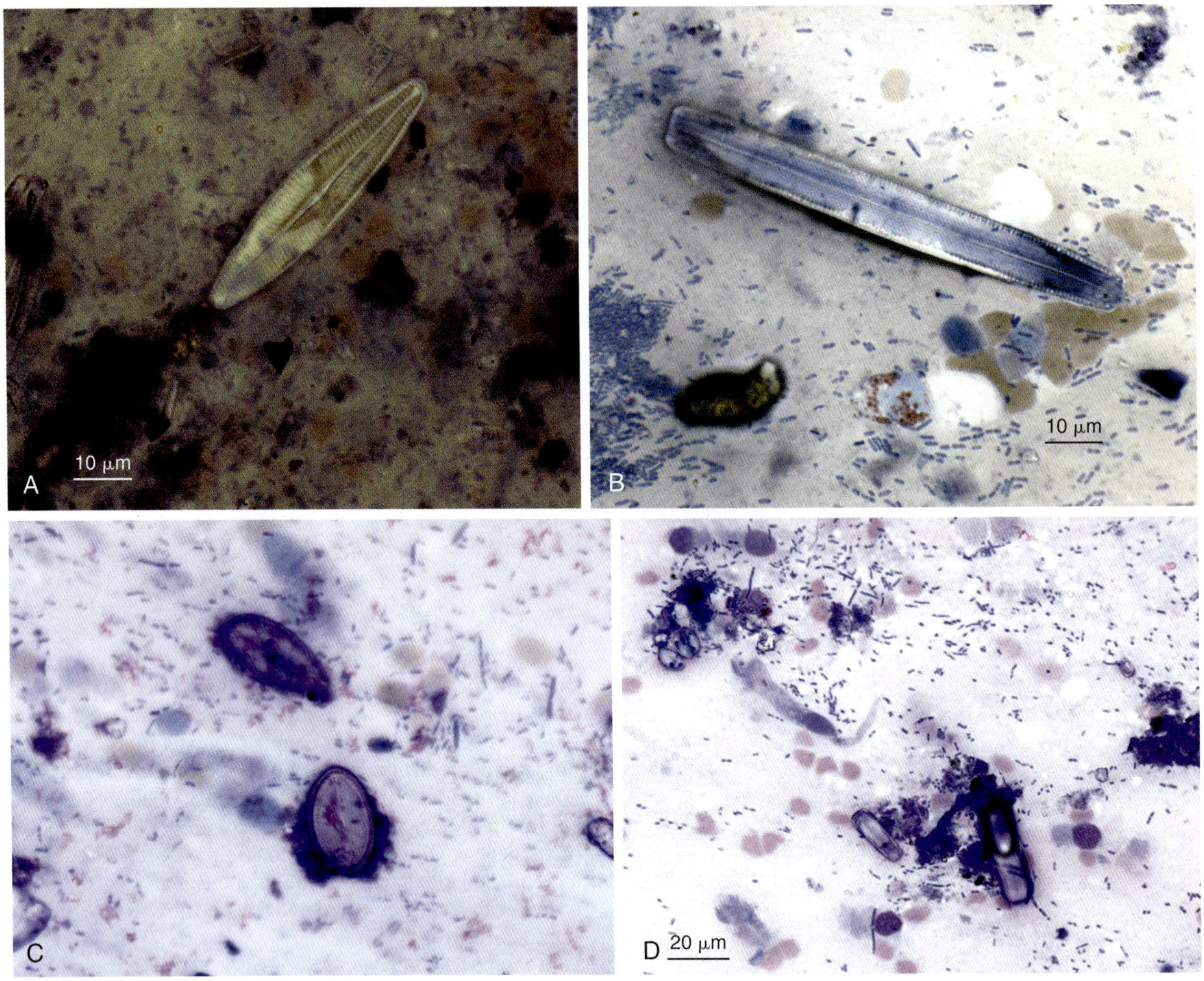

■ **FIGURE 5.55 Diatom aspiration. Postmortem respiratory fluid. Squash prep. Dog. A,** One fusiform diatom (silica-coated unicellular algae) with a central core and lateral striations measuring 60 × 10 μm appears against a background of mixed bacteria, *Navicula tripuncata*. (Wright-Giemsa, HP oil.) **B,** There is one elongate diatom measuring 100 × 10 μm having blunted ends and striated borders. (Wright-Giemsa, HP oil.) **C,** Two diatoms are ovoid to teardrop-shaped measuring 16 × 10 μm. (Wright-Giemsa, HP oil.) **D,** Several diatoms along with columnar respiratory epithelium against a background containing erythrocytes and mixed background. The presence of diatoms supported drowning in this case. (Wright-Giemsa, IP oil.) (Courtesy Johanna Rigas et al., Utah State University. Presented at the 2015 ASVCP case review session.)

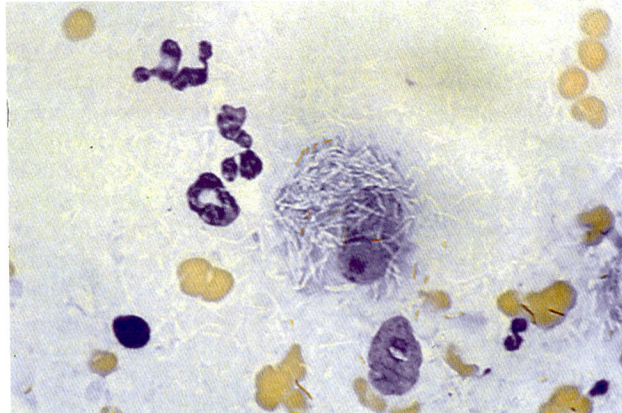

■ **FIGURE 5.56 Mycobacterial pneumonia.** Negative-staining, rod-shaped bacteria located intracellular and in the background consistent with *Mycobacterium* spp. (Wright-Giemsa; HP oil.)

Bacterial infections may be a primary disease of the lung but are also commonly seen secondary to viral infections, mucosal irritation, and decreased mucociliary clearance (Anderton et al., 2004) such as occurs in *Bordetella bronchiseptica* infection (see Fig. 5.51), fungal infections, and neoplasia. Gram-negative bacteria of enteric origin are reported in dogs and cats requiring positive-pressure ventilation, and these isolates tend to be resistant to commonly used antimicrobials (Epstein et al., 2010). In general, microbiologic culture and sensitivity is suggested if bacteria are seen because cytopathologic classification of bacteria based on morphology is unreliable. Several recent reports highlighted outbreaks of the gram-positive cocci *Streptococcus equi* subsp. *zooepidemicus* in dogs in shelters that have been linked to fatal, often hemorrhagic pneumonia (Byun et al., 2009; Priestnall et al., 2010). The presence of filamentous rods suggests infection with either *Nocardia* or *Actinomyces* spp. or rarely *Fusobacterium*. Because these species require special culture techniques, the laboratory should be alerted if such organisms are suspected.

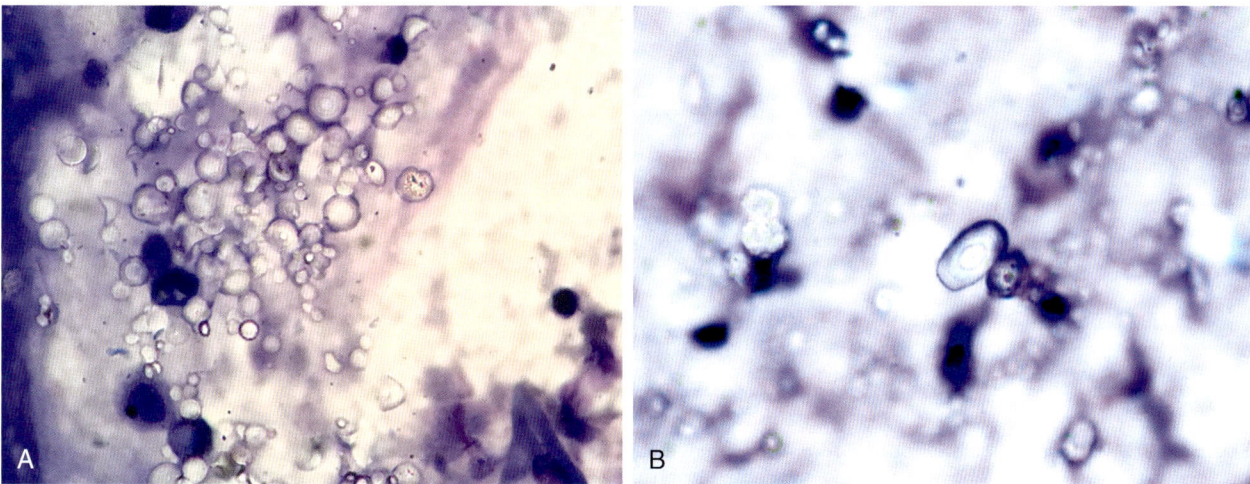

■ **FIGURE 5.57 Calcospherite bodies. Chronic broncholithiasis. Bronchoalveolar lavage. Cat.** Same case in A and B. **A,** Multiple spherical structures that appear clear and refractile against the mucus. The patient presented with increased respiratory effort over several weeks. Radiographs display a severe miliary pattern, and cytopathology revealed a mixed inflammatory response. Test results for mycobacterial infection were negative. (Modified Wright; HP oil.) **B,** Higher magnification view of the mineral structure to demonstrate the lamination. (Modified Wright: HP oil.) (Courtesy Eilidh Wilson, TDDS, Exeter, UK.)

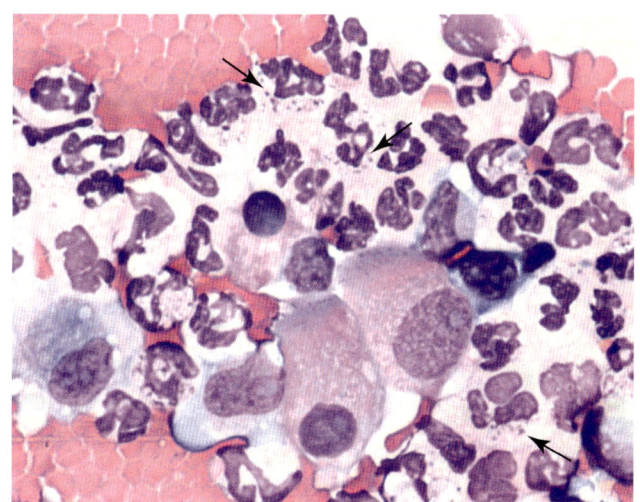

■ **FIGURE 5.58 Feline respiratory disease complex. *Mycoplasma*. Bronchoalveolar lavage. Cat.** Suppurative inflammation; within neutrophils are tiny, pleomorphic bacteria *(arrows)* confirmed by polymerase chain reaction as *Mycoplasma felis*. Two ciliated respiratory epithelium are present in the center of the field. (Wright; HP oil.) (Courtesy Andrew Torrance, TDDS, Exeter, UK.)

Mycoplasma spp. has been described in a TW from a 4-month-old dog. Small basophilic coccoid structures (0.3–0.9 μm in diameter) were observed in low to moderate numbers within neutrophils and adherent to epithelial cells in a direct smear using Wright-Giemsa stain (Williams et al., 2006). Infectious pneumonia is often uncommon in cats. Feline respiratory disease complex may less commonly involve *Mycoplasma felis*. In these cases, small, pleomorphic bacteria may be observed within background mucus or phagocytized by neutrophils in respiratory fluid cytopathologic specimens (Fig. 5.58).

Cats with infectious pneumonia may not exhibit clinical signs, and this disease has been associated with varied etiologies. Bacterial infection was the most common at 50%; viral causes were 25%; and the remainder was from fungal, protozoal, parasitic, or mixed causes. The white blood differential count and thoracic radiographs may be normal even though systemic infection exists. Therefore, clinicians should evaluate the respiratory tract with other techniques such as BAL when infection is detected in other organ systems (Macdonald et al., 2003).

Although *Yersinia pestis* is an uncommon inhabitant of the respiratory tract, the pneumonic form of plague in cats has a high zoonotic potential, thus making identification of the organism crucial. *Y. pestis* is a gram-negative bacillus cytopathologically recognizable as bipolar coccobacilli present both intra- and extracellularly with large numbers of degenerate neutrophils. Pneumonic plague accounts for approximately 10% of feline cases and can be seen with or without the classic bubonic presentation (Eidson et al., 1991).

Dogs infected with leptospirosis may also develop a pulmonary hemorrhagic syndrome similar to that seen in humans. Although cytopathologic findings have not been reported, histopathologically, these cases present with marked pulmonary hemorrhage, minimal extravascular fibrin, and an absence of inflammatory cell infiltrates (Klopfleisch et al., 2010).

Fungi

Mycotic pneumonia. Systemic mycoses spreading to the lungs are more likely to be found in the pulmonary interstitium than in the airways or alveoli. Thus, although mycotic agents may be detected by airway washes (Fig. 5.59) (Hawkins and DeNicola, 1990), FNA of the pulmonary parenchyma has increased sensitivity for detection of these organisms (see Table 5.1).

Blastomyces dermatitidis is a dimorphic fungus that can infect numerous tissues, but the lung is the most frequently involved organ in primary infection. Pulmonary lesions consist

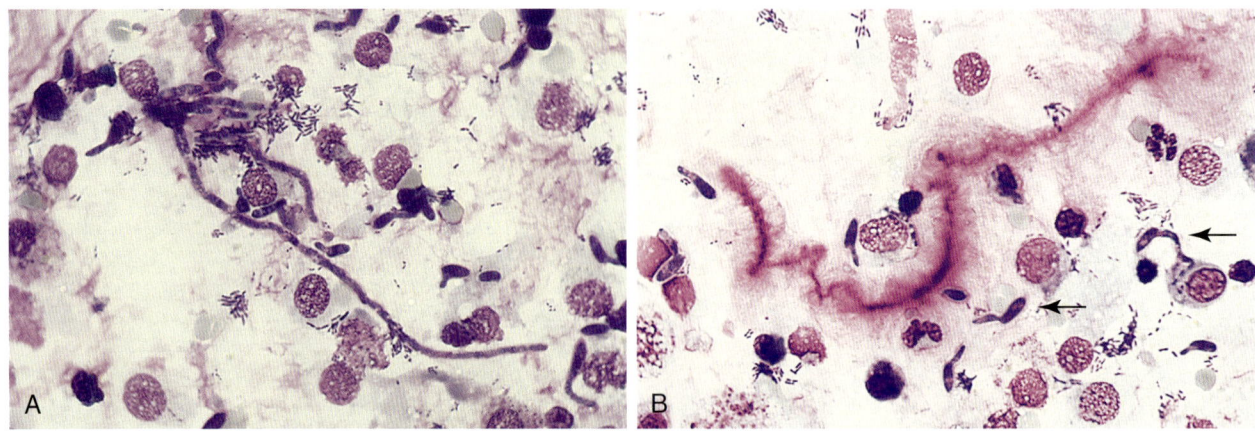

FIGURE 5.59 Mycotic and bacterial pneumonia. Bronchoalveolar lavage. Dog. A, Hyphae and microconidia. Mixed-cell inflammation is present along with mixed bacterial bacilli, branching and septate hyphae of *Fusarium* spp., and oval to curved microconidia of *Fusarium* spp. (Romanowsky stain; HP oil.) **B, Curschmann's spiral and microconidia.** Magenta-staining spiral-shape mucus plug considered to come from subepithelial mucous gland ducts of diseased bronchi such as chronic bronchitis as associated with this chronic fungal infection. *Arrows* demonstrate microconidia with slender germ tube projections. (Methanolic Romanowsky stain; HP oil.) (Courtesy Janice Andrews et al., Ohio State University. Presented at the 1991 ASVCP case review session.)

of multiple, variably sized nodules dispersed through all lung fields. Infection usually occurs in young, large-breed dogs. The prevalence is less in cats than dogs; however, Siamese cats seem especially susceptible. Organisms can be readily retrieved via TW or BAL in animals with radiographic evidence of disease (see Table 5.1). Usually, the yeast form of the organism is observed; however, the rare hyphal stage may be seen. The extracellular yeast forms are dark blue, round, and 5 to 20 μm in diameter, with a thick, biconcave wall having a granular internal structure (Fig. 5.60A). Broad-based budding may be seen and best detected using PAS stain (Fig. 5.60B–C). The organisms are likely found in aggregates of mucus and necrotic debris, so squash preparations are vital for organism identification. Pyogranulomatous or granulomatous inflammation is the rule.

Cryptococcosis is frequently associated with the nasal cavity; however, approximately 30% of affected cats also have pulmonary lesions. The capsule material of *Cryptococcus* species organisms can give the sample a mucinous texture. The presence of an inflammatory response varies seemingly related to the thickness of the capsule. Microscopically, *Cryptococcus* spp. are narrow-based budding yeast surrounded by a wall and nonstaining capsule (Fig. 5.61).

H. capsulatum is also a dimorphic fungus that infects both cats and dogs. Pulmonary disease is common in affected cats. In addition to systemic histoplasmosis seen in both species, a self-limiting syndrome of pulmonary histoplasmosis is also seen in dogs. The small, yeastlike organisms are round to oval and 1 to 4 μm in diameter with a purple nucleus and lightly basophilic protoplasm surrounded by a thin, clear halo (Fig. 5.62). Organisms are seen within macrophages and neutrophils as well as extracellularly. Macrophages may be packed with organisms. *Histoplasma* infection induces a mixed to pyogranulomatous reaction.

Coccidioides spp. is primarily a respiratory pathogen found in arid regions with *C. immitis* in California and *C. posadasii* in Arizona. Animals within endemic areas are frequently infected, but development of clinical signs is relatively uncommon. Disseminated disease occurs after primary lung infection, especially in dogs. Boxers and Doberman pinschers may be predisposed to disseminated disease. Respiratory involvement occurs in approximately 25% of cats with coccidioidomycosis (Greene and Troy, 1995). Coccidioidomycosis is associated with pyogranulomatous or granulomatous inflammation. *Coccidioides* spp. spherules (sporangium) are large organisms seen extracellularly (Fig. 5.63). Spherules range in size from 10 to 100 μm in Romanowsky-stained preparations and contain a thick, double-contoured wall with finely granular, blue-green protoplasm. Occasionally, internal endospores of 2 to 5 μm may be seen. The organism's size and internal structure are easier to appreciate on wet-mount preparations because the fixing and staining process results in shrinkage and distortion of the organism. Organisms are scarce in cytologic preparations, and multiple slides may need to be examined to find the organism. TW or BAL rarely reveals these organisms. Because of the organism's large size, scanning is best done with a scanning objective (e.g., 10×). Mycelia may rarely be seen in tissue.

Pneumocystis carinii (better called *Pneumocystis* spp. to reflect the canine variants or *Pneumocystis canis*) is most commonly reported in young dogs, primarily miniature Dachshunds (Lobetti, 2001), but has also been reported in Cavalier King Charles spaniels (Sukura et al., 1996; English et al., 2001; Watson et al., 2006) and a Yorkshire terrier (Cabanes et al., 2000). Several immune defects have been identified that may predispose some dogs to *Pneumocystis* spp., including hypogammaglobulinemia related to decreased IgG, decreased lymphocyte proliferation, and reduced numbers of B lymphocytes (Lobetti, 2000; Watson et al., 2006). Infection results in a diffuse interstitial pneumonia. The abundant foamy fluid present in the alveoli often contain trophozoites and cyst forms. Cysts are extracellular, approximately 5 μm in diameter, and contain four to eight round, 1 to 2 μm basophilic bodies (Fig. 5.64A–C). Trophozoites are pleomorphic, ranging from 2 to 7 μm in length (see Fig. 5.64B–C). Although trophozoites stain positive with Romanowsky stain, Gram stain, and hematoxylin and eosin, cyst walls stain positive with Grocott methenamine silver (GMS), PAS, toluidine blue, Gram stain, and calcofluor white (Fig. 5.64D). When organisms are suspected but not seen, the

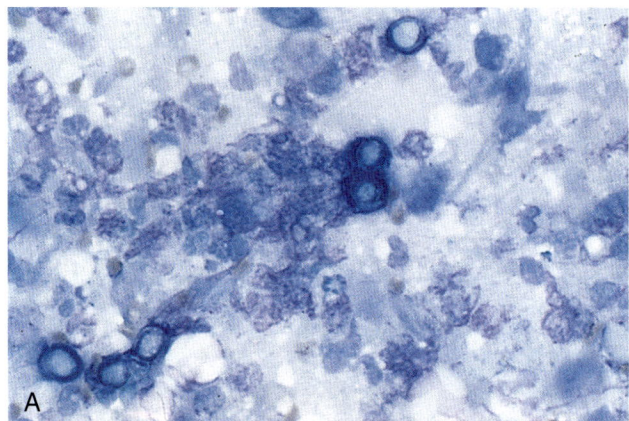
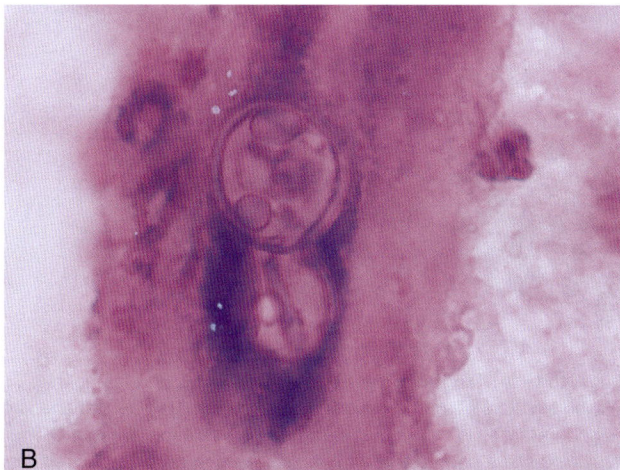
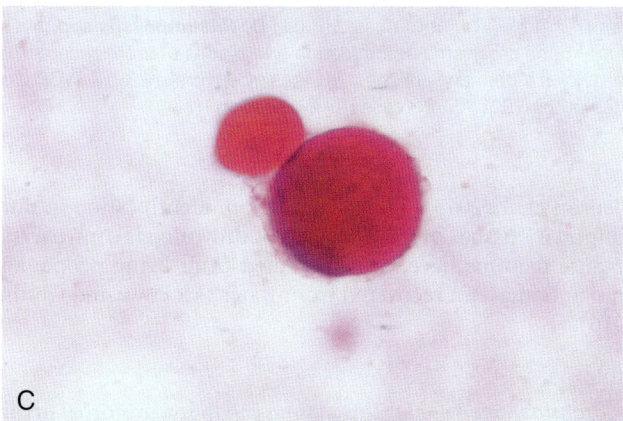

■ **FIGURE 5.60 Blastomycosis. A, Tissue aspirate.** Several thick-walled, deeply basophilic yeast forms of *Blastomyces dermatitidis* are embedded in a necrotic cellular background. (Wright-Giemsa; HP oil.) Same case in B and C. **B, Lung aspirate. Dog.** Thick double-walled capsule in a broad-based budding form of *Blastomyces dermatitidis*. (NMB; HP oil.) **C, Lung aspirate, Dog.** A "snowman" appearance is recognized related to the broad-based budding form. (PAS; HP oil.)

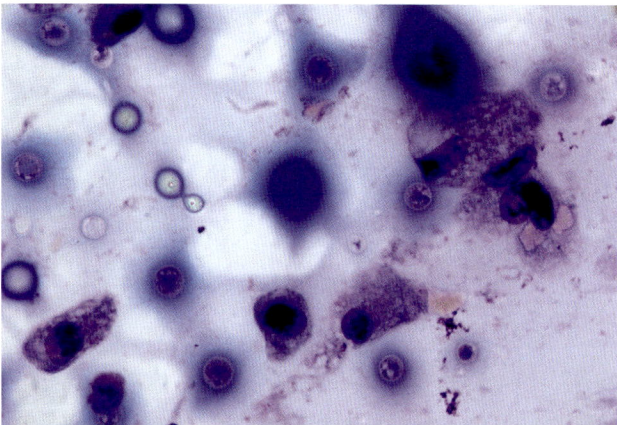

■ **FIGURE 5.61 Cryptococcosis. Lung imprint.** *Cryptococcus gattii* yeast exhibit narrow-based budding. Organisms are separated by poorly staining to nonstaining capsules. Species identification was performed by polymerase chain reaction. (Wright-Giemsa; HP oil.)

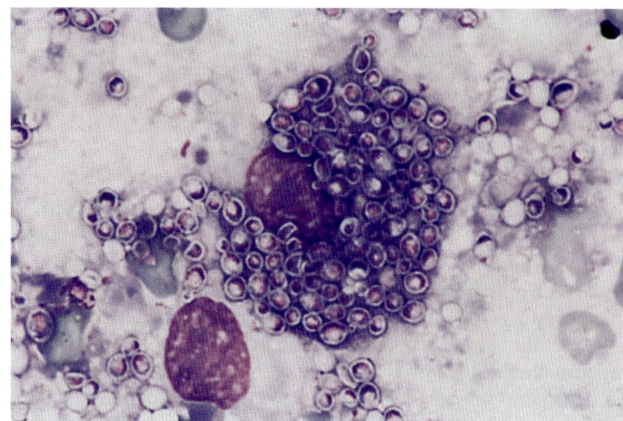

■ **FIGURE 5.62 Histoplasmosis. Tissue aspirate.** The macrophage is filled with numerous *Histoplasma capsulatum* organisms along with many extracellular organisms from a ruptured macrophage as denoted by the pink-staining free nucleus. Note the small size and thin capsule of the yeast form; admixed misshapen bluish-gray staining erythrocytes can be used estimate relative size. (Wright-Giemsa; HP oil.)

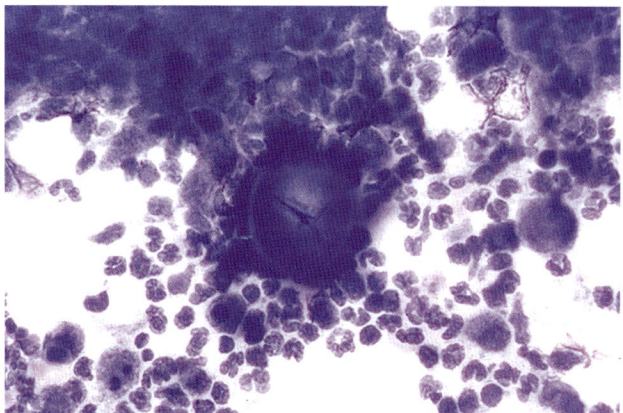

■ **FIGURE 5.63 Coccidioidomycosis. Tissue aspirate.** Huge *Coccidioides immitis* spherule with thick, double-contoured wall surrounded by numerous neutrophils, a frequent observation, which can be used to demonstrate the large size of the organism. (Wright-Giemsa; HP oil.)

diagnosis may be confirmed by a PCR assay (Hagiwara et al., 2001; Okine et al., 2018).

Sporothrix schenckii are uncommonly identified in the pulmonary parenchyma of dogs and cats. When present, large numbers of organisms are often, but not always, seen in infected cats, whereas organisms are relatively rare in other species

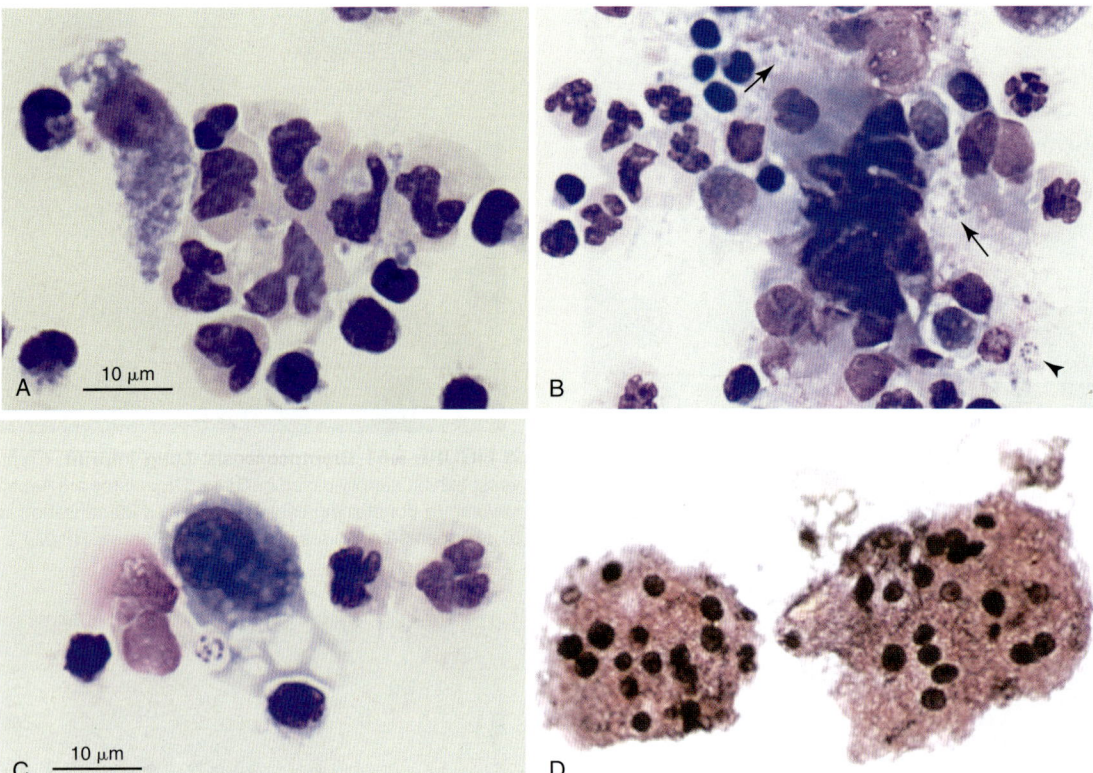

■ **FIGURE 5.64 Pneumocystis. Bronchoalveolar lavage. Dog.** Same case in A to C. **A, Trophozoites.** This Cavalier King Charles spaniel dog presented with a progressive severe dyspnea of 3 to 4 weeks' duration and displayed a mixed inflammatory response. Numerous free and one large cluster of trophozoites are intermixed among an equal mix of small lymphocytes and neutrophils in this cytocentrifuge preparation. (Wright-Giemsa; HP oil.) **B, Trophozoites and cyst.** Several individual and groups of trophozoites *(arrows)* are seen along with a pale-staining cyst *(arrowhead)* containing eight basophilic spores. (Wright-Giemsa; HP oil.) **C. Cyst.** Two neutrophils, two small lymphocytes, and a free pink-staining free nucleus are present. Note the 5 μm cyst containing a tight cluster of individual sporozoites (1–2 μm). (Wright-Giemsa; HP oil.) **D, *Pneumocystis* spp. cysts. Bronchoalveolar lavage. Horse.** Black-brown positive staining of the walls of the round organisms embedded in two islands of proteinaceous cell debris. (Grocott methenamine silver; HP oil.) (A–C, Courtesy Kate English et al., Royal Veterinary College, UK. Presented at the 2010 ASVCP case review session. D, Courtesy Amy MacNeill et al., University of Florida. Presented at the 2001 ASVCP case review session.)

(Crothers et al., 2009). Round to oval to cigar-shaped 2 × 7 μm organisms with a thin, clear halo, slightly eccentric purple nucleus, and lightly basophilic cytoplasm are observed both within macrophages and extracellularly. The presence of cigar-shaped organisms differentiates sporotrichosis from histoplasmosis.

Lycoperdonosis, or puffball mushroom toxicosis, results from the inhalation of spores from the mature puffball mushroom, which appears in North America and Europe from summer to late fall. These brown fruiting mushrooms (Fig. 5.65A) induce a marked pyogranulomatous, suppurative, or eosinophil-rich mixed cell inflammation (Fig. 5.65B–C) present in tracheal washes, bronchoalveolar washes, or lung aspirates. Lycoperdon spores can be found in macrophages of the lungs and draining lymph nodes as 3 to 5 μm round structures with a pale green coloration (Fig. 5.65D), a clear central area, and thin, dark wall (Alenghat et al., 2010). Less severe cases appear to respond to corticosteroids alone without antifungal medication, suggesting this condition can present as a hypersensitivity reaction (Buckeridge et al., 2011).

Algae

Aspiration pneumonia. Respiratory fluid from animals that have aspirated from standing bodies of water may contain diatom algae (see Fig 5.55) in addition to neutrophils, mixed bacteria, and foreign material more typical of aspiration pneumonia (Benson et al., 2013). The use of diatom identification in nonpulmonary tissues in the diagnosis of drowning is controversial because diatoms have been recovered from living people and human bodies not recovered from water (McEwen and Gerdin, 2016).

Protozoa

Protozoal pneumonia. *Toxoplasma gondii* is a protozoal organism that can cause interstitial pneumonia in dogs and cats. Cytopathologic examination of TW or BAL samples reveals an increase in the numbers of nondegenerate neutrophils. *T. gondii* tachyzoites are 1 to 4 μm, crescent-shaped bodies with lightly basophilic cytoplasm and a central metachromatic nucleus (Fig. 5.66) (see Table 5.1). Organisms may be found intracellularly (primarily within macrophages) and extracellularly. These organisms may occasionally be retrieved by BAL and rarely by TW samples (Hawkins et al., 1997; Bernsteen et al., 1999). However, because toxoplasmosis causes an interstitial pneumonia and these procedures focus on the airways, it may be difficult to retrieve these organisms unless disease is marked. Absence of organisms in a suspect patient does not negate the possibility of infection. A case of feline toxoplasmosis involving lung aspiration reported the use of immunohistochemical staining for definitive diagnosis (Poitout et al., 1998).

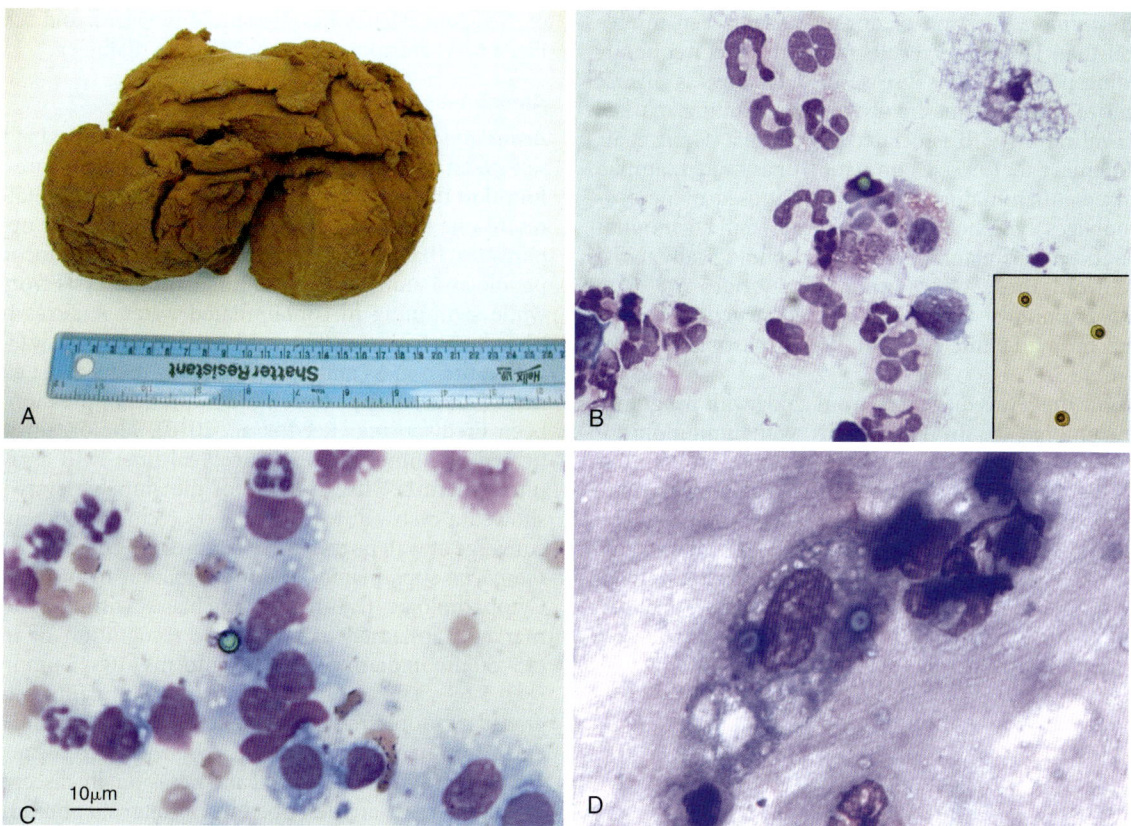

■ **FIGURE 5.65 Puffball mushroom toxicosis (lycoperdonosis).** Same case in A and B. **A, Puffball mushroom.** Spore-rich, degenerate, and deflated olive-green specimen of *Calvatia gigantea* from the family Lycopodiaceae considered responsible for respiratory distress in a dachshund. **B, Lycoperdonosis. Bronchoalveolar lavage. Dog.** Mixed inflammatory response composed predominately of neutrophils; not seen were lesser numbers of eosinophils admixed. One intracellular bluish-green stained round spore is observed near center. (Wright; HP oil.) *Inset*: Close-up view of green-yellow spores taken directly from the mushroom of approximate size of the organism in the BAL. (Unstained; HP oil.) **C, Suspected puffball mushroom toxicosis. Lung aspirate. Dog.** This 6-month-old puppy presented with a 4-day history of dyspnea. There were a diffuse, miliary to nodular, interstitial pattern on radiographs and a marked mixed cell inflammatory response on cytopathology. The neutrophils are mostly nondegenerate. A macrophage with oblong nucleus contains an intracellular round bluish-green stained spore. With focus directed to the spore, a scale indicates this spore measures approximately 5 μm in diameter, slightly smaller than the nearby erythrocytes. A lighter center with a wall rim is consistent among the spores found. A row of basophilic respiratory epithelial cells present. (Methanolic Romanowsky; HP oil.) **D, Lycoperdonosis. Endotracheal wash. Dog.** *Lycoperdon pyriforme* was the best DNA sequence match in this case of pneumonitis. Note the two light green spores with the macrophage embedded in bluish-gray mucin. (A–B, Courtesy David Buckeridge and Andy Torrance, TDDS, Exeter, UK. C, Courtesy Christine Olver, Colorado State University. D, Courtesy Karen Jackson, University of Pennsylvania.)

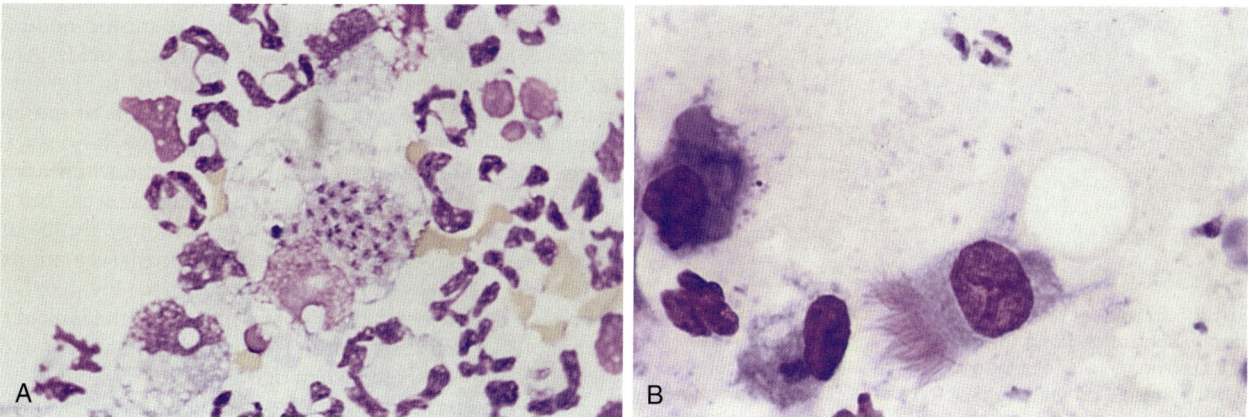

■ **FIGURE 5.66 Toxoplasmosis. A, Tissue aspirate.** Numerous neutrophils surround a faintly stained macrophage that has phagocytized numerous *Toxoplasma gondii* organisms. (Wright-Giemsa; HP oil.) **B, Lung imprint. Dog.** Same case as in Figure 5.50. Located in the upper part of the photomicrograph are banana-shaped organisms with a metachromatic central nucleus typical of *Toxoplasma gondii* tachyzoites. *Neospora* spp. can have a similar morphologic appearance and can be confirmed only by immunohistochemistry. (Romanowsky stain; HP oil.)

Neospora caninum infection of dogs is usually seen in animals younger than 1 year and results in progressive, frequently fatal, ascending paralysis. The disease in older dogs is diverse but characterized by systemic involvement, including marked pulmonary infiltration with associated pneumonia (Greig et al., 1995; Ruehlmann et al., 1995). Examination of aspirated samples reveals a mixed inflammatory response composed of neutrophils, macrophages, lymphocytes, plasma cells, and eosinophils with intra- and extracellular tachyzoites morphologically indistinguishable from those of *T. gondii*. Tachyzoites are 1 to 5 μm × 5 to 7 μm, oval to crescent-shaped structures with a central metachromatic nucleus and lightly basophilic cytoplasm (see Table 5.1).

Sarcocystis neurona was diagnosed from a dog with pyogranulomatous pneumonia by strong reactivity with immunohistochemistry and consistent with DNA sequencing (Fig. 5.67). Definitive hosts such as opossums become infected after ingestion of muscle sarcocysts within intermediate hosts such as raccoons and skunks (Dubey et al., 2006) or grass, soil, or water contaminated with sporocysts. The rosette pattern of radial arrangement of merozoites (see Fig. 5.67A) has not been found with *Toxoplasma* or *Neospora*. Merozoites measure 2 by 5 μm, and schizonts (see Fig. 5.67A) are approximately 20 μm in diameter.

Amoebae

Acanthamoeba spp. are free-living amoebae found in fresh water, salt water, soil, dust, and sewage. They are more commonly found in the southeastern portion of the United States and represent one form that can infect animals. They are opportunistic parasites that can affect the lungs of immunocompromised people and animals through inhalation of cysts from the air or while swimming in contaminated water. A Texas puppy with respiratory signs and neurologic dysfunction was diagnosed with a brain mass and granulomatous pneumonia caused by an *Acanthamoeba* spp. infection; immunosuppression may have been predisposing (Reed et al., 2010). The organism was confirmed by immunofluorescence, real-time PCR assays, and cyst ultrastructure. Ultrastructure of the amoebic cysts in this case showed a cyst wall with two layers (ectocyst and endocyst that converge at wall pores); these features are characteristic of *Acanthamoeba* spp., helping to differentiate it from other amoebae. Cytopathologic features of amebiasis within a necrotic and markedly inflamed tissue include recognition of trophozoites (15–50 μm in diameter) and cyst forms (10–25 μm in diameter) (Fig. 5.68). The trophozoite contains abundant vacuolated and granular cytoplasm with a small, round nucleus and single large and prominent nucleolus. The cyst with 1 to 3 μm thick walls contains granulated material and occasionally discernible nucleoli. Single cases are described in German shepherd dogs, akitas, Labrador retrievers, and mixed breed dogs (Greene et al., 2012).

Multicellular Parasites

Numerous helminths are capable of infestation of the respiratory tract of dogs and cats. TW and BAL can be helpful in identifying either the larvae or the egg; however, the etiologic agent is not always present in the sample. An increase in airway eosinophils should be accompanied by heartworm and fecal testing.

Aelurostrongylus abstrusus (Fig. 5.69) is a feline metastrongyloid lungworm that is generally considered asymptomatic but may induce coughing. Adults live in respiratory bronchioles and alveoli and lay eggs in alveolar spaces, which hatch to release larvae (Table 5.5). The ova and larvae, not the adults, induce the inflammatory reaction (see Fig. 5.69A–C). Eosinophils and neutrophils found in TW or BAL samples characterize the early infection associated with the nodules. Similar to conditions found in *Filaroides* spp. infection, parasitic nodules are more commonly seen in the peripheral lung fields. As such, adult nematodes are typically not observed in TW or BAL samples but may be observed on tissue imprints or fine-needle aspirate biopsy of the lung nodules. With time, however, fibromuscular hyperplasia occurs, and the reaction appears more fibroblastic. Most typically, the larval stage is seen, but occasionally morulated and coiled larvated ova may also be identified (see Fig. 5.69B). The pale or unstained larvae are usually coiled on themselves or may be uncoiled (see Fig. 5.69C). The tail has a double bend and a dorsal spine with the kinked tail as a major characteristic feature of this larvae (see Fig. 5.69D), which is often obscured when tightly coiled.

Paragonimus kellicotti is a trematode primarily seen in cats and, less commonly, dogs, in North America, whereas *Paragonimus westermanii* is more common in Asia (see Table 5.5) (Palić et al., 2011; Lawson, 2020). The caudal lung lobes, particularly those of the right side, are frequently affected by this

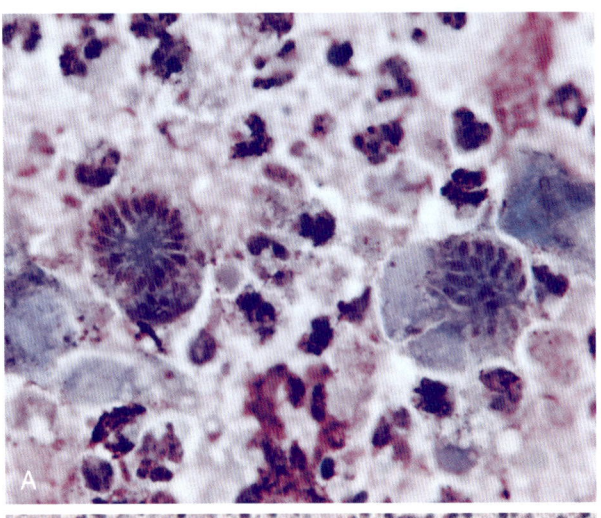

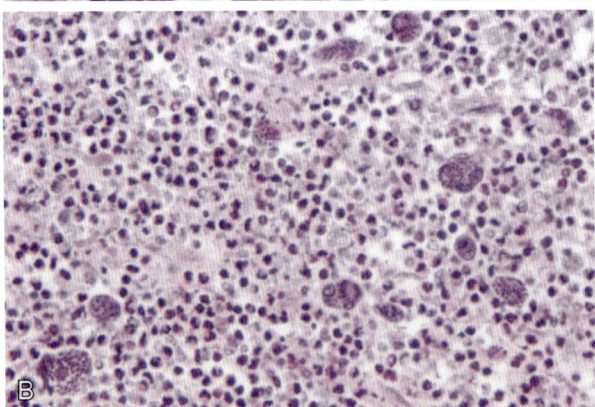

■ **FIGURE 5.67 Sarcocystosis.** Same case in A and B. **A, *Sarcocystis neurona* schizonts. Lung imprint. Dog.** Note two schizonts with magenta staining merozoites that appear to radiate from the center of the schizont; the left formation is denoted as a radial arrangement and the right formation as a haphazard arrangement. (Modified Wright; HP oil.) **B, *S. neurona* schizonts. Lung nodule. Dog.** The nine relatively huge schizonts are embedded in a mass of neutrophils. (H&E; IP.) (Courtesy Charlotte Hollinger et al., Michigan State University. Presented at the 2010 ASVCP case review session.)

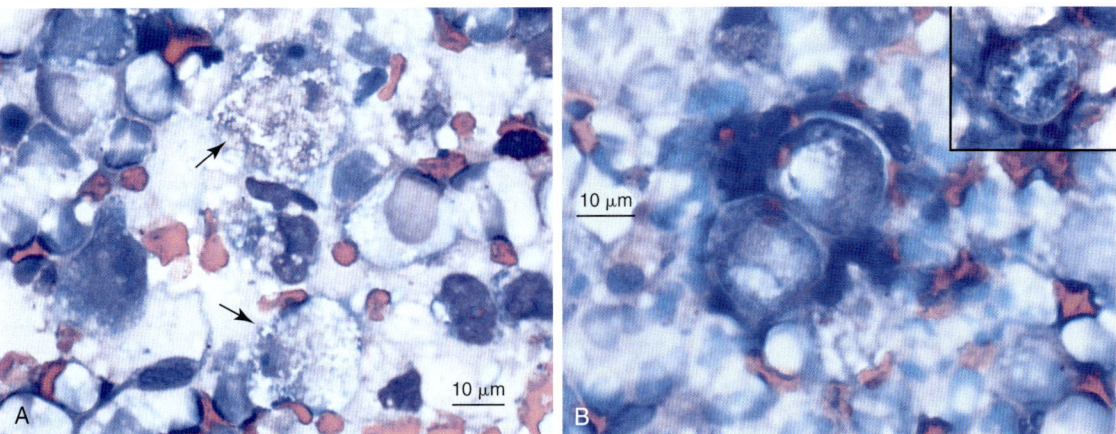

FIGURE 5.68 Acanthamoebiasis. Lung imprint. Dog. Same case in A and B. **A,** *Acanthamoeba* **spp. trophozoites.** Numerous macrophages and lymphocytes are shown along with two trophozoites *(arrows)*. This puppy concurrently had canine distemper virus and canine adenovirus-2 infections. (Modified Wright; HP oil.) **B,** *Acanthamoeba* **spp. cysts.** Two round cysts each contain a discernible nucleus with single prominent nucleolus. *Inset*: One cyst with distinct large basophilic cytoplasmic granules and thick colorless circumscribed wall. (Modified Romanowsky; HP oil.) (Courtesy Katie Boes et al., Purdue University. Presented at the 2010 ASVCP case review session.)

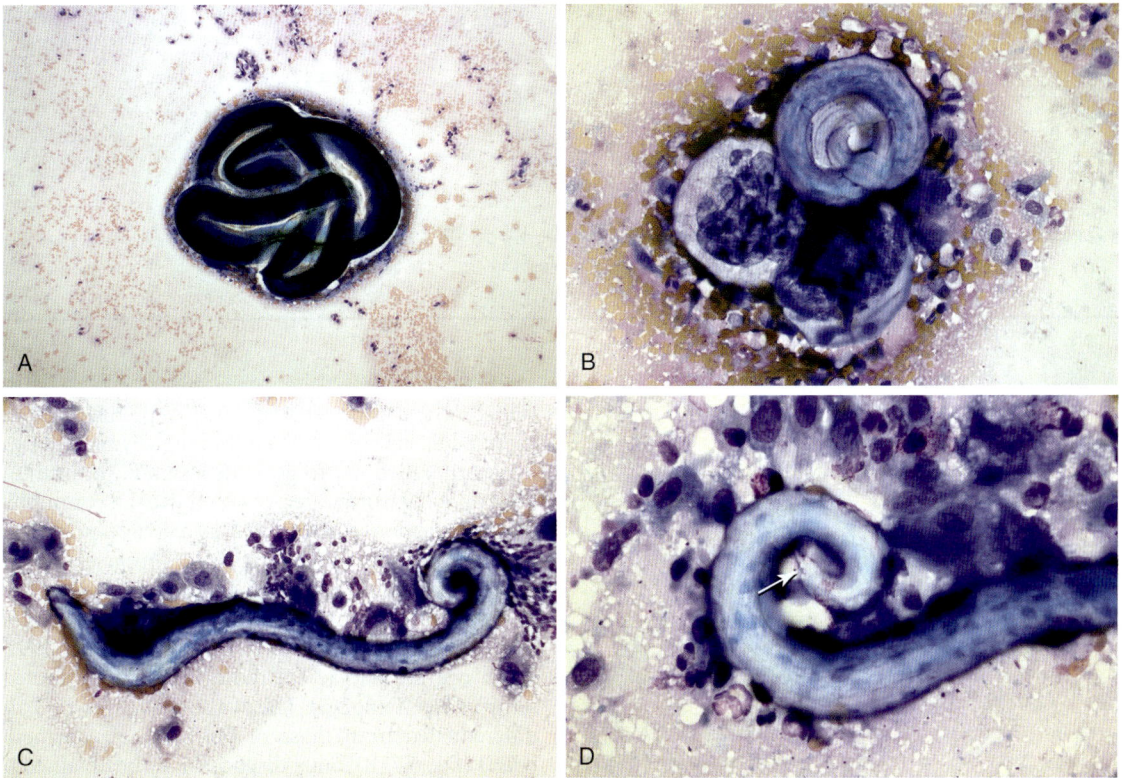

FIGURE 5.69 Aelurostrongyliasis. Lung imprint. Cat. Same case in A to D. **A, Adult.** A coiled fragment of an *Aelurostrongylus abstrusus* adult nematode is surrounded by respiratory epithelial cells and mixed inflammatory cells. (Wright-Giemsa; LP.) **B, Ova.** Three ova are surrounded by mixed inflammatory cells. Morulated eggs *(left)* develop into larvated eggs *(top right)* (Wright-Giemsa; IP.) **C, Larva.** Larvated eggs hatch to release first-stage larvae. (Wright-Giemsa; IP.) **D, Larval tail.** First-stage larvae have coiled tails that often obscure the distal tail kink *(arrow)*. (Wright-Giemsa; HP oil.) (Courtesy Katie Boes and D. Phillip Sponenberg, Virginia Tech University. Presented at the 2012 ASVCP case review session.)

lung fluke. This focal location within the caudal lung lobe makes cytopathologic viewing of the ova via TW or BAL difficult (Fig. 5.70); however, the eggs can be readily identified by fecal examination using either Baermann apparatus or flotation. Cytopathologic examination of the inflammatory cysts demonstrates numerous eosinophils with concurrent neutrophilic and macrophagic inflammation.

Eucoleus aerophilus (formerly *Capillaria aerophila*) is a parasite of dogs, foxes, and cats that lives in the trachea and bronchi but also can be found in the nasal passages. Parasite eggs may be observed in bronchial washings (Leissinger et al., 2016) (see Table 5.5).

The canine lungworm *Filaroides hirthi* lives in the alveoli and bronchioles (Rebar et al., 1992). Both embryonated ova and larvae

TABLE 5.5 Multicellular Parasites Found in Airway Samples From Dogs and Cats

PARASITE	DEFINITIVE HOST	ADULT LOCATION	ADULT MORPHOLOGY	OVA MORPHOLOGY	LARVA MORPHOLOGY
Nematodes					
Aelurostrongylus abstrusus	Cats	Bronchioles / Lung parenchyma	4–7 mm (M) / 9–10 mm (F)	80 × 70 μm / Morulated or larvated	360–400 μm / Kinked tail
Angiostrongylus vasorum	Dogs	Right heart / Pulmonary arteries	14–21 mm	50–60 μm / Morulated or larvated	310–400 μm / Kinked tail / Cephalic button
Crenosoma vulpis	Dogs	Trachea / Bronchi, bronchioles	3.5–8 mm (M) / 12–16 mm (F)	40–70 μm / Morulated or larvated	200–300 μm / Straight, pointed tail / Cephalic button
Filaroides hirthi	Dogs	Bronchioles / Lung parenchyma	2–3 mm (M) / 6–13 mm (F)	80 × 50 μm / Larvated	240–290 μm / Kinked tail
Oslerus (Filaroides) osleri	Dogs	Trachea / Bronchi	5 mm (M) / 9–15 mm (F)	80 × 50 μm / Larvated	232–266 μm / Kinked tail
Eucoleus (Capillaria) aerophilus	Dogs and cats	Trachea / Bronchi	15–25 mm (M) / 20–40 mm (F)	58–80 × 30–40 μm / Brown / Asymmetric bipolar opercula	—
Eucoleus (Capillaria) boehmi	Dogs	Nasal passages / Sinuses	15–40 mm in length	54–60 × 30–35 μm / Golden / Asymmetric bipolar opercula / Finely pitted surface	—
Dirofilaria immitis	Dogs and cats	Right heart / Pulmonary arteries	12–6 cm (M) / 25–30 cm (F)	—	290–330 μm / Tapered head / Straight tail
Trematodes					
Paragonimus kellicotti	Dogs and cats	Lung parenchyma	7–16 × 4–8 μm / Red-brown	75–118 × 42–67 μm / Yellow-brown / Single operculum	—

F, Female; *M*, male.

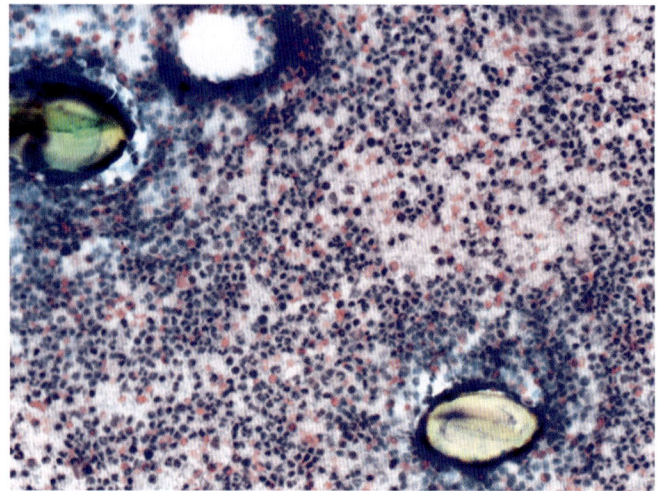

■ **FIGURE 5.70 Paragonimiasis. Lung mass aspirate. Cat.** Two light yellow-brown to translucent 100 × 50 μm ova are seen in a background of marked cellularity embedded in a massive sea of neutrophils, eosinophils, erythrocytes, and necrotic debris. The organism typically induces a strong eosinophilic and mixed cell inflammation. Fecal examination identified the parasite as *Paragonimus kellicotti*. (Wright-Giemsa; IP.) (Courtesy Linda Berent et al., University of Illinois. Presented at the 2001 ASVCP case review session.)

(Fig. 5.71A) can be retrieved by TW or BAL (see Table 5.5). *F. hirthi* adults live in alveoli and respiratory bronchioles. Although live worms tend not to generate a significant immune response, dead or dying worms are associated with an eosinophilic granulomatous reaction characterized by variable numbers of eosinophils, macrophages, and fibroblasts. *F. hirthi* larvae are more likely to incite a suppurative reaction than an eosinophilic reaction. Cytopathologic identification of adults or larvae is rare in samples obtained by FNA (Andreasen and Carmichael, 1992). Embryonated ova and larvae are more commonly detected by airway samples (see Table 5.5). The ova and larvae of *F. hirthi* cannot be differentiated from those of *Oslerus osleri* (formerly *Filaroides osleri*) (Fig. 5.71B), but a diagnosis may be obtained by localizing the infection to the pulmonary parenchyma or tracheobronchial tree (see Table 5.5). *F. hirthi* can be found in subpleural pulmonary nodules, whereas *O. osleri* forms tracheal nodules. There are fewer reports of *Filaroides milksi* infection in dogs. The two *Filaroides* species are differentiated based on subtle differences in adult worm size and morphology and not ova or egg morphology.

Crenosoma vulpis is a nematode lungworm of red foxes that also infects dogs (Matos et al., 2016). *C. vulpis* infection can be identified using BAL (Unterer et al., 2002). Inflammation with a predominance of eosinophils is most commonly found (Shaw et al., 1996); however, eosinophils with neutrophils as well as primarily neutrophilic inflammations are found rarely. Adult, ova, and larval stage of *C. vulpis* can be identified in TW or BAL fluid (Fig. 5.72). Fecal examination using Baermann technique

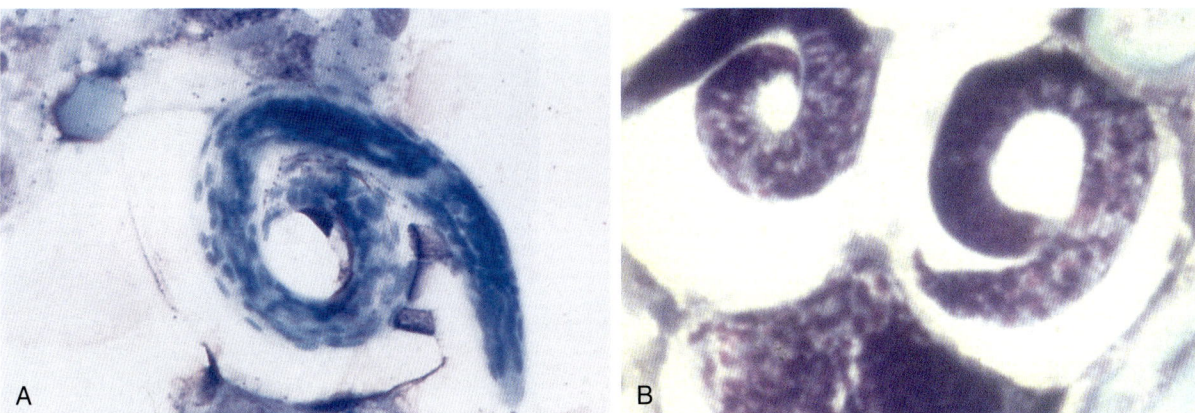

■ **FIGURE 5.71 Lungworm larvae. A,** *Filaroides hirthi* **larva. Bronchoalveolar lavage (BAL). Dog.** The larva is morphologically similar to those of *Aelurostrongylus* spp. and *Oslerus* spp. and can be distinguished by its kinked tail and finding characteristic larvae in the feces or BAL. (Wright-Giemsa; HP oil.) **B,** *Oslerus osleri* **larvae. Transtracheal wash. Dog.** A 10-month-old puppy was presented with a 3-month history of episodic labored breathing. Thoracic radiographs indicated a nodule on the trachea ventral wall that was confirmed by bronchoscopic examination. Two larvae are coiled, which obscures the distal tail kink. (B, Courtesy Bruce LeRoy and Gary Kociba, The Ohio State University. Presented at the 1995 ASVCP case review session.)

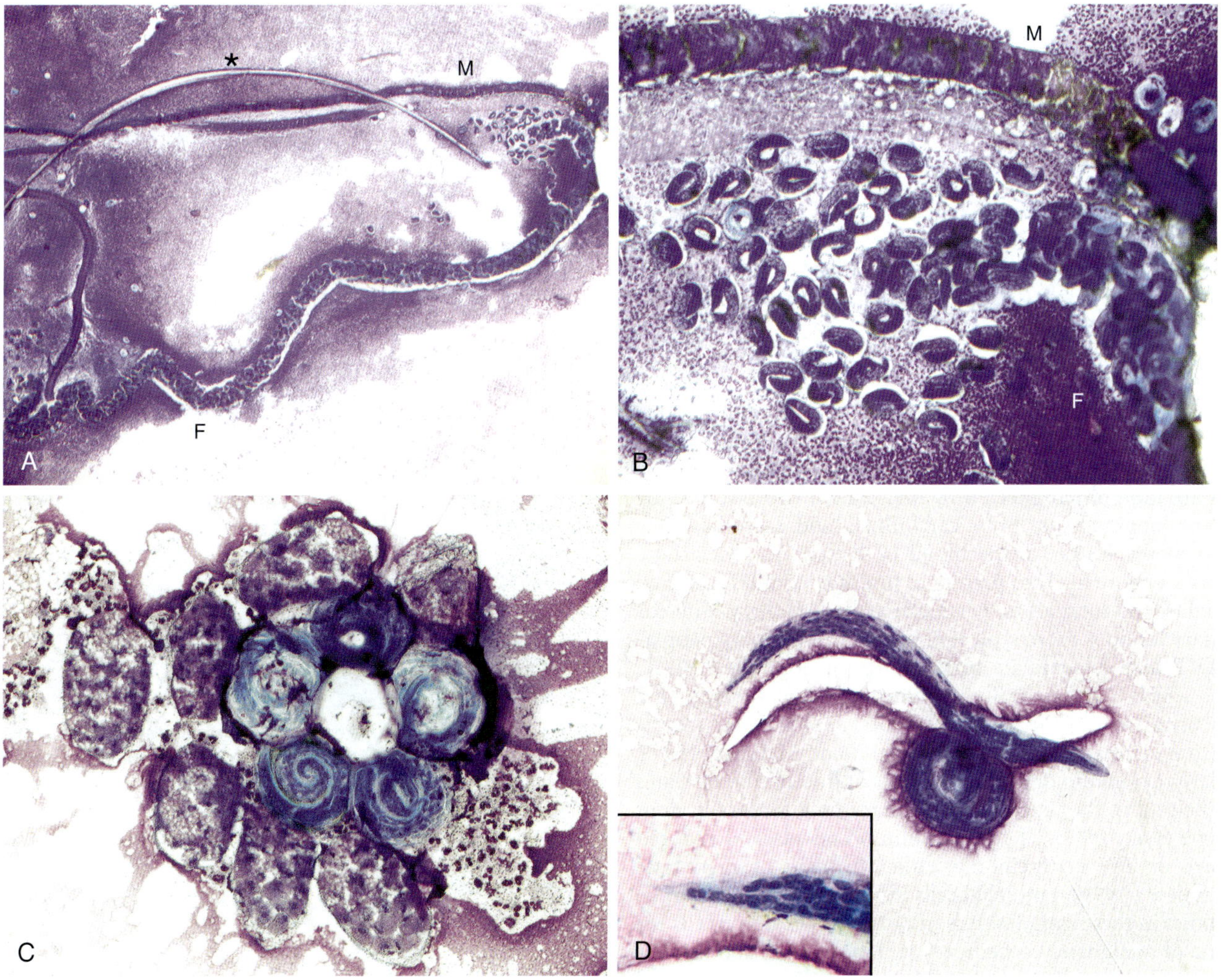

■ **FIGURE 5.72 Crenosomosis. Endotracheal wash. Dog.** Same case in A to D. **A,** Because of their large size, adult *Crenosoma vulpis* nematodes are best observed using low magnification. There are fragments of adult male (M) and female (F) nematodes. The female nematode is wider than the male and contains many oval eggs. A single, elliptical, nonstaining hair fragment *(asterisk)* is also present. (Wright-Giemsa; LP.) **B,** Fragments of male (M) and female (F) nematodes are surrounded by numerous degenerate neutrophils. The female is partially ruptured, allowing better visualization of the larvated eggs. (Wright-Giemsa; IP.) **C,** Five larvated eggs are surrounded by seven morulated eggs and degenerate neutrophils. (Wright-Giemsa; HP oil.) **D,** One larvated egg and one first-stage larva. (Wright-Giemsa; HP oil.). *Inset:* The larva has a smooth, pointed tail with a slight deflection. (Wright-Giemsa; HP oil.) (Courtesy Nicole Weinstein, University of Pennsylvania.)

is the most sensitive method for diagnosis (Unterer et al., 2002; McGarry and Morgan, 2009).

Angiostrongylus vasorum is a metastrongyloid nematode found in Europe and parts of North America, primarily throughout Atlantic Canada. Also known as the fox lungworm and French heartworm, the adults are found in the right side of the heart and pulmonary arteries of dogs. Eggs hatch quickly, and first-stage larvae migrate through the capillary beds into the bronchioles, bronchi, and trachea (Fig. 5.73). The most common respiratory signs include gagging, coughing and dyspnea, and bleeding in severe cases. Alveolar, interstitial, or mixed patterns are often detected in the peripheral lung fields by radiography; however, the disease presentation, as well as the presence of peripheral eosinophilia and BAL eosinophilic inflammation, is variable (Morgan and Shaw, 2010; Schnyder et al., 2010). Diagnosis depends on the identification of first-stage larvae in the feces via the Baermann test or direct fecal smears or in the respiratory tract fluids via either BAL or TW cytopathology (Conboy, 2004; Barçante et al., 2008; Morgan and Shaw, 2010; Morgan et al., 2010). However, negative larval identification does not rule out disease, and ELISA for circulating antibody detection or PCR on BAL material should be considered (Canonne et al., 2018). Another report used a commercial in-clinic detection test for an antigen released by *A. vasorum* adults in plasma or serum specimens, which has a relative sensitivity of 98.1% and a relative specificity of 99.4% compared with the Baermann technique (Palić et al., 2017). *A. vasorum* first-stage larvae can be differentiated from *C. vulpis* larvae based on the morphology of their tails. The tails of *A. vasorum* larvae are longer than those of other species and have an indentation on both the dorsal and ventral surface as well as a dorsal spine, whereas the tails of *C. vulpis* larvae are pointed and lack indentations (McGarry and Morgan, 2009).

Neoplastic Tumors

Primary as well as metastatic neoplasia of the lung and respiratory tree can be diagnosed through bronchial washings and lung aspiration. In dogs and cats, especially young animals, the lungs are more often affected by metastatic neoplasia than by primary lung tumors. Both carcinomas and sarcomas may spread to the lungs via the blood or lymphatics. Metastatic tumors are more likely to present as multiple nodules scattered throughout all lung lobes, particularly the periphery, whereas a solitary lesion is more typical of primary pulmonary neoplasia. TVT may disseminate to the lungs of dogs (Park et al., 2006), which may be readily identified by cytopathology. In a study of cats with primary lung tumors, 38 of 45 were identified from cytopathologic samples (Hahn and McEntee, 1997). Similarly, cytopathologic examinations of fine-needle aspirates were helpful in the diagnosis of primary lung tumors in dogs (Ogilvie et al., 1989). The most common neoplasia diagnosed by BAL or TW is carcinoma, either primary or metastatic (Rebar et al., 1992). Epithelial cells exfoliate readily and can be identified in these samples. It is important to examine cells for criteria of malignancy, specifically variation in cell and nuclear size, prominent nucleoli, multiple nuclei and/or nucleoli, and nuclear molding (Fig. 5.74). Dysplastic or metaplastic changes to epithelial cells secondary to inflammation can complicate the diagnosis, so the sample should be scrutinized for evidence of inflammation.

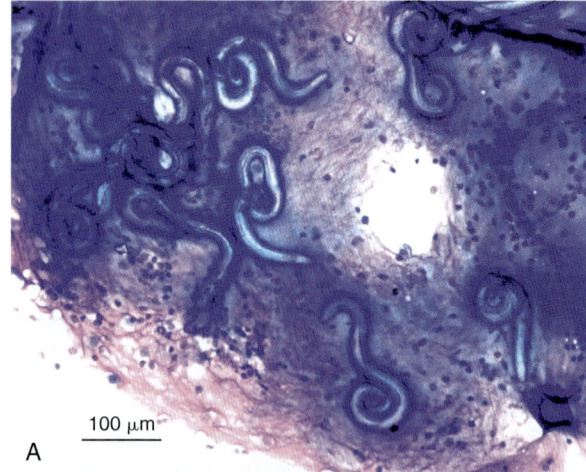
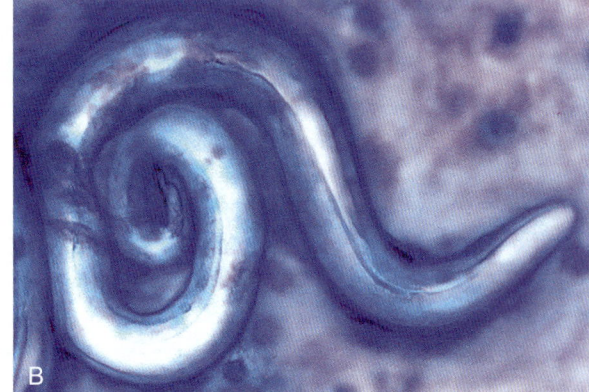
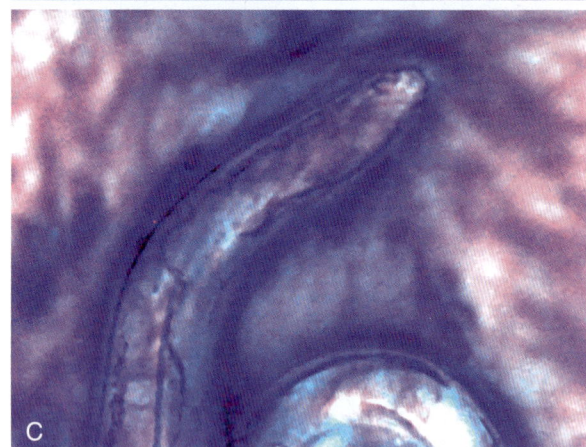

■ **FIGURE 5.73 Angiostrongyliasis. Bronchoalveolar lavage. Dog.** Same case in A to C. **A,** Many *Angiostrongylus* spp. larvae have coiled tails. (Methanolic Romanowsky; IP.) **B,** *Angiostrongylus* spp. larva with a coiled tail that terminates with a distal tail kink. (Methanolic Romanowsky, HP oil.) **C,** *Angiostrongylus* spp. larval head showing a button projection. (Methanolic Romanowsky; HP oil.) (Courtesy Pierre Deshuillers, Toulouse, France.)

Epithelial Neoplasia

Multiple types of lung carcinomas have been identified in dogs and cats. Adenocarcinomas of bronchogenic or bronchiolar/alveolar origin are most prevalent; however, carcinomas can arise from any level of the respiratory epithelium (Figs. 5.75 and 5.76).

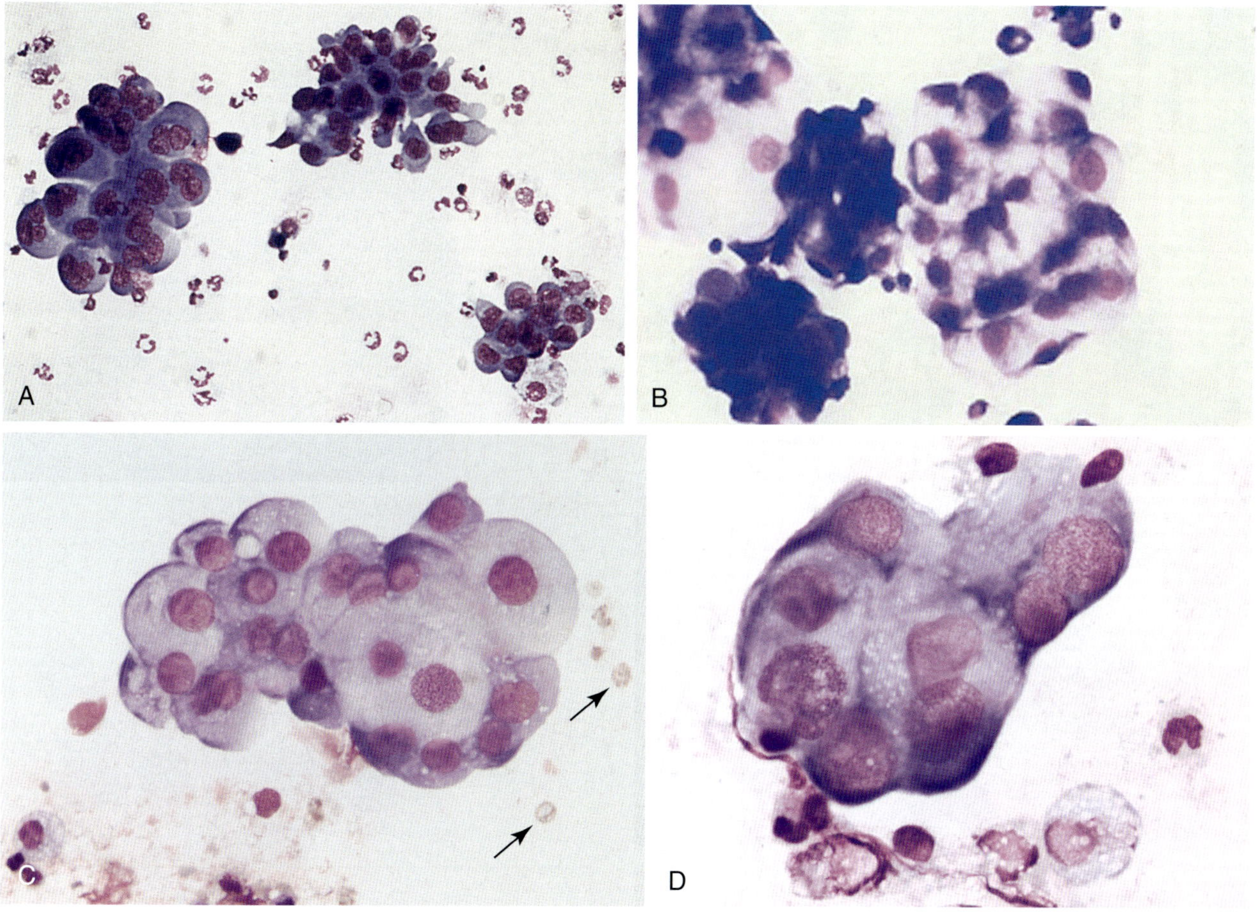

■ **FIGURE 5.74 A, Pulmonary carcinoma. Bronchoalveolar lavage. Dog.** Large clusters of cohesive pleomorphic epithelium that appear to form acinar structures, suggestive of an adenocarcinoma, are surrounded by neutrophils. Multinucleated forms are noted. Neutrophils can be used to appreciate the relative size of the neoplastic cells if present. (Methanolic Romanowsky; IP.) **B, Carcinoma. Transtracheal wash (TTW). Dog.** Clusters of cohesive variably sized epithelial cells some with dark basophilic cytoplasm and some with pale, abundant cytoplasm, which suggests a secretory function of an adenocarcinoma. (Wright-Giemsa; IP.) **C, Carcinoma. TTW. Dog.** Cluster of very large, lightly basophilic cohesive variably sized epithelial cells with finely stippled chromatin and indistinct nucleoli. Erythrocytes (arrows) can be used to appreciate the relative size of the neoplastic cells. (Wright-Giemsa; HP oil.) **D, Carcinoma. TTW. Dog.** Cohesive cluster of anaplastic epithelial cells. A neutrophil and macrophage in the lower right can be used to appreciate the relative size of the neoplastic cells. (Wright-Giemsa; HP oil.) (A, Courtesy Robert King, University of Florida.)

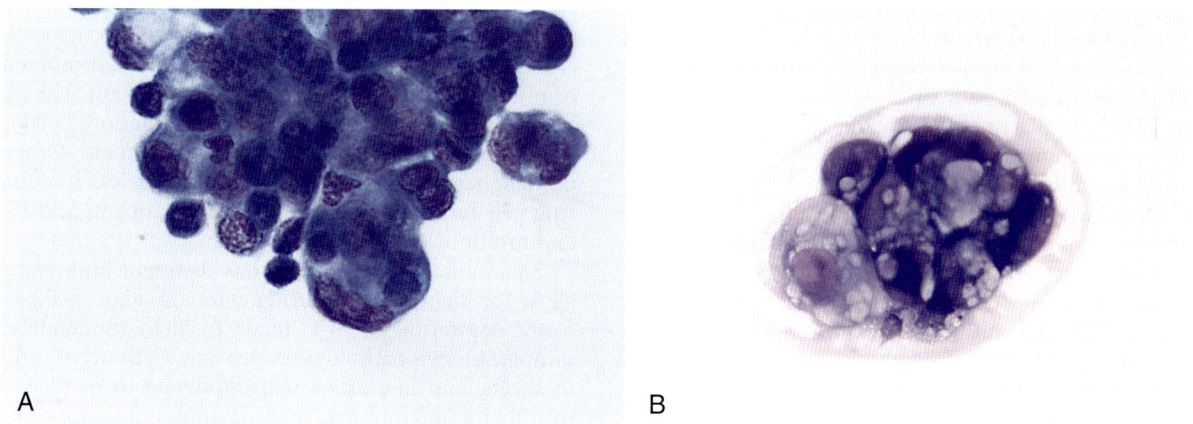

■ **FIGURE 5.75 Bronchogenic carcinoma. A,** Cohesive cluster of basophilic pleomorphic epithelial cells with high nucleocytoplasmic ratios. (Wright-Giemsa; IP.) **B, Pleural fluid. Dog.** Cells from bronchogenic carcinomas that exfoliate into the thoracic fluid may have prominent vacuolation due to the fluid environment or secretory function. (Wright-Giemsa; HP oil.)

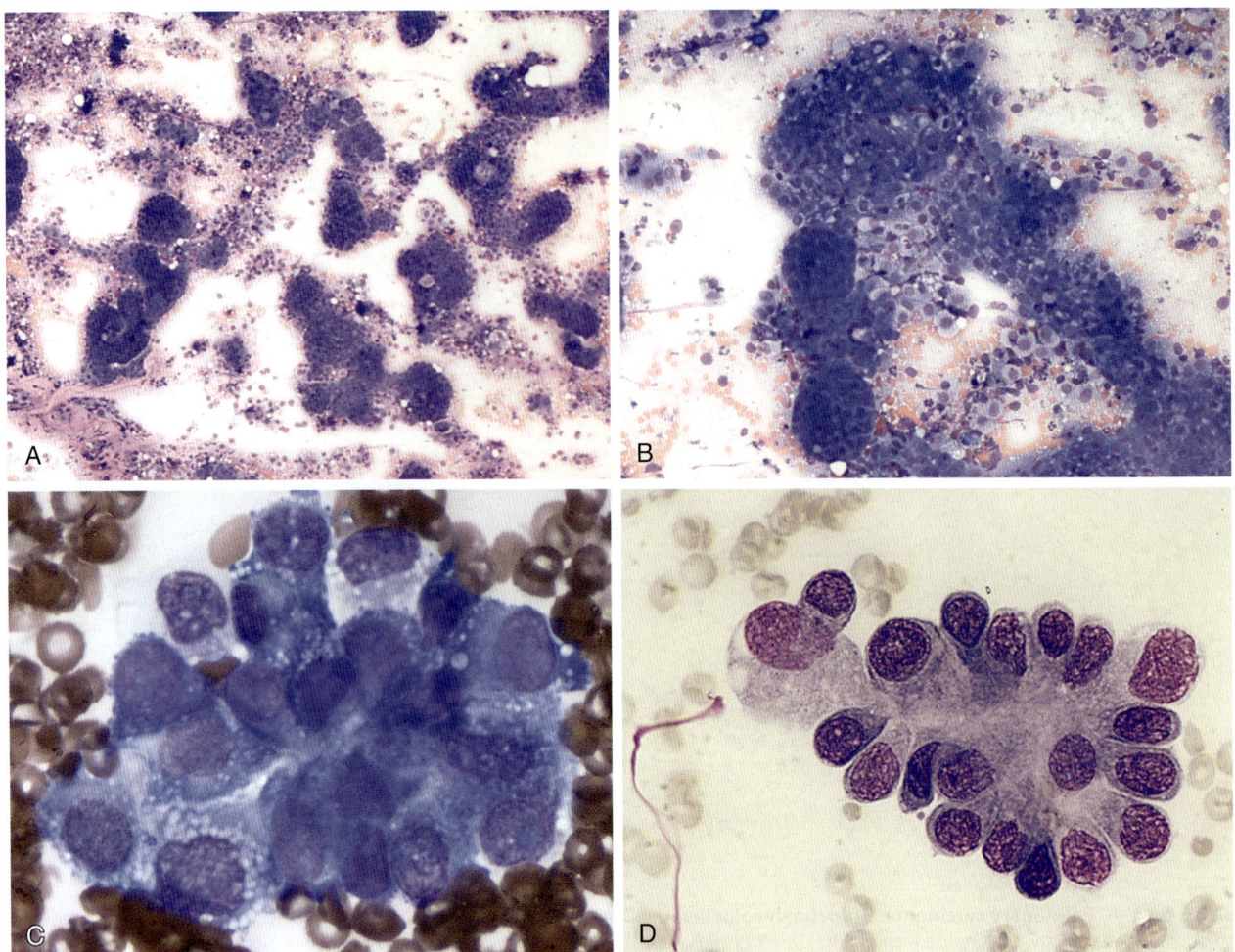

■ **FIGURE 5.76 Adenocarcinoma. Lung. Dog.** Same case in A to C. **A,** Dense sheets and trabecular pattern appear at low magnification. (Wright-Giemsa; LP) **B,** Balls of densely populated cohesive basophilic cells and attendant rows of neoplastic cells suggestive of tubular formation. (Wright-Giemsa; IP) **C,** Cohesive, acinar-like arrangement of cells containing numerous punctate cytoplasmic vacuoles. (Wright-Giemsa; HP oil.) **D,** Acinar formation with nuclei around the circumference suggests glandular origin. (Wright-Giemsa; HP oil.) (D, Courtesy Rose Raskin, University of Florida.)

Cytopathologic differentiation is not possible. Lung carcinomas most typically present as multifocal nodules seen in the periphery of the lung lobes; however, they may involve the entire lung lobe or be present only in the hilar region. Eosinophilic infiltrates may occur in association with bronchoalveolar carcinoma in dogs (Fig. 5.77A). Papillary patterns are identified by cytopathology and may be accompanied by significant mixed neutrophilic and macrophagic inflammation (Fig. 5.77B–D).

Numerous carcinomas metastasize to the pulmonary parenchyma, such as mammary carcinomas and carcinomas of the urinary bladder, prostate, and endocrine glands. cytopathologic preparations from primary and metastatic carcinomas are similar, and the two are difficult to definitively differentiate by cytologic evaluation alone (Figs. 5.78 and 5.79).

Aspirates contain moderate numbers of epithelial cells in sheets, aggregates, and clusters with fewer numbers of individualized cells. Individual cells may appear round and can be confused with discrete cell neoplasia, but they are typically larger than those from discrete cell tumors and can be distinguished by finding cell-to-cell association. Acinar formation indicates glandular origin, suggesting an adenocarcinoma. Moderate to marked pleomorphism between clumps of cells, as well as within cells of the same cluster, is common in pulmonary carcinomas. Nuclei are round and frequently eccentrically placed and contain coarsely clumped chromatin and prominent, single to multiple nucleoli. Anisokaryosis is common. The cytoplasm is deeply basophilic, and punctate vacuolation, particularly in the perinuclear region, is frequently prominent. Other criteria of malignancy that may be seen include nuclear molding, signet ring cell formation, cell or nuclear gigantism, and binucleate and multinucleate cells.

Squamous cell carcinoma has distinguishing features that allow for identification during cytopathologic evaluation (Fig. 5.80). Aspiration of SCC tends to yield moderately cellular samples for cytopathologic evaluation. Cells occur individually, in sheets, and in clusters with moderate to marked variation in cell size, nuclear size, nucleocytoplasmic ratios, amount of cytoplasm, and degree of keratinization. Individual cell morphology ranges from basal squamous cells with little or no keratinization to fully keratinized squamous cells. The basal cells are cuboidal to round with deeply basophilic cytoplasm, large central nuclei, coarse chromatin, and prominent nucleoli.

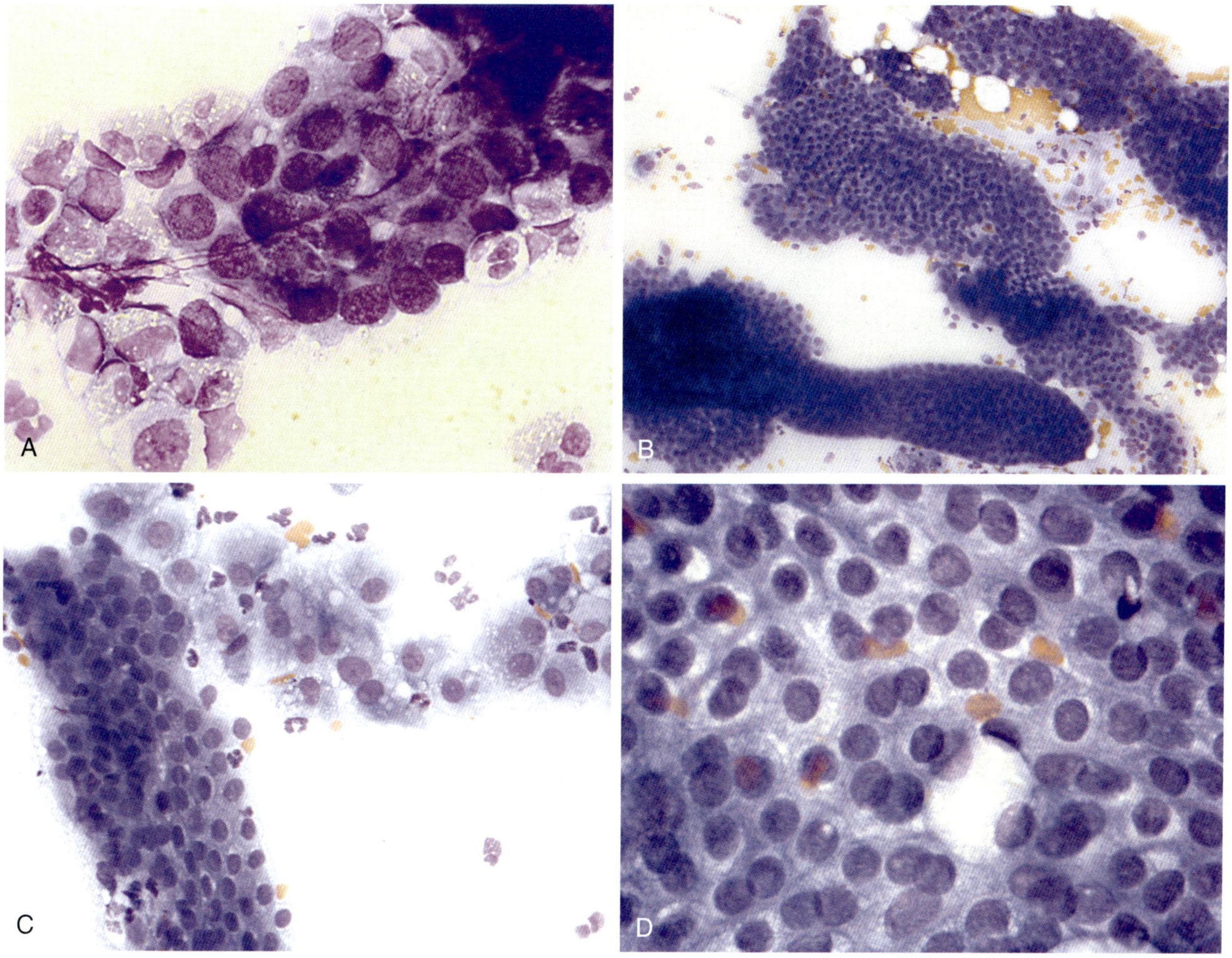

FIGURE 5.77 Lung adenocarcinoma. A, Eosinophilic infiltrate. Lung mass imprint. Dog. Malignant epithelial cell cluster along with numerous eosinophils that surround and penetrate the neoplasm. Many eosinophils appear vacuolated, but granules are found in other cells. Peripheral eosinophilia was not noted in this case. (Wright-Giemsa; HP oil.) **Papillary adenocarcinoma with mixed-cell inflammation. Lung mass aspirate. Dog.** Same case in B to D. **B,** Large 5 × 5 × 5 cm right caudal lung mass exfoliates with high cellularity. On scanning at low magnification, a papillary or tubular pattern becomes evident. (Wright-Giemsa; IP.) **C,** Papillary formation with epithelial cells lining up along the edge. Numerous large foamy and vacuolated macrophages infiltrate along with nondegenerate neutrophils. (Wright-Giemsa; HP oil.) **D,** Sheet of epithelium displaying minimal characteristics of malignancy. These cells have moderate amounts of basophilic foamy or vacuolated cytoplasm. Binucleation is common along with mild anisokaryosis supporting a low grade of malignancy. (A, Courtesy Karen Young and Richard Meadows, University of Wisconsin. Presented at the 1992 ASVCP case review session. B–D, Courtesy Rose Raskin, University of Florida.)

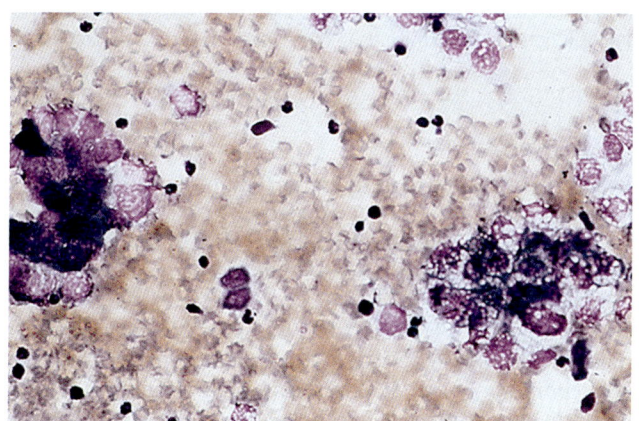

FIGURE 5.78 Metastatic carcinoma. Lung. Dog. A metastatic lesion to the lung was suspected to have originated from a urethral carcinoma. (Wright-Giemsa; HP oil.) (Courtesy Rose Raskin, University of Florida.)

Mature squamous cells are large with abundant homogenous cytoplasm and pyknotic or karyorrhectic nuclei. Asynchrony of cytoplasmic and nuclear maturation is common in SCC.

Squamous metaplasia may occur with chronic inflammation, and caution should be taken when differentiating squamous metaplasia from neoplasia (see Fig. 5.46). However, SCC of the lung typically originates from areas of squamous metaplasia of the bronchial epithelium, suggesting that metaplasia may readily proceed to neoplasia in the lower respiratory tract. Bronchogenic tumors frequently contain both glandular and squamous components. Recent classification of lung tumors in humans and veterinary medicine uses histologic patterns without reference to possible cell of origin (Wilson, 2017).

Mesenchymal Neoplasia

Tumors arising from the pulmonary connective tissue are relatively rare in dogs and cats. These include osteosarcoma,

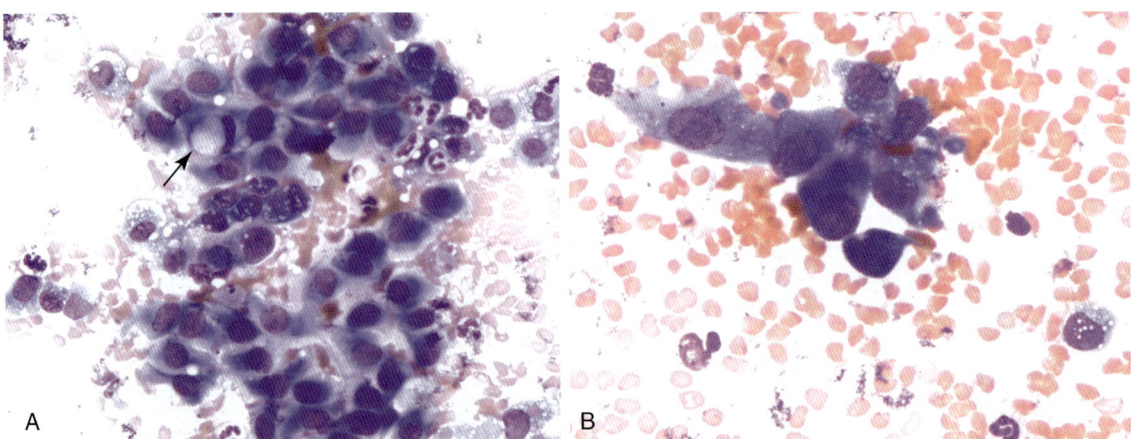

■ **FIGURE 5.79 Anaplastic carcinoma. Dog.** Same case in A and B. **A,** Dense clusters of epithelial cells with moderate to marked pleomorphism. Some cells appear cohesive, whereas others have wispy, spindled borders and others appear round in shape. The origin of this neoplasia was not determined. A large secretory vacuole giving a signet ring appearance is seen in the upper cluster of cells *(arrow)*. Note the large size of the neoplastic cells relative to the neutrophils. (Wright-Giemsa; HP oil.) **B,** Note the spindle-shaped appearance of the cells in this cluster even though histopathology confirmed the diagnosis of an anaplastic carcinoma. (Wright-Giemsa; HP oil.)

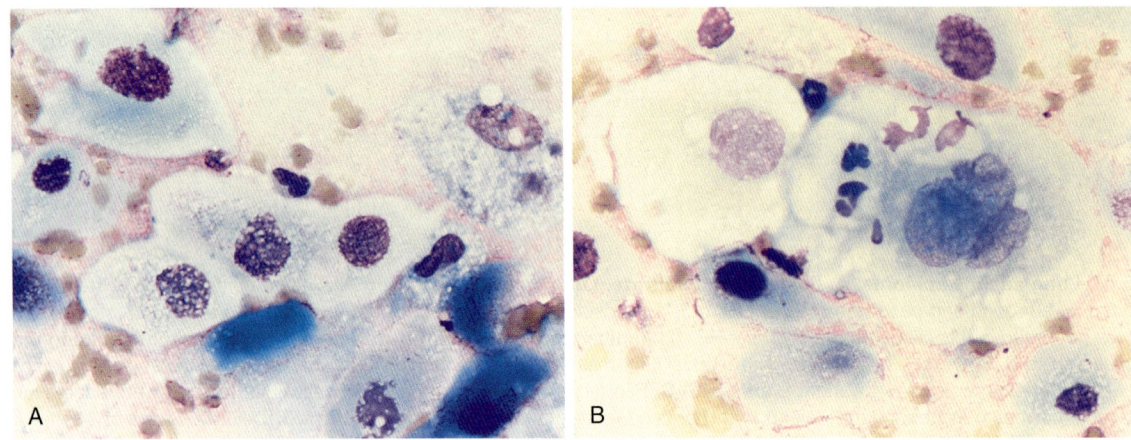

■ **FIGURE 5.80 Squamous cell carcinoma. Cat. A,** Multiple squamous cells in various stages of keratinization, including aqua blue staining anuclear keratin flakes. A macrophage is located in the *upper right*. (Wright-Giemsa; HP oil.) **B,** Very large squamous epithelial cells. The cell on the *far right* has multiple nucleoli that exhibit emperipolesis involving neutrophils. Emperipolesis is the presence of an intact cell within the cytoplasm of another cell. Emperipolesis is unlike phagocytosis in which the engulfed cell is killed by the lysosomal enzymes of the macrophage. Instead, the engulfed cell remains viable within the other and can exit at any time without causing structural or functional abnormalities in either cell. The biological process has no known diagnostic importance. (Wright-Giemsa; HP oil.)

chondrosarcoma, hemangiosarcoma, fibrosarcoma, rhabdomyoma, rhabdomyosarcoma, and schwannoma. When reported, the neoplastic cell population resembles those seen in the more common sites (Fig. 5.81). Metastatic neoplasms such as hemangiosarcoma or melanoma may be found in the lung (Figs. 5.82 and 5.83).

Hemolymphatic Neoplasia

Hemolymphatic neoplasia may disseminate throughout the parenchyma, resulting in diffuse infiltrative disease or as discrete nodules. Several round cell cytomorphologic types have been identified, including lymphoma and histiocytic sarcoma. These are more commonly reported in dogs than in cats (Fig. 5.84).

Lymphoma. Bronchoalveolar lavage samples have been shown to be more sensitive than radiographs in diagnosing malignant multicentric lymphoma (Fig. 5.85) (Hawkins et al., 1993, 1995; Yohn et al., 1994). However, BAL is likely only important for staging this neoplasm because primary lung lymphoma has not been reported to occur in animals, as it has in humans. The degree of involvement by a monomorphic population of lymphoid cells is helpful in distinguishing between a reactive population of lymphocytes, especially when malignant features are minimal (Fig. 5.86A). Histopathology with immunophenotyping may be

CHAPTER 5 Respiratory System

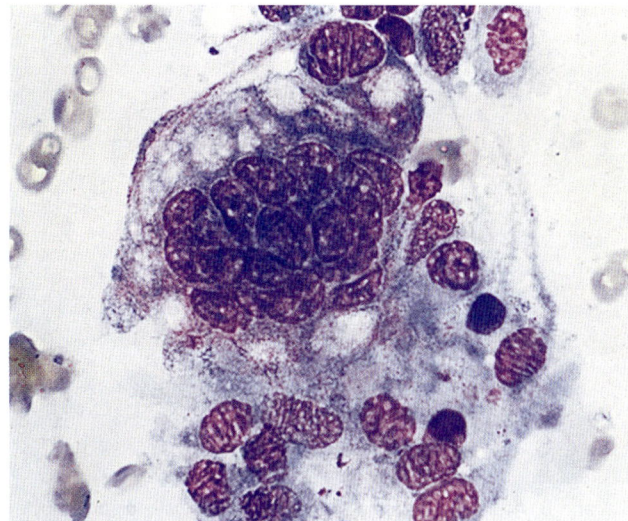

■ **FIGURE 5.81 Giant cell sarcoma. Lung mass. Dog.** Multinucleate giant cell with attendant spindle-shaped sarcoma cells with stippled nuclear chromatin and minimal pale staining cytoplasm. Surrounding erythrocytes can be used to appreciate the relatively gigantic size of the neoplastic cell, which appears morphologically similar to a megakaryocyte. (Wright-Giemsa; HP oil.) (Courtesy Rick Alleman, University of Florida.)

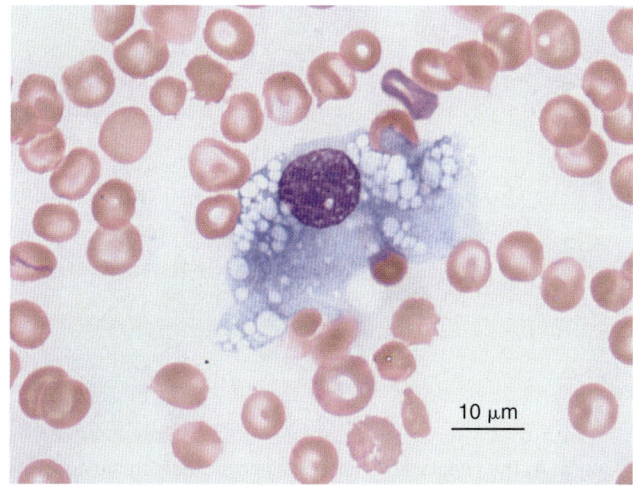

■ **FIGURE 5.82 Disseminated hemangiosarcoma. Lung aspirate biopsy. Dog.** A single neoplastic endothelial cell is characterized by a large round nucleus containing multiple prominent nucleoli and coarse chromatin. The abundant wispy lightly basophilic cytoplasm contains several variably sized punctate vacuoles. Necropsy with histopathology confirmed a widespread involvement of the lungs, kidney, and heart. (Wright-Giemsa; HP oil.) (Courtesy Rose Raskin, University of Florida.)

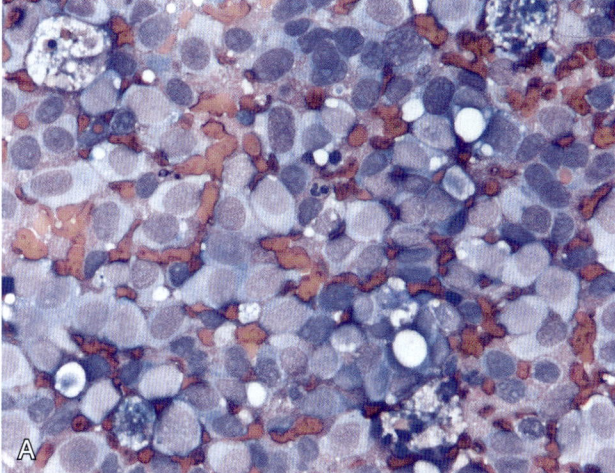

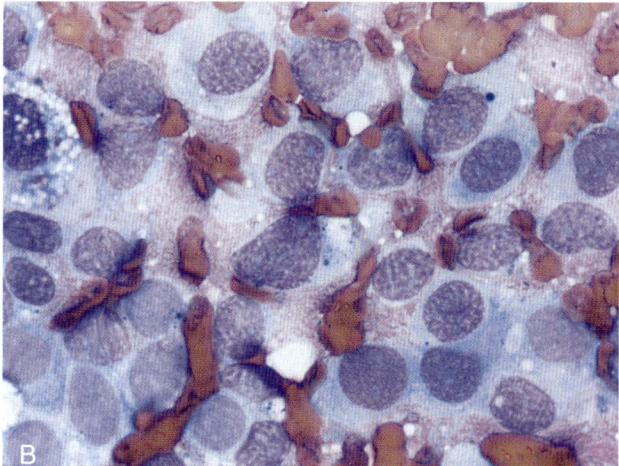

■ **FIGURE 5.83 Metastatic amelanotic melanoma. Lung aspirate. Dog.** Same case in A and B. **A,** Pleomorphic individualized cells with high nuclear to cytoplasm ratio and scant to moderate pale-staining cytoplasm. Erythrocytes can be used to determine their relatively large size. There are four vacuolated macrophages with ingested debris, some of which may be black melanin pigment; hence they would be termed melanophages. (Wright-Giemsa; IP.) **B,** Higher magnification to demonstrate the rare melanin granules (center cell). Partial view of a foamy macrophage with phagocytized debris to the *left*. (Wright-Giemsa; HP oil.)

helpful in establishing the malignant nature of the lymphoid population (Fig. 5.86B–D).

Histiocytic sarcoma. The lung is one of the primary sites of infiltration in histiocytic sarcoma of both dogs and cats. Early reports suggested a predisposition in Bernese mountain dogs, rottweilers, golden retrievers, and flat-coated retrievers. Recent reports show that miniature schnauzers in the United States and Pembroke Welsh corgis in Japan have a high risk and more commonly have localized lung involvement (Takahashi et al., 2014). Histiocytic neoplasia in dogs has been defined as a spectrum of diseases characterized by proliferation of Langerhans dendritic cells, interstitial dendritic cells, or macrophages (Affolter and Moore, 2000, 2002; Moore et al., 2006; Mastrorilli et al., 2012; Moore, 2014). Histiocytic sarcoma occurs in cats, primarily affecting the liver, spleen, and bone marrow more commonly than the lung (Walton et al., 1997; Kraje et al., 2001; Busch et al., 2008). The cell of origin in cat appears variable because one report suggests that at least in some cases, histiocytic sarcoma in cats may originate in the skin similar to Langerhans cells; however, another report characterizes a case of macrophage origin (Affolter and Moore, 2006; Busch et al., 2008; Friedrichs and Young, 2008). Malignant histiocytes are large, often markedly pleomorphic discrete cells that contain abundant, often vacuolated, deeply basophilic cytoplasm. Nuclei are oval to reniform with lacy or coarsely stippled chromatin and prominent multiple nucleoli (Figs. 5.87 and 5.88). A

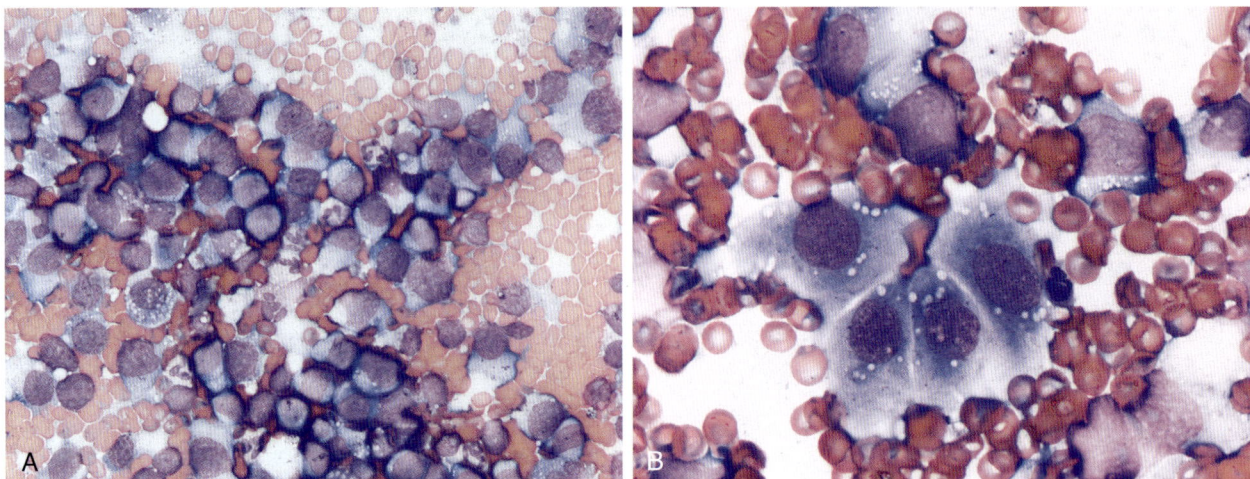

■ **FIGURE 5.84 Pulmonary lymphoma. Lung aspirate. Dog.** Same case in A and B. **A,** Large lymphoid cells with occasionally distinct nucleoli and scant to moderate amounts of lightly staining basophilic cytoplasm. (Wright-Giemsa; IP.) **B,** Four reactive hyperplastic cohesive respiratory epithelial cells with basophilic cytoplasm surrounding a round to oval nucleus with granular chromatin are located beneath three neoplastic lymphocytes. Surrounding erythrocytes can be used to appreciate the relative size of the nucleated cell types. There is scattered pink staining free nuclear protein. (Wright-Giemsa; HP oil.)

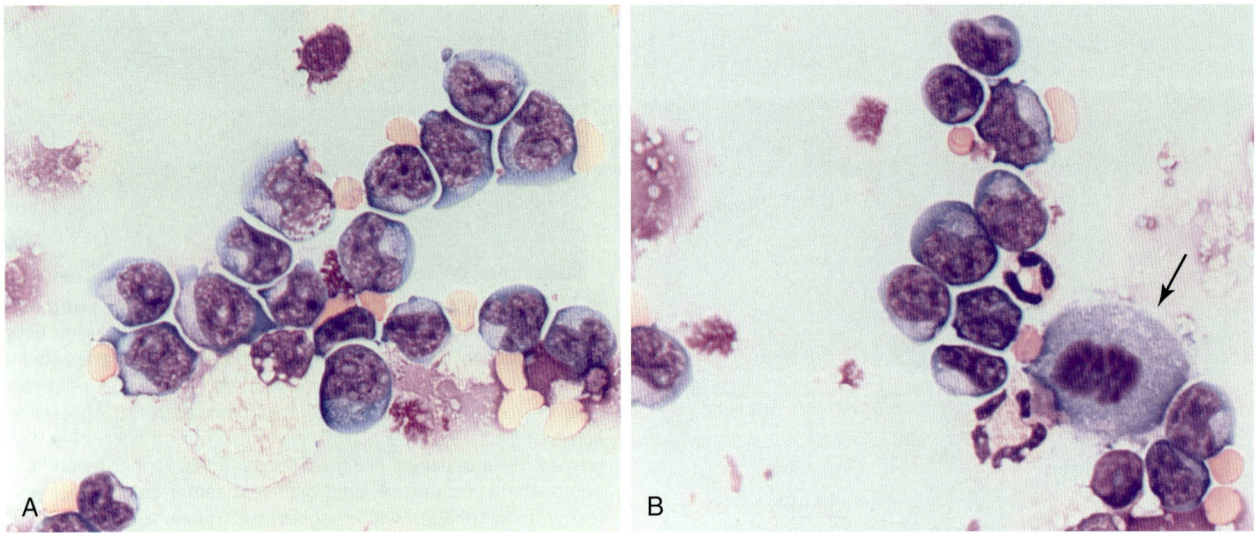

■ **FIGURE 5.85 Lymphoma. Bronchoalveolar lavage. Dog.** Same case in A and B. **A,** The neoplastic lymphocytes have pleomorphic nuclei that are oval to oblong to kidney bean shaped; some contain a bluish nucleoli set in a clumped chromatin nucleus. A perinuclear unstained area is apparent in many cells that contain faint azurophilic granules (not visible), a morphologic feature of unknown significance. (Wright-Giemsa; HP oil.) **B,** Mitotic figure (arrow). Large size of the neoplastic lymphocytes can be appreciated by comparison with the two neutrophils. (Wright-Giemsa; HP oil.) (Courtesy Michel Desnoyers et al., University of Montreal. Presented at the 2001 ASVCP case review session.)

continuum between discrete histiocytic cells and spindled mesenchymal cells is seen; the appearance frequently varies in masses from the same animal and may even vary from different sites of the same mass. Multinucleated cells are frequently present, but the number seen is variable (see Fig. 5.87B). Cells may also exhibit phagocytosis of erythrocytes and leukocytes, which helps to suggest a macrophagic origin; however, phagocytosis is not a consistent feature. Histiocytic sarcoma can be cytopathologically difficult to differentiate from granulomatous inflammation, large cell anaplastic carcinoma, large cell T-cell lymphoma, and plasmacytoma or extramedullary myeloma.

Positive immunoreactivity to lysozyme, CD1a, CD18, CD163, CD204, MAC387, MHC class II, and Iba1 have been used to identify histiocytic (dendritic and macrophagic) conditions (Brown et al., 1994; Mastrorilli et al., 2012; Moore, 2014; Pierezan et al., 2014). Transmission electron microscopy has been able to demonstrate intracytoplasmic organelles consistent with Birbeck granules of Langerhans cells in the pulmonary histiocytes in the cat (Busch et al., 2008).

*"**Lymphomatoid Granulomatosis.**"* Pulmonary lymphomatoid granulomatosis is an uncommon pleocellular lymphoid neoplasia that has been reported primarily in young to middle-aged

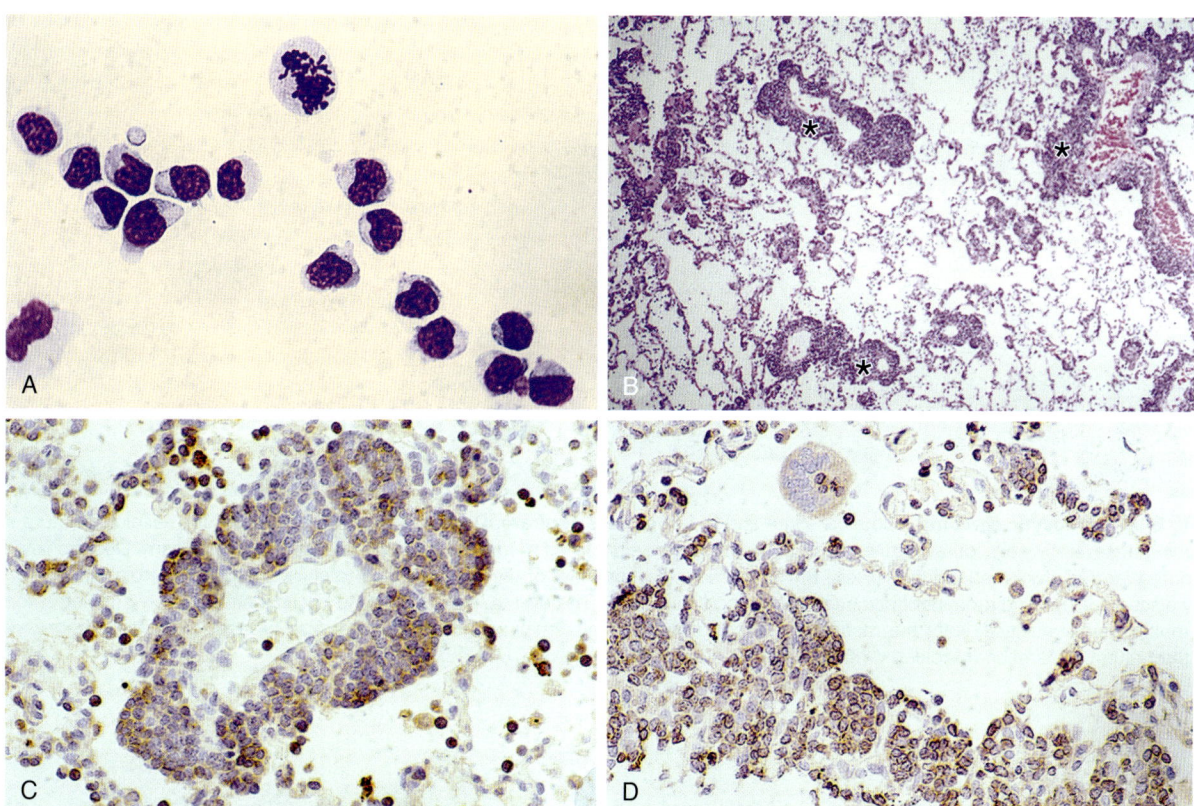

■ **FIGURE 5.86 Pulmonary lymphoma. Dog.** Same case in A to D. **A, Bronchoalveolar lavage.** Increased fluid cell count (945 cells/µL) with 79% medium-sized lymphocytes having a uniform appearance. Note the atypical mitotic figure in *top center*. (Wright-Giemsa; HP oil.) **B, Lung section.** Neoplastic lymphocytes were present primarily as a cuff around blood vessels and bronchioles *(asterisks)*. Evidence for vascular invasion and destruction was absent. This dog presented with only respiratory signs, suggesting a possible primary pulmonary lymphoma. (H&E; LP.) **C, Lung section.** Positive immunoreactivity confirming the presence of T-lymphocytes around a blood vessel and occasionally dispersed within alveolar septae. (anti-CD3/diaminobenzidine Chromagen; HP oil.) **D, Pulmonary lymphoma. Lung section.** Dense reactivity by cuffed lymphoid cells with a T-cell marker. Note the negative reaction of the multinucleated giant cell at the *top center* with intracellular T-lymphocytes. (anti-CD3/diaminobenzidine Chromagen; HP oil.) (Courtesy Rose Raskin, University of Florida.)

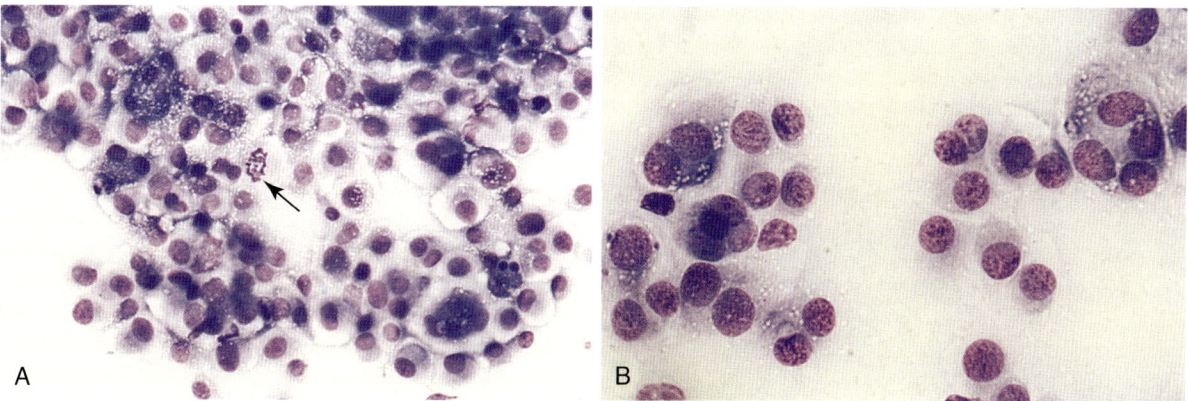

■ **FIGURE 5.87 Histiocytic sarcoma.** Same case in A and B. **A, Lung imprint. Dog.** Highly cellular collection of atypical cells with round nuclei and moderate clear to basophilic cytoplasm with occasional punctate vacuoles. Note the mitotic figure *(arrow)*. (Modified Wright; HP oil.) **B,** Frequent binucleate and multinucleate forms are present in this field. Nuclei are often eccentrically located with distinct to indistinct cytoplasmic borders. Immunoreactivity (not shown) for a histiocytic marker (anti-CD18 antigen) was positive to confirm cell origin. (Modified Wright; HP oil.)

dogs (Postorino et al., 1989; Fitzgerald et al., 1991; Bain et al., 1997). The term *lymphomatoid granulomatosis* is controversial because it actually describes the pattern of disease seen with several different types of lymphoma and inflammatory diseases. Typically, extensive infiltration of one or more lung lobes occurs with angiocentric and angiodestructive features. The morphology is characterized by variable numbers of large, pleomorphic, mononuclear cells that range from lymphoid to plasmacytoid to histiocytic in appearance; binucleate cells and mitoses are common (Fig. 5.89). Neoplastic cells may comprise

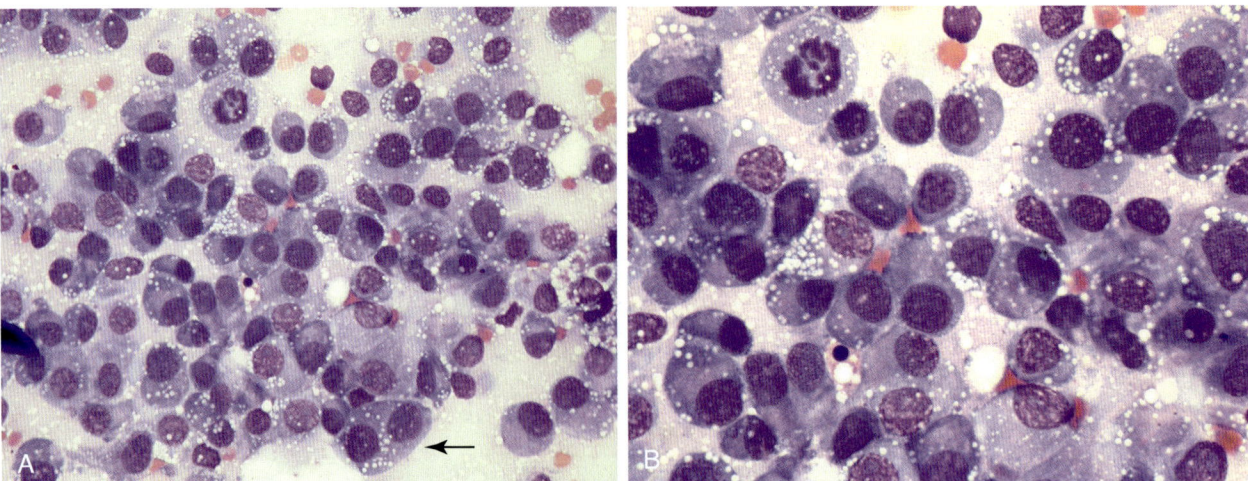

■ **FIGURE 5.88 Histiocytic sarcoma.** Same case in A and B. **Lung mass aspirate. Dog. A,** Sample taken from a 10-year-old miniature schnauzer with coughing of several weeks' duration. Dense collection of round cells having moderate amounts of basophilic cytoplasm. Occasional multinucleate cells noted *(arrow)*. (Modified Wright; HP oil.) **B,** Higher magnification view of the previous field to show the plasmacytoid features with an eccentrically placed nucleus and prominent paranuclear clearing (Golgi zone). The oval to irregularly round nucleus has coarsely stippled chromatin and contains multiple small nucleoli. Note the moderate number of cytoplasmic small punctate vacuoles. Also present is a mitotic figure, which was frequent throughout the smear. (Modified Wright; HP oil.) (Courtesy Rose Raskin, TDDS, Exeter, UK.)

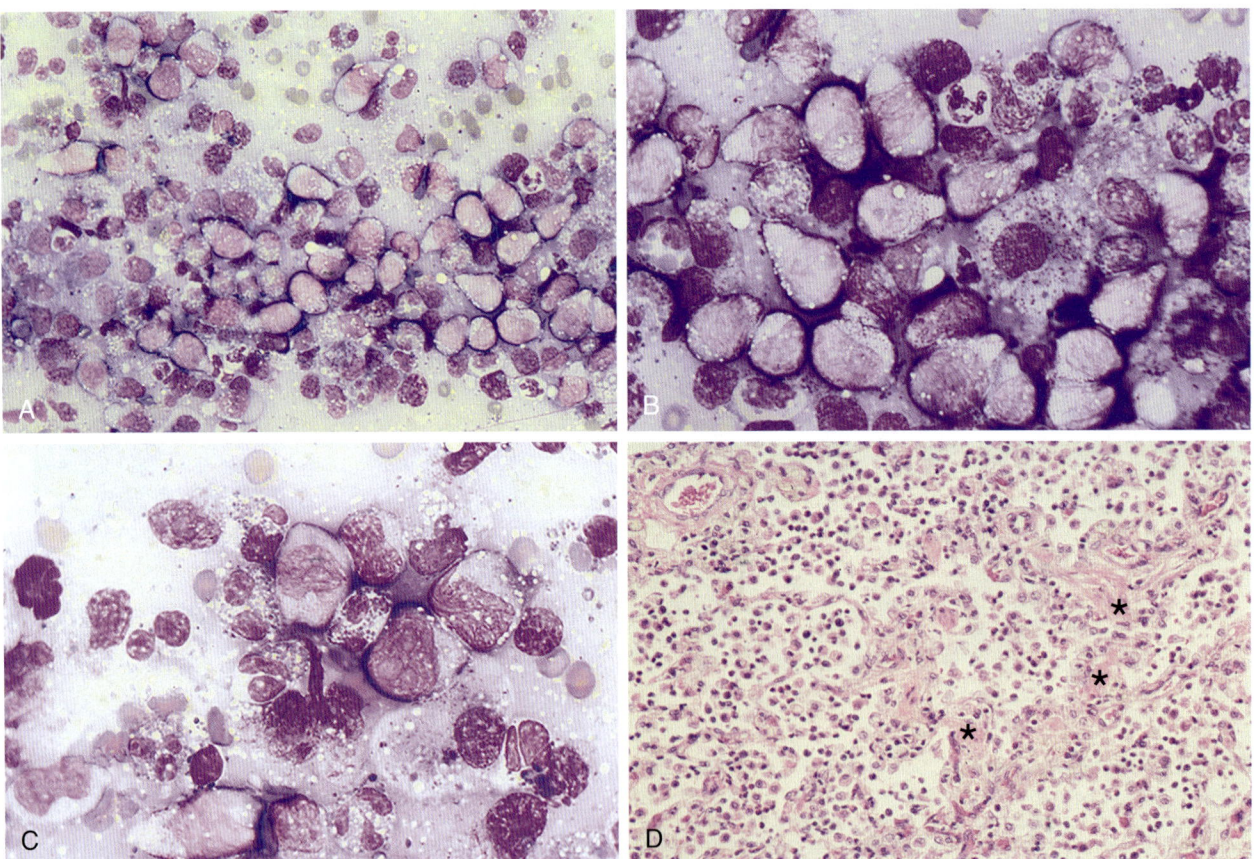

■ **FIGURE 5.89 "Lymphomatoid granulomatosis." Dog.** Same case in A to D. **A, Lung imprint.** Highly cellular sample with many large, poorly differentiated mononuclear cells. (Wright-Giemsa; HP oil.) **B, Lung imprint.** Intermixed between the large mononuclear cells are eosinophils, neutrophils, and small lymphocytes. A reactive T-cell population was supported by antibody markers. (Wright-Giemsa; HP oil.) **C, Lung imprint.** In some areas, eosinophils are the predominant cell type and normal histiocytes may be found in addition to the neoplastic lymphoid cells that appear larger than the surrounding eosinophils. (Wright-Giemsa; HP oil.) **D, Tissue section. Lung.** Neoplastic lymphocytes and a mixed inflammatory infiltrate fill alveoli and bronchioles. Eosinophilic, fibrillar protein accumulates along the alveolar walls (hyaline membranes; *asterisks*), indicating pulmonary parenchymal injury. Necropsy confirmed only the lungs were involved. (H&E; IP.) (Courtesy Rose Raskin, University of Florida.)

the minority of the cell population present and are admixed with numerous small lymphocytes, eosinophils, and plasma cells. Peripheral basophilia and canine dirofilariasis have been inconsistently associated with lymphomatoid granulomatous. Grossly and cytopathologically, this condition may be confused with eosinophilic granulomatosis, which is an inflammatory condition that consists of a pleocellular population of epithelioid cells, macrophages, eosinophils, and lymphocytes. What distinguishes them is the presence of vascular and airway invasion and destruction seen in lymphomatoid granulomatosis but lacking in eosinophilic granulomatosis. Immunophenotyping assists to confirm the lymphoid origin of the large mononuclear cell population. One study found three dogs with variable CD3 expression by the atypical cells (Smith et al., 1996). Molecular clonality evaluation will also assist in diagnosis of lymphoma but it is best appreciated on histopathology and should not be made by cytopathology alone.

Mast cell tumor. Mast cell tumors rarely metastasize to the lungs or originate from intrathoracic structures (Cartagena-Albertus et al., 2019). Primary pulmonary mast cell tumors appear cytopathologically similar to those arising from more common sites, such as the skin.

Naked Nuclei Cytomorphology Neoplasms

Further discussion of lung masses having a naked nuclei cytomorphology or neuroendocrine origin such as carcinoids is found in Chapter 17.

REFERENCES

Affolter VK, Moore PF. Canine cutaneous and systemic histiocytosis: reactive histiocytosis of dermal dendritic cells. *Am J Dermatopathol.* 2000;22: 40-48.

Affolter VK, Moore PF. Localized and disseminated histiocytic sarcoma of dendritic cell origin in dogs. *Vet Pathol.* 2002;39:74-83.

Affolter VK, Moore PF. Feline progressive histiocytosis. *Vet Pathol.* 2006;43: 646-655.

Alenghat T, Pillitteri CA, Bemis DA, et al. Lycoperdonosis in two dogs. *J Vet Diagn Invest.* 2010;22:1002-1005.

Anderton TL, Maskell DJ, Preston A. Ciliostasis is a key early event during colonization of canine tracheal tissue by Bordetella bronchiseptica. *Microbiology.* 2004;150:2843-2855.

Andreasen CB. Bronchoalveolar lavage. *Vet Clin North Am Small Anim Pract.* 2003;33:69-88.

Andreasen CB, Carmichael P. What is your diagnosis? Lung aspirate and transtracheal wash from a 1-year-old dog with dyspnea. *Vet Clin Pathol.* 1992;21:77-78.

Bain PJ, Alleman AR, Sheppard BJ, et al. What is your diagnosis? Lung mass from an 18-month-old Boxer. *Vet Clin Pathol.* 1997;26(55):91-92.

Baldwin F, Becker AB. Bronchoalveolar eosinophilic cells in a canine model of asthma: two distinctive populations. *Vet Pathol.* 1993;30:97-103.

Barçante JMP, Barçante TA, Ribeiro VM, et al. Cytological and parasitological analysis of bronchoalveolar lavage fluid for the diagnosis of *Angiostrongylus vasorum* infection in dogs. *Vet Parasitol.* 2008;158:93-102.

Barnhart K, Lewis B. Laryngopharyngeal mass in a dog with upper airway obstruction. *Vet Clin Pathol.* 2000;29:47-50.

Bauer NB, O'Neill E, Sheahan BJ, et al. Calcospherite-like bodies and caseous necrosis in tracheal mucus from a dog with tuberculosis. *Vet Clin Pathol.* 2004;33:168-172.

Benjamino KP, Birchard SJ, Niles JD, et al. Pharyngeal mucoceles in dogs: 14 cases. *J Am Anim Hosp Assoc.* 2012;48:31-35.

Benson CJ, Edlund MB, Gray S, et al. The presence of diatom algae in a tracheal wash from a German Wirehaired Pointer with aspiration pneumonia. *Vet Clin Pathol.* 2013;42:221-226.

Bernsteen L, Gregory CR, Aronson LR, et al. Acute toxoplasmosis following renal transplantation in three cats and a dog. *J Am Vet Med Assoc.* 1999;215:1123-1126.

Billen F, Peeters D, Peters IR, et al. Comparison of the value of measurement of serum galactomannan and Aspergillus-specific antibodies in the diagnosis of canine sino-nasal aspergillosis. *Vet Microbiol.* 2009;133:358-365.

Blum S, Elad D, Zukin N, et al. Outbreak of *Streptococcus equi* subsp. *Zooepidemicus* infections in cats. *Vet Microbiol.* 2010;144:236-239.

Bottero E, Melega M, Dimartino ER, et al. Diagnosis of feline mesenchymal nasal hamartoma by squash preparation cytology. *Vet Clin Pathol.* 2018;47:629-633.

Britton AP, Davies JL. Rhinitis and meningitis in two shelter cats caused by *Streptococcus equi* subspecies *zooepidemicus*. *J Comp Pathol.* 2010; 143:70-74.

Brosinski K, Janik D, Polkinghorne A, et al. Olfactory neuroblastoma in dogs and cats – a histological and immunohistochemical analysis. *J Comp Pathol.* 2012;146:152-159.

Brown DE, Thrall MA, Getzy DM, et al. Cytology of canine malignant histiocytosis. *Vet Clin Pathol.* 1994;23:118-123.

Brummer DG, French TW, Cline JM. Microlithiasis association with chronic bronchopneumonia in a cat. *J Am Vet Med Assoc.* 1989;194(8):1061-1064.

Buckeridge D, Torrance A, Daly M. Puffball mushroom toxicosis (lycoperdonosis) in a two-year-old dachshund. *Vet Rec.* 2011;168:304.

Burgener DC, Slocombe RF, Zerbe CA. Lymphoplasmacytic rhinitis in five dogs. *J Am Anim Hosp Assoc.* 1987;23:565-568.

Burgess KE, Greem EM, Wood RD, et al. Angiofibroma of the nasal cavity in 13 dogs. *Vet Comp Oncol.* 2011;9:304-309.

Burton SA, Honor DJ, Horney BS, et al. What is your diagnosis? Transtracheal aspirate from a dog. *Vet Clin Pathol*, 1992;21:112-113.

Busch MDM, Reilly CM, Luff JA, et al. Feline pulmonary Langerhans cell histiocytosis with multiorgan involvement. *Vet Pathol.* 2008;45:816-824.

Byun JW, Yoon SS, Woo GH, et al. An outbreak of fatal hemorrhagic pneumonia caused by *Streptococcus equi* subsp. *zooepidemicus* in shelter dogs. *J Vet Sci.* 2009;10:269-271.

Cabanes FJ, Roura X, Majo N, et al. *Pneumocystis carinii* pneumonia in a Yorkshire terrier dog. *Med Mycol.* 2000;38:451-453.

Cafarchia C, Sasanelli M, Lia RP, et al. Lymphocutaneous and nasal sporotrichosis in a dog from southern Italy: case report. *Mycopathologia.* 2007;163:75-79.

Calvert CA, Mahaffey MB, Lappin MR, et al. Pulmonary and disseminated eosinophilic granulomatosis in dogs. *J Am Anim Hosp Assoc.* 1988;24: 311-320.

Camus M, Cazzini P, Beck J, et al. What is your diagnosis? An endotracheal wash from a dyspneic 3-month-old female Labrador retriever. *Vet Clin Pathol.* 2013;42:527-528.

Camus MS, Farris JE. What is your diagnosis? Transtracheal wash in a cat. *Vet Clin Pathol.* 2020;49:681-683.

Caniatti M, Roccabianca P, Scanziani E, et al. Nasal rhinosporidiosis in dogs: four cases from Europe and a review of the literature. *Vet Rec.* 1998;142: 334-338.

Caniatti M, da Cunha NP, Avallone G, et al. Diagnostic accuracy of brush cytology in canine chronic intranasal disease. *Vet Clin Pathol.* 2012;41: 133-140.

Canonne AM, Billen F, Losson B, et al. Angiostrongylosis in dogs with negative fecal and in-clinic rapid serological tests: 7 cases (2013-2017). *J Vet Intern Med.* 2018;32:951-955.

Carswell JL, Williams KJ. Respiratory system. In: Maxie MG, ed. *Jubb, Kennedy, and Palmer's Pathology of Domestic Animals.* Philadelphia: Saunders; 2007:523-653.

Cartagena-Albertus JC, Moise A, Moya-Garcia S, et al. Presumptive primary intrathoracic mast cell tumours in two dogs. *BMC Vet Res.* 2019;15: 204-210.

Caudill MN, Stilwell JM, Howerth EW, et al. Chronic granulomatous pneumonia and lung rupture secondary to aspiration of activated charcoal in a French bulldog. *Vet Clin Pathol.* 2019;48:67–70.

Cazzini P, Bęczkowski P, Millins C, et al. What is your diagnosis? Fine-needle aspirate from a nasal mass in a dog. *Vet Clin Pathol.* 2019;48:367-369.

Clercx C, Wallon J, Gilbert S, et al. Imprint and brush cytology in the diagnosis of canine intranasal tumours. *J Small Anim Pract.* 1996;37:423-427.

Colledge SL, Messick JB, Huang A. What is your diagnosis? Transtracheal wash fluid in a dog. *Vet Clin Pathol* 42:238-239, 2013.

Conboy G. Natural infections of *Crenosoma vulpis* and *Angiostrongylus vasorum* in dogs in Atlantic Canada and their treatment with milbemycin oxime. *Vet Rec.* 2004;155:16-18.

Crawford PC, Dubovi EJ, Castleman WL, et al. Transmission of equine influenza virus to dogs. *Science.* 2005;310:482-485.

Crothers SL, White SD, Ihrke PJ, et al. Sporotrichosis: a retrospective evaluation of 23 cases seen in northern California (1987-2007). *Vet Dermatol.* 2009;20:249-259.

Curran M, Boothe DM, Hathcock TL, Lee-Fowler T. Analysis of the effects of storage temperature and contamination on aerobic bacterial culture results of bronchoalveolar lavage fluid. *J Vet Intern Med.* 2020;34(1):160-165.

Day MJ, Henderson SM, Belshaw Z, et al. An immunohistochemical investigation of 18 cases of feline nasal lymphoma. *J Comp Pathol.* 2004;130:152-161.

De Lorenzi D, Bonfanti U, Masserdotti C, et al. Diagnosis of canine nasal aspergillosis by cytological examination: a comparison of four different collection techniques. *J Small Anim Pract.* 2006a;47:316-319.

De Lorenzi D, Bonfanti U, Masserdotti C, et al. Nasal melanosis in three dogs. *J Small Anim Pract.* 2006b;47:682-685.

De Lorenzi D, Masserdotti C, Bertoncello D, et al. Differential cell counts in canine cytocentrifuged bronchoalveolar lavage fluid: a study on reliable enumeration of each cell type. *Vet Clin Pathol.* 2009;38:532-536.

de Vos J, Ramos Vega S, Noorman E, et al. Primary frontal sinus squamous cell carcinoma in three dogs treated with piroxicam combined with carboplatin or toceranib. *Vet Comp Oncol.* 2012;10:206-213.

Dehard S, Bernaerts F, Peeters D, et al. Comparison of bronchoalveolar lavage cytospins and smears in dogs and cats. *J Am Anim Hosp Assoc.* 2008;44:285-294.

DeHeer HL, McManus P. Frequency and severity of tracheal wash hemosiderosis and association with underlying disease in 96 cats: 2002-2003. *Vet Clin Pathol.* 2005;34:17-22.

Dennis JC, Allgier JG, Desouza LS, et al. Immunohistochemistry of the canine vomeronasal organ. *J Anat.* 2003;203:329-338.

Dirscherl P, Beisker W, Kremmer E, et al. Immunophenotyping of canine bronchoalveolar and peripheral blood lymphocytes. *Vet Immunol Immunopathol.* 1995;48:1-10.

Doughty RW, Brockman D, Neiger R, et al. Nasal oncocytoma in a domestic shorthair cat. *Vet Pathol.* 2006;43:751-754.

Dubey JP, Chapman JL, Rosenthal BM, et al. Clinical *Sarcocystis neurona*, *Sarcocystis canis*, *Toxoplasma gondii*, and *Neospora caninum* infection in dogs. *Vet Parasitol.* 2006;137:36-49.

Duncan C, Stephen C, Lester S, et al. Sub-clinical infection and asymptomatic carriage of *Cryptococcus gattii* in dogs and cats during an outbreak of cryptococcosis. *Med Mycol.* 2005;43:511-516.

Dye JA, McKiernan BC, Rozanski EA, et al. Bronchopulmonary disease in the cat: historical, physical, radiographic, clinicopathologic, and pulmonary functional evaluation of 24 affected and 15 healthy cats. *J Vet Intern Med.* 1996;10:385-400.

Eidson M, Thilsted JP, Rollag OJ. Clinical, clinicopathologic, and pathologic features of plague in cats: 119 cases (1977-1988). *J Am Vet Med Assoc.* 1991;199:1191-1197.

Elie M, Sabo M. Basics in canine and feline rhinoscopy. *Clin Tech Small Anim Pract.* 2006;21:60-63.

English K, Peters SE, Maskell DJ, et al. DNA analysis of *Pneumocystis* infecting a Cavalier King Charles spaniel. *J Eukaryot Microbiol.* 2001;48(suppl 1):106S.

Epstein SE, Mellema MS, Hopper K. Airway microbial culture and susceptibility patterns in dogs and cats with respiratory disease of varying severity. *J Vet Emerg Crit Care (San Antonio).* 2010;20:587-594.

Euzéby J. Validation of publication of new names and new combinations previously effectively published outside the IJSEM, validation list no. 104 (*Conchiformibius* corrig., gen. nov.). *Int J Syst Evol Microbiol.* 2005;55: 1395-1397.

Fitzgerald SD, Wolf DC, Carlton WW. Eight cases of canine lymphomatoid granulomatosis. *Vet Pathol.* 1991;28:241-245.

Flatland B, Greene RT, Lappin MR. Clinical and serologic evaluation of cats with cryptococcosis. *J Am Vet Med Assoc.* 1996;209:1110-1113.

Flórez MM, Pedraza F, Grandi F, et al. Letter to the editor: cytologic subtypes of canine transmissible venereal tumor. *Vet Clin Pathol.* 2012;41:3-5.

French TW. The use of cytology in the diagnosis of chronic nasal disorders. *Compend Contin Educ Pract Vet.* 1987;9:115-121.

Friedrichs KR, Young KM. Histiocytic sarcoma of macrophage origin in a cat: case report with a literature review of feline histiocytic malignancies and comparison with canine hemophagocytic histiocytic sarcoma. *Vet Clin Pathol.* 2008;37:121-128.

Gaschen L, Kircher P, Lang J. Endoscopic ultrasound instrumentation, applications in humans, and potential veterinary applications. *Vet Radiol Ultrasound.* 2003;44:665-680.

Gaspar LF, Ferreira I, Colodel MM, et al. Spontaneous canine transmissible venereal tumor: cell morphology and influence on p-glycoprotein expression. *Turk J Vet Anim Sci.* 2010;34:447-454.

Gori S, Scasso A. Cytologic and differential diagnosis of rhinosporidiosis. *Acta Cytol.* 1994;38:361-366.

Greene CE, Howerth EW, Kent M. Nonenteric amebiasis: acanthamebiasis, hartmannelliasis, and balamuthiasis. In: Greene CE, ed. *Infectious Diseases of the Dog and Cat.* 4th ed. Philadelphia: Elsevier; 2012:802-806.

Greene RT, Troy GC. Coccidioidomycosis in 48 cats: a retrospective study (1984-1993). *J Vet Intern Med.* 1995;9:86-91.

Greig B, Rossow KD, Collins JE, et al. Neospora caninum pneumonia in an adult dog. *J Am Vet Med Assoc.* 1995;206:1000-1001.

Grotheer M, Hirschberger J, Hartmann K, et al. Comparison of signalment, clinical, laboratory and radiographic parameters in cats with feline asthma and chronic bronchitis. *J Feline Med Surg.* 2020;22(7):649-655.

Hagiwara Y, Fujiwara S, Takai H, et al. *Pneumocystis carinii* pneumonia in a Cavalier King Charles Spaniel. *J Vet Med Sci.* 2001;63:349-351.

Hahn KA, McEntee MF. Primary lung tumors in cats: 86 cases (1979-1994). *J Am Vet Med Assoc.* 1997;211:1257-1260.

Harder TC, Vahlenkamp TW. Influenza virus infection in dogs and cats. *Vet Immunol Immunopathol.* 2010;134:54-60.

Hawkins EC, Davidson MG, Meuten DJ, et al. Cytologic identification of *Toxoplasma gondii* in bronchoalveolar lavage fluid of experimentally infected cats. *J Am Vet Med Assoc.* 1997;210:648-650.

Hawkins EC, DeNicola DB. Collection of bronchoalveolar lavage fluid in cats, using an endotracheal tube. *Am J Vet Res.* 1989;50:855-859.

Hawkins EC, DeNicola DB. Cytologic analysis of tracheal wash specimens and bronchoalveolar lavage fluid in the diagnosis of mycotic infections in dogs. *J Am Vet Med Assoc.* 1990;197:79-83.

Hawkins EC, DeNicola DB, Kuehn NF. Bronchoalveolar lavage in the evaluation of pulmonary disease in the dog and cat. State of the art. *J Vet Intern Med.* 1990;4:267-274.

Hawkins EC, DeNicola DB, Plier ML. Cytological analysis of bronchoalveolar lavage fluid in the diagnosis of spontaneous respiratory tract disease in dogs: a retrospective study. *J Vet Intern Med.* 1995;9:386-392.

Hawkins EC, Kennedy-Stoskopf S, Levy J, et al. Cytologic characterization of bronchoalveolar lavage fluid collected through an endotracheal tube in cats. *Am J Vet Res.* 1994;55:795-802.

Hawkins EC, Kennedy-Stoskopf S, Levy JK, et al. Effect of FIV infection on lung inflammatory cell populations recovered by bronchoalveolar lavage. *Vet Immunol Immunopathol.* 1996;51:21-28.

Hawkins EC, Morrison WB, DeNicola DB, et al. Cytologic analysis of bronchoalveolar lavage fluid from 47 dogs with multicentric malignant lymphoma. *J Am Vet Med Assoc.* 1993;203:1418-1425.

Hawkins EC, Rogala AR, Large EE, et al. Cellular composition of bronchial brushings obtained from healthy dogs and dogs with chronic cough and cytologic composition of bronchoalveolar lavage fluid obtained from dogs with chronic cough. *Am J Vet Res.* 2006;67:160-167.

Henderson SM, Bradley K, Day MJ, et al. Investigation of nasal diseases in the cat—a retrospective study of 77 cases. *J Feline Med Surg.* 2004;6: 245-257.

Hicks DG, Fidel JL. Intranasal malignant melanoma in a dog. *J Am Anim Hosp Assoc.* 2006;42:472-476.

Hirt R, Tektas OY, Carrington SD, et al. Comparative anatomy of the human and canine efferent tear duct system—impact of mucin MUC5AC on lacrimal drainage. *Curr Eye Res.* 37:961-970.

Holt DE, Goldschmidt MH. Nasal polyps in dogs: five cases (2005-2011). *J Small Anim Pract.* 2011;52:660-663.

Hyde D, Orthoefer J, Dungworth D, et al. Morphometric and morphologic evaluation of pulmonary lesions in beagle dogs chronically exposed to high ambient levels of air pollutants. *Lab Invest.* 1978;38:455-469.

Jelínek F, Vozková D, Kosáková D, et al. Giant cell tumor of bone located in the concha of a cat. *Veterinární Lékař.* 2008;6:5-9.

Jerram RM, Guyer CL, Braniecki A, et al. Endogenous lipid (cholesterol) pneumonia associated with bronchogenic carcinoma in a cat. *J Am Anim Hosp Assoc.* 1998;34:275-280.

Johnson LR, Clarke HE, Bannasch MJ, et al. Correlation of rhinoscopic signs of inflammation with histologic findings in nasal biopsy specimens of cats with or without upper respiratory tract disease. *J Am Vet Med Assoc.* 2004;225:395-400.

Johnson LR, De Cock HE, Sykes JE, et al. Cytokine gene transcription in feline nasal tissue with histologic evidence of inflammation. *Am J Vet Res.* 2005;66:996-1001.

Johnson LR, Drazenovich TL. Flexible bronchoscopy and bronchoalveolar lavage in 68 cats (2001-2006). *J Vet Intern Med.* 2007;21:219-225.

Johnson LR, Drazenovich TL, Herrera MA, et al. Results of rhinoscopy alone or in conjunction with sinuscopy in dogs with aspergillosis: 46 cases (2001-2004). *J Am Vet Med Assoc.* 2006;228:738-742.

Johnson LR, Johnson EG, Hulsebosh SE, et al. Eosinophilic bronchitis, eosinophilic granuloma, and eosinophilic bronchopneumopathy in 75 dogs (2006-2016). *J Vet Intern Med.* 2019;33(5):2217-2226.

Johnson LR, Vernau W. Bronchoscopic findings in 48 cats with spontaneous lower respiratory tract disease (2002-2009). *J Vet Intern Med.* 2011;25:236-243.

Johnson LR, Vernau W. Bronchoalveolar lavage fluid lymphocytosis in 104 dogs (2006-2016). *J Vet Intern Med.* 2019;33(3):1315-1321.

Jones DJ, Norris CR, Samii VF, et al. Endogenous lipid pneumonia in cats: 24 cases (1985-1998). *J Am Vet Med Assoc.* 2000;216:1437-1440.

Jones JC, Ober CP. Computed tomographic diagnosis of nongastrointestinal foreign bodies in dogs. *J Am Anim Hosp Assoc.* 2007;43:99-111.

Jordan HL, Cohn LA, Armstrong PJ. Disseminated *Mycobacterium avium* complex infection in three Siamese cats. *J Am Vet Med Assoc.* 1994;204:90-93.

Kano R, Ishida R, Nakae S, et al. The first reported case of canine subcutaneous *Cryptococcus flavescens* infection. *Mycopathologia.* 2012;173:179-182.

King RR, Greiner EC, Ackerman N, et al. Nasal capillariasis in a dog. *J Am Anim Hosp Assoc.* 1990;26:381-385.

Klopfleisch R, Kohn B, Plog S, et al. An emerging pulmonary haemorrhagic syndrome in dogs: similar to the human leptospiral pulmonary haemorrhagic syndrome? *Vet Med Int.* 2010;2010:928541.

Koehler JW, Weiss RC, Aubry OA, et al. Nasal tumor with widespread cutaneous metastases in a Golden Retriever. *Vet Pathol.* 2012;49:870-875.

Kraje AC, Patton CS, Edwards DF. Malignant histiocytosis in 3 cats. *J Vet Intern Med.* 2001;15:252-256.

Kuehn NF. Nasal computed tomography. *Clin Tech Small Anim Pract.* 2006;21:55-59.

Kuiken T, Rimmelzwaan G, van Riel D, et al. Avian H5N1 influenza in cats. *Science.* 2004;306:241.

Lana SE, Withrow SJ. Tumors of the respiratory system—nasal tumors. In: Withrow SJ, MacEwen EG, eds. *Small Animal Clinical Oncology.* Philadelphia: Saunders; 2001:370-377.

Lawson CA. What is your diagnosis? Endotracheal tube wash from a Labrador retriever. *Vet Clin Pathol.* 2020;49(1):156-157.

Lawson MJ, Craven BA, Peterson EG, et al. A computational study of odorant transport and deposition in the canine nasal cavity: implications for olfaction. *Chem Senses.* 2012;37:553-566.

Lecuyer M, Dube PG, DiFruscia R, et al. Bronchoalveolar lavage in normal cats. *Can Vet J.* 1995;36:771-773.

Leissinger M, Pipe-Martin H, Acierno M. What is your diagnosis? Tracheobronchial lavage from a dog. *Vet Clin Pathol.* 2016;45:511-512.

Leme LR, Schubach TM, Santos IB, et al. Mycological evaluation of bronchoalveolar lavage in cats with respiratory signs from Rio de Janeiro, Brazil. *Mycoses.* 2007;50:210-214.

Lenz JA, Furrow E, Craig LE, et al. Histiocytic sarcoma in 14 miniature schnauzers—a new breed predisposition? *J Small Anim Pract.* 2017;58:461-467.

Lester SJ, Malik R, Bartlett KH, et al. Cryptococcosis: update and emergence of *Cryptococcus gattii*. *Vet Clin Pathol.* 2011;40:4-17.

Llanos-Cuentas EA, Roncal N, Villaseca P, et al. Natural infections of *Leishmania peruviana* in animals in the Peruvian Andes. *Trans R Soc Trop Med Hyg.* 1999;93:15-20.

Lobetti R. Common variable immunodeficiency in miniature dachshunds affected with *Pneumocystis carinii* pneumonia. *J Vet Diagn Invest.* 2000;12:39-45.

Lobetti RG. *Pneumocystis carinii* infection in miniature dachshunds. *Compend Contin Educ Pract Vet.* 2001;23:320-324.

Lopez A. Respiratory system, thoracic cavity, and pleura. In: Thomson RG, McGavin MD, Carlton WW, et al. *Thomson's Special Veterinary Pathology.* Philadelphia: Mosby; 2000:125-195.

Macdonald ES, Norris CR, Berghaus RB, et al. Clinicopathologic and radiographic features and etiologic agents in cats with histologically confirmed infectious pneumonia: 39 cases (1991-2000). *J Am Vet Med Assoc.* 2003;223:1142-1150.

Masserdotti C, De Lorenzi D. Le figurazioni non cellulari in citologia diagnostic [Non-cellular structures in diagnostic cytology]. *Veterinaria.* 2000;14:51-55.

Mastrorilli C, Spangler EA, Chrisopherson PW, et al. Multifocal cutaneous histiocytic sarcoma in a young dog and review of histiocytic cell immunophenotyping. *Vet Clin Pathol.* 2012;41:412-418.

Matos B, Colella V, Alho AM, et al. *Crenosoma vulpis* infection in a four-month old puppy. *Helminthologia.* 2016;53:276-280.

McCauley M, Atwell RB, Sutton RH, et al. Unguided bronchoalveolar lavage techniques and residual effects in dogs. *Aust Vet J.* 1998;76:161-165.

McEwen BJ, Gerdin J. Veterinary forensic pathology: drowning and bodies recovered from water. *Vet Pathol.* 2016;53:1049-1056.

McGarry JW, Morgan ER. Identification of first-stage larvae of metastrongyles from dogs. *Vet Rec.* 2009;165:258-261.

McKay JS, Cox CL, Foster AP. Cutaneous alternariosis in a cat. *J Small Anim Pract.* 2001;42:75-78.

Meier WA, Meinkoth JH, Brunker J, et al. Cytologic identification of immature endospores in a dog with rhinosporidiosis. *Vet Clin Pathol.* 2006;35:348-352.

Meler E, Dunn M, Lecuyer M. A retrospective study of canine persistent nasal disease: 80 cases (1998-2003). *Can Vet J.* 2008;49:71-76.

Mercier E, Peters IR, Day MJ, et al. Toll- and NOD-like receptor mRNA expression in canine sino-nasal aspergillosis and idiopathic lymphoplasmacytic rhinitis. *Vet Immunol Immunopathol.* 2012;145:618-624.

Meuten DJ, Calderwood-Mays MB, Dillman RC, et al. Canine laryngeal rhabdomyoma. *Vet Pathol.* 1985;22:533-539.

Michiels L, Day MJ, Snaps F, et al. A retrospective study of non-specific rhinitis in 22 cats and the value of nasal cytology and histopathology. *J Feline Med Surg.* 2003;5:279-285.

Mills PC, Litster A. Using urea dilution to standardise cellular and non-cellular components of pleural and bronchoalveolar lavage (BAL) fluids in the cat. *J Feline Med Surg.* 2006;8:105-110.

Moore AS, Ogilvie GK. Tumors of the respiratory tract. In: Moore AS, Ogilvie GK, eds. *Feline Oncology: A Comprehensive Guide to Compassionate Care.* Trenton, NJ: Veterinary Learning Systems; 2001:368-384.

Moore PF. A review of histiocytic diseases of dogs and cats. *Vet Pathol.* 2014;51:167-184.

Moore PF, Affolter VK, Vernau W. Canine hemophagocytic histiocytic sarcoma: a proliferative disorder of CD11d+ macrophages. *Vet Pathol.* 2006;43:632-645.

Morgan ER, Jeffries R, van Otterdijk L, et al. *Angiostrongylus vasorum* infection in dogs: presentation and risk factors. *Vet Parasitol.* 2010;173:255-261.

Morgan E, Shaw S. *Angiostrongylus vasorum* infection in dogs: continuing spread and developments in diagnosis and treatment. *J Small Anim Pract.* 2010;51:616-621.

Mukaratirwa S, van der Linde-Sipman JS, Gruys E. Feline nasal and paranasal sinus tumours: clinicopathological study, histomorphological description and diagnostic immunohistochemistry of 123 cases. *J Feline Med Surg.* 2001;3:235-245.

Nagata K, Lamb M, Goldschmidt MH, et al. The usefulness of immunohistochemistry to differentiate between nasal carcinoma and lymphoma in cats: 140 cases (1986–2000). *Vet Comp Oncol.* 2014;12:52-57.

Ninomiya F, Suzuki S, Tanaka H, et al. Nasal and paranasal adenocarcinomas with neuroendocrine differentiation in dogs. *Vet Pathol.* 2008;45:181-187.

Oakes MG, McCarthy RJ. What is your diagnosis? Soft-tissue mass within the lumen of the larynx, caudal to the epiglottis. *J Am Vet Med Assoc.* 1994;204:1891-1892.

Ogilvie GK, Haschek WM, Withrow SJ, et al. Classification of primary lung tumors in dogs: 210 cases (1975-1985). *J Am Vet Med Assoc.* 1989;195:106-108.

Okine AAK, Chapman S, Hostutler RA, et al. Diagnosis of pneumocystis pneumonia in a 2-year-old King Charles Cavalier Spaniel using the polymerase chain reaction. *Vet Clin Pathol.* 2018;47:146-149.

Padrid P, Amis TC. Chronic tracheobronchial disease in the dog. *Vet Clin North Am Small Anim Pract.* 1992;22:1203-1229.

Padrid PA, Feldman BF, Funk K, et al. Cytologic, microbiologic, and biochemical analysis of bronchoalveolar lavage fluid obtained from 24 healthy cats. *Am J Vet Res.* 1991;52:1300-1307.

Palić J, Busch K, Unterer S, et al. What is your diagnosis? Fine-needle aspirate of a lung nodule and bronchoalveolar lavage from a dog. *Vet Clin Pathol.* 2017;46:533-534.

Palić J, Hostetter S, Riedesel E, et al. What is your diagnosis? Aspirate of a lung nodule in a dog. *Vet Clin Pathol.* 2011;40:99-100.

Papazoglou LG, Koutinas AF, Plevraki AG, et al. Primary intranasal transmissible venereal tumour in the dog: a retrospective study of six spontaneous cases. *J Vet Med A Physiol Pathol Clin Med.* 2001;48:391-400.

Park MS, Kim Y, Kang MS, et al. Disseminated transmissible venereal tumor in a dog. *J Vet Diagn Invest.* 2006;18:130-133.

Patnaik AK. Histologic and immunohistochemical studies of granular cell tumors in seven dogs, three cats, one horse, and one bird. *Vet Pathol.* 1993;30:176-185.

Patnaik AK, Ludwig LL, Erlandson RA. Neuroendocrine carcinoma of the nasopharynx in a dog. *Vet Pathol.* 2002;39:496-500.

Peeters D, Peters IR, Helps CR, et al. Distinct tissue cytokine and chemokine mRNA expression in canine sino-nasal aspergillosis and idiopathic lymphoplasmacytic rhinitis. *Vet Immunol Immunopathol.* 2007;117:95-105.

Pereira SA, Menezes RC, Gremião ID, et al. Sensitivity of cytopathological examination in the diagnosis of feline sporotrichosis. *J Feline Med Surg.* 2011;13:220-223.

Petite AF, Dennis R. Comparison of radiography and magnetic resonance imaging for evaluating the extent of nasal neoplasia in dogs. *J Small Anim Pract.* 2006;47:529-536.

Pierezan F, Mansell J, Ambrus A, et al. Immunohistochemical expression of ionized calcium binding adapter molecule 1 in cutaneous histiocytic proliferative, neoplastic and inflammatory disorders of dogs and cats. *J Comp Pathol.* 2014;151(4):347-351.

Piperisova I, Neel JA, Tarigo J. What is your diagnosis? Nasal discharge from a dog. *Vet Clin Pathol.* 2010;39:121-122.

Piva S, Zanoni RG, Specchi S, et al. Chronic rhinitis due to *Streptococcus equi* subspecies *zooepidemicus* in a dog. *Vet Rec.* 2010;167:177-178.

Poitout F, Weiss DJ, Dubey JP. Lung aspirate from a cat with respiratory distress. *Vet Clin Pathol.* 1998;27:10.

Postorino NC, Wheeler SL, Park RD, et al. A syndrome resembling lymphomatoid granulomatosis in the dog. *J Vet Intern Med.* 1989;3:15-19.

Poth T, Seibold M, Werckenthin C, et al. First report of *Cryptococcus magnus* infection in a cat. *Med Mycol.* 2010;48:1000-1004.

Priestnall S, Erles K. *Streptococcus zooepidemicus*: an emerging canine pathogen. *Vet J.* 2011;188:142-148.

Priestnall SL, Erles K, Brooks HW, et al. Characterization of pneumonia due to *Streptococcus zooepidemicus* subsp. *zooepidemicus* in dogs. *Clin Vaccine Immunol.* 2010;17:1790-1796.

Raya AI, Fernandez-de Marco M, Nunez A, et al. Endogenous lipid pneumonia in a dog. *J Comp Pathol.* 2006;135:153-155.

Rebar AH, Hawkins EC, DeNicola DB. Cytologic evaluation of the respiratory tract. *Vet Clin North Am Small Anim Pract.* 1992;22:1065-1085.

Reed LT, Miller MA, Visvesvara GS, et al. Diagnostic exercise: cerebral mass in a puppy with respiratory distress and progressive neurologic signs. *Vet Pathol.* 2010;47(6):1116-1119.

Reichle JK, Wisner ER. Non-cardiac thoracic ultrasound in 75 feline and canine patients. *Vet Radiol Ultrasound.* 2000;41:154-162.

Reinero CR, Masseau I, Grobman M, et al. Perspectives in veterinary medicine: description and classification of bronchiolar disorders in cats. *J Vet Intern Med.* 2019;33(3):1201-1221.

Roy PE, Magnan-Lapointe F, Huy ND, et al. Chronic inhalation of marijuana and tobacco in dogs: pulmonary pathology. *Res Commun Chem Pathol Pharmacol.* 1976;14:305-317.

Rudorf H, Brown P. Ultrasonography of laryngeal masses in six cats and one dog. *Vet Radiol Ultrasound.* 1998;39:430-434.

Ruehlmann D, Podell M, Oglesbee M, et al. Canine neosporosis: a case report and literature review. *J Am Anim Hosp Assoc.* 1995;31:174-183.

Rutherford S, Whitbread T, Ness M. Idiopathic osseous hyperplasia of the nasal turbinates in a Welsh terrier. *J Small Anim Pract.* 2011;52:492-496.

Sako T, Shimoyama Y, Akihara Y, et al. Neuroendocrine carcinoma in the nasal cavity of ten dogs. *J Comp Pathol.* 2005;133:155-163.

Salazar I, Sanchez Quinteiro P, Cifuentes JM, et al. The vomeronasal organ of the cat. *J Anat.* 1996;188(Pt 2):445-454.

Santagostino SF, Mortellaro CM, Boracchi P, et al. Feline upper respiratory tract lymphoma: site, cyto-histology, phenotype, FeLV expression, and prognosis. *Vet Pathol.* 2015;52:250-259.

Schnyder M, Fahrion A, Riond B, et al. Clinical, laboratory, and pathological findings in dogs experimentally infected with *Angiostrongylus vasorum*. *Parasitol Res.* 2010;107:1471-1480.

Shaw DH, Conboy GA, Hogan PM, Horney BS. Eosinophilic bronchitis caused by *Crenosoma vulpis* infection in dogs. *Can Vet J.* 1996;37(6):361-363.

Silva V, Pereira CN, Ajello L, et al. Molecular evidence for multiple host-specific strains in the genus Rhinosporidium. *J Clin Microbiol.* 2005;43:1865-1868.

Silverstein D, Greene C, Gregory E, et al. Pulmonary alveolar proteinosis in a dog. *J Vet Intern Med.* 2000;14:546-551.

Singh MK, Johnson LR, Kittleson MD, et al. Bronchomalacia in dogs with myxomatous mitral valve degeneration. *J Vet Intern Med.* 2012;26:312-319.

Smallwood LJ, Zenoble RD. Biopsy and cytological sampling of the respiratory tract. *Semin Vet Med Surg (Small Anim).* 1993;8(4):250-257.

Smith KC, Day MJ, Shaw SC, et al. Canine lymphomatoid granulomatosis: an immunophenotypic analysis of three cases. *J Comp Pathol.* 1996;115:129-138.

Spoor MS, Royal AB, Berent LM. The elusive globule leukocyte. *Vet Clin Pathol.* 2011;40:136.

Sukura A, Saari S, Järvinen AK, et al. *Pneumocystis carinii* pneumonia in dogs—a diagnostic challenge. *J Vet Diagn Invest.* 1996;8:124-130.

Sykes JE, Malik R. Cryptococcosis. In: Greene CE, ed. *Infectious Diseases of the Dog and Cat.* 4th ed. Philadelphia: Elsevier; 2012:621-634.

Szatmári V, Teske E, Nikkels PGJ, et al. Pulmonary alveolar proteinosis in a cat. *BMC Vet Res.* 2015;11:302.

Takahashi M, Tomiyasu H, Hotta E, et al. Clinical characteristics and prognostic factors in dogs with histiocytic sarcomas in Japan. *J Vet Med Sci* 2014;76(5):661-666.

Tang KN, Mansell JL, Herron AJ, et al. The histologic, ultrastructural, and immunohistochemical characteristics of a thyroid oncocytoma in a dog. *Vet Pathol.* 1994;31:269-271.

Tasker S, Foster DJ, Corcoran BM, et al. Obstructive inflammatory laryngeal disease in three cats. *J Feline Med Surg.* 1999a;1:53-59.

Tasker S, Knottenbelt CM, Munro EA, et al. Aetiology and diagnosis of persistent nasal disease in the dog: a retrospective study of 42 cases. *J Small Anim Pract.* 1999b;40:473-478.

Tennant K, Patterson-Kane J, Boag AK, et al. Nasal mycosis in two cats caused by Alternaria species. *Vet Rec.* 2004;155:368-370.

Teske E, Stokhof AA, van den Ingh TSGAM, et al. Transthoracic needle aspiration biopsy of the lung in dogs with pulmonic diseases. *J Am Anim Hosp Assoc.* 1991;27:289-294.

Trivedi SR, Sykes JE, Cannon MS, et al. Clinical features and epidemiology of *Cryptococcus* in cats and dogs in California: 93 cases (1988-2010). *J Am Vet Med Assoc.* 2011;239:357-369.

Unterer S, Deplazes P, Arnold P, et al. Spontaneous *Crenosoma vulpis* infection in 10 dogs: laboratory, radiographic and endoscopic findings. *Schweiz Arch Tierheilkd.* 2002;144:174-179.

Vail DM, Mahler PA, Soergel SA. Differential cell analysis and phenotypic subtyping of lymphocytes in bronchoalveolar lavage fluid from clinically normal dogs. *Am J Vet Res.* 1995;56:282-285.

Vanda B, de Buen N, Jasso R, et al. Inflammatory cells and ferruginous bodies in bronchoalveolar lavage in urban dogs. *Acta Cytologica.* 1998;42:939-944.

Viitanen SJ, Lappalainen A, Rajamäki MM. Co-infections with respiratory viruses in dogs with bacterial pneumonia. *J Vet Intern Med.* 2015;29:544-551.

Walton RM, Brown DE, Burkhard MJ, et al. Malignant histiocytosis in a domestic cat: cytomorphologic and immunohistochemical features. *Vet Clin Pathol.* 1997;26:56-60.

Watson PJ, Wotton P, Eastwood J, et al. Immunoglobulin deficiency in Cavalier King Charles spaniels with *Pneumocystis* pneumonia. *J Vet Intern Med.* 2006;20:523-527.

White ME, Jaffey JA, Finley A, et al. What is your diagnosis? Impression smears of a nasopharyngeal nodule in a cat. *Vet Clin Pathol.* 2021;50:89-91.

Whittemore JC, Webb CB. Successful treatment of nasal sporotrichosis in a dog. *Can Vet J.* 2007;48:411-414.

Wiedmeyer CE, Whitney MS, Dvorak LD, et al. Mass in the laryngeal region of a dog. *Vet Clin Pathol.* 2003;32(1):37-39.

Williams M, Olver C, Thrall MA. Transtracheal wash from a puppy with respiratory disease. *Vet Clin Pathol.* 2006;35:471-473.

Wilson DW. Tumors of the respiratory tract. In: Meuten DJ, ed. *Tumors in Domestic Animals.* 5th ed. Ames, IA: John Wiley & Sons, Inc; 2017:467-498.

Windsor RC, Johnson LR, Herrgesell EJ, et al. Idiopathic lymphoplasmacytic rhinitis in dogs: 37 cases (1997-2002). *J Am Vet Med Assoc.* 2004;224:1952-1957.

Witham AI, French AF, Hill KE. Extramedullary laryngeal plasmacytoma in a dog. *N Z Vet J.* 2012;61:61-64.

Wood EF, O'Brien RT, Young KM. Ultrasound-guided fine-needle aspiration of focal parenchymal lesions of the lung in dogs and cats. *J Vet Intern Med.* 1998;12:338-342.

Workman HC, Bailiff NL, Jang SS, et al. *Capnocytophaga cynodegmi* in a rottweiler dog with severe bronchitis and foreign-body pneumonia. *J Clin Microbiol.* 2008;46:4099-4103.

Xie C-H, Yokato A. Phylogenetic analysis of *Alysiella* and related genera of *Neisseriaceae*: proposal of *Alysiella crassa* comb. nov., *Conchiformibium steedae* gen. nov., comb. nov., *Conchiformibium kuhniae* sp. nov. and *Bergeriella denitrificans* gen. nov., comb. nov. *J Gen Appl Microbiol.* 2005;51:1-10.

Ybarra WL, Johnson LR, Drazenovich TL, et al. Interpretation of multisegment bronchoalveolar lavage in cats (1/2001–1/2011). *J Vet Intern Med.* 2012;12:1281-1287.

Yohn SE, Hawkins EC, Morrison WB, et al. Confirmation of a pulmonary component of multicentric lymphosarcoma with bronchoalveolar lavage in two dogs. *J Am Vet Med Assoc.* 1994;204:97-101.

6 CHAPTER

Body Cavity Fluids

Katie M. Boes

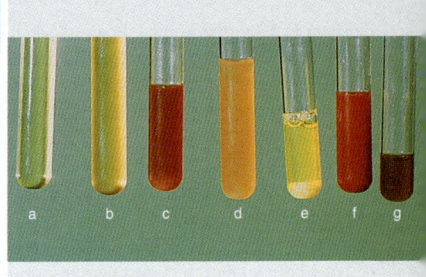

Typically, there is little fluid (<5 mL) present in the peritoneal, pleural, and pericardial cavities, and thus they are considered potential spaces. Detailed physiologic descriptions of serous body cavity homeostasis are available (Dempsey and Ewing, 2011). These serous body cavities are lined by specialized cells, termed *mesothelial cells*. Increased accumulation of fluid (effusion) in these potential spaces results from an imbalance in fluid production and removal or vessel leakage. Clinical signs of the presence of increased amounts of fluid include abdominal distension (ascites), abdominal pain, dyspnea with an obstructive breathing pattern, muffled heart sounds, and cardiac arrhythmias. Collection and evaluation of fluid from these sites may be therapeutic as well as diagnostic for the presence of inflammatory, hemorrhagic, neoplastic, or lymphatic conditions. Further diagnostic tests may be indicated as per the cytopathologic characteristics. Removal and examination of fluid is a relatively low-risk procedure, particularly for the diagnostic yield that can be produced.

SAMPLE COLLECTION AND TECHNIQUE

The fluid should be collected into a lavender-top tube (ethylenediaminetetraacetic acid [EDTA] anticoagulant) for evaluation of both nucleated cells and red blood cells (RBCs). A portion of the sample should also be placed in a red-top tube (or any sterile tube without additives) for biochemical assays such as potassium, creatinine, lactate, and glucose. Finally, a portion of the fluid should be placed in a sterile tube for aerobic, anaerobic, mycoplasma, and fungal cultures. Samples intended for culture should not be refrigerated and processed within 24 hours of obtaining. Tubes that contain EDTA should not be used for bacterial culture because EDTA is bacteriostatic (Songer and Post, 2005). When sent to a diagnostic laboratory, the tubes should be sent by express mail or courier and kept cooled, not frozen, to prevent in vitro changes, along with freshly prepared slides. This allows the clinical pathologist evaluating the sample to compare the cellularity and appearance of the cells in the sample submitted with those in the tube at the time of collection.

Peritoneal Fluid Collection

Place the patient in left lateral recumbency and restrain. Clip and surgically prepare an area (e.g., 10 × 10 inches square) with the umbilicus in the center. The urinary bladder should be emptied before performing paracentesis. Infiltrate a small area with a local anesthetic, if desired. Use a 20- to 22-gauge needle or over-the-needle catheter to penetrate the abdomen. Attempt to obtain fluid in four quadrants, allowing the fluid to flow freely by gravity and capillary action. If needed, gentle suction with a 3 or 6 mL syringe can be used. For a complete description of the technique, readers are referred elsewhere (Walters, 2003). Allow the animal to rest quietly while fluid is being removed. Moving the animal or allowing the patient to move while the needle is in the abdomen can result in laceration or puncture of organs. Some investigators prefer to have the patient standing for fluid removal; however, it is more likely that the omentum will occlude the needle in this position.

If an adequate sample is not obtained using the traditional four-quadrant abdominocentesis, a diagnostic peritoneal lavage (DPL) may be used. This technique is identical to that described earlier; however, a catheter is used over a needle. After removing the stylet, 10 to 20 mL/kg of warmed isotonic fluids is introduced via an intravenous fluid set. The animal is then gently rolled from side to side, walked briefly, and massaged to distribute the fluid throughout the abdomen. The sample is then obtained using the four-quadrant approach. Detailed descriptions of this technique can be found elsewhere (Walters, 2003). Using the DPL technique doubles the accuracy of a straight-needle abdominocentesis (Crowe, 1984). A significant drawback of using this technique is the undeterminable effect of dilution on the total nucleated cell count and total protein.

Pleural Fluid Collection

For removal of fluid from the thorax, the patient should be in standing or in ventral or sternal recumbency. Clip the hair and surgically prepare the thoracic wall from the 5th to the 11th intercostal space. Infiltrate a small area at the 7th to 8th intercostal space at the level of the costochondral junction with local anesthetic. It is best to attach extension tubing to the hub of the needle or over-the-needle catheter and a three-way stopcock for removal of pleural fluid. Insert the needle or catheter into the chest wall at the surgically prepared site, taking care to avoid the intercostal vessels located just caudal to each rib. For a complete description of this technique, readers are referred elsewhere (Tseng and Waddell, 2000).

Pericardial Fluid Collection

For removal of fluid from the pericardial sac, sedate the patient if necessary. Surgically prepare an area over the lower to mid 5th to 7th intercostal space bilaterally. Place the patient in left lateral or sternal recumbency. Attach electrocardiogram leads to monitor for dysrhythmias during the procedure. Infiltrate an area at the costochondral junction, or near where the lower and midthorax meet, with local anesthetic. Use a 16- to 18-gauge over-the-needle catheter with a three-way valve to which a 30 or 60 mL syringe is attached. Always maintain negative pressure on the syringe as the chest wall is punctured. Carefully advance the needle into the fourth intercostal space through a nick incision in the direction of the heart. Advance the needle until resistance is met (from the pericardium). A release will be felt as the needle enters the pericardial sac, and a flash of blood is often seen. Thread the tubing or catheter so that it is securely within the pericardial sac. For a complete description of this technique, readers are referred elsewhere (Gidlewski and Petrie, 2005; Shaw and Rush, 2007).

FLUID SAMPLE HANDLING

Fluid Physical Characteristics

Note the color and turbidity of the fluid initially upon removal (Fig. 6.1). If the fluid is clear initially and then turns red, iatrogenic blood contamination is likely. Conversely, if a sample is red throughout collection, hemorrhagic fluid should be suspected. The color and turbidity of the fluid should be reevaluated after centrifugation. Turbidity is stated as clear, hazy, cloudy, or opaque and can help to detect cellular or particle contributions to the fluid. Samples can be spun for 3 to 5 minutes at 450 g (~1500–2000 rpm) to obtain the pellet.

Fluid Slide Preparation

For cytopathologic examination, make both a direct nonconcentrated smear by a compression spread (squash) or blood film spread technique and smears from the pellet of a centrifuged sample using either a blood film spread or compression-spread technique. Refer to Chapter 1 for more details. From the resulting supernatant or from a spun microhematocrit tube, total protein should be measured by refractometry. The remaining pellet is reconstituted using an equal amount of remaining liquid by flicking the tube with a finger or using a stir stick. A small amount of unspun fluid may additionally be placed in a cytocentrifuge if available, and a cytocentrifuged preparation is produced for improved visibility of cytoplasmic features. Alternative devices have been suggested to concentrate fluid materials, such as a salad spin mixer (Marcos et al., 2016). Fluid may additionally be prepared as a cell block (Marcos et al., 2017) and submitted for histopathology (see Appendix 5). After cytopathologic slide preparation, methanolic Romanowsky stains such as Wright stain or an aqueous Romanowsky stain can be applied for immediate in-clinic evaluation.

The remaining unstained smears and an EDTA and serum tube filled with fluid may be submitted to the laboratory for complete diagnostic evaluation. Maher et al. (2010) showed that after 24 and 48 hours of storage, there are a significant decrease in the total nucleated cell count, a decrease in the number of neutrophils and neoplastic cells, and an increase in the number of unrecognizable cells. In addition, bacteria that were seen in fresh samples were no longer found at 24 and 48 hours (Maher et al., 2010).

> **KEY POINT** Direct smears should be prepared and left unstained to send with the fluid when submitting to a laboratory if a delay of several hours is anticipated before evaluation.

Fluid Protein Quantitation

Protein quantitation is typically done via refractometry from the supernatant; however, some institutions determine protein via spectrophotometry or automated analysis. Both methods offer accurate readings in a wide range of protein concentrations (Braun et al., 2001; George, 2001; George and O'Neill, 2001). However, some refractometer protein scales do not show values below 2.5 g/dL. It has been shown with canine effusions that refractometry underestimates the protein content when the spectophometric concentration is less than 2.0 g/dL and that spectrophotometry using the biuret method is more accurate when there is high protein content (Braun et al., 2001). Others have found that refractometry can be used accurately down to 1.0 g/dL (George and O'Neill, 2001). A similar finding of underestimating the protein content in feline effusions with refractometry may also occur (Papasouliotis et al., 2002). In that same study, a dry chemistry analyzer produced increased globulins concentration and therefore a lower albumin/globulin (A:G) ratio compared with a reference wet analyzer using the same biuret and bromocresol green methodologies. This finding is particularly important because a decreased A:G ratio supports a diagnosis of feline infectious peritonitis (FIP) (Hartmann et al., 2003; Shelly et al., 1988). A more recent study (Hetzel et al., 2012) showed acceptable results for total protein were produced using a VetScan (Zoetis) tabletop analyzer, whereas the VetTest (IDEXX Laboratories) and SpotChem (Arkray) analyzers were determined to be unacceptable for evaluating total protein in canine effusions.

For cloudy or turbid samples and bloody samples, the fluid should be centrifuged and the protein measured on the supernatant. Turbidity may interfere with evaluation of protein by either refractometry or spectrophotometry. The protein content is used along with the nucleated cell count and cellular content to assist in classifying the effusion and help formulate a list of possible etiologies (Fig. 6.2).

> **KEY POINT** The measurement of specific gravity using a standard refractometer has not been validated for use with body cavity fluids, only urine. Therefore, the use of specific gravity values in low-protein fluids should be regarded with caution (George, 2001).

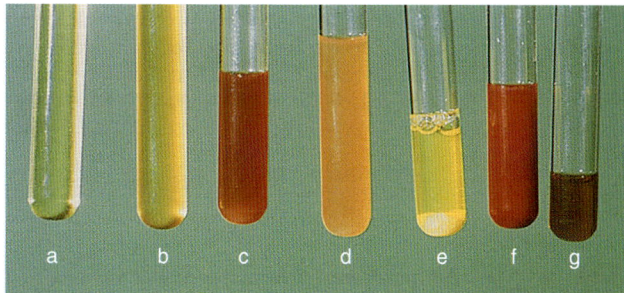

■ **FIGURE 6.1 Effusion color and turbidity.** Gross appearance of various effusions. *Left to right,* These are likely (a) colorless and clear—transudate; (b) yellow and hazy—modified transudate; (c) orange-red and cloudy—hemorrhagic (hemolyzed) or bilious; (d) orange and cloudy—exudate with hemorrhage; (e) yellow and cloudy with sediment—exudate; (f) red and opaque—hemorrhagic or iatrogenic blood contamination; and (g) brown and cloudy—bilious, gastrointestinal rupture, or chronic hemorrhagic.

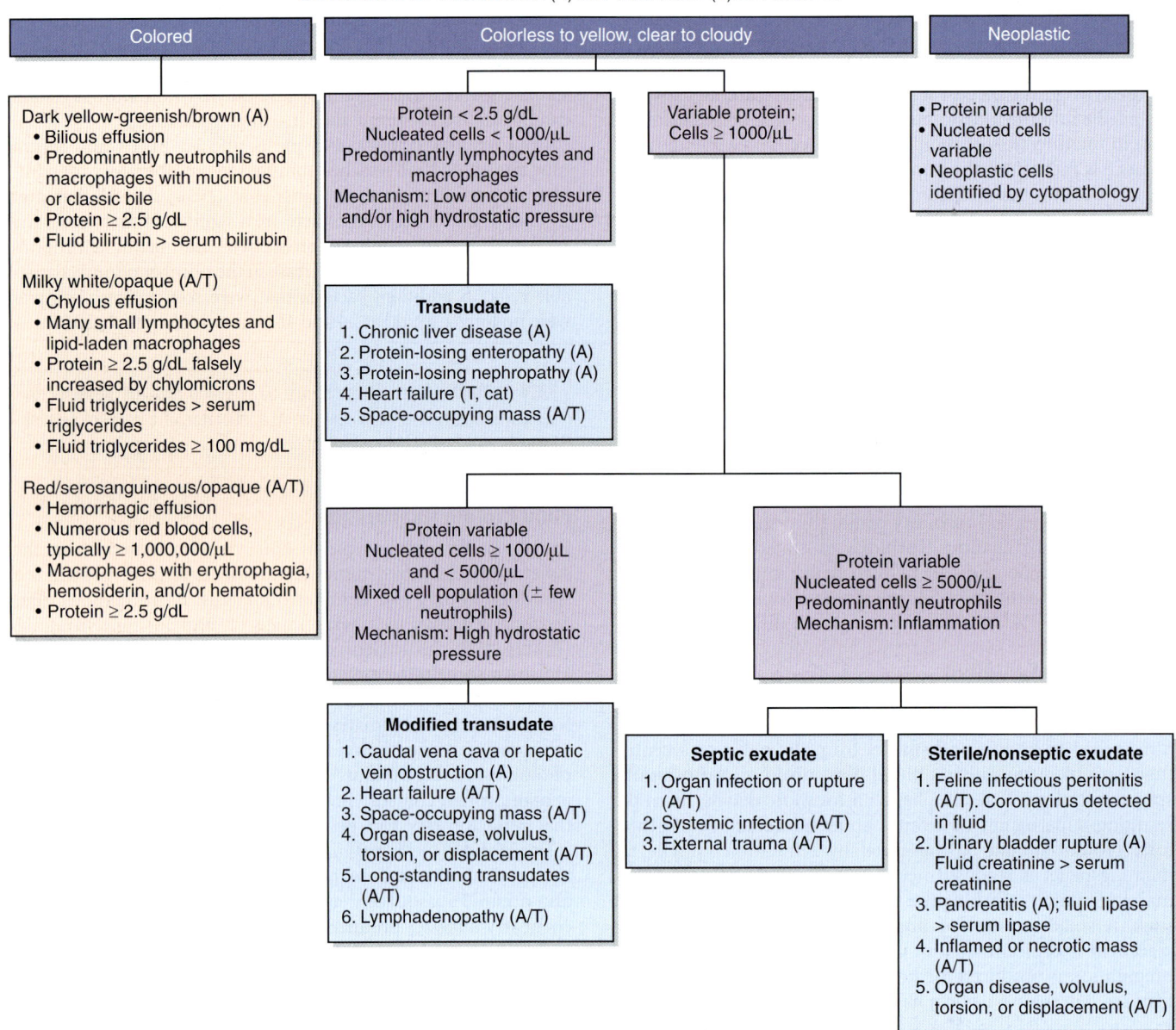

■ FIGURE 6.2 **Algorithm for effusion classification.** Abdominal (A) and thoracic (T) effusions are easily classified by color and content. Attempt to first classify the effusion by looking for evidence of bile, chyle, blood, or neoplasia. For other conditions that produce colorless or minimally colored fluids, use protein concentration and cell types to further classify these effusions as pure transudates (low protein), modified transudates (high protein), or exudates (high nucleated cells). Transudation often results from increased hydrostatic pressure within blood and lymphatic vessels. Exudation of significant numbers of neutrophils, macrophages, or both from injured lymphatic and blood vessels (exudate) results from infectious or noninfectious etiologies. (Modified from Meyer DJ, Harvey JW. *Veterinary Laboratory Medicine—Interpretation and Diagnosis.* 3rd ed. Elsevier; 2004.)

Fluid Red Blood Cell and Total Nucleated Cell Counts

Although an initial impression of the cellularity and amount of blood can usually be made by visual inspection of the sample, knowledge of the actual cell counts for erythrocytes and nucleated cells is important for further classification of the type of fluid. With this information, one can begin to narrow the list of possible causes for the abnormal fluid accumulation. For samples being submitted to a reference laboratory, placing some of the sample in a lavender-top tube (EDTA) and some in a red-top tube (no additive) is recommended. The lavender-top tube contains anticoagulant that prevents the sample from clotting if there is a high protein content or blood contamination.

The RBC count and total nucleated cell count (TNCC) are easily obtained with an automated hematology analyzer (Gorman et al., 2009; Pinta da Cunha et al., 2009); however, automated nucleated cell differential counts are less reliable. Flocculent or clotted fluids or fluids with high fibrinogen content in the fluid may produce erroneous cell counts or clog the internal tubing of the analyzer, and automated fluid analysis may be declined for these samples.

If an automated hematology analyzer is not available, the RBC mass can be estimated by spinning a microhematocrit tube with fluid and measuring the packed cell volume (PCV). This is mainly applicable to fluids that are red and semitranslucent to opaque. Although traditional, the hemacytometer method for determining the TNCC is slow, laborious, and inherently inaccurate. Similarly, estimation of TNCC can be performed for overall evaluation from well-made direct smears. Each microscope differs in magnification, but often the estimate can be accomplished by counting nucleated cells from an average field in the monolayer and multiplying the count by the square of the lens objective. For example, if an average of 6 nucleated cells is observed using the 40× objective, the calculation would be 6 nucleated cells/field × 40^2 = 6 nucleated cells/field × 1600 = 9600 nucleated cells/µL.

> **KEY POINT** Do not use gel-containing serum separator tubes for submission of fluid to a reference laboratory. Cells may bind to the gel in these tubes and result in an artifactual low cell count.

Fluid Nucleated Cell Differential

Standard procedures for performing a differential of the nucleated cells vary among laboratories. Some laboratories perform no cell differential, some perform a three-part differential of 100 cells (large mononuclear cells, small mononuclear cells, and granulocytes), and yet others provide a 100-cell differential of all cell types observed. Automated differentials have been evaluated and shown to only have modest concordance with human observations and are likely best used as a screening tool (Pinta da Cunha et al., 2009; Bauer and Moritz, 2012). The cell differential provides a relative picture of the types and numbers of cells and aids in establishing a list of potential causes of the fluid accumulation. A differential is not a substitute for a complete cytopathologic evaluation because microscopic examination of a smear also includes the noncellular components of the smear. The cytopathologic evaluation is performed in an attempt to determine a specific diagnosis.

NORMAL CYTOLOGY AND ARTIFACTS

Normal fluid is clear and colorless (see Fig. 6.1, a), and the background appears lightly eosinophilic or basophilic with Romanowsky staining. Several types of cells may be found in body cavity effusions, and their relative proportions vary depending on the cause of the fluid accumulation. Cells expected to be in normal fluid include mesothelial cells, mononuclear phagocytes, lymphocytes, and rare neutrophils.

Mesothelial Cells

In most cases, the cytopathologist will find mesothelial cells in body cavity fluids. These are included as large mononuclear cells for the purpose of the three-part cell differential. Mesothelial cells may be seen as individualized cells (Fig. 6.3) or in variably sized sheets (Fig. 6.4). They have a moderate amount of homogeneous medium-blue cytoplasm and occasionally cytoplasmic blebs.

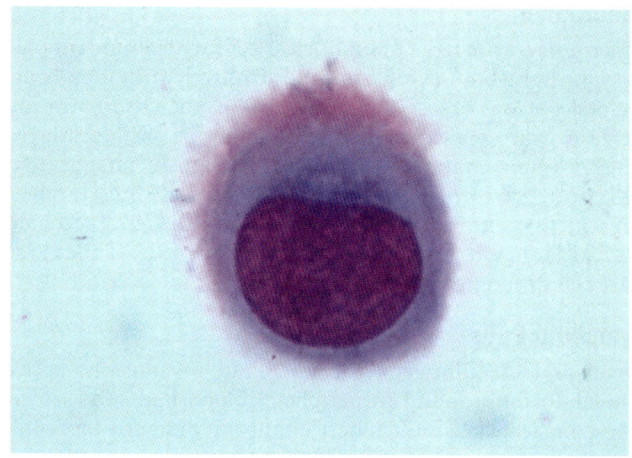

■ **FIGURE 6.3 Normal mesothelial cell. Cavitary effusion smear.** The exfoliated cell shows its characteristic pink fringe (glycocalyx) along the cytoplasmic border. (Wright-Giemsa; HP oil.) (From Meyer DJ, Franks PT. Classification and cytologic examination. *Compend Contin Educ Pract Vet*. 1987;9:123–129.)

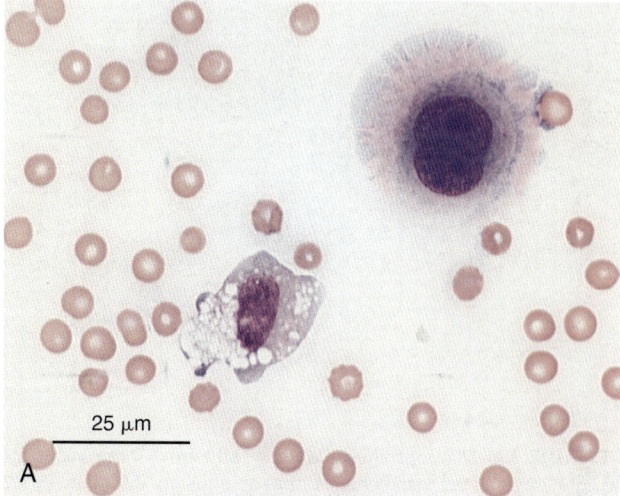

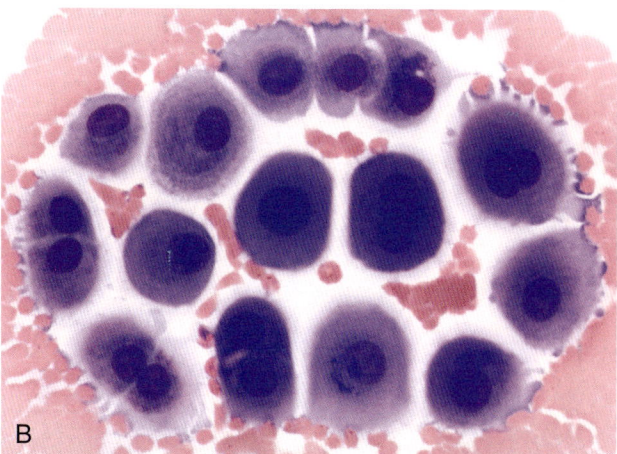

■ **FIGURE 6.4 Reactive mesothelial cells. Cavitary effusion. A,** There are an exfoliated binucleate mesothelial cell (*upper right*) and vacuolated macrophage (*lower left*). The mesothelial cell has a characteristic pink fringe (glycocalyx) along the cytoplasmic border. (Modified Wright; HP oil.) **B,** Group of reactive mesothelial cells are at the feathered edge of a smear. Several cells contain paranuclear dark granules of unknown significance. (Modified Wright; HP oil.)

Macrophages

Macrophages are large mononuclear cells with abundant pale-gray to light-blue cytoplasm and a round to kidney bean–shaped nucleus (Fig. 6.5; see Fig. 6.4A). The chromatin may be fine, and small, round nucleoli may be visible. Macrophages often contain vacuoles or previously phagocytized cells or debris if there is inflammation or if the fluid has been present for a long time (Fig. 6.6). Macrophages are considered as large mononuclear cells for the purpose of the three-part cell differential.

Lymphoid Cells

Small and medium lymphocytes found in effusions appear similar to those found in peripheral blood and solid tissues. These nucleated cells often have a thin rim of lightly basophilic cytoplasm and a round nucleus. Lymphocytes are considered small mononuclear cells for the purpose of the three-part cell differential. In normal fluids, they are present in higher proportions in cats than in dogs. The nucleus nearly fills the cell, producing a uniformly high nucleocytoplasmic (N:C) ratio. The chromatin is finely stippled to evenly clumped; nucleoli are typically not visible (Fig. 6.7).

Neutrophils

Neutrophils appear similar to those found in peripheral blood. They are medium-sized cells with pale to clear cytoplasm and a segmented nucleus. Neutrophils should be absent or present in very low numbers in normal fluid, but they are found in increased numbers with chronic effusions or with inflammation (see Figs. 6.6 and 6.7B).

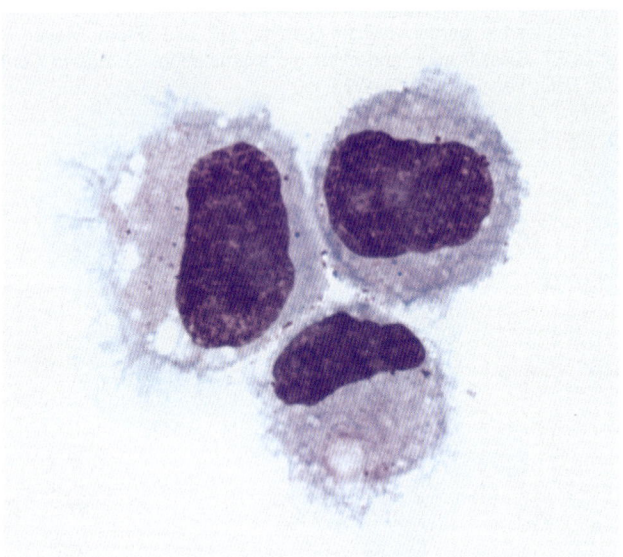

■ **FIGURE 6.5 Macrophages. Cavitary effusion.** Three vacuolated and lightly granulated macrophages from an effusion. (Modified Wright; HP oil.)

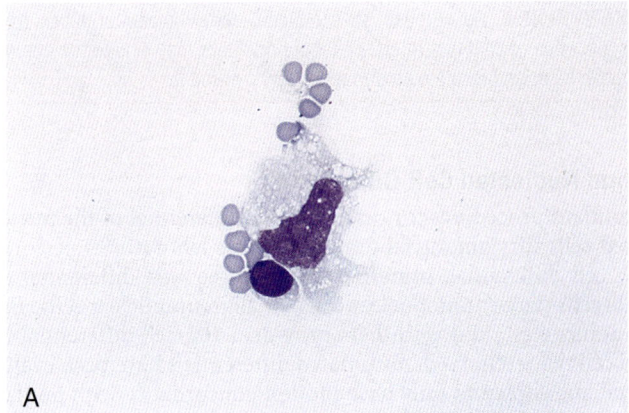

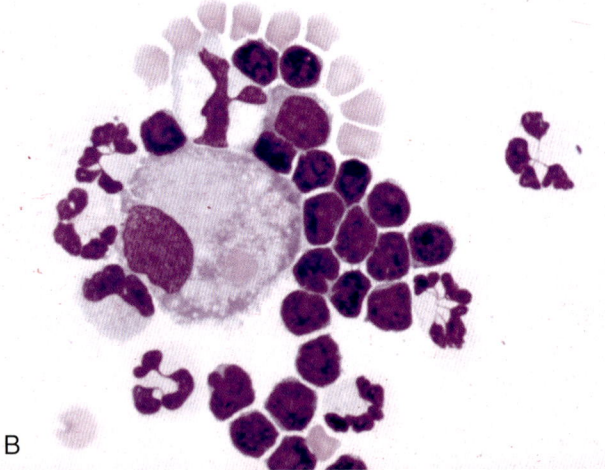

■ **FIGURE 6.7 Transudates. Cavitary effusion. A, Pure transudate.** A macrophage, a small lymphocyte, and 10 erythrocytes. Normal fluid and transudates generally have a nucleated cell count of <1000/µL and a protein concentration of <2.5 g/dL. (Methanolic Romanowsky; HP oil.) **B, Modified transudate.** Pleural fluid from a cat with hypertrophic cardiomyopathy had 2.5 g protein/dL and 4000 nucleated cells/µL. There are numerous small lymphocytes, nondegenerate neutrophils, and erythrocytes surrounding a large macrophage. The macrophage has phagocytized a red blood cell indicative of acute hemorrhage. Mild hemorrhage by diapedesis may occur with congestive disorders, such as cardiac failure. (Methanolic Romanowsky; HP oil.)

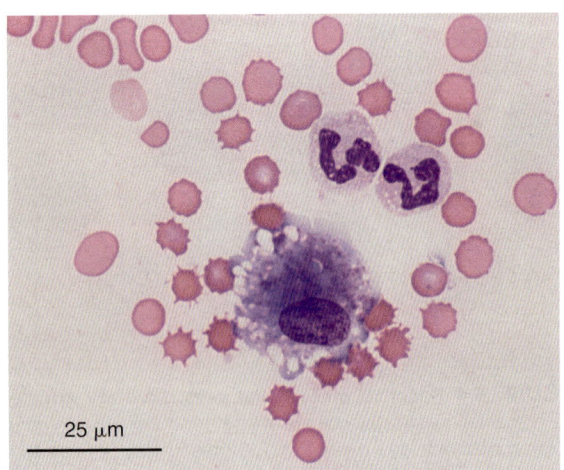

■ **FIGURE 6.6 Macrophage and neutrophils. Cavitary effusion.** A vacuolated and basophilic macrophage and two nondegenerate neutrophils are surrounded by erythrocytes. (Modified Wright; HP oil.)

CELLULAR AND FLUID RESPONSES TO INJURY

Effusion is the accumulation of fluid within the peritoneal, pleural, or pericardial space. The pathogenesis of an effusion may occur through one or more processes that disrupt vascular pressure (transudation), permeability (exudation), or integrity (blood or lymphatic vessel rupture) or a process that leads to rupture of a fluid-filled organ. Mesothelium easily becomes hyperplastic or reactive when an effusion or inflammation is present.

Mesothelial Cell Hyperplasia

Hyperplastic mesothelial cells are large (12–30 μm) with homogeneous deep-blue cytoplasm and may display a pink to red "fringed" glycocalyx cytoplasmic border (see Fig. 6.4). This feature helps identify these cells as mesothelial cells rather than macrophages or other large mononuclear cells. These cells may contain one or more nuclei of equal size (see Fig. 6.4B). Nucleoli may be visible, and occasional mitotic figures may be evident.

Cholesterol Crystals

Cholesterol crystals are rarely observed in cavitary fluid and are thought to result from release and aggregation of cholesterol from necrotic cell membranes. These fluids typically appear turbid and milky with a predominance of lymphocytes and a fluid cholesterol-to-triglyceride ratio greater than 1 (Lama et al., 2016). Such fluids grossly resemble chyle and had been classified as "pseudochylous effusions" (a term no longer used). Cholesterol crystals are colorless rhomboid or rectangular structures, often with notched edges (Fig. 6.8). Rarely, they may be elongated (MacGregor et al., 2004). Cholesterol crystals have been observed in a dog with ascites and sclerosing encapsulating peritonitis, a dog with pericardial effusion and aortic thromboembolism, and humans with tuberculosis or rheumatoid arthritis (MacGregor et al., 2004; Lama et al., 2016).

Transudation

Transudative effusions result from increased vascular hydrostatic pressure or decreased blood vascular oncotic pressure, as described by Starling principles (O'Brien and Lumsden, 1988; Stewart, 2000; Dempsey and Ewing, 2011). Because there is not a strong inflammatory stimulus within the cavity, the TNCCs tend to be lower than those of exudates with fewer neutrophils. However, a transudate's fluid protein concentration may vary depending on the pathogenesis and chronicity of the effusion. Transudates are subcategorized as a pure transudate also known as *transudate* (protein-poor transudate) and a *modified transudate* (protein-rich transudate) based on the protein content and TNCC.

Fluid transudation occurs with increased blood and lymphatic hydrostatic pressures. Pressure in blood and lymphatic vessels may increase with hypertensive or congestive disorders, resulting in increased net flow of fluid out of blood vessels and decreased net removal of fluid via the lymphatics. Causes of systemic hypertension include congestive heart failure, renal failure, and excessive fluid administration. Localized or regional venous congestion may occur with right-sided heart failure, left-sided heart failure, hepatitis or hepatopathy, venous thrombus, compressive mass or mass-like lesions, or organ torsion or volvulus. In these cases, vascular leakage occurs in the "upstream" vessels of lowest resistance and highest porosity, typically postcapillary venules or sinusoidal (discontinuous) capillaries. The characteristics of the effusion are therefore partially dependent on the fluid characteristics typical of the congested tissue. Because portal blood contains lower protein than hepatic sinusoidal blood, leakage of portal blood tends to produce peritoneal effusions with lower protein concentrations than effusions because of hepatic sinusoidal leakage. Disorders of the heart and veins that drain the hepatic sinusoids, such as congestive heart failure, right-sided heart failure, and Budd-Chiari–like syndrome, are therefore expected to cause high-protein transudates (modified transudate) from protein-rich hepatic lymph, whereas periportal and portal vein disorders tend to produce low-protein transudates (pure transudate) from low protein intestinal lymph (Fig. 6.9). Examples of the latter include idiopathic hepatic fibrosis, canine chronic hepatitis, vacuolar hepatopathy, portal vein hypoplasia, and portal vein thrombosis (James et al., 2008; Buob, 2011).

In addition to presinusoidal portal hypertension, decreased oncotic blood pressure caused by marked hypoalbuminemia

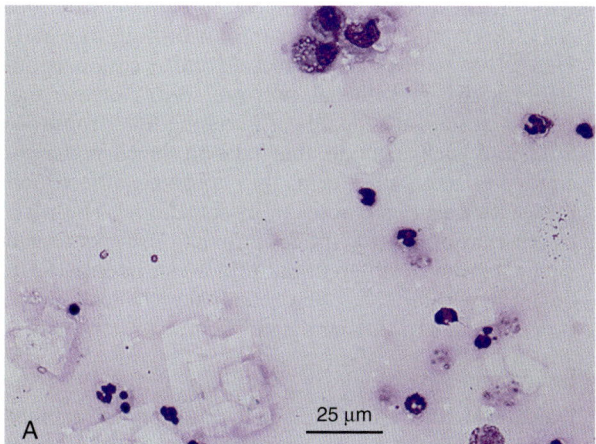
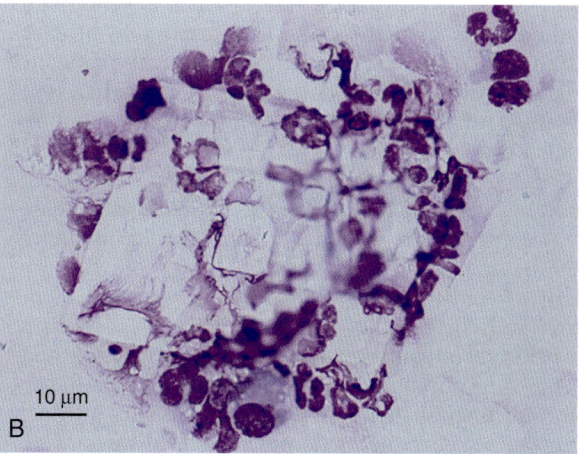

FIGURE 6.8 Cholesterol crystals. Peritoneal fluid. Dog. Same case in A and B. **A,** Rectangular and rhomboidal crystals are outlined by a faint eosinophilic background. (Romanowsky; HP oil.) **B,** Neutrophils and free nuclear protein surround numerous colorless rectangular crystals. (Romanowsky; HP oil.) Sclerosing encapsulating peritonitis was diagnosed at necropsy. (Courtesy Tara Arndt, University of California-Davis. Presented at the 2010 ASVCP case review session.)

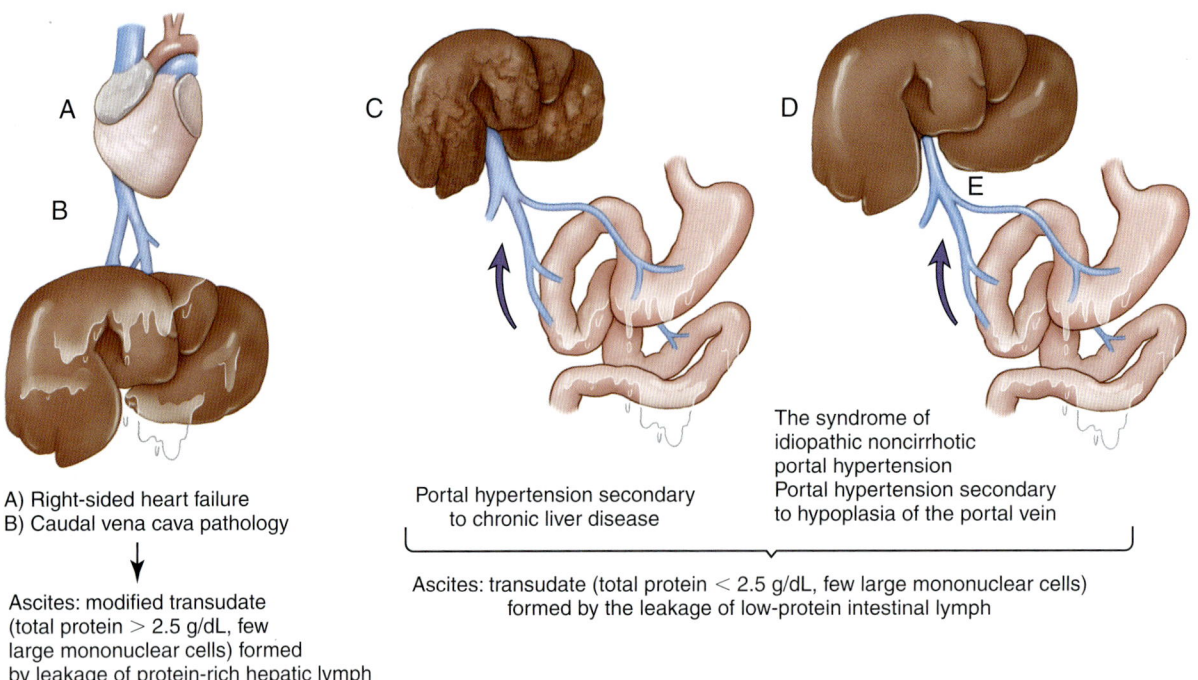

■ **FIGURE 6.9 Pathophysiology of transudate formation.** (Modified from Meyer DJ, Harvey JW. *Veterinary Laboratory Medicine—Interpretation and Diagnosis*. 3rd ed. Elsevier; 2004.)

(serum albumin <1.5 g/dL) is another pathogenesis for a pure transudate (protein-poor transudate). Potential hypoalbuminemic disorders include protein-losing nephropathy, protein-losing enteropathy, and hepatic failure. These fluids have a low protein content and a low total nucleated cell count (protein <2.5 g/dL and cells <1000/μL). The cells commonly found in pure transudates are similar to those in normal fluid, which are mostly mononuclear cells consisting of macrophages, small lymphocytes, and nonreactive mesothelial cells (see Fig. 6.7A). Nondegenerate neutrophils may make up a small proportion of the population.

Pure transudates may transition to modified transudates if there is a chronic effusion. The accumulation of fluid in a body cavity causes increased cavitary pressure, which is irritating to the mesothelial cells lining the space. They respond by proliferating and sloughing into the effusion. With time, the sloughed mesothelial cells die, and in so doing release chemoattractants that draw small numbers of phagocytes into the effusion to remove cellular debris. The result is a mild increase in both total protein (>2.5 g/dL) and variable TNCC (often <5000/μL). Thus, modified transudates may represent pure transudates that have been present long enough to elicit a mild inflammatory reaction (see Fig. 6.7B).

Similarly, chemoattractants increase the proportion of inflammatory cells in chronic modified transudates. In these cases, the principal inflammatory cell is the nondegenerate neutrophil. Over time, modified transudates gradually become cytologically indistinguishable from nonseptic exudates in which the neutrophil becomes the predominant cell. In cases of extended duration, modified transudates can have a cloudy or milky appearance. The gross appearance of these fluids is the result of high lipid content (caused by higher cholesterol content than serum) but is in no way related to a true chylous effusion because no triglycerides or chylomicrons are present (Hillerdal, 1997; Fossum et al., 1986b; Meadows and MacWilliams, 1994). The phagocytes attracted to remove cellular debris from transudates are rich in enzymes that digest protein but are virtually devoid of enzymes that will break down complex lipids. Consequently, although most of the constituents of dying cells are removed by phagocytosis, the lipid content of the cells simply accumulates in the effusion. Effusions formed in this manner are easily distinguished cytologically from true chylous effusions (Fossum et al., 1986b).

A common cellular constituent of the modified transudate is the reactive mesothelial cell (see Fig. 6.4A). Because of the ability of mesothelial cells to respond to irritation by proliferation, the presence of increased numbers of mesothelial cell clusters and rafts is a common finding in reactivity (see Fig. 6.4B). Mitoses are increased, and occasional multinucleated reactive mesothelial cells are seen. Reactive mesothelial cells in clusters are capable of imbibing lipid from the effusion fluid, and when they do, they take on the characteristics of secretory cells. In this form, they must be differentiated from metastatic adenocarcinoma or mesothelioma. This may be done by critically evaluating the cell populations for criteria of malignancy. However, differentiation between neoplasia and mesothelial hyperplasia can be occasionally challenging to the less experienced, and further diagnostic testing may be necessary.

Exudation

Exudates are the result of increased vascular permeability secondary to inflammation. An exudative fluid usually contains both increased protein and an increased TNCC. The total protein concentration is usually greater than 3.0 g/dL, along with cell counts greater than 5000/μL. Infectious causes for exudates include viruses, bacteria (Fig. 6.10), fungi, protozoa, and helminths.

Noninfectious causes involve organ inflammation such as pancreatitis (Figs. 6.11 and 6.12), gastritis or enteritis, torsion or volvulus, steatitis, inflammatory neoplasia, and irritants such as bile, urine, keratin, and sperm. Cytopathologic evaluation is useful to determine an underlying cause in cases of exudative effusions.

Inflammatory effusions are classified according to the standard rules for inflammation as neutrophilic, mixed, or macrophagic. The terms *granulomatous* and *pyogranulomatous* are not generally applied to effusions because granuloma is a solid structure and thus not applicable to a fluid environment. In exudates, neutrophils (either nondegenerate or degenerate) often comprise more than 50% of the inflammatory cells seen (Alonso, 2021). Mixed reactions are characterized by the

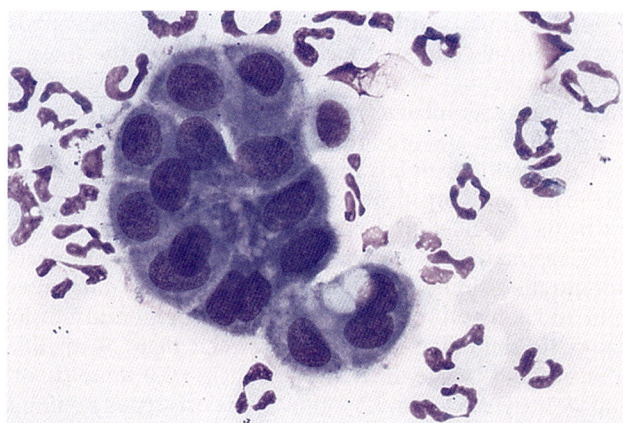

■ **FIGURE 6.11 Nonseptic exudate. Pancreatitis. Peritoneal fluid. Dog. Fluid smear.** Fluid from a dog with acute pancreatitis had 3.0 g protein/dL and 8000 nucleated cells/µL, compatible with an exudate. Note the sheet of reactive mesothelial cells and degenerative and nondegenerative neutrophils. Nonspecific exudates often require further testing, such as ultrasonography, radiographs, or fluid and serum chemistry testing, to determine the specific cause of the effusion. (Romanowsky; HP oil.)

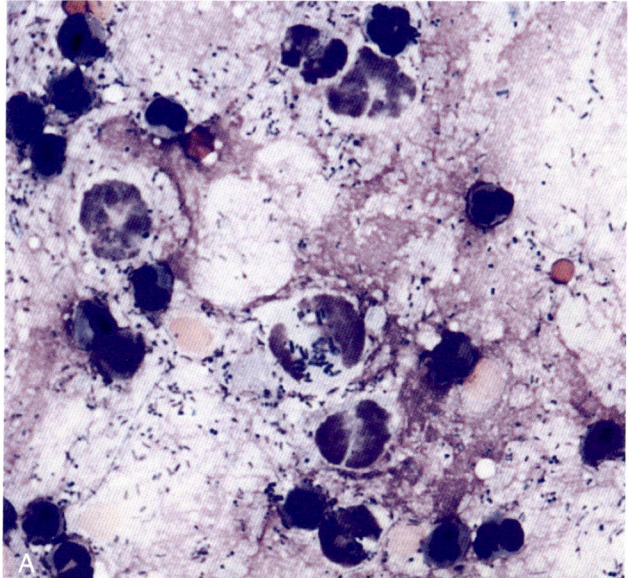

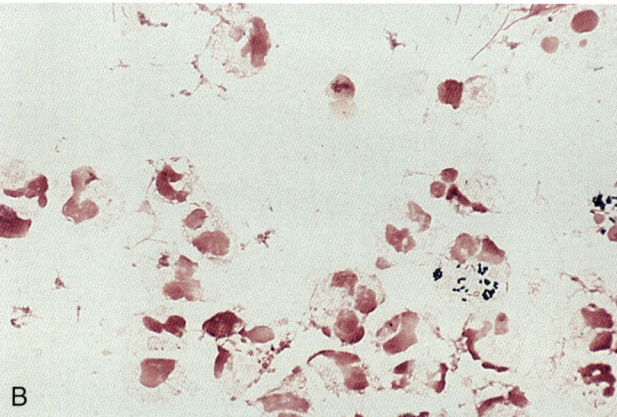

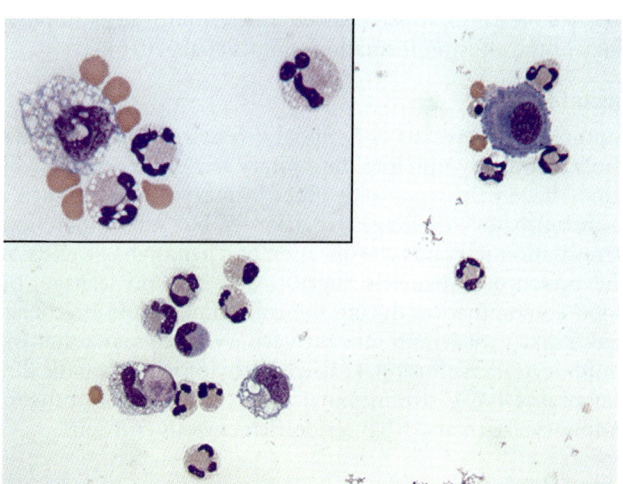

■ **FIGURE 6.12 Nonseptic exudate. Pancreatitis. Peritoneal fluid. Dog. Fluid smear.** Pink/turbid fluid with 28.12×10^9/L total nucleated cell count. The diagnosis of pancreatitis is made from clinical presentation, biochemical data, and serum canine pancreatic lipase immunoreactivity (PLI) test >2000 µg/L (reference interval 0-200 µg/L). The fluid consists mostly of nondegenerate neutrophils and vacuolated macrophages. One reactive mesothelial cell is shown. (Wright; HP oil.) *Inset:* The three neutrophils contain several colorless punctate vacuoles that are suggestive of lipid. The macrophage contains variably sized colorless vacuoles. Suspicion for steatitis relates to the presence of frequent cytoplasmic vacuoles within the inflammatory cells. (Wright; HP oil.) (Courtesy Rose Raskin, University of Bristol, UK.)

■ **FIGURE 6.10 Exudates. Bacterial sepsis. A, Peritoneal fluid. Dog.** A degenerate neutrophil (center) has ingested numerous bacteria and is surrounded by many extracellular bacteria and other inflammatory cells embedded in a granular eosinophilic proteinaceous background. A ruptured pancreatic abscess was diagnosed. (Modified Wright; HP oil.) **B, Pleural fluid. Cat.** This sample contains many nucleated cells (>100,000 cells/µL) and greater than 3.0 g/dL protein, compatible with an exudate. The degenerate neutrophils are swollen with foamy or vacuolated cytoplasm (hydropic change) and contain enlarged, hyposegmented, pale nuclei (karyolysis). Note the presence of small, gram-positive, pleomorphic bacterial bacilli. Aerobic and anaerobic cultures are recommended in cases of pyothorax. (Gram; HP oil.)

presence of neutrophils and macrophages. In histiocytic inflammation, macrophages are the prevalent cell seen.

On cytopathology, most inflammatory effusions are nonspecific in terms of an etiologic diagnosis. However, as with inflammatory responses elsewhere, cytomorphology provides significant clues as to the underlying cause. Neutrophilic inflammatory effusions indicate severe active irritation. If neutrophils are degenerate, an effort should be made to identify bacterial organisms within phagocytes (primarily neutrophils). This is generally easiest at the feathered edge of the smear. If organisms are not seen, the fluid should still be cultured. Mixed and macrophagic inflammatory effusions reflect less severe irritation and are found with resolving acute effusions or in association with less irritating etiologic agents than bacteria (e.g., fungal organisms or foreign bodies).

Chemical evaluation of effusion fluid is also useful in recognizing sepsis. Measuring blood and fluid lactate and glucose concentrations in dogs with peritonitis may help differentiate septic and nonseptic effusions. In dogs with peritoneal effusion, a blood-to-fluid glucose difference greater than 20 mg/dL, a blood-to-fluid lactate difference less than −2.0 mmol/L, or a fluid lactate greater than 2.5 mmol/L supports septic peritonitis (Bonczynski et al., 2003; Levin et al., 2004). These measurements are less reliable in cats (Bonczynski et al., 2003; Levin, 2004) and are unreliable for detecting postsurgical sepsis in dogs (Szabo et al., 2011). A study that evaluated measurement of lactate dehydrogenase (LDH) in effusion fluid of dogs and cats found enzyme concentration to be significantly higher in exudates compared with transudates. However, researchers noted that LDH activity should not be used as a substitute for standard effusion analysis based on the physical and cytopathologic fluid features, which can better determine the pathophysiology of the effusion formation (Smuts et al., 2016).

Vessel Rupture

Ruptured blood vessels or lymphatic vessels result in escape of whole blood or lymph into the cavitary space, respectively. Mild hemorrhage may occur with other primary disorders, such as an inflammatory or congestive disorder, but substantial blood extravasation warrants classification of a hemorrhagic effusion. The presence of platelets suggests active blood leakage, but blood contamination during the collection should be considered. Leakage of lymph into the cavitary space may result in a lymphocyte-rich effusion. Leakage of chyle-rich lymphatic fluid that drains the gastrointestinal (GI) tract typically causes a lymphocyte-rich and triglyceride-rich chylous effusion.

Organ Rupture

Rupture of a fluid-filled organ, such as the esophagus, GI tract, gallbladder, urinary bladder, or reproductive tract, results in movement of the organ's luminal contents into the surrounding cavitary space. Peracute ruptures contain relatively low protein and nucleated cell counts, which then increase as inflammation develops over the acute and subacute phases. The erythrocyte count is variable, depending on the extent of blood vessel injury that occurs during the rupture. Cytopathologic identification of noncellular substances, such as bile, urinary crystals, or digesta, may aid in a diagnosis.

PERITONEAL EFFUSIONS

Noninfectious (Nonseptic) Exudates

A nonseptic exudate is an inflammatory effusion without the visual detection of infectious agents via cytopathologic examination. More common causes of nonseptic exudates include pancreatitis (see Figs. 6.11 and 6.12) and bile peritonitis in dogs and FIP and alimentary large cell lymphoma in cats. However, substantial inflammation of any organ within the peritoneal cavity could result in a nonseptic exudate, regardless of whether the primary disease is inflammatory, infectious, neoplastic, or degenerative. Although the inciting cause of the inflammation is often not observed on cytopathologic examination, the inflammatory cell types seen in the fluid may help prioritize differential diagnoses. Nonseptic exudates caused by ruptured "sterile organs," such as the gallbladder and urinary bladder, are described in the Organ Rupture sections. Neoplastic causes of nonseptic exudates are presented in the Neoplastic Effusions section.

Feline Infectious Peritonitis

FIP is unique among the causes of exudates in that the fluid is usually high in protein and relatively low in cellularity (Norris et al., 2005; Fischer et al., 2012). FIP has been noted to cause 18% of pleural (Davies and Forrester, 1996), 9.8% of pericardial (Davidson et al., 2008), and 5% of peritoneal (Wright et al., 1999) effusions. Classification of the effusion as inflammatory is based primarily on the presence of high total protein (often >4.5 g/dL), which is a reflection of a similar elevation in serum protein, as well as the product of vasculitis and increased vascular permeability. As such, the fluid is often yellow and hazy or cloudy because of the high protein concentration (Fig. 6.13), with or without grossly visible fibrin aggregates. Cytopathologically, these fluids are usually relatively low in cell number (<5000/μL) (Tasker, 2018) and inconsistent with regard to the cell types present. In a majority of cases, the predominant cell is the nondegenerate neutrophil (Fig. 6.14A). However, activated macrophages are commonly observed (Fig. 6.14B) (Paltrinieri et al., 1999; Norris et al., 2005). In rare cases, the lymphocyte is prevalent, and the effusion can even appear chyle-like (Savary et al., 2001). Regardless of the predominant cell type, slides in all cases have a bluish-gray to purple granular

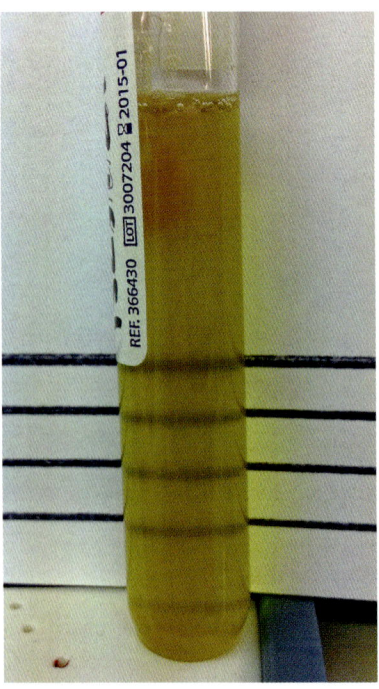

■ **FIGURE 6.13** Feline infectious peritonitis. Peritoneal fluid. Cat. **Tube with fluid.** The fluid is yellow and cloudy because of a high protein concentration (4.8 g/dL). Note the dark yellow fibrin clot below the fluid-air interface.

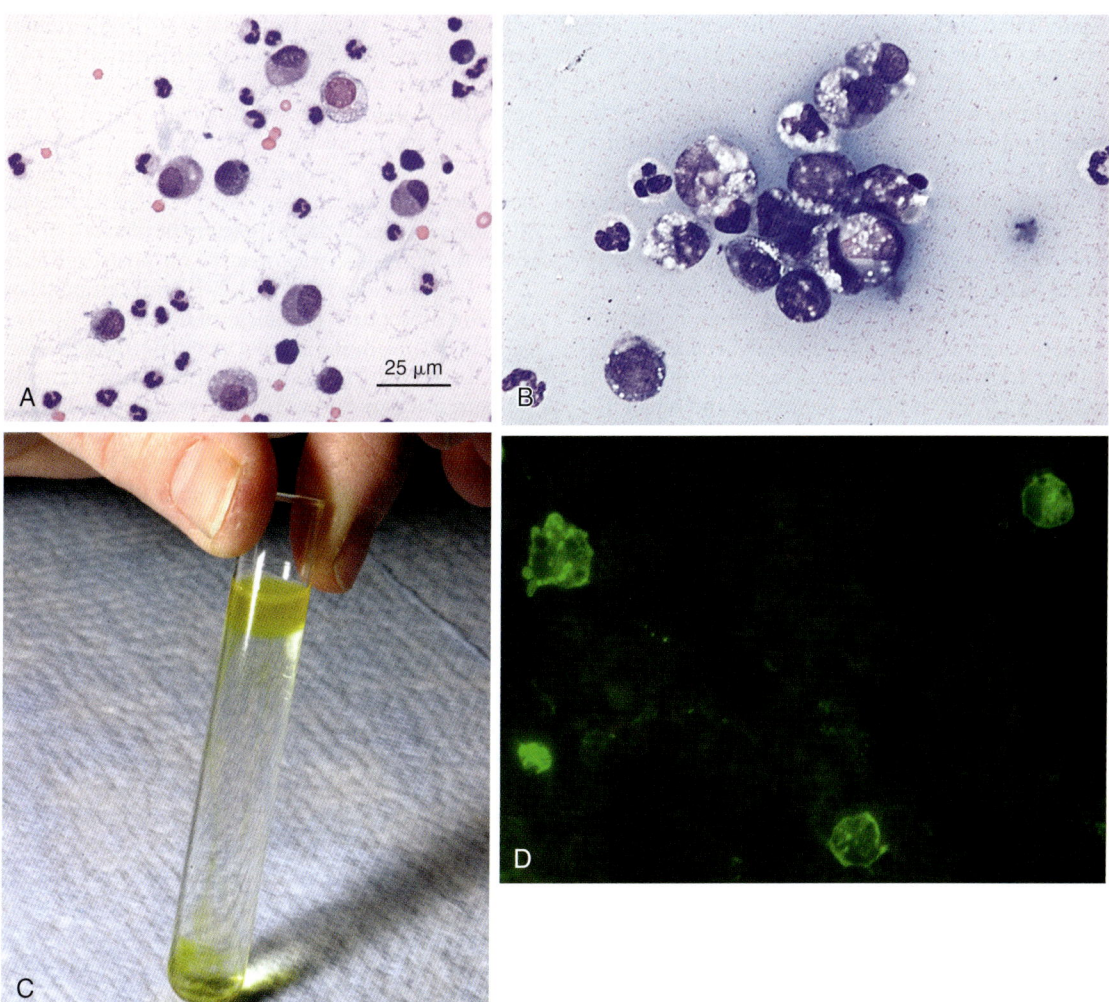

■ **FIGURE 6.14 Feline infectious peritonitis (FIP). Peritoneal fluid. Cat. A, Concentrated smear.** Nondegenerative neutrophils and macrophages present within a faint granular proteinaceous background. The lack of a visible infectious agent and inflammatory cell population support the cytopathologic diagnosis of nonseptic exudate. (Modified Wright; HP oil.) **B, Cytopathologic preparation.** Vacuolated macrophages and neutrophils appear against a faint granular basophilic proteinaceous background. Lymphocytes may be intermediate in size and appear reactive in some cases of FIP. (Methanolic Romanowsky; HP oil.) **C, Rivalta test.** A layer of gel on top of the acetic acid solution indicates a positive test. Fluid is from a cat with polymerase chain reaction–confirmed FIP. Note the yellow streaks of gel in the middle of the tube from partially floating material. **D. Feline coronavirus (FCoV) immunofluorescence test.** Demonstration of intracellular FCoV within effusion macrophages by immunofluorescence is a specific test for FIP. There are three immunofluorescent-positive (green) macrophages. Stain artifact lower left. (FCoV immunofluorescence; HP oil.) (C, Courtesy Sam Royer, Purdue University. D, Courtesy Jacqueline Norris, University of Sydney, Australia.)

background that results from the high protein content (see Fig. 6.14), and clumps and strands of fibrin may be observed.

Electrophoresis of either the effusion fluid or the serum reveals a polyclonal gammopathy (Tasker, 2018). The total protein, A:G ratio, and percent globulins in effusions have all been evaluated as a tool for diagnosing FIP from effusions. Paltrinieri et al. (1999) found that a total protein greater than 3.5 g/dL alone had a sensitivity of 87.1% and a specificity of 60%. Shelly et al. (1988) found that a gamma globulin concentration greater than or equal to 32% had a 100% positive predictive value (PPV). This same study found an A:G ratio greater than 0.81 had a negative predictive value (NPV) of 100%. Sparkes et al. (1994) found a 94% PPV and 100% NPV for FIP when the total protein of an effusion was greater than 3.5 mg/L at the same time globulins made up greater than 50% of the protein.

An additional test that can help rule out FIP is the Rivalta test. To perform this relatively simple test, place one drop of 98% acetic acid into 5 mL distilled water and mix well in a clear reagent tube. Slowly layer one drop of the effusion fluid to the surface of the acetic acid solution. A positive test result requires that the drop of effusion retain its form on the surface or slowly sink to the bottom as a droplet or jellyfish-like shape (see Fig. 6.14C). The positive reaction to the acetic acid is due to the presence of a high concentration of proteins, including fibrinogen and other acute phase proteins, which visibly clot upon contact with acids. A study reported no major differences using acetic acid, distilled white vinegar, and wine vinegar (Fischer et al., 2013). This same study showed that refrigerated storage for up to 21 days did not affect results. This test has a reported PPV of 58.4% to 88.4% and NPV of 66.7% to 93.4% (Fischer et al., 2012) in contrast to PPV of 86% and NPV of 97%

in an earlier study (Hartmann et al., 2003). The sensitivity and specificity of the Rivalta test are reported to be 91.3% and 65.5%, respectively (Fischer et al., 2012). The effect of clot formation in the Rivalta test is similar for the measurement of effusion TNCC by an automated hematologic analyzer such as Sysmex, which uses two channels: DIFF (white blood cell differential) and BASO (basophil) for TNCC calculation. The DIFF channel classifies cells based on complexity and nucleic acid content. The BASO channel classifies cells based on volume and the complexity of cells after contact with an acidic reagent that collapses all the nucleated cells except basophils. In FIP cases, there is a lower count in the BASO channel related to increased cell clumping within fibrin. One study found that when the ratio of DIFF to BASO is greater than 1.7, FIP is highly suggestive, and when it is greater than 3.4 (3400/μL), it is considered diagnostic for FIP (Giordano et al., 2015). Other supportive tests include α1-acid glycoprotein (AGP) greater than 1.5 g/L based on acute phase proteins circulating in blood or greater than 1.55 mg/mL in the effusion support a diagnosis of FIP (Tasker, 2018).

The most specific fluid testing for FIP is the detection of feline coronavirus (FCoV) within effusion macrophages via direct immunofluorescence (DIF) or immunochemistry as well as within the effusion via reverse transcriptase polymerase chain reaction (RT-PCR) testing. Positive DIF staining of effusion macrophages (see Fig. 6.14D) has high specificity (71%–100%) for FIP and is often considered diagnostic (Hartmann et al., 2003; Litster et al., 2013). Unfortunately, a negative result does exclude FIP because the NPV is low (57%–66%) (Parodi et al., 1993; Hartmann et al., 2003). Detection of FCoV in effusions via RT-PCR is 69% to 89% sensitive and 96% to 100% specific for FIP (Doenges et al., 2017; Felten et al., 2017), and analysis of effusion samples has a higher sensitivity for FIP diagnosis compared with analysis of serum or blood samples (Doenges et al., 2017; Felten et al., 2017). However, the detection of FCoV by RT-PCR should be used along with other tests for confirmation such as histologic examination of affected tissue specimens. A study that evaluated multiple diagnostic tests for FIP in blood, effusion, and tissue comparing cytopathology, AGP, molecular tests, and DIFF/BASO found cytopathology, RT-PCR, and DIFF/BASO may confirm a clinical diagnosis on effusions (Stranieri et al., 2018). In addition, they suggested that for effusions, evaluating the cytopathology and DIFF/BASO would provide high diagnostic power.

> **KEY POINT** Demonstration of FCoV antigen by immunostaining in effusions or tissues together with typical cytopathologic or histopathologic features of FIP provides a definitive diagnosis of FIP. Furthermore, detection of FCoV RNA by RT-PCR at high levels in effusions supports a diagnosis of FIP.

Postoperative Exudates

Intraabdominal surgery is expected to alter peritoneal fluid characteristics in the absence of detectable sepsis (Botte and Eberhard, 1983). In dogs, peritoneal lavage fluid collected within 3 days after uncomplicated intestinal resection and anastomoses were turbid and pink to red with increased TNCC. Microscopically, there was a predominance of neutrophils with both nondegenerate and degenerate forms. The TNCCs were 500 to 3000/μL on postsurgical day 1, 616 to 2050/μL on postsurgical day 2, and 3600 to 10,500/μL on postsurgical day 3,

whereas lavage fluids from control dogs contained 17 to 52 nucleated cells/μL. The RBC counts were less than 40,000/μL in all postsurgical lavage fluids and 185 to 1900/μL in control lavage fluids. Bacteria were not detected by cytopathology or culture in any lavage fluids.

Postoperative peritoneal drain fluid characteristics have been documented in dogs after experimental celiotomy and silicone peritoneal drain placement (Szabo et al., 2011). The drain fluid volume was greatest on postsurgical day 1 (mean, 2.8 mL/kg per day; range, 1.2–5.2 mL/kg per day), decreased over the subsequent postsurgical days, and lowest on postsurgical day 7 (mean, 0.6 mL/kg per day; range, 0–1.5 mL/kg per day). Increased TNCCs were observed in drain fluids on all 7 postsurgical days and were highest on postsurgical days 3 and 4. Values were as follows:

Day 1: mean, 15,100/μL; range, 300 to 43,200/μL
Day 2: mean, 3200/μL; range, 300 to 13,400/μL
Day 3: mean, 13,300/μL; range, 500 to 149,800/μL
Day 4: mean, 14,500/μL; range, 400 to 84,100/μL
Day 5: mean, 8500/μL; range, 1300 to 27,500/μL
Day 6: mean, 4800/μL; range, 400 to 12,000/μL
Day 7: mean, 7700/μL; range, 1300 to 29,000/μL

The highest TNCCs in postsurgical days 3 to 5 were seen in a dog that developed incisional inflammation. Microscopically, degenerate neutrophils predominated in drain fluids from all dogs on all postsurgical days. Intracellular and extracellular bacteria were observed in drain fluid from 4 of the 10 dogs and were considered drain contaminants versus peritoneal infections.

Studies are lacking in dogs and cats on the effects of repeated abdominocentesis in normal and diseased patients. Because postsurgery produces an expected inflammatory response, it is conceivable that numbers and percentages of nondegenerate neutrophils from a recent prior paracentesis might rise (Fig. 6.15).

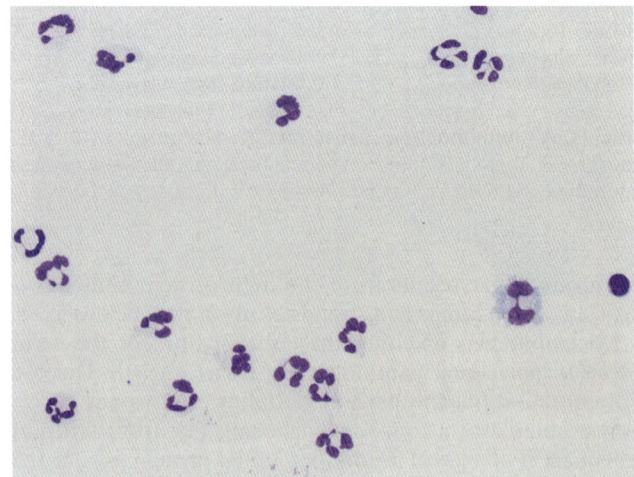

■ **FIGURE 6.15 Mild neutrophilic inflammation. Peritoneal fluid. Cat. Cytocentrifuged specimen.** Color/transparency: yellow/hazy; protein <2.0 g/dL; total nucleated cell count <1000/μL. Cell count and protein suggest a transudate, but the cell differential consisting of 92% neutrophils, 7% mononuclear phagocytes, and 1% lymphocytes supports an inflammatory response. History indicated that an abdominocentesis occurred 2 days earlier, which may have contributed to the mild neutrophilic response. (Wright-Giemsa; HP oil.) (Courtesy Rose Raskin, University of Florida.)

Eosinophilic Exudates

An inflammatory effusion with more than 10% eosinophils is termed an *eosinophilic exudate* or a *mixed-cell exudate with eosinophils* depending on the percentages of other inflammatory cell types. Effusions with low protein content and TNCC and more than 10% eosinophils may be termed *eosinophilic effusion* to denote the absence of a strong inflammatory presence. With large numbers of eosinophils, the fluid grossly may have a green tint (Fig. 6.16). An increased eosinophil percentage is more commonly seen as a component of chylous or neoplastic effusions, which would warrant the cytopathologic diagnosis to emphasize the primary chylous or neoplastic process: chylous effusion with eosinophilic exudate or neoplastic effusion with paraneoplastic eosinophilic exudate.

Lymphoma and systemic mastocytosis are common causes of eosinophilic exudates in dogs and cats (Fossum et al., 1993; Peaston and Griffey, 1994; Bounous et al., 2000; Barrs et al., 2002; Cowgill and Neel, 2003; Tomiyasu et al., 2010; Gupta et al., 2013; Harris et al., 2013). Other disorders that may cause peritoneal eosinophilic exudates include peritoneal cestodiasis, coccidioidomycosis, systemic sarcocystosis, feline eosinophilic GI sclerosing fibroplasia (Fig. 6.17), and pneumothorax (Miller et al., 1984; Fossum et al., 1993; Allison et al., 2006; Craig et al., 2009, Patten et al., 2013; Piech et al., 2020). One study identified disorders in dogs and cats with eosinophilic exudates but did not specify which cavity contained the effusion. These animals had hemangiosarcoma, allergic airway disease, lung lobe torsion, bite wound causing intestinal perforation, feline leukemia virus, pulmonary or intestinal parasitism, or heartworm disease (Fossum et al., 1993). The presence of eosinophils in the absence of an underlying cause does not provide a specific diagnosis, and the cause is often unknown in these cases.

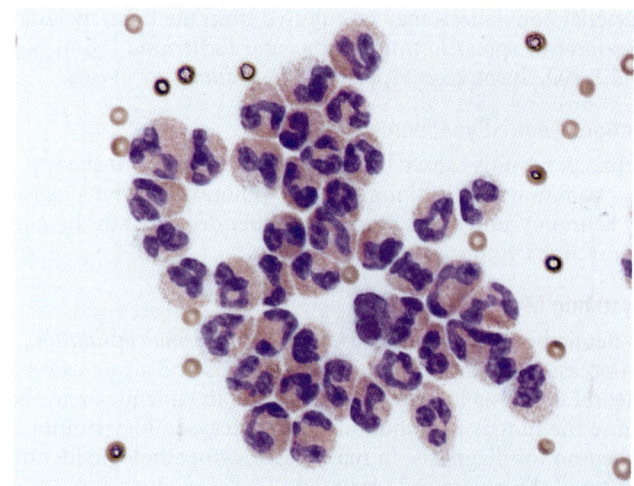

■ **FIGURE 6.17 Eosinophilic exudate. Peritoneal fluid. Cat. Fluid smear.** Many eosinophils in a peritoneal effusion from a cat with feline gastrointestinal eosinophilic sclerosing fibroplasia. (Courtesy Sarah Beatty et al., University of Florida. Presented at the 2013 ASVCP case review session.)

Infectious (Septic) Exudates
Primary Bacterial Peritonitis

Primary bacterial peritonitis, also known as spontaneous bacterial peritonitis, is defined as a bacterial infection of the peritoneal cavity without an obvious source for the infection. Suspected routes of infection include hematogenous or lymphogenous spread and bacterial translocation across devitalized GI, urinary, or biliary tracts. The expected cytopathologic findings are an exudate with degenerate neutrophils and intracellular bacterial without evidence of organ perforation (Fig. 6.18). One to several

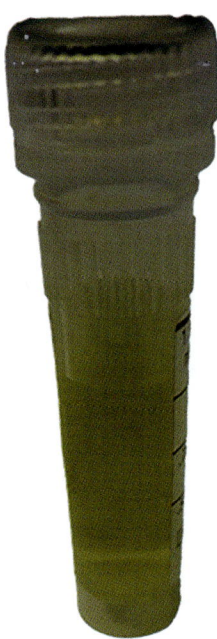

■ **FIGURE 6.16 Eosinophilic effusion. Peritoneal fluid. Cat. Tube with fluid.** The fluid appears grossly yellow-green. Estimated total nucleated cell count is 1400/μL, and the cell differential consists of 87% eosinophils, 10% neutrophils, 2% lymphocytes, and 1% large mononuclear cells. The green hue is likely related to the large presence of unstained eosinophils, (Courtesy Rose Raskin, TDDS, Exeter, UK.)

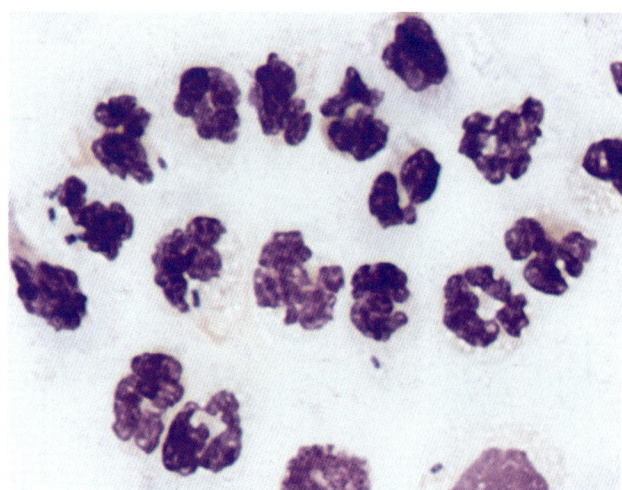

■ **FIGURE 6.18 Primary bacterial peritonitis. Peritoneal fluid. Dog. Fluid smear.** Fluid from a dog with septicemia contained 77,000 nucleated cells/μL, 2.8 g protein/dL, and 89,000 red blood cells/μL. Note degenerate and nondegenerate neutrophils with extracellular and intracellular monomorphic bacterial bacilli without evidence of organ perforation. Bacterial culture of the fluid identified *Escherichia coli*.

bacterial populations may be cultured from the fluid, including *Enterococcus* spp., *Clostridium* spp., and *Escherichia coli* in dogs and *E. coli*, *Streptococcus* spp., and *Clostridium* spp. in cats.

Actinomycotic Pyoabdomen

Septic peritonitis caused by *Actinomyces* spp. or *Nocardia* spp. is less common than actinomycotic pyothorax. Effusions caused by actinomycotic bacteria will be further described in the Actinomycotic Pyothorax section.

Systemic Mycoses

Systemic histoplasmosis, caused by *Histoplasma capsulatum*, is an occasional cause of peritoneal effusions and a rare cause of pleural effusions in dogs and cats living in endemic areas. Because the fungus is ubiquitous in the area, serology cannot be relied on for diagnosis. In many cases, cytopathologic identification of the organism is essential.

Effusions caused by histoplasmosis present in a variety of ways. On the basis of physical characteristics, the fluid has been reported as a pure transudate (Stickle and Hribernik, 1978), a modified transudate (Dillon et al., 1982; VanSteenhouse and DeNovo, 1986), and an exudate (Kowalewich et al., 1993). On cytopathology, these effusions have inflammatory characteristics with a mixture of neutrophils and macrophages. Histoplasmosis is considered to be disseminated when observed in effusions and can be found in the lungs, liver, spleen, bone marrow, rectal wall, and peripheral blood.

Demonstration of the organism is best done within macrophages (Fig. 6.19) at the feathered edge of sediment or direct smears. *Histoplasma* organisms measure approximately 2 to 4 μm in diameter, appear round to slightly ovoid in shape, and have a single basophilic nucleus surrounded by a thick, colorless cell wall (pseudocapsule). In fluids, it is common to see individual organisms free in the background. Two other organisms have similar cytomorphology. One organism is *Sporothrix*, but it differs in size (3–5 μm in diameter) and shape (elongated to cigar shaped), and the infection is usually restricted to the skin (see Figs. 3.59 and 3.60); disseminated disease has been described in cats and dogs. The other organism is *Leishmania*; however, it is distinguished by the presence of an internal kinetoplast, which gives it the appearance of having two nuclei (see Fig. 3.64).

If there is uncertainty in the cytopathologic diagnosis, a urine antigen test is available. This test detects a glycoprotein antigen released from viable *Histoplasma* yeast and excreted ultimately into the urine (Kauffman, 2007; Cook et al., 2012). A similar test has been evaluated for the detection of *Blastomyces* spp. infections in dogs (Spector et al., 2008). The test cross-reacts with antigens from *Histoplasma* spp. and may prove to be a useful tool in detecting disease as well as monitoring resolution or recurrence.

Other systemic mycoses, including blastomycosis (Fig. 6.20), cryptococcosis (Fig. 6.21), coccidioidomycosis (Fig. 6.22), and aspergillosis (Fig. 6.23) may rarely involve the serosal cavities and induce pericarditis, pleuritis, or peritonitis.

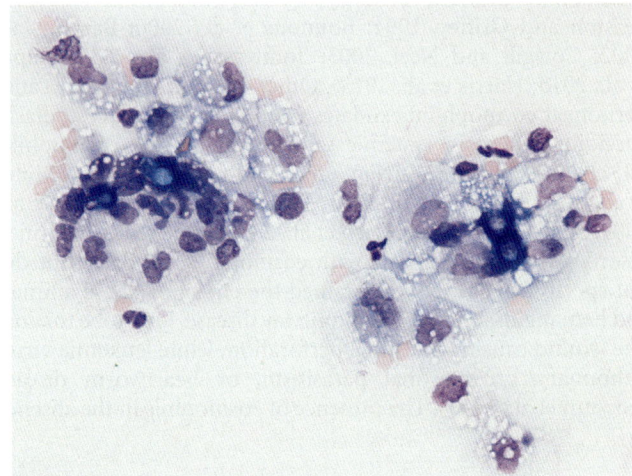

FIGURE 6.20 Blastomycosis. Pericardial fluid. Dog. Within the feathered edge of a direct smear, many vacuolated macrophages and a few degenerate neutrophils surround several dark blue, thick-walled yeast consistent with *Blastomyces dermatitidis*. (Wright-Giemsa; IP.) (Courtesy Rose Raskin, Purdue University.)

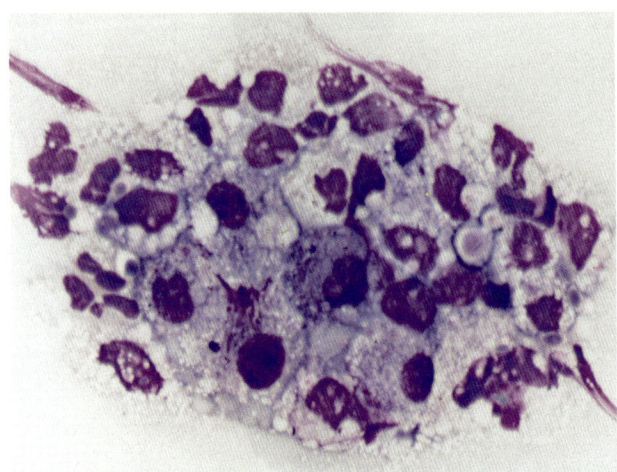

FIGURE 6.21 Cryptococcosis. Peritoneal fluid. Cat. Macrophages and neutrophils aggregate at the feathered edge of the smear. There are several small round to oval, poorly encapsulated, narrow-based budding *Cryptococcus neoformans* yeast toward the left and right sides of the aggregated leukocytes. Diagnosis confirmed on culture. (Courtney Nelson et al., University of Illinois. Presented at the 2017 ASVCP case review session, bonus case.)

FIGURE 6.19 Histoplasmosis. Cavitary fluid. Dog. Fluid smear. A macrophage has phagocytized oval 2 to 3 μm yeast organisms consistent with *Histoplasma capsulatum*. (Modified Wright; HP oil.)

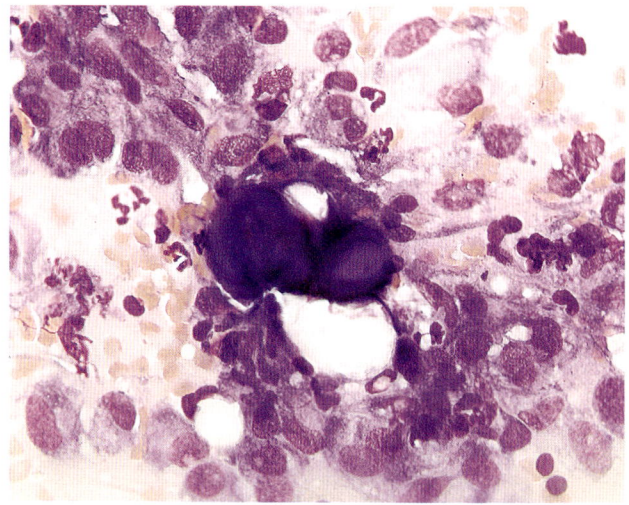

■ **FIGURE 6.22 Coccidioidomycosis. Dog. Pericardial imprint.** Two *Coccidioides* spp. spherules surrounded by fusiform macrophages (epithelioid macrophages) and a few neutrophils. (Wright-Giemsa; HP oil.)

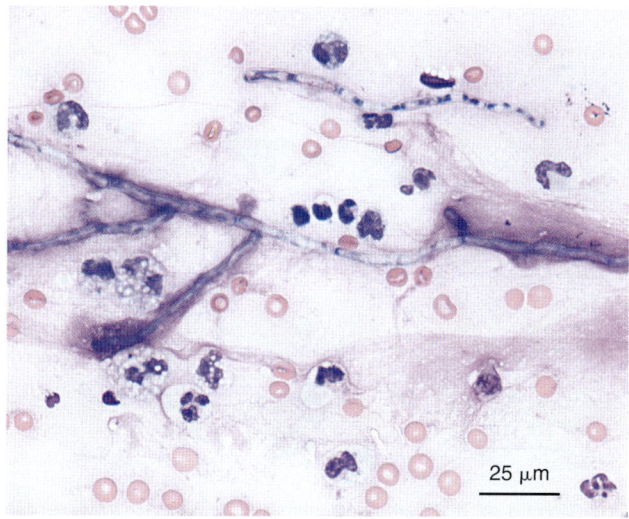

■ **FIGURE 6.23 Aspergillosis. Pericardial fluid. Dog. Fluid smear.** Degenerative neutrophils and vacuolated macrophages surround septate, branching hyphae of *Aspergillus* spp., as confirmed by fungal culture. Neutrophils and erythrocytes can be used to appreciate the size of the hyphae. (Modified Wright; HP oil.) (Courtesy Rose Raskin, Purdue University.)

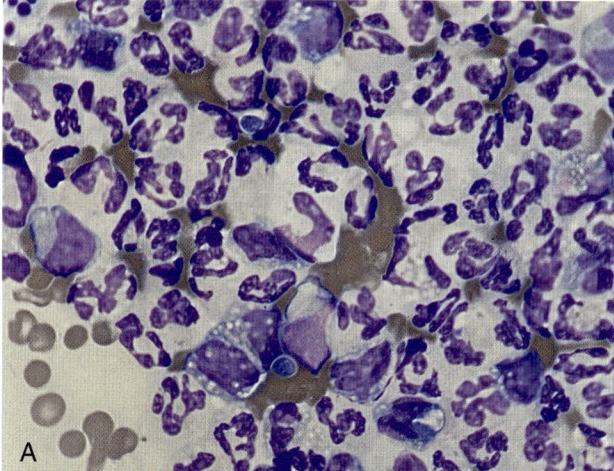

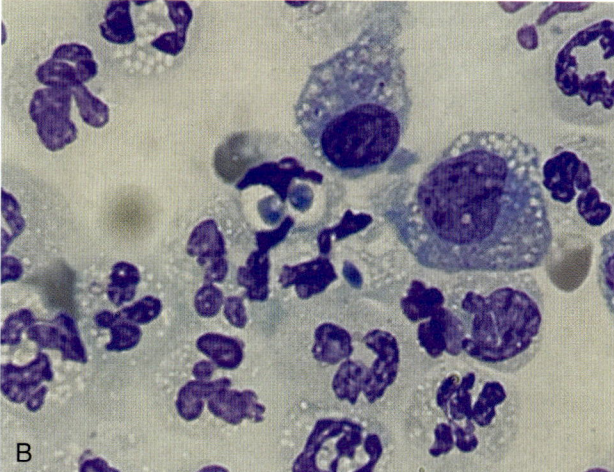

■ **FIGURE 6.24 Candidiasis. Peritoneal fluid. Dog. Cytocentrifuge specimen.** Same case in A and B. Red and opaque before centrifugation, colorless or clear after centrifugation; total nucleated cell count is 51,602/uL, hematocrit (fluid) is <3%, and protein is 4.1 g/dL. **A,** Two oval basophilic yeast organisms 5 μm in length with a distinct clear halo are found between neutrophils and macrophages. (Modified Wright; HP oil.) **B,** Three yeasts are present with two engulfed by a neutrophil. Two macrophages are shown. This mixed-cell but predominantly neutrophilic exudate followed a recent surgical history of intestinal resection and anastomosis. (Modified Wright; HP oil.) (Courtesy of Rose Raskin, Kansas State University.)

Candida Peritonitis

Yeast organisms such as *Candida albicans* and *Candida glabrata* have been associated with a marked inflammatory reaction. Associated conditions include intestinal resection and anastomosis, intestinal perforation, gallbladder rupture, other intestinal surgery, or use of broad-spectrum antimicrobial therapy (Bradford et al., 2013). *Candida* spp. are commensal organisms within the alimentary, upper respiratory, and lower urogenital tracts that are opportunistic when the patient is immunocompromised or the mucosal membrane barrier has been damaged. The prognosis is guarded as sometimes there is a good response to antifungals, but often euthanasia is elected related to a poor response. The cytopathologic diagnosis involves the presence of a mixed-cell exudate with or without concurrent bacterial infection. The extracellular or intracellular yeast within degenerate neutrophils and macrophages are round to oval, basophilic, measuring between 3 and 8 μm with a clear, thin halo and occasional narrow based budding (Fig. 6.24).

Systemic Protozoonosis

Toxoplasmosis (Fig. 6.25), neosporosis (Fig. 6.26), sarcocystosis, and leishmaniasis are rare causes of effusions in cats and dogs (Allison et al., 2006; Barrs et al., 2006; Holmberg et al., 2006; Dell'Orco et al., 2009). When present, effusions may be classified as modified transudates, exudates, or eosinophilic exudates. Exudates may contain intracellular or extracellular tachyzoites diagnostic for protozoal infection. However, speciation is best achieved with serum antibody titers or fluid PCR.

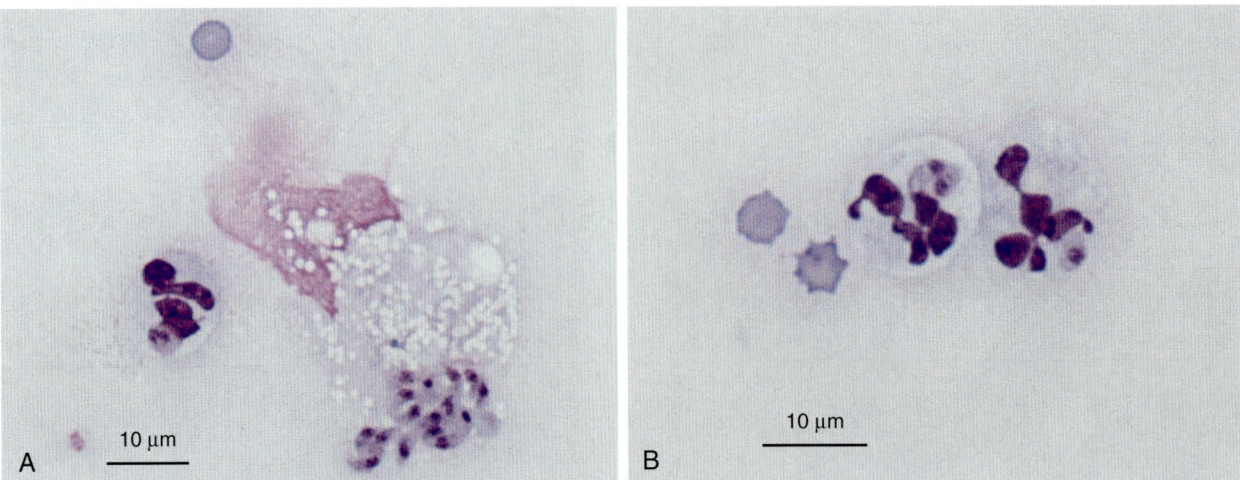

■ **FIGURE 6.25 Toxoplasmosis. Pleural fluid. Cat. Fluid smear.** Same case in A and B. **A,** Note banana-shaped tachyzoites released from the rupture macrophage; the size can be appreciated relative to the nondegenerative neutrophil, which appears to have phagocytized a tachyzoite. (Wright-Giemsa; HP oil.) **B,** Neutrophils contain intracellular tachyzoites. (Wright-Giemsa; HP oil.) (Courtesy Deborah Davis et al., IDEXX, West Sacramento, CA. Presented at the 2004 ASVCP case review session.)

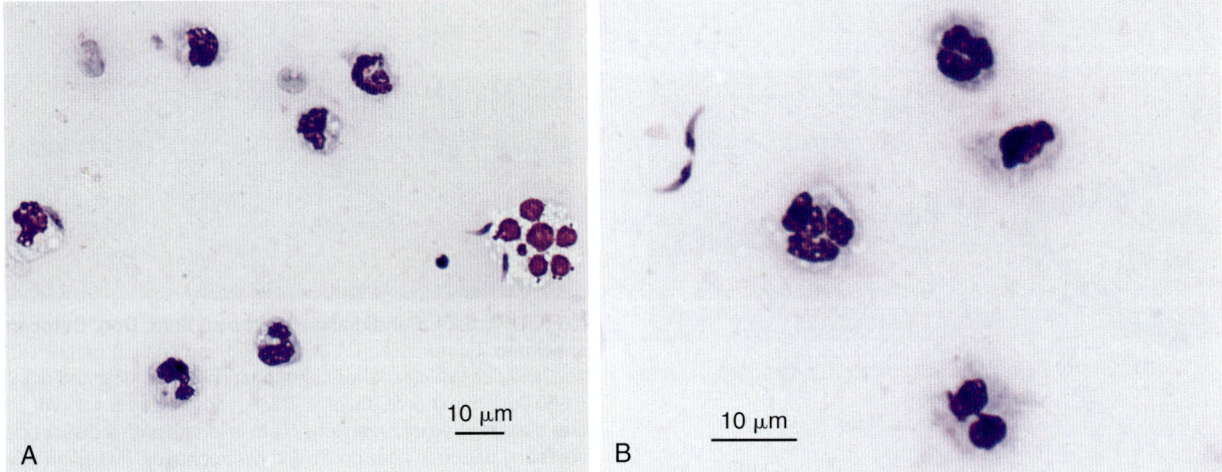

■ **FIGURE 6.26 Neosporosis. Peritoneal fluid. Dog. Fluid smear.** Same case in A and B. **A,** There are neutrophils and two extracellular crescent-shaped tachyzoites measuring approximately 7 μm long *(right side)*. (Wright-Giemsa; HP oil.) **B,** Four degenerate neutrophils and two elongated extracellular tachyzoites containing a prominent eccentric nucleus. Definitive differentiation from toxoplasmosis requires serology and/or polymerase chain reaction. (Wright-Giemsa; HP oil.) (Courtesy Tara Holmberg et al., University of California. Presented at the 2005 ASVCP case review session.)

Peritoneal Cestodiasis

In a small number of dogs with ascites, often from western North America, the etiology is aberrant cestodiasis associated with *Mesocestoides* infection (Stern et al., 1987; Crosbie et al., 1998; Caruso et al., 2003; Patten et al., 2013). Additionally, *Echinococcus multilocularis* infection has been associated with this disease in Europe and Canada (Brosinski et al., 2012; Oscos-Snowball et al., 2015). This disease has been termed *canine peritoneal larval cestodiasis* (Patten et al., 2013). Pleural involvement has also been reported (Toplu et al., 2004). Rare reports of infection involve cats (Eleni et al., 2007; Jabbar et al., 2012; Venco et al., 2005). Peritoneal aspirates from anorexic, ascitic dogs have the gross appearance of tapioca pudding or cream of wheat (Fig. 6.27A). Motile cestodes can be seen in fluid with the unaided eye. Microscopically, the fluid is usually a suppurative exudate (Caruso et al., 2003); however, mild eosinophilic inflammation has also been described (Patten et al., 2013). Microscopic examination may reveal partially intact metacestodes with visible tetrathyridia, a unique larval form having four suckers that represents the asexual reproductive form of *Mesocestoides* spp. infection (Fig. 6.27B). However, larvae are more commonly ruptured, revealing fragments of loose parenchyma with calcareous corpuscles (Fig. 6.28), which may be seen in nonspecific cestode infections. Cestode ova are not usually found in the feces (Crosbie et al., 1998). Molecular testing is necessary for identification of the different cestode species (Crosbie et al., 2000). Cases of this parasitic disease have been reported in Italy, Germany, and Japan (Bonfanti et al., 2004; Wirtherle et al., 2007; Kashiide et al., 2014). Presentation of the cestode cysts or masses are discussed later under Nodular Cestodiasis.

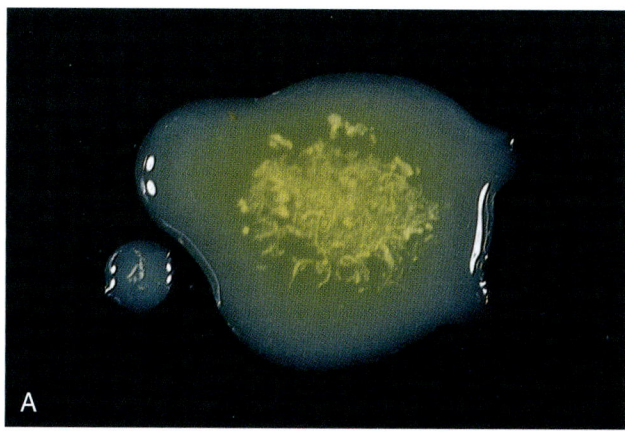 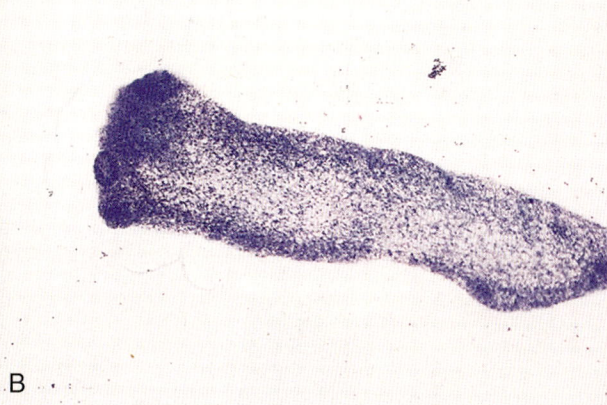

■ **FIGURE 6.27 Cestodiasis. Peritoneal fluid. Dog.** Same case in A and B. **A, Macroscopic fluid.** Gross view of the ascitic fluid revealed a tapioca pudding appearance. Motility of these granules may be observed with the unaided eye. **B, Tetrathyridia larva.** Note the oval structures at the left end that represent suckers and identify the parasite as *Mesocestoides* spp. (Aqueous Romanowsky; LP.) (Courtesy of Jocelyn Johnsrude, IDEXX, West Sacramento, CA.)

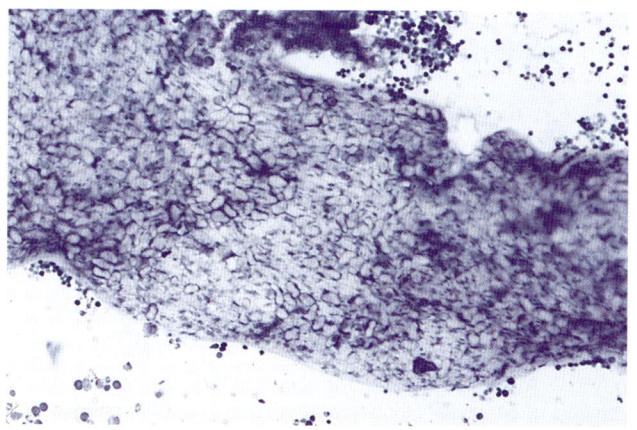

■ **FIGURE 6.28 Cestodiasis. Calcareous corpuscles. Peritoneal fluid. Dog.** Irregularly ovoid, colorless mineral-containing structures (calcareous corpuscles) are suspended within loose parenchymal tissue. Tiny dark dots representing inflammatory cells surround the large structure. (Aqueous Romanowsky; LP.)

Vessel Rupture and Lymphatic Hypertension

Hemoperitoneum (Hemoabdomen)

Hemorrhagic effusions can occur in any of the major body cavities, including the peritoneal cavity. These effusions are serosanguineous to red (Fig. 6.29A) depending on the duration of the effusion and the extent of the hemorrhage. Physical evaluation reveals a protein concentration slightly less than that of peripheral blood. PCVs of effusions are often the same or slightly less than that of peripheral blood (Mandell and Drobatz, 1995; Mongil et al., 1995; Culp et al., 2010), and direct fluid smears often resemble those of anemic peripheral blood smears (Fig. 6.29B).

Hemoperitoneum is generally divided into traumatic and nontraumatic (spontaneous), with the former being subdivided into blunt trauma (e.g., motor vehicle accident) and penetrating (e.g., gunshot wound). Malignant neoplasia was the final diagnosis in 68.3% to 80% of canine cases of acute nontraumatic hemoperitoneum (Pintar et al., 2003; Aronsohn et al., 2009). Of them, 63.3% to 88% were determined to be hemangiosarcoma. Other causes of canine hemoperitoneum include hematomas, torsion (liver and splenic), and coagulopathies such as rodenticide intoxication (Pintar et al., 2003; Beal et al., 2008; Aronsohn et al., 2009). Similar studies in cats implicate malignant neoplasia as the etiology in feline hemoperitoneum in 44% to 46% of cases (Mandell and Drobatz, 1995; Culp et al., 2010). Hemangiosarcoma composed 28% and 60% of these tumors. Other causes include coagulopathies, hepatic necrosis, ruptured urinary bladder, hepatic torsion, hepatic rupture secondary to amyloidosis, and FIP-associated lesions of the liver and kidney (Mandell and Drobatz, 1995; Swann and Brown, 2001; Culp et al., 2010).

Cytopathology can differentiate true hemorrhagic effusions from sample contamination at the time of collection. Hemorrhagic effusions contain predominantly RBCs with relatively few numbers of leukocytes compared with that in peripheral blood. Noteworthy is the microscopic observation of macrophages containing phagocytized red cells (erythrophagocytosis) and/or hemosiderin, which confirms the effusion as hemorrhagic (Fig. 6.30A; see Fig. 6.29C). These cells are best observed at the feathered edge of sediment smears. Hemorrhagic effusions do not contain platelets; if observed, an indication that the effusion was contaminated by peripheral blood during collection. A positive Prussian blue stain confirms the iron-rich pigment as hemosiderin (Fig. 6.30B).

Chyloabdomen (Chylous Ascites)

Chyloabdomen is the accumulation of chyle in the peritoneal cavity caused by rupture or leakage of lymphatic vessels that drain the GI tract. Chyloabdomen is less common than chylothorax, with an incidence of 0.002% in one study (Hatch et al., 2018). The most common causes for chyloabdomen are malignant neoplasia (carcinomatosis, lymphoma, or other), cardiac disease, and lymphangiectasia (Hatch et al., 2018), and concurrent chylothorax is expected in 47% of patients (Hatch et al., 2018). Less common causes of chyloabdomen include pancreatitis, inflammatory bowel disease, FIP, steatitis, biliary cirrhosis, postoperative accumulation following ligation of the thoracic duct, and congenital lymphatic abnormalities

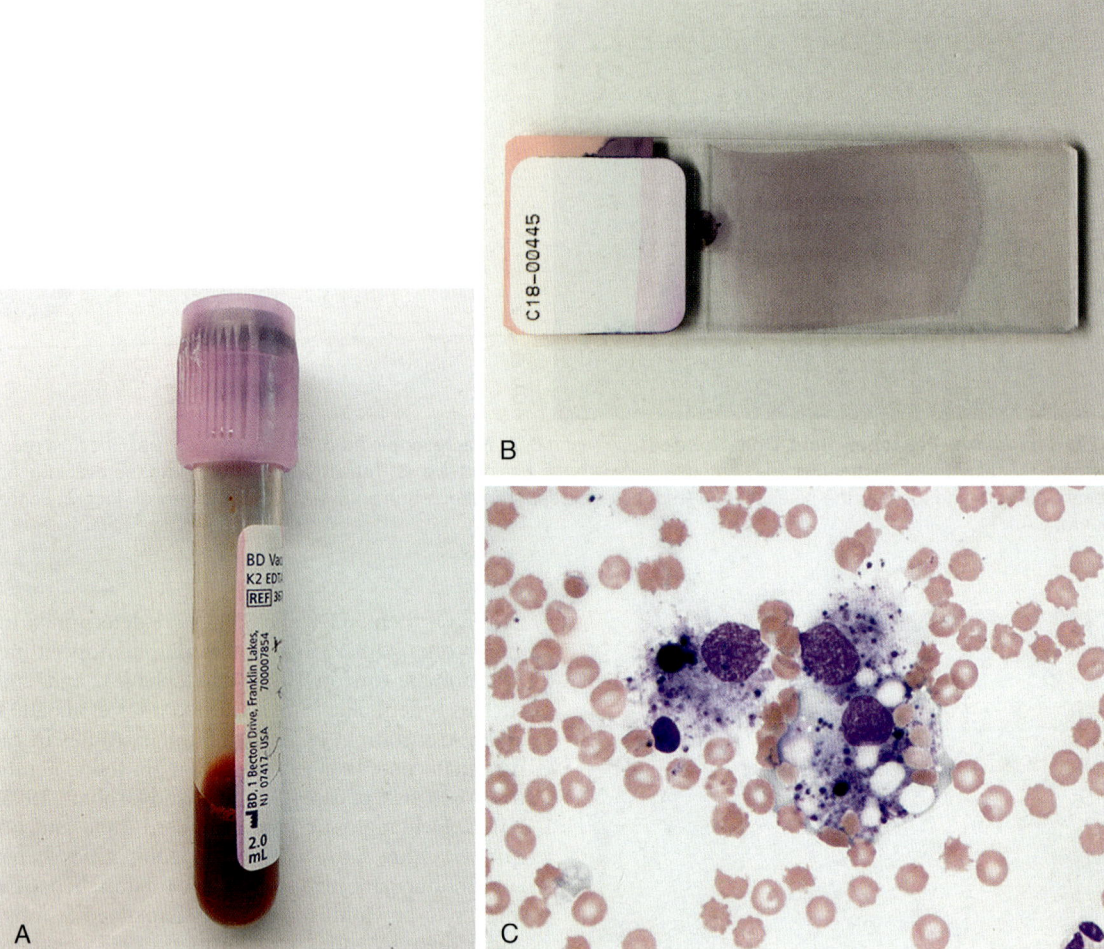

■ **FIGURE 6.29 Hemorrhagic effusion. Peritoneal fluid. Dog.** Same case in A to C. **A, Tube with fluid.** Hemorrhagic fluids are red and opaque. **B, Macroscopic direct smear.** Direct smears of hemorrhagic fluids resemble smears of peripheral blood. (Wright-Giemsa.) **C, Microscopic direct smear.** Three macrophages contain a dark, granular pigment (hemosiderin), and one macrophage exhibits erythrophagia. There are many erythrocytes, resembling the monolayer of a peripheral blood smear. Platelets are absent. (Wright-Giemsa; HP oil.)

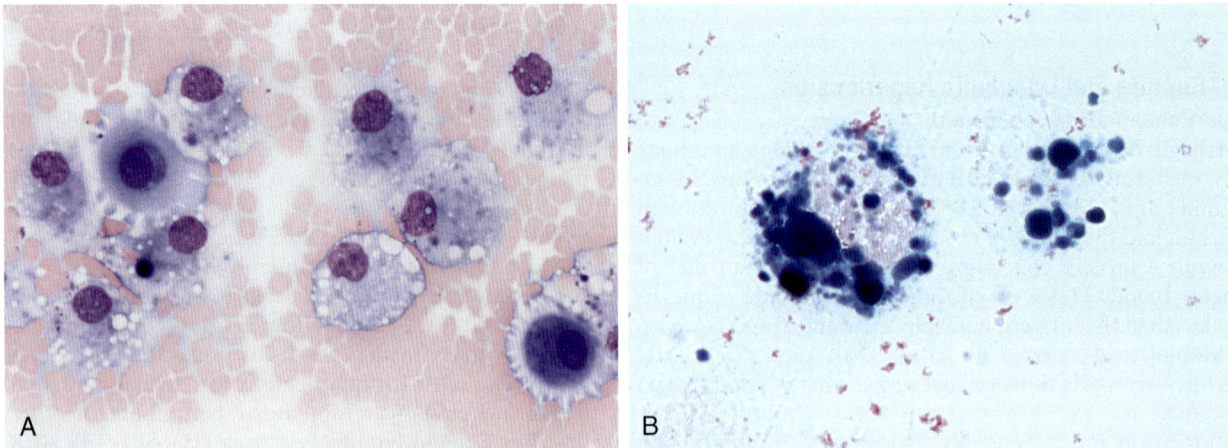

■ **FIGURE 6.30 Hemorrhagic effusion. Cat.** Same case in A and B. **A,** Vacuolated macrophages contain variable amounts of blue-gray, finely granular pigment (hemosiderin). Two basophilic reactive mesothelial cells are admixed. (Modified Wright; HP oil.) **B,** Two hemosiderin-laden macrophages contain Prussian blue–positive material (iron stored as hemosiderin); cell morphology is faint because of the type of stain. (Prussian blue; HP oil.)

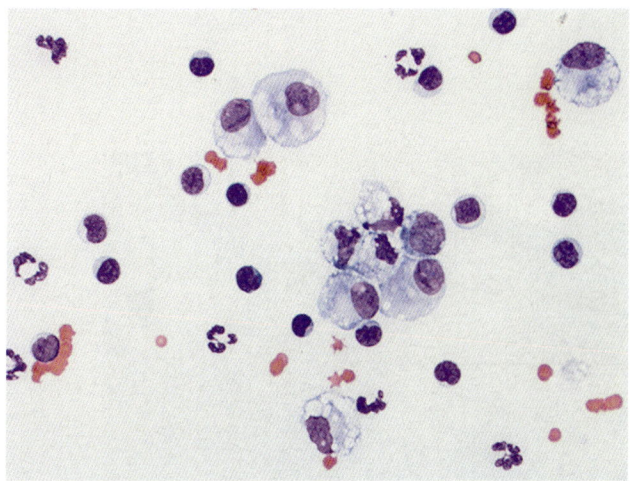

■ **FIGURE 6.31 Nonchylous lymphocyte-rich transudate. Peritoneal fluid. Cat. Cytocentrifuged specimen smear.** Light yellow/hazy; protein is 5.4 g/dL; total nucleated cell count is less than 1000/μL; fluid triglycerides are 38 mg/dL (abnormal fluid triglyceride concentrations considered greater than 100 mg/dL); 48% mostly small lymphocytes; 37% large mononuclear cells (macrophages); 15% nondegenerate neutrophils. (Wright-Giemsa; HP oil.) (Courtesy Rose Raskin, University of Florida.)

(Fossum et al., 1992; Gores et al., 1994; Hatch et al., 2018; Nelson, 2001; Savary et al., 2001).

Reported chyloabdomen fluid characteristics are high protein content (cats: mean, 4.3 g/dL; range, 1.7–7.2 g/dL; dogs: mean, 3.1 g/dL; range, 1.1–5.6 g/dL), high triglyceride concentrations (cats: median, 1404 mg/dL; range, 41–7170 mg/dL; dogs: median, 155 mg/dL; range, 13–3024 mg/dL), and low cholesterol concentrations (cats and dogs: mean, 77 mg/dL; range, 11–149 mg/dL) (Hatch et al., 2018). Expected cytopathologic findings are a predominance of nondegenerate neutrophils with or without small lymphocytes or macrophages (Hatch et al., 2018). Neoplastic cells may be observed in cases of lymphoma or carcinomatosis. Chylous effusions are further discussed in the Chylothorax section.

Nonchylous Lymphocyte-Rich Transudate

Uncommon is the finding of lymphocyte-rich nonchylous transudate with high protein (modified transudate) (Fig. 6.31) in a peritoneal effusion. Cytopathologic diagnosis may be given as modified transudate (transudate with high protein). Similar etiologies are expected to those in the pleural cavity (see later discussion). Considering the abdominal location, cardiac conditions such as feline hypertrophic cardiomyopathy and abdominal neoplasia are especially considered.

Organ Rupture
Gastrointestinal Perforation

More common causes of GI perforation in dogs and cats include trauma, dehiscence of a prior surgical site, gastric ulcers, nonsteroidal antiinflammatory drug administration, GI neoplasia, and ingested foreign bodies. Depending on the extent of the perforation, the effusion may be hazy, cloudy, flocculent, or opaque and yellow, tan, white, brown, green, orange, or red (Fig. 6.32A). The fluid protein content and TNCCs are typically classified as an exudate, but these concentrations may be low in peracute perforations or if there is concurrent pathology or mechanisms, such as hypoalbuminemia or recent peritoneal lavage. Cytopathologic examination of the fluid often reveals digesta, such as keratin, hair fragments, muscle fragments or amorphous brown material, degenerate neutrophils, intracellular and extracellular mixed bacteria and yeast, and digesta-laden macrophages (Fig. 6.32B–D). The inflammatory cells may aggregate around the digesta as part of a foreign body response (Figs. 6.32B and 6.33A). Larger fragments of digesta may not be observed with small or fibrin-covered perforations. If a barium radiographic contrast agent was administered with GI perforation present, crystalline foreign material may be seen within neutrophils, macrophages, and the background (see Fig. 6.33) (Renschler et al., 2008).

Bilious Effusion

Rupture of the gallbladder or common bile duct may occur in any species secondary to direct trauma or disease of the biliary tree. Causes such as gastric dilation and volvulus, cholelithiasis, gunshot wounds, and iatrogenic secondary to fine-needle aspiration or surgery have all been reported. In addition, it is an infrequent accompaniment to diaphragmatic hernia from any cause in dogs and cats. When the results of direct trauma are mainly in the biliary system, leakage of bile is virtually always restricted to the peritoneal cavity, with a resulting peritonitis. When associated with diaphragmatic hernia, leakage of bile occurs when liver is trapped in the diaphragmatic rent and there is rupture or necrosis of the gallbladder or common bile duct. In this circumstance, both peritonitis and pleuritis can result. Bile is a very irritating substance; its presence quickly elicits an inflammatory response. Grossly, the fluid may be initially brown (Fig. 6.34), orange, yellow, or green; however, as the response becomes more and more cellular, this discoloration may become masked. Large volumes of fluid can usually be obtained. Based on physical characteristics, these effusions are usually exudates (Ludwig et al., 1997; Owens et al., 2003).

Cytopathologically, the striking feature of bilious effusion is the presence of bile in the smear. Frequently, bile is seen as yellow to green to blue-black granular material scattered in the slide background and in the cytoplasm of neutrophils, reactive mesothelial cells, and macrophages (Figs. 6.35 and 6.36). In reactions of greater duration, bile granules may have all been converted to rhomboidal to amorphous golden crystals of bile pigment. When such crystals are found in the cytoplasm of effusion phagocytes in the absence of evidence of prior hemorrhage (e.g., erythrophagocytosis), the possibility of bilious effusion should be strongly considered. In addition to the typical appearance of bilious effusions, acellular, amorphous, fibrillar blue-grey, mucinous material (Fig. 6.37) has been associated with biliary tree rupture, particularly of the common bile duct in dogs (Owens et al., 2003). It is suspected that this bile-free material is produced by biliary and gallbladder epithelium as a consequence to extrahepatic biliary obstruction with regurgitation of normal bile into hepatic lymph and venous blood. This material has been termed "white bile" (Owens et al., 2003).

The inflammatory response to bile is generally composed of nondegenerate neutrophils—84% to 98% of TNCC (Ludwig et al., 1997) (see Fig. 6.37B–D). Varying numbers of macrophages and reactive mesothelial cells can be admixed depending on duration of contact with the bile irritant. Fluid bilirubin

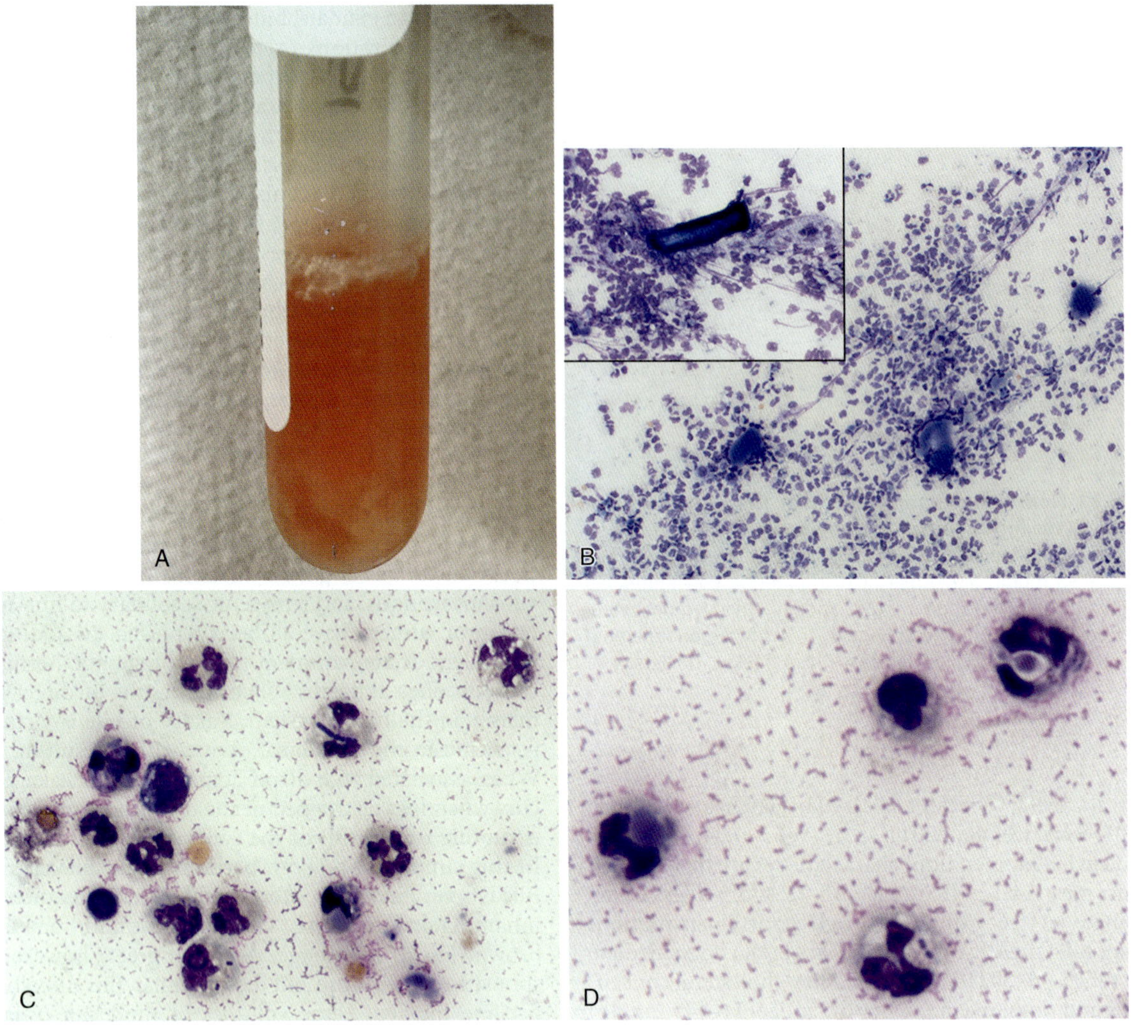

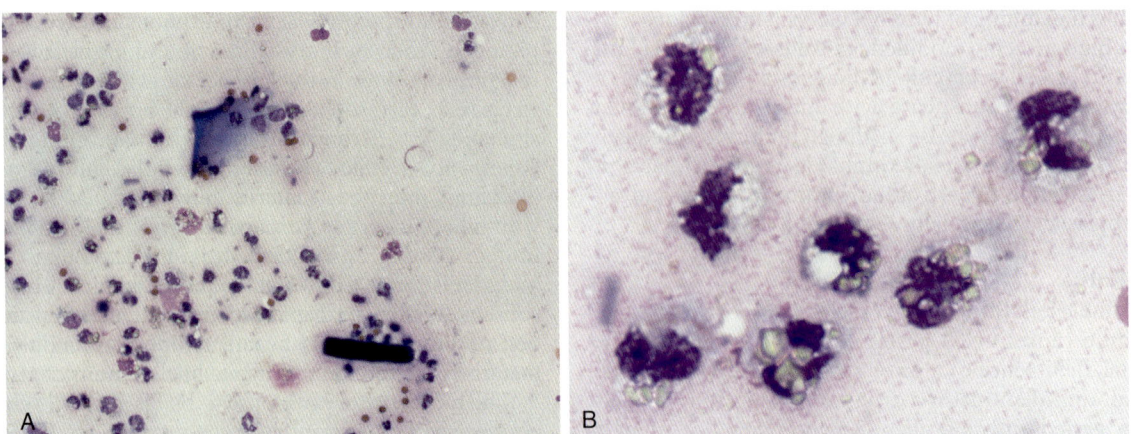

■ **FIGURE 6.32 Intestinal perforation. Peritoneal fluid. Cat.** Same case in A to D. **A, Tube with fluid.** The effusion is orange-red with tan flocculent aggregates of leukocytes and fibrin. **B, Fluid smear.** Several large, blue-green, amorphous structures (digesta) are surrounded by a myriad of degenerate neutrophils. (Wright-Giemsa; IP.) *Inset*: An elongated dark blue-green fragment is surrounded by aggregates of degenerate neutrophils and faint granular amorphous debris in the background (digesta). (Wright-Giemsa, HP.) **C. Fluid smear.** Several degenerate neutrophils contain phagocytized bacterial bacilli, bacterial cocci, or amorphous material (digesta). (Wright-Giemsa, HP oil.) **D, Fluid smear.** The neutrophils contain a phagocytized amorphous blue material digesta (*left*), narrow-based budding yeast (*top right*), or bacteria (*bottom*). Necropsy diagnosed intestinal large cell lymphoma as the cause of the intestinal perforation. (Wright-Giemsa, HP oil.)

■ **FIGURE 6.33 Intestinal perforation. Peritoneal fluid. Dog.** Same case in A and B. Two days prior to fluid collection, the dog underwent a gastrointestinal barium contrast study and an intestinal resection and anastomoses for foreign body removal. **A, Digesta.** A keratinocyte (*top*) and an unidentifiable, blue-black elongated fragment of digesta are both surrounded by inflammatory cells. (Wright-Giemsa, IP.) **B, Barium crystals.** Many degenerate neutrophils contain a pale yellow-green crystalline material (barium). (Wright-Giemsa, HP oil.)

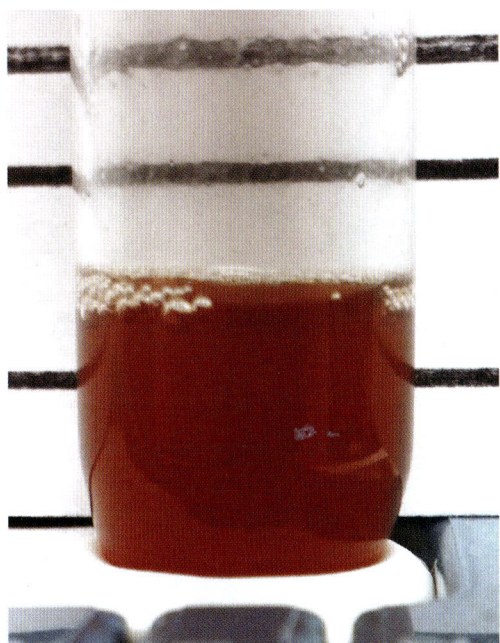

■ **FIGURE 6.34 Bilious effusion. Peritoneal fluid. Dog. Tube with fluid.** The fluid is red-brown because of the presence of hemorrhage (red) and bile (brown).

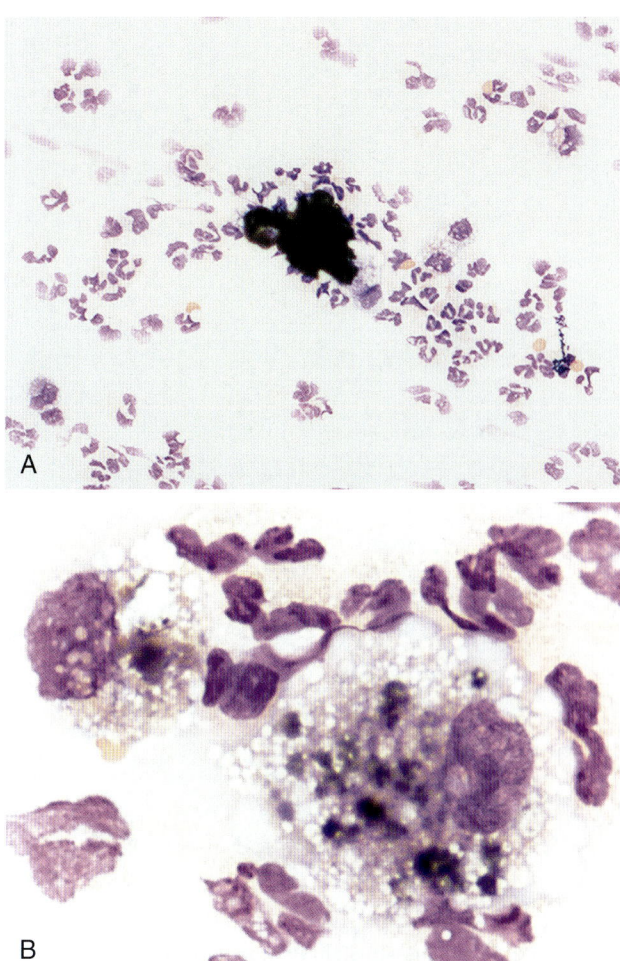

■ **FIGURE 6.35 Bilious effusion. Peritoneal fluid. Dog.** Same case in A and B. **Fluid smear. A,** Degenerate neutrophils surround dark, brown to black amorphous bile. (Wright-Giemsa; HP oil.) **B,** Two macrophages contain a phagocytized brown-black granular material (bile) and are surrounded by several degenerate neutrophils. (Wright-Giemsa; HP oil.)

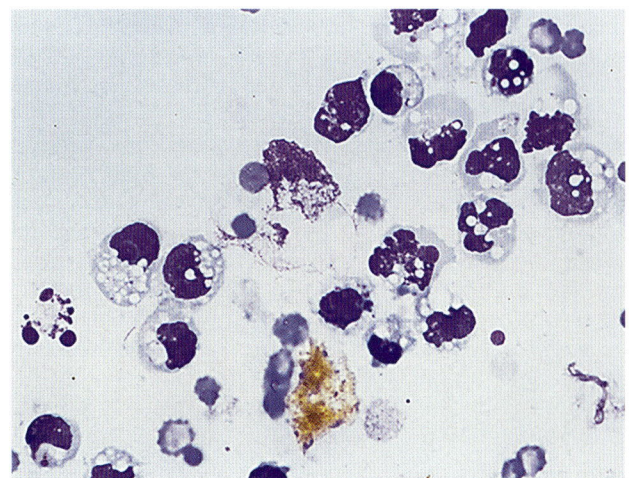

■ **FIGURE 6.36 Bilious effusion. Peritoneal fluid. Dog. Fluid smear.** Total nucleated cell count is 20,000/μL and protein is 3.5 g/dL. Note extracellular gold-brown crystalline material, vacuolated neutrophils, and macrophages. Some of the neutrophils contain pyknotic nuclei and others contain karyolytic nuclei. (Romanowsky; HP oil.)

concentrations are several times higher than serum concentrations, a finding that is 100% diagnostic (Ludwig et al., 1997; Owens et al., 2003). Effusion bilirubin is usually elevated twice serum levels, but rarely in the white bile cases studied was the fluid bilirubin not increased (Owens et al., 2003). There is a poor survival rate when the bilious effusion is also septic (Ludwig et al., 1997).

Uroperitoneum (Uroabdomen)

Uroperitoneum in cats and dogs is frequently seen secondary to a ruptured bladder, although compromise of any of the urinary tract that lies within the peritoneal cavity can produce uroperitoneum. The most common cause of a ruptured bladder is trauma (Aumann et al., 1998). Sources of trauma include blunt abdominal trauma (e.g., vehicular), aggressive catheterization, or palpation or expression. Urine in the peritoneal space results in chemical irritation. The protein content and total nucleated cell count may be variable owing to dilution from the urine. Initially, a mononuclear cell population may predominate, suggestive of a modified transudate. Later, the neutrophil is usually the predominant cell type as the effusion becomes an exudate. Bacteria may or may not be present. Neutrophils exposed to the irritant material undergo necrosis or apoptosis and may show karyorrhexis, pyknosis (karyopyknosis), or karyolysis with ragged nuclear borders (Figs. 6.38 and 6.39). In some cases, urinary crystals are found on cytopathologic examination, which supports the diagnosis of uroperitoneum. In cats, the creatinine and potassium concentrations in the effusion were found to be higher than serum concentrations (generally a ratio of 2:1) (Aumann et al., 1998). A higher effusion creatinine concentration vs. serum creatinine concentration tends to persist longer than a higher effusion urea nitrogen (BUN) concentration versus serum BUN concentration because creatinine equilibrates more slowly than urea nitrogen. One study found that

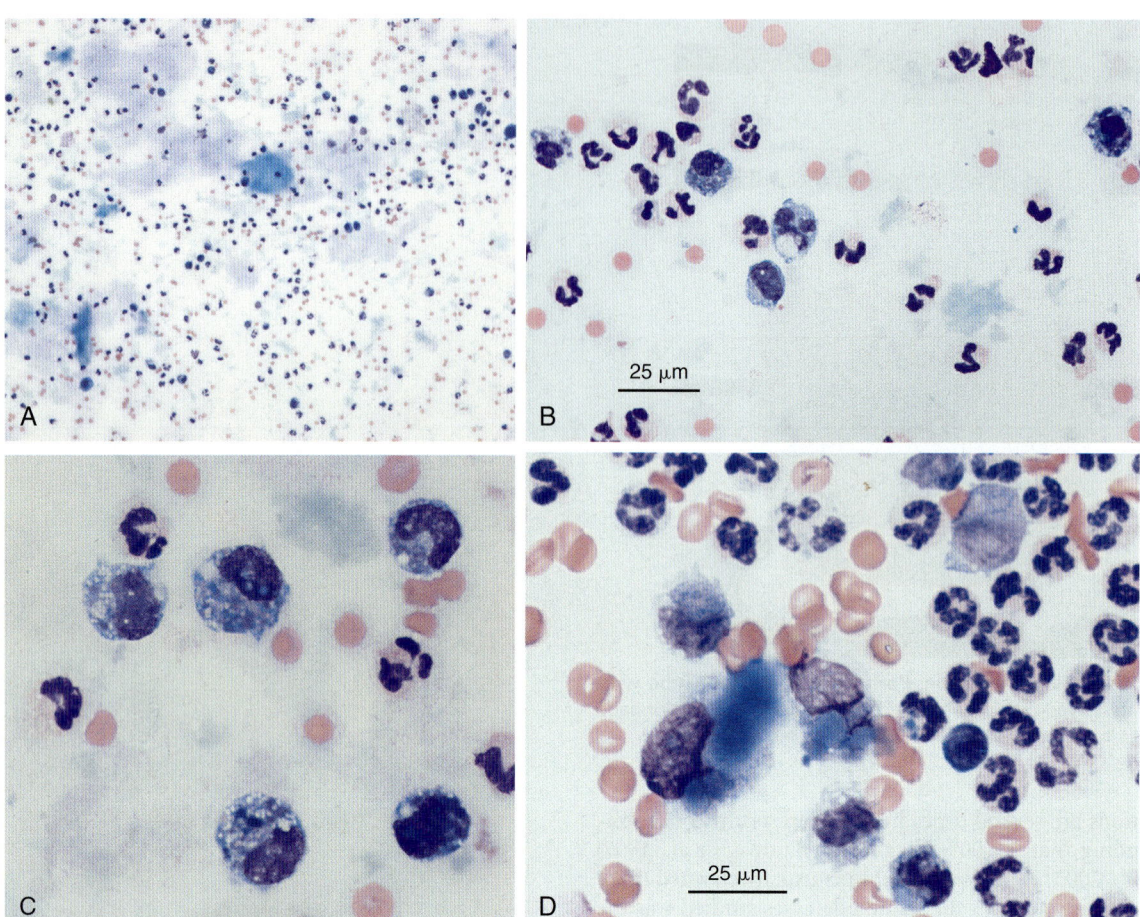

FIGURE 6.37 Bilious effusion. Peritoneal fluid. Dog. Same case in A to C. **Concentrated specimens. A,** Fluid from a dog with a ruptured gallbladder. Note the numerous neutrophils and lakes of blue-gray amorphous mucinous material ("white bile") throughout the background. (Modified Wright; IP.) **B,** Variably degenerate neutrophils, vacuolated macrophages, and amorphous blue-gray mucinous material. (Modified Wright; HP oil.) **C,** Neutrophils and vacuolated macrophages that contain light blue to dark blue debris (bile) are shown. The background contains faint blue mucinous protein. (Modified Wright; HP oil.) **D,** In peritoneal fluid from another case of bilious effusion, two macrophages (*lower left*) and one neutrophil next to them have phagocytized dense, hyalinized blue amorphous bilious mucus. (Modified Wright; HP oil.) (D, Courtesy Rose Raskin, Purdue University.)

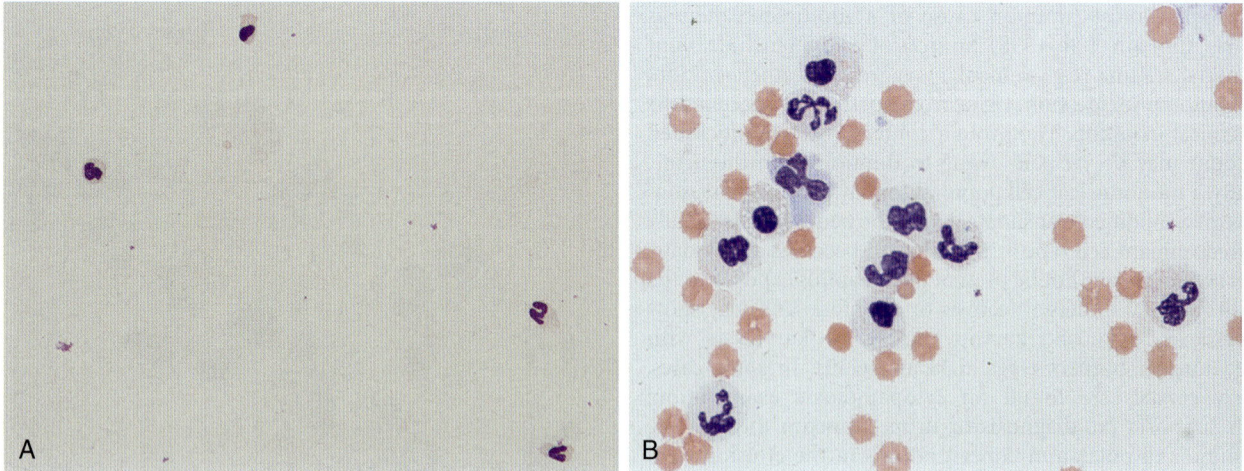

FIGURE 6.38 Uroperitoneum. Peritoneal fluid. Dog. Same case in A and B. The patient presented with lethargy 2 days after vehicle trauma. Abdominocentesis indicated red/cloudy fluid with protein <2 g/dL, total nucleated cell count of 2240/μL, red blood cells 50,000/μL, K^+ (mEq/L) fluid/blood 15.77/.33 (blood K^+ reference interval [RI], 3.98–4.41), and creatinine (mg/dL) fluid/blood ratio >12/5.1 (blood creatine RI, 0.8–1.5). Cell differential: 92% neutrophils, 5% mononuclear phagocytes, 3% lymphocytes. **A, Direct smear.** Fluid is very dilute, resembling a transudate, but the high percentage of neutrophils supports an exudate. (Wright-Giemsa; HP oil.) **B, Cytocentrifuge specimen.** Neutrophils display mild karyolysis and pyknosis. (Wright-Giemsa; HP oil.) (Courtesy Rose Raskin, University of Florida.)

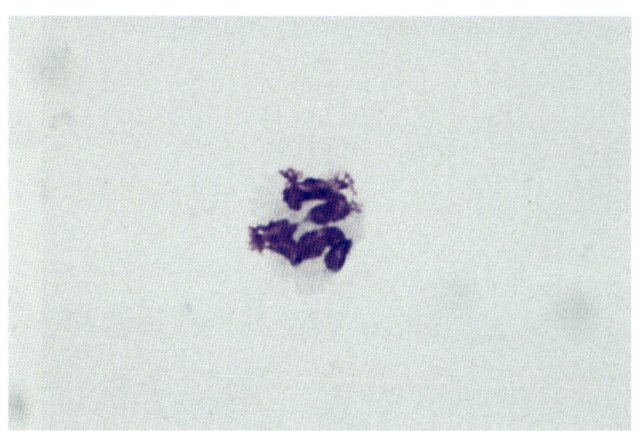

■ **FIGURE 6.39** **Uroperitoneum. Peritoneal fluid. Dog. Fluid smear.** Degenerative neutrophil. Urine is a chemical irritant, causing karyolytic changes to cells. (Wright-Giemsa; HP oil.) (Courtesy Rose Raskin, University of Florida.)

85% of dogs with uroperitoneum had an abdominal fluid/serum creatinine ratio greater than 2:1 (all these dogs had an effusion creatinine concentration that was four times the serum concentration), and 100% had an abdominal fluid/serum potassium ratio greater than 1.4:1 (Schmiedt et al., 2001). In addition, serum Na:K also tends to be decreased in cases of uroabdomen (Aumann et al., 1998). Cases of urothorax have been described in a dog and a cat (Störk et al., 2003; Klainbart et al., 2011).

Reproductive Tract Tears

Infrequent occurrences of sperm have been detected in the peritoneal fluid in dogs (Slater et al., 2004; DiDomenico et al., 2020). This usually occurs secondary to uterine or vaginal tears from traumatic breeding or rarely from complications of an intraabdominal surgical vasectomy. As sperm induce an inflammatory response, nondegenerate neutrophils are present, which may phagocytize the sperm over time along with macrophages. The sperm heads are most notable on cytopathology with Romanowsky staining as pale blue oval structures with or without tails (Fig. 6.40). The presence of sperm within the peritoneal cavity is termed *seminoperitoneum*.

One uncommon finding was the presence of ciliated columnar cells arising from an oviductal hamartoma as described in the abdominal fluid from a dog (Fry et al., 2003).

Non-neoplastic Nodules and Masses
Gossypiboma (Textiloma)

Gossypibomas, also known as textilomas, are intracavitary granulomas that form as a result of a retained foreign object, typically a surgical sponge (Krimer et al., 2010; Putwain and Archer, 2010). These masses may be incidental findings or may result in urinary incontinence, fistula formation, or neoplastic transformation (Haddad et al., 2010). Cytopathologic evaluation of the lesions reveal multinucleated giant cells with phagocytized basophilic shards of the degraded surgical sponge fibers (Fig. 6.41A). These fibers exhibit birefringence under polarized light (Fig. 6.41B).

Nodular Cestodiasis

In addition to parasitic ascites discussed previously, peritoneal cestodiasis may present as nodules or cavernous masses in the absence of effusion from *Mesocestoides* spp. or *Echinococcus* spp. (Brosinski et al., 2012; Oscos-Snowball et al., 2015). The cytopathologic findings of these larvae are similar to those found in peritoneal fluid and may include fragments of loose to cohesive parenchyma or prominent large irregular-shaped, hyaline membrane–like cystic structures from *E. multilocularis* measuring 100 to 200 μm in diameter. Both parasites produce 5 to 10 μm round to oval nonstaining crystalline particles consistent in appearance with calcareous corpuscles (Fig. 6.42). Calcareous corpuscles are concretions composed of Ca, Mg, P, CO_2, and organic components.

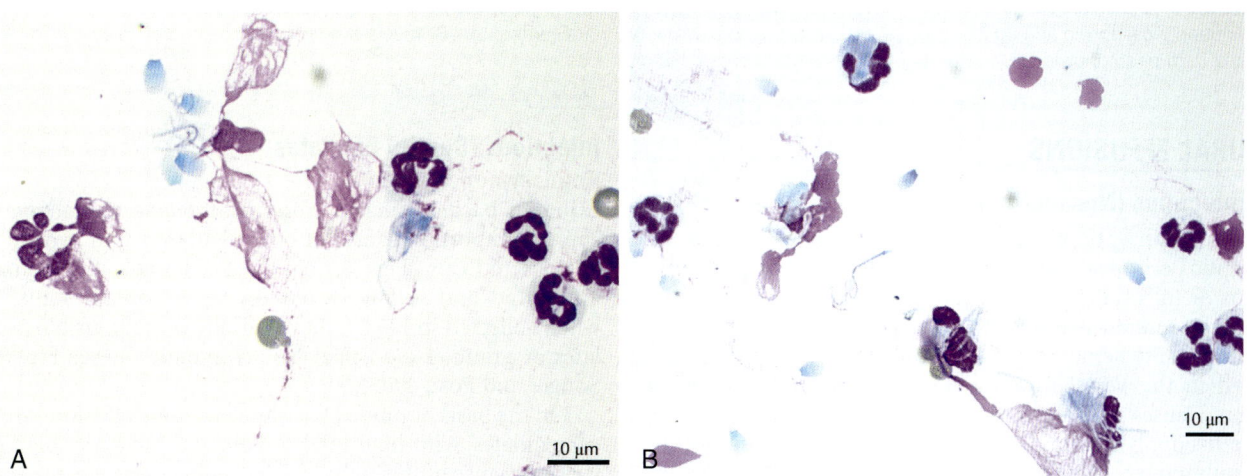

■ **FIGURE 6.40** **Seminoperitoneum. Peritoneal fluid. Dog. Direct smear.** Same case in A and B. **A,** Mildly degenerate neutrophils predominate along with numerous pale blue sperm heads measuring approximately 5 μm in length against a background containing nuclear debris. **B,** Neutrophils exhibit phagocytosis of spermatozoa heads and tails. The condition occurred as a complication of vasectomy. (Modified Wright-Giemsa; HP oil.) (Courtesy Amy DiDomenico, North Carolina State University.)

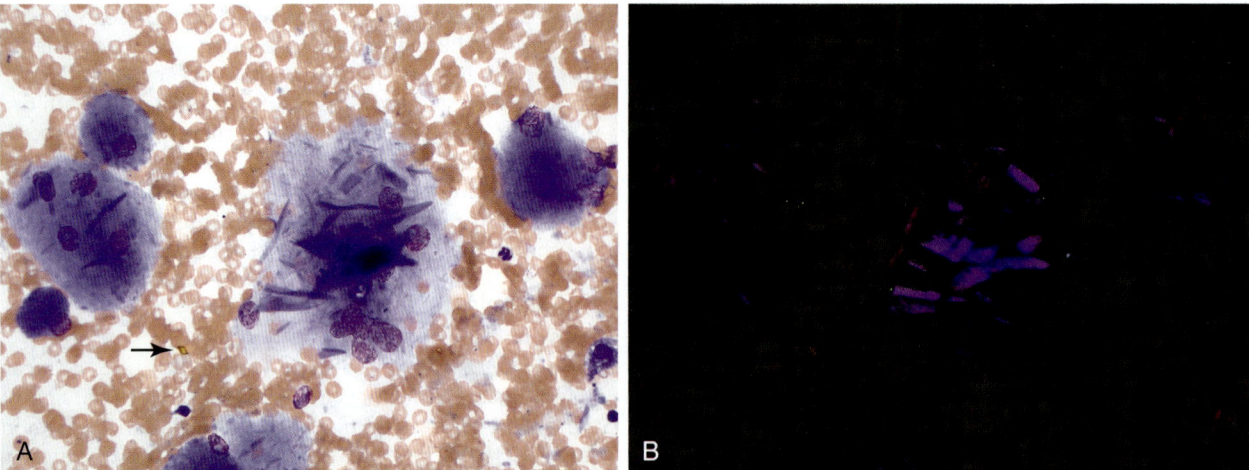

FIGURE 6.41 Gossypiboma. Peritoneal mass. Dog. Same specimen in A and B. **A, Nonpolarized slide.** Several multinucleated giant cells and macrophages contain variably basophilic, shard-like fibers and light basophilic, amorphous material. There is one small extracellular hematoidin crystal *(arrow)* indicative of chronic hemorrhage. (Wright-Giemsa; HP oil.) **B, Polarized slide.** Using the same field of view as A, the shard-like fibers are birefringent under polarized light. (Wright-Giemsa; HP oil.) This gossypiboma was an incidental finding in a 5-year-old castrated male dog that underwent a laparotomy at 5 months of age to remove an ingested foreign body.

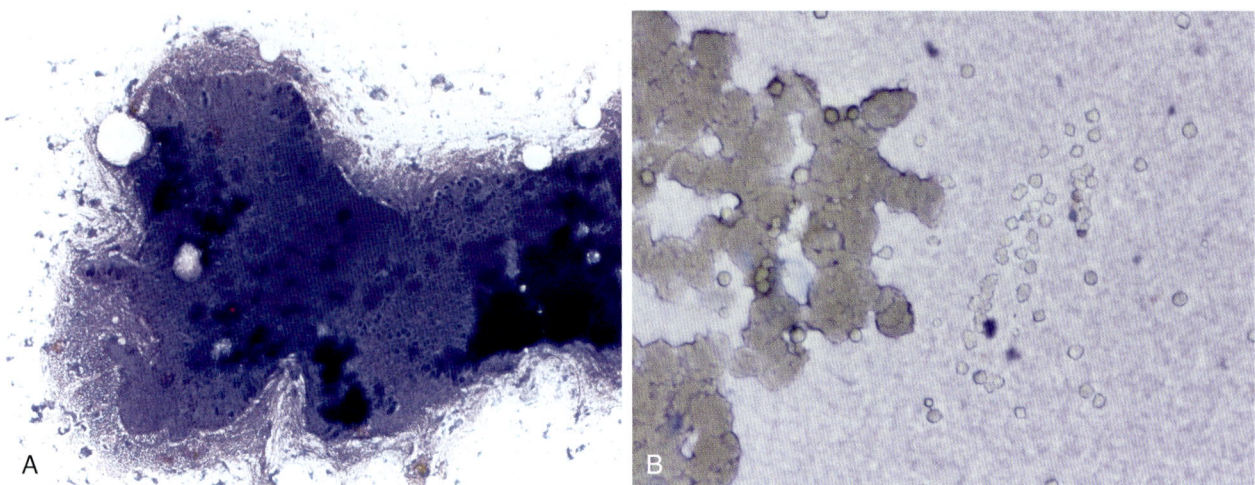

FIGURE 6.42 Peritoneal cestodiasis. Peritoneal nodule. Dog. Cytopathologic specimen. Same case in A and B. **A,** Fragment of a cestode larva is deeply basophilic and contains loose, reticulated parenchyma. (Wright-Giemsa; LP.) **B,** Yellow-brown calcareous corpuscles are in thick aggregates *(left)* or are individually scattered *(right)*. (Wright-Giemsa; HP oil.)

PLEURAL EFFUSIONS

Noninfectious (Nonseptic) Exudates

Causes of nonseptic pleural exudates are similar to those of nonseptic peritoneal exudates and include nonexfoliating neoplasms or infections, FIP, and causes of eosinophilic exudate. Lung lobe torsion may result in a combination of nonseptic exudation and hemorrhagic effusion, which are further described in the Vessel Rupture and Lymphatic Hypertension section. Causes of pleural eosinophilic exudates include chylous effusion, lymphoma, systemic mastocytosis, pneumothorax, pulmonary parasitism, and caudal venal caval surgery (Miller et al., 1984; Fossum et al., 1993; Allison et al., 2006). Other disorders likely include allergic airway disease, lung lobe torsion, feline leukemia virus, and heartworm disease (Fossum et al., 1993).

Infectious (Septic) Exudates
Actinomycotic Pyothorax

Complex bacteria such as *Nocardia asteroides* and *Actinomyces* spp. are important causes of both pyothorax and pyoabdomen in dogs and cats (Figs. 6.43 and 6.44). Grossly, these effusions are turbid and yellow to blood-tinged "tomato soup." Even when collected in EDTA, they typically contain visible particulates or granules (so-called "sulfur granules") (see Fig. 6.43A; Songer and Post, 2005).

On the basis of physical parameters, these effusions are typical exudates, with high total protein and markedly high cellularity. Because of the high cellularity, direct smears are generally adequate for cytopathologic examination. If particles are observed in the fluid, it is important to make compression-spread (squash) preparations of these particles in addition to making smears of the fluid alone.

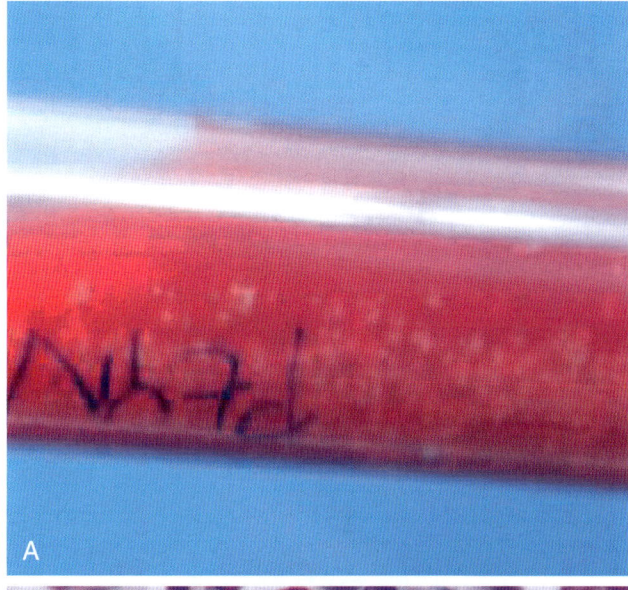
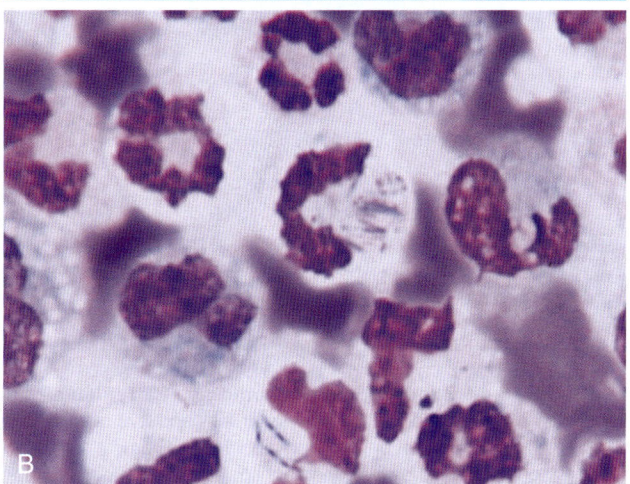

■ **FIGURE 6.43 Actinomycotic pyothorax. Pleural fluid. Cat.** Same case in A and B. **A, Tube with fluid.** The gross appearance indicates the presence of blood with numerous light-yellow particles (sulfur granules). **B, Fluid smear.** Two neutrophils have phagocytized the slender rod-shaped, often beaded bacteria. (Aqueous Romanowsky; HP oil.) (Courtesy Janina Łukaszewska, Wrocław, Poland.)

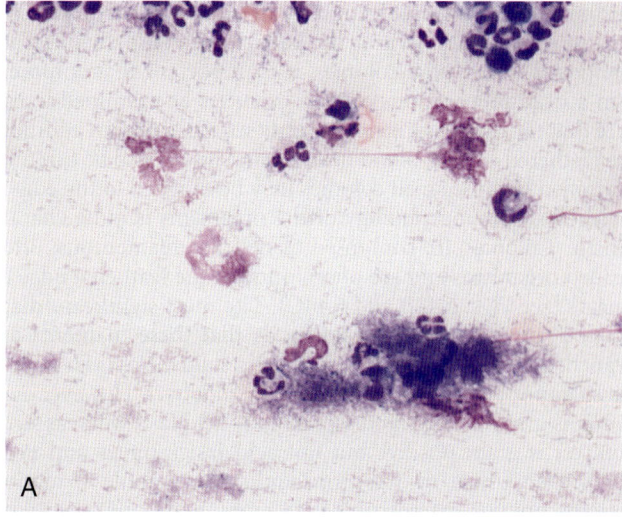
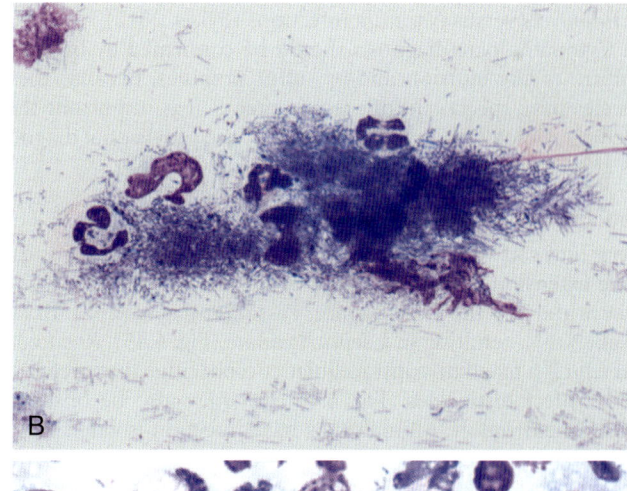
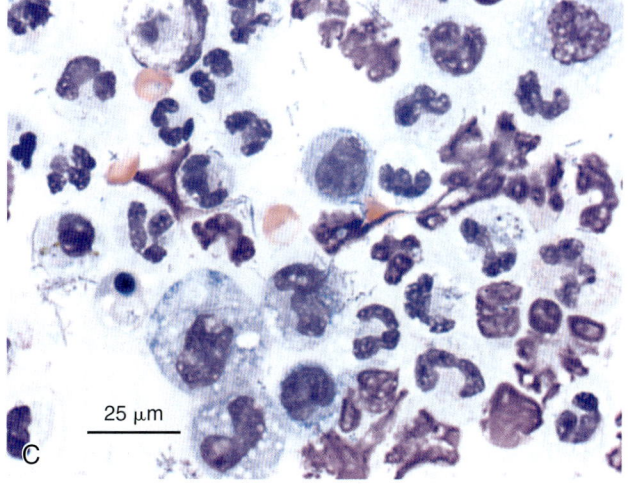

■ **FIGURE 6.44 Actinomycotic pyothorax. Pleural fluid. Direct smear. Dog.** Same case in A to C. **A,** A bacterial colony (sulfur granule) appears along with neutrophils and eosinophilic nuclear material. The bacterial colonies are often located at the feathered edge of the smear. (Modified Wright; IP.) **B,** Higher magnification of the same colony as in A. The colony of *Actinomyces* bacteria appears pleomorphic and includes filamentous forms. (Modified Wright; HP oil.) **C,** Nondegenerate and degenerate neutrophils as well as vacuolated macrophages appear with intra- and extracellular slender rod-shaped bacteria. (Modified Wright; HP oil.)

Microscopically, nocardial and actinomycotic infections are characterized by neutrophilic to mixed inflammation, probably dependent on the duration of the disease. In the more chronic reactions, there is generally a significant reactive mesothelial cell component to the response. A striking feature of the inflammatory response is the morphology of neutrophils. Whereas most cases of septic pleuritis and peritonitis are signaled by the presence of predominantly degenerating neutrophils, in nocardial and actinomycotic effusions, the majority of the neutrophils away from the organisms are nondegenerate or show signs of aging (hypersegmentation) or apoptosis (karyorrhexis and/or pyknosis [karyopyknosis]). Degenerating neutrophils are only seen immediately in the vicinity of the bacterial organisms because these agents, in contrast to most other bacteria, produce only weak local toxins. The net effect of this phenomenon is that smears in these cases may be easily misinterpreted as noninfectious, particularly if the organisms are not widespread. Because the particles seen grossly often are composed of bacterial colonies, it is important that compression-spread preparations of these particles be examined to ensure that the diagnosis is not missed (see Fig. 6.44). In addition, the feathered edge of blood film smears should also be carefully examined because small colonies may be dragged to the edge.

Microscopic morphology of the organisms is quite characteristic. Colonies are composed of delicate, filamentous, often beaded organisms and are often found at the feathered edge of smears (see Figs. 6.43B and 6.44C). The most significant diagnostic feature of these organisms is that these filaments are branched. Using standard hematologic stains, *Nocardia* organisms cannot be differentiated from *Actinomyces*. However, *Nocardia* is gram positive and segmentally acid fast, whereas *Actinomyces* is gram positive but not acid fast (Songer and Post, 2005). Dense mats of organisms and sulfur granule formation (microscopic or macroscopic) are more commonly seen with *Actinomyces* versus *Nocardia* infections (Sykes, 2012).

Cytopathologic diagnosis should be confirmed by bacterial culture of the effusion and/or sulfur granules. Because these species have special culture requirements, it is important that the bacteriology laboratory be aware of the provisional diagnosis at the time of sample submission.

Rhodococcal Pleuropneumonia

Dogs and cats with respiratory *Rhodococcus equi* infections can have extension of the bacterial pneumonia onto the overlying pleura and into the pleural space (Passamonti et al., 2011; Bryan et al., 2017), resulting in a septic exudate (Fig. 6.45). *Rhodococcus equi* is a facultative intracellular coccobacillus that preferentially infect histiocytes (Fig. 6.46) but may also be observed within neutrophils. Animals may have infection isolated to the lungs and pleural cavity or may show signs of systemic infection, such as endophthalmitis or endocarditis (Passamonti et al., 2011; Bryan et al., 2017).

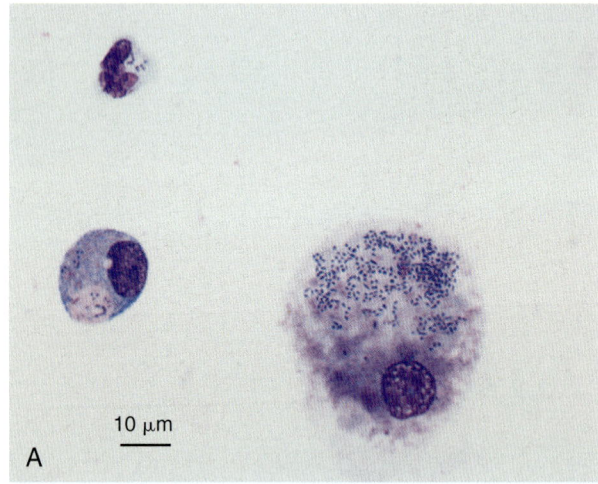
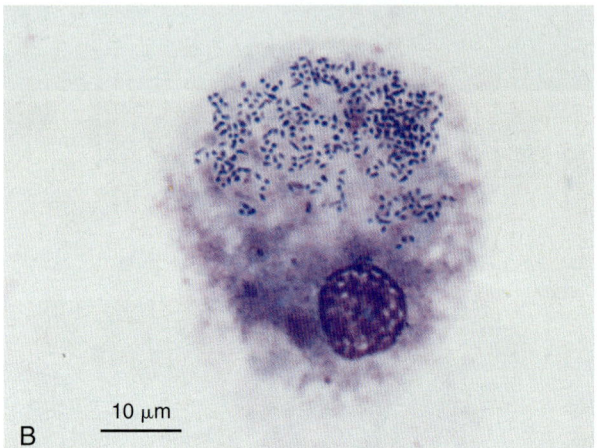

■ **FIGURE 6.46 Rhodococcosis. Pyothorax. Cat. Pleural fluid smear.** Same case in A and B. **A**, One neutrophil and two macrophages contain a uniform population of bacteria. (Wright-Giemsa; HP oil.) **B**, Higher magnification shows a macrophage that contains a uniform population of coccobacilli. (Wright-Giemsa; HP oil.) A diagnosis of *Rhodococcus equi* was confirmed by culture. (Courtesy Eric Morissette et al., University of Florida. Presented at the 2007 ASVCP case review session.)

Systemic Mycoses and Protozoonosis

Any systemic or pulmonary mycotic or protozoal infection has the potential to cause pleural effusion. These effusions are described in the Peritoneal Effusions section.

Vessel Rupture and Lymphatic Hypertension
Hemothorax

Hemothorax is associated with a variety of causes (Mellanby et al., 2002). In dogs, these include rodenticide intoxication, neoplasia (Slensky et al., 2003), parasitic infestation (Sasanelli et al., 2008; Chikweto et al., 2012), and iatrogenic (Cohn et al., 2003). Feline hemothorax has been associated with rodenticide intoxication and fat embolism (Sierra et al., 2007). The fluid characteristics are similar to those of hemoperitoneum discussed previously.

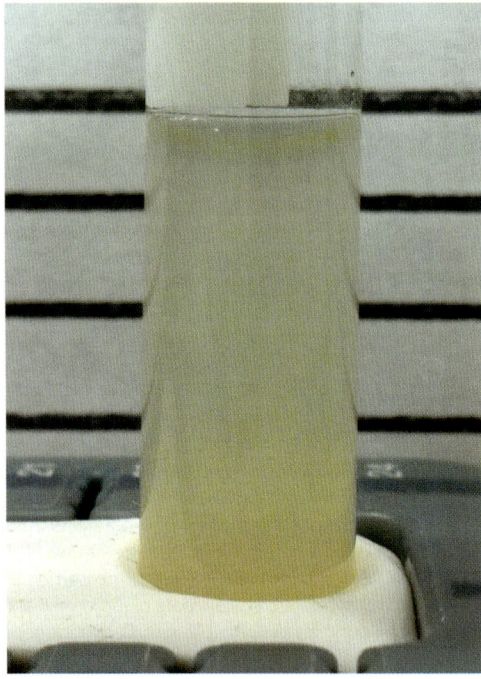

■ **FIGURE 6.45 Rhodococcosis. Pyothorax. Cat. Tube with pleural fluid.** The color and clarity are tan and opaque, consistent with an exudate.

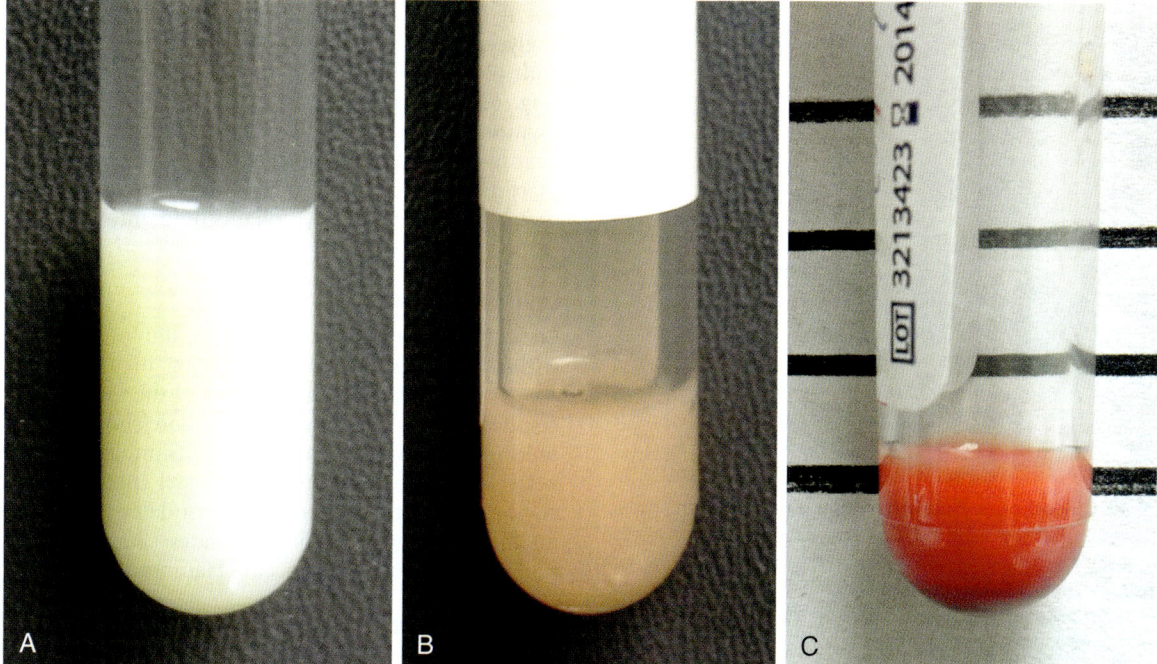

FIGURE 6.47 Chylous effusion. Cat. Multiple tubes with pleural fluid. **A,** White and opaque (milky) fluid is related to the high triglycerides concentration without significant hemorrhage. **B,** Pink and opaque appearance indicates a mild hemorrhagic component. **C,** Red fluids may occur with substantial hemorrhage that can obscure the milky appearance. This fluid contained a 4200 total nucleated cell count/µL, 1,210,000 red blood cells/µL, 5.6 g protein/dL, and 205 mg triglycerides/dL. Note the white triglyceride lipid layer that has accumulated at the top of the fluid.

Chylothorax

Chyle is a mixture of lymph and chylomicrons. Triglyceride-rich chylomicrons are derived from dietary lipids processed in the intestine and transported via lymphatics. Historically, chylous effusions were thought to be primarily a result of thoracic duct rupture. It is now known that thoracic duct hypertension with transudation of chyle is more common than rupture of the thoracic duct. Causes of chylous effusions in the thoracic cavity include cardiovascular disease, neoplasia (e.g., lymphoma, thymoma, and lymphangiosarcoma), heartworm disease, diaphragmatic hernia, lung torsion, mediastinal fungal granulomas, chronic coughing, vomiting, primary lymphedema, iatrogenic, or idiopathic (Fossum et al., 1986a, 1991; Waddle and Giger, 1990; Forrester et al., 1991; Kerpsack et al., 1994; Neath et al., 2000; Small et al., 2008; Singh and Brisson, 2010; Mclane and Buote, 2011; Schuller et al., 2011; Meakin et al., 2013). In one study (Fossum et al., 1986a), Afghan hounds had a higher incidence of chylothorax than other breeds of dogs. This may be because Afghan hounds are overrepresented in cases of lung lobe torsion (Neath et al., 2000). Purebred cats were overrepresented in a retrospective study by Fossum et al. (1991). Chylous pleural effusions are more prevalent in cats (30.5%) than dogs (18.9%) (Davies and Forrester, 1996; Mellanby et al., 2002); however, the prevalence of chylothorax in the Mellanby study may be underestimated because mediastinal effusions were also included in that study. Chylomediastinum has not been described in animals.

Grossly, chylous effusions often have a milky to pink-white to red appearance, depending on the quantity of dietary fat content and the presence or absence of hemorrhage (Fig. 6.47). However, chylous effusions may be clear or serosanguineous depending on the diet. Chylous effusions have a triglyceride concentration that is greater than the serum triglycerides concentration; often the effusion/serum ratio is greater than 3:1 (Meadows and MacWilliams, 1994). In addition, a cholesterol-to-triglyceride (C:T) ratio of less than 1 was proposed to be characteristic of a chylous effusion. However, another study found it to be less reliable (Waddle and Giger, 1990). Based on lipoprotein electrophoretic studies, pleural chylous effusions can be better identified by fluid triglyceride concentrations greater than 100 mg/dL (1.1 mmol/L) and nonchylous effusions by concentrations less than 100 mg/dL (Waddle and Giger, 1990).

Cell counts and protein concentrations are typically increased versus pure transudate parameters. Therefore, chylous effusions generally fit into modified transudate or, more frequently, exudate categories depending on the degree of chronicity (Fossum et al., 1986a, 1986b, 1991). Notably, the total protein measured by refractometry can be very high because of artifactual interference by the lipid in the solution (George, 2001).

Initially, the chylous effusion is characterized by predominantly small lymphocytes (Fig. 6.48) (Fossum et al., 1991). Chyle is an irritant, and over time, neutrophils and/or macrophages become prominent (Fig. 6.49A), although small lymphocytes with lesser numbers of reactive lymphocytes are readily observed as are reactive mesothelial cells. "Smeared" nuclear material from ruptured lymphocytes may also be admixed (Fossum et al., 1986a, 1986b; Small et al., 2008; Schuller et al., 2011). In addition, the inflammatory cells may contain phagocytized lipid, which appear as multiple discrete, colorless vacuoles within the cytoplasm (Fig. 6.49B).

Lymphocyte-Rich Transudate

A lymphocyte-rich transudate has been used to describe feline pleural effusions that contain predominantly small lymphocytes

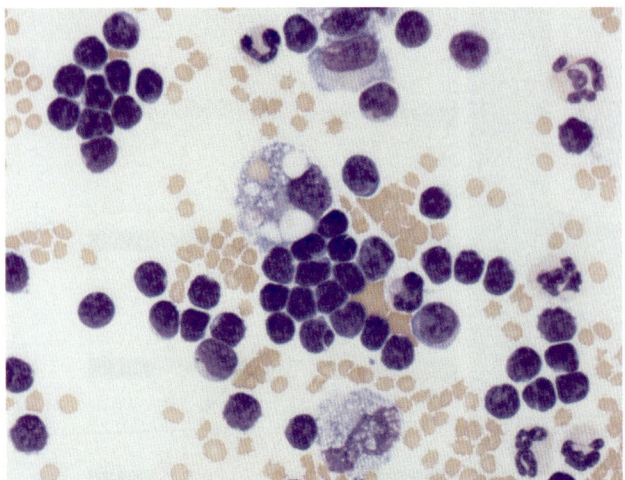

■ **FIGURE 6.48** Chylothorax. Pleural fluid. Cat. Concentrated smear. The fluid has 4200 total nucleated cell count/µL, 20,000 red blood cells/µL, and 3.5 g protein/µL with many small lymphocytes and fewer neutrophils and macrophages. Two macrophages contain colorless, discrete, punctate to large cytoplasmic vacuoles (lipid), and one macrophage exhibits erythrophagia. (Modified Wright; HP oil.)

but if it is greater than 100 mg/dL, it is less than the blood triglyceride concentration (Probo et al., 2018). Most cats with pleural lymphocyte-rich transudates have cardiac disease (Fig. 6.50), mediastinal neoplasia (lymphoma, carcinoma, or thymoma), or intrathoracic masses that may result in pulmonary hypertension (Probo et al., 2018). Therefore, it is likely that there are decreased pulmonary lymphatic drainage and transudation of pulmonary lymphatic fluid into the pleural cavity (Probo et al., 2018).

Lung Lobe Torsion

Lung lobe torsion results in compression of vessels and airways within the twisted pedicle, resulting in emphysema, edema, congestion, ischemia, and necrosis of the torsed lung lobe. The resulting pleural effusion may therefore show characteristics of pulmonary congestion and hypertension, inflammation, blood vessel injury, and/or lymphatic vessel injury. Most fluids are chylous effusions or modified transudates (Neath et al., 2000), but hemorrhagic effusions, exudates (Fig. 6.51), and eosinophilic exudates may also occur (Hambrook et al., 2012).

Organ Rupture
Esophageal Perforation

Esophageal perforation in dogs is most commonly a result of foreign body ingestion and lodgment in the esophagus. If the perforation communicates with the pleural space, it may result in pneumothorax, hemothorax, and/or septic exudate. Cytopathologic findings therefore may include many degenerate neutrophils and erythrocytes, intracellular and extracellular mixed bacteria, and hemosiderin-laden macrophages and erythrophagocytic macrophages. Because the esophageal lining is squamous epithelium, squamous epithelial cells may exfoliate into the fluid. These cells may be nonkeratinized or keratinized and surrounded by neutrophils (Fig. 6.52).

Spirocercosis produces an esophageal nodule predominantly in dogs that may rupture into the pleural cavity, producing an inflammatory effusion with the presence of characteristic ova

but do not contain chylomicrons or have the gross milky appearance of a chylous effusion (Probo et al., 2018). The terms *nonchylous lymphorrhagic effusion* and *lymphocyte-rich effusion* have also been used to describe this effusion type. Lymphocyte-rich transudates are colorless, yellow, or pink and clear or turbid with or without fibrin aggregates (Probo et al., 2018). Typical fluid characteristics are low cell counts (TNCC: mean, 5051/µL; range, 200–25,680/µL; RBC: mean, 112,375/µL; range, 10,000–480,000/µL), variable protein content (mean, 3.2 g protein/dL; range, 1.5–5.1 g protein/dL), and predominantly small lymphocytes (mean, 79%; range, 42%–100%) (Probo et al., 2018). The fluid triglyceride concentration is usually less than 100 mg/dL,

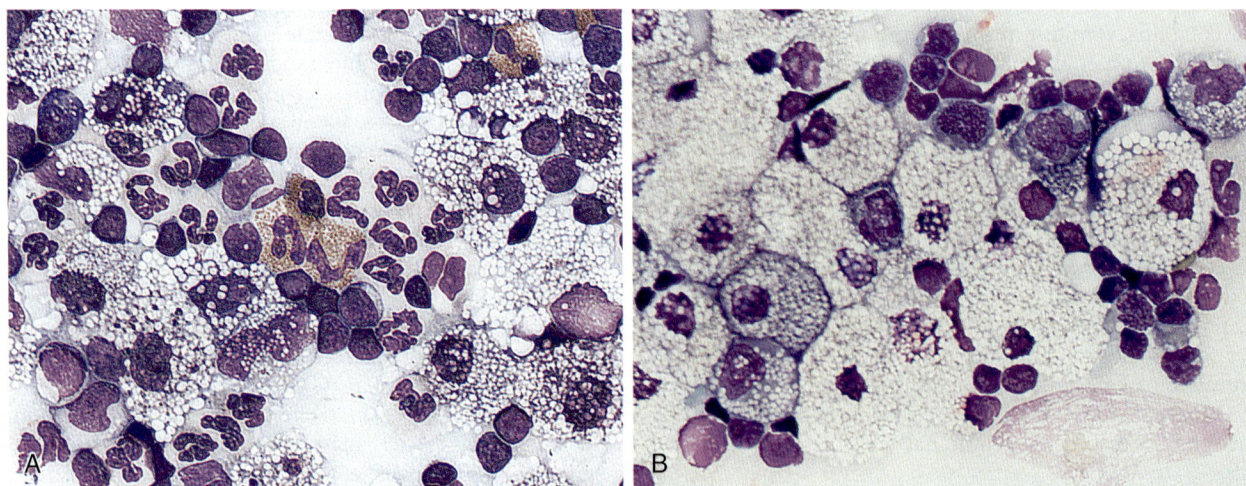

■ **FIGURE 6.49** Chylothorax. Pleural fluid. Cat. Concentrated smear. Same case as in Figure 6.47A. **A,** With chronicity, chyle incites secondary inflammation. In this case, neutrophils outnumber small lymphocytes. This fluid also contained lipid-laden macrophages and increased percentages of eosinophils (center and top right) and plasma cells (top left, eccentric nucleus and deep basophilic cytoplasm). (Modified Wright; HP oil.) **B,** Note the mixture of small lymphocytes and macrophages with numerous colorless, discrete, punctate cytoplasmic vacuoles (lipid). Several cells are ruptured (*bottom right*; faint amorphous eosinophilic material) because of the lipolytic effect of the triglycerides on cell membranes. (Modified Wright; HP oil.)

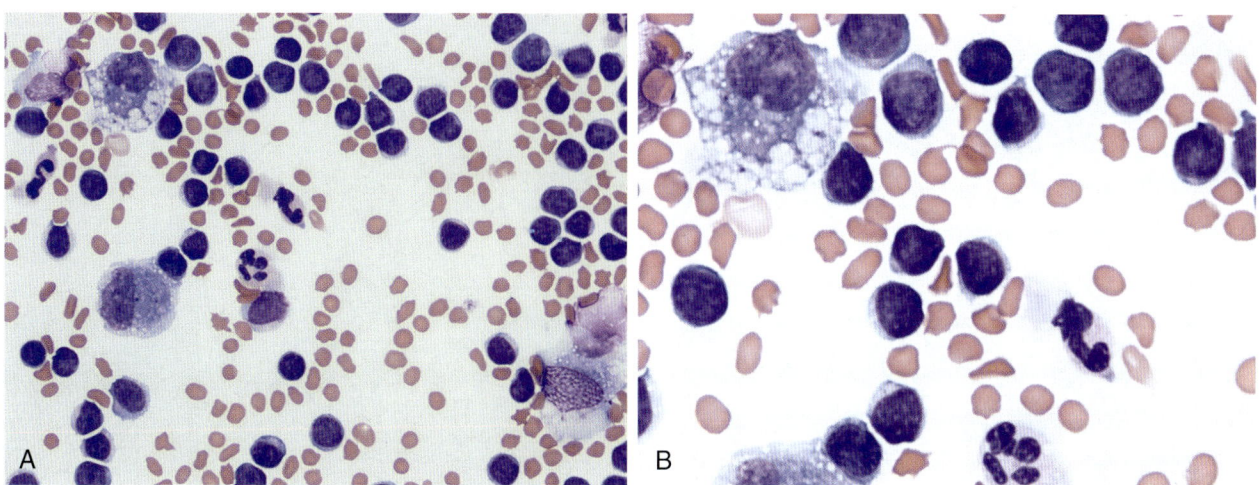

FIGURE 6.50 Lymphocyte-rich transudate. Pleural fluid. Cat. Concentrated smear. Same case in A and B. The patient presented with bicavitary effusion after a 1-month history of respiratory effort. Clinical diagnosis was hypertrophic cardiomyopathy. Pleural fluid was pink and slightly hazy before centrifugation and colorless and clear after centrifugation with protein of 3.1 g/dL and total nucleated cell count of 3778/µL. **A,** Cell differential of the fluid was 75% lymphocytes, 20% neutrophils, and 5% large mononuclear cells. (Wright; HP oil.) **B,** Lymphocytes present were both small and medium. Fluid represents a nonchylous effusion related to lymphatic hypertension as a result of cardiac disease. (Wright; HP oil.) (Courtesy Rose Raskin, Michigan State University.)

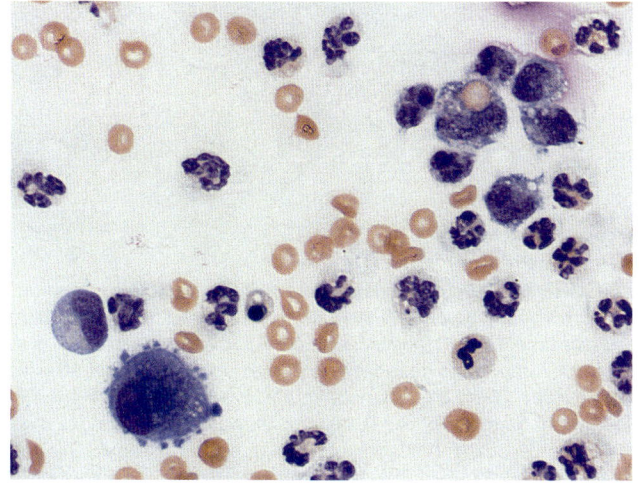

FIGURE 6.51 Lung lobe torsion. Pleural fluid. Dog. Fluid smear. This fluid was red and opaque compatible with a hemorrhagic effusion. Microscopically, the estimated nucleated cellularity was 100,000/µL with 82% neutrophils, 18% macrophages, and rare lymphocytes and reactive mesothelial cells. The image shows many erythrocytes and neutrophils and fewer macrophages, and one exhibits erythrophagia indicative of recent hemorrhage (*upper right*). There is a reactive mesothelial cell with cytoplasmic blebs (*lower left*), and one cell is undergoing apoptosis with a pyknotic nuclei (*center*). The fluid was interpreted as a hemorrhagic effusion and nonseptic exudate. Lung lobectomy and histopathology identified aspiration pneumonia with lung lobe torsion. (Modified Wright; HP oil.)

(Chikweto et al., 2012; Ravanbakhsh et al., 2021) (Fig. 6.53). More disease description is given in Chapter 7.

Lung Rupture

Effusion characteristics in animals with lung perforations vary depending on the underlying cause of the perforation, such as migrating foreign bodies, vehicle accidents, surgical complications, or aspiration pneumonia (Frendin et al., 1997). Effusions may therefore exhibit characteristics of transudates, exudates, or hemorrhagic effusions. Cytopathologic support to specifically diagnose lung perforation is rarely observed, and a diagnosis is typically accomplished with radiographic evidence of pneumothorax. However, the identification of activated charcoal in pleural fluid from a dog with aspiration pneumonia aided in the diagnosis of lung rupture in one case (Fig. 6.54) (Caudill et al., 2018).

PERICARDIAL EFFUSIONS

Pericardial effusions may also be classified as pure transudates, modified transudates, nonseptic and septic exudates, hemorrhagic effusions (hemopericardium), and chylous effusions (chylopericardium), and the fluid characteristics are similar to those previously discussed regarding peritoneal and pleural effusions. Incidental presence of *Dirofilaria repens* microfilariae has been reported in a couple of dogs (Paździor-Czapula et al., 2018).

In dogs, most pericardial effusions are hemorrhagic (90%), and fewer fluids are neoplastic (Fig. 6.55) (4.6%), septic exudates (3.1%), chylous (1.2%), nonseptic exudates (0.4%), pure transudates (0.4%), or modified transudates (0.4%) (Cagle et al., 2014). The incidence of pericardial effusions associated with neoplasia in dogs varies between 38% and 71% (Berg and Wingfield, 1984; Sisson et al., 1984; Kerstetter et al., 1997; MacDonald et al., 2009). The incidence of pericarditis without an identifiable cause (idiopathic) varies between 19% and 67% (Berg and Wingfield, 1984; Sisson et al., 1984; Kerstetter et al., 1997; Atencia et al., 2013). Other infrequent reported causes include bacterial and fungal infections, cardiac insufficiency, uremia, trauma, foreign body, coagulopathy, hernia, parasitic, and left atrial rupture (Berg and Wingfield, 1984; Aronson and Gregory, 1995; Petrus and Henik, 1999; Shubitz et al., 2001; Peterson et al., 2003; Paździor-Czapula et al., 2018).

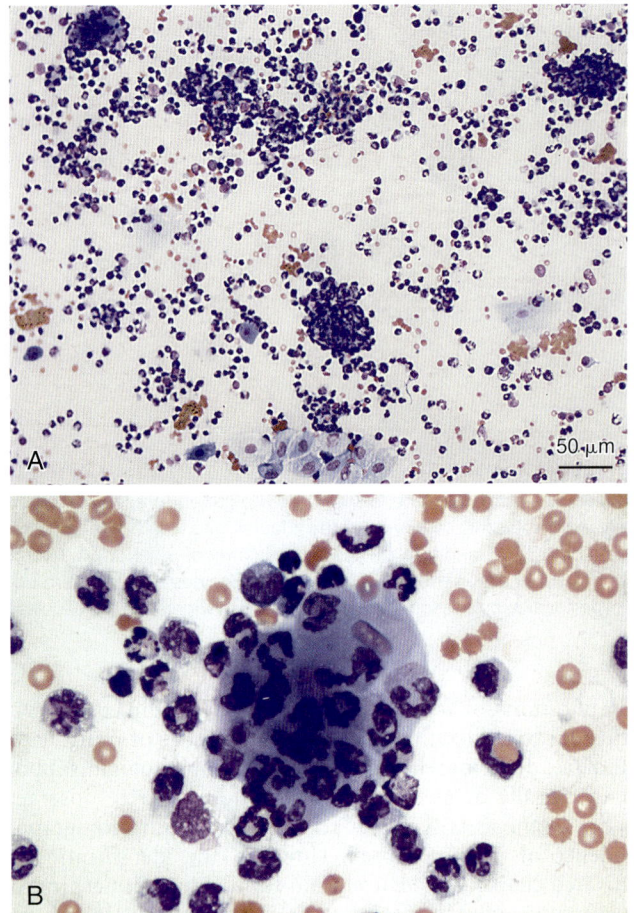

FIGURE 6.52 Esophageal perforation. Pleural fluid. Dog. Same case in A and B. **A,** Several cell aggregates appear against a background of neutrophils. A sheet of squamous epithelial cells (*bottom center*) is present along with scattered individualized intermediate to basal squamous cells. (Modified Wright; IP.) **B,** Many erythrocytes and neutrophils compatible with a hemorrhagic effusion and exudate. The neutrophils aggregate around a well-differentiated oval, basophilic keratinocyte that has exfoliated from the epithelium of the esophageal lumen. One neutrophil is undergoing karyorrhexis (*upper left*), and another neutrophil exhibits erythrophagia (*lower right*). (Modified Wright; HP oil.) (Courtesy Rose Raskin, Purdue University.)

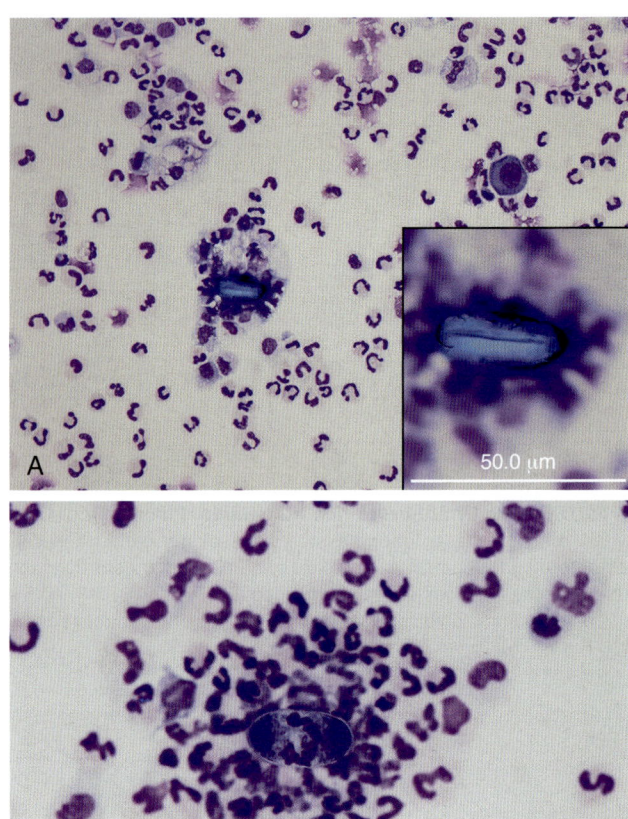

FIGURE 6.53 Spirocercosis. Pleural fluid. Dog. Same case in A and B. This young dog from Peru with respiratory distress had a caudal esophageal nodule and thoracic effusion. **A,** *Spirocerca lupi* ovum is surrounded by numerous neutrophils and macrophages. (Wright-Giemsa; HP oil.) *Inset:* Ovum has a smooth surface with a central longitudinal fold. (Wright-Giemsa; HP oil.) **B,** Neutrophils aggregate around an ovum with a thin capsule and internal purple aggregated material. Ova measure approximately 35 to 38 μm in length and 15 μm in width. Ova are released from a likely ruptured nodule that incites an acute inflammatory response. (Wright-Giemsa; HP oil.) (Courtesy Arefeh Ravanbakhsh, PDS Inc., University of Saskatchewan.)

Pericardial effusions are rare in cats, and most (75%) are attributed to congestive heart failure (Rush et al., 1990; Hall et al., 2007). Other causes of feline pericardial effusions are neoplasia (5.4%–18%), idiopathic (4.1%), uremia or fluid overload (3.4%), thyrotoxic cardiomyopathy (2.1%), FIP (0.7%), and diaphragmatic hernia (0.7%) (Rush et al., 1990; Hall et al., 2007). Most neoplastic effusions are lymphoma, typically of T-cell origin (Rush et al., 1990; Hall et al., 2007; Amati et al., 2014).

Obtaining a diagnosis of neoplasia via cytopathologic evaluation of pericardial effusions may be challenging because of the high frequency reactive mesothelial cells and the low frequency of neoplastic cell exfoliation. The pericardial effusion is often associated with moderate to marked mesothelial hyperplasia, which mimics carcinoma cells. The mesothelial cells are very large with dark basophilic cytoplasm and are often binucleated with prominent nucleoli (see Fig. 6.4B). Mitotic figures that are occasionally bizarre may mimic carcinoma. Consequently, cytopathology often cannot reliably differentiate mesothelial cell hyperplasia from neoplasia. Unlike lymphoma, which may exfoliate many large neoplastic round cells, other neoplasms of mesenchymal origin typically do not shed neoplastic cells into effusions. To underscore the difficulty in diagnosis, 74% of 19 neoplastic effusions were not detected with cytopathology, and 13% of 31 nonneoplastic effusions were falsely reported as neoplastic. In another study that evaluated 47 pericardial effusions, cytopathology identified the cause in only 6 (12.8%); 5 were infectious, and 1 was lymphoma (MacDonald et al., 2009).

Exudates

Pericardial exudates are rare in dogs and cats, making up fewer than 5% of all pericardial effusions (MacDonald et al., 2009;

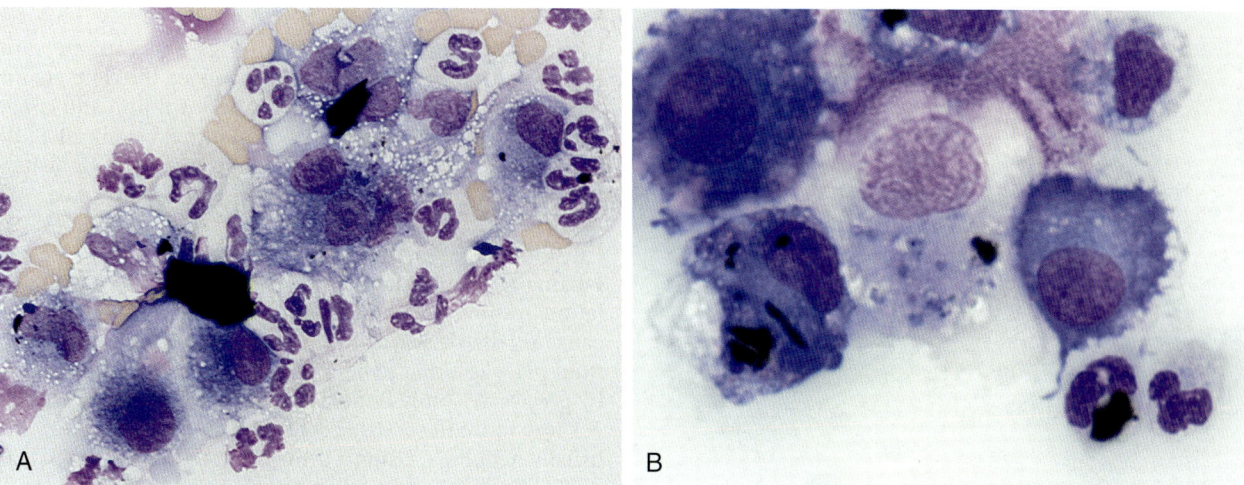

FIGURE 6.54 Lung rupture. Pleural fluid. Dog. Same case in A and B. **A,** Degenerate neutrophils and macrophages (one binucleated) admixed with extracellular and phagocytized black angular to granular material (carbon). (Modified Wright; HP oil.) **B,** Macrophages and a neutrophil contain a black angular material (carbon); reactive mesothelial cell is at *right*. (Modified Wright; HP oil.) The dog developed aspiration pneumonia and lung lobe rupture after being administered activated charcoal for toxicosis therapy. (Courtesy Megan Caudill et al., University of Georgia. Presented at the 2018 ASVCP case review session.)

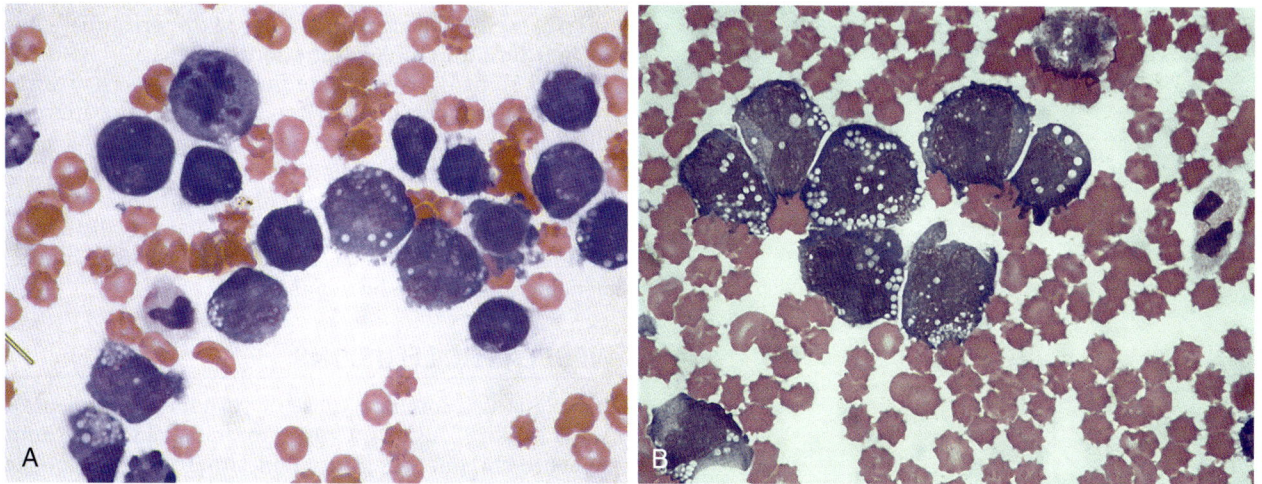

FIGURE 6.55 Neoplastic effusion. T-cell lymphoma. Pericardial fluid. Dog. Sedimented preparation. Same case in A and B. **A,** Fluid is described grossly as bloody. The nucleated cell count estimate is 3500/µL. Cell differential indicated 92% large mononuclear cells, 5% nondegenerate neutrophils, and 3% small lymphocytes. The large mononuclear cells are large, approximately 4 × RBC diameter, deeply basophilic, containing numerous punctate vacuoles. A mitotic figure with abnormal dispersed chromatin. (Wright; HP oil.) **B,** Nuclei appear very irregular with multiple deep indentations. Nucleoli are prominent and multiple. Most cells display punctate vacuolation. Polymerase chain reaction for antigen receptor rearrangement testing of the fluid indicated the presence of a clonal T-lymphocyte population. (Wright; HP oil.) (Courtesy Rose Raskin, Synlab/VPG/TDDS, Exeter, UK.)

Cagle et al., 2014). Potential etiologies include FIP, neoplasia, or infection. Septic exudates may result from migrating foreign bodies, such as foxtail awns, or systemic bacterial, mycotic, or protozoal infections (MacDonald et al., 2009).

Vessel Rupture and Lymphatic Hypertension
Hemopericardium

Hemorrhagic effusion is the most common pericardial effusion in dogs. Most causes of hemopericardium are neoplastic, regardless of whether or not neoplastic cells are observed in the effusion (Cagle et al., 2014). Hemangiosarcoma and mesothelioma are the most common cardiac and pericardial tumors in dogs followed by less frequent occurrences of lymphoma (see Fig. 6.55), neuroendocrine tumors, and thyroid follicular adenocarcinomas (MacDonald et al., 2009). Cytopathologic features of hemopericardium are similar to those of hemoperitoneum and hemothorax except that reactive mesothelial cells are more common in hemopericardium (Fig. 6.56). Hemorrhagic pericardial effusions are less likely to be diagnostic via cytopathology compared with other pericardial effusion types because a cytopathologic diagnosis is only made in 7.7% of pericardial effusions with a fluid PCV of 10% or greater versus a 20.3% cytopathologic diagnostic rate when the fluid PCV is less than 10% (Cagle et al., 2014).

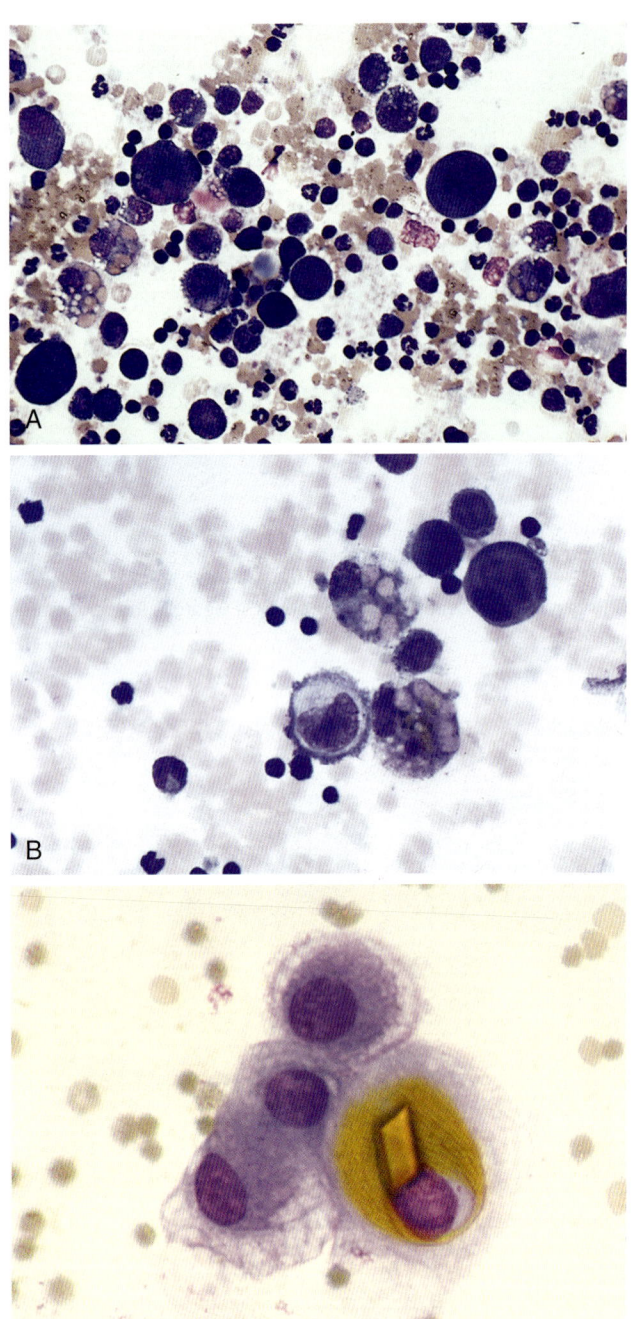

■ **FIGURE 6.56 Hemopericardium. Pericardial fluid. Dog. A, Buffy-coat preparation.** This fluid was red and turbid with 5 million red blood cells/μL, 7000 nucleated cells/μL, and protein of 4.0 g/dL. The leukocytes present are comprised of neutrophils, lymphocytes, erythrophages (*left edge*), and variably sized deeply basophilic reactive mesothelial cells. (Romanowsky; HP oil.) **B, Fluid smear.** A few small lymphocytes and macrophages and three reactive mesothelial cells with deeply basophilic cytoplasm. One macrophage (*top center*) exhibits erythrophagia (partially digested erythrocytes), and a second macrophage contains granular brown hemosiderin pigment (*center right*, next to the pale-staining mesothelial cell). (Romanowsky; HP oil.) **C,** Four mesothelial cells are present, one of which contains a cytoplasmic golden rhomboid hematoidin crystal encircled by fine bilirubin crystals. (Wright-Giemsa; HP oil.) (C, Courtesy Rose Raskin, University of Florida.)

Chylopericardium

Chylous pericardial effusions in dogs and cats are rare. Reported causes include neoplasms involving the right atrium and cranial vena cava, idiopathic chylopericardium, and congestive heart failure (Peaston et al., 1990; Mansfield et al., 2000; Boston et al., 2006; Hall et al., 2007). The cytopathologic features of chylopericardium are similar to those of chylothorax.

Pericardial Ancillary Diagnostics

Further testing is often required (e.g., ultrasonography, coagulation testing, pericardiectomy) to determine the underlying cause of the pericardial effusion. Measurement of pericardial fluid pH was found to be diagnostically helpful when measured by precise instrumentation (Edwards, 1996). A pH greater than 7.3 was more likely associated with noninflammatory disease, usually neoplasia. Using a urine dipstick to measure pH, a pericardial fluid pH greater than or equal to 7.0 was associated with neoplasia in 93% of the cases, whereas a value less than 7.0 was more often associated with nonneoplastic disease. Other studies using the urine dipstick to measure the pH of pericardial effusions generally found that there was too much overlap for it to be diagnostically reliable (Fine et al., 2003; de Laforcade et al., 2005).

Serum cardiac troponin I (cTnI) and cardiac troponin T (cTnT) were evaluated in 37 dogs with pericardial effusions. Higher serum cTnI concentrations (mean, 2.77 ng/dL; range, 0.09–47.18 ng/dL) were more frequently associated with effusions related to hemangiosarcoma than with idiopathic pericardial effusions (mean, 0.05 ng/dL; range, 0.03–0.09 ng/dL). Serum cTnT was not diagnostically useful (Shaw et al., 2004). In another study, a plasma cTnI concentration greater than 0.25 ng/mL had a sensitivity of 81% and specificity of 100% in identifying pericardial effusions associated with cardiac hemangiosarcoma (Chun et al., 2010).

NEOPLASTIC EFFUSIONS

Neoplasia is a common cause of peritoneal and pleural effusions in dogs and cats. Gross appearance and cell count and total protein concentration parameters are generally not helpful in classifying neoplastic effusions. The salient cytopathologic characteristic is the microscopic observation of neoplastic cells.

In dogs and cats, the common causes of neoplastic effusions are lymphoma (pleural) and adenocarcinoma or carcinoma (pleural and peritoneal), with mesothelioma and other hematopoietic neoplasms being less common. Sarcomas rarely exfoliate into effusions regardless of whether they are the cause of the effusion.

Diagnostic cells may not be evident in an effusion, so if a mass is present, fluid analysis along with fine-needle aspiration cytopathology of the mass increases the likelihood of identifying neoplasia. In one study, detection of malignant tumors in abdominal and thoracic fluids had a sensitivity of only 64% for dogs and 61% for cats; however, the specificities were high at 99% for dogs and 100% for cats (Hirschberger et al., 1999). One study found that telomerase activity had only 50% sensitivity and 83% specificity; the test was not recommended as a stand-alone diagnostic tool (Spangler et al., 2000). Cytopathology had a diagnostic accuracy of 94% and 99% in diagnosing ovarian carcinoma in effusions, as determined using two different cytopathologists (Bertazzolo et al., 2012).

Carcinoma and Adenocarcinoma

Effusions associated with carcinomas and adenocarcinomas may be the result of either an intracavitary or an extracavitary neoplasm. Primary neoplasms within the abdominal cavity are gastric, colonic, or intestinal adenocarcinoma (Fig. 6.57); urothelial cell carcinoma (previously transitional cell carcinoma); cholangiocarcinoma; pancreatic adenocarcinoma; ovarian adenocarcinoma (Fig. 6.58); and prostatic carcinoma. In the thorax, the predominant neoplasm is pulmonary adenocarcinoma (Figs. 6.59 and 6.60). Neoplastic effusions caused by extracavitary metastatic disease include urothelial cell carcinoma (previously transitional cell carcinoma), mammary carcinoma, and prostatic carcinoma. Tumor cells may be present in the peritoneal and pleural fluids by invading either into parenchymal blood vessels and lymphatics or by invading directly through the overlying mesothelial surface.

On cytopathology, these tumors are morphologically similar, and the organ of origin usually cannot be determined (Clinkenbeard, 1992). Effusions associated with carcinomas contain rafts (see Figs. 6.59A and 6.60A) and acinar arrangements (see Figs. 6.59B and 6.60B) of round to polygonal cells with variable amounts of often extremely basophilic cytoplasm. Cytoplasmic basophilia may be so intense as to obscure nuclear detail. Inflammation may or may not be present, but reactive mesothelial cells are often present.

Carcinoma cells can resemble reactive mesothelial cells and be a challenge to differentiate. Generally, a diagnosis of malignant neoplasia can be made if the cell population in question

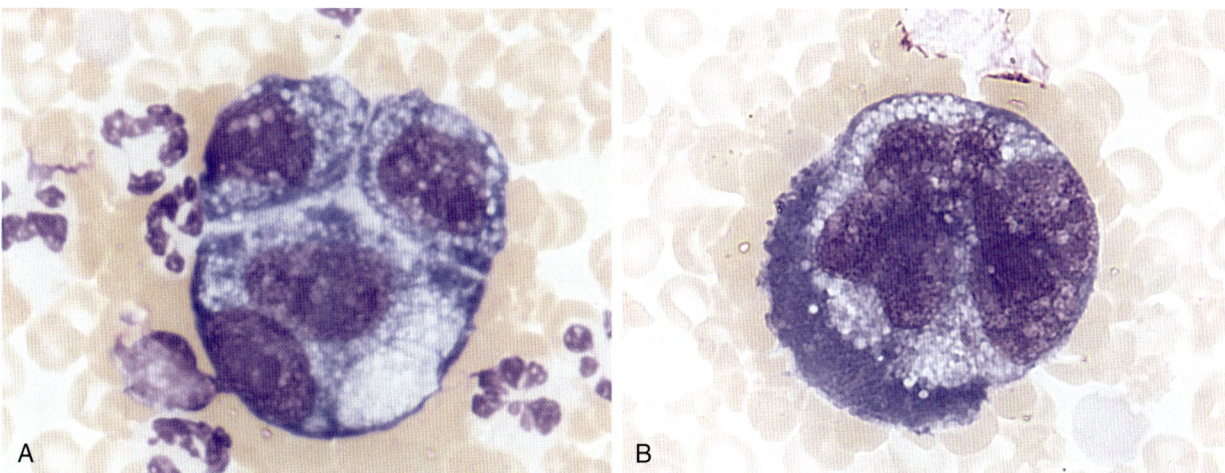

FIGURE 6.57 Neoplastic effusion. Colonic adenocarcinoma. Peritoneal fluid. Dog. Same case in A and B. **A,** This dog was presented for bloody diarrhea, and a rectal mass was identified via palpation and ultrasound. Although the fluid characteristics were that of a transudate (1.9 g protein/dL, 2230 nucleated cells/ μL, 140,000 erythrocytes/μL), neoplastic cells were observed on cytocentrifuged preparations. Three carcinoma cells exhibit criteria of malignancy: anisocytosis, anisokaryosis, binucleation, one to two nucleoli, and stippled chromatin. Cytoplasmic vacuolization suggests glandular origin. (Wright-Giemsa; HP oil.) **B,** Multinucleated carcinoma cell contains four nuclei. (Wright-Giemsa; HP oil.)

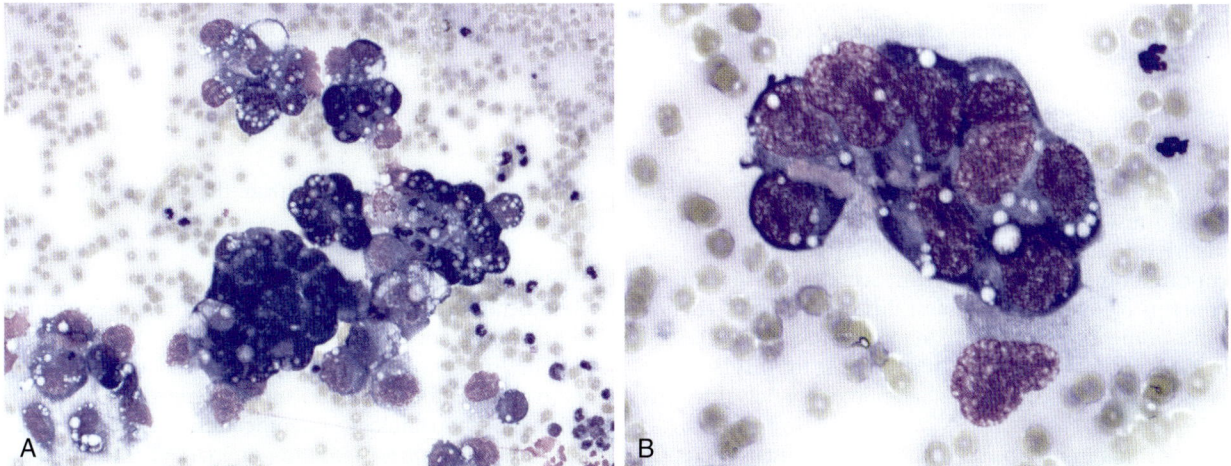

FIGURE 6.58 Neoplastic effusion. Anaplastic ovarian carcinoma. Peritoneal fluid. Dog. Same case in A and B. **A,** Tight clusters of cohesive round to polygonal cells surrounded by erythrocytes, neutrophils, and rare lymphocytes and macrophages. Neutrophils infiltrate the cluster of tumor cells to right of center. Surrounding neutrophils demonstrate the large size of the neoplastic cells. (Wright-Giemsa; IP.) **B,** Carcinoma cells display anisocytosis, anisokaryosis, pleomorphic nuclei, clumped chromatin, and multiple nucleoli and are associated with a pink eosinophilic, extracellular material (matrix or thickened basement membrane) most notable at *left*. (Wright-Giemsa; HP oil.) (Courtesy Ruth Houseright, University of Wisconsin. Presened at the 2014 ASVCP case review session.)

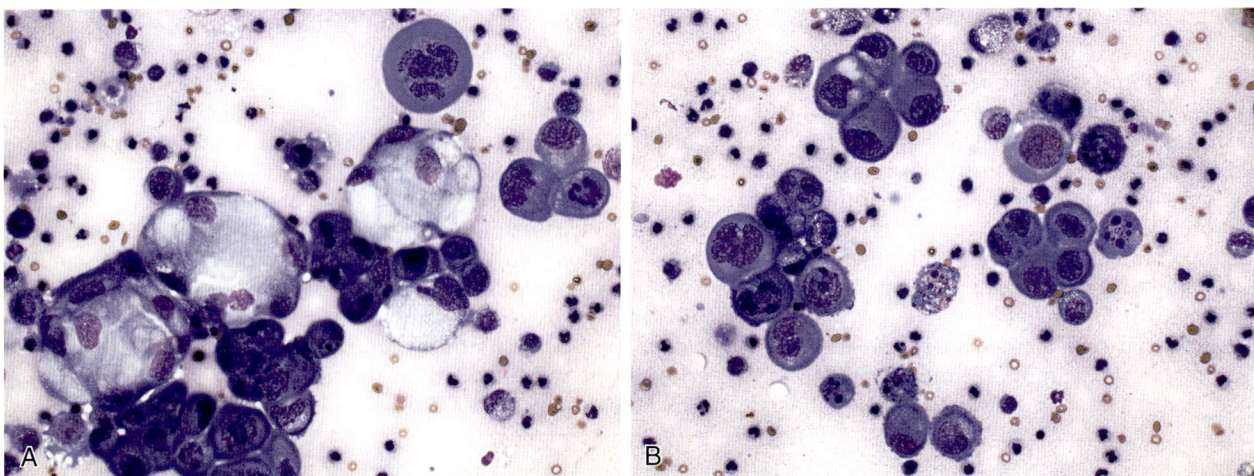

■ **FIGURE 6.59 Neoplastic effusion. Pulmonary adenocarcinoma. Pleural fluid. Cat.** Same case in A and B. **A,** This highly proteinaceous (5.8 g/dL) and cellular (24,100 nucleated cells/μL, 59,000 erythrocytes/μL) fluid contained many neutrophils and clusters of variably vacuolated carcinoma cells that exhibit marked criteria of malignancy, including multinucleation (*top*) and mitotic figures (*right*). Surrounding neutrophils emphasize the relatively large size of the neoplastic cells. (Wright-Giemsa; IP.) **B,** Note the carcinoma cells arranged in an acinar formation (*top* and *right*). Several carcinoma cells exhibit karyorrhexis (*center* and *bottom center*). Interpretation was a neoplastic effusion with secondary nonseptic exudate. (Wright-Giemsa; IP.)

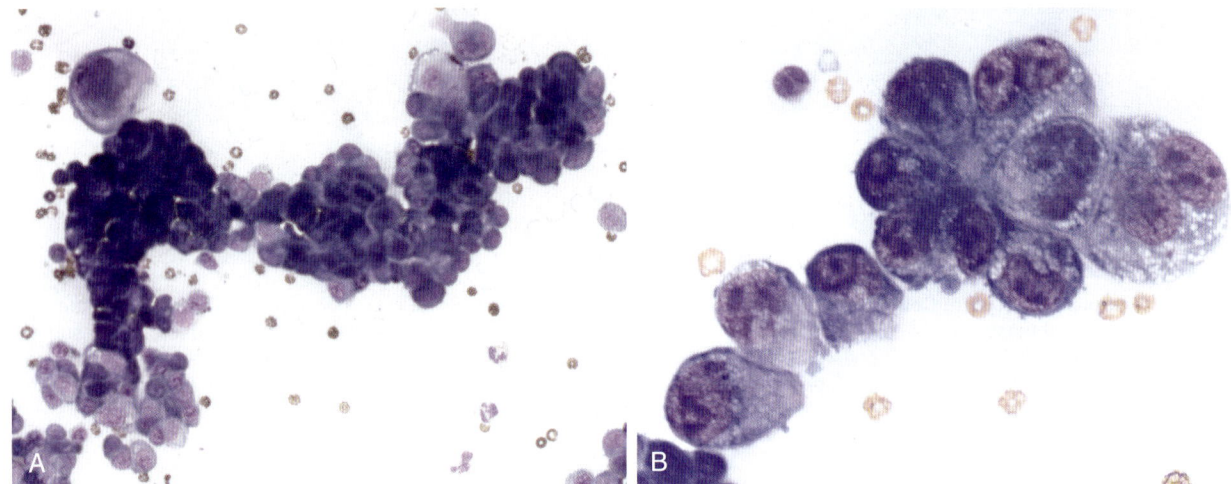

■ **FIGURE 6.60 Neoplastic effusion. Pulmonary adenocarcinoma. Pleural fluid. Dog.** Same case in A and B. **A,** Neoplastic effusion with secondary nonseptic exudate (4.7 g protein/dL, 43,170 nucleated cells/μL, and 80,000 erythrocytes/μL). Note the raft of cohesive round to polygonal epithelial cells, suggestive of tubular gland formation, with occasional marked anisocytosis and anisokaryosis (*top left*). (Wright-Giemsa; IP.) **B,** Neoplastic cells form an acinus. (Wright-Giemsa; HP oil.)

fulfills five strong nuclear criteria. Areas where nuclear detail can be seen must be found. When there is still cytopathologic ambivalence, additional diagnostic tests may be necessary.

Adenocarcinomas are formed from secretory tissue, which often contains cytoplasmic vacuoles; this differentiates adenocarcinoma from other types of carcinoma. In some cells, the amount of secretory product is sufficient to displace the nucleus peripherally, forming a balloon or signet ring cell (Figs. 6.59A and 6.61).

Mucinous effusions may be encountered with mucus-secreting carcinomas that rupture and leak into the cavitary fluids (de Brito Galvao et al., 2009; Tropf et al., 2015) or from myxosarcoma (Riegel et al., 2008). A viscous fluid with mucin lakes in the background and cytochemically confirmed mucin within neoplastic cells helps identify cases of mucinous gastric carcinoma and mucinous pulmonary papillary adenocarcinoma (Fig. 6.62). Stains such as Alcian blue, periodic acid–Schiff, and mucicarmine help to demonstrate the presence of mucins (see Appendix 2).

Mesothelioma

Mesothelioma is an uncommon tumor that arises from the mesothelial lining of the serous body cavities. One report involving five dogs suggested that mesotheliomas can arise in dogs secondary to chronic idiopathic pericardial hemorrhage (Machida et al., 2004). On cytopathology, mesothelioma is extremely challenging to differentiate from carcinoma or marked reactive mesothelial hyperplasia. Mesothelioma cells are generally round to slightly polygonal in shape and are arranged primarily in clusters; however, spindle shapes have also been observed. This variation in cytomorphology likely arises from the multiple histologic subtypes, including a granular cell morphology, deciduoid (Morini et al., 2006), epithelioid (Leisewitz and Nesbit, 1992), cystic, sclerosing (Geninet et al., 2003), and even a lipid-rich form (Avakian

CHAPTER 6 Body Cavity Fluids 275

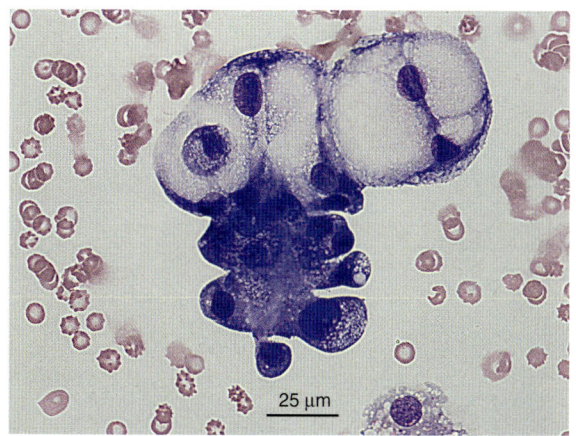

■ **FIGURE 6.61 Neoplastic effusion. Signet ring formation. Adenocarcinoma. Pleural fluid. Dog. Fluid smear.** Marked anisocytosis and anisokaryosis are present with the same cell cluster. Abundant secretory product appears as colorless material expanding the cytoplasm and forcing the nucleus to the periphery. (Modified Wright; HP oil.) (Courtesy Rose Raskin, Purdue University.)

et al., 2008). Nuclei are hyperchromic and located centrally. Often nuclei of adjacent cells within a cluster appear to press against each other, resulting in deformation of nuclei (nuclear molding). Because of the difficulty of differentiating mesothelioma from reactive mesothelial hyperplasia, caution must be used when evaluating suspect populations for criteria of malignancy. As with effusions associated with carcinomas, at least five strong nuclear criteria of malignancy (see Table 2.1) must be seen before a presumptive diagnosis is made. When there is still cytopathologic ambivalence, a second opinion is recommended, especially related to the variable cytopathologic morphology of mesothelioma (Figs. 6.63 to 6.65).

After the diagnosis of malignancy has been established, cytopathology cannot further differentiate mesothelioma from carcinoma. A presumptive diagnosis of carcinoma is logical based on the relative frequency of their occurrence. One tool to attempt to diagnose mesothelioma is the dual expression of cytokeratin and vimentin immunomarkers (Geninet et al., 2003; Bacci et al., 2006; Morini et al., 2006; Avakian et al., 2008; Gumber et al., 2011) (Fig. 6.66). A case of mesothelioma has been recognized by

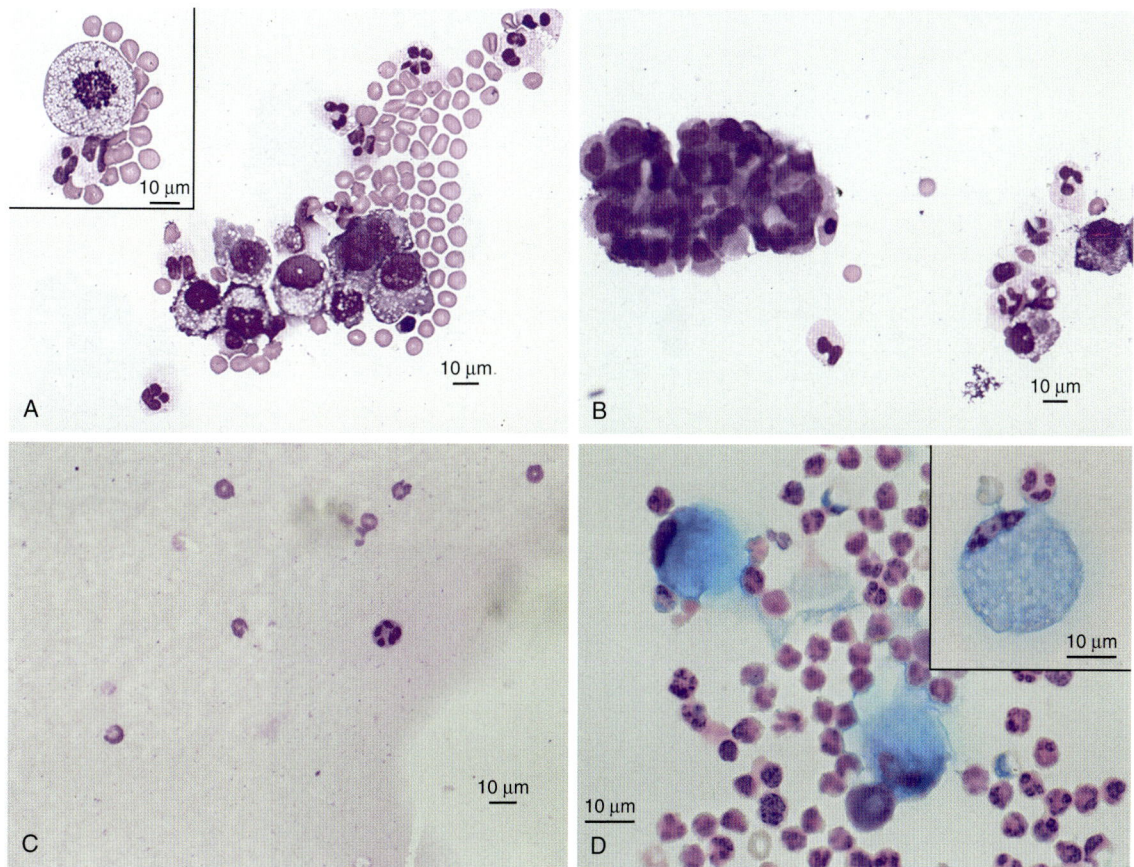

■ **FIGURE 6.62 Mucinous and neoplastic effusion. Mucinous gastric carcinoma. Peritoneal fluid. Dog.** Same case in A to D. The patient presented with chronic vomiting. **A, Cytocentrifuge specimen.** Pale orange, cloudy fluid became pale yellow and clear after centrifugation. Protein is 2.5 g/dL, nucleated cells are 3200/μL, and red blood cells (RBCs) are <30,000/μL with a cell differential of 73% nondegenerate neutrophils, 23% large mononuclear cells, and 4% lymphocytes. Neoplastic cells compose most of the large mononuclear cells. Nuclei measure 3 to 5 × RBC diameter. Cytoplasm is deeply basophilic and highly vacuolated. *Inset:* High magnification of neoplastic cell in mitosis with numerous punctate vacuoles filling the cytoplasm. (Wright; HP oil.) **B, Cytocentrifuge specimen.** One large cluster of reactive mesothelial cells (*left*) admixed with neutrophils and neoplastic cells (20 μm in diameter). (Wright; HP oil.) **C, Direct smear.** One neutrophil with several erythrocytes appears against a dense eosinophilic proteinaceous background. (Wright; HP oil.) **D, Sediment smear.** Two mucin-containing cells appear against a mucin-rich background along with numerous neutrophils. *Inset:* One mucin-rich (blue stain) cell contains a nucleus compressed against the periphery. (Alcian blue; HP oil.) Cytopathologic evaluation expressed concern for neoplasia, although the cell type could not be precisely determined. Histopathologic examination from surgical specimens diagnosed mucinous gastric carcinoma with metastasis to the spleen and mesentery, the latter accounting for the mucinous effusion. (Courtesy of Rose Raskin, Purdue University.)

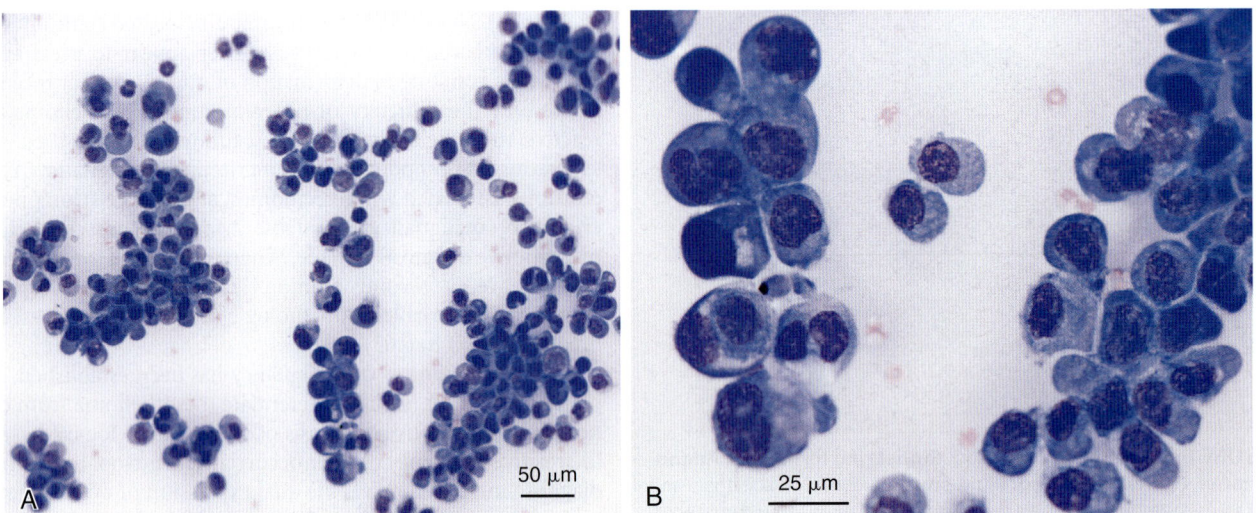

■ **FIGURE 6.63 Neoplastic effusion. Mesothelioma. Pleural fluid. Cat.** Same case in A and B. **A,** Large cell clusters with papillary formations (fingerlike projections) make up the majority of the nucleated cell population. (Modified-Wright; IP.) **B,** Malignant features include anisokaryosis, multinucleation, high and variable nucleocytoplasmic ratio, coarse chromatin, and prominent nucleoli. (Modified-Wright; HP oil.) The diagnosis confirmed by immunochemical expression of cytokeratin, vimentin, and calretinin, a prerequisite to differentiate from a carcinoma. (Courtesy of Cheryl Swenson et al., Michigan State University. Presented at the 2005 ASVCP case review session.)

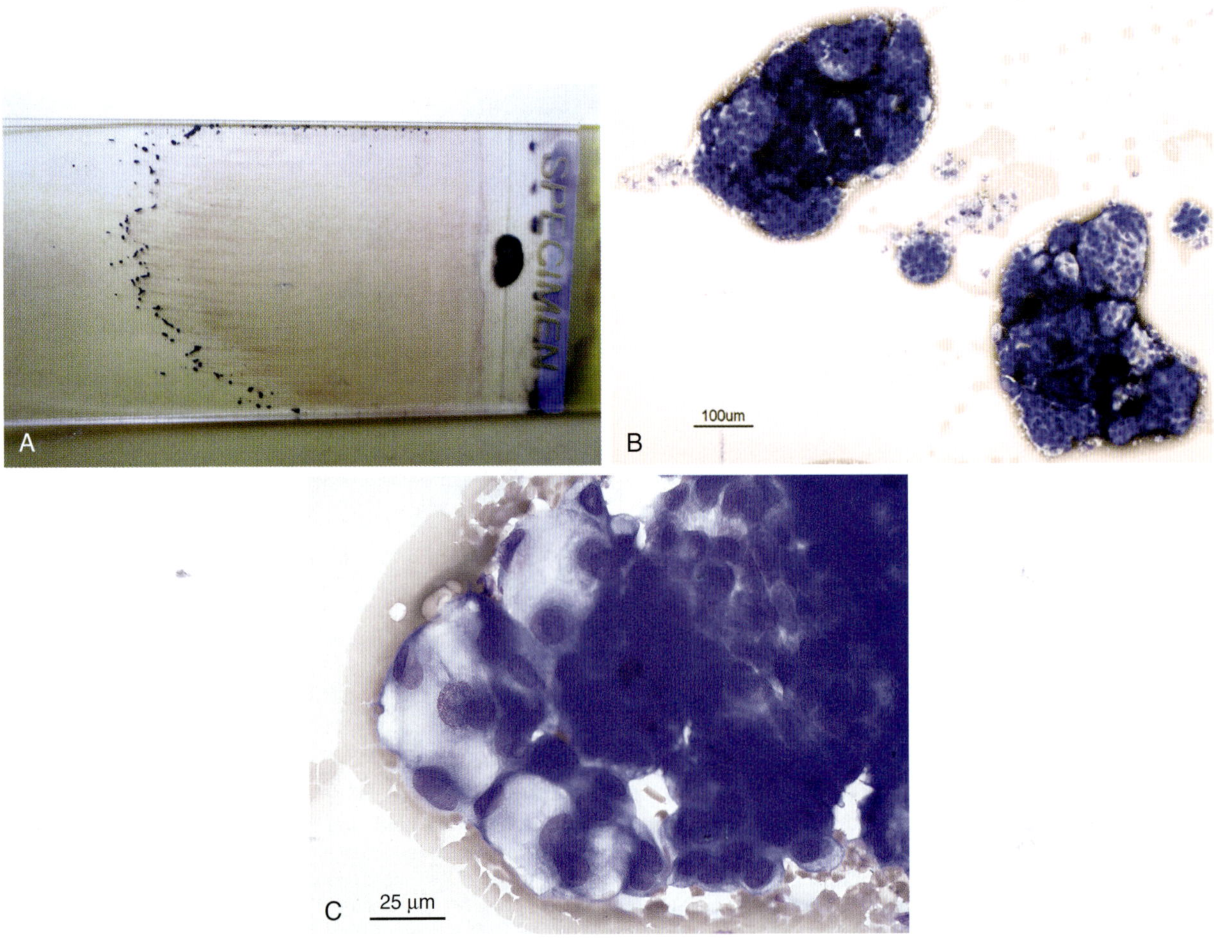

■ **FIGURE 6.64 Neoplastic effusion. Mesothelioma. Peritoneal fluid. Dog.** Same case in A to C. **A, Macroscopic slide.** Large cell clusters are grossly visible at the feathered edge of a direct smear. **B, Direct smear.** One small cluster of reactive mesothelium is shown in comparison appearing between two large neoplastic cell clusters. (Wright-Giemsa; LP.) **C, Direct smear.** Cell clusters are variable in size with prominent cytoplasmic vacuolation. Morphology is indistinguishable from that of secretory adenocarcinoma. Histopathology or immunohistochemistry is a prerequisite for definitive diagnosis. (Wright-Giemsa; HP oil.) (Courtesy Sarah Hammond et al., Virginia Polytechnic Institute and State University. Presented at the 2012 ASVCP case review session.)

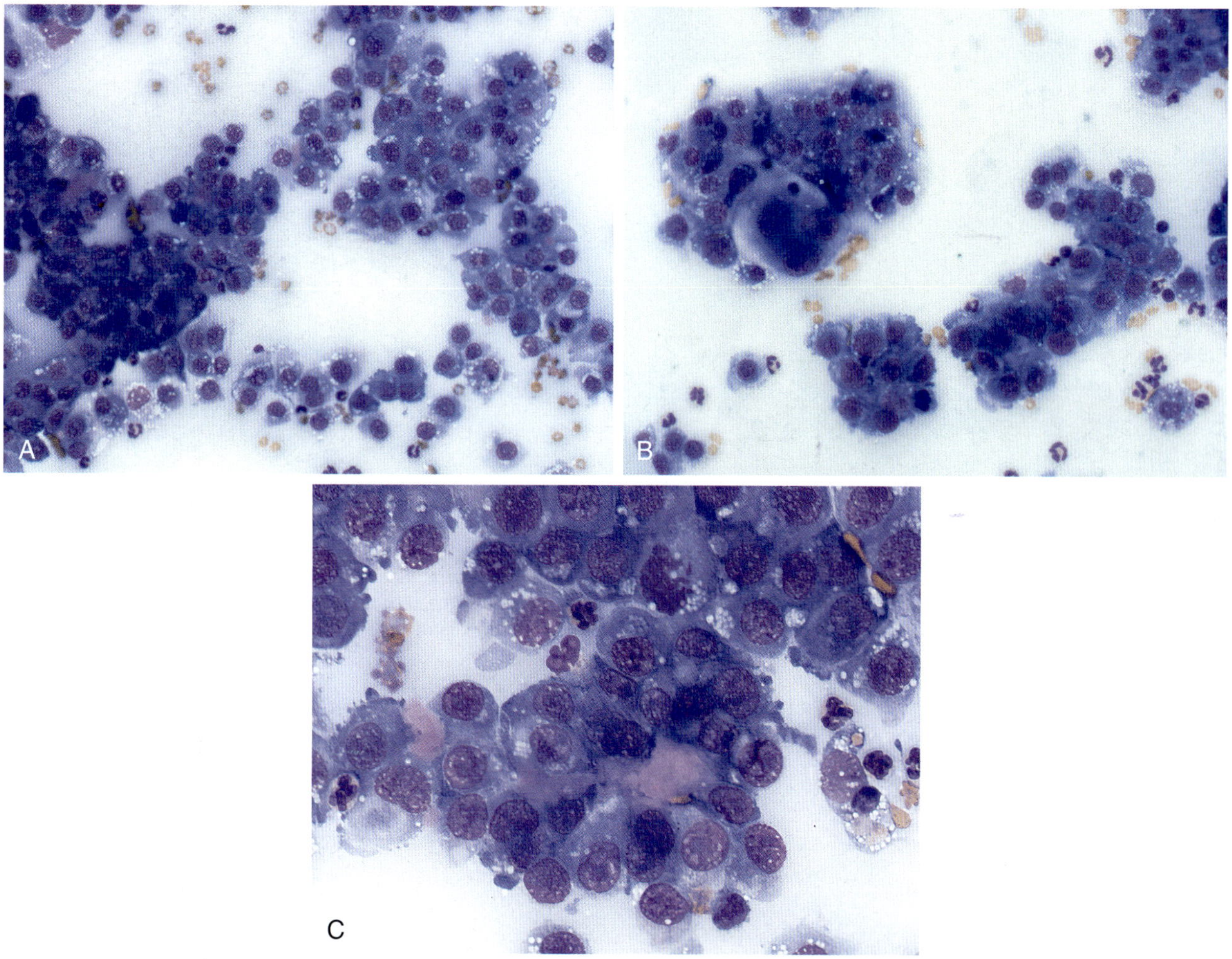

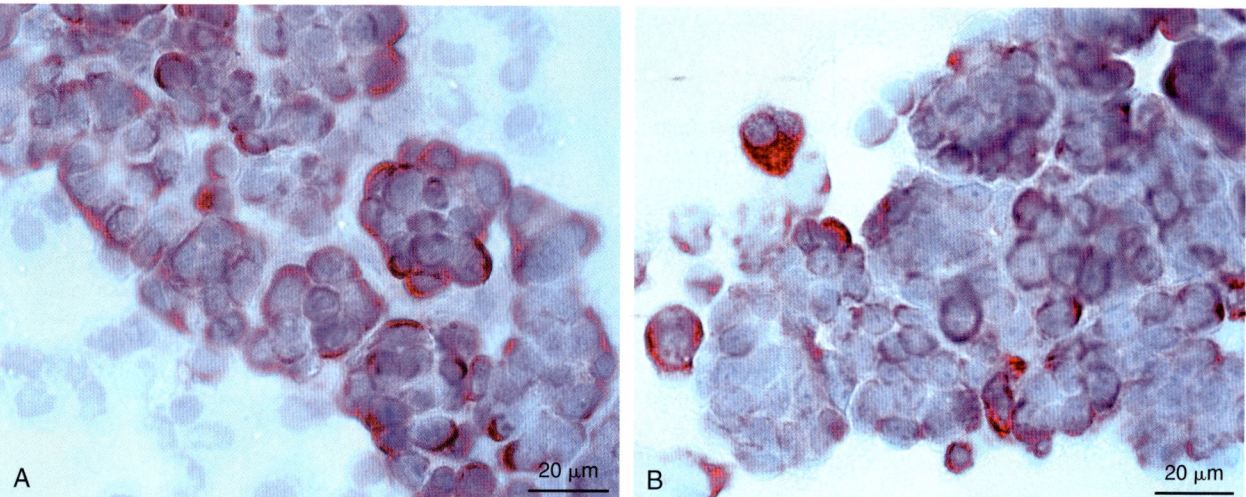

■ **FIGURE 6.65** **Neoplastic effusion. Mesothelioma. Pleural fluid. Dog.** Same case in A to C. **A,** Sheets and clusters of irregularly round cells with punctate cytoplasmic vacuoles and occasional surface blebs. (Wright-Giemsa; IP.) **B,** Malignant features include anisokaryosis, anisocytosis, multinucleation, and multiple, prominent nucleoli. Mild neutrophilic inflammation is present. (Wright-Giemsa; IP.) **C,** These cells aggregate around pink eosinophilic, intercellular material that mimics an adenocarcinoma. A mitotic figure is located at top center. Histopathology or immunohistochemistry is a prerequisite for definitive diagnosis. (Wright-Giemsa, HP oil.)

■ **FIGURE 6.66** **Neoplastic effusion. Mesothelioma. Cavitary fluid. Dog. Immunocytochemistry of fluid smear.** Same case in A and B. **A,** Many neoplastic cells display strong, diffuse, cytoplasmic immunoreactivity for the epithelial cell marker, pancytokeratin. (Pancytokeratin antibody; HP oil.) **B,** The neoplastic cells also demonstrate strong, focal to diffuse, cytoplasmic immunoreactivity for the mesenchymal cell marker, vimentin. (Vimentin antibody; HP oil.) Co-expression of vimentin and cytokeratin support mesothelial cell origin in this case. Histopathologic diagnosis was mesothelioma. (Courtesy Kansas State University.)

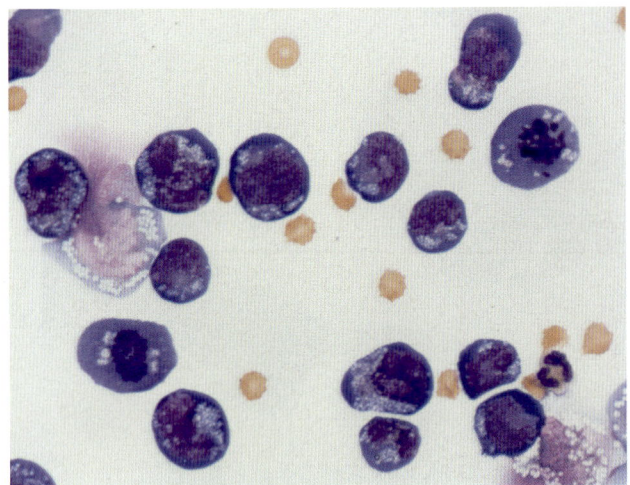

■ **FIGURE 6.67** Neoplastic effusion. Lymphoma. Peritoneal fluid. Dog. Fluid smear. Cellularity of this sample is 19,160 nucleated cells/µL with a protein of 1.6 g/dL. Note the individual large round cells with high nucleocytoplasmic ratios, irregularly round nuclei, two mitotic figures (*upper right, lower left*), and moderately abundant basophilic punctate vacuolated cytoplasm that resembles carcinoma cells. Several erythrocytes and one neutrophil gauge the relative size of the neoplastic lymphoid cells. The light-purple, smudged structures are free nuclei from lysed cells (*upper left, lower right corner*). (Wright-Giemsa; HP oil.)

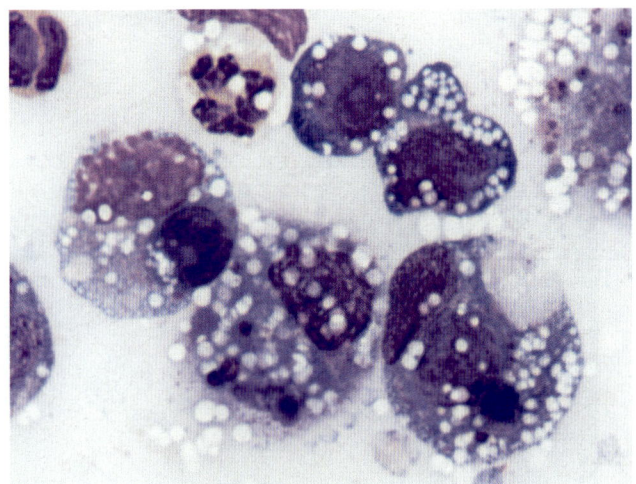

■ **FIGURE 6.69** Neoplastic effusion. Lymphoma Pleural fluid. Dog. Fluid smear. Note the three macrophages (bottom three cells) and two neoplastic lymphoid cells with punctate vacuolation (*upper right*), next to a nondegenerate neutrophil. The macrophages have phagocytized dark basophilic cellular debris and one has phagocytized a round cell (*left*). (Wright-Giemsa; HP oil.)

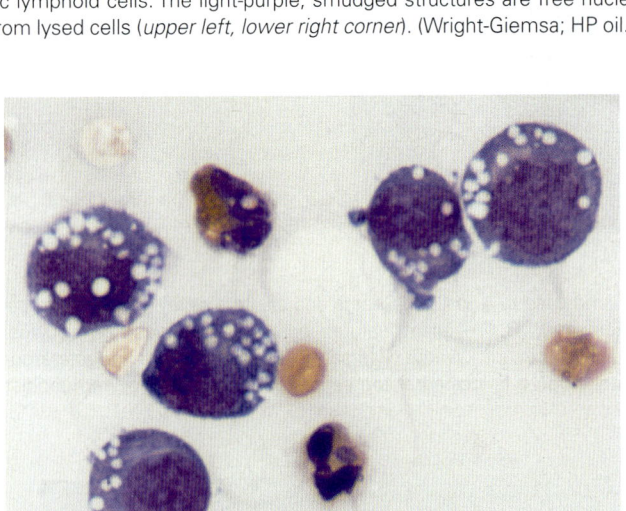

■ **FIGURE 6.68** Neoplastic effusion. Lymphoma. Pleural fluid. Dog. Fluid smear. Note five individual large lymphoid cells with punctate vacuolation, one eosinophil, one nondegenerate neutrophil, and four erythrocytes. A few faint gray protein crescents are also present in the background reflecting the high fluid protein concentration (3.6 g/dL). (Wright-Giemsa; HP oil.)

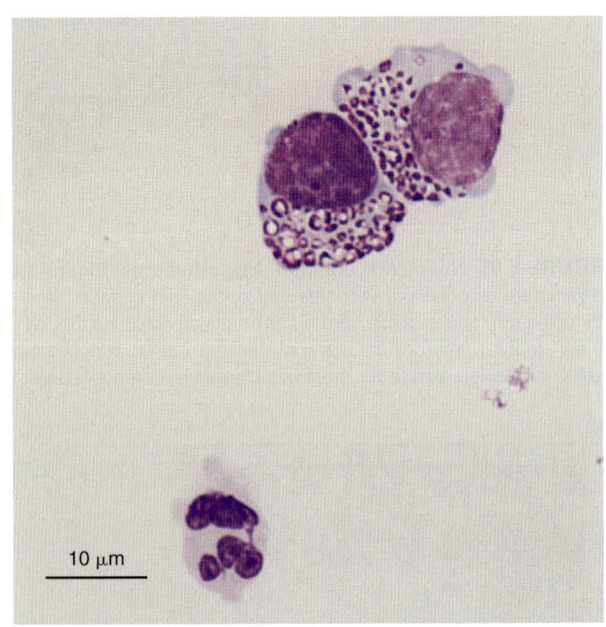

■ **FIGURE 6.70** Neoplastic effusion. Granular cell lymphoma. Pleural fluid. Cat. This fluid was light yellow and hazy with a protein of 4.2 g/dL and nucleated cell count of 5600/µL. In addition, 63% of nucleated cells were densely granulated as shown. Granules varied from fine to coarse (as shown) and were frequently eccentrically placed to one side of the cell. Nondegenerate neutrophils (one shown), small lymphocytes, and occasional mononuclear were admixed. (Wright-Giemsa; HP oil.) (Courtesy Rose Raskin, University of Florida.)

the use of the immunohistochemical marker calretinin in a horse (Stoica et al., 2004). Although calretinin has been used to diagnose mesothelioma in humans and one horse, this immunomarker has consistently been shown to be negative in dogs and cats (Geninet et al., 2003; Bacci et al., 2006; Morini et al., 2006).

Lymphoma

Effusions associated with lymphoma are generally highly cellular and contain an immature population of discrete round cells that are morphologically consistent with lymphocytes (Figs. 6.55 and 6.67 to 6.69). The neoplastic cells have high N:C; scant to moderate amounts of cytoplasm; and often scattered, small, colorless cytoplasmic vacuoles. Occasionally, granular lymphocytes are the predominant neoplastic cell (Figs. 6.70 to 6.72). Moderate numbers of mitoses are observed.

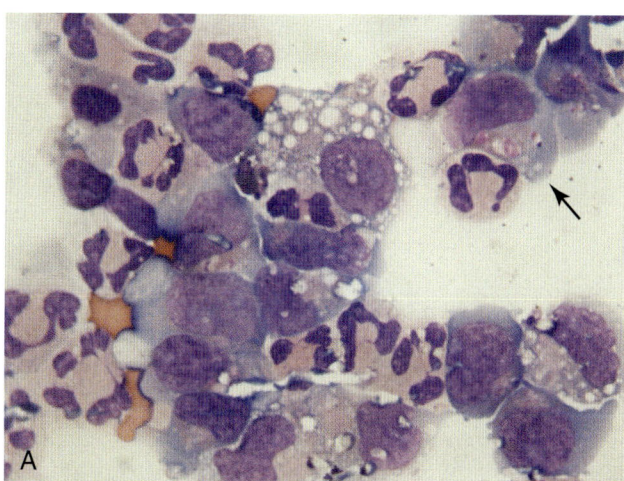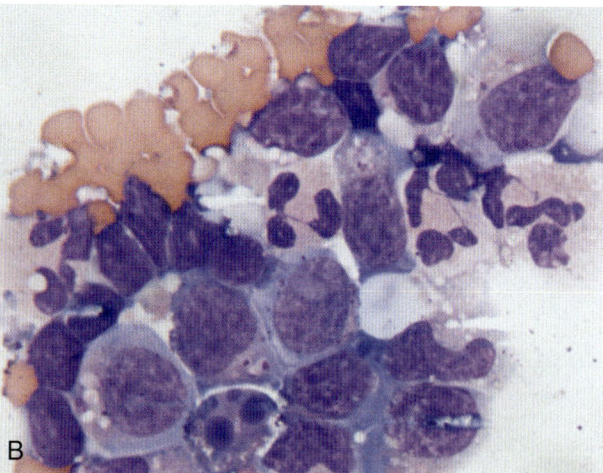

■ **FIGURE 6.71 Neoplastic effusion. Granular cell lymphoma. Peritoneal fluid. Concentrated smear.** Same case in A and B. Yellow, mildly turbid fluid. The nucleated cell count was 1.7×10^9/L with a cell differential of 59% lymphocytes, 24% nondegenerate neutrophils, and 17% large mononuclear phagocytes. About one-third of lymphocytes contain fine cytoplasmic granulation. **A,** Mixed-cell population with 11 lymphoid cells, several of which contain fine eosinophilic granules *(arrow)*. The nuclear size is approximate to that of the neutrophil, indicating a medium-sized lymphocyte. (Wright; HP oil.) **B,** Several lymphoid cells appear to contain a prominent nucleus. (Wright; HP oil.) (Courtesy Rose Raskin, University of Bristol, UK.)

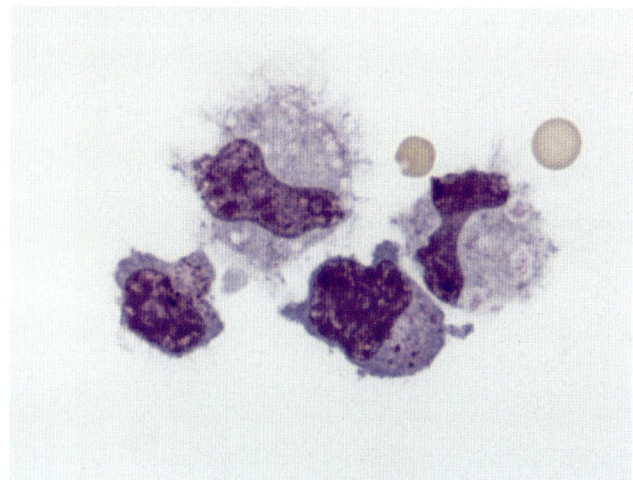

■ **FIGURE 6.72 Neoplastic effusion. Granular cell lymphocytes. Peritoneal fluid. Cat. Cytocentrifuged smear.** Effusion was light yellow and hazy with low protein (2.3 g/dL) and low cellularity (120 nucleated cells/μL). There are two granular lymphocytes (lower two cells) and two macrophages with elongate nuclei and rarefied cytoplasm (upper two cells). The two erythrocytes help gauge the size of the lymphocytes. (Wright-Giemsa; HP oil.)

Variable number of RBCs, reactive mesothelial cells, and inflammatory cells may be admixed.

Chyle can be associated with lymphoma (Fossum et al., 1986b; Fossum et al., 1991; Gores et al., 1994), which is detected by the presence of large immature lymphocytes. Rare cases of lymphoma have cells that are morphologically similar to normal small lymphocytes. These cases are problematic, and cytopathology can only suggest the possibility of lymphoma. In these cases, additional diagnostic testing is required (Ridge and Swinney, 2004).

Evaluation of the types of lymphoid cells found within the fluid by immunocytochemistry or flow cytometry may provide useful information. A monotypic population of medium and/or large lymphocytes is more likely associated with neoplasia (Figs. 6.73A and 6.74A; see Figs. 6.55B, 6.67, and 6.68) than with a reactive process. Immunocytochemistry with antibodies against the molecules CD3 (T cell) and CD79a or CD20 (B cell) is helpful in these cases for minimal phenotyping (see Figs. 6.73B and 6.74B). Additional information is found in Chapter 18.

Other Neoplasms

Other tumor cells are rarely observed in effusions. These include neoplastic cells of neuroendocrine carcinoma (Fig. 6.75), malignant melanoma (Fig. 6.76), myxosarcoma (Fig. 6.77), systemic mastocytosis (Fig. 6.78), and malignant plasmacytoma (Fig. 6.79) (de Souza et al., 2001; Riegel et al., 2008; Morges and Zaks, 2011; Sommerey et al., 2012). Myxosarcoma has an extensive background of dense, mucinous matrix, which often an induces windrowing of the cells within the sample.

BICAVITARY EFFUSIONS

Concurrent pleural and peritoneal effusions in dogs and cats typically indicate generalized or multisystemic disease. Most animals are diagnosed with malignant neoplasia (40%) or cardiovascular disease (see Fig. 6.50) (27%) (Steyn et al., 1993; Moore et al., 2016). Less common causes of bicavitary effusions include infectious disease, pancreatitis, protein-losing enteropathy (Fig. 6.80), coccidiomycosis, and non-neoplastic liver disease (Steyn et al., 1993; Piech et al., 2020).

EFFUSION ANCILLARY DIAGNOSTICS

In some instances, other laboratory testing of effusions may contribute useful information for differential diagnosis. A summary of previously described tests is shown in Table 6.1.

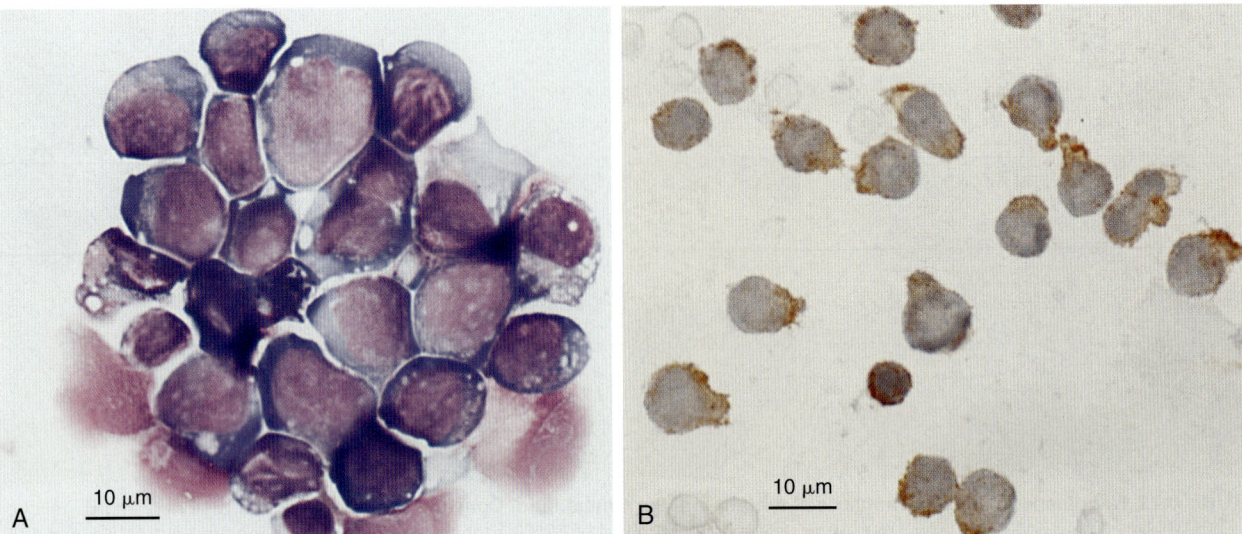

■ **FIGURE 6.73 Neoplastic effusion. T-cell lymphoma. Pleural fluid. Dog.** Same case in A and B. **A, Cytocentrifuged specimen.** Variably sized round cell population having scant to moderate basophilic cytoplasm, fine to moderately coarse chromatin with occasional prominent nucleoli, and variable nucleocytoplasmic ratios. Cells are aggregated with an acinar appearance related to cytocentrifugation. (Modified Wright; HP oil.) **B, Sediment smear.** Immunostaining displays positive cell surface immunoreactivity in all lymphoid cells for the CD3 antigen, which supports a single population of T lymphocytes. Note the small, round immunoreactive stained cell just below center, which is likely a normal T lymphocyte, for comparison. (CD3 antibody; HP oil.) (Courtesy Rose Raskin, Purdue University.)

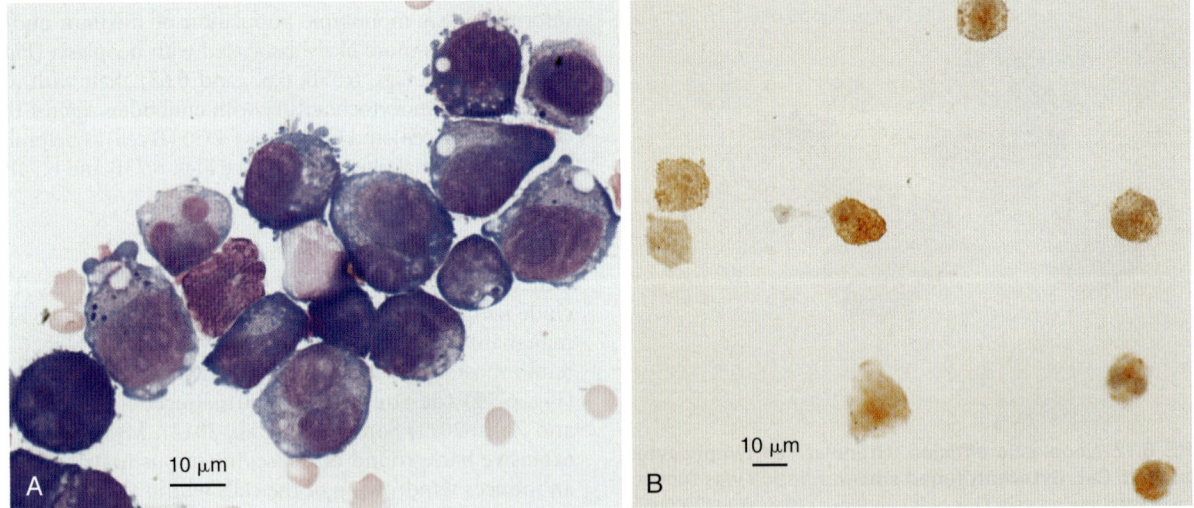

■ **FIGURE 6.74 Neoplastic effusion. B-cell lymphoma. Pleural fluid. Cat.** Same case in A and B. **A, Cytocentrifuged specimen.** Round cells with marked pleomorphism are shown. Neoplastic lymphoid cells have one to two nuclei with large prominent nucleoli surrounded by scant to moderate basophilic cytoplasm. Cells with surface blebbing may be lymphoid or mesothelial in origin. (Modified Wright; HP oil.) **B, Sediment smear.** All of the large round cells were immunoreactive for the CD79a antigen, supporting B-cell origin. CD3 antigen was absent on all cells (not shown). (CD79a antibody; HP oil.) (Courtesy Rose Raskin, Purdue University.)

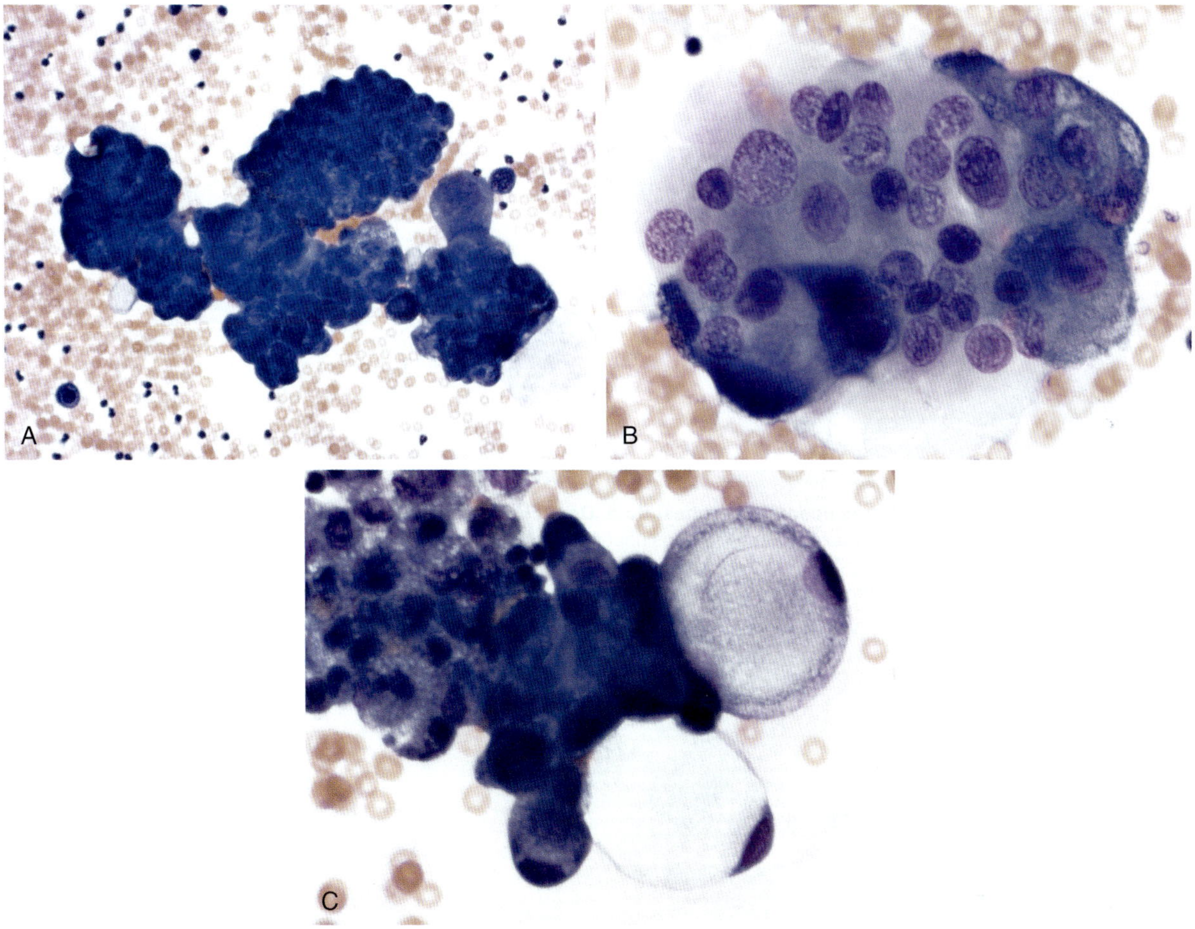

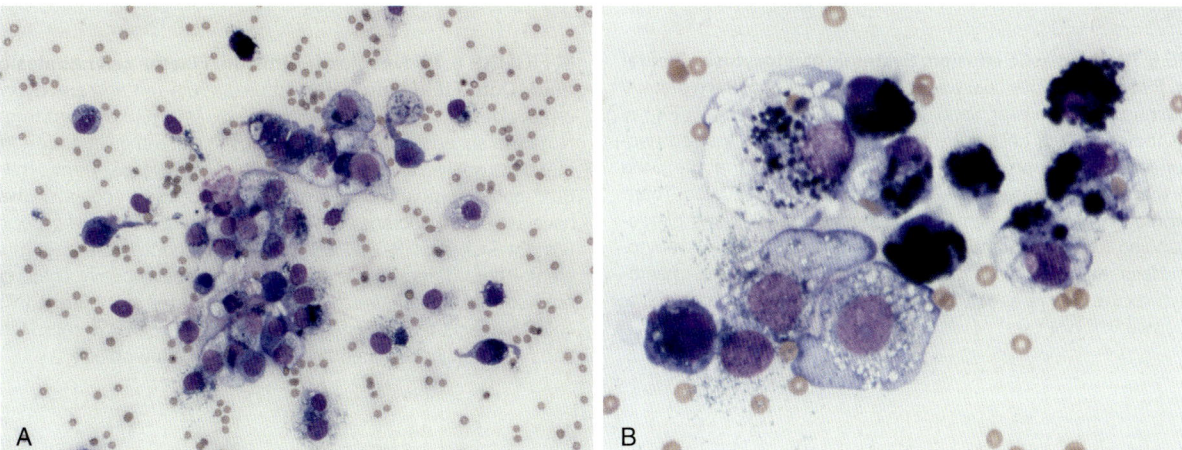

■ **FIGURE 6.75 Neoplastic effusion. Neuroendocrine carcinoma. Pleural fluid. Dog.** Same case in A to C. **Fluid smear. A,** A branching cluster of tightly cohesive, deeply basophilic, round to polygonal cells. (Wright-Giemsa; IP.) **B,** Within the less dense sheets, these cells contain a moderate amount of light eosinophilic or basophilic cytoplasm with indistinct cell borders. Nuclei have reticulated chromatin containing large and prominent nucleoli. Anisokaryosis is marked. (Wright-Giemsa; HP oil.) **C,** Two large cells exhibit signet ring morphology owing to large cytoplasmic vacuoles that displace and compress their respective nuclei peripherally. Erythrocytes serve as a reference size for the neoplastic cells. The diagnosis was supported by coexpression of cytokeratin and chromogranin A. (Wright-Giemsa; HP oil.) (Courtesy Mary Leissinger et al., Louisiana State University. Presented at the 2013 ASVCP case review session.)

■ **FIGURE 6.76 Neoplastic effusion. Malignant melanoma. Pleural fluid. Cat.** Fluid smear. Same case in A and B. **A,** Loosely cohesive or individualized, round, spindle-shaped or stellate cells contain few to many dark green, cytoplasmic granules (melanin). (Wright-Giemsa; IP.) **B,** Two neoplastic melanocytes with nuclei containing prominent nucleoli surrounded by voluminous faint basophilic cytoplasm with punctate vacuoles (*bottom* and *left*) and several melanomacrophages; one is large and foamy (*upper left*), and the others are packed with dark melanin pigment. Compared with the two melanocytes, the melanomacrophages contain variably sized, multifocal aggregates of melanin caused by collection of the granules within phagosomes and phagolysosomes. The macrophages also exhibit erythrophagia. (Wright-Giemsa; HP oil.) (Courtesy Danielle Gordon et al., University of Illinois. Presented at the 2018 ASVCP case review session.)

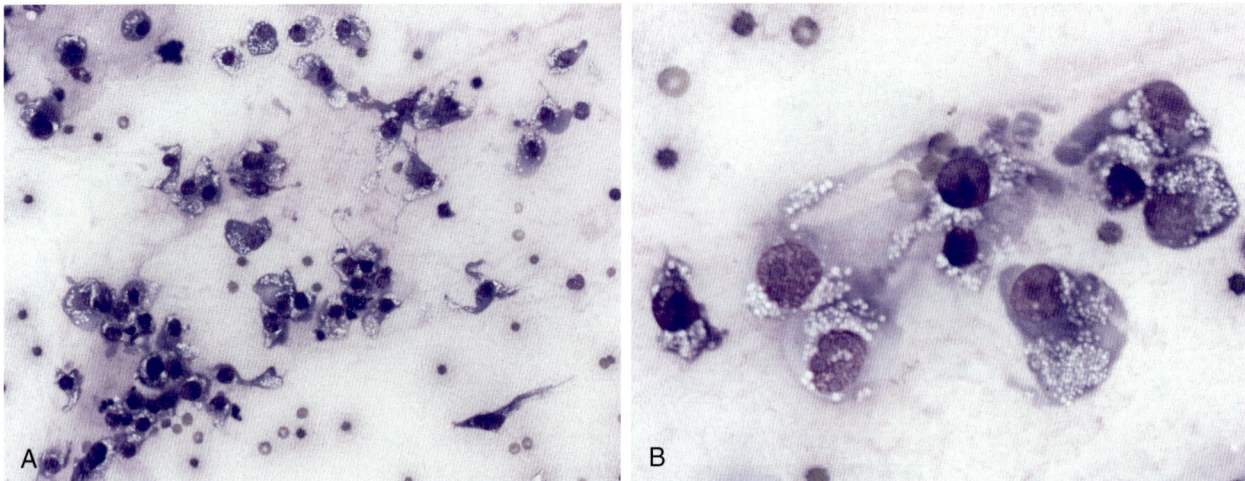

■ **FIGURE 6.77 Neoplastic effusion. Myxosarcoma. Peritoneal fluid. Dog. Fluid smear.** Same case in A and B. **A,** Note the individualized and loosely aggregated spindle to stellate cells admixed with a faint eosinophilic, fibrillar proteinaceous matrix. (Modified Wright; IP.) **B,** Neoplastic cells contain a moderate amount of variably basophilic cytoplasm with many discrete and colorless vacuoles, round nuclei, reticular chromatin, and one to multiple prominent nucleoli. (Wright-Giemsa; HP oil.) (Courtesy April White, Colorado State University. Presented at the 2013 ASVCP case review session.)

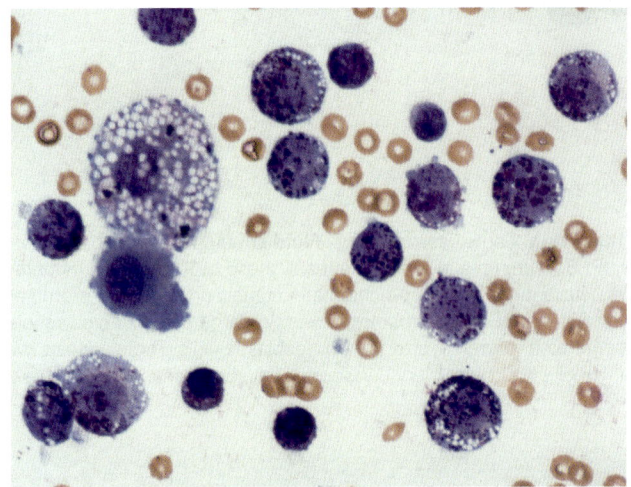

■ **FIGURE 6.78 Neoplastic effusion. Systemic mastocytosis. Pleural fluid. Dog. Fluid smear.** This fluid was red and opaque with 3.8 g protein/dL, 64,740 nucleated cells/µL, and 220,000 erythrocytes/µL. Eighty percent of the nucleated cells were individualized, variably sized neoplastic round cells with purple cytoplasmic granules often aggregated located in scant to moderate cytoplasm with punctate vacuoles. There are a large macrophage with numerous punctate vacuoles and phagocytized granules (*upper left*) and a reactive mesothelial cell with cytoplasmic surface blebs immediately below and touching the macrophage. Erythrocytes serve as reference for size of the neoplastic cells. (Wright-Giemsa; HP oil.)

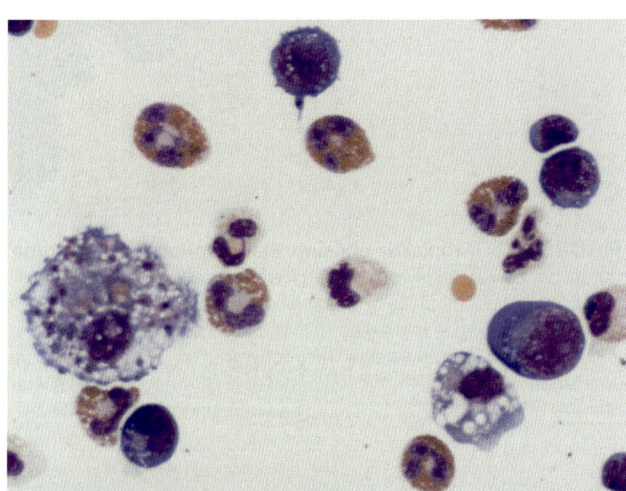

■ **FIGURE 6.79 Neoplastic effusion. Plasma cell neoplasia. Pleural fluid. Dog. Fluid smear.** This effusion was tan and cloudy with 4.3 g protein/dL, 22,430 nucleated cells/µL, and <10,000 erythrocytes/µL. Note the six eosinophils, five neoplastic plasma cells, four nondegenerate neutrophils, and one macrophage. The large foamy macrophage (*left*) contains phagocytized debris. Two of the neoplastic plasma cells have a cleaved nucleus with a perinuclear halo (*lower left, upper right*). (Wright-Giemsa; HP oil.) PCR for antigen receptor rearrangement on the pleural fluid detected a clonal immunoglobulin heavy chain gene rearrangement, and pleural fluid flow cytometry identified CD45+ large cells that lacked expression of markers for T cells, B cells, monocytes, and neutrophils, compatible with plasma cell neoplasia.

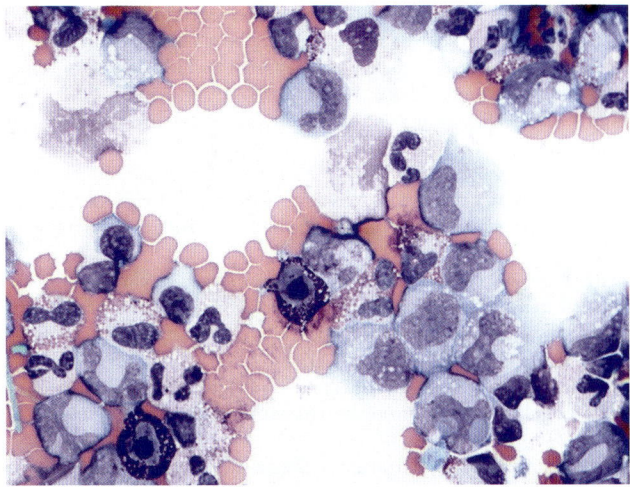

FIGURE 6.80 Bicavitary effusion. Protein-losing enteropathy. Peritoneal fluid. Dog. Concentrated specimen. Fluid was colorless/clear becoming colorless to clear upon centrifugation with protein <2.5 g/dL and 667 nucleated cells/μL, consistent with a pure transudate. Cell differential indicated 55% mononuclear phagocytes, 14% segmented neutrophils, 13% eosinophils, 12% small lymphocytes, and 6% mast cells, suggesting mild mixed-cell inflammation. (Wright; HP oil.) This dog was reported to have a history over several years of diarrhea, a 1-week history of respiratory effort, exercise intolerance, and bicavitary space effusion. Histopathologic diagnosis was mild neutrophilic and lympho-plasmacytic enteritis (ileum) with lacteal dilation. These changes, together with the clinical finding of panhypoproteinemia, suggest protein-losing enteropathy. (Courtesy Rose Raskin, Michigan State University.)

TABLE 6.1 Biochemical, Immunologic, and Molecular Tests Used to Evaluate Specific Effusions

SUSPECTED EFFUSION	TEST	SUPPORTIVE RESULTS
Bilious effusion	Bilirubin	Fluid bilirubin > serum bilirubin
Cholesterol-rich (nonchylous) effusion	Cholesterol	Fluid cholesterol/triglyceride ratio >1
	Triglyceride	Fluid cholesterol > serum cholesterol
Chylous effusion	Cholesterol	Fluid cholesterol/triglyceride ratio <1
	Triglyceride	Fluid triglycerides > serum triglycerides
		Fluid triglycerides >100 mg/dL
Feline infectious peritonitis	Total protein	Fluid TP >3.5 g/dL
	Albumin	Fluid TP >3.5 g/dL and A:G ratio <1
	Globulins	Fluid A:G ratio <0.81
	FCoV antigen	Fluid coronavirus DIF positive
		Fluid coronavirus PCR positive
	Rivalta test	Fluid Rivalta test positive
Neoplastic pericardial effusion (dogs)	pH	Fluid pH >7.3
Pancreatitis with nonseptic peritonitis	Amylase	Fluid amylase > serum amylase
	Lipase	Fluid lipase > serum lipase
Septic peritonitis (dogs)	Glucose	Blood glucose − fluid glucose >20 mg/dL
	Lactate	Blood lactate − fluid lactate <−2.0 mmol/L
		Fluid lactate >2.5 mmol/L
Uroperitoneum	Creatinine	Fluid creatinine > serum creatinine
	Potassium	Fluid potassium > serum potassium

A:G, Albumin to globulin; *DIF*, direct immunofluorescence; *FCoV*, feline coronavirus; *PCR*, polymerase chain reaction; *TP*, total protein.

REFERENCES

Allison R, Williams P, Lansdowne J, et al. Fatal hepatic sarcocystosis in a puppy with eosinophilia and eosinophilic peritoneal effusion. *Vet Clin Pathol.* 2006;35(3):353-357.

Alonso FH, Christopher MM, Paes PRO. The predominance and diagnostic value of neutrophils in differentiating transudates and exudates in dogs. *Vet Clin Pathol.* 2021;50:384-393.

Amati M, Venco L, Roccabianca P, et al. Pericardial lymphoma in seven cats. *J Feline Med Surg.* 2014;16:507-512.

Aronsohn MG, Dubiel B, Roberts B, et al. Prognosis for acute nontraumatic hemoperitoneum in the dog: a retrospective analysis of 60 cases (2003-2006). *J Am Anim Hosp Assoc.* 2009;45(2):72-77.

Aronson LR, Gregory CR. Infectious pericardial effusion in five dogs. *Vet Surg.* 1995;24(5):402-407.

Atencia S, Doyle RS, Whitley NT. Thoracoscopic pericardial window for management of pericardial effusion in 15 dogs. *J Small Anim Pract.* 2013;54(11):564-569.

Aumann M, Worth LT, Drobatz KJ. Uroperitoneum in cats: 26 cases (1986-1995). *J Am Anim Hosp Assoc.* 1998;34:315-324.

Avakian A, Alroy J, Rozanski E, et al. Lipid-rich pleural mesothelioma in a dog. *J Vet Diagn Invest.* 2008;20(5):665-667.

Bacci B, Morandi F, De Meo M, et al. Ten cases of feline mesothelioma: an immunohistochemical and ultrastructural study. *J Comp Pathol.* 2006;134(4):347-354.

Barrs VR, Beatty JA, McCandlish IA. Hypereosinophilic paraneoplastic syndrome in a cat with intestinal T cell lymphosarcoma. *J Small Anim Pract.* 2002;43:401-405.

Barrs VR, Martin P, Beatty JA. Antemortem diagnosis and treatment of toxoplasmosis in two cats on cyclosporine therapy. *Aust Vet J.* 2006;84:30-35.

Bauer N, Moritz A. Flow cytometric analysis of effusions in dogs and cats with the automated haematology analyser ADVIA 120. *Vet Rec.* 2012;156(21):674-678.

Beal MW, Doherty AM, Curcio K. Peliosis hepatis and hemoperitoneum in a dog with diphacinone intoxication. *J Vet Emerg Crit Care.* 2008;18:388-392.

Berg RJ, Wingfield W. Pericardial effusion in the dog: a review of 42 cases. *J Am Anim Hosp Assoc.* 1984;30(5):721-730.

Bertazzolo W, Bonfanti U, Mazzotti S, et al. Cytologic features and diagnostic accuracy of analysis of effusions for detections of ovarian carcinoma in dogs. *Vet Clin Pathol.* 2012;41(1):127-132.

Bonczynski JJ, Ludwig LL, Barton LJ, et al. Comparison of peritoneal fluid and peripheral blood pH, bicarbonate, glucose, and lactate concentrations as a diagnostic tool for septic peritonitis in dogs and cats. *Vet Surg.* 2003;32:161.

Bonfanti U, Bertazzolo W, Pagliaro L, et al. Clinical, cytological and molecular evidence of *Mesocestoides* sp. infection in a dog from Italy. *J Vet Med A Physiol Pathol Clin Med.* 2004;51:435-438.

Boston SE, Moens NM, Martin DM. Idiopathic primary chylopericardium in a dog. *J Am Vet Med Assoc.* 2006;229:1930-1933.

Botte RJ, Eberhard R. Cytology of peritoneal effusion following intestinal anastomosis and experimental peritonitis. *Vet Surg.* 1983;12:20-23.

Bounous DI, Bienzle D, Miller-Liebl D. Pleural effusion in a dog. *Vet Clin Pathol.* 2000;29:55-58.

Bradford K, Meinkoth J, McKeirnen K, et al. *Candida* peritonitis in dogs: report of 5 cases. *Vet Clin Pathol.* 2013;42:227-233.

Braun JP, Guelfi JF, Pagès JP, et al. Comparison of four methods for determination of total protein concentrations in pleural and peritoneal fluid from dogs. *Am J Vet Res.* 2001;62:294.

Brosinski K, Gutbrod A, Venzin C, et al. What is your diagnosis? Peritoneal fluid from a dog with abdominal pain. *Vet Clin Pathol.* 2012;41(2):297-298.

Bryan LK, Clark SD, Diaz-Delgado J, et al. Rhodococcus equi infection in dogs. *Vet Pathol.* 2017;54:159-163.

Buob S. Portal hypertension: pathophysiology, diagnosis and treatment. *J Vet Intern Med.* 2011;25(2):169-186.

Cagle LA, Epstein SE, Owens SD, et al. Diagnostic yield of cytologic analysis of pericardial effusion in dogs. *J Vet Intern Med.* 2014;28(1):66-71.

Caruso KJ, James MP, Fisher D, et al. Cytologic diagnosis of peritoneal cestodiasis in dogs caused by *Mesocestoides sp*. *Vet Clin Pathol.* 2003;32(1):50-60.

Caudill MN, Stilwell JM, Howerth EW, et al. Chronic granulomatous pneumonia and lung rupture secondary to aspiration of activated charcoal in a French bulldog. *Vet Clin Pathol.* 2019;48:67-70.

Chikweto A, Bhaiyat MI, Tiwari KP, et al. Spirocercosis in owned and stray dogs in Grenada. *Vet Parasitol.* 2012;190(3-4):613-616.

Chun R, Kellihan HB, Henik RA, et al. Comparison of plasma cardiac troponin I concentrations among dogs with cardiac hemangiosarcoma, noncardiac hemangiosarcoma, other neoplasms, and pericardial effusion of nonhemangiosarcoma origin. *J Am Vet Med Assoc.* 2010;237(7):806-811.

Clinkenbeard KD. Diagnostic cytology: carcinomas in pleural effusions. *Compend Contin Educ Pract Vet.* 1992;14(2):187-194.

Cohn LA, Stoll MR, Branson KR, et al. Fatal hemothorax following management of an esophageal foreign body. *J Am Anim Hosp Assoc.* 2003;39(3):251-256.

Cook AK, Cunningham LY, Cowell AK, et al. Clinical evaluation of urine *Histoplasma capsulatum* antigen measurement in cats with suspected disseminated histoplasmosis. *J Feline Med Surg.* 2012;14:512-515.

Cowgill E, Neel J. Pleural fluid from a dog with marked eosinophilia. *Vet Clin Pathol.* 2003;32(3):147-149.

Craig LE, Hardam EE, Hertzke DM, et al. Feline gastrointestinal eosinophilic sclerosing fibroplasia. *Vet Pathol.* 2009;46:63-70.

Crosbie PR, Boyce WM, Platzer EG, et al. Diagnostic procedures and treatment of eleven dogs with peritoneal infections caused by *Mesocestoides* spp. *J Am Vet Med Assoc.* 1998;213:1578-1583.

Crosbie PR, Platzer EG, Nadler SA, et al. Molecular systematics of *Mesocestoides* spp. (Cestoda: Mesocestoididae) from domestic dogs (*Canis familiaris*) and coyotes (*Canis latrans*). *J Parasitol.* 2000;82:350-357.

Crowe DT. Diagnostic abdominal paracentesis techniques: clinical evaluation in 129 dogs and cats. *J Am Anim Hosp Assoc.* 1984;20(2):223-230.

Culp WT, Weisse C, Kellogg ME, et al. Spontaneous hemoperitoneum in cats: 65 cases (1994-2006). *J Am Vet Med Assoc.* 2010;236(9):978-982.

Davidson BJ, Paling AC, Lahmers SL, et al. Disease association and clinical assessment of feline pericardial effusion. *J Am Anim Hosp Assoc.* 2008;44(1):5-9.

Davies C, Forrester SD. Pleural effusion in cats: 82 cases (1987 to 1995). *J Small Anim Pract.* 1996;37(5):217-224.

de Brito Galvao JF, Pressler BM, Freeman LJ, et al. Mucinous gastric carcinoma with abdominal carcinomatosis and hypergastrinemia in a dog. *J Anim Hosp Assoc.* 2009;45:197-202.

de Laforcade AM, Freeman LM, Rozanski EA, et al. Biochemical analysis of pericardial fluid and whole blood in dogs with pericardial effusion. *J Vet Intern Med.* 2005;19(6):833-836.

Dell'Orco M, Bertazzolo W, Paccioretti F. What is your diagnosis? Peritoneal effusion from a dog. *Vet Clin Pathol.* 2009;38(3):367-369.

Dempsey SM, Ewing PJ. A review of the pathophysiology, classification, and analysis of canine and feline cavitary effusions. *J Am Anim Hosp Assoc.* 2011;47(1):1-11.

de Souza ML, Torres LF, Rocha NS, et al. Peritoneal effusion in a dog secondary to visceral mast cell tumor. A case report. *Acta Cytol.* 2001;45(1):89-92.

DiDomenico AE, Stowe DM, Lynch AM. What is your diagnosis? Abdominal fluid from a dog. *Vet Clin Pathol.* 202049(1):164-166.

Dillon AR, Teer PA, Powers RD, et al. Canine abdominal histoplasmosis: a report of four cases. *J Am Anim Hosp Assoc.* 1982;18(3):498-502.

Doenges SJ, Weber K, Dorsch R, et al. Comparison of real-time reverse transcriptase polymerase chain reaction of peripheral blood mononuclear cells, serum and cell-free blood cavity effusion for the diagnosis of feline infectious peritonitis. *J Feline Med Surg.* 2017;19:344-350.

Edwards NJ. The diagnostic value of pericardial fluid pH determination. *J Am Anim Hosp Assoc.* 1996;32:63-67.

Eleni C, Scaramozzino P, Busi M, et al. Proliferative peritoneal and pleural cestodiasis in a cat caused by metacestodes of *Mesocestoides* sp. Anatomohistopathological findings and genetic identification. *Parasite.* 2007;14(1):71-76.

Felten S, Leutenegger CM, Balzer HJ, et al. Sensitivity and specificity of real-time reverse transcriptase polymerase chain reaction detecting feline coronavirus mutations in effusions and serum/plasma of cats to diagnose feline infectious peritonitis. *BMC Vet Res.* 2017;13:288.

Fine DM, Tobias AH, Jacob KA. Use of pericardial fluid pH to distinguish between idiopathic and neoplastic effusions. *J Vet Intern Med.* 2003;17(4):525-529.

Fischer Y, Sauter-Louis C, Hartmann K. Diagnostic accuracy of the Rivalta test for feline infectious peritonitis. *Vet Clin Pathol.* 2012;41(4):558-567.

Fischer Y, Weber K, Sauter-Louis C, et al. The Rivalta's test as a diagnostic variable in feline effusions—evaluation of optimum reaction and storage conditions. *Tierarztliche Praxis Kleintiere.* 2013;41(5):297-303.

Forrester SD, Fossum TW, Rogers KS. Diagnosis and treatment of chylothorax associated with lymphoblastic lymphosarcoma in four cats. *J Am Vet Med Assoc.* 1991;198:291-294.

Fossum TW, Birchard SJ, Jacobs RM. Chylothorax in 34 dogs. *J Am Vet Med Assoc.* 1986a;188:1315-1318.

Fossum TW, Forrester SD, Swenson CL, et al. Chylothorax in cats: 37 cases (1969-1989). *J Am Vet Med Assoc.* 1991;198(4):672-678.

Fossum TW, Hay WH, Boothe HW, et al. Chylous ascites in three dogs. *J Am Vet Med Assoc.* 1992;200:70-76.

Fossum TW, Jacobs RM, Birchard SJ. Evaluation of cholesterol and triglyceride concentrations in differentiating chylous and nonchylous pleural effusions in dogs and cats. *J Am Vet Med Assoc.* 1986b;188:49-51.

Fossum TW, Wellman M, Relford RL, et al. Eosinophilic pleural or peritoneal effusions in dogs and cats: 14 cases (1986-1992). *J Am Vet Med Assoc.* 1993;202:1873-1876.

Frendin J, Obel N. Catheter drainage of pleural fluid collections and pneumothorax. *J Small Anim Pract.* 1997;38:237-242.

Fry MM, DeCock HEV, Greeley MA, et al. Abdominal fluid from a dog. *Vet Clin Pathol.* 2003;32:77-80.

Geninet C, Bernex F, Rakotovao F, et al. Sclerosing peritoneal mesothelioma in a dog - a case report. *J Vet Med A Physiol Pathol Clin Med.* 2003;50(8):402-405.

George JW. The usefulness and limitations of hand-held refractometers in veterinary laboratory medicine: an historical and technical review. *Vet Clin Pathol.* 2001;30(4):201-210.

George JW, O'Neill SL. Comparison of refractometer and biuret methods for total protein measurement in body cavity fluids. *Vet Clin Pathol.* 2001;30(1):16-18.

Gidlewski J, Petrie JP. Therapeutic pericardiocentesis in the dog and cat. *Clin Tech Small Anim Pract.* 2005;20(3):151-155.

Giordano A, Stranieri A, Rossi G, et al. High diagnostic accuracy of the Sysmex XT-2000iV delta total nucleated cells on effusions for feline infectious peritonitis. *Vet Clin Pathol.* 2015;44:295-302.

Gores BR, Berg J, Carpenter JL, et al. Chylous ascites in cats: nine cases (1978-1993). *J Am Vet Med Assoc.* 1994;205:1161-1164.

Gorman ME, Villarroel A, Tornquist SJ, et al. Comparison between manual and automated total nucleated cell counts using the ADVIA 120 for pleural and peritoneal fluid samples from dogs, cats, horses, and alpacas. *Vet Clin Pathol.* 2009;38:388-391.

Gumber S, Fowlkes N, Cho DY. Disseminated sclerosing peritoneal mesothelioma in a dog. *J Vet Diagn Invest.* 2011;23:1046-1050.

Gupta A, Fowlkes N, Evans ED, et al. What is your diagnosis? Abdominal fluid from a dog. *Vet Clin Pathol.* 2013;42:113-114.

Haddad JL, Goldschmidt MH, Patel RT. Fibrosarcoma arising at the site of a retained surgical sponge in a cat. *Vet Clin Pathol.* 2010;39:241-246.

Hall DJ, Shofer F, Meier CK, et al. Pericardial effusion in cats: a retrospective study of clinical findings and outcome in 146 cats. *J Vet Intern Med*. 2007;21(5):1002-1007.

Hambrook LE, Kudnig ST. Lung lobe torsion in association with chronic diaphragmatic hernia and haemorrhagic pleural effusion in a cat. *J Feline Med Surg*. 2012;14:219-223.

Harris BJ, Constantino-Casas F, Archer J, et al. Loeffler's endocarditis and bi-cavity eosinophilic effusions in a dog with visceral mast cell tumour and hypereosinophilia. *J Comp Pathol*. 2013;149(4):429-433.

Hartmann K, Binder C, Hirschberger J, et al. Comparison of different tests to diagnose feline infectious peritonitis. *J Vet Intern Med*. 2003;17:781-790.

Hatch A, Jandrey KE, Tenwolde MC, et al. Incidence of chyloabdomen diagnosis in dogs and cats and corresponding clinical signs, clinicopathologic tests results, and outcomes: 53 cases (1984-2014). *J Am Vet Med Assoc*. 2018;253:886-892.

Hetzel N, Papasouliotis K, Dodkin S, et al. Biochemical assessment of canine body cavity effusions using three bench-top analysers. *J Small Anim Pract*. 2012;53(8):459-464.

Hillerdal G. Chylothorax and pseudochylothorax. *Eur Respir J*. 1997;10(5):1157-1162.

Hirschberger J, DeNicola DB, Hermanns W, et al. Sensitivity and specificity of cytologic evaluation in the diagnosis of neoplasia in body fluids from dogs and cats. *Vet Clin Pathol*. 1999;28:142-146.

Holmberg TA, Vernau W, Melli AC, et al. Neospora caninum associated with septic peritonitis in an adult dog. *Vet Clin Pathol*. 2006;35(2):235-238.

Jabbar A, Papini R, Ferrini N, et al. Use of a molecular approach for the definitive diagnosis of proliferative larval mesocestoidiasis in a cat. *Infect Genet Evol*. 2012;12(7):1377-1380.

James FE, Knowles GW, Mansfield CS, et al. Ascites due to pre-sinusoidal portal hypertension in dogs: a retrospective analysis of 17 cases. *Aust Vet J*. 2008;86(2):180-186.

Kashiide T, Matsumoto J, Yamaya Y, et al. Case report: first confirmed case of canine peritoneal larval cestodiasis caused by *Mesocestoides vogae* (syn. *M. corti*) in Japan. *Vet Parasitol*. 2014;201:154-157.

Kauffman CA. Histoplasmosis: a clinical and laboratory update. *Clin Microbiol Rev*. 2007;20(1):115-132.

Kerpsack SJ, McLouglin MA, Graves TK, et al. Chylothorax associated with lung lobe torsion and a peritoneopericardial diaphragmatic hernia in a cat. *J Am Anim Hosp Assoc*. 1994;30(4):351-354.

Kerstetter KK, Krahwinkel DJ, Millis DL, et al. Pericardiectomy in dogs: 22 cases (1978-1994). *J Am Vet Med Assoc*. 1997;211:736-740.

Klainbart S, Merchav R, Ohad DG. Traumatic urothorax in a dog: a case report. *J Small Anim Pract*. 2011;52(10):544-546.

Kowalewich N, Hawkins EC, Skowronek AJ, et al. Identification of Histoplasma capsulatum organisms in the pleural and peritoneal effusions of a dog. *J Am Vet Med Assoc*. 1993;202(3):423-426.

Krimer PM, Duval JM. Pathology in practice. *J Am Vet Med Assoc*. 2010;236:1181-1183.

Lama A, Ferreiro L, Toubes ME, et al. Characteristics of patients with pseudochylothorax—a systematic review. *J Thorac Dis*. 2016;8:2093-2101.

Leisewitz AL, Nesbit JW. Malignant mesothelioma in a seven-week-old puppy. *J S Afr Vet Assoc*. 1992;63(2):70-73.

Levin GM, Bonczynski JC, Ludwig LL, et al. Lactate as a diagnostic test for septic peritoneal effusions in dogs and cats. *J Am Anim Hosp Assoc*. 2004;40(5):364-371.

Litster AL, Pogranichniy R, Lin TL. Diagnostic utility of a direct immunofluorescence test to detect feline coronavirus antigen in macrophages in effusive feline infectious peritonitis. *Vet J*. 2013;198(2):362-366.

Ludwig LL, McLoughlin MA, Graves TK. Surgical treatment of bile peritonitis in 24 dogs and 2 cats: a retrospective study (1987–1994). *Vet Surg*. 1997;26(2):90-98.

MacDonald KA, Cagney O, Magne ML. Echocardiographic and clinicopathologic characterization of pericardial effusion in dogs: 107 cases (1985–2006). *J Am Vet Med Assoc*. 2009;235(12):1456-1461.

MacGregor JM, Rozanski EA, McCarthy RJ, et al. Cholesterol-based pericardial effusion and aortic thromboembolism in a 9-year-old mixed-breed dog with hypothyroidism. *J Vet Intern Med*. 2004;18:354-358.

Machida N, Tanaka R, Takemura N, et al. Development of pericardial mesothelioma in golden retrievers with a long-term history of idiopathic haemorrhagic pericardial effusion. *J Comp Pathol*. 2004;131(2-3):166-175.

Maher I, Tennant KV, Papasouliotis K. Effect of storage time on automated cell count and cytological interpretation of body cavity effusions. *Vet Rec*. 2010;167(14):519-522.

Mandell DC, Drobatz K. Feline hemoperitoneum 16 cases (1986-1993). *J Emerg Crit Care*. 1995;5(2):93-97.

Mansfield CS, Callanan JJ, McAllister H. Intra-atrial rhabdomyoma causing chylopericardium and right-sided congestive heart failure in a dog. *Vet Rec*. 2000;147:264-267.

Marcos R, Santos M, Marrinhas C, et al. Cytocentrifuge preparation in veterinary cytology: a quick, simple, and affordable manual method to concentrate low cellularity fluids. *Vet Clin Pathol*. 2016;45:725-731.

Marcos R, Santos M, Marrinhas C, et al. Cell tube block: a new technique to produce cell blocks from fluid cytology samples. *Vet Clin Pathol*. 2017;46:195-201.

Mclane MJ, Buote NJ. Lung lobe torsion associated with chylothorax in a cat. *J Feline Med Surg*. 2011;13(2):135-138.

Meadows RL, MacWilliams PS. Chylous effusions revisited. *Vet Clin Pathol*. 1994;23:54-62.

Meakin LB, Salonen LK, Baines SJ, et al. Prevalence, outcome and risk factors for postoperative pyothorax in 232 dogs undergoing thoracic surgery. *J Small Anim Pract*. 2013;54(6):313-317.

Mellanby RJ, Villiers E, Herrtage ME. Canine pleural and mediastinal effusions: a retrospective study of 81 cases. *J Small Anim Pract*. 2002;43:447-451.

Miller BH, Roudebush P, Ward HG. Pleural effusion as a sequel to aelurostrongylosis in a cat. *J Am Vet Med Assoc*. 1984;185(5):556-557.

Mongil CM, Drobatz K, Dendricks JC. Traumatic hemoperitoneum in 28 cases: a retrospective review. *J Am Anim Hosp Assoc*. 1995;31(3):217-222.

Morges MA, Zaks K. Malignant melanoma in pleural effusion in a 14-year-old cat. *J Feline Med Surg*. 2011;13(7):532-535.

Moore AR, Coffey E, Leavell SE, et al. Canine bicavitary carcinomatosis with transient needle tract metastasis diagnosed by multiplex immunocytochemistry. *Vet Clin Pathol*. 2016;45:495-500.

Morini M, Bettini G, Morandi F, et al. Deciduoid peritoneal mesothelioma in a dog. *Vet Pathol*. 2006;43(2):198-201.

Neath PJ, Brockman DJ, King LG. Lung lobe torsion in dogs: 22 cases (1981–1999). *J Am Vet Med Assoc*. 2000;217(7):1041-1044.

Nelson KL. Chyloabdomen in a mature cat. *Can Vet J*. 2001;42(5):381-383.

Norris JM, Bosward KL, White JD, et al. Clinicopathological findings associated with feline infectious peritonitis in Sydney, Australia: 42 cases (1990-2002). *Aust Vet J*. 2005;83(11):668-673.

O'Brien PJ, Lumsden JH. The cytologic examination of body cavity fluids. *Semin Vet Med Surg (Small Anim)*. 1988;3(2):140-156.

Oscos-Snowball A, Tan E, Peregrine AS, et al. What is your diagnosis? Fluid aspirated from an abdominal mass in a dog. *Vet Clin Pathol*. 2015;44(1):167-168.

Owens SD, Gossett R, McElhaney MR, et al. Three cases of canine bile peritonitis with mucinous material in abdominal fluid as the prominent cytologic finding. *Vet Clin Pathol*. 2003;32:114-120.

Paltrinieri S, Parodi MC, Cammarata G. In vivo diagnosis of feline infectious peritonitis by comparison of protein content, cytology, and direct immunofluorescence test on peritoneal and pleural effusions. *J Vet Diagn Invest*. 1999;11(4):358-361.

Papasouliotis K, Murphy K, Dodkin S, et al. Use of the Vettest 8008 and refractometry for determination of total protein, albumin, and globulin concentrations in feline effusions. *Vet Clin Pathol*. 2002;31:162-166.

Parodi MC, Cammarata G, Paltrinieri S, et al. Using direct immunofluorescence to detect coronaviruses in peritoneal and pleural effusions. *J Small Anim Pract*. 1993;34(12):609-613.

Passamonti F, Leptri E, Coppola G, et al. Pulmonary rhodococcosis in a cat. *J Feline Med Surg*. 2011;13:283-285.

Patten PK, Rich LJ, Zaks K, et al. Cestode infection in 2 dogs: cytologic findings in liver and mesenteric lymph node. *Vet Clin Pathol*. 2013;42(1):103-105.

Paździor-Czapula K, Otrocka-Domagał I, Myrdek P, et al. *Dirofilaria repens*—an etiological factor or an incidental finding in cytologic and histopathologic biopsies from dogs. *Vet Clin Pathol*. 2018;47(2):307-311.

Peaston AE, Church DB, Allen GS, et al. Combined chylothorax, chylopericardium, and cranial vena cava syndrome in a dog with thymoma. *J Am Vet Med Assoc.* 1990;197:1354-1356.

Peaston AE, Griffey SM. Visceral mast cell tumour with eosinophilia and eosinophilic peritoneal and pleural effusions in a cat. *Aust Vet J.* 1994;71(7):215-217.

Peterson PB, Miller MW, Hansen EK, et al. Septic pericarditis, aortic endarteritis, and osteomyelitis in a dog. *J Am Anim Hosp Assoc.* 2003;39(6):528-532.

Petrus DJ, Henik RA. Pericardial effusion and cardiac tamponade secondary to brodifacoum toxicosis in a dog. *J Am Vet Med Assoc.* 1999;215:647-648.

Piech TL, Jaffey JA, Hostnik ET, et al. Bicavitary eosinophilic effusion in a dog with coccidioidomycosis. *J Vet Intern Med.* 2020;34(4):1582-1586.

Pinta da Cunha N, Giordano A, Caniatti M, et al. Analytical validation of the Sysmex XT-2000iV for cell counts in canine and feline effusions and concordance with cytologic diagnosis. *Vet Clin Pathol.* 2009;38(2):230-241.

Pintar J, Breitschwerdt EB, Hardie EM, et al. Acute nontraumatic hemoabdomen in the dog: a retrospective analysis of 39 cases (1987-2001). *J Am Anim Hosp Assoc.* 2003;39(6):518-522.

Probo M, Valenti V, Venco L, et al. Pleural lymphocyte-rich transudates in cats. *J Feline Med Surg.* 2018;20(8):767-771.

Putwain S, Archer J. What is your diagnosis? Intra-abdominal mass aspirate from a spayed dog with abdominal pain. *Vet Clin Pathol.* 2009;38:253-256.

Ravanbakhsh A, Munasinghe L, Acuna C, et al. What is your diagnosis? Thoracic fluid from a dog. *Vet Clin Pathol.* 2021;50(1):84-85.

Renschler J, Tarigo J, Neel J, Grindem C. What is your diagnosis? Particulate material in peritoneal fluid from a dog. *Vet Clin Pathol.* 2008;37:129-132.

Ridge L, Swinney G. Angiotrophic intravascular lymphosarcoma presenting as bi-cavity effusion in a dog. *Aust Vet J.* 2004;82(10):616-618.

Riegel CM, Stockham SL, Patton KM, et al. What is your diagnosis? Muculent pleural effusion from a dog. *Vet Clin Pathol.* 2008;37(3):353-356.

Rush JE, Keene BW, Fox PR. Pericardial disease in the cat: a retrospective evaluation of 66 cases. *J Am Anim Hosp Assoc.* 1990;26(1):39-46.

Sasanelli M, Paradies P, Otranto D, et al. Haemothorax associated with *Angiostrongylus vasorum* infection in a dog. *J Small Anim Pract.* 2008;49(8):417-420.

Savary KCM, Sellon RK, Law JH. Chylous abdominal effusion in a cat with feline infectious peritonitis. *J Am Anim Hosp Assoc.* 2001;37(1):35-40.

Schmiedt C, Tobias KM, Otto CM. Evaluation of abdominal fluid: peripheral blood creatinine and potassium ratios for diagnosis of uroperitoneum in dogs. *J Vet Emerg Crit Care.* 2001;11(4):275-280.

Schuller S, Garreres AL, Remy I, et al. Idiopathic chylothorax and lymphedema in 2 whippet littermates. *Can Vet J.* 2011;52(11):1243-1245.

Shaw SP, Rozanski EA, Rush JE. Cardiac troponins I and T in dogs with pericardial effusion. *J Vet Intern Med.* 2004;18(3):322-324.

Shaw SP, Rush JE. Canine pericardial effusion: diagnosis, treatment, and prognosis. *Compend Contin Educ Vet.* 2007;29(7):405-411.

Shelly SM, Scarlett-Kranz J, Blue JT. Protein electrophoresis on effusions from cats as a diagnostic test for feline infectious peritonitis. *J Am Anim Hosp Assoc.* 1988;24:495-500.

Shubitz LF, Matz ME, Noon TH, et al. Constrictive pericarditis secondary to *Coccidioides immitis* infection in a dog. *J Am Vet Med Assoc.* 2001;218(4):537-540.

Sierra E, Rodríguez F, Herráez P, et al. Post-traumatic fat embolism causing haemothorax in a cat. *Vet Rec.* 2007;161(5):170-172.

Singh A, Brisson BA. Chylothorax associated with thrombosis of the cranial vena cava. *Can Vet J.* 2010;51(8):847-852.

Sisson D, Thomas WP, Ruehl WW, et al. Diagnostic value of pericardial fluid analysis in the dog. *J Am Vet Med Assoc.* 1984;184:51-55.

Slater LA, Davidson AP, Dahlinger J. Vet med today: theriogenology question of the month. *J Am Vet Med Assoc.* 2004;225:1535-1537.

Slensky KA, Volk SW, Schwarz T, et al. Acute severe hemorrhage secondary to arterial invasion in a dog with thyroid carcinoma. *J Am Vet Med Assoc.* 2003;223(5):649-653.

Small MT, Atkins CE, Gordon SG, et al. Use of a nitinol gooseneck snare catheter for removal of adult Dirofilaria immitis in two cats. *J Am Vet Med Assoc.* 2008;233(9):1441-1445.

Smuts CM, Mills JN, Gaál T. Transudate or exudate: can lactate dehydrogenase activity in canine and feline effusions help to differentiate between the 2? *Vet Clin Pathol.* 2016;45:680-688.

Sommerey CC, Borgeat KA, Hetzel U, et al. Intrathoracic myxosarcoma in a dog. *J Comp Pathol.* 2012;147(2-3):199-203.

Songer JG, Post KW. *Veterinary Microbiology: Bacterial and Fungal Agents of Animal Disease*. St. Louis: Saunders; 2005:10-12, 55-59, 83-86.

Spangler EA, Rogers KS, Thomas JS, et al. Telomerase enzyme activity as a diagnostic tool to distinguish effusions of malignant and benign origin. *J Vet Intern Med.* 2000;14(2):146-150.

Sparkes AH, Gruffydd-Jones TJ, Harbour DA. An appraisal of the value of laboratory tests in the diagnosis of feline infectious peritonitis. *J Am Anim Hosp Assoc.* 1994;30(4):345-350.

Spector D, Legendre AM, Wheat J, et al. Antigen and antibody testing for the diagnosis of blastomycosis in dogs. *J Vet Intern Med.* 2008;22(4):839-843.

Stern A, Walder EJ, Zontine WJ, et al. Canine *Mesocestoides* infections. *Compend Contin Educ Pract Vet.* 1987;9:223-231.

Stewart RH. Editorial: the case for measuring plasma colloid osmotic pressure. *J Vet Intern Med.* 2000;14(5):473-474.

Steyn PF, Wittum TE. Radiographic, epidemiologic, and clinical aspects of simultaneous pleural and peritoneal effusions in dogs and cats: 48 cases (1982-1991). *J Am Vet Med Assoc.* 1993;202:307-312.

Stickle JE, Hribernik TN. Clinicopathologic observations in disseminated histoplasmosis in dogs. *J Am Anim Hosp Assoc.* 1978;14(1):105-110.

Stoica G, Cohen N, Mendes O, et al. Use of immunohistochemical marker calretinin in the diagnosis of a diffuse malignant metastatic mesothelioma in an equine. *J Vet Diagn Invest.* 2004;16(3):240-243.

Störk CK, Hamaide AJ, Schwedes C, et al. Hemiurothorax following diaphragmatic hernia and kidney prolapse in a cat. *J Feline Med Surg.* 2003;5(2):91-96.

Stranieri A, Giordano A, Paltrinieri S, et al. Comparison of the performance of laboratory tests in the diagnosis of feline infectious peritonitis. *J Vet Diagn Invest.* 2018;30(3):459-463.

Swann HM, Brown DC. Hepatic lobe torsion in 3 dogs and a cat. *Vet Surg.* 2001;30(5):482-486.

Sykes JE. Actinomycosis and nocardiosis. In: Greene CE, ed. *Infectious Diseases of the Dog and Cat*. 4th ed. St. Louis: Elsevier Saunders; 2012:484-520.

Szabo SD, Jermyn K, Neel J, et al. Evaluation of postceliotomy peritoneal drain fluid volume, cytology, and blood-to-peritoneal fluid lactate and glucose differences in normal dogs. *Vet Surg.* 2011;40:444-449.

Tasker S. Diagnosis of feline infectious peritonitis: update on evidence supporting available tests. *J Feline Med Surg.* 2018;20(3):228-243.

Tomiyasu H, Fujino Y, Ugai J, et al. Eosinophilia and eosinophilic infiltration into splenic B-cell high-grade lymphoma in a dog. *J Vet Med Sci.* 2010;72(10):1367-1370.

Toplu N, Yildiz K, Tunay R. Massive cystic tetrathyridiosis in a dog. *J Small Anim Pract.* 2004;45(8):410-412.

Tropf M, Sellon R, Paulson K, et al. Mucinous pleural effusion in a dog with a pulmonary adenocarcinoma and carcinomatosis. *J Am Anim Hosp Assoc.* 2015;51:311-314.

Tseng LW, Waddell LS. Approach to the patient in respiratory distress. *Clin Tech Small Anim Pract.* 2000;15(2):53-62.

VanSteenhouse JL, DeNovo RC. Atypical Histoplasma capsulatum infection in a dog. *J Am Vet Med Assoc.* 1986;188(5):527-528.

Venco L, Kramer L, Pagliaro L, et al. Ultrasonographic features of peritoneal cestodiasis caused by *Mesocestoide*s sp. in a dog and in a cat. *Vet Radiol Ultrasound.* 2005;46(5):417-422.

Waddle JR, Giger U. Lipoprotein electrophoresis differentiation of chylous and nonchylous pleural effusions in dogs and cats and its correlation with pleural effusion triglyceride concentration. *Vet Clin Pathol.* 1990;19:80-85.

Walters JM. Abdominal paracentesis and diagnostic peritoneal lavage. *Clin Tech Small Anim Pract.* 2003;18(1):32-38.

Wirtherle N, Wiemann A, Ottenjann M, et al. First case of canine peritoneal larval cestodosis caused by *Mesocestoides lineatus* in Germany. *Parasitol Int.* 2007;56:317-320.

Wright KN, Gompf RE, DeNovo RC Jr. Peritoneal effusion in cats: 65 cases (1981-1997). *J Am Vet Med Assoc.* 1999;214(3):375-381.

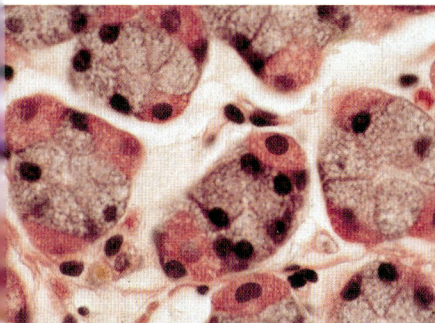

CHAPTER 7

Oral Cavity, Gastrointestinal Tract, and Associated Structures

Shannon Jones Hostetter

Endoscopy has facilitated increased access to the mucosal surface of the gastrointestinal (GI) tract and enhanced the application of diagnostic cytopathology for its evaluation. It is an especially useful adjunct procedure when combined with the histologic examination of tissue for the complete assessment of GI tract. The cytologic and histologic findings tend to be disparate when (1) the specimens are obtained from different sites, (2) the lesion is deeply located in the lamina propria or submucosa precluding exfoliation, (3) surface-associated findings are lost during processing of the histologic sample, and (4) cell or tissue distortion (artifact) is present in either the cytologic or the histologic specimen.

Specimen imprint and brushing cytologic preparations can each provide useful information when concurrently examined with the histologic specimen (Jergens et al., 1998). Brushing procedures tend to exfoliate more cells but also have the potential to induce hemorrhage and introduce leukocytes that may be mistaken for inflammation. Brushing technique often represents pathology of the deeper lamina propria compared with imprints, which reflect the surface and mucosal changes. The criteria that differentiate between benign and malignant lesions of the epithelium must be carefully evaluated when examining esophageal and GI cytopathologic specimens because the cellular atypia associated with epithelial hyperplasia and regeneration related to inflammation can mimic epithelial neoplasia.

ORAL CAVITY

The most common reason for the cytopathologic examination of the oral cavity is for the evaluation of a mass or an ulcerative lesion. Radiographic findings are useful to indicate if there is bone involvement.

Normal Cytology

Superficial and intermediate squamous epithelial cells that comprise the mucosa are the commonly exfoliated cell type for the buccal cavity, gingiva, and the surface of the tongue (Fig. 7.1). These may be normally keratinized as in the hard palate, tongue, and gingiva. A variety of oropharyngeal bacteria can be seen in samples from the oral cavity. Noteworthy is *Conchiformibius* (basionym: *Simonsiella*) spp. (Fig. 7.2). Neutrophils are normally lost via transmigration through the mucous membranes into the oral cavity and may be observed in low numbers.

Other cell types expected from deeper harvesting include lymphoid cells from tonsils, skeletal muscle from the tongue, and stromal tissue within the submucosa. Tonsils are found in crypts or grooves at the dorsolateral aspect of the caudal oropharynx and are part of the mucosa-associated lymphoid tissues that include nasal, bronchial, and GI sites such as Peyer's patches. The lymphoid cell population is similar to other lymphoid organs, such as lymph nodes, but is covered by stratified squamous epithelium.

Hyperplasia

Hyperplastic lesions of the oral cavity are common, especially in dogs, with gingival hyperplasia accounting for more than 20% of biopsied oral masses in a recent retrospective (Mikiewicz et al., 2019). Cytopathologically, gingival hyperplasia may be difficult to diagnose because the lesion is often caused by proliferation of fibrous connective tissue rather than epithelium and therefore may not exfoliate readily (Murphy et al., 2020). Additionally, lymphoplasmacytic inflammation may be associated with the lesion, particularly in cats.

Inflammation

Inflammatory diseases that can affect the oral cavity include immune-mediated diseases such as pemphigus vulgaris and bullous pemphigoid; foreign body reactions; dental disease; systemic manifestations of uremia; and bacterial, viral, algal, and fungal infections. The inflammatory exudate can be composed of leukocytes, necrotic debris, and bacterial flora. Specific localized inflammation should be termed glossitis, gingivitis, or tonsillitis. Tonsillitis begins within the squamous epithelium with an infiltration of neutrophils, whereas the lymphoid cell population shows reactivity (Fig. 7.3)

Inflammatory lesions are more frequently diagnosed in cats, comprising over 50% of the histopathologic diagnoses from lesions within the oral cavity. In dogs, inflammatory lesions are diagnosed less commonly than hyperplastic and neoplastic lesions (Wingo, 2018; Mikiewicz et al., 2019); however, green lingual masses in the dog have been associated with infection from *Chlorella*, an alga (Fig. 7.4A). Cytopathology is diagnostic with green spherical sporangia along with inflammatory cells, but the chlorophyll color is lost during processing for histopathology, so cytologic examination is quite helpful (Fig. 7.4B–D).

Feline chronic gingivostomatitis (FCG) is a common cause of oral inflammation in cats (Lommer, 2013). Lesions are classically bilateral and present as erythematous, friable, proliferative, or ulcerated areas that can be either localized or more extensive within the oral cavity. Extension of the inflammation into either the caudal oral cavity or oropharynx is a classic

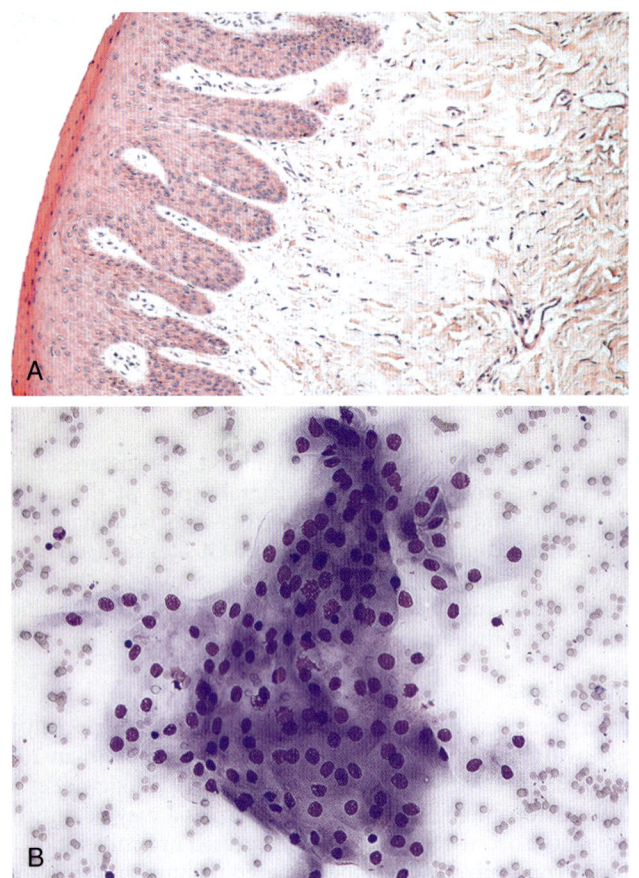

■ **FIGURE 7.1 Oral cavity. Normal epithelium. Dog. A, Gingiva.** Keratinized stratified squamous epithelium forms papillary projections of the lamina propria (connective tissue). (H&E; LP.) **B, Tongue.** A sheet of uniform epithelial cells obtained by fine-needle aspirate biopsy. (Wright; HP oil.) (A, Courtesy Rose Raskin, Purdue University.)

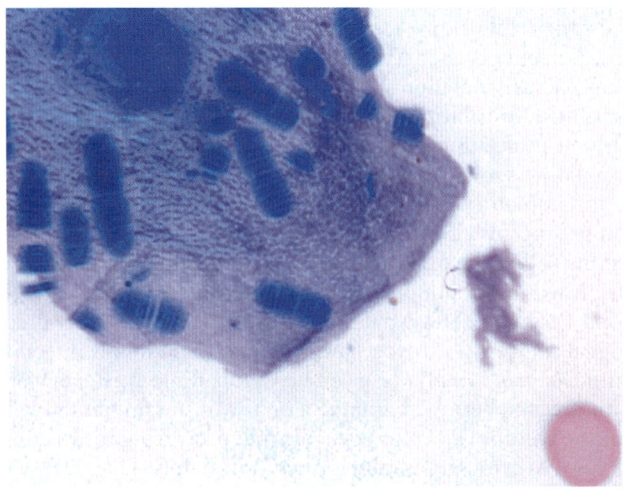

■ **FIGURE 7.2 Oral cavity. Normal epithelium with flora. Dog.** One intermediate squamous epithelial cell is covered with *Conchiformibius* (basionym: *Simonsiella*) spp. (rounded rectangular structures with cross striations). A single erythrocyte is present in the *lower right* for size comparison. (Wright; HP oil.) (Courtesy Rose Raskin, Purdue University.)

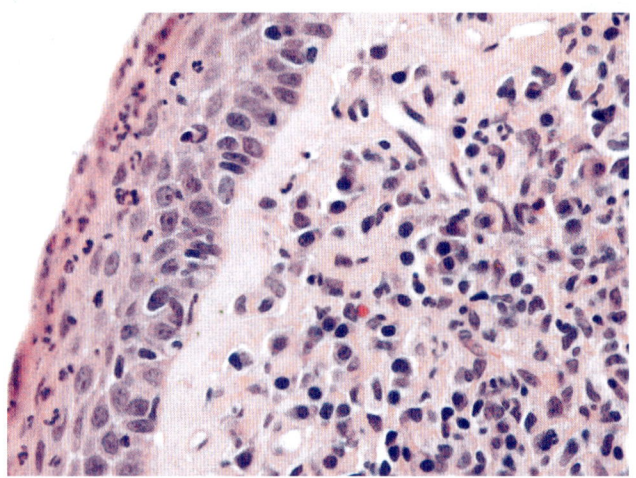

■ **FIGURE 7.3 Neutrophilic tonsillitis with lymphoid reactivity. Histology. Dog.** Inflammatory cells permeate the superficial mucosal layer in response to local necrosis. Lymphoid cells are small with many plasma cells throughout the lamina propria. (H&E; IP.) (Courtesy Rose Raskin, Purdue University.)

feature of FCG, and recent reports highlight cases in which the inflammation extends into the esophagus. The inflammatory infiltrate is classically composed predominantly of plasma cells, lymphocytes, and sometimes neutrophils (Kouki et al., 2017).

Some raised plaque-like oral lesions with ulcerated surface contain a pure eosinophilic population or are mixed with eosinophils and neutrophils. Oral eosinophilic granuloma, also referred to as ulcerative eosinophilic stomatitis, has been reported in dogs and may have a higher prevalence in certain breeds such as Cavalier King Charles spaniels and may represent a hypersensitivity response (Fig. 7.5) (Joffe and Allen, 1995; German et al., 2002). The lesions often resolve with either conservative management or allergy therapy (Mendelsohn et al., 2019).

Calcinosis circumscripta is another non-neoplastic condition that occasionally affects the oral cavities of dogs and cats. The lesion typically presents as a raised white mass on underside of the tongue related to dystrophic mineralization with concurrent macrophagic to granulomatous inflammation and fibroplasia in the more advanced stages. Cytopathologically, the lesions contain variable amounts of fine to coarse, extracellular, crystalline material composed of calcium salts that may appear within macrophages (Fig. 7.6). Calcium within the crystalline material can be confirmed with von Kossa stain (Fig. 7.7) or Alizarin red S (Marcos et al., 2006).

Foreign body reactions are another common cause of inflammatory lesions in the oral cavity. Multinucleated giant cells and reactive fibroblasts are additional features of some lesions (Fig. 7.8). Evidence of chronic inflammation, such as lymphocytes, plasma cells, and macrophages, can be present (Fig. 7.9).

Cysts

Reports have identified cystic swellings (odontogenic keratocysts) within the gingiva of a cat and dog, respectively, composed numerous parakeratotic squamous cells or dysplastic granular squamous epithelium (McEntire et al., 2015; Kwon et al., 2019). Excision is curative.

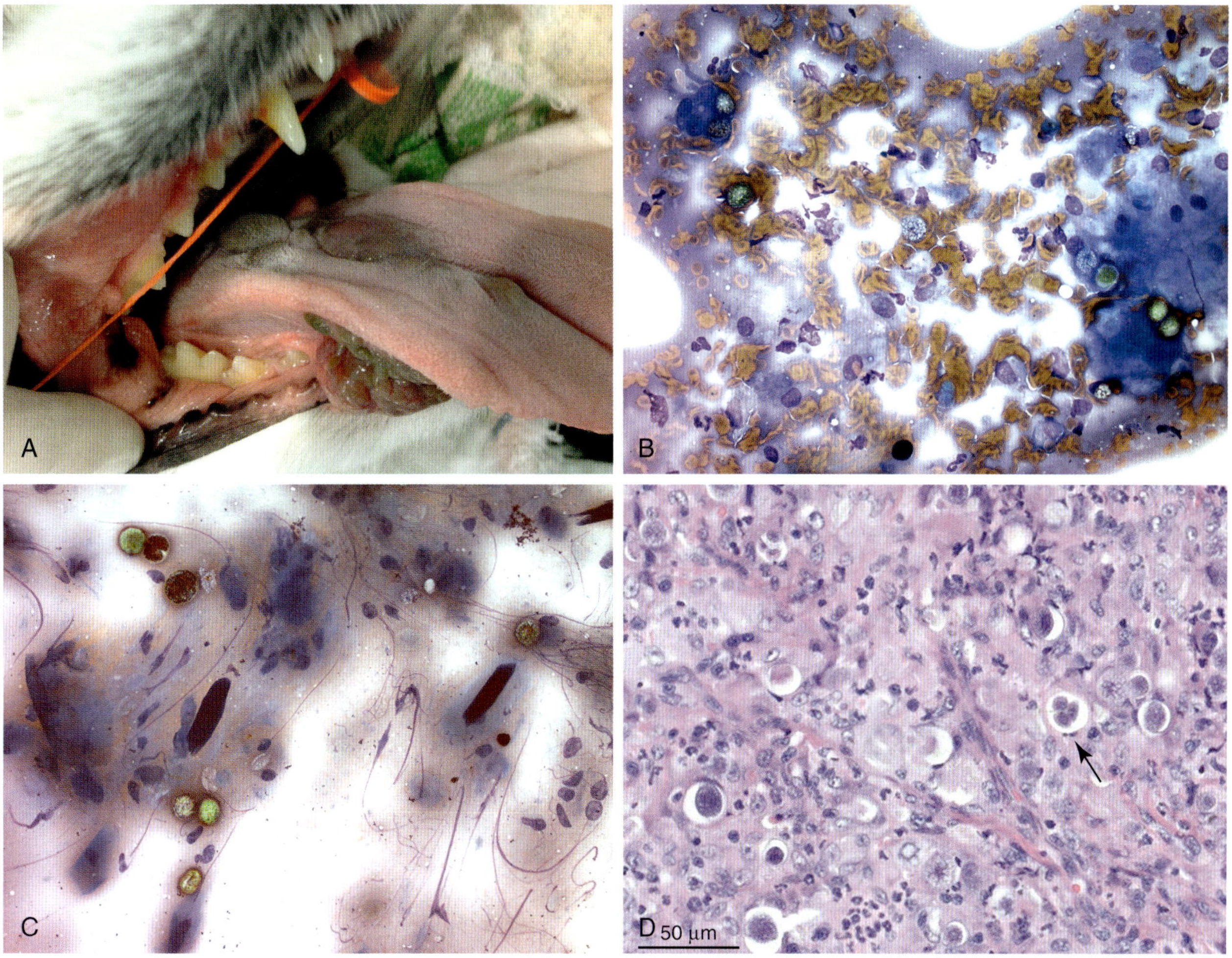

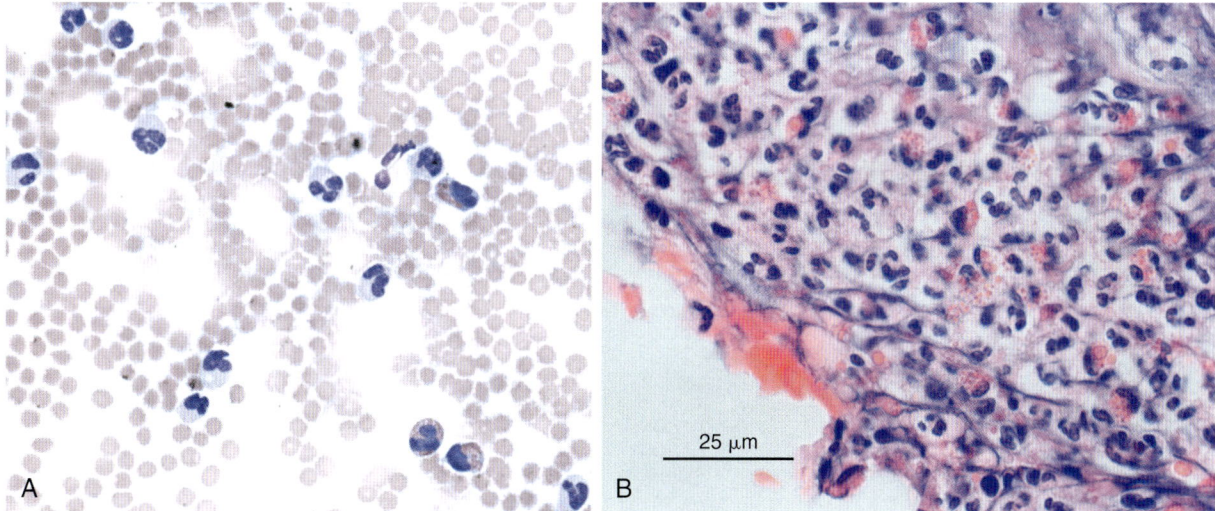

FIGURE 7.4 Oral cavity. Chlorellosis. Tongue. Dog. Same case in A to D. **A,** Multiple green masses on the surface and underside of the tongue from a dog known to be a pond swimmer. **B** and **C, Aspirate.** Variable numbers of inflammatory cells and squamous epithelium are admixed with green spherical granular sporangia. (Romanowsky; HP oil.) **D, Histology.** One organism displays endosporulation *(arrow)* appearing to divide into three parts. Mixed neutrophilic and macrophagic inflammation is present. (H&E; IP.) (Courtesy of Natalie Hoepp, IDEXX.)

FIGURE 7.5 Oral cavity. Soft palate. Dog. Same case in A and B. **A, Eosinophilic and neutrophilic stomatitis. Imprint.** This nonpainful 2 × 2 cm raised plaque-like lesion with ulcerated surface appeared on the soft palate of a Cavalier King Charles spaniel. A mixed population of mainly nondegenerate neutrophils and eosinophils appears against a hemodilute background. Both cell types were within normal reference ranges in circulation. (Wright; HP oil.) **B, Ulcerative eosinophilic stomatitis. Histology.** The ulcerated surface is densely infiltrated with a mixture of neutrophils and eosinophils. Adjacent to this area (not shown) was granulation tissue. However, granuloma formation was not observed. (H&E; IP.) (Courtesy Rose Raskin, Purdue University.)

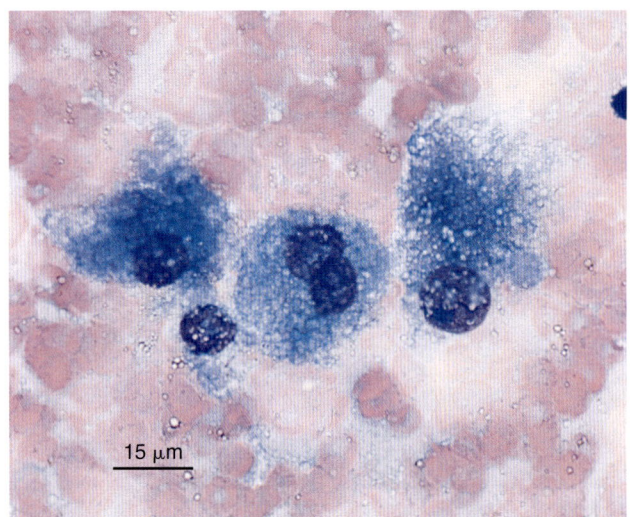

FIGURE 7.6 **Tongue. Calcinosis circumscripta. Aspirate. Dog.** A white bump on the middle of this canine tongue was present for 6 months. Four highly vacuolated and foamy macrophages appear against a refractile and granular background along with erythrocytes producing granulomatous inflammation. (Wright; HP oil.) (Courtesy Rose Raskin, Purdue University.)

Neoplasia

Epithelial, mesenchymal, and round cell neoplasia can involve the oral cavity. The correlation between cytopathologic interpretation and histopathologic diagnosis is very high for oral neoplastic lesions when the cytology samples are acquired via fine-needle insertion, aspiration biopsy, or section impression (Bonfanti et al., 2015).

Round cell neoplasms can occur within the oral cavity or at the mucocutaneous junction and include lymphoma (Fig. 7.10), plasmacytoma (Fig. 7.11), mast cell tumor (Fig. 7.12), transmissible venereal tumor, and histiocytoma. Extramedullary plasmacytomas (EMPs) can involve the oral mucous membranes, tongue, tonsil, or mucosa of the digestive tract (Iwaki et al., 2018). EMPs represent approximately 5% of canine oral tumors and are typically solitary masses, although multicentric tumors have been reported (Wright et al., 2008; Smithson et al., 2012). These neoplasms are considered benign, although they can be locally invasive. Aspirates from oral EMP typically reveal a monomorphic population of round cells with the classic morphologic appearance of plasma cells.

Epithelial neoplasms also occur in dogs and cats. Squamous cell carcinoma (SCC) is the most commonly diagnosed oral neoplasm in cats and is also common in dogs (Mikiewicz et al.,

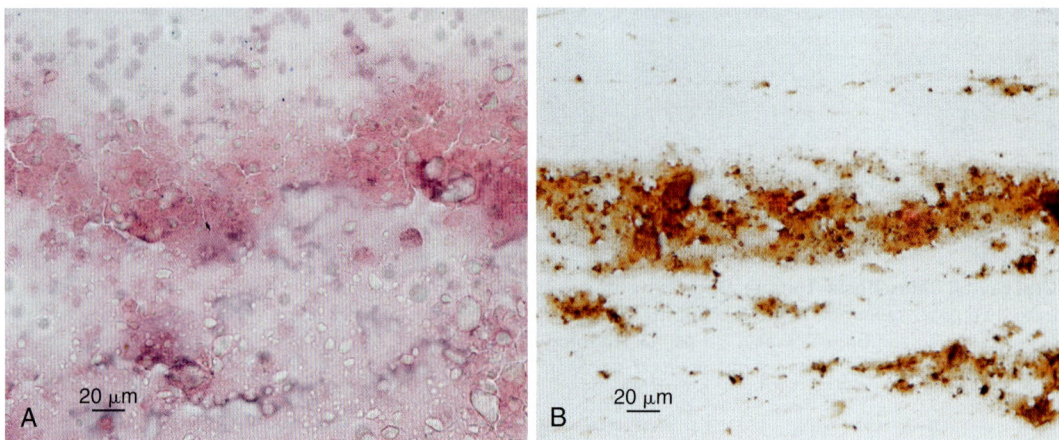

FIGURE 7.7 **Tongue. Calcinosis circumscripta. Imprint. Dog.** Same case in A and B. **A,** Large coarse clear refractile granules are prominent in the background. (Wright-Giemsa; IP.) **B,** Same magnification as in A. Brown-staining granules confirm calcium mineralization. (von Kossa; IP.) (Courtesy Rose Raskin, University of Florida.)

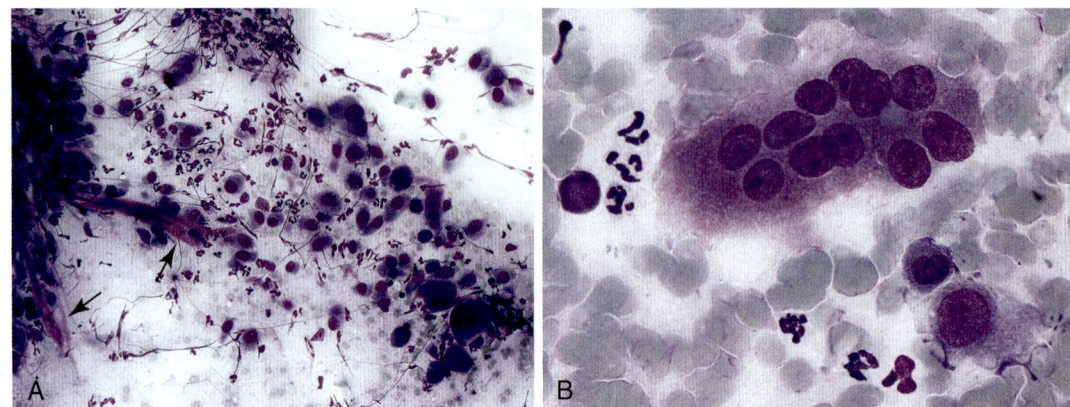

FIGURE 7.8 **Oral cavity inflammation. mucosa aspirate. Dog.** Same case in A and B. **A,** This patient had an oral foreign body with a marked inflammatory response. Neutrophils and macrophages predominate with scattered erythrocytes and a pale proteinaceous background. Streaming nuclear debris and bright eosinophilic extracellular matrix material *(arrows)* are present. (Wright, IP.) **B,** Multinucleated giant cells can be seen with foreign body reactions. (Wright, HP oil.)

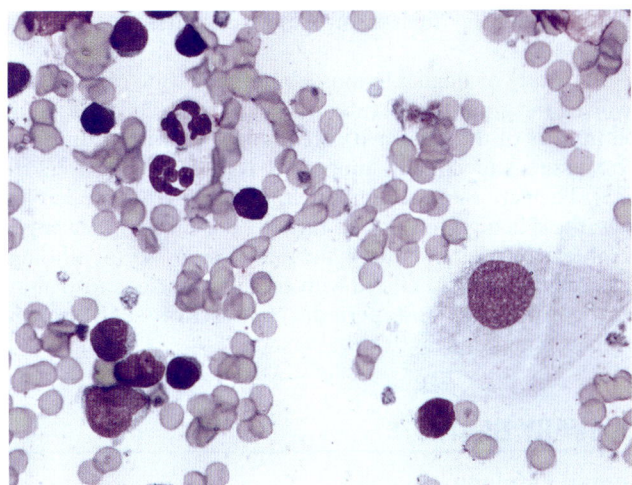

■ **FIGURE 7.9 Oral cavity chronic inflammation. Tongue aspirate. Dog.** Mixed inflammation, composed of small and medium lymphocytes and nondegenerate neutrophils. An intermediate squamous epithelial cell is located in the lower right. (Wright, HP oil.)

2019). SCC can occur anywhere in the oral cavity, although the sublingual, maxillary, and mandibular areas are common locations in cats versus the oral mucosa and tonsils in dogs (Munday et al., 2017; Murphy et al., 2020). Cytopathologic and histopathologic features of SCC in both species include variably pleomorphic, angular, epithelial cells that typically exhibit some degree of keratinization. Perinuclear cytoplasmic vacuolization of the neoplastic cells commonly occurs, and neutrophilic inflammation is usually present with emperipolesis (Fig. 7.13). Metastasis to regional lymph nodes is a potential sequela. Adenocarcinomas of the submucosal glands are infrequently diagnosed in dogs and cats but display the classic features of epithelial malignancy (Fig. 7.14).

Odontogenic tumors are best recognized by histopathology, and the palisading orientation of the cuboidal to columnar basal epithelium is important to distinguish hyperplastic gingival epithelium from odontogenic epithelium. Cytopathologic features include dense parabasal squamous epithelium (Fig. 7.15). Odontogenic epithelium often forms visible bridges between cells, and keratinization is common (Figs. 7.16 and 7.17). Feline inductive odontogenic tumors are classified as expansive tumors of odontogenic epithelium with odontogenic mesenchyme, which appear as dense sheets of palisading squamous epithelium along with spindle mesenchymal cells admixed with pink extracellular matrix (Leite-Filho et al., 2017). This tumor has recently been termed *infiltrative inductive ameloblastic fibroma* to be similar to other species (Munday et al., 2017). This an infrequent dental tumor of young kittens, generally in cats up to 3 years of age, with most animals being younger than 18 months. The firm, smooth, well-circumscribed, pink mass is most often found on the rostral maxilla, occasionally causing tooth loss. Surgical excision prevents reoccurrence and metastasis is not usual. Peripheral giant cell granuloma (PGCG), formerly called giant cell epulis, is a gingival lesion that occurs in both dogs and cats. PGCG is composed of multinucleate giant cells and stromal cells (Fig. 7.18). These are typically considered benign non-neoplastic lesions that are cured with surgical excision, although some lesions can be locally invasive with extension into bone (Desoutter et al., 2012; Murphy et al., 2020).

Oral melanomas often are malignant and infiltrative, may contain abundant or only minimal pigment (amelanotic melanomas), and may metastasize to the regional lymph nodes (Figs. 7.19 and 7.20). Overall, the accuracy of cytopathology in the diagnosis of oral melanoma is good; however, the cytopathologic diagnosis of amelanotic melanomas can be more challenging because minimal cytoplasmic melanin pigment (often described as a fine dusting rather than distinct granules) may be present. Additionally, the neoplastic melanocytes can be individualized or cohesive, and many cell shapes (round, fusiform, spindle) can be found within the same preparation. In cases in which the diagnosis is in question, either immunocytochemistry or histopathology with immunohistochemistry (IHC) can be used (Przezdziecki et al., 2015; Munday et al., 2017).

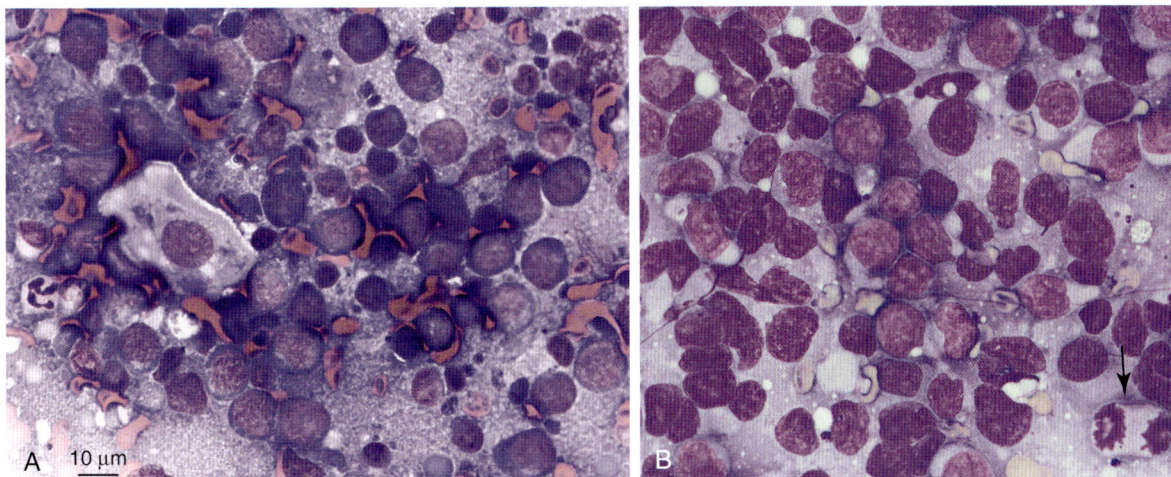

■ **FIGURE 7.10 Oral cavity neoplasms. Lymphoma. Dog. A, Tonsil. Tissue imprint.** Clinical signs consisted of coughing, wheezing, and lethargy. The enlarged tonsil was removed. Cytopathology displayed a mixed lymphoid cell population; however, large lymphocytes predominated. Histopathologic correlation confirmed lymphoma. Note the large squamous epithelial cell, likely of mucosal origin. (Modified Wright; HP oil.) **B, Tongue. Aspirate.** Large lymphocytes with an immature chromatin pattern predominate in this lesion. (Erythrocytes within the lesion may be used for size comparison.) A mitotic figure is present in the lower right *(arrow)*. (Modified Wright, HP oil.) (A, Courtesy Rose Raskin, Purdue University.)

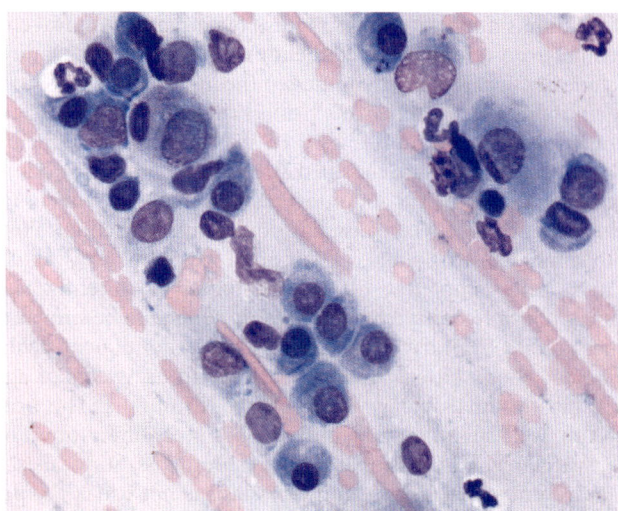

■ **FIGURE 7.11 Oral plasmacytoma. Buccal mucosa aspirate. Cat.** An ulcerated area on the mandible near the molars demonstrated a pleomorphic population of plasma cells. Note the moderate anisokaryosis with occasional binucleation. Leukocytes and erythrocytes are present in rows related to the saliva content of the sample. (Modified Wright; HP oil.) (Courtesy Rose Raskin, Purdue University.)

Fibrosarcoma, chondrosarcoma, and osteosarcoma (Figs. 7.21 and 7.22) are mesenchymal tumors that commonly involve the oral cavity. Fibroma, hemangiosarcoma, and liposarcoma are less frequent (Piseddu et al., 2011). Fibrosarcomas of the mandible and maxilla occasionally can have cytologic and histologic benign morphologic features but demonstrate aggressive biologic behavior (Ciekot et al., 1994). Neoplasia detected in the soft or hard palate may be an extension from the nasal cavity. The tongue is a site for muscle origin tumors, such as rhabdomyoma and rhabdomyosarcoma, which have a pleomorphic population containing granular cells, spindle cells, or both. Striations may be seen, but the diagnosis often requires immunochemistry such as myoglobin and desmin (Chapman et al., 2008).

In a study of lingual lesions, about 4% of the cases in dogs involved the granular cell tumor (Dennis et al., 2006). Granular cell tumors of the oral cavity are thought to arise from neural crest tissue and contain numerous lysosomes (Figs. 7.23 to 7.25). They are more commonly found on the tongue in older dogs; these benign tumors are rare in cats. Grossly, they appear as solitary or multiple raised, firm, red lesions. Cytopathologically, cells are individualized with eccentric nucleus with abundant eosinophilic and periodic acid–Schiff (PAS)-positive cytoplasmic granules.

SALIVARY GLAND

Normal Cytology

Cytopathologic evaluation of salivary gland disease is diagnostically rewarding. The salivary gland also may be sampled accidentally when attempting to aspirate the mandibular lymph node. The salivary gland contains uniform secretory epithelial cells that are clustered and/or individual with eccentric, dark basophilic nuclei, and clear, vacuolated to foamy cytoplasm (Figs. 7.26 to 7.29). The cytoplasmic staining of the cells differs between serous cells (distinguishable) and mucous cells (may appear clear). Individual epithelial cells can be difficult to differentiate from macrophages; however, they have uniformly clear to finely vacuolated cytoplasm and do not contain phagocytized material. Eosinophilic or lightly basophilic-staining mucus is commonly observed and when present may cause erythrocytes to "stream" or line up in parallel rows (Fig. 7.30).

Hyperplasia

Hyperplasia is suspected when there is glandular enlargement and the epithelial cells appear relatively normal cytologically. The cells may be surrounded by abundant mucus. A differential consideration would be a sialocele. However, ptyalism, vomiting,

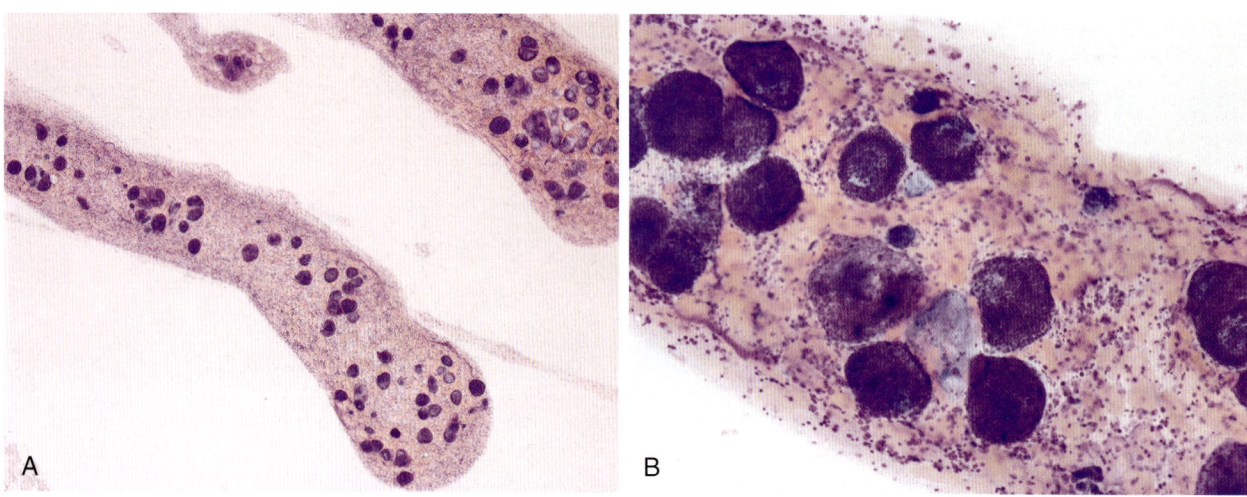

■ **FIGURE 7.12 Oral cavity neoplasm. Mast cell tumor. Tongue. Aspirate. Dog.** Same case in A and B, **A,** This patient presented with dysphagia. An aspirate of a focal tongue mass revealed numerous individualized round cells with scattered erythrocytes on a pale background containing free granules. (Modified Wright, IP.) **B,** Higher magnification highlights the cytoplasmic granulation that often prevents adequate visualization of nuclear detail. (Modified Wright, HP oil.)

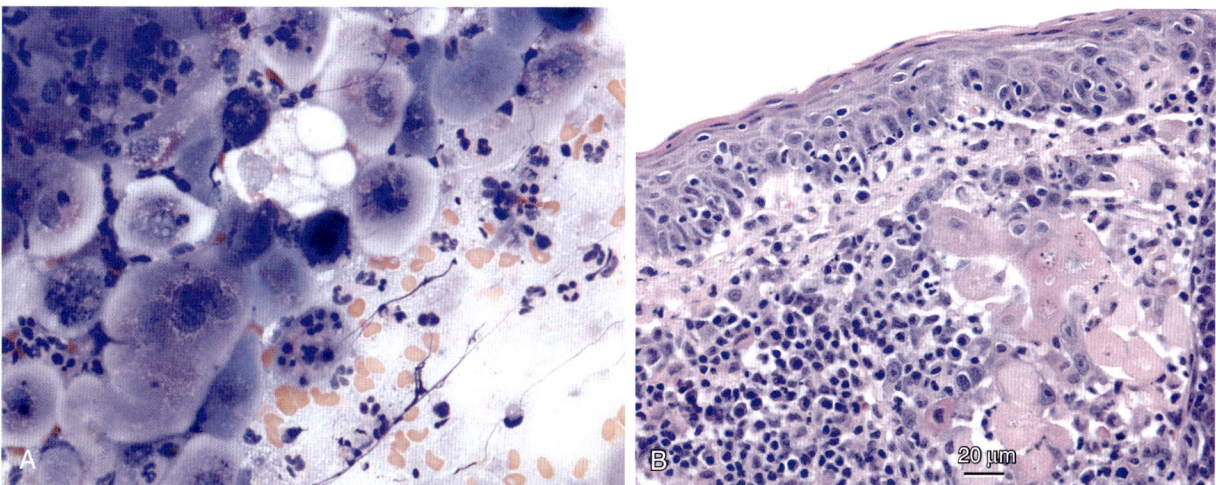

FIGURE 7.13 Oral cavity neoplasms. Squamous cell carcinoma. Dog. A, Oral mass aspirate. Dyskeratosis with neutrophilic inflammation. Malignant criteria include variable nucleocytoplasmic ratios, multinucleation, and variable staining. Many cells also exhibit perinuclear vacuolization of the cytoplasm and variable keratinization. Keratinized squamous cells often induce neutrophilic inflammation. (Modified Wright; HP oil.) **B, Tonsil. Histology.** Dyskeratotic and anaplastic squamous cells infiltrate into the lymphoid aggregates within the lamina propria. (H&E; IP.) (Courtesy Rose Raskin, Purdue University.)

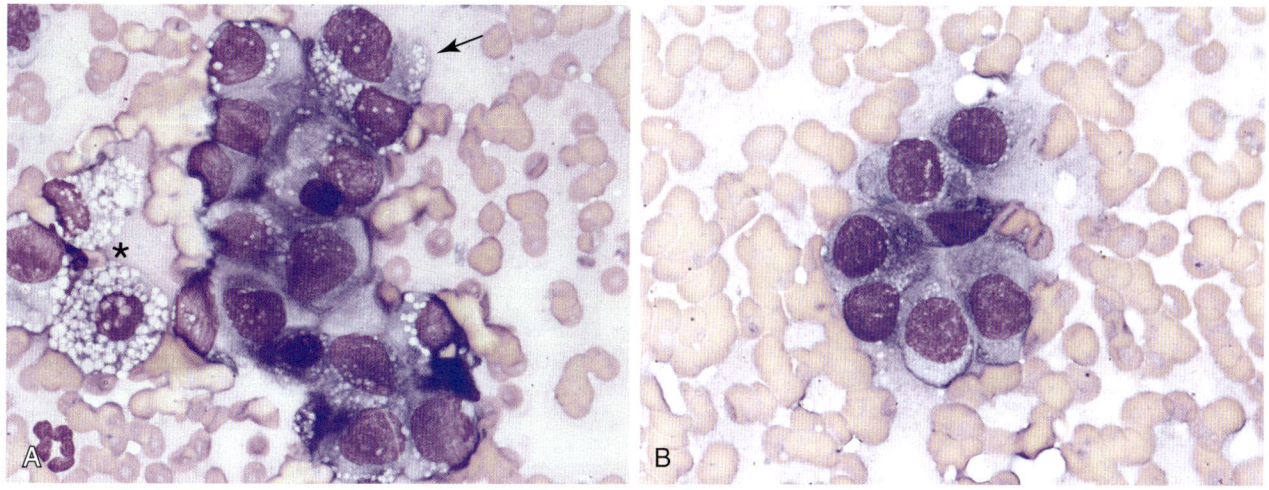

FIGURE 7.14 Adenocarcinoma. Epiglottal mass. Tissue imprint. Dog. Same case in A and B. **A,** A mass was discovered during intubation in a middle-aged Shih Tzu presenting with respiratory distress. Cohesive round to polygonal cells form a tubular structure. These cells have a high to moderate nucleocytoplasmic ratio, exhibit moderate anisokaryosis, and often have perinuclear vacuoles. A binucleated cell in present at the top of the structure *(arrow)*. A clump of three individualized macrophages *(asterisk)* with cytoplasmic vacuoles is present. (Modified Wright, HP oil.) **B,** Acinar formation is evident by the circular alignment of nuclei. (Modified Wright, HP oil.)

retching, and gulping along with the presence of nonpainful bilateral salivary gland enlargement, usually involving the mandibular region with cytopathology revealing normal to hyperplastic salivary gland epithelium without evidence of inflammation, suggests a phenobarbital-responsive sialadenosis (Boydell et al., 2000; Alcoverro et al., 2014).

Inflammation

Inflammation of the salivary gland (sialadenitis) may occur secondary to trauma, sialoliths, or ascending infection or in association with salivary secretions that collect in areas outside the gland or associated ducts. A sialocele is an accumulation of salivary secretions in non–epithelial-lined cavities (pseudocysts) adjacent to the duct. A ranula is a similar cystic distension filled with salivary secretions that occurs below the tongue on the floor of the mouth. Although the cause is not known, trauma plus a developmental predisposition is proposed. The accumulated saliva stimulates an inflammatory reaction that changes over time. The initial inflammatory influx is composed of neutrophils and macrophages along with secretory epithelial cells set in an eosinophilic to basophilic mucus background (Figs. 7.30 and 7.31). Bilateral sialadenitis may relate to an immune-mediated response or viral infection (Fig. 7.32). Lymphocytes and plasma cells replace the neutrophilic component and can become a prominent feature. Although the foamy macrophages can appear morphologically

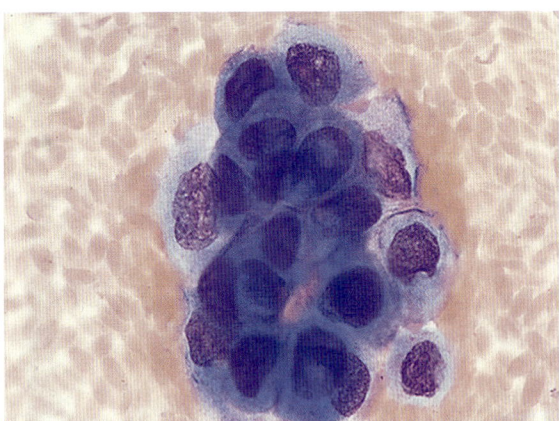

■ **FIGURE 7.15 Oral epithelial odontogenic tumor. Imprint.** An impression of an epithelial cell neoplasm can be made based on the general morphology of the clustered interdigitating neoplastic epithelial cells. They show mild to moderate anisocytosis and anisokaryosis, and the nuclei show mild to moderate shape variation. The morphologic features are suggestive of an epithelial cell malignancy. The cytoplasm contains fine eosinophilic granules. (Wright; HP oil.)

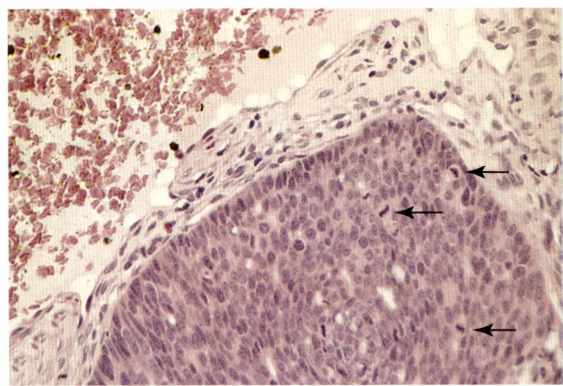

■ **FIGURE 7.16 Oral epithelial odontogenic malignancy. Histology.** The dense neoplastic epithelial cell population shows mild central swirling with palisading cuboidal to columnar epithelial cells located at the periphery. Mitotic figures are present *(arrows)*. The neoplastic cells are surrounded by a less-dense (pale pink) fibrovascular stroma. (H&E; IP.)

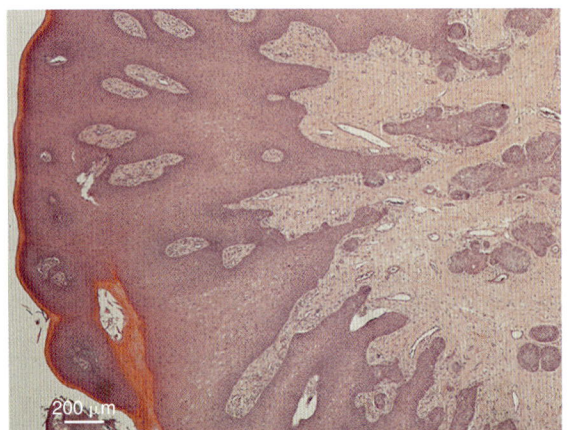

■ **FIGURE 7.17 Gingiva. Canine acanthomatous ameloblastoma. Histology.** Dense cords of thickened (acanthomatous) odontogenic epithelium extend into the submucosa of this infiltrative tumor. A layer of keratinizing epithelium is present at *left*. (H&E; LP.) (Courtesy Rose Raskin, Michigan State University.)

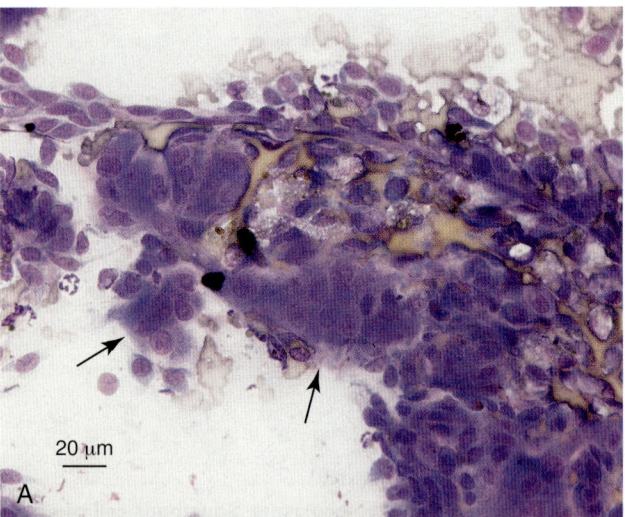

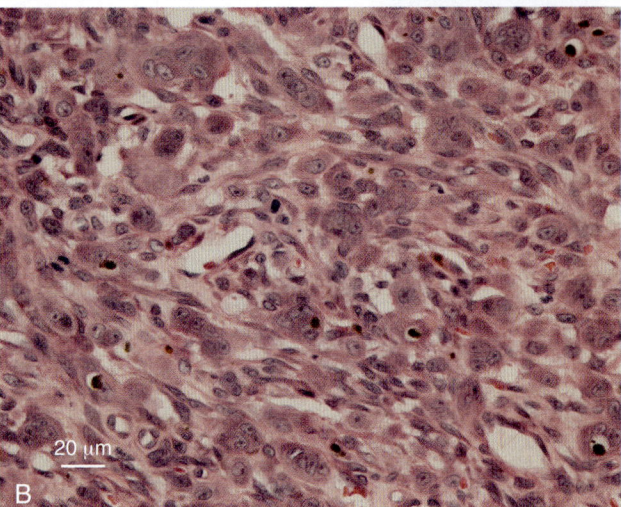

■ **FIGURE 7.18 Gingiva. Peripheral giant cell granuloma. Dog.** Same case in A and B. **A, Aspirate.** Aggregates of inflammatory cells composed of multinucleate histiocytes *(arrows)* and individualized macrophages are prominent. Fibrovascular stroma creates a linear form *(upper half)*. (Wright-Giemsa; IP.) **B, Histology.** Frequent anaplastic nuclear features are present in this solid mass of multinucleate cells with minimal stroma. (H&E; LP.) (Courtesy Rose Raskin, Purdue University.)

similar to the plump secretory epithelial cells, differentiation is not necessary when formulating the cytopathologic impression. Chronic inflammation of a sialocele may result in osseous metaplasia (O'Connell et al., 2016).

In dogs ranging in age from 3 to 10 years, necrotizing sialometaplasia typically involves the mandibular salivary gland. Canine necrotizing sialometaplasia may be associated with gland swelling, marked pain, vomiting, retching, ptyalism, and anorexia with a progressive course. Cytopathologic findings range from no abnormalities to hyperplasia with mononuclear inflammation. Mild neutrophilic inflammation with squamous metaplasia and pleomorphic mesenchymal proliferation may be seen as well (Duncan et al., 1999).

Neoplasia

Salivary gland neoplasia is uncommon in dogs and cats. The majority of tumors arise from the parotid and mandibular

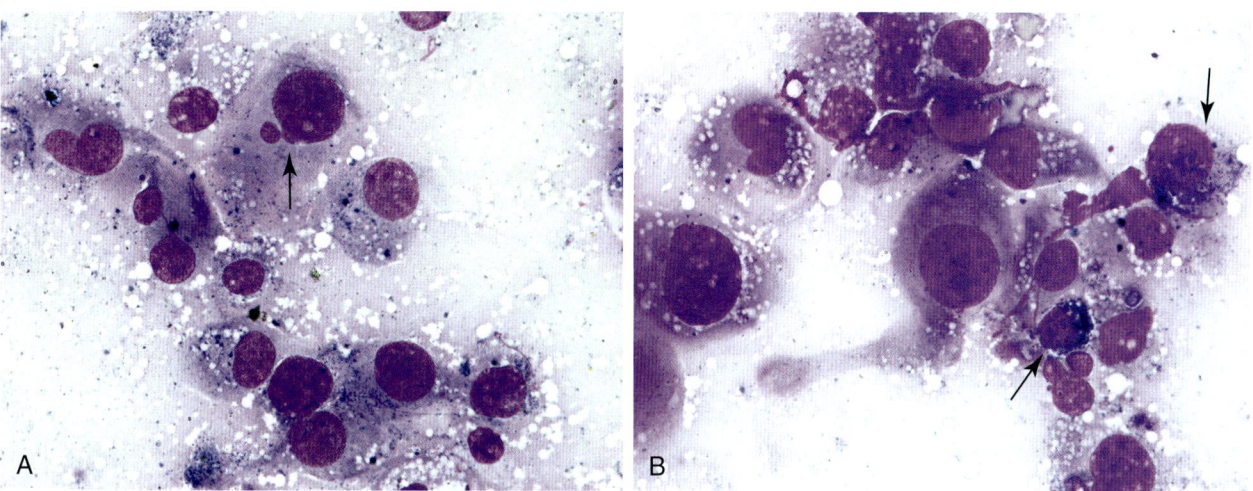

■ **FIGURE 7.19 Oral malignant melanoma. Tongue aspirate. Dog.** Same case in A and B. **A,** Pleomorphic round to polygonal to fusiform cells exhibiting criteria of malignancy including variable nucleocytoplasmic ratios, anisocytosis, anisokaryosis, and nuclear pleomorphism, including blebbing (*arrow*). Most neoplastic cells contain some cytoplasmic dark pigment (melanin). (Wright; HP oil.) **B,** Abundant intracytoplasmic melanin is noted in a few cells (*arrows*). Most of the other cells do not contain obvious pigment (amelanotic) and can be easily confused with neoplastic epithelial cells or pleomorphic round cells. (Wright; HP oil.)

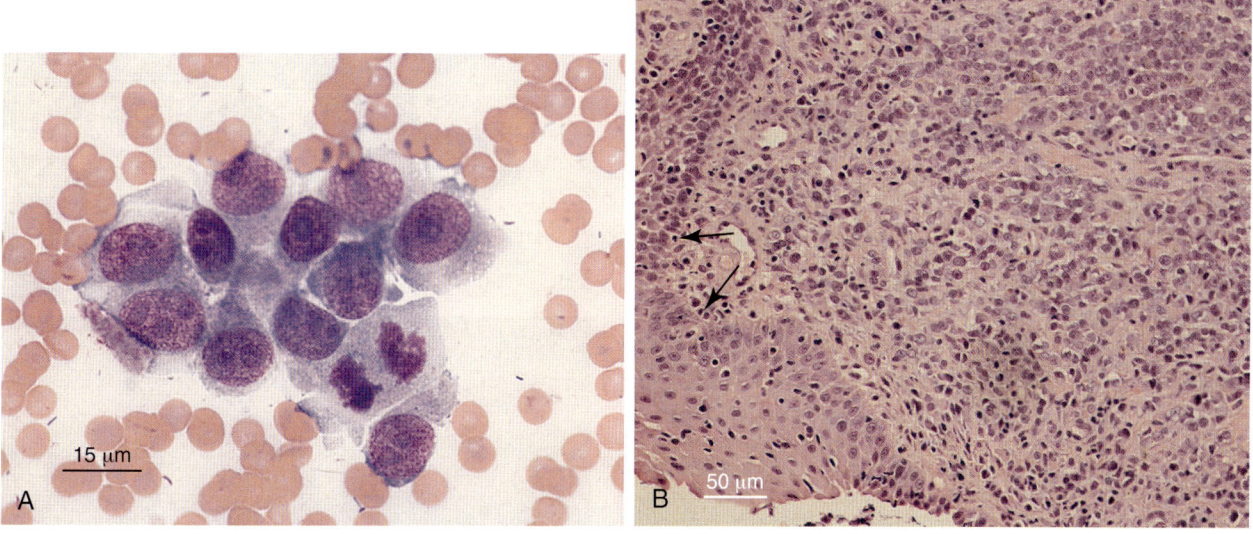

■ **FIGURE 7.20 Buccal wall amelanotic melanoma. Dog.** Same case in A and B. **A, Imprint.** Against a background of erythrocytes and bacteria is an aggregate of neoplastic cells displaying variable and high nucleocytoplasmic ratio, coarse chromatin, multiple prominent nucleoli, anisokaryosis, and a mitotic figure (*lower right*). Rare fine granules are present within the cytoplasm, but granulation is not significant. (Wright; HP oil.) **B, Histology.** Poorly granulated individualized cells with pale open nuclei infiltrate the submucosa with some displaying junctional activity by their presence within the basal layer of the epithelium (*between arrows*) support the diagnosis of melanoma. Hyperchromatic cells noted are neutrophils. (H&E; IP.) (Courtesy Rose Raskin, Purdue University.)

salivary glands, are of epithelial origin, and are malignant. Classification of these neoplasms can be complicated because of variations in histologic subtypes, and cytopathologic evaluation may not reliably predict biological behavior (Munday et al., 2017). Salivary carcinomas demonstrate the general characteristics of epithelial malignancy that may range from relatively well-differentiated to marked pleomorphism (Figs. 7.33 and 7.34). The neoplastic epithelial cells can form acinar structures, and some of the cells can have abundant retained cytoplasmic secretions that displace the nucleus to the periphery, forming a cell that appears similar to a signet ring. In rare cases, salivary gland carcinoma may appear bilateral (Mazzullo et al., 2005). Psammoma bodies (spherical concentric lamellae of nonpolarizing calcium apatite crystals) have been found in association with salivary carcinoma, possibly secondary to tissue damage or as a precursor to malignancy (Allen et al., 2018). Mixed salivary neoplasms are rare and contain both neoplastic epithelial cell and mesenchymal cell components that can include bone and cartilage.

The second most common salivary gland neoplasm (acinic cell carcinoma) primarily involves the serous salivary glands

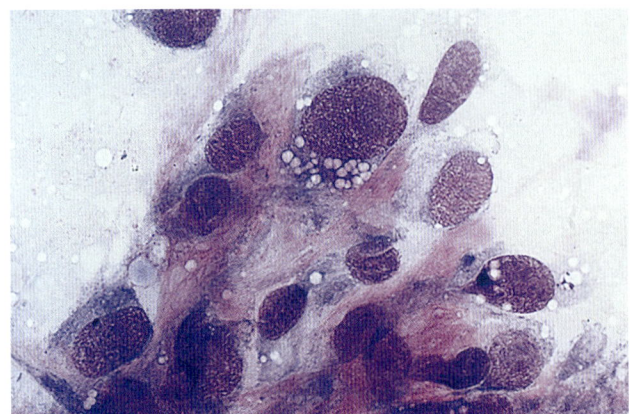

■ **FIGURE 7.21 Oral osteosarcoma. Imprint. Dog.** Pleomorphic mesenchymal cells show marked anisocytosis and anisokaryosis. The nuclei have stippled nuclear chromatin that contains multiple faintly stained variably sized nucleoli and are surrounded by moderately abundant basophilic cytoplasm with indistinct cell borders. The swirls of intercellular eosinophilic matrix produced by the neoplastic cells supports the cytopathologic impression of a malignant bone tumor. (Wright; HP oil.)

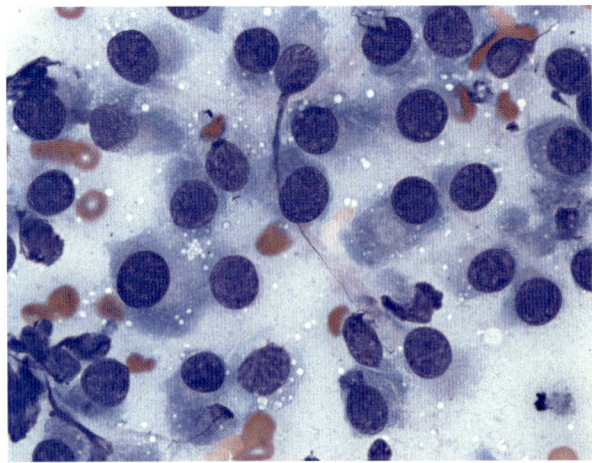

■ **FIGURE 7.22 Oral mass involving mandible. Osteosarcoma. Aspirate. Dog.** This patient had an additional affected site (proximal humerus) in addition to the mandibular mass. Note the plasmacytoid appearance (eccentric nuclei, basophilic cytoplasm with perinuclear clearing) that is evidence in many of the neoplastic osteoblasts. Eosinophilic extracellular matrix also is present, although it is less prominent than in Figure 7.21. (Modified Wright, HP oil.)

(Newman et al., 2018). The epithelial cells had low to moderate nucleocytoplasmic ratios, indistinct cell borders, and basophilic cytoplasm that contained variable numbers of small dull-pink cytoplasmic granules and small punctate vacuoles. These acinar cells stain PAS-positive and diastase resistant, indicating neutral mucopolysaccharides. Mucous salivary glands would be expected to be positive for Alcian blue and mucicarmine, indicating acid mucopolysaccharides.

ESOPHAGUS

Normal Cytology

The mucosal layer of the esophagus has a stratified squamous epithelium that contains openings for the ducts of the esophageal

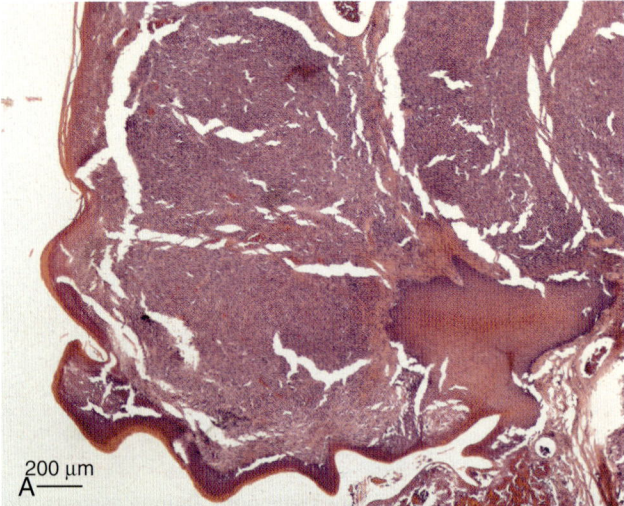
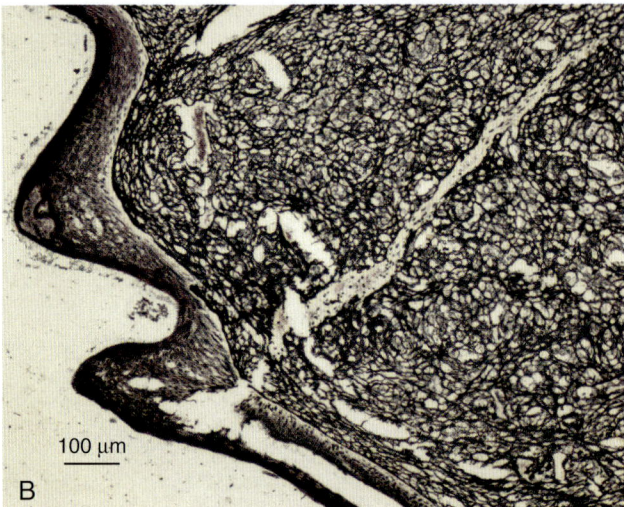
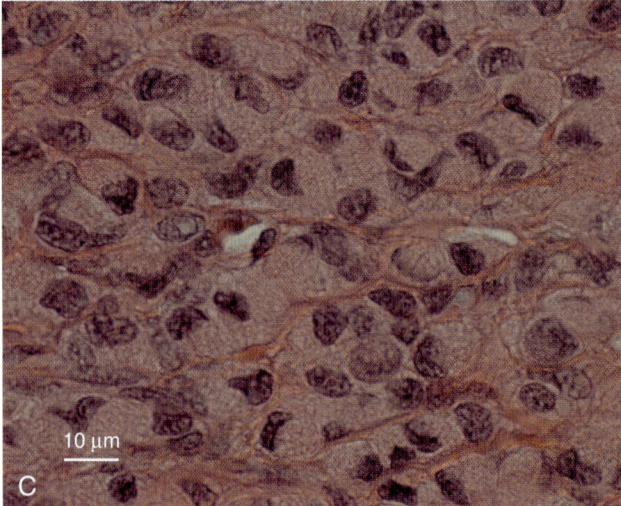

■ **FIGURE 7.23 Tongue. Granular cell tumor. Histology. Cat.** Same case in A to C. **A,** Low magnification of a small raised lingual mass showing dense cellularity. (H&E; LP.) **B,** Dense network of stromal fibers separate the cells into small aggregates. (Reticulin; LP.) **C,** Stromal fibers create cords of individualized cells that have abundant granular eosinophilic cytoplasm and a hyperchromatic eccentric nucleus. (H&E; HP oil.) (Courtesy Rose Raskin, Michigan State University.)

mucous glands. Exfoliated stratified squamous epithelial cells can either appear angular or have the rounded shape of intermediate epithelial cells and basal cells with eccentric nuclei. Large numbers of basal epithelial cells can indicate trauma, inflammation, or erosion. The stromal cells and glandular cells usually do not exfoliate. Samples from the gastroesophageal region may contain squamous epithelium mixed with gastric columnar epithelium. Ingesta with oropharyngeal flora consisting of a mixed bacterial population of rods, cocci, and *Conchiformibius* (basionym: *Simonsiella*) spp. may be noted in esophageal samples (see Fig. 7.2).

Inflammation

Gastroesophageal reflux esophagitis occurs in both dogs and cats, most commonly involving the distal esophagus. It is caused by the action of regurgitated gastric (pepsin and acid) and possibly duodenal (bile acids and pancreatic enzymes) secretions that have a corrosive effect on the stratified squamous epithelium. General anesthesia is a known cause of reflux esophagitis in dogs and cats, and antibiotic therapy (clindamycin and doxycycline)

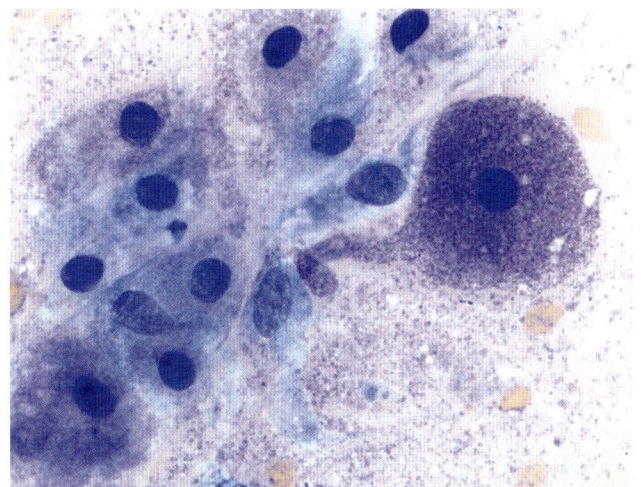

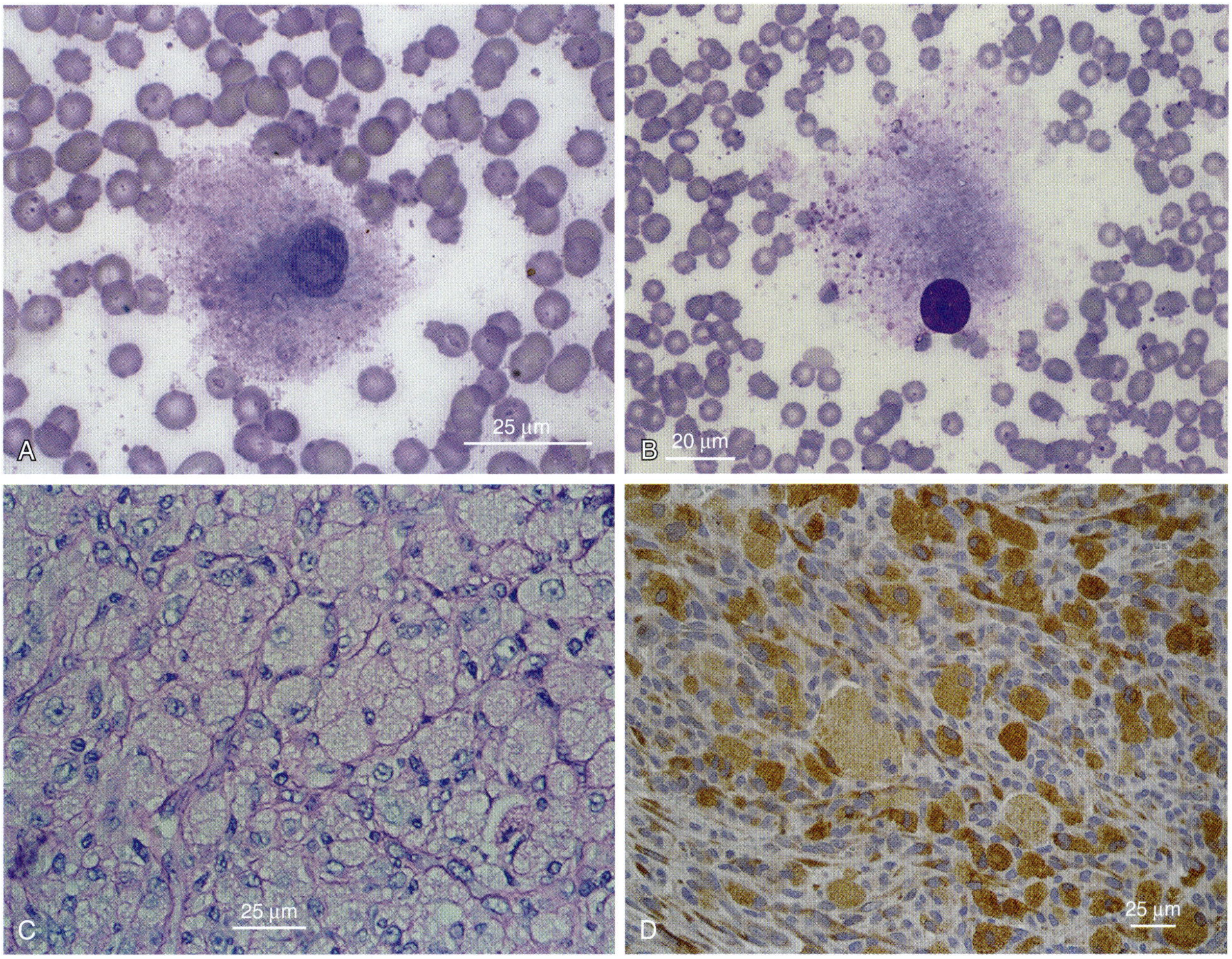

FIGURE 7.24 Tongue. Granular cell tumor. Tissue aspirate. Dog. Granular cells have abundant cytoplasm containing numerous fine deeply eosinophilic to purple stained presumed lysosomal granules. Free granules also are present within the background. (Modified Wright; HP oil.)

FIGURE 7.25 Hard Palate. Granular cell tumor. Dog. Same case in A to D. **A and B, Aspirate.** A 2-year-old German shepherd dog presented for evaluation of a 4 cm mass on the hard palate. A population of individualized cells measuring 25 to 100 μm with cytoplasm containing numerous small lavender granules. The cells had round to ovoid nuclei with a finely stippled chromatin and a single prominent nucleolus. (Wright; HP oil.) **C, Histology.** The granular cytoplasm stain variably positive for glycogen. (PAS; HP oil.) **D, Histology.** Cells are immunoreactive to neuron-specific enolase, a marker for neuroendocrine tissue. (NSE/benzidine; IP.) (Courtesy Mara Varvil, Purdue University.)

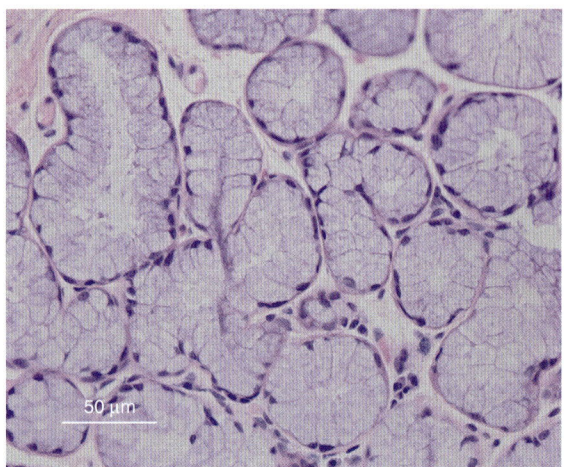

■ **FIGURE 7.26 Normal salivary gland tissue. Histology.** Mucus-containing salivary gland epithelium is arranged in acinar structures. The small dense nuclei are compressed to the periphery by the pale foamy mucus. (H&E; IP.) (Courtesy Rose Raskin, Purdue University.)

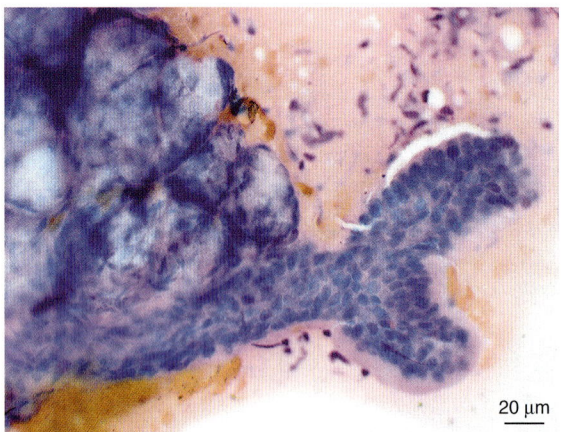

■ **FIGURE 7.27 Normal salivary gland. Retropharyngeal area. Aspirate. Dog.** Clusters of foamy and lightly basophilic salivary gland epithelium are associated with a tubular structure, consistent with a duct. The ductular epithelium have high nucleocytoplasmic ratios that line the length of the duct. (Wright; HP oil.) (Courtesy Rose Raskin, North Carolina State University.)

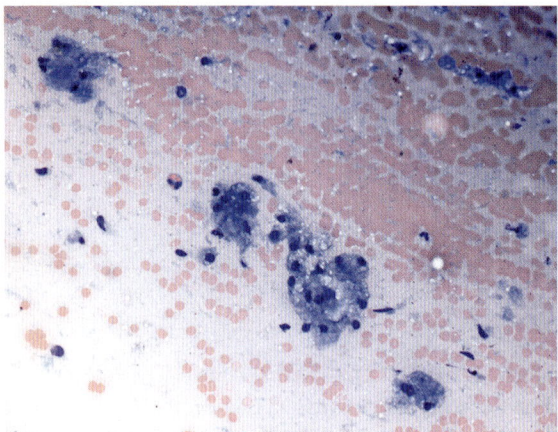

■ **FIGURE 7.28 Salivary gland epithelium. Normal. Aspirate.** Several basophilic cell clusters and erythrocytes appear in windrow fashion within the eosinophilic to amphophilic mucous background. (Modified Wright; IP.)

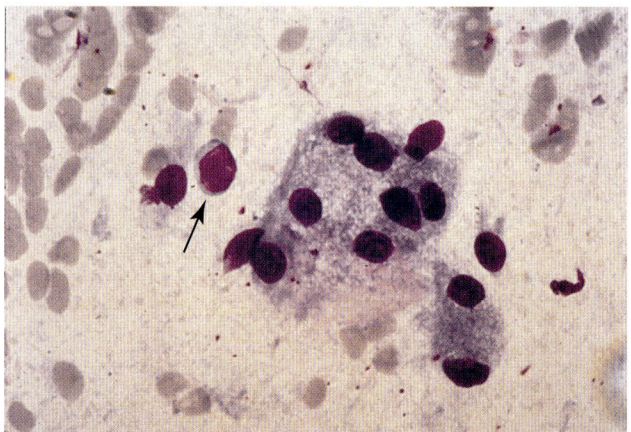

■ **FIGURE 7.29 Salivary gland epithelium. Normal. Imprint.** The epithelial cells that make up this small cluster have abundant basophilic, granular-appearing cytoplasm associated with a dense, often eccentric nucleus. Cytoplasmic vacuolization is often present. A medium-sized lymphocyte with a small rim of lightly basophilic cytoplasm *(arrow)* and a free round nucleus is noted. The surrounding erythrocytes help to judge the size of the nucleated cells. (Modified Wright; HP oil.)

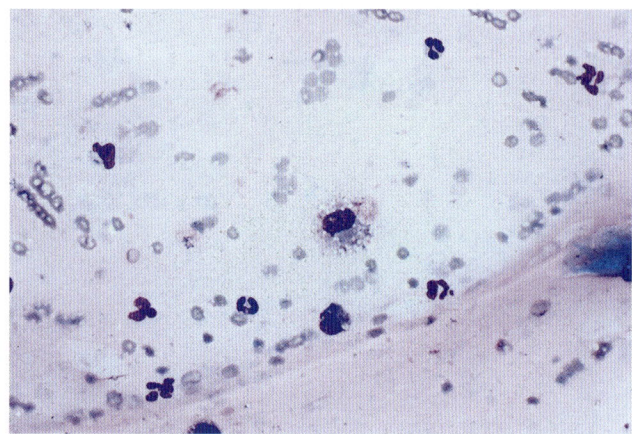

■ **FIGURE 7.30 Sialocele (salivary mucocele). Aspirate.** This specimen is from a fluctuant submandibular swelling. The pink-blue mucus and occasional foamy macrophage along with a low number of neutrophils and erythrocytes are indicative of a sialocele. The windrowing of erythrocytes (linear arrangement) suggests the presence of mucus. (Wright; HP oil.)

has been associated with esophageal injury in cats (Beatty et al., 2006). Esophageal inflammation from mucosal injury has a prominent neutrophilic component (Fig. 7.35), and the epithelial cells show reactive hyperchromasia or nuclear and cytoplasmic degenerative changes.

Esophageal foreign bodies are another cause of inflammation, arising from either pressure necrosis of the mucosa or secondary bacterial infection (Bongard et al., 2019). Stricture formation is a potential sequela to esophageal inflammation. Esophageal inflammation is suggested if oropharyngeal contamination is not present and the site sampled appears inflamed endoscopically. Less commonly encountered causes of esophageal inflammation include oomycosis (*Lagenidium* spp. and *Pythium* spp., both described in dogs; see discussion under Stomach) and eosinophilic esophagitis in cats (Helman and

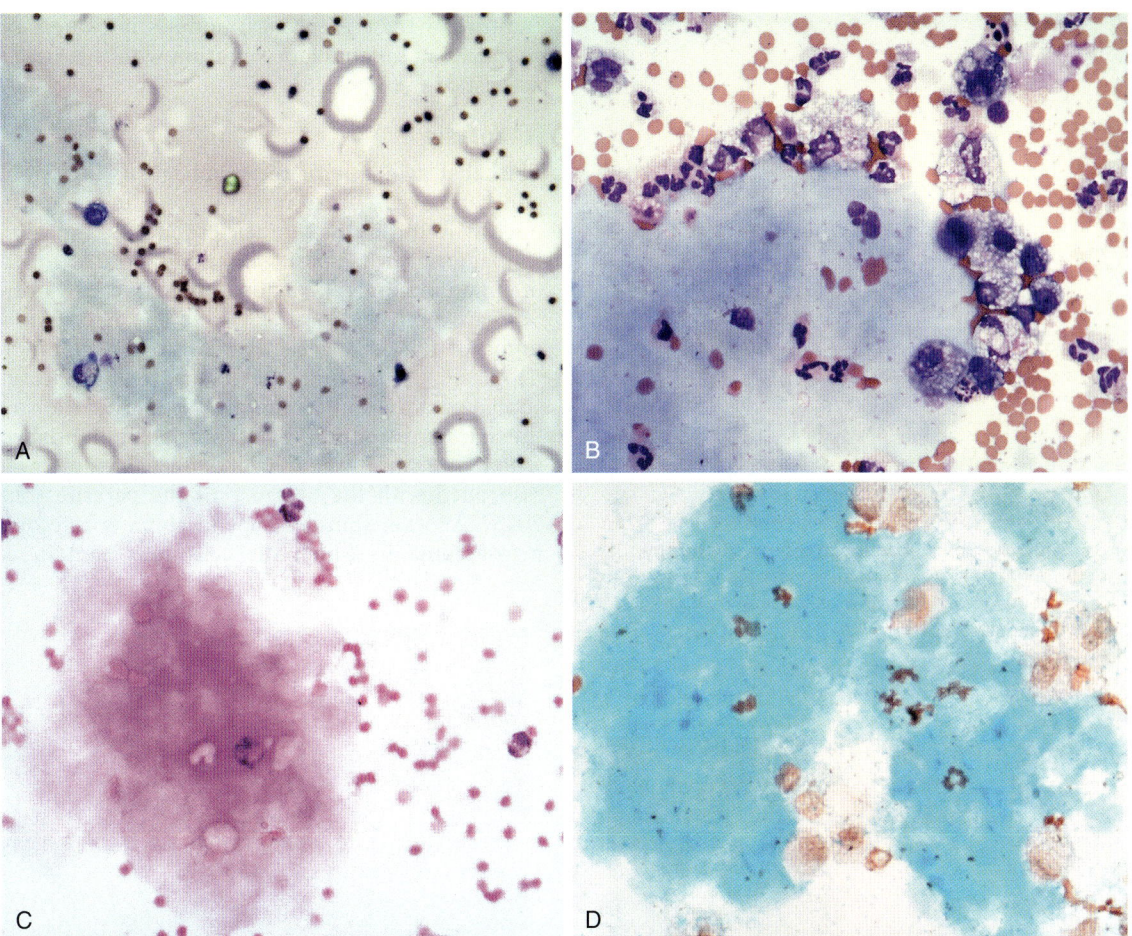

■ **FIGURE 7.31 Sialocele fluid. Aspirate. Dog.** Same case in A to D. **A,** Fluid-filled swelling on the patient's ventral neck was aspirated; aspirate was markedly cloudy and yellow-orange, with a total solids >3.0 g/dL. The nucleated cell count was approximately 4000/μL. This is a direct smear showing a low nucleated cellularity, low to moderate numbers of erythrocytes (no windrowing), and two macrophages on a light pink-grey background with abundant protein crescents. Small lakes of light blue material are noted in the background. (Wright; HP oil.) **B,** Cytocentrifuged smear reveals 78% nondegenerate neutrophils, some hypersegmented, and 22% vacuolated macrophages with rare lymphocytes noted. Dense blue lakes of suspected mucin are present. (Wright; HP oil.) **C,** Positive reaction to PAS staining supporting glycogen, carbohydrates, or mucoproteins is present. (PAS; HP oil.) **D,** Strong positive reaction supports the presence of acid mucins. (Alcian blue; HP oil.) (Courtesy Rose Raskin, Royal Veterinary College, UK.)

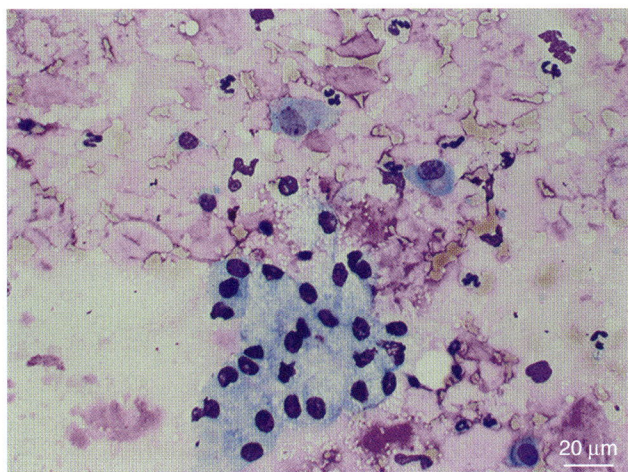

■ **FIGURE 7.32 Mandibular salivary gland. Sialadenitis. Aspirate. Dog.** Bilateral enlargement of both mandibular salivary glands reveals a mostly neutrophilic inflammatory response. Infectious agents are not noted. (Wright; HP oil.) (Courtesy Rose Raskin, North Carolina State University.)

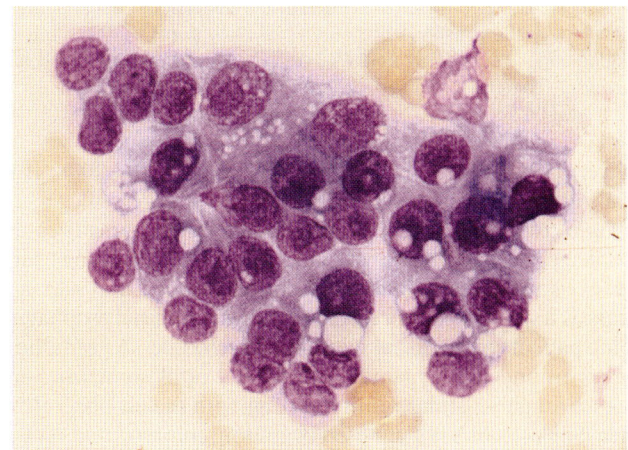

■ **FIGURE 7.33 Parotid salivary gland. Adenocarcinoma. Aspirate. Cat.** A cluster of immature cells displays moderate anisokaryosis, coarse chromatin, prominent nucleolus, and high nucleocytoplasmic ratio. Histopathology confirmed the malignant appearance. (Wright; HP oil.) (Courtesy Rick Alleman, University of Florida.)

Rupture of these esophageal nodules into the thoracic cavity produces an inflammatory effusion with the presence of characteristic ova (Fig. 7.36).

Neoplasia

Epithelial neoplasia of the esophagus is uncommon in dogs and cats. SCC occurs rarely in cats and dogs, is most frequently found in the thoracic esophagus, and can be difficult to diagnose with superficial sampling of the mucosa because of inflammation. The cytopathologic features of esophageal SCC are similar to oral SCC (see Fig. 7.13). An adenocarcinoma of the esophageal glands is a less common epithelial neoplasm. Its location and cytopathologic features can be similar to a thyroid carcinoma. Neoplastic transformation of the *Spirocerca*-induced granuloma is a potential consequence with lesion chronicity. In fact, esophageal sarcomas are usually associated with the presence of the parasite (Shipov et al., 2015). Another spindle-shape sarcoma is an esophageal leiomyosarcoma in which the cells may contain eosinophilic

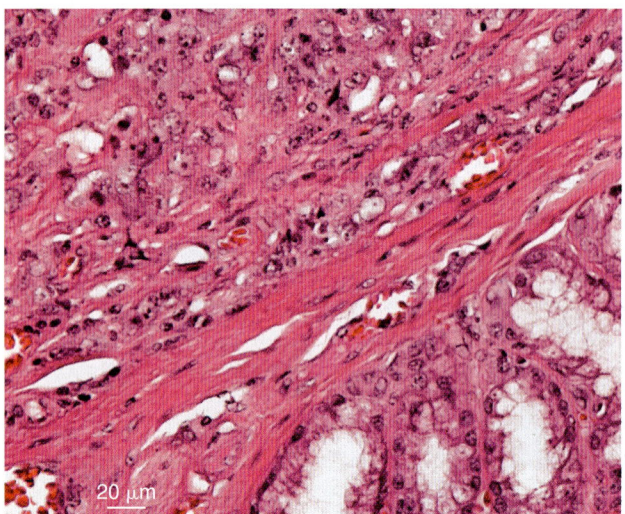

■ **FIGURE 7.34 Salivary gland. Adenocarcinoma. Histology.** Salivary gland tissue from the tonsillar region demonstrates marked distortion of architecture (above pink connective tissue line) compared with the normal glandular structure (*lower right*). (H&E; IP.) (Courtesy Rose Raskin, Michigan State University)

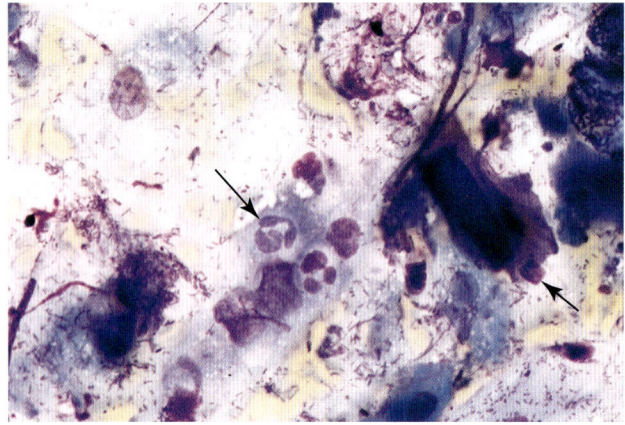

■ **FIGURE 7.35 Esophagitis. Brushing.** This specimen was obtained endoscopically from an inflamed site in the esophagus. Esophagitis is indicated by the presence of neutrophils *(long arrow)*. Other findings include angular squamous epithelial cells, keratin bar *(short arrow)*, and numerous bacteria (oral flora). (Wright; HP oil.)

Oliver, 1999; Grooters et al., 2003; Berryessa et al., 2008; Pera et al., 2017).

Spirocerca lupi is a spiruroid nematode that parasitizes the esophageal wall of dogs in warm climates where the dung beetle serves as the intermediate host. Endoscopically, the mass appears as a smooth, nonulcerated nodule in the distal esophagus; some patients may present with multiple nodules. A granuloma forms around the nematode, and adult worms sometimes appear through a fistula communicating with the esophageal lumen. Spirocercosis is diagnosed by finding embryonated eggs in a fecal flotation or in esophageal nodules. Aspiration of nodules may show neutrophilic and macrophagic inflammation along with the presence of oval ova measuring 30 × 15 μm containing variably dense material and having a thick capsule, which has a smooth or longitudinal fold (De Lorenzi and Furlanello, 2010).

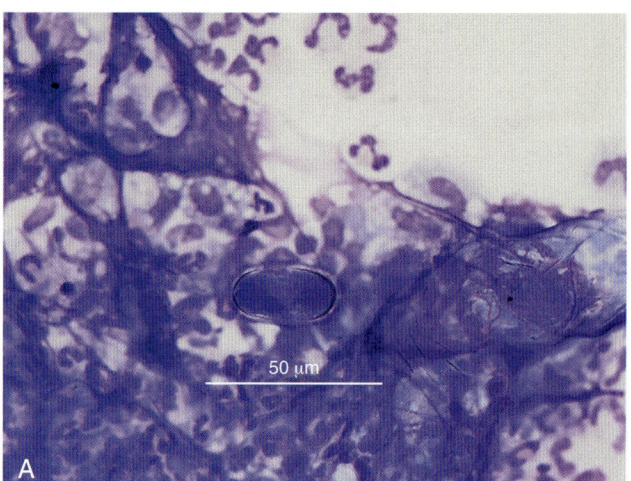
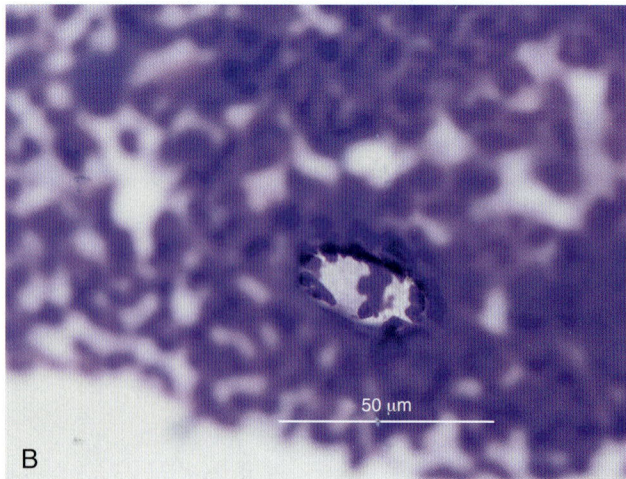

■ **FIGURE 7.36** *Spirocerca lupi* **ova. Esophageal nodule. Dog.** Same case in A and B. **A,** Young dog from Peru had a caudal esophageal nodule and thoracic effusion. Eggs from likely ruptured nodule are shown from the fluid. Ovum displaying a thin capsule and diffuse basophilic stain uptake. (Wright-Giemsa; HP oil.) **B,** Ovum containing internal purple aggregated material. (Wright-Giemsa; HP oil.) (Courtesy Arefeh Ravanbakhsh, PDS Inc., University of Saskatchewan.)

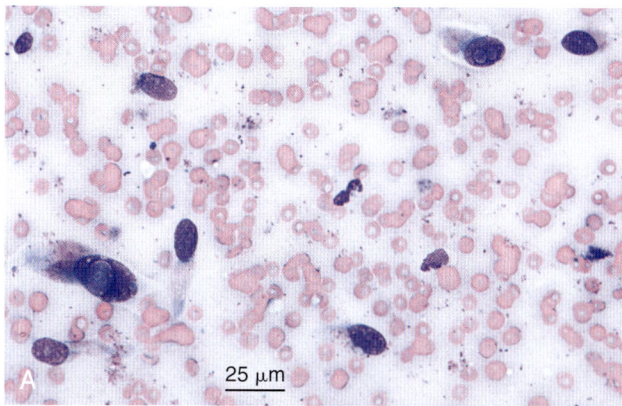

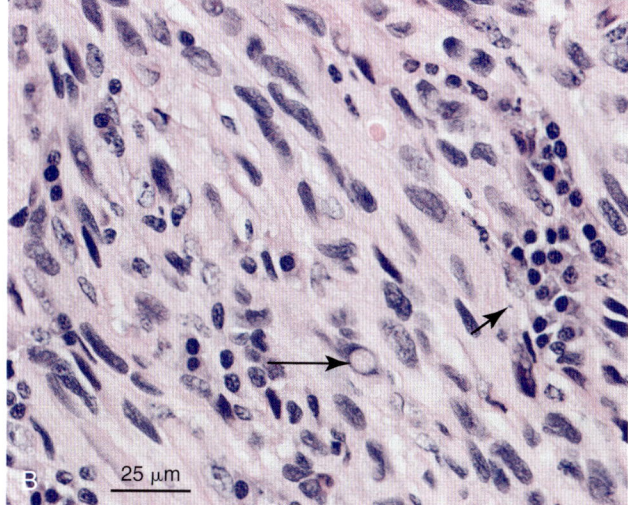

■ **FIGURE 7.37 Esophagus. Leiomyosarcoma. Dog.** Same case in A and B. **A, Imprint.** Several spindle-shaped cells with indistinct cell borders of variable cell size, variable nucleocytoplasmic ratio, and anisokaryosis are present along with hemodilution. Eosinophilic granulation is prominent, ranging from fine to coarse in the cytoplasm of some of the mesenchymal cells as well as within the background. Intranuclear glycogen appears as single or multiple vacuoles, a finding usually associated with hepatocytes but may be found in neoplastic cells with glycogen synthetase activity. (Wright; IP) **B, Histology.** This esophageal mass is composed of haphazardly arranged spindle cells with multifocal perivascular aggregates of lymphocytes and plasma cells *(short arrow)*. Neoplastic cells have marked variation in nuclear shape and size with oval or spindle-like or bizarre shaped nuclei with clumped chromatin, vacuolar inclusions *(long arrow)*, and frequent mitotic figures. The cell margins are indistinct and cell cytoplasm and/or intercellular matrix is sparse to abundant, eosinophilic, and slightly fibrillar. Smooth muscle actin was present on immunohistochemistry supporting the diagnosis. (H&E; HP oil.) (Courtesy Rose Raskin, Purdue University.)

cytoplasmic granules as well as nuclear glycogen vacuoles and pleomorphism (Fig. 7.37).

GASTROINTESTINAL CYTOPATHOLOGY

Gastrointestinal cytopathology can be performed during endoscopic evaluation of patients with chronic or severe GI signs as a rapid and reliable diagnostic tool. The correlation between GI cytopathology and histopathology results is high, and the short turnaround time for results can provide clinicians with more time to implement treatments (Jergens et al., 1998; Ruiz et al., 2017). Intraoperative cytopathologic evaluation of GI lesions may also be useful to determine if resection of the lesion can improve the clinical outcome (Tidd et al., 2019). Additionally, cytopathologic evaluation of endoscopic GI samples can reveal superficial mucosal organisms and inflammation more effectively than histopathology because structures such as spiral bacteria may be lost in the fixation and embedding process. Fibrosis and lesions deep to the lamina propria, however, are usually not detected with superficial endoscopic cytopathology.

The patient's history, endoscopic appearance of the lesion, and endoscopic site sampled are vital for formulating an accurate interpretation of GI cytopathologic specimens. Adequate assessment of these cytopathologic specimens is relatively time consuming and labor intensive. Cytology and histology are complementary processes for the evaluation of GI disease and should be interpreted in conjunction with other diagnostic test results. However, one should not be discouraged if pathology is not detected either cytologically or histologically. In one study, the majority of gastric specimens, 25% of intestinal samples, and 33% of colonic samples were classified as normal even though GI disease was suspected (Jergens et al., 1998). Several grading schemes have been developed to help increase the diagnostic utility of GI cytopathology. For pathologists who frequently evaluate GI cytopathology from dogs and cats, implementation and utilization of one of these grading schemes may help improve their diagnostic consistency and accuracy (Jergens et al., 2016a; Maeda et al., 2017).

STOMACH

Normal Cytology

Gastric mucosal epithelial cells are columnar and appear as uniform cell clusters with oval to round nuclei and moderate amounts of lightly basophilic to light eosinophilic cytoplasm (Fig. 7.38). There can be a mucin vacuole at the luminal surface of the columnar cells. The columnar morphology is more obvious in large cell clusters. The variable amount of mucus in the cytopathologic specimen has variable staining characteristics. Cytopathologically, fundic glandular epithelium consists of rounded parietal cells (lightly eosinophilic cytoplasm) and chief cells (granular to microvesicular basophilic cytoplasm) and may be seen in oval to elliptical clusters (Fig. 7.39). The tinctorial characteristic of the cell appears to be affected by the amount of mucus present. Intranuclear inclusions, when present, appear within the parietal cells of dogs and are composed of PAS-positive, diastase-sensitive glycogen; their significance is unknown (Silvestri et al., 2017). Cardiac glands and pyloric glands also secrete mucus but do not contain parietal and chief cells.

The presence of oropharyngeal flora such as *Conchiformibius* (basionym: *Simonsiella*) spp., along with mucus, pyknotic neutrophils, mixed bacterial flora, and digesta debris, is a common finding in gastric samples from nondiseased stomachs. Mucin granules are large, coarse, and dark purple and should not be mistaken for bacterial cocci or free mast cell granules (Fig. 7.40). Pyknotic neutrophils probably represent blood cells that are continually lost through the mucous membranes of the GI tract. Neutrophils that are not associated with oropharyngeal or esophageal digesta may represent true gastritis. Again, the endoscopic visualization of an inflamed area corroborates the cytopathologic impression of gastritis.

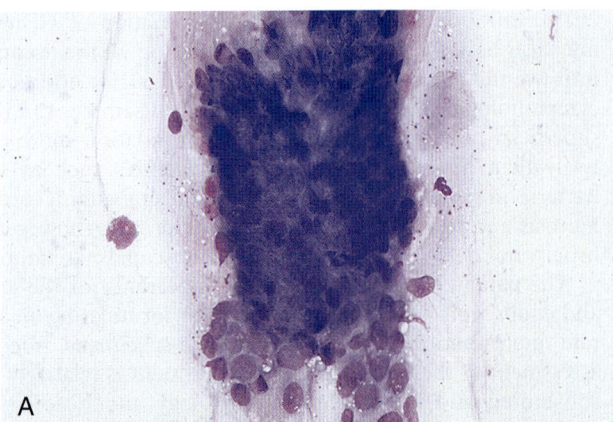
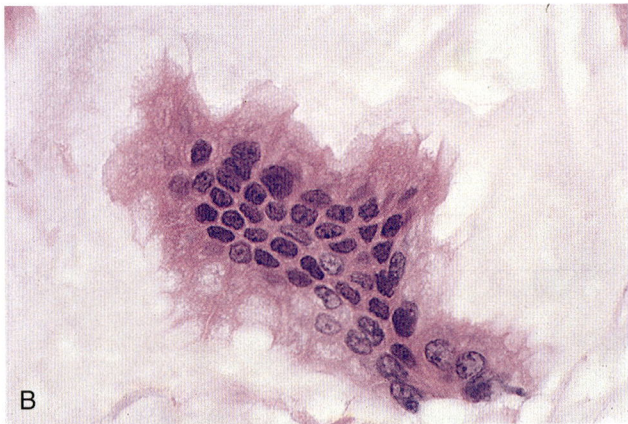

■ **FIGURE 7.38** Gastric mucosal epithelial cells. **A, Normal. Imprint.** The epithelial cells in this specimen are relatively uniform with round to oval nuclei containing dispersed chromatin and moderate amounts of basophilic cytoplasm. The features can be observed at the periphery of the cell cluster where the cells are in a monolayer, emphasizing the importance of proper sample management. Free purple mucin granules are observed in the background adjacent to the cell cluster. (Wright; HP oil.) **B, Histology.** Note the relatively uniform morphologic features and the absence of leukocytes and bacteria. The jagged border of the tissue is an artifact. (H&E; HP oil.)

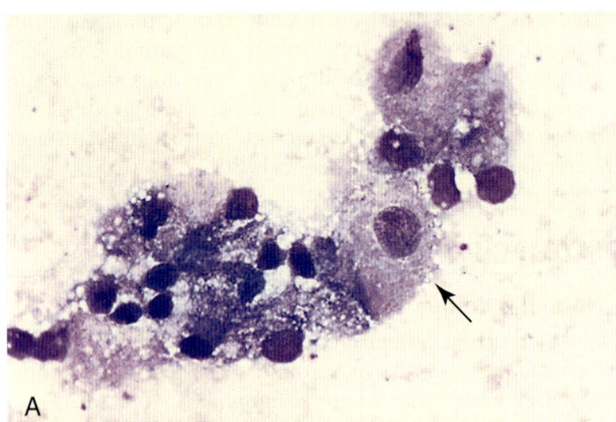
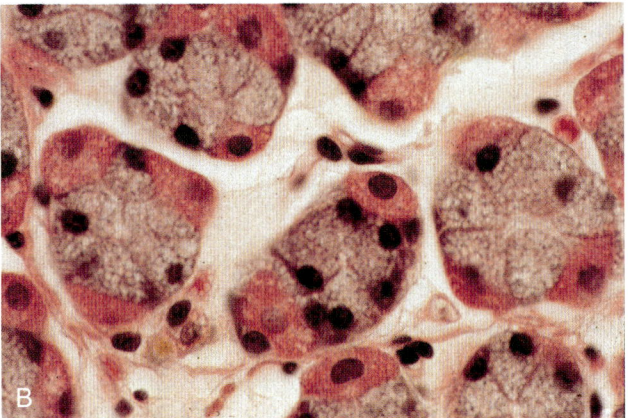

■ **FIGURE 7.39 A, Gastric fundic glandular epithelial cells. Imprint.** Two epithelial cell populations are present. The larger epithelial cells *(arrow)* with abundant, homogeneous, lightly eosinophilic cytoplasm are consistent with parietal cells. The smaller epithelial cells with granular-like or microvesicular basophilic cytoplasm are consistent with chief cells. Both cell types make up the fundic glands of the stomach. (Wright; HP oil.) **B, Gastric fundic glands. Histology.** The oval-shaped fundic glands are composed of two epithelial cell types. The parietal cells stain intensively eosinophilic, and the pale-staining chief cells have microvesicular cytoplasm. (H&E; HP oil.)

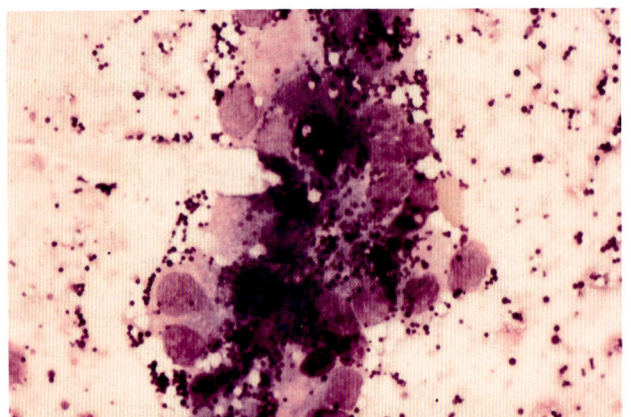

■ **FIGURE 7.40 Gastric imprint biopsy with mucin granules. Imprint.** There is a dense cluster of mucin-producing epithelial cells that are identified by the presence of numerous large coarse dark purple mucin granules that appear similar to bacterial cocci. These cells should not be confused with mast cells, whose metachromatic granules are smaller. (Wright; HP oil.)

Gastric spiral bacteria (i.e., gastric helicobacters) often are associated with mucus (Fig. 7.41) and are more consistently observed in brushing cytologic specimens. They measure in length approximately the diameter of a canine erythrocyte. They are routinely observed in dogs and cats with and without gastric disease. *Helicobacter felis* bacteria and *Helicobacter heilmannii* bacteria cannot be differentiated by light microscopy, and at times lymphocytic inflammation is absent on cytopathology but present on histopathology (Fig. 7.42). In 96 gastric samples, 48% contained gastric spiral organisms (Jergens et al., 1998). The Warthin-Starry stain accentuates the identification of the organism within gastric mucus or in the mucosa. Fluorescence in situ hybridization (FISH) techniques using molecular probes, which target the 16S rRNA bacterial gene, specifically identifies intact bacteria within tissues (Fig. 7.43). Culture is needed to identify specific types of spiral bacteria. The importance of spiral bacteria as a cause of gastric disease in dogs and cats requires additional clarification because these organisms are common in animals without clinical disease or histologic abnormalities and

CHAPTER 7 Oral Cavity, Gastrointestinal Tract, and Associated Structures

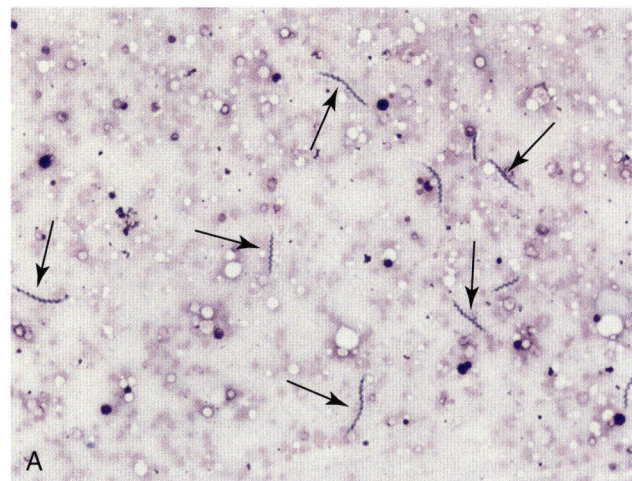

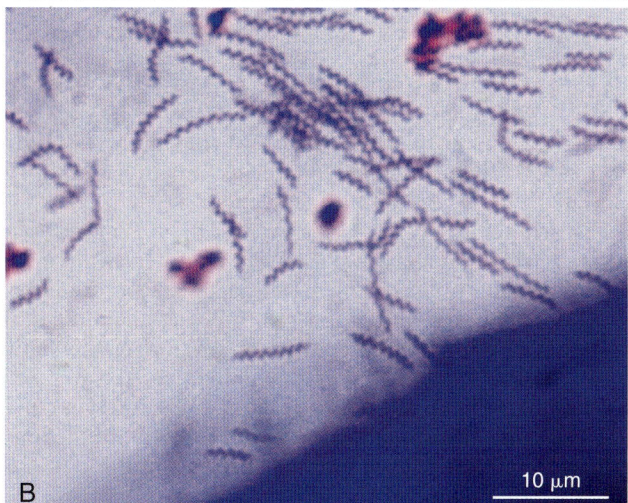

FIGURE 7.41 Spiral-shaped bacteria. Imprint. A, Numerous *Helicobacter*-like or *Gastrospirillum*-like spiral-shaped bacteria *(arrows)* are embedded in the mucus. Spiral-shaped organisms are commonly observed cytologically in both nondiseased and diseased stomachs of dogs and cats (Wright; HP oil.) **B, Dog.** Close-up of spiral organisms from another case showing a variable size in length from 5 to 10 μm. (Wright; HP oil.) (B, Courtesy Rose Raskin, Purdue University.)

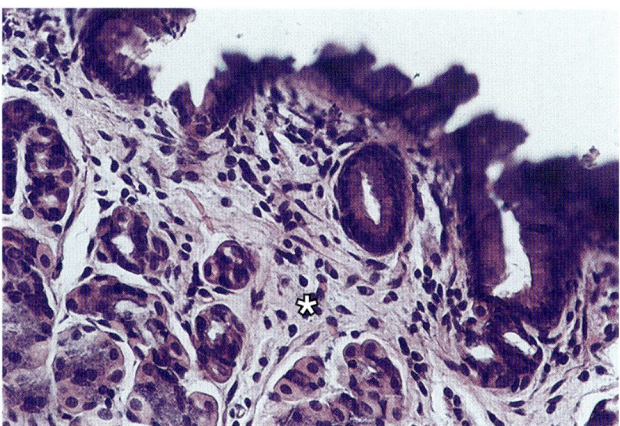

FIGURE 7.42 Lymphocytic gastritis. Histology. Although no inflammatory cells were observed in the cytopathologic specimen, there was mild increase in lymphocytes, stromal fibrosis, and edema around the gastric glands *(asterisk)*. Microscopic examination of a biopsy is generally required to determine the presence or absence of inflammation. Only a rare spiral-shaped organism was observed (not shown) on the mucosal surface, probably because of the absence of the mucous layer. A Warthin-Starry stain can be used to identify the organism in tissue. (H&E; HP oil.)

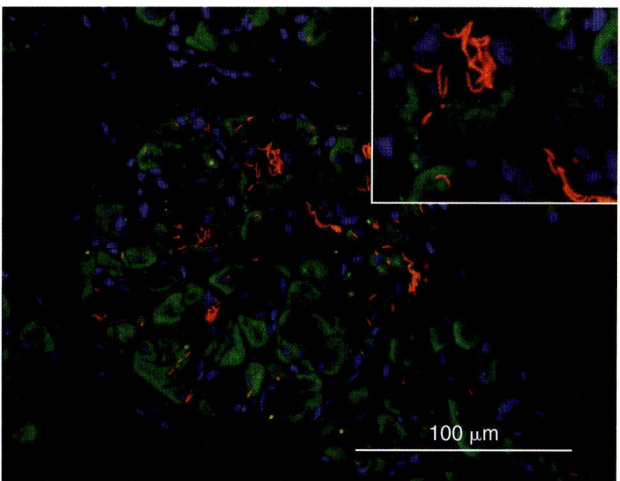

FIGURE 7.43 Fluorescent in situ hybridization. This molecular technique shows invasive *Helicobacter* spp. within a gastric mucosal biopsy specimen obtained from a dog with chronic vomiting. *Inset:* Higher magnification displays the orange fluorescent (Cy-3 labeled) spirochete bacteria in a cluster.

do not alter gastric function experimentally (Hermanns et al., 1995; Happonen et al., 1996; Simpson et al., 1999; Neiger and Simpson, 2000). In other studies, however, an association between gastric pathology and the presence of helicobacters has been found (Amorim et al., 2015).

Cyniclomyces guttulatus (formerly *Saccharomycopsis guttulata*) is a yeast occasionally identified in canine gastric, intestinal, and colonic samples (Fig. 7.44). This is a common yeast residing in the GI tracts of rabbits and may be seen in dogs after consuming rabbit fecal pellets. Although generally considered nonpathogenic in dogs, there is some evidence it can serve as an opportunistic pathogen in some circumstances (Winston et al., 2016).

Hyperplasia

The cytopathologic impression of mucosal and secretory hyperplasia is subjective. Increased numbers of mucosal secretory cells or goblet cells with attendant diffuse mucin granules (globules) may indicate mucosal secretory hyperplasia. A definitive diagnosis requires histology.

Inflammation

Neutrophils, along with other inflammatory cells, are associated with gastric ulcers (Fig. 7.45). As indicated above, the presence of oropharyngeal flora or digesta admixed with neutrophils tempers the cytopathologic impression of true inflammation. Lymphocytic or lymphoplasmacytic inflammation is associated with chronic gastritis (Fig. 7.46). *Physaloptera* spp. is one specific cause of chronic inflammation that can be observed endoscopically (Fig. 7.47). Other parasites that cause gastritis, especially in cats, are Ollulanus and Gnathostoma. Parasites or

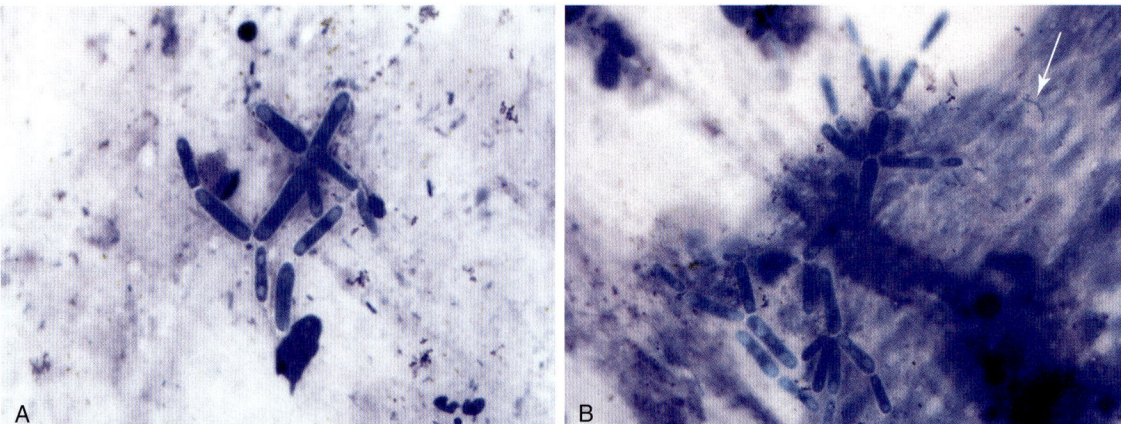

■ **FIGURE 7.44** *Cyniclomyces guttulatus.* **Endoscopic gastric imprint. Dog. A,** Oval to cylindrical branching and short chains of yeast structures (5–7 μm × 20 μm) surrounded by a thin, unstained (clear) cell wall are morphologically consistent with *C. guttulatus* and can be confirmed by culture. The characteristic arrangement of the yeast resembles "balloon animals." (Wright; HP oil.) **B,** In addition to the *C. guttulatus* organisms, a spiral bacterium *(arrow)* is seen on top of a faint sheet of uniform epithelial cells. (Wright; HP oil.)

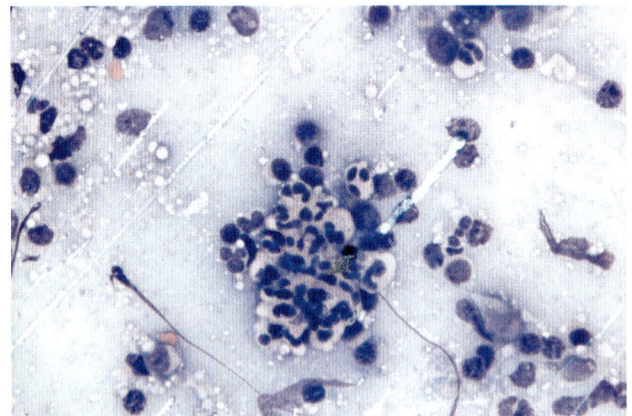

■ **FIGURE 7.45 Gastric inflammation. Neutrophilic gastritis. Brushing. Dog.** Increased neutrophils (notable clump located at the center of the image) and lesser numbers of lymphocytes were present in this cytopathology specimen from a dog presenting with chronic vomiting. Ulcerative and erosive lesions were observed endoscopically. (Modified Wright; HP oil.)

parasite fragments are rarely seen on cytopathology (Jergens et al., 1998). Gastric nodular lymphocytic inflammation can be associated with *Helicobacter* spp. infection.

Gastric phycomycosis or zygomycosis can be associated with severe gastric inflammation. Prolonged treatment with antibiotics or immunosuppression may lead to gastric candidiasis (Fig. 7.48). The oral and esophageal mucous membranes are additional sites for candidiasis. PAS or Gomori methenamine silver (GMS) stains can be used to highlight yeast, true fungal, and oomycetal *(Pythium)* organisms (Fig. 7.49). A discussion of additional organisms that may be found throughout the intestinal tract, including the stomach, is present in the section on inflammation in the colon.

In recent years, an inflammatory condition affecting the stomach and/or intestine and resulting in chronic GI signs has been described in cats. *Feline gastrointestinal eosinophilic sclerosing fibroplasia* (FGESF) typically causes a solitary mass lesion composed of eosinophilic to mixed cell inflammation, collagen, and necrosis (Fig. 7.50). Bacteria are frequently associated with the inflammation. Common locations for FGESF lesions are the

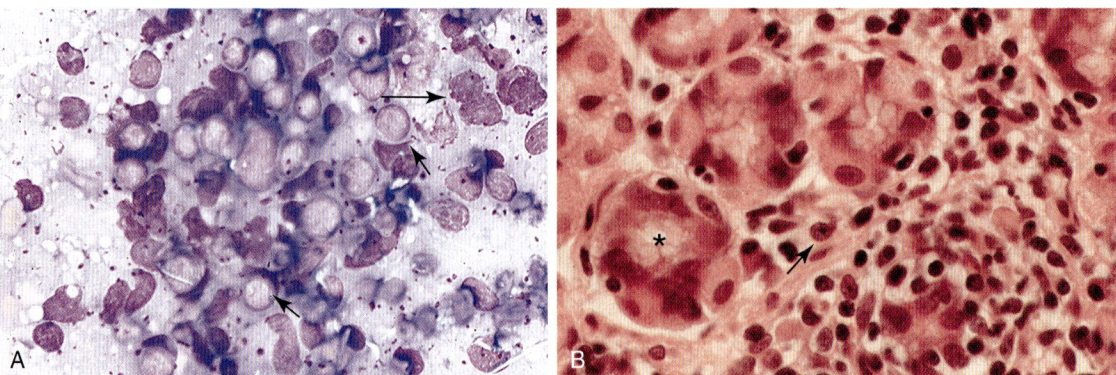

■ **FIGURE 7.46 Lymphocytic gastritis. Imprint. Dog. A,** A dense population of lymphocytes is a notable feature. The predominant cell type is a medium to large lymphocyte with a nucleus that is composed of smooth chromatin surrounded by minimal cytoplasm *(short arrows)*. There are frequent irregular formations of free nuclear protein from ruptured cells *(long arrow)* and numerous granules that represent mucin granules. The differential considerations include lymphocytic gastritis or gastric lymphoma. (Wright; HP oil.) **B, Histology.** A heterogeneous population of lymphocytes *(arrow)* surrounds the gastric glands *(asterisk)*. A small number of plasma cells were admixed (not shown), resulting in a morphologic diagnosis of lymphoplasmacytic gastritis. (H&E; HP oil.)

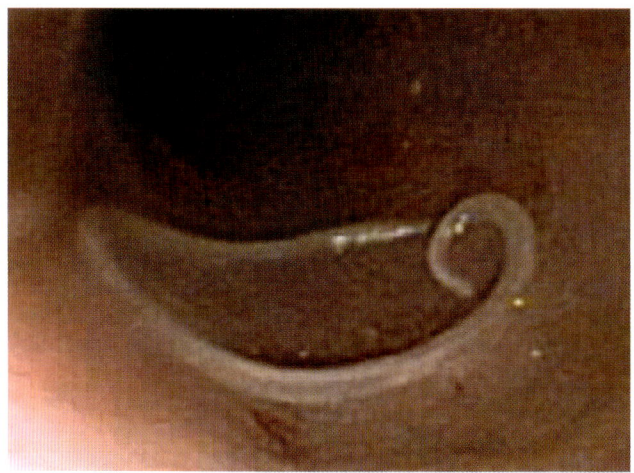

■ **FIGURE 7.47** ***Physaloptera*. Gastric endoscopic view.** An approximate 2 cm long, white nematode consistent with *Physaloptera* was endoscopically observed in the fundus of a dog with recurrent vomiting. It is one cause (uncommon) of chronic gastritis.

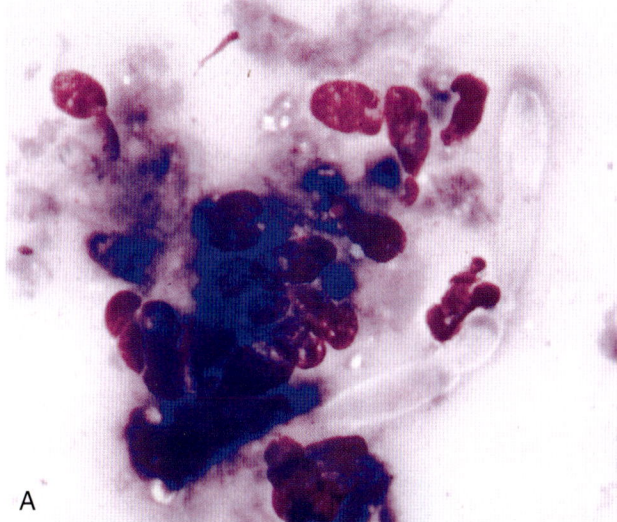

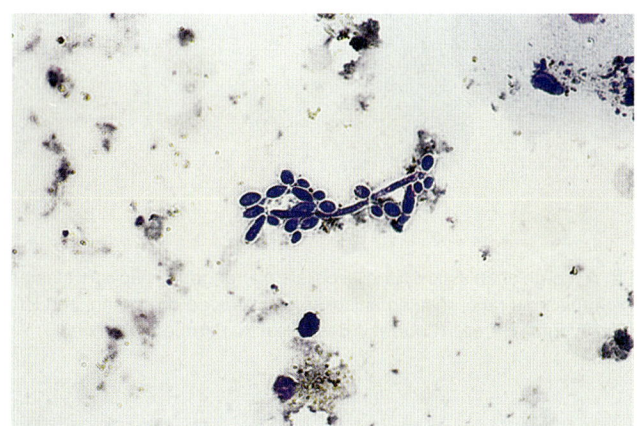

■ **FIGURE 7.48 Gastric candidiasis. Brushing.** Numerous basophilic pseudohyphae and blastospores of *Candida* spp. A silver stain (Gomori methenamine stain) can be used to highlight the organism in tissue. (Wright; HP oil.)

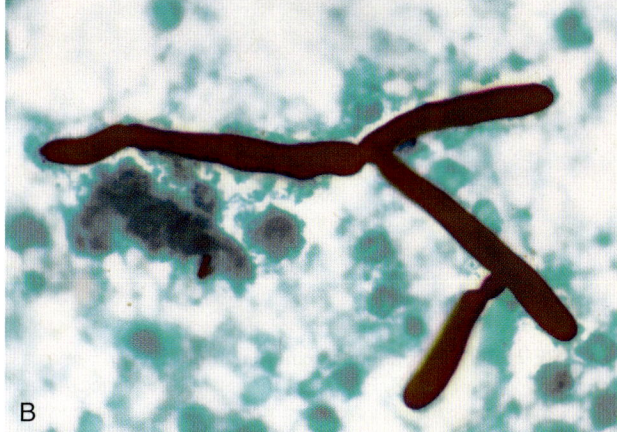

■ **FIGURE 7.49 Gastric pythiosis. Imprint. Dog. A, Romanowsky stain.** Inflammatory cells aggregate around a barely visible hyphal structure that is highlighted by the basophilic proteinaceous background. (Wright-Giemsa; HP oil.) **B, Silver stain.** The cell wall of this water mold is highlighted by the use of this stain. (GMS; HP oil.) (Courtesy Rose Raskin, Purdue University.)

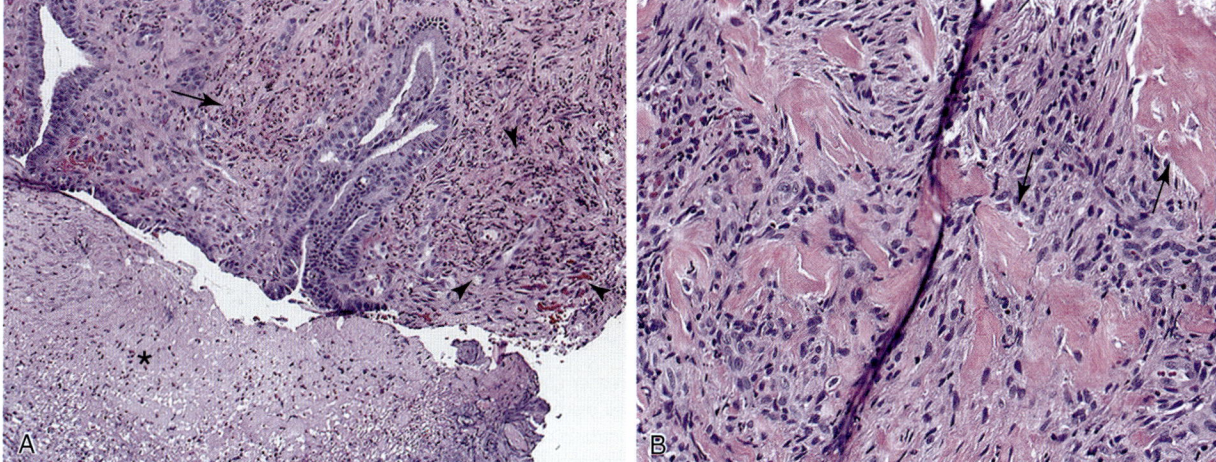

■ **FIGURE 7.50 Feline gastrointestinal eosinophilic sclerosing fibroplasia. Mass near pyloric sphincter. Endoscopic biopsy. Histology. Cat.** Same case in A and B. **A,** The mass consisted of an expanded lamina propria caused by fibrous tissue proliferation *(arrowheads)* and eosinophilic infiltration *(arrow)*. There was surface ulceration, and a coagulum of inflammatory cells and debris was located on the mucosal surface *(asterisk)*. (H&E, LP.) **B,** Trabecula of dense hyalinized collagen *(arrows)* were bordered by immature mesenchymal cells in some areas of the lesion. (H&E, IP.)

pyloric sphincter, ileocecocolic junction, and colon, although extraintestinal lesions within the draining lymph nodes and liver also have been described (Craig et al., 2009; Linton et al., 2015).

Neoplasia

Gastric neoplasms are uncommon in dogs and cats. Gastric adenocarcinoma is the most commonly diagnosed gastric neoplasm in dogs but is rare in cats. It can be more difficult to diagnose cytopathologically when it is located in the submucosa or muscularis. In addition, the occasional development of reactive fibrosis adds an additional barrier that precludes exfoliation of the neoplastic cells. Malignant cells usually exfoliate readily when gastric ulceration is present. On cytopathology, gastric adenocarcinoma cells typically have a high nucleocytoplasmic ratio, exhibit variable anisocytosis and anisokaryosis, and may contain abundant punctate vacuolization (Fig. 7.51). In some neoplasms, the neoplastic cells may lose their cohesiveness, making them difficult to distinguish from lymphoma or other round cell tumors. Gastric adenocarcinomas may metastasize to draining lymph nodes or distant sites such as the liver (see Chapter 9) (Munday et al., 2017).

Lymphoma is the most commonly diagnosed gastric neoplasm in cats, also occurs in dogs, and readily exfoliates cells for cytopathologic evaluation (Fig. 7.52). On cytopathology,

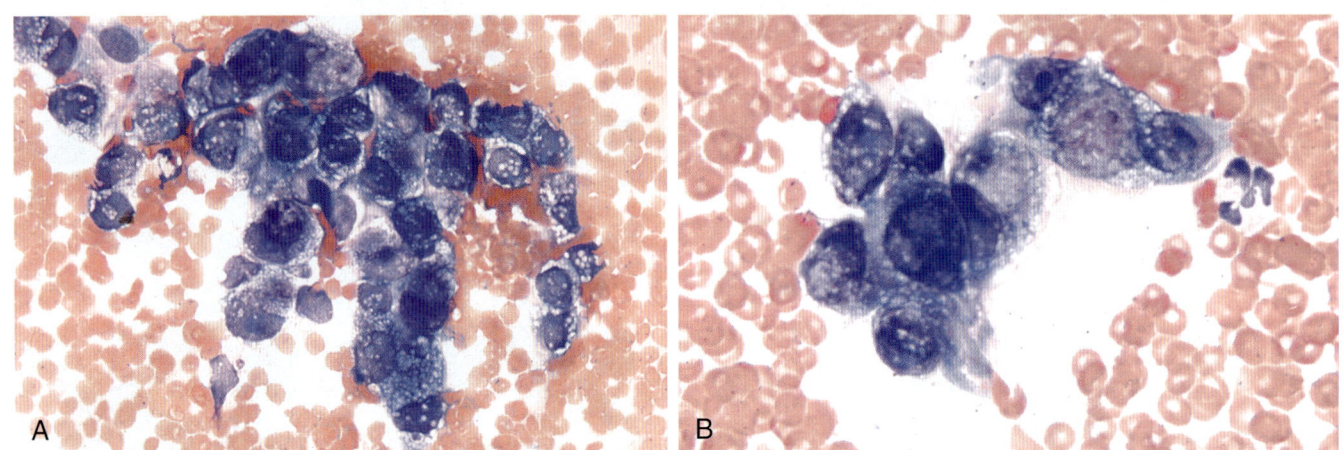

■ **FIGURE 7.51 Gastric adenocarcinoma. Imprint. Dog.** Same case in A and B. **A,** Large anaplastic epithelial cells are arranged in papillary clusters. (Modified Wright; HP oil.) **B,** Prominent malignant features include a high nucleocytoplasmic ratio, marked anisokaryosis, coarse chromatin, and large nucleoli. The cytoplasm is filled with numerous small punctate vacuoles. (Modified Wright; HP oil.) (Courtesy Rose Raskin, Purdue University.)

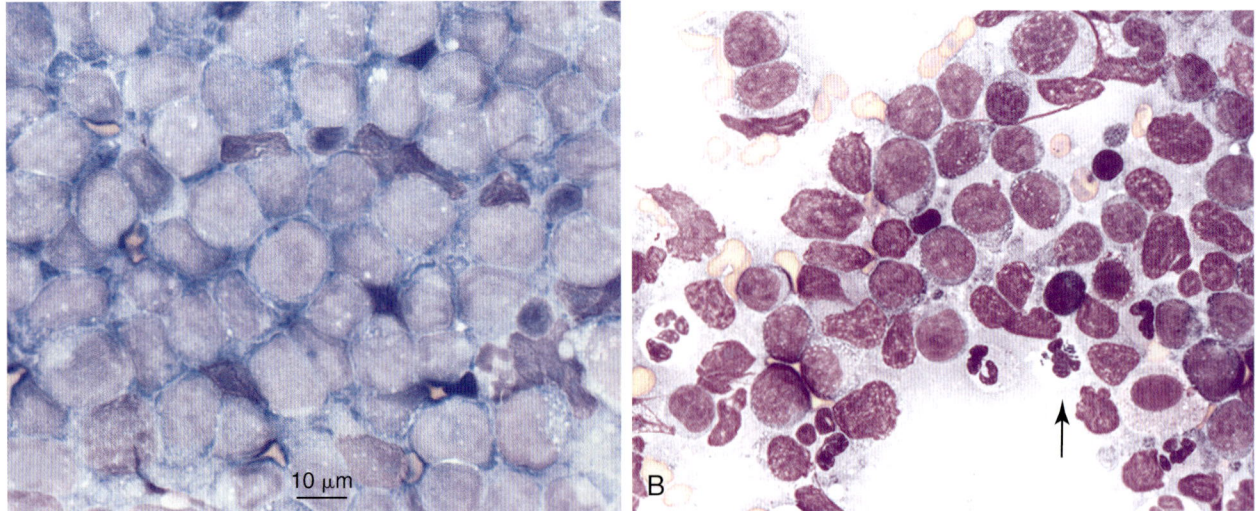

■ **FIGURE 7.52 Gastric lymphoma. A, Imprint. Cat.** The mass at the greater curvature is highly cellular with a monomorphic population of large lymphoid cells having nuclei measuring three to four times the red blood cell diameter. The round nuclei have one or more prominent nucleoli. Cells have scant deeply basophilic cytoplasm with occasional small punctate vacuoles. (Modified Wright; HP oil.) **B, Brushing. Cat.** In a separate case, mucosal ulceration occurred secondary to lymphoma. In addition to the monomorphic population of immature mostly intermediate lymphocytes, scattered neutrophils that occasionally contain phagocytosed bacteria *(arrow)* are present. (Modified Wright, HP oil.) (A, Courtesy Rose Raskin, Purdue University.)

unless large numbers of predominantly immature lymphocytes are present, lymphoma can be difficult to differentiate from severe lymphocytic inflammation. Small cell lymphoma (well-differentiated lymphocytes) usually cannot be confidently diagnosed with cytopathology and requires histopathology with subsequent immunophenotyping or molecular studies (i.e., polymerase chain reaction for antigen receptor rearrangement performed on tissue DNA or flow cytometry) to confirm a diagnosis. Other round cell tumors, including EMP and mast cell neoplasia, occur less commonly (Munday et al., 2017).

INTESTINE

Normal Cytology

The intestinal mucosal epithelium is columnar, and crypts are present. The duodenum is the region most commonly sampled endoscopically, although sampling of the ileum also is recommended for diagnosing enteropathies in dogs and cats (Jergens et al., 2016b). Mucosal cell types that can be observed in cytopathologic specimens include columnar epithelial cells and mucus-producing goblet cells (Figs. 7.53 and 7.54). The duodenum is the region most commonly sampled endoscopically, which has unique submucosal mucous glands (Brunner's glands) (Fig. 7.54B–C). Low numbers of lamina propria and interepithelial mucosal mast cells, the latter termed *globule leukocytes*, may be found in the GI tract (Figs. 7.55 and 7.56) (Takeuchi et al., 1969). The mucosal epithelial cells contain basophilic round to oval nuclei with moderate amounts of light basophilic cytoplasm and chromatin that is smooth to finely stippled (less aggregated than that observed in lymphocytes) and indistinct nucleoli. Mucus may be diffuse or seen as distinct basophilic to purple granules (Fig. 7.57A). These structures should not be confused with the irregularly shaped granular magenta-stained particles of lubricant products that are common contaminants (Fig. 7.57B). Paneth cells within the mucosal glands contain coarse eosinophilic granular cytoplasm and can be difficult to distinguish from mucus-producing cells.

Aggregated lymphoid follicles (Peyer's patches) are scattered in the mucosa of the antimesenteric wall of the small intestine. Endoscopically, they appear as oval to elongated mucosal depressions that are several millimeters to 1 cm in diameter (Fig. 7.58). They may project slightly above the mucosal surface when activated or appear as slight depressions and be mistaken for an ulcerlike lesion. The follicular aggregate of B lymphocytes is covered by a mixed population of T and B lymphocytes extending into the lamina propria in rounded mucosal projections. An erroneous cytopathologic impression of lymphocytic inflammation or even lymphoma is possible if a follicle is unknowingly sampled or if the endoscopist does not communicate her or his observations with the cytopathologist. A heterogeneous lymphocyte population generally comprises a lymphoid follicle or inflammatory reaction, and this variability aids in differentiation from the homogeneous lymphocyte population characteristic of lymphoma. Low numbers of lymphocytes and plasma cells may be seen cytopathologically, but they are less frequent than one might anticipate based on the number present histologically in tissue without pathology. Granular lymphocytes may be normally observed in low numbers, especially in cats (Fig. 7.59). Bacteria are usually not observed in the small intestine or are only present in low numbers as a heterogeneous population.

Hyperplasia

A cytopathologic impression sample of hyperplastic tissue is based on prominent numbers of mucus-secreting epithelial cells and/or a marked increase in goblet cells. It is important to differentiate changes of epithelial hyperplasia or metaplasia caused by reparative lesions from relatively well-differentiated neoplasia. Criteria for hyperplasia include preservation of polarity, uniformity of cell size with minimal anisocytosis, and cohesiveness of cells. Correlation with the histologic findings is recommended when there are problematic cytopathologic findings.

Inflammation

Monomorphic populations of bacteria, especially if observed in patients with clinical signs, could indicate infection or overgrowth

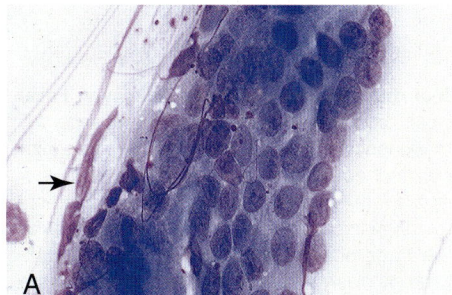 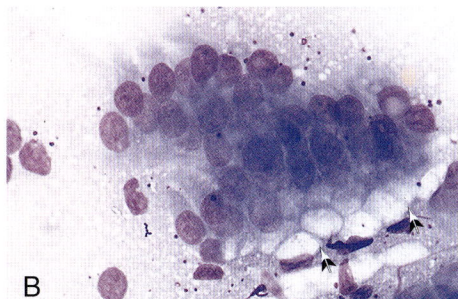 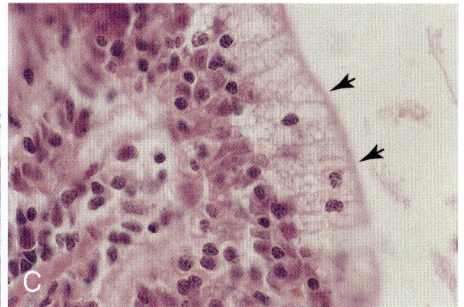

■ **FIGURE 7.53 Intestinal mucosal epithelial cells. Normal. A, Imprint.** Cluster of uniform epithelial cells with round to oval nuclei and confluent basophilic cytoplasm. Streaks of free nuclear protein are noted on the left *(arrow)*. (Wright; HP oil.) **B, Imprint.** The columnar epithelial cells have large clear cytoplasmic vacuoles *(arrows)* that represent apical mucous vacuoles. The cells have indistinct cell borders, and a few mucin granules are scattered around them. (Wright; HP oil.) **C, Histology.** The columnar epithelial cells contain basilar nuclei and show cytoplasmic rarefaction (increased lucency) at the apical end *(arrows)* because of their cytoplasmic mucus content. (H&E; HP oil.)

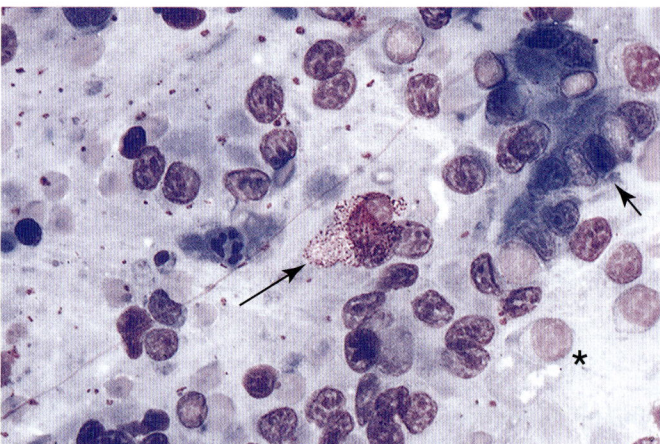

FIGURE 7.55 Intestinal mucosal cells. Normal epithelium and mast cell. Imprint. In the center is a single well-granulated, slightly distorted mast cell likely from the lamina propria. The oval nucleus with ropy chromatin is surrounded by a moderately abundant cytoplasm containing small metachromatic stained granules *(long arrow)*. An occasional mast cell is a normal finding in an intestinal cytologic specimen. Basophilic epithelial cells *(short arrow)* and lightly stained medium-sized lymphocytes with round nucleus, diffuse chromatin, and scant to moderate rim of lightly basophilic cytoplasm are present *(asterisk)*. Free nuclei that retain clumped chromatin pattern are scattered through the field. (Wright; HP oil.)

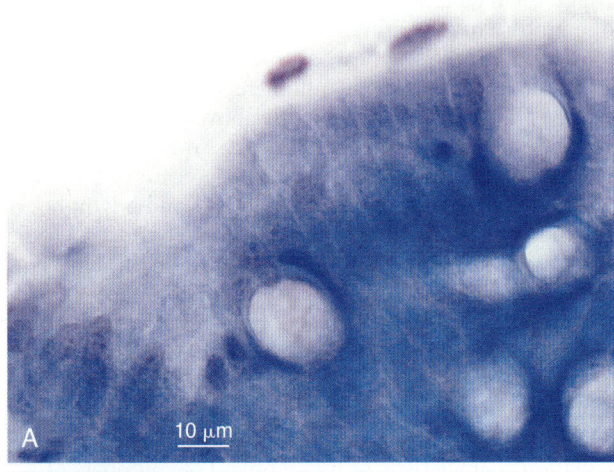
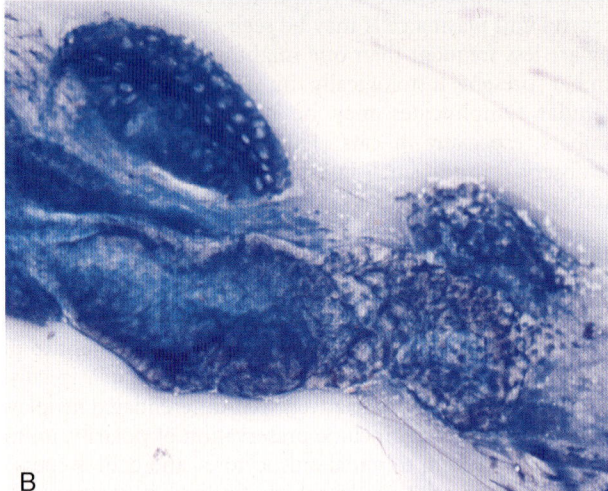
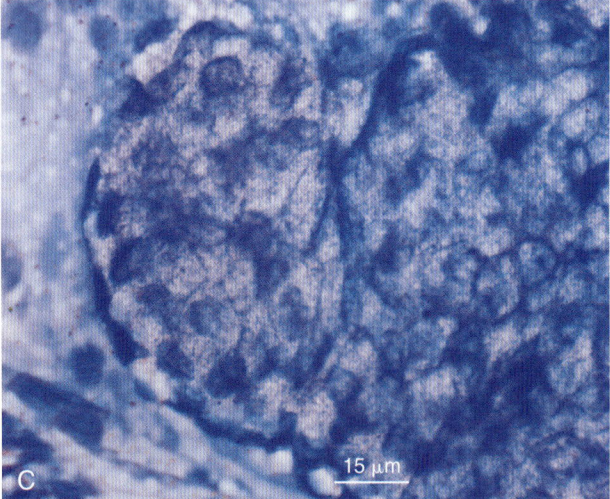

FIGURE 7.54 Duodenal epithelium. Normal. Imprint. Dog. Same case in A to C. **A,** Columnar epithelium arranged in palisading fashion with interspersed round pale goblet cells. The apical border has a translucent layer of mucus. (Modified Wright; HP oil.) **B,** Lower magnification shows on the left side mucosal epithelium with prominent speckled regions of goblet cells. The right side reveals the submucosa mucus glands called Brunner's glands, unique in the duodenum. (Modified Wright; IP.) **C,** High magnification of the submucosal Brunner's glands. The pale foamy cytoplasm resembles salivary gland tissue. (Modified Wright; HP oil.) (Courtesy Rose Raskin, Purdue University.)

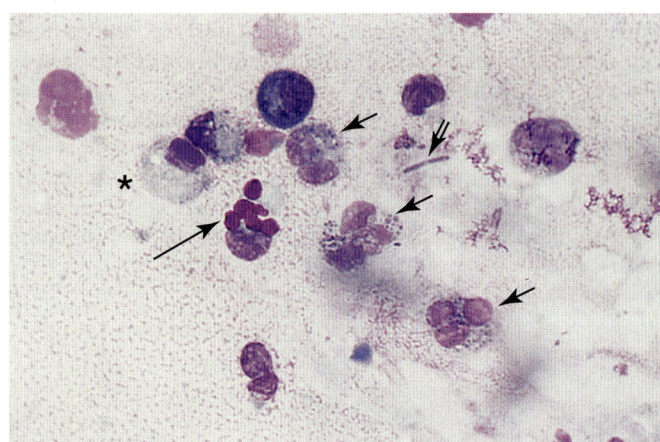

FIGURE 7.56 Intestinal mucosal cells. Globule leukocyte. Fecal smear. The mononuclear cell *(long arrow)* has a round to oval eccentric nucleus composed of homogeneous chromatin, light blue-gray cytoplasm that is packed with large distinct eosinophilic granules. The globule leukocyte normally resides in the interepithelial region of the lining intestinal mucosa or seldom in the lamina propria and are considered a type of mast cell. Also present are three eosinophils *(short arrows)* with pink-brown cytoplasmic granules, a plasma cell with dark blue cytoplasm *(top)*, and a poorly staining globule leukocyte *(asterisk)* with blue-gray cytoplasm containing spherical outlines of globules. A large rod-shaped bacterium *(double arrow)* is present. The presence of abundant eosinophils suggests eosinophilic colitis. The histopathologic morphologic diagnosis from a colonic tissue biopsy was eosinophilic colitis. (Wright; HP oil.)

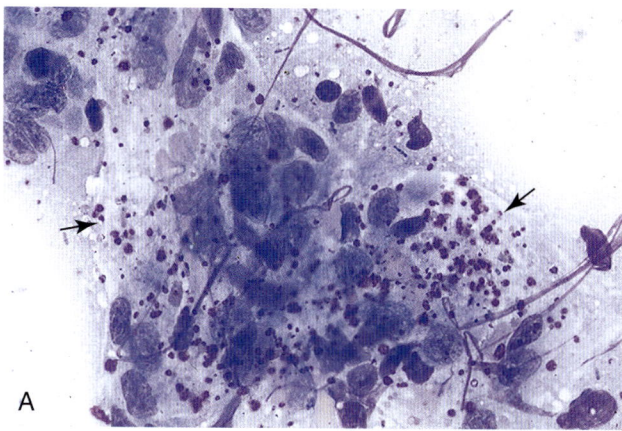 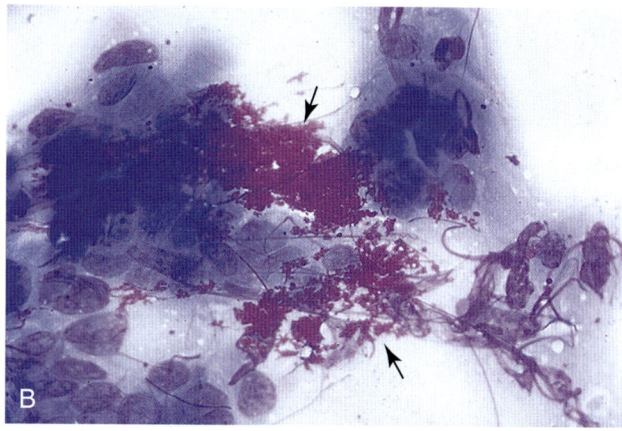

FIGURE 7.57 **Background material. A, Intestinal epithelial cells. Normal. Mucin granules. Imprint.** Numerous variably sized mucin secretory granules cover a dense cluster of uniform intestinal epithelial cells *(arrows)*. The cellular distortion is an artifact of the preparation. Streaks of free nuclear protein are noted. (Wright; HP oil.) **B, Intestinal epithelial cells. Normal. Gel lubricant. Imprint.** In the center of these dense clumps of intestinal epithelial cells are irregularly shaped homogeneous islands of magenta-stained material that represent the gel used for lubrication of the endoscope *(arrows)*. (Wright; HP oil.)

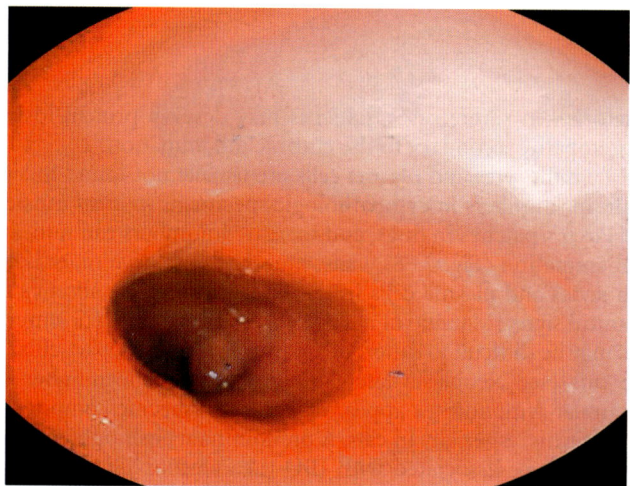 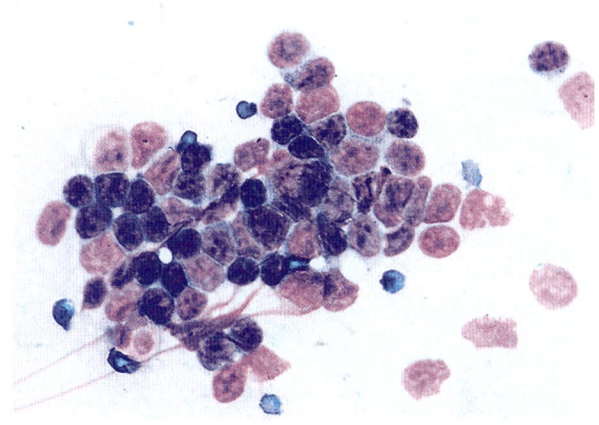

FIGURE 7.58 Duodenum. Lymphoid aggregate. Endoscopy. The proximal canine duodenum showing a well-defined lymphoid aggregate along the right lateral mucosal wall. Note the distinct follicular appearance (white-gray patches), which suggests antigenic stimulation. Evaluation of histopathologic and cytopathologic specimens from this dog confirmed the presence of lymphocytic-plasmacytic enteritis.

FIGURE 7.59 Intestinal aggregated lymphoid follicle (Peyer's patch). Brushing. This densely packed cluster of lymphocytes is composed of small (darkest stained) and medium lymphocytes (lightest stained with visible rim of lightly basophilic cytoplasm). Four free nuclei are located to the far right. (Wright; HP oil.)

of pathogenic bacteria. In such cases, additional diagnostics such as FISH or culture may be indicated. Epithelial-adherent bacteria are an abnormal finding in small intestinal cytopathologic specimens (Fig. 7.60). Additional diagnostics, such as culture, polymerase chain reaction, and FISH are recommended to rule out infection with pathogenic bacteria (e.g., virulent *Escherichia coli*, *Clostridium*) if adherent bacteria are observed in association with clinical signs. Mucosal ulceration can lead to neutrophilic inflammation and secondary bacterial infection. In these cases, the bacterial population is typically heterogeneous (Fig. 7.61).

The presence of neutrophils is abnormal in small intestinal cytopathology samples and is indicative of neutrophilic inflammation. Neutrophilic inflammation can occur with mucosal erosion or ulceration from any cause (Fig. 7.62), as well as together with macrophages in certain infectious diseases, including viral diseases such as feline infectious peritonitis (Fig. 7.63) and fungal diseases such as histoplasmosis (Fig. 7.64). When neutrophilic or macrophagic inflammation is present, PAS or GMS stains can be used to highlight fungal and protozoal agents along with serum or urine antigen testing for specific pathogens when obvious etiologic agents are absent.

Giardiasis can be diagnosed by finding the trophozoites in duodenal specimens. *Giardia* trophozoites appear as binucleate, pear-shaped organisms with four pairs of flagella (Fig. 7.65). Infection with coccidian parasites (e.g., *Toxoplasma, Hammondia, Neospora, Isospora*) is infrequently associated with clinical signs in dogs, and zoites may be identified in GI cytopathology samples (Fig. 7.66) (Palic et al., 2012). Fungal agents, such as *Candida* spp., *Cryptococcus* spp., *Cokeromyces* spp., or *Blastomyces* spp. may

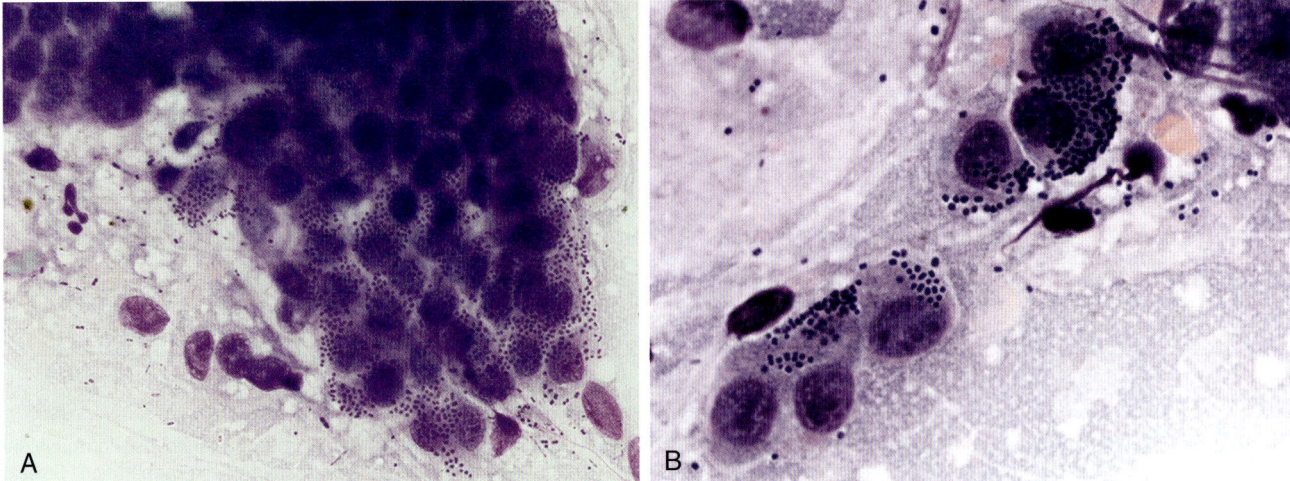

FIGURE 7.60 Abnormal bacteria in small intestinal samples. Ileum. Imprint. Dog. Same case in A and B. **A,** This patient presented with chronic diarrhea. Mild to moderate mixed inflammation (lymphoplasmacytic and neutrophilic) was identified on histopathology. Cytopathology revealed occasional inflammatory cells (a neutrophil is seen to the left of the epithelial cluster in the image), as well as a monomorphic population of bacteria intimately associated with the epithelial cells. Bacteria adhered to the surface of intestinal epithelial cells could be mistaken for mucin granules. (Modified Wright, HP oil.) **B,** The adherent bacteria are more distinct with individualized epithelial cells. (Modified Wright, HP oil.)

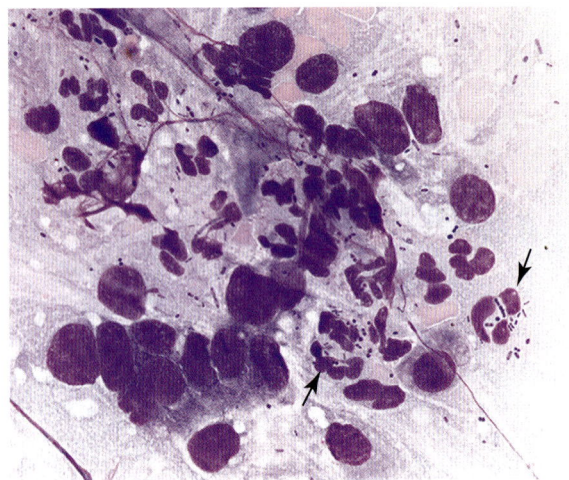

FIGURE 7.61 Neutrophilic enteritis with phagocytized bacteria. Ileum. Brushing. Dog. Neutrophilic inflammation with bacterial infection is a common finding in patients with mucosal ulceration. Note the increased numbers of neutrophils that sometimes contain engulfed bacteria of mixed morphology *(arrows)*. Extracellular mixed bacteria also are present, as well as a row of epithelial cells in the lower left. (Modified Wright, HP oil.)

be secondary to immunosuppression or present in some cases of severe mucosal damage (Fig. 7.67). A predominance of eosinophils may be associated with an intestinal *Candida* granuloma (Duchaussoy et al., 2015). A variety of other infectious agents can be found in the intestine as well as the colon, and many of these are discussed under the section on inflammation of the colon.

Lymphoplasmacytic or eosinophilic inflammation is frequently observed in small intestinal samples from patients with chronic enteritis. The presence of chronic enteric inflammation, in addition to clinical signs, is used to diagnose inflammatory bowel disease (IBD) in dogs and cats. The etiology of IBD is the subject of much research and debate but is likely multifactorial. In severe cases, patients may develop protein-losing enteropathy secondary to the chronic inflammation.

Lymphocytes and plasma cells are usually not found in significant numbers in cytopathologic specimens in areas outside of Peyer's patches in dogs, and increased numbers can indicate inflammation (Fig. 7.68). Cats, however, may have more lymphocytes and plasma cells in the GI mucosa in the absence of clinical signs (Marsilio et al., 2019). Severe lymphocytic enteritis may be difficult to differentiate from lymphoma, particularly in cats (see Neoplasia later). An increase in the number of granular lymphocytes appears to be a nonspecific component of enteritis, especially in cats. A predominant eosinophilic infiltrate may be associated with IBD (i.e., eosinophilic gastroenteritis) or occur secondarily as a host response to parasitic or dietary antigens (Fig. 7.69). FGESF, discussed earlier under gastric inflammation (see Fig. 7.50), may appear similar to these eosinophilic conditions. In addition to eosinophils, fibroblasts are also present and contribute to the severe intestinal fibrosis (Fig. 7.70). In more than half of the FGESF cases, intralesional bacteria may be found (Craig et al., 2009).

Neoplasia

Neoplasia of the intestine in dogs and cats is usually malignant and is more commonly diagnosed in cats than dogs (Munday et al., 2017). The ability to detect neoplasia by cytopathology depends on the extent of infiltration and the presence of ulceration. Lymphoma is the most prevalent and second most prevalent intestinal neoplasm in cats and dogs, respectively. Cats are typically diagnosed with low-grade, small cell lymphoma of T-cell origin, which is believed to be a progression from chronic lymphocytic enteritis (type 2 enteropathy-associated T-cell lymphoma [EATL]). Distinguishing between IBD and type 2 EATL in cats, particularly in the earlier phases of the neoplastic transformation, can be diagnostically challenging on histopathology, let alone cytopathology. Histopathology, IHC, and clonality testing are recommended to help confirm the diagnosis in suspected

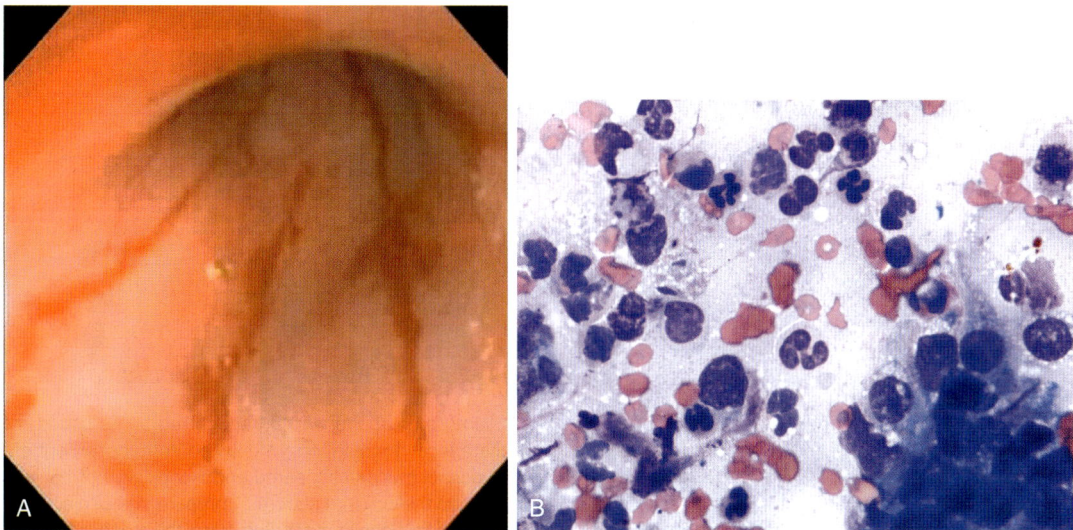

■ **FIGURE 7.62 Duodenal erosion and inflammation. Dog. A, Erosive surface. Endoscopic view.** Visible are multiple linear erosions along the duodenal mucosa. Imprint and brushing cytologic specimens often reveal the neutrophil to be the predominant inflammatory cell in association with superficial mucosal injury as shown in B. **B, Neutrophilic enteritis. Brushing.** Neutrophils and a dense clump of epithelial cells (*lower right*), plus red cells are embedded in a blue-gray mucinous background. (Modified Wright; HP oil.)

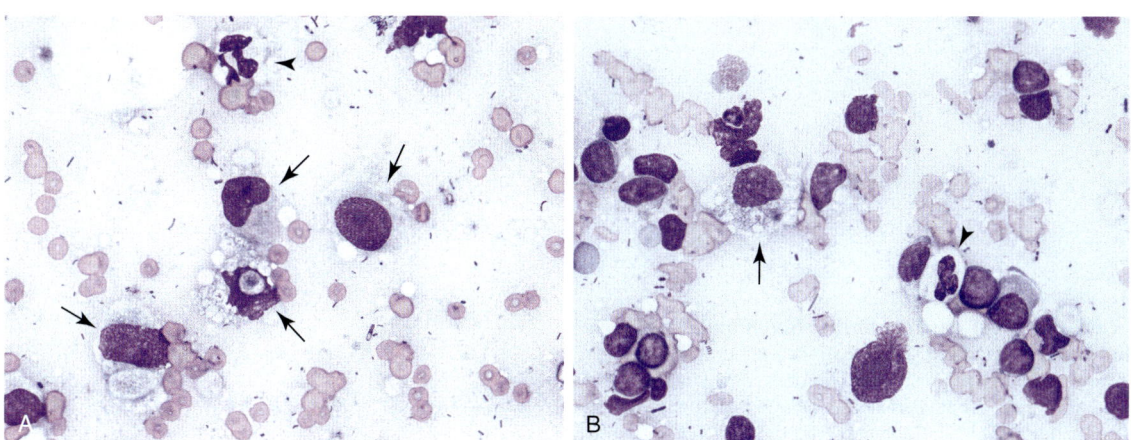

■ **FIGURE 7.63 Chronic inflammation due to feline infectious peritonitis. Ileum. Brushing. Cat.** Same case in A and B. **A,** Increased numbers of foamy macrophages *(arrows)* indicate chronic inflammation, as was found in this cat with feline infectious peritonitis. Neutrophils *(arrowhead)* also were present in increased numbers, as well as mixed extracellular bacteria. **B,** In some areas such as this field, lymphocytes and plasma cells predominated, although occasional macrophages *(arrow)* and neutrophils *(arrowhead)* were still present. (Modified Wright, HP oil.)

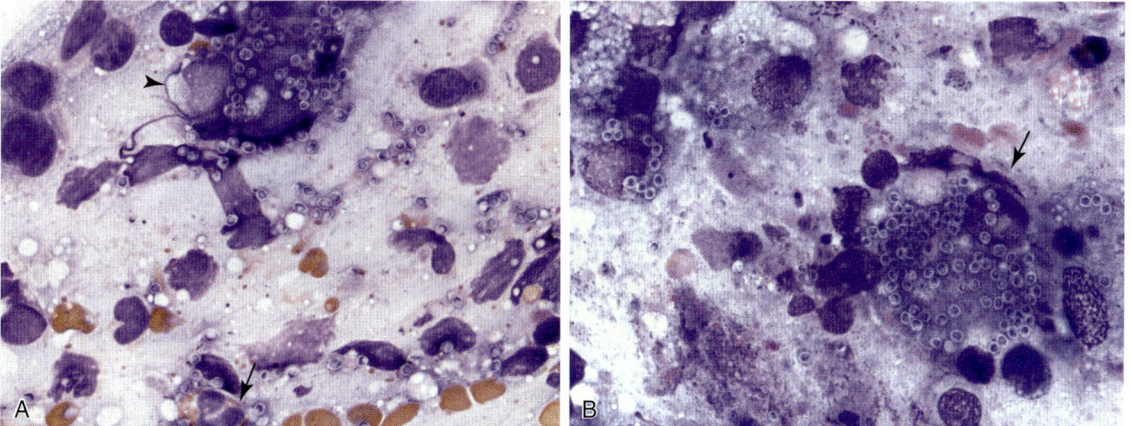

■ **FIGURE 7.64 Chronic inflammation due to histoplasmosis. Duodenum. Brushing. Dog.** Same case in A and B. **A,** In addition to the numerous extracellular yeast morphologically consistent with *Histoplasma capsulatum*, increased inflammatory cells, including eosinophils *(arrow)* and lymphocytes *(arrowhead)*, were identified in this sample from a dog with chronic diarrhea and weight loss. **B,** Macrophages also were increased and often had increased amounts of cytoplasm containing phagocytized organisms *(arrow)*. (Modified Wright, HP oil.)

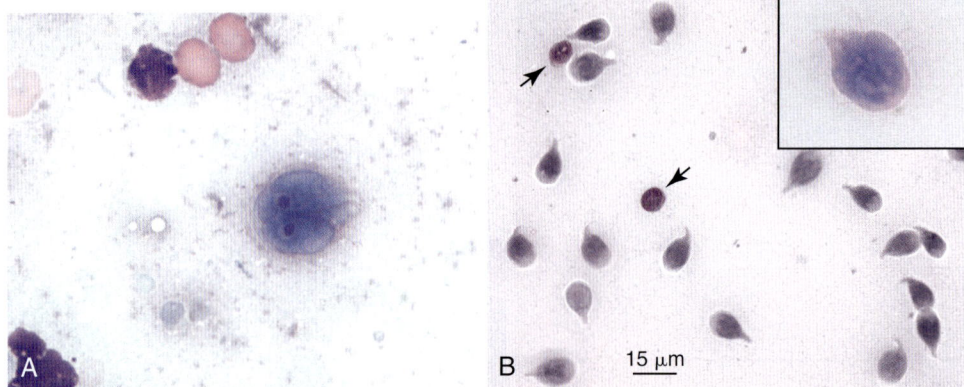

■ **FIGURE 7.65 Giardiasis. Dog. A, Duodenal imprint.** *Giardia intestinalis* (*lamblia* or *duodenalis*) is recognized by its paired metachromatically stained nuclei and multiple flagella. The diagnosis also can be made by zinc sulfate fecal flotation, enzyme-linked immunosorbent assay, or immunofluorescence fecal tests. (Modified Wright; HP oil.) **B, Duodenal imprint.** The duodenal mucosa appeared endoscopically normal in this dog presenting with hypoproteinemia. Numerous trophozoites were present in association with epithelium (not shown). Compare size of giardial trophozoites with the two small lymphocytes *(arrows)*. (Modified Wright; HP oil.) *Inset:* Note the multiple flagella extending from the trophozoite. (B, Courtesy Rose Raskin, Purdue University.)

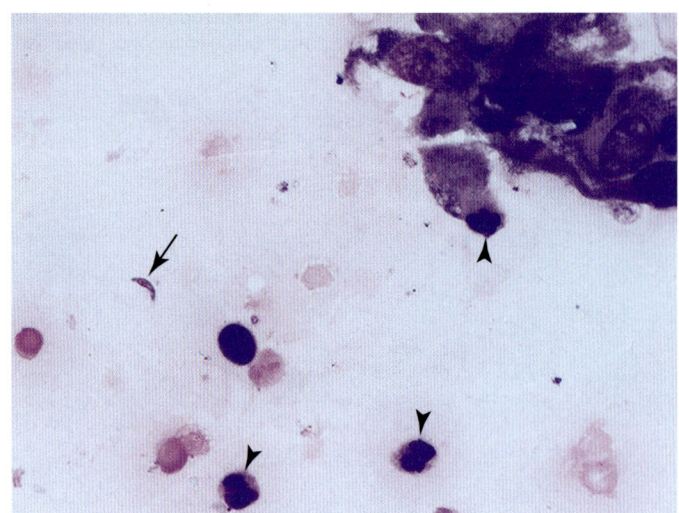

■ **FIGURE 7.66 Protozoal gastroenteritis. *Hammondia heydorni* infection. Duodenum. Brushing. Dog.** Extracellular protozoal zoites *(arrow)* and inflammatory cells (indistinct neutrophils, *arrowheads*) were found in this sample from an adult Italian greyhound with chronic anorexia, vomiting, and weight loss. (Modified Wright, HP oil.)

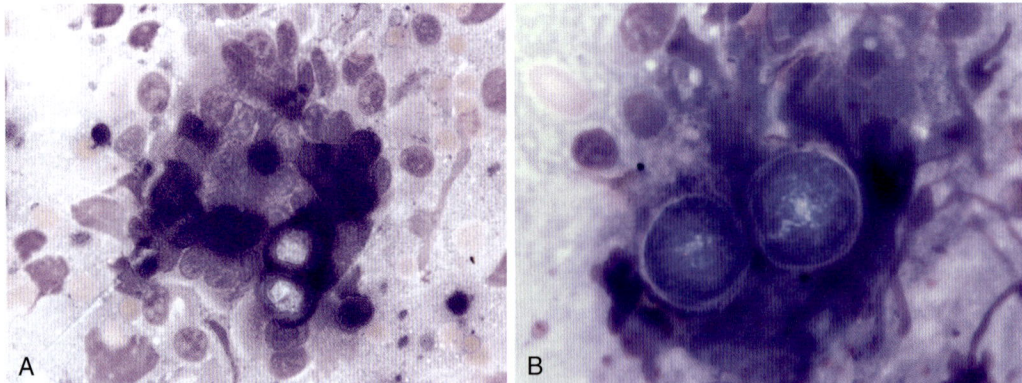

■ **FIGURE 7.67 Mycotic infections. A, Duodenum. Brushing. Dog.** *Cokeromyces recurvatus.* Two basophilic, round, thick-walled structures with pale blue centers approximately 15 μm in diameter, consistent with a fungus, are associated with an epithelial cluster in the center of the image. These likely represent daughter buds of a larger primary yeast based on their size. The uncommon pathogenic fungus morphologically resembles the relatively more common fungal pathogen, *Blastomyces dermatitidis,* and requires culture for identification. Free nuclei and scattered erythrocytes are present within the background. (Modified Wright; HP oil.) **B, *Blastomyces dermatitidis*. Endoscopic duodenal cytologic specimen.** Embedded in a purple meshwork of free nuclear protein are two large round deeply basophilic yeast with less densely stained centers. The relatively large size (approximately 20 μm diameter) can be estimated by comparison with the compressed red cell and adjacent small lymphocytes. Their thick wall likely results in the clear space around the organism. (Modified Wright; HP oil.) (B, Courtesy of Heather Flaherty, Iowa State University.)

CHAPTER 7 Oral Cavity, Gastrointestinal Tract, and Associated Structures

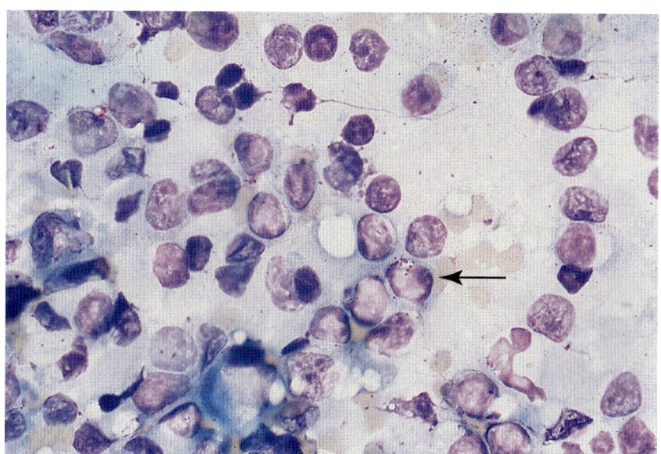

FIGURE 7.68 Lymphocytic enteritis. Granular lymphocyte. Imprint. Cat. Medium lymphocytes are prominent admixed with scattered small lymphocytes. A granular lymphocyte is located slightly to the right of center *(arrow)*. In other areas, occasional neutrophils and macrophages contributed to the inflammatory reaction. (Wright; HP oil.)

cases (Sabattini et al., 2016; Munday et al., 2017). Large cell T-cell lymphoma is less frequently encountered in cats, as well as large granular lymphocyte (LGL) lymphoma, a distinct and uncommon type of T-cell lymphoma. LGL lymphoma is derived from cytotoxic T cells or natural killer cells; often involves the intestinal tract, spleen, and draining lymph nodes; and tends to follow an aggressive clinical course (Fig. 7.71). (Finotello et al., 2018). LGL lymphoma also occurs rarely in dogs (Snead, 2007). The majority of primary intestinal lymphomas in dogs are T-cell lymphomas, with EATL large cell type (type 1) being the most common (Fig. 7.72) (Noland and Kiupel, 2018). Some EATL may coexpress both CD3 and CD20 molecules (Noland and Kiupel, 2018; Matsumoto et al., 2019a). Eosinophils may be associated with the neoplastic T lymphocytes in some cases (Ozaki et al., 2006). The distinction between intestinal inflammation and lymphoma in dogs can sometimes be challenging with cytopathology, particularly in cases of lymphoma with a small cell phenotype. Although there appears to be excellent sensitivity for detecting lymphoma on cytopathology, the specificity is not as high (Maeda et al., 2017). Histopathology, followed by additional diagnostics such as IHC, Ki67 index, and clonality testing, are recommended for confirmation of the diagnosis in suspected cases (Carrasco et al., 2015). One study on canine intestinal T-cell lymphoma suggests large cell transformation of small cell lymphoma may occur rather than the existence of two distinct entities (Matsumoto et al., 2019a). Other round cell tumors, including mast cell neoplasia, may involve the small intestine (Fig. 7.73).

Intestinal adenocarcinoma is the most commonly diagnosed intestinal neoplasm in dogs and the second most commonly diagnosed tumor in cats. On cytopathology, these cells have the general characteristics of neoplastic epithelial cells from other sites (Fig. 7.74). In our experience, other intestinal neoplasms (e.g., leiomyosarcoma, leiomyoma, and fibrosarcoma) are difficult to diagnose cytopathologically because of their deeper location and decreased tendency to exfoliate; they also occur far less commonly than lymphoma and adenocarcinoma.

COLON, CECAL, AND RECTUM

Normal Cytology

Colonic and cecal cytopathologic specimens consist of groups or sheets of uniform columnar epithelial cells with a higher frequency than the small intestine of goblet cells that contain mucin and basilar nuclei (Fig. 7.75). A prominent mixed bacterial flora is a common finding. Rectal scrapings contain columnar epithelial clusters and fecal material. Aggregated lymphoid follicles are present in the colon and a mixture of small, medium, and large lymphocytes are observed cytologically. Fecal cytopathology is covered in detail in Chapter 10.

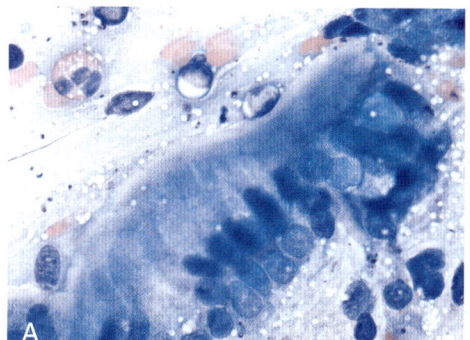
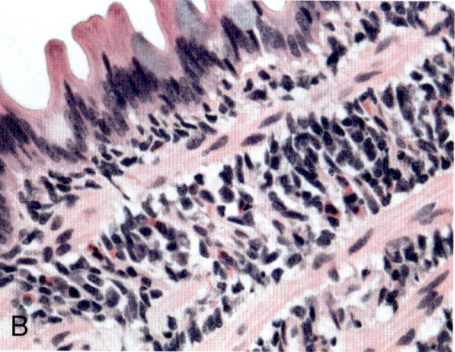
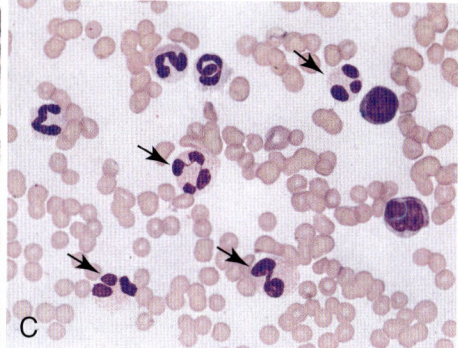

FIGURE 7.69 Enteritis. A, Eosinophilic enteritis. Dog. Imprint. Two medium-sized lymphocytes and an eosinophil *(upper left)* are associated with a row of uniform epithelial cells embedded in a blue-gray mucinous background. (Modified Wright; HP oil.) **B, Eosinophilic enteritis. Endoscopic biopsy histology. Dog.** Increased numbers of eosinophils are present within the lamina propria. (H&E; HP oil.) **C, Eosinophilic, neutrophilic, and lymphocytic enteritis. Ileum. Brushing. Cat.** This patient presented with chronic diarrhea and weight loss. Increased numbers of eosinophils *(arrows)*, neutrophils, and lymphocytes were noted on the specimen, as well as moderate hemodilution; however, complete blood count data were within reference intervals at the time of sample collection. Inflammatory bowel disease was suspected as the cause of the inflammation by histopathology. (Modified Wright; HP oil.)

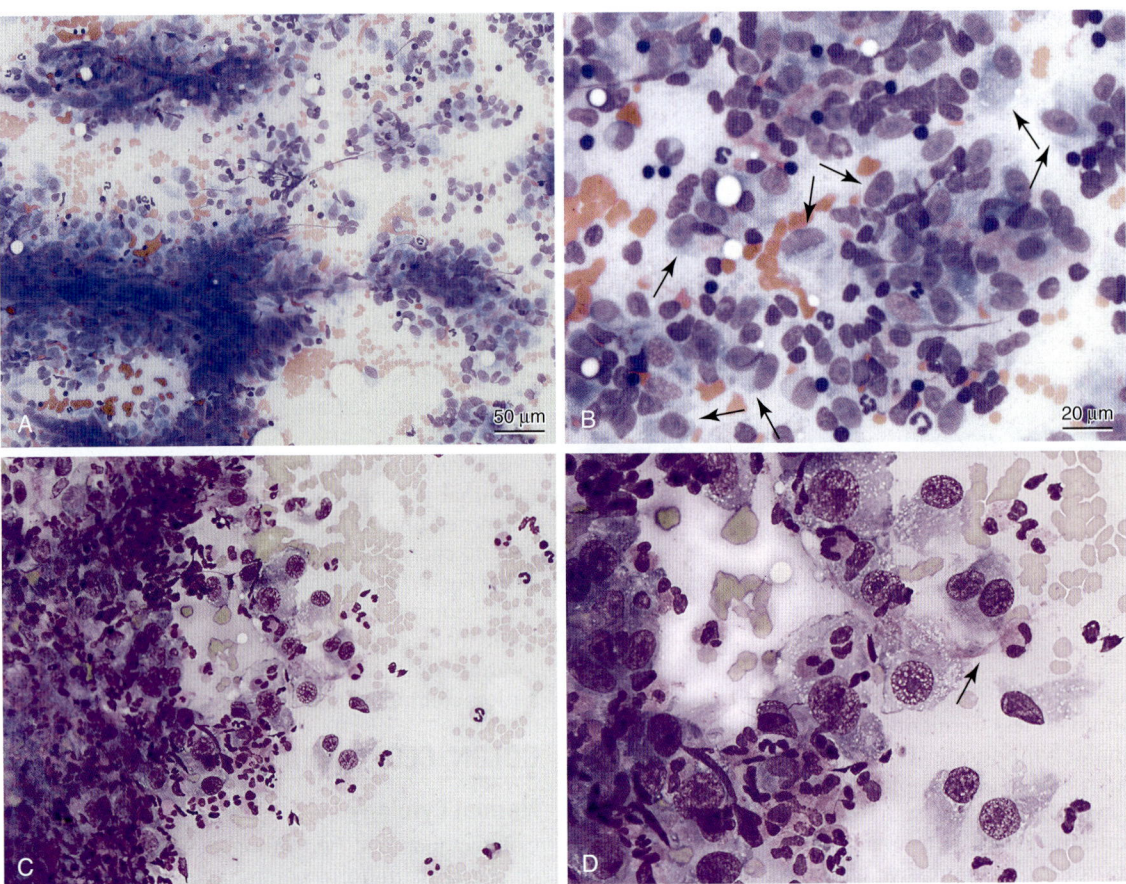

■ **FIGURE 7.70 Feline gastrointestinal eosinophilic sclerosing fibroplasia (FGESF). Jejunal aspirate. Cat.** Same case in A and B. **A,** Highly cellular specimen composed of atypical mesenchymal cells, small lymphocytes, and occasional neutrophils. Eosinophils not shown. Mesenchymal cells present as loose aggregates or storiform fashion. (Wright-Giemsa; IP.) **B,** Mildly to moderately atypical mesenchymal cells *(arrows)* predominate and appear individually or in small aggregates admixed with bright eosinophilic matrix material. These cells are fusiform or stellate with wispy indistinct cytoplasmic borders and a moderate amount of medium basophilic cytoplasm occasionally containing few clear punctate vacuoles. Histopathology is warranted to rule out other inflammatory or neoplastic conditions. (Wright-Giemsa; HP oil.) **Presumptive FGESF. Jejunal lymph node. Aspirate. Cat.** Same case in C and D. **C,** Dense collections of eosinophils with lesser numbers of neutrophils and atypical spindle cells were present in some areas. (Wright, HP oil.) **D,** Higher magnification to show amorphous, eosinophilic matrix material *(arrow)* associated with the spindle cells. Numerous eosinophils with atypical spindle mesenchymal cells were present in aspirates from the corresponding jejunal mass in this patient. (Wright; HP oil.)

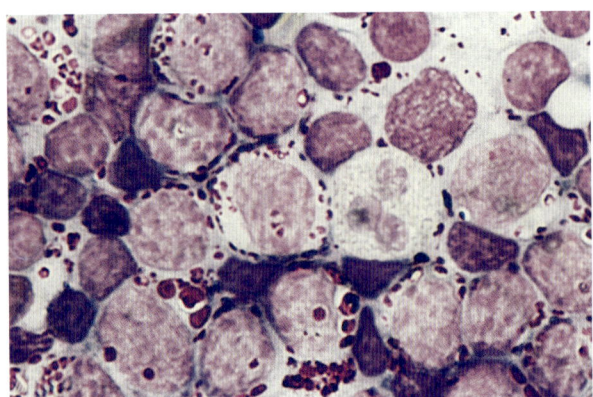

■ **FIGURE 7.71 Large granular lymphoma. Abdominal mass. Aspirate. Cat.** This monomorphic population is composed of lymphoid cells with a round to oval nucleus and ropy chromatin surrounded by a minimal to moderate amount of lightly basophilic cytoplasm that contains prominent coarse variably sized metachromatic granules. Darkly stained small lymphocytes are sandwiched among the neoplastic cells, and a segmented eosinophil with faintly stained granules is centrally located. At surgery, the confluent mass involved the lymph nodes and small intestine. (Wright; HP oil.)

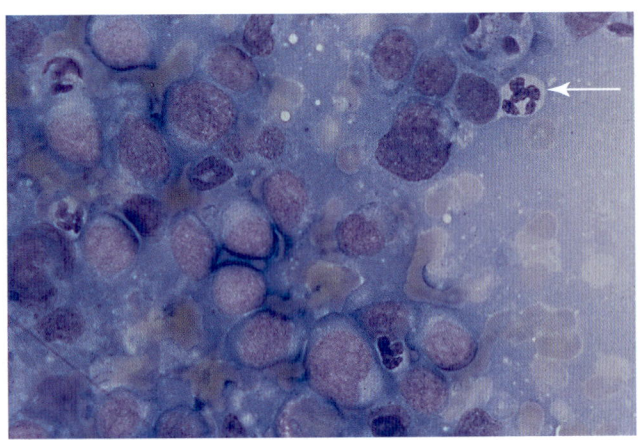

■ **FIGURE 7.72 Intestinal lymphoma. Imprint. Dog.** Numerous medium and large lymphoid cells are embedded in basophilic stained mucus. These immature lymphocytes have an oval to irregularly shaped nucleus composed of homogeneous, pale-staining chromatin surrounded by minimal to moderately abundant lightly basophilic cytoplasm. Their size can be appreciated by comparison with the neutrophil *(arrow)* and adjacent erythrocyte. (Wright; HP oil.) (Courtesy Denny Meyer, University of Florida.)

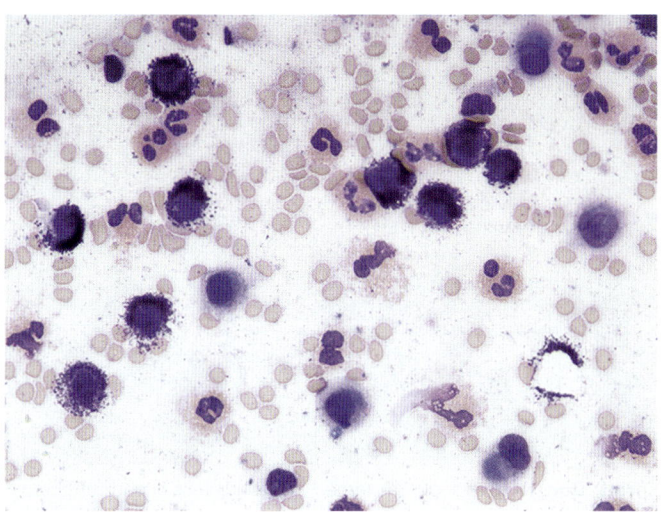

■ **FIGURE 7.73 Mast cell neoplasia. Jejunal mass. Aspirate. Cat.** Numerous well-granulated mast cells and eosinophils predominate in this aspirate from a feline mast cell tumor involving the small intestine. (Modified Wright; IP.)

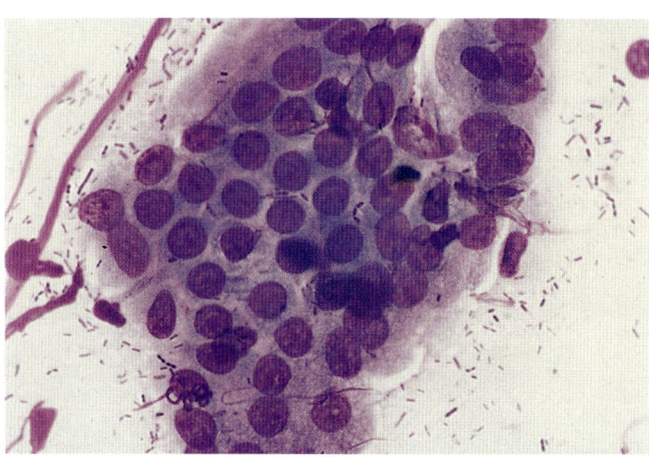

■ **FIGURE 7.75 Normal colonic epithelial cells. Imprint.** The sheet of epithelial cells demonstrates uniform cytomorphologic features and staining. Numerous bacteria of varying size and shapes are a normal finding. (Wright; HP oil.)

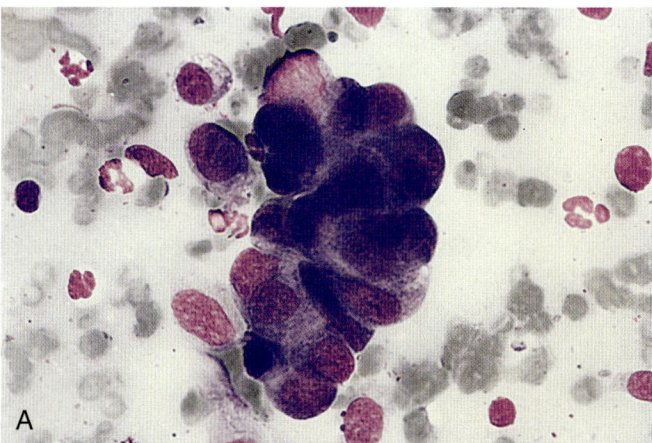

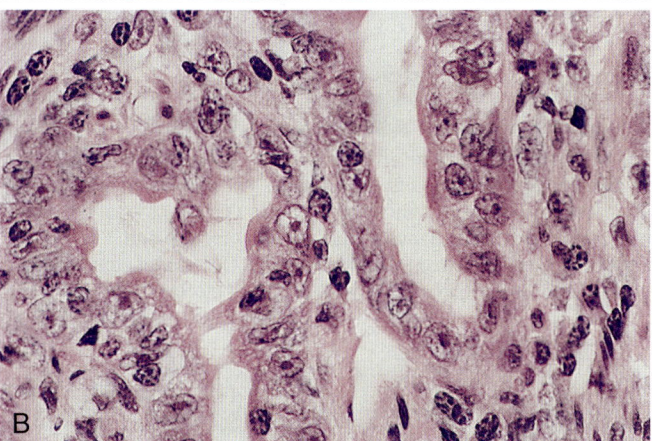

■ **FIGURE 7.74 Intestinal adenocarcinoma. A, Imprint.** Epithelial cells in this dense cluster demonstrate increased basophilia, marked anisocytosis and anisokaryosis, variable nucleocytoplasmic ratios, and overgrowth of neighboring cells. Their large size is appreciated by comparison with the neutrophils. (Wright; HP oil.) **B, Histology.** Disorganized epithelial tubules are formed by cells that demonstrate moderate to marked anisocytosis and anisokaryosis, variable nuclear chromatin patterns, prominent nucleoli, and variable nucleocytoplasmic ratios. (H&E; HP oil.)

Hyperplasia

Observing a relatively normal-appearing mucosa endoscopically combined with a cytopathologic finding of a uniform population of epithelial cells supports a diagnosis of mucosal hyperplasia (polyp) or adenoma. Hyperplastic epithelial cells can have mild cellular atypia and distinct nucleoli, especially associated with rectal mucosal hyperplasia (Fig. 7.76).

Inflammation

The finding of neutrophils indicates active inflammation involving the colon, rectum, or both because neutrophils entering the more proximal intestinal lumen would be rapidly destroyed (Fig. 7.77A). Possible infectious causes of neutrophilic colitis include bacteria (*Clostridium perfringens*; Fig. 7.77B), *Campylobacter jejuni*, *Salmonella* spp., an enterotoxic strain of *E. coli*, and parasites (*Trichuris vulpis*) (Fig. 7.78). A relationship between infection with *Clostridium perfringens* type A and acute hemorrhagic diarrhea syndrome in dogs (formerly known as *canine hemorrhagic gastroenteritis*) has been suggested (Leipig-Rudolph et al., 2018). The presence of small to medium lymphocytes with or without plasma cells is consistent with a generic morphologic impression of chronic colitis (Fig. 7.79). Macrophagic inflammation can be found in some forms of IBD, specifically granulomatous colitis. Traditionally known as a cause of hematochezia and weight loss in boxer dogs and more recently attributed to infection with an adherent and invasive strain of *E. coli*, a similar syndrome has also been described in cats (Simpson et al., 2006; Matsumoto et al., 2019b). Hemorrhage induced by sampling is common in colonic and rectal sampling. Leukocytes in the blood can confound the cytopathologic interpretation, especially if there is a concurrent leukocytosis.

The identification of either neutrophilic or macrophagic inflammation in colonic or rectal samples can also be associated with infectious causes of colitis. These samples can be used to detect infectious agents such as *Prototheca* spp. (rectum), *Histoplasma capsulatum* (intestine, rectum), *Balantidium coli* (rectum), *Blastocystis hominis* (rectum), and *Cryptococcus neoformans* (intestine) (Chapman et al., 2009). *Prototheca* spp. are

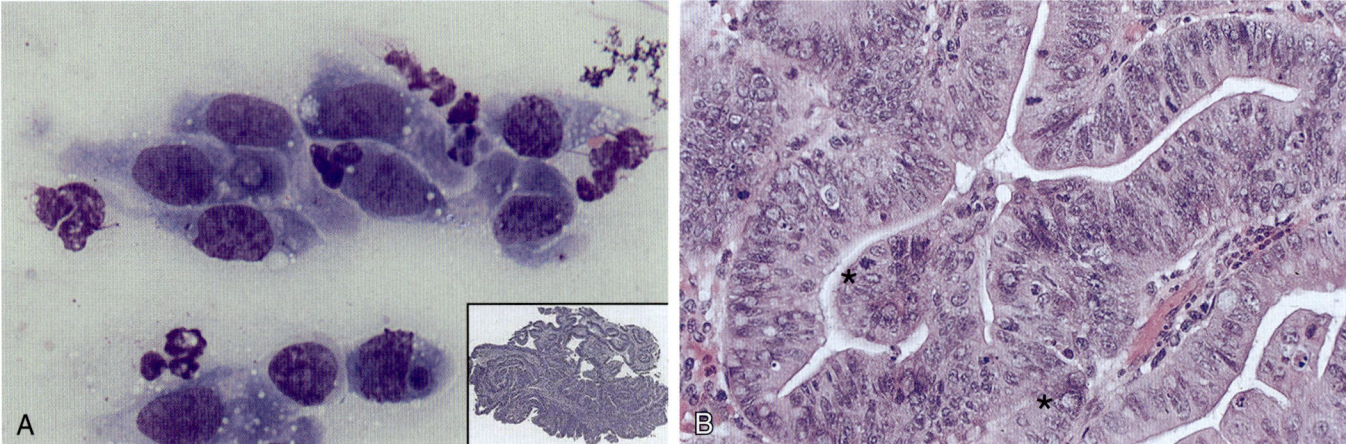

■ **FIGURE 7.76 Hyperplastic colonic epithelial cells. A, Colon mass imprint. Dog.** A 12-year-old rat terrier with a 1.5-year history of chronic diarrhea and hematochezia was found to have a polypoid mass on ultrasound. Cytopathologic differential considerations for this mass lesion are polyp, adenoma, or well-differentiated carcinoma. (Modified Wright; HP oil.) *Inset:* Subgross histology reveals a poorly delineated mass within the mucosa. Cells are arranged in gland and ductlike structures supported by a fine fibrovascular stroma. Mitoses are not seen. There are scattered lymphocytes and other inflammatory cells. Histopathologic diagnosis is colonic mucosal polyp, adenoma, and hyperplasia with mild multifocal lymphocytic infiltrates (H&E; LP.) **B, Histology.** A second case example with papillary projections *(asterisks)* covered by hyperplastic columnar mucosal epithelial cells with basilar nuclei, coarse chromatin, and prominent nucleoli. The tissue architecture is consistent with a benign lesion. (H&E; IP.) (A, Courtesy Karena Tang, Purdue University. Inset, Courtesy Mark Ackermann.)

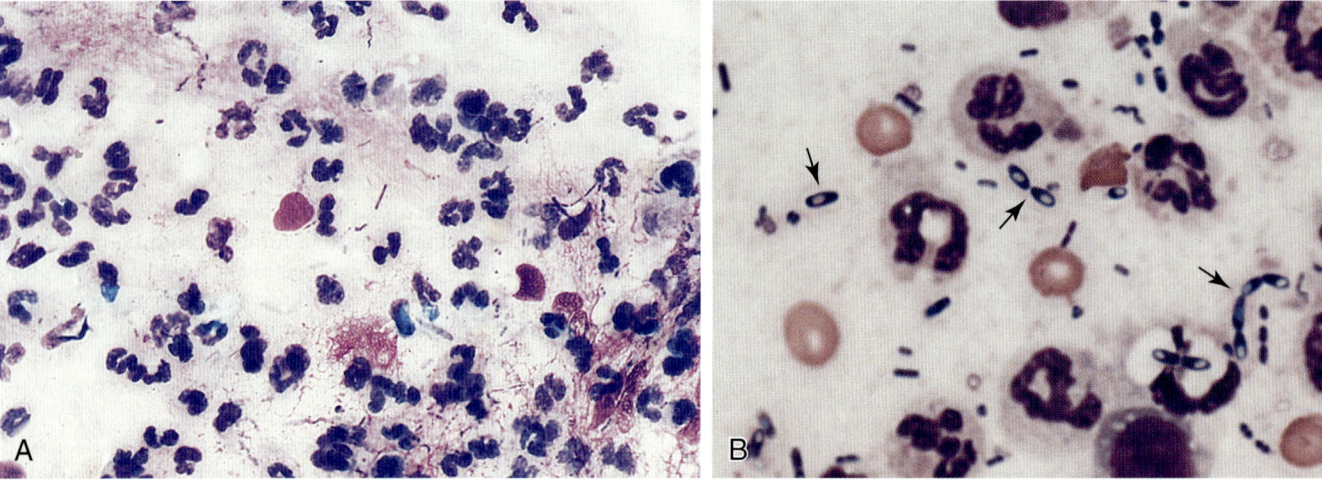

■ **FIGURE 7.77 Neutrophilic colitis. A, Scraping.** Neutrophils are the predominant inflammatory cell. Colonic bacterial flora is admixed. Differential diagnostic considerations include infections by *Campylobacter*, *Salmonella*, *Clostridium*, and *Trichuris*. A cause was not determined in this case. (Wright; HP oil.) **B, Clostridial colitis. Rectal smear.** Numerous neutrophils are the predominant inflammatory cell in this direct fecal smear. An increased number of large rod-shaped bacterial endospores with a clear center and an increased density predominantly on one end ("safety pin" appearance) are the notable feature *(short arrows)*. The bacterial morphology is consistent with *Clostridium perfringens*. Occasional organisms can be normally seen, but greater than 5 organisms per 1000× oil field is considered abnormal. (Wright; HP oil.) (B, Courtesy Rose Raskin, Purdue University.)

colorless algae (1.3–13.4 μm wide × 1.3–16.1 μm long) with basophilic granular cytoplasm, a clear cell wall, and a small nucleus (Fig. 7.80). Endosporulation may be noted. Systemic fungal infections can be initially detected by a rectal scraping. These include *H. capsulatum* (2–4 μm), which is often located within macrophages, and *C. neoformans* (yeast, 3.5–7 μm) with its microscopic hallmark of a prominent clear, nonstaining capsule. Although *H. capsulatum* traditionally exists in yeast form, it rarely can also have a hyphae-like morphology (Schumacher et al., 2013) (Fig. 7.81). *Balantidium coli* (40–80 μm × 25–45 μm to 30–300 μm × 30–100 μm) is a ciliated protozoan that infects dogs ingesting pig feces. It is thought that damage to the colonic mucosa by trichuriasis may predispose to *B. coli* infection. *Blastomyces dermatitidis* (yeast, 7–15 μm) may be found as a refractile, deeply basophilic yeast with a thick cell wall in the stomach, intestine, and/or colon (see Fig. 7.67B). *Pythium insidiosum*, a

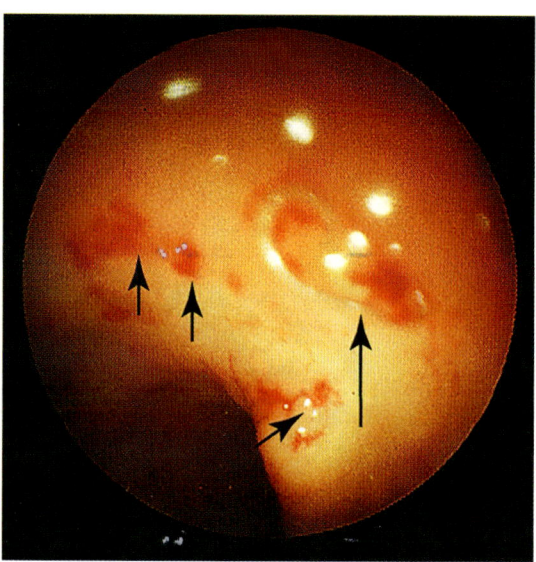

■ **FIGURE 7.78** ***Trichuris vulpis*-induced colitis. Endoscopic view.** *T. vulpis* is attached to a hemorrhagic colonic mucosal site *(long arrow)*. Several other areas of mucosal inflammation and hemorrhage are present *(short arrows)*. A moderate number of neutrophils were observed in a fecal smear (not shown). (Courtesy Colin Burrows and Denny Meyer, University of Florida.)

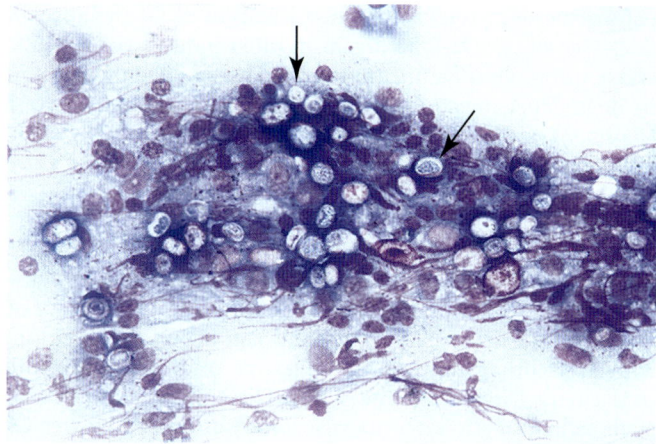

■ **FIGURE 7.80** ***Prototheca* spp. Colonic imprint.** The algae appear as variably sized, oval clear structures with eosinophilic to basophilic stippling *(arrows)*. The organisms are embedded in a dense sheet of epithelial cells. (Wright; HP oil.)

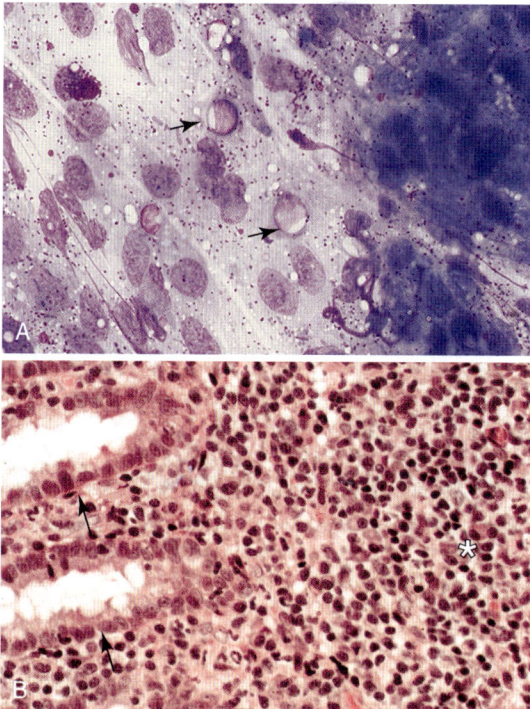

■ **FIGURE 7.79 Lymphocytic colitis. A, Imprint.** An increased number of small to medium-sized lymphocytes having a round to oval nucleus with homogeneous chromatin and a small rim of clear to lightly basophilic cytoplasm is present *(arrows)*. Dense basophilic clusters of epithelial cells *(far right)* and abundant mucin granules suggestive of mucosal hyperplasia are set in a lightly basophilic background of mucus. (Wright; HP oil.) **B, Histology.** There is a moderate to marked increase in small to medium-sized lymphocytes that invade the deeper mucosal region *(asterisk)*. Hypertrophic mucosal glands *(arrows)* are lined by prominent goblet cells with large clear mucous–filled vacuoles. (H&E; HP oil.)

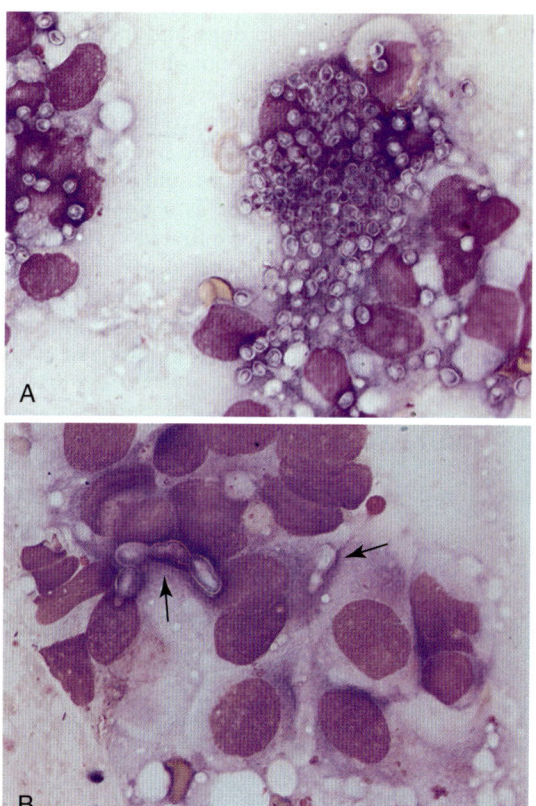

■ **FIGURE 7.81 *Histoplasma capsulatum*. Colon brushing. Dog.** Same case in A and B. **A,** This patient had significant inflammatory enteritis and colitis (predominantly macrophagic and lymphoplasmacytic) and numerous oval yeast present both within macrophages and free within the background. The morphology of the yeast depicted in this image is classic for *H. capsulatum*, and similar yeast were found in the small intestinal cytopathologic specimens as well. (Modified Wright, HP oil.) **B,** In addition to the more classic yeast forms; in some areas of the colonic samples, the yeast appeared to form hyphae *(arrows)*. This is an uncommon yet previously documented morphology of the organism. (Modified Wright; HP oil.)

pathogenic oomycete, is the causative agent of GI pythiosis in dogs (see Fig. 7.49). The organism often induces eosinophilic and neutrophilic inflammation and can be confined to the colon in dogs. Dual infections with *Pythium* and pathogenic yeast (*Blastomyces*, *Basidiobolus*) have been reported (Connolly et al., 2012; Parambeth et al., 2019).

Neoplasia

Colonic carcinoma/adenocarcinoma and lymphoma (Figs. 7.82 and 7.83) are most commonly diagnosed and appear cytopathologically similar to those described in other parts of the intestinal tract. Plasmacytomas can occur in the colon, as well as other areas of the digestive tract, including the oral cavity (Figs. 7.84 and 7.85). Disseminated neoplasia, such as histiocytic sarcoma, also rarely affects the lower GI tract (Fig. 7.86).

Gastrointestinal stromal tumor (GIST) may occur in dogs and is thought to be derived from the interstitial cells of Cajal (Munday et al., 2017). These tumors may affect the stomach, intestines, and cecum. Differentials for GIST should include leiomyosarcoma but are generally more aggressive with a higher rate of metastasis. Only the spindle-shaped and epithelioid variants have been recognized in dogs, and the most common GIST are spindle shaped. If a tumor does not express KIT (CD117) using immunochemistry, then GIST should be ruled out. Around 75% of canine GISTs also contain detectable S100 expression with variable expression of smooth muscle actin, desmin, neuron-specific enolase, CD34, and protein gene product 9.5. Histologically, they appear as a poorly demarcated, nonencapsulated, expansive to infiltrative proliferation of neoplastic mesenchymal cells arranged in streams, whorls, and interwoven bundles supported by fine fibrous or myxomatous stroma. Neoplastic cells are spindle shaped with indistinct cell borders and contain small to moderate amounts of cytoplasm.

Nuclei are ovoid to elongate, finely stippled to vesiculated, and often contain one distinct nucleolus. Anisokaryosis is moderate, and mitotic figures are frequent. On cytopathology, the background may contain abundant dense eosinophilic myxoid matrix (Fig. 7.87). Therapy for GIST involves use of a tyrosine kinase inhibitor drug.

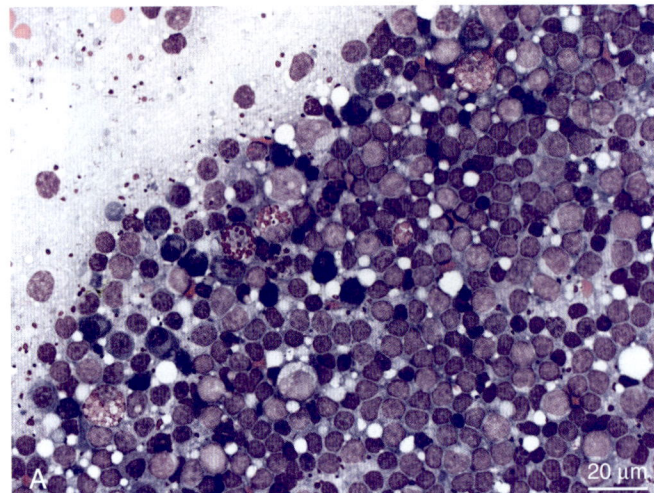
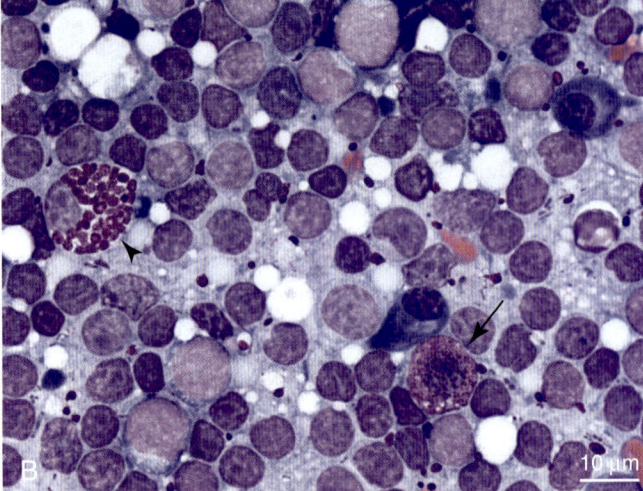

■ **FIGURE 7.83 B-cell lymphoma. Cecal mass. Imprint. Cat.** Same case in A and B. **A,** This cat had lymphocytosis, weight loss, thickened bowel loops, and abdominal lymphadenomegaly. **A,** The lymphoid cells were numerous and consisted of a heterogeneous population. Scattered among these cells are a low to moderate number of globule leukocytes identified by a small round nucleus (size of an erythrocyte) with abundant clear cytoplasm containing numerous large round variably stained magenta granules. (Wright-Giemsa; HP oil.) **B,** Small lymphocytes predominate with an expanded number of intermediate lymphocytes and plasma cells along with a mild increase in large lymphoid cells. One well-differentiated mast cell *(arrow)* with small granules is seen along with a globule leukocyte *(arrowhead)*. These cells have a low to moderate nucleocytoplasmic ratio. Cytopathology considered a reactive lymphoid cell population and suggested further diagnostics. Histopathology identified expansion of the lymphoid cells from the lamina propria and subsequent polymerase chain reaction for antigen receptor rearrangement testing supported a clonal B-cell population. (Wright-Giemsa; HP oil.) (Courtesy Rose Raskin, University of Florida.)

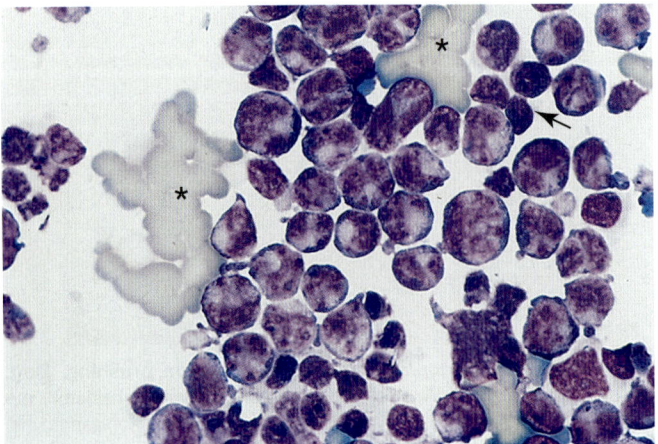

■ **FIGURE 7.82 Colonic lymphoma. Imprint.** Pleomorphic medium to large lymphoid cells composed of irregularly shaped to reniform to convoluted nuclei surrounded by moderately abundant dark basophilic cytoplasm are the notable abnormal microscopic finding. Their anaplastic morphology makes them difficult to recognize as a lymphoid cell type. A few small lymphocytes with dense nuclei and minimal cytoplasm are admixed *(arrow)*. Two small islands of yellow-green erythrocytes are present *(asterisks)*. (Wright; HP oil.)

CHAPTER 7 Oral Cavity, Gastrointestinal Tract, and Associated Structures

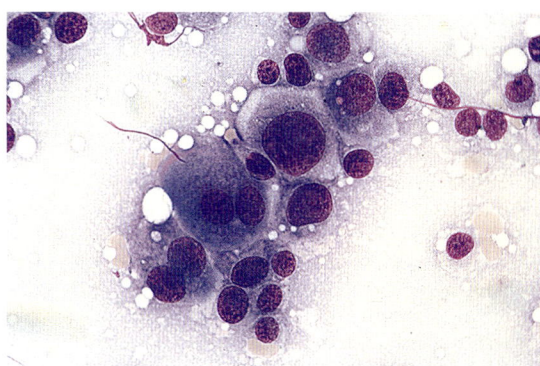

■ **FIGURE 7.84 Colonic plasmacytoma. Imprint. Dog.** These cells demonstrate characteristics of malignancy that include marked anisocytosis and anisokaryosis and variable nucleocytoplasmic ratio. Although they have morphologic features that are consistent with an anaplastic carcinoma, the eccentric nucleus and basophilic cytoplasm is also suggestive of a plasma cell derivation. Histopathology along with immunohistochemical staining of the tissue biopsy confirmed a plasmacytoma. (Wright; HP oil.)

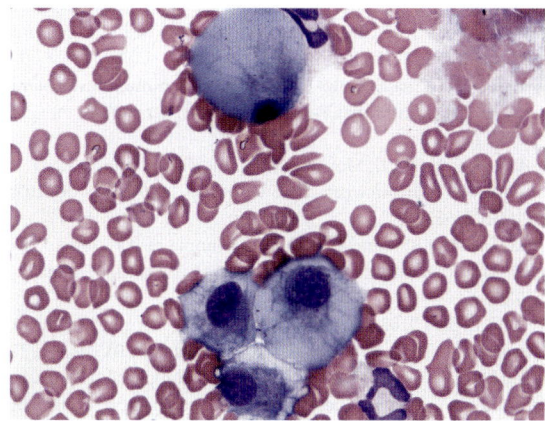

■ **FIGURE 7.85 Colonic plasmacytoma. Scraping. Dog.** The neoplastic plasma cells had a Mott cell morphology with cytoplasm distended with indistinct Russell bodies (immunoglobulin). Numerous erythrocytes and a single neutrophil *(lower right)* also are shown. (Modified Wright; HP oil.)

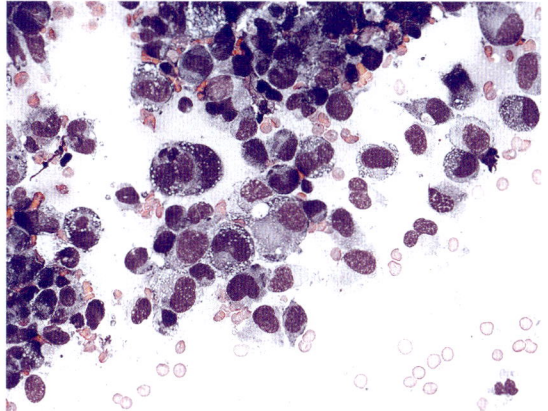

■ **FIGURE 7.86 Histiocytic sarcoma. Colon brushing. Dog.** Depicted are numerous pleomorphic, individualized, round to spindle-shaped cells from a patient with disseminated histiocytic sarcoma. Many cells have a reniform nucleus and clear cytoplasmic vacuoles. Some cells are multinucleated. (Modified Wright, IP.)

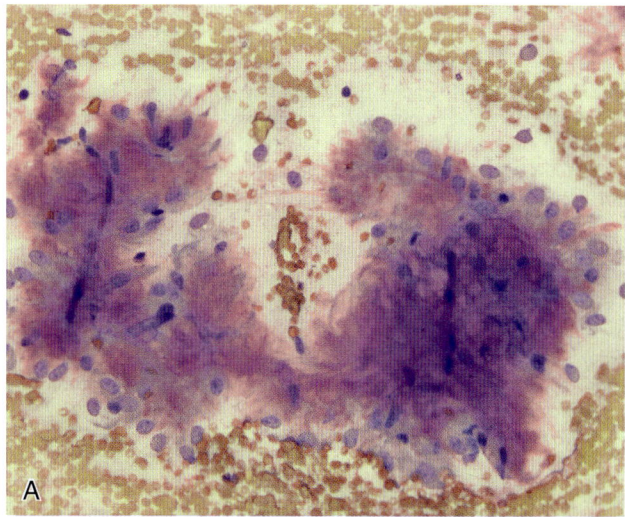

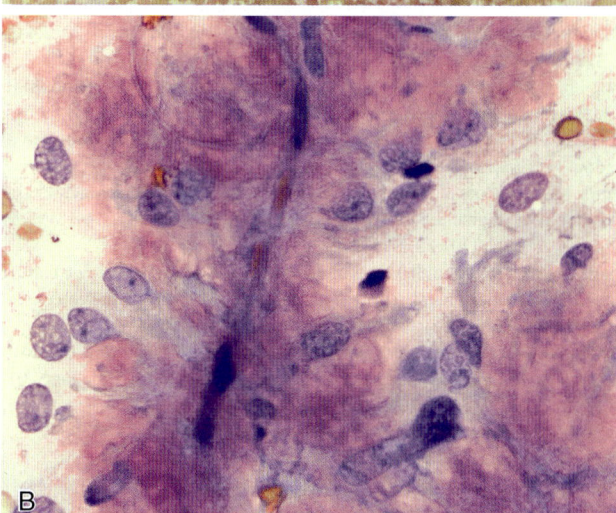

■ **FIGURE 7.87 Gastrointestinal stromal tumor (GIST). Cecal mass. Aspirate. Dog.** Same case in A and B. **A,** There was history of chronic vomiting, diarrhea, hematochezia, and tenesmus related to the intestinal mass. Abundant amounts of fibrillar pink extracellular matrix are present with enclosed capillaries and low numbers of intact spindle cells. (Wright-Giemsa; IP.) **B,** The intact spindle cells have an oval nucleus with stippled chromatin and one to two small nucleoli. There were small to moderate amounts of light blue cytoplasm. Anisocytosis and anisokaryosis were mild. On histopathology, a spindle cell tumor was diagnosed and about 90% of the neoplastic cells had weak to strong cytoplasmic labeling for KIT (CD117) confirming the diagnosis of a GIST. (Wright-Giemsa; HP oil.) (Courtesy Rose Raskin, Michigan State University.)

REFERENCES

Alcoverro E, Tabar MD, Lloret A. Phenobarbital-responsive sialadenosis in dogs: case series, *Top Companion Anim Med*. 2014;29(4):109-112.

Allen J, Talley AM, Grindem CB, et al. What is your diagnosis? Submandibular mass in a dog. *Vet Clin Pathol*. 2018;47:676-678.

Amorim I, Smet A, Alves O, et al. Presence and significance of *Helicobacter* spp. in the gastric mucosa of Portuguese dogs. *Gut Pathog*. 2015;7:12.

Beatty JA, Swift N, Foster DJ, et al. Suspected clindamycin-associated oesophageal injury in cats: five cases. *J Feline Med Surg*. 2006;8(6):412-419.

Berryessa NA, Marks SL, Pesavento PA, et al. Gastrointestinal pythiosis in 10 dogs from California. *J Vet Intern Med*. 2008;22(4):1065-1069.

Bonfanti U, Bertazzolo W, Gracis M, et al. Diagnostic value of cytological analysis of tumours and tumour-like lesions of the oral cavity in dogs and cats: a prospective study on 114 cases. *Vet J.* 2015;205(2):322-327.

Bongard AB, Furrow E, Granick JL. Retrospective evaluation of factors associated with degree of esophagitis, treatment, and outcomes in dogs presenting with esophageal foreign bodies (2004-2014): 114 cases. *J Vet Emerg Crit Care.* 2019;29(5):528-534.

Boydell P, Pike R, Crossley D. Sialadenosis in dogs. *J Am Vet Med Assoc.* 2000; 216:872-874.

Carrasco V, Rodriguez-Bertos A, Rodriguez-Franco F, et al. Distinguishing intestinal lymphoma from inflammatory bowel disease in canine duodenal endoscopic biopsy samples. *Vet Pathol.* 2015;52(4):668-675.

Chapman S, Nabity M, Calise D. What is your diagnosis? Lingual mass in a dog. *Vet Clin Pathol.* 2008;37(1):133-139.

Chapman S, Thompson C, Wilcox A, et al. What is your diagnosis? Rectal scraping from a dog with diarrhea. *Vet Clin Pathol.* 2009;38(1):59-62.

Ciekot PA, Powers BE, Withrow SJ, et al. Histologically low-grade, yet biologically high-grade, fibrosarcomas of the mandible and maxilla in dogs: 25 cases (1982-1991). *J Am Vet Med Assoc.* 1994;204(4):610-615.

Connolly SL, Frank C, Thompson CA, et al. Dual infection with *Pythium insidiosum* and *Blastomyces dermatitidis* in a dog. *Vet Clin Pathol.* 2012;41(3): 419-423.

Craig LE, Hardam EE, Hertzke DM, et al. Feline gastrointestinal eosinophilic sclerosing fibroplasia. *Vet Pathol.* 2009;46(1):63-70.

De Lorenzi D, Furlanello T. What is your diagnosis? Esophageal nodules in a dog. *Vet Clin Pathol.* 2010;39:391-392.

Dennis MM, Ehrhart N, Duncan CG, et al. Frequency of and risk factors associated with lingual lesions in dogs: 1,196 cases (1995-2004). *J Am Vet Med Assoc.* 2006;228(10):1533-1537.

Desoutter AV, Goldschmidt MH, Sanchez MD. Clinical and histologic features of 26 canine peripheral giant cell granulomas (formerly giant cell epulis). *Vet Pathol.* 2012;49(6):1018-1023.

Duchaussoy AC, Rose A, Talbot JJ, et al. Gastrointestinal granuloma due to *Candida albicans* in an immunocompetent cat. *Med Mycol Case Rep.* 2015; 10:14-17.

Duncan RB, Feldman BF, Saunders GK, et al. Mandibular salivary gland aspirate from a dog. *Vet Clin Pathol.* 1999;28(3):97-99.

Finotello R, Vasconi ME, Sabattini S, et al. Feline large granular lymphocyte lymphoma: an Italian Society of Veterinary Oncology (SIONCOV) retrospective study. *Vet Comp Oncol.* 2018;16(1):159-166.

German AJ, Holden DJ, Hall EJ, et al. Eosinophilic diseases in two Cavalier King Charles spaniels. *J Small Anim Pract.* 2002;43(12):533-538.

Grooters AM, Hodgin EC, Bauer RW, et al. Clinicopathologic findings associated with *Lagenidium* sp. infection in 6 dogs: initial description of an emerging oomycosis. *J Vet Intern Med.* 2003;17(5):637-646.

Happonen I, Saari S, Castren L, et al. Comparison of diagnostic methods for detecting gastric *Helicobacter*-like organisms in dogs and cats. *J Comp Pathol.* 1996;115(2):117-127.

Helman RG, Oliver J. Pythiosis of the digestive tract in dogs from Oklahoma. *J Am Anim Hosp Assoc.* 1999;35(2):111-114.

Hermanns W, Kregel K, Breuer W, et al. *Helicobacter*-like organisms: histopathological examination of gastric biopsies from dogs and cats. *J Comp Pathol.* 1995;112(3):307-318.

Iwaki Y, Monahan C, Smedley R, et al. Tonsillar plasmacytoma in a dog. *Can Vet J.* 2018;59(8):851-854.

Jergens AE, Andreasen CB, Hagemoser WA, et al. Cytologic examination of exfoliative specimens obtained during endoscopy for diagnosis of gastrointestinal tract disease in dogs and cats. *J Am Vet Med Assoc.* 1998;213(12):1755-1759.

Jergens AE, Hostetter SJ, Andreasen CB. Oral cavity, gastrointestinal tract, and associated structures. In: Raskin RE, Meyer DJ, eds. *Canine and Feline Cytology. A Color Atlas and Interpretation Guide.* 3rd ed. St. Louis: Elsevier; 2016a:231.

Jergens AE, Willard MD, Allenspach K. Maximizing the diagnostic utility of endoscopic biopsy in dogs and cats with gastrointestinal disease. *Vet J.* 2016b;214:50-60.

Joffe DJ, Allen AL. Ulcerative eosinophilic stomatitis in three Cavalier King Charles spaniels. *J Am Anim Hosp Assoc.* 1995;31(1):34-37.

Kouki MI, Papadimitriou SA, Psalla D. Chronic gingivostomatitis with esophagitis in cats. *J Vet Intern Med.* 2017;31(6):1673-1679.

Kwon SJ, Hong YJ, Choi US. What is your diagnosis? Gingival mass in a cat. *Vet Clin Pathol.* 2019;48:361-363.

Leipig-Rudolph M, Busch K, Prescott JF, et al. Intestinal lesions in dogs with acute hemorrhagic diarrhea syndrome associated with netF-positive *Clostridium perfringens* type A. *J Vet Diagn Invest.* 2018;30(4):495-503.

Leite-Filho RV, Tagliari NJ, Grandi F, et al. Cytologic features of a feline inductive odontogenic tumor. *Vet Clin Pathol.* 2017;46(3):516-519.

Linton M, Nimmo JS, Norris JM, et al. Feline gastrointestinal eosinophilic sclerosing fibroplasia: 13 cases and review of an emerging clinical entity. *J Feline Med Surg.* 2015;17(5):392-404.

Lommer MJ. Oral inflammation in small animals. *Vet Clin North Am Small Anim Pract.* 2013;43(3):555-571.

Maeda S, Tsuboi M, Sakai K, et al. Endoscopic cytology for the diagnosis of chronic enteritis and intestinal lymphoma in dogs. *Vet Pathol.* 2017;54(4):595-604.

Marcos R, Santos M, Oliveira J, et al. Cytochemical detection of calcium in a case of calcinosis circumscripta in a dog. *Vet Clin Pathol.* 2006;35(2): 239-242.

Marsilio S, Ackermann MR, Lidbury JA, et al. Results of histopathology, immunohistochemistry, and molecular clonality testing of small intestinal biopsy specimens from clinically healthy client-owned cats. *J Vet Intern Med.* 2019;33(2):551-558.

Matsumoto I, Nakashima K, Goto-Koshino Y, et al. Immunohistochemical profiling of canine intestinal T-cell lymphomas. *Vet Pathol.* 2019a;56(1):50-60.

Matsumoto I, Nakashima K, Morita H, et al. *Escherichia coli*-induced granulomatous colitis in a cat. *JFMS Open Rep.* 2019b;5(1). doi:10.1177/2055116919836537.

Mazzullo G, Sfacteria A, Iannelli N, et al. Carcinoma of the submandibular salivary glands with multiple metastases in a cat. *Vet Clin Pathol.* 2005;34:61-64.

McEntire MC, Rigas JD, Farnsworth RK, et al. What is your diagnosis? Oral soft tissue and cystic lesion in a dog. *Vet Clin Pathol.* 2015;44(2):327-328.

Mendelsohn D, Lewis JR, Scott KI, et al. Clinicopathological features, risk factors and predispositions, and response to treatment of eosinophilic oral disease in 24 dogs (2000-2016). *J Vet Dent.* 2019;36(1):25-31.

Mikiewicz M, Pazdzior-Czapula K, Gesek M, et al. Canine and feline oral cavity tumours and tumour-like lesions: a retrospective study of 486 cases (2015-2017). *J Comp Pathol.* 2019;172:80-87.

Munday JS, Löhr CV, Kiupel M. Tumors of the alimentary tract. In: Meuten DJ, ed. *Tumors in Domestic Animals.* 5th ed. Ames, IA: John Wiley & Sons Inc.; 2017:499-601.

Murphy BG, Bell CM, Soukup JW. *Veterinary Oral and Maxillofacial Pathology.* Hoboken, NJ: Wiley-Blackwell; 2020.

Neiger R, Simpson KW. *Helicobacter* infection in dogs and cats: facts and fiction. *J Vet Intern Med.* 2000;14(2):125-133.

Newman AW, Asakawa MG, Stokol T. What is your diagnosis? Mandibular mass in a cat. *Vet Clin Pathol.* 2018;47:501-502.

Noland EL, Kiupel M. Coexpression of CD3 and CD20 in canine enteropathy-associated T-cell lymphoma. *Vet Pathol.* 2018;55(2):241-244.

O'Connell K, Leach J, Berman K, et al. What is your diagnosis? Salivary gland mass in a dog. *Vet Clin Pathol.* 2016;45(2):389-390.

Ozaki K, Yamagami T, Nomura K, et al. T-cell lymphoma with eosinophilic infiltration involving the intestinal tract in 11 dogs. *Vet Pathol.* 2006; 43(3):339-344.

Palic J, Parker VJ, Fales-Williams AJ, et al. What is your diagnosis? Duodenal brush preparation from a dog. *Vet Clin Pathol.* 2012;41(3):431-432.

Parambeth JC, Lawhon SD, Mansell J, et al. Gastrointestinal pythiosis with concurrent presumptive gastrointestinal basidiobolomycosis in a boxer dog. *Vet Clin Pathol.*2019;48(1):83-88.

Pera J, Palma D, Donovan TA. Eosinophilic esophagitis in a kitten. *J Am Anim Hosp Assoc.* 2017;53(4):214-220.

Piseddu E, De Lorenzi D, Freeman K, et al. Cytologic, histologic, and immunohistochemical features of lingual liposarcoma in a dog. *Vet Clin Pathol.* 2011;40(3):393-397.

Przezdziecki R, Czopowicz M, Sapierzynski R. Accuracy of routine cytology and immunocytochemistry in preoperative diagnosis of oral amelanotic melanomas in dogs. *Vet Clin Pathol.* 2015;44(4):597-604.

Ruiz G, Verrot L, Laloy E, et al. Diagnostic contribution of cytological specimens obtained from biopsies during gastrointestinal endoscopy in dogs and cats. *J Small Anim Pract.* 2017;58(1):17-22.

Sabattini S, Bottero E, Turba ME, et al. Differentiating feline inflammatory bowel disease from alimentary lymphoma in duodenal endoscopic biopsies. *J Small Anim Pract.* 2016;57(8):396-401.

Schumacher LL, Love BC, Ferrell M, et al. Canine intestinal histoplasmosis containing hyphal forms. *J Vet Diagn Invest.* 2013;25(2):304-307.

Shipov A, Kelmer G, Lavy E, et al. Long-term outcome of transendoscopic oesophageal mass ablation in dogs with *Spirocerca lupi*-associated oesophageal sarcoma. *Vet Rec.* 2015;177(14):365.

Silvestri S, Lepri E, Dall'Aglio C, et al. Nuclear glycogen inclusions in canine parietal cells. *Vet Pathol.* 2017;54(3):520-526.

Simpson KW, Dogan B, Rishniw M, et al. Adherent and invasive *Escherichia coli* is associated with granulomatous colitis in boxer dogs. *Infect Immun.* 2006;74(8):4778-4792.

Simpson KW, Strauss-Ayali D, McDonough PL, et al. Gastric function in dogs with naturally acquired gastric *Helicobacter* spp. infection. *J Vet Intern Med.* 1999;13:507-515.

Smithson CW, Smith MM, Tappe J, et al. Multicentric oral plasmacytoma in 3 dogs. *J Vet Dent.* 2012;29(2):96-110.

Snead EC. Large granular intestinal lymphosarcoma and leukemia in a dog. *Can Vet J.* 2007;48(8):848-851.

Takeuchi A, Jervis HR, Sprinz H. The globule leucocyte in the intestinal mucosa of the cat: a histochemical, light and electron microscopic study. *Anat Rec.* 1969;164:79-100.

Tidd KS, Durham AC, Brown DC, et al. Outcomes in 40 cats with discrete intermediate- or large-cell gastrointestinal lymphoma masses treated with surgical mass resection (2005-2015). *Vet Surg.* 2019;48(7):1218-1228.

Wingo K. Histopathologic diagnoses from biopsies of the oral cavity in 403 dogs and 73 cats. *J Vet Dent.* 2018;35(1):7-17.

Winston JA, Piperisova I, Neel J, et al. Cyniclomyces guttulatus infection in dogs: 19 cases (2006-2013). *J Am Anim Hosp Assoc.* 2016;52(1):42-51.

Wright ZM, Rogers KS, Mansell J. Survival data for canine oral extramedullary plasmacytomas: a retrospective analysis (1996-2006). *J Am Anim Hosp Assoc.* 2008;44(2):75-81.

8 CHAPTER

Pancreas (Exocrine and Endocrine)

Julie Allen

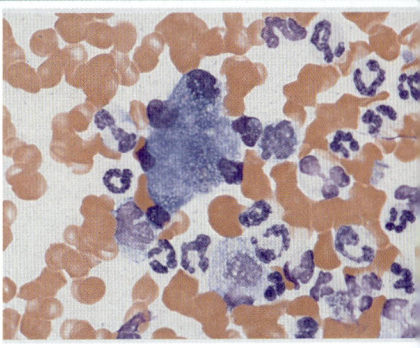

Diagnosing pancreatic disease can be challenging because of the nonspecific clinical presentation of pancreatic diseases, the lack of sensitive and specific serologic tests, and the challenges in imaging and sampling the pancreas. With the exception of exocrine pancreatic insufficiency (EPI), symptomatic exocrine pancreatic disease typically manifests the same spectrum of clinical signs, such as anorexia, vomiting, and lethargy, regardless of the underlying cause. The increasing use of fine-needle aspiration (FNA) biopsy has been advantageous, particularly now that the initial fears of inducing pancreatitis have been abated (Cordner et al., 2010; Crain et al., 2015). Similar to evaluation of other organs, pancreatic cytopathology is not always definitive because it may be difficult to differentiate nodular hyperplasia and well-differentiated neoplasia or to discriminate the primary process in some patients with concurrent disease, such as pancreatic carcinoma with secondary pancreatitis. The gold standard for the diagnosis of pancreatic disease has long been histopathology; however, even histopathology has its limitations, such as lack of standardization and advocacy for attaining multiple tissue biopsies.

NORMAL ANATOMY AND HISTOLOGY

The pancreas is a tubuloalveolar glandular organ composed predominantly of exocrine tissue (~95%–98%) with small amounts of scattered endocrine tissue, termed *pancreatic islets* (Tsuchitani, 2016). The organ is composed of three parts, the right lobe, body, and left lobe, which lie between the duodenum, stomach, and spleen. The distal end of the feline pancreas terminates in a hooklike structure (Mansfield and Jones, 2001). Many smaller ducts converge to form the larger pancreatic ducts, of which dogs typically have two, one entering at the major duodenal papilla and the other at the minor duodenal papilla. Most cats have only one pancreatic duct, which combines with the bile duct before entering the duodenum. This anatomic variation contributes to the predisposition in cats to develop triaditis (i.e., inflammation within the intestine, liver, and pancreas) (Fragkou et al., 2016).

The exocrine portion is composed of tubuloacinar structures that secrete inactive digestive enzymes (zymogens), which are activated by trypsin (via enterokinase) within the intestinal lumen. Bicarbonate is also produced and excreted into the duodenum to neutralize the incoming gastric contents and provide an optimal pH for digestive enzyme reactions. Furthermore, the pancreas also produces intrinsic factor, which is vital for the absorption of cobalamin (vitamin B_{12}). Consequently, patients with EPI often require vitamin B_{12} supplementation.

The endocrine cells are composed of four different cell types that each secrete different pancreatic polypeptides (PPs). The beta (β) cells that produce insulin and amylin (amyloid polypeptide) are the most numerous, making up 60% to 75% of islet cells, followed by the alpha (α) cells that produce glucagon and involve 20% to 25%. There are low numbers of delta (δ) and PP cells that produce somatostatin and PPs, respectively (Brown et al., 2017).

Histologically, the acinar cells are arranged around central lumens (Fig. 8.1), which are lined by flattened duct cells, termed *centroacinar cells* (Munday et al., 2017). Intercalated ducts originate from the acinar lumens and transport the secreted zymogens into the intralobular ducts along with the bicarbonate and water produced by the duct cells. The acinar cells contain round, basilar nuclei and occasional nucleoli. Their cytoplasm has differential staining; it is deeply basophilic toward the base and eosinophilic toward the apex (where the zymogen granules are stored) (see Fig. 8.1). The centroacinar cells are slightly paler with less cytoplasm. The intercalated ducts converge to form large interlobular ducts embedded within denser connective tissue. Goblet cells are occasionally observed between the epithelial cells of these larger ducts. Both the intercalated and intralobular ducts are lined by simple cuboidal epithelial cells, whereas the interlobular duct epithelial cells are more columnar. The interlobular ducts empty their contents into the pancreatic ducts. The islet cells scattered throughout the exocrine tissue are typically paler staining and smaller than the acinar cells (Fig. 8.2). The pancreas is surrounded by a thin collagenous capsule that extends septae into the parenchyma forming lobules. Capillaries are often embedded within the stroma. Pacinian corpuscles are present in the normal cat pancreas. These structures resemble onions with lamellae of flattened cells around a central nerve fiber surrounded by a fine capsule. Their exact function is unknown, but they are mechanoreceptors with perhaps a role in regulation of blood flow (Standop et al., 2001).

SAMPLE COLLECTION

Cytopathologic samples are usually obtained via ultrasound guidance. Although ultrasound is useful for identifying abnormalities in the pancreas, the organ is difficult to image because of its thin structure (6–8 mm in dogs and 4–6 mm in cats), similar ultrasonographic appearance to adjacent mesenteric

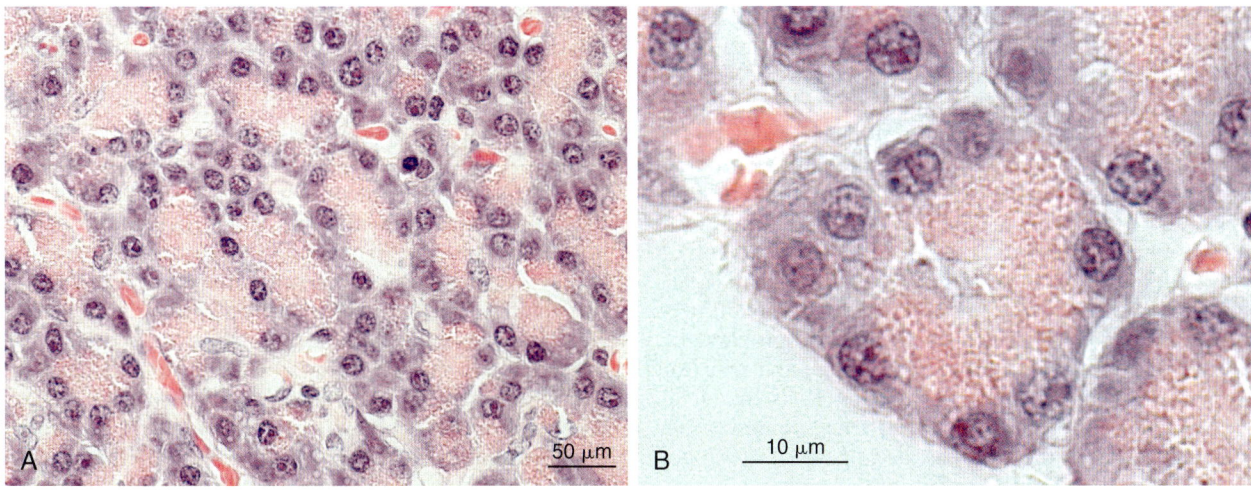

FIGURE 8.1 Normal exocrine pancreas. Histology. Dog. Same case in A and B. **A,** Packeting of epithelium in acinar arrangement with the nuclei forming a ring of cells. (H&E; HP oil.) **B,** Higher magnification of a single pancreatic acinus. Note the basilar location of the nuclei and abundant cytoplasm containing eosinophilic zymogen granules that empty their enzyme products from the apical edge into the center. (H&E; HP oil.) (Courtesy Rose Raskin, Purdue University.)

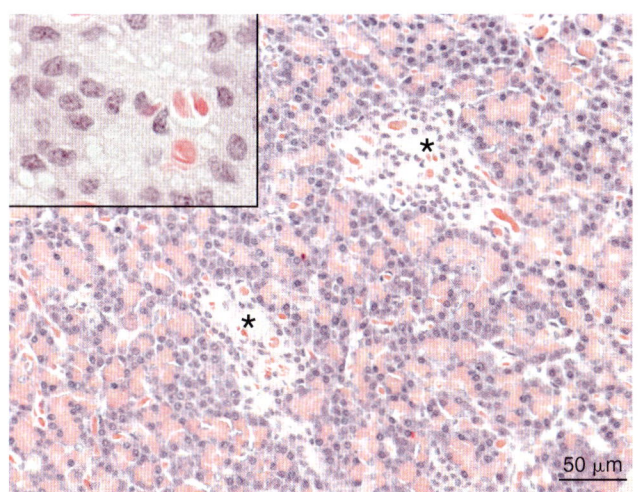

FIGURE 8.2 Normal endocrine pancreas. Histology. Dog. Acinar structures of eosinophilic granular cells comprise the exocrine pancreas. Two pale staining islets *(asterisks)* of endocrine pancreas are shown. (H&E; IP.) *Inset:* High magnification of islet cells showing uniform nuclei with abundant pale and vacuolated cytoplasm that are intermingled with capillaries. (H&E; HP oil.) (Courtesy Rose Raskin, Purdue University.)

adipose tissue, and close association with the gastrointestinal (GI) tract. Additionally, the ultrasonographic appearance of different lesions often appears similar, necessitating cytopathologic and/or histopathologic biopsies for further characterization. In human medicine, most pancreatic sampling occurs via endoscopic ultrasound (EUS) guidance, which has been shown to be more sensitive than transabdominal ultrasound and computed tomography. EUS-guided FNA has been performed safely in dogs but is not yet widely practiced (Kook et al., 2012). Impression smears of tissues can also be performed intraoperatively.

The acquisition of ultrasound-guided cytopathologic samples of the pancreas is similar to that of other organs. A study in humans showed no difference between 22- and 25-gauge needles (Lee et al., 2009), and several other studies have also demonstrated that a larger gauge needle does not necessarily equate to a better sample. On the contrary, larger gauge needles may be associated with more hemorrhage, although this is unlikely to be clinically relevant. Although nonaspiration techniques often are less hemodiluted, aspiration techniques are preferred for sampling the pancreas. Four to five aspirates should be performed, and one to two slides should be stained and assessed for adequate cellularity before submission to a diagnostic laboratory (Liffman and Courtman, 2017). Of 94 dogs that underwent pancreatic FNA, 73.5% were diagnosed, with inflammation being the most common diagnosis, followed by neoplasia, normal-appearing pancreatic tissue, hyperplasia, cyst formation, and necrosis (Cordner et al., 2015). Only 11 cases had concurrent histopathology performed, and the concordance between cytopathology and histopathology was 91%. Adverse effects from the procedure were seen in 7.4% of the dogs, and these were usually related to concurrent disease, the performance of an accompanying procedure, or both (Cordner et al., 2015). In a study of ultrasound-guided FNA of the pancreas in 73 cats, 67% samples were of diagnostic quality, and the correlation with histopathology was 86% (Crain et al., 2015). Although 11% of the pancreatic aspiration group had postprocedural complications, such as hemorrhage or hypotension, they were typically because these patients also underwent liver aspiration or had nonpancreatic comorbidities. The complication rate was similar to cats undergoing FNA of other organs and cats not undergoing aspiration. Additionally, there was no difference in mortality rate between cats with or without pancreatic aspiration (Crain et al., 2015).

One of the concerns of transabdominal FNA of cancer is the potential for tumor transplantation in the abdominal wall. In dogs, urothelial carcinoma (also known as transitional cell carcinoma) is well documented for potential seeding, but in human medicine, transplantation of pancreatic neoplasms is most common (Liffman and Courtman, 2017). A more recent study in humans; however, found that EUS FNA for pancreatic cancer was not associated with an increased rate of seeding or mortality and was therefore deemed safe (Kim et al., 2018).

As mentioned earlier, histopathology is considered the benchmark for diagnosis; however, multiple biopsies of the pancreas are indicated to increase the likelihood of an accurate diagnosis in dogs (Newman et al., 2006), and evaluation of the entire pancreas is often necessary in cats due to their multifocal lesion distribution (Bazelle and Watson, 2014). Consequently, a negative result on histopathology does not always exclude pancreatic pathology. Incidentally, this also makes interpretation of studies using histopathology as the gold standard problematic. Pancreatic tissue biopsy is an invasive procedure and may lead to postoperative complications. A study by Pratschke et al. (2015) found that 10 of 43 dogs and cats had complications after surgical biopsy of the pancreas, half of which developed pancreatitis. However, the risk was diminished with good surgical technique. If ascites is present in a patient with suspected pancreatic disease, abdominocentesis and fluid cytopathology may be helpful. An exudative effusion is often observed with acute pancreatitis, and neoplastic cells may exfoliate with pancreatic cancers. Chyloabdomen has also been reported secondary to pancreatic carcinoma in a cat (Véran et al., 2018).

NORMAL CYTOLOGY AND ARTIFACTS

Fine-needle aspiration biopsy of the healthy pancreas is often unrewarding, with samples being of low nucleated cellularity and hemodiluted and consequently of insufficient diagnostic quality (Cordner et al., 2010). However, cytopathologic biopsies of the diseased pancreas are often more fruitful. When adequately cellular, the main cell population consists of clusters of exocrine pancreatic acinar cells that form acini and tubules on a background of blood or light pink proteinaceous material. Acinar cells are small to medium in size and polygonal with low to moderate nucleocytoplasmic (N:C) ratios. Their nuclei are round and basally located, having stippled to reticulated chromatin, with occasional single, small, prominent nucleoli (see Fig. 8.1B). Cells have moderate amounts of basophilic, grainy cytoplasm filled with small, eosinophilic zymogen granules. The cells display minimal anisocytosis and anisokaryosis. Duct epithelial cells are cuboidal and often have higher N:C ratios, ovoid nuclei, and stippled chromatin. Epithelial cells lining larger ducts are columnar and may have cilia. With excessive pressure or poor sample handling, the epithelial cells may be individualized or disrupted with cell-free zymogen granules in the background. Intercalated between the exocrine pancreatic cells are rare small islets of endocrine cells. By cytopathology, the islet cells display the typical naked nuclei appearance of endocrine cells: round and uniform nuclei embedded within lightly basophilic cytoplasm having indistinct cell borders. When intact, the cells have high N:C ratios with small amounts of basophilic cytoplasm. The nuclei contain finely stippled chromatin and occasionally single, prominent nucleoli.

Scattered leukocytes may also be noted on pancreatic cytopathologic specimens. These cells should be interpreted in association with the degree of hemodilution and the peripheral white blood cell count. Mesothelial cells can also be inadvertently sampled and visualized. Extramedullary hematopoiesis has been described in other textbooks, but this is not clearly documented in the peer-reviewed literature. The author postulates as to whether these cells, when previously described, may have emanated from the rare incidences of intrapancreatic ectopic splenic tissue (see later).

PANCREATIC CYSTIC LESIONS

Cystic lesions of the pancreas include congenital cysts, acquired retention cysts, and pseudocysts. Congenital cysts occur mainly in cats and are usually observed in association with polycystic kidney disease or hepatic cysts (Lafuente et al., 2018). These variably sized, occasionally multiloculated cysts are hypoechoic with thin walls on ultrasound. Aspiration yields thin, clear fluid. As true cysts, a single flat layer of cuboidal to attenuated epithelium lines them. Retention cysts form secondary to pancreatic duct obstruction such as occurs secondary to pancreatoliths. Over time, these cysts can compress the surrounding tissue, leading to compression atrophy and loss of function.

Pseudocysts are the most common cystlike lesion and are a sequela to pancreatitis, and consequently their presenting clinical signs and clinicopathologic changes are similar (VanEnkevort et al., 1999). Release of pancreatic enzymes into the pancreatic parenchyma causes necrosis, inflammation, and fibrosis. When contiguous with a duct, these can lead to dilation and cyst formation. Pseudocysts appear more irregular with a thicker wall and more echogenic contents on ultrasound compared with true cysts. Because pseudocysts form secondary to pancreatitis, they lack a true epithelial lining, and the margins are formed by granulation tissue (Munday et al., 2017). Their contents range from clear in color to turbid and bloody. On cytopathology, all the aforementioned structures appear similar to cystic lesions seen elsewhere. They are typically of high protein and low nucleated cellularity, composed of occasional reactive macrophages and rare nondegenerate neutrophils on an eosinophilic to purple, stippled, proteinaceous background (Fig. 8.3). Abundant crystalline debris and cholesterol crystals may be seen. Hemorrhage may be observed in the form of erythrophagia (Fig. 8.3B) or hemosiderin-laden macrophages. The key reason to aspirate these lesions is to differentiate them from abscesses or cystic neoplasms (36% of cats with pancreatic neoplasia have cystic tumors) (Törner et al., 2019). Measurement of pseudocyst fluid lipase may be helpful because pseudocyst fluids typically have higher enzyme activity compared with serum; measurement of amylase activity is less reliable (VanEnkevort et al., 1999). Pancreatic pseudocysts are usually managed conservatively via serial monitoring along with treatment of the pancreatitis. However, percutaneous drainage or ethanol ablation as well as surgical intervention (cystogastrostomy, omentalization, or debridement) may be performed if there is evidence of obstruction or the lesion continues to enlarge (Sadler et al., 2016).

TISSUE INJURY (NECROSIS, MINERALIZATION)

Release of pancreatic enzymes from the damaged pancreatic parenchyma causes acute cellular death (necrosis) and possible inflammation, and if chronic, fibrosis may occur. Necrosis is most often associated with pancreatitis and pancreatic malignancy (Fig. 8.4). There may be saponification of surrounding fat with the presence of secondary calcium deposits and mild inflammation (Fig. 8.5A). Use of polarized light is helpful to visualize the mineralization, which may also appear refractile (Fig. 8.5B).

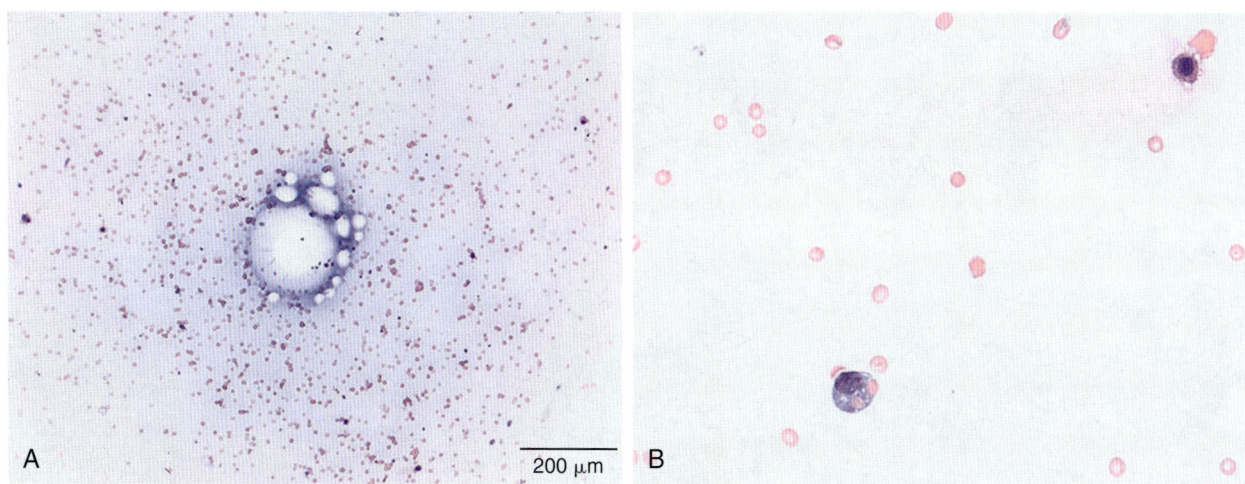

■ **FIGURE 8.3 Pancreatic pseudocyst (presumed). Tissue aspirate. Dog.** Same case in A and B. **A,** Low cellularity consisting of inflammatory cells on a proteinaceous background with mild hemodilution. (Romanowsky; LP.) **B,** Inflammatory cells are predominantly macrophages. Note the erythrophagocytic macrophage and granulated mast cell. No epithelial cells are seen. (Romanowsky; HP oil.)

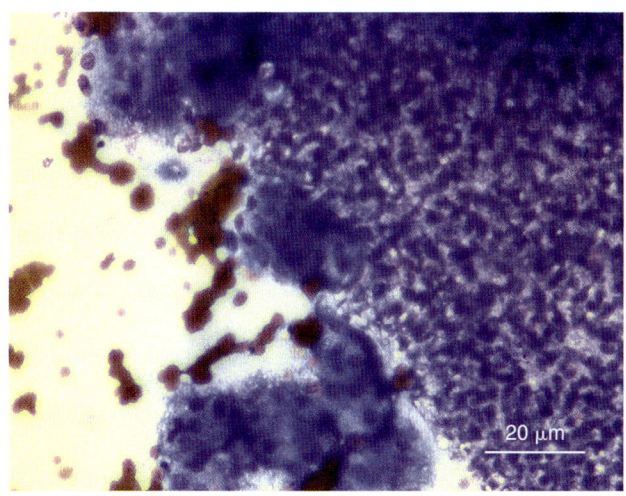

■ **FIGURE 8.4 Pancreatic necrosis. Tissue aspirate. Dog.** Specimen contains clumps of dark purple amorphous necrotic material along with moderately atypical pancreatic epithelium present in variably sized, cohesive sheets. These cells appear indistinct, suggestive of cellular necrosis. These display a moderate nucleocytoplasmic ratio, moderate anisokaryosis, and occasional bi- or trinucleation and nuclear molding. (Wright-Giemsa; IP.) (Courtesy Rose Raskin, University of Florida.)

PANCREATIC NODULAR HYPERPLASIA

Nodular hyperplasia is a common incidental finding in older dogs and cats (Newman et al., 2005). The lesions are generally not considered preoplastic or a result of prior inflammation, although if they occur in younger animals, prior injury is suspected. The nodules involve predominantly the acinar cells, with ductal hyperplasia occurring less commonly. Clinically, the condition is often asymptomatic with multiple (rarely single), variably sized (usually <1–2 cm) nodules detected upon ultrasound examination performed for an unrelated reason (Hecht et al., 2007). Grossly, the nodules give an irregular texture to the organ with normal tissue interposed between hyperplastic, raised, smooth, firm nodules that appear white or tan on cut section. Histologically, the nodules are unencapsulated and appear similar to normal pancreas with cuboidal cells seen in clusters (Newman et al., 2005). In dogs, the nodules can cause surrounding atrophy and fibrosis and have been associated with lymphocytic inflammation.

On aspiration, the samples are typically of high cellularity and composed of numerous cohesive clusters of uniform acinar cells with low N:C ratios, small round basilar nuclei, stippled chromatin, and abundant cytoplasm. They may contain fine, clear vacuoles. In some cases of hyperplasia, the cells may be larger with higher N:C ratios, increased cytoplasmic basophilia, and fewer granules. There may be a slight increase in anisocytosis and anisokaryosis with some binucleation noted and rare mitotic figures (Figs. 8.6 to 8.8). The hyperplastic cells may have higher nucleocytoplasmic ratios and fewer zymogen granules. This lesion must be differentiated from well-differentiated pancreatic neoplasia (adenoma or carcinoma) by histopathology. The presence of multiple nodules and their relatively small size, resemblance to normal pancreas, and lack of capsule aid in diagnosis of nodular hyperplasia (Munday et al., 2017).

> *Cytopathologic differential diagnosis:* pancreatic adenoma, well-differentiated pancreatic adenocarcinoma, normal pancreas.

NONINFECTIOUS INFLAMMATORY DISORDERS

Pancreatitis

Pancreatitis is the most common condition affecting the pancreas. Middle-aged to older animals predominate, but any age animal can be affected. In dogs, there are several breed predispositions, including miniature schnauzers, boxers, border collies, cocker spaniels, cavalier King Charles spaniels, and various terriers (Watson et al., 2007). It was suggested that Siamese cats may be overrepresented, but several more recent studies have not supported this (De Cock et al., 2007). In a study of 115 cats

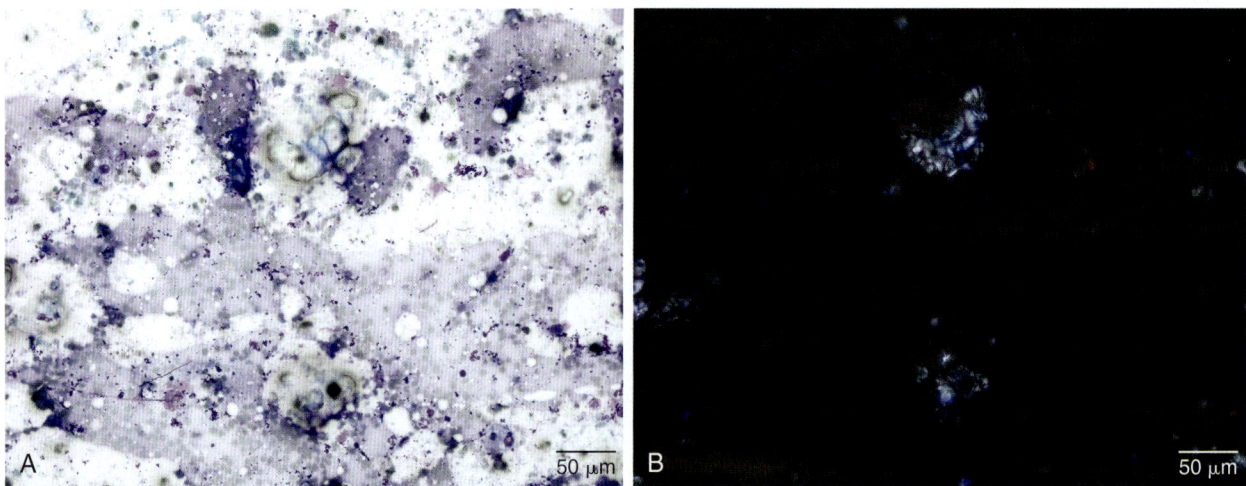

■ **FIGURE 8.5 Peripancreatic fat saponification. Tissue aspirate. Cat.** Same case in A and B. **A,** Ultrasound examination revealed a 1.2 × 0.6 cm oval, centrally hyperechoic structure adjacent to the pancreatic body. Basophilic background contains ample free, nonstaining lipid and abundant fragments of clear refractile material. (Wright-Giemsa; IP oil.) **B,** Polarized view reveals the presence of mineral, likely calcium. This cat had a history of diabetes mellitus and a recent episode of vomiting and inappetence. Biochemical data supported a diagnosis of pancreatitis, as did a markedly elevated Precision PSL test result. (Polarized Wright-Giemsa; IP oil.) (Courtesy Francisco Conrado, University of Florida.)

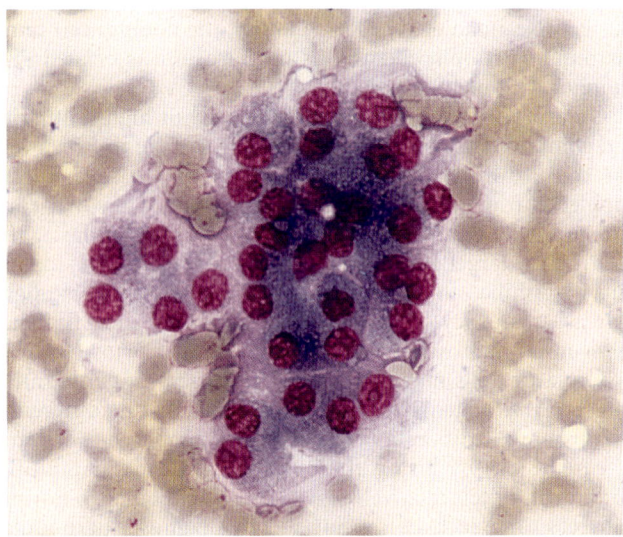

■ **FIGURE 8.6 Hyperplastic nodule of the exocrine pancreas. Tissue aspirate. Dog.** Ultrasound examination indicated a hypoechoic mass. Nucleocytoplasmic ratio is higher than normal epithelium along with increased cytoplasmic basophilia with frequent binucleation. (Wright-Giemsa; HP oil.) (Courtesy Rose Raskin, University of Florida.)

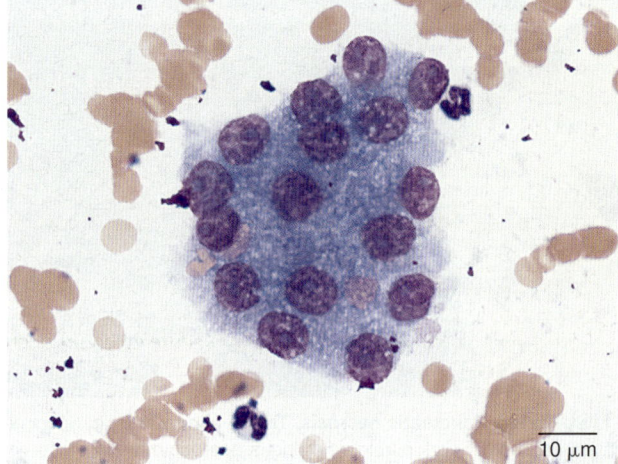

■ **FIGURE 8.7 Hyperplastic pancreatic nodule. Tissue aspirate. Cat.** Ultrasound study found a moderately enlarged, lobular, and hypoechoic pancreas with numerous, well-defined, round, hypoechoic nodules. The background contains magenta granular material (ultrasound coupling gel). A single cluster consists of polygonal cells with variably distinct cytoplasmic borders and a moderate amount of basophilic granular cytoplasm. The round nucleus is paracentral measures 1.5 to 2 × RBC diameter and has coarsely stippled chromatin with a single, round distinct nucleolus. Anisocytosis and anisokaryosis among this population is mild, and the nucleocytoplasmic ratio is increased. (Wright-Giemsa; HP oil.) (Courtesy Rose Raskin, University of Florida.)

at necropsy, only 33% had no evidence of pancreatic inflammation (De Cock et al., 2007).

Pancreatitis is typically classified as acute or chronic. This distinction may be clinical, based on the onset and duration of clinical signs, or histologic, by identifying the type of inflammatory cell infiltrate, the presence or absence of fibrosis, or atrophy. The histologic definition is likely the most accurate, but not all cases of pancreatitis will have histologic assessment. Acute pancreatitis often presents as a clinically acute problem with high risk of systemic complications, such as disseminated intravascular coagulation (DIC) or multiple organ dysfunction syndrome. On cytopathology and histopathology, acute pancreatitis is characterized by suppurative inflammation, edema, and necrosis, but these changes are typically reversible with no permanent damage to the pancreas. In contrast, chronic pancreatitis tends to be clinically milder or subclinical (Bazelle and Watson, 2014). The characteristic feature of histopathology is the permanence and irreversibility of the lesions, characterized by fibrosis and atrophy with or without lymphocytic

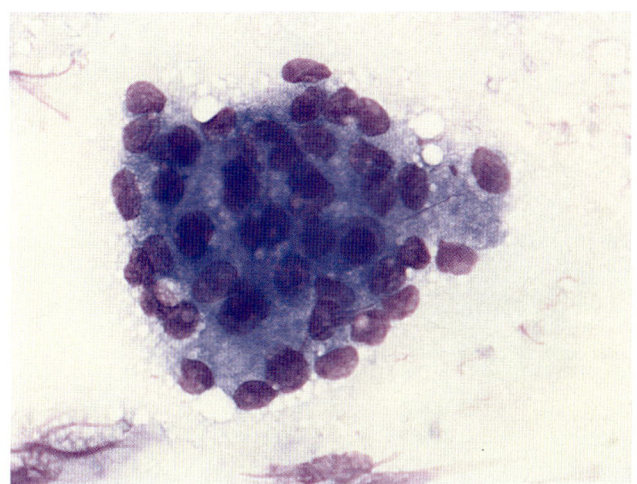

FIGURE 8.8 Hyperplastic pancreatic parenchyma. Tissue aspirate. Dog. Ultrasound examination indicated an enlarged, hypoechoic and lobular pancreas with clinical signs of pancreatitis. The field shows a dense cluster of exocrine pancreatic epithelium. These cells are round to oval and have variably distinct cytoplasmic borders and a low to moderate amount of basophilic foamy cytoplasm that typically contains several distinct and indistinct vacuoles. The round or oval nucleus is paracentral to eccentric, measures roughly 1.5 to 2 × RBC diameter, has clumped chromatin, and one or two small discernible nucleoli. Overall anisocytosis and anisokaryosis are mild to moderate, and nucleocytoplasmic ratio is often high. (Wright-Giemsa; HP oil.) (Courtesy Rose Raskin, University of Florida.)

infiltrates. If there is greater than 80% to 90% pancreatic atrophy, then EPI and diabetes mellitus (DM) may develop. Trypsin-like immunoreactivity (TLI) remains the test of choice for the diagnosis of EPI and has excellent sensitivity and specificity (Mansfield, 2013). However, there is overlap between acute and chronic pancreatitis, with some acute episodes occurring on a background of subclinical or clinically managed chronic pancreatitis. If there is fibrosis, the disease process is chronic, even if there is concurrent neutrophilic inflammation and necrosis. The cause of pancreatitis is often unknown, although various etiologies have been described, including the ingestion of high-fat foods, genetics, hyperlipidemia, trauma, and certain drugs, such as azathioprine.

Acute Pancreatitis

Affected dogs often present with the classic signs of pancreatitis, including anorexia, vomiting, diarrhea (small and large bowel), and abdominal pain, although sometimes the signs can be subtler. Cats often display nonspecific signs, such as anorexia and lethargy (Xenoulis, 2015). As mentioned earlier, patients with severe pancreatitis may present in shock, with DIC, or with multiorgan failure with death occurring within hours.

Routine laboratory work may reveal anemia of inflammation or relative polycythemia, an inflammatory leukogram, thrombocytopenia (particularly if there is concurrent DIC), increased serum hepatic and pancreatic enzyme activities, hyperbilirubinemia, hypocalcemia (caused by saponification and mineralization of fat), hypoalbuminemia, hyperglycemia or hypoglycemia, hyperlipidemia, and a variety of electrolyte changes (Xenoulis, 2015).

Abdominal radiographs typically reveal nonspecific findings, such as decreased contrast or opacity in the cranial abdomen; however, they are useful for eliminating other differential diagnoses for acute abdomen, such as intestinal foreign bodies. Ultrasound is very operator dependent, but when pancreatitis is noted, the pancreas appears enlarged, hypoechoic, and poorly defined, often with free fluid and hyperechoic fat. Dilation with or without obstruction of the bile duct may be observed, along with corrugation of the adjacent duodenal mucosa (Xenoulis, 2015).

In the past, measurement of amylase and lipase on routine biochemical panels was used for the diagnosis of pancreatitis; however, these assays have been found to lack sensitivity and specificity, particularly in cats. Consequently, various serologic markers have been developed to assess for pancreatic inflammation including TLI, trypsin activation peptide, and pancreas-specific lipase immunoreactivity (PLI) (Mansfield, 2013). The latter test, the PLI, is specific for the pancreas and remains the most sensitive and specific of the developed tests, although it still has its limitations. Widely available immunoassays include the laboratory-based enzyme-linked immunosorbent assay tests Spec fPL and Spec cPL (Texas A&M University) for cats and dogs, respectively. A recently marketed point-of-care immunoassay is the semiquantitative VetScan cPL Rapid Test (Zoetis Services) for dogs, which showed unacceptable variability in intra- and inter-assay runs (Steiner et al., 2019). The in-house SNAP cPL Test (IDEXX Laboratories) provides only a negative or positive result and has a high negative predictive value with any positive results requiring additional confirmatory testing. More sensitive lipase assays, including the DGGR-based assay (used in the Precision PSL Test [Antech Diagnostics]), measure total serum lipase but appear less specific for the pancreas. A recent study compared these four tests and found their diagnostic performance to be similar under laboratory settings (Cridge et al., 2018).

Aspiration of a suspected inflamed pancreas is not usually indicated unless there is a mass lesion or failure to respond to appropriate therapy. If the affected organ is aspirated, the typical cytopathologic findings are inflammatory cells and fewer epithelial cells. In acute pancreatitis, neutrophils predominate with fewer vacuolated, phagocytic macrophages, and lymphocytes (Figs. 8.9 and 8.10). Hemosiderin-laden macrophages and hematoidin crystals may be seen as a result of prior hemorrhage. Occasionally, the neutrophils may aggregate or enmesh within necrotic debris (see Fig. 8.10B). The acinar cells, although uniform, may also show signs of degeneration or hyperplasia. Degenerative changes include cell swelling, pale cytoplasm, foamy cytoplasm (hydropic change), and loss of zymogen granules. Hyperplastic changes may include increased N:C ratios, increased cytoplasmic basophilia, and loss of zymogen granules (see Fig. 8.10A). In some situations, acinar cells can display significant atypia, and as always, caution should be used in overinterpreting these changes as neoplasia in the face of considerable inflammation. However, pancreatitis can occur as a sequela to neoplasia, so repeat imaging and aspiration could be considered in cases with pancreatic masses. In acute pancreatitis, there are often variable amounts of necrosis of both the pancreatic parenchyma and surrounding adipose tissue. This is visualized by cytopathology as scattered amorphous purple material in the background with interspersed necrotic cells with glassy nuclei. Dystrophic mineralization can also occur, and consequently, calcified material can be seen (see Fig. 8.10B). In

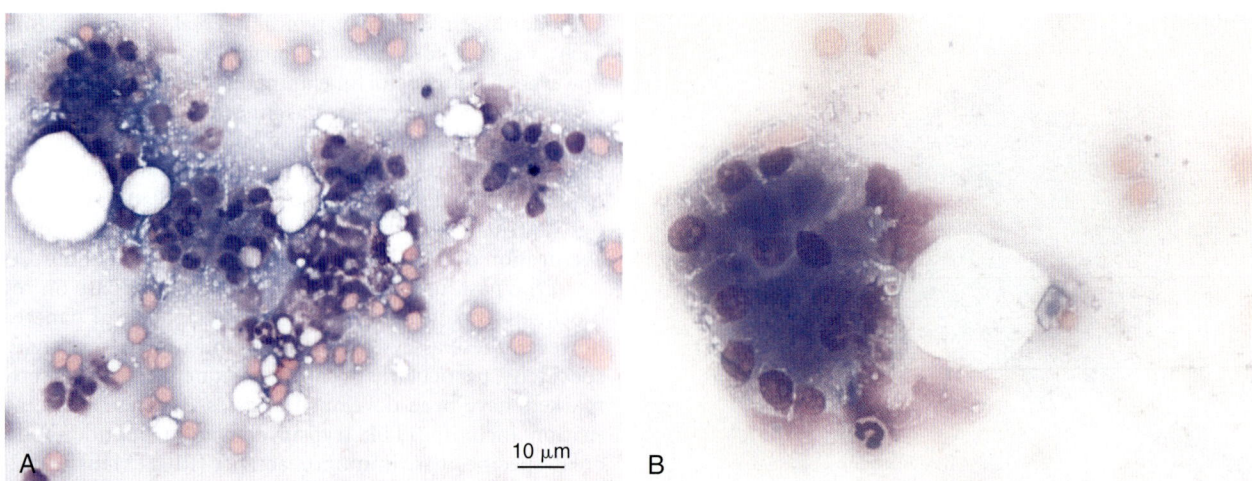

■ **FIGURE 8.9 Acute pancreatitis. Tissue aspirate. Dog.** Same case in A and B. **A,** Local peritonitis was detected by ultrasound, coincident with a history of eating a sausage. Dense cell clusters with associated neutrophils display the loss of intact borders, suggesting tissue necrosis. (Modified Wright; HP oil.) **B,** Higher magnification of an intact acinus displays an indistinct appearance to the cells at the periphery. (Modified Wright; HP oil.) (Courtesy Cheryl Moller, Murdoch University.)

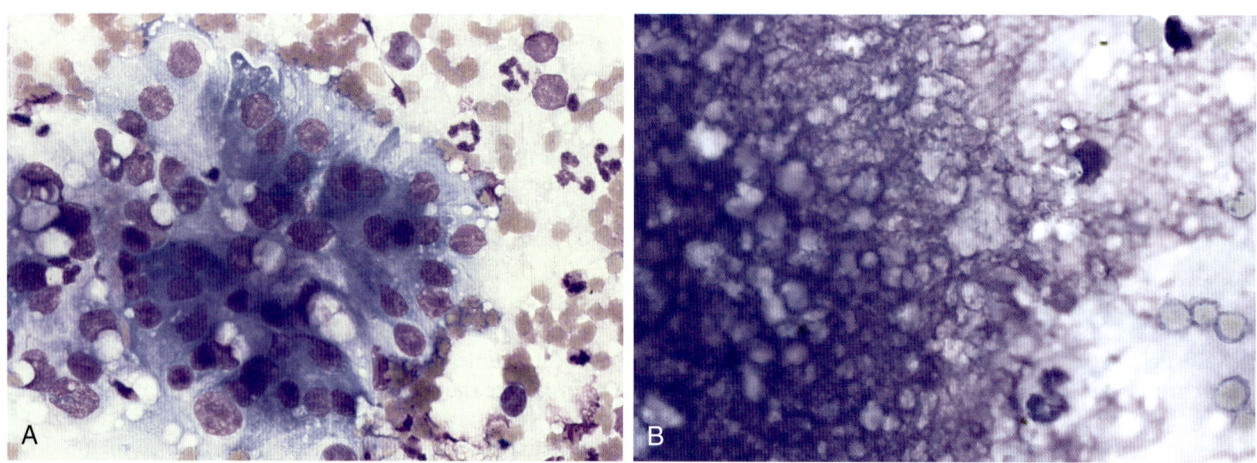

■ **FIGURE 8.10 Acute pancreatitis. Tissue aspirate. Dog.** Same case in A and B. **A,** Numerous neutrophils surround hyperplastic and atypical epithelium characterized by several features of malignancy. (Modified Wright; HP oil.) **B,** In addition to necrosis, there is mineralization with refractile clear crystals throughout the deep basophilic background. (Modified Wright; HP oil.) (Courtesy Rose Raskin, Purdue University.)

some patients, particularly cats, necrosis can predominate with minimal inflammation. Both dogs and cats can also develop acute or chronic pancreatitis with mixed inflammation noted on cytopathology.

Gross evaluation of the pancreas is not reliable for the diagnosis of pancreatitis because focal or multifocal lesions can be missed. Although the gold standard for diagnosis of pancreatitis is histopathology, the lack of gross lesions can hamper the ability to obtain diagnostic tissue biopsies. When present, gross lesions may include focal, multifocal, or diffuse areas of swelling (edema), hemorrhage, softening (necrosis), chalky areas of mineralization, and fibrinous peritonitis with adhesions. Studies have also shown that single tissue biopsies are inadequate, and multiple tissue biopsies are required to optimize lesion detection (Xenoulis, 2015). However, this is often not clinically feasible. On histopathology of acute pancreatitis, the inflammation, edema, necrosis, and mineralization can be observed; however, there is no standardized technique for tissue biopsy, and there is no consensus for disease diagnosis. Histopathology does remain helpful in differentiating inflammatory from neoplastic disease, identifying acute versus chronic inflammation, and documenting the presence or absence of irreversible changes, such as fibrosis.

Acute pancreatitis may lead to hypovolemia and renal ischemia secondary to systemic inflammation and oxidative stress. Affected patients may develop acute kidney injury with anuria and azotemia, which are associated with poorer outcomes in dogs with acute pancreatitis (Gori, 2019). A recent study also noted the occurrence of immune-medicated hemolytic anemia (IMHA) and pancreatitis in cats (Zoia and Drigo, 2017). It was not clear if one condition triggered the other or if the two disorders shared a common immune-mediated pathogenesis.

Panniculitis, polyarthritis, and osteomyelitis have also been noted in dogs with pancreatitis; however, many of these patients were later discovered to have underlying pancreatic neoplasia (Mellanby et al., 2003).

> **KEY POINT** Pancreatitis can be associated with significant comorbidities, including but not limited to acute kidney injury, polyarthritis, panniculitis, pancreatic neoplasia, and IMHA.

Chronic Pancreatitis

As mentioned previously, chronic pancreatitis can be difficult to recognize because of its milder presentation or complete lack of clinical signs (Bostrom et al., 2013). If patients do display signs, it is usually as a response to an acute exacerbation of the chronic pancreatitis. The clinical signs are even more vague, and intermittent GI signs often prevail, including colitis (related to the proximity of the transverse colon and left limb of the pancreas).

Clinicopathologic abnormalities include increased serum liver enzyme activities, hyperbilirubinemia, and hypercholesterolemia. Some dogs have concurrent hepatobiliary, endocrine disease, and chronic enteropathy or inflammatory bowel disease (IBD). A distinct form of chronic hepatitis has been observed in English cocker spaniels and resembles IgG4RD in humans (Watson et al., 2011). Affected dogs have chronic pancreatic inflammation (often presenting as masses), keratoconjunctivitis sicca, xerostomia, and proteinuria. This immune-mediated disease is characterized by many periductal and perivascular, IgG4-positive plasma cells (Watson, 2017). Cats often have chronic pancreatitis in conjunction with hepatobiliary disorders (hepatic lipidosis, cholangiohepatitis) or intestinal disease as well as DM. *Triaditis* is used to describe concurrent inflammation of the pancreas, liver, and small intestine (Fragkou et al., 2016). The exact pathogenesis of the triaditis is unclear.

Cytopathologic evaluation typically yields lower cellularity samples compared with those of acute pancreatitis. Lymphocytes and plasma cells predominate with few reactive macrophages. Occasionally, eosinophilic strands consistent with collagen may be noted (Fig. 8.11). If necrosis and neutrophils are also seen, then they likely represent an acute inflammatory process. Hyperplastic acinar cells may be observed. Histologically, there are proliferative lobules of pancreatic tissue separated by abundant, eosinophilic, fibrous tissue along with pancreatic atrophy. Clinical differentiation of acute and chronic pancreatitis can be particularly challenging in cats without histopathology.

> **KEY POINT** The diagnosis of pancreatitis relies on a combination of signalment, history, physical examination, and blood testing with supportive cytopathology and histopathology.

Miscellaneous Noninfectious Inflammatory Disorders

Pancreatolithiasis has been reported in cats, although pancreatoliths have not been described by cytopathology (Plesman et al., 2014). Given the merging of the pancreatic and common bile ducts, biliary obstruction and rupture are possible sequelae.

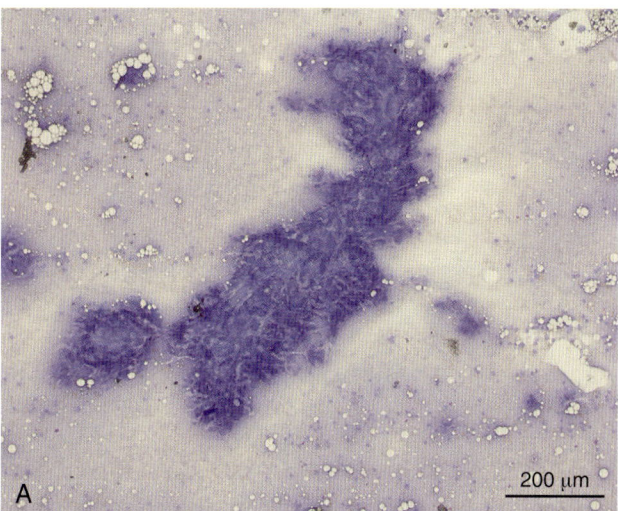
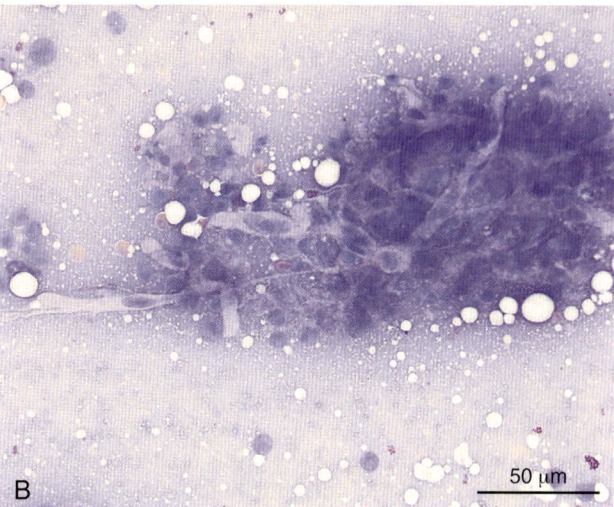

FIGURE 8.11 Chronic pancreatitis. Tissue aspirate. Cat. Same case in A and B. **A,** Clusters of basophilic pancreatic epithelial cells with intersecting fibrovascular stroma are present against a basophilic, proteinaceous background with cell-free lipid and mild hemodilution. (Romanowsky; LP.) **B,** Pancreatic acinar cells contain basophilic cytoplasm and light, uniform zymogen granules, which are more easily discernable in the background protein as cell-free granules released from ruptured cells. There are several spindle cells with associated light pink, fibrillar, extracellular matrix intersecting between the exocrine pancreatic epithelial cells (presumed fibrosis). (Romanowsky; HP oil.) *Not shown:* In other areas of the slide, low numbers of small and large lymphocytes with rare plasma cells are scattered between the pancreatic epithelial cells.

INFECTIOUS INFLAMMATORY DISORDERS

Pancreatic Abscess

Pancreatic abscesses are uncommon and often sequelae to pancreatitis. In one study, miniature schnauzers were overrepresented (6 of 36 dogs) (Anderson et al., 2008). Lesions may occur as single masses or affect the pancreas diffusely. Ultrasound often demonstrates cavitary lesions with variably thick walls and mixed echogenicity contents. Cytopathology reveals numerous, degenerate neutrophils with fewer foamy, vacuolated macrophages (activated) and small lymphocytes on a background of disrupted cells and debris. Pancreatic origin may be confirmed

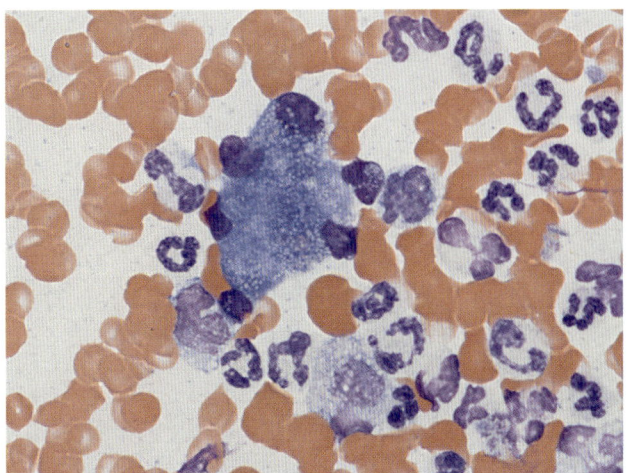

■ **FIGURE 8.12 Pancreatic abscess. Pancreatic parenchyma. Tissue aspirate. Dog.** Ultrasound noted an enlarged pancreas with lobular appearance in this patient with clinical signs of pancreatitis. A small cluster of pancreatic exocrine epithelium is shown along with many degenerate and nondegenerate neutrophils and few macrophages. Not shown but found in the specimen were neutrophils containing phagocytized bacteria (bacilli). (Wright-Giemsa; HP oil.) (Courtesy Rose Raskin, University of Florida.)

by the observance of acinar cells. Bacteria may or may not be detected (Fig. 8.12). Cultures are frequently negative (sterile), although one case report confirmed *Staphylococcus aureus* as the etiologic agent in one cat (Nemoto et al., 2017). Infection can originate from the bloodstream, GI tract, or biliary tree. Pancreatic abscessation can be challenging to differentiate from acute pancreatitis in the absence of organisms or ultrasonographic findings. In humans, the term *phlegmon* is used to describe noninfected, defined masses of inflammation associated with pancreatitis; this term may be more applicable to most of the reported cases of pancreatic abscessation in veterinary medicine. An increased blood urea nitrogen concentration, increased serum alkaline phosphatase activity, and rising serum total carbon dioxide concentration had a negative association with survival in 36 dogs with pancreatic abscesses (Anderson et al., 2008). This study also documented a 71% mortality rate. Surgical intervention is often required for drainage, omentalization, and closure or open peritoneal drainage. Antimicrobial therapy is often used despite the sterility of most lesions.

Pancreatic Flukes

Pancreatic flukes *(Eurytrema procyonis)* can infect foxes, raccoons, and occasionally domestic cats (Hoffman et al., 2017). When present, they are more often found in the tail of the pancreas in cats. Adult flukes have a predilection for the pancreatic and bile ducts and gallbladder, occasionally causing inflammation, hyperplasia, and fibrosis (Vyhnal et al., 2008). Although infected animals are often asymptomatic, heavy burdens of flukes can lead to pancreatitis, pancreatic atrophy, and EPI, but the flukes rarely seem to induce pancreatic damage in cats (Köster et al., 2017). Adult flukes are often fragmented on cytopathology, but suckers within cellular parenchymal fragments may be observed (Fig. 8.13). The fluke eggs stain green to brown, measure 45 to 53 μm long, 29 to 36 μm wide, and are longitudinally symmetrical with a single operculum (see Fig. 8.13C).

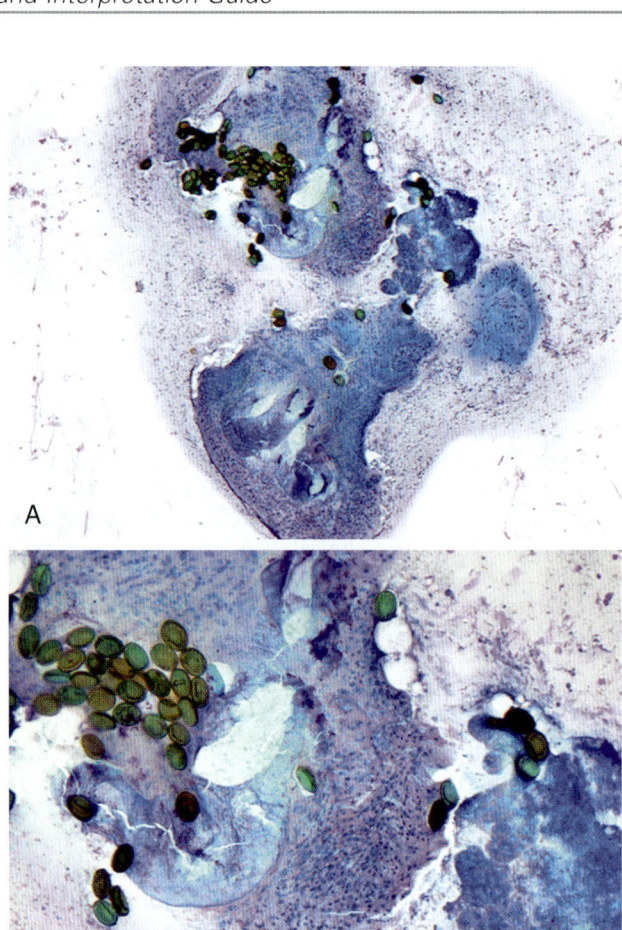

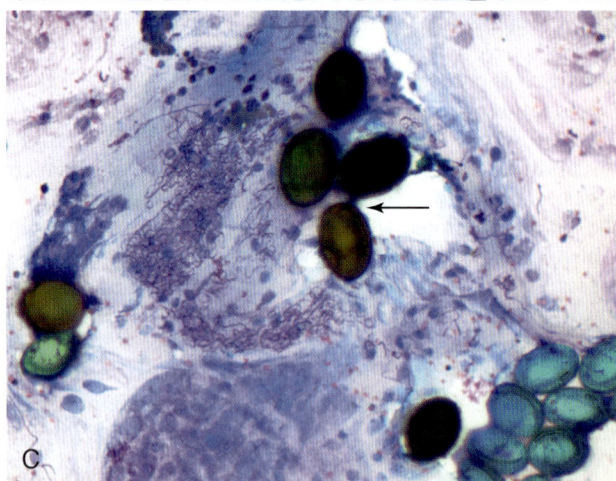

■ **FIGURE 8.13 Pancreatic trematodiasis. Tissue aspirate. Cat.** Same case in A and C. **A,** Fragments of adult *Eurytrema procyonis* flukes containing presumed suckers and cellular, internal parenchyma. Green fluke ova are also present. (Wright-Giemsa; LP.) **B,** Higher magnification of the adult fluke parenchyma, testes (dark blue clusters at *right*), and presumed cuticle (pale blue in *center*), along with green to brown ova. (Wright-Giemsa; LP.) **C,** Green to brown fluke ova are ovoid, approximately 30 × 50 μm, and have a slightly flattened end *(arrow)* on one side. (Wright-Giemsa; IP.) (Courtesy Angela Royal, University of Missouri.)

Miscellaneous Infectious Inflammatory Disorders

Other primary infections of the pancreas are rare. The pancreas can occasionally be affected in diffuse systemic diseases, such as toxoplasmosis, schistosomiasis, pythiosis, mycobacteriosis, and cryptococcosis (Duncan et al., 2000; Gow and Gow, 2008; Rodriguez et al., 2014; Dycus et al., 2015; Tangeman et al., 2015). Pancreatic necrosis has been observed in cats with systemic calicivirus infection (Pesavento et al., 2004). Increased canine pancreas-specific lipase concentrations have been reported in dogs infected with parvovirus, babesiosis, and monocytic ehrlichiosis, but these increases had no effect on outcome, and dogs with ehrlichiosis displayed no overt signs of pancreatitis (Mylonakis et al., 2014; Köster et al., 2015; Kalli et al., 2017). Hyperinsulinemic hypoglycemia syndrome has been reported in dogs with bartonellosis and nesidioblastosis, presumably caused by pancreatic hyperplasia (Breitschwerdt et al., 2014; Polansky et al., 2018).

MISCELLANEOUS NONNEOPLASTIC TUMORS

Ectopic splenic tissue has been observed within the pancreases of dogs and cats (Ramírez et al., 2013). Additionally, there has been a single case report of a pancreatic choristoma (mass of normal tissue found in an abnormal location) within the gallbladder of a dog (Abou Monsef et al., 2019).

NEOPLASTIC TUMORS

Pancreatic Adenoma

Pancreatic adenomas are benign exocrine epithelial tumors that are often incidental findings. They are most commonly of acinar origin and less often ductular; regardless, there is no difference in behavior. Adenomas do not metastasize and do not have the propensity to develop into adenocarcinomas. Histologically, adenomas are usually small (<1 cm), single masses that are partially or fully encapsulated with or without compression and atrophy of the surrounding parenchyma. Some tumors may be cystic. Ductal adenomas display tubular and ductular formations of cuboidal to columnar cells, with occasional pseudostratification and cyst formation noted within some ductal adenomas. Some of the ductular columnar cells may display mild vacuolation apically, whereas some of the acinar cells may lack zymogen granulation. Acinar adenomas are, not surprisingly, in acinar formation, uniform, and intercalated by fibrovascular stroma. The lack of invasion and atypia differentiate adenomas from well-differentiated adenocarcinomas (Munday et al., 2017). On cytopathology, cohesive clusters of cuboidal to columnar epithelial cells are seen with ductular origin cells, whereas acinar formations are seen with acinar tumors. The cells have round nuclei with single nucleoli and moderate amounts of basophilic cytoplasm. Mild anisocytosis and anisokaryosis and rare mitotic figures may be appreciated. The neoplastic cells appear similar to those of normal tissue, hyperplastic nodules, and some well-differentiated adenocarcinomas (Munday et al., 2017).

Pancreatic Carcinoma

Although uncommon in dogs and cats, pancreatic adenocarcinoma is the most common tumor of the exocrine pancreas. There is an increasing incidence with age, but no breed or sex predispositions have been described. Clinical signs are nonspecific, and include weight loss, vomiting, anorexia, and abdominal pain. Some animals are icteric because of secondary biliary obstruction. Routine laboratory data abnormalities are similar to those of pancreatitis; however, extremely increased serum lipase activities (>10,000 IU/mL) are suggestive of pancreatic carcinoma (Quigley et al., 2001). In one study, 15% of cats with exocrine pancreatic carcinoma had concurrent DM (Linderman et al., 2013). On ultrasound, pancreatic carcinomas may appear as solitary or multiple hypoechoic masses, although they may be diffuse in the cat. Some tumors may be cystic. A single pancreatic mass larger than 2 cm in diameter is more likely to be malignant in cats (Hecht et al., 2007). Tumors often invade adjacent tissues and can lead to biliary obstruction. Metastases may be observed within the liver, regional lymph nodes, mesentery, and distant sites (Chang et al., 2007). Most patients have metastases at the time of diagnosis. Concurrent pancreatitis and steatitis may also be noted. Consequently, pancreatic carcinomas have a poor prognosis.

There are several histologic subtypes of pancreatic carcinoma: ductal adenocarcinoma, acinar adenocarcinoma, hyalinizing pancreatic carcinoma, mixed exocrine–endocrine carcinoma, undifferentiated pancreatic carcinoma, colloidal (or mucinous noncystic) carcinoma, and squamous cell carcinoma (Gebbie et al., 2012; Hagiwara et al., 2017; Munday et al., 2017; Luo et al., 2019). Ductal and acinar adenocarcinomas are most common in dogs and cats (Fig. 8.14). The histologic appearance varies depending on the degree of differentiation. Well-differentiated tumors typically are easily identifiable as pancreatic. The cells are uniform and often retain zymogen granulation. They have low N:C ratios. In contrast, poorly differentiated tumors have higher N:C ratios, enlarged nuclei, and coarse chromatin. The degree of atypia and mitotic index correlate with the degree of differentiation with poorly differentiated tumors having increased pleomorphism and frequent mitoses. Hyalinizing pancreatic adenocarcinoma has only been described in dogs. This variant is characterized by aggregates of brightly eosinophilic hyaline material within the stroma and ductal lumens. The exact composition of this material is unclear as various immunohistochemical and histochemical stains are negative (Dennis et al., 2008).

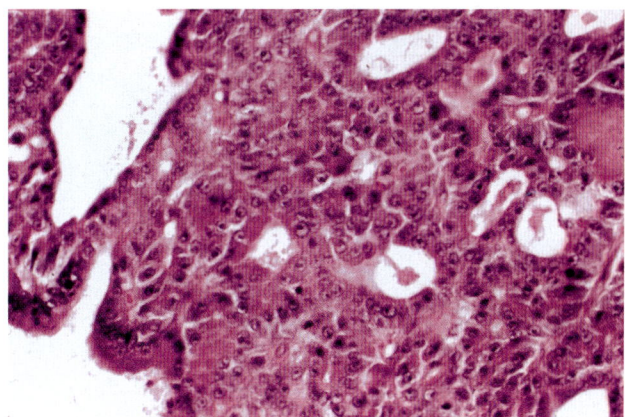

■ **FIGURE 8.14** **Pancreatic adenocarcinoma. Pancreatic mass. Histology. Dog.** Papillary (elongated clump) and cluster formation of pancreatic exocrine epithelial cells that are forming disorganized glandular and ductular structures. (H&E; IP.) (Courtesy Claire Andreasen, Iowa State University.)

Colloidal (or mucinous noncystic) carcinoma has been reported in a cat (Hagiwara et al., 2017). The tumor was gelatinous grossly with large amounts of periodic acid–Schiff–positive and Alcian blue–positive mucin interspersed between the neoplastic epithelial cells. Squamous cell carcinoma of presumed pancreatic duct origin has also been reported in a cat with carcinomatosis (Gebbie et al., 2012).

Cytopathologic evaluation of pancreatic masses correlates well with histopathology in human and veterinary medicine. However, differentiation of well-differentiated adenocarcinomas from adenomas and hyperplasia is challenging (Munday et al., 2017). Poorly differentiated or undifferentiated carcinomas are often easily distinguished. They appear similar to carcinomas elsewhere and often do not provide identifying features of their underlying pancreatic origin. Aspirates of pancreatic adenocarcinoma are usually highly cellular with clusters, rows, and sheets of epithelial cells (Figs. 8.15 to 8.17). Acinar or tubular structures (or both) may be seen (Fig. 8.18). The neoplastic cells are often markedly pleomorphic with pronounced anisocytosis and anisokaryosis. Karyomegaly and increased N:C ratios are observed. The nuclear chromatin is reticular to coarsely clumped; nuclear margins may be irregular, leading to angular or polygonal nuclei; and molding may be appreciated. Nuclei often have single to multiple, variably shaped, prominent nucleoli of varying sizes. Abnormal mitotic figures may be noted, which increases the confidence in diagnosis of malignancy. Increased cytoplasmic basophilia and occasional vacuolation may also be appreciated. Zymogen granules may be seen in well-differentiated acinar adenocarcinomas. The neoplastic cells are often within a background of mixed inflammation, hemorrhage, or necrosis.

In human pathology, various cytopathologic criteria are used to aid in the diagnosis of well-differentiated pancreatic adenocarcinoma. No such criteria exist in veterinary medicine, but the human criteria may be extrapolated for use in dogs and cats. The criteria include anisokaryosis (variation in nuclear size greater than four times in the same epithelial group); nuclear membrane irregularity (deep notches or grooves, crumpled nuclei, and so on) and nuclear crowding, overlapping or three-dimensionality, and karyomegaly (single nuclei >2.5 times the diameter of a red blood cell) (Lin and Staerkel, 2003).

Paraneoplastic alopecia has occasionally been described in association with pancreatic exocrine (and rarely endocrine) neoplasia in addition to hepatocellular carcinomas, metastatic intestinal carcinoma, cholangiocarcinoma, and hepatosplenic plasma cell neoplasia in veterinary medicine (Sharpe et al.,

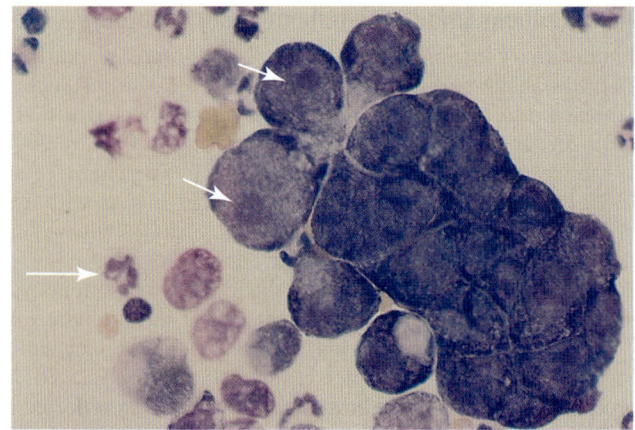

FIGURE 8.16 Pancreatic adenocarcinoma. Pancreatic mass. Tissue imprint. Cat. A dense, slightly elongated basophilic epithelial cell cluster shows marked anisocytosis and anisokaryosis. The cytoplasm is not easily observed because the nucleocytoplasmic ratio is markedly increased. Gigantic nucleoli are observed in some cells *(short arrows)*. The cells at the upper end of the cluster appear to be forming a disorganized acinar structure. The inappropriately large size of the neoplastic cells can be appreciated by comparison with a neutrophil *(long arrow)*. (Wright; HP oil.) (Courtesy Claire Andreasen, Iowa State University.)

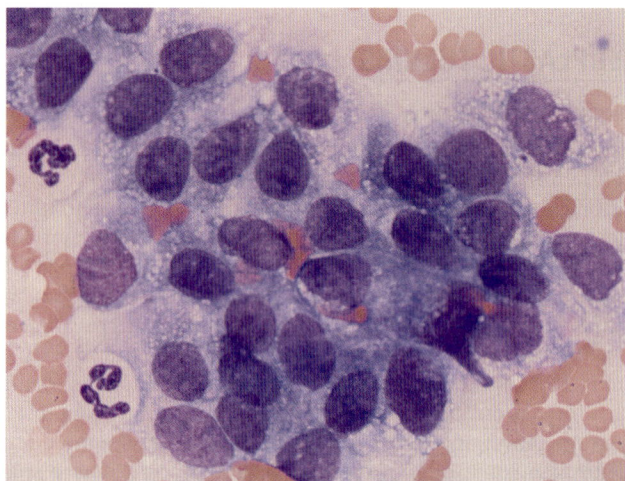

FIGURE 8.17 Pancreatic adenocarcinoma. Aspirate. Cat. A nodule measuring 0.6 × 0.8 cm on the right lobe of pancreas was biopsied, revealing a sheet of atypical cohesive cells. These cells are polygonal with distinct cellular borders and a moderate amount of pale basophilic cytoplasm that often contains many fine colorless vacuoles. The round to oval nuclei measure 3 to 4 × RBC diameter and has coarse chromatin with one to three round to oval, distinct nucleoli. Binucleation is occasional. Anisocytosis and anisokaryosis are moderate. The animal had multifocal pulmonary nodules presumed to be metastatic from the pancreas. (Wright-Giemsa; HP oil.) (Courtesy Rose Raskin, University of Florida.)

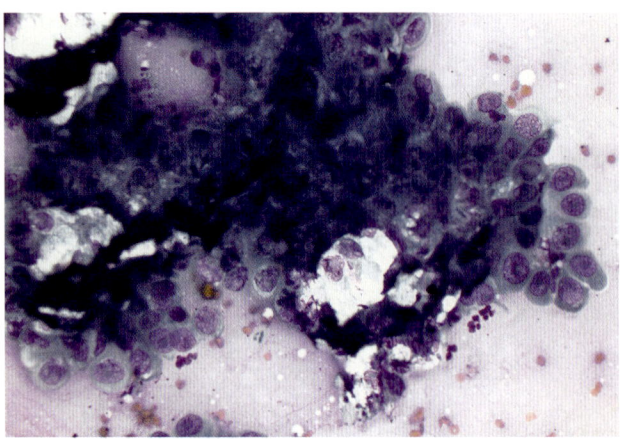

FIGURE 8.15 Pancreatic adenocarcinoma. Pancreatic mass. Tissue aspirate. Cat. A honeycomb-like sheet with peripheral rows of cuboidal neoplastic epithelial cells. Their nuclei are round with reticular chromatin and a central, prominent nucleolus. (Wright-Giemsa; HP oil.) (Courtesy Katie Boes, Virginia Tech.)

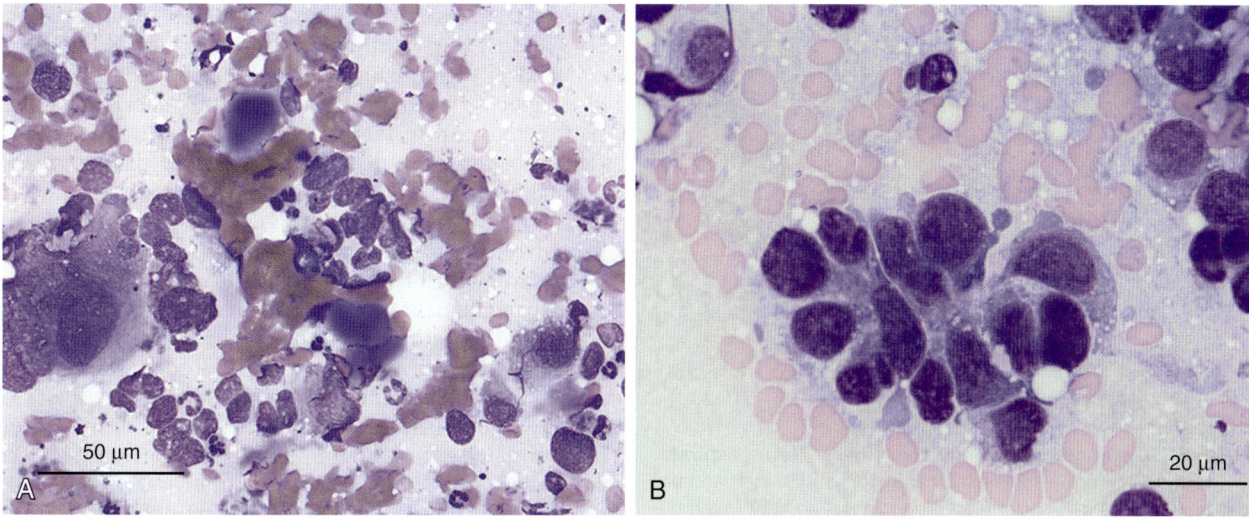

FIGURE 8.18 Pancreatic adenocarcinoma. Aspirate. Dog. Same case in A and B. **A,** There are few neoplastic cells and amorphous basophilic necrotic material and mixed, predominantly neutrophilic, inflammation. Several neoplastic cells are ruptured, but the lysed nuclei still show epithelial arrangement (rows) and criteria of malignancy (nuclear gigantism). (Romanowsky; HP oil.) **B,** Epithelial cells form a crude acinus and show criteria of malignancy, including karyomegaly, anisokaryosis, and nuclear molding. (Romanowsky; HP oil.)

2014; Caporali et al., 2016). The alopecia is typically bilaterally symmetrical and nonpruritic with a smooth (glabrous) appearance and easy epilation. Pruritis may occur if there is secondary infection, such as may occur with *Malassezia* spp. overgrowth. The alopecia is typically reversible with complete resection of the primary tumor. Lymphocytic mural folliculitis is potentially another cutaneous manifestation of pancreatic neoplasia in cats (Lobetti, 2015).

> **KEY POINT** Paraneoplastic glabrous alopecia and lymphocytic mural folliculitis have been seen in association with pancreatic adenocarcinoma in cats. The etiology of these concurrent disorders is unclear.

In dogs, pancreatic tumors may also cause the paraneoplastic syndrome panniculitis, polyarthritis, and pancreatic neoplasia (PPP) (Gear et al., 2006). Panniculitis is believed to be the result of high levels of circulating activated pancreatic enzymes released from the diseased pancreas, leading to widespread necrosis and inflammation of adipose tissue with subsequent hemorrhage and mineralization. The polyarthritis is likely caused by extension of the panniculitis into the joint or bone, as well as primary inflammation of the perimyseal and bone marrow adipose tissue (Gear et al., 2006).

Pancreatic Endocrine Tumors

As mentioned earlier, the pancreatic endocrine cells form the islets of Langerhans in the pancreas and are surrounded by exocrine cells (see Fig. 8.2). The α-, β-, δ-, and PP-secreting cells are included in this group (Figs. 8.19 to 8.24). A neoplasm arising from one of these pancreatic endocrine cells is termed *pancreatic endocrine tumor* (PET) or *islet cell tumor* (Table 8.1), which includes benign (islet cell adenoma) and malignant (islet cell carcinoma) variants.

The most frequently diagnosed PET is a β-cell tumor, also known as an insulin-secreting tumor, which includes insulinoma

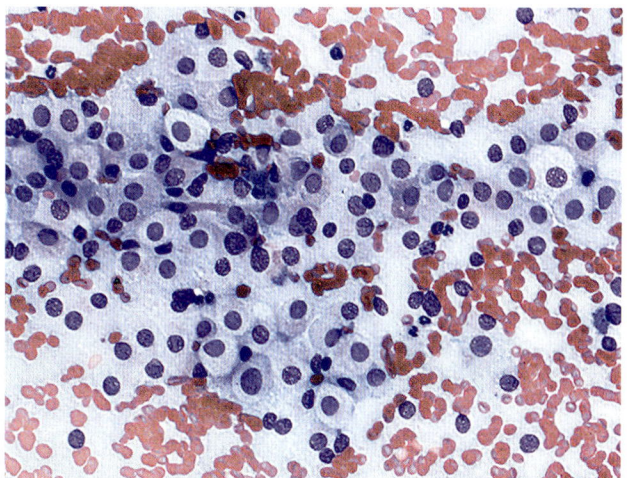

FIGURE 8.19 Insulinoma (β-cell tumor). Pancreatic mass. Tissue aspirate. Dog. Pancreatic mass in a severely hypoglycemic dog shows loosely cohesive sheets of uniform neoplastic cells. Cytoplasm of several cells appears pinkish-blue. (Romanowsky; IP.) (Courtesy Katie Boes, Virginia Tech.)

(β-cell adenoma) and malignant insulinoma (β-cell carcinoma) (see Figs. 8.19 to 8.21). In domestic animals, β-cell tumors are most commonly diagnosed in dogs, generally large breeds with median age between 8.5 and 10 years (Goutal et al., 2012; Rosol and Meuten, 2017). Commonly affected breeds include boxers, German shepherds, Irish setters, poodles, fox terriers, collies, and Labrador retrievers, but these results may be biased by their breed popularities (Goutal et al., 2012; Rosol and Meuten, 2017). These tumors are rare in the cat (Cervone et al., 2019). A single case report of osseous metaplasia was described in association with an insulinoma (Pieczarka et al., 2014).

Most β-cell tumors actively secrete inappropriate amounts of insulin, resulting in clinical hypoglycemia and clinical signs including generalized weakness, hind-limb weakness, ataxia, muscle tremors, seizures, and peripheral neuropathy (Hess, 2013). Most dogs with β-cell tumors exhibit Whipple's triad: (1) clinical signs associated with hypoglycemia, (2) fasting blood glucose less than 40 mg/dL, and (3) alleviation of clinical signs with dextrose administration. A tentative diagnosis of β-cell tumor can be made by demonstrating hypoglycemia with a normal or increased serum insulin concentration. A decreased serum fructosamine concentration, an indicator of chronic hypoglycemia, may also aid in diagnosis.

Less frequent PETs include gastrin-secreting tumor (gastrinoma or malignant gastrinoma), glucagon-producing islet cell adenoma (α islet cell adenoma, glucagonoma), somatostatin-producing islet cell adenoma (δ islet cell adenoma, somatostatinoma), PP-secreting islet cell carcinoma, and other PETs secreting an assortment of hormones different from pancreatic hormones. Gastrin-secreting tumors are derived from ectopic pancreatic amine precursor uptake and decarboxylase (APUD) cells that produce excessive gastrin, resulting in a Zollinger-Ellison–like syndrome (see Figs. 8.22 and 8.23). Affected animals show clinical signs of gastric ulceration, including vomiting, anorexia, progressive weight loss, intermittent diarrhea,

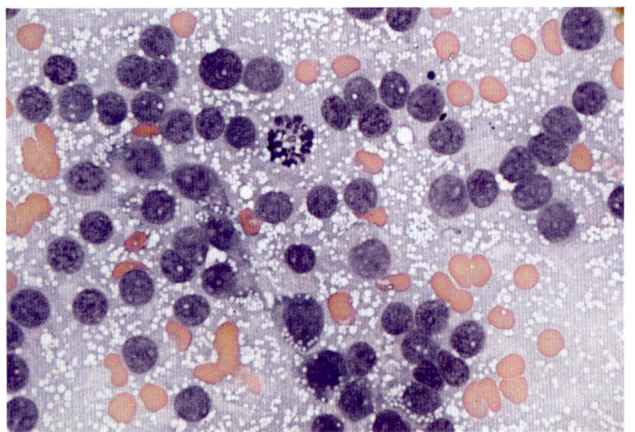

■ **FIGURE 8.20 Islet cell carcinoma. Liver mass. Tissue aspirate. Dog.** Cytopathology from a metastatic hepatic mass (shown) and primary pancreatic mass (not shown) revealed rows of uniform round nuclei on a light basophilic background with many colorless vacuoles. Intact cells contain light eosinophilic or basophilic cytoplasm with the same colorless vacuoles. Note the mitotic figure. Results for immunohistochemical staining for insulin were negative. (Wright-Giemsa; HP oil.)

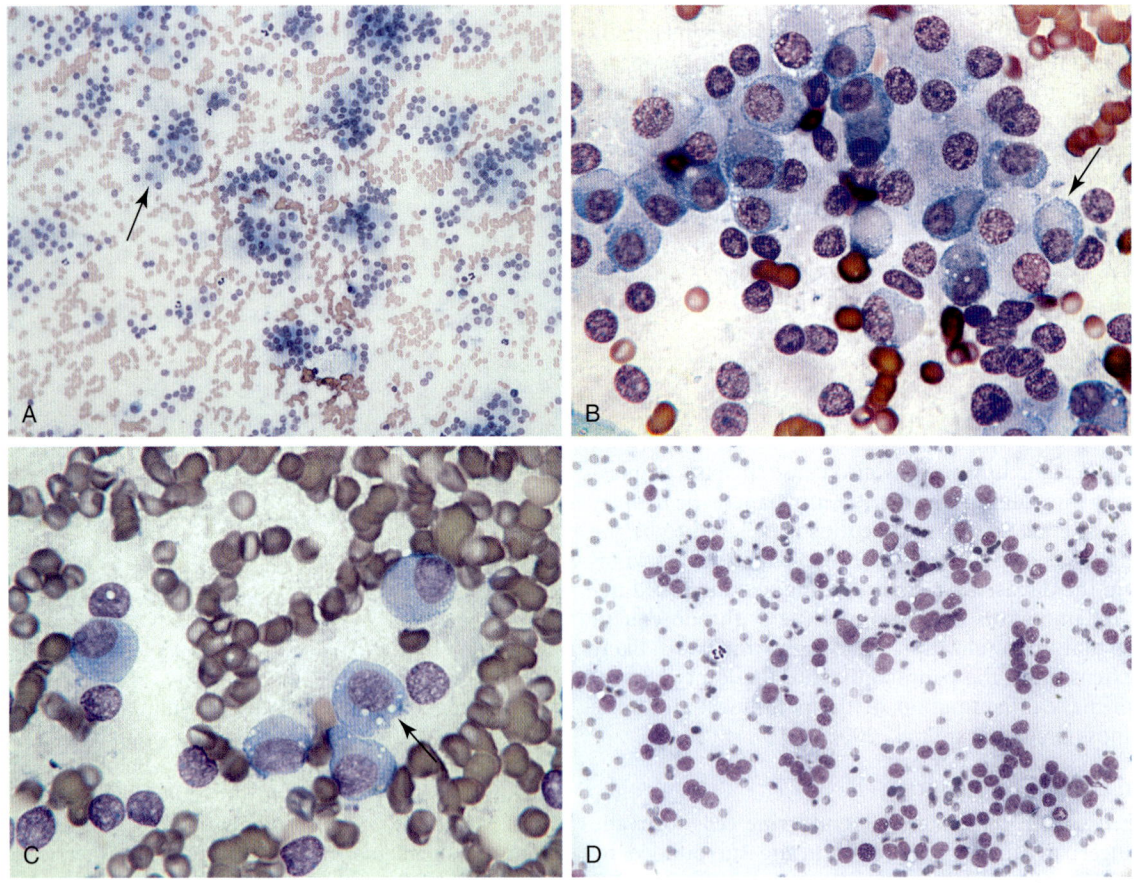

■ **FIGURE 8.21 Insulinoma (β-cell tumor). Tissue aspirate. Dog.** Same case in A and D. **A, Pancreatic mass.** Cytopathology of an abdominal mass located in the pancreas of this severely hypoglycemic dog shows loose cell clusters *(arrow)*. (Aqueous Romanowsky; LP.) **B, Pancreatic mass.** Higher magnification displays a population of round to loosely cohesive polygonal cells. Nuclei are round with coarsely stippled chromatin and a prominent nucleolus. The moderate anisokaryosis is excessive for an endocrine population, which warrants concern for malignant insulinoma. Note the light pink to basophilic cytoplasm *(arrow)* and presence of small punctate clear cytoplasmic vacuoles. (Aqueous Romanowsky; HP oil.) **C, Pancreatic mass.** Several intact individualized cells show distinct cytoplasmic borders, and cells contain frequent punctate, clear vacuoles *(arrow)*. (Aqueous Romanowsky; HP oil.) **D, Lymph node.** The pancreatic lymph node contains rows of uniform, lysed nuclei. The absence of lymphocytes suggests effacement of the lymph node by neoplastic cells. (Aqueous Romanowsky; IP.) (From Choi US. *Practical Guide to Diagnostic Cytology of the Dog and Cat.* OKVET; 2012.)

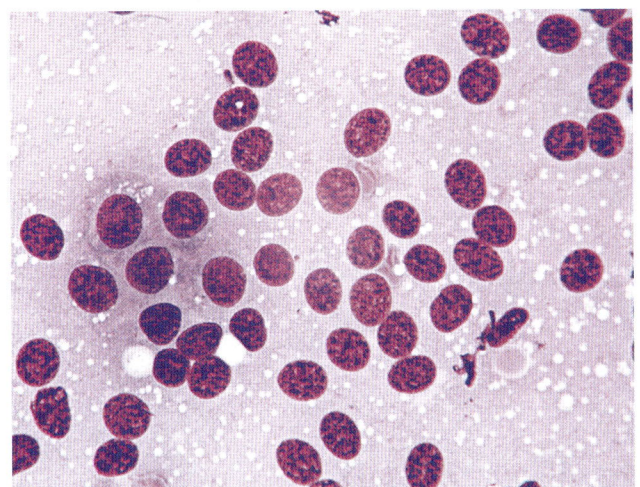

■ **FIGURE 8.22 Gastrin-secreting tumor. Pancreatic mass. Dog.** Numerous naked nuclei and punctate clear vacuoles are scattered in the background along with few cells having distinct cytoplasmic borders. (Hemacolor; HP oil.) (Courtesy Walter Bertazzolo, Italy.)

and dehydration (Gal et al., 2011). Serum gastrin concentrations are often increased, termed *hypergastrinemia*. One dog with a malignant gastrinoma also had a concomitant pancreatic somatostatinoma (Hoenerhoff and Kiupel, 2004). Glucagonoma typically causes hyperglycemia via glucagon secretion and is less frequently associated with superficial necrolytic dermatitis or necrolytic migratory dermatitis (Oberkirchner et al., 2010). Superficial necrolytic dermatitis has also been reported in a dog with malignant insulinoma (Isidoro-Ayza et al., 2014).

> **KEY POINT** Paraneoplastic phenomena associated with some PETs include superficial necrolytic dermatitis and peripheral neuropathy.

Tumors of the endocrine pancreas are often very cellular and share the typical cytopathologic features of neoplasms of endocrine and neuroendocrine cells. Cytopathologic preparations often appear as naked nuclei or free nuclei embedded in a background of pale cytoplasm with few distinct cytoplasmic borders (see Figs. 8.19 to 8.24) (Cruz Cardona et al., 2010).

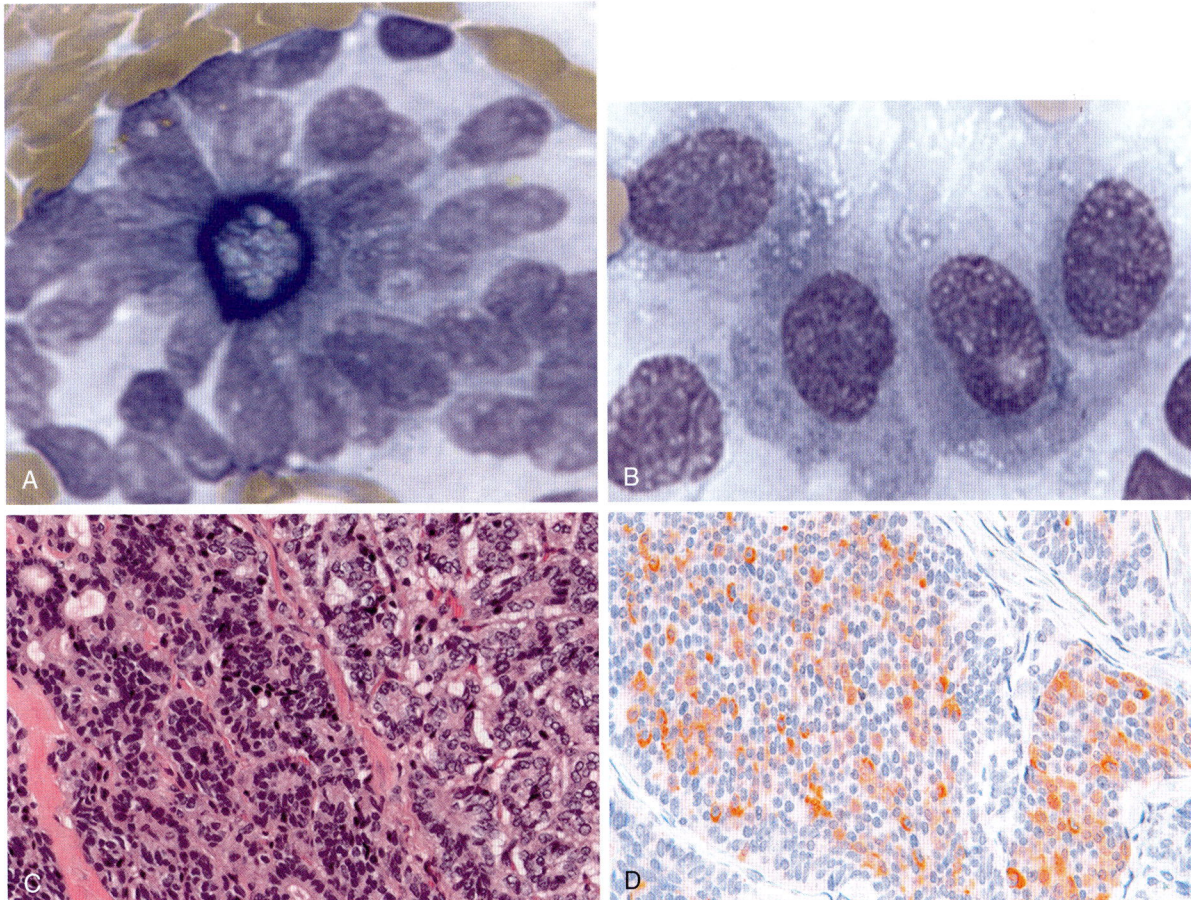

■ **FIGURE 8.23 Gastrin-secreting tumor. Lymph node. Dog.** Same case in A to D. **A, Tissue imprint.** Cytopathology of mass from nearly effaced abdominal lymph node displays a pseudorosette structure with a crystalline center identified histochemically as calcium. (Wright; HP oil.) **B, Tissue imprint.** Higher magnification of tumor cells shows the poorly defined cell borders and faint cytoplasmic granularity. (Wright; HP oil.) **C, Histology.** Several rosettes are present, especially in the *upper left corner*. The centers of the rosettes frequently stained periodic acid–Schiff positive and occasionally contained mineral. (H&E; IP.) **D, Immunohistology.** More than half of the cells expressed gastrin. Immunohistochemistry for gastrin was performed at the Minnesota Veterinary Diagnostic Laboratory. In addition, the majority of cells reacted to pancytokeratins, synaptophysin, and chromogranin A (not shown). Primary clinical signs were chronic vomiting, extreme lethargy, diarrhea, and progressive loss of appetite. (Gastrin antibody; IP.) (Courtesy Sarah Johnson, Purdue University. Presented at the 2011 ASVCP case review session.)

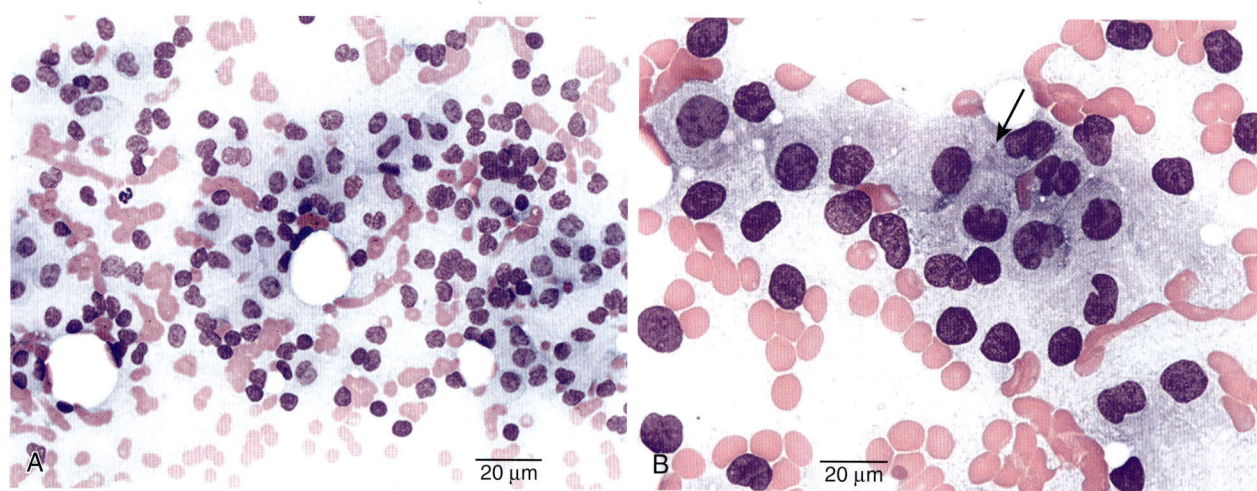

■ **FIGURE 8.24** Pancreatic polypeptide–secreting tumor or metastatic islet cell carcinoma. Mesenteric lymph node. Tissue aspirate. Dog. Same case in A and B. **A,** Loose cluster of epithelial cells with indistinct cytoplasmic borders are mixed with numerous naked or free nuclei, typical of neuroendocrine tumors. (Wright-Giemsa; IP.) **B,** Higher magnification hints at the presence of an eosinophilic granule in the cytoplasm, which may be secretory material *(arrow)*. Nuclear shape is round, lobulated, or reniform, and the chromatin is finely reticular or clumped. Nucleoli are indistinct. Approximately 98% of the tumor cells were immunoreactive for pancreatic polypeptide. Histologically, the tumor appeared malignant. The dog was presented for chronic (1-year) nonspecific clinical signs, including intermittent vomiting and watery diarrhea. (Wright-Giemsa; HP oil.) (Courtesy of Janice Cruz Cardona, University of Florida.)

TABLE 8.1 Cell of Origin and Clinical Aspects of Pancreatic Endocrine Tumors

PANCREATIC ENDOCRINE TUMORS	CELL OF ORIGIN	CLINICAL ASPECTS
Insulinoma Malignant insulinoma	β Islet cell	Hypoglycemia with normal or increased serum insulin concentration Low serum fructosamine concentration Whipple's triad of hypoglycemia, signs of hypoglycemia, and alleviation of signs with dextrose administration
Gastrinoma Malignant gastrinoma	Non-β islet cell	Increased fasting serum gastrin concentration Zollinger-Ellison–like syndrome, resulting in chronic vomiting
Glucagonoma	α Islet cell	Hyperglycemia with hyperglucagonemia Associated syndrome is superficial necrolytic dermatitis or necrolytic migratory dermatitis
PP-secreting islet cell carcinoma	PP-secreting islet cell	Absent or nonspecific clinical signs Has been associated with intermittent vomiting and watery diarrhea
Other PETs (somatostatinoma, VIP adenoma)	δ Islet cell (somatostatinoma) or other islet cell	PETs usually secrete more than one hormone and can secrete hormones not normally secreted such as VIP, ACTH, or chromogranin

ACTH, Adrenocorticotropic hormone; *PET,* pancreatic endocrine tumor; *PP,* pancreatic polypeptide; *VIP,* vasoactive intestinal peptide.

This appearance often results from the fragile nature of the cells from these tissues. This cytopathologic feature should not be confused with poorly prepared samples from other tissues, where cell lysis occurs when excessive pressure is applied to the slides during sample preparation. In the latter case, cell damage such as nuclear lysis and nuclear streaming will also be evident. In some instances, the cytoplasm may contain fine, eosinophilic granules (see Figs. 8.19 and 8.24); small, punctate, colorless vacuoles (see Figs. 8.20 and 8.21); or rosette-like formations centered on mineral (see Fig. 8.23A). There may be mild to moderate anisokaryosis, and nuclei may contain a single prominent nucleolus. Nuclei are typically round; however, indented nuclei may be encountered infrequently (see Fig. 8.24). Although most PETs in dogs are carcinomas, nuclear features of malignancy are inconsistently seen; similar to other endocrine tumors, it is often difficult to predict the biologic behavior of these lesions based on cytomorphology alone (Rosol and Meuten, 2017). If the criteria for malignancy are met, a diagnosis of islet cell carcinoma can be reliably made; however, the lack of criteria of malignancy cannot be used by itself to diagnose islet cell adenoma. Often these lesions are identified simply as islet cell tumors unless there is sufficient criteria of malignancy, tissue or vascular invasion, or metastatic disease, warranting diagnosis of islet cell carcinoma. Microscopic features are similar among the various PETs; therefore, determination of the specific islet cell origin requires immunohistochemistry or measurement of plasma analyte or hormone concentrations relevant to the patient's clinical signs.

> **KEY POINT** The presence of numerous intact free or naked nuclei aids in the identification of the tumor as of endocrine origin; however, it can be difficult to predict biologic behavior based on cytopathological findings alone because aggressive tumors may appear benign.

The biologic behavior of PETs in dogs is well characterized. Most are carcinomas that tend to be locally invasive with poor long-term prognosis. Metastasis is via lymphatics, with involvement of liver and regional lymph nodes, which occurs in about 50% of the cases (Hess, 2013) (see Figs. 8.20 and 8.21D). Tumor thrombosis and venotomy has been reported in two dogs; the surgeries had no negative effect on prognosis (Hambrook and Kudnig, 2012). Given the challenge in prognosticating these tumors, tissue microarray analysis has been used. On univariate analysis, the presence of nuclear atypia was significantly predictive of disease-free intervals for canine insulinoma, whereas tumor size, tumor, node, metastasis (TNM) stage; necrosis; and Ki67 index were significant in terms of prognosis (both disease-free interval and survival time). On multivariate analysis, tumor size and Ki67 index were still predictive for survival time, as was tumor size for disease-free interval (Buishand et al., 2014). Ki67 has previously been used as a biomarker for insulinoma. One study discovered that stromal fibrosis in addition to Ki67 was significantly predictive of survival (Buishand et al., 2010).

Confirmation can be made by exploratory celiotomy or ultrasound-guided FNA if a pancreatic lesion is large enough. Tobin et al. (1999) suggest that after a tentative diagnosis is made, exploratory celiotomy and partial pancreatectomy are indicated in dogs because surgery can significantly increase the mean survival time from 74 days (medical or dietary management) to 381 days (surgery plus medical or dietary management). Despite widespread metastasis or incomplete surgical excision, prolonged survival times have been noted in response to medical management, most recently, a combination of prednisone and toceranib phosphate (Flesner et al., 2019).

Miscellaneous Pancreatic Neoplasia

The pancreas can be a site of metastasis, namely lymphoma or histiocytic sarcoma (Arnold et al., 2012; Ueno et al., 2014), or local tissue invasion, such as with gastric or intestinal adenocarcinoma. There are rare reports of pancreatic mesenchymal tumors, including lymphangiosarcoma and carcinosarcoma (Hecht et al., 2007; Yamamoto et al., 2012). Carcinoids may also affect the pancreas and are discussed in detail in Chapter 17.

REFERENCES

Abou Monsef Y, Atalay Vural S, Kutsal O. Pancreatic choristoma in a canine gallbladder. *J Comp Pathol.* 2019;166:17-19.

Anderson JR, Cornell KK, Parnell NK, et al. Pancreatic abscess in 36 dogs: a retrospective analysis of prognostic indicators. *J Am Anim Hosp Assoc.* 2008;44(4):171-179.

Arnold E, Pressler B, Heng, HG. What is your diagnosis? Histiocytic sarcoma. *J Am Vet Med Assoc.* 2012;240(7):821-823.

Bazelle J, Watson P. Pancreatitis in cats: is it acute, is it chronic, is it significant? *J Feline Med Surg.* 2014;16(5):395-406.

Bostrom BM, Xenoulis PG, Newman SJ, et al. Chronic pancreatitis in dogs: a retrospective study of clinical, clinicopathological, and histopathological findings in 61 cases. *Vet J.* 2013;195(1):73-79.

Breitschwerdt EB, Goldkamp C, Castleman W, et al. Hyperinsulinemic hypoglycemia syndrome in 2 dogs with bartonellosis. *J Vet Intern Med.* 2014;28:1331-1335.

Brown DL, Van Wettere JA, Cullen JM. Hepatobiliary system and exocrine pancreas. In: Zachary JF, ed. *Pathologic Basis of Veterinary Disease.* 6th ed. St. Louis: Elsevier; 2017:412-470.

Buishand FO, Kik M, Kirpensteijn J. Evaluation of clinico-pathological criteria and the Ki67 index as prognostic indicators in canine insulinoma. *Vet J.* 2010;185(1):62-67.

Buishand FO, Visser J, Kik M, et al. Evaluation of prognostic indicators using validated canine insulinoma tissue microarrays. *Vet J.* 2014;201(1):57-63.

Caporali C, Albanese F, Binanti D, et al. Two cases of feline paraneoplastic alopecia associated with a neuroendocrine pancreatic neoplasia and a hepatosplenic plasma cell tumour. *Vet Dermatol.* 2016;27(6):508-512.

Cervone M, Harel M, Ségard-Weisse E, et al. Use of contrast-enhanced ultrasonography for the detection of a feline insulinoma. *JFMS Open Rep.* 2019;23:5(2):2055116919876140.

Chang SC, Liao JW, Lin YC, et al. Pancreatic acinar cell carcinoma with intracranial metastasis in a dog. *J Vet Med Sci.* 2007;69(1):91-93.

Cordner AP, Armstrong PJ, Newman SJ, et al. Effect of pancreatic tissue sampling on serum pancreatic enzyme levels in clinically healthy dogs. *J Vet Diagn Invest.* 2010;22:702-707.

Cordner AP, Sharkey LC, Armstrong PJ, et al. Cytologic findings and diagnostic yield in 92 dogs undergoing fine-needle aspiration of the pancreas. *J Vet Diagn Invest.* 2015;27(2):236-240.

Crain SK, Sharkey LC, Cordner AP, et al. Safety of ultrasound-guided fine-needle aspiration of the feline pancreas: a case-control study. *J Feline Med Surg.* 2015;17(10):858-863.

Cridge H, MacLeod AG, Pachtinger GE, et al. Evaluation of SNAP cPL, Spec cPL, VetScan cPL Rapid Test, and Precision PSL assays for the diagnosis of clinical pancreatitis in dogs. *J Vet Intern Med.* 2018;32(2):658-664.

Cruz Cardona JA, Wamsley HL, Farina LL, et al. Metastatic pancreatic polypeptide-secreting islet cell tumor in a dog. *Vet Clin Pathol.* 2010;39:371-376.

De Cock HE, Forman MA, Farver TB, et al. Prevalence and histopathologic characteristics of pancreatitis in cats. *Vet Pathol.* 2007;44(1):39-49.

Dennis MM, O'Brien TD, Wayne T, et al. Hyalinizing pancreatic adenocarcinoma in six dogs. *Vet Pathol.* 2008;45(4):475-483.

Duncan RB, Lindsay D, Chickering WR, et al. Acute primary toxoplasmic pancreatitis in a cat. *Feline Pract.* 2000;28(1):6-8.

Dycus DL, Fisher C, Butler R. Surgical and medical treatment of pyloric and duodenal pythiosis in a dog. *J Am Anim Hosp Assoc.* 2015;51(6):385-391.

Flesner BK, Fletcher JM, Smithee T, et al. Long-term survival and glycemic control with toceranib phosphate and prednisone for a metastatic canine insulinoma. *J Am Anim Hosp Assoc.* 2019;55(1):e55105.

Fragkou FC, Adamama-Moraitou KK, Poutahidis T, et al. Prevalence and clinicopathological features of triaditis in a prospective case series of symptomatic and asymptomatic cats. *J Vet Intern Med.* 2016;30(4):1031-1045.

Gal A, Ridgway MD, Fredrickson RL. An unusual clinical presentation of a dog with gastrinoma. *Can Vet J.* 2011;52(6):641-644.

Gear RN, Bacon NJ, Langley-Hobbs S, et al. Panniculitis, polyarthritis and osteomyelitis associated with pancreatic neoplasia in two dogs. *J Small Anim Pract.* 2006;47(7):400-404.

Gebbie RC, Hardcastle MR, Hunter SA, et al. Transcoelomic spread and metastasis of a squamous cell carcinoma of presumed pancreatic duct origin in a cat. *N Z Vet J.* 2012;60(2):154-159.

Gori E, Lippi I, Guidi G, et al. Acute pancreatitis and acute kidney injury in dogs. *Vet J.* 2019;245:77-81.

Goutal CM, Brugmann BL, Ryan KA. Insulinoma in dogs: a review. *J Am Anim Hosp Assoc.* 2012;48(3):151-163.

Gow AG, Gow DJ. Disseminated *Mycobacterium avium* complex infection in a dog. *Vet Rec.* 2008;162:594-595.

Hagiwara K, Michishita M, Yoshimura H, et al. Pancreatic colloid carcinoma in an elderly cat. *J Comp Pathol.* 2017;157(4):266-269.

Hambrook LE, Kudnig ST. Tumor thrombus formation in two dogs with insulinomas. *J Am Vet Med Assoc.* 2012;241(8):1065-1069.

Hecht S, Penninck DG, Keating JH. Imaging findings in pancreatic neoplasia and nodular hyperplasia in 19 cats. *Vet Radiol Ultrasound.* 2007;48(1):45-50.

Hess RS. Insulinoma in dogs. In: Rand J, ed. *Clinical Endocrinology of Companion Animals.* Ames, IA: Wiley-Blackwell; 2013:229-239.

Hoenerhoff M, Kiupel M. Concurrent gastrinoma and somatostatinoma in a 10-year-old Portuguese water dog. *J Comp Pathol.* 2004;130(4):313-318.

Hoffman DA, Piech TL, Taylor HL, et al. What is your diagnosis? Pancreatic aspirate from a cat. *Vet Clin Pathol.* 2017;46(3):540-541.

Isidoro-Ayza M, Lloret A, Bardagí M, et al. Superficial necrolytic dermatitis in a dog with an insulin-producing pancreatic islet cell carcinoma. *Vet Pathol.* 2014;51(4):805-808.

Kalli IV, Adamama-Moraitou KK, Patsika MN, et al. Prevalence of increased canine pancreas-specific lipase concentrations in young dogs with parvovirus enteritis. *Vet Clin Pathol.* 2017;46(1):111-119.

Kim SH, Woo YS, Lee KH, et al. Preoperative EUS-guided FNA: effects on peritoneal recurrence and survival in patients with pancreatic cancer. *Gastrointest Endosc.* 2018;88(6):926-934.

Kook P, Baloi P, Ruetten M, et al. Feasibility and safety of endoscopic ultrasound-guided fine needle aspiration of the pancreas in dogs. *J Vet Intern Med.* 2012;26:513-517.

Köster LS, Shell L, Ketzis J, et al. Diagnosis of pancreatic disease in feline platynosomosis. *J Feline Med Surg.* 2017;19(12):1192-1198.

Köster LS, Steiner JM, Suchodolski JS, et al. Serum canine pancreatic-specific lipase concentrations in dogs with naturally occurring *Babesia rossi* infection. *J S Afr Vet Assoc.* 2015;86(1):E1-E7.

Lafuente S, Fresno L, Anselmi C, et al. Complete laparoscopic excision of a hepatic cyst and omentopexy in a Persian cat. *JFMS Open Rep.* 2018;4(2):2055116918817631.

Lee JH, Stewart J, Ross WA, et al. Blinded prospective comparison of the performance of 22-gauge and 25-gauge needles in endoscopic ultrasound-guided fine needle aspiration of the pancreas and peri-pancreatic lesions. *Dig Dis Sci.* 2009;54(10):2274-2281.

Liffman R, Courtman N. Fine needle aspiration of abdominal organs: a review of current recommendations for achieving a diagnostic sample. *J Small Anim Pract.* 2017;58(11):599-609.

Lin F, Staerkel G. Cytologic criteria for well differentiated adenocarcinoma of the pancreas in fine-needle aspiration biopsy specimens. *Cancer.* 2003;99:44-50.

Linderman MJ, Brodsky EM, de Lorimier LP, et al. Feline exocrine pancreatic carcinoma: a retrospective study of 34 cases. *Vet Comp Oncol.* 201311(3):208-218.

Lobetti R. Lymphocytic mural folliculitis and pancreatic carcinoma in a cat. *J Feline Med Surg.* 2015;17(6):548-550.

Luo G, Fan Z, Gong Y, et al. Characteristics and outcomes of pancreatic cancer by histological subtypes. *Pancreas.* 2019;48(6):817-822.

Mansfield C. Practical interpretation and application of exocrine pancreatic testing in small animals. *Vet Clin North Am Small Anim Pract.* 2013;43(6):1241-1260.

Mansfield CS, Jones BR. Review of feline pancreatitis part one: the normal feline pancreas, the pathophysiology, classification, prevalence and aetiologies of pancreatitis. *J Feline Med Surg.* 2001;3(3):117-124.

Mellanby RJ, Stell A, Baines E, et al. Panniculitis associated with pancreatitis in a cocker spaniel. *J Small Anim Pract.* 2003;44(1):24-28.

Munday JS, Löhr CV, Kiupel M. Tumors of the alimentary tract. In: Meuten DJ, ed. *Tumors in Domestic Animals.* 5th ed. Ames, IA: Wiley Blackwell; 2017:597-601.

Mylonakis ME, Xenoulis PG, Theodorou K, et al. Serum canine pancreatic lipase immunoreactivity in experimentally induced and naturally occurring canine monocytic ehrlichiosis (*Ehrlichia canis*). *Vet Microbiol.* 2014;169(3-4):198-202.

Nemoto Y, Haraguchi T, Miyama TS, et al: Pancreatic abscess in a cat due to *Staphylococcus aureus* infection, *J Vet Med Sci* 79(7):1146-1150, 2017.

Newman SJ, Steiner JM, Woosley K, et al. Correlation of age and incidence of pancreatic exocrine nodular hyperplasia in the dog. *Vet Pathol.* 2005;42(4):510-513.

Newman SJ, Steiner JM, Woosley K, et al. Histologic assessment and grading of the exocrine pancreas in the dog. *J Vet Diagn Invest.* 2006;18(1):115-118.

Oberkirchner U, Linder KE, Zadrozny L, et al. Successful treatment of canine necrolytic migratory erythema (superficial necrolytic dermatitis) due to metastatic glucagonoma with octreotide. *Vet Dermatol.* 2010;21(5):510-516.

Pesavento PA, MacLachlan NJ, Dillard-Telm L, et al. Pathologic, immunohistochemical, and electron microscopic findings in naturally occurring virulent systemic feline calicivirus infection in cats. *Vet Pathol.* 2004;41(3):257-263.

Pieczarka EM, Russell DS, Santangelo KS, et al. Osseous metaplasia within a canine insulinoma. *Vet Clin Pathol.* 2014;43:89-93.

Plesman RL, Norris A, Ringwood PB. What is your diagnosis? Pancreatolithiasis. *J Am Vet Med Assoc.* 2014;244(6):647-649.

Polansky BJ, Martinez SA, Chalkley MD. Resolution of hyperinsulinemic hypoglycemia following partial pancreatectomy in a dog with nesidioblastosis. *J Am Vet Med Assoc.* 2018;253(7):893-896.

Pratschke KM, Ryan J, McAlinden A, et al. Pancreatic surgical biopsy in 24 dogs and 19 cats: postoperative complications and clinical relevance of histological findings. *J Small Anim Pract.* 2015;56(1):60-66.

Quigley KA, Jackson ML, Haines DM. Hyperlipasemia in 6 dogs with pancreatic or hepatic neoplasia: evidence for tumor lipase production. *Vet Clin Pathol.* 2001;30(3):114-120.

Ramírez GA, Altimira J, García-González B, et al. Intrapancreatic ectopic splenic tissue in dogs and cats. *J Comp Pathol.* 2013;148(4):361-364.

Rodriguez JY, Lewis BC, Snowden KF. Distribution and characterization of *Heterobilharzia americana* in dogs in Texas. *Vet Parasitol.* 2014;203(1-2):35-42.

Rosol TJ, Meuten DJ. Tumors of the endocrine glands. In: Meuten DJ, ed. *Tumors in Domestic Animals.* 5th ed. Ames, IA: Wiley Blackwell; 2017:822-827.

Sadler RA, Fields EL, Whittemore JC. Attempted ultrasound-guided ethanol ablation of a suspected pancreatic pseudocyst in a dog. *Can Vet J.* 2016;57(11):1169-1174.

Sharpe SJ, Meadows RL, Senter DA, et al. Pathology in practice. Liver malignancy and paraneoplastic alopecia in a cat. *J Am Vet Med Assoc.* 2014;244(11):1265-1267.

Standop J, Ulrich A, Schneider MB, et al. Pacinian corpuscle in the human pancreas. *Pancreas.* 2001;23(1):36-39.

Steiner JM, Guadiano P, Gomez RR, et al. Partial analytical validation of the VetScan cPL rapid test. *Vet Clin Pathol.* 2019;48:683-690.

Tangeman L, Davignon D, Patel R, et al. Abdominal cryptococcosis in two dogs: diagnosis and medical management. *J Am Anim Hosp Assoc.* 2015;51(2):107-113.

Tobin RL, Nelson RW, Lucroy MD, et al. Outcome of surgical versus medical treatment of dogs with beta cell neoplasia: 39 cases (1990-1997). *J Am Vet Med Assoc.* 1999;215(2):226-230.

Törner K, Aupperle-Lellbach H, Staudacher A, et al. Primary solid and cystic tumours of the exocrine pancreas in cats. *J Comp Pathol.* 2019;169:5-19.

Tsuchitani M, Sato J, Kokoshima H. A comparison of the anatomical structure of the pancreas in experimental animals. *J Toxicol Pathol.* 2016;29:147-154.

Ueno H, Miyoshi K, Fukui S, et al. Extranodal lymphoma with peripheral nervous system involvement in a dog. *J Vet Med Sci.* 2014;76(5):723-727.

VanEnkevort BA, O'Brien RT, Young KM. Pancreatic pseudocysts in 4 dogs and 2 cats: ultrasonographic and clinicopathologic findings. *J Vet Intern Med.* 1999;13(4):309-313.

Véran E, Gallay-Lepoutre J, Gory G, et al. Chyloabdomen in a cat with pancreatic carcinoma. *Open Vet J.* 2018;8(4):452-457.

Vyhnal KK, Barr SC, Hornbuckle WE, et al. *Eurytrema procyonis* and pancreatitis in a cat. *J Feline Med Surg.* 2008;10(4):384-387.

Watson P. Canine breed-specific hepatopathies. *Vet Clin North Am Small Anim Pract.* 2017;47(3):665-682.

Watson PJ, Roulois AJ, Scase T, et al. Prevalence and breed distribution of chronic pancreatitis at post-mortem examination in first-opinion dogs. *J Small Anim Pract.* 2007;48(11):609-618.

Watson P, Roulois A, Scase T, et al. Characterization of chronic pancreatitis in English cocker spaniels. *J Vet Intern Med.* 2011;25(4):797-804.

Xenoulis PG. Diagnosis of pancreatitis in dogs and cats. *J Small Anim Pract.* 2015;56(1):13-26.

Yamamoto R, Suzuki K, Uchida K, et al. Pancreatic carcinosarcoma in a cat. *J Comp Pathol.* 2012;147(2-3):223-226.

Zoia A, Drigo M. Association between pancreatitis and immune-mediated haemolytic anaemia in cats: a cross-sectional study. *J Comp Pathol.* 2017;156(4):384-388.

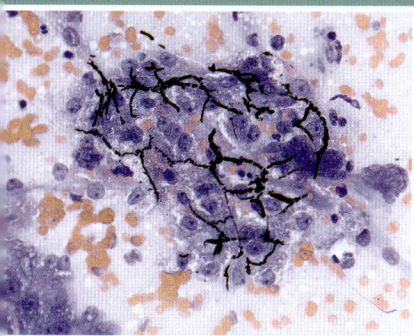

CHAPTER 9

Hepatobiliary System

Laureen M. Peters and Denny J. Meyer

Cytopathologic and histopathologic examination of liver specimens correlates best for diffuse diseases that cause hepatomegaly. The evaluation of focal lesions with fine-needle aspiration biopsy (FNAB) is more diagnostically rewarding with the guidance of ultrasound (Roth, 2001; Bahr et al., 2013). The diagnosis of certain liver pathologies, including fibrosis, regenerative nodules, and well-differentiated hepatocellular tumors, relies on tissue architecture, which cannot be easily assessed on FNAB (Bahr et al., 2013).

SAMPLE COLLECTION AND TECHNIQUE

Indications and Contraindications

Aspiration of the liver is often the next diagnostic step if a hepatopathy is suspected based on clinical history, physical examination, hematologic and biochemical changes, or abnormalities identified on diagnostic imaging studies. Examples include jaundice, high liver enzyme activities, abnormal liver function test results, hepatomegaly, abnormal echogenicity, and identification of masses.

Hemostasis should be assessed before FNAB is performed to rule out thrombocytopenia, thrombocytopathia, and abnormal coagulation times; the latter is particularly important because decreased liver function and biliary disease can lead to reduced synthesis or activation of clotting factors (Prins et al., 2010). A thorough history to rule out administration of drugs inhibiting coagulation or recent bleeding episodes should also be taken. If the indications for FNAB of the liver are considered to offset the risk of bleeding with findings of inadequate hemostasis, careful monitoring of the animal for significant abdominal hemorrhage after sampling is mandatory. Aspiration of a large cavitated lesion may pose a relative contraindication for FNAB when hemangiosarcoma is suspected because obtaining a suitable sample for a cytopathologic diagnosis is unlikely, and there is potential for rupturing a necrotic capsule and causing a life-threateningly hemorrhage. In human literature, tumor seeding through the needle tract is described as another potential risk. However, there are no studies documenting this event in the veterinary literature (Klopfleisch et al., 2011).

> **KEY POINT** Liver cytopathology is most rewarding for diffuse conditions such as vacuolar hepatopathy, inflammation, and round cell neoplasia. However, histopathology for assessment of tissue architecture may be warranted for the diagnosis of fibrosis, nodular regeneration, well-differentiated hepatocellular and cholangiocellular neoplasia, cavitated lesions, and focal inflammation.

Liver Sampling

Sampling the liver is typically conducted with ultrasonographic guidance. The need for chemical restraint depends on the disposition of the patient, but adequate immobilization is critical because of the risk of vessel laceration. Choice of needle size ranges from 1 to 3 inches in length, 20 to 22 gauge, depending on the indication and the size of the animal. If a needle with a stylet is used, the stylet is left in place until the liver is entered to reduce contamination from skin and mesenteric fat as it is penetrated. When the needle is within the hepatic parenchyma, it is quickly advanced and withdrawn two or three times. Acquisition of the specimen can be obtained by either nonaspiration procedure ("capillary" sampling) or aspiration using a 5 to 12 mL syringe (see Chapter 1). In general, the nonaspiration approach should be tried first and was determined in one study to be superior to aspiration with greater cellularity, less hemodilution, and better cytologic preservation (Fleming et al., 2019). If the specimen is nondiagnostic, the aspiration technique can be attempted. For more details on slide preparation, see Chapter 1. Protection from formalin fumes during sampling, storage, and shipping is critical to preserve morphologic detail. At least one unfixed cytologic slide preparation should be saved for potential special stains such as Ziehl-Neelsen, rhodanine, Perls Prussian blue, Congo red, or immunocytochemical stains.

Bile Sampling

Puncture of the gallbladder to sample bile for cytopathologic examination is indicated when an inflammatory biliary disease is suspected but is contraindicated when extrahepatic bile duct obstruction is present to avoid potential iatrogenic rupture of the gallbladder. It is recommended to remove as much bile as possible during aspiration to minimize the risk of bile peritonitis. Some ultrasonographers may favor the transhepatic approach for the same reason, although others suggest any approach is safe (Rothuizen and Twedt, 2009). The patient should be monitored for bile leakage, preferably ultrasonically, 1 to 2 hours after the procedure even though the incidence appears low (Peters et al., 2016).

Bile, like any other fluid obtained, should be submitted in both an ethylenediaminetetraacetic acid (EDTA) tube for optimal cellular preservation and in a sterile plain tube for other diagnostic tests, including bacterial culture. Making a fresh direct smear is advisable, particularly if sample processing is delayed, because cells deteriorate quickly when exposed to the inhospitable conditions in bile. Because bile is a low-protein specimen and does not avidly stick to a glass surface, several direct smears, concentrated smears, and the cytocentrifuge preparation (the most rewarding technique) are recommended for optimal results. After smears are made, bile aspirates can be submitted to the microbiology laboratory in a Luer lock capped syringe for culture and for the cytocentrifuge preparation.

NORMAL CYTOLOGY AND ARTIFACTS

Liver

Hepatocytes constitute the predominant cell type of a normal liver (Fig. 9.1). They are typically present in sheets, where they are polygonal to rounded when found individualized, with a diameter of 25 to 30 μm (3–4 × RBC diameter). They contain a centrally placed, round nucleus with coarse chromatin and often a single small but prominent centrally placed nucleolus. The cytoplasm is abundeant and pale basophilic, containing numerous pale pink granules caused by the varying tinctorial properties of the different organelles. This cytoplasmic appearance is typically described as amphophilic related to being both blue and pink. Binucleation is occasional (see Fig. 9.1B–C) and is more frequently seen in older dogs; cellular (but not nuclear) size also seems to increase with age (Stockhaus et al., 2002). Low numbers of mixed leukocytes are also found in aspirates of clinically unremarkable livers, including low numbers of neutrophils and small lymphocytes, as well as occasional macrophages and well-differentiated mast cells (see Fig. 9.1B). Mature hepatocytes may accumulate lipofuscin pigment (see Hepatic Pigments) from breakdown of organelles forming green or dark cytoplasmic granules (see Fig. 9.1D).

Few dense clusters of smaller, cuboidal biliary epithelial cells with a high nucleocytoplasmic (N:C) ratio can occasionally be observed and may contain punctate cytoplasmic vacuoles (Fig. 9.2). Larger bile ducts, including the common bile duct, are lined by ciliated columnar epithelial cells (Figs. 9.3 and 9.4).

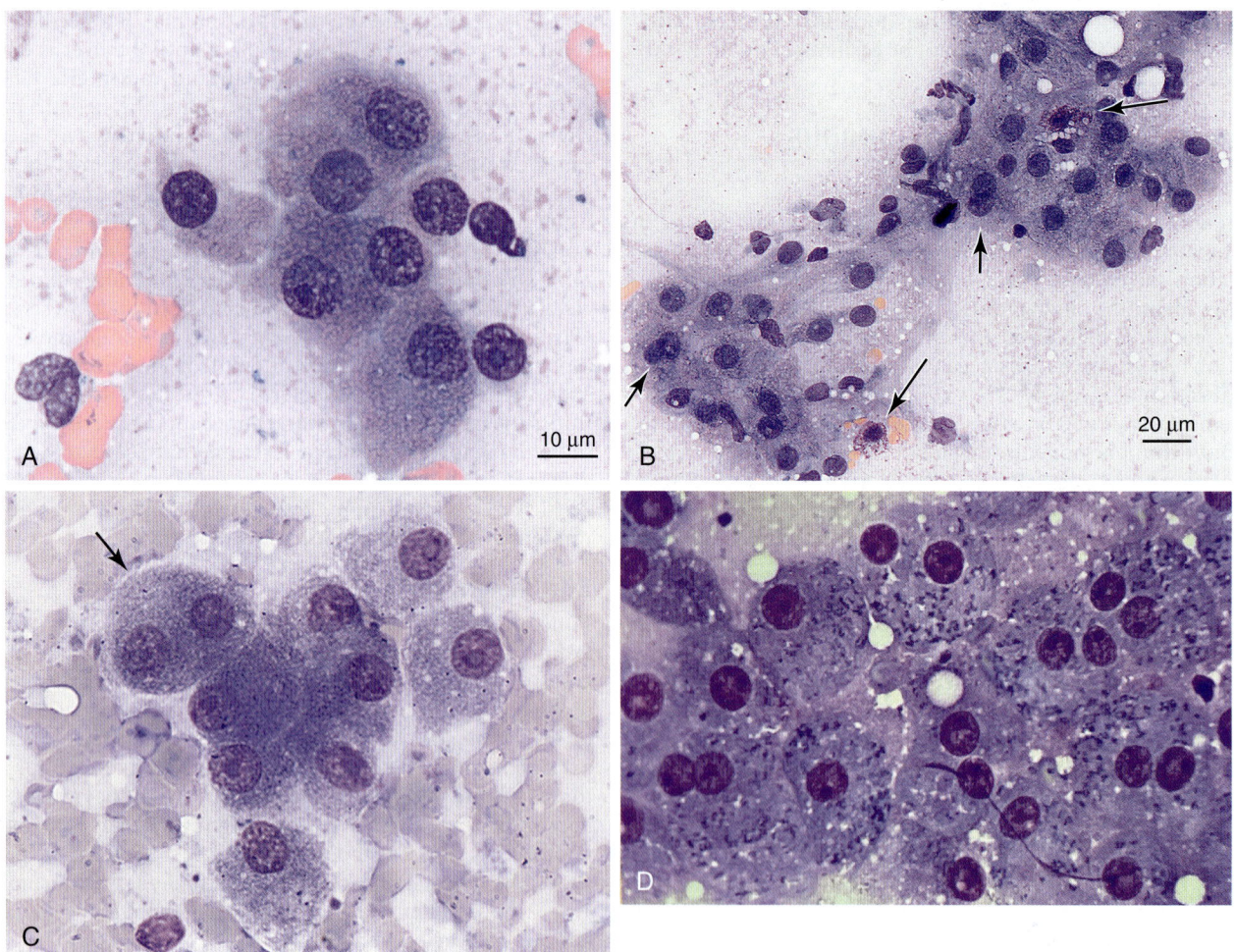

■ **FIGURE 9.1 Normal hepatocytes. Liver aspirate. A,** A small sheet of polygonal hepatocytes with characteristic blue-pink ("amphophilic"), granular cytoplasm and a round nucleus, typically containing a single distinct nucleolus. (Modified Wright; HP oil.) **B,** Scattered mast cells *(long arrows)* and occasional binucleated hepatocytes *(short arrows)* are normal findings. The mast cell granules may not stain vividly. (Modified Wright; HP oil.) Contrast this image with an example of a hepatic mast cell neoplasia (see Fig. 9.79). **C,** An occasional binucleate cell *(arrow)* is a normal finding. (Wright-Giemsa; HP oil.) **D, Dog.** The hepatocytes arranged in a sheet have one or two nuclei with a single prominent nucleolus. The cytoplasm contains frequent green-black granules consistent with lipofuscin, a normal "wear and tear" pigment. (Aqueous Romanowsky; HP oil.) (D, Courtesy Rose Raskin, University of Florida.)

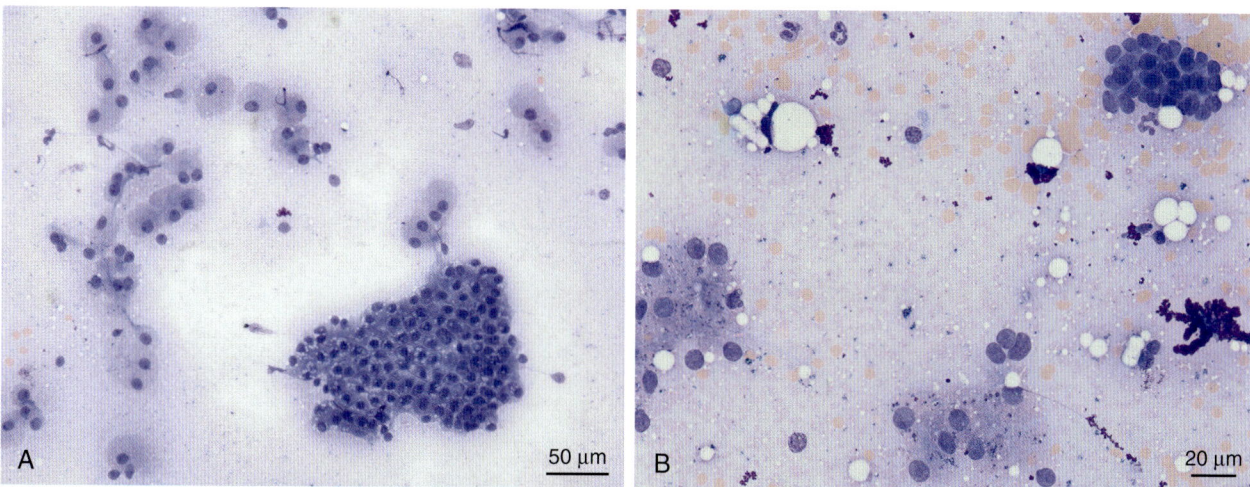

■ **FIGURE 9.2 Normal biliary epithelium. Liver aspirate. A, Dog.** A large, dense sheet of biliary epithelial cells is present in the right bottom corner, alongside less cohesive hepatocytes. Compared with hepatocytes, the biliary epithelial cells have much less cytoplasm, giving the cells a higher nucleocytoplasmic ratio. Note the mild cytoplasmic vacuolation, a feature commonly found in biliary epithelium, which is unlikely to be of clinical significance. (Modified Wright; IP.) **B, Cat.** A dense tubular cluster of normal biliary ductal cells is present in the *top right corner*, along with small sheets of hepatocytes containing lipofuscin. (Modified Wright; HP oil.)

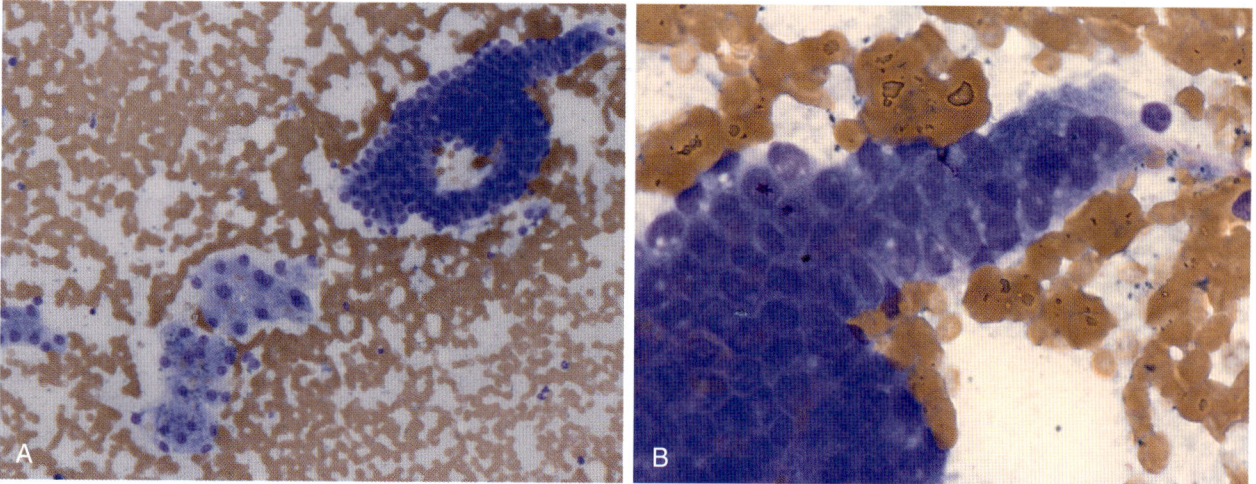

■ **FIGURE 9.3 Normal biliary ductal epithelium. Liver aspirate. Dog.** Same case in A and B. **A,** One tubular cluster of uniform biliary epithelial cells is shown. (Wright-Giemsa; IP.) **B,** Higher magnification reveals the columnar to cuboidal shape with a pale apical region of the cells. There is generally a high nucleocytoplasmic ratio. The round or oval nucleus is approximately 1 to 1.5 times the size of an erythrocyte in diameter with finely stippled chromatin and indistinct nucleoli. (Wright-Giemsa; HP oil.) (Courtesy Rose Raskin, University of Florida.)

Other cells potentially observed during the sampling procedure of the liver are sheets of mesothelial cells, which should not be mistaken for biliary epithelium or a neoplastic cell population (Fig. 9.5).

Bile

The basic components of bile are bile acids, cholesterol, lecithin, bilirubin, inorganic salts, water, and mucin. Bile from the gallbladder grossly appears yellow to dark green but appears shiny golden yellow on an unstained smear on a glass slide. With Romanowsky staining, the fluid smear is basophilic and microscopically displays a green-gray, finely granular appearance (Fig. 9.6) with occasional biliary epithelial cells (Fig. 9.7). These cells may be more likely to exfoliate under hyperplastic conditions (Fig. 9.8) and are often poorly preserved after prolonged in vitro exposure to bile.

Although bile from healthy animals is generally sterile, a low incidence of transient, self-limiting bactibilia (presence of bacteria in bile) has been reported in clinically healthy dogs undergoing repeated cholecystocentesis, with no increased incidence of bactibilia associated with hypercortisolism in that study (Kook et al., 2010).

RESPONSES TO TISSUE INJURY

Nuclear Changes

One or more rectangular nuclear crystalloid inclusions, also called *brick bodies* (Fig. 9.9), are occasionally noted in a low proportion of hepatocytes in aspirates of clinically healthy dogs

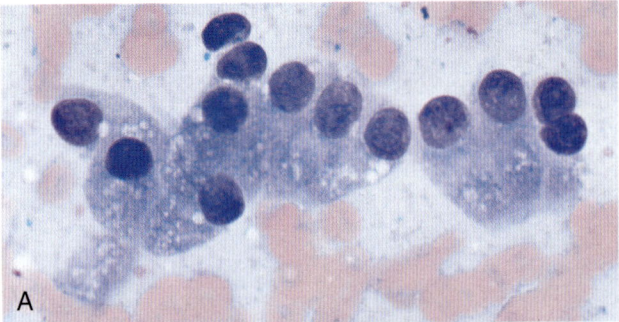

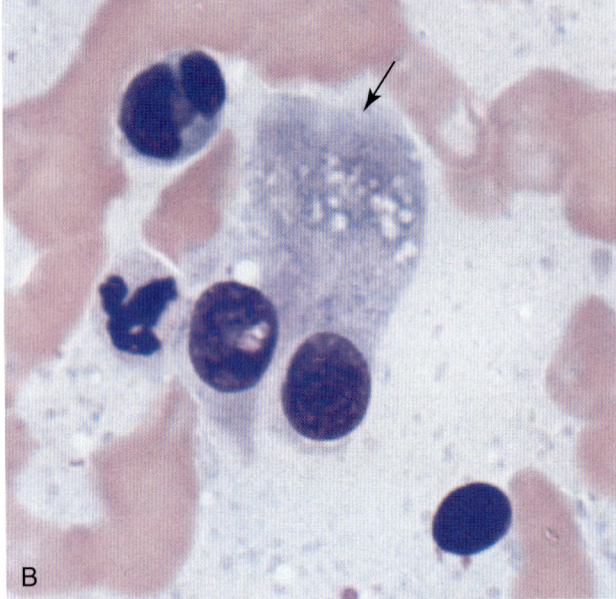

■ **FIGURE 9.4 Normal biliary epithelium. Liver imprint. Dog.** Same case in A and B. **A,** A row of columnar epithelium with vacuolated and finely granulated cytoplasm from a patient with thickened gallbladder. Note the basilar location of the nuclei. (Wright; HP oil.) **B,** Two biliary cells display a ciliated brush border *(arrow)*. (Wright; HP oil.) (Courtesy of Rose Raskin, Purdue University.)

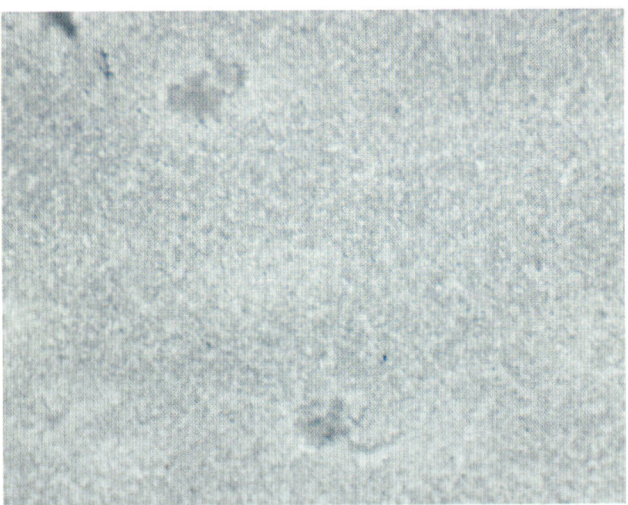

■ **FIGURE 9.6 Normal bile. Gallbladder fluid smear. Cat.** This aspirated gallbladder fluid was dark green with protein of 12.8 g/dL. Note the finely granular to amorphous character of mucinous bile that stains green-gray. Bacteria are not commonly present. (Wright; HP oil.) (Courtesy Rose Raskin, Purdue University.)

of all ages with an unknown diagnostic significance (Stockhaus et al., 2002). Although found occasionally in normal dogs, they appear more frequent in older dogs (Cullen and Stalker, 2016) and hyperplastic hepatocytes. Studies indicate these inclusions consist of proteins possibly produced in excess of release from the nucleus (Richter et al., 1965). Less commonly, intranuclear cytoplasmic invaginations can be observed (Fig. 9.10). Their significance is not fully established, but they have been reported in neoplastic cells of dogs and cats, including hepatocellular carcinoma, but also in non-neoplastic diseases such as cholangiohepatitis (Attipa and Szladovits, 2019). These invaginations can be difficult to distinguish from true cytoplasmic inclusions, such as glycogen (Fig. 9.11) or viral inclusions. The latter are

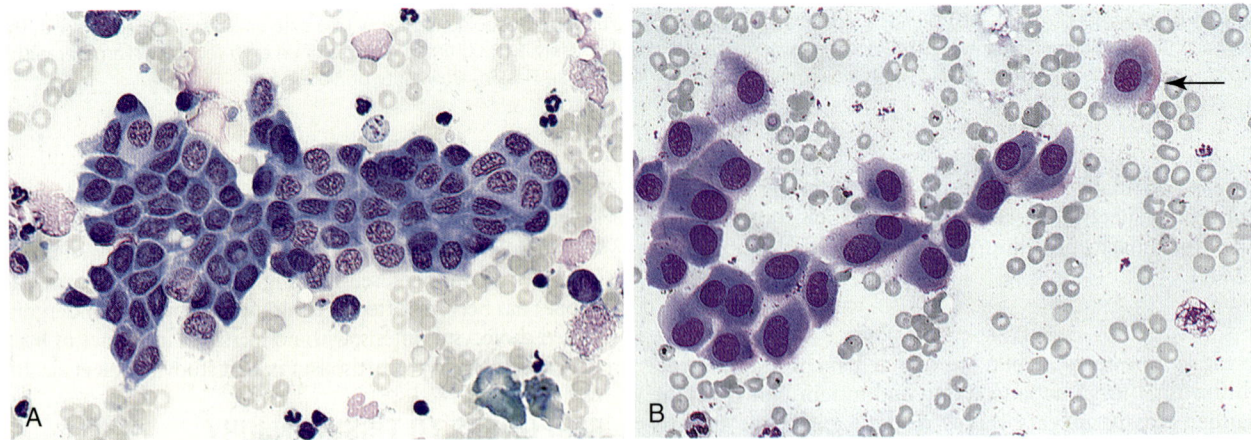

■ **FIGURE 9.5 Mesothelium. Liver. Cytopathologic specimen. A,** Their angular shape (fish scale–like) identifies a sheet of mesothelial cells, probably scraped off during the sampling procedure. They should not be mistaken for a metastatic neoplasm or biliary epithelium. Note the cell size relative to the brownish-stained erythrocytes that surround the sheet of cells. (Wright-Giemsa; HP oil.) **B,** A classic mesothelial cell *(arrow)* has an oval appearance that is surrounded by a pink fringe (glycocalyx) at the cytoplasmic border. Numerous green-gray stained erythrocytes surround the mesothelial cells serve as a micrometer for cell size. (Wright-Giemsa; HP oil.)

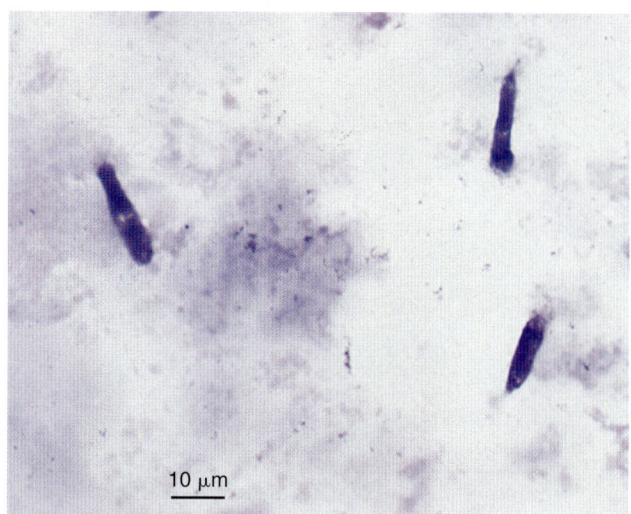

■ **FIGURE 9.7 Biliary epithelium in bile. Fluid smear. Dog.** Three shrunken ciliated columnar epithelial cells appear within the lightly mucinous and proteinaceous background. (Wright; HP oil.) (Courtesy Rose Raskin, Purdue University.)

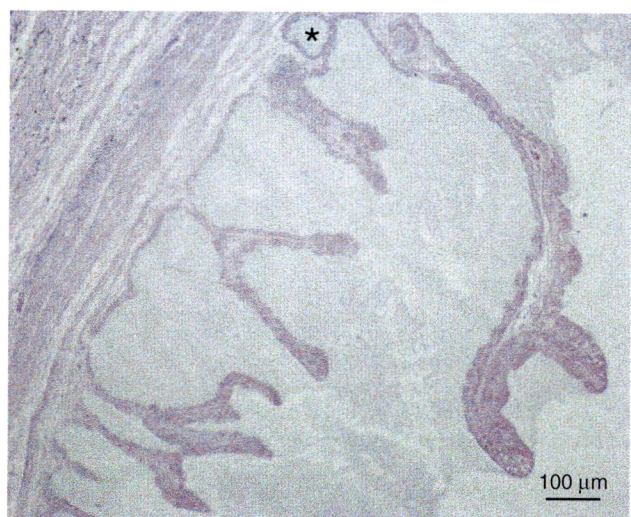

■ **FIGURE 9.8 Gallbladder. Cystic mucinous hyperplasia. Histology. Dog.** Note the enlarged mucosal projections with dense lightly basophilic mucus between projections. There is a small mucosal cyst in the top center of the image *(asterisk)*. The enlarged gallbladder was an incidental finding at necropsy unrelated to the primary condition. (H&E; LP.) (Courtesy Rose Raskin, Purdue University.)

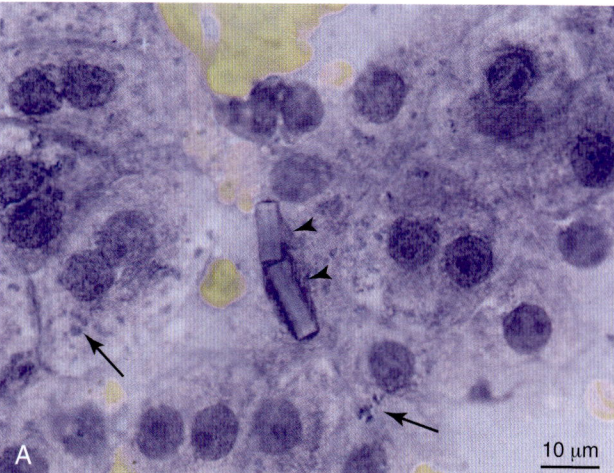

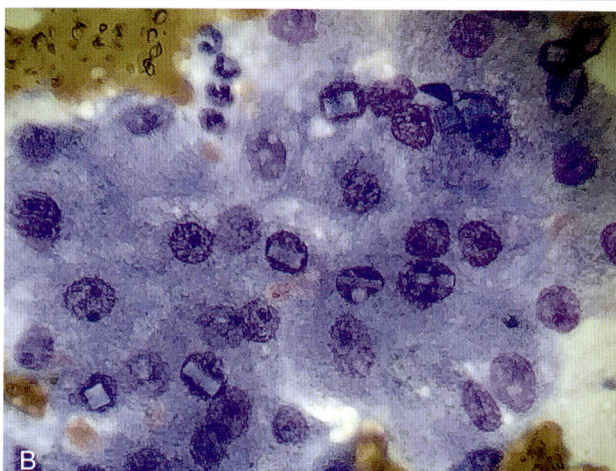

■ **FIGURE 9.9 Nuclear crystalloid inclusions. A. Liver cytologic preparation.** One or two rectangular crystals are occasionally observed in the nuclei of hepatocytes *(arrowheads)*, an incidental finding of no known diagnostic importance. The cytoplasm contains green to blue-black pigment consistent with lipofuscin *(arrows)* and is occasionally mildly rarefied. (Modified Wright; HP oil.) **B, Dog. Liver aspirate.** Patient with chronic vomiting, increased liver enzyme activities, and a 7-cm hyperechoic liver mass. There are numerous variably sized rectangular to square intranuclear crystals. Mild chronic active hepatitis was diagnosed. (Wright-Giemsa; HP oil.) (B, Courtesy Rose Raskin, University of Florida.)

caused by canine adenovirus 1 and canid alpha herpesvirus 1 infection and appear as variably sized, magenta, homogenous, intranuclear structures. The viral inclusions typically cause margination of the chromatin, leading to the appearance of a thickened nuclear membrane (Fig. 9.12) (van den Ingh et al., 2006). Glycogen inclusions may be determined by periodic acid–Schiff (PAS) staining with and without diastase. Glycogen is sensitive to diastase, and inclusions become PAS negative.

Hepatotoxicity can arise from drug therapy, including lomustine. Animals receiving this drug for various neoplastic diseases such as lymphoma, mast cell neoplasia, histiocytic sarcoma, and brain tumors may develop hepatic disease, producing histopathologic changes such as multifocal sinusoidal and portal aggregates of hemosiderin-laden Kupffer cells, hepatocytes with karyomegaly, multifocal mild to moderate cytoplasmic hepatocellular vacuolization, mild to moderate neutrophilic and lymphoplasmacytic periportal inflammation, and bridging fibrosis (Kristal et al., 2004). Cytopathology can recognize many of these histopathologic changes such as karyomegaly (Fig. 9.13), which occurred in 8 of 10 dogs examined by needle-cut biopsy.

Cytoplasmic Changes

Hepatocellular cytoplasmic changes are commonly observed in association with metabolic disease and secondary to cellular

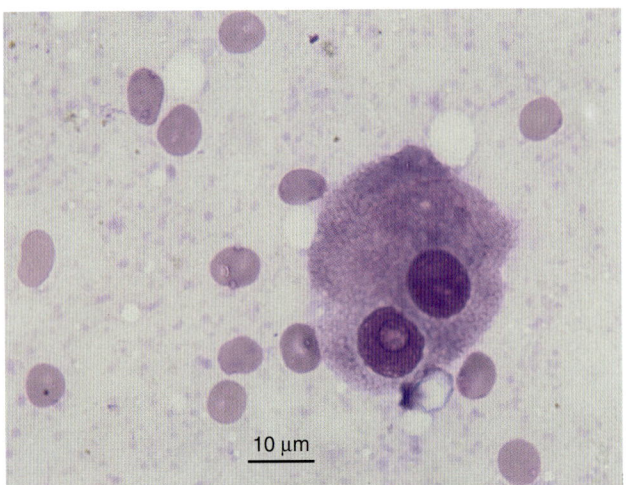

FIGURE 9.10 Intranuclear cytoplasmic invagination. Cytopathologic specimen. Dog. Binucleated hepatocyte with an intranuclear cytoplasmic invagination in one nucleus *(bottom left)*, an incidental finding in a liver aspirate from a dog with cholangiohepatitis (not depicted). (Modified Wright; HP oil.) (Courtesy Charalampos Attipa, The Royal Veterinary College, UK.)

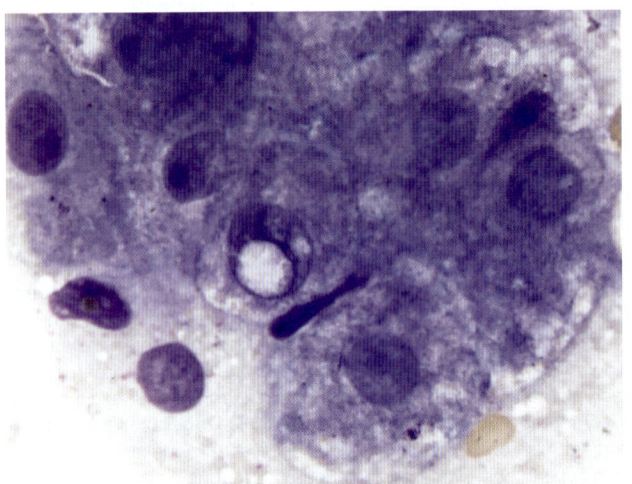

FIGURE 9.11 Intranuclear glycogen inclusion. Liver aspirate. Cat. This patient presented with a 1-year history of weight loss with recent hyperbilirubinemia. Focally to diffuse numbers of hepatocytes displayed mild to moderate indistinct cytoplasmic vacuolar degeneration, consistent with glycogen deposition. Occasionally, nuclei contained a single clear to finely granular vacuole not similar to the cytoplasm. To confirm glycogen, PAS staining with diastase is recommended. (Wright; HP oil.) (Courtesy Rose Raskin, Michigan State University.)

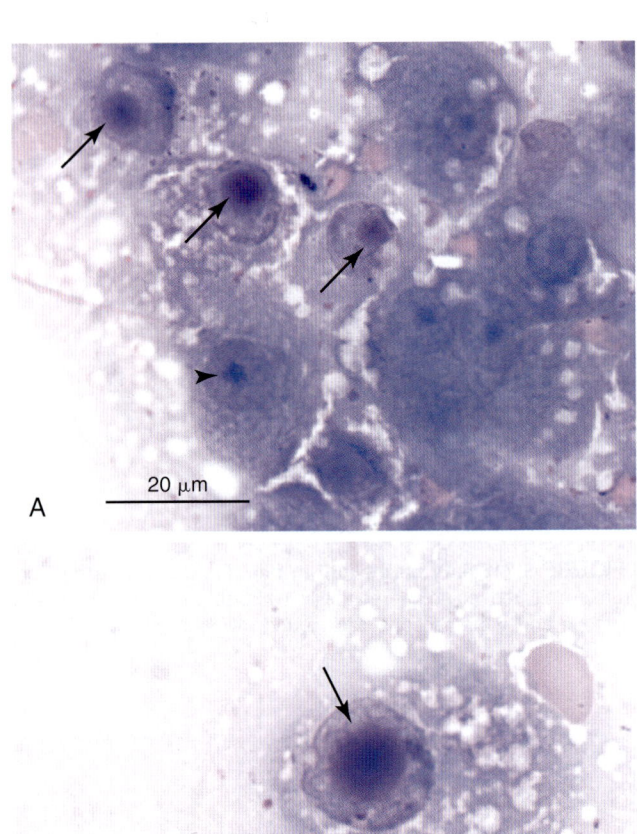

FIGURE 9.12 Nuclear viral inclusion. Infectious canine hepatitis. Liver aspirate. Dog. Same case in A and B. **A,** Infectious canine hepatitis produced vacuolar changes in addition to nuclear inclusions. Here there is a comparison between normal basophilic nucleoli *(arrowhead)* and three nuclei with variably sized magenta round intranuclear inclusions *(arrows)*. (Wright; HP oil.) **B,** Notice the single hepatocyte with large magenta nuclear inclusion with chromatin margination, leaving a pale area between the inclusion and the nuclear membrane *(arrow)*. (Wright; HP oil.) (Courtesy Rose Raskin, Purdue University.)

injury. The terms *hepatocellular vacuolation, vacuolar change, vacuolar hepatopathy,* and *vacuolar degeneration* are often used as umbrella terms to refer to lipid, glycogen, and water accumulation. Discrete, well-demarcated cytoplasmic vacuoles represent accumulation of lipid (triglycerides) that has been cleared during the staining process (Figs. 9.14 to 9.16). Excess accumulation of lipid in the liver is referred to as *lipidosis, steatosis,* or *fatty liver*. The terms *microvacuolar (microvesicular)* and *macrovacuolar (macrovesicular)* lipidosis are used to describe vacuoles that are smaller or larger than the nucleus, respectively.

The presence of lipids may be identified using an air-dried slide and placing one drop of oil red-O (ORO) stain and one drop of new methylene blue on the specimen. After a few minutes, place a coverslip on top of the mixture and tilt the slide touching a paper towel to drain the bulk of the stain. When observed through the microscope, the ORO-stained lipid is a dull orange-red color that fills the vacuoles (see Fig. 9.16C). The free lipid is bright red and outside the cells.

Hepatic lipidosis (steatosis) is the abnormal accumulation of lipid in the liver that can be associated with negative energy balance (e.g., starvation, diabetes mellitus, ketosis) or secondary to hypoxic and toxic hepatocellular injury (e.g., caused by cyanide, aflatoxin, or tetracycline) (Cullen et al., 2006; Newman et al., 2007; Cullen and Stalker, 2016). In cats, FNAB is effective for the definitive diagnosis of feline hepatic lipidosis when the increased

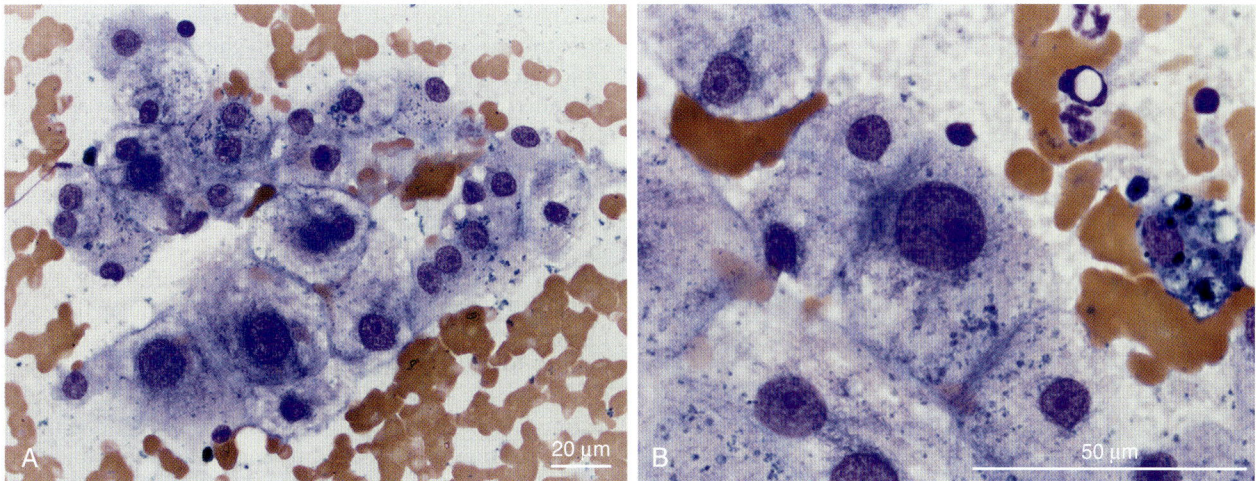

■ **FIGURE 9.13 Karyomegaly. Suspected hepatotoxicity. Liver aspirate. Dog.** Same case in A and B. This patient with histiocytic sarcoma presented with hepatic parenchyma mottled with ill-defined nodules on ultrasound. As the animal received chemotherapy, lomustine hepatotoxicity was suspected. **A,** There are two hepatocytes with a single giant nucleus that is approximately twice the size of normal hepatocytes. Six pairs of binucleated hepatocytes appear in one field, which suggests regeneration. The cytoplasm contains frequent sprinkling of lipofuscin granules. (Wright-Giemsa; HP oil.) **B,** One giant nucleus measured 17 μm in diameter. Note the presence of a hemosiderin-laden macrophage. (Wright-Giemsa; HP oil.) (Courtesy Rose Raskin, University of Florida.)

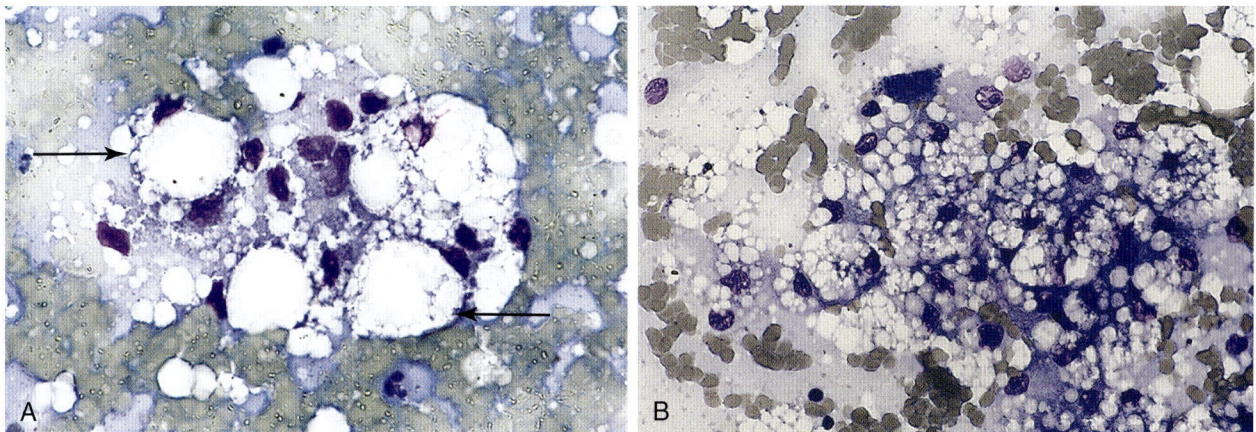

■ **FIGURE 9.14 Lipidosis. Liver aspirate. Cat.** Same case in A and B. **A,** The patient was an icteric 5-year-old cat with a markedly increased serum alkaline phosphatase value and hepatomegaly. The cytoplasm of the hepatocytes is markedly distended by large, clear vacuoles (macrovesicular) that cause nuclear margination or a "signet ring" appearance *(arrows)* and make the hepatocyte difficult to recognize. (Wright-Giemsa; IP.) **B,** Sometimes the hepatocellular cytoplasm is distended by small, variably sized vacuoles (microvesicular). Both cytomorphologic findings of fatty change are consistent with a diagnosis of the feline hepatic lipidosis syndrome. (Wright-Giemsa; IP.)

bilirubin is accompanied by a normal to minimally increased gamma glutamyltransferase (GGT) activity relative to the moderately to markedly increased alkaline phosphatase (ALP) activity, coupled with diffuse hepatic hyperechogenicity (Center et al., 1993). The majority of the hepatocytes typically have macrovacuolation or a mixture of both microvacuolation and macrovacuolation. Secondary lipidosis may be associated with underlying diseases such as congenital portosystemic shuts, pancreatitis, diabetes mellitus, neoplasia, or cholangiohepatitis (Sepesy et al., 2006; Hunt et al., 2013; Cullen and Stalker, 2016).

Microvacuolation may be indicative of mitochondrial injury (Fig. 9.17) (Cullen and Stalker, 2016). A rare cause of microvacuolar hepatopathy in young cats is lysosomal storage disease, such as Niemann Pick disease type C (Brown et al., 1994) (see Fig. 9.17B).

Accidental aspiration of mesenteric or subcutaneous fat, or hyperplasia of hepatic stellate cells or Ito cells (also called or lipocytes) should not be mistaken as hepatic lipidosis (Figs. 9.18 and 9.19). Hepatic stellate or Ito cells are important for storage of vitamin A, participation in hepatic fibrosis, and acting as liver-associated antigen-presenting cells.

Hepatocellular cytoplasmic rarefaction refers to a reduction in the density of the cytoplasm, often giving the cytoplasm a reticulated appearance. The change can be caused by increased glycogen or water content (Fig. 9.20). Glycogen accumulation is often seen in dogs exposed to excess endo- or exogenous glucocorticoids (Fig. 9.21) and is termed *steroid hepatopathy* (Schaer and Ginn, 1999; Cullen and Stalker, 2016). Hepatocytes may be markedly enlarged (up to 10-fold in extreme cases), leading to generalized hepatomegaly, and ALP activity is commonly

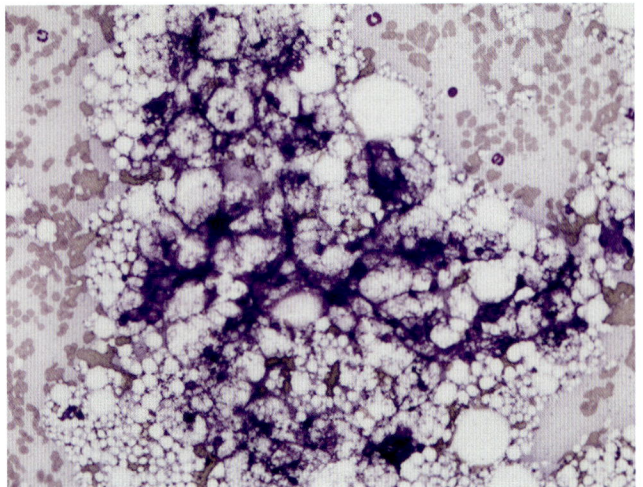

FIGURE 9.15 Lipidosis. Liver aspirate. Cat. Highly vacuolated cells are poorly distinguishable as hepatocytes. (Wright-Giemsa; IP.) (Courtesy Dave Edwards, University of Tennessee.)

concomitantly increased mildly to markedly. When hyperadrenocorticism and treatment with glucocorticoid medications (injectable, oral, and topical) have been eliminated, a search for an underlying cause of a stress-induced hypercortisolemia such as neoplasia, primary hepatobiliary disease, pancreatitis, or gastrointestinal pathology is warranted (Sepesy et al., 2006). Various types of hepatocellular injury such as cholestasis, toxic insults, and hypoxia can alter the integrity of the cell membrane and cytoplasmic organelles, resulting in increased cellular water content referred to as hydropic degeneration, which may also be referred to as hepatocellular degeneration histologically (Fig. 9.22). This cytoplasmic change cannot be confidently distinguished microscopically from the changes associated with increased cytoplasmic glycogen without special staining. PAS staining of unfixed slides, with and without diastase digestion, can be used to confirm cytoplasmic glycogen accumulation. Glycogen stains positive with PAS but is removed by diastase digestion, giving a negative reaction to PAS on diastase treated slides, whereas change caused by hydropic degeneration does not stain with PAS. Neutral mucin is also

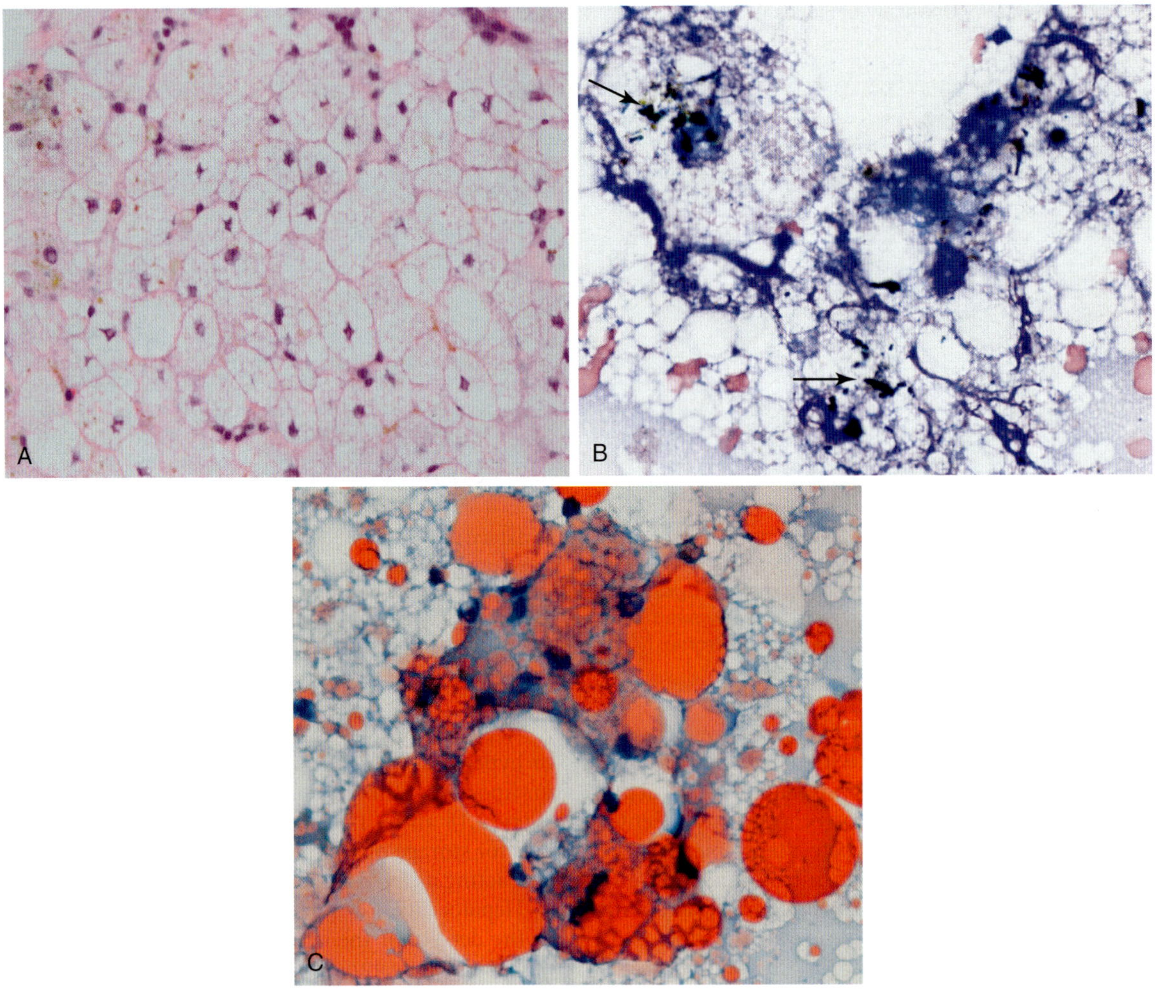

FIGURE 9.16 Lipidosis. Liver. Cat. Same case in A and C. **A, Histology.** Tissue section demonstrates the highly vacuolated appearance of hepatocytes in an advanced stage of lipidosis. (H&E; IP.) **B, Romanowsky specimen.** Notice the dark pigmented material consistent with retained bile or lipofuscin *(arrows)* in the hepatocytes with both microvesicular and macrovesicular vacuolation. (Wright; HP oil.) **C, Wet mount specimen.** The concurrent application of new methylene blue (NMB) and oil red O (ORO) demonstrates stained nuclei and lipoid substances, respectively. Lipids with an affinity for the dye present within microvesicular vacuoles stain dull orange compared with the large free droplets of ORO, which stain brightly orange. (NMB/ORO; IP.) (Courtesy Rose Raskin, Purdue University.)

CHAPTER 9 Hepatobiliary System 347

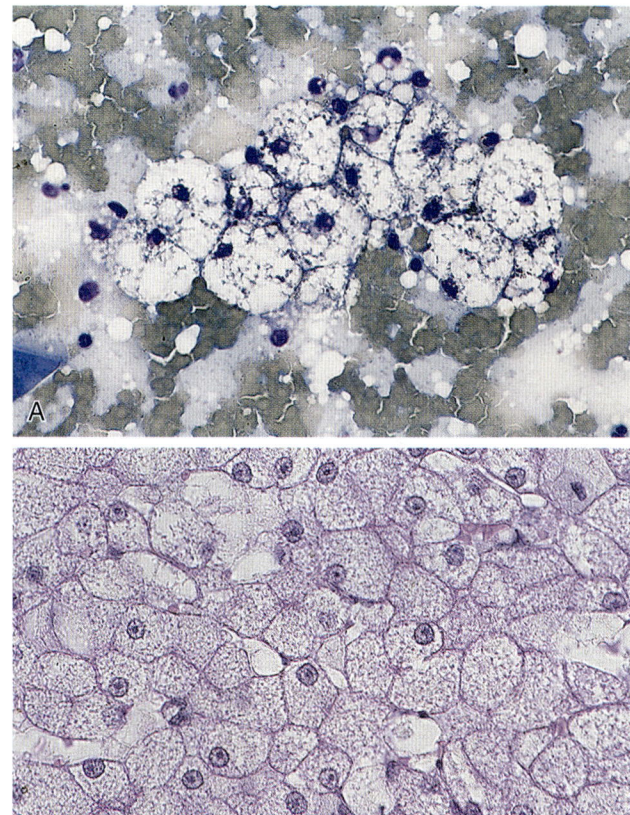

FIGURE 9.17 Microvesicular vacuolation. A, Liver aspirate. Dog. Fine-droplet (microvesicular) lipidosis in an aspirate from a puppy with hepatomegaly and ascites is suggestive of a lipid storage disease; the diagnosis was not confirmed. (Wright-Giemsa; IP.) **B, Lipid storage disease. Cat. Liver histology.** Note the cytopathologic features observed in A are similar to a histopathologic specimen from a kitten with documented lipid storage disease, Niemann-Pick disease type C. (H&E; HP oil.) (B, Courtesy Diane Brown, Colorado State University.)

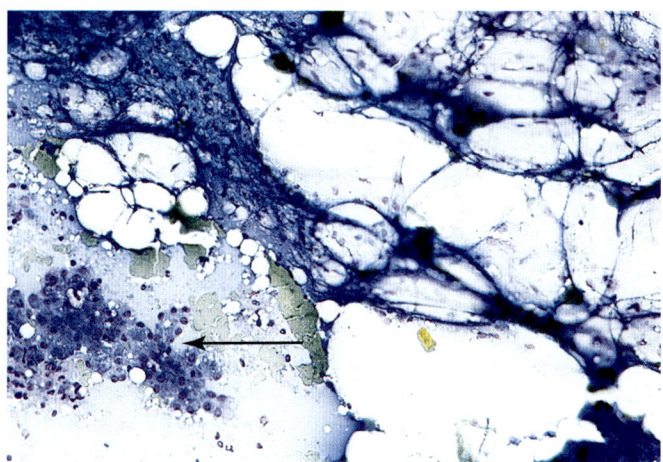

FIGURE 9.18 Mesenteric fat. Occasionally, mesenteric fat is aspirated, which could be confused with hepatic lipidosis. Comparison with a clump of hepatocytes *(arrow)* is helpful in providing a perspective of the much larger size of the mesenteric adipocytes. (Wright-Giemsa; LP.)

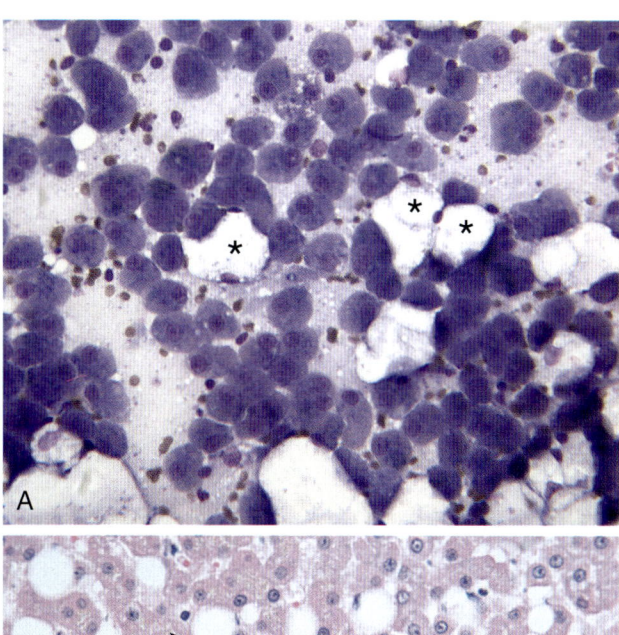

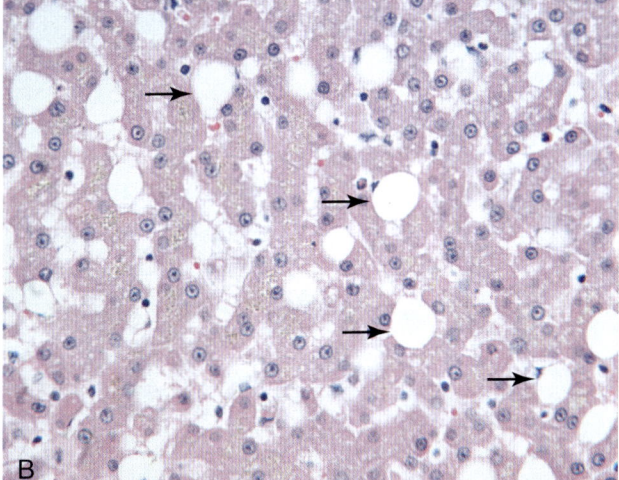

FIGURE 9.19 Hepatic stellate cell or Ito cell (formerly fat-storing cell, lipocyte) hyperplasia. Cat. Same case in A and B. **A, Cytopathologic specimen.** Hyperplastic basophilic and binucleated liver cells with frequent hepatic stellate (Ito) cells *(asterisks)* are scattered among the hepatocytes. Although commonly observed in cats, there is no known diagnostic interpretation. (Romanowsky; HP oil.) **B, Histology.** Histologic correlate of this incidental finding in an aged cat shows individual lipocytes *(arrows)*. (H&E; IP.) (Courtesy Lorenzo Ressel, University of Liverpool, UK.)

resistant to diastase treatment. In contrast, lipid vacuoles stain positive with Sudan stains (e.g., Sudan Black B, Sudan III, or ORO) when applied to unfixed slides (see Fig. 9.16C). See Appendix 2 for protocol information.

Hepatocellular vacuolation caused by both lipid and glycogen accumulation can be seen in regenerative hyperplastic nodules (Fig. 9.23) and in benign and malignant hepatocellular tumors.

> **KEY POINT** Well-defined cytoplasmic vacuolation indicates lipid accumulation, whereas poorly circumscribed cytoplasmic rarefaction is consistent with either glycogen or water deposition. Lipid accumulation is seen secondary to negative energy balance or hypoxic or toxic liver insults. Glycogen storage commonly reflects excess corticosteroid levels, and water is accumulated secondary to sublethal cell injury.

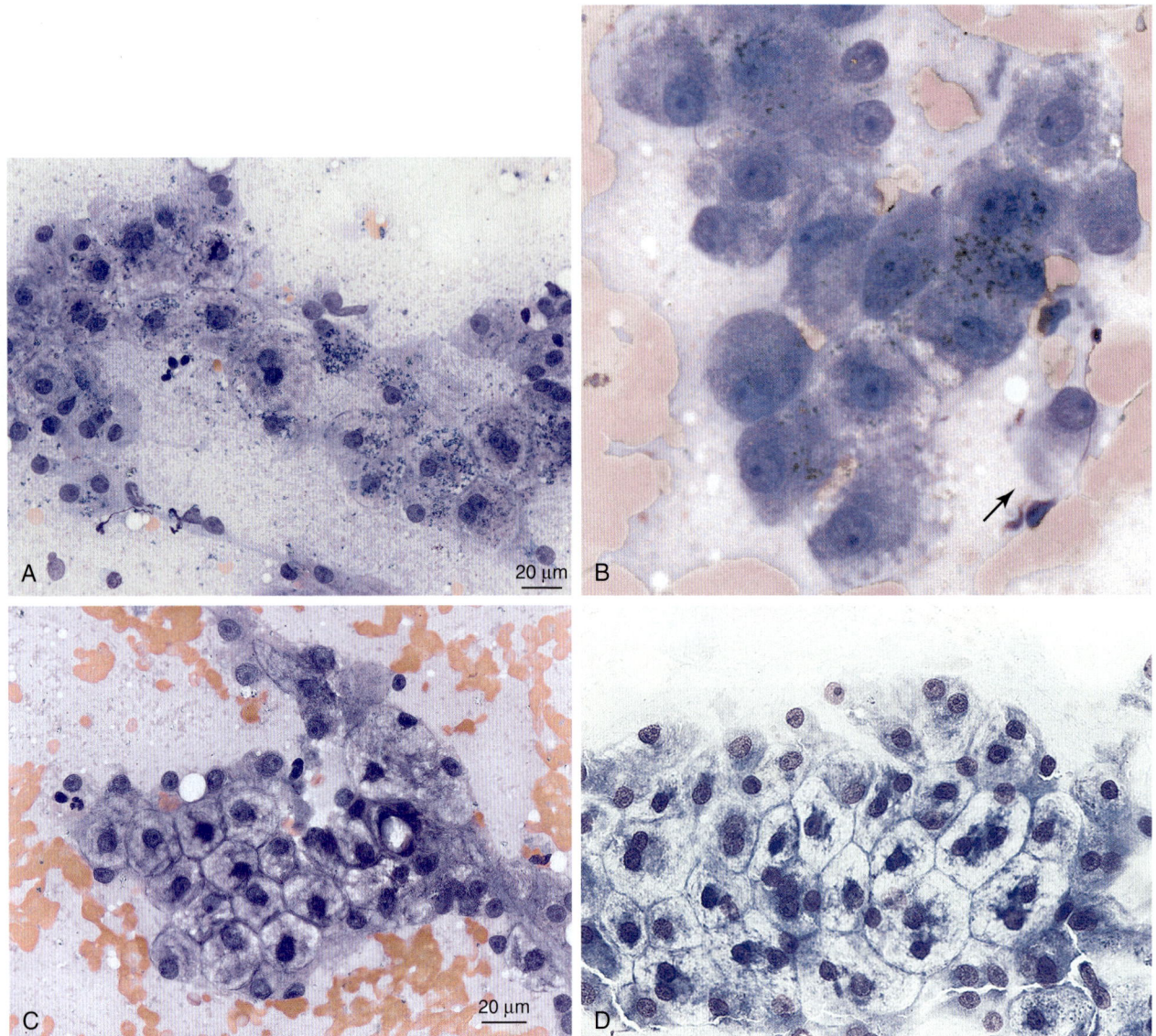

■ **FIGURE 9.20 Cytoplasmic rarefaction. Glycogen deposition. Cytopathologic specimen. Dog. A,** Hepatocytes display mild rarefaction beginning at the periphery of the cells. Note the abundant lipofuscin accumulation in this 13-year-old dog. Several binucleated hepatocytes are present. (Modified Wright; HP oil.) **B,** Hepatocytes in this imprint specimen display mild peripheral cytoplasmic rarefaction with mild lipofuscin pigmentation in this suspected case of chronic active hepatitis. Note the single columnar biliary cell *(arrow)*. (Wright; HP oil.) **C,** Uniform sheet of hepatocytes with moderate cytoplasmic rarefaction from a dog with hepatomegaly and increased serum alkaline phosphatase (ALP) activity. The finding is consistent with excess glycogen storage, which is typically associated with the administration of exogenous corticosteroids and endogenous hypercortisolemia (hyperadrenocorticism). Note how the paler cytoplasm makes the cell borders stand out, emphasizing the hexagonal shape of the hepatocytes. (Modified Wright; HP oil.) **D,** A sheet of hepatocytes displaying marked cytoplasmic rarefaction (lacy cytoplasm) from a dog with hepatomegaly, markedly increased serum ALP activity, and normal serum bilirubin concentration. Steroid-induced hepatopathy was suspected. (Wright-Giemsa; IP.) (B, Courtesy Rose Raskin, Purdue University.)

Hepatic Pigments

The main types of pigment encountered in hepatocytes are lipofuscin, bile, copper, hemosiderin, and ceroid (Table 9.1).

Lipofuscin

Lipofuscin is the most common pigment observed in hepatocytes (Scott and Buriko, 2005; Scott, 2006) and appears as small blue-green to green-black granules within the cytoplasm (see Figs. 9.1D, 9.13A, 9.16B, and 9.20A). Histologically, it has a yellow-brown color with hematoxylin and eosin stain (H&E) and is often located in the cytoplasm of hepatocytes in the centrilobular region. It represents lysosomes filled with indigestible lipid-containing residues from autophagy of membranous organelles, which accumulate as a normal aging product of cell breakdown; hence, it is commonly referred to as "wear and tear" pigment (Cullen and Stalker, 2016). Lipofuscin exhibits autofluorescence when an unfixed specimen is examined under ultraviolet light and stains with the Schmorl ferric-ferricyanide reduction stain and Long Ziehl-Neelsen stain. Other stains for lipofuscin include Sudan black B or ORO for lipids, as well as PAS.

CHAPTER 9 Hepatobiliary System

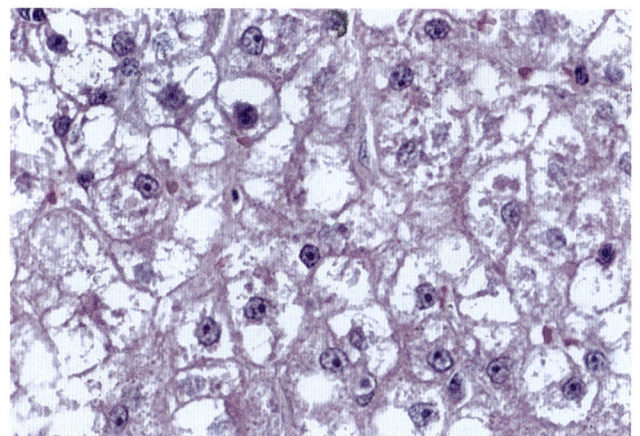

■ **FIGURE 9.21 Glycogen deposition and steroid hepatopathy. Histology. Dog.** Hepatocytes display marked glycogen deposition with cytoplasmic rarefaction in this patient with corticosteroid-induced hepatopathy. Note the similarities to the cytopathologic specimen in Figure 9.20D. (H&E; HP oil.)

Bile Pigment

Retention of bile pigment indicates cholestasis, which is a consequence of liver pathology, resulting in hepatocellular or canalicular accumulation. The accumulation of bile in the liver is easiest to see with Romanowsky staining as dark green-black plugs within bile canaliculi, but it can also be found as dark green-blue to blue-black, variably sized granules within hepatocytes (Fig. 9.24). Bilirubin crystals may appear in bile as golden yellow needle forms. Histologically, the color can range from yellow to brown to green with H&E. Liver bilirubin is converted to biliverdin and stains positive using the Hall's staining method with van Gieson counterstain.

Hemosiderin

Hemosiderin is an insoluble, iron-containing protein produced by the phagocytic digestion of heme. It is mainly found in Kupffer cells and other macrophages but can also be observed in hepatocytes. On cytopathology, it appears as variably sized granules and clumps ranging from golden brown to blue-black

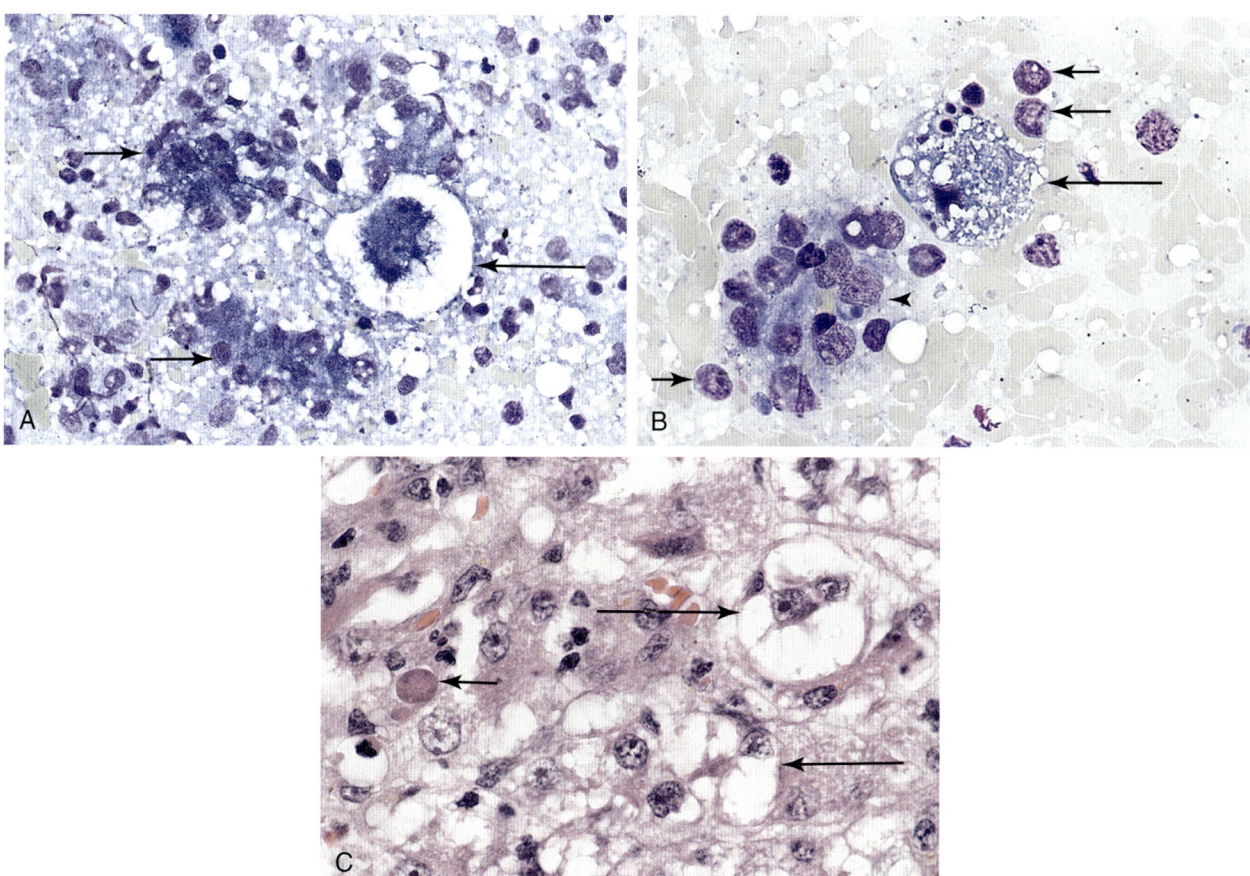

■ **FIGURE 9.22 Hydropic or ballooning degeneration.** Same case in A and B. **Cytopathologic specimen. A,** One markedly swollen binucleated hepatocyte demonstrates hydropic (ballooning) degeneration *(long arrow)*. Other hepatocytes *(short arrows)* show less cytoplasmic alteration or appear morphologically normal. Also present are a moderate number of inflammatory cells (difficult to recognize as lymphocytes and neutrophils) surrounded by a bluish-gray background ("dirty" appearance), which is suggestive of necrotic debris. (Wright-Giemsa; IP.) **B,** In another field, a hepatocyte is undergoing apoptosis, as illustrated by nuclear condensation and fragmentation within a granular, microvacuolated cytoplasm *(long arrow)*. A few inflammatory lymphocytes are in close proximity *(short arrows)*. A small clump of hepatocytes *(arrowhead)* demonstrates regenerative changes consisting of mild anisocytosis and anisokaryosis. The findings along with moderately increased serum alanine aminotransferase and aspartate aminotransferase values, a mild rise in the serum bilirubin concentration, and only a slight increase in the serum alkaline phosphatase value support a morphologic diagnosis of acute liver injury (hepatitis) (e.g., toxin, drug induced). (Wright-Giemsa; HP oil.) **C, Ballooning degeneration. Dog. Histology.** Note histomorphologic similarities to a specimen of acute liver injury from carprofen administration. Swollen hepatocytes caused by ballooning degeneration *(long arrows)* are admixed with lesser affected hepatocytes. A dense-staining eosinophilic structure *(short arrow)* represents a hepatocyte undergoing apoptosis. (H&E; HP oil.)

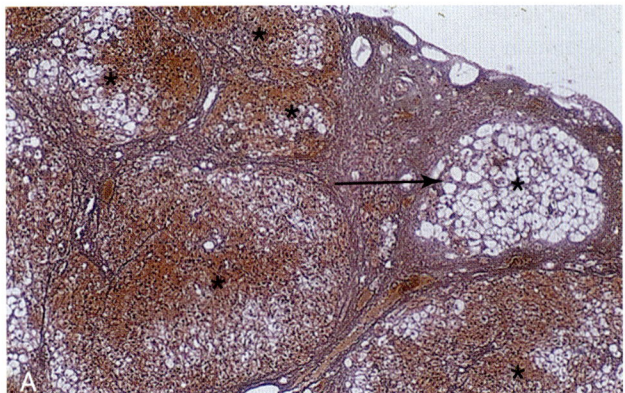
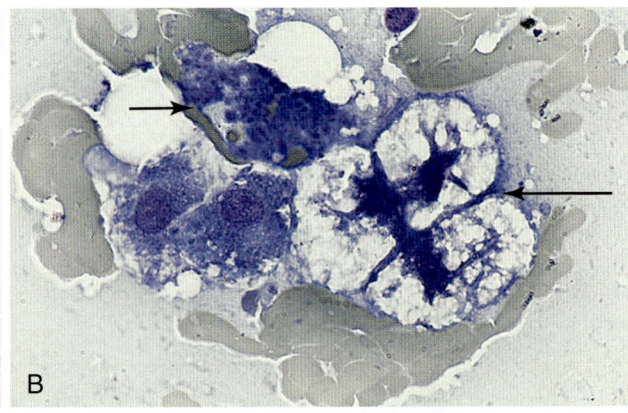

■ **FIGURE 9.23** **Nodular hyperplasia with vacuolar change. Liver. Dog. A, Histology.** Six nodules of varying size *(asterisks)* can be seen in this wedge biopsy specimen from a clinically healthy 12-year-old mixed breed dog with mildly raised serum liver enzyme values and numerous hepatic nodules observed at surgery. Note the dramatic variation in hepatocyte morphology among the nodules. If the nodule located to the upper right *(arrow)* was examined cytopathologically or histopathologically, the findings would be consistent with "vacuolar hepatopathy," suggestive of a metabolic disease. (Gordon & Sweets reticulin; LP.) **B, Cytopathologic specimen.** Shown are hepatocytes with morphologic characteristics that range from near normal to marked cytoplasmic rarefaction *(long arrow)*. A dense clump of platelets *(short arrow)* is a common artifact and should not be confused with a multinucleated cell or infectious agents. (Wright-Giemsa; HP oil.)

TABLE 9.1 Identification of Liver Cell Pigments[a]

	LIPOFUSCIN	BILE	COPPER	HEMOSIDERIN	CEROID
Cytopathology (Romanowsky)	Blue-green to green-black granules	Dark green-blue granules Dark green-black in canaliculi	Crystalline, refractile blue-green to pale blue gray	Golden brown to dark blue-black granules	Golden brown to green-yellow granules
Histopathology (H&E)	Yellow-brown to dark brown granules	Yellowish-brown to yellow to green	Orange to golden-brown Green-black (rubeanic acid) Red to orange-red (rhodanine)	Golden brown	Brown to golden brown
Cytochemical stains	Long Ziehl-Neelsen + Schmorl reaction + PAS Sudan black B	Hall[b]	Rubeanic acid Rhodanine	Prussian blue	Long Ziehl-Neelsen positive Schmorl reaction negative
Interpretation	Normal aging	Cholestasis	Abundant amount with chronic hepatitis or metabolic disease	Hemolytic anemia Focal hemorrhage or congestion Portosystemic shunt Recent transfusion	Hepatocellular injury
Examples	Fig. 9.1D Fig. 9.9A Fig. 9.13A Fig. 9.20A Fig. 9.27	Fig. 9.24 Fig. 9.27	Fig. 9.27 Fig. 9.28 Fig. 9.29 Fig. 9.30	Fig. 9.25 Fig. 9.26	Fig. 9.34B

[a]All pigments are typically located in the cytoplasm of hepatocytes except ceroid, which is mostly located in macrophages. Hemosiderin also may be observed in macrophages, and bile is often prominent in canaliculi between hepatocytes.
[b]Hall stain is best for liver bilirubin, staining it green because of biliverdin content; bile from gallbladder or hematoidin is unlikely to react.
H&E, Hematoxylin and eosin; *PAS,* periodic acid–Schiff; *Rho,* rhodanine; *Rub,* rubeanic acid.

(Figs. 9.25 and 9.26A). Histologically, the granules are refractile and have a golden-brown color with H&E. A Prussian blue stain stains the granules dark blue (Fig. 9.26B). Hepatic hemosiderin accumulation is associated with excessive erythrocyte breakdown (e.g., hemolysis, focal hemorrhage), increased iron (e.g., after transfusions or excessive iron supplementation), or decreased iron utilization (e.g., shunts or markedly decreased erythropoiesis) but also in areas of severe congestion.

Copper

Copper appears as coarse, variably sized, refractile, light blue seafoam green granules within the hepatocyte cytoplasm (Figs. 9.27 to 9.30). On histologic sections, copper stains as orange to golden brown granules (see Fig. 9.30B). Copper can be difficult to identify on Romanowsky stained slides and H&E sections, thereby requiring rhodanine and rubeanic acid stains, which are specific for detecting copper. One study

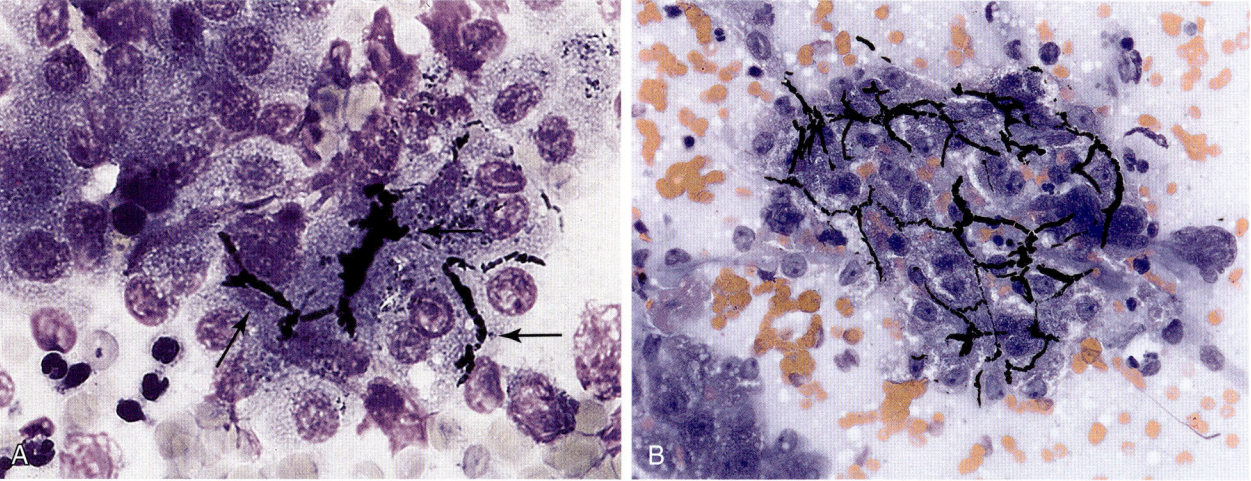

■ **FIGURE 9.24 Cholestasis. Liver. Cytopathologic specimen. Dog. A,** Cholestasis is indicated by green-black ribbons of inspissated bile forming casts of the biliary canaliculi that course between hepatocytes *(arrows)*. Within some hepatocytes is a fine granular dark material considered to be bile or lipofuscin. (Wright-Giemsa; HP oil.) **B,** Marked cholestasis is present alongside mild cytoplasmic rarefaction. (Modified Wright; HP oil.)

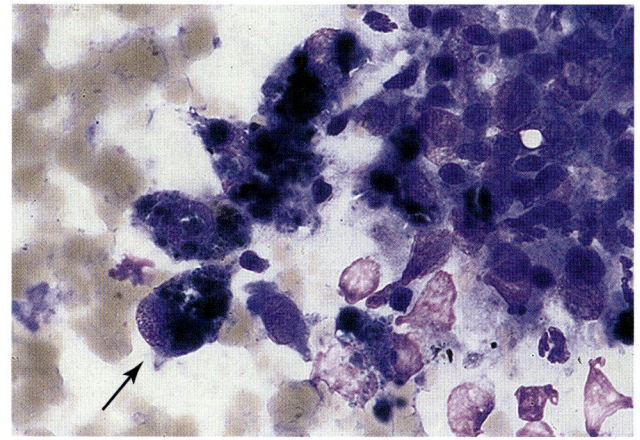

■ **FIGURE 9.25 Hemosiderin. Liver. Cytopathologic specimen.** Several macrophages, including the one indicated *(arrow)*, contain dense, bluish-black material that stained intensively for iron with Prussian blue stain (not shown). (Wright-Giemsa; HP oil.)

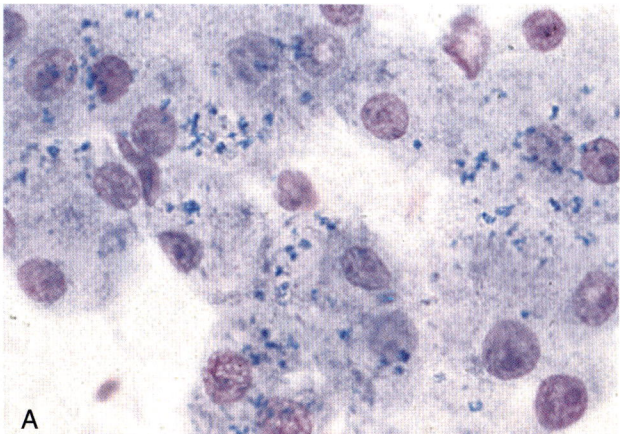

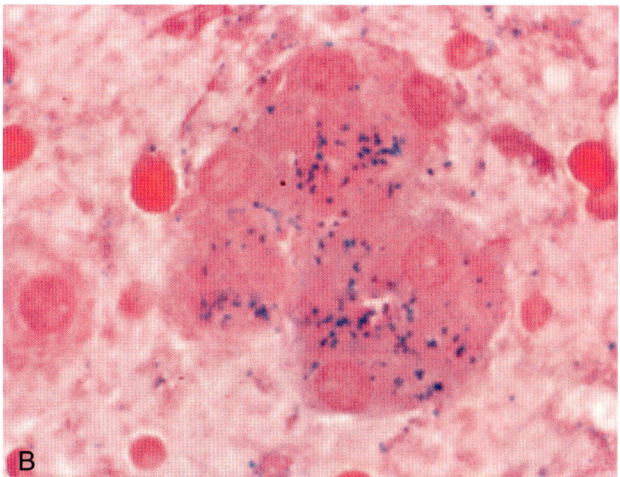

■ **FIGURE 9.26 Iron overload. Dog.** Same case in A and B. **A,** The cytoplasm of the hepatocytes contains abundant, variably sized blue-black granules consistent with iron or another pigment. (Wright-Giemsa; HP oil.) **B, Iron stain.** The granules stain dark blue in this cytopathologic specimen, confirming iron. (Prussian blue; HP oil.) (Courtesy Rose Raskin, University of Florida.)

proposed a protocol for the semiquantitative grading of rhodanine-stained cytopathologic specimens for copper content and demonstrated acceptable diagnostic performance (Moore et al., 2016).

Prolonged staining with rubeanic acid (72 hours) was shown to be the effective in detecting copper within canine liver (Thornburg et al., 1985). Copper granules stain blue-green to green-black with rubeanic acid stain and orange-red with rhodanine stain (see Figs. 9.28B, 9.29B, and 9.30B, *inset*). Marked copper accumulation is seen in Bedlington terriers with autosomal recessive copper-associated hepatitis, in which copper accumulation typically begins in the centrilobular area of the liver. Other predisposed breeds include Labrador retrievers, Dobermann pinschers, West Highland white terriers, dalmatians, and possibly Skye terriers (Dirksen and Fieten, 2017; Strickland et al., 2018). Mutations in the copper transporters have been shown to be associated with the attenuation

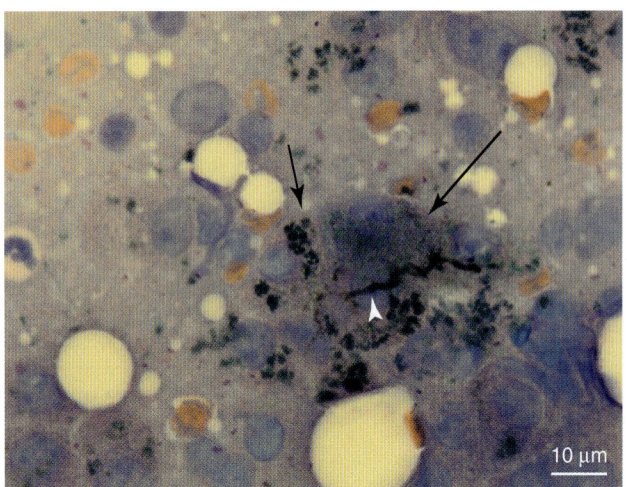

■ **FIGURE 9.27 Copper accumulation. Liver cytopathologic specimen. Dog.** The cytoplasm of the hepatocyte in the center of the image contains turquoise-green refractile, angular crystal-like structures, consistent with copper granules *(long arrow)*. Other cells contain dark green lipofuscin *(short arrow)*, and a bile cast is also present *(arrowhead)*. (Modified Wright; HP oil.)

Ceroid

Ceroid is a pigment that is rich in oxidized lipids and is generally found in macrophages clearing up after an event of cellular injury (e.g., secondary to severe malnutrition, vitamin E deficiency, or irradiation). It can also accumulate in hepatocytes and may be deleterious to the cell if present in large quantities. The granular pigment, which may appear in clumps, has a golden brown to greenish-yellow color with Romanowsky staining and golden brown to brown color with H&E staining. Like lipofuscin, which represents a later, more advanced form of oxidized lipid, ceroid stains positive with the long Ziehl-Neelsen stain method, but it does not stain with Schmorl ferric-ferricyanide reduction stain despite exhibiting autofluorescence.

Hemosiderin and ceroid are also observed within lipogranulomas, which are aggregates of Kupffer cells and other macrophages containing abundant lipid and brown pigment; these have been associated with portosystemic shunts and feline lymphocytic cholangitis/cholangiohepatitis along with other liver pathologies (Isobe et al., 2008; Warren et al., 2011).

Cystic Lesions

Aspiration of cavitated lesions, such as cysts or hemangiosarcomas, typically have too low a cell yield to allow a definitive cytopathologic confirmation (Roth, 2001). Light-yellow fluid can be obtained from cystic lesions, which are especially prominent in cats. These may be congenital in origin. Cysts are typically acellular or poorly cellular (Fig. 9.31). Chronic hemorrhage may be present in some cysts with the presence of hemosiderin-laden macrophages. Obtaining clear to whitish mucinous fluid from a cavitational lesion suggests a cystadenoma.

Extramedullary Hematopoiesis

Although fetal hematopoiesis shifts from the liver to the spleen and later to the bone marrow before birth, the liver remains favorable for hematopoiesis throughout life (Johns and Christopher, 2012). Extramedullary hematopoiesis (EMH) of all three lineages can be seen secondary to bone marrow failure, as a response to increased peripheral demand of blood cells (e.g., secondary to

and enhancement of copper accumulation in Labrador retrievers and possibly Dobermann pinschers (Wu et al., 2019). Copper accumulation caused by a genetic or metabolic (primary) defect that causes hepatic disease tends to be located in the centrilobular area of the liver with concentrations generally of greater than 2000 μg/g (ppm) of liver dry weight, whereas copper accumulation because of hepatic disease (secondary) tends to have a random patchy distribution or to be located in the periportal area of the liver with a dry weight copper measurement of less than 2000 μg/g (Smedley et al., 2009). However, a hepatic copper concentration of 1000 μg/g is speculated to be a concentration at which hepatic injury is likely (Strickland et al., 2018).

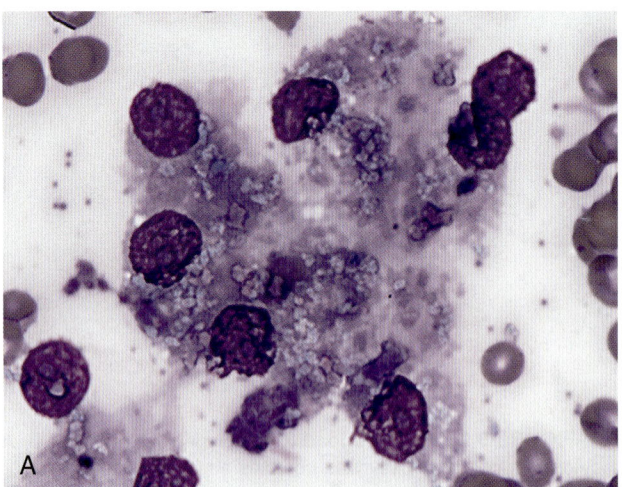
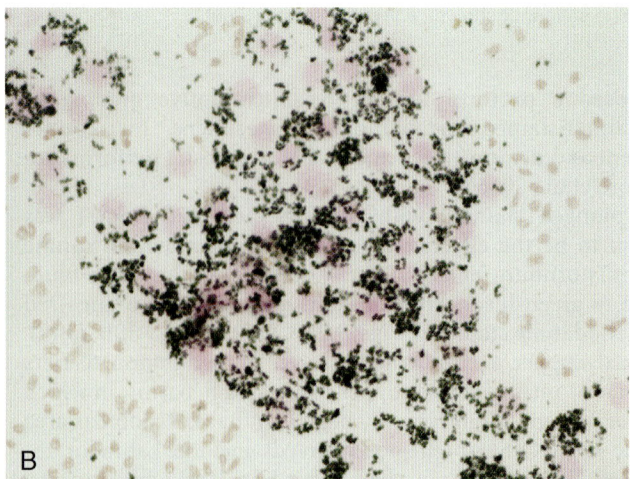

■ **FIGURE 9.28 Copper granules. Liver cytopathologic specimen.** Same case in A and B. **Dog. A,** The cytoplasm of the hepatocytes contains blue-grey angular crystalline structures, consistent with copper granules. (Wright-Giemsa; HP oil.) **B,** Copper granules stain black, indicating a positive reaction with rubeanic acid stain. (Rubeanic acid; IP.) (Courtesy Dave Edwards, University of Tennessee.)

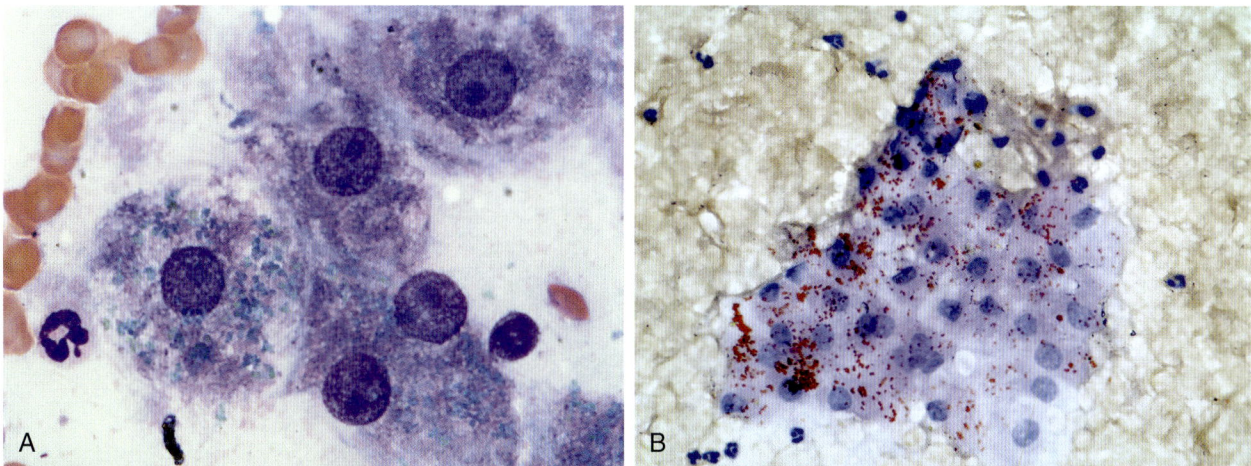

■ **FIGURE 9.29 Copper accumulation. Dog. Liver cytopathologic specimen.** Same case in A and B. **A,** Copper (lighter turquoise-green) and lipofuscin (darker green-blue) granules are observed in the bottom two hepatocytes, which also display mild cytoplasmic rarefaction. (Modified Wright; HP oil.) **B,** A sheet of hepatocytes containing numerous orange-brown granules, indicative of copper accumulation (Rhodanine, IP.) (Courtesy Emma Holmes, The Royal Veterinary College, UK.)

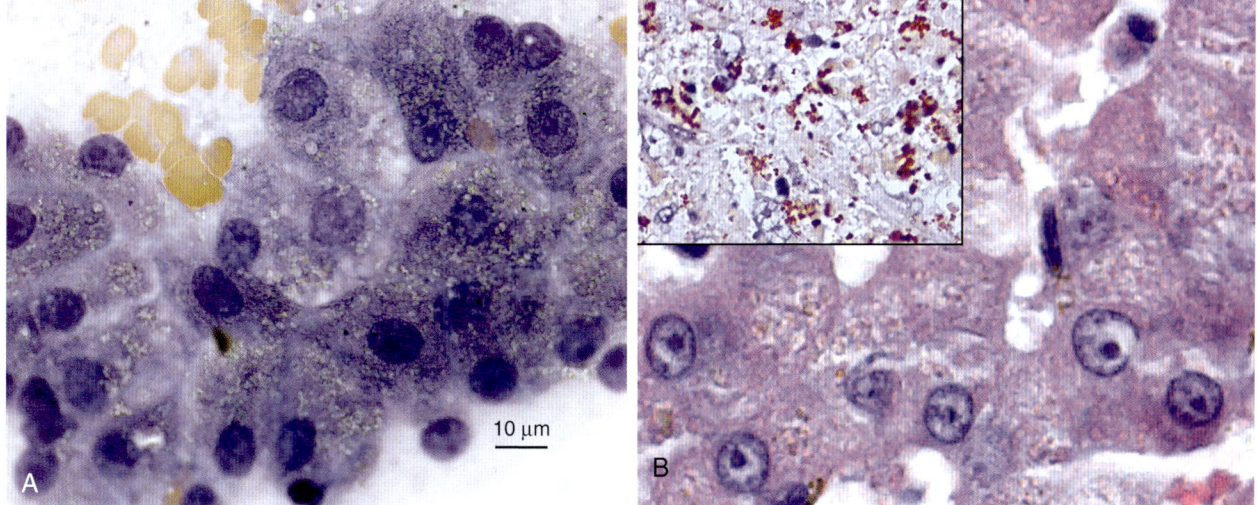

■ **FIGURE 9.30 Copper hepatopathy. Dog. Same case A and B. A, Liver aspirate.** Numerous refractile blue-green to colorless crystals are noted within hepatocytes. (Wright; HP oil.) **B, Histology.** Golden brown to orange refractile crystals fill the hepatocytes in this adult dog with chronic cholestasis. There was a lymphoplasmacytic and suppurative hepatitis (not shown). Copper levels measured from the liver dry weight were found to be at toxic levels 5860 ppm compared with normal of 120 to 400 ppm. (H&E; HP oil.) *Inset:* Liver section example of positive copper stain reaction. (Rhodanine; HP oil.) (Courtesy of Kristin Nunez, Purdue University.)

immune-mediated destruction or inflammation), or within foci of tissue inflammation, injury, and repair. Occasionally, the distinction between myeloid hematopoiesis and neutrophilic inflammation in such lesions can be challenging. EMH can also be found within hyperplastic or regenerative nodules (Fig. 9.32) or as part of myelolipomas, in which hematopoietic precursors are found admixed with adipose tissue. Regardless of the lineages observed, EMH should be composed of mainly late stages with fewer early precursors; the predominance of a uniform population of immature hematopoietic precursors suggests leukemia rather than a benign proliferation.

Amyloidosis

Hepatic amyloid deposition is associated with excessive synthesis of the acute-phase protein serum amyloid A (SAA) secondary to an underlying inflammatory condition and thus classified as reactive or secondary systemic amyloidosis. Cytopathologically, amorphous, wispy swirls of eosinophilic material are observed in close proximity to hepatocytes (Fig. 9.33A) and in macrophages (Neo-suzuki et al., 2017). Histochemical staining with Congo red examined by a polarizing filter to detect an apple-green birefringence is helpful to diagnose the presence of amyloid (Figs. 9.33B–C). Clinically, amyloid deposition can lead to significant hepatomegaly and friable hepatic parenchyma, which can culminate in spontaneous rupture and clinically relevant hemorrhage, particularly in cats (Beatty et al., 2002). Familial disease has been reported in Shar-Pei dogs and Abyssinian, Oriental shorthair, and Siamese cats (DiBartola et al., 1986; van der Linde-Sipman et al., 1997; Flatland et al., 2007; Segev et al., 2012; Paltrinieri et al., 2015). A history of chronic comorbid disease,

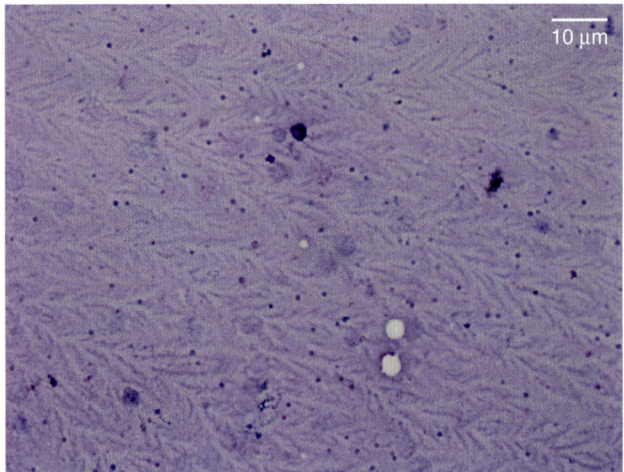

■ **FIGURE 9.31 Hepatic cyst. Liver aspirate. Dog.** This patient presented for workup for a limb lesion, and a 3.0 cm cavitated liver mass was found. The specimen was poorly cellular with rare mononuclear cells against a dense basophilic proteinaceous background with a ferning pattern suggestive of mucinous nature. (Wright-Giemsa; HP oil.) (Courtesy Rose Raskin, University of Florida.)

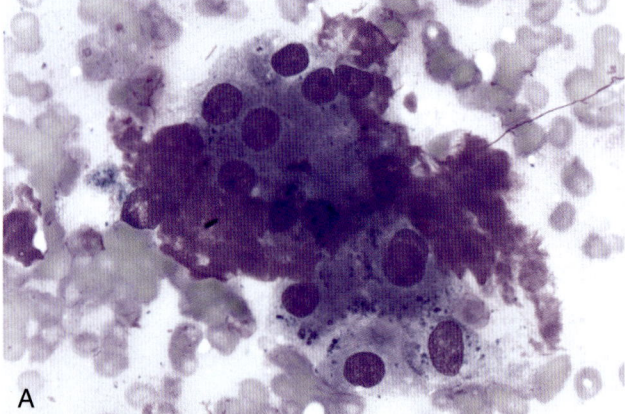

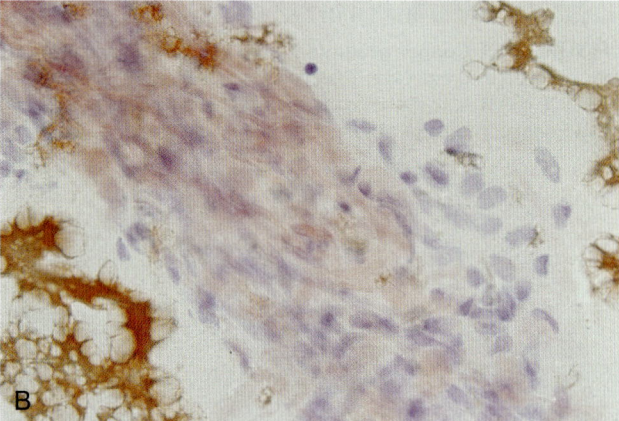

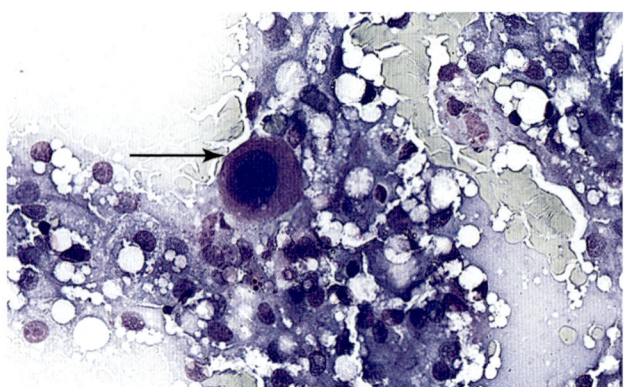

■ **FIGURE 9.32 Extramedullary hematopoiesis. Liver cytopathologic specimen. Dog.** Megakaryocyte *(arrow)*, not to be confused with a multinucleated giant cell, is observed in this cytopathologic specimen from a 10-year-old Labrador retriever mixed breed dog with nodular hyperplasia confirmed histologically. Many of the hepatocytes contain variably sized cytoplasmic vacuoles consistent with lipid. (Wright-Giemsa; IP.)

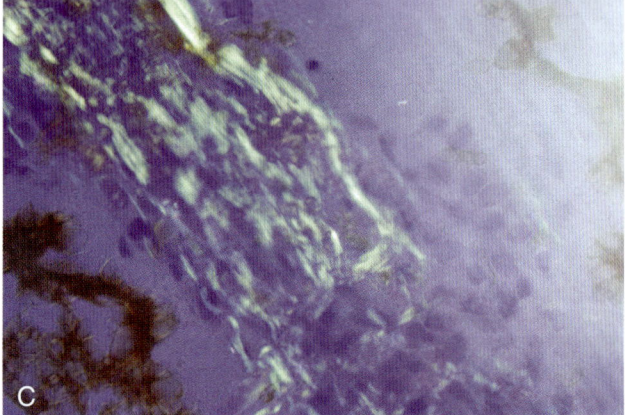

■ **FIGURE 9.33 Hepatic amyloidosis. Cytopathologic specimen. Dog.** Same case in A and C. **A,** A Chinese Shar-Pei dog presented with hepatomegaly and abnormal liver test results. Amyloid appears as swirls of eosinophilic material, which courses between hepatocytes. Hepatocytes have pigmented granules consistent with lipofuscin. (Wright-Giemsa; HP oil.) **B,** Amyloid stains orange-red. (Congo red; IP.) **C,** When a polarizing filter is used with a specimen stained with Congo red stain, the amyloid material appears birefringent. (Congo red/polarized; IP.) (Courtesy Dave Edwards, University of Tennessee.)

including neoplastic and inflammatory (infectious and noninfectious), was present in most Shar-pei and non–Shar-pei dogs with clinical signs attendant to the underlying disease (Segev et al., 2012). Decreased albumin and increased urea nitrogen and creatinine were present in almost all of the dogs at the time of presentation. Renal amyloidosis was the most common histologic finding in both Shar-pei and non–Shar-pei dogs, with the liver and spleen the most common extrarenal organs with amyloid deposition (Segev et al., 2012).

Nodular and Regenerative Hepatocellular Hyperplasia

Nodular hepatocellular hyperplasia is a commonly and often incidentally found pathology of unknown cause in the older dog, generally older than 8 years, but is less common in cats. The number of nodules range from a few to numerous, and the size varies from microscopic to macroscopic (≤3 cm in diameter) and may cause distortion of the hepatic surface (see Fig. 9.23A). Hepatocytes in hyperplastic nodules often contain cytoplasmic vacuolation, reflecting glycogen or lipid accumulation (Fig. 9.34; see also Fig. 9.32). This can lead to a grossly visible light brown

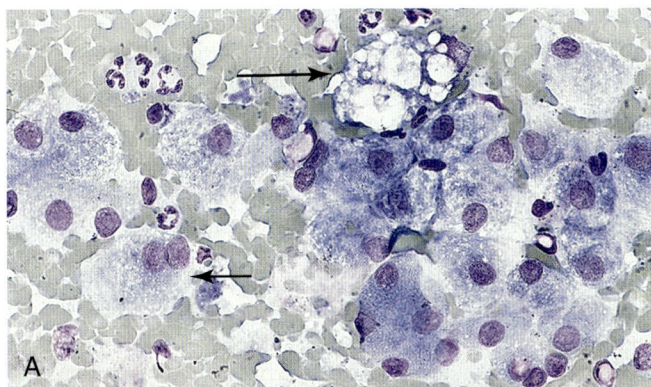

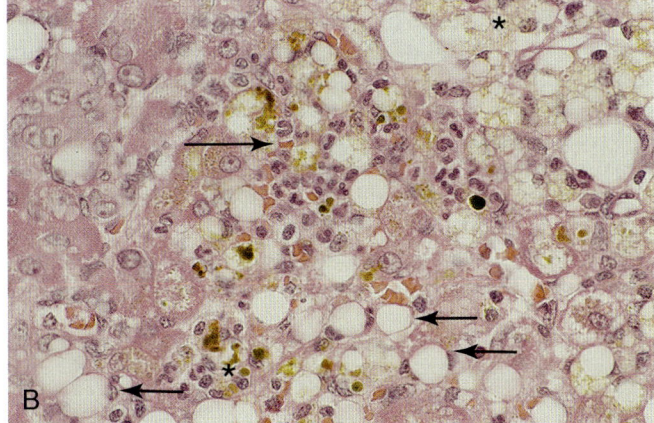

■ **FIGURE 9.34 Nodular hyperplasia. Liver. Dog.** Same case in A and B. **A, Cytopathologic biopsy.** An 11-year-old mixed-breed dog presented with a mildly increased serum alanine aminotransferase activity, moderately increased serum alkaline phosphatase activity, and variable echogenicity with possible nodules noted by ultrasound. Approximately equal numbers of neutrophils and lymphocytes are scattered among the hepatocytes, and there is a clump of foamy (vacuolated) macrophages present *(long arrow)*. Hepatocytes show mild cytoplasmic rarefaction, and some are binucleated *(short arrow)*. These findings are nonspecific but compatible with nodular or regenerative hyperplasia. (Wright-Giemsa; IP.) **B, Histology.** Diagnosis was confirmed with a subsequent wedge biopsy. Notable microscopic findings include a foci of extramedullary hematopoiesis (granulopoiesis) that is composed of segmented, band, and metamyelocyte neutrophils *(long arrow)*, hypertrophy of hepatic stellate cells (Ito cell, lipocyte, fat-storage cell) *(short arrows)*, and foci of macrophages filled with golden brown material consistent with ceroid pigment *(asterisks)*, some of which are vacuolated (upper right) similar to those observed in the cytopathologic biopsy. (H&E; IP.)

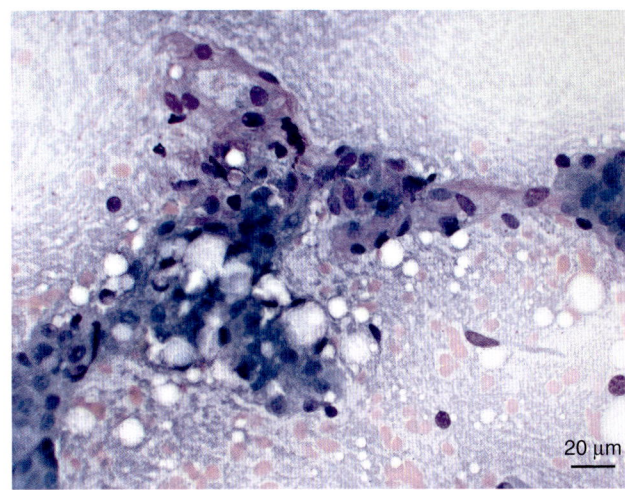

■ **FIGURE 9.35 Nodular hyperplasia with fibrosis. Liver mass aspirate. Dog.** An 11-year-old dog presented on wellness check with significantly elevated enzymes. On ultrasound, a 9 cm liver mass was determined and sampled for cytopathology. Hepatocytes displayed mild atypia with increased nucleocytoplasmic ratio and cytoplasmic basophilia. Also noted was the presence of multiple spindle mesenchymal cells associated with eosinophilic amorphous fibrillar matrix. (Wright; HP oil.) (Courtesy Rose Raskin, North Carolina State University.)

to yellow discoloration compared with the surrounding normal hepatic parenchyma and is reflected in mild, nonspecific increases in liver enzyme activity, most commonly ALP activity. Cytopathologically, hyperplastic hepatocytes may not be easily differentiated from normal hepatic parenchyma, but a mild increase in cellular and nuclear size, mild anisocytosis and anisokaryosis, mildly increased N:C, increased numbers of binucleated cells, or increased cytoplasmic basophilia may be seen; mitotic figures are uncommonly observed (Cullen, 2017). Other features occasionally seen within hyperplastic nodules include foci of mixed inflammation, lipogranulomas, and EMH (see Figs. 9.32 and 9.34). Necrosis or areas of hemorrhage are uncommon in hyperplastic nodules. Hyperplastic nodules cannot be differentiated from regenerative nodules on cytopathology. The latter are a consequence of typically chronic hepatocellular injury, often with loss of normal architecture within and around the nodules and accompanied by fibrosis (Fig. 9.35) or cirrhosis on histology, whereas hyperplastic nodules typically retain normal lobular arrangement on histology (Charles et al., 2006; Cullen and Stalker, 2016). Furthermore, regenerative and hyperplastic nodules cannot be confidently differentiated from adenomas and well-differentiated hepatocellular carcinomas with cytopathology generally. Consequently, when nodules are detected on ultrasound or during an exploratory laparotomy, histopathology for the assessment of tissue architecture may be needed to rule out a neoplastic process with certainty.

Biliary Sludge and Gallbladder Mucoceles

Mucoceles and sludge are detected by ultrasound of the gallbladder and can result in cholestasis and gallbladder rupture if untreated (Owens et al., 2003). Biliary sludge appears hyperechogenic and grossly is dark sandlike material. *Sludge* refers to a dense viscous mixture of cholesterol crystals, calcium products, mucin, and other materials resulting from delayed excretion (Figs. 9.36 and 9.37A). Sandlike particles may contain calcium crystals or microspheroliths (Fig. 9.37B). Mucoceles on ultrasound have kiwi‚Äêlike or stellate patterns and appear black and jelly-like related to excessive secretion of mucin from gallbladder epithelium. The rates of bacterial infection of the gallbladder were 10.0% for biliary sludge and 14.3% for gallbladder mucoceles with almost all of the bacterial species identified being intestinal flora. Their conclusion was biliary sludge may be the stage preceding the appearance of gallbladder mucoceles (Mizutani et al., 2017). The presence of microspheroliths ranging in size from 5 to 15 μm and composed of calcium carbonate have been demonstrated in bile, which may precede to the formation of gallstones (Wells and Camus,

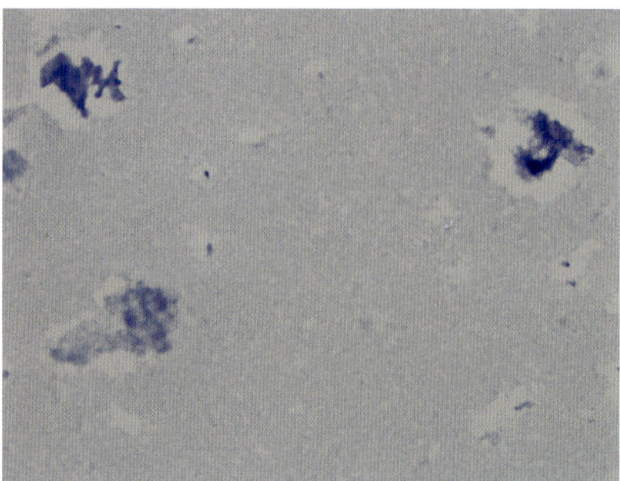

■ **FIGURE 9.36 Bile sludge. Bile fluid smear. Cat.** The patient was determined to have mild to moderate elevations in alanine aminotransferase and aspartate aminotransferase activities plus mild hyperbilirubinemia. Ultrasound of the gallbladder indicated sludge. An aspirate of the fluid was green and turbid. The direct smear was composed of fine granular gray-blue background material with many large dense blue-gray mucoid aggregates dispersed throughout. (Wright-Giemsa; HP oil.) (Courtesy Rose Raskin, University of Florida.)

2017). These calcium carbonate microspheroliths are yellow to light brown, refractile sandlike particles and birefringent using polarized light (Fig. 9.37C–D).

Hepatic Cell Death and Fibrosis

Injury to the liver may result in cell death in the form of apoptosis or necrosis (oncosis) (Cullen and Staker, 2016). There are morphologic differences between the two cellular disturbances. Apoptosis is a form of programmed cell death without much leakage of internal contents producing initially shrinkage of chromatin, cellular detachment, and intact rounded cellular borders (Fig. 9.38). An early response to hypoxia, ischemia, or toxic injury is coagulative necrosis, which refers to the denaturation of cytoplasmic proteins that produces an intense cytoplasmic staining with an intact but distorted nucleus (Fig. 9.39). With more severe cell death, denaturation of nuclear proteins occurs, and necrosis is commonly recognized with cellular swelling, loss of cytoplasmic and nuclear membrane integrity, and reduced mitochondrial function causing release of lysosomal enzymes (Fig. 9.40; see also Fig. 9.39). This incites an inflammatory response and leads to a rise in liver enzymes detected in the blood.

In response to hepatic injury, there is production of fibrosis through activation of hepatic stellate cells, resulting in production

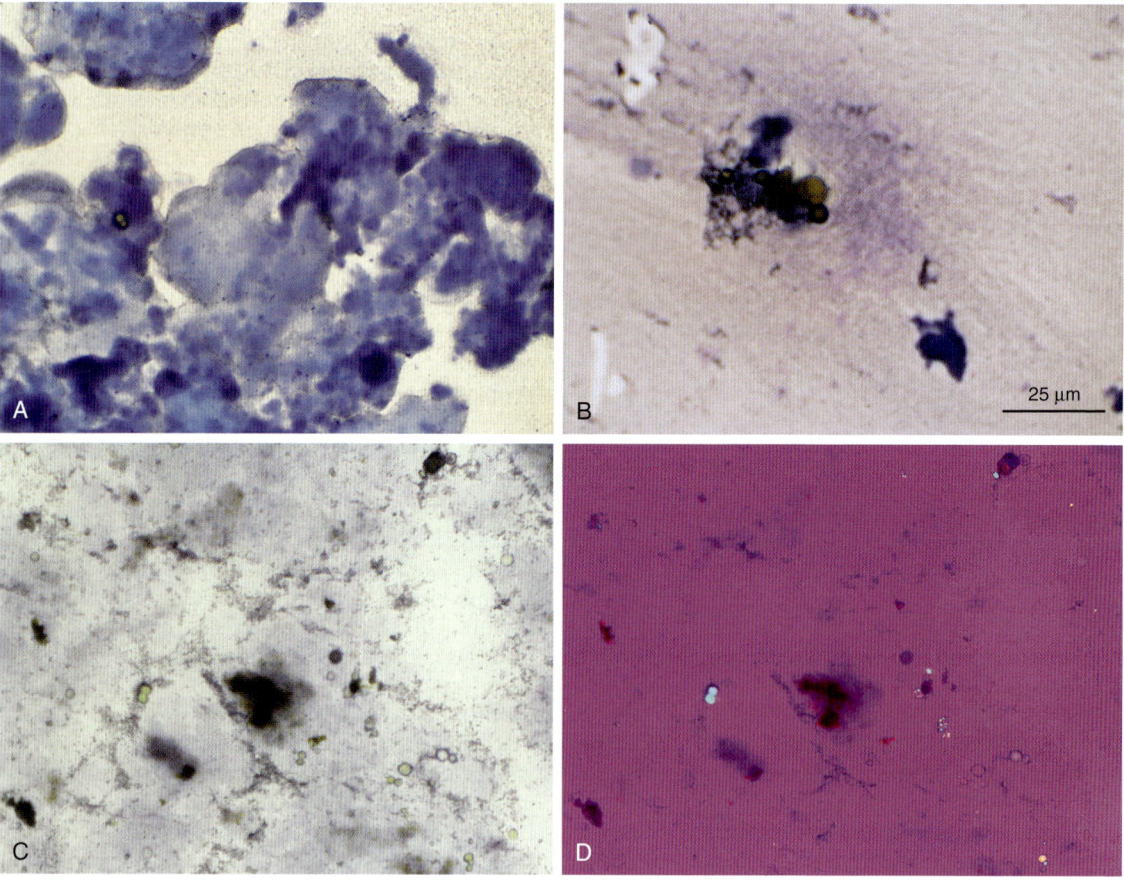

■ **FIGURE 9.37 Bile microspheroliths. Bile fluid smear. Dog.** Same case in A and D. The patient presented for workup of elevated liver enzymes and concern for hyperadrenocorticism. **A,** Large aggregates of blue-gray mucoid material (sludge) containing few small yellow crystals. (Modified Wright; HP oil.) **B,** Several yellow-brown round crystals, likely composed of calcium carbonate, are admixed with mucoid blue-gray material. (Modified Wright; HP oil.) **C,** Indistinguishable crystalline particles are present without polarization. (Modified Wright; HP oil.) **D,** Same field as in C, which when polarized easily reveals the refractile birefringent calcium carbonate crystals. (Modified Wright/Polarized; HP oil.) (Courtesy Mara Varvil, Purdue University.)

INFLAMMATION AND INFECTION

The assessment of hepatic inflammation by FNAB often provides an incomplete picture of the pathology because of the inability to assess the lobular distribution and the magnitude of the inflammatory and degenerative or necrotic changes. Reported sensitivity of liver cytopathology for the presence of inflammation varies from 25% to 100%, depending on the type of inflammation and study design (Roth, 2001; Weiss et al., 2001; Wang et al., 2004). Focal inflammation may be missed by the needle at sampling, and mild inflammation can be difficult to distinguish from hemodilution, particularly if the patient has a peripheral leukocytosis. If inflammatory cells are found in obvious excess of peripheral concentrations, are present in clumps, are closely admixed with hepatobiliary epithelium, or mainly composed of cells not commonly expected in peripheral blood (e.g., macrophages or plasma cells), true inflammation is likely. Furthermore, neutrophils displaying degenerate changes or nuclear streaming are also strongly suggestive of true intrahepatic inflammation, and evidence of any underlying causes, such as infectious organisms, necrosis, or neoplastic cells, is further supportive. Although infectious agents, autoimmune diseases, and toxin or drug effects can cause inflammation, the underlying etiology of acute and chronic inflammation often remains undetermined except for in breeds predisposed to copper accumulation (Poldervaart et al., 2009; Dirksen and Fieten, 2017; Strickland et al., 2018). Mild, nonspecific, reactive hepatitis can be seen secondary to inflammatory bowel disease and, notably, pancreatitis, and sinusoidal leukocytosis may be observed with corticosteroid excess in dogs (Cullen and Staker, 2016).

Neutrophilic Inflammation

Finding increased numbers of neutrophils admixed with sheets of hepatocytes or biliary epithelium is consistent with neutrophilic inflammation (Figs. 9.42 and 9.43). If only few (or no)

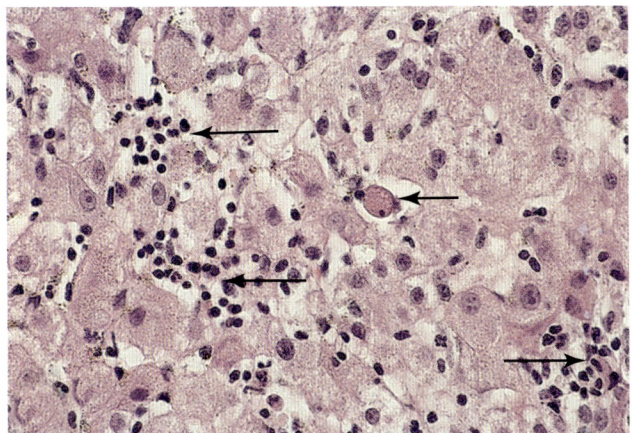

■ **FIGURE 9.38 Apoptosis. Chronic hepatic disease. Dog. Histology.** Histopathology confirmed the presence of chronic progressive liver disease and defined the extent of the inflammation, bridging necrosis, and fibrotic changes. These are important prognostic criteria that cannot be assessed cytopathologically. Notable histopathologic findings in this photomicrograph include severe piecemeal necrosis defined as lymphocytes *(long arrows)* streaming from the portal tracts into the surrounding parenchyma and associated hepatocellular necrosis, increased fibrosis, and apoptosis *(short arrow)*. The dog died of liver failure 7 months later. See Figure 9.48 for cytopathology from this case. (H&E; IP.)

of extracellular matrix (Fig. 9.41; see also Fig. 9.35). One study determined that the number of spindle cells and mast cells could help diagnose hepatic fibrosis. The optimal cutoff point for the spindle cells to hepatocytes ratio was 1 spindle cell per 10 hepatocytes with 95.5% sensitivity and 100% specificity. The optimal cutoff point for the mast cells to hepatocytes ratio was 4 mast cells per 100 hepatocytes with 86.4% sensitivity and 90% specificity (Masserdotti and Bertazzolo, 2016).

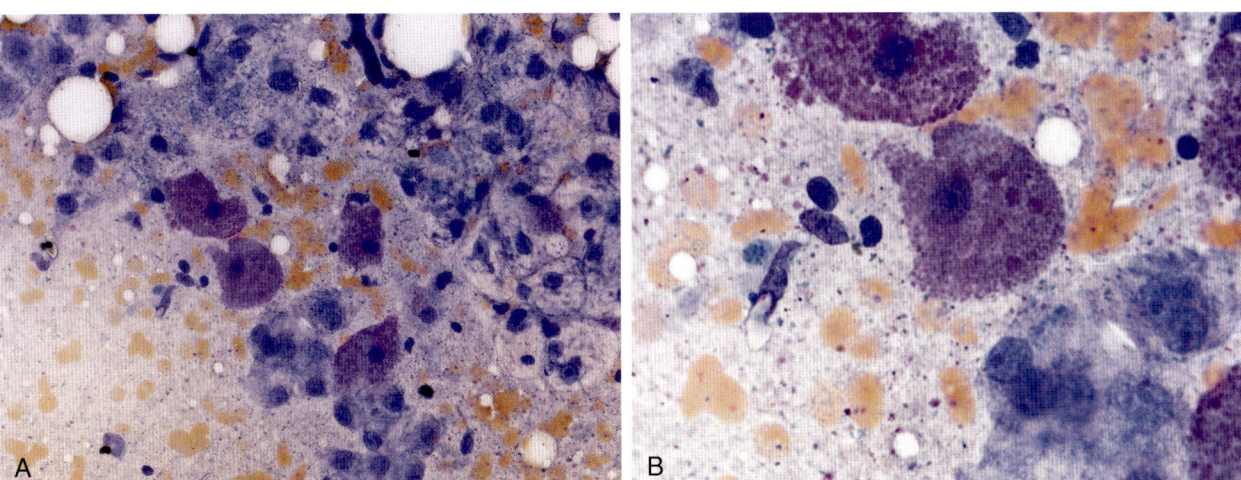

■ **FIGURE 9.39 Granular hepatocytes. Liver aspirate. Dog.** Same case in A and B. A 10-year-old canine patient presented for staging workup of cutaneous mast cell tumor. Noted were an elevated serum alanine aminotransferase level and hyperechoic liver nodules on abdominal ultrasound. **A,** Four dissociated eosinophilic cells with condensed nucleus and distinct cytoplasmic outlines are admixed with sheets and clusters of hepatocytes having diffuse cytoplasmic rarefaction. (Wright-Giemsa; HP oil.) **B,** Higher magnification demonstrates the similarity of the nucleus to that of hepatocytes in size and single nucleolus. The cytoplasm contains diffuse and aggregated eosinophilic granules. The significance of these cells is unknown, but the intense staining and accumulation of cytoplasmic organelles is suggestive of hepatocytes exhibiting early cell death. (Wright-Giemsa; HP oil.) (Courtesy of Christina Jeffries, Colorado State University.)

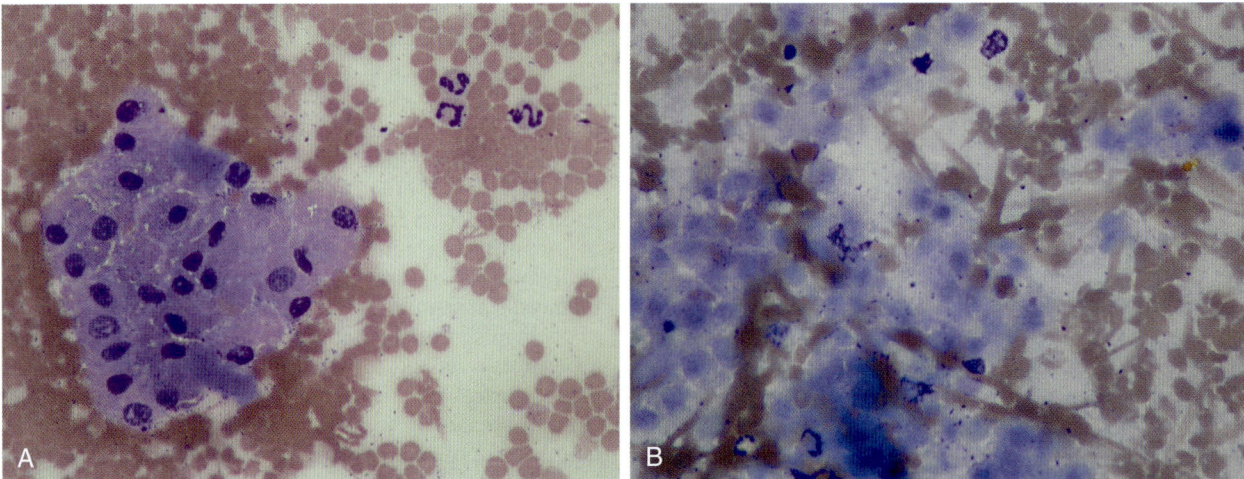

■ **FIGURE 9.40 Necrosis. Liver aspirate. Dog. A,** Hepatocytes are arranged in sheets. Hepatocyte nuclei are fragmented and occasionally condensed. There are large cytoplasmic fragments that are amorphous, basophilic, and finely granular consistent with mild necrosis. (Wright; HP oil.) **B,** The patient has been jaundiced for 2 to 3 weeks, and ultrasound shows a blocked bile duct with an irregular liver mass. Nearly all cells in the specimen are poorly distinct replaced by an amorphous pale blue cytoplasm suggestive of severe necrosis. As a result of red cell lysis and recrystallization, the hemoglobin appears as needles in the background. (Wright; HP oil.) (Courtesy Rose Raskin, Synlab/VPG/TDDS, Exeter, UK.)

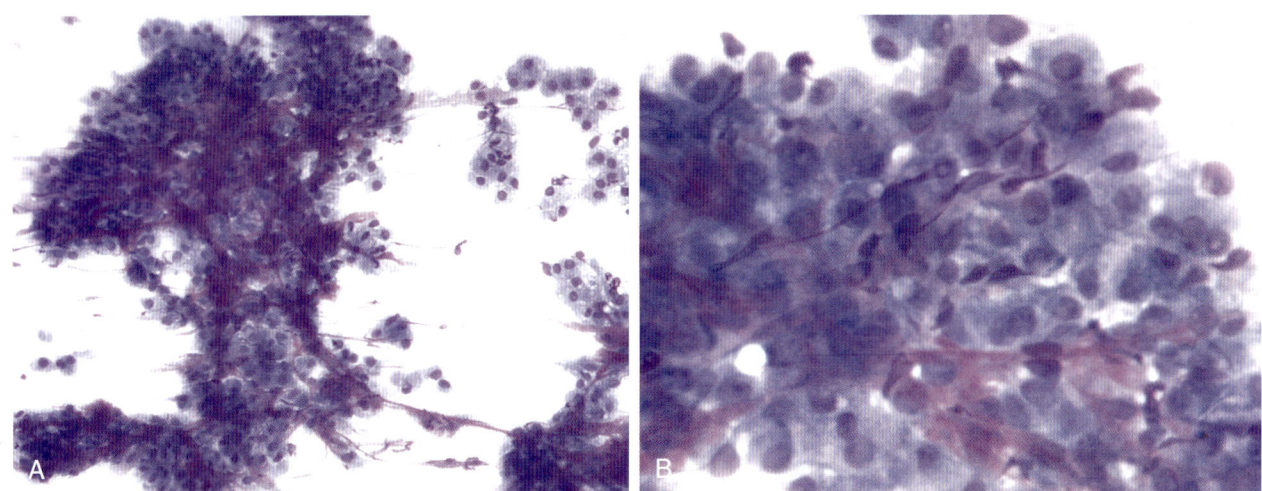

■ **FIGURE 9.41 Fibrosis. Liver aspirate. Dog.** Same case in A and B. The patient was diagnosed with hyperadrenocorticism and liver enzyme abnormalities. The patient had a 1-year history of allergy medicine (oclacitinib) administration. Ultrasound detected a 5.15 × 3.63 cm hypoechoic liver mass, which was sampled. **A,** Hepatocytes are arranged in variably sized cohesive sheets that are frequently disorganized and often admixed with a moderate amount of bright eosinophilic extracellular matrix. (Wright-Giemsa; IP.) **B,** Occasional spindle cells are recognized between the eosinophilic fibrotic material. (Wright-Giemsa; HP oil.) (Courtesy Rose Raskin, University of Florida.)

hepatocytes are found alongside high numbers of degenerate or necrotic neutrophils and streaming nuclear material, then a hepatic abscess is likely, provided the aspirates are truly representative of the liver. Sampling a solitary hypoechoic structure in the hepatic parenchyma in association with neutrophilia or fever should be considered carefully because of the potential of rupturing the abscess and inducing peritonitis.

The neutrophils and surrounding tissue should be carefully examined for infectious agents (Figs. 9.44 and 9.45). Neutrophilic cholangitis and cholangiohepatitis is more common in cats than dogs (Fig. 9.46; see Fig. 9.43B). The most common bacteria include *Escherichia coli* and *Enterococcus* spp., which are hypothesized to ascend from the gastrointestinal tract (Harrison et al., 2018), however hematogenous spread is also possible. Concurrent conditions, such as pancreatitis (see Fig. 9.43A), inflammatory bowel disease (see Fig. 9.43B), or bile duct obstruction should be considered as underlying causes of neutrophilic inflammation. Viral infections associated with neutrophilic inflammation include feline infectious peritonitis, canine adenovirus 1, and alpha herpesvirus. Toxins and drugs that cause hepatocellular necrosis may have an attendant neutrophilic inflammation.

The anatomic location of the neutrophilic infiltration in the lobule cannot be determined by cytopathology, precluding

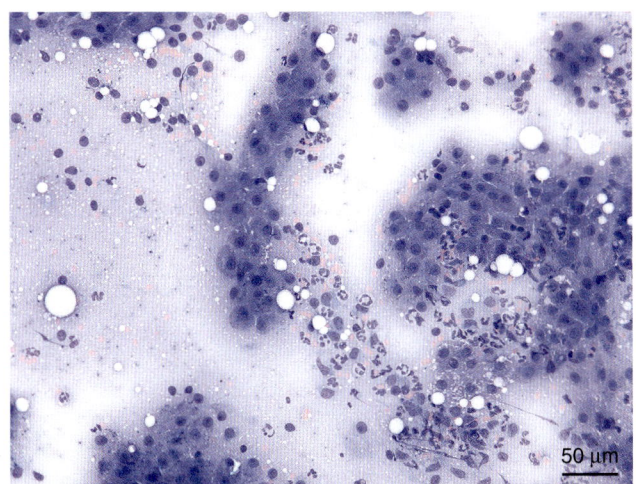

■ **FIGURE 9.42 Neutrophilic inflammation. Liver cytopathologic specimen. Cat.** Increased numbers of nondegenerate neutrophils and occasional macrophages are found in clumps closely associated and admixed with sheets of hepatocytes and low numbers of lipid vacuoles. (Modified Wright; IP.)

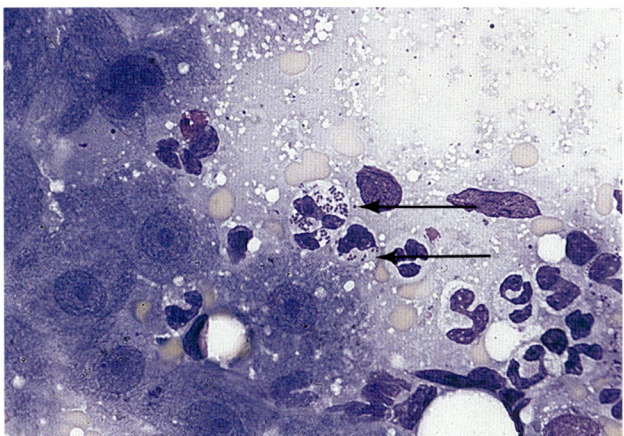

■ **FIGURE 9.44 Bacterial infection. Suppurative hepatitis. Cytopathologic specimen. Cat.** The presence of neutrophils intimately associated with hepatocytes is indicative of suppurative hepatitis. Note the paucity of erythrocytes, which indicates that the majority of the neutrophils are not a component of blood contamination. Two neutrophils are packed with bacteria (arrows). This cat also had moderately increased serum alanine aminotransferase and aspartate aminotransferase values, a slightly increased serum alkaline phosphatase value, a mild rise in the serum bilirubin concentration, and a mild neutrophilia. (Wright-Giemsa; HP oil.)

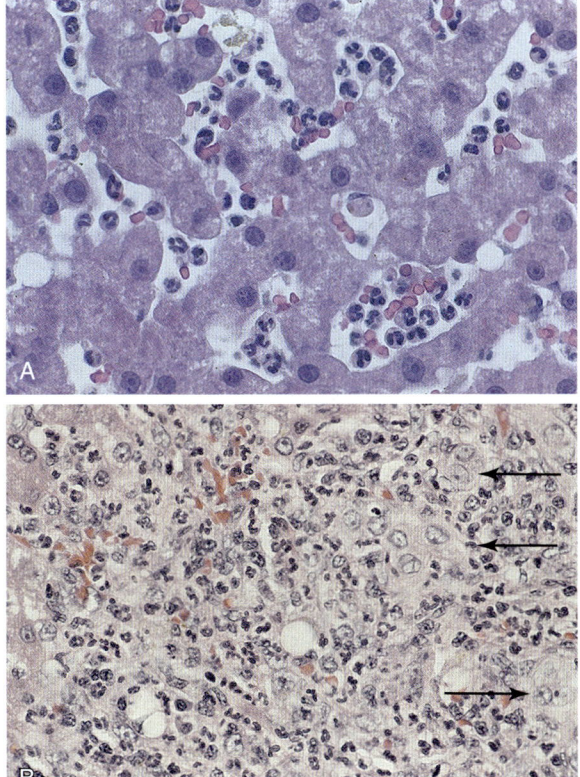

■ **FIGURE 9.43 Suppurative inflammation. Histology.** Contrast the following histologic findings in two icteric cats with moderately increased serum liver enzyme values. **A, Suppurative hepatitis in a cat.** This specimen primarily involves the parenchyma (sinusoidal leukostasis). The inflammation in was secondary to acute pancreatitis that was presumptively diagnosed by ultrasonography. (H&E; HP oil.) **B, Suppurative cholangiohepatitis in cat.** In contrast, this specimen involves primarily bile duct inflammation (cholangitis or cholangiohepatitis). Hyperplastic bile ductular epithelial cells are indicated (arrows). Severe enteritis was diagnosed by histopathology and associated with the cholangitis/cholangiohepatitis. (H&E; IP.)

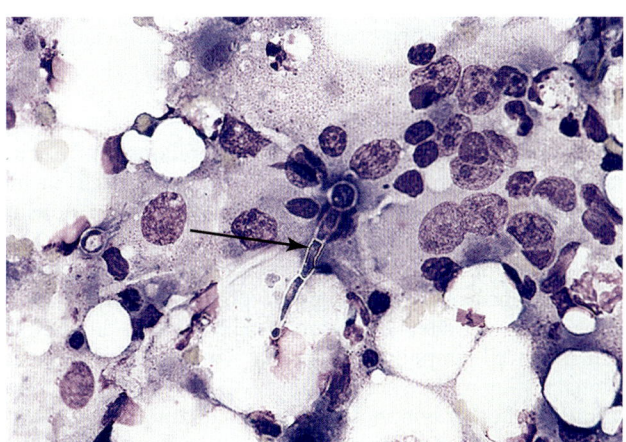

■ **FIGURE 9.45 Mycotic infection. Suppurative hepatitis. Cytopathologic specimen. Dog.** Neutrophils were prominent in areas (not shown) of this aspirate from a dog with moderately increased liver enzyme tests and hypoechoic foci with ultrasound examination. A mycotic agent (arrow) was discovered after additional searching. A diagnosis of hepatic hyalohyphomycosis, a term applied to opportunistic infections caused by nonpigmented fungi with hyaline hyphal elements as the basic tissue form, was subsequently made based on the culture of *Paecilomyces* spp. from the tissue obtained at surgery. (Wright-Giemsa; HP oil.)

differentiation between primarily parenchymal inflammation (hepatitis) versus primarily inflammation of the bile ducts (cholangitis) (see Fig. 9.43). Linking the morphologic assessment with the biochemical findings can be of value. An ALP or GGT activity markedly higher than that of serum alanine aminotransferase (ALT) activity is more consistent with cholangitis or cholangiohepatitis, especially if the serum bilirubin concentration is concomitantly increased. This generalization of course

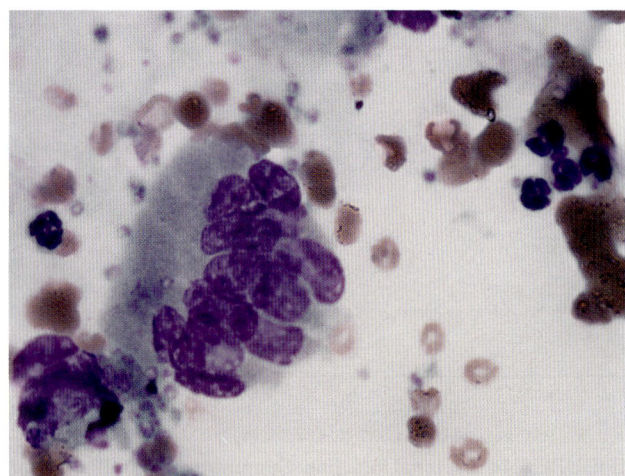

■ **FIGURE 9.46 Suppurative cholangitis. Bile duct mass. Mass aspirate. Cat.** A mass near major duodenal papilla measured 1.4 × 0.97 cm. A cluster of mildly atypical columnar epithelial cells with moderate amount of pale or medium basophilic cytoplasm and a clear rim of microvilli are consistent with bile duct origin. Small groups of nondegenerate neutrophils are also shown. (Wright-Giemsa; HP oil.) (Courtesy Rose Raskin, University of Florida.)

does not apply to the differential diagnosis of the feline lipidosis syndrome, primarily a hepatocellular disease, in which the serum ALP activity is often dramatically raised in association with hyperbilirubinemia.

Lymphocytic Inflammation

The occurrence of increased numbers of predominantly small, mature lymphocytes with or without a few plasma cells or medium lymphocytes, is consistent with lymphocytic or nonsuppurative inflammation (Figs. 9.47 and 9.48; see also Fig. 9.38). It can usually be distinguished from large cell lymphoma based on the absence of a monomorphic population of immature lymphocytes (see later) but is more challenging to differentiate from small cell lymphoma or chronic lymphoid leukemia; additional testing may be needed, such as a complete blood count, aspiration of other lymphoid organs, histopathology, immunophenotyping, or polymerase chain reaction for clonality (see Chapter 18).

Lymphocytic inflammation is more commonly observed in cats with lymphocytic cholangitis, also referred to as lymphocytic cholangitis/cholangiohepatitis or lymphocytic portal hepatitis and is not necessarily associated with clinical signs (Weiss et al., 1995). This is typically a chronic disease, with slow progression; an immune-mediated pathogenesis has been proposed (Day, 1998; Warren et al., 2011; Cullen and Stalker, 2016).

The cytopathologic finding of predominantly small lymphocytes is not common in the dog and should be followed by histologic examination for chronic progressive hepatitis (see Figs. 9.38 and 9.48). Testing for levels in the liver or staining liver slides aids in evaluating secondary copper accumulation.

Mixed Inflammation

Finding a mixture of neutrophils and lymphocytes, with or without macrophages in a feline liver cytopathology specimen, suggests feline infectious peritonitis (Fig. 9.49) or a more

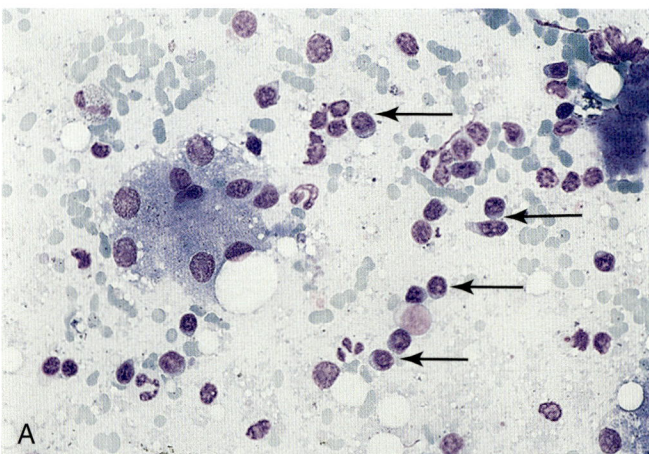
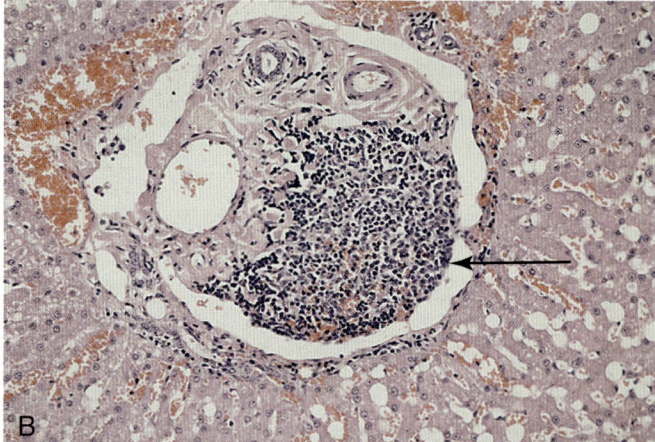
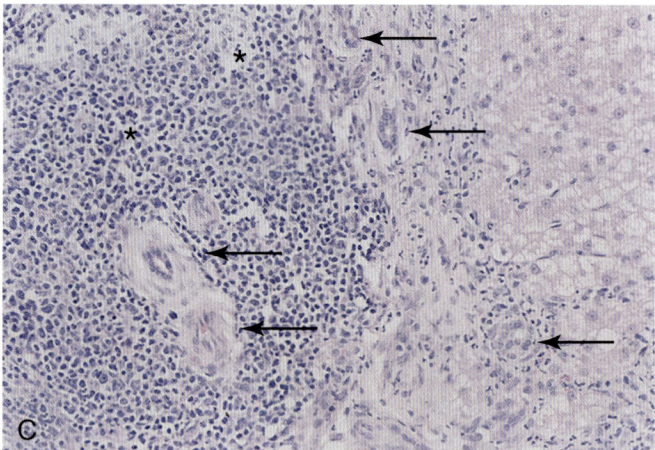

■ **FIGURE 9.47 Lymphocytic portal hepatitis. Liver. Cat. A, Cytopathologic specimen.** Predominance of predominantly small, inflammatory lymphocytes *(arrows)* from an aged cat with unknown cause. (Wright-Giemsa; IP.) **B, Histology.** There is a prominent lymphocytic infiltrate that is confined to the portal area *(arrow)* (H&E; LP.) **C, Histology.** Occasionally, extensive lymphocytic infiltration (portal-to-portal bridging) is observed. In this specimen, there are marked bile duct proliferation *(arrows)*, moderate fibrous tissue, and a dense lymphocytic infiltrate in the portal area that extends upward to connect to another portal tract *(asterisks)*. (H&E; LP.) (B, From Weiss DJ, Gagne JM, Armstrong PJ. Characterization of portal lymphocytic infiltrates in feline liver. *Vet Clin Pathol*. 1995;24:91-95.)

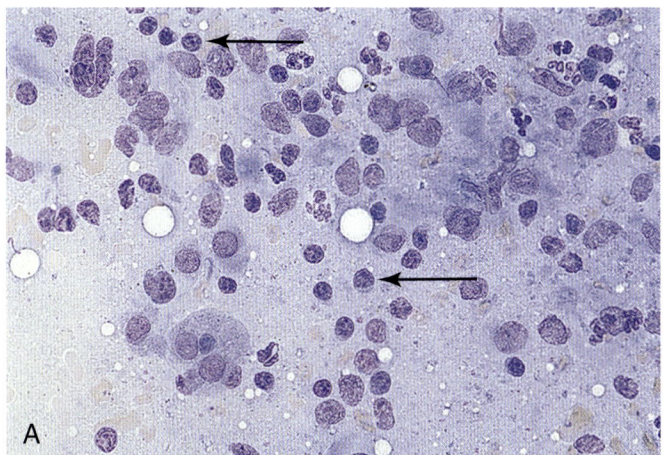

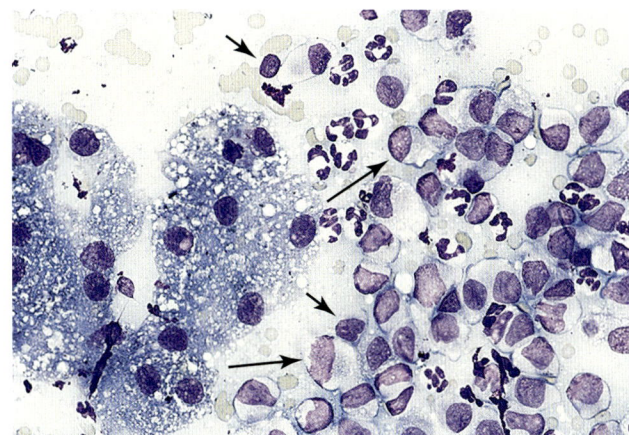

FIGURE 9.49 **Mixed cell inflammation. Liver imprint. Cat.** Neutrophils and histiocytes may be a prominent component of the mixed cell inflammation in cats with feline infectious peritonitis (FIP) involving the liver. This specimen is from one of several small white foci on the surface of the liver. The histiocytes are the large mononuclear cells in contrast to the neutrophils, with oval to reniform nuclei composed of bland homogenous chromatin and surrounded by a moderate amount of blue-gray cytoplasm *(long arrows)*. A lesser number of small mononuclear cells (lymphocytes) are admixed *(short arrows)*. Similar lesions were located on the kidney and in the mesentery in this case of noneffusive FIP confirmed histologically. (Wright-Giemsa; HP oil.)

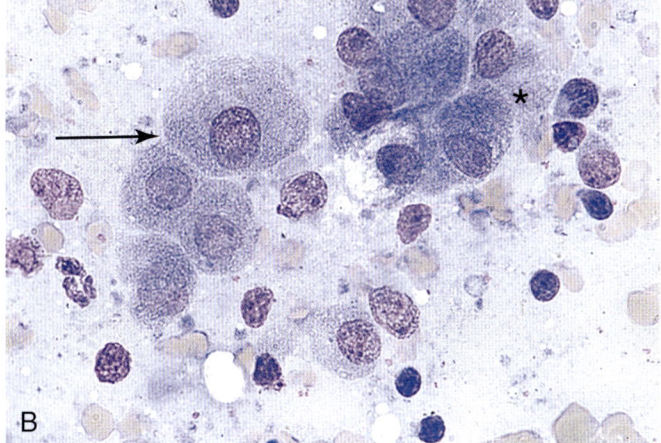

FIGURE 9.48 **Lymphocytic inflammation. Liver. Cytopathologic specimen. Dog.** Same case in A and B. **A,** A 5-year-old Labrador retriever presented with clinical lethargy, reduced appetite, and persistent mild to moderate abnormal alanine aminotransferase and aspartate aminotransferase values documented several times over 6 weeks. Small lymphocytes are the predominant inflammatory cell *(arrows)*. (Wright-Giemsa; IP.) **B,** Lymphocytes are intimately associated with the hepatocytes *(asterisk)*. Lesser numbers of neutrophils are also present. The mild to moderate hepatocellular anisocytosis and anisokaryosis *(arrow)* are suggestive of a regenerative (reparative) response. See Figure 9.38 for the histology from this case. (Wright-Giemsa; HP oil.)

Eosinophilic Inflammation

Small numbers of eosinophils may be a constituent of nonspecific mixed inflammatory cell reactions in dogs and cats. A prominent eosinophilic component has been reported in patients with parasitic disease, such as the liver fluke *Metorchis conjunctus*, and *Sarcocystis canis* (Watson and Croll, 1981; Allison et al., 2006). High numbers of eosinophils can also be observed in patients with hypereosinophilic syndrome, eosinophilic enteritis, and as part of tumor-associated inflammation and paraneoplastic infiltration.

Bile Infection

Cytopathologic examination of bile is inexpensive and yields diagnostically relevant information that precedes and complements bacterial culture for both canine and feline bile (Figs. 9.53 to 9.56). Interestingly, the presence of microorganisms was detected more frequently on cytopathologic examination than by culture, and the concurrence of inflammatory cells was often not present (see Fig. 9.54) (Peters et al., 2016; Pashmakova et al., 2017). Consequently, concurrent microscopic examination and bacterial culture of bile samples are recommended for all cats and dogs evaluated for hepatobiliary disease. Agreement between microscopic examination and bacterial culture of bile samples for detection of bactibilia is optimized when dogs and cats are not receiving antimicrobials at least 24 hours before the time of sample collection (Pashmakova et al., 2017). The majority of the animals with bactibilia had concurrent hepatobiliary, pancreatic, or gastrointestinal disease with a significant positive correlate with increased canine pancreatic lipase immunoreactivity concentration (cPLI) (Peters et al., 2016; Pashmakova et al., 2017). Other microorganisms, such as protozoa or yeast,

chronic form of neutrophilic cholangiohepatitis that may be associated with a variety of extrahepatic diseases. In dogs, chronic hepatitis may present with a mixed inflammatory response (Fig. 9.50). In aged dogs, mixed cell inflammation is commonly encountered in association with nodular hyperplasia. In both dogs and cats, mixed inflammation can be associated with infectious organisms, including protozoa (e.g., *Cytauxzoon felis*; Fig. 9.51), *Toxoplasma gondii*, *Neospora caninum*, *Leishmania* spp., *Sarcocystis* spp.), cestodes [e.g., *Mesocestoides* spp. (Patten et al., 2013), *Echinococcus* spp. (Stock et al., 2018)], trematodes (e.g., *Heterobilharzia americana*; Fig. 9.52) (Le Donne et al., 2016), fungi (e.g., coccidioidomycosis, aspergillosis), and mycobacteria. Special stains, such as PAS for fungal elements or Ziehl-Neelsen for acid-fast bacteria can aid in their recognition.

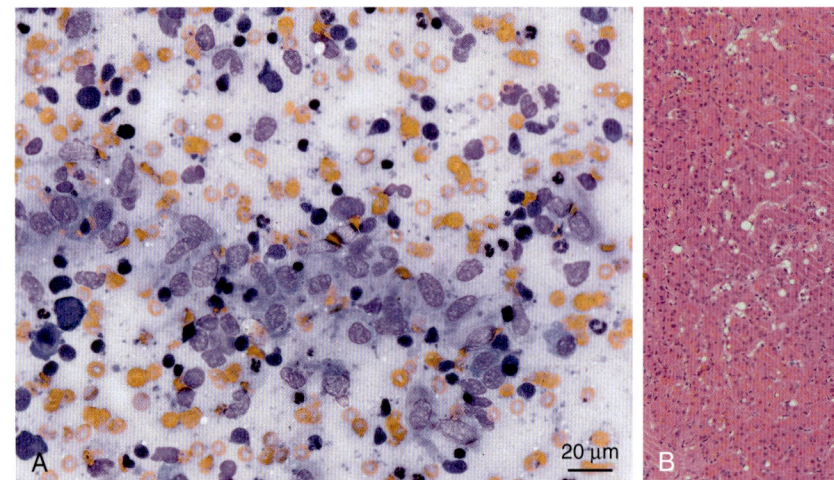
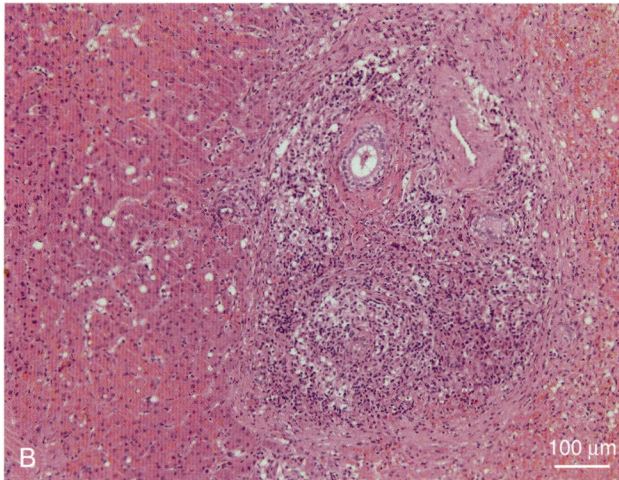

■ **FIGURE 9.50 Mixed cell inflammation. Liver. Dog.** Same case in A and B. **A, Aspirate.** Clumps of macrophages and mixed lymphocytes, with lower numbers of nondegenerate neutrophils are found in the liver from an adult pug with hepatomegaly, ascites, and increased liver enzyme activities. Although inflammatory liver disease is identified, the lobular location and the magnitude of the inflammation cannot be determined. (Modified Wright; HP oil.) **B, Histology.** The portal triad is markedly distended by a mixed cell inflammation, predominated by aggregates of macrophages and lymphocytes, with lower numbers of neutrophils and evidence of fibrosis (H&E; LP). The morphologic diagnosis of this specimen was chronic active, multifocal to coalescing, pyogranulomatous cholangitis; no underlying cause was found, but ascending enteric bacterial infection was suspected.

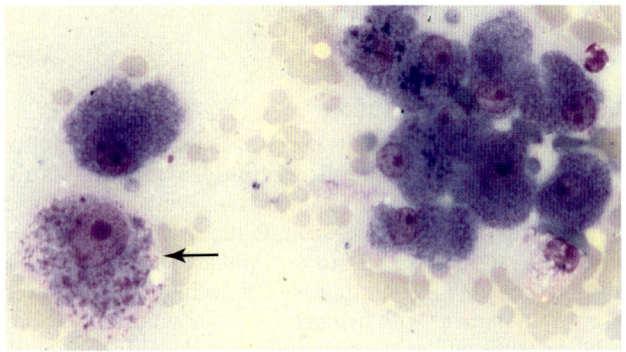

■ **FIGURE 9.51 Cytauxzoonosis schizont. Liver imprint. Cat.** This specimen was taken at necropsy from the liver of an infected cat. Several of the hepatocytes contain coarse pigmented granules suggestive of bile or lipofuscin. A single schizont of intermediate stage of maturation is present with developing merozoites (purple granules) within a macrophage *(arrow)*. Note the prominent nucleolus of the infected macrophage. (Wright-Giemsa; HP oil.) (Courtesy Rose Raskin, University of Florida.)

have been reported in bile, including *Cystoisospora* spp. (Fig. 9.57), *Toxoplasma* spp., *Hammondia* spp., and *Cyniclomyces guttulatus* (Neel et al., 2006; Irvine et al., 2016; Peters et al., 2016; Palić, 2017).

Trematode ova may be present in bile or bile ducts of the liver. One type in cats is *Amphimerus pseudofelineus* (Fig. 9.58), which produces nonsuppurative pericholangitis, bile duct hyperplasia, pericholangial fibrosis, and cholestasis. The operculated pear-shaped ova measure approximately 30 × 15 μm. Another trematode in cats is *Platynosomum fastosum*, which causes suppurative inflammation in bile fluid along with the presence of ova (Fig. 9.59). Ova are described as yellow-brown, oval operculated thick-walled structures measuring approximately 30 to 45 μm × 20 to 30 μm (Flatland, 2009; Stern et al., 2020).

NEOPLASIA

The liver is an uncommon site of primary neoplasia in dogs and cats; the majority of tumors found in this organ are metastatic. Of primary hepatic tumors, cholangiocellular origin is more common in cats, whereas hepatocellular origin is more frequently seen in dogs (van Sprundel et al., 2014).

Hepatocellular Neoplasia

Hepatocytes can give rise to hepatocellular adenomas or carcinomas, and very rarely, hepatoblastomas develop from hepatic progenitor cells. By cytopathology, hepatocellular adenomas and well-differentiated hepatocellular carcinomas may not be easily differentiated from normal hepatic parenchyma, hyperplastic, and regenerative nodules. If overt criteria of malignancy are lacking on cytopathology, a tissue biopsy may be needed to assess the architecture histopathologically. The cytopathologic evaluation of liver together with Ki-67 immunochemistry (a marker of cell proliferation) can improve the diagnostic accuracy of cytopathology alone and rule in or out liver neoplasia (Neumann and Kaup, 2005).

The hepatocellular adenoma is usually a single mass involving one liver lobe, which can grow as large as 12 to 15 cm. It is composed of relatively normal-appearing hepatocytes that can demonstrate mild anisocytosis and anisokaryosis, as well as slightly more prominent nucleoli or increased cytoplasmic basophilia.

Hepatocellular carcinomas occur in three different forms, namely massive, nodular, and diffuse, in descending order of frequency. If cells display multiple overt criteria of malignancy, such as moderate to marked anisokaryosis, karyomegaly, multinucleation, nucleolar atypia, high N:C, and numerous mitotic figures, a cytopathological diagnosis of hepatocellular

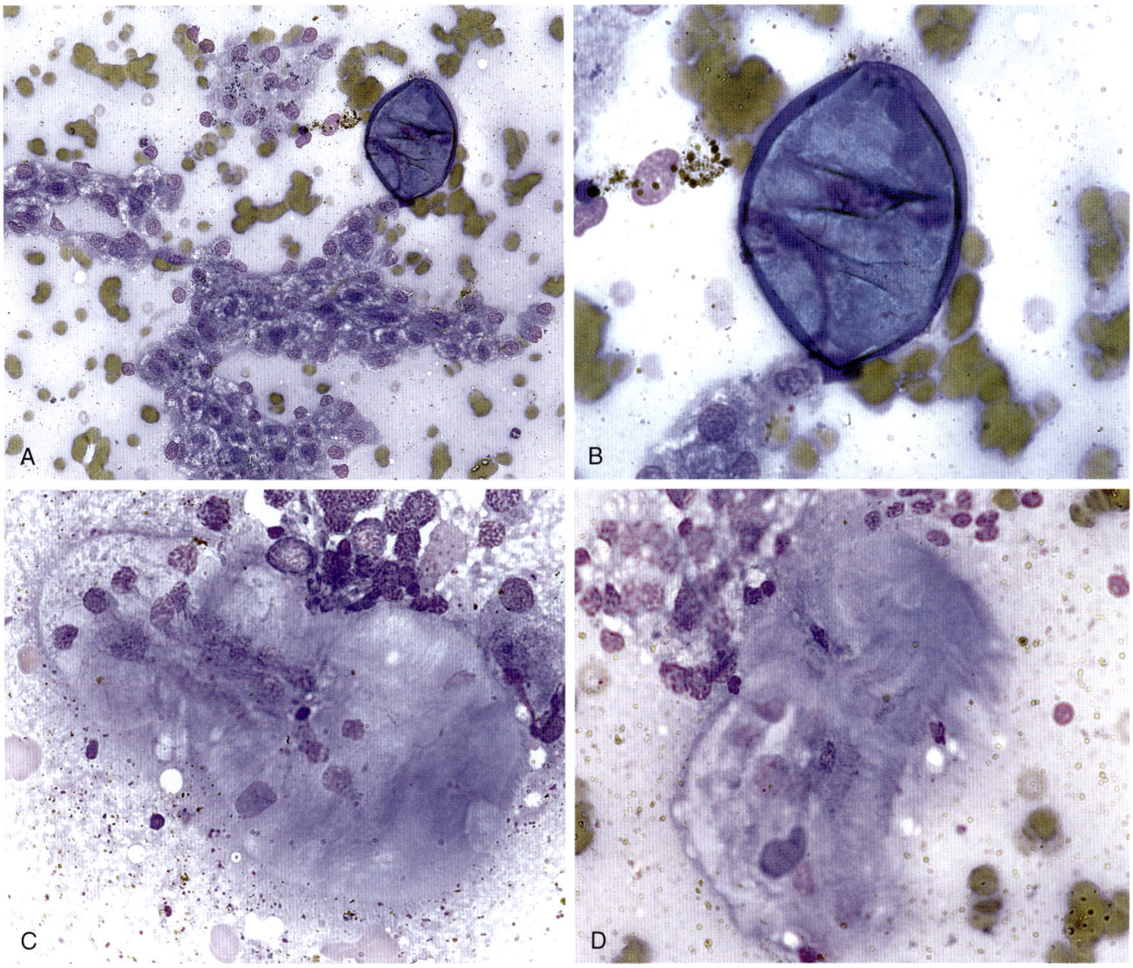

FIGURE 9.52 Blood fluke infection. Heterobilharzia americana. Liver aspirate. Dog. Same case in A to D. **A,** A single collapsed basophilic eggshell against the background of hepatocytes showing marked vacuolar changes consistent with glycogen deposition. Mild neutrophilic and eosinophilic inflammation was present (not shown). **B,** Higher magnification of the empty eggshell. Macrophage with hemosiderin lies to the left of the ovum. **C,** A pear-shaped structure intact, ciliated miracidium is shown with internal nuclear structures. **D,** A ruptured miracidium showing the once internal nuclear structures. The peripheral cilia are clearly visible particularly along the top and right side of the miracidium. Polymerase chain reaction testing of the feces confirmed the diagnosis. (Courtesy Rose Raskin, Kansas State University.)

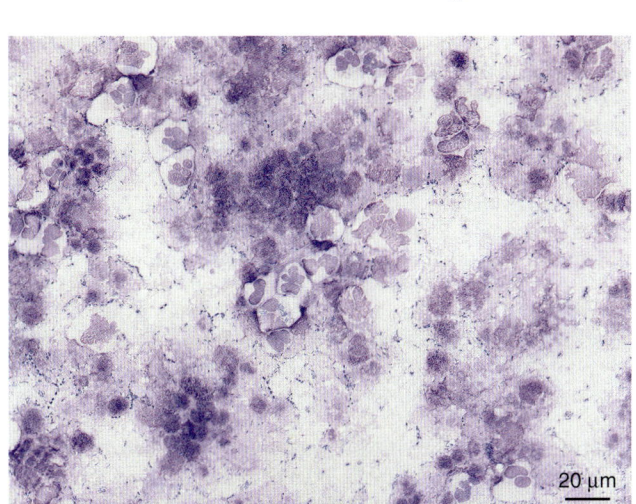

FIGURE 9.53 Bactibilia with neutrophilic inflammation. Bile fluid smear. Cat. High numbers of degenerate and necrotic neutrophils are found in this gallbladder aspirate, containing mixed intra- and extracellular bacteria (Modified Wright; HP oil.)

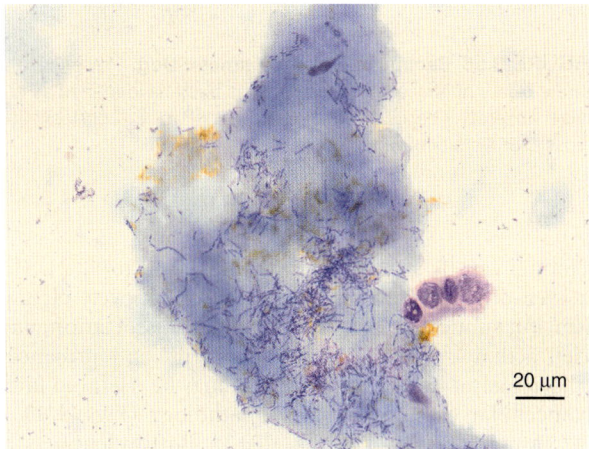

FIGURE 9.54 Bactibilia, Bile fluid smear. Cat. Numerous large spore-forming rods, cultured as *Clostridium* spp., are found in the mucinous bile of a 10-year-old cat with chronic vomiting and diarrhea. Note the absence of an inflammatory response and the presence of golden bilirubin crystals, as well as a row of poorly preserved, short columnar biliary epithelial cells. (Modified Wright; HP oil.).

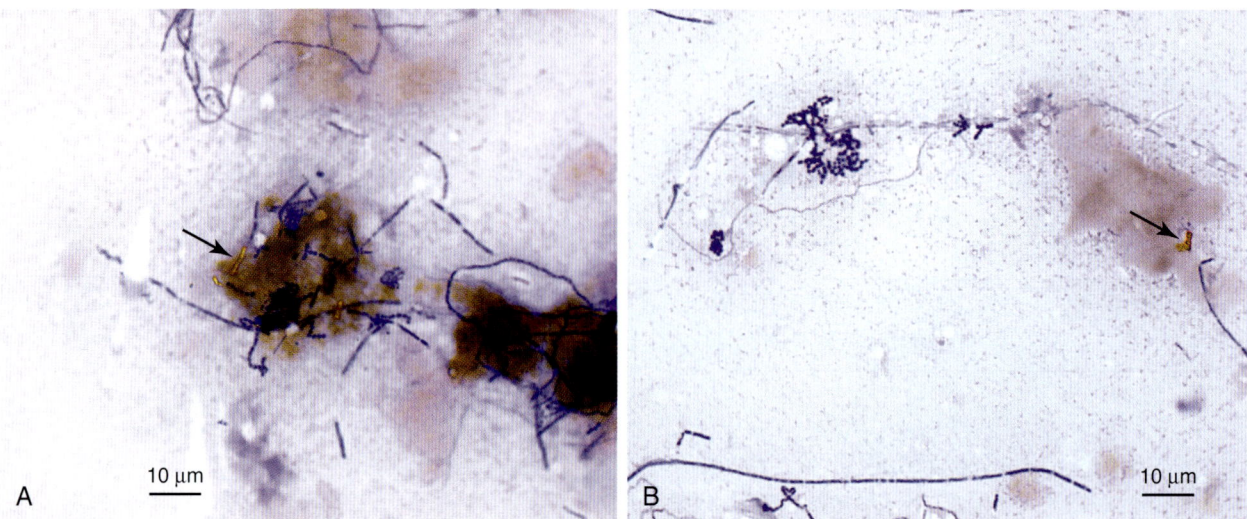

■ **FIGURE 9.55 Bactibilia. Bile fluid smear. Cat.** Same case in A and B. **A,** This dark green gallbladder fluid contains large dark orange material with gold-yellow bilirubin crystals *(arrow)*. (Wright; HP oil.) **B,** Bacteria range in shape from short rods and cocci to filamentous forms. Note bilirubin crystal *(arrow)*. Culture grew alpha-hemolytic *Streptococcus* and *Clostridium perfringens*. (Wright; HP oil.) (Courtesy Rose Raskin, Purdue University.)

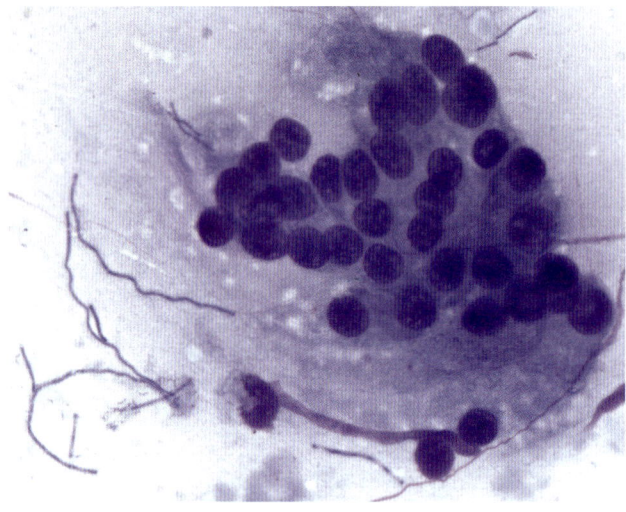

■ **FIGURE 9.56 Bactibilia. Bile fluid smear. Dog.** Presence of degenerate biliary epithelium and filamentous bacteria identified as gram-positive anaerobic bacilli. (Wright-Giemsa; HP oil.) (Courtesy Justin Breitbach, University of Florida.)

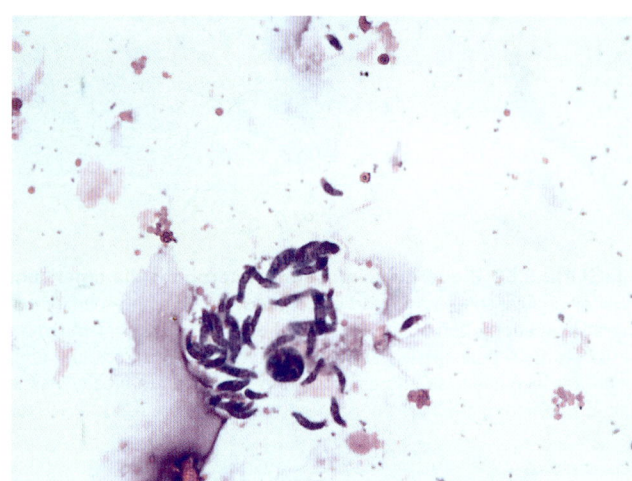

■ **FIGURE 9.57 Protozoan infection. Cystoisospora spp. (formerly Isospora spp.). Bile fluid. Direct smear. Dog.** A 10-month-old basenji presented with chronic intermittent vomiting and diarrhea. The banana-shaped organisms (merozoites) are approximately 3 × 10 μm with deeply basophilic cytoplasm and contain a central to paracentral variably staining round nucleus and eosinophilic globular material. One round meront, approximately 7 to 10 μm (in diameter) structure, contains multiple merozoites. Polymerase chain reaction and amplicon sequencing from bile supported the diagnosis, whereas serology for *Neospora* and *Toxoplasma* was negative. (Modified Wright; HP oil.). (Courtesy Laureen Peters et al., The Royal Veterinary College, UK. Presented at the 2013 ASVCP case review session.)

carcinoma can be straightforward (Figs. 9.60 to 9.62). However, well-differentiated carcinomas may lack overt pleomorphism, but subtle changes such as cellular dissociation, naked nuclei, acinar or palisading arrangement, and presence of capillaries admixed with hepatocytes may be useful to favor a hepatocellular carcinoma by cytopathology (Figs. 9.63 and 9.64) (Masserdotti and Drigo, 2012). Both adenomas and carcinomas can contain areas of EMH, dilated sinusoids, cystic or cavernous spaces, and cytoplasmic accumulation of glycogen or lipid; vacuolation is particularly prominent in the rare clear cell variant of hepatocellular carcinoma. Histologic features of local infiltration, vascular invasion, and detection of focal or distant metastasis are used on a tissue biopsy to help distinguish a well-differentiated carcinoma from an adenoma for a definitive diagnosis of malignancy. Rarely, paraneoplastic hypoglycemia in association with hepatocellular carcinoma has been attributed to secretion of insulin-like growth factor type II (see Fig. 9.62) (Zini et al., 2007).

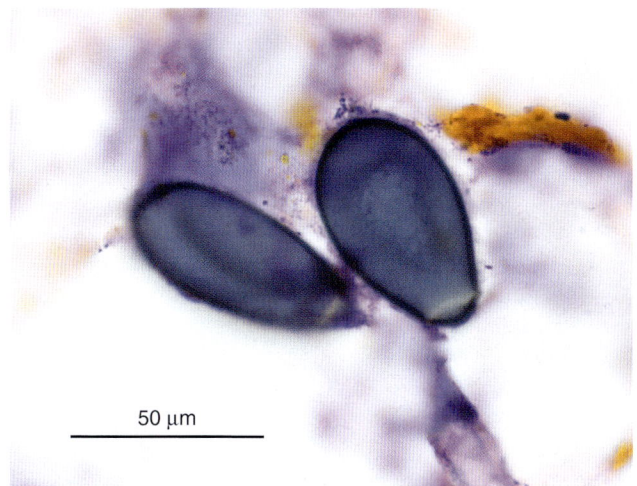

■ **FIGURE 9.58 Trematode infection. Amphimerus pseudofelineus. Liver aspirate. Cat.** Bile-stained ova from bile ducts within the liver appear in a cat that presented for icterus, weight loss, and elevated liver enzyme activities. Ultrasound indicated an anechoic cystic structure in the liver, distension of intrahepatic bile ducts, and enlarged gallbladder. Note the single operculated end of the pear-shaped ova. (Wright; HP oil.) (Courtesy Denise Bounous, Louisiana State University. Presented at the 1989 ASVCP case review session.)

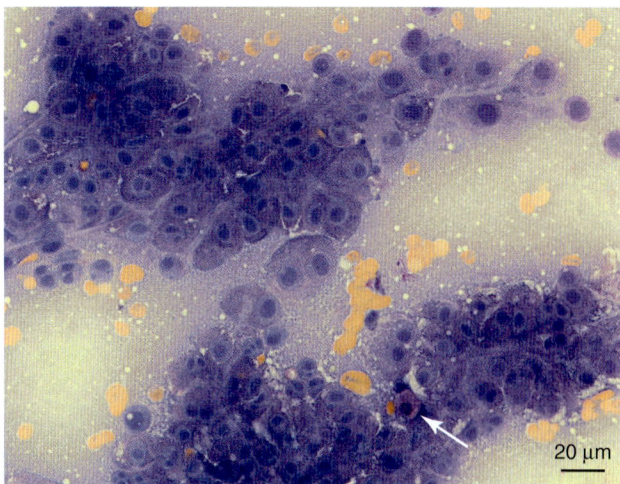

■ **FIGURE 9.60 Hepatocellular carcinoma. Liver cytopathologic specimen. Dog.** Clusters of hepatocytes display marked pleomorphism, including prominent anisocytosis, anisokaryosis, binucleation and trinucleation, nucleoli of variable number and size, including frequent macronucleoli. Note how the cytoplasm retains its characteristic granular amphophilic properties, identifying these cells as hepatocytes despite the marked nuclear atypia. Cells in the lower right corner also display mild cytoplasmic rarefaction, and there is a single necrotic cell *(arrow)*. (Modified Wright; HP oil).

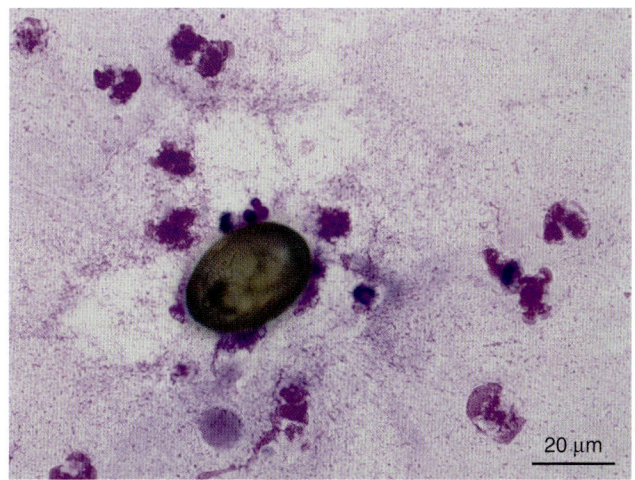

■ **FIGURE 9.59 Trematode infection. Platynosomum fastosum. Bile fluid smear. Cat.** An adult cat presented with inappetence and increased serum liver enzyme activities. Ultrasound indicated the gallbladder and common bile duct were mildly distended with thickened walls. Color and transparency of the bile fluid is amber and turbid. Numerous degenerate neutrophils surround a single yellow-brown, oval structure measuring approximately 30 × 20 µm in size with a thin dark brown rim and granular embryonated internal structure. (Wright-Giemsa; HP oil.) (Courtesy Jere Stern, University of Florida.)

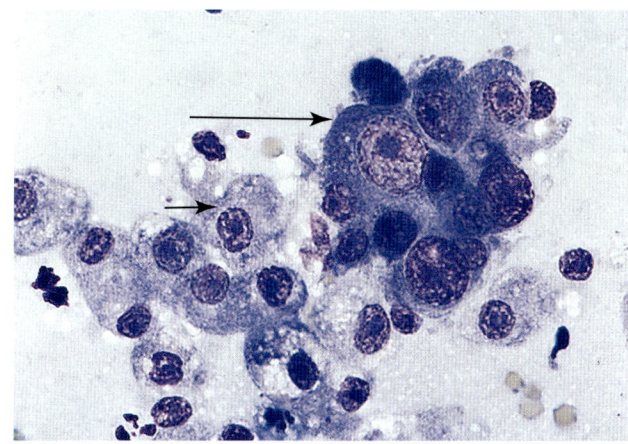

■ **FIGURE 9.61 Hepatocellular carcinoma. Liver cytopathologic specimen. Dog.** Specimen from a patient with large mass confined to one liver lobe on imaging. The malignant neoplasm may be relatively well differentiated, which was confirmed histologically. Normal-sized hepatocytes *(short arrow)* are contrasted with more anaplastic hepatocytes *(long arrow)*. (Wright-Giemsa; HP oil.)

> **KEY POINT** Hyperplastic or regenerative nodules, hepatocellular adenomas, and well-differentiated hepatocellular carcinomas can be difficult to distinguish by cytopathology alone.

Biliary Neoplasia

Most biliary tumors arise within the hepatic parenchyma; extrahepatic bile duct tumors are rare. Cholangiocellular adenomas are typically solitary masses, composed of small cystic spaces lined by a single layer of well-differentiated biliary epithelium and supported by variable amounts of stroma. However, when they are primarily cystic composed of clear acellular fluid, the term *biliary cystadenoma* may be applied (Adler and Wilson, 1995) (Fig. 9.65). These cystic masses are often impossible to distinguish from congenital cystic lesions, and it is suspected that most cases considered to be cholangiocellular cystadenomas in cats may be in fact non-neoplastic cystic structures (van

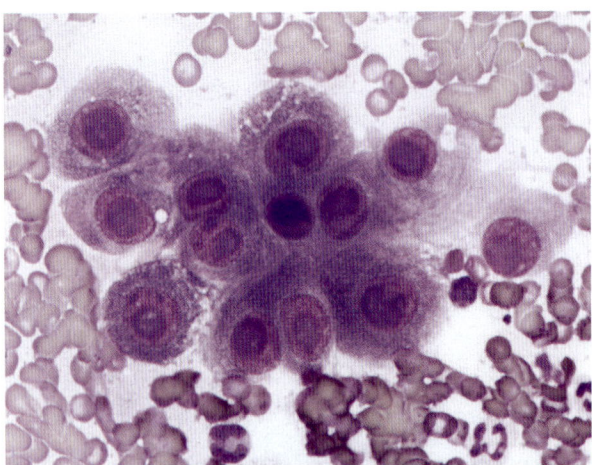

■ **FIGURE 9.62 Hepatocellular carcinoma. Liver cytopathologic specimen. Dog.** This patient had hypoglycemia with relatively uniform hepatocyte size and only mild to moderate anisocytosis and anisokaryosis, but the nuclei contain gigantic nucleoli. The large cell and nucleolar size can be appreciated by comparing each with the size of the neutrophils. The paraneoplastic hypoglycemia has been ascribed to insulinlike growth factor type II. (Romanowsky; HP oil.)

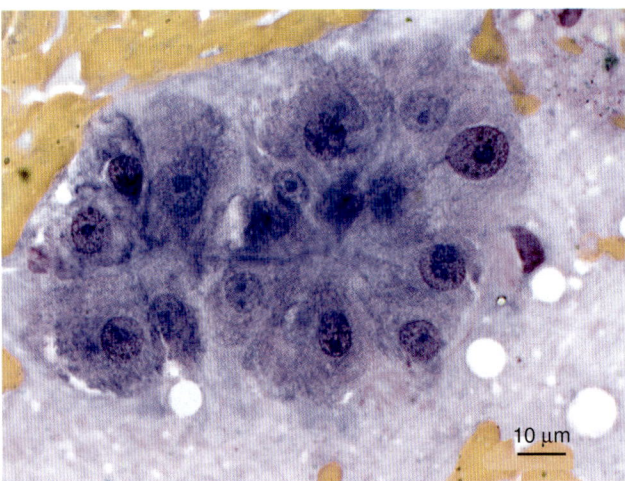

■ **FIGURE 9.64 Presumptive hepatocellular carcinoma. Pseudoacinar formation. Liver aspirate. Dog.** A 10-year-old dog presented with ultrasound findings of heterogeneous liver with nodules. Cytopathology noted atypical hepatocytes with moderate to marked anisokaryosis and papillary formations. The presence of pseudoacinar formation as shown here supported hepatocellular neoplasia and histopathology was suggested. (Aqueous Romanowsky; HP oil.) (Courtesy Rose Raskin, North Carolina State University.)

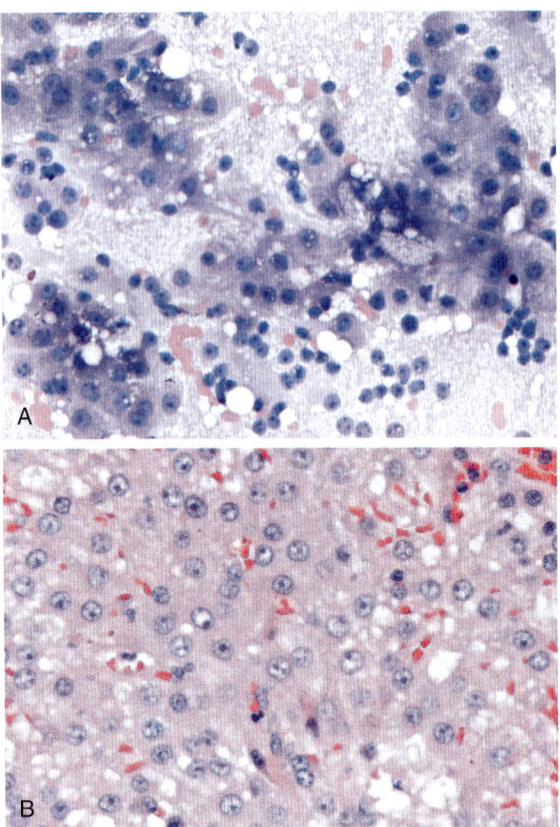

■ **FIGURE 9.63 Well-differentiated hepatocellular carcinoma. Liver. Dog.** Same case in A and B. **A, Cytopathologic specimen.** Cytopathologic features suggestive of malignancy include dissociation of hepatocytes, palisading of nuclei, many free nuclei, anisokaryosis, increased nucleocytoplasmic ratio, and multiple nucleoli. (Wright; IP.) **B, Histology.** There is a lack of organization with multiple cell layers of cells within cords and absence of portal tracts, prominent nucleoli, and increased nucleocytoplasmic ratio from this mass that measured 14 × 10 cm. (H&E; IP.) (Courtesy of Rose Raskin, Purdue University.)

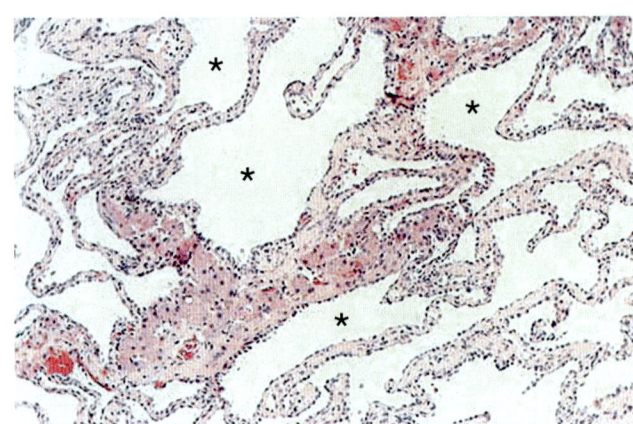

■ **FIGURE 9.65 Cystadenoma. Liver. Cat. Histologic specimen.** This liver specimen is from a 12-year-old cat with oral disease but otherwise clinically healthy. Mildly increased serum liver enzyme tests were noted on a preanesthetic examination. Multiple fluid-filled lesions were noted on ultrasound examination and clear, acellular fluid was aspirated with ultrasound guidance. A cystadenoma was diagnosed histologically. Note multiple cystic spaces *(asterisks)*, lined by a single layer of cuboidal biliary epithelium. (H&E; IP.)

Sprundel et al., 2014); clinically, there is no difference between these two processes (Cullen, 2017). Cytopathologically, cholangiocellular adenomas are composed of relatively normal-appearing, small cuboidal to columnar biliary epithelial cells, with scant amounts of pale basophilic cytoplasm, exfoliating in small, dense sheets and clusters and occasionally in tubular or acinar formations. When cystic spaces are aspirated, the fluid can either have a bile-like appearance or a mucinous character, and epithelial cells may be scant on these smears, precluding a definitive diagnosis of an underlying tumor.

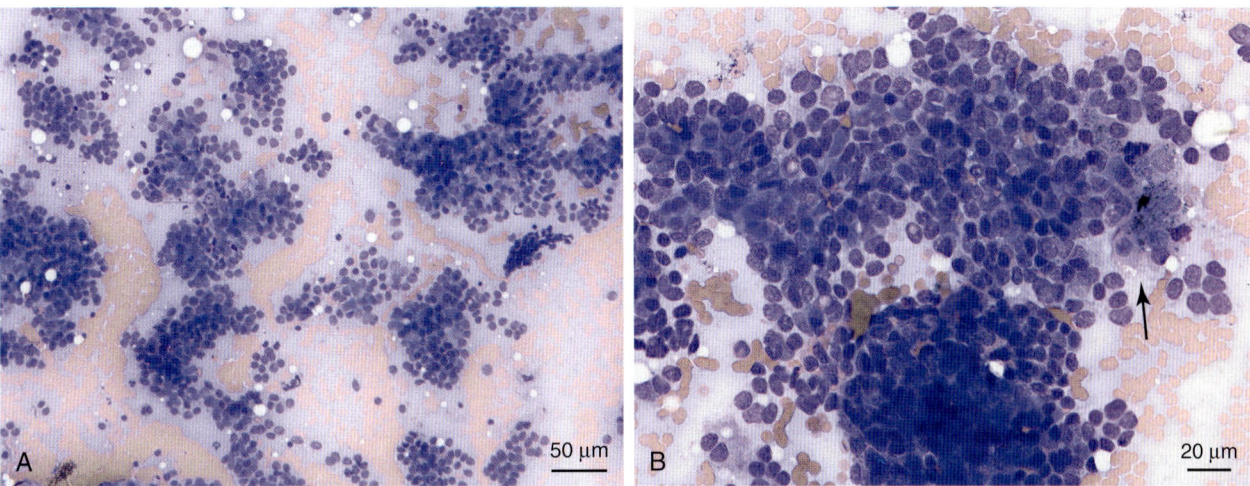

■ **FIGURE 9.66 Cholangiocellular carcinoma. Liver. Cytopathologic specimen. Cat.** Same case in A and B. **A,** This biliary carcinoma appears as multiple dense clusters of biliary epithelial cells with minimal cytoplasm. (Modified Wright; IP.) **B,** The cells often do not show obvious cytopathologic criteria of malignancy other than inappropriate large size and overgrowth of neighboring cells; see hepatocytes at the right edge of B *(arrow)*. (Modified Wright; HP oil.)

Cholangiocellular carcinoma is commonly multinodular and may be composed of cystic spaces (cholangiocellular cystadenocarcinomas). The cytopathologic picture in well-differentiated carcinomas can be very similar to that of cholangiocellular adenomas, and thus histopathologic examination is often necessitated for differentiation and prognostication (Figs. 9.66 to 9.68). Some malignant forms can, however, display prominent cellular pleomorphism or anaplastic features, with high numbers of mitotic figures and rarely also squamous differentiation. Carcinomas are also more likely to cause hepatocellular necrosis in the surrounding tissue and elicit reactive fibroplasia, although

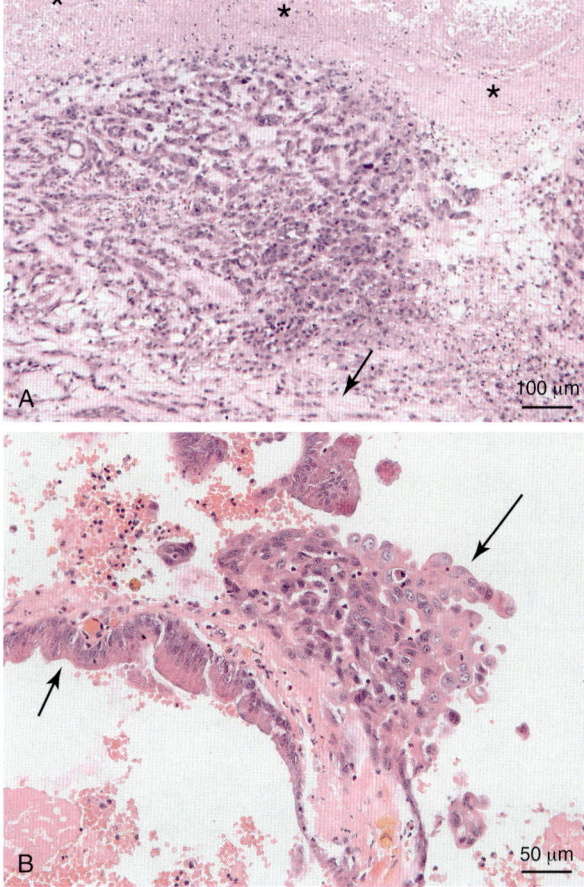

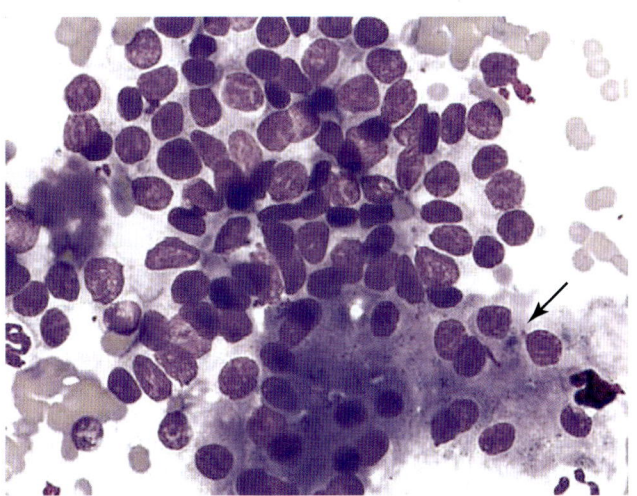

■ **FIGURE 9.67 Cholangiocellular carcinoma. Liver. Cytopathologic specimen. Cat.** The cells comprising this biliary carcinoma have large nuclei with a scant rim of pale-staining cytoplasm. Despite only demonstrating mild to moderate anisocytosis and anisokaryosis, the abnormally large size is indicative of neoplasia; contrast their inappropriate size to the hepatocytes in the lower part of the specimen *(arrow)*. The fine bluish granules in the cytoplasm of the hepatocytes are consistent with lipofuscin pigment. (Romanowsky; HP oil.) (Courtesy Dave Edwards, University of Tennessee.)

■ **FIGURE 9.68 Biliary cystadenocarcinoma. Liver Dog. Histology. A,** Photomicrograph from a large cystic liver mass in a 12-year-old Labrador retriever. The neoplasm is composed of variably organized tubules of neoplastic biliary epithelium at the margins of the mass. Note also abundant necrosis *(asterisks)* and fibrous stroma *(arrow)* (H&E; LP). **B,** Neoplastic epithelial cells lining the central cystic spaces range from cuboidal to columnar *(short arrow)* to squamous *(long arrow)*. (H&E; IP). (Courtesy of Jonathan Williams, The Royal Veterinary College, UK.)

the latter typically does not exfoliate well with a FNAB. Biliary carcinomas can be difficult to distinguish cytopathologically from metastatic adenocarcinomas to the liver.

Hepatic Neuroendocrine Carcinoma (Carcinoid)

In a study of 10 dogs with hepatic neuroendocrine carcinoma, most exhibited anorexia, vomiting, polydipsia and polyuria, icterus, lethargy, and weight loss (Patnaik et al., 2005). Neuroendocrine cells scattered throughout the intrahepatic and extrahepatic biliary system, including the gallbladder, can give rise to neuroendocrine carcinomas, also called *hepatic carcinoids*. Although they may present as benign neoplasms, most of these are aggressive and malignant in behavior. Cytopathologically, these tumors appear very similar to other neuroendocrine tumors (see Chapter 17), with high proportions of free nuclei, occasionally arranged in acini and palisades (Figs. 9.69, 9.70, and 9.71A). Because the intrahepatic form of this tumor often displays a diffuse to multinodular growth pattern (Meachem and Wobeser, 2016), it can also easily be confounded with metastatic neuroendocrine tumors (e.g., insulinoma, pheochromocytoma). Other differential considerations include cholangiocellular tumors, particularly in specimens with a higher proportion of intact cells. A silver stain (e.g., Grimelius or Churukian-Schenk method) is helpful to demonstrate the fine neuroendocrine granules (Fig. 9.71B), but immunochemistry with antibodies against neuron-specific enolase, synaptophysin, or chromogranin A may be needed for confirmation of neuroendocrine origin (Patnaik et al., 2005).

Round Cell Tumors

Lymphoma is the most common neoplasm involving the liver of dogs and cats, often causing a uniform hepatomegaly. The diffuse neoplastic infiltration and ease of exfoliation make FNAB diagnostically rewarding. Finding high numbers of relatively monomorphic, immature lymphocytes is diagnostic for

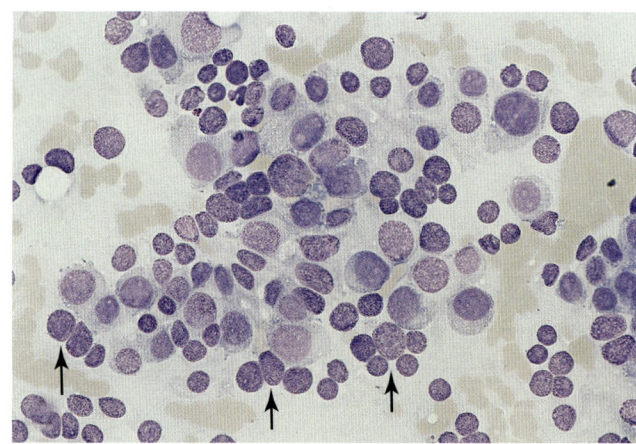

■ **FIGURE 9.70 Hepatic neuroendocrine carcinoma (carcinoid). Cytopathologic specimen.** These round to oval cells, obtained from a solitary hepatic mass, have features consistent with a hepatic carcinoid, a neuroendocrine tumor characterized by a naked nuclei cytomorphology. There is moderate to marked anisocytosis, anisokaryosis, and variable nucleocytoplasmic ratio. The nucleus is composed of delicate chromatin surrounded generally by scant amounts of clear to lightly basophilic cytoplasm often with indistinct cytoplasmic borders. Their fragile nature is suggested by frequent free nuclei located at the periphery *(arrows)*, giving them a small lymphocyte-like appearance. (Romanowsky; HP oil.)

lymphoma (Fig. 9.72). However, small cell lymphoma can be on cytopathology indistinguishable from lymphocytic hepatitis, and further diagnostics, such as histopathology or clonality testing (see Chapter 18), may be needed for a definitive diagnosis (Figs. 9.73 and 9.74). Hepatic lymphoma is often a component of multicentric lymphoma, and the liver is commonly aspirated as part of disease staging. However, hepatic lymphoma without involvement of peripheral nodes does occur, including hepatosplenic and hepatocytotropic T-cell lymphoma (Figs. 9.75 and 9.76) (Fry et al., 2003; Cienava et al., 2004; Keller et al., 2013; Masserdotti et al., 2016). These are of γδ T-cell origin and typically contain magenta cytoplasmic granules (see Fig. 9.75B). In hepatosplenic lymphoma, neoplastic lymphocytes can display erythrophagia, whereas in hepatocytotropic lymphoma, neoplastic lymphocytes may be found within the cytoplasm of hepatocytes and rarely within biliary epithelial cells (Fig. 9.77; see also Fig. 9.76).

Acute myeloid or lymphoid leukemia can infiltrate the liver, causing diffuse hepatomegaly (Fig. 9.78). Additional examination of the peripheral blood, bone marrow, or immunophenotyping may be necessary to differentiate myeloid from lymphoid leukemia and from lymphoma. Occasionally, plasma cell tumors involve the liver.

Liver aspirates are performed as part of mast cell tumor staging, both for high-grade cutaneous and visceral forms of mast cell tumors. Low numbers of individually scattered mast cells are a normal finding (Stockhaus et al., 2002; Masserdotti, 2013), whereas high numbers of mast cells, particularly if observed in clumps or exhibiting decreased granulation and cellular pleomorphism, are suspicious for mast cell neoplasia (Fig. 9.79). Mild increases in hepatic mast cell number may be observed in association with reactive mastocytosis (Stockhaus et al., 2004).

Disseminated histiocytic sarcoma is another round cell tumor that can involve both canine and feline livers (Figs. 9.80

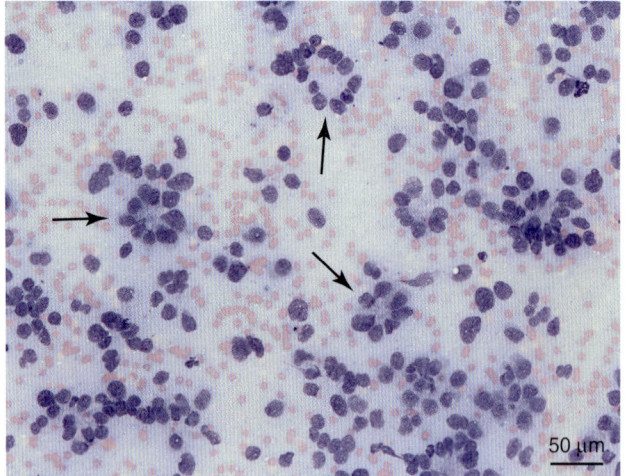

■ **FIGURE 9.69 Hepatic neuroendocrine carcinoma. Liver aspirate. Dog.** Specimen is from a 10-year-old Greyhound with multifocal hepatic nodules. High numbers of free nuclei are found in acinar arrangements *(arrows)*, characteristic for neuroendocrine tumors. Where intact, cells are cuboidal to rounded, with a round to oval nucleus, high nucleocytoplasmic ratio, and scant amounts of clear to lightly basophilic cytoplasm often with indistinct cytoplasmic borders. (Modified Wright stain, IP.)

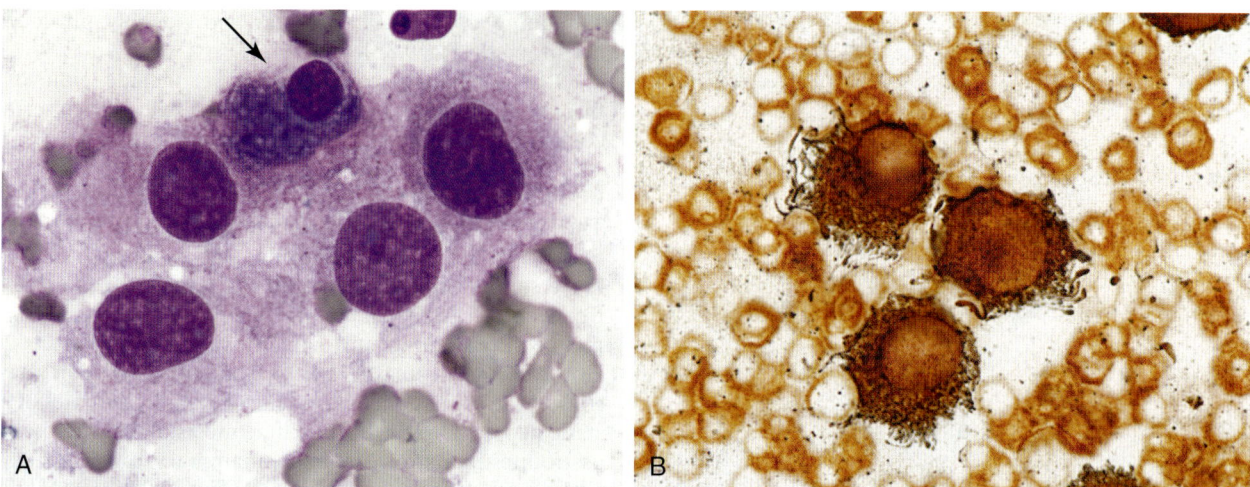

■ **FIGURE 9.71 Carcinoid. A, Metastatic liver mass imprint.** These large round cells with round nuclei composed of delicate, open chromatin surrounded by confluent cytoplasm are from a heart base tumor that metastasized to the liver. Noteworthy are the abundant, fine eosinophilic neuroendocrine granules located in the cytoplasm. A hepatocyte at the top center *(arrow)* of the cell cluster contrasts with the large size of the neoplastic cells. (Romanowsky; HP oil.) **B, Hepatic carcinoid.** Cells react positively to an argyrophilic (silver) stain, which demonstrates the neuroendocrine granules. (Silver stain; HP oil.) (Courtesy Dave Edwards, University of Tennessee.)

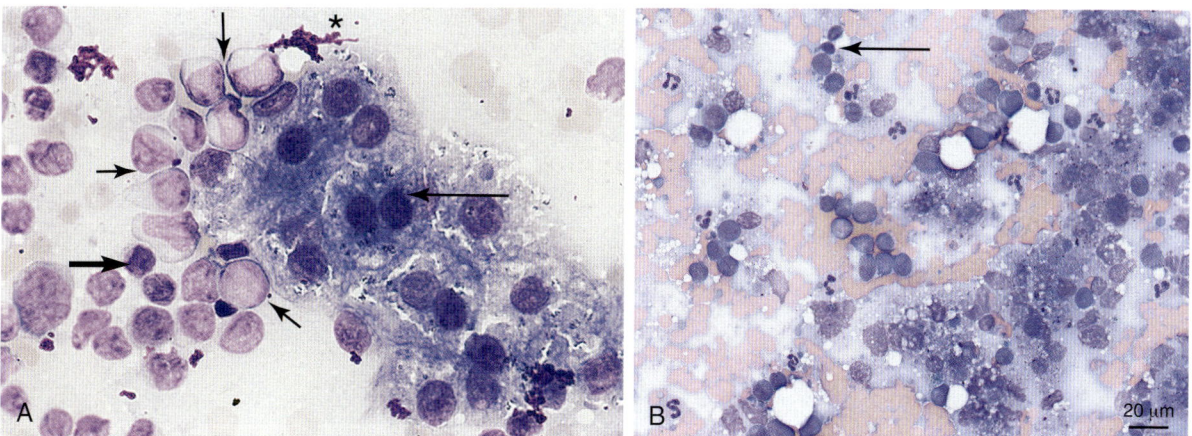

■ **FIGURE 9.72 Lymphoma. Liver. Dog. A, Aspirate.** Specimen from a 3-year-old Labrador retriever with icterus, hepatomegaly, mildly elevated liver enzyme activities, and total bilirubin of 3.1 mg/dL (normal <0.6 mg/dL). Lymphoma is indicated by the presence of numerous medium to large lymphocytes *(short arrows)*. A small, dark-staining lymphocyte *(thick arrow)* is a useful micrometer for assessing size and immature morphologic features of the neoplastic cells. The binucleated hepatocyte *(long arrow)* contains a small amount of blue-black granular pigment consistent with lipofuscin or bile. Small globs of irregularly shaped, metachromatically stained material represent ultrasound gel *(asterisks)*. (Wright-Giemsa; HP oil.) **B, Cytopathologic specimen.** High numbers of medium to large lymphocytes are found closely admixed with vacuolated and necrotic hepatocytes. Erythrocytes, small lymphocytes *(arrow)*, and neutrophils can be used as micrometers to determine the size of the neoplastic cells. (Modified Wright; HP oil.).

and 9.81). Neoplastic cells are typically large, with a round to oval nucleus and high amounts of pale basophilic cytoplasm, which may contain cytoplasmic vacuoles. In disseminated histiocytic sarcoma, which is derived from dendritic cells identified by CD1 surface antigen, there is usually marked cellular pleomorphism, with prominent anisocytosis and anisokaryosis, macrocytosis and karyomegaly, frequent multinucleation, and high numbers of mitotic figures (see Fig. 9.80). Hemophagocytic histiocytic sarcoma, a distinct subtype, arises from CD11d+ macrophages and displays prominent erythrophagia and occasionally phagocytosis of other hemic cells (see Fig. 9.81) (Moore, 2014). However, these tumors may lack overt criteria of malignancy, in which case they can be difficult to distinguish from non-neoplastic macrophages, particularly in cases of immune-mediated hemolytic anemia.

Mesenchymal Tumors

Hemangiosarcoma is one of the most common metastatic tumors in the liver, but it can also arise as a primary neoplasm from intrahepatic endothelial cells. Cytopathologic features are identical to splenic hemangiosarcomas (see Chapter 4), typically with poorly exfoliating pleomorphic spindle cells, often

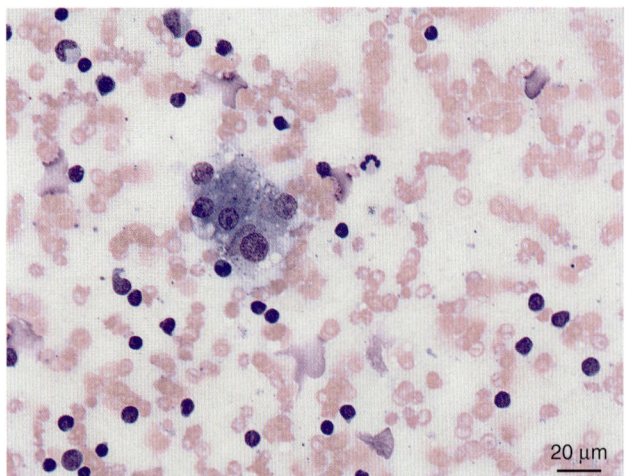

■ **FIGURE 9.73** **Small cell lymphoma. Liver cytopathologic specimen. Dog.** High numbers of small, mature lymphocytes surround a small sheet of mildly vacuolated hepatocytes, containing lipofuscin. Small cell lymphoma involving the liver was histologically confirmed, and absence of a peripheral lymphocytosis ruled out spillover from a chronic lymphocytic leukemia. (Modified Wright; HP oil.)

containing cytoplasmic vacuoles and possibly phagocytosed erythrocytes (Fig. 9.82).

Other primary sarcomas in the liver include leiomyosarcomas, fibrosarcomas, myelolipomas, and extraskeletal osteosarcomas (Cullen, 2017).

Metastatic Neoplasia

The liver is a frequent site for metastatic neoplasia of epithelial, mesenchymal, or hematopoietic origins. Lymphoma is the more common round cell tumor, hemangiosarcoma the more frequent mesenchymal tumor, and pancreatic carcinoma the main epithelial tumor involving the canine liver (Cullen, 2017). However, the neoplastic cell type identified may or may not suggest the primary neoplastic site of origin. Examples of metastatic neoplasia to the liver include metastatic leiomyosarcoma, gastrointestinal stromal tumor, mammary carcinoma, gastric adenocarcinoma, and insulinoma (Figs. 9.83 to 9.88). Therefore, the objective of cytopathology is to identify a neoplastic lesion as part of a staging process or prompt additional diagnostic efforts if the primary lesion was not readily detectable on initial examination.

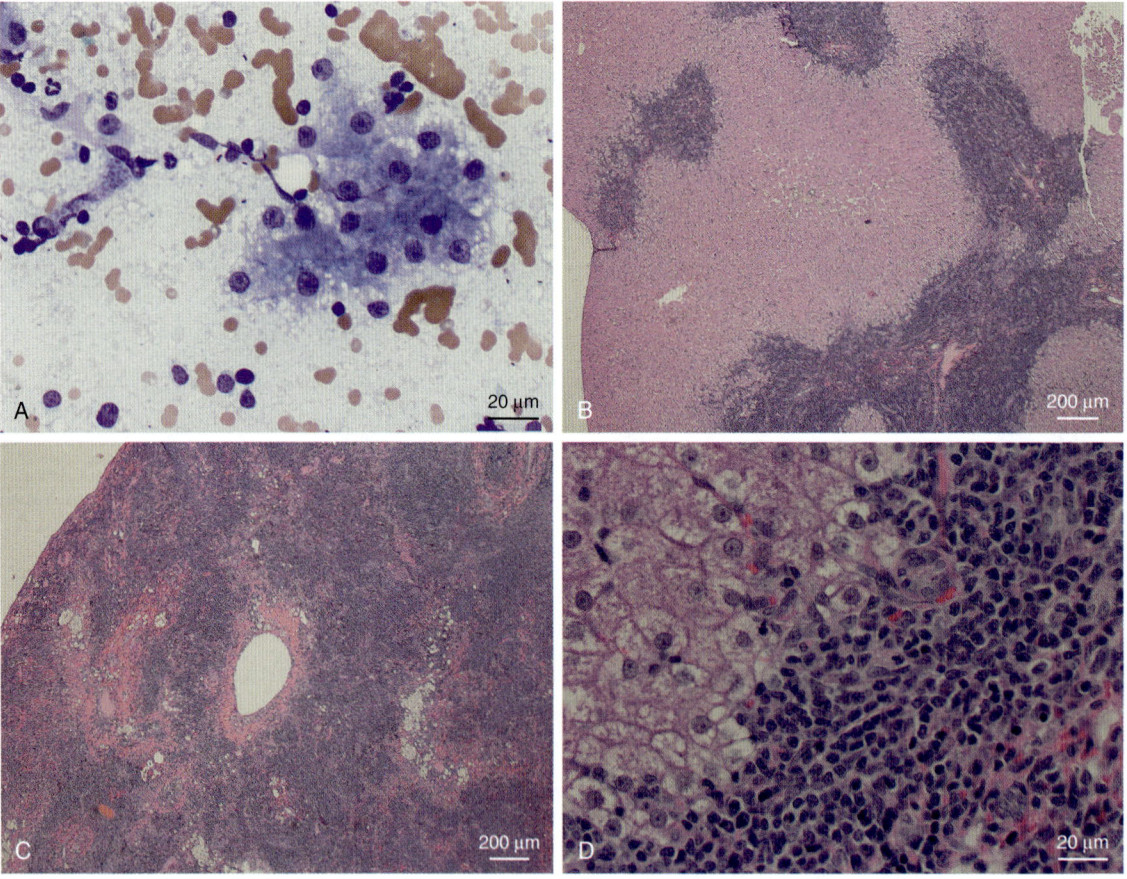

■ **FIGURE 9.74** **Lymphoma. Liver. Cat.** Same case in A and D. **A, Aspirate.** Hepatocytes display mild to moderate distinct cytoplasmic vacuolization and cytoplasmic rarefaction. A heterogeneous lymphoid population is present in moderate numbers composed mostly of small well-differentiated lymphocytes, fewer intermediate and large-sized lymphocytes, and plasma cells. (Wright-Giemsa; HP oil.) **B, Histology.** In some areas, there is a monomorphic population of round cells infiltrating and expanding into periportal and midzonal areas as well as around hyperplastic biliary ducts. (H&E; LP.) **C, Histology.** Other areas appear more diffusely infiltrated by a neoplastic round cell population. (H&E; LP.) **D, Histology.** Higher magnification demonstrates the uniformity of the round cell population. The cells are medium to large with variably discrete cellular borders and contain a scant amount of cytoplasm. The nuclei are irregularly round to oval, small to medium, and occasionally large (1.5–4 × RBC diameter) with finely stippled to hyperchromatic chromatin and contain one or two purple variably discrete, small nucleoli. (H&E; HP oil.) (A–D, Courtesy Rose Raskin, University of Florida.)

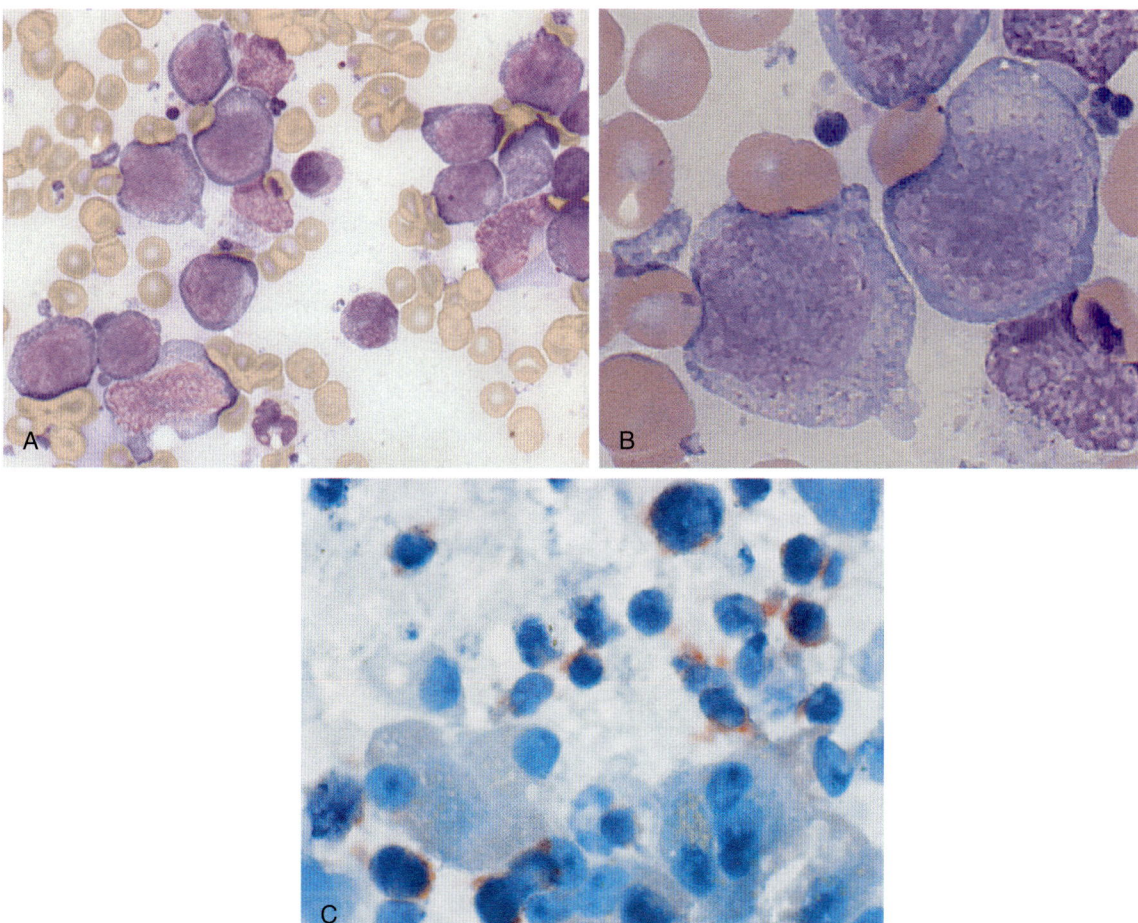

■ **FIGURE 9.75 Hepatosplenic lymphoma. Liver cytopathologic specimen. Dog.** Same case in A to C. **A,** A monomorphic population of large mononuclear cells that measure more than three times the diameter of an erythrocyte. Nuclei are round with occasional indentation, and the cytoplasm is generally scant and moderately basophilic. Nucleoli are prominent and frequently multiple. The large size and nuclear irregularly suggest a histiocytic appearance. (Wright; HP oil.) **B,** Higher magnification shows few fine eosinophilic granules within the perinuclear clear zone. (Wright; HP oil.) **C,** Notice the positive-stained large and medium sized gamma-delta T-cells along with negative-stained hepatocytes. (AEC, anti-TCRγδ; HP oil.) (Courtesy Rose Raskin, Purdue University.)

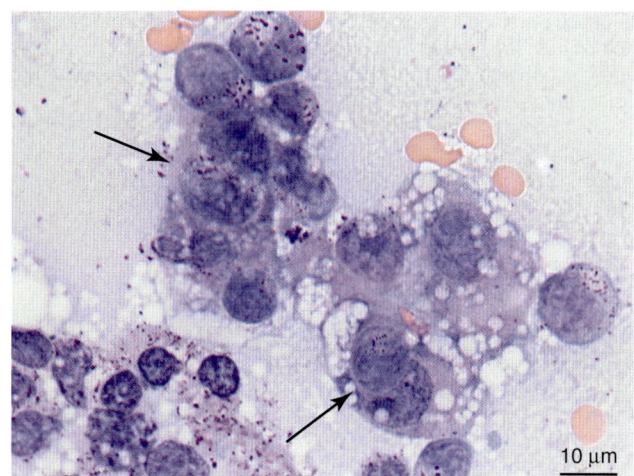

■ **FIGURE 9.76 Lymphoma of granular lymphocytes. Liver cytopathologic specimen. Cat.** Large lymphocytes contain prominent magenta cytoplasmic granules. Note occasional neoplastic lymphocytes within intact (and vacuolated) hepatocytes *(arrows)*, molding into the nucleus, suggestive of hepatocytotropic lymphoma. (Modified Wright; HP oil.)

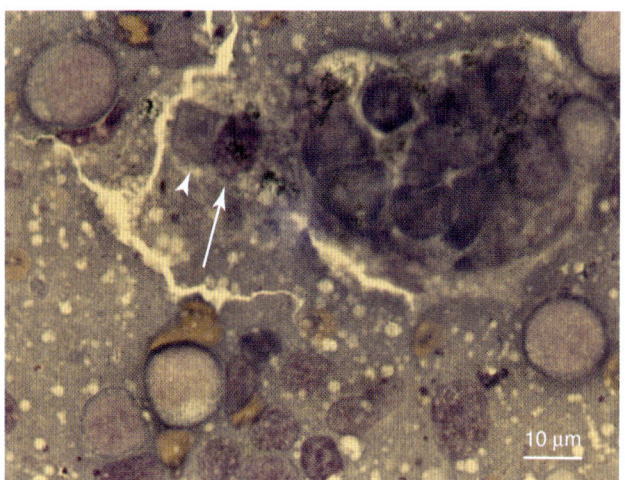

■ **FIGURE 9.77 Hepatocytotropic lymphoma. Liver cytopathologic specimen. Dog.** Medium to large lymphoid cells appear in the background and within hepatocytes, recognized by the granules within the cytoplasm. One lymphoid cell *(arrow)* is readily visible within a hepatocyte *(arrowhead)*, noting the prominent single nucleolus as is typical for hepatocytes. (Courtesy Yvonne Wikander, Kansas State University.)

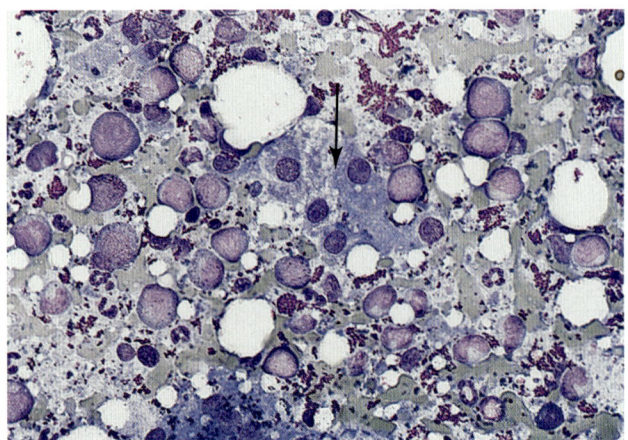

■ **FIGURE 9.78 Acute myelogenous leukemia. Liver aspirate. Cat.** Large, round to oval, immature discrete cells outnumber hepatocytes *(arrow)*. This patient presented with hepatomegaly, nonregenerative anemia, and neutropenia. The cytopathologic features are most consistent with an immature cell type of hematopoietic origin. Similar cells were found in the aspirate from the bone marrow and cytochemical stains were used to confirm a diagnosis of acute myelogenous leukemia. A large amount of variably sized, irregular clumps of metachromatic material (ultrasound gel) is located among the cells. The large clear spaces are consistent with extracellular lipid that was probably admixed with the specimen from the mesenteric fat during the sampling procedure. (Wright-Giemsa; IP.)

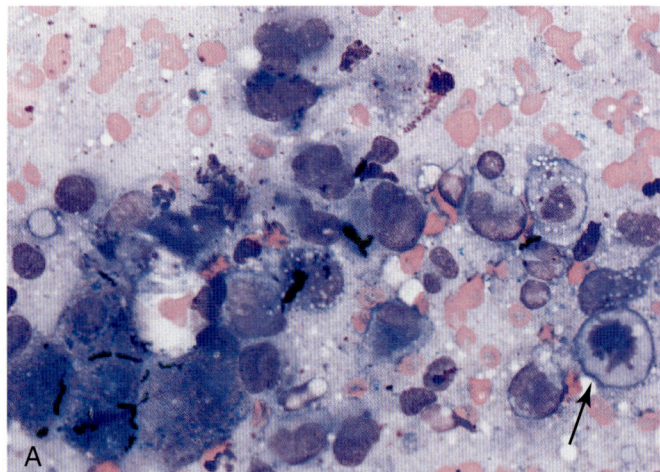

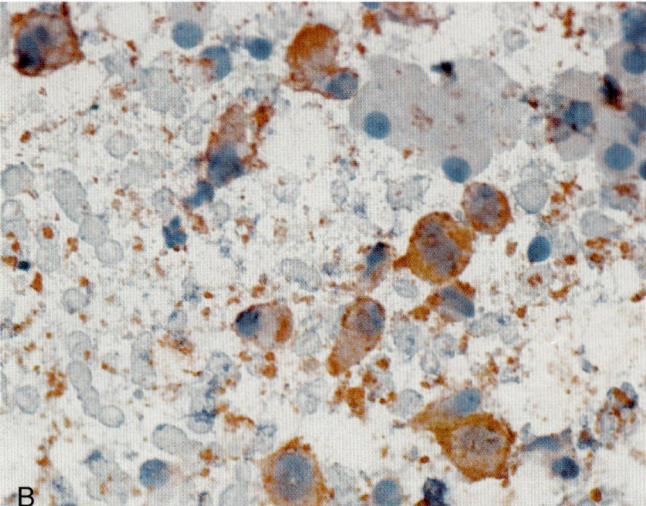

■ **FIGURE 9.80 Histiocytic sarcoma. Liver. Cytopathologic specimen. Dog. A,** A pleomorphic population of irregularly shaped large round cells is present alongside hepatocytes that display marked cholestasis as indicated by the prominent black-green canaliculi. Indented and multilobulated nuclear shapes are common as well as an abnormal mitotic figure on the right lower edge *(arrow)*. (Wright; HP oil.) **B,** Notice the positive-stained large pleomorphic round cells and negative-stained hepatocytes. The reaction along with other immunocytochemical stains supports dendritic origin. (AEC, anti-CD1a; HP oil.) (Courtesy Rose Raskin, Purdue University.)

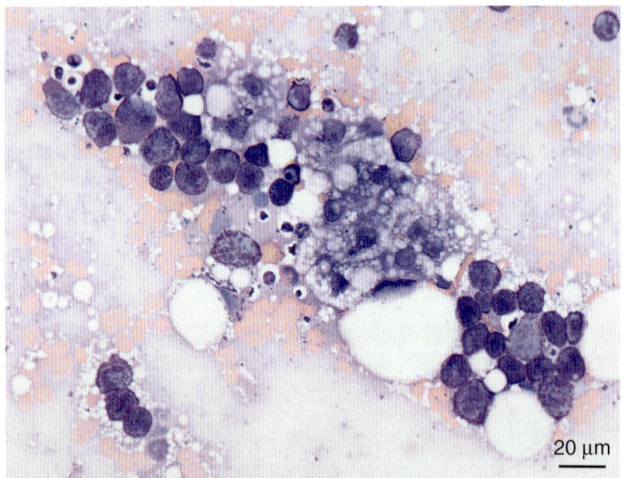

■ **FIGURE 9.79 Mast cell tumor. Liver aspirate. Dog.** High numbers of mast cells surround hepatocytes in this patient with metastasis from a cutaneous mast cell tumor. Note the prominent anisocytosis and anisokaryosis between mast cells. Hepatocytes display vacuolar change, mainly lipid vacuoles, but occasionally also rarefaction. (Modified Wright; HP oil.)

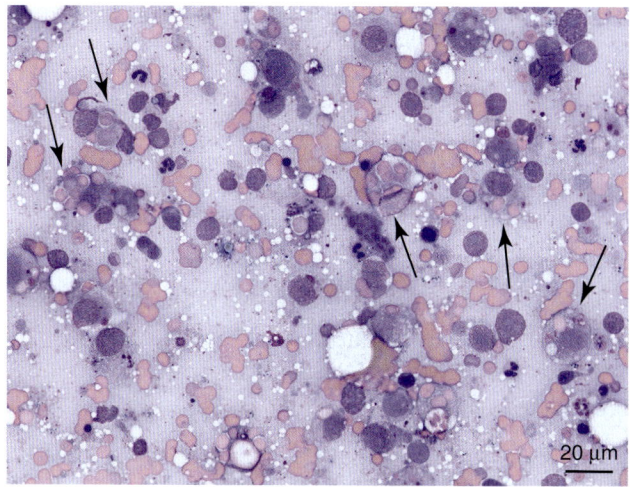

■ **FIGURE 9.81 Hemophagocytic histiocytic sarcoma. Liver. Cytopathologic specimen. Cat.** This case of histiocytic sarcoma involved the liver in a cat with severe anemia and hepatomegaly. Note the prominent erythrophagia by neoplastic cells *(arrows)*, consistent with a hemophagocytic histiocytic sarcoma, indicating macrophage origin. (Modified Wright; HP oil.)

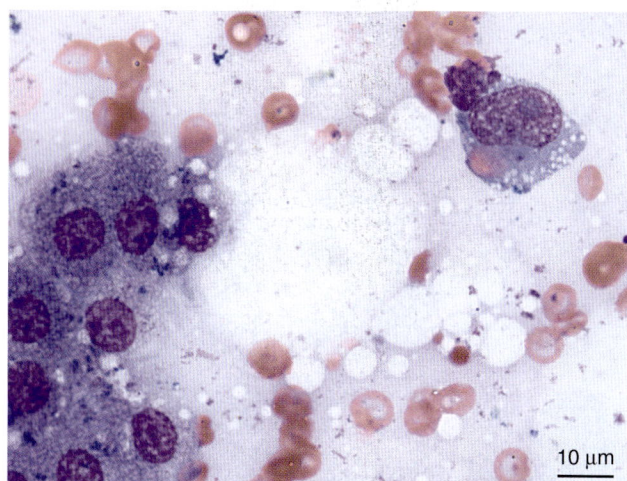

■ **FIGURE 9.82 Hemangiosarcoma. Liver aspirate. Dog.** A 6-year-old golden retriever presented for examination of a 3.5 cm liver mass. The specimen contained markedly atypical mesenchymal cells found individually and in variably sized dense aggregates. These spindle-shaped to oval cells have variably distinct cellular borders and a moderate to large amount of medium basophilic cytoplasm that contains a few colorless punctate vacuoles. The nucleus contained multiple distinct nucleoli. Only one neoplastic cell is shown which displays erythrophagia. Hepatocytes appeared minimally affected, with ample amounts of lipofuscin. (Wright-Giemsa; HP oil.) (Courtesy Rose Raskin, University of Florida.)

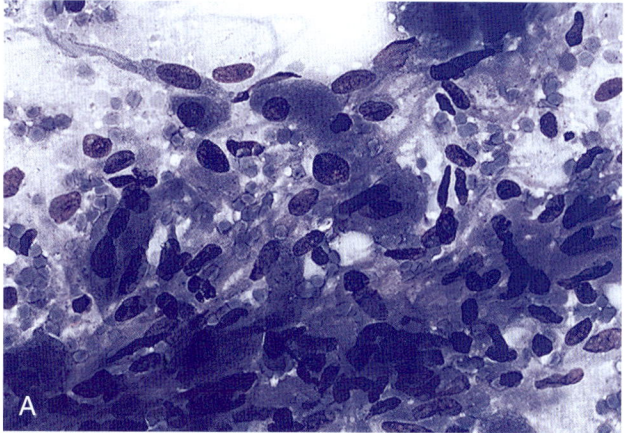
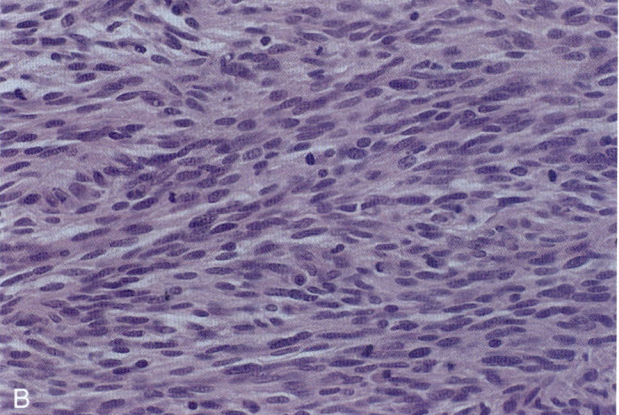
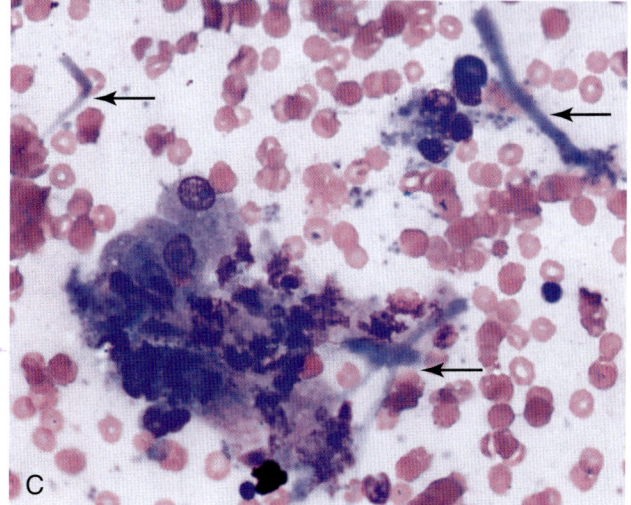

■ **FIGURE 9.83 Metastatic leiomyosarcoma. Liver. Dog.** Same case in A and B. **A, Aspirate.** Spindle-shaped cells were the only cell type present in this liver specimen from a dog with anorexia, weight loss, microcytic anemia, normal serum liver enzyme activities, and variable echogenicity on ultrasound examination. A metastatic spindle cell tumor was diagnosed by cytopathology. (Wright-Giemsa; IP.) **B, Histology.** An ulcerated intestinal mass was found at surgery and histopathology determined it to be a leiomyosarcoma. (H&E; IP.) **C, Cytopathologic specimen.** A second case shows the basophilic strands of smooth muscle cytoplasm mixed with a cluster of hepatocytes. The site of tumor origin was the jejunum. (Wright; HP oil.) (C, Courtesy Rose Raskin, Purdue University.)

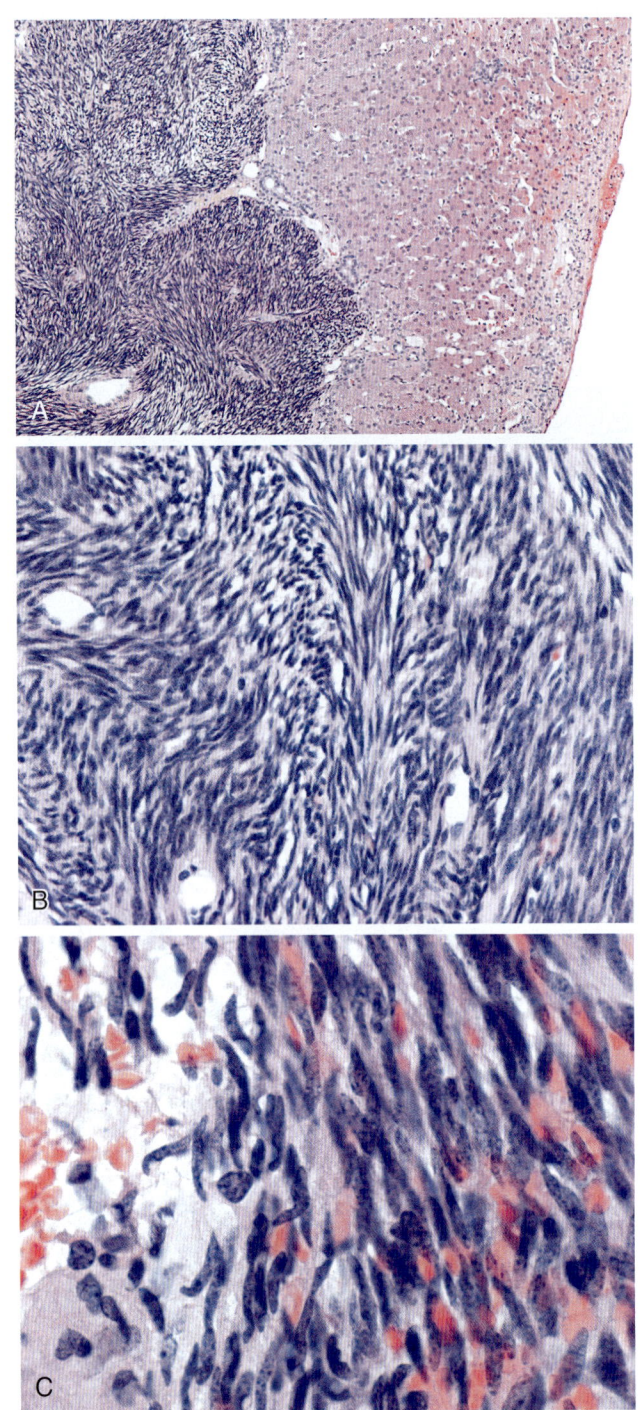

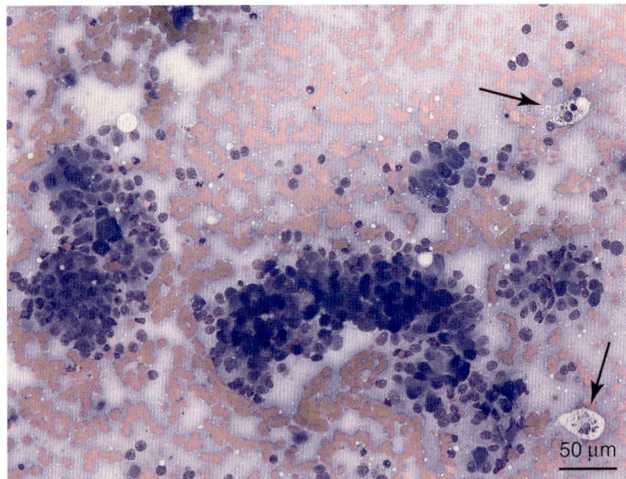

FIGURE 9.85 Metastatic mammary carcinoma. Liver aspirate. Dog. An 11-year-old female spayed cocker spaniel, previously diagnosed with a mammary carcinoma, presented with a liver mass. The specimen was predominated by high numbers of metastatic epithelial cells, found in loose tubular arrangements, with only few hepatocytes remaining (not depicted) and occasional phagocytic macrophages *(arrows)*; the hepatic lymph node was completely effaced by neoplastic cells. The cell of origin cannot be reliably determined from cytopathology alone. (Modified Wright; IP.)

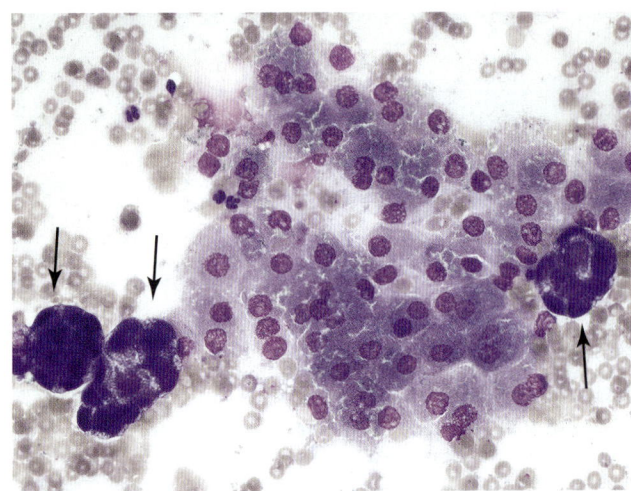

FIGURE 9.86 Metastatic gastric adenocarcinoma. Liver aspirate. Dog. Cohesive clusters of deeply basophilic polygonal cells with a high nucleocytoplasmic ratio and cytoplasmic vacuolization *(arrows)* noticeably contrast in appearance to the sheets of well-differentiated hepatocytes at the center of the image. (Modified Wright, HP oil.) (Courtesy Shannon Hostetter, Iowa State University.)

FIGURE 9.84 Metastatic gastrointestinal stromal tumor. Liver. Histology. Dog. Same case in A and C. **A,** Low magnification of a non-encapsulated, dark, solid, mesenchymal mass that invaded the liver from a primary mass located in the midabdomen with the small intestine. (H&E; LP.) **B,** Higher magnification to show the interlacing bundles of spindle cells in an intersecting manner. (H&E; IP.) **C,** Isolated spindle cells display elongated nucleus with scant cytoplasm. Neoplastic cells were strongly positive for vimentin, CD117 (c-kit), and S-100 but negative for desmin. (H&E; HP oil.) (Courtesy Parrula MCM, et al., The Ohio State University. Presented at the 2007 ASVCP case review session.)

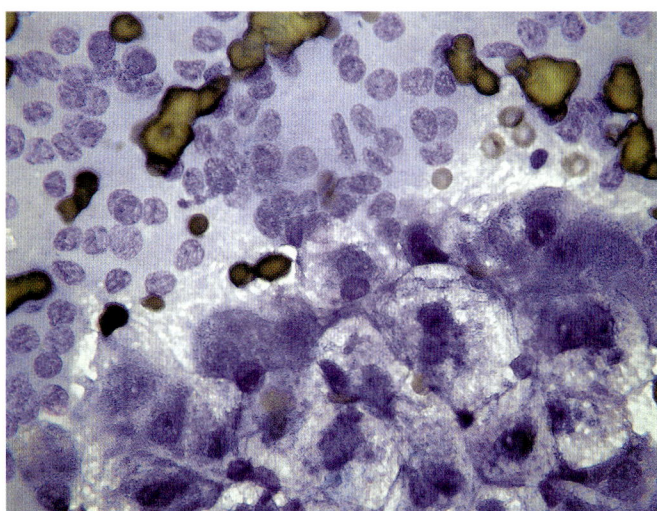

■ **FIGURE 9.87 Metastatic insulinoma. Liver cytopathologic specimen. Dog.** The upper left area contains neoplastic pancreatic islet cells with indistinct cytoplasmic borders and mild anisokaryosis. The lower right area contains hepatocytes that display vacuolar change. (Aqueous Romanowsky; HP oil.) (From Choi US. Practical Guide to Diagnostic Cytology of the Dog and Cat. OKVET; 2012.)

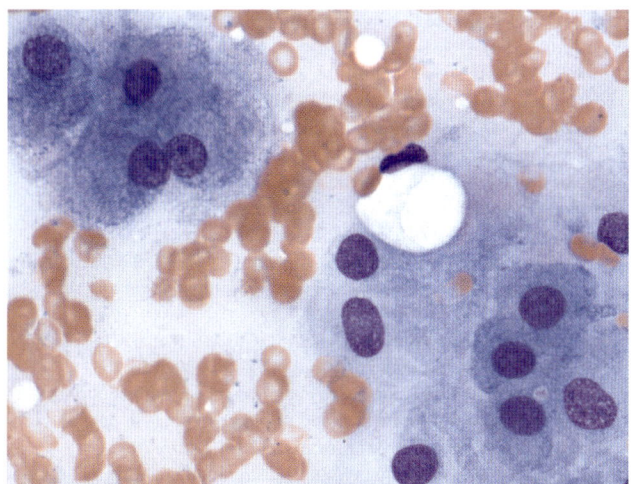

■ **FIGURE 9.88 Metastatic insulinoma. Liver aspirate. Dog.** Aspirate of a hepatic nodule displays several sheets and clusters of mildly atypical epithelial cells that often have indistinct cytoplasmic borders appearing as naked nuclei embedded in a lake of cytoplasm as shown on the lower right side. When cell borders are visible, the cells appear round or polygonal with a small to moderate amount of finely basophilic granules. The round or oval paracentral nucleus is approximately 1 to 1.5 × or rarely 3 × RBC diameter with coarse chromatin and one to three, small round or oval distinct nucleoli. Anisocytosis and anisokaryosis are mild with occasional karyomegaly noted. Mildly atypical hepatocytes are shown in the upper left side. (Wright-Giemsa; HP oil.) (Courtesy Rose Raskin, University of Florida.)

REFERENCES

Adler R, Wilson DW. Biliary cystadenoma of cats. *Vet Pathol.* 1995;32:415-418.

Allison R, Williams P, Lansdowne J, et al. Fatal hepatic sarcocystosis in a puppy with eosinophilia and eosinophilic peritoneal effusion. *Vet Clin Pathol.* 2006;35:353-357.

Attipa C, Szladovits B. Intranuclear cytoplasmic invaginations in small animals: a retrospective study of 18 cases [abstract]. *Vet Clin Pathol.* 2019;48:526.

Bahr KL, Sharkey LC, Murakami T, et al. Accuracy of US-guided FNA of focal liver lesions in dogs: 140 Cases (2005–2008). *J Am Anim Hosp Assoc.* 2013;49(3):190-196.

Beatty JA, Barrs VR, Martin PA et al. Spontaneous hepatic rupture in six cats with systemic amyloidosis. *J Small Anim Pract.* 2002;43:355-363.

Brown DE, Thrall MA, Walkley SU, et al. Feline Niemann-Pick disease type C. *Am J Pathol.* 1994;144(6):1412-1415.

Center SA, Crawford MA, Guida L, et al. A retrospective study of 77 cats with severe hepatic lipidosis: 1975-1990. *J Vet Intern Med.* 1993;7(6):349-359.

Charles JA, Cullen JM, Van den Ingh TSGAM, et al. Morphological classification of neoplastic disorders of the canine and feline liver. In: WSAVA liver Standardization Group, ed. *WSAVA Standards for Clinical and Histological Diagnosis of Canine and Feline Liver Diseases*. Philadelphia: Elsevier; 2006: 117-124.

Cienava EA, Barnhart KF, Brown R, et al. Morphologic, immunohistochemical, and molecular characterization of hepatosplenic T-cell lymphoma in a dog. *Vet Clin Pathol.* 2004;33:105-110.

Cullen JM, Van den Ingh TSGAM, Van Winkle T, et al. Morphological classification of parenchymal disorders of the canine and feline liver: 1. Normal histology, reversible hepatocytic injury and hepatic amyloidosis. In WSAVA liver Standardization Group, ed. *WSAVA Standards for Clinical and Histological Diagnosis of Canine and Feline Liver Diseases*. Philadelphia: Elsevier; 2006:77-84.

Cullen JM, Stalker MJ. Liver and biliary system. In: Maxie MG, ed. *Jubb, Kennedy, and Palmer's Pathology of Domestic Animals.* 6th ed. Vol 2. Philadelphia: Elsevier; 2016:258-352.

Cullen JM. Tumors of the liver and gallbladder. In: Meuten DJ, ed. *Tumors in Domestic Animals.* 5th ed. Ames, IA: Wiley Blackwell; 2017:602-631.

Day MJ. Immunohistochemical characterization of the lesions of feline progressive lymphocytic cholangitis/cholangiohepatitis. *J Comp Pathol.* 1998;119:135-147.

DiBartola SP, Tarr MJ, Benson MD. Tissue distribution of amyloid deposits in Abyssinian cats with familial amyloidosis. *J Comp Pathol.* 1986;96:387-398.

Dirksen K, Fieten H. Canine copper-associated hepatitis. *Vet Clin Small Anim Pract.* 2017;47:631-644.

Flatland B. If you have the gall…. *Vet Clin Pathol.* 2009;38:280.

Flatland B, Moore RR, Wolf CM, et al. Liver aspirate from a Shar Pei dog. *Vet Clin Pathol.* 2007;36:105-108.

Fleming KL, Howells EJ, Villiers EJ, et al. A randomised controlled comparison of aspiration and non-aspiration fine-needle techniques for obtaining ultrasound-guided cytological samples from canine livers. *Vet J.* 2019;252:105372.

Fry MM, Vernau W, Pesavento PA, et al. Hepatosplenic lymphoma in a dog. *Vet Pathol.* 2003;40:556-562.

Harrison JL, Turek BJ, Brown DC, et al. Cholangitis and cholangiohepatitis in dogs: a descriptive study of 54 cases based on histopathologic diagnosis (2004–2014). *J Vet Intern Med.* 2018;32:172-180.

Hunt GB, Luff JA, Daniel L, et al. Evaluation of hepatic steatosis in dogs with congenital portosystemic shunts using oil red O staining. *Vet Pathol.* 2013; 50(6):109-115.

Irvine KL, Walker JM, Friedrichs KR. Sarcocystid organisms found in bile from a dog with acute hepatitis: a case report and review of intestinal and hepatobiliary Sarcocystidae infections in dogs and cats. *Vet Clin Pathol.* 2016;45(1):57-65.

Isobe K, Matsunaga S, Nakayama H, et al. Histopathological characteristics of hepatic lipogranulomas with portosystemic shunts in dogs. *J Vet Med Sci.* 2008;70(2):133-138.

Johns JL, Christopher MM. Extramedullary hematopoiesis. A new look at the underlying stem cell niche, theories of development, and occurrence in animals. *Vet Pathol.* 2012;49:508-523.

Keller SM, Vernau W, Hodges J, et al. Hepatosplenic and hepatocytotropic T-cell lymphoma: two distinct types of T-cell lymphoma in dogs. *Vet Pathol.* 2013;50:281-290.

Klopfleisch R, Sperling C, Kershaw O, et al. Does the taking of biopsies affect the metastatic potential of tumours? A systematic review of reports on veterinary and human cases and animal models. *Vet J.* 2011;190:e31-e42.

Kook PH, Schellenberg S, Grest P, et al. Microbiologic evaluation of gallbladder bile of healthy dogs and dogs with iatrogenic hypercortisolism: a pilot study. *J Vet Intern Med.* 2010;24:224-228.

Kristal O, Rassnick KM, Gliatto JM, et al. Hepatotoxicity associated with CCNU (lomustine) chemotherapy in dogs. *J Vet Intern Med.* 2004;18:75-80.

Le Donne V, McGovern DA, Fletcher JM, et al. Cytologic diagnosis of *Heterobilharzia americana* infection in a liver aspirate from a dog. *Vet Pathol.* 2016;53(3):633-636.

Masserdotti C. Proportion of mast cells in normal canine hepatic cytologic specimens: comparison of 2 staining methods. *Vet Clin Pathol.* 2013;42(4):522-525.

Masserdotti C, Bertazzolo W. Cytologic features of hepatic fibrosis in dogs: a retrospective study on 22 cases. *Vet Clin Pathol.* 2016;45:361-367.

Masserdotti C, Drigo M. Retrospective study of cytologic features of well-differentiated hepatocellular carcinoma in dogs. *Vet Clin Pathol.* 2012;41:382-390.

Masserdotti C, Salemi GP, Gigli E, et al. What is your diagnosis? Hepatomegaly in a cat. *Vet Clin Pathol.* 2016;45(1):199-200.

Meachem MD, Wobeser BK. What's Your Diagnosis? Multiple hepatic masses in a cat. *Vet Clin Pathol.* 2016;45(3):509-510.

Mizutani S, Torisu S, Kaneko Y, et al. Retrospective analysis of canine gallbladder contents in biliary sludge and gallbladder mucoceles. *J Vet Med Sci.* 2017;79(2):366-374.

Moore AR, Coffey E, Hamar D. Diagnostic accuracy of Wright-Giemsa and rhodanine stain protocols for detection and semi-quantitative grading of copper in canine liver aspirates. *Vet Clin Pathol.* 2016;45(4):689-697.

Moore PF. A Review of histiocytic diseases of dogs and cats. *Vet Pathol.* 2014;51(1):167-184.

Neel JA, Tarigo J, Grindem CB. Gallbladder aspirate from a dog. *Vet Clin Pathol.* 2006;35:467-470.

Neo-suzuki S, Mineshige T, Kamiie J, et al. Hepatic AA amyloidosis in a cat: cytologic and histologic identification of AA amyloid in macrophages. *Vet Clin Pathol.* 2017;46(2):331-336.

Neumann S, Kaup F. Usefulness of Ki-67 proliferation marker in the cytologic identification of liver tumors in dogs. *Vet Clin Pathol.* 2005;34:132-136.

Newman SJ, Smith JR, Stenske KA, et al. Aflatoxicosis in nine dogs after exposure to contaminated commercial dog food. *J Vet Diagn Invest.* 2007;19:168-175.

Owens SD, Gossett R, McElhaney MR, et al. Three cases of canine bile peritonitis with mucinous material in abdominal fluid as the prominent cytologic finding. *Vet Clin Pathol.* 2003;32:114-120.

Palić J. Laboratory medicine: yesterday, today, tomorrow: the beauty of bile. *Vet Clin Pathol.* 2017;46(4):549-550.

Paltrinieri S, Sironi G, Giori L, et al. Changes in serum and urine SAA concentrations and qualitative and quantitative proteinuria in Abyssinian cats with familial amyloidosis: a five-year longitudinal study (2009-2014). *J Vet Intern Med.* 2015;29:505-512.

Pashmkova MB, Piccione J, Bishop MA, et al. Agreement between microscopic examination and bacterial culture of bile samples for detection of bactibilia in dogs and cats with hepatobiliary disease. *J Am Vet Med Assoc.* 2017;250:1007-1013.

Patnaik AK, Newman SJ, Scase T, et al. Canine hepatic neuroendocrine carcinoma: an immunohistochemical and electron microscopic study. *Vet Pathol.* 2005;42:140-146.

Patten P, Rich LJ, Zaks K, et al. Cestode infection in 2 dogs: cytologic findings in liver and a mesenteric lymph node. *Vet Clin Pathol.* 2013;42(1):103-108.

Peters LM, Glanemann B, Garden OA, et al. Cytological findings of 140 bile samples from dogs and cats and associated clinical pathological data. *J Vet Intern Med.* 2016;30(1):123-131.

Poldervaart JH, Favier RP, Penning LC, et al. Primary hepatitis in dogs: a retrospective review (2002-2006). *J Vet Intern Med.* 2009;23:72-80.

Prins M, Schellens CJMM, van Leeuwen MW, et al. Coagulation disorders in dogs with hepatic disease. *Vet J.* 2010;185:163-168.

Richter WR, Stein RJ, Rdzok EJ, et al. Ultrastructural studies of intranuclear crystalline inclusions in the liver of the dog. *Am J Pathol.* 1965;47(4):587-599.

Roth L. Comparison of liver cytology and biopsy diagnoses in dogs and cats: 56 cases. *Vet Clin Pathol.* 2001;30:35-38.

Rothuizen J, Twedt DC. Liver biopsy techniques. *Vet Clin North Am Small Anim Pract.* 2009;39:469-480.

Schaer M, Ginn PE. Iatrogenic Cushing's syndrome and steroid hepatopathy in a cat. *J Am Anim Hosp Assoc.* 1999;35:48-51.

Scott M. Laboratory medicine: yesterday, today, tomorrow: bye-bye bile, hello lipofuscin? *Vet Clin Pathol.* 2006;35(1):5.

Scott M, Buriko K. Characterization of the pigmented cytoplasmic granules common in canine hepatocytes. *Vet Clin Pathol.* 2005;34:281-282.

Segev G, Cowgill LD, Jessen S, et al. Renal amyloidosis in dogs: a retrospective study of 91 cases with comparison of the disease between Shar-Pei and Non-Shar-Pei dogs. *J Vet Intern Med.* 2012;26:259-268.

Sepesy LM, Center SA, Randolph JF, et al. Vacuolar hepatopathy in dogs: 336 cases (1993-2005). *J Am Vet Med Assoc.* 2006;229:246-252.

Smedley R, Mullaney T, Rumbeiha W. Copper-associated hepatitis in Labrador retrievers. *Vet Pathol.* 2009;46:484-490.

Stern JK, Walden HDS, Marshall K, et al. What is your diagnosis? Bile from a cat. *Vet Clin Pathol.* 2020;49:354-355.

Strickland JM, Buchweitz JP, Smedley RC, et al. Hepatic copper concentrations in 546 dogs (1982-2015). *J Vet Intern Med.* 2018;32:1943-1950.

Stock G, Pantchev N, Globokar M. What is your diagnosis? Generalized nodular change in a canine liver. *Vet Clin Pathol.* 2018;47:511-512.

Stockhaus C, Teske E, Van Den Ingh T, et al. The influence of age on the cytology of the liver in healthy dogs. *Vet Pathol.* 2002;39:154-158.

Stockhaus C, Van Den Ingh T, Rothuizen J, et al. A multistep approach in the cytologic evaluation of liver biopsy samples of dogs with hepatic disease. *Vet Pathol.* 2004;41:461-470.

Thornburg LP, Beissenherz M, Dolan M, et al. Histochemical demonstration of copper-associated protein in the canine liver. *Vet Pathol.* 1985;22:327-332.

Van den Ingh TSGAM, Van Winkle T, Cullen JM, et al. Morphological classification of parenchymal disorders of the canine and feline liver. 2. Hepatocellular death, hepatitis and cirrhosis. In: WSAVA liver Standardization Group, ed. *WSAVA Standards for Clinical and Histological Diagnosis of Canine and Feline Liver Diseases.* Philadelphia: Elsevier; 2006:85-102.

Van der Linde-Sipman JS, Niewold TA, Tooten PCJ, et al. Generalized AA-amyloidosis in Siamese and oriental cats. *Vet Immunol Immunopathol.* 1997;56:1-10.

Van Sprundel RGHM, Van den Ingh TSGAM, Guscetti F, et al. Classification of primary hepatic tumours in the cat. *Vet J.* 2014;202:255-266.

Wang KY, Panciera DL, Al-Rukibat RK, et al. Accuracy of ultrasound-guided fine-needle aspiration of the liver and cytologic findings in dogs and cats: 97 cases (1990-2000). *J Am Vet Med Assoc.* 2004;224:75-78.

Warren A, Center SA, McDonough S, et al. Histopathologic features, immunophenotyping, clonality, and eubacterial fluorescence in situ hybridization in cats with lymphocytic cholangitis/cholangiohepatitis. *Vet Pathol.* 2011;48(3):627-641.

Watson TG, Croll NA. Clinical changes caused by the liver fluke *Metorchis conjunctus* in cats. *Vet Pathol.* 1981;18:778-785.

Weiss DJ, Blauvelt M, Aird B. Cytologic evaluation of inflammation in canine liver aspirates. *Vet Clin Pathol.* 2001;30:193-196.

Weiss DJ, Gagne JM, Armstrong PJ. Characterization of portal lymphocytic infiltrates in feline liver. *Vet Clin Pathol.* 1995;24:91-95.

Wells B, Camus MS. Laboratory medicine: yesterday, today, tomorrow: gallbladder rocks! *Vet Clin Pathol.* 2017;46(3):387-388.

Wu X, Mandigers JJP, Watson AL, et al. Association of the canine ATP7A and ATP7B with hepatic copper accumulation in Dobermann dogs. *J Vet Intern Med.* 2019;33:1646-1652.

Zini E, Glaus TM, Minuto F, et al. Paraneoplastic hypoglycemia due to an insulin-like growth factor type-II secreting hepatocellular carcinoma in a dog. *J Vet Intern Med.* 2007;21:193-195.

CHAPTER 10

Fecal and Rectal Cytopathology

Francisco O. Conrado

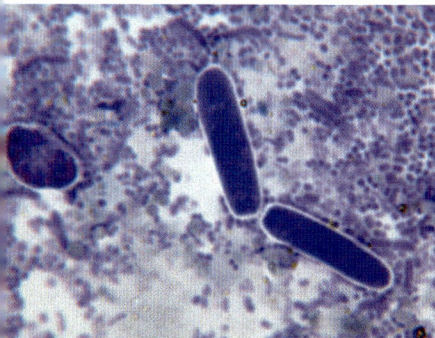

Multiple fecal diagnostic tests are available for complete evaluation of patients with gastrointestinal (GI) signs. These include wet-mount fecal cytopathology, dry-mount fecal cytopathology, bacterial culture, fecal antigen detection methods, fecal flotation, fecal sedimentation, and the Baermann technique, which are detailed elsewhere (Broussard, 2003). This chapter focuses on dry-mount fecal cytopathology (air-dried stained smear) for the diagnostic evaluation of patients with GI signs and highlights its utility for the identification of infectious agents, inflammation, and neoplasia (Frezoulis et al., 2017). Dry-mount fecal cytopathology can provide a definitive diagnosis or help rule out selected causes of diarrhea by complementing other diagnostic tests, such as wet-mount fecal cytopathology, bacterial culture, and fecal antigen detection (e.g., polymerase chain reaction [PCR]).

When evaluating dry-mount fecal cytopathology, it is most effective to use a systematic approach for assessment of background flora, the presence of abnormal eukaryotic cells, and pathogenic microorganisms (Box 10.1). Cytopathologic features are unevenly distributed in preparations from fecal material, necessitating diligent examination of the entire slide using the 40× and 100× oil objectives.

SAMPLE COLLECTION AND PROCESSING

Fecal sample collection method significantly affects the numbers of certain cytopathologic features, and each method differs in their sensitivity to demonstrate abnormalities (Frezoulis et al., 2017). This occurs because of the different parts of the rectum that are represented in the sample (i.e., luminal, mucosal, or both), as well as the cellular (eukaryotic and prokaryotic) components present.

Sampling methods for fecal cytopathology include collection of unadulterated fecal material, rectal saline lavage, and rectal scraping. A small amount of fresh feces may be obtained during digital rectal examination. A saline-moistened, cotton-tipped applicator or fecal loop is used if a rectal examination is not possible. Voided feces may be used, if collected immediately, although they are more representative of the luminal portion of the rectum and are not ideal for cytopathologic evaluation. Voided feces are preferred for other diagnostic tests (e.g., fecal flotation, fecal sedimentation, Baermann technique) because it may be rich in parasitic eggs and cysts (Broussard, 2003) (Figs. 10.1 to 10.3).

BOX 10.1 Guidelines for Systematic Dry-Mount Fecal Cytopathology Evaluation

1. 10× or 20× objectives
    Evaluate overall cellularity (eukaryotic cells), background, degree of blood contamination, and noncellular components (e.g., plant material, keratinized debris)
2. 20×, 40×, or 50× objectives[a]
    Evaluate cellular components:
    a. Inflammatory cells (fecal leukocytes): types and quantity
    b. Epithelial cells (host cells): normal, hyperplastic, or neoplastic
    c. Other atypical cells (e.g., large lymphoid cells)
3. 100× oil objective[a]
    Evaluate the background flora:
    a. Heterogeneity and predominance of bacilli vs. bacterial overgrowth
    b. Presence of a few fecal yeast vs. yeast overgrowth
    c. Presence and number of spore-forming bacteria
4. 40×, 50×, or 100× oil objectives[a]
    Examine the smear for other potential pathogens:
    a. Algal (e.g., *Prototheca* spp., *Chlorella* spp.)
    b. Bacterial (e.g., gull-wing–shaped and spiriliform bacteria)
    c. Fungal (e.g., *Histoplasma* spp., *Aspergillus* spp., *Blastomyces* spp., *Candida* spp., *Cryptococcus* spp.)
    d. Oomycetal (e.g., *Pythium* spp., *Lagenidium* spp.)
    e. Protozoal (e.g., *Cryptosporidium* spp., *Giardia* spp., *Entamoeba* spp., *Tritrichomonas* spp., *Balantidium* spp.)
    f. Rare findings (e.g., parasitic ova, oocyst, larvae)

[a]A coverslip is recommended for examination.

Usually, for fecal material obtained during digital examination or using a saline-moistened applicator, a gloved finger or cotton tip of the applicator is gently rolled on the glass slide to prepare a direct thin film. For dry feces, a dilution may be used to prepare a thin film by placing a drop of sterile saline on a clean glass slide, adding a small amount of fecal material, mixing with a sterile wooden applicator, and spreading using a squash or blood-smear technique.

Rectal saline lavage enriches collection of mucosal material, including mucus, motile protozoa, and bacteria because lavage fluid contains relatively less luminal fecal material (Broussard, 2003). However, it may be a less sensitive collection method for the detection of fecal leukocytes and host epithelial cells, as well

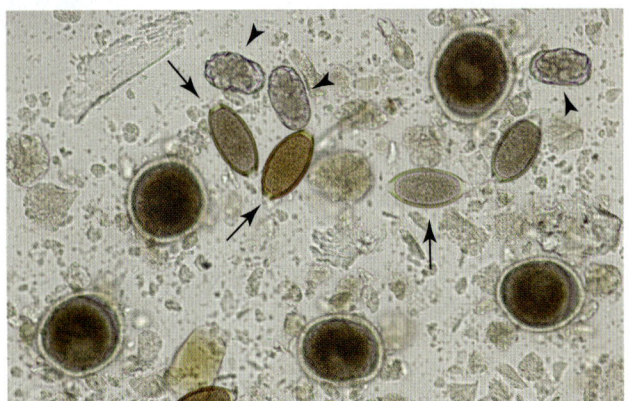

FIGURE 10.1 **Nematode ova. Feces. Dog.** Several common types of ova are shown: *Toxocara canis* (large, dark, and round), *Trichuris vulpis* *(arrows)*, and *Ancylostoma caninum* *(arrowheads)*. (Unstained wet mount; IP.) (Courtesy Rose Raskin, Purdue University.)

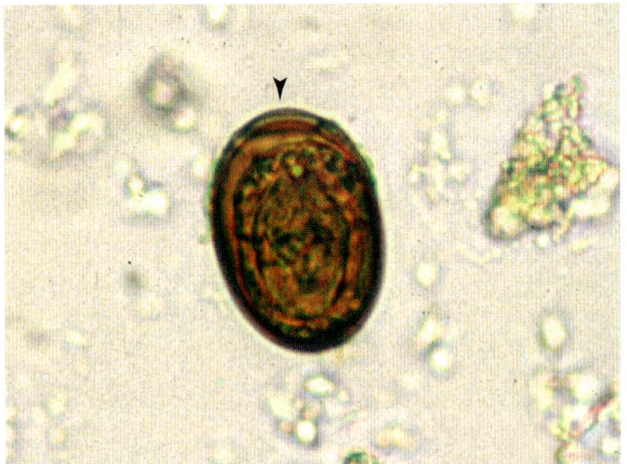

FIGURE 10.2 **Trematode ovum. Feces. Cat.** *Platynosumum fastosum (concinnum)*. Ova measure 34.0 to 50.0 μm × 20.0 to 35.0 μm with a thick wall and an operculated end *(arrowhead)*. (Unstained wet mount; LP.) (Courtesy Rose Raskin, University of Florida.)

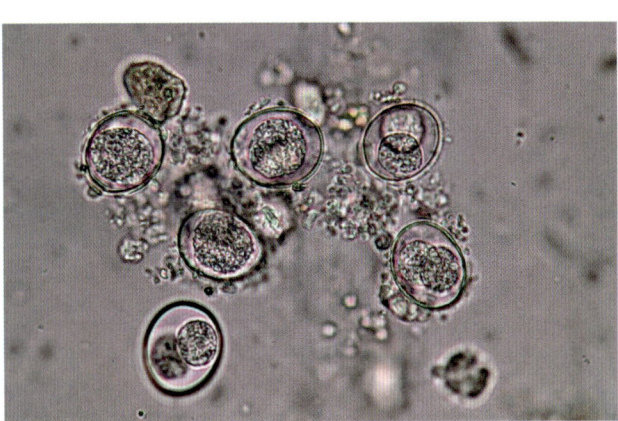

FIGURE 10.3 **Coccidia oocysts. Feces. Dog.** Oval oocysts with a clear outer wall and one or two internal cells (sporonts). (Unstained wet mount; HP oil.)

as neoplastic infiltrates (Frezoulis et al., 2017). Properly collected lavage fluid should have a mud-like consistency, and a single drop can be used to prepare a thin film.

Material obtained by rectal scraping is often submitted as a sample for dry-mount fecal cytopathology, though feces and rectal scrape material are not synonymous. A rectal scraping is a more invasive method, performed by direct scraping of the rectal mucosa. This is typically done using a saline-moistened cotton-tipped applicator, a blunt spatula, or the tip of the collector's gloved finger. A rectal scraping is typically required to identify infections localized to the deeper portion of the mucosa or to characterize mucosal cellular infiltrates. Independent of collection method, examination of a fresh sample (<5 minutes old) that is representative of the mucosal surface is paramount. Care should be taken to prepare a thin film that is not excessively dense (Fig. 10.4). Dense areas of fecal smear preparations are prone to detachment from the slide during staining and may obscure cytologic detail. Because the cellular content of fecal material is dynamic and will likely continue to change after sample collection, immediate examination after collection is recommended.

KEY POINT Preparation of a thin film of freshly collected fecal material is recommended. A glass coverslip protects the 40× and 60× dry objectives from bacterial contamination and is essential for proper focusing.

KEY POINT Results of dry-mount fecal cytopathology should be interpreted in the context of the patient's clinical presentation and results of other diagnostic tests.

KEY POINT Fecal material may detach from the slide during the staining process and contaminate stain solutions. It is critically important to change the stain solution after staining the fecal slides if a dip technique is used or stain at the end of a batch run if an automated station is used. These precautions prevent bacterial contamination of subsequent nonfecal specimens.

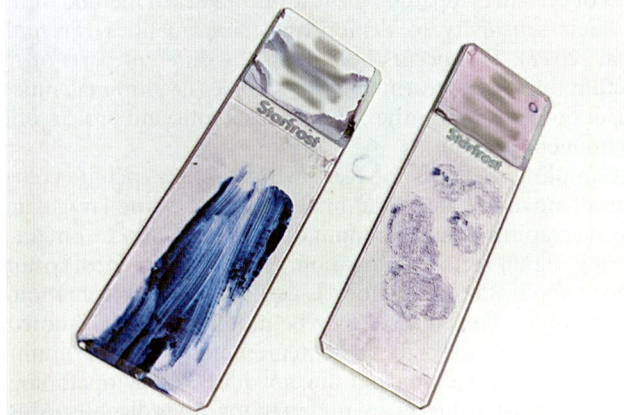

FIGURE 10.4 **Rectal scraping preparations**. A slide that is too dense to examine effectively *(left)* and a thin, well-prepared smear *(right)*.

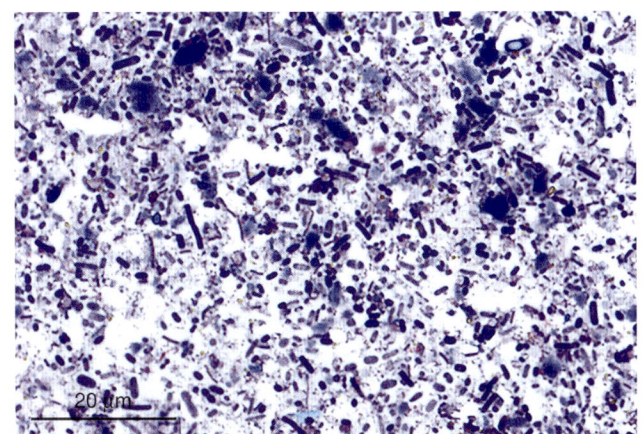

FIGURE 10.5 Normal bacterial flora. Dog. Rectal scrape from a 3-year-old whippet presented for diarrhea. A highly heterogeneous bacterial flora is present, comprising predominantly mixed bacilli on a pale basophilic background with amorphous debris and lacking host cells. No pathogen was observed. (Wright-Giemsa; HP oil.)

NORMAL OR INCIDENTAL MICROSCOPIC FINDINGS

The background microbial flora should be predominantly composed of a heterogeneous population of bacilli (Fig. 10.5). Notably, there should be fewer than three to five spore-forming bacilli per 100× oil objective field (Broussard, 2003; Marks et al., 2011). Cocci should be absent or rarely observed. A few extracellular, round or oval, 5.0 to 10.0 μm in diameter, finely stippled, variably basophilic yeast with a thin, colorless capsule may be seen (Fig. 10.6). These may sometimes show narrow-based budding. Although these yeast organisms are frequently found in diarrheal stools, it is not certain whether there is a direct causal relationship (Suchodolski, 2011).

The yeast *Cyniclomyces guttulatus* (formerly known as *Saccharomycopsis guttulata*) is part of the normal intestinal flora of some rodents and lagomorphs (rabbits, guinea pigs, and chinchillas) (Zierdt et al., 1988). Occasionally, a low number of individual or groupings of *Cyniclomyces* organisms may be observed as an incidental finding in canine feces and are thought to represent a nonpathogenic result of coprophagia (Fig. 10.7). However, there is uncertainty about whether this yeast is entirely nonpathogenic in dogs. A few studies have associated this yeast with clinical cases of chronic diarrhea (Houwers and Blankenstein, 2001; Winston et al., 2016), although shedding a large number of the organism is typically related with other causes of diarrhea in dogs (Mandigers et al., 2014), suggesting that *C. guttulatus* may have a role as an opportunistic agent in some cases. A large number of *C. guttulatus*, both individually and in mats of budding organisms, may be seen in the feces of dogs with diarrhea (Figs. 10.7 and 10.8). The presence of many budding organisms in a fresh fecal sample may represent a factor contributing to the ongoing diarrhea or may simply represent abnormal flora caused by underlying disease, physiologic processes, or prior antimicrobial treatments. In this context, this observation should be denoted as an abnormal finding.

It is common to see a variable amount of irregularly shaped, colorless or amber material and green-blue material with parallel cell walls, representing digesta and ingested plant matter, respectively (Fig. 10.9). The background also commonly contains a variable amount of amorphous basophilic material, consistent with mucus (Fig. 10.10). The amount of mucus observed depends on whether the underlying disease is associated with excessive rectal secretion of mucus or the sampling method is more representative of the rectal mucosa or rectal lumen (e.g., samples obtained by saline lavage or scraping may contain more mucus).

Well-differentiated epithelial cells, including squamous or rectal columnar epithelial cells, may be present in variable

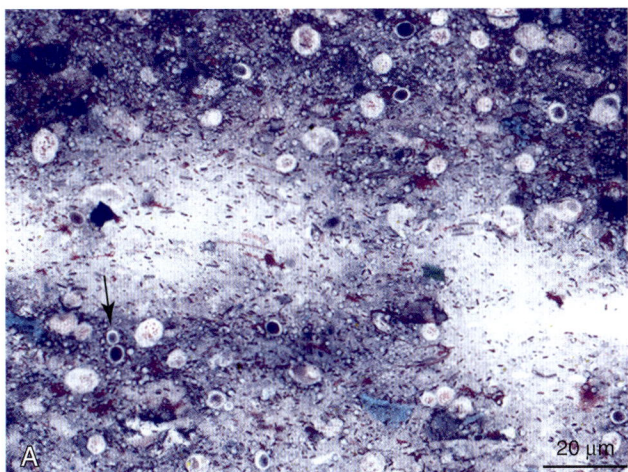 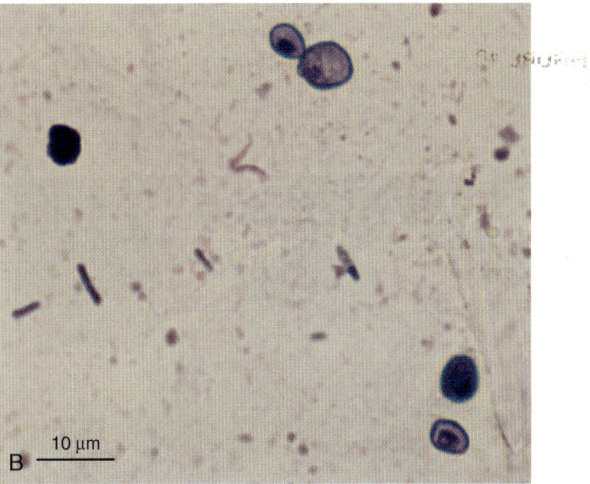

FIGURE 10.6 Incidental yeast. Cat. A, Fecal cytopathology from an 8-year-old domestic shorthair cat presented for large bowel diarrhea. The cat was receiving probiotics containing *Saccharomyces cerevisiae*. Numerous round or oval, 5.0 to 10.0 μm in diameter, finely stippled, variably basophilic yeasts are seen extracellularly. (Wright-Giemsa; HP oil.) Occasional organisms exhibit narrow-based budding *(arrow)*. **B,** This cat presented with diarrhea. Yeasts appear both as single and budding forms with both clear and focally dense staining areas within the structure. The significance of the yeast is unknown in causing the diarrhea; however, yeasts occur more commonly in watery stools, possibly because of the wash effect that releases the organisms more readily. (Wright; HP oil.) (Courtesy Rose Raskin, Purdue University.)

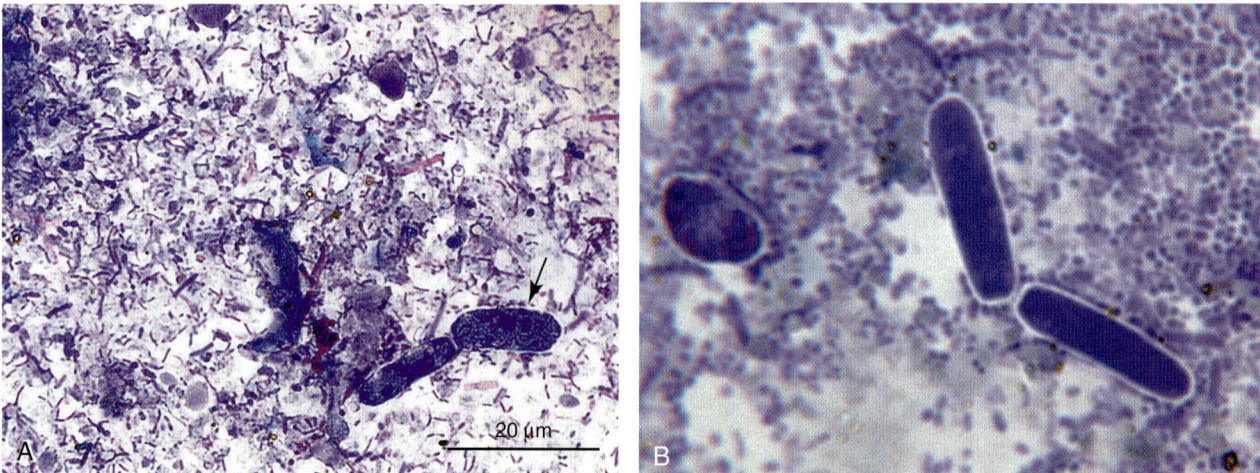

■ **FIGURE 10.7 Yeast.** *Cyniclomyces guttulatus.* **A, Dog.** Rectal scraping from a 1-year-old German shepherd presented for chronic diarrhea. The bacterial flora consists of mixed bacilli on a pale basophilic background containing amorphous debris and one budding *Cyniclomyces guttulatus* organism *(arrow)*. No pathogen is observed. (Wright-Giemsa; HP oil.) **B,** Abnormal bacterial flora containing numerous diplococci is present on a pale basophilic background that contains a single incidental, extracellular fecal yeast *(left)* and two *Cyniclomyces* organisms *(right)* that measure approximately 5 × 10–15 μm. (Wright-Giemsa; HP oil.)

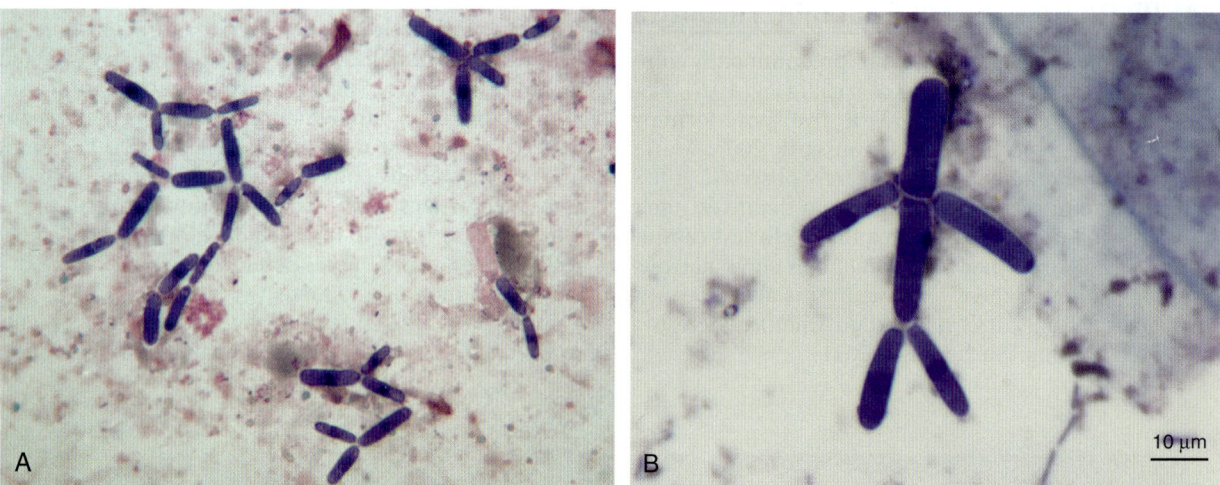

■ **FIGURE 10.8 Yeast.** *Cyniclomyces guttulatus.* **Dog. A,** Several budding organisms observed in the feces of a dog with chronic diarrhea. (Wright-Giemsa; IP.) **B,** Higher magnification of budding yeast showing multiple budding projections. (Modified Wright; HP oil.) (B, Courtesy Kristin Fisher, Purdue University.)

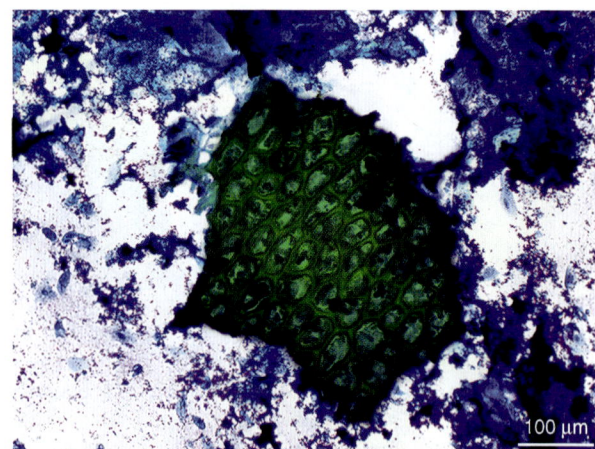

■ **FIGURE 10.9 Plant material.** Rectal scraping from a 12-year-old Louisiana Catahoula leopard dog. Green-blue ingested plant matter with parallel cell walls is commonly seen in canine and feline fecal smears. (Wright-Giemsa; IP.)

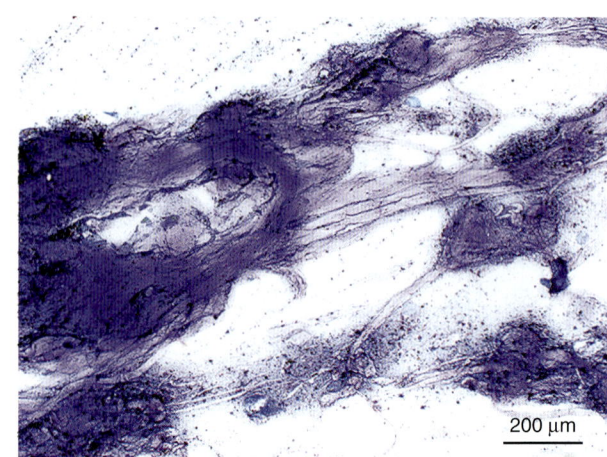

■ **FIGURE 10.10 Mucus. Dog.** Rectal scraping from a 15-year-old rat terrier. Abundant amorphous to streaming, variably basophilic mucus is present admixed with basophilic debris and a mixed bacterial population. (Wright-Giemsa; LP.)

CHAPTER 10 Fecal and Rectal Cytopathology

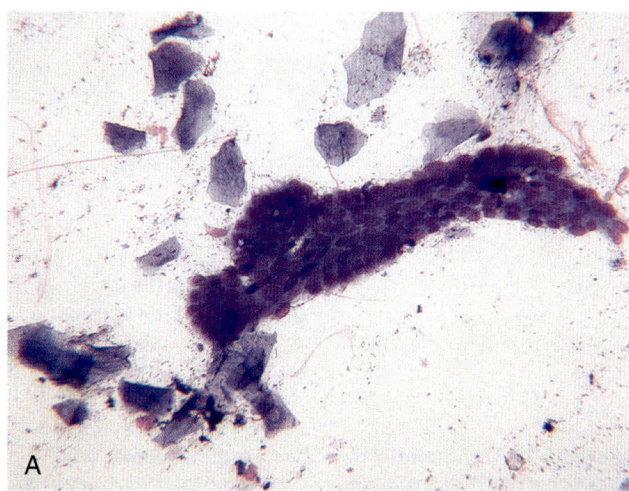

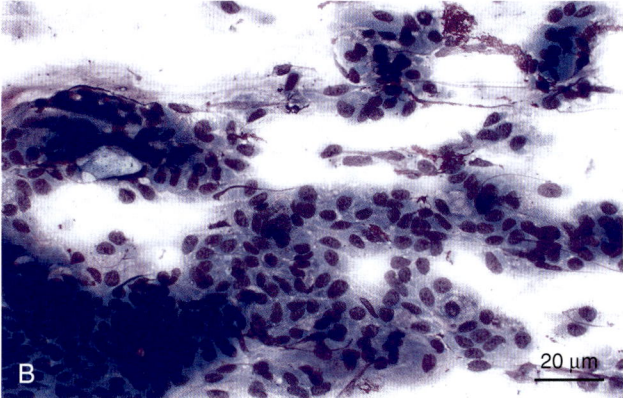

■ **FIGURE 10.11 A, Rectal epithelium and anucleated squamous epithelial cells.** A single large, tightly cohesive, multicellular sheet of low columnar epithelial cells is present in a rectal scrape, surrounded by individualized anucleated, keratinized squamous epithelial cells and scant streaming nuclear material from lysed cells. (Wright-Giemsa; IP.) **B, Columnar rectal epithelium. Dog.** Rectal scraping from a 10-year-old Belgian Malinois presented for increased frequency of defecation. A large cluster of uniform-appearing columnar epithelial cells is present. (Wright-Giemsa; HP oil.)

numbers depending on the sample collection method and underlying disease (Fig. 10.11A). With atraumatic sample collection methods, low numbers of well-differentiated epithelial cells may be present individually or in small sheets. With more invasive collection methods that may abrade the mucosa (i.e., rectal scraping or catheterization for saline lavage), the number and sheet size of epithelial cells are expected to be increased (Fig. 10.11B). In samples collected atraumatically, observation of many epithelial cells in large, multicellular sheets should not be considered normal and should raise concern for underlying mucosal pathology involving sloughing of apical epithelial cells (Fig. 10.12). Squamous epithelial cells are suggestive of concurrent sampling of epithelium from the perianal area.

Other incidental finding includes variable amounts of amorphous, globular to streaming, pink-magenta material consistent with lubricant. Lubricant should not be used when collecting samples by digital examination or rectal scraping for fecal cytopathology because large amounts of lubricant will likely obscure cytologic detail and prevent adequate staining (Fig. 10.13). Saline solution should be used for lubrication instead.

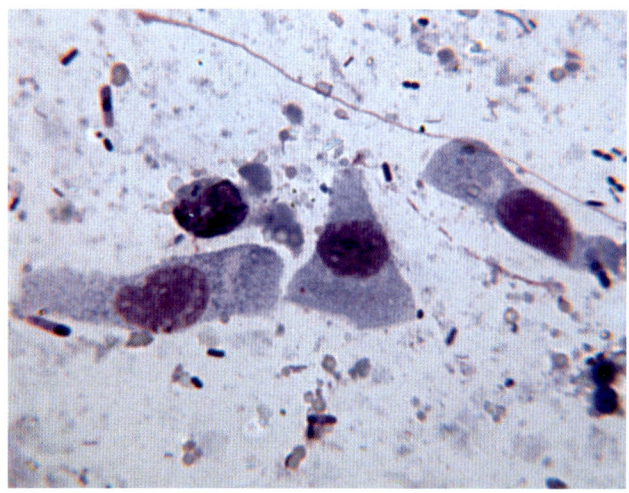

■ **FIGURE 10.12 Columnar epithelium. Dog.** A single small lymphocyte *(top left)* and three well-differentiated epithelial cells are present in the fecal smear in a patient with diarrhea. The pale basophilic background contains a pleomorphic bacterial population composed mostly of small bacilli. (Wright-Giemsa; HP oil.)

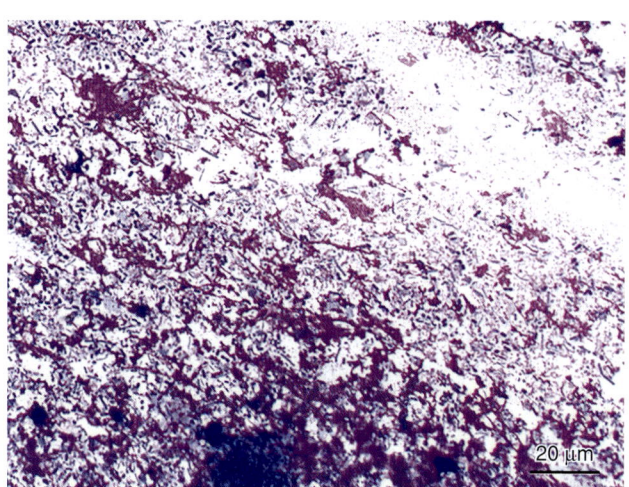

■ **FIGURE 10.13 Lubricant.** Rectal scraping from a 10-year-old vizsla. An abundant amount of amorphous to streaming, pink-magenta material consistent with lubricant is present. The mixed bacterial population and a few neutrophils are poorly visible related to the copious amount of lubricant present. (Wright-Giemsa; HP oil.)

> **KEY POINT** Amorphous basophilic debris (ingesta) and green-blue material (plant material) are commonly seen in the feces of dogs and cats. Epithelial cells are expected in variable number, depending on the collection method. Lubricant should not be used because it obscures cytologic detail.

ABNORMAL MICROSCOPIC FINDINGS

Abnormal Flora

Overgrowth of microorganisms is often accentuated by a prominent population of monomorphic or oligomorphic bacilli, an increased number of cocci, or an increased number of yeast (e.g., *Candida*) (Figs. 10.14 to 10.20). It is typically a secondary, nonspecific finding and a consequence of an underlying

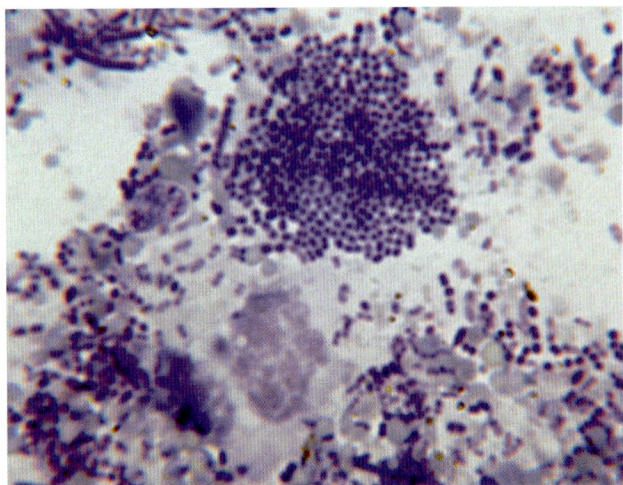

■ **FIGURE 10.14 Abnormal flora. Predominance of cocci.** An abnormal bacterial flora containing numerous diplococci and a microcolony (top center) of diplococci is present along with a single poorly preserved karyolytic neutrophil. (Wright-Giemsa; HP oil.)

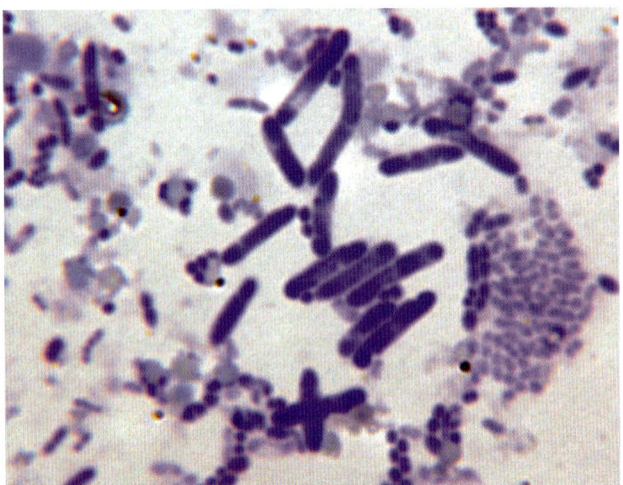

■ **FIGURE 10.15 Abnormal flora. Large bacilli.** Overgrowth of large, plump bacilli along with an increased number of diplococci. (Wright-Giemsa; HP oil.)

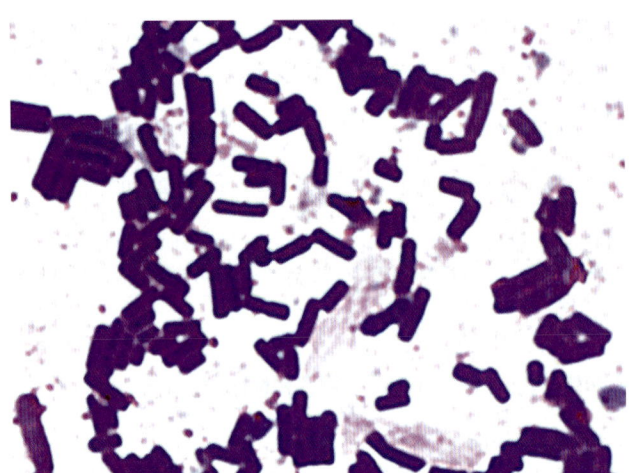

■ **FIGURE 10.16 Abnormal flora. Large bacilli. Dog.** Rectal scraping from a 7-year-old Labrador retriever presented for small bowel diarrhea. A monomorphic population of large, plump bacilli predominates. (Wright-Giemsa; HP oil.)

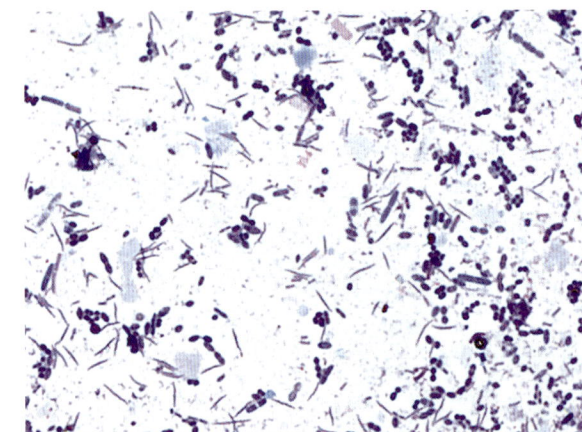

■ **FIGURE 10.17 Abnormal flora. Cocci and thin bacilli. Dog.** Rectal scraping from a 12-year-old boxer dog presented for chronic intermittent mixed-bowel diarrhea. Numerous small, plump cocci are admixed with a monomorphic population of long, thin bacilli. (Wright-Giemsa; HP oil.)

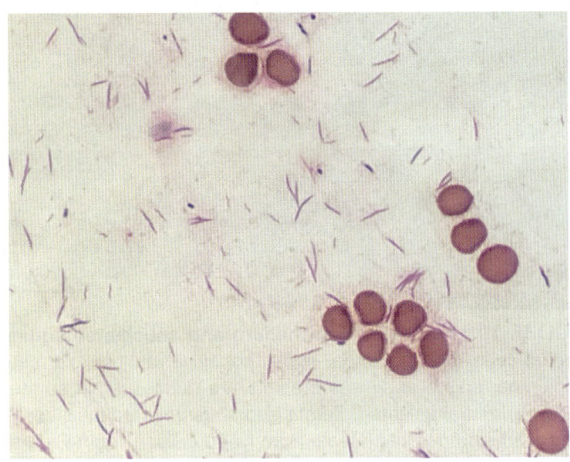

■ **FIGURE 10.18 Abnormal flora. Slender bacilli. Cat.** Direct smear from the red jelly-like (mucoid) fecal material from a 5-month-old domestic shorthair cat that presented with blood in feces. In addition to the erythrocytes, there is a predominance of long slender bacilli measuring approximately 6 μm in length. A second population of shorter curved bacilli is also present. Fecal floatation test was negative for ova, as was a fecal PCR test for *Campylobacter* spp. See Fig. 10.22 for follow-up. (Wright; HP oil.) (Courtesy Rose Raskin, Purdue University.)

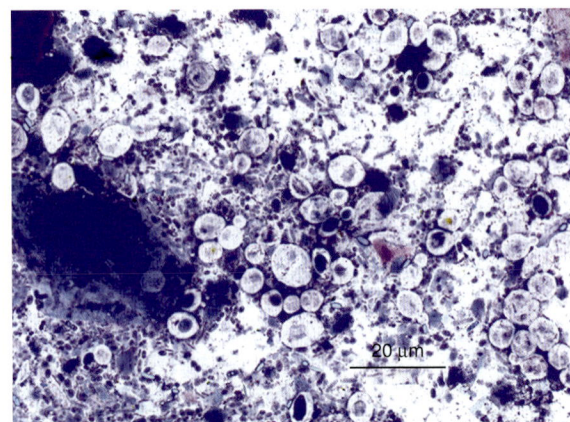

■ **FIGURE 10.19 Abnormal flora. Yeast overgrowth. Cat.** Rectal swab from a 6-year-old domestic shorthair cat. Numerous yeast organisms present are considered to represent overgrowth caused by antibiotic therapy. (Wright-Giemsa; HP oil.)

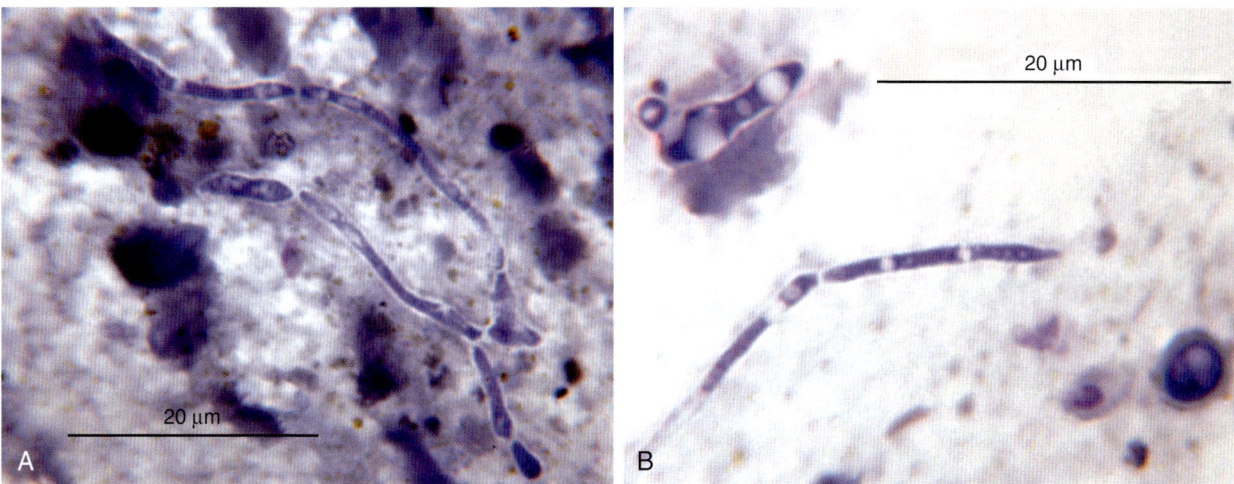

■ **FIGURE 10.20 Abnormal flora. Candidiasis. Dog.** Same case in A and B. **A,** *Candida* spp. pseudohyphae are present in fecal material collected from a dog with chronic gastrointestinal signs after recent exploratory laparotomy. The pale basophilic background, devoid of the usual bacterial flora, contains a moderate amount of incidental irregularly shaped, refractile, amber material and deeply basophilic mucus. (Wright-Giemsa; HP oil.) **B,** *Candida* spp. pseudohyphae and blastospore (dark round structure at lower right.) (Wright-Giemsa; HP oil.)

disease, recent enteric surgical procedures, pathophysiology, or antimicrobial administration. The latter may have effects on the intestinal microbiota that persists for months (Yoon and Yoon, 2018). Although microbial overgrowth may exacerbate underlying pathology, it is not likely the primary cause of GI disease per se; an exception is spore-forming bacteria (discussed later).

> **KEY POINT** Overgrowth of background flora is usually the consequence of an underlying disease, pathophysiology, or previous antimicrobial treatment.

FECAL LEUKOCYTES

Conspicuous numbers of fecal neutrophils should prompt consideration of distal colitis or proctitis (Figs. 10.21 to 10.24) or bacterial enteritis, such as salmonellosis, clostridial colitis, enteric colibacillosis, campylobacteriosis, and infection by other

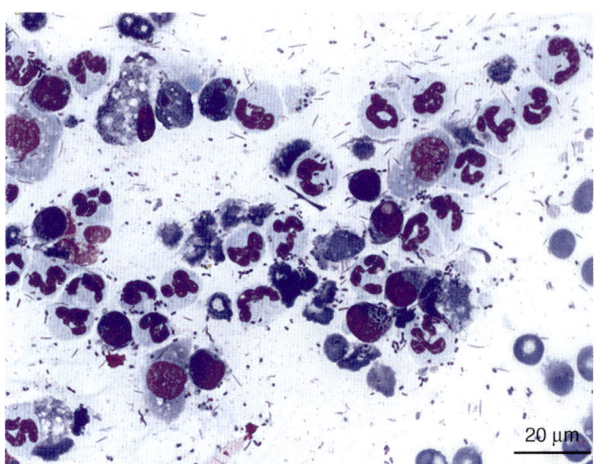

■ **FIGURE 10.21 Mixed inflammation, bacterial infection (colitis). Dog.** Rectal scraping from a 6-month-old mastiff presented for large-bowel diarrhea and hematochezia. Numerous nondegenerate to mildly degenerate neutrophils are found, some containing phagocytized bacteria. A few small, well-differentiated and intermediate-sized lymphocytes are present along with rare karyorrhectic or pyknotic cells. (Wright-Giemsa; HP oil.)

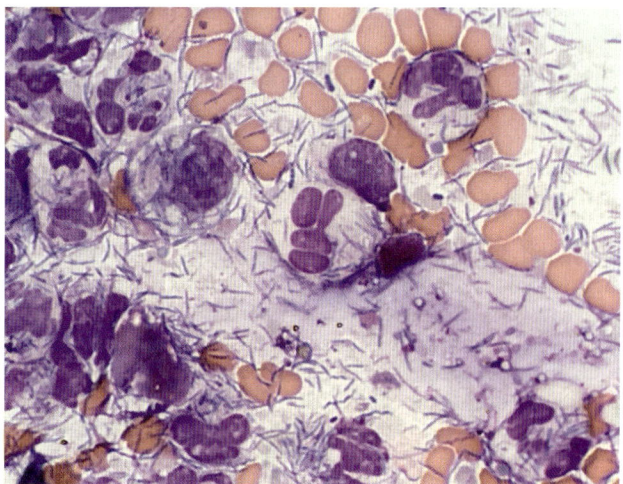

■ **FIGURE 10.22 Neutrophilic bacterial colitis. Fecal smear. Cat.** Sample taken from mucoid feces that persisted for 2 weeks after initial presentation shown in Figure 10.18. Direct smear reveals substantial increase in numbers of similar previous slender bacteria occurring both extracellularly and intracellularly within mildly karyolytic neutrophils. Normal consistency and appearance of feces returned after a course of metronidazole administration, supporting the pathogenic nature of the bacteria. (Wright; HP oil.) (Courtesy Rose Raskin, Purdue University.)

invasive or enterotoxigenic bacteria (Broussard, 2003). Current recommendations for additional diagnostic testing to confirm GI infection, such as culture or molecular techniques for detecting bacterial agents or toxins, vary depending on the specific organism and are described elsewhere (Marks et al., 2011). The diagnostic laboratory should be contacted regarding submission of feces for bacterial culture. Other considerations for the presence of prominent fecal neutrophils include whipworm infestation, which often has concomitant hemorrhagic, mucoid diarrhea; primary inflammatory bowel disease (IBD), which often has accompanying lymphocytes or plasma cells; and distal intestinal tissue necrosis, such as ulcerated neoplasm. An occasional neutrophil and lymphocyte have been reported in clinically healthy dogs but not the observation of macrophages or eosinophils (Frezoulis et al., 2017).

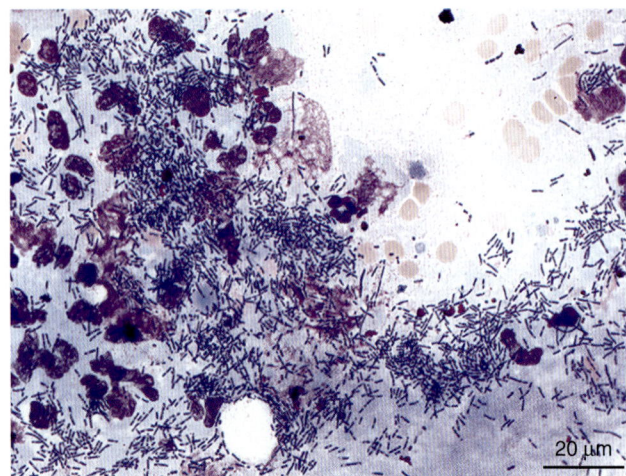
■ **FIGURE 10.23 Neutrophilic bacterial colitis. Cat.** Rectal scraping from a 12-year-old domestic shorthair cat. Abnormal bacterial flora with a predominance of bacilli and diplococci. Several mildly to moderately degenerate (karyolytic) neutrophils are admixed with bacteria. (Wright-Giemsa; HP oil.)

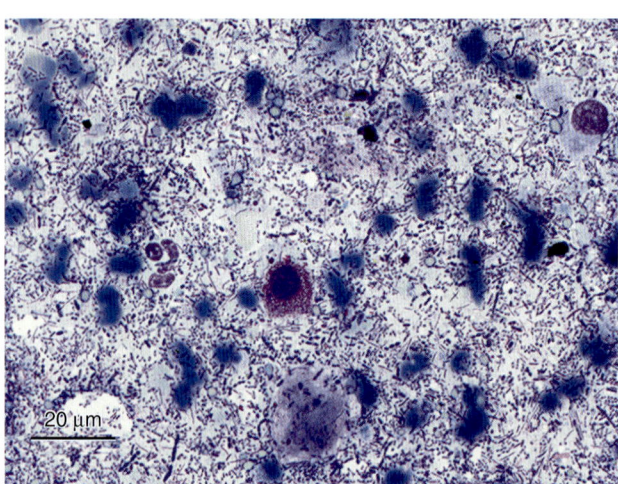
■ **FIGURE 10.24 Mixed cell colitis with mast cells. Dog.** Rectal scraping from a 12-year-old Bouvier des Flandres presented for diarrhea and hematochezia. A degenerate neutrophil and a well-granulated mast cell *(center left)* are shown against a background of red blood cells and bacteria. (Wright-Giemsa; HP oil.)

The presence of fecal eosinophils is suggestive of eosinophilic enteritis or eosinophilic colitis; mast cells may be concomitantly observed (Evans et al., 2006; Kleinschmidt et al., 2007) (see Fig. 10.24). Eosinophilic enteritis or colitis may occur in dogs or cats of any breed or age. However, it is more common in young adult animals, and boxers, Doberman pinschers, and German shepherds appear to be predisposed. The diagnosis of eosinophilic enteritis or colitis is possible after other causes of eosinophilic inflammation have been excluded (Hall and German, 2005). Cats with eosinophilic enteritis commonly have concomitant peripheral eosinophilia (Tucker et al., 2014). Eosinophils appear as a component of the mixed inflammatory response to certain infections (e.g., fungal, oomycetal, algal), nematode parasites, foreign body reactions, or neoplasms (Fig. 10.25).

Conspicuous numbers of small and intermediate-sized lymphocytes with or without plasma cells occur with lymphoplasmacytic enteritis and colitis (Figs. 10.26 and 10.27). Lymphoplasmacytic enteritis typically occurs in older animals with increased incidence in German shepherds, Chinese Shar-Peis, and purebred cats. Distinct forms of IBD include immunoproliferative (lymphoplasmacytic) enteropathy in basenjis and hereditary protein-losing enteropathy in soft-coated wheaten terriers in which the predominant inflammatory infiltrate is lymphoplasmacytic (Littman et al., 2000; Hall and German, 2005). The morphology of the small lymphocyte cannot differentiate between lymphocytic inflammatory enteritis and small cell lymphoma when it is the only population on intestinal sample for cytopathologic evaluation. One of the most important differential diagnoses of intestinal lymphoma is lymphoplasmacytic enteritis and, in

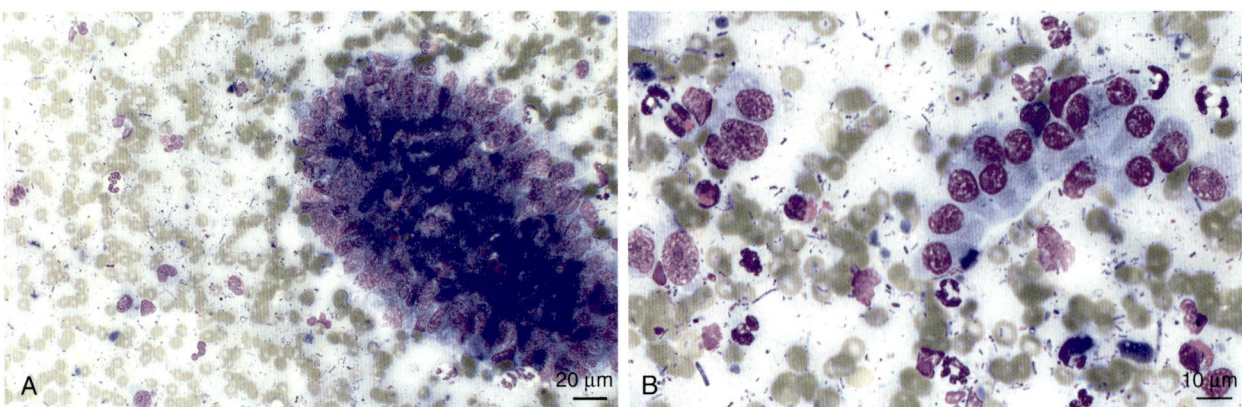
■ **FIGURE 10.25 Eosinophilic colitis. Dog.** Rectal scraping from a 2-year-old Great Dane presented for hematochezia and lethargy later diagnosed with gastrointestinal pythiosis. **A,** Several eosinophils are found in close association to a cluster of rectal epithelium. (Wright-Giemsa; HP oil.) **B,** Eosinophils are seen scattered throughout the preparation, along with a few neutrophils. A small cluster of uniform-appearing rectal epithelial cells is seen on the *upper right*. (Wright-Giemsa; HP oil.)

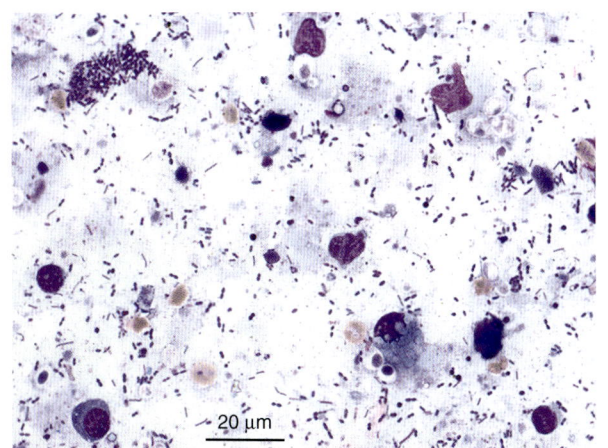

■ **FIGURE 10.26 Lymphoplasmacytic colitis. Dog.** Rectal scraping from a 1-year-old mixed-breed dog presented for intermittent mixed-bowel diarrhea. Several small, well-differentiated and intermediate-sized lymphocytes are seen admixed with a mixed bacterial flora, along with a few yeast organisms. A mature plasma cell *(lower left)* and a Mott cell *(center right)* are also noted. (Wright-Giemsa; HP oil.)

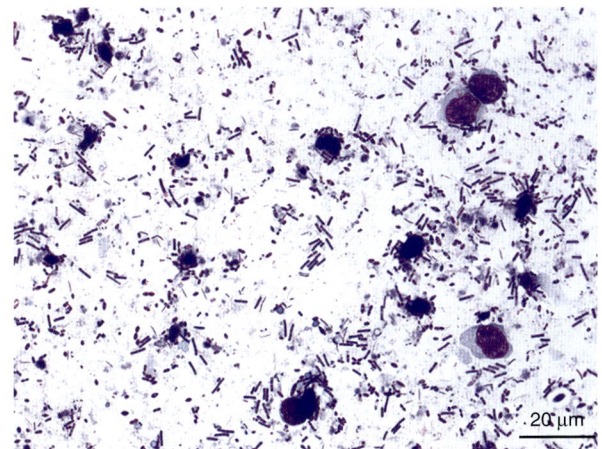

■ **FIGURE 10.27 Lymphocytic colitis with abnormal flora. Dog.** Rectal scraping from a 9-year-old English setter. Small, well-differentiated and intermediate-sized lymphocytes, including a granular lymphocyte, are seen with an abnormal flora composed of mixed bacilli bacteria. (Wright-Giemsa; HP oil.)

many cases, the only certain way to diagnose a neoplastic infiltration of the intestinal wall is to demonstrate the transmural spread of the neoplastic lymphoid cells. Studies in dogs and cats indicate endoscopic biopsies are unreliable for differentiating between IBD and intestinal lymphoma and clearly demonstrate the advantage of the transmural (i.e., full-thickness) histopathologic biopsy for the diagnosis of intestinal small cell lymphoma (Evans et al., 2006; Kleinschmidt et al., 2006). For the differentiation of feline IBD and small cell alimentary lymphoma, clonality analysis can increase the possibility of correctly diagnosing small cell alimentary lymphoma in the duodenal endoscopic biopsy when the companion cytopathologic specimen is predominantly small lymphocytes (Sabattini et al., 2016). The diagnostic metrics for chronic enteropathy in cats is further confounded by a study that demonstrated that the integrated results from histopathology, immunohistochemistry, and clonality testing were interpreted as consistent with small cell lymphoma or lymphocytic enteritis in a large number of clinically healthy cats (Marsilio et al., 2019). Lastly, an occasional lymphocyte may be seen in the fecal material of healthy dogs, particularly if collected by rectal scraping, and may represent exfoliated lymphocytes from the colonic lymphoid follicles (Frezoulis et al., 2017).

The presence of macrophages in fecal material is abnormal and indicates chronic inflammation. When associated with an infectious (e.g., fungal, oomycetal, or algal) causation, intracellular microorganisms may be identified. Granulomatous colitis is an inflammatory disease that primarily affects young adult boxers and French bulldogs. The disease is characterized by the presence of large macrophages that are strongly periodic acid–Schiff (PAS) positive (Fig. 10.28) (German et al., 2000; Conrado et al., 2021). Granulomatous colitis has been associated with mucosal invasion by *Escherichia coli*, and treatment with antimicrobials can induce lasting clinical remission (Hostutler et al., 2004; Craven et al., 2011; Manchester et al., 2013).

> **KEY POINT** Conspicuous numbers of fecal neutrophils should prompt consideration of bacterial enteritis such as salmonellosis, clostridial colitis, enteric colibacillosis, or campylobacteriosis. The cytologic morphology of small lymphocytes cannot reliably differentiate between lymphocytic enteritis and small cell alimentary lymphoma. Large macrophages with PAS-positive cytoplasm are indicative of granulomatous colitis of boxers and French bulldogs.

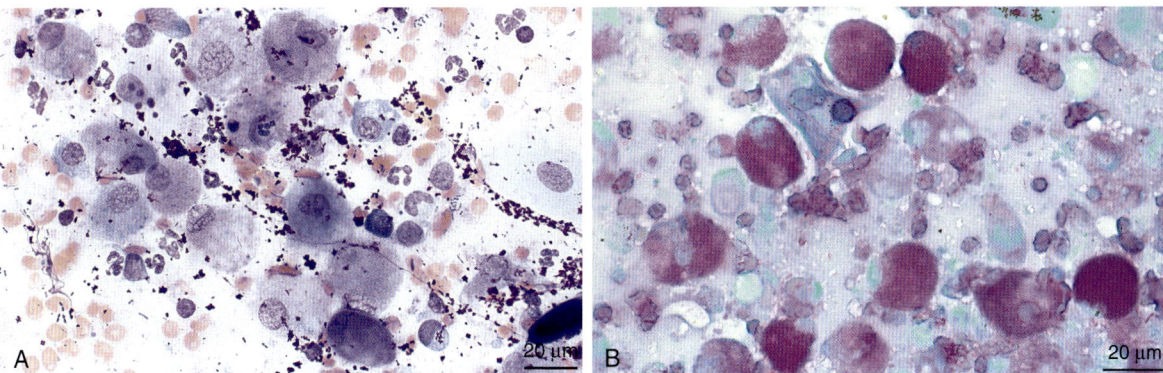

■ **FIGURE 10.28 Granulomatous colitis. Dog.** Rectal scraping from a 1.5-year-old French bulldog presented for chronic diarrhea and hematochezia. Granulomatous colitis was confirmed by the presence of numerous periodic acid–Schiff–positive macrophages on cytopathology and histopathology and detection of mucosal invasive *Escherichia coli* using fluorescence in situ hybridization. **A,** Numerous large macrophages with abundant amphophilic cytoplasm appear with neutrophils, lymphocytes, plasma cells, and bacteria. (Wright-Giemsa; HP oil.) **B,** Large macrophages are intensely positive staining. (PAS; HP oil.)

OTHER CELL TYPES

The number of epithelial cells observed in a sample depends on the collection method and the presence of underlying mucosal pathology with sloughing of apical epithelial cells. If inflammation is absent, epithelial cells should appear well differentiated. Criteria for assessment of atypia in epithelial cells are similar to those in other tissues; inflammation can induce a hyperplastic response associated with cytoplasmic or nuclear changes that mimic those observed with neoplasia (Figs. 10.29 and 10.30). In such cases, histopathology may provide definitive diagnosis. The cytopathologic identification of neoplasms such as lymphoma (Fig. 10.31), mast cell tumor, and GI mesenchymal tumor is enhanced by collecting the specimen via a rectal scraping.

Globule leukocytes may appear in rectal scrapes from dogs and cats (Fig. 10.32). Increased numbers of these cells have been associated with several disease processes, including parasitism and neoplasia, and they are thought to represent a specific type of interepithelial mucosal mast cell (Spoor et al., 2011; Vogel et al., 2018).

Creatorrhea is the presence of undigested muscle fibers in feces. It may be seen with diseases that cause maldigestion or hypermotility (Mundt and Shanahan, 2011), and may be observed on either wet-mount or dry-mount fecal cytopathology preparations (Fig. 10.33). Fecal material from animals with

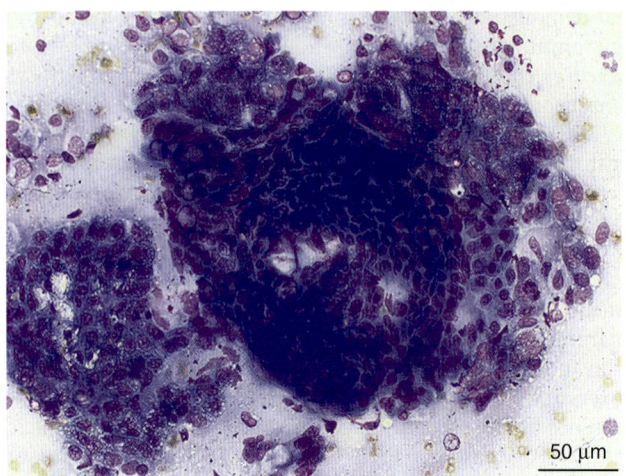

■ **FIGURE 10.29 Atypical rectal epithelium, colitis. Dog.** Rectal scraping from a 3-year-old dachshund presented for regurgitation, tenesmus, and large bowel diarrhea. A large cluster of mildly to moderately atypical rectal epithelial cells appears consistent with dysplastic or hyperplastic changes and is associated with a mixed inflammatory infiltrate that is secondary to bacterial infection. The dog was diagnosed with angiocentric B-cell lymphoma at necropsy with no evidence of intestinal epithelial neoplasia. (Wright-Giemsa; IP.)

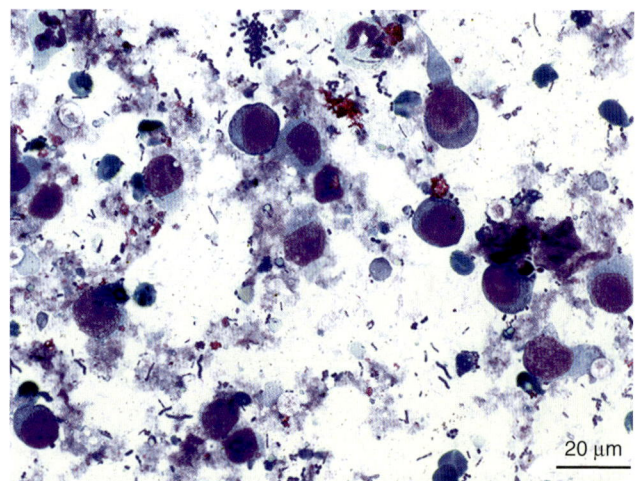

■ **FIGURE 10.31 Large cell lymphoma. Dog.** Rectal scraping from a 16-year-old shih tzu presented for hematochezia and dyschezia. Several large lymphoid cells are present along with a mixed bacterial flora. These cells are round or oval, with discrete cytoplasmic borders, a high nucleocytoplasmic ratio, and discernible nucleoli. (Wright-Giemsa; HP oil.)

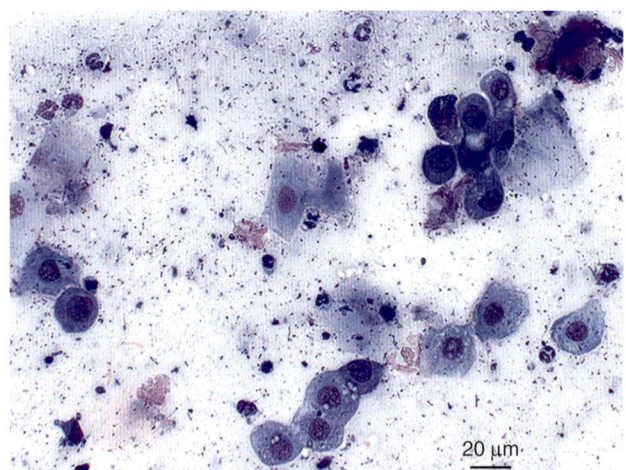

■ **FIGURE 10.30 Hyperplastic squamous epithelium, colitis. Dog.** Rectal scraping from a 7-year-old golden retriever. A mixture of squamous epithelial cells and neutrophils is present along with mixed bacterial flora. Few atypical squamous epithelial cells exhibit increased nucleocytoplasmic ratio and cytoplasmic basophilia, consistent with hyperplastic changes induced by inflammation. (Wright-Giemsa; HP oil.)

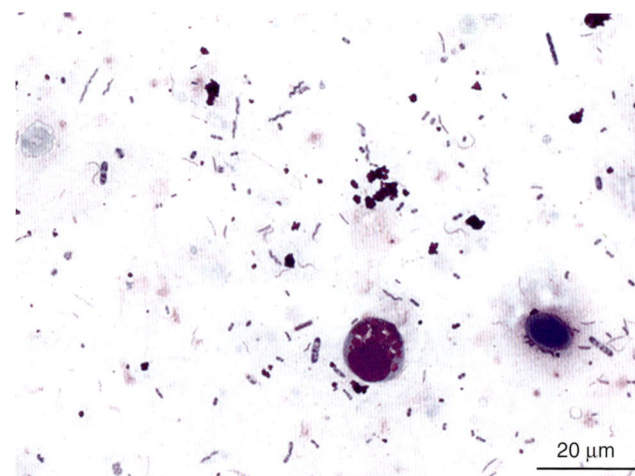

■ **FIGURE 10.32 *Campylobacter*-like bacteria and globule leukocyte. Dog.** Rectal scraping from a 12-year-old mixed-breed dog presented for chronic loose stools and hematochezia. A single globule leukocyte (off center) contains several large, magenta cytoplasmic globules. Numerous spiriliform bacteria appear in the background. (Wright-Giemsa; HP oil.)

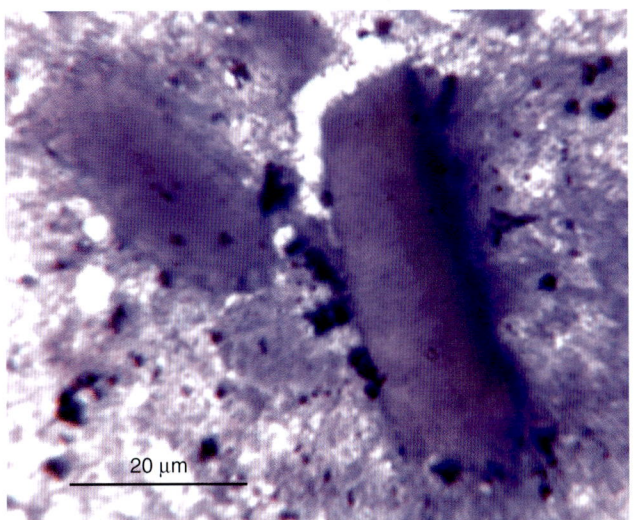

FIGURE 10.33 Creatorrhea. Dog. Two fragments of undigested skeletal muscle appear on a background of mixed bacteria in a rectal scraping from a dog with chronic diarrhea and hematochezia. The fragment at the right shows striations typical of skeletal muscle. This finding may be seen in patients with maldigestion or hypermotility disorders. (Aqueous Romanowsky; HP oil.)

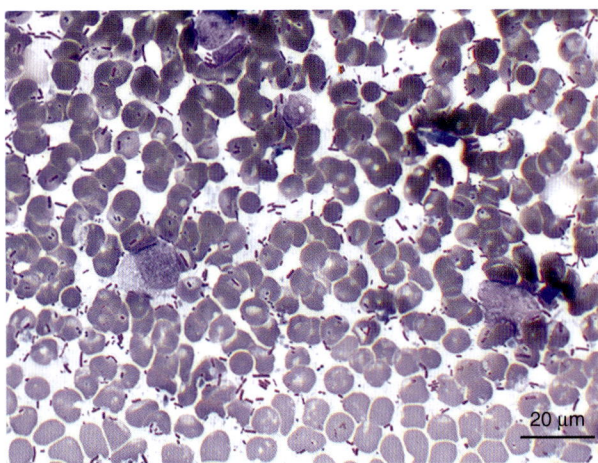

FIGURE 10.35 Trauma-induced bleeding. Dog. Rectal scraping from a 2-year-old otterhound. Numerous red blood cells are present along with a mixed bacterial flora. The erythrocytes are likely associated with the sampling technique. (Wright-Giemsa; HP oil.)

conditions resulting in maldigestion may also contain poorly preserved adipocytes, suggestive of undigested fat (Fig. 10.34).

The presence of erythrocytes is considered generally abnormal in fecal material; a small amount can be associated with traumatic sampling (Fig. 10.35). Microscopic evidence of acute and chronic hemorrhage typically consists of the observation of frank blood or hemoglobin crystals (Fig. 10.36) or hemoglobin breakdown products (Fig. 10.37), respectively.

Potential Microbial Pathogens

In addition to the microbial flora that is expected in feces, potential pathogens may also be present. In some instances, definitive cytopathologic diagnosis of GI infectious disease is

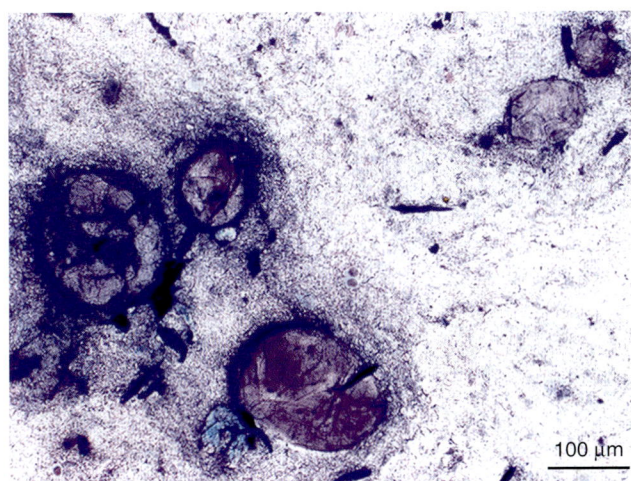

FIGURE 10.34 Undigested fat. Dog. Rectal scrape from an 11-year-old Old English sheepdog presented for hematochezia. Large, poorly preserved, globoid cells, consistent with adipocytes, appear individualized and in variably sized clusters, suggestive of undigested fat. (Wright-Giemsa; IP.)

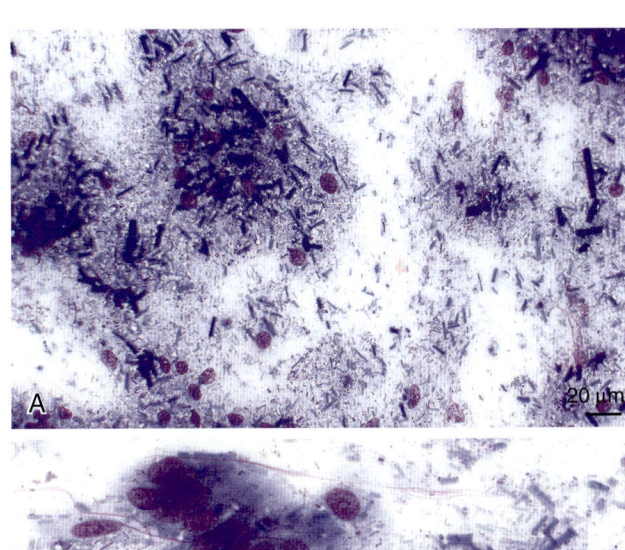

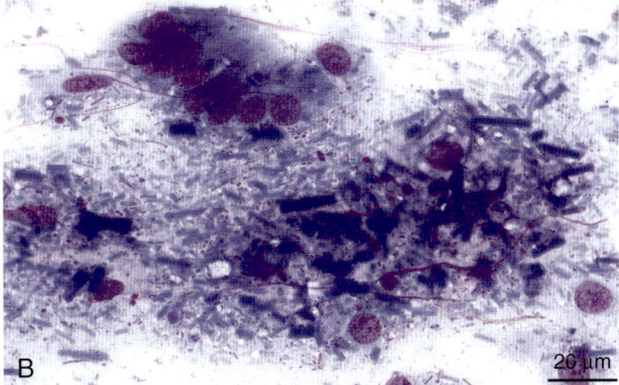

FIGURE 10.36 Hemoglobin crystals. Dog. Rectal scraping from an 8-year-old Weimaraner presented for hematochezia. **A,** Numerous, variably sized, rectangular to elongated, gray-blue hemoglobin crystals appear along with a mixed bacterial flora, consistent with hemorrhage. (Wright-Giemsa; HP.) **B,** Hemoglobin crystals are seen associated with a small cluster of well-differentiated rectal epithelium. (Wright-Giemsa; HP oil.)

possible (e.g., fungal, algal, oomycetal, protozoal). However, by dry-mount fecal cytopathology alone, pathogenic bacteria can be morphologically indistinguishable from incidental nonpathogenic organisms. For bacterial culture of feces, the referral laboratory should be contacted because unique sample collection,

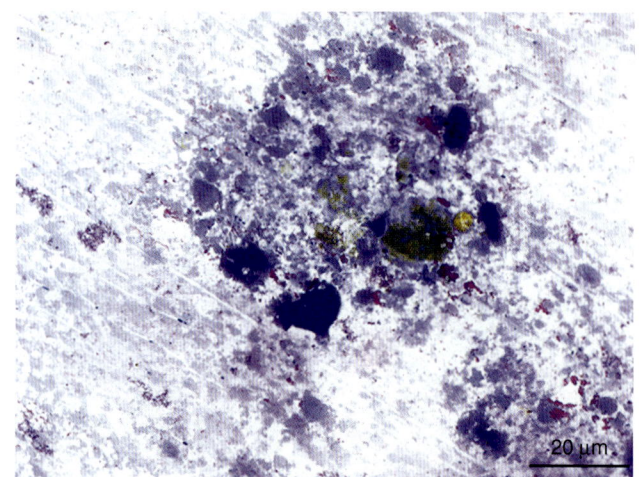

FIGURE 10.37 Heme breakdown products. Dog. Rectal scraping from a 15-year-old miniature schnauzer presented for hematochezia. A moderate amount of amorphous golden yellow material, consistent with normal or abnormal catabolism of blood, is present along with bacteria. (Wright-Giemsa; HP oil.)

handling, and culture conditions are essential for enteric pathogen detection (Broussard, 2003; Marks et al., 2011).

Small numbers of spore-forming bacteria can be an incidental finding in feces (Fig. 10.38). However, conspicuously large numbers of spore-forming bacteria is an abnormal finding, and concurrent fecal neutrophils further support bacteria-induced diarrhea (Figs. 10.39 and 10.40). *Clostridium perfringens* is a gram-positive spore-forming rod. The optimal diagnostic approach for suspected canine *C. perfringens*–associated diarrhea is the use of a positive enzyme-linked immunosorbent assay (ELISA) to detect *C. perfringens* enterotoxin in conjunction with PCR to detect enterotoxigenic strains (Marks et al., 2011). Because sporulation is correlated with enterotoxin production, fecal endospore counting of Romanowsky or Gram-stained fecal smears (≥5 spores per high power field) was suggested initially as a screening tool for diagnosis (Broussard, 2003). Several studies subsequently reported no association between fecal endospore counts and the presence of diarrhea or between spore counts and the detection of *C. perfringens* enterotoxin in fecal specimens. Furthermore, it has been demonstrated that sporulation of enterotoxigenic strains continually occurs in

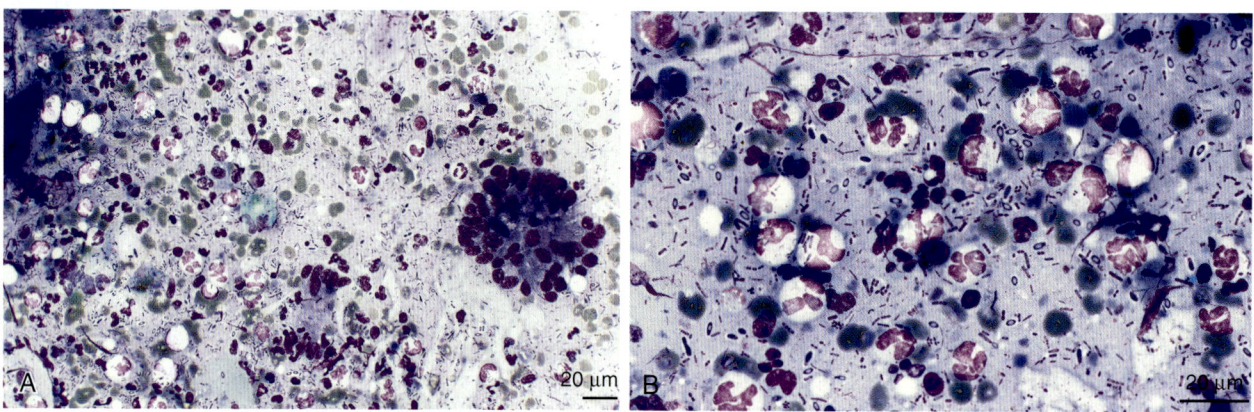

FIGURE 10.38 Mixed-cell colitis with spore-forming bacilli. Dog. Rectal scraping from a 2.5-year-old German shorthair pointer presented for hematochezia, weight loss, tenesmus, and anorexia. **A,** A predominance of neutrophils appears with a mixed bacterial flora having increased numbers of spore-forming bacilli and bacterial endospores. A small cluster of mildly atypical or hyperplastic rectal epithelium appears at *right*. (Wright-Giemsa; HP.) **B,** Numerous degenerate (karyolytic) neutrophils are noted along with spore-forming bacilli. (Wright-Giemsa; HP oil.)

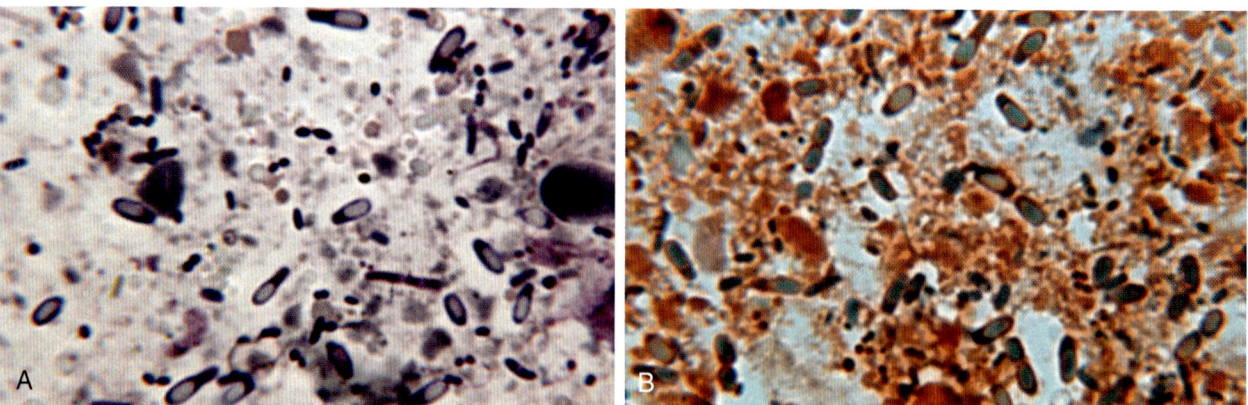

FIGURE 10.39 Spore-forming bacilli. Dog. Same case in A and B. Numerous spore-forming bacilli are present in the feces of a dog with diarrhea, suggestive of *Bacillus* spp. or *Clostridium* spp. organisms. **A,** Individualized spores are visible along with the sporulated bacilli, often containing a terminally located spore that renders a tennis racket appearance. When the spores are centrally located, sporulated bacilli may have a safety pin appearance. (Wright-Giemsa; HP oil.) **B,** Malachite green is a microbiologic stain used to identify the presence of bacterial spores, such as in *Bacillus* spp. or *Clostridium* spp. Steam is included in the staining process to permeabilize the hard, dehydrated, multilamellar spore walls. A pink safranin counterstain helps to distinguish the spores. (Malachite green/Safranin; HP oil.)

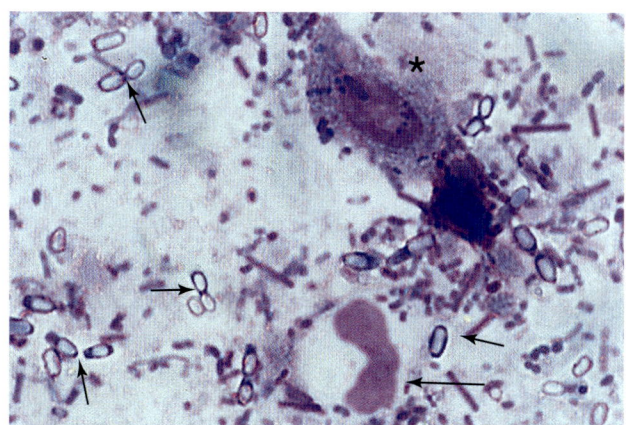

FIGURE 10.40 Clostridial colitis. Fecal smear. Numerous neutrophils were present upon scanning of this direct smear. An increased number of large, rod-shaped bacterial endospores with a clear center and an increased density predominantly on one end ("safety pin") are the notable feature *(short arrows)*. The bacterial morphology is consistent with *Clostridium perfringens*. Confirmation involved measurement of the enterotoxin in the feces. A degenerate neutrophil *(long arrow)* and epithelial cell *(asterisk)* are shown. (Wright; HP oil.) (Courtesy Denny Meyer and Dave Twedt, Colorado State University.)

both nondiarrheic and diarrheic dogs (Marks et al., 2011). The lack of correlation is likely because of the possible presence of nonpathogenic spore-forming bacteria or the presence of spore-forming *Clostridium* spp. that do not produce enterotoxin (Marks et al., 2002; Broussard, 2003). In fecal samples from dogs with acute hemorrhagic diarrhea, a *C. perfringens* type A strain has been identified by real-time polymerase chain reaction for *netE* and *netF* genes (Sindern et al., 2019). Smear of fresh feces should be made quickly because nonpathogenic spore-forming bacteria may form spores during a delay in sample processing, especially at room temperature.

Pleomorphic fecal bacteria that exhibit gull-wing and spiral morphology on dry-mount fecal cytopathology include treponeme-like bacteria, *Serpulina* spp., *Helicobacter* spp., *Anaerobiospirillum* spp., and *Campylobacter* spp. (Figs. 10.41 to 10.45). It is unusual to observe pleomorphic gull-wing and spiral-shaped bacteria in routine dry-mount fecal preparations, and this is an abnormal finding when observed in large numbers (see Figs. 10.44 and 10.45). *Campylobacter* spp. are gram-negative, microaerophilic, curved, motile rods. They are best observed with 100× oil with coverslip in thin areas or areas that contain mucus because they tend to localize on the mucus-rich mucosal surface. There are many species in the genus; most are considered to be nonpathogenic. A direct gram-stained smear of feces is used to identify *Campylobacter*-like organisms. Detection of small (0.5–1.0 × 5.0–10.0 μm) curved or gull wing–shaped bacteria only suggests the presence of *Campylobacter*-like organisms. This should not be used as the sole method to diagnose campylobacteriosis. The inability to differentiate between organisms of similar morphology such as *Arcobacter* or nonpathogenic campylobacters requires other tests. Culture via selective media is helpful to confirm the diagnosis. In addition, commercial PCR molecular techniques are available to identify and differentiate *Campylobacter* spp. if further characterization is necessary. Diarrhea has been associated with fecal isolation of

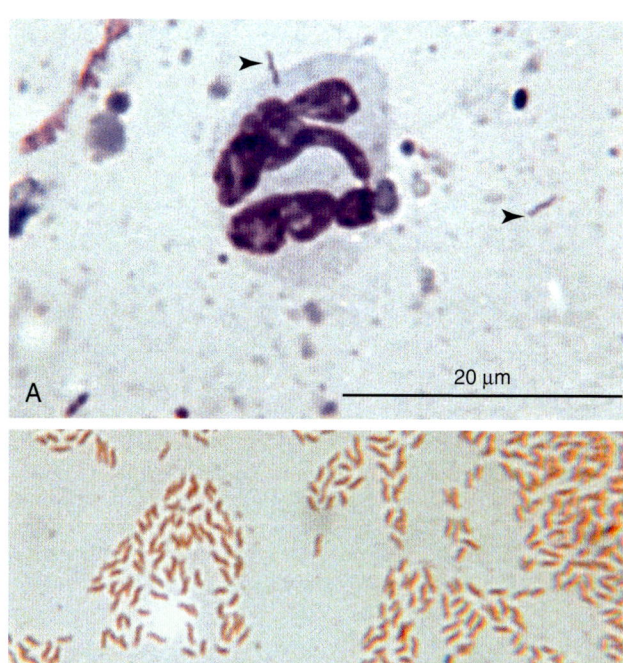

FIGURE 10.41 Campylobacteriosis. Dog. Same case in A and B. **A,** A neutrophil is seen along with two small, pleomorphic, gull-wing–shaped bacteria *(arrowheads)* in a fecal smear from a dog with diarrhea. *Campylobacter* spp. was isolated by bacterial culture. (Wright-Giemsa; HP oil.) **B,** Gram stain of *Campylobacter* spp. cultured from the feces indicates that the bacteria are gram-negative bacilli. (Gram stain; HP oil.)

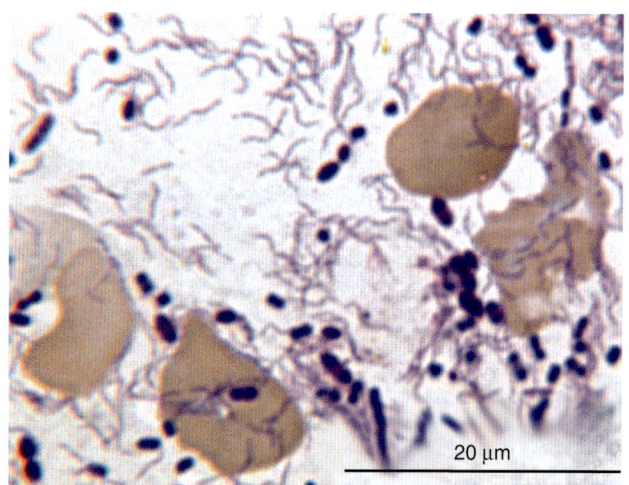

FIGURE 10.42 Spiriliform bacteria. Dog. Numerous fine, pleomorphic, gull-wing–shaped, and spiriliform fecal bacteria consistent with *Serpulina* spp. are larger than those shown in Figure 10.40. The dog presented with chronic mucoid diarrhea. The large number of spiriliform bacteria in this sample may reflect the mucoid nature of the diarrhea because this morphology of bacteria tends to occur within mucoid gastrointestinal secretions. (Wright-Giemsa; HP oil.)

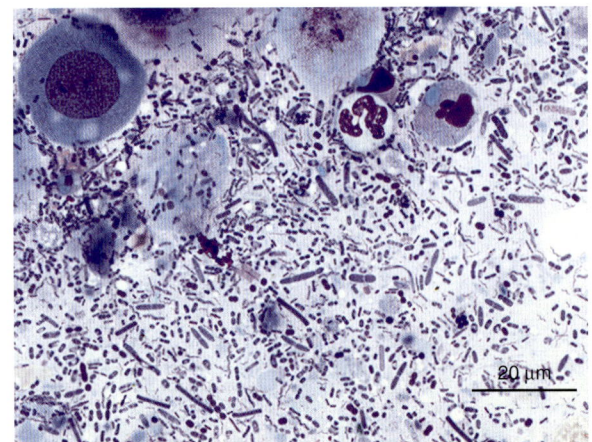

FIGURE 10.43 Spiriliform bacteria, colitis. Dog. Rectal scraping from a 3-year-old Doberman pinscher presented for large bowel diarrhea. Mixed bacterial flora is present containing increased numbers of thin and plump spiriliform bacteria. Neutrophilic inflammation and hyperplastic epithelial cells are also present. (Wright-Giemsa; HP oil.)

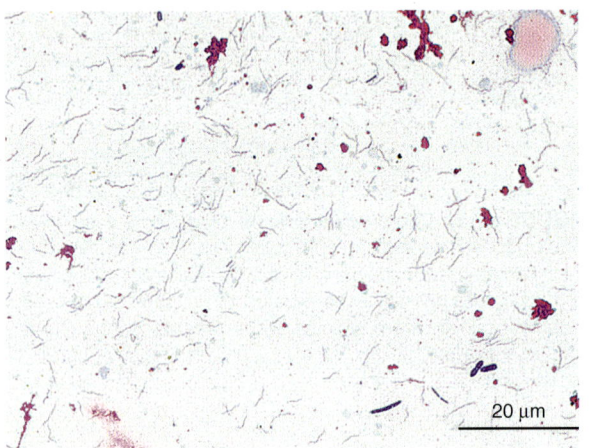

FIGURE 10.44 Spiriliform bacteria. Dog. Rectal scraping from a 14-year-old Pomeranian presented for chronic large bowel diarrhea. The bacterial flora consists predominantly of small, thin, spiriliform bacteria. (Wright-Giemsa; HP oil.)

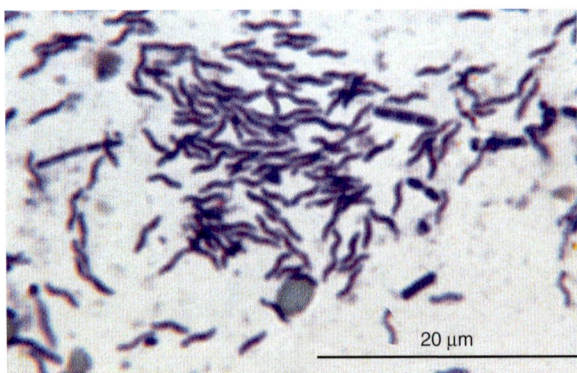

FIGURE 10.45 Treponeme-like bacteria. Dog. Numerous darkly stained, spiriliform bacteria that exhibit several complete convolutions are seen in the fecal smear of a dog with diarrhea. These bacteria are larger than those shown in Figure 10.41. Examination of a fecal wet mount may help identify conclusively these as a nonpathogenic treponeme-like bacterium, which exhibits very rapid forward motility in the fluid medium. (Wright-Giemsa; HP oil.)

bacteria from the aforementioned genera. Additionally, all these genera have been isolated from the feces of asymptomatic dogs and cats (Malnick et al., 1990; Broussard, 2003; De Cock et al., 2004; Misawa et al., 2002; Bender et al., 2005; Rossi et al., 2008). Concurrent observation of fecal neutrophils would support a diarrheal causal relationship.

> **KEY POINT** The finding of large numbers of spore-forming rods in association with diarrhea should be followed up by an ELISA to detect *C. perfringens* enterotoxin in conjunction with PCR to detect enterotoxigenic strains. A direct Romanowsky or Gram stain smear of feces is used to identify *Campylobacter*-like organisms and, when present in large numbers, should be followed by culture or PCR for confirmation.

Protozoal, fungal, or pseudofungal (i.e., algal and oomycetal) infections are occasionally diagnosed using dry-mount fecal cytopathology (Baumgardner and Paretsky, 1997; Graves et al., 2005; Chapman et al., 2009; Vince et al., 2014). Feline *Tritrichomonas foetus* (proposed new name *T. blagburni*) is a flagellate protozoan (Figs. 10.46 to 10.48) that colonizes portions of the large intestine of cats worldwide and causes chronic and recurrent large-bowel diarrhea with mucus and fresh blood (Yao and Köster, 2015; Gookin et al., 2017). Trichomonads may be observed extracellularly in direct smears or wet mounts with iodine stain of fresh feces from cats, but flotation solutions destroy trophozoites (Payne and Artzer, 2009). *Tritrichomonas* spp. may be difficult to distinguish from *Giardia* spp. and *Pentatrichomonas hominis* based on morphology alone, so additional diagnostic testing (e.g., culture, PCR) must be used for confirmation (Yao and Köster, 2015). Polymerase chain reaction testing for the presence of *T. foetus* rDNA in feces is considered to be the most sensitive means for diagnosis of infection in cats. However, PCR

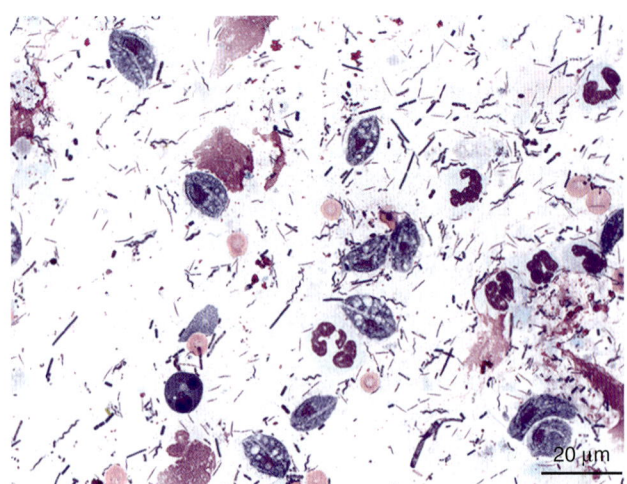

FIGURE 10.46 Tritrichomonosis or tritrichomoniasis, colitis. Cat. Rectal scraping from a 7-year-old Maine coon cat presented for chronic diarrhea. Several *Tritrichomonas* spp. trophozoites are present, admixed with a mixed bacterial flora containing several spiriliform bacteria. Fecal neutrophils are also common, indicating concurrent inflammation. (Wright-Giemsa; HP oil.)

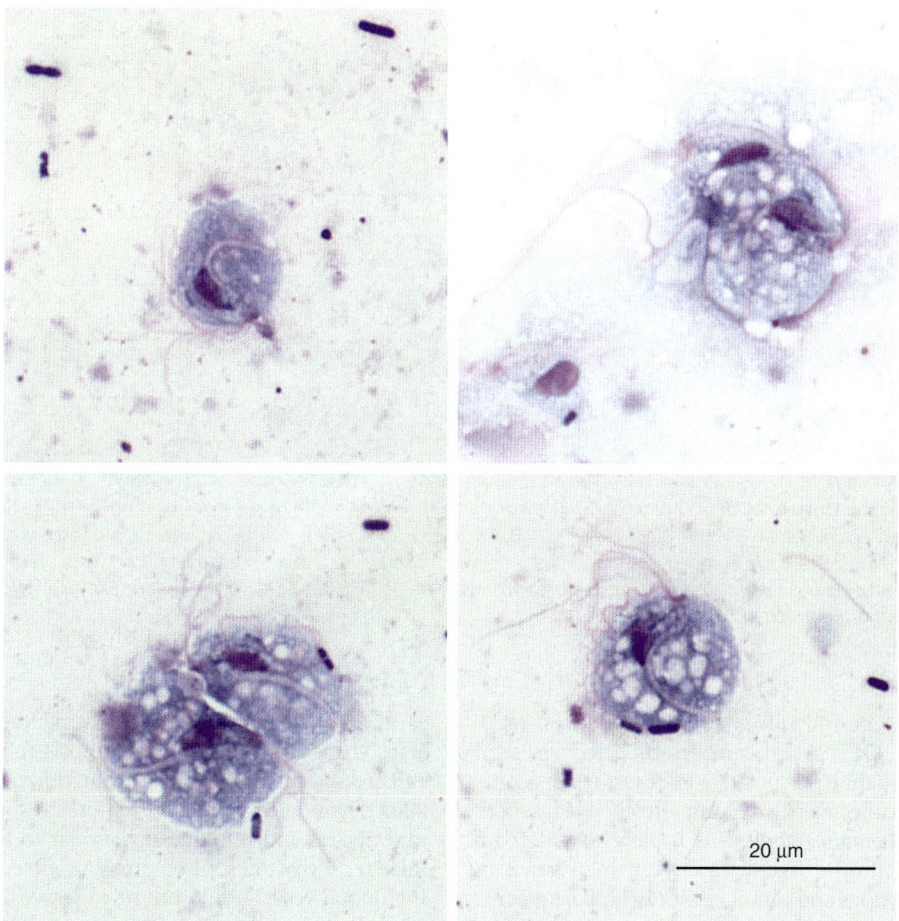

■ **FIGURE 10.47 Tritrichomonosis or tritrichomoniasis. Cat.** Rectal scraping from a 1-year-old domestic longhair presented for chronic diarrhea. *Tritrichomonas* spp. trophozoites appear admixed with mixed bacilli. These organisms have a central axostyle, an undulating membrane, a posterior flagellum, and three anterior flagella. (Wright-Giemsa; HP oil.)

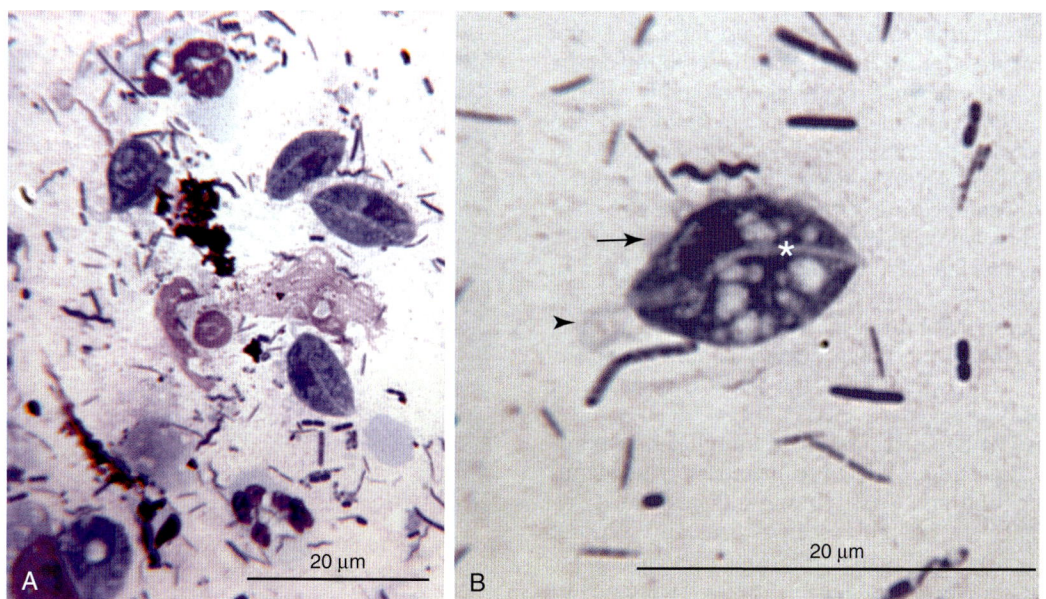

■ **FIGURE 10.48 Tritrichomonosis or tritrichomoniasis. Cat.** Same case in A and B. **A,** Several trophozoites are shown along with two intact neutrophils that appear to contain phagocytized bacteria. This patient had a negative ELISA test result for *Giardia* spp. antigen and responded well to ronidazole treatment for *Tritrichomonas* spp. (Wright-Giemsa; HP oil.) **B,** *Tritrichomonas* spp. is shown with a central axostyle *(asterisk)*, an undulating membrane *(arrow)*, and three anterior flagella *(arrowhead)*.

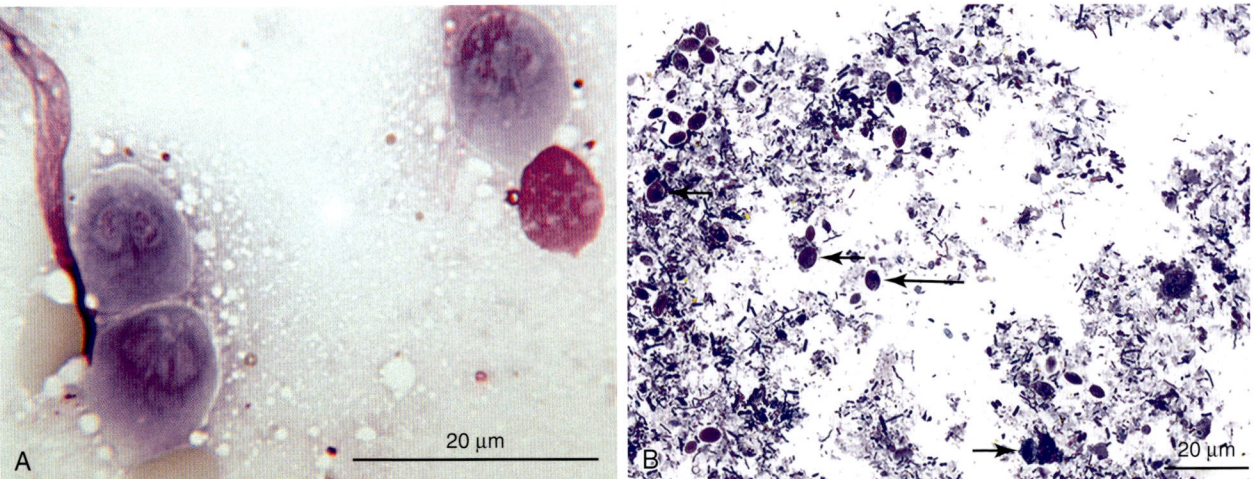

■ **FIGURE 10.49 Giardiasis. Dog. A,** *Giardia* spp. trophozoites are shown from the feces of a dog with diarrhea. These flagellate protozoan organisms are pyriform with two apical nuclei. (Wright-Giemsa; HP oil.) **B,** Fecal smear from a 2-month-old intact male Yorkshire terrier dog presented for liquid diarrhea. Several presumptive *Giardia* spp. cysts *(arrows)* are seen admixed with a mixed bacterial flora. Cysts were found on a fecal flotation test, and a fecal antigen test was positive for *Giardia* spp. *Giardia* spp. cysts are usually not detected by dry-mount fecal cytopathology; fecal flotation is usually required for this purpose. (Wright-Giemsa; HP oil.)

test results are likely to be influenced by fecal collection technique (Gookin et al., 2017). Fecal samples collected via fecal loop had increased probability of positive PCR test results compared with samples collected by colonic flush (Hedgespeth et al., 2020). *Pentatrichomonas hominis* is usually considered a commensal and opportunistic agent, rarely causing disease in immunocompromised dogs and cats (Li et al., 2014; Bastos et al., 2018).

It is uncommon to diagnose giardiasis using fecal cytopathology (Fig. 10.49). *Giardia* trophozoites are more easily identified in fresh fecal wet mounts, although care should be taken to distinguish them from trichomonads. Their movement is described as a "falling leaf," but they may be observed fluttering in place by using their flagella. Giardia trophozoites are usually 12 to 18 μm by 10 to 12 μm in size (see Fig. 10.49A). As opposed to *Giardia* spp. cysts, trophozoites shed in feces are labile and rapidly die on exposure to air. Adding immunofluorescence techniques to fecal flotation tests increases the sensitivity of diagnosing giardiasis in dogs and cats (Saleh et al., 2019). Recognition of cysts in direct fecal smears is difficult because of the presence of yeasts, plant material, and debris with similar appearance (see Fig. 10.49B). *Giardia* spp. cysts are ellipsoidal and measure 8 to 12 μm by 7 to 10 μm in size with a thick refractile wall best recovered by zinc sulfate centrifugation technique (Dryden et al., 2006). The small size and the intermittent shedding further complicate correct diagnosis, thereby supporting use of the SNAP *Giardia* test in veterinary clinics (Uehlinger et al., 2017).

Protothecosis is a disease caused by a unicellular, achlorophyllic, aerobic algae closely related to members of the genus *Chlorella*. Canine protothecosis is typically a disseminated disease with an inevitably fatal course. Dogs generally show GI signs as well as ocular or neurologic abnormalities. In cats, the disease usually manifests as a cutaneous disease (Stenner et al., 2007). The round, oval, or reniform organisms measuring 3 to 20 μm in diameter are often seen in rectal scrapes from dogs with protothecosis (Rallis et al., 2002; Stenner et al., 2007; Vince et al., 2014). They occasionally contain several endospores (Figs. 10.50 to 10.52), but diagnosis may also be achieved by culture and histopathologic evaluation of lesions (Stenner et al., 2007). Nonendosporulated *Prototheca* spp. cells (see Fig. 10.50) may appear morphologically similar to the incidental extracellular fecal yeast described previously (see Figs. 10.6 and 10.19). Incidental yeast should not be observed intracellularly, whereas *Prototheca* may be seen within macrophages and extracellularly (see Figs. 10.51 and 10.52).

Other potential pathogens identified on dry-mount fecal cytopathology include the ameba *Entamoeba* spp. (Fig. 10.53),

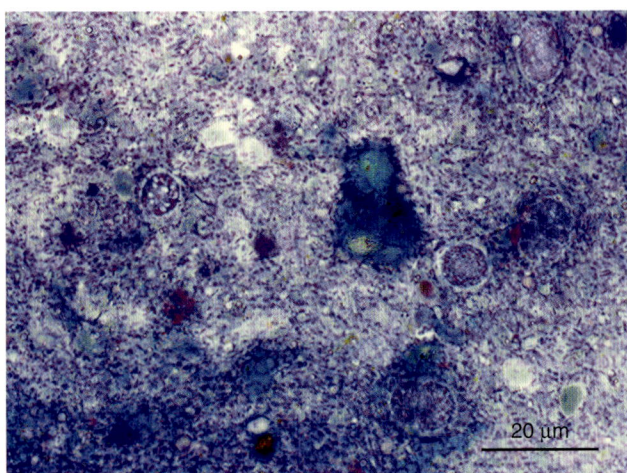

■ **FIGURE 10.50 Protothecosis, colitis. Dog.** Rectal scraping from a 2-year-old boxer presented for chronic, mucoid diarrhea, hematochezia, and acute blindness. Numerous round, oval, or reniform *Prototheca* spp. organisms measure approximately 5.0 to 10.0 μm × 10.0 to 20.0 μm. They have a thin, colorless capsule. Shown are nonendosporulated single-cell forms. (Wright-Giemsa; HP oil.)

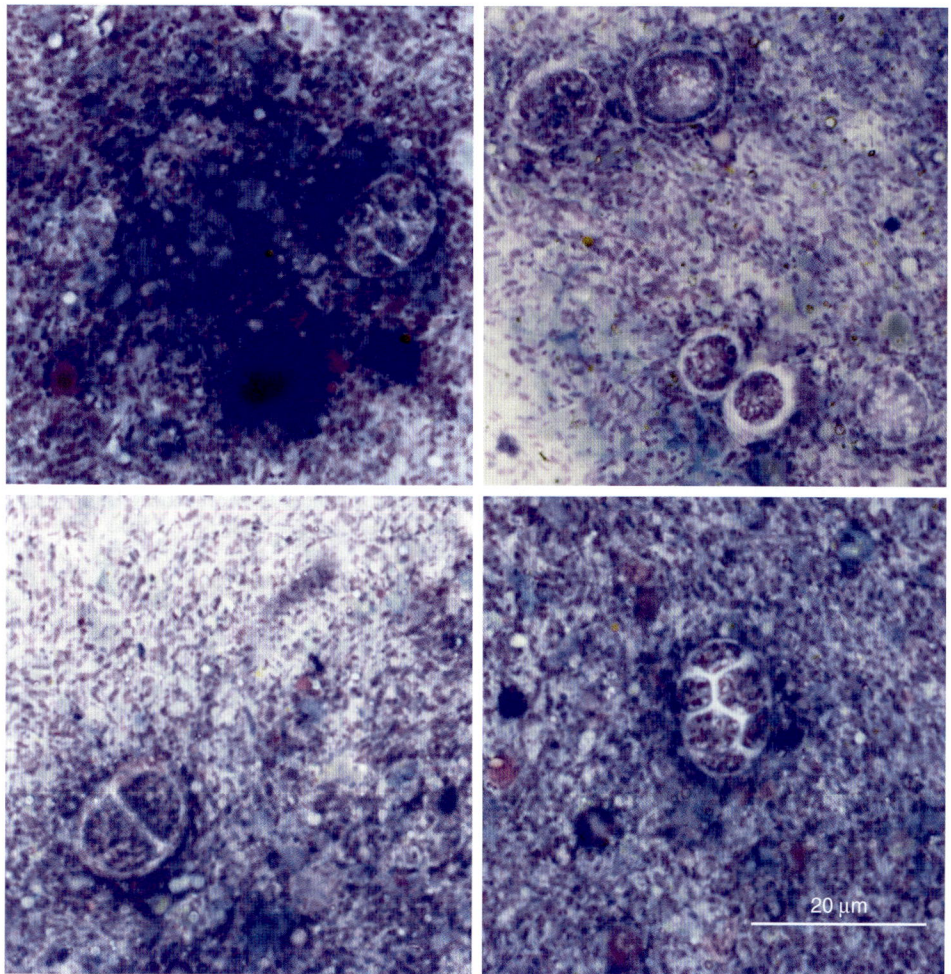

■ **FIGURE 10.51 Protothecosis, colitis. Dog.** Same case as in Figure 10.50. *Prototheca* spp. contain a granular central nucleus or two to six endospores. (Wright-Giemsa; HP oil.)

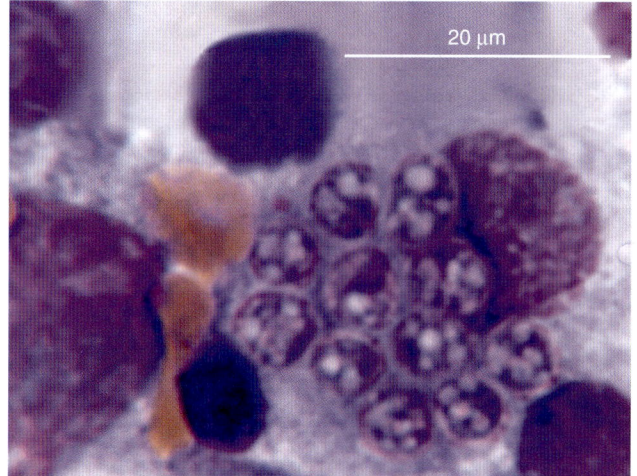

■ **FIGURE 10.52 Protothecosis, colitis. Dog.** Several single-cell *Prototheca* spp. organisms are found within a macrophage in the rectal scrape of a dog with diarrhea. (Wright-Giemsa; HP oil.)

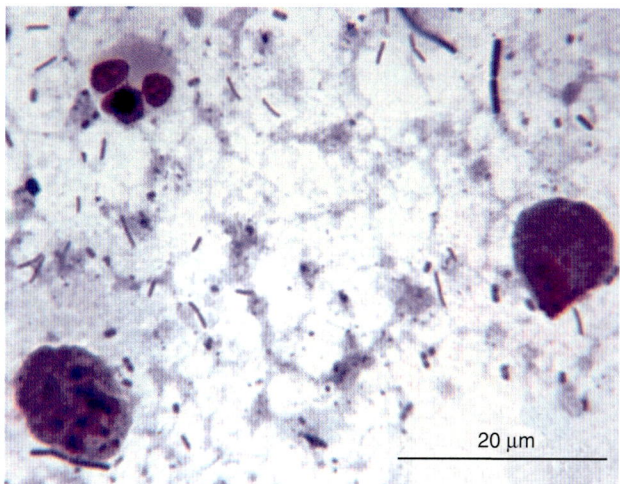

■ **FIGURE 10.53 Entamoebiasis. Dog.** Two *Entamoeba histolytica* protozoal organisms are present along with a single neutrophil *(upper left)* in the feces of a dog with diarrhea. (Wright-Giemsa; HP oil.) (Courtesy Rick Alleman, University of Florida.)

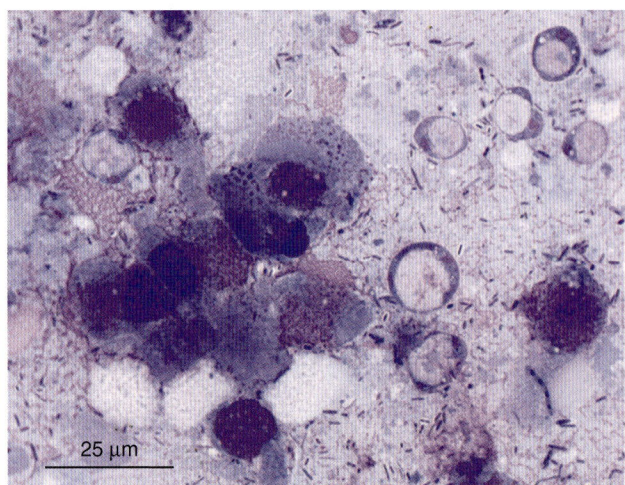

■ **FIGURE 10.54 Blastocystosis. Dog.** Rectal scraping from a dog with diarrhea. Several organisms and well-differentiated epithelial cells are present in a background of mixed bacterial flora. The intestinal organism is most consistent with *Blastocystis* spp., an algal-like protist (stramenopile). The binucleated forms support this identification rather than *Iodamoeba bütschlii*, which can look similar. (Aqueous Romanowsky; HP oil.) (Courtesy Craig Thompson, Purdue University.)

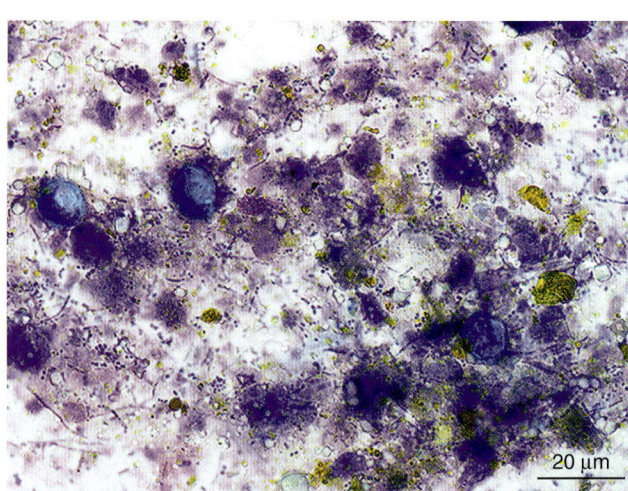

■ **FIGURE 10.56 Blastomycosis. Dog.** Rectal scraping from a 2-year-old Old English sheepdog presented for anorexia, vomiting, and lethargy. Three round or oval *Blastomyces dermatitidis* organisms appear with a mixed bacterial flora and golden yellow heme-pigmented debris. They measure approximately 10.0 to 15.0 μm and have a double-contoured wall with a deeply basophilic internal structure. (Wright-Giemsa; HP oil.) (Courtesy Russell Moore, University of Illinois.)

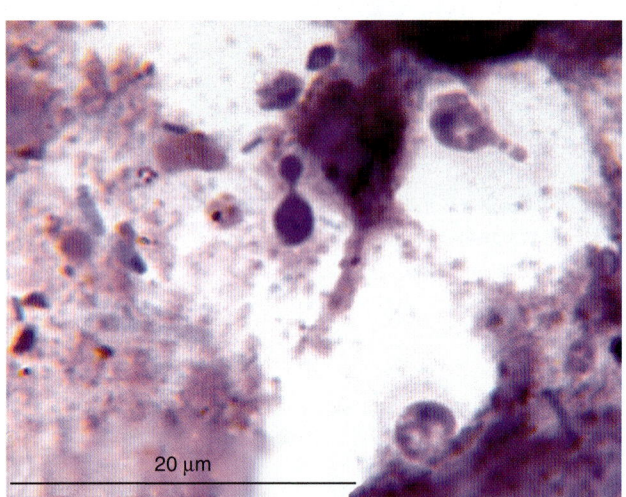

■ **FIGURE 10.55 Cryptococcosis. Dog.** Three budding *(top)* and one nonbudding *(lower right) Cryptococcus* organisms are present with a few bacilli in the feces of a dog with diarrhea. Most forms of *Cryptococcus* develop a thick, polysaccharide capsule that does not stain and is represented by the wide, colorless area surrounding the narrow-based budding, purple yeast. (Wright-Giemsa; HP oil.)

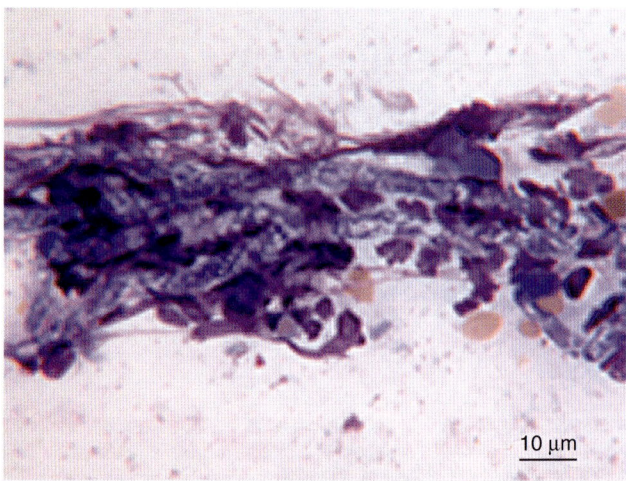

■ **FIGURE 10.57 Oomycosis, colitis. Dog.** A branching oomycete appears surrounded by neutrophils, nucleoproteinaceous material, and erythrocytes in this rectal scraping from a dog with a history of bloody, mucoid diarrhea and inappetence. Other cytopathologic findings not shown consisted of marked mixed inflammation, which was primarily neutrophilic with lesser macrophagic and eosinophilic inflammation. An oomycete, consistent with *Pythium* spp. or *Lagenidium* spp., was cultured. (Wright-Giemsa; HP oil.)

the protist *Blastocystis* spp. (Fig. 10.54), the fungi *Cryptococcus* spp. (Fig. 10.55) and *Blastomyces* spp. (Fig. 10.56), and the oomycete *Pythium* spp. (Fig. 10.57). Of these, *Blastocystis* spp. is unlikely to represent a primary enteric pathogen because approximately 70% of dogs and cats may be carriers without exhibiting intestinal disease (Ruaux and Stang, 2014).

Although dry-mount fecal cytopathology is not the preferred method for the diagnosis of intestinal parasites, ova or oocysts from multicellular parasites and coccidia are occasionally seen in fecal material from affected animals (Figs. 10.58 to 10.61). Other diagnostic tests are usually necessary for confirmation and speciation.

CHAPTER 10 Fecal and Rectal Cytopathology

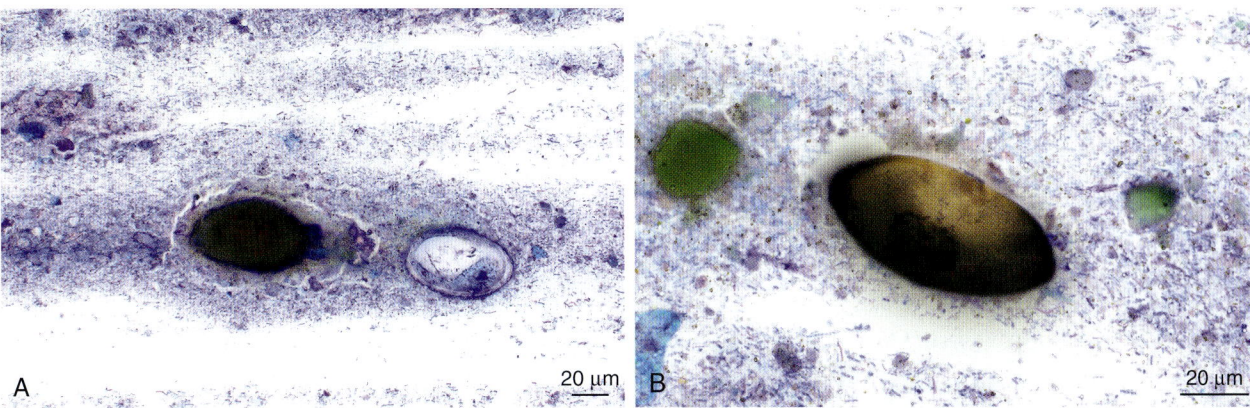

FIGURE 10.58 Nematode ova. Dog. Fecal smear from a 6-year-old mixed-breed dog presented for trauma from a car. **A,** Fecal flotation revealed numerous *Trichuris* spp. *(left)* and *Ancylostoma* spp. *(right)* ova, which were seen on a direct fecal smear. (Wright-Giemsa; HP oil.) **B,** Close-up of a *Trichuris* spp. ovum. (Wright-Giemsa; HP oil.)

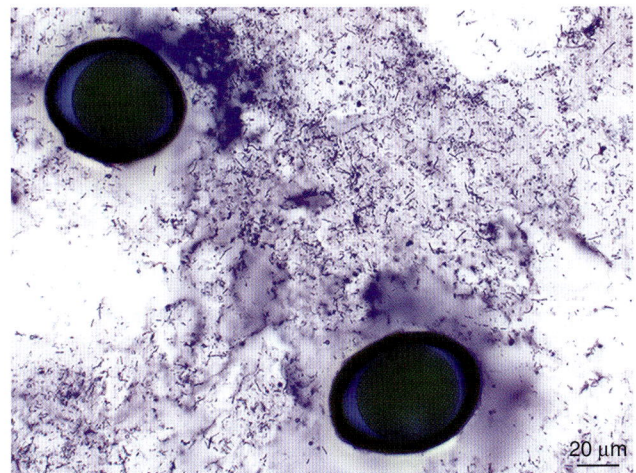

FIGURE 10.59 *Toxocara* spp. ova. Cat. Fecal smear from a 7-year-old domestic shorthair cat. Fecal flotation test revealed numerous *Toxocara* spp. ova that appeared on a fecal smear. (Wright-Giemsa; HP oil.)

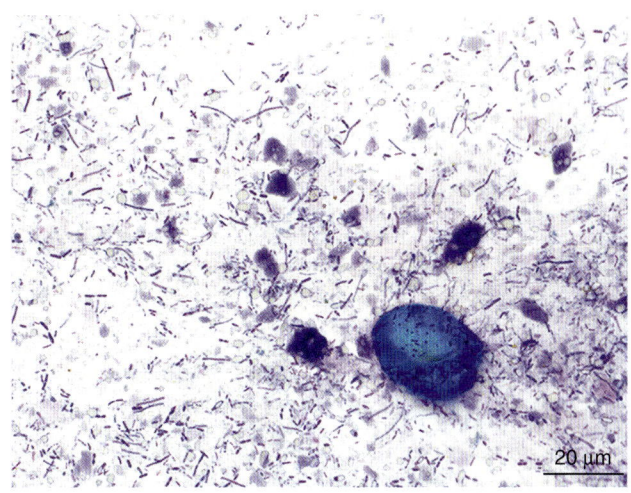

FIGURE 10.61 *Isospora* spp. oocyst. Dog. Fecal smear from a 6-month-old chihuahua presented for bloody diarrhea. *Isospora* spp. oocysts were present on a fecal flotation test and in a fecal smear. (Wright-Giemsa; HP oil.)

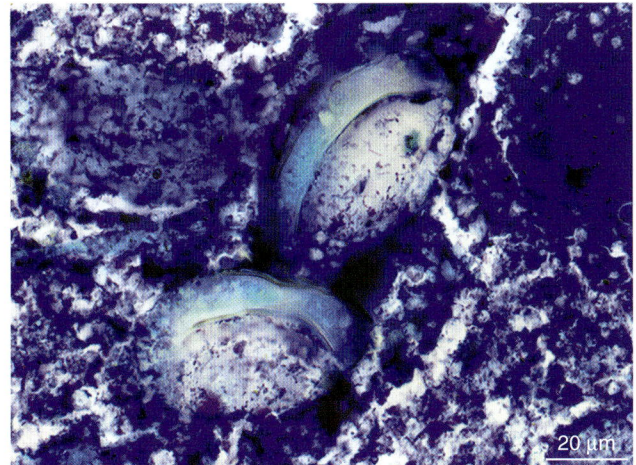

FIGURE 10.60 *Spirometra* spp. ova. Cat. Rectal scraping from a 11-year-old domestic shorthair cat presented for chronic, mixed-bowel diarrhea. Several *Spirometra* spp. ova are found scattered throughout the preparation, which were identified on fecal flotation. (Wright-Giemsa; HP oil.)

REFERENCES

Bastos BF, Brener B, de Figueiredo MA, et al. Pentatrichomonas hominis infection in two domestic cats with chronic diarrhea. *JFMS Open Rep.* 2018;4(1).

Baumgardner DJ, Paretsky DP. Identification of *Blastomyces dermatitidis* in the stool of a dog with acute pulmonary blastomycosis. *J Med Vet Mycol.* 1997;35(6):419-421.

Bender JB, Shulman SA, Averbeck GA, et al. Epidemiologic features of *Campylobacter* infection among cats in the upper Midwestern United States. *J Am Vet Med Assoc.* 2005;226(4):544-547.

Broussard JD. Optimal fecal assessment. *Clin Tech Small Anim Pract.* 2003;18(4):218-230.

Chapman S, Thompson C, Wilcox A, et al. What is your diagnosis? Rectal scraping from a dog with diarrhea. *Vet Clin Pathol.* 2009;38(1):59-62.

Conrado FO, Jones EA, Graham E. Cytologic, histopathologic, and clinical features of granulomatous colitis in a French bulldog. *Vet Clin Pathol.* 2021. Epub ahead of print.

Craven M, Mansfield CS, Simpson KW. Granulomatous colitis of boxer dogs. *Vet Clin North Am Small Anim Pract.* 2011;41(2):433-445.

De Cock HE, Marks SL, Stacy BA, et al. Ileocolitis associated with *Anaerobiospirillum* in cats. *J Clin Microbiol.* 2004;42(6):2752-2758.

Dryden MW, Payne PA, Smith V. Accurate diagnosis of *Giardia* spp. and proper fecal examination procedures. *Vet Ther.* 2006;7(1):4-14.

Evans SE, Bonczynski JJ, Broussard JD, et al. Comparison of endoscopic and full-thickness biopsy specimens for diagnosis of inflammatory bowel disease and alimentary tract lymphoma in cats. *J Am Vet Med Assoc.* 2006;229(9):1447-1450.

Frezoulis PS, Angelidou E, Diakou A, et al. Optimization of fecal cytology in the dog: comparison of three sampling methods. *J Vet Diagn Invest.* 2017;29(5):767-771.

German AJ, Hall EJ, Kelly DF, et al. An immunohistochemical study of histiocytic ulcerative colitis in boxer dogs. *J Comp Pathol.* 2000;122(2-3):163-175.

Gookin JL, Hanrahan K, Levy MG. The conundrum of feline trichomonosis. *J Feline Med Surg.* 2017;19(3):261-274.

Graves TK, Barger AM, Adams B, et al. Diagnosis of systemic cryptococcosis by fecal cytology in a dog. *Vet Clin Pathol.* 2005;34:409-412.

Hall EJ, German AJ. Diseases of the small intestine. In: Ettinger SJ, Feldman EC, eds. *Textbook of Veterinary Internal Medicine.* 6th ed. St. Louis: Elsevier; 2005:1367-1373.

Hedgespeth BA, Stauffer SH, Robertson JB, et al. Association of fecal sample collection technique and treatment history with *Tritrichomonas foetus* polymerase chain reaction test results in 1717 cats. *J Vet Intern Med.* 2020;34:734-741.

Hostutler RA, Luria BJ, Johnson SE, et al. Antibiotic-responsive histiocytic ulcerative colitis in 9 dogs. *J Vet Intern Med.* 2004;18(4):499-504.

Houwers DJ, Blankenstein B. *Cyniclomyces guttulatus* and diarrhea in dogs. *Tijdschr Diergeneeskd.* 2001;126(14-15):502.

Kleinschmidt S, Meneses F, Nolte I, et al. Retrospective study on the diagnostic value of full-thickness biopsies from the stomach and intestines of dogs with chronic gastrointestinal disease symptoms. *Vet Pathol.* 2006;43(6):1000-1003.

Kleinschmidt S, Meneses F, Nolte I, et al. Characterization of mast cell numbers and subtypes in biopsies from the gastrointestinal tract of dogs with lymphocytic-plasmacytic or eosinophilic gastroenterocolitis. *Vet Immunol Immunopathol.* 2007;120(3-4):80-92.

Li WC, Gong PT, Ying M, et al. *Pentatrichomonas hominis*: first isolation from the feces of a dog with diarrhea in China. *Parasitol Res.* 2014;113(5):1795-1801.

Littman MP, Dambach DM, Vaden SL, et al. familial protein-losing enteropathy and protein-losing nephropathy in soft coated wheaten terriers: 222 cases (1983–1997). *J Vet Intern Med.* 2000;14(1):68-80.

Malnick H, Williams K, Phil-Ebosie J, et al. Description of a medium for isolating *Anaerobiospirillum* spp., a possible cause of zoonotic disease, from diarrheal feces and blood of humans and use of the medium in a survey of human, canine, and feline feces. *J Clin Microbiol.* 1990;28(6):1380-1384.

Manchester, AC, Hill S, Sabation B, et al. Association between granulomatous colitis in French bulldogs and invasive *Escherichia coli* and response to fluoroquinolone antimicrobials. *J Vet Intern Med.* 2013;27(1):56-61.

Mandigers PJ, Duijvestijn MB, Ankringa N, et al. The clinical significance of *Cyniclomyces guttulatus* in dogs with chronic diarrhoea, a survey and a prospective treatment study. *Vet Microbiol.* 2014;172(1-2):241-247.

Marks SL, Kather EJ, Kass PH, et al. Genotypic and phenotypic characterization of *Clostridium perfringens* and *Clostridium difficile* in diarrheic and healthy dogs. *J Vet Intern Med.* 2002;16(5):533-540.

Marks SL, Rankin SC, Byrne BA, et al. Enteropathogenic bacteria in dogs and cats: diagnosis, epidemiology, treatment, and control. *J Vet Intern Med.* 2011;25(6):1195-1208.

Marsilio S, Ackermann MR, Lidbury J, et al. Results of histopathology, immunohistochemistry, and molecular clonality testing of small intestinal biopsy specimens from clinically healthy client-owned cats. *J Vet Intern Med.* 2019;33(2):551-555.

Misawa N, Kawashima K, Kondo F, et al. Isolation and characterization of *Campylobacter, Helicobacter,* and *Anaerobiospirillum* strains from a puppy with bloody diarrhea. *Vet Microbiol.* 2002;87(4):353-364.

Mundt LA, Shanahan K. Fecal analysis. In: *Graff's Textbook of Routine Urinalysis and Body Fluids.* Philadelphia: Lippincott Williams & Wilkins; 2011:281.

Payne PA, Artzer M. The biology and control of *Giardia* spp. and *Tritrichomonas foetus.* *Vet Clin North Am Small Anim Pract.* 2009;39(6):993-1007.

Rallis TS, Tontis D, Adamama-Moraitou KK, et al. Protothecal colitis in a German shepherd dog. *Aust Vet J.* 2002;80(7):406-408.

Rossi M, Hänninen ML, Revez J, et al. Occurrence and species level diagnostics of *Campylobacter* spp., enteric *Helicobacter* spp. and *Anaerobiospirillum* spp. In healthy and diarrheic dogs and cats. *Vet Microbiol.* 2008;129(3-4):304-314.

Ruaux CG, Stang BV. Prevalence of blastocystis in shelter-resident and client-owned companion animals in the US Pacific Northwest. *PLoS One.* 2014;9(9):e107496.

Sabattini S, Bottero E, Turba ME, et al. Differentiating feline inflammatory bowel disease from alimentary lymphoma in duodenal endoscopic biopsies. *J Small Anim Pract.* 2016;57(8):396-401.

Saleh MN, Heptinstall JR, Johnson EM, et al. Comparison of diagnostic techniques for detection of *Giardia duodenalis* in dogs and cats. *J Vet Intern Med.* 2019;33(3):1272-1277.

Sindern N, Suchodolski JS, Leutenegger CM, et al. Prevalence of *Clostridium perfringens* netE and netF toxin genes in the feces of dogs with acute hemorrhagic diarrhea syndrome. *J Vet Intern Med.* 2019;33(1):100-105.

Spoor MS, Royal AB, Berent LM. The elusive globule leukocyte. *Vet Clin Pathol.* 2011;40(2):136.

Stenner VJ, Mackay B, King T, et al. Protothecosis in 17 Australian dogs and a review of the canine literature. *Med Mycol.* 2007;45(3):249-266.

Suchodolski JS. Intestinal microbiota of dogs and cats: a bigger world than we thought. *Vet Clin North Am Small Anim Pract.* 2011;41(2):261-272.

Tucker S, Penninck DG, Keating JH, et al. Clinicopathological and ultrasonographic features of cats with eosinophilic enteritis. *J Feline Med Surg.* 2014;16(12):950-956.

Uehlinger FD, Naqvi SA, Greenwood SJ, et al. Comparison of five diagnostic tests for *Giardia duodenalis* in fecal samples from young dogs. *Vet Parasitol.* 2017;244:91-96.

Vince AR, Pinard C, Ogilvie AT, et al. Protothecosis in a dog. *Can Vet J.* 2014;55(10):950-954.

Vogel P, Janke L, Gravano DM, et al. Globule leukocytes and other mast cells in the mouse intestine. *Vet Pathol.* 2018;55(1):76-97.

Winston JA, Piperisova I, Neel J, et al. *Cyniclomyces guttulatus* infection in dogs: 19 cases (2006–2013). *J Am Anim Hosp Assoc.* 2016;52(1):42-51.

Yao C, Köster LS. *Tritrichomonas foetus* infection, a cause of chronic diarrhea in the domestic cat. *Vet Res.* 2015;46:35.

Yoon MY, Yoon SS. Disruption of the gut ecosystem by antibiotics. *Yonsei Med J.* 2018;59(1):4-12.

Zierdt CH, Detlefson C, Muller J, et al. *Cyniclomyces guttulatus (Saccharomycopsis guttulata)*-culture, ultrastructure and physiology. *Antonie Van Leeuwenhoek.* 1988;54(4):357-366.

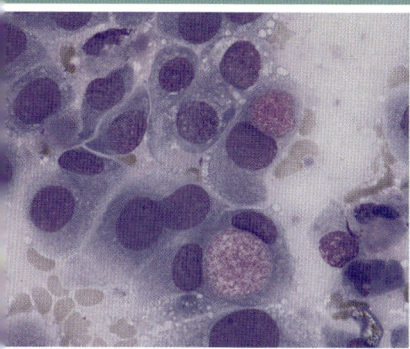

CHAPTER 11

Urinary System

Laura Snyder and Davis Seelig

KIDNEYS

Normal Anatomy and Histology

The urinary system is composed of kidneys, ureters, urinary bladder, and urethra. The kidney has four basic morphologic components: glomeruli, tubules, interstitium, and blood vessels (Fig. 11.1). The functional unit of the kidney is the nephron. Each nephron is composed of a glomerulus and renal tubule system. The glomerulus is a capillary tuft lined by fenestrated endothelium that is intimately associated with tubule epithelial cells. Components of the glomerulus (Fig. 11.2), including the endothelium, basement membrane, and specialized epithelial cells known as podocytes, make up the filtration barrier of the kidney.

The renal tubule is divided into distinct functional segments, including the proximal convoluted tubule, loop of Henle (ascending and descending limbs), distal convoluted tubule, and collecting ducts. Reflective of function, the epithelial cells lining the tubules vary from a single layer of cuboidal cells with a brush border in the proximal convoluted tubules to columnar epithelium with no brush border in the distal convoluted segments (Fig. 11.3). Caudate urothelial cells line the renal pelvis and calyces. Similarly, the mucosa of the ureters, urinary bladder, and urethra are lined almost exclusively by urothelial epithelial cells that allow stretching. Renal interstitial tissue is composed of connective tissue (mesenchymal cells), an extensive capillary network, lymphatic tissue, and smooth muscle cells (Borjesson, 2003). Periodic acid–Schiff (PAS) staining helps to differentiate the proximal tubule (positive) from the distal tubule (negative) on histopathology. The distal tubules have a prominent lumen compared with the distal tubule, which is nearly completely filled. Capillaries are identified by compressed dense nuclei along a lumen often filled with erythrocytes (see Fig. 11.3).

Specialized Renal Collection Techniques

Renal tissue biopsy is frequently indicated in dogs and cats with glomerular disease (and proteinuria) or acute kidney injury (Nowicki et al., 2010). Tissue biopsy can be performed under ultrasound guidance or using surgical methods (Debruyn et al., 2012). The increased risks associated with tissue biopsy include the transection of blood vessels or renal pelvis with resultant hemorrhage, hydronephrosis, or hematuria (Borjesson, 2003). A multi-institutional study found complication rates for renal tissue biopsy of dogs and cats at 13.4% and 18.5%, respectively (Vaden et al., 2005; Nowicki et al., 2010). The most common complication was hemorrhage. There have been a number of recent published reviews comparing renal tissue biopsy methods to optimize specimen procurement and minimize complications (Rawlings et al., 2003; Rawlings and Howerth, 2004; Vaden, 2004; Vaden, 2005; Vaden et al., 2005).

For fine-needle aspirate biopsy (FNAB), manual kidney immobilization, and blind percutaneous aspiration can be used to obtain samples for cytopathologic review, especially in cats. However, this technique is best reserved for diffuse lesions that result in renomegaly because focal lesions may be missed, and there is an increased risk of inadvertent puncture or laceration of major blood vessels. Ultrasound-guided FNAB is recommended because it is minimally invasive and has a low complication rate (Debruyn et al., 2012). In the two largest cases, representing 100 dogs and 93 cats, the overall diagnostic yield of ultrasound-guided FNAB cytopathology samples was considered good (72% for dogs and 68% for cats) but did vary according to specific renal ultrasonographic characteristics (McAloney et al., 2018a, 2018b). In the dog, FNAB samples that were obtained from kidneys with ultrasonographic pelvic dilation, unclear corticomedullary interface, or an infiltrative or nodular appearance had the highest diagnostic yields (McAloney et al., 2018a). In cats, FNAB samples that were obtained from kidneys with ultrasonographic subcapsular renal infiltrate, diffuse renal enlargement, or an infiltrative or nodular appearance had the highest diagnostic yields (McAloney et al., 2018b). The primary potential complication is hemorrhage; therefore, a platelet count, clotting profile, and inquiry regarding administration of blood thinners are considered prudent and recommended. However, in the two case series referenced previously, no complications (including hemorrhage) were reported.

> **KEY POINT** Ultrasonographic findings that are most frequently associated with obtaining a diagnostic renal FNAB sample are:
> - Dogs: pelvic dilation, unclear corticomedullary interface, an infiltrative or nodular appearance
> - Cats: subcapsular renal infiltrate, diffuse renal enlargement, an infiltrative or nodular appearance

For ultrasound-guided FNAB, the patient is maintained in dorsal recumbency. If changes are bilateral, aspiration of the caudal pole of left kidney is recommended because it decreases the risk of inadvertent aspiration of bowel and pancreas. The needle is directed from the cortex of the caudal pole, ventral to

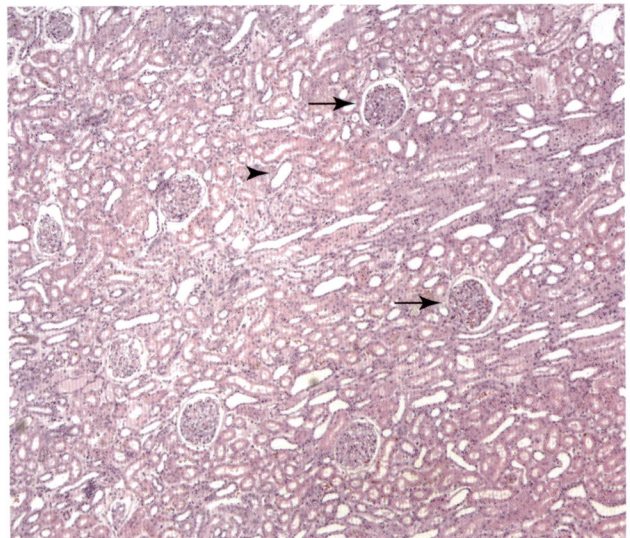

■ **FIGURE 11.1 Normal kidney. Histology. Dog.** Glomeruli *(arrows)* are found amid renal tubules *(arrowhead)* sectioned longitudinally. Typically, a single layer of cuboidal epithelial cells lines the tubules. (H&E; IP.)

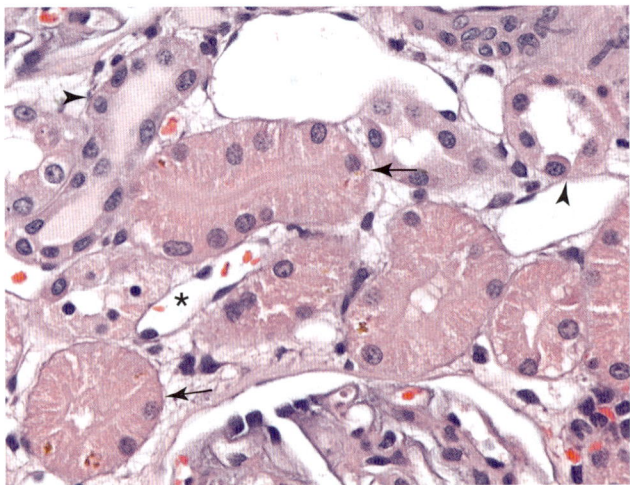

■ **FIGURE 11.3 Normal kidney cortex. Renal tubules. Histology. Dog.** Note proximal tubules *(arrows)* with the characteristic pink, thick brush border lining the tubular lumen and nearby distal tubules *(arrowheads)* with a single layer of epithelial cells and no brush border. Periodic acid–Schiff staining is positive for the proximal tubules and negative for the distal tubules (not shown). The flattened layer of endothelial cells and the presence of erythrocytes within the lumen easily identify a capillary *(asterisk)*. (H&E; HP oil.)

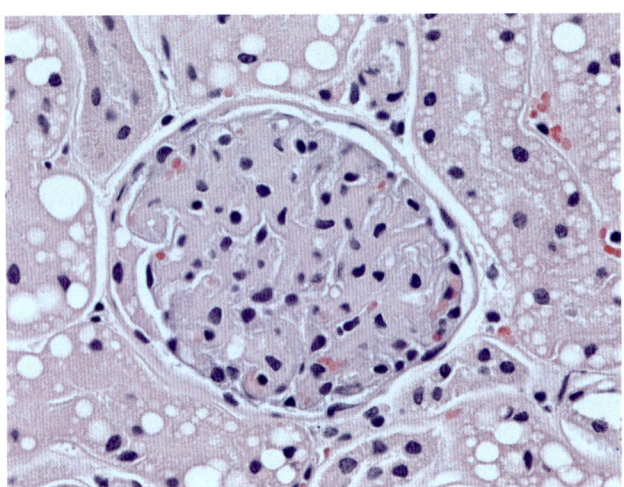

■ **FIGURE 11.2 Normal kidney cortex. Glomerulus. Histology. Cat.** Magnification of a single glomerulus with a central capillary tuft lined by fenestrated endothelium (not demonstrated). Normal feline renal tubular cells with intracytoplasmic lipid vacuoles surround the glomerulus. (H&E; HP oil.)

dorsal. The needle can be angled from medial to lateral to avoid hitting a large renal vessel. Care should be taken to avoid hitting the renal pelvis, which could result in hematuria. Begin with a 25- to 27-gauge, 1½-inch needle. If sample of adequate cellularity is not obtained, a larger bore needle can be used. The best results are obtained if multiple preparations are made and one slide is rapidly stained with either a Romanowsky stain or new methylene blue stain to assess sample adequacy (Borjesson, 2003).

Regardless of the type of mass, aspiration of both the central and peripheral areas is recommended because the center of a mass may consist of necrotic debris or inflammatory cells, resulting in a misleading or nondiagnostic sample. Although purulent inflammation and necrosis can be associated with malignancy, abundance of either may mask the primary disorder. Thus, multiple aspirations in different areas of the mass are generally recommended to maximize cellular yield and diagnostic potential as well as to differentiate between primary and secondary inflammation (Borjesson, 2003). If fluid is obtained, a direct smear can be made immediately and the remaining fluid can be placed into ethylenediaminetetraacetic acid (EDTA) to prevent clotting. Both sediment and cytocentrifuged smears can then be prepared, especially if the sample is of low cellularity. Finally, impression smears can be made from renal tissue biopsy specimens. Cytopathologic evaluation of impression smears can aid in rapid diagnosis of infection or neoplasia (Borjesson, 2003).

Normal Renal Cytology

Renal aspirates are typically of low cellularity and usually contain small tubules and clusters of renal tubular cells admixed with blood. Because the kidneys are highly vascular, the presence of blood is to be expected and generally considered iatrogenic. Tubular cells generally exfoliate singly or in small clusters of round, oval, cuboidal, or columnar cells. They have abundant basophilic, occasionally vacuolated cytoplasm that surrounds a uniform, round, often eccentrically placed nucleus (Fig. 11.4). Feline tubular cells are cytologically similar except that cats normally have lipid deposition within their renal tubules. Lipid droplets appear as prominent, variably sized, intracytoplasmic, colorless, punctate vacuoles (Figs. 11.5 and 11.6). Fully intact renal tubules arranged in cohesive linear structures may also be present (Fig. 11.7). Tubular cells can also contain dark, intracytoplasmic granules of lipofuscin that should not be confused with a well-differentiated melanocyte tumor (Fig. 11.8). Glomeruli may exfoliate singly or in dense, deeply basophilic, rounded clusters and have very uniform round to oval nuclei (Fig. 11.9). Uncommonly, melanin may be found in a normal kidney but may result from chronic injury

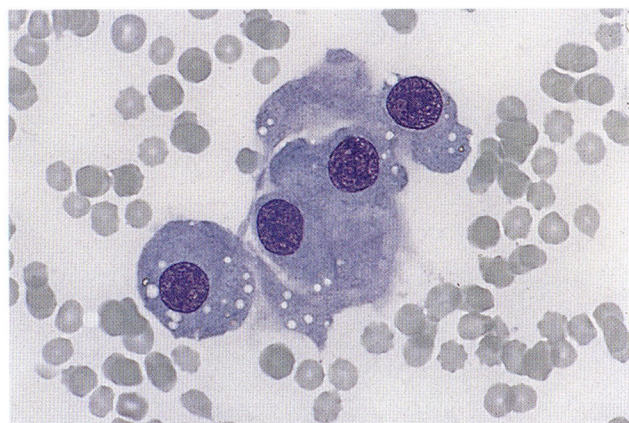

■ **FIGURE 11.4 Renal tubular epithelial cells. Cytologic specimen. Dog.** Depicted is a small group of renal tubular cells that vary from round to columnar in appearance. The background erythrocytes provide a perspective on cell size. (Wright-Giemsa; HP oil.)

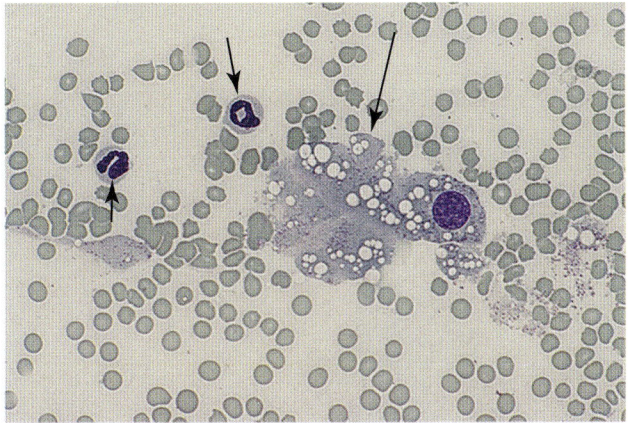

■ **FIGURE 11.5 Renal tubular epithelial cells. Cytology specimen. Cat.** Note the variably sized intracytoplasmic lipid droplets that appear as clear, punctate vacuoles within the renal tubule cells. Free vacuolated cytoplasm from a ruptured cell is also present *(long arrow)*. The size of the tubular cells can be compared with the neutrophils present *(short arrows)*. (Wright-Giemsa; HP oil.)

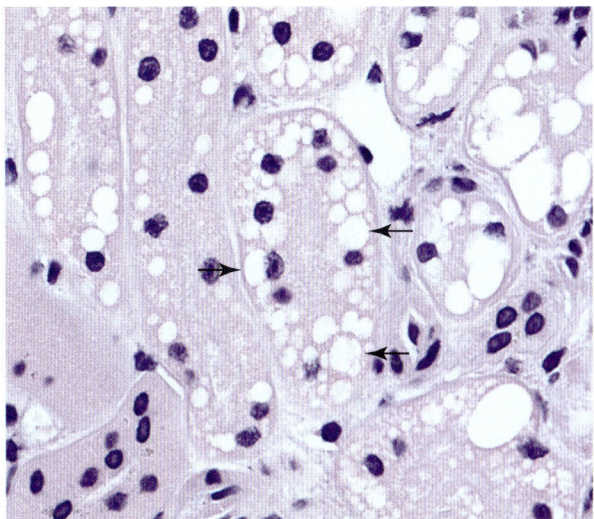

■ **FIGURE 11.6 Renal tubules. Histology. Cat.** Note the variably sized intracytoplasmic lipid droplets that appear as clear, punctate vacuoles within these proximal renal tubule cells. A cross-section of a single tubule is demonstrated *(arrows)*. (H&E; HP oil.)

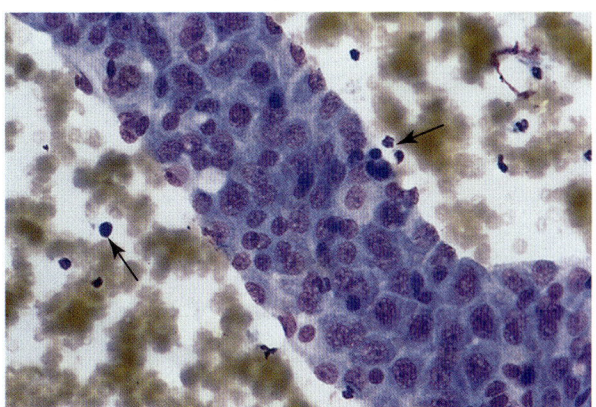

■ **FIGURE 11.7 Intact renal tubule. Cytologic specimen.** Cells within the tubule are minimally pleomorphic. Cell nuclei are round and uniform with small regular nucleoli. The large size is suggestive of a collecting duct or distal tubule. Leukocytes *(arrows)* provide a perspective of size of the structure. (Wright-Giemsa; HP oil.)

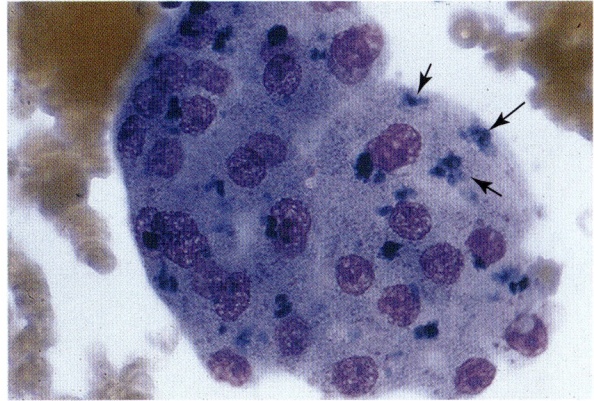

■ **FIGURE 11.8 Renal tubule. Lipofuscin pigmentation. Cytopathologic specimen.** The dark intracytoplasmic granules of lipofuscin *(arrows)* of the cells composing this segment of a tubule indicate the ascending loop of Henle or distal tubules as the site of origin. The possibility of a well-differentiated melanocyte tumor could be an initial misleading impression. (Wright-Giemsa; HP oil.)

and should not be confused with neoplasia (Cooper, 2002) (Fig. 11.10).

Noninfectious Inflammatory Disorders
Crystals

Crystals are rarely noted in cytopathologic preparations from renal aspirates. However, their presence can be very useful to diagnose nephrotoxicosis or tissue damage. Oxalic acid, a metabolite of ethylene glycol, can precipitate in renal tubules as calcium oxalate crystals (Fig. 11.11). Cytopathologically, these crystals appear clear and colorless, with barely perceptible ragged to linear borders (Fig. 11.12A). These crystals are readily visualized under polarized light (Fig. 11.12B).

Acute kidney injury and intratubular crystals have also been associated with outbreaks of nephrotoxicosis caused by ingestion of contaminated pet food (Puschner and Reimschuessel, 2011). Pale green to golden yellow, round to dumbbell-shaped crystals have been identified on renal histopathology (Fig. 11.13) and in urine sediment cytopathology. These crystals are suggestive of

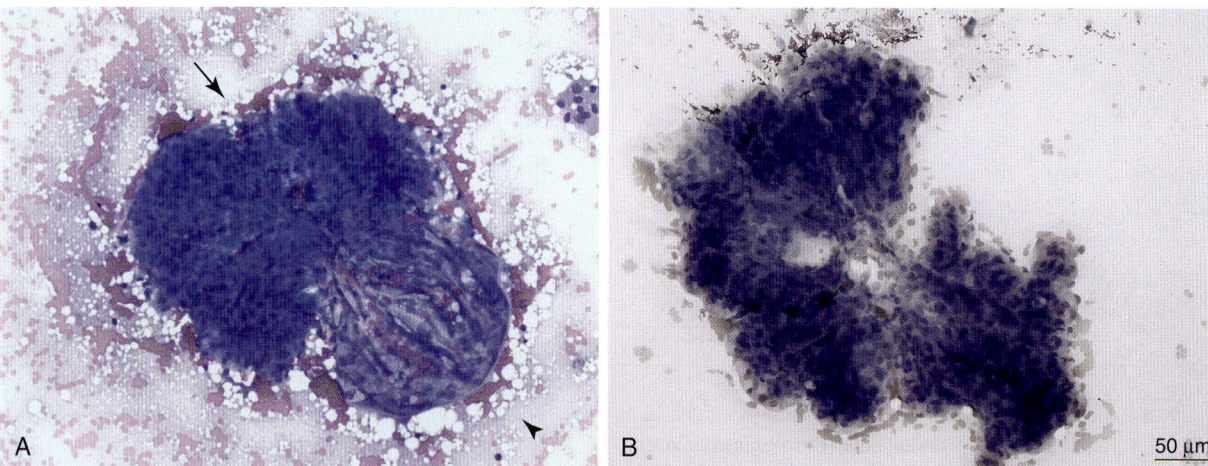

FIGURE 11.9 Glomeruli. Renal cortex. Aspirate. A, Intact. A single intact glomerulus with one end *(arrowhead)* consisting of a capillary tuft with linear vascular endothelium and the opposite end *(arrow)* consisting of tubule epithelial cells. (Wright-Giemsa; IP.) **B, Partially intact. Cat.** The patient presented with multiple round, well-defined, anechoic, enhancing structures. In addition to tubular structures (not shown), a rare dense tuft of cells, consistent with a glomerulus, is found. The glomerulus is partially ruptured, a more common finding relative to the integrity of glomeruli in cytopathologic preparations. (Wright-Giemsa; IP.) (A, From Friedrichs KR. Laboratory medicine—yesterday, today, tomorrow: renal resplendence. *Vet Clin Pathol* 2007;36:7. B, Courtesy Rose Raskin, University of Florida.)

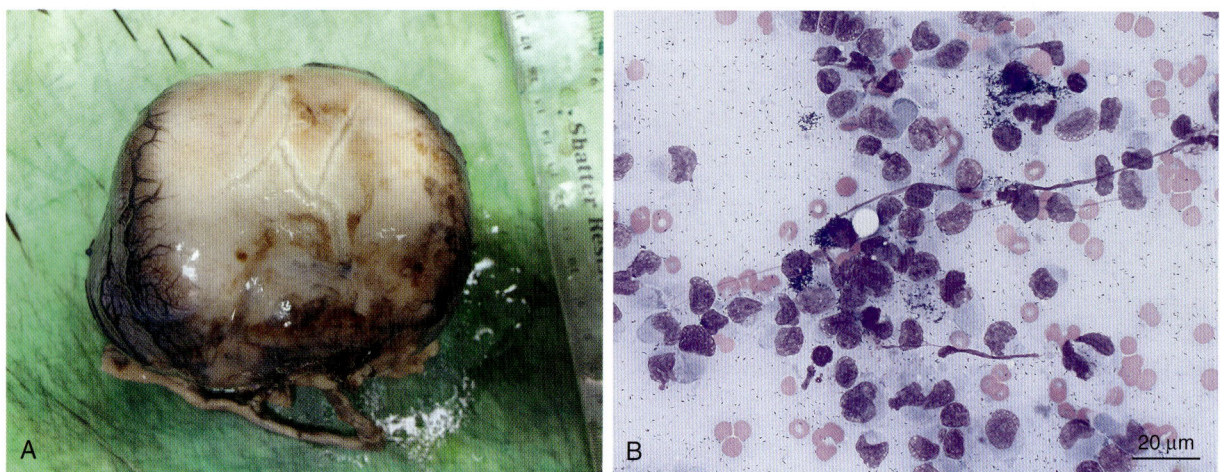

FIGURE 11.10 Melanosis. Kidney. Dog. Same case in A and B. **A, Macroscopic.** The overall pale tan color of the kidney is the result of histologically confirmed diffuse lymphoma infiltration. In addition, brown patches over the surface and especially surrounding blood vessels are related to melanin deposition, likely secondary to kidney disease. **B, Microscopic.** Present between low numbers of neoplastic lymphocytes are individualized melanocytes that contain fine black granules. Initial concern was given to a diagnosis of melanoma, especially in areas of dense melanocyte presence. However, melanocytic neoplasia was not histologically confirmed. (Wright-Giemsa; HP oil.) (Courtesy Rose Raskin, University of Florida.)

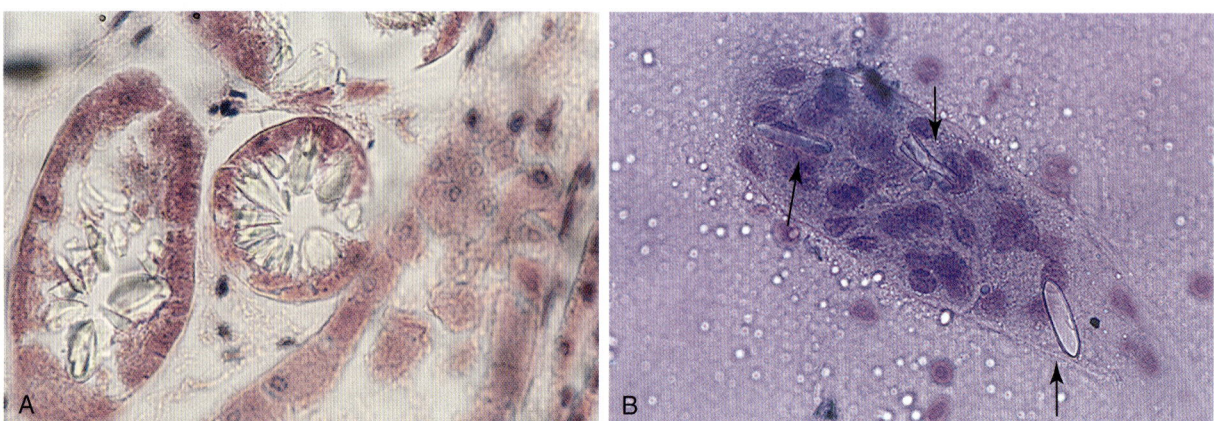

FIGURE 11.11 Ethylene glycol toxicosis. Renal tubules. Dog. Same case in A and B. **A, Histology.** Calcium oxalate monohydrate crystals are imbedded in two renal tubules taken at necropsy. (H&E; HP oil.) **B, Touch imprint.** Calcium oxalate monohydrate crystals are imbedded in the renal tubules *(arrows)*. (NMB; HP oil.) (Courtesy Denny Meyer.)

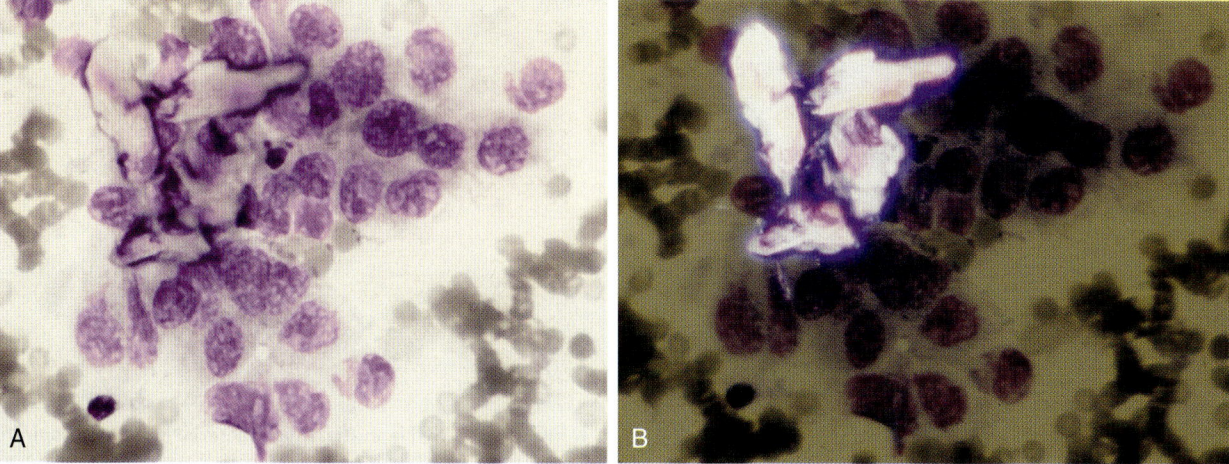

■ **FIGURE 11.12 Ethylene glycol toxicosis. Kidney aspirate. Cat.** Same case in A and B. **A, Nonpolarized.** Irregularly shaped crystals were present within renal tubular epithelium from an animal diagnosed histologically with oxalate crystals at necropsy. (Wright-Giemsa; HP oil.) **B, Polarized.** The polarizing filter demonstrates that the irregularly shaped crystals present within renal tubular epithelium were refractive as expected for calcium oxalate. (Wright-Giemsa; HP oil.) (Courtesy Rose Raskin, University of Florida.)

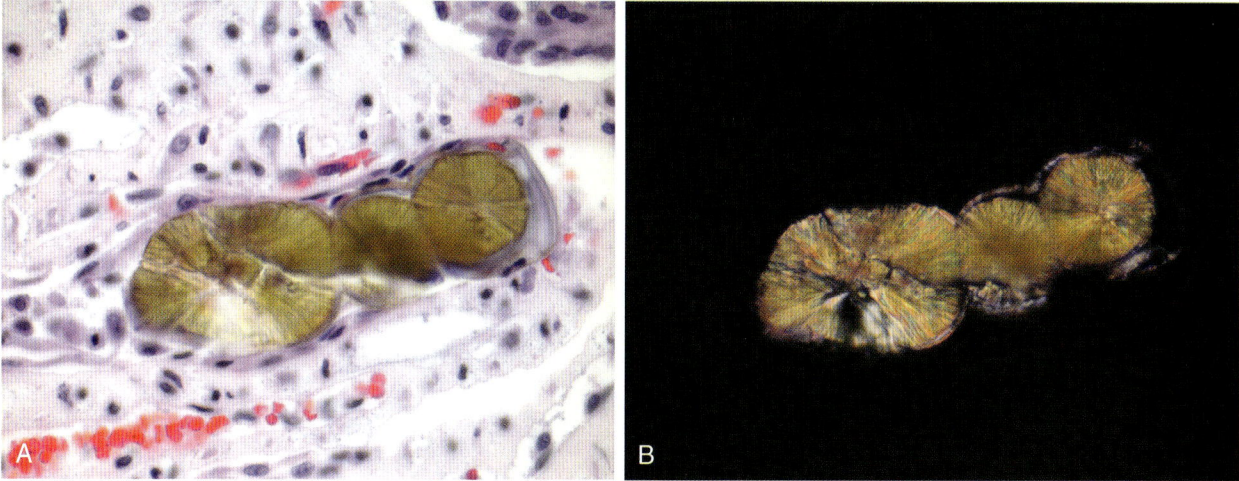

■ **FIGURE 11.13 Pet food toxicosis. Renal tubules. Histology. Dog.** Same case in A and B. **A, Nonpolarized.** Note the large, yellow to golden, round to oval crystals filling this renal tubule and compressing renal tubule epithelial cells. These crystals are presumed to form secondary to melamine and cyanuric acid precipitation associated with consumption of tainted dog food in 2007. Acute tubular necrosis is present but not depicted here. **B, Polarized.** This filter demonstrates a colorful refractivity of crystals within the tubules. (Courtesy Jessica Hoane, Michigan State University.)

those formed from the combined precipitation of melamine and cyanuric acid and may be readily misclassified as green-tinged calcium carbonate crystals or smooth ammonium biurate crystals.

Calcification as dystrophic mineralization may result after tissue necrosis from inflammation, degeneration, or thrombosis or as metastatic mineralization from hypercalcemia and/or hyperphosphatemia (Fig. 11.14).

Infectious Inflammatory Disorders

Pyelonephritis is an inflammatory tubulointerstitial disease that often results from an ascending infection of the lower urinary tract. Hematogenous spread of infectious agents with specific tropism for renal tubules, such as in canine leptospirosis, is less common. Marked suppurative inflammation is easily diagnosed cytopathologically and is characterized by increased numbers of neutrophils with scattered activated macrophages (Fig. 11.15). When the underlying etiology is bacterial infection, intracytoplasmic bacteria can be noted such as *Mycobacterium* spp. (Fig. 11.16). Bacterial culture and sensitivity are recommended even if bacteria are not observed. Similarly, systemic algal (e.g., *Prototheca zopfii*), fungal (e.g., *Cryptococcus neoformans*, *Aspergillus* spp., and phaeohyphomycosis) (Giri et al., 2011), protozoal (e.g., *Leishmania* spp.) (Zatelli et al., 2003), and amebic (e.g., *Balamuthia mandrillaris*) (Foreman et al., 2004) infections can localize in the kidneys and be readily diagnosed cytopathologically. Cytopathology of these lesions is characterized by mixed inflammation, clusters of renal tubular cells, and the presence of organisms. Samples obtained by FNAB can also be submitted for fungal culture or other diagnostic techniques (e.g., polymerase chain reaction [PCR]). Feline infectious peritonitis involving the kidney is uncommonly diagnosed using cytopathology (Giordano et al., 2005). However, the aspirates are characterized by pyogranulomatous inflammation (refer to Figs. 6.14B and 9.49). The cytopathologic finding complements a presumptive diagnosis predicated on the cat's history, presenting symptoms, examination of cavitary effusion if it is present,

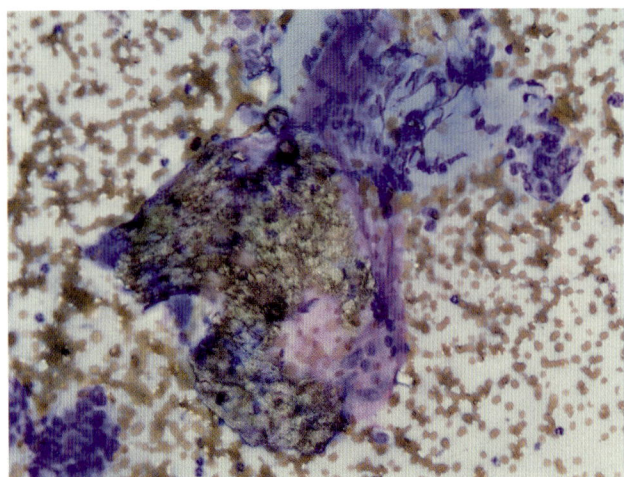

■ **FIGURE 11.14 Calcification. Renal aspirate. Cat.** The patient presented with acute kidney injury with enlarged kidneys having reduced corticomedullary definition. The refractile granular material is associated with the glomerular capillary tufts (pink bands) and most likely represents calcification given this patient's calcium × phosphorus product was 147 (normal <70). This could result from either dystrophic or metastatic calcification. (Wright; IP.) (Courtesy Rose Raskin, Royal Veterinary College, UK.)

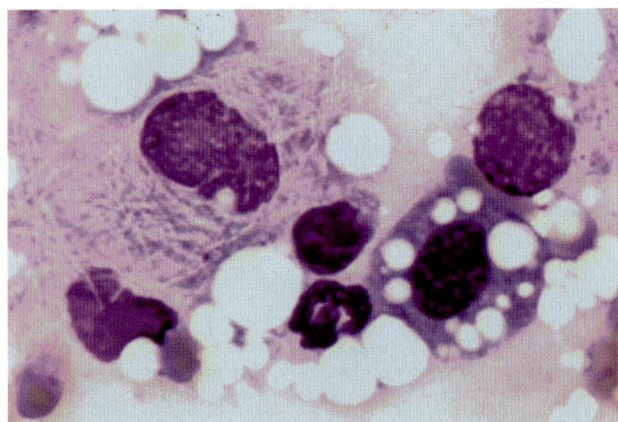

■ **FIGURE 11.16 Nephritis. Mycobacterial infection. Aspirate. Cat.** One intact macrophage contains *Mycobacterium* spp. as demonstrated by negative-staining streaks within the cytoplasm. Also present is a typical feline renal tubular epithelial cell having multiple discrete lipid cytoplasmic vacuoles along with a neutrophil and a small lymphocyte *(center)*. This animal had a systemic infection. (Wright-Giemsa; HP oil.) (Courtesy Rose Raskin, University of Florida.)

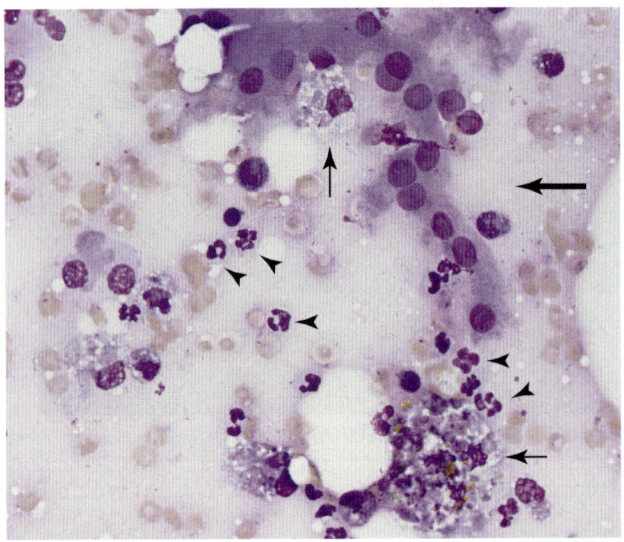

■ **FIGURE 11.15 Nephritis. Kidney. Cytopathologic specimen.** Note the small, cohesive cluster of basophilic renal tubular cells *(larger arrow)* admixed with a population of nondegenerate neutrophils *(arrowheads)*. Large, foamy macrophages *(small arrows)* containing smooth, blue cellular debris are also present. Pyelonephritis was suspected. (Wright-Giemsa; HP oil.)

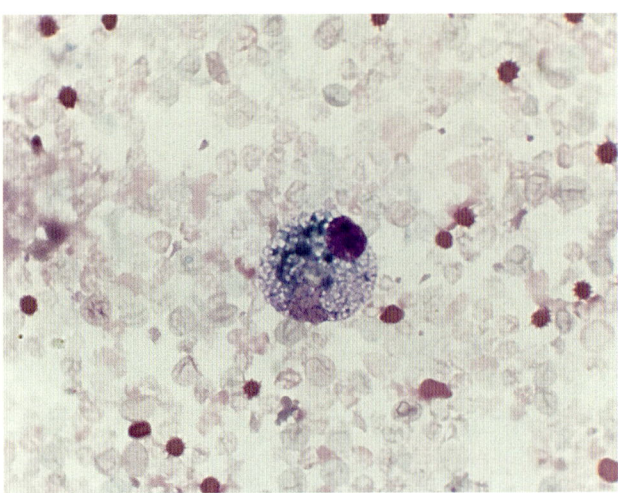

■ **FIGURE 11.17 Renal cyst. Aspirate. Fluid smear.** Cystic fluid is often of low cellularity with a proteinaceous background. Macrophages typically predominate and exhibit erythrophagia or contain heme breakdown products when hemorrhage is present, such as hemosiderin in this image. (Aqueous Romanowsky; HP oil.)

and the results of supporting laboratory tests, including a positive coronavirus PCR or immunofluorescence assay result.

Non-neoplastic Tumors
Cysts and Pseudocysts

Renal cysts may be acquired or congenital and single or multiple. They are thin walled, lined by flattened or cuboidal epithelium, and filled with watery, clear to yellow-tinged fluid. Clinical history and ultrasonographic evaluation may be sufficient to diagnose polycystic kidney disease; however, cytopathologic evaluation may be valuable to rule out abscesses and neoplasia. Renal cysts have variable cellularity composed predominantly of macrophages on a stippled proteinaceous background (Fig. 11.17).

Blood is often present, and erythrophagia or macrophages containing hemosiderin or hematoidin crystals may be observed (Borjesson, 2003).

Perinephric pseudocysts are not lined by epithelium and therefore are not true cysts. Rather, these are collections of fluid that develop between the renal capsule and the renal reflection of the peritoneum. Cats are more commonly affected than dogs and may have coexisting chronic renal disease. Pseudocyst fluid is often watery, clear, and of low very cellularity with low numbers of small lymphocytes.

Note that some renal neoplasms may have a cystic component. Neoplastic cells may or may not exfoliate into the accumulated fluid. Aspiration of solid components associated with a cystic structure or mass should be performed if present.

Neoplastic Tumors

Primary renal tumors are uncommon in dogs and cats (Henry et al., 1999; Bryan et al., 2006). Tumors can arise from epithelial tissue, mesenchymal tissue, or embryonal tissue of mixed origin. Several paraneoplastic syndromes, including polycythemia, leukocytosis, hypertrophic osteopathy, and hypercalcemia, have been described secondary to renal tumors (Peeters et al., 2001; Chiang et al., 2007; Gajanayake et al., 2010; Durno et al., 2011; Johnson and Lenz, 2011; Petterino et al., 2011). Most primary renal tumors in both dogs and cats consist of malignant epithelial tumors (renal carcinoma, urothelial carcinoma [previously known as transitional cell carcinoma], and adenocarcinoma) (Henry et al., 1999; Ramos-Vara et al., 2003; Bryan et al., 2006). Renal carcinomas frequently are immunoreactive to both cytokeratin and vimentin antibodies (Gil da Costa et al., 2011). Other tumors include renal adenoma, urothelial papilloma (previously termed transitional cell papilloma), fibroma, sarcoma (including hemangiosarcoma, fibrosarcoma, leiomyosarcoma, and osteosarcoma) (Sato et al., 2003), and nephroblastoma. Renal lymphoma, a common entity in cats, may represent primary renal neoplasia or be a manifestation of multicentric disease (Snead, 2005; Breshears et al., 2011).

Renal Adenoma and Carcinoma

Renal adenoma and carcinoma are benign and malignant neoplastic proliferations of tubular cell origin and comprise 10% and 65% of primary renal neoplasms in dogs, respectively (Baskin and DePaoli, 1977). Renal adenomas are often round, well-circumscribed, compressive, and unencapsulated cortical nodules measuring 0.5 to 2.0 cm in diameter. Although renal adenomas are typically incidental findings, dogs with renal carcinoma are often presented for progressive weight loss and hematuria. Renal carcinomas tend to be large, firm, solitary masses measuring 1 to 22 cm in diameter with a 56% metastatic rate to the lungs, liver, serosal surfaces, or other sites.

Malignant renal epithelial neoplasms often exfoliate well for cytopathologic evaluation. In general, renal carcinomas are characterized by high cellularity with many cells observed in variably sized, loose aggregates to poorly cohesive clusters (Figs. 11.18 to 11.20). Because of the number of single, occasionally round cells present in renal carcinomas, they can be mistaken for nephroblastomas, round cell tumors, or neuroendocrine tumors.

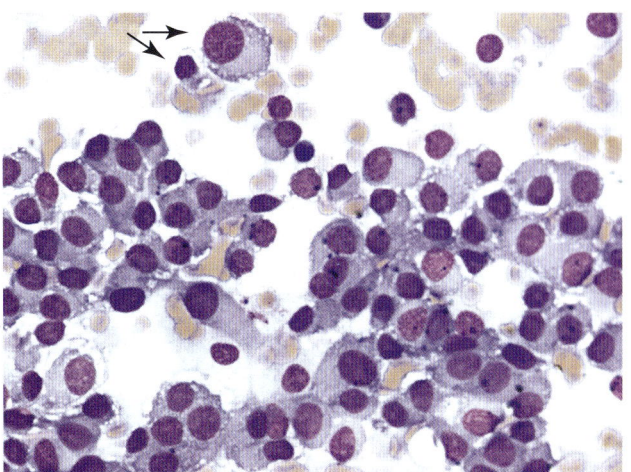

FIGURE 11.19 Renal carcinoma. Cytopathologic specimen. This cluster of poorly cohesive cuboidal cells shows moderately increased nucleocytoplasmic ratios with mild to occasionally marked anisocytosis and anisokaryosis *(arrows)*. Erythrocytes admixed can be used to denote size of the neoplastic cells. (Wright-Giemsa; HP oil.)

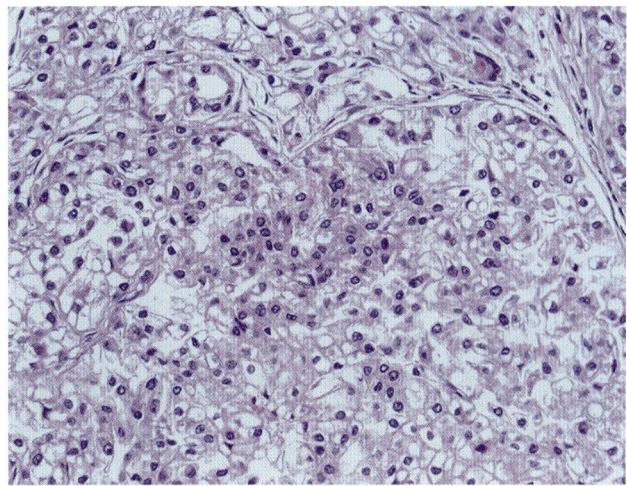

FIGURE 11.20 Renal carcinoma. Histology. Dog. The mass is composed of haphazard tubules and structures lined by polygonal cells supported by a fibrovascular stroma. Individual cells have centrally located round to oval nuclei with dispersed chromatin and occasional prominent nucleoli. Cytoplasm is abundant and varies from clear to eosinophilic and granular. Anisokaryosis is moderate. (H&E; HP oil.)

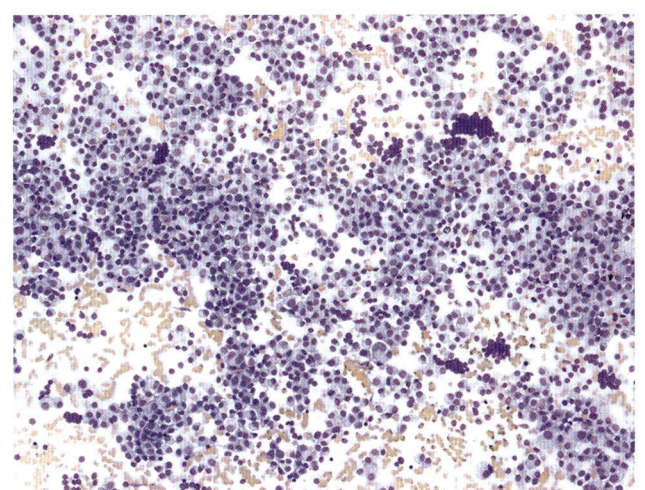

FIGURE 11.18 Renal carcinoma. Cytopathologic specimen. Note the high cellularity. Neoplastic cells are found individually and in loose clusters or sheets. Cells are only minimally pleomorphic. With renal tumors, it can be difficult to differentiate between poorly cohesive carcinomas (depicted here), nephroblastomas, and round cell tumors. (Wright-Giemsa; IP.)

Individual cells are generally cuboidal with mild to occasionally marked anisocytosis and anisokaryosis (see Fig. 11.19). The cells in general have variable nucleocytoplasmic (N:C) ratios with a moderate amount of often deep-blue cytoplasm and round to polygonal nuclei. Hyaline globules were demonstrated in a canine case of renal carcinoma that appeared as magenta amorphous extracellular hyalinized material that has been shown to consist of basement membrane lamellae (Collicutt et al., 2013) (Fig. 11.21). As highlighted in a recent canine case series, renal carcinoma and renal epithelial hyperplasia can have similar cytomorphology requiring histopathology for differentiation (McAloney et al., 2018a).

The cytopathologic appearance in a cat of a rare renal oncocytoma revealed a lightly granular cell similar to the appearance of renal carcinoma being arranged in sheets and papillary clusters, along with abundant single cells (Lee et al., 2017).

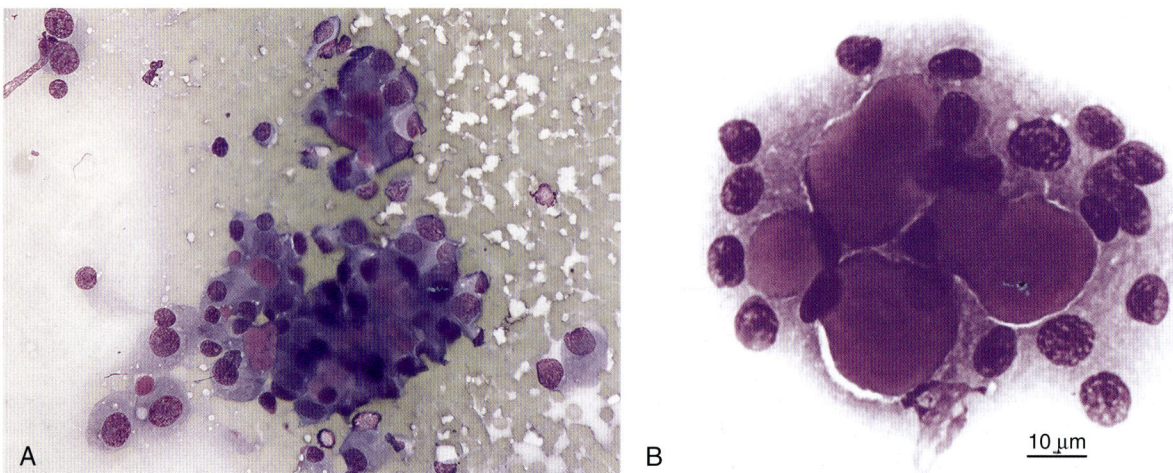

FIGURE 11.21 Renal carcinoma with hyaline globules. Renal mass imprint. Dog. Same case in A and B. Ultrasound indicated a mass measuring at least 9 × 14 cm involving the left kidney. **A,** Cohesive sheets of round to polygonal epithelial cells with variably distinct cytoplasmic borders. The cytoplasm was lightly basophilic and rarely contained a few clear vacuoles. The nuclei were round to oval with stippled chromatin and occasional nucleoli. Admixed between these cells was an extracellular, eosinophilic, globular material. (Wright; HP oil.) **B,** Higher magnification showing the distinct eosinophilic globular material, which is composed of lamellae of basement membranes produced in excess by the neoplastic cell population. (Wright; HP oil.) (Courtesy Nancy Collicutt, University of Georgia. Presented at the 2012 ASVCP case review session.)

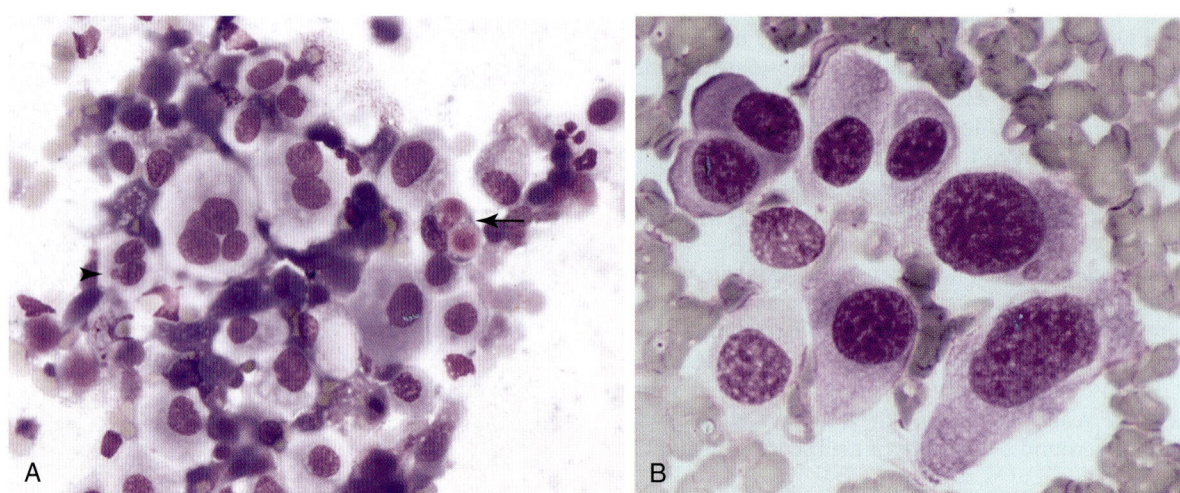

FIGURE 11.22 Urothelial cell carcinoma. Cytopathologic specimen. A, Site unknown. This cluster of urothelial cells contains numerous criteria of malignancy, including marked anisocytosis and anisokaryosis, variable nucleocytoplasmic (N:C) ratio, pleomorphic and multiple nuclei, and micronuclei *(arrowhead)*. Note the characteristic pink cytoplasmic inclusions, termed *Melamed-Wolinska bodies (arrow)*. (Wright-Giemsa; HP oil.) **B, Urinary bladder. Dog.** This group of urothelial cells appeared individualized with marked anisocytosis and anisokaryosis, variable N:C ratio, and pleomorphic nuclei. Erythrocytes admixed can be used to denote size of the neoplastic cells. (Wright-Giemsa; HP oil.) (B, Courtesy Rick Alleman, University of Florida.)

Key findings reported positive cytokeratin immunoreactivity and numerous cytoplasmic mitochondria seen by ultrastructure (Lee et al., 2017). Diagnosis of renal oncocytoma requires histopathology, electron microscopy, and immunochemistry for confirmation (Buergelt and Adjiri-Awere, 2000; Lee et al., 2017). On histopathology, these renal neoplastic cells are eosinophilic and densely granular and are PAS positive (Buergelt and Adjiri-Awere, 2000).

Renal Urothelial Carcinoma

Urothelial carcinomas that arise from the renal pelvis may exfoliate in small sheets, in loose aggregates, or as individual cells. Single cells are large and can be cuboidal, polygonal, or even spindle shaped. Urothelial cells often have marked anisocytosis and anisokaryosis, variable N:C, pleomorphic nuclei, and prominent and multiple nucleoli (Fig. 11.22). Characteristic pink homogeneous to granular cytoplasmic inclusions, termed *Melamed-Wolinska bodies*, are often noted (see Fig. 11.22A). They contain mucopolysaccharides, represent degenerating cells, and may be lysosomal in origin (Arya et al., 2012).

Renal Nephroblastoma

Renal nephroblastomas involve 6% and 18% of canine and feline renal tumors, respectively (Meuten and Meuten, 2017).

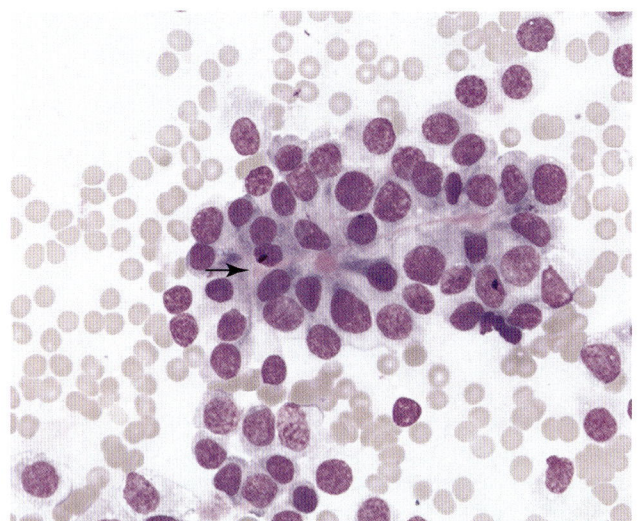

■ **FIGURE 11.23 Nephroblastoma. Kidney. Cytopathologic specimen.** This cluster of polygonal to cuboidal cells shows high nucleocytoplasmic ratios with mild anisocytosis and anisokaryosis. Note the pink extracellular matrix material (stroma or basement membrane) coursing through the cluster *(arrow)*. Nuclei are round to polygonal, chromatin is stippled, and nucleoli are not obvious. (Wright-Giemsa; HP oil.)

polygonal to cuboidal with typically a high N:C ratio, a scant amount of pale blue cytoplasm, and mild anisokaryosis and anisocytosis. Nucleolar criteria of malignancy are generally absent. Histopathology and immunohistochemistry are often necessary for definitive characterization. Nephroblastomas are characterized by positive vimentin immunoreactivity of mesenchymal cells and positive cytokeratin immunoreactivity of the epithelial cells within the tumor.

Nephroblastomas have been associated with the thoracolumbar region of the spinal cord where ectopic renal blastemal cells are thought to incorporate into the dura during embryonic life (Neel and Dean, 2000). They display pseudorosettes as well as dense cell clusters similar to the renal location.

Renal Lymphoma

Renal lymphoma aspirates generally contain a homogeneous population of discrete round cells with cytomorphologic features consistent with large, immature lymphocytes. There can be numerous lysed cells in the background. Neoplastic lymphocytes often show moderate to marked pleomorphism, have nuclei composed of homogeneous smooth chromatin, and have a small to moderate amount of basophilic cytoplasm (Fig. 11.25A). Occasionally, prominent nucleoli can be seen, and rarely, the neoplastic lymphocytes may contain bright pink cytoplasmic granules (Fig. 11.25B). Canine renal T-cell lymphoma, confirmed with histopathology, was diagnosed using urine sediment microscopy with flow cytometry and PCR for antigen receptor rearrangement (PARR). Therefore, urine flow cytometry or PARR can be performed on urine-derived cells as a quick and cost-effective means to aid in the diagnosis of urinary tract lymphoma (Witschen et al., 2020).

Renal Sarcoma

They are composed of mixed cell populations, including blastemal, epithelial, and mesenchymal elements (Henry et al., 1999; Michael et al., 2013). Cytopathologically, the predominant cell types are usually the blastemal or epithelial components as cells tend to exfoliate singly or in loose aggregates and sheets (Figs. 11.23 and 11.24). Similar to renal carcinomas, nephroblastoma cells can mimic round cell neoplasia (e.g., lymphoma) or tumors of neuroendocrine origin. They may form immature glomerular (see Fig. 11.24A) and pseudorosette structures (see Figs. 11.23 and 11.24B). The nephroblastoma cells are generally

Renal sarcomas often exfoliate poorly. They are composed of oval- to spindle-shaped cells observed individually or in variably sized aggregates. The N:C ratio is high, with small amounts

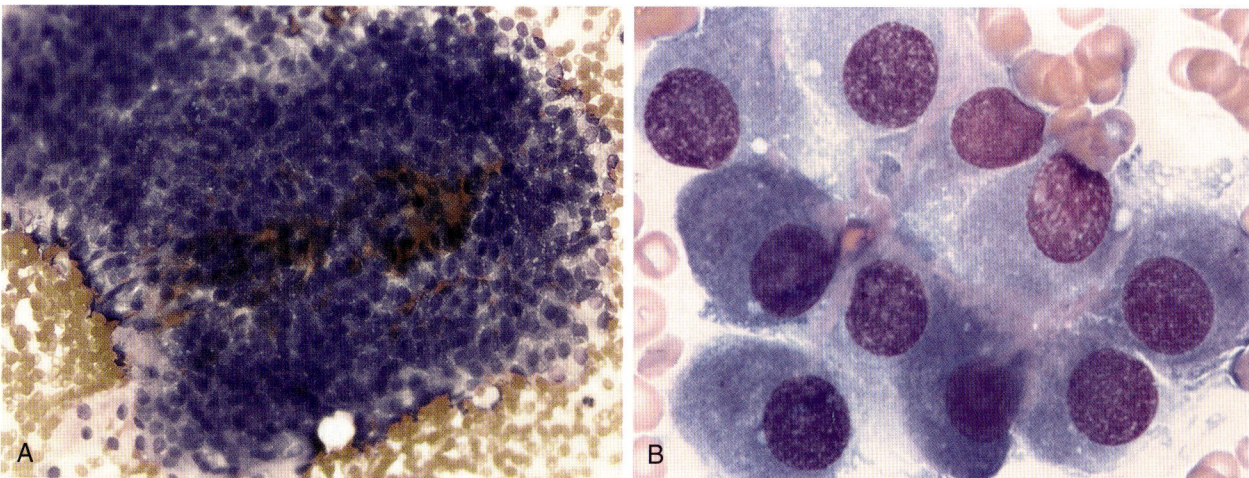

■ **FIGURE 11.24 Nephroblastoma. Kidney. Mass aspirate. Dog.** Same case in A and B. **A,** Multiple large renal masses are present. The specimen contains a large cell cluster resembling an immature tubular structure or glomerulus with dense cellularity. (Modified Wright; IP.) **B,** Cells were present individually and in small clusters of cells with variably distinct cell borders. More distinct cell borders are shown. The cytoplasm is basophilic and variably abundant. Admixed between the pseudorosette formations is a fibrillar eosinophilic matrix. (Modified Wright; HP oil.) (Courtesy Rose Raskin, Michigan State University.)

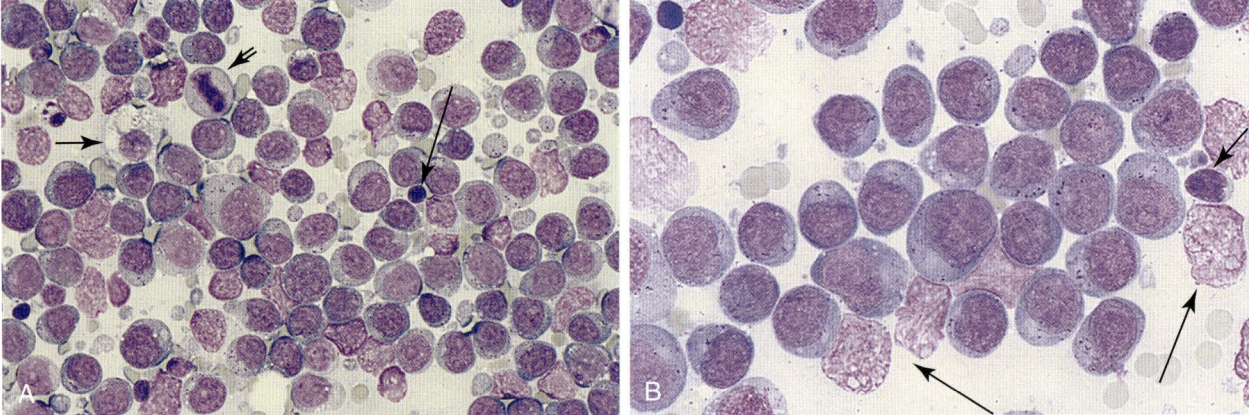

■ **FIGURE 11.25 Lymphoma. Kidney. Aspirate. A,** This sample contains a dense population of discrete cells with cytomorphologic features consistent with large lymphocytes. Note the marked pleomorphism; smooth, homogeneous nuclear chromatin; and relatively abundant basophilic cytoplasm compared with a small lymphocyte *(long arrow).* The presence of pink cytoplasmic granules is a less common feature of lymphoma. These cells are differentiated from renal tubular cells by their abundance and high nucleocytoplasmic ratio as well as the presence of many cytoplasmic fragments (lymphoglandular bodies) within the background. An activated macrophage *(short arrow)* and a mitotic figure *(double arrow)* are also seen. (Wright-Giemsa; HP oil.) **B,** A relatively normal, small lymphocyte *(short arrow)* accentuates the atypical features of the neoplastic lymphocytes. In addition to the features described in A, prominent nucleoli can be seen in some of the malignant cells, and the pink cytoplasmic granules are more readily observed. Five or six lacy, pink, ovoid formations sometimes referred to as "basket cells," represent free nuclear chromatin from lysed cells *(long arrows).* This is a frequent finding in aspirates from tissues composed of fragile cells, such as neoplastic lymphocytes. Smaller, light basophilic cytoplasmic fragments (lymphoglandular bodies) are also present. (Wright-Giemsa; HP oil.)

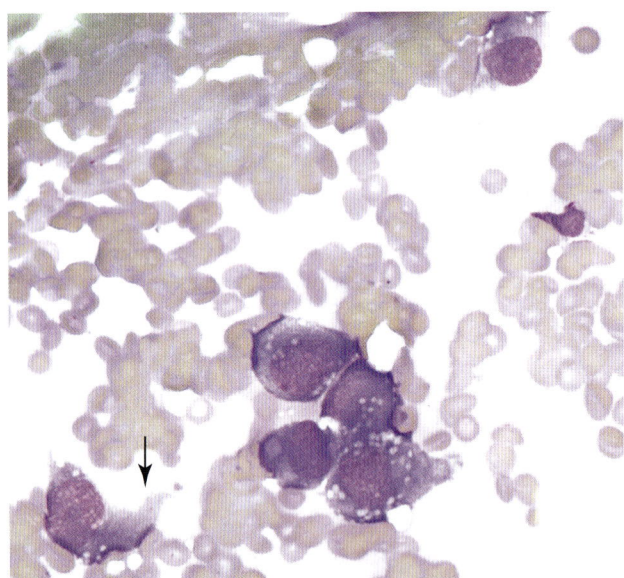

■ **FIGURE 11.26 Sarcoma. Kidney. Cytopathologic specimen.** Cells of mesenchymal neoplasia tend to exfoliate singly or in small aggregates rather than cohesive clusters. Cell shape may vary from round to oval to spindle shaped. A cytopathologic impression of mesenchymal cells is denoted by finding cells with wispy tails *(arrow).* Malignancy is characterized by variable, often high nucleocytoplasmic ratios, moderate to deep blue, wispy cytoplasm that often contains numerous uniform punctate vacuoles, cellular pleomorphism, and moderate anisokaryosis. (Wright-Giemsa; HP oil.)

> **KEY POINT** Sensitivity and specificity for renal FNAB diagnosis of neoplasia:
> - Canine renal carcinoma: 67% sensitivity, 90% specificity (McAloney et al., 2018a).
> - Feline renal round cell neoplasia and carcinoma: 100% sensitivity, 100% specificity (McAloney et al., 2018b).

URETERS

The ureter is a tube connecting each kidney to the urinary bladder. It is lined by urothelium or transitional epithelium, which is sequentially circumscribed by layers of lamina propria, smooth muscle, and fibroelastic adventitia. Because of their small diameter and uncommon primary pathology, the ureters are rarely directly sampled unless substantially enlarged by a focal lesion. Primary ureteral neoplasia is rare, with ureteral invasion by neoplastic processes originating from the urinary bladder (especially urothelial carcinoma) more common. Primary ureter neoplasia in dogs includes benign neoplasms, notably fibroepithelial polyps (Deschamps et al., 2007). Figure 11.27 demonstrates the cytopathologic and histopathologic features of a fibroepithelial polyp in a dog that produced unilateral renomegaly and hematuria (Etzioni et al., 2020). Cytopathologic features of an anaplastic sarcoma with giant cells affecting the ureter have been described (Rigas et al., 2012).

URINARY BLADDER AND URETHRA

Normal Anatomy and Histology

of moderate to deep-blue wispy cytoplasm, often with punctate vacuoles, surrounding round to oval nuclei with prominent nucleoli. Anisocytosis and anisokaryosis are often marked (Fig. 11.26). Cytopathology alone cannot distinguish between metastatic sarcomas and sarcomas arising from renal vessels or smooth muscle.

The urinary bladder is a saclike structure lined sequentially by stratified or transitional epithelial mucosa, submucosa, two inner and outer longitudinal layers and one circular layer of muscle, and a thin serosal surface of fibroelastic adventitia and mesothelium. The urinary bladder voids urine into the urethra, which is a long, tubelike structure also lined

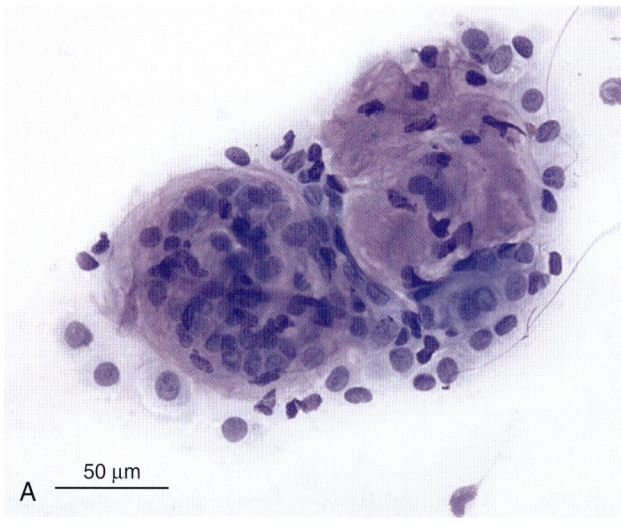

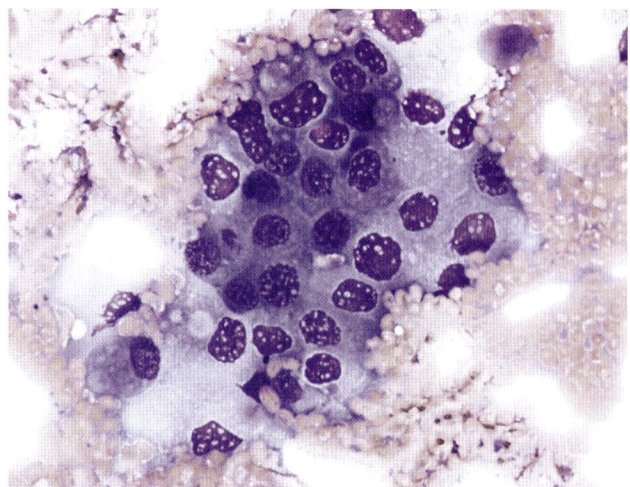

■ **FIGURE 11.28** **Degenerate urothelial cells. Urinary bladder. Cytopathologic specimen.** Prolonged exposure to urine causes mild to marked cellular disruption, inhibiting definitive cytopathologic characterization. Common alterations include coarse chromatin, clear vacuoles within the cytoplasm or nucleus (or both), and irregular nuclear margins. (Wright-Giemsa; HP oil.)

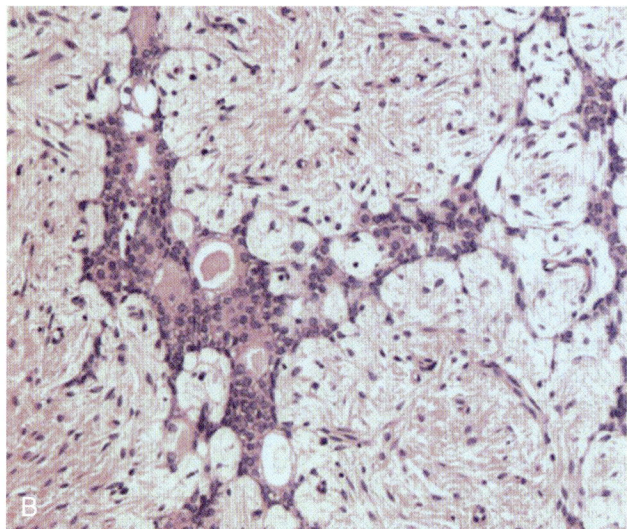

■ **FIGURE 11.27** **Fibroepithelial polyp. Ureter. Dog.** Same case in A and B. **A, Mass imprint.** Cytopathologic features include benign urothelium surrounding an oval, cellular blood vessel *(left)* and eosinophilic mucinous spindle cells with abundant wispy cytoplasm *(right)*. (Modified Wright; HP oil.) **B, Histology.** Shown is marked proliferation of benign fibrovascular and myxomatous elements, the latter being Alcian blue positive. Uniform urothelium surrounds blood vessels and the surface of the mass (not shown). (H&E; LP.) (Courtesy of Athema Etzioni, Purdue University.)

by urothelium (transitional urinary epithelium) leading to the external environment.

Specialized Collection Techniques

Collection techniques remain controversial as to the best and safest method (Wycislo and Piech, 2019). Cells from masses within the urinary bladder or urethra can be readily obtained using ultrasound-guided FNAB or traumatic urethral catheterization. Occasionally, tumor cells can be noted in urine sediment; however, the submission of urine for cytopathology rarely results in a definitive diagnosis of neoplasia because of poor cellular preservation or low cellularity. Traumatic urethral catheterization can provide adequate and diagnostic samples; however, many of the cells obtained may be superficial or reactive urothelial cells. As such, traumatic catheterization can result in a misleading cytopathologic assessment because the subjacent pathology has not been sampled. Although a few cases of tumor implantation along the ventral abdominal wall after direct FNAB of urinary bladder masses have been reported, this complication is infrequent and more commonly associated with surgical invention for tumor removal or debulking (Nyland et al., 2002; Higuchi et al., 2013). Thus, ultrasound-guided FNAB may remain the best method for obtaining tissue-associated cells and maximizing cellular yield for cytopathologic review.

Normal Cytology and Artifacts

Normal urothelial cells are most commonly observed upon urine sediment examination during a complete urinalysis (see Chapter 12). Urothelial cells are round to irregularly round cells arranged individually or in pavement-like sheets. These cells contain a moderate amount of lightly basophilic cytoplasm with poorly distinct cell borders. Their nuclei are round or slightly ovoid, centrally placed, and fill one-third to one-quarter of the cell volume. Chromatin is coarse, and anisocytosis and anisokaryosis are minimal to mild. Prolonged exposure to urine within the urinary bladder or within a sample container may result in cellular and nuclear degeneration, termed *urine scalding* (Fig. 11.28).

Inflammatory Disorders

Urinary cystitis may occur secondary to infection (e.g., bacterial cystitis, mycotic cystitis), trauma (e.g., cystoliths), hemorrhagic diathesis (e.g., vasculitis), hypersensitivity, or stress, or the cause may not be identified (e.g., feline idiopathic cystitis). Infectious agents may be observed on cytopathology in cases of infectious cystitis (Fig. 11.29). Regardless of the underlying cause, urinary cystitis may result in urothelial hyperplasia with or without urothelial atypia. The urothelial hyperplastic response may result in grossly flat, papillary, or polypoid lesions, the latter of which may mimic neoplasia. Polypoid cystitis is characterized by inflammation, epithelial proliferation, and development of a non-neoplastic mass. Similar to most urinary bladder diseases, affected dogs present with hematuria or recurrent urinary tract

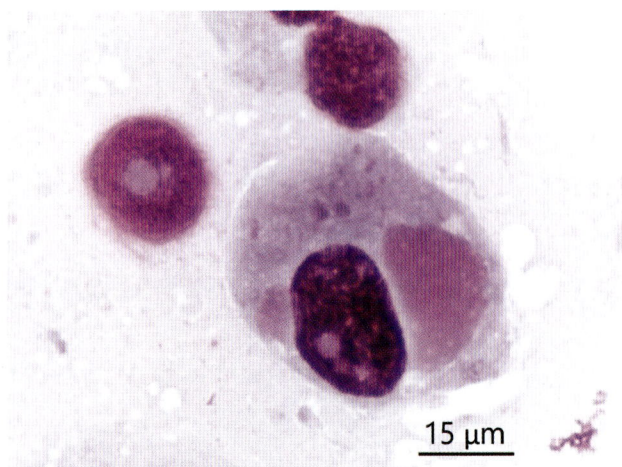

■ **FIGURE 11.29 Canine distemper virus inclusion. Urinary bladder imprint. Dog.** A urothelial cell contains two homogeneous, fuchsia, variably sized, intracytoplasmic canine distemper viral inclusions flanking the cell's nucleus. Bar = 15 μm. (Aqueous Romanowsky; HP oil.) (Courtesy Katie Boes and Thomas Cecere, Virginia Tech and State University.)

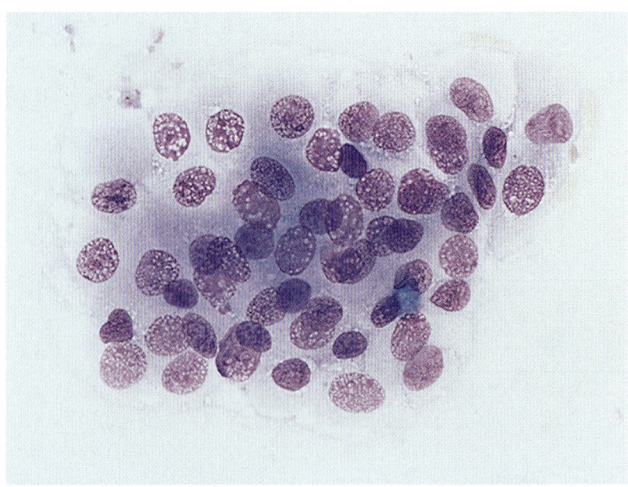

■ **FIGURE 11.31 Urothelial hyperplasia or benign polyp. Urinary bladder. Cytopathologic specimen.** The urothelial cells within this epithelial cluster have round to oval uniform nuclei. The chromatin is coarse (a common cytomorphologic feature of urothelial cells) without obvious nucleoli. Cell borders are often readily observed and there is only mild pleomorphism. (Wright-Giemsa; HP oil.)

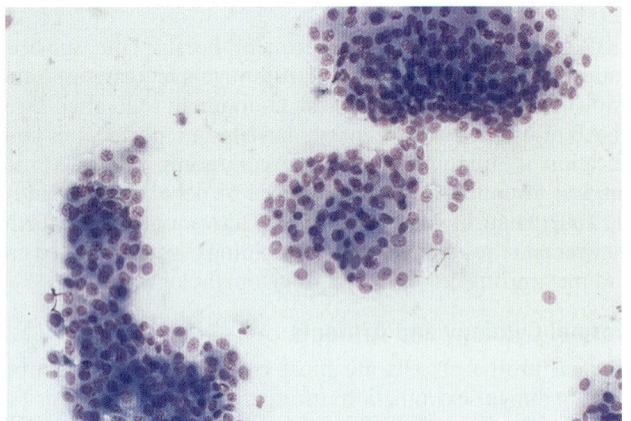

■ **FIGURE 11.30 Urothelial hyperplasia or benign polyp. Urinary bladder. Cytopathologic specimen.** Epithelial hyperplasia or polyp formation is distinguished from malignant epithelial neoplasia by the distinctive, regular clustering pattern and uniform appearance of the epithelial cells. (Wright-Giemsa; IP.)

infection. However, unlike urothelial neoplasia, these masses are most frequently located cranioventrally in the urinary bladder rather than in the trigone region (Martinez et al., 2003). Urothelial hyperplasia may exfoliate in large cellular sheets with mild pleomorphism (Fig. 11.30); nuclei are generally uniform with coarse, ragged chromatin patterns (Fig. 11.31).

Non-neoplastic Tumors
Fibroepithelial Polyp
Fibroepithelial polyp is histopathologically characterized by an exophytic growth of abundant fibrovascular stroma that is lined by urothelium and attached to the urinary bladder or urethra by a narrow stalk. Cytopathologically, this lesion is indistinguishable from urothelial hyperplasia or cystitis, urothelial papilloma, and low-grade urothelial carcinoma.

Inflammatory Pseudotumors
A rare tumorous condition in dogs was described in which single or multiple, polypoid, firm masses, measuring 1 to 7 cm were associated with mixed inflammatory cells within a dense stromal submucosa (Böhme et al., 2010). Hematuria was the main clinical sign, often associated with dysuria and crystalluria. Histologically, the masses were well delineated with an expansive submucosa infiltrated by a mixed inflammatory cell component covered by a thin cap of benign hyperplastic urothelium. The stromal cells in the submucosa were spindle shaped and arranged in a swirling pattern. Immunochemistry revealed these stromal cells were vimentin and variably desmin and actin positive, helping to term them myofibroblastic cells. Cytopathologic preparations are often limited to the surface urothelium and inflammatory cells, as the stromal cells exfoliate poorly (Fig. 11.32).

Neoplastic Tumors
Tumors of the urinary bladder and urethra are occasionally encountered. Epithelial tumors include carcinomas, papillomas, and adenomas. Carcinomas include urothelial carcinoma, squamous cell carcinoma, adenocarcinoma, and undifferentiated carcinoma. Approximately 90% of urinary bladder and urethral tumors are epithelial in origin, and the majority are malignant. Of these, urothelial carcinoma is most common (Norris et al., 1992; Mutsaers et al., 2003; Wilson et al., 2007).

Urothelial Papilloma
Urothelial papillomas are characterized by varying size clusters of uniform urothelial cells. These cells are cuboidal to polyhedral and show mild anisokaryosis, with an increased N:C ratio (Fig. 11.33). These tumors are cytopathologically similar to urothelial hyperplasia or cystitis, fibroepithelial polyp, and low-grade urothelial carcinoma.

Urothelial Carcinoma
Urothelial carcinoma is of urinary epithelial cell origin. In dogs, it most commonly occurs in the trigone region of the urinary bladder, whereas urothelial carcinoma more commonly involves the urinary bladder wall distant from the trigone in cats (Mutsaers et al., 2003; Wilson et al., 2007). Neutered male dogs have a significantly increased risk of developing urolithial carcinoma

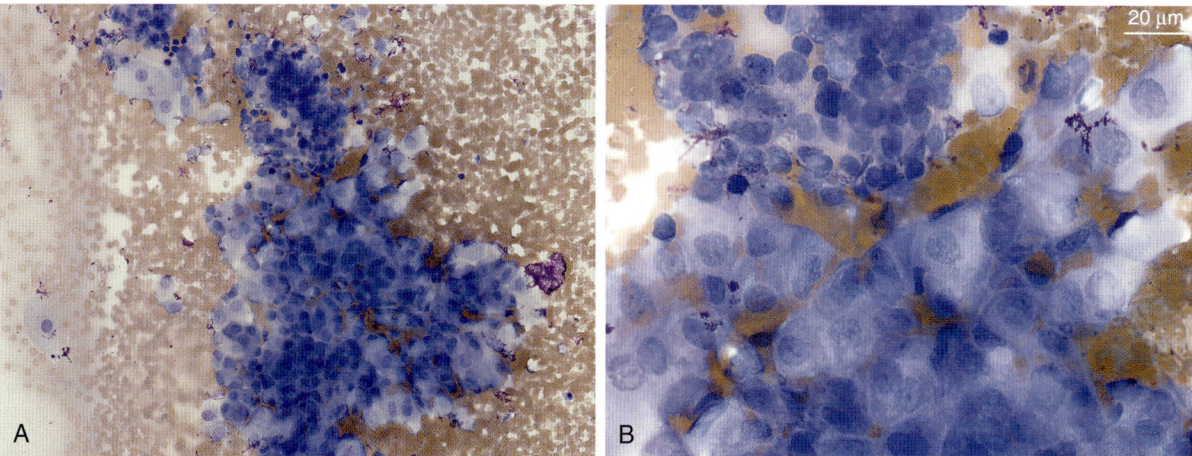

■ **FIGURE 11.32 Inflammatory pseudotumor. Urinary bladder. Needle-cut biopsy imprint. Dog.** Same case in A and B. Multiple bladder masses are found on ultrasound examination. **A,** A dense cell cluster with urothelial cells and several squamous epithelial cells are present. Sprinkled throughout are several small, condensed lymphocytes. The background contains occasional magenta ultrasound gel. (Modified Wright; IP.) **B,** Higher magnification demonstrates a mildly atypical urothelial cell population and several mononuclear cell infiltrates representing lymphocytes and macrophages. Histopathology confirmed a non-neoplastic mass with ulcerated urothelium lacking nuclear atypia and a submucosal proliferation of spindle cells in an edematous extracellular matrix (stromal polyp). (Modified Wright; HP oil.) (Courtesy Rose Raskin, Purdue University.)

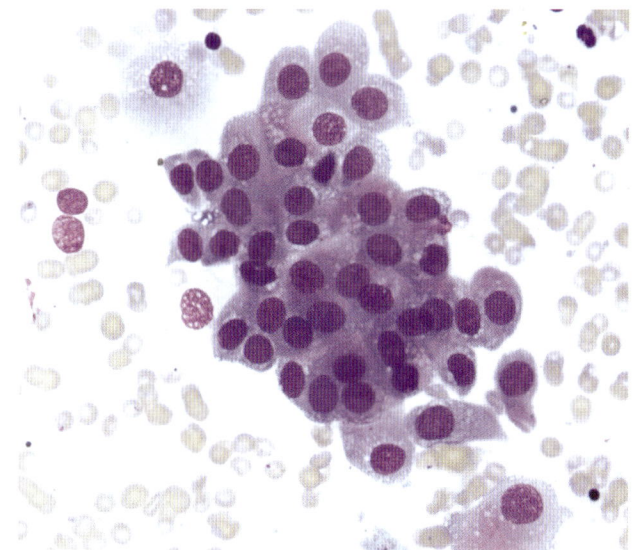

■ **FIGURE 11.33 Urothelial papilloma. Urinary bladder. Cytopathologic specimen.** Epithelial polyp formation or hyperplasia is distinguished from malignant epithelial neoplasia by the uniform appearance of the epithelial cells. These cells show mild anisokaryosis and anisocytosis with a mildly increased nucleocytoplasmic ratio. Note the cytoplasmic vacuoles that can be seen in urothelial cells. (Wright-Giemsa; HP oil.)

compared with unneutered male dogs (Bryan et al., 2007). Scottish terriers are at significantly increased risk for urothelial carcinoma. Shetland sheepdogs, West Highland white terriers, fox terriers, and beagles also appear to be overrepresented (Meuten and Meuten, 2017).

Urothelial carcinoma may be diagnosed cytopathologically (Figs. 11.34 and 11.35A) and appears similar to urothelial carcinoma of the kidney (see description in the renal section). The eosinophilic cytoplasmic inclusion (Melamed-Wolinska body) is found within a degenerating benign or malignant urothelial cell and, when present outside of the urinary system, metastatic urothelial carcinoma is suspected. The diagnosis of canine urothelial carcinoma can often be made cytopathologically because the cells tend to readily exfoliate and show many characteristics of malignancy (Mutsaers et al., 2003). The proliferation may be papillary or solid with cystic degeneration and progression into the submucosa or muscle layers (Fig. 11.35B–D). Concurrent or secondary bacterial cystitis may confound the diagnosis. In cases of equivocal cytopathologic findings, collection of fresh urine or cells or tissues by other sampling methods, such as traumatic catheterization, ultrasound-guided FNAB, or tissue biopsy, may yield a diagnosis.

Identification of a unique mutation in the *BRAF* gene in canine urothelial carcinoma and prostatic carcinoma has led to the development of a PCR-based liquid biopsy test that can reliably detect the mutant allele in urine samples (CADET *BRAF*, Antech Diagnostics) (Mochizuki et al., 2015). This mutation, which is a thymine-to-adenine transversion in exon 15 of chromosome 16 and results in the substitution of the amino acid valine to glutamic acid (V595E), is reported in the tumor cells of 65% to 85% of dogs with urothelial carcinoma and 85% of dogs with prostatic carcinoma (Decker et al., 2015; Mochizuki et al., 2015; Aupperle-Lellbach et al., 2018). Notably, there may be breed-specific factors to consider as a higher prevalence of the *BRAF* mutation has been reported in terriers as compared with non-terrier breeds (Pantke, 2018; Grassinger et al., 2019). Initial studies have reported moderate sensitivity (71%–75%) and excellent specificity (100%) for *BRAF* testing in differentiating dogs with urothelial carcinoma from healthy dogs and dogs with cystitis (Mochizuki et al., 2015; Aupperle-Lellbach H et al., 2018; Wiley et al., 2019). CADET *BRAF* PLUS detects DNA copy number changes and is used for dogs with clinical signs of urothelial carcinoma that are not associated with a *BRAF* mutation.

This genetic approach has largely supplanted a previous noninvasive diagnostic assay, the veterinary urinary bladder tumor antigen test (V-BTA; Alidex Inc.). Although this test has been shown suitable in screening for urothelial carcinoma in dogs in the absence of moderate to marked hematuria, pyuria, glucosuria, or proteinuria (Borjesson et al., 1999), the specificity of the test declines rapidly if dogs have non–urothelial carcinoma urinary tract disease (Borjesson et al., 1999; Henry et al., 2003). Cyclooxygenase-2, uroplakin III, and cytokeratin 7 show promise as useful immunohistochemical stains to verify tumors of urothelial origin in histopathology sections, if needed

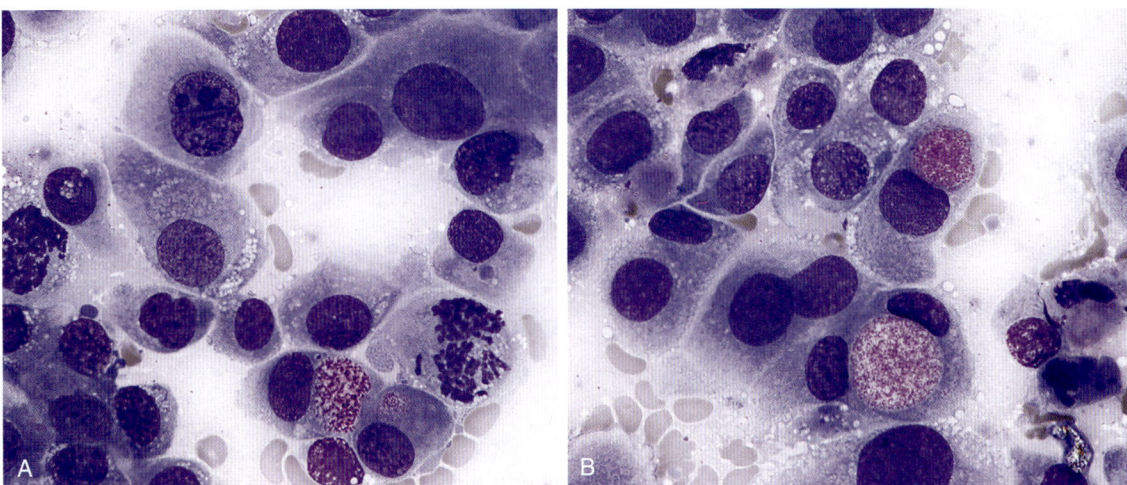

■ **FIGURE 11.34 Urothelial cell carcinoma. Urethra. Aspirate. Dog.** Same case in A and B. A 2-year-old Labrador retriever presented with a urethral mass. **A,** Round to ovoid epithelial cells appear individually and in cohesive sheets with distinct cell borders. Nuclei have round, ovoid to irregular, scalloped borders. Nuclear chromatin is often coarsely stippled with one to five small to large prominent round nucleoli. Anisocytosis, anisokaryosis, and anisonucleosis are moderate to marked. There are frequent binucleated cells, and one abnormal mitotic figure is shown having lag chromatin. (Modified Wright; HP oil.) **B,** In addition to similar cytomorphology as in A, there are two large round pink granular cytoplasmic inclusions consistent with Melamed-Wolinska bodies. (Modified Wright; HP oil.) (Courtesy Rose Raskin, Kansas State University.)

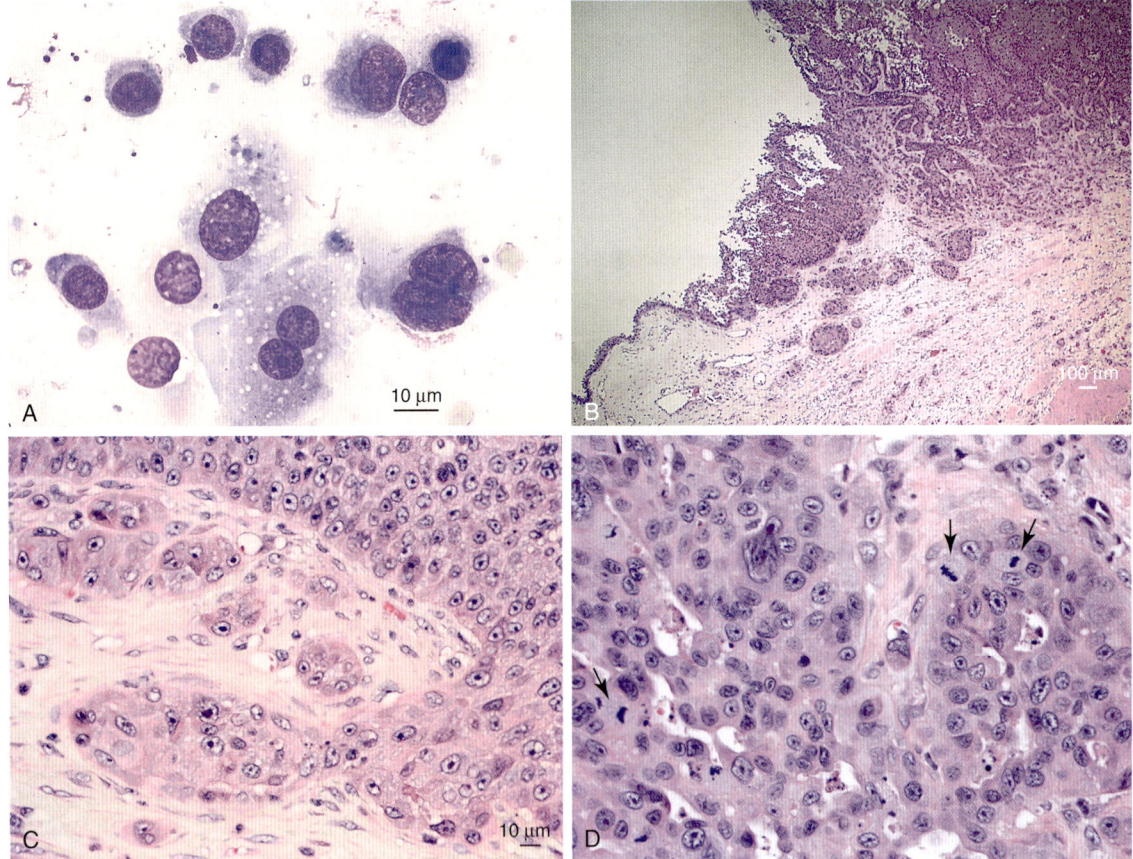

■ **FIGURE 11.35 Urothelial cell carcinoma. Urinary bladder. Cat.** Same case in A to D. An 18-year-old patient presented with hematuria and stranguria. The bladder mucosa has multiple, variably pale and firm plaques with an overall thickened bladder mucosa. **A, Aspirate.** The urothelial cell population is pleomorphic with frequent binucleation, moderate to marked anisokaryosis and anisocytosis, coarse chromatin, and prominent nucleoli. Cytoplasm is occasionally vacuolated. (Modified Wright; HP oil.) **B, Histology.** A demarcation is seen between the normal mucosa of a few cell layers and the progressively thicker neoplastic region. The neoplastic cells invade all layers of the bladder wall (not shown). (H&E; LP.) **C, Histology.** The neoplastic cells extend into the submucosa in areas where there is mucosal layer disorganization with a lack of distinct umbrella and basal cell layers. (H&E; IP.) **D, Histology.** Neoplastic cells are polygonal with abundant eosinophilic to amphophilic cytoplasm. Nuclei are large, round, and vesicular with variably sized nucleoli. Several mitotic figures are present *(arrows)*. The pattern is solid with frequent areas of central necrosis (eosinophilic debris within spaces). (H&E; IP.) (Courtesy Rose Raskin, Purdue University.)

(Khan et al., 2000; Ramos-Vara et al., 2003; Knottenbelt et al., 2006).

Mesenchymal Tumors

Mesenchymal tumors of the urinary bladder include leiomyoma (Fig. 11.36), leiomyosarcoma, and rhabdomyosarcoma (Fig. 11.37) (Alleman et al., 1991). Urinary bladder leiomyoma and leiomyosarcoma may appear morphologically similar on cytopathology. Both are typically characterized by elongated spindle cells with oval nuclei, variable amounts of pink matrix, and minimal pleomorphism. Histologic assessment of tissue architecture is necessary to distinguish these neoplasms. Rhabdomyosarcomas are rare and appear to be more common in younger animals. The morphology of neoplastic cells is highly variable; however, strap cells, multinucleated cells, and muscle fiber striations may be observed in some cases.

Lymphoma

Urinary bladder lymphoma may be metastatic, or rarely, primary (Fig. 11.38).

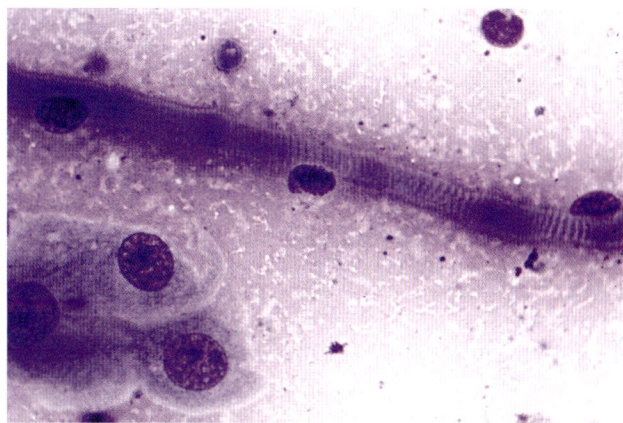

■ **FIGURE 11.37 Rhabdomyosarcoma. Urinary bladder. Aspirate. Dog.** A single muscle fiber with striations is present along with three hyperplastic urothelial cells. A lymphocyte *(upper right)* denotes the relatively large size of the neoplastic myocyte. Histopathology confirmed the diagnosis of a rhabdomyosarcoma. (Wright-Giemsa; HP oil.) (Courtesy Rose Raskin, University of Florida.)

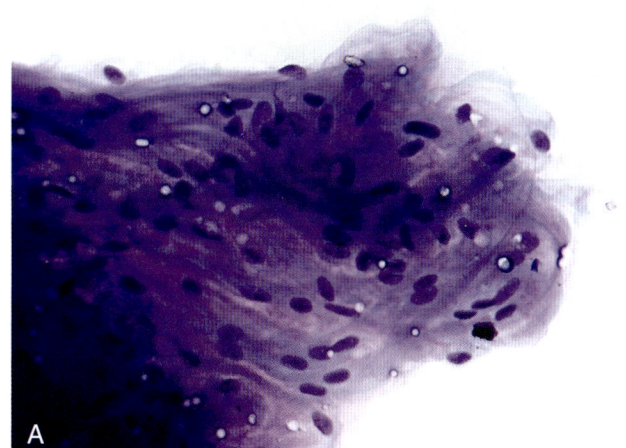
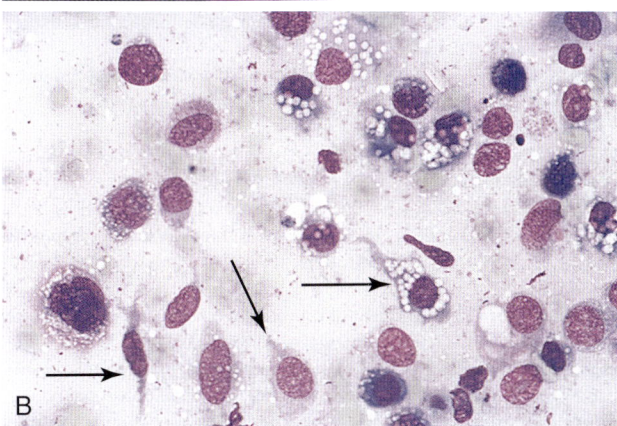

■ **FIGURE 11.36 Smooth muscle neoplasms. Urinary bladder. Cytopathologic specimen. A, Leiomyoma.** Neoplastic smooth muscle cells are elongated with abundant cytoplasm surrounding an oval nucleus composed of homogeneous chromatin and single nucleolus and embedded in an amorphous metachromatic-staining intercellular matrix creating a palisading, wavelike pattern. The benign appearance is characterized by uniform cell and nuclear size. Histopathology is necessary to distinguish leiomyoma from leiomyosarcoma when minimal to mild anisocytosis or anisokaryosis is observed. (Aqueous Romanowsky; HP oil.) **B, Leiomyosarcoma.** Neoplastic mesenchymal cells tend to sparsely exfoliate or in small aggregates. Cell shape varies from round to oval to spindle with wispy tails *(arrows)*. Malignancy is characterized by moderate to marked anisokaryosis, anisocytosis, and variable nucleocytoplasmic ratios. The cells have a round to oval nucleus comprised of a stippled chromatin pattern with a lightly stained nucleolus. There is a minimal amount of variably stained vacuolated cytoplasm often with indistinct cell borders, which are accentuated by a pink-blue proteinaceous, intercellular matrix background. (Wright-Giemsa; HP oil.)

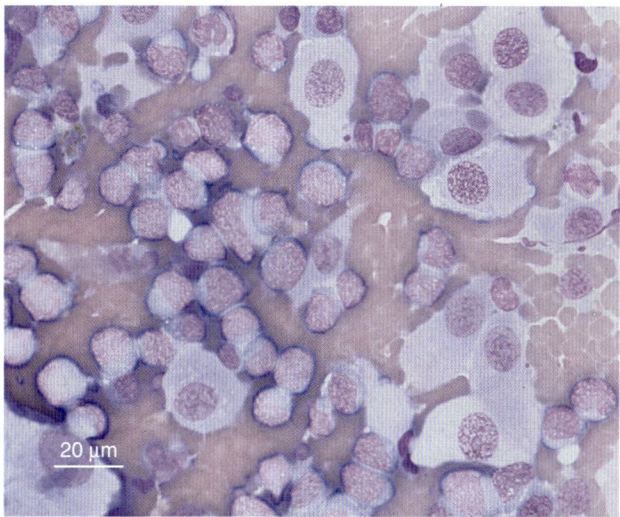

■ **FIGURE 11.38 B-cell lymphoma. Urinary bladder. Imprint. Dog.** Traumatic urinary catheterization resulted in tissue pieces that were imprinted for cytopathologic examination. Two nucleated cell populations are observed. The largest cells with abundant light basophilic cytoplasm are normal urothelial cells. The predominant cell type is variably sized, round to oval, neoplastic, large lymphoid cells (3 × RBC diameter) with a small amount of basophilic cytoplasm, eccentric nuclei, reticular chromatin, and indistinct nucleoli. Immunocytochemistry demonstrated CD3-negative and CD79a-positive lymphoid cells, supportive of B-cell origin. (Wright-Giemsa; HP oil.) (Courtesy Rose Raskin, University of Florida.)

REFERENCES

Alleman AR, Raskin RE, Uhl EW, et al. What is your diagnosis? Bladder mass from an 11-month-old dog. *Vet Clin Pathol*. 1991;20:44, 49-50.

Ayra P, Khalbuss WE, Monaco SE, et al. Melamed-Wolinska bodies. *Diagn Cytopathol*. 2012;40(2):150-151.

Aupperle-Lellbach H, Grassinger J, Hohloch, C, et al. Diagnostic value of the BRAF variant V595E in urine samples, smears and biopsies from canine transitional cell carcinoma. *Tierarztl Prax Ausg K Kleintiere Heimtiere*. 2018;46(5):289-295.

Baskin GB, DePaoli A. Primary renal neoplasms of the dog. *Vet Pathol*. 1977;14:591-605.

Böhme B, Ngendahayo P, Hamaideet A, et al. Inflammatory pseudotumours of the urinary bladder in dogs resembling human myofibroblastic tumours: a report of eight cases and comparative pathology. *Vet J*. 2010;183:89-94.

Borjesson DL. Renal cytology. *Vet Clin North Am Small Anim Pract*. 2003;33(1):119-134.

Borjesson DL, Christopher MM, Ling GV. Detection of canine transitional cell carcinoma using a bladder tumor antigen urine dipstick test. *Vet Clin Pathol*. 1999;28(1):33-38.

Breshears MA, Meinkoth JH, Stern AW, et al. Pathology in practice. Renal lymphoma. *J Am Vet Med Assoc*. 2011;238(2):167-169.

Bryan JN, Keeler MR, Henry CJ, et al. A population study of neutering status as a risk factor for canine prostate cancer. *Prostate*. 2007;67(11):1174-1181.

Bryan JN, Henry CJ, Turnquist SE, et al. Primary renal neoplasia of dogs. *J Vet Intern Med*. 2006;20(5):1155-1160.

Buergelt CD, Adjiri-Awere A. Bilateral renal oncocytoma in a greyhound dog. *Vet Pathol*. 2000;37:188-192.

Chiang YC, Liu CH, Ho SY, et al. Hypertrophic osteopathy associated with disseminated metastases of renal cell carcinoma in the dog: a case report. *J Vet Med Sci*. 2007;69(2):209-212.

Collicutt NB, Garner BC, Brown C, et al. What is your diagnosis? Renal mass in a dog. *Vet Clin Pathol*. 2013;42(3):389-390, 2013.

Cooper BJ. Disease at the cellular level. In: Slauson DO, Cooper BJ, eds. *Mechanisms of Disease: A Textbook of Comparative General Pathology*. 3rd ed. St. Louis, MO: Mosby; 2002:68.

Debruyn K, Haers H, Combes A, et al. Ultrasonography of the feline kidney: technique, anatomy and changes associated with disease. *J Feline Med Surg*. 2012;14(11):794-803.

Decker B, Parker HG, Dhawan D, et al. Homologous mutation to human BRAF V600E is common in naturally occurring canine bladder cancer—evidence for a relevant model system and urine-based diagnostic test. *Mol Cancer Res*. 2015;13(6):993-1002.

Deschamps JY, Roux FA, Fantinato M, et al. Ureteral sarcoma in a dog. *J Small Anim Pract*. 2007;48(12):699-701.

Durno AS, Webb JA, Gauthier MJ, et al. Polycythemia and inappropriate erythropoietin concentrations in two dogs with renal T-cell lymphoma. *J Am Anim Hosp Assoc*. 2011;47(2):122-128.

Etzioni AL, Raskin RE, Van Alstine WG, et al. The cytologic and histologic diagnosis of ureteral fibroepithelial polyp in a dog. *Vet Clin Pathol*. 2020;49:646-651.

Foreman O, Sykes J, Ball L, et al. Disseminated infection with *Balamuthia mandrillaris* in a dog. *Vet Pathol*. 2004;41(5):506-510.

Gajanayake I, Priestnall SL, Benigni L, et al. Paraneoplastic hypercalcemia in a dog with benign renal angiomyxoma. *J Vet Diagn Invest*. 2010;22(5):775-780.

Gil da Costa RM, Oliveira JP, Saraiva AL, et al. Immunohistochemical characterization of 13 canine renal cell carcinomas. *Vet Pathol*. 2011;48(2):427-432.

Giordano A, Paltrinieri S, Bertazzolo W, et al. Sensitivity of Tru-cut® and fine needle aspiration biopsies of liver and kidney for diagnosis of feline infectious peritonitis. *Vet Clin Pathol*. 2005;34(4):368-374.

Giri DK, Sims WP, Sura R, et al. Cerebral and renal phaeohyphomycosis in a dog infected with *Bipolaris* species. *Vet Pathol*. 2011;48(3):754-757.

Grassinger JM, Merz S, Aupperle-Lellbach H, et al. Correlation of BRAF variant V595E, breed, histological grade and cyclooxygenase-2 expression in canine transitional cell carcinomas. *Vet Sci*. 2019;6(1):1-15.

Henry CJ, Tyler JW, McEntee MC, et al. Evaluation of a bladder tumor antigen test as a screening test for transitional cell carcinoma of the lower urinary tract in dogs. *Am J Vet Res*. 2003;64(8):1017-1020.

Henry CJ, Turnquist SE, Smith A, et al. Primary renal tumours in cats: 19 cases (1992-1998). *J Feline Med Surg*. 1999;1(3):165-170.

Higuchi T, Burcham GN, Childress MO, et al. Characterization and treatment of transitional cell carcinoma of the abdominal wall in dogs: 24 cases (1985-2010). *J Am Vet Med Assoc*. 2014;242(4):499-506.

Johnson RL, Lenz SD. Hypertrophic osteopathy associated with a renal adenoma in a cat. *J Vet Diagn Invest*. 2011;23(1):171-175.

Khan KNM, Knapp DW, Denicola DB, et al. Expression of cyclooxygenase-2 in transitional cell carcinoma of the urinary bladder in dogs. *Am J Vet Res*. 2000;61(5):478-481.

Knottenbelt C, Mellor D, Nixon C, et al. Cohort study of COX-1 and COX-2 expression in canine rectal and bladder tumours. *J Small Anim Pract*. 2006;47(4):196-200.

Lee S, Choi HJ, Lee HB, et al. Renal oncocytoma in a cat with chronic renal failure. *JFMS Open Rep*. 2017;3:1–5.

Martinez I, Mattoon JS, Eaton KA, et al. Polypoid cystitis in 17 dogs (1978-2001). *J Vet Intern Med*. 2003;17(4):499-509.

McAloney CA, Sharkey LC, Feeney DA, et al. Evaluation of the diagnostic utility of cytologic examination of renal fine-needle aspirates from dogs and the use of ultrasonographic features to inform cytologic diagnosis. *J Am Vet Med Assoc*. 2018a;252(10):1247-1256.

McAloney CA, Sharkey LC, Feeney DA, et al. Diagnostic utility of renal fine-needle aspirate cytology and ultrasound in the cat. *J Feline Med Surg*. 2018b;20(6):544-553.

Meuten DJ, Meuten TLK. Tumors of the urinary system. In: Meuten DJ, ed. *Tumors in Domestic Animals*. 5th ed. Ames: John Wiley and Sons; 2017:632-688.

Michael HT, Sharkey LC, Kovi RC, et al. Pathology in practice. Renal nephroblastoma in a young dog. *J Am Vet Med Assoc*. 2013;242(4):471-473.

Mochizuki H, Shapiro SG, Breen M. Detection of BRAF Mutation in urine DNA as a molecular diagnostic for canine urothelial and prostatic carcinoma. *PLoS One*. 2015;10(12):e0144170.

Mutsaers AJ, Widmer WR, Knapp DW. Canine transitional cell carcinoma. *J Vet Intern Med*. 2003;17(2):136-144.

Neel J, Dean GA. A mass in the spinal column of a dog [nephroblastoma]. *Vet Clin Pathol*. 2000;29:87-89.

Norris AM, Laing EJ, Valli VEO, et al. Canine bladder and urethral tumors: a retrospective study of 115 cases (1980-1985). *J Vet Intern Med*. 1992;6(3):145-153.

Nowicki M, Rychlik A, Nieradka R, et al. Usefulness of laparoscopy guided renal biopsy in dogs. *Pol J Vet Sci*. 2010;13(2):363-371.

Nyland TG, Wallack ST, Wisner ER. Needle-tract implantation following US-guided fine-needle aspiration biopsy of transitional cell carcinoma of the bladder, urethra, and prostate. *Vet Radiol Ultrasound*. 2002;43(1):50-53.

Pantke P. Diagnosis and treatment of transitional cell carcinoma of the lower urinary tract in the dog. *Kleintierpraxis*. 2018;63(2):76-92.

Peeters D, Clercx C, Thiry A, et al. Resolution of paraneoplastic leukocytosis and hypertrophic osteopathy after resection of a renal transitional cell carcinoma producing granulocyte-macrophage colony-stimulating factor in a young bull terrier. *J Vet Intern Med*. 2001;15(4):407-411.

Petterino C, Luzio E, Baracchini L, et al. Paraneoplastic leukocytosis in a dog with a renal carcinoma. *Vet Clin Pathol*. 2011;40(1):89-94.

Puschner B, Reimschuessel R. Toxicosis caused by melamine and cyanuric acid in dogs and cats: uncovering the mystery and subsequent global implications. *Clin Lab Med*. 2011;31(1):181-199.

Ramos-Vara JA, Miller MA, Boucher M, et al. Immunohistochemical detection of uroplakin III, cytokeratin 7, and cytokeratin 20 in canine urothelial tumors. *Vet Pathol*. 2003;40(1):55-62.

Rawlings CA, Howerth EW. Obtaining quality biopsies of the liver and kidney. *J Am Anim Hosp Assoc*. 2004;40(5):352-358.

Rawlings CA, Diamond H, Howerth EW, et al. Diagnostic quality of percutaneous kidney biopsy specimens obtained with laparoscopy versus ultrasound guidance in dogs. *J Am Vet Med Assoc*. 2003;223(3):317-321.

Rigas JD, Smith TJ, Gorman ME, et al. Primary ureteral giant cell sarcoma in a Pomeranian. *Vet Clin Pathol*. 2012;41(1):141-146.

Sato T, Aoki K, Shibuya H, et al. Leiomyosarcoma of the kidney in a dog. *J Vet Med A Physiol Pathol Clin Med*. 2003;50(7):366-369.

Snead EC. A case of bilateral renal lymphosarcoma with secondary polycythaemia and paraneoplastic syndromes of hypoglycaemia and uveitis in an English springer spaniel. *Vet Comp Oncol.* 2005;3(3):139-144.

Vaden SL. Renal biopsy: methods and interpretation. *Vet Clin North Am Small Anim Pract.* 2004;34(4):887-908.

Vaden SL. Renal biopsy of dogs and cats. *Clin Tech Small Anim Pract.* 2005;20(1):11-22.

Vaden SL, Levine JF, Lees GE, et al. Renal biopsy: a retrospective study of methods and complications in 283 dogs and 65 cats. *J Vet Intern Med.* 2005;19(6):794-801.

Wiley C, Wise C, Breen M. Novel noninvasive diagnostics. *Vet Clin North Am Small Anim Pract.* 2019;49(5):781-791.

Wilson HM, Chun R, Larson VS, et al. Clinical signs, treatments, and outcome in cats with transitional cell carcinoma of the urinary bladder: 20 cases (1990-2004). *J Am Vet Med Assoc.* 2007;231(1):101-106.

Witschen PM, Sharkey LC, Seelig DM, et al. Diagnosis of canine renal lymphoma by cytology and flow cytometry of the urine. *Vet Clin Pathol.* 2020;49:137-142.

Wycislo KL, Piech TL. Urinary tract cytology. *Vet Clin North Am Small Anim Pract.* 2019;49:247-260.

Zatelli A, Borgarelli M, Santilli R, et al. Glomerular lesions in dogs infected with *Leishmania* organisms. *Am J Vet Res.* 2003;64(5):558-561.

12 CHAPTER

Urine

Jessica Anne Hokamp and Denny J. Meyer

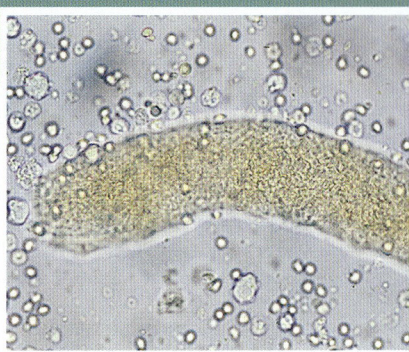

COMPLETE URINALYSIS

The complete urinalysis helps evaluate the health and function of the entire urinary tract when performed in conjunction with complete bloodwork. A complete urinalysis is part of the baseline data that should be collected for patients presented for general diagnostic evaluation but is essential when clinical signs of stranguria, pollakiuria, polyuria and polydipsia, discolored urine, anorexia, vomiting, or a mass or lesion in the bladder or distal urinary tract are present (Vap and Shropshire, 2017).

Automated urine chemistry and sediment analyzers are currently available to practitioners, but few studies have evaluated their accuracy and precision, and to date results are not without error (Hernandez et al., 2019). Thus, practitioners and pathologists must know how to accurately perform and interpret a complete urinalysis. Fortunately, after a standardized urinalysis protocol is established, it is not technically difficult or generally cost prohibitive.

The complete urinalysis includes a macroscopic and microscopic exam. The macroscopic examination includes assessment of color and clarity, measurement of urine-specific gravity (USG) to determine renal concentrating ability, and chemical analysis using a reagent test strip. The microscopic examination includes examination of insoluble components of the urine, ideally as a combination of wet mounts and air-dried, stained cytology smears. The results of the reagent test strip analysis might guide the practitioner to perform additional confirmatory or quantitative diagnostic testing. Details of interpretation of the macroscopic examination and chemical analysis of urine are beyond the scope of this chapter, and readers are referred to other resources (Stockham and Scott, 2008; Callens and Bartges, 2015). Refer to Box 12.1 for a standardized urinalysis procedure.

URINE COLLECTION

The primary reason for evaluation of urine should be considered when deciding the timing and method of urine collection. A first-morning sample is best for measurement of the USG to assess tubular function because it is most concentrated (Reppas and Foster, 2016a). For evaluation of insoluble particles, cellular components, and infectious agents, a freshly formed midday sample is recommended (Reppas and Foster, 2016a).

Cystocentesis, catheterization, and voided (free catch) are methods used for urine collection. Cystocentesis should be considered when bacterial or fungal culture are planned. Microscopic hematuria may be introduced while sampling and can be exacerbated in patients with preexisting bladder inflammation. Thus, if monitoring a patient for recurrent hematuria, a voided sample is recommended (Reppas and Foster, 2016a). A midstream sample is recommended for voided collection, and the collection method should be reported to the microbiologist (Callens and Bartges, 2015; Reppas and Foster, 2016a). Urine collected from a table can have a false-positive reagent test strip protein reaction if a quaternary ammonium disinfectant or chlorhexidine is present on the table surface (Stockham and Scott, 2008; Reppas and Foster, 2016a).

SPECIMEN PROCESSING AND SLIDE PREPARATION

Urine collection containers should be clean, sterile, nonbreakable, and leakproof (Vap and Shropshire, 2017). Urine is a volatile substance and should be evaluated as soon as possible after collection, ideally within 30 minutes or practically within 1 hour of collection at room temperature (Albasan et al., 2003; Gunn-Christie et al., 2012; Reppas and Foster, 2016a). If this is not possible, urine should be immediately stored at 4°C until examination to slow bacterial growth and cell degradation. Urine should not be stored longer than 6 to 12 hours before examination to avoid bacterial proliferation, degeneration, or decreased numbers of casts, erythrocytes, leukocytes, and epithelial cells, or formation or dissolution of crystals. A refrigerated specimen should be allowed to warm to room temperature before evaluation because cold temperature can interfere with chemical reagent strip readings, falsely increase the USG, cause substances to precipitate, and promote crystal formation (Sturgess et al., 2001; Albasan et al., 2003; Callens and Bartges, 2015; Reppas and Foster, 2016a, 2016b; Vap and Shropshire, 2017). Urine pH is minimally affected if preserved by refrigeration for up to 24 hours (Raskin et al., 2002; Albasan et al., 2003). If there is concern for crystalluria, the urine should not be refrigerated but instead should be evaluated within 30 minutes of collection at room temperature. Urine should not be frozen before microscopic examination because sediment constituents will be altered (Vap and Shropshire, 2017).

Wet-Mount Preparation

The most routine method to examine the urine sediment is via a wet-mount slide. This may be most commonly as an unstained preparation or, if necessary, via staining to assist in cell identification and morphologic features.

BOX 12.1 Recommended Steps in Performing a Complete Urinalysis Manually

1. **Collection:** Obtain a standard volume of urine (e.g., 6 mL) in a conical tube. Always use the same volume of urine between and among patients. Cystocentesis is the preferred collection method except when trying to avoid iatrogenic hematuria. Evaluate samples within 30–60 minutes after collection to avoid artifactual changes.
2. **Physical characteristics:** If urine has been refrigerated, allow it to rewarm to room temperature. Cold urine will appear turbid. Observe and record the color and degree of transparency before and after centrifugation. Color and transparency are best appreciated using a clean glass tube with 1 mL of well-mixed urine.
3. **Chemical reagent strip:** Follow manufacturer instructions on how to saturate each reagent pad (either rapidly place one drop on each pad by pipet or dip the reagent strip into the urine tube). It is critical to interpret results in the proper order and time sequence as prescribed by the manufacturer. Because reagent strips are labile, strictly observe the expiration date, limit exposure of direct light, and monitor environmental temperature.
4. **Confirmatory and quantitative diagnostic tests:** Confirmatory tests or additional diagnostic tests might be considered based on the results of the chemistry analysis.
   - *Ictotest*: This test is more sensitive and easier to interpret than the dipstick. It is used to confirm the presence of bilirubin.
   - *Acetest*: This has a lower detection limit than some reagent pads and can be used to confirm trace or questionable ketone reactions on reagent pads. However, the manufacturer recently discontinued this test.
   - *Sulfosalicylic acid test*: Perform this test to evaluate total protein, especially when urine pH is strongly alkaline. The procedure is more sensitive than reagent strips and specific for all proteins, not just albumin, which is predominantly detected by the protein pad. This test is becoming less common in many reference laboratories in favor of performing a urine protein:creatinine ratio.
   - *Urine protein:creatinine ratio* (UPC): This test quantifies proteinuria standardized to urine creatinine concentration. Normal UPC is <0.2 in dogs and cats.
   - *Urine protein gel electrophoresis*: Laboratories that perform urine protein gel electrophoresis are limited, but this test is used to determine if renal proteinuria is primarily glomerular or tubular in origin (Hokamp et al., 2018).
5. **Centrifugation:** Pipet the remaining 5 mL of urine (2 mL minimum) into a conical tube, and centrifuge it for 5 minutes at 400–450 $\times$ g. Remember to convert the relative centrifugal force to the appropriate revolutions per minute on the centrifuge depending on the rotor radius. Note the amount of sediment and presence or absence of lipid on the top of the urine. Remove the supernatant by pipet to achieve a standard sediment concentration for your laboratory (e.g., 10% or 20%).

   Using 20% standard:
   - Total of 5 mL: Remove 4.0 mL supernatant and resuspend in the remaining 1.0 mL.
   - Total of 4 mL: Remove 3.2 mL supernatant and resuspend in the remaining 0.8 mL.
   - Total of 3 mL: Remove 2.4 mL supernatant and resuspend in the remaining 0.6 mL.
   - Total of 2 mL: Remove 1.6 mL supernatant and resuspend in the remaining 0.4 mL.
6. **Specific gravity:** Pipet a drop of whole urine or supernatant onto a distilled water-calibrated refractometer and record measurement. If refractometer measurement is hazy or unreadable due to insoluble components in the whole urine sample, use supernatant only for specific gravity. If specific gravity extends off the scale, dilute the urine 1:1 with distilled water and reread, doubling the last two digits (e.g., 1.024 to 1.048).
7. **Microscopic preparation (wet mount):** Place one drop of the resuspended sediment on a microscope glass slide for viewing the unstained sediment. A second drop can be placed in an adjacent spot on the same slide with one drop of new methylene blue stain or urine sediment stain, mixed with a wooden applicator stick. Place a coverslip on each of the urine drops and allow the particles to settle before examination.
8. **Microscopic examination (wet mount):** Scan urine drop with lowered condenser.
   Under low-power magnification (10× objective), record the types and numbers of casts and squamous or nonsquamous epithelial cells per low-power field.
   Under high-dry magnification (40×, high power field) observe and record the following:
   - Bacteria: description of morphology and amount seen (few, many)
   - Crystals: type and amount (none, few, moderate, many)
   - Erythrocytes: numbers per high-power field (normal, 0–5/hpf)
   - Leukocytes: numbers per high-power field (normal 0–5/hpf)
   - Lipid droplets: positive or negative
   - Mucous threads: positive or negative
   - Parasites, fungi: type seen and morphology
   - Sperm: positive or negative (may be normal when seen)
9. **Microscopic examination (dry mount):** Prepare one or more sediment smears and allow them to air dry. Stain with Romanowsky stain and examine the morphology of blood cells, normal or neoplastic epithelial cells, and infectious agents if present.

Unstained Sediment Preparation

A standardized volume of urine in a sealed, conical tube should be used for sedimentation. A 5 mL aliquot of urine is centrifuged at a low speed (400–450 $\times$ g) as the relative centrifugal force (RCF) for 5 minutes to pellet nonsoluble components (Callens and Bartges, 2015; Vap and Shropshire, 2017). Longer times or higher force can damage cells and casts. Relative centrifugal force can be converted to revolutions per minute (RPM) with the following equation:

$$RPM = \sqrt{[RCF / (r \times 1.118)]} \times 1000$$

where r is the rotational radius of the centrifuge rotor in millimeters.

Most of the supernatant is removed using a pipette, leaving a standardized amount in contact with the pelleted sediment to achieve a sediment concentration of approximately 10% to 20%. Resuspend the sediment in the remaining supernatant using a bulb pipette or by gently inverting the tube, place a drop onto a glass slide, and add a coverslip (Fig. 12.1). The volume of the drop and size and thickness of the glass slide and coverslip should always remain the same.

Stained Sediment Preparation

Commercial urine sediment stain or new methylene blue is frequently used for the microscopic examination of the sediment when there is difficulty identifying structures in the wet mount (Fig. 12.2). It is recommended that the microscopic examination of an unstained sediment precede examination of the stained sample to avoid misinterpretation because of stain-contaminated with bacteria, yeast, or fungus as well as stain precipitate. Stains

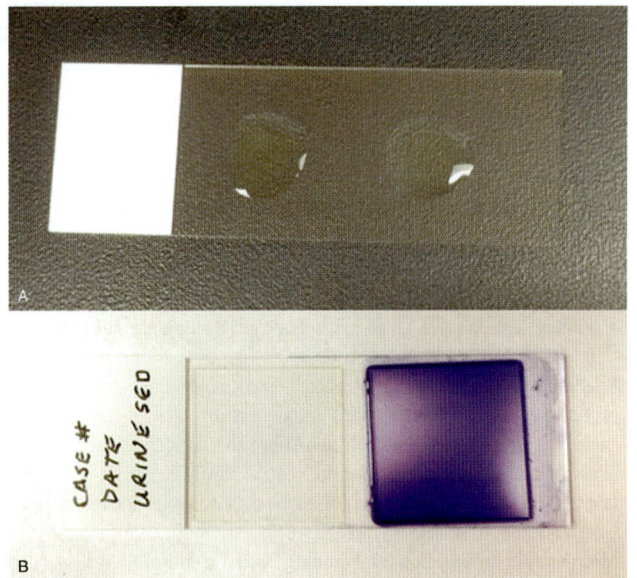

FIGURE 12.1 Urine sediment. Wet-mount preparation. A, Application of two adjacent sediment drops. **B,** Coverslip preparations. The left coverslip is unstained for viewing all sediment constituents and recording their presence semiquantitatively. The right coverslip contains an additional drop of 0.5% new methylene blue for closer inspection of cells and infectious agents. If seen in the stained sample, crystals and castlike structures should be ignored as possible artifacts from the stain. Excess fluid may be removed by touching edges to an absorbent paper. (Courtesy Rose Raskin, Purdue University.)

may be filtered before use as shown in Fig. 1.18B to minimize precipitate.

Dry-Mount Preparation

Some insoluble particles are more difficult to identify or classify in wet mounts than in dry mounts or Romanowsky-stained cytopathology smears (Fig. 12.3). These elements include bacteria and specific leukocyte or epithelial cell types owing to the osmotic and pH changes in urine and presence of bacterial toxins that alter the size, structure, and transparency of particles.

MICROSCOPIC EXAMINATION AND REPORTING

When examining a wet mount, microscope settings need to be modified to increase contrast (see Fig. 12.2A). This is achieved by lowering the condenser or partially closing the illumination diaphragm. Examine the wet mount at both low power (10× objective) and high dry power (40× objective) and evaluate at least 10 fields at each magnification. Results are reported semiquantitatively or with subjective descriptors. Erythrocytes and leukocytes are reported as a range per high-power field (#–#/hpf). Large epithelial cells and casts, including description of the type of cell or cast, are typically reported as a range per low-power field (#–#/lpf) (Vap and Shropshire, 2017). Alternatively, number of small epithelial cells may be reported per high-power field. Crystals (including type), infectious agents (including type), lipid droplets, and spermatozoa are reported using subjective descriptors (positive/negative or rare, few, moderate, or many).

The urine sediment can be evaluated by manual microscopy or by an automated instrument. Hernandez et al. (2019) found that one automated analyzer of canine and feline urine sediment, IDEXX SediVue Dx, had similar clinical interpretations of the results as manual microscopy for two crystal types and most cellular elements, with the exception for the identification of epithelial cells.

An alternative but less commonly used method to enumerate insoluble urine particles is by means of a counting chamber. The whole urine sample is mixed gently but not centrifuged, and a standardized volume is pipetted into a well of a counting chamber with a microscopic grid. All particles in a defined area are counted, and results are expressed as particles per volume of urine rather than per low- or high-power field (Reppas and Foster, 2016b). A modification of this method was evaluated using a small standardized volume (60 μL) of unspun urine quality control material in a microtiter well without a coverslip

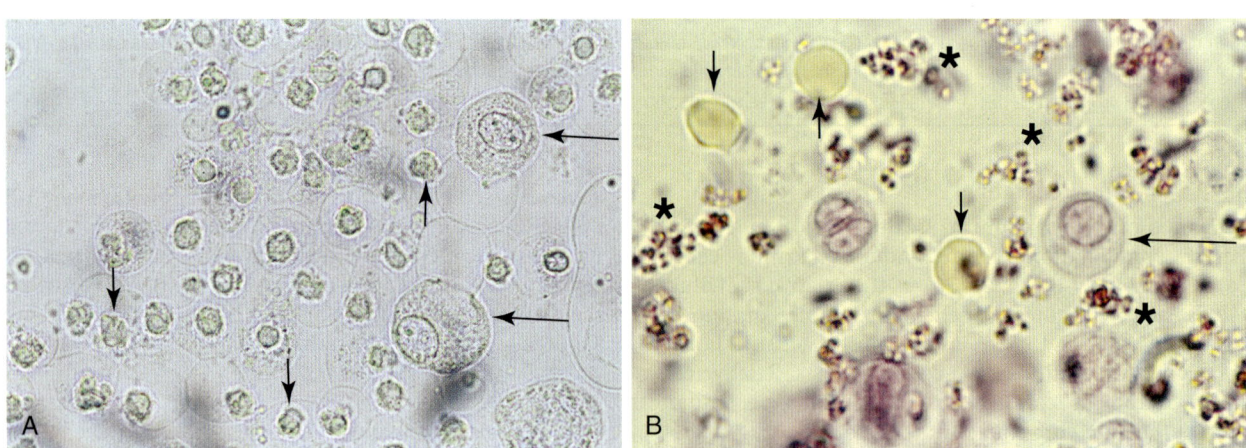

FIGURE 12.2 Urine sediment. Wet mount. Same case in A and B. **A, Unstained specimen.** This unstained urine sediment illustrates the enhanced contrast of the cellular constituents when the microscope's condenser is lowered. Crenated erythrocytes are predominant *(short arrows)*, and two plump epithelial cells with granular-appearing cytoplasm are present *(long arrows)*. (Unstained; HP oil.) **B, Stained specimen.** Applying stain to the specimen highlights cellular detail. An epithelial cell *(long arrow)* and erythrocytes *(short arrows)* are present. The stain should be free of precipitate via periodic filtration or replacement. As illustrated in this photomicrograph, the stain particles are distracting and give the misleading impression of bacteria *(asterisks)*. (Sedi-Stain; HP oil.)

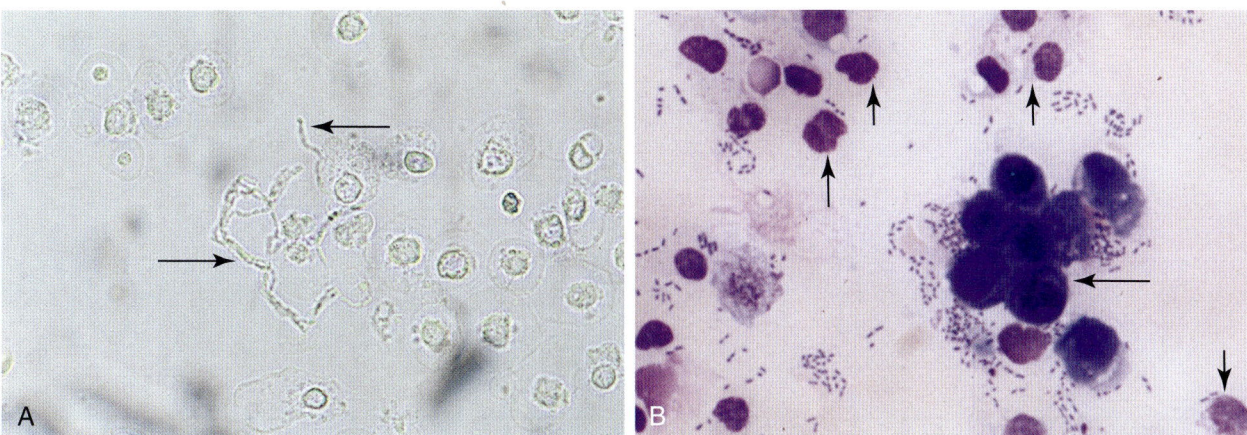

■ **FIGURE 12.3 Bacterial cystitis. Urine sediment. A, Wet mount.** Chains of bacteria *(arrows)* and unidentified cells (presumed degenerate neutrophils with a mononuclear cell appearance and crenated erythrocytes) are observed in this unstained urine sediment obtained by percutaneous cystocentesis. Identification of the cell type is not important in this setting and, in fact, may be impossible owing to changes induced by the physiochemical nature of the urine. (Unstained; HP oil.) **B, Dry mount.** Romanowsky-stained cytopathologic preparation of an infected urine specimen highlights the bacteria and a clump of uniform epithelial cells *(long arrow)*. Most cells, presumably neutrophils, have swollen, rounded nuclei or have lysed owing to the hostile environment and cannot be identified *(short arrows)*. In other fields, some of these cells retained slight segmentation, and many were observed to contain bacteria, supporting their classification as a neutrophil. Again, identification of the cell type is not important in this setting. These figures further illustrate that the Romanowsky-stained urine sediment definitively accentuates identification of bacteria compared with unstained preparations. (Wright; HP oil.)

(Chase et al., 2018). This study demonstrated the effects of centrifugation on reproducibility of leukocyte and erythrocyte counts and frequency of morphologic changes.

KEY POINT To accentuate the constituents in the unstained urine sediment, the iris diaphragm is partially closed and the substage condenser of the microscope is lowered. This is a dynamic process conducted while viewing the specimen to improve contrast or resolution.

Cellular Components
Erythrocytes

Fewer than 5 erythrocytes/hpf are considered normal in dogs and cats, especially if the urine has been collected by cystocentesis or catheterization. More than 5/hpf is considered hematuria (Callens and Bartges, 2015; Vap and Shropshire, 2017) (Fig. 12.4). Hematuria can be iatrogenic (damage from bladder palpation, cystocentesis, or catheterization) or pathologic (trauma or inflammation of the genitourinary tract, or coagulopathies). Voided

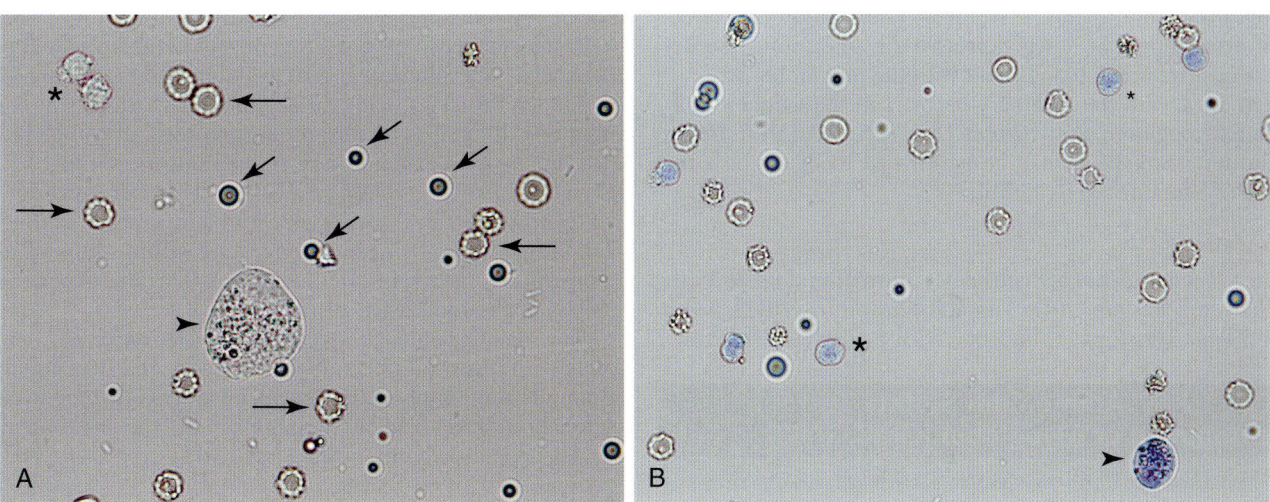

■ **FIGURE 12.4 Bacterial cystitis. Urine sediment. Wet mount.** Same case in A and B. **A, Unstained.** Urine collected by cystocentesis from a dog with hematuria, pyuria, and bacteriuria. Erythrocytes *(arrows)* are predominantly crenated but still maintain a biconcave appearance. Fewer leukocytes *(asterisk)* are identified by their slightly larger size and granular cytoplasm. A single nonsquamous epithelial cell (presumed urothelial cell) is present and contains a larger amount of granular cytoplasm *(arrowhead)*. Infrequent bacterial rods occasionally in pairs are seen in the background as well as lipid droplets *(short arrows)*. (Unstained; IP.) **B, Stained.** The leukocytes *(asterisks)* are easier to identify in this image, staining pale purple. The nonsquamous epithelial cell *(arrowhead)* is clearly visible. Erythrocytes appear mildly crenated and stain pale orange. (Sedi-Stain; IP.)

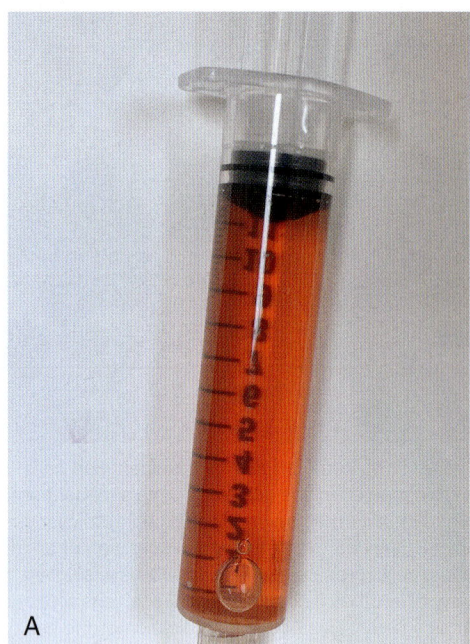 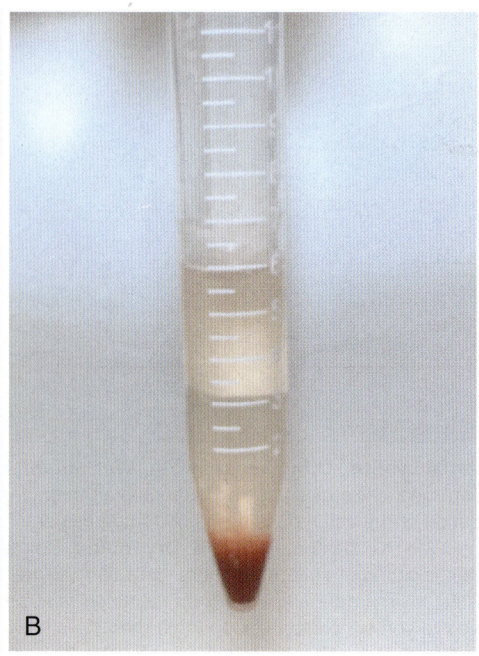

FIGURE 12.5 Hematuria. Macroscopic. Dog. Same case in A and B. **A, Original submission.** Urine appeared red and clear with few intact erythrocytes. **B, After ammonium sulfate testing.** To determine the source of color and rule out myoglobinuria, ammonium sulfate was added to the urine and centrifuged as per instructions (see Box 12.2). Hemoglobin has precipitated leaving a clear to pale yellow supernatant. A red supernatant would have suggested myoglobin. (Courtesy Rose Raskin, Kansas State University.)

urine samples from dogs in estrus might also be hematuric due to genital tract hemorrhage (Stockham and Scott, 2008).

Erythrocytes are approximately 5 to 7 μm in diameter, round, and refractile and vary from colorless to pale yellow to orange and might appear biconcave. Erythrocytes crenate and may have a granular appearance in hypertonic or aged urine and should not be confused with leukocytes, which have a granular appearance but are approximately twice the diameter of an erythrocyte. Erythrocytes swell and appear as colorless smooth balloons or rings in hypotonic or alkaline urine and are subject to lysis within a few hours. Thus, if sediment examination is delayed, erythrocytes might be falsely decreased due to osmotic lysis despite a positive occult blood result with the reagent test strip.

Red urine with few or no erythrocytes in the sediment may contain hemoglobin or myoglobin (Fig. 12.5A). An ammonium sulfate test (Box 12.2) may be performed to distinguish the source of hematuria (Fig. 12.5B).

Leukocytes

Up to 5 leukocytes/hpf are considered normal in dogs and cats (Callens and Bartges, 2015; Vap and Shropshire, 2017). More than 5 leukocytes/hpf is abnormal with pyuria (pus in urine)

BOX 12.2 Ammonium Sulfate Test for Hemoglobin or Myoglobin (Graff, 1983)

1. Dissolve by mixing 2.8 g of analytical grade ammonium sulfate into 5 mL of urine to produce an 80% saturated solution of ammonium sulfate at 20°–25°C. (The final volume should be 6.5 mL.)
2. Centrifuge the solution at approximately 2000 × g for 15 min.

Interpretation: Hemoglobin will precipitate out, leaving a clear to pale yellow supernatant, but myoglobin will stay in solution (colored supernatant).

---

most often involving neutrophils and macrophages to a lesser degree (see Fig. 12.3). Leukocytes in a voided urine sample or collected via catheterization should be considered to have originated from anywhere along the genitourinary tract. Leukocytes in a urine sample collected by cystocentesis should be considered to have originated from the kidneys, ureters, bladder, or proximal urethra. Leukocyturia may indicate inflammation, which may result from infection (bacteria, fungi, parasites) or other pathology such as neoplasia, urolithiasis, and trauma. Gross hemorrhage can secondarily increase urine leukocyte numbers in the absence of true inflammation.

Leukocyte types are not differentiated in the urine sediment. Leukocytes are spherical and 10 to 14 μm in diameter, twice the size of erythrocytes, with variably granular cytoplasm. Nuclei might be difficult to discern on wet mounts but can be identified on air-dried Romanowsky-stained smears (see Fig. 12.3B). Crenation, swelling, pyknosis, and lysis can occur dependent on USG, urine pH, and storage time and temperature, with up to half of leukocytes lysing or deteriorating within 1 hour at room temperature in alkaline, dilute urine (Stockham and Scott, 2008; Reppas and Foster, 2016b).

The majority of leukocytes in the urine are generally neutrophils with lesser numbers of macrophages and occasional eosinophils and lymphocytes (Stockham and Scott, 2008). Rarely, exfoliation from bladder lymphoma into the urine demonstrates neoplastic lymphocytes (Fig. 12.6).

Epithelial Cells

Epithelial cells, up to 0 to 2/lpf, are normal in canine and feline urine sediment. It may be very difficult to morphologically distinguish renal tubular epithelial cells from urothelial cells, and simply categorizing them as squamous versus nonsquamous may be appropriate (Vap and Shropshire, 2017).

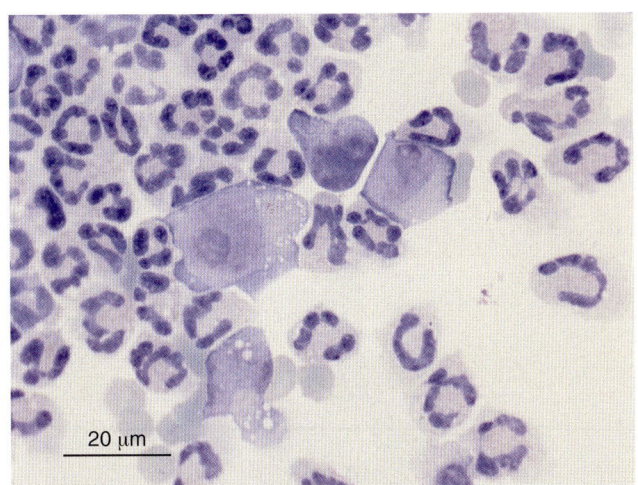

FIGURE 12.6 Neoplastic lymphoid cells. Urine sediment. Dry mount. Dog. The presence of abnormal leukocytes suggested a stained sediment smear be made from a dry mount. Many nondegenerate neutrophils are present along with four large round cells, each with a prominent nucleus and scant to moderate punctate basophilic cytoplasm. A bladder mass diagnosed as lymphoma was the source of the neoplastic cell population. (Modified Wright; HP oil.) (Courtesy Rose Raskin, Purdue University.)

Urothelial cells, previously known as transitional epithelial cells, line the renal pelvis, ureters, bladder, and most of the urethra. They have a moderate to large amount of grainy cytoplasm and a single round, central to paracentral nucleus. Urothelial cells are relatively large and vary from 20 to 40 μm in diameter depending on their site of origin. They vary in shape from round to pear, polygonal, or caudate (Fig. 12.7). On a Romanowsky-stained cytopathologic specimen, urothelial cells may contain one or more bright magenta cytoplasmic vacuoles, called Melamed-Wolinska bodies (Fig. 12.8), which are periodic acid–Schiff and uroplakin positive and likely represent degenerative change (see Chapter 11). Normal urothelial cells may swell with protracted exposure to urine altering their appearance; therefore, they are best examined in a midday fresh sample along with an air-dried Romanowsky-stained preparation if large cells are initially observed during a routine urinalysis (Reppas and Foster, 2016b; Vap and Shropshire, 2017).

Increased numbers of urothelial cells are suggestive of inflammation or urothelial carcinoma, previously termed transitional cell carcinoma, the latter being of greater concern when cells are clustered and there is a concomitant radiographic finding of a mass in the lower urinary tract (Figs. 12.9 and 12.10). Inflamed mucosa can shed hyperplastic or dysplastic urothelial

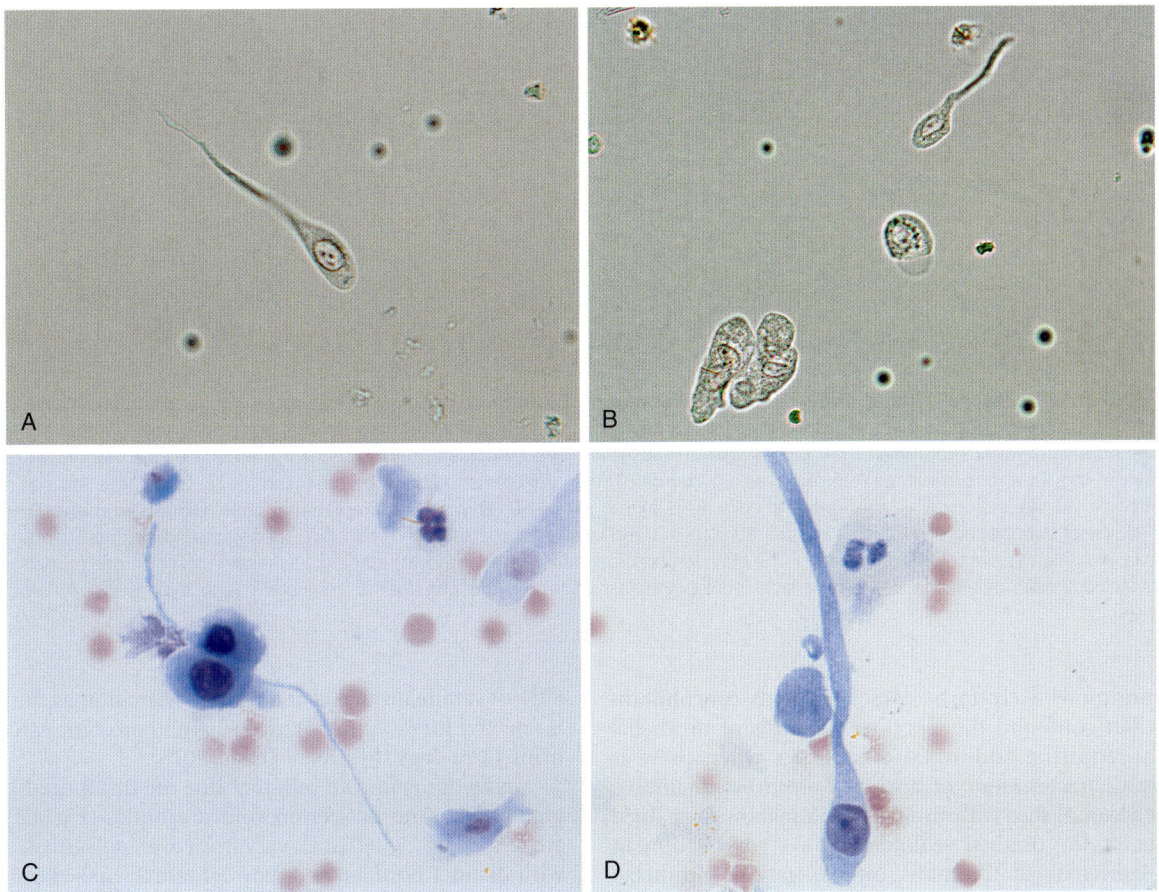

FIGURE 12.7 Caudate urothelial cells. Urine sediment. Dog. Same case in A to D. **A, Unstained.** Single tadpole-like cell with round nucleus containing several small nucleoli. The cytoplasm extends from the cell as a single projection or tail. (Unstained; IP.) **B, Unstained.** One epithelial cell cluster, a single round epithelial cell, and one caudate urothelial cell are present. (Unstained; IP.) **C, Stained.** Two epithelial cells with long thin cytoplasmic extensions appear along with two large squamous-like epithelial cells and one neutrophil. (Wright-Giemsa; HP oil.) **D, Stained.** One urothelial cell with a long cytoplasmic projection or tail appears next to a neutrophil and a cytoplasmic remnant. The caudate-shaped cells may represent urothelium from the renal pelvis, but this is unproven. (Wright-Giemsa; HP oil.) (Courtesy Rose Raskin, University of Florida.)

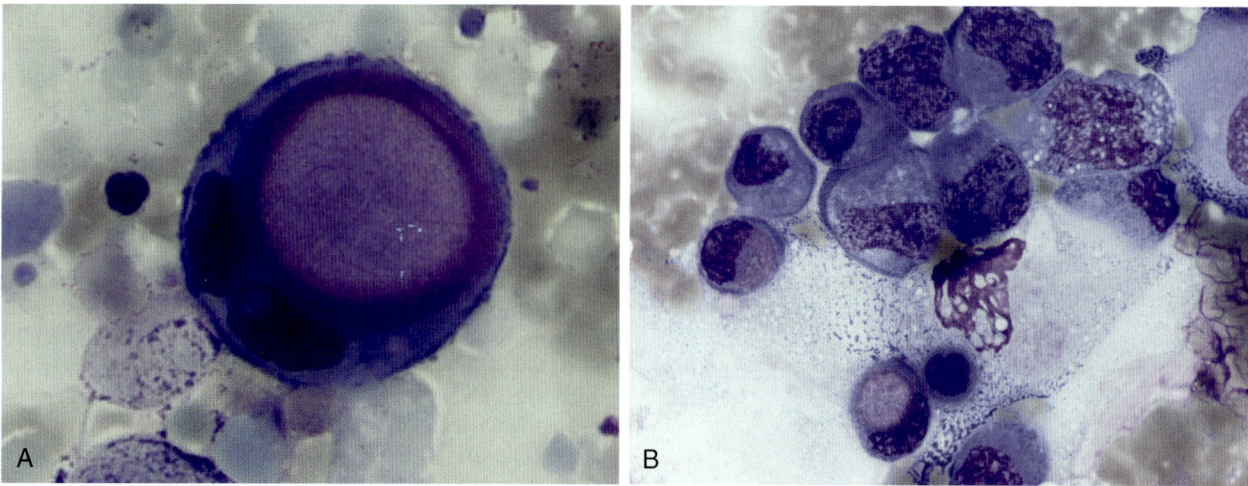

■ **FIGURE 12.8 Urothelial carcinoma. Urine sediment. Dry mount. Dog. A,** A single urothelial cell with binucleation and a Melamed-Wolinska body, a pink granular vacuole creating a signet ring–like appearance of the cell. (Wright; HP oil.) **B,** A cluster of urothelial cells displays anisocytosis, anisokaryosis, and Melamed-Wolinska bodies. (Wright; HP oil.) (A, Courtesy Mackenzie Long, The Ohio State University. B, Courtesy Susan Smith and Mackenzie Long, The Ohio State University.)

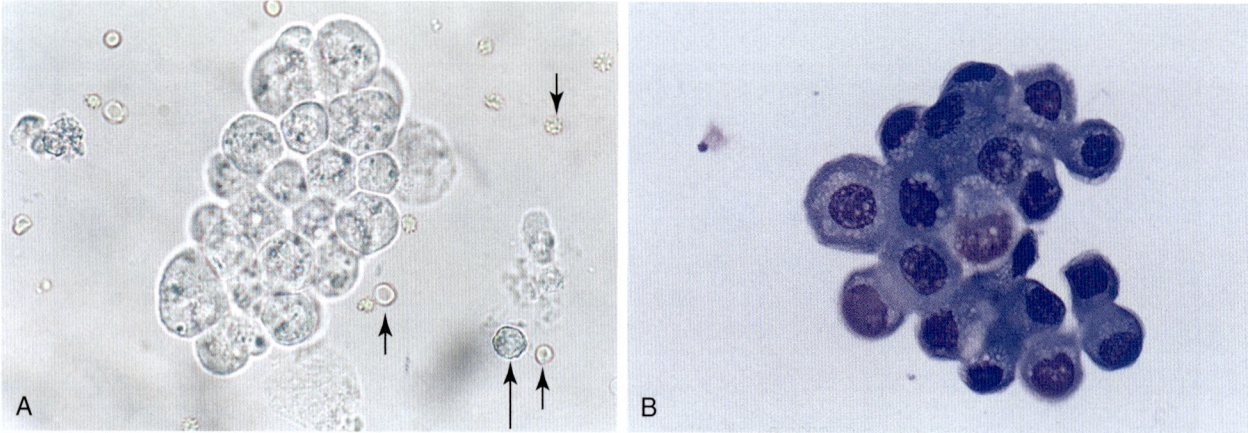

■ **FIGURE 12.9 A, Epithelial cell cluster. Urine sediment. Wet mount.** Epithelial cells demonstrate mild to moderate anisocytosis (20–40 μm in diameter). Erythrocytes (~5–7 μm in diameter, *short arrows*), some with a smooth surface and some with a crenated appearance, and a leukocyte (presumed neutrophil) (~10–12 μm in diameter, *long arrow*) are observed. The cytoplasmic granules of the presumed neutrophil were in random motion (brownian movement); sometimes referred to as a *glitter cell*. These granules should not be mistaken for bacteria. Note the size relationship of the erythrocyte vs. the leukocyte vs. the epithelial cells. (Unstained; HP oil.) **B, Hyperplastic epithelial cells. Urine sediment. Dry mount.** A drop of the sediment was placed on a glass slide (the surface of which was first coated with a thin layer of serum and air dried), spread, air dried, and stained as a routine cytopathologic preparation. The stained preparation facilitates the cytopathologic assessment for criteria of malignancy. Mild to moderate anisocytosis, anisokaryosis, and variable nucleocytoplasmic ratio were considered consistent with hyperplasia of urothelial cells. (Wright; HP oil.)

cells and are more likely to be associated with concomitant leukocytes but confound the tentative diagnosis of urothelial carcinoma, requiring additional diagnostics when there is uncertainty. Characterization of suspected urothelial carcinoma cells can be accomplished with an air-dried Romanowsky-stained preparation of the original sediment or a second sediment specimen collected via traumatic catheterization. Urothelial carcinoma cells display anisocytosis, anisokaryosis, anisonucleoliosis, abnormal mitotic figures, multiple nucleoli, multinucleation, or nuclear molding. The *BRAF* mutation assay is suggested as an additional diagnostic test for confirmation or when cytopathologic identification of urothelial carcinoma cells is uncertain. The *BRAF* V595E mutation was found in approximately 80% of canine urothelial and prostatic carcinomas, and the assay is sensitive for detection of urothelial and prostatic carcinomas in urine from dogs (Mochizuki et al., 2015).

Squamous epithelial cells that line the distal urethra and vagina are commonly seen in voided samples (Fig. 12.11). They are large cells (30–60 μm); vary from oval, polygonal, or angular with distinct borders; and may contain a small round nucleus. When found, foam cells suggest vaginal origin in a voided urine sample (Fig. 12.12).

Renal tubular epithelial cells may be present in low numbers in urine. They are slightly larger than leukocytes, appear round to cuboidal to columnar (Fig. 12.13), and have a large round nucleus (Graff, 1983). An air-dried, Romanowsky-stained

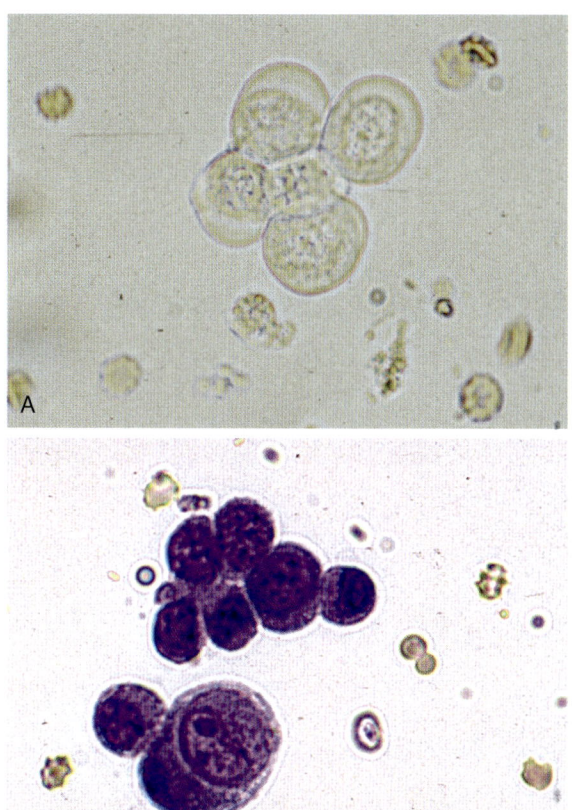

■ **FIGURE 12.10 Carcinoma. Urine sediment.** Same case in A and B. **A, Unstained.** Epithelial cells demonstrate more variability in cell size and nucleocytoplasmic ratio. Atypical cell clusters should be investigated further with a cytopathologic preparation of the sediment stained with a Romanowsky stain. (Unstained; HP oil.) **B, Stained.** The cytopathologic criteria for malignancy are more evident in the stained preparation, which, in this epithelial cell cluster, include high and variable nucleocytoplasmic ratios, prominent nucleoli, and coarse chromatin. Urothelial cell carcinoma was suspected by cytopathology. (Wright-Giemsa; HP oil.) (Courtesy Rose Raskin, University of Florida.)

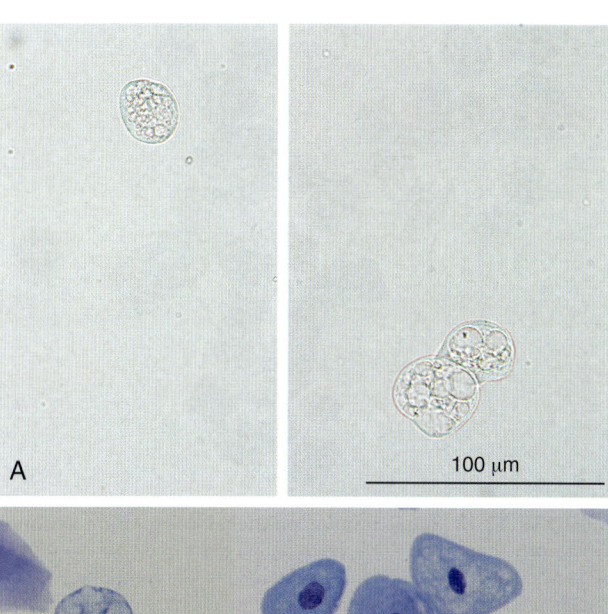

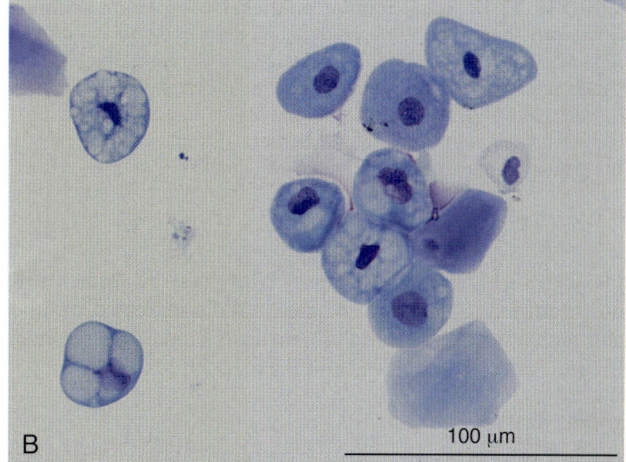

■ **FIGURE 12.12 Foam squamous cells. Urine sediment. Female dog.** Same case in A and B. **A, Unstained.** Large round cells, one on the left and two on the right, are present in a free catch or voided urine sample. Present are multiple intracellular, clear, circular vacuoles within these cells. (Unstained; HP.) **B, Stained.** From a cytocentrifuge preparation, the majority of the squamous cells display cytoplasmic vacuolation either as small or large nonstaining vacuoles. The cells range from intermediate to anucleate squames with the majority as superficial squamous epithelium. (Wright-Giemsa; HP oil.) (Courtesy Francisco Conrado, University of Florida.)

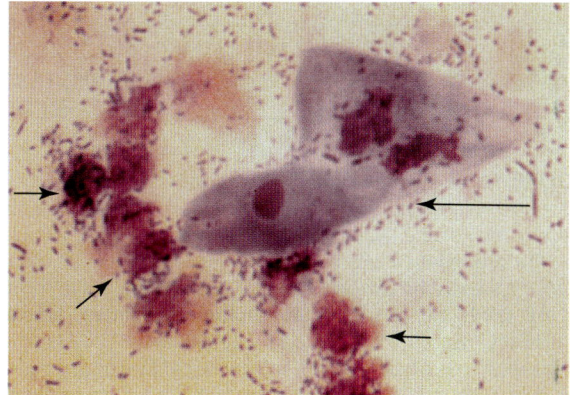

■ **FIGURE 12.11 Contaminated urine specimen. Free catch.** Frequent extracellular bacterial rods are seen in the background. The presence of a mature squamous epithelial cell *(long arrow)* with only a small number of leukocytes *(short arrows)* suggests the bacteria is likely from contamination. No bacteria or neutrophils were observed in a second specimen obtained via percutaneous cystocentesis. (Wright; HP oil.)

cytopathologic preparation can be used to differentiate these cells from leukocytes or other epithelial cells.

Casts

Casts are elongated, cylindrical structures that form via precipitation of Tamm-Horsfall mucoprotein, which is secreted by renal tubule cells, and by albumin when there is concomitant proteinuria. Cast formation is pronounced in environments favoring protein denaturation and precipitation (low flow, concentrated salts, low pH). Casts dissolve rapidly and should be evaluated immediately after collection. Casts are enumerated per low-power field and differentiated by their type.

Hyaline Casts

Hyaline casts, representing solidified Tamm-Horsfall mucoprotein, are colorless and transparent with parallel sides and rounded

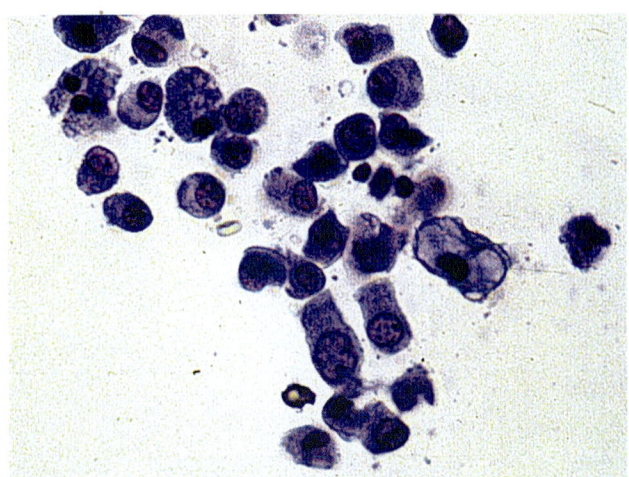

■ **FIGURE 12.13 Renal tubular epithelial cells. Urine sediment. Dry mount.** These cells are approximately the same size as inflammatory leukocytes but have a round nucleus with clumped chromatin. The cytoplasm ranges from round to cuboidal to columnar. The cuboidal and columnar cells appear to have a fringed apical end, suggestive of the proximal tubular ends with brush borders. (Wright-Giemsa; HP oil.) (Courtesy University of Florida Cytology Collection.)

ends (Fig. 12.14). Low numbers (<2/lpf) may be seen in urine from healthy dogs and cats, whereas mildly increased numbers occur with fever, exercise, and protein-losing renal disease (Stockham and Scott, 2008; Callens and Bartges, 2015).

Cellular Casts

Cellular casts are produced by the entrapment of epithelial cells, leukocytes, or erythrocytes into tubular matrix (Callens and Bartges, 2015). These casts reflect the underlying renal disease. Epithelial cell casts reflect tubular degeneration and sloughing of tubular epithelial cells caused by necrosis, toxicity, or renal ischemia (Fig. 12.15). Leukocyte casts are indicative of inflammation or infection, notably pyelonephritis. Erythrocyte casts (Fig. 12.16) are indicative of glomerular or tubular hemorrhage, renal infarction, or immune-mediated renal disease. Hemoglobin and myoglobin casts are red to brown and granular and are associated with hemoglobinuria or myoglobinuria (Fig. 12.17).

Granular Casts

Granular casts result either from the breakdown of cellular casts or the inclusion of aggregates of plasma proteins (e.g., albumin) or immunoglobulin light chains. Depending on the size of inclusions, they can be classified as coarse or fine, though the distinction has no diagnostic significance. It has been proposed that there is an evolution in the granular cast over time from coarse to fine owing to ongoing degeneration of the cast within the tubules (Osborne and Stevens, 1999). Low numbers (<2/lpf) may be seen in urine from healthy animals (Fig. 12.18). Increased numbers suggest renal tubular damage (Callens and Bartges, 2015). Occasionally, lipid droplets may be incorporated into the cast (Fig. 12.19). Fatty casts are formed by the breakdown of lipid-rich epithelial cells and are associated with renal ischemia, the nephrotic syndrome, or disorders of lipid metabolism (Callens and Bartges, 2015).

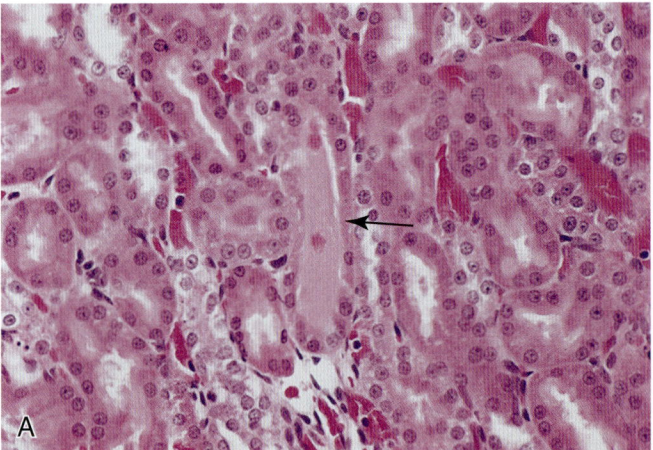
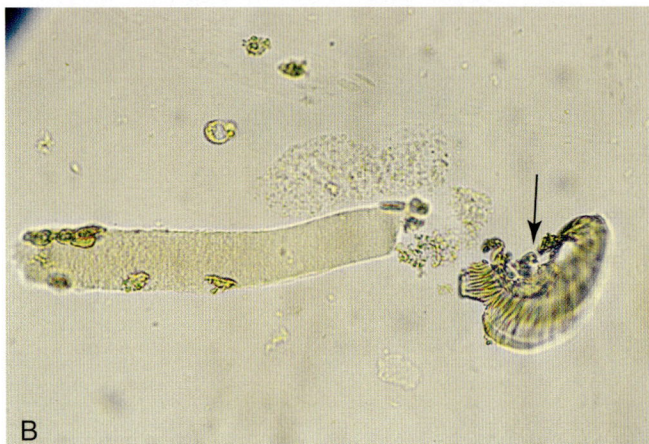
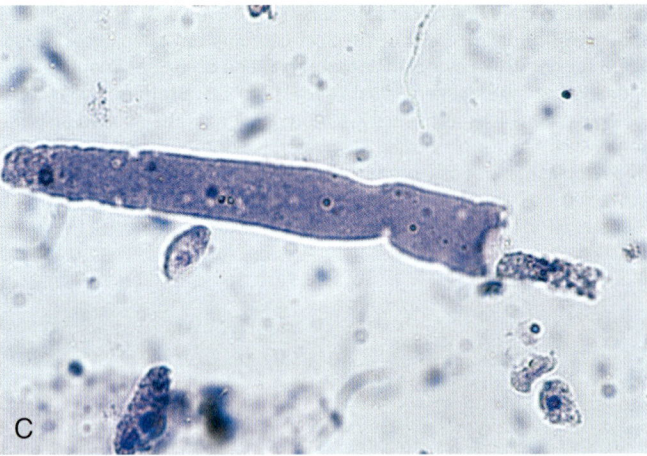

■ **FIGURE 12.14 Hyaline cast. A, Histology.** Casts form in the renal tubules *(arrow)* (ascending limb of the loop of Henle and distal tubule) and reflect their shape. Acidity, solute concentration, and flow rate facilitate the precipitation and solidification of Tamm-Horsfall mucoprotein, which is secreted by renal tubule cells resulting in the formation of a cast. (H&E; HP oil.) **B, Cytopathologic specimen. Unstained with artifact.** Hyaline casts are clear and colorless. They rapidly dissolve, especially in alkaline urine. An occasional hyaline cast per low-power field is normal. Cast formation is increased in association with albuminuria. Increased numbers are associated with strenuous exercise, fever, congestive heart failure, diuretic treatment, and primary glomerular diseases. A chip of collection container, likely plastic, is present *(arrow)*. (Unstained; HP oil.) **C, Cytopathologic specimen. Stained.** Note the smooth, homogenous appearance of the hyaline cast. (Sedi-Stain; HP oil.)

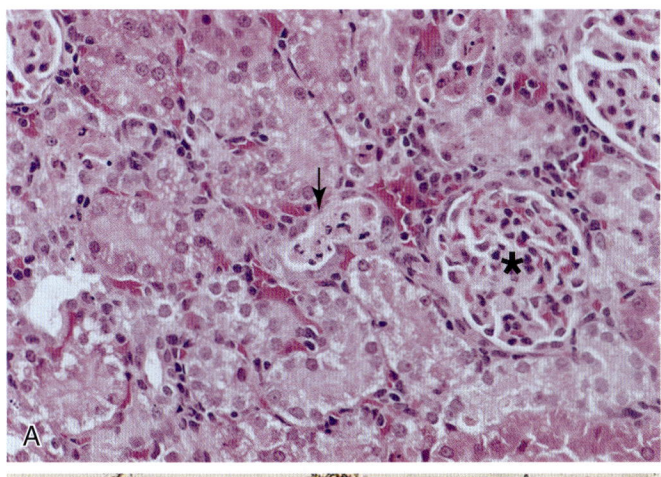

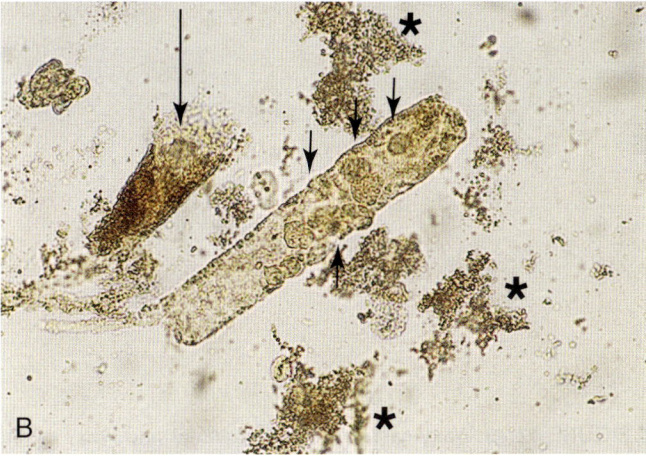

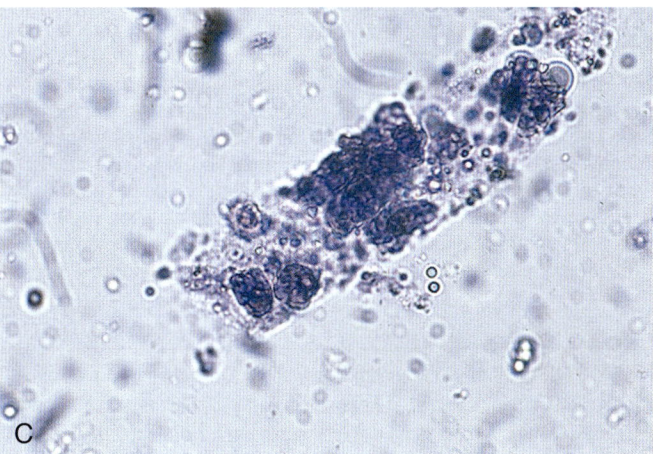

■ **FIGURE 12.15 Cellular cast. A, Histology.** Pyelonephritis has resulted in the formation of a cellular cast *(arrow)*. The pink protein matrix contains dark-staining neutrophil nuclei and unidentified nuclear debris. A glomerulus is present *(asterisk)*. (H&E; HP oil.) **B, Cytopathologic specimen. Unstained.** Cells, most consistent morphologically with epithelial cells, can be seen embedded in the cast matrix *(short arrows)*. The finding is suggestive of acute tubular necrosis. A fragmented granular cast *(long arrow)* and amorphous debris (unrecognizable granular material) *(asterisks)* are observed. (Unstained; HP oil.) **C, Cytopathologic specimen. Stained.** A stained specimen further supports the identity of cells in the cast as epithelial cells (when focused up and down). A few lipid droplets are observed. (Sedi-Stain; HP oil.)

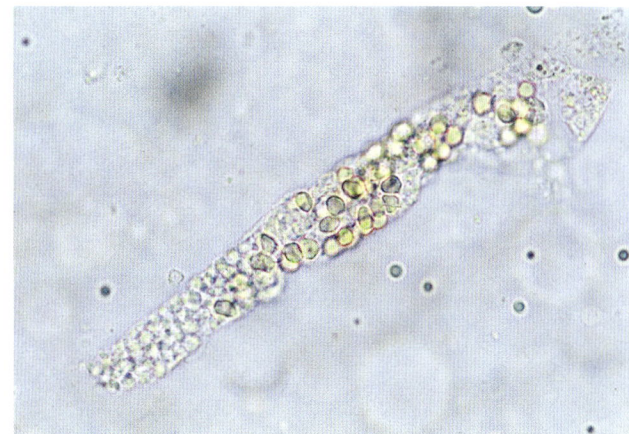

■ **FIGURE 12.16 Red cell cast.** A fragile and uncommon finding, red cell casts indicate acute intrarenal injury. The urine specimen is from a dog that had sustained a traumatic injury (hit by car). A few lipid droplets are present in the background. Note that the lipid droplets are more refractile than erythrocytes and vary in size. (Unstained; HP oil.)

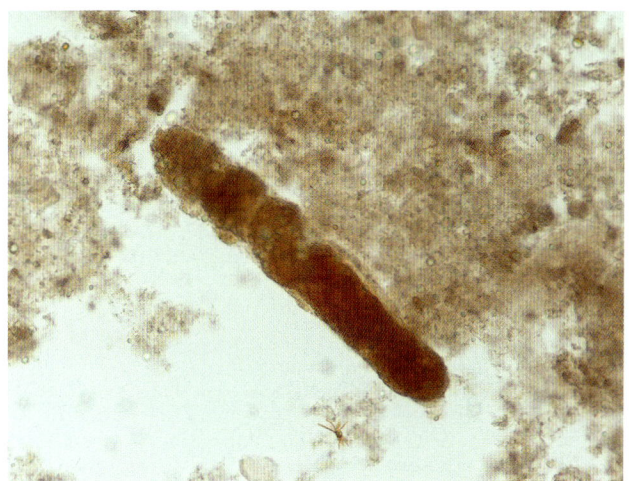

■ **FIGURE 12.17 Myoglobin cast.** A dog with pigmentary nephropathy and myoglobinuria shed numerous granular, brownish-red myoglobin casts into the urine. (Unstained; IP.)

Waxy Casts

Waxy casts represent the final product of cast evolution formed in association with very low urine flow from severe chronic kidney disease (Osborne and Stevens, 1999). They are significantly larger than hyaline casts due to urine stasis and their formation in diseased, dilated renal tubules. They are cylindrical, possess a high refractive index, and have fractures, sharp edges, and broken-off ends (Figs. 12.20 and 12.21).

Crystals

Crystals in the urine (crystalluria) are described and enumerated per low-power field. Crystalluria is common in canine and feline urine, and although some crystals do provide an increased risk for urolithiasis, crystalluria alone is not necessarily pathologic nor does it always indicate urolithiasis (Callens and Bartges, 2015). The type of crystal depends on urine pH and temperature, concentration of crystallogenic materials in the

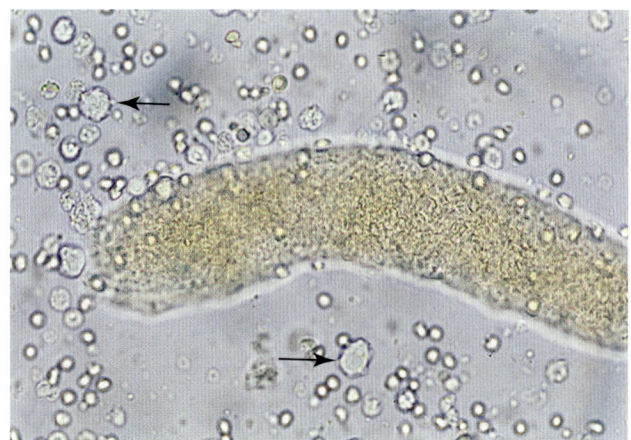

■ **FIGURE 12.18 Granular cast.** Granular casts represent degraded cellular material from injured renal tubular epithelial cells or, less often, inflammatory cells, embedded in a protein matrix. The granularity is sometimes further categorized as fine or coarse; however, the type of granularity is not of diagnostic importance. Nephrotoxins (e.g., gentamicin sulfate, amphotericin B), nephritis, and ischemia are pathologic events that result in their formation. Moderate numbers of epithelial cells *(arrows)*, leukocytes, and erythrocytes (inconspicuous) are present. Marked numbers of brightly refractile lipid droplets are prominent in this specimen. The lipiduria was attributed to the lubricant used to facilitate catheterization. (Unstained; HP oil.)

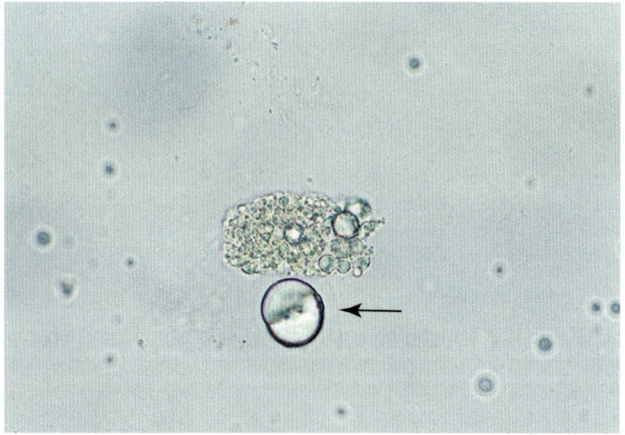

■ **FIGURE 12.19 Granular cast with lipid droplets (fatty cast).** This cast was present in the urine of a dog with nephrotic syndrome. They can be seen in association with diabetes mellitus and in cats with renal tubular injury. A moderate number of lipid droplets (out of focus) are present. A starch granule (glove powder) is located beneath the cast *(arrow)*. (Unstained; HP oil.)

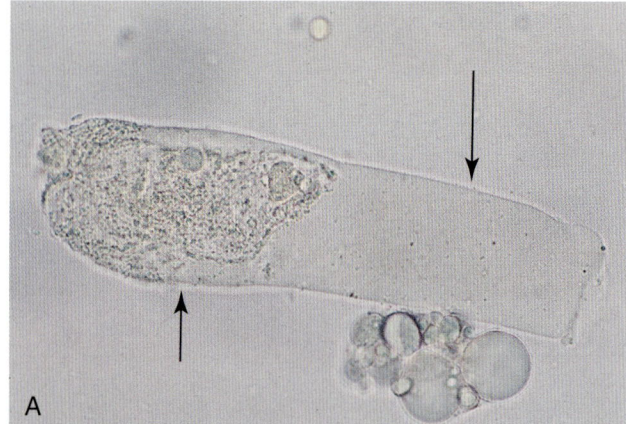

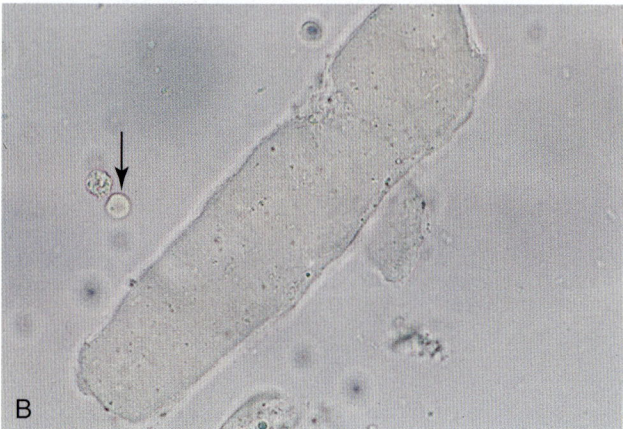

■ **FIGURE 12.20 Waxy casts. A,** Mixed granular and waxy casts. Waxy casts are thought to represent progressive development from granular casts as illustrated by this cast that has both granular cast *(short arrow)* and waxy cast *(long arrow)* characteristics. (Unstained; HP oil.) **B, Waxy cast.** These casts indicate chronic tubular pathology because additional time is required for their formation. Implicit in the pathogenesis of their formation is localized tubular obstruction. One sequela is dilation of the tubular lumen resulting in a wide cast. The word "broad" is sometimes added as a descriptive adjective when the width is two to four times that of a hyaline or granular cast. The magnitude of its width is apparent when contrasted to an erythrocyte *(arrow)*. A fracture or crack is often observed *(top right)*. (Unstained; HP oil.)

> **KEY POINT** If there is concern for crystalluria, use freshly formed urine (not a first morning sample) and examine it within 30 minutes of collection. It is best to maintain the sample at room temperature without refrigeration, which will cause crystals to form or dissolve.

urine, and the amount of time elapsed between urine collection and examination (Table 12.1). Evaluation for crystalluria should be performed within 30 minutes to 1 hour of urine collection for accuracy. Any crystals detected in urine that has been stored for longer than 1 hour should be reevaluated in a freshly collected urine sample (Albasan et al., 2003). Urine samples should remain at room temperature because refrigeration causes rapid formation or dissolution of crystals, causing erroneous results (Reppas and Foster, 2016b).

Acid Urine Crystals

Urine with a neutral or acidic pH tends to favor the formation of amorphous urates, sodium urate, uric acid, calcium oxalate, bilirubin, cystine, xanthine, calcium hydrogen phosphate dihydrate (brushite), sulfa, allantoin, and tyrosine crystals (Figs. 12.22 to 12.35).

Urates and uric acid crystals (see Figs. 12.22 to 12.25) occur in a variety of shapes such as amorphous granules, needles, rhombi, bricks, and barrels. They have similar significance to the presence of ammonium urate crystalluria usually indicative

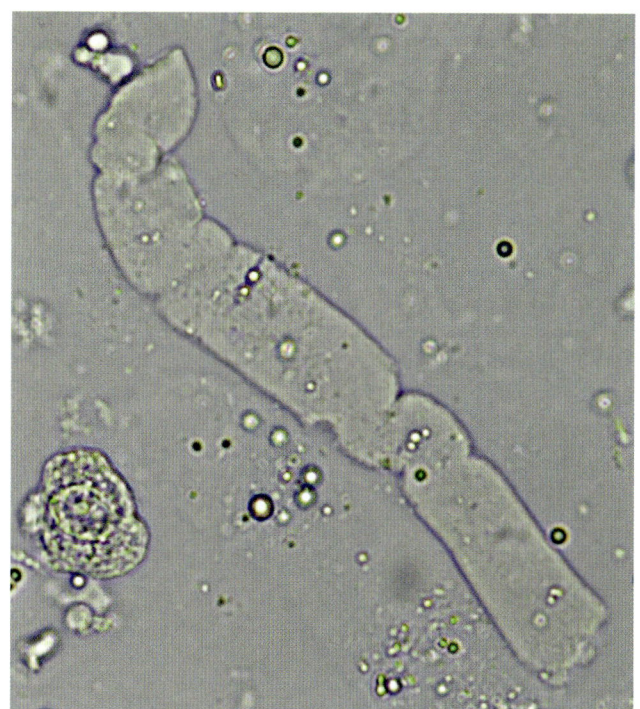

■ **FIGURE 12.21 Waxy cast and hyaline cast.** This waxy cast demonstrates the presence of squared ends and multiple fractures. A faint hyaline cast is seen parallel and just below the waxy cast with indistinct edges and embedded lipid droplets. A nonsquamous epithelial cell (presumed urothelial cell) is also present. (Unstained; IP.)

of liver insufficiency. The presence of abundant amorphous urate crystals was documented in a dog after L-asparaginase treatment for lymphoma related to tumor lysis syndrome and purine metabolism (Tvedten et al., 2019). Hyperuricosuria is normal for several breeds such as dalmatians, bulldogs, and Russian terriers, among others, that have a genetic mutation related to uric acid metabolism in which there is no conversion to allantoin.

Calcium oxalate crystalluria (see Figs. 12.26 to 12.29) can occur with hypercalciuric disorders or hyperoxaluric disorders, such as calcium oxalate urolithiasis or ethylene glycol toxicity. Calcium oxalate dihydrate (weddellite) forms frequently develop with storage and refrigeration. They occur as dipyramidal crystals appearing as squares with intersecting diagonal lines or "envelope" appearance. Calcium oxalate monohydrate crystals (whewellite) are more commonly associated with ethylene glycol toxicity (Osborne and Stevens, 1999). The monohydrate form often takes the appearance of a picket fence with rounded ends compared with the pointed ends of struvite. In addition, the monohydrate form can appear as dumbbell or spindle shapes singly or crisscross. A recent report in a cat found the whewellite form appeared as round to slightly oblong, light golden brown, with radial striations that were insoluble in 5% acetic acid and 1 M sodium hydroxide but soluble in hydrochloric acid (Parambeth et al., 2018). Oxalate crystals similar to urate crystals polarize but unlike urates are soluble in hydrochloric acid (Box 12.3).

Low numbers of bilirubin crystals (see Fig. 12.30) can be seen in healthy dogs, but larger numbers are associated with liver disease or hemolytic anemia. These crystals appear as golden yellow needles that easily disintegrate with exposure to light.

Cystine crystalluria (see Fig. 12.31) can indicate a proximal tubular defect in amino acid reabsorption but have been reported with hereditary cystinuria in several breeds of dogs, including dachshunds, Newfoundland dogs, English bulldogs, and Scottish terriers, but rarely in cats (Callens and Bartges, 2015). They appear as colorless hexagonal plates. Cystine crystalluria can predispose to urolithiasis in acidic urine.

Xanthine crystalluria can develop secondary to excessive administration of allopurinol; however, hereditary xanthine crystalluria and urolithiasis have been reported in Cavalier King Charles spaniels, dachshunds, and cats (Osborne et al., 1996; Kucera et al., 1997; Schweighauser et al., 2009; Davis and Grindem, 2015; Furman et al., 2015). These crystals appear as yellow-brown spherules in an acid or occasional neutral urine pH.

Sulfonamide administration with insufficient hydration may result in the formation of yellow crystals (see Figs. 12.33 and 12.34A) resembling bundles of wheat sheaves or spherical forms with radiating lines similar to calcium carbonate. An acid urine pH is a helpful guide in diagnosis as well as a confirmatory lignin test (see Fig. 12.34B) (Box 12.4).

Allantoin is infrequently noted as a cause of crystalluria because it is more soluble than uric acid and is normally found as an end product of purine metabolism. In one dog with acute myeloid leukemia, it was conjectured that the increased tumor burden produced the urine crystals without obvious clinical significance (Meichner et al., 2015). The crystals appear as long, needle-shaped, and colorless to slightly yellow-brown, occurring singly and in bundles, sheaves, and fans. Crystals dissolved in 1 N sodium hydroxide but were insoluble in 5% acetic acid.

Melamine and cyanuric acid-induced crystalluria with associated urolithiasis and nephrotoxicity (see Chapter 11) have been reported in dogs and cats because of exposure to pet foods contaminated with melamine and cyanuric acid (Cianciolo et al., 2008). In urine, they appear as spherical yellow-brown crystals with radial striations (Osborne et al., 2009) (see Fig. 12.35).

Alkaline Urine Crystals

Struvite (magnesium ammonium phosphate), amorphous phosphate, calcium phosphate, ammonium urate (also referred to as *ammonium biurate*), and calcium carbonate crystals tend to form in neutral pH or alkaline urine (Figs. 12.36 to 12.41).

Struvite crystals (see Figs. 12.36 and 12.37) can be seen in healthy animals without urolithiasis. In dogs, the crystals can be associated with bacterial urinary tract infection (UTI) and can be associated with struvite uroliths in cats (Osborne et al., 1996; Callens and Bartges, 2015).

Amorphous phosphates (see Fig. 12.38) appear similar in size and shape to amorphous urates but differ in the urine pH in which they form. Calcium phosphate (see Fig. 12.39) appear as colorless needle-shaped crystals.

Ammonium urate crystals (see Fig. 12.40) are uncommon in healthy dogs and cats. An exception are the same breeds with inborn errors for uric acid metabolism such as dalmatians and English bulldogs. These breeds lack uricase to convert uric acid to allantoin, resulting in hyperuricosuria and consequent predisposition to ammonium urate and uric acid crystalluria. In

TABLE 12.1 Characteristics and Solubility Properties of Urine Crystals

CRYSTAL	MORPHOLOGY OR EXAMPLE	SIGNIFICANCE	FEATURES	SOLUBLE	INSOLUBLE
Found Primarily in Acid Urine					
Allantoin	Long needle-like, colorless to slightly yellow-brown	Associated with a high tumor burden (e.g., acute myeloid leukemia)	Occurs singly and in bundles, sheaves, and fans	1 N sodium hydroxide	5% acetic acid
Amorphous urates	Fig. 12.22A	May be found in healthy dalmatians; in other breeds indicate liver insufficiency	Fine yellow-brown granules; may be found in neutral pH	Heated alkali	Acetic acid
Bilirubin	Fig. 12.30	Normal in concentrated urine from male dogs; increased formation or decreased metabolism of bilirubin	Light sensitive; bilirubinuria precedes bilirubinemia; amber-colored needles	Acid, alkali, or acetone	Alcohol or ether
Calcium hydrogen phosphate dihydrate (brushite)	Fig. 12.32	May be found in apparently normal dogs or associated with calcium-containing uroliths	Lath-shaped colorless prisms; "French fries"; present in weakly acid urine	Citric acid	
Calcium oxalate dihydrate (weddellite)	Fig. 12.26	May be normal in dogs and cats or present in ethylene glycol toxicity	May be present in neutral or rarely alkaline urine; "envelope"	HCl	Acetic acid
Calcium oxalate monohydrate (whewellite)	Figs. 12.27 to 12.29	Associated with ethylene glycol toxicity	May be present in neutral or rarely alkaline urine; hemp seed or dumbbell shape	HCl	5% acetic acid
Cholesterol	Colorless flat plates with notched edge	Suggest tissue breakdown or may be found in healthy dogs	Similar to those found in tissues; may be found in neutral pH	Hot alcohol or ether	Alcohol
Cystine	Fig. 12.31	High risk for uroliths; Newfoundlands, Labrador retrievers, dachshunds, mastiffs, French bulldogs, Australian cattle dogs, basset hounds, cats	May be seen in neutral or rarely alkaline urine; screen with sodium cyanide–nitroprusside test; hereditary	HCl, alkali (ammonia)	Boiling water, acetic acid, alcohol
Sodium urate	Fig. 12.22B–D	May be associated with uroliths		Heated	
Sulfonamides	Figs. 12.33 and 12.34	Associated with reduced water intake while receiving medication	Lignin test helps differentiate from calcium carbonate (see Box 12.4)	Acetone	
Tyrosine	Fine, highly refractile, colorless, clumped needles	May be associated with liver disease	Infrequent occurrence	Ammonium hydroxide, HCl, dilute mineral oil	Acetic acid, alcohol
Uric acid	Figs. 12.23 to 12.25	May be found in healthy dalmatians, bulldogs, and black Russian terriers, as well as birds and reptiles	Polarize with a variety of colors; rhombi, barrel shape	Sodium hydroxide	Alcohol, HCl, acetic acid
Xanthine	Yellow-brown spherules	Associated with allopurinol treatment; hereditary in Cavalier King Charles spaniels, dachshunds, and cats	Occasionally found in neutral pH urine	1 N sodium hydroxide	Acetic acid, HCl
Melamine and cyanuric acid crystals	Fig. 12.35	Associated with uroliths and nephrotoxicity; contamination of pet foods with melamine and cyanuric acid	Green to yellow to brown, circular, with radiating striations	Sodium citrate	
Found Primarily in Alkaline Urine					
Ammonium urate (biurate)	Fig. 12.40	May be found in healthy dalmatians and English bulldogs; in other breeds indicates liver insufficiency	Found also in neutral and acid pH; sodium hydroxide liberates ammonia; thorn-apple or mite shape	Heated alkali	10% acetic acid converts crystals to uric acid
Amorphous phosphate	Fig. 12.38	May be found in healthy dog and cat urine	May be found in neutral pH	Acetic acid	
Calcium carbonate	Fig. 12.41	Normal in horses, rabbits, guinea pigs, and goat urine	Not seen in dogs and cats; misdiagnosed for sulfonamides and calcium oxalate monohydrate	Acetic acid–induced effervescence	
Calcium phosphate	Fig. 12.39	Associated with nephrolithiasis	Colorless long needles	Dilute acetic acid	
Magnesium ammonium phosphate (struvite)	Figs. 12.36 and 12.37	May be normal in dogs and cats, associated with uroliths in infected or sterile urine	Sharp edges, prism-like coffin-lid shape	Dilute acetic acid	

HCl, Hydrochloric acid.

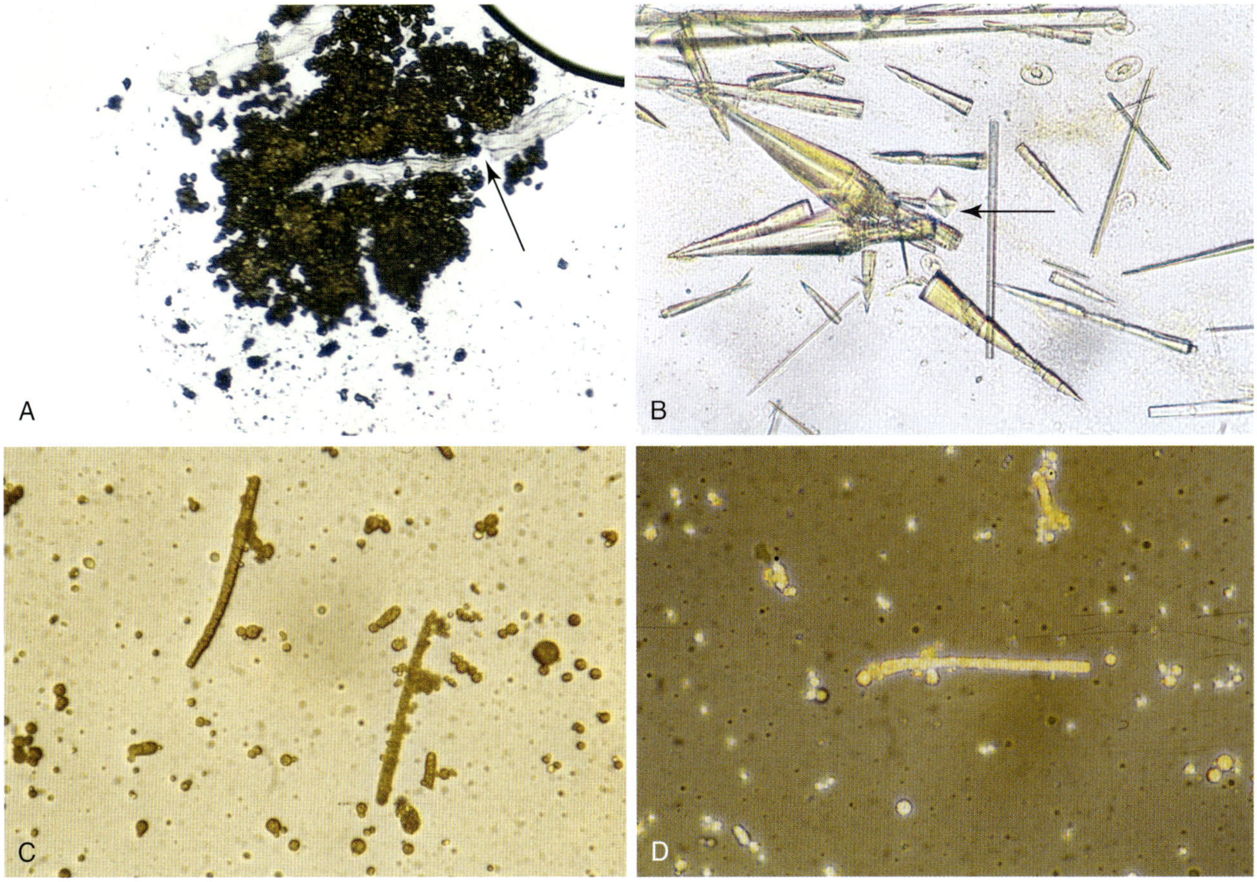

CHAPTER 12 Urine

■ FIGURE 12.22 Urate crystals. Urine sediment. A, Amorphous urate crystals and cotton fiber. Sodium, potassium, magnesium, and calcium urate salts form a granular precipitate that is yellowish to dark brown. They can appear similar to amorphous phosphate crystal precipitates. A congenital extrahepatic portosystemic shunt was diagnosed. A cotton fiber is trapped within the crystals *(arrow)*. (Unstained; HP oil.) B, Sodium urate crystals. These crystals were observed in association with ammonium urate uroliths in a bulldog. A calcium oxalate dihydrate crystal is also observed *(arrow)*. (Unstained; HP oil.) Same case in C and D. Sodium urate crystals. pH 6.0. Unstained. Dog. C, Nonpolarized. Two forms of sodium urate crystals are shown from the urine of a dalmatian. The stick shapes and round spheres changed after a short period into rhomboid uric acid forms (not shown). (Unstained; HP oil.) D, Polarized. Dog. Under polarized light, these crystals were highly reflective, consistent with urates. (Unstained; HP oil.) (C–D, Courtesy Rose Raskin, Purdue University.)

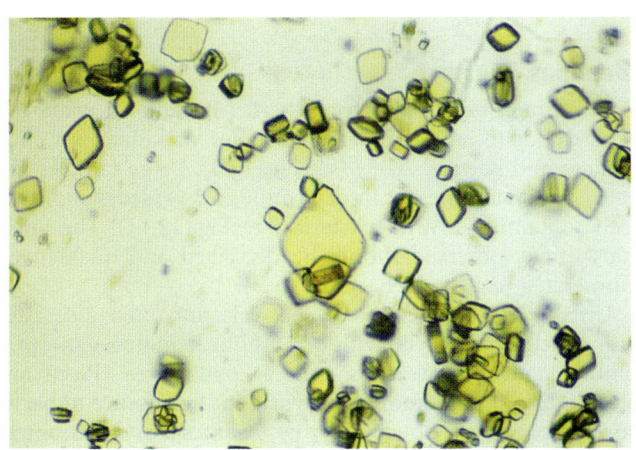

■ FIGURE 12.23 Uric acid crystals. Rhomboid. Urine sediment. These crystals are uncommonly observed in dogs and cats but are common in humans owing to the difference in purine metabolism. They have the same associations as listed for ammonium urate crystals. (Unstained; HP oil.)

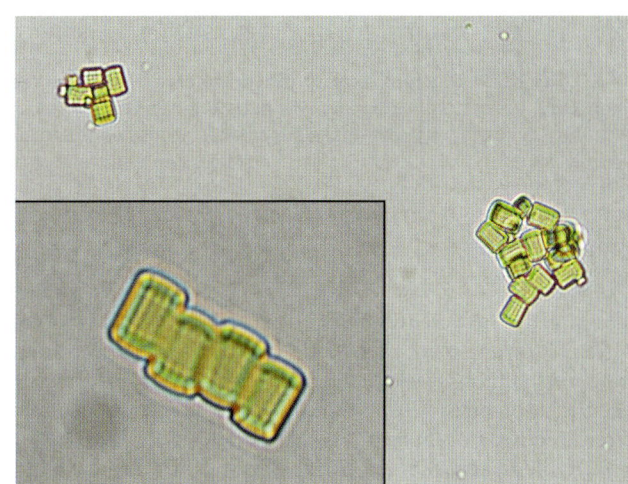

■ FIGURE 12.24 Uric acid crystals. Brick. Urine sediment. Dog. Urine with a pH of 6.3 shows a cluster of uniform brick-shaped rectangular crystals. *Inset:* A row of four brick crystals with a regular stippled pattern. Identity of the crystals involved solubility testing noting the crystals were insoluble in 1 N hydrochloric acid, consistent with uric acid crystals. (Unstained; HP oil.) (Courtesy Rose Raskin, Michigan State University.)

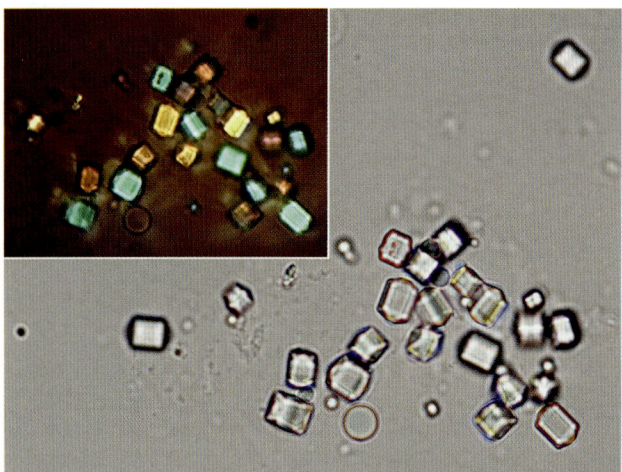

■ **FIGURE 12.25 Uric acid crystals. Barrel. Urine sediment. Dog.** Urine with a pH of 6.0 from a dog. Unstained crystals are colorless, multifaceted, and barrel shaped with pointed ends. Crystals were insoluble in hydrochloric acid with some crystal dissolution using sodium hydroxide. (Unstained; HP oil.) *Inset:* Polarized crystals exhibit birefringence with various colors. (Polarized; HP oil.) (Courtesy Rose Raskin, University of Florida.)

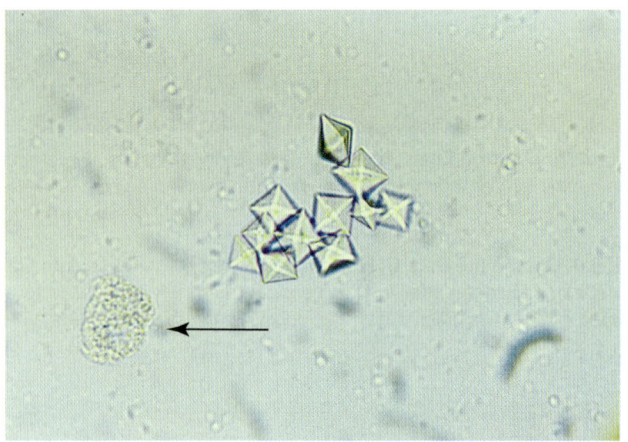

■ **FIGURE 12.26 Calcium oxalate dihydrate crystals. Urine sediment. Dog.** This photomicrograph illustrates the classical "envelope" form. They can be found in the urine of apparently healthy dogs and cats and in association with calcium oxalate urolithiasis and ethylene glycol toxicity. The latter should be promptly considered in a dog or cat with acute renal failure. A fragment of a granular cast is located to the lower left *(arrow)*. (Unstained; HP oil.)

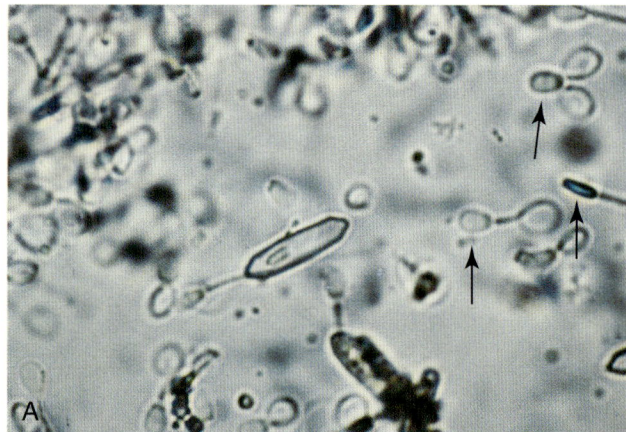

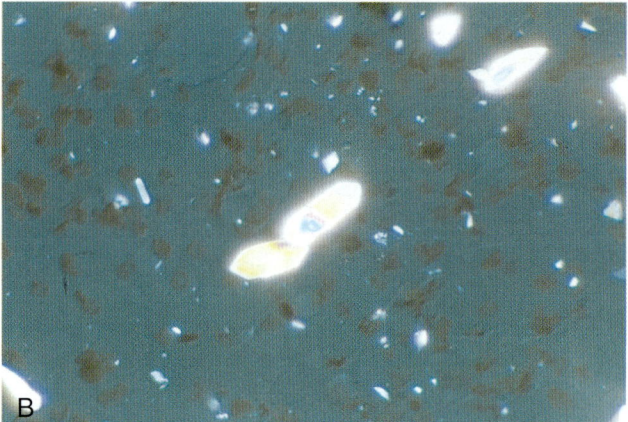

■ **FIGURE 12.27 Calcium oxalate monohydrate crystals and spermatozoa. Urine sediment. Dog.** Same case in A and B. **A,** These crystals have been erroneously referred to as hippuric acid. These crystals, alone or in combination with the dihydrate form, are observed in association with ethylene glycol toxicity. They have pointed ends (hippuric acid–like appearance) and often have a small, raised projection observed on one end. Numerous spermatozoa are observed *(arrows)*. Spermatozoa can be observed in the urine of male dogs collected by cystocentesis. (Unstained; HP oil.) **B, Polarized.** Polarization accentuates the raised projection noted on one end of the crystal. (Polarized; HP oil.)

other breeds, the water-soluble product allantoin that is formed is excreted in the urine (see Acid Urine Crystals). Ammonium urate crystalluria is associated with congenital portosystemic vascular anomalies (shunts) and liver insufficiency secondary to reduced hepatocellular mass (e.g., cirrhosis) (Osborne et al., 1996; Callens and Bartges, 2015). Crystals are brown with a spiculated (thorn apple) or mite (ginger) appearance.

Calcium carbonate is not detected in canine and feline urine, but crystals appearing similar to these spherules with radiating lines or dumbbell shape are more likely to be calcium oxalate monohydrate or sulfonamide crystals (Osborne et al., 1996) (see Fig. 12.41).

Infectious Agents

Urine formed by the kidneys is sterile. Bacteria in urine collected by cystocentesis indicates bladder or kidney infection (Callens and Bartges, 2015) (see Fig. 12.3). Urine samples collected via cystocentesis can determine if a voided sample has been contaminated with bacteria (see Fig. 12.11). The infectious agents observed should be described and qualitatively enumerated (e.g., many bacterial rods).

Urinary tract infections by bacteria are often associated with concurrent pyuria, with or without hematuria and proteinuria, and clinical signs such as pollakiuria (Piech and Wycislo, 2019). The finding of pyuria in the absence of bacteriuria, especially if obtained by cystocentesis or concomitant clinical signs of a UTI, is an indication to culture the urine sample. Air-dried Romanowsky-stained smears of urine sediment improve the identification of bacteria when evaluated concurrently with wet mounts (Swenson et al., 2004; O'Neil et al., 2013) (see Fig. 12.3).

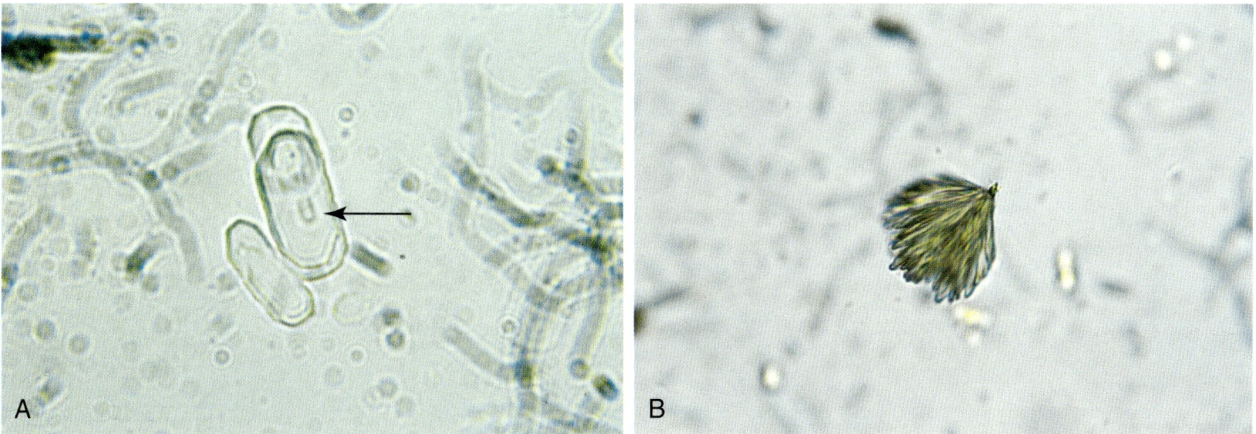

■ **FIGURE 12.28 Calcium oxalate monohydrate crystals. Urine sediment. A, Cat.** This crystal is associated with ethylene glycol toxicity. The calcium oxalate monohydrate in cats is wider than the canine counterpart with rounded ends; a raised projection on the larger of the two crystals is noted *(arrow)*. The out-of-focus elongated material is artifact (dust in the camera optics). (Unstained; HP oil.) **B, Dog.** Fan-shaped aggregate of calcium oxalate monohydrate crystals was associated with calcium oxalate uroliths. Fan-shaped crystals are also associated with the use of sulfa-containing antibacterials. (Unstained; HP oil.)

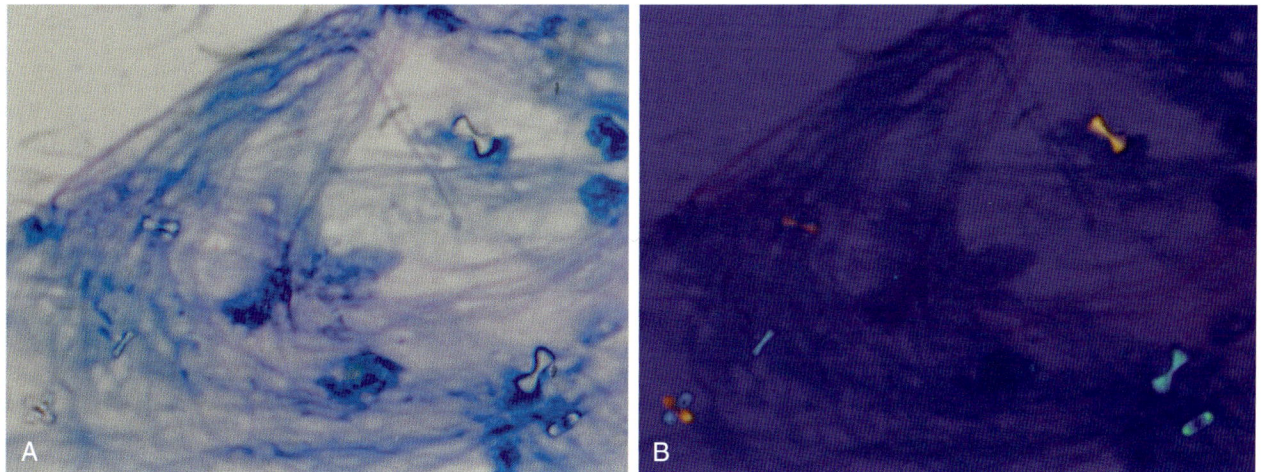

■ **FIGURE 12.29 Calcium oxalate monohydrate crystals. Urine sediment stained. Dog.** Same case in A and B. **A, Direct.** In this case of acute renal failure with nephrotoxicosis on necropsy likely from ethylene glycol toxicity, the urine revealed several colorless crystals with varying shape ranging from flat hexagonal to spindle-shaped admixed with inflammatory cells, bacteria, and erythrocytes. Shown is a clot with several of the spindle-shaped crystals. (Wright-Giemsa; HP oil.) **B, Polarized.** The crystals exhibit birefringence under polarized light. (Polarized Wright-Giemsa; HP oil.) (Courtesy Rose Raskin, University of Florida.)

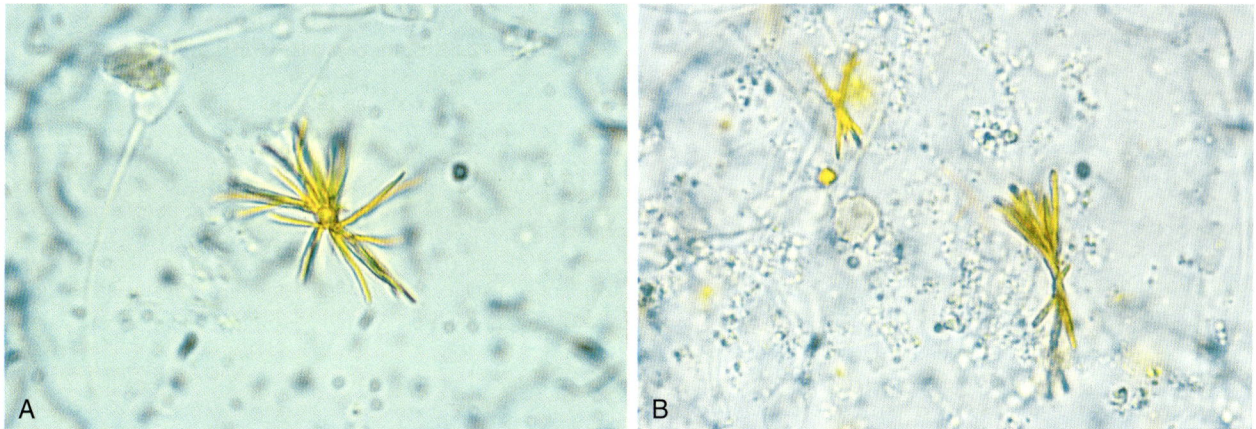

■ **FIGURE 12.30 Bilirubin crystals. A–B, Urine sediment.** Bilirubin can crystallize in association with bilirubinuria. Crystals are golden yellow with needle shapes and dissolve readily with exposure to light. (Unstained; HP oil.)

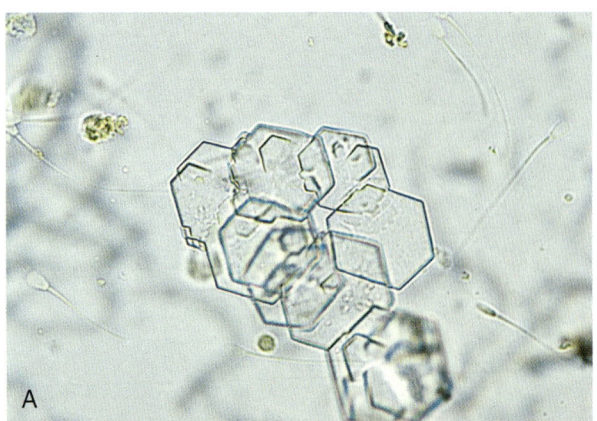
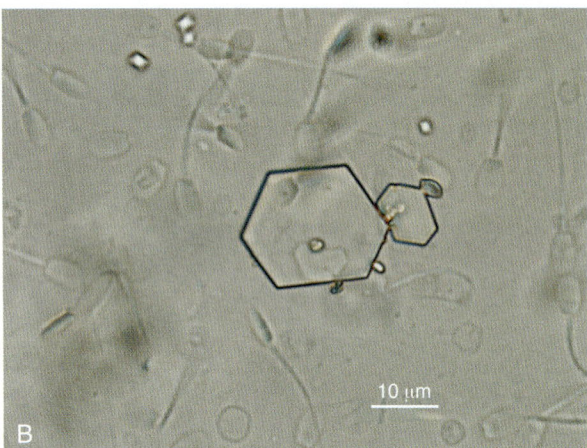

■ **FIGURE 12.31 Cystine crystals and spermatozoa. Urine sediment. A,** Cystine crystalluria is always an abnormal finding and indicates the metabolic disorder of cystinuria. Occasional spermatozoa are seen in the background. Cystine crystalluria may or may not be associated with cystine uroliths. (Unstained; HP oil.) **B,** This urine is from another animal. This mastiff had multiple cystine uroliths in the urinary bladder and one in the urethra that was confirmed by stone analysis. The urine also contained spermatozoa. The crystal has a very regular hexagon plate appearance. (Unstained; HP oil.) (B, Courtesy Rose Raskin, University of Florida.)

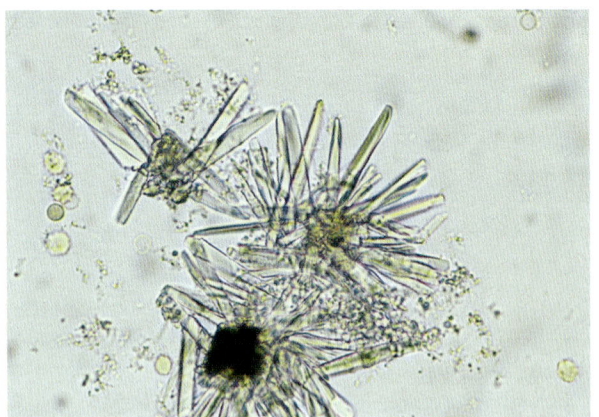

■ **FIGURE 12.32 Calcium hydrogen phosphate dihydrate (brushite) crystals.** This form of calcium phosphate crystals is observed in urine specimens from apparently healthy dogs and in association with calcium phosphate uroliths and calcium phosphate and calcium oxalate uroliths. They tend to form in urine with an acidic pH. The long lath-shaped prisms are colorless. (Unstained; HP oil.)

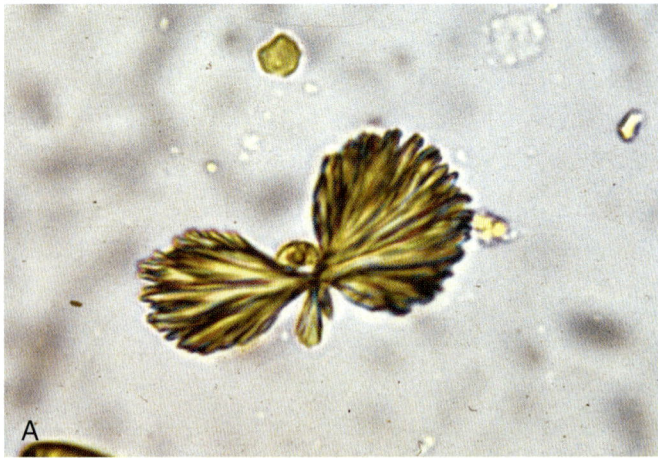
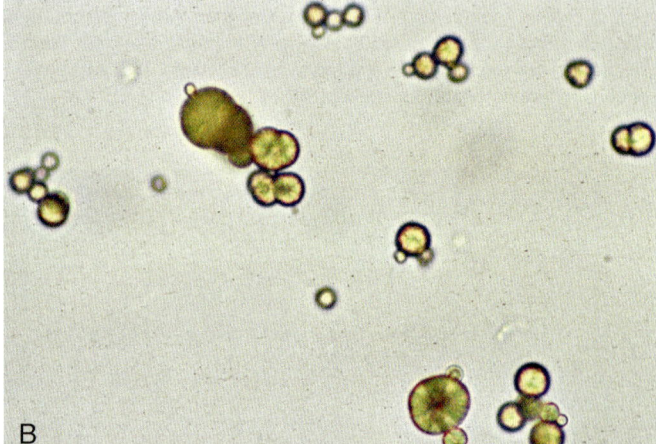
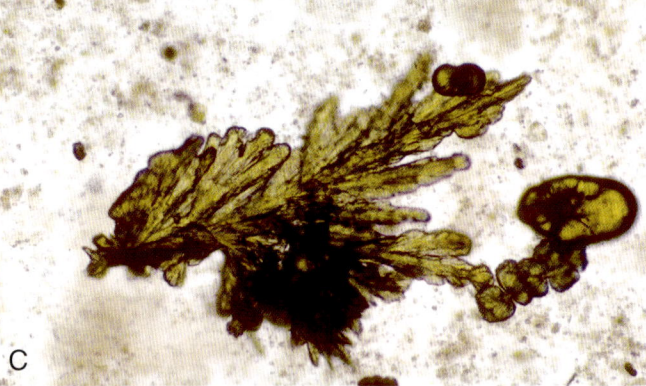

■ **FIGURE 12.33 Sulfa crystals. Urine sediment. A,** One form of sulfa crystals that may result from sulfonamide administration is shown. These yellow crystals resemble bundles or wheat sheaves. The result of a lignin test used as a screening test for sulfonamides was positive in this case. (Unstained; HP oil.) **B,** Another form of sulfa crystals resembles calcium carbonate crystals; however, they are more yellow in color. Spherical forms with radiating streaks appear singly or attached. The result of a lignin test was positive for this sample. (Unstained; HP oil.) **C,** This sample demonstrates both bundles and spherical forms of sulfa crystals in the same field. (Unstained; HP oil.) (Courtesy Rose Raskin, University of Florida.)

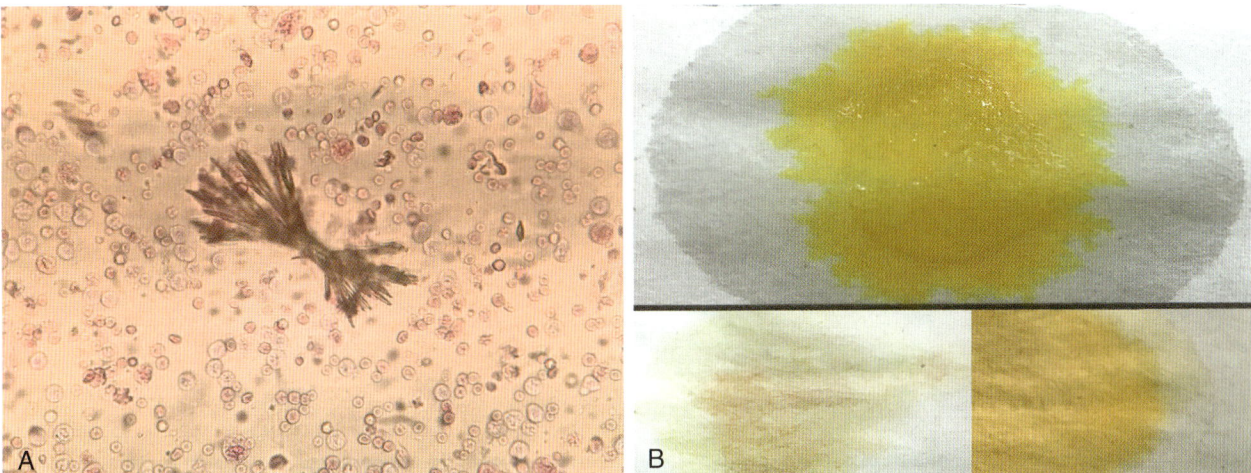

■ **FIGURE 12.34 Sulfa crystals with lignin testing. Dog. Catheterized urine with a pH of 6.8.** Same case in A and B. **A, Microscopic. Wet mount.** Admixed with numerous leukocytes and erythrocytes is an aggregate in the form of wheat sheaves. (Unstained; IP.) **B, Macroscopic. Lignin test.** A sheet of newspaper is the base on which a drop of urine is placed along with a drop of concentrated hydrochloric acid. *Top:* The immediate bright yellow reaction of the patient is positive for the presence of sulfonamides. The patient had begun trimethoprim-sulfamethoxazole 4 days before the urinalysis for a history of dysuria and stranguria. *Bottom left:* Control urine from another dog shows minimal color change. *Bottom right:* The patient sample after drying still shows a dark golden color compared with the dried control urine. (Courtesy Rose Raskin, University of Bristol, UK.)

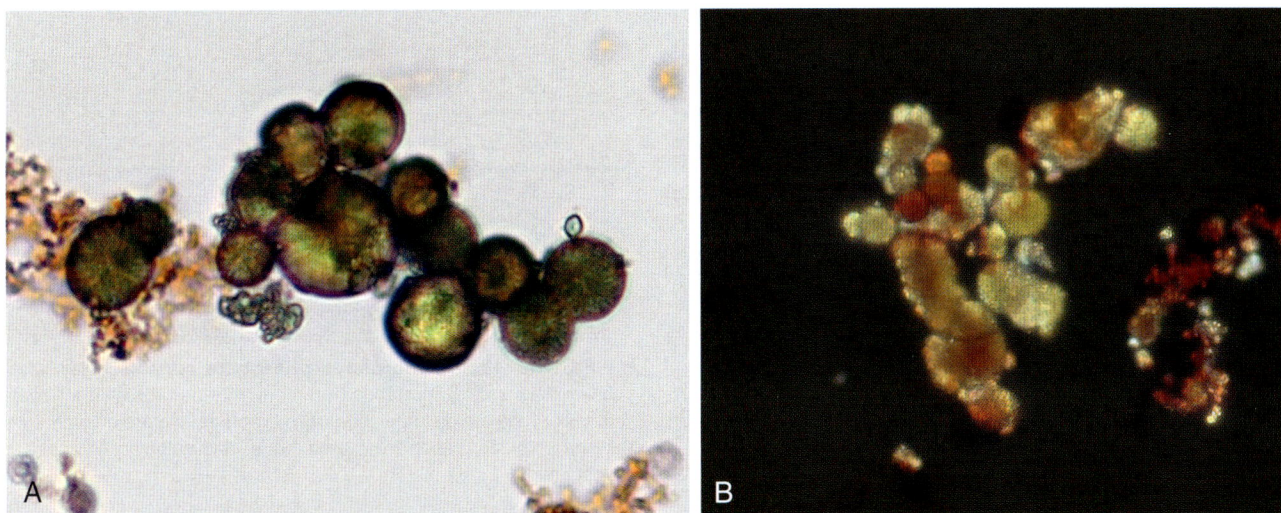

■ **FIGURE 12.35 Melamine and cyanuric acid crystals. Urine sediment.** Same case in A and B. **A, Direct.** The patient had ingested pet food contaminated with melamine and cyanuric acid. The spherical green-yellow-brown circular crystals have radiating striations. (Unstained, IP.) **B, Polarized.** Melamine and cyanuric acid crystals are refractile and enhanced with polarization, which help distinguish them from sulfa crystals, as does a negative lignin test result. (Unstained, IP).

BOX 12.3 Performing the Crystal Solubility Tests

When the identity of the crystal is unknown, use of solubility properties along with urine pH is helpful. This is performed by adding to the specimen while on the stage of the microscope (or to the tube containing the sediment) a few drops of a chemical reagent, which is known to dissolve the crystals under investigation. For example, whereas calcium oxalate is soluble in hydrochloric acid, uric acid is not soluble. Reagents can be stocked in dropper bottles for ease of use during urinalysis.

BOX 12.4 Performing the Lignin Test for Sulfonamides in Urine (Graff, 1983)

1. Place a few urine drops on a blank strip of newspaper or paper towel. (Do not use filter paper or bond quality paper.)
2. Add one drop of 25% hydrochloric acid in the center of the moistened area.

Interpretation: A bright yellow to orange reaction within 15 minutes indicates a positive reaction.

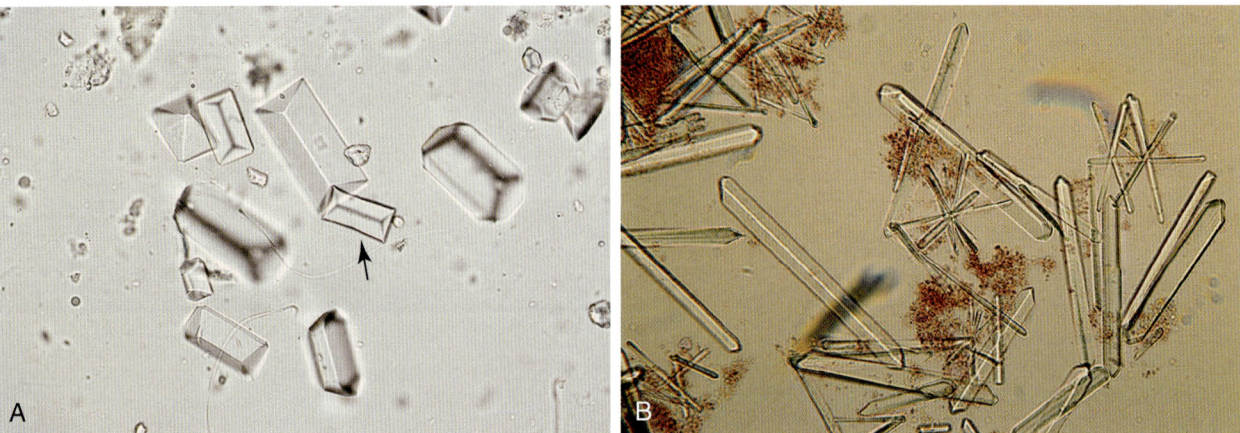

■ **FIGURE 12.36 Magnesium ammonium phosphate (struvite) crystalluria. A, Coffin lid appearance.** These crystals have been previously misnamed as triple phosphates. The small crystal in the center *(arrow)* illustrates the form that has been referred to as a coffin lid appearance (closed casket as viewed from the top). They can be a normal finding in dogs and cats or be associated with struvite uroliths (sterile and infected). They tend to be found in urine with a pH > 7. (Unstained; HP oil.) **B, Rod shape.** Present are a variety of shapes, including a rodlike shape in this specimen and a "fern leaf" appearance (not shown). Small islands of reddish-stained amorphous phosphates are present. (Sedi-Stain; HP oil.)

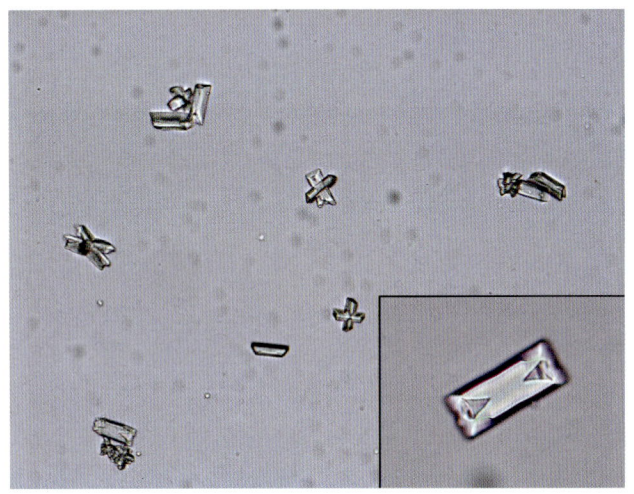

■ **FIGURE 12.37 Struvite crystals. Urine sediment. Urine pH 8. Cat.** Several rectangular and intersecting rod-shaped crystals are present that were soluble in acetic acid. (Unstained; IP) *Inset:* A single coffin lid variety is shown. (Unstained; HP oil.) (Courtesy Rose Raskin, University of Florida.)

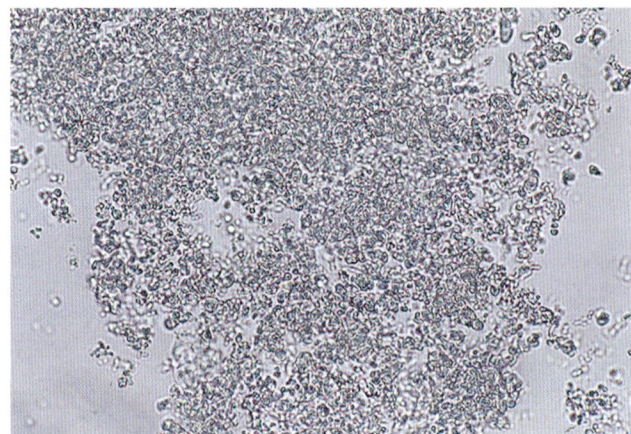

■ **FIGURE 12.38 Amorphous phosphate crystals.** They have no known diagnostic importance but should not be mistaken for bacterial colonies. They are distinguished from amorphous urate crystals by their lack of color, formation in alkaline urine, and solubility in acetic acid. (Unstained; HP oil.)

Other infectious agents (Figs. 12.42 to 12.45) that might be observed in the urine and can possibly indicate local or systemic pathology include yeasts (e.g., *Candida* spp., *Blastomyces dermatitidis*), fungal hyphae (e.g., *Aspergillus* spp.), opportunistic fungi (e.g., *Schizophyllum commune*), and algae (e.g., *Prototheca* spp.) (Pressler et al., 2005). *Candida* spp. are 2 to 7 μm × 3 to 8 μm spherical to ovoid organisms that may be individualized or budding (Vap and Shropshire, 2017). *Candida* spp. form pseudohyphae, which are approximately 3 μm × 10 to 15 μm with clear septae-like connections between segments (see Figs. 12.42 and 12.43). A true infection may relate to excessive antibiotic usage, long-term corticosteroids, or immune-compromised conditions. Yeast and fungi in urine sediments may be contaminants, especially if a stain has been used; therefore, the stain should be examined for evidence of fungi (see Fig. 1.18).

Parasites such as *Pearsonema plica* and *Pearsonema feliscati* ova (canine and feline bladder worm) (Fig. 12.46) are occasionally found in urine. The dog or cat may acquire infection after ingesting infected earthworms or earthworm-associated material. Adult *Pearsonema* spp. develop in the urinary bladder mucosa and may cause minor irritation with subsequent cystitis. The football-shaped eggs may appear in the urine within 2 months of infection. This form of urinary nematode appears to be more common in the southeastern United States. Dogs and rarely cats that scavenge on fish or frogs are susceptible to develop hematuria and pass into the urine ova of *Dioctophyma renale* (giant kidney worm of dogs). These ova appear brown, barrel-shaped, and thick shelled, with a rough surface and bipolar plugs (Fig. 12.47).

Dirofilaria immitis microfilaria can be observed due to bleeding into the urine (Fig. 12.48). A mixed population of

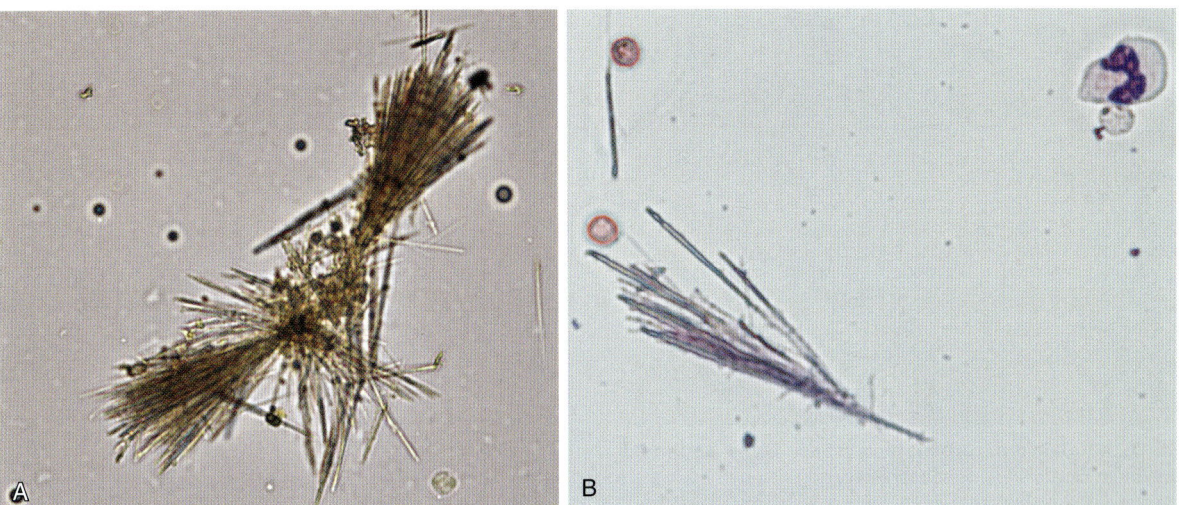

■ **FIGURE 12.39 Calcium phosphate crystals. pH of 8.5. Dog.** Same case in A and B. **A, Wet mount.** These clusters of colorless, long, needle-shaped crystals were present from an Airedale terrier with elevated liver enzymes and anemia. (Unstained; IP.) **B, Dry mount.** This stained preparation demonstrates the intact needle-shaped crystals, two erythrocytes, and one neutrophil. (Modified Wright; IP.) (Courtesy of Rose Raskin, Purdue University.)

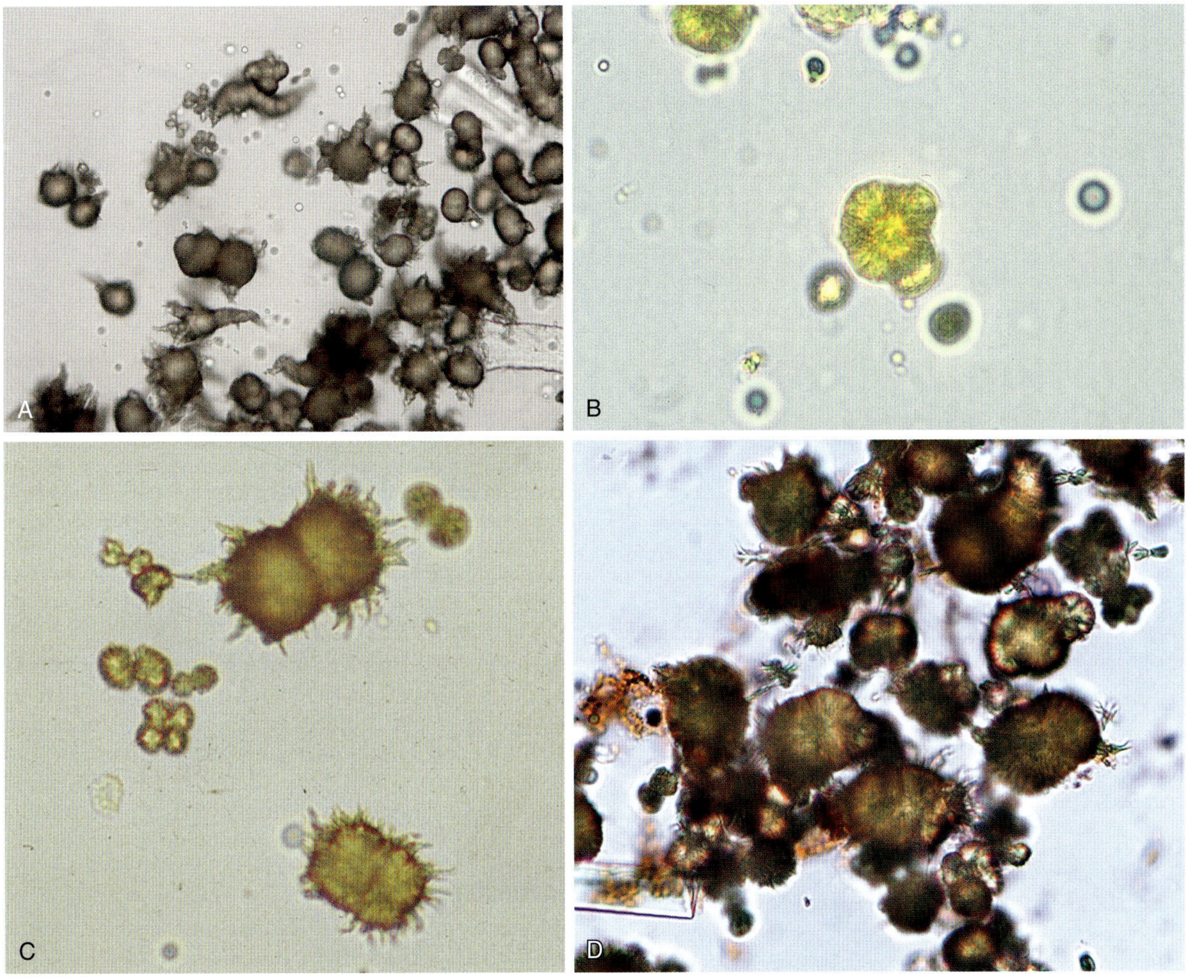

■ **FIGURE 12.40 Ammonium urate (ammonium biurate) crystals. Urine sediment. A, Dog. Urine pH of 7.8.** These crystals from a free catch specimen appear dark and resemble a mite or ginger with few spiny processes but rather elongate projections. The animal presented with increased hepatic enzyme activities. (Unstained; IP.) **B, Cat.** Spheroid aggregates of crystals with smooth surfaces are common in the cat and were associated with a single congenital extrahepatic portosystemic shunt. A few out-of-focus lipid droplets are observed, a normal finding in cats. (Unstained; HP oil.) **C,** These brown crystals are spherical with spines (thorn apple) and were associated a congenital extrahepatic portosystemic shunt. (Unstained; HP oil.) **D, Dog.** These crystals are yellow-brown and appear more rounded to smooth in appearance with fewer prominent thornlike projections. A struvite crystal is present in the lower left side. (Unstained; IP.) (A, Courtesy Rose Raskin, University of Bristol. C, Courtesy Rick Alleman, University of Florida.)

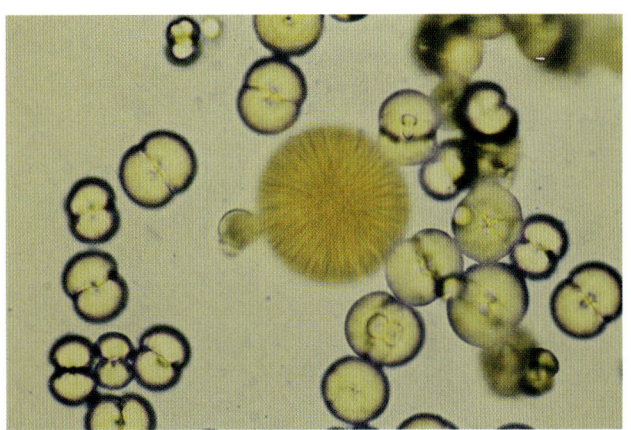

■ **FIGURE 12.41** Calcium carbonate crystals. Urine sediment. Calcium carbonate crystals are not observed in dog or cat urine but are observed in the urine of horses, rabbits, and guinea pigs. (Unstained; HP oil.)

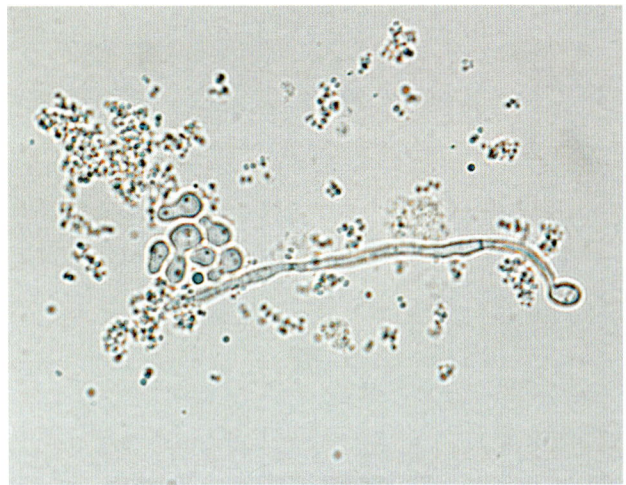

■ **FIGURE 12.42** *Candida albicans* infection. Urine sediment. Wet mount. Dog. Urine pH was 7.5, and there are hyphal-like structures of variable length. These structures have roughly parallel walls, measure approximately 1 μm in diameter, and are occasionally septate. Right-angle branching and terminal yeastlike budding structures are occasionally noted. The granular material on the left side is extracellular bacteria that are frequently form microcolonies. Diagnosis was confirmed by culture. (Unstained; HP oil.)

bacteria or *Cyniclomyces guttulatus* yeasts suggests contamination with feces (e.g., inadvertent puncture of the intestine during cystocentesis) (Fig. 12.49) (Winston et al., 2016).

> **KEY POINT** Examination of air-dried, stained cytology smears of urine sediment improves the sensitivity and specificity of bacteriuria detection. If a UTI is suspected, it is recommended to immediately centrifuge recently formed urine (not first morning urine) and prepare air-dried smears for Romanowsky-stained cytopathologic examination.

Lipid Droplets

Lipid droplets are a normal finding and likely originate from renal tubular epithelial cells, particularly in cats (Fig. 12.50).

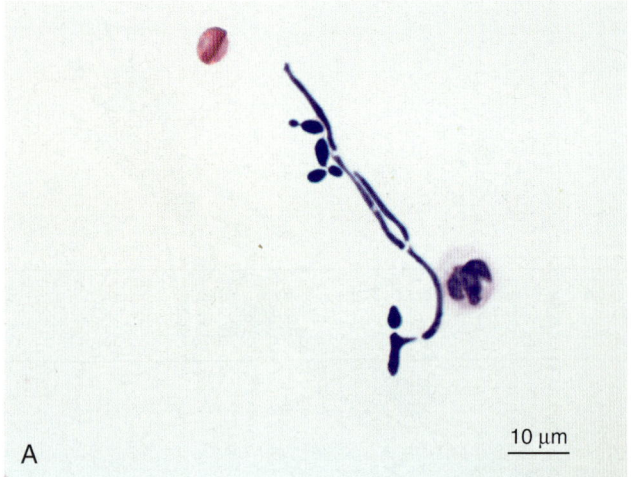

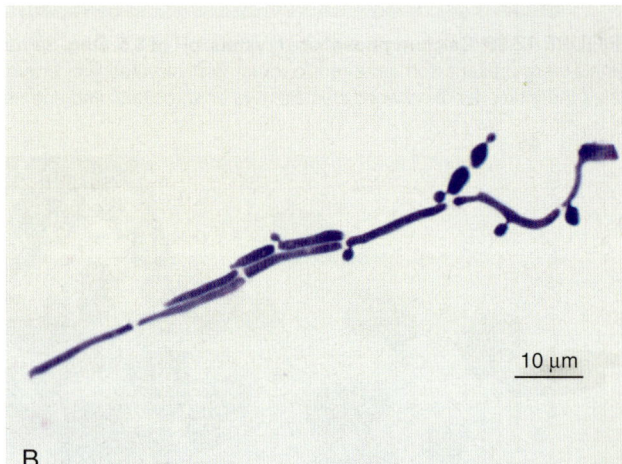

■ **FIGURE 12.43** *Candida albicans* infection. Urine sediment. Dry mount. Dog. The patient was treated for an immune-mediated anemia and thrombocytopenia with immunosuppressants and corticosteroids. Urine culture confirmed the diagnosis. **A,** Pseudohyphal structures with budding forms are compared with an erythrocyte and neutrophil. (Modified Wright; HP oil.) **B,** The spacing between segments is irregular, supporting the fact these are not true hyphae. Note the budding arises from the terminal end of the hyphal-like structure. (Modified Wright; HP oil.) (Courtesy Priscila Beatriz Da Silva Serpa, Purdue University.)

However, lipid droplets may also result from contaminating lubricants. Grossly, they form a milky surface after urine centrifugation. Lipid droplets have a refractile appearance with a dark ring and variable size, and they resemble erythrocytes by light microscopy (see Figs. 12.4A, 12.18, and 12.40B). Lipid droplets incorporated into tubular matrix are termed fatty casts (see Fig. 12.19). See previous discussion under Granular Casts.

Spermatozoa

Spermatozoa are commonly seen in the urine sediment from intact males, especially in voided urine (see Figs. 12.27A and 12.31). High numbers in a sample collected via cystocentesis or catheterization might be indicative of retrograde ejaculation (Vap and Shropshire, 2017). Females may have spermatozoa in their urine after breeding (Osborne and Stevens, 1999). Spermatozoa have an oval, spatulate head with a tail. If the head and tail are separated during the collection procedure or sample

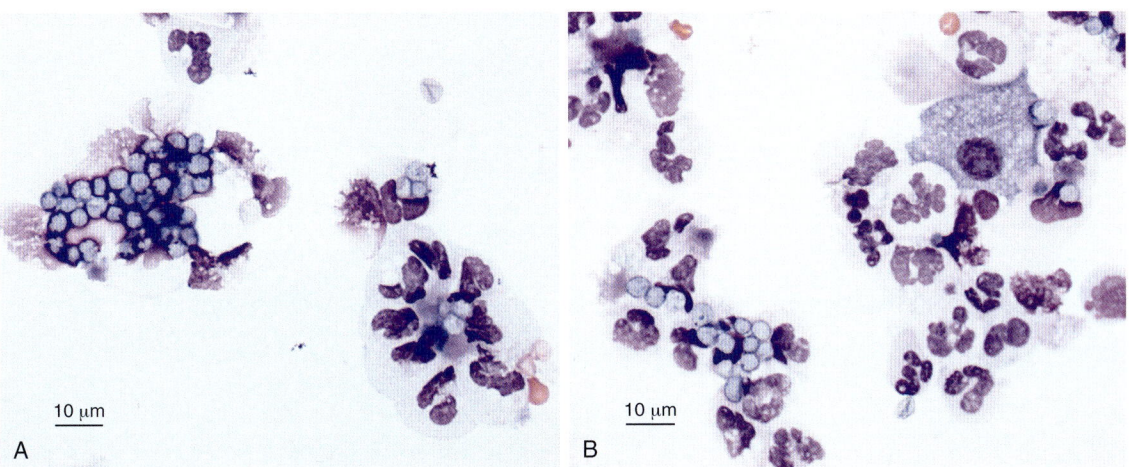

■ **FIGURE 12.44** ***Schizophyllum commune* infection. Urine sediment. Dry mount. Cat.** Sample taken from a subcutaneous ureteral bypass port for a 6-month urine evaluation after surgery. This opportunistic fungus was identified via PCR testing. **A,** Many neutrophils appear in association with aggregates of fungal basidiospores. These round structures measure approximately 4 to 5 μm in diameter. (Modified Wright; HP oil.) **B,** Many neutrophils and a single macrophage are present. The fungal basidiospores are often associated with the neutrophils and are occasionally phagocytized. (Modified Wright; HP oil.) (Courtesy Andrea Pires dos Santos, Purdue University.)

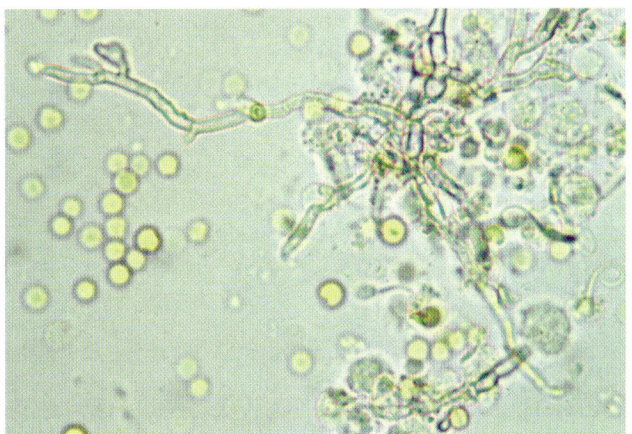

■ **FIGURE 12.45** ***Aspergillus* spp. infection. Urine sediment. Wet mount. Dog.** Septate hyphal forms are present in the urine of an animal with disseminated *Aspergillus* spp. infection. Diagnosis was confirmed by urine culture. A group of red cells is seen at the left, but large, clear, slightly granular leukocytes are closely associated with the infectious agent. (Unstained; IP.) (Courtesy Rose Raskin, University of Florida.)

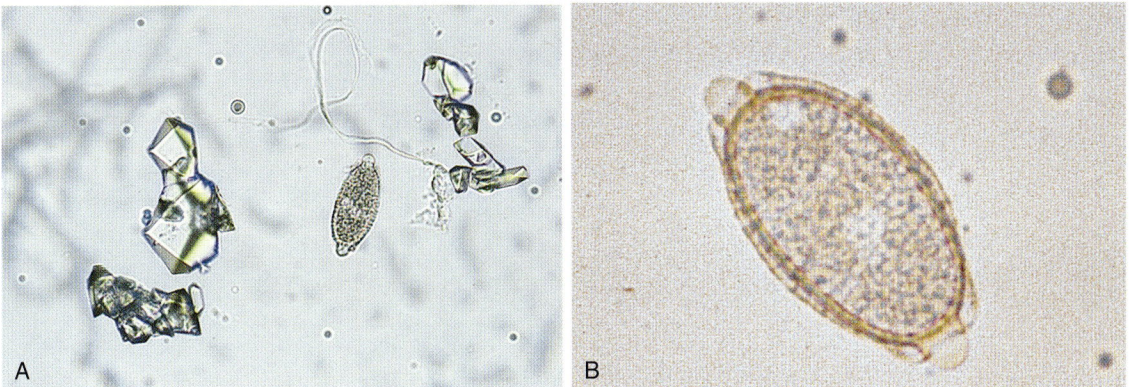

■ **FIGURE 12.46** ***Pearsonema* spp. infection. Urine sediment. Wet mount. A, *Pearsonema plica* ovum.** The ovum of the bladder worm of dogs and cats has slightly tipped bipolar plugs and a granular appearance. These features help distinguish it from pollen grain contaminants. Aggregates of magnesium ammonium phosphates crystals are also observed. (Unstained, IP.) **B, *Pearsonema feliscati* ovum. Cat.** Close-up magnification demonstrates the tilted terminal plugs, which help identify the ovum. No clinical signs were associated with this animal. The ovum measures approximately 40 × 65 μm. (Unstained; HP oil.) (B, Courtesy Rose Raskin, University of Florida.)

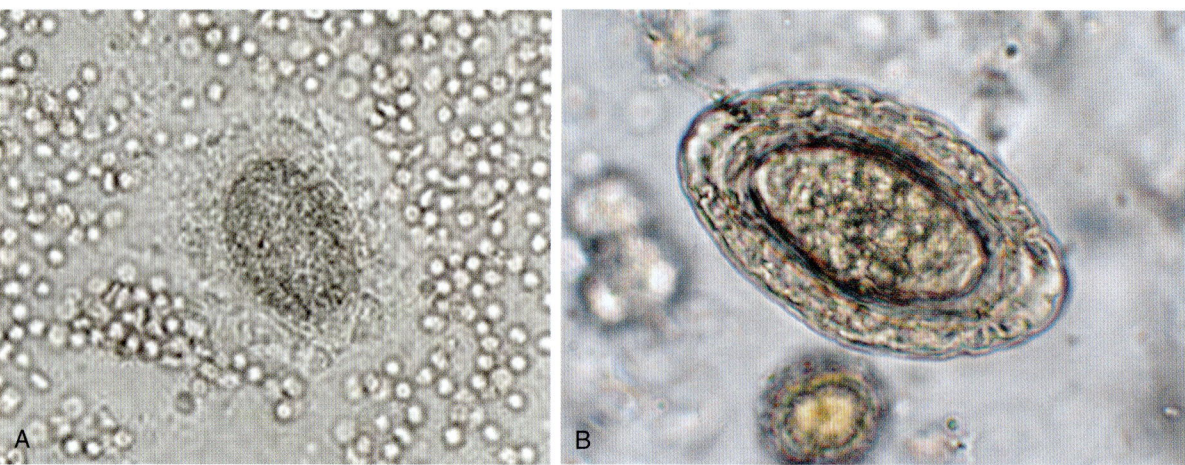

■ **FIGURE 12.47** *Dioctophyma renale* **ovum. Dog. A,** Hematuria is evident related to the presence of the giant kidney worm. Note the size difference between erythrocytes and the ovum that is approximately 70 × 50 μm. (Unstained, HP oil.) **B,** *Dioctophyma renale* **ovum. Maned wolf.** The detail of the ovum in this urine sample demonstrates the barrel shape with a thick rough and pitted shell that has bipolar plugs on opposite ends. The size of this ovum is approximately 65 × 45 μm. (Unstained, HP oil.) (A, Courtesy Juliana Pereira Matheus, Porto Alegre, Brazil. B, Courtesy Thomas Nolan, University of Pennsylvania.)

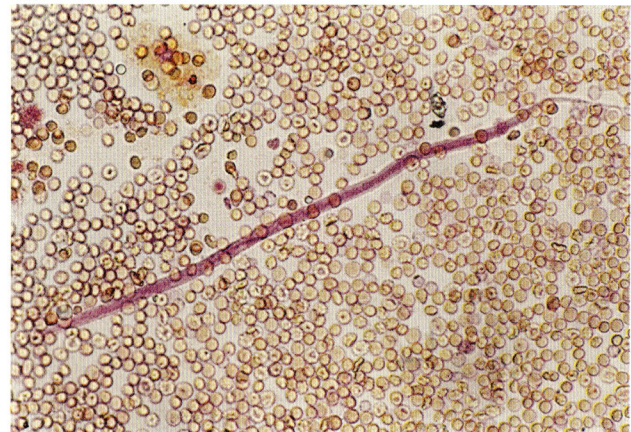

■ **FIGURE 12.48** *Dirofilaria immitis* **microfilaria. Urine sediment. Wet mount.** The microfilaria was an incidental finding in this dog with hemorrhagic cystitis. Numerous erythrocytes are observed. (NMB; IP.)

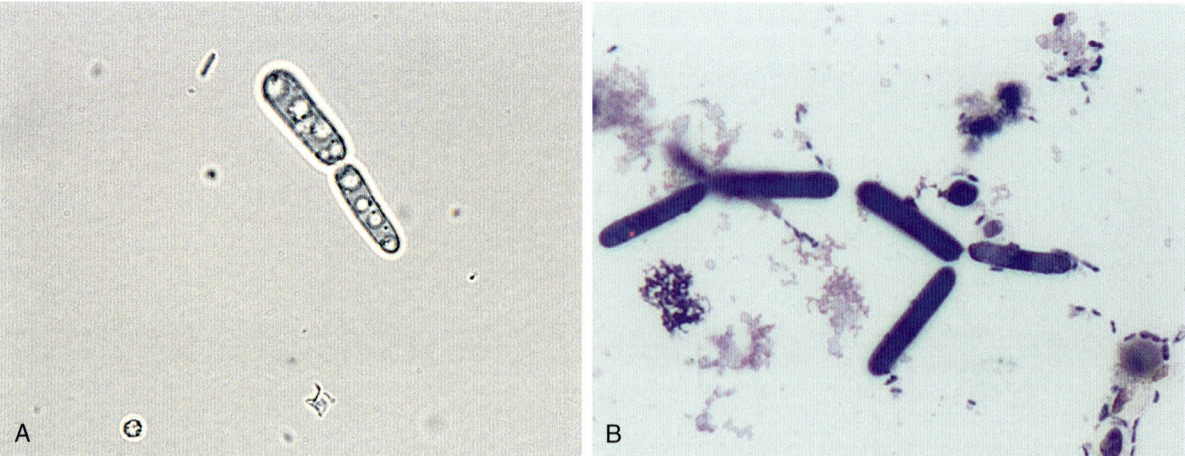

■ **FIGURE 12.49** *Cyniclomyces guttulatus* **yeast. Urinary sediment. Dog. A,** Two budding forms against a background containing occasional bacterial rods and cocci were found in the urine from inadvertent enterocentesis during a cystocentesis procedure. Notice the presence of multiple vacuoles within the organism. (Unstained; HP oil.) **B,** This free-catch urine sample from a dog was contaminated with mixed bacteria and yeast, which are occasionally found in canine fecal samples, and suggested to be caused by ingestion of rabbit feces. The presence of these yeasts in the urine sediment indicates fecal contamination. (Sedi-Stain, HP oil.)

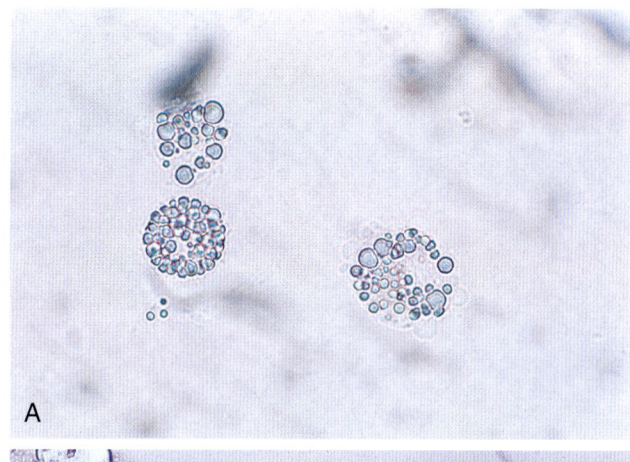

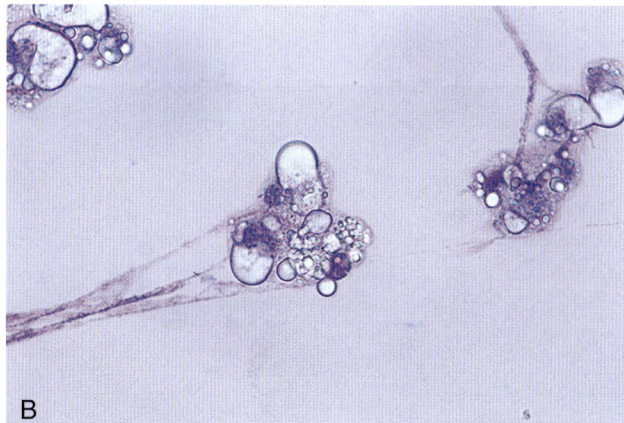

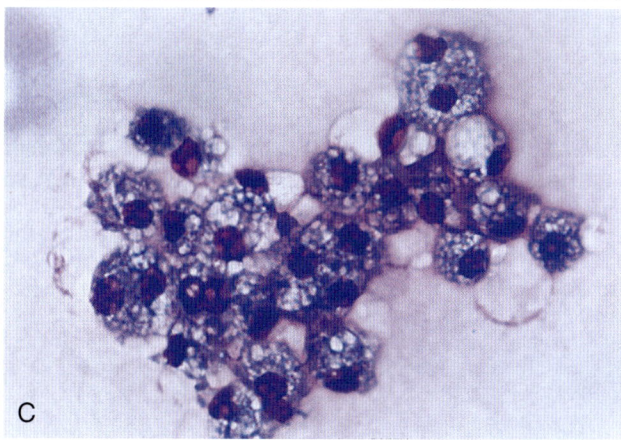

■ **FIGURE 12.50 Lipid droplets. Urine sediment.** Lipid vacuoles in epithelial cells may be a prominent cytomorphologic feature in feline urine sediments. They are identified by their size variation and refractile nature when focusing up and down. **A, Unstained.** (HP oil.) **B, New methylene blue.** (HP oil.) **C, Dry mount.** The methanolic Romanowsky stain dissolves the lipid droplets, resulting in punctate holes in the cytoplasm of the cells. (Wright; HP oil.)

preparation, the heads might resemble yeastlike organisms and the tails as hyphal-like organisms upon perusal at low power.

Artifacts

Incidental findings in the urine can include plastic (see Fig. 12.14B), dye crystals (Fig. 12.51), starch granules (Fig. 12.52), plant fibers (Fig. 12.53; see also Fig. 12.22A), pollen (Fig. 12.54), and mannitol crystals (Fig. 12.55).

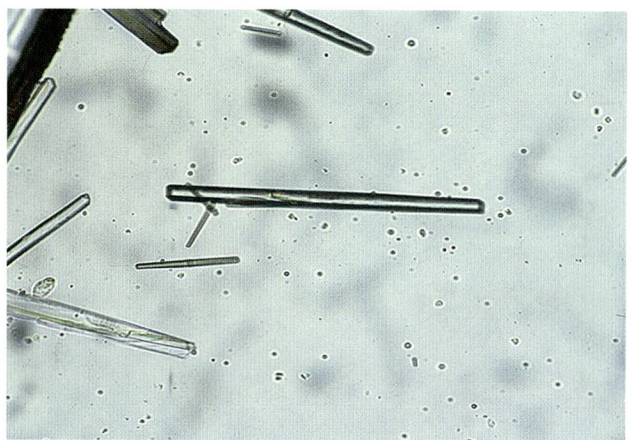

■ **FIGURE 12.51 Urine artifact. Radiopaque contrast dye crystals. wet mount.** These needle-shaped crystals were observed in association with the use of an iodinated radiopaque contrast agent for an excretory urogram. (Unstained; HP oil.)

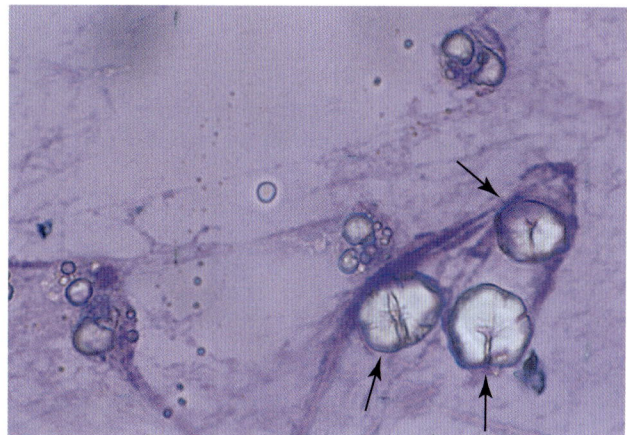

■ **FIGURE 12.52 Urine artifact. Starch granules. Wet mount.** These glove powder structures *(arrows)* are contaminants. An "X" with a central depression can be observed by focusing up and down on the granules. Poorly formed wisps of mucus stain but variably sized refractile lipid droplets do not stain with the water-based stain. (NMB; HP oil.)

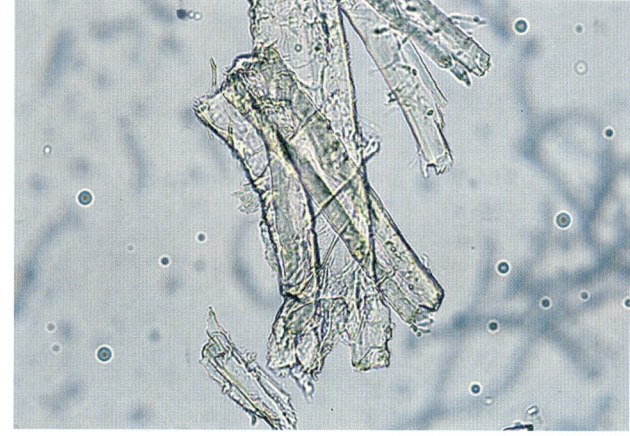

■ **FIGURE 12.53 Urine artifact. Cotton fibers. Wet mount.** Plant fibers such as cotton from clothing or gauze pads can mimic hyaline or granular casts or crystals. (Unstained; HP oil.)

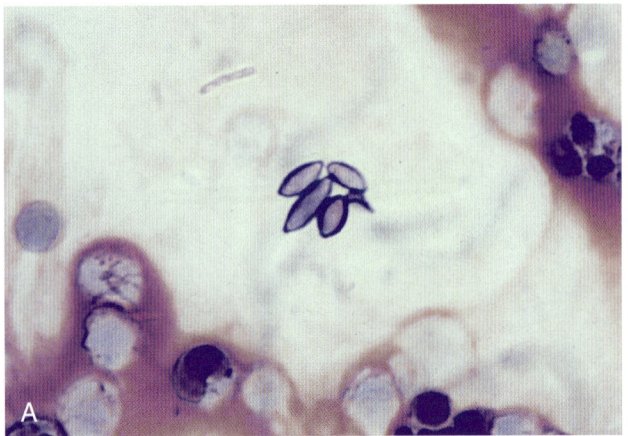
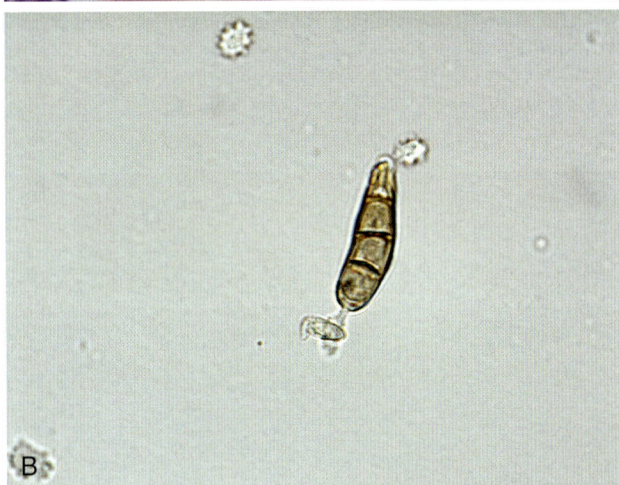
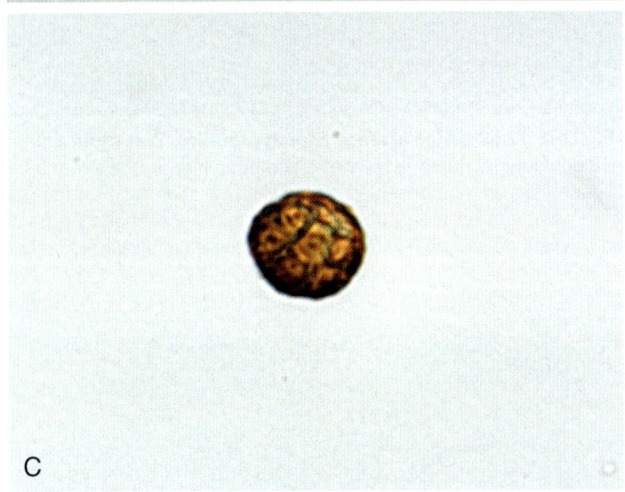

■ **FIGURE 12.54 Urine artifact. Pollen grains. Wet mount.** Pollen grains of various sizes and morphology can contaminate urine. They are often ovoid, elliptical, or round. **A,** Four football-shaped green pollen grains measure about the size of the neutrophils shown at the periphery. (NMB; HP oil.) **B,** The single brown fungal spore is elliptical with four segmentations. (Unstained; HP oil.) **C,** A single round brown pollen grain has circular divisions on its surface. (Unstained; HP oil.)

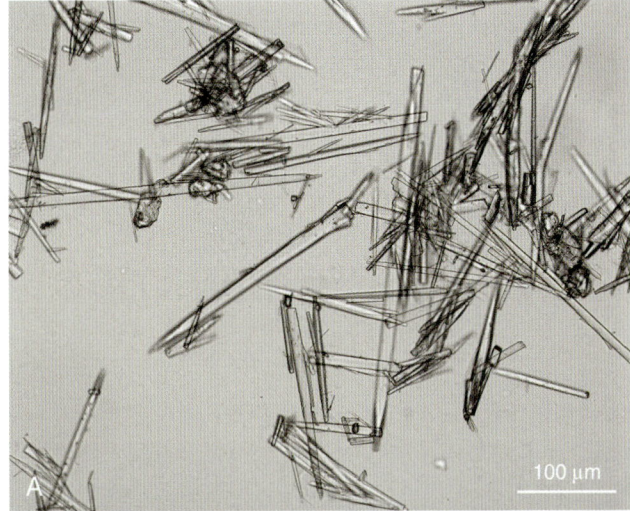
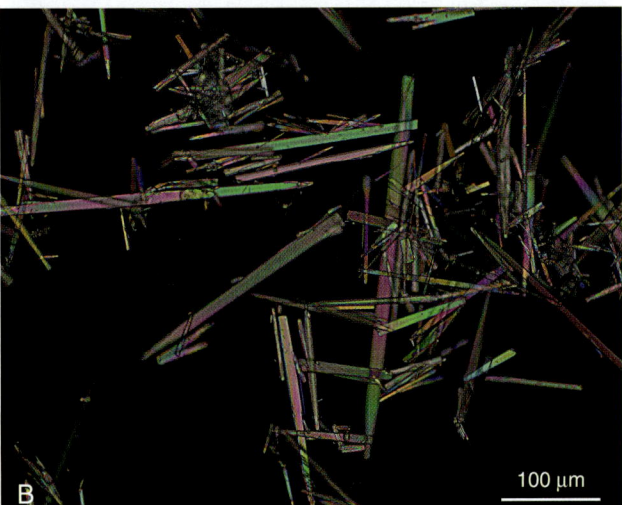

■ **FIGURE 12.55 Urine artifact. Mannitol crystals. pH of 7. Wet mount. Cat.** Same case in A and B. **A, Unstained.** A 1-month-old kitten received 0.5 g/kg of mannitol intravenously over 20 minutes about 8 hours before urine submission. On presentation, the patient was stuporous, and the initial differentials were intracranial disease or traumatic brain injury. Colorless crystals have sharp pointed variably sized shapes that resemble clustered sticks. (Unstained; IP.) **B, Polarized.** The crystals show a birefringence common with mannitol. (Polarized; IP.) (Courtesy Bill Vernau and BinXi Wu, University of California, Davis.)

REFERENCES

Albasan H, Lulich JP, Osborne CA, et al. Effects of storage time and temperature on pH, specific gravity, and crystal formation in urine samples from dogs and cats. *J Am Vet Med Assoc.* 2003;222:176-179.

Callens AJ, Bartges JW. Urinalysis. *Vet Clin Small Animt.* 2015;45:621-637.

Chase J, Hammond J, Bilbrough G, et al. Urine sediment examination: potential impact of red and white blood cell counts using different sediment methods. *Vet Clin Pathol.* 2018;47:608-616.

Cianciolo RE, Bischoff K, Ebel JG, et al. Clinicopathologic, histologic, and toxicologic findings in 70 cats inadvertently exposed to pet food contaminated with melamine and cyanuric acid. *J Am Vet Med Assoc.* 2008;233:729-737.

Davis KU, Grindem CB. What is your diagnosis? Urine crystals in a dog. *Vet Clin Pathol.* 2015;44(2):331-332.

Furman E, Hooijberg EH, Leidinger E, et al. Hereditary xanthinuria and urolithiasis in a domestic shorthair cat. *Comp Clin Path.* 2015;24:1325-1329.

Graff SL. *A Handbook of Routine Urinalysis.* Philadelphia: JB Lippincott; 1983:69-132.

Gunn-Christie RG, Flatland B, Friedrichs KR, et al. ASVCP quality assurance guidelines: control of preanalytical, analytical, and postanalytical factors for urinalysis, cytology, and clinical chemistry in veterinary laboratories. *Vet Clin Pathol.* 2012;41(1):18-26.

Hernandez AM, Bilbrough GEA, DeNicola DB, et al. Comparison of the performance of the IDEXX SediVue Dx(R) with manual microscopy for the detection of cells and 2 crystal types in canine and feline urine. *J Vet Intern Med.* 2019;33(1):167-177.

Hokamp JA, Leidy SA, Gaynanova I, et al. Correlation of electrophoretic urine protein banding patterns with severity of renal damage in dogs with proteinuric chronic kidney disease. *Vet Clin Pathol.* 2018;47:425-434.

Kucera J, Bulkova T, Rychla R, et al. Bilateral xanthine nephrolithiasis in a dog. *J Small Anim Pract.* 1997;38:302-305.

Meichner K, Olsson SA, Stewart DR, et al. What is your diagnosis? Urine crystals in a dog. *Vet Clin Pathol.* 2015;44(4):613-614.

Mochizuki H, Shapiro SG, Breen M. Detection of BRAF mutation in urine DNA as a molecular diagnostic for canine urothelial and prostatic carcinoma. *PLoS One.* 2015;10(12):e0144170.

O'Neil E, Horney B, Burton S, et al. Comparison of wet-mount, Wright-Giemsa and Gram-stained urine sediment for predicting bacteriuria in dogs and cats. *Can Vet J.* 2013;54:1061-1066.

Osborne CA, Lulich JP, Ulrich LK, et al. Feline crystalluria. Detection and interpretation. *Vet Clin North Am Small Anim Pract.* 1996;26:369-391.

Osborne CA, Lulich JP, Ulrich LK, et al. Melamine and cyanuric acid-induced crystalluria, uroliths, and nephrotoxicity in dogs and cats. *Vet Clin North Am Small Anim Pract.* 2009;39:1-14.

Osborne CA, Stevens JB. *Urinalysis: A Clinical Guide to Compassionate Patient Care.* Shawnee Mission, KS: Bayer Corporation; 1999:125-179.

Parambeth JC, Hernandez AM, Nabity MB, et al. What is your diagnosis? Unusual urinary crystals from a cat. *Vet Clin Pathol.* 2018;47:507-508.

Piech TL, Wycislo KL. Importance of urinalysis. *Vet Clin North Am Small Anim Pract.* 2019;49:233-245.

Pressler BM, Gookin JL, Sykes JE, et al. Urinary tract manifestations of protothecosis in dogs. *J Vet Intern Med.* 2005;19:115-119.

Raskin RE, Murray KA, Levy JK. Comparison of home monitoring methods for feline urine pH measurement. *Vet Clin Pathol.* 2002;31:51-55.

Reppas G, Foster SF. Practical urinalysis in the cat: 1: urine macroscopic examination 'tips and traps'. *J Feline Med Surg.* 2016a;18:190-202.

Reppas G, Foster SF. Practical urinalysis in the cat: 2: urine microscopic examination 'tips and traps'. *J Feline Med Surg.* 2016b;18:373-385.

Schweighauser A, Howard J, Malik Y, et al. Xanthinuria in a domestic shorthair cat. *Vet Rec.* 2009;164:91-92.

Stockham SL, Scott MA. Urinary system. In: *Fundamentals of Veterinary Clinical Pathology.* 2nd ed. Ames, IA: Blackwell Publishing; 2008:415-494.

Sturgess CP, Hesford A, Owen H, et al. An investigation into the effects of storage on the diagnosis of crystalluria in cats. *J Feline Med Surg.* 2001;3:81-85.

Swenson CL, Boisvert AM, Kruger JM, et al. Evaluation of modified Wright-staining of urine sediment as a method for accurate detection of bacteriuria in dogs. *J Am Vet Med Assoc.* 2004;224:1282-1289.

Tvedten H, Lilliehöök I, Rönnberg H, et al. Massive uric acid crystalluria and cylinduria in a dog after L-asparaginase treatment for lymphoma. *Vet Clin Pathol.* 2019;48:425-428.

Vap LM, Shropshire SB. Urine cytology: collection, film preparation, and evaluation. *Vet Clin North Am Small Anim Pract.* 2017;47:135-149.

Winston JA, Piperisova I, Neel J, et al. *Cyniclomyces guttulatus* infection in dogs: 19 cases (2006–2013). *J Am Anim Hosp Assoc.* 2016;52:42-51.

13 CHAPTER

Reproductive System

Laia Solano-Gallego and Carlo Masserdotti

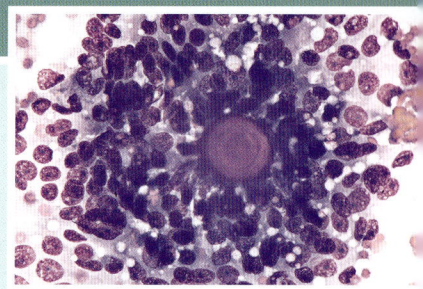

FEMALE REPRODUCTIVE SYSTEM

The focus of this section is the mammary glands, ovaries, uterus, and vagina of dogs and cats involving normal anatomy, cytopathology, and histopathology. The lesions discussed include duct ectasia, cysts, hyperplasia, inflammation, and neoplasia.

Mammary Glands

Mammary gland lesions are common in female dogs and cats. Important information in the investigation of mammary gland disease includes history, breed, and age; whether the gland was intact or older when the dog or cat was neutered; date of last estrus, pregnancy, or hormone therapy; size, number, and consistency of lesion(s); attachment to underlying tissue; rate of growth; presence of ulceration; and evidence of metastasis. Ancillary diagnostic tests used to evaluate mammary lesions include a thorough evaluation of health status involving a complete physical examination, complete blood count (CBC), serum biochemical profile, urinalysis or coagulation profile, imaging, cytopathology, and histopathology. The ease of obtaining cytopathologic specimens from mammary lesions, low invasive nature, moderate to good diagnostic accuracy, and relatively small expense make exfoliative cytopathology a useful diagnostic tool in the evaluation of mammary disease. When combined with history, signalment, and clinical findings, cytopathologic examination of mammary aspirates is particularly useful for differentiation between neoplastic disease, cystic lesions, and mastitis.

Collection Techniques

Exfoliative cytopathology is also useful for evaluation of regional lymph nodes, distant metastatic sites, and neoplastic effusions associated with mammary malignancies. Unfortunately, use of cytopathology to evaluate mammary neoplasms can be difficult, and definitive diagnoses may not always be possible. Some of these difficulties are related to sample collection, and others are simply inherent in the nature of mammary neoplasia. With an understanding of the potential difficulties of mammary cytopathology, the cytopathologist can provide useful diagnostic information concerning mammary gland disease.

Cytopathologic samples from mammary lesions may be obtained by expressing material from the gland, imprints, fine-needle aspiration (FNA), or fine-needle capillary sampling (FNCS) of the affected area. Proper sample collection is particularly important for cytopathology to be useful in the evaluation of mammary tumors. There is considerable tissue heterogeneity, such as both solid and cystic areas within canine mammary tumors; therefore, sampling of multiple solid areas within a single tumor and similar samplings of additional tumors are essential. In contrast to dogs, feline tumors are uniformly distributed. Furthermore, areas of inflammation within the parenchyma of some neoplasms must be correctly interpreted. In large neoplasms, the proliferative tissue can range from benign to malignant structures, and consequently, the interpretation of cytopathologic examination is directly related to the sampling area. Care should also be taken to aspirate the periphery of a mammary mass as opposed to fluctuant areas within a solid lesion or the center of large tumors. These areas tend to yield fluid of low intact cellularity or necrosis, resulting in a nondiagnostic or poorly diagnostic sample.

Normal Anatomy and Histology

Mammary glands are compound tubuloalveolar glands that are believed to be extensively modified sweat glands. In dogs and cats, five pairs of mammary glands are arranged as bilaterally symmetrical rows extending from the ventral thorax to the inguinal region. During pregnancy and lactation, the mammary glands undergo marked hyperplasia and hypertrophy to produce immunoglobulin-containing colostrum followed by milk (Foster, 2017a).

Histologically, mammary glands are composed of a secretory component consisting of alveolar secretory epithelial cells and the initial portion of the intralobular ducts (Figs. 13.1 to 13.3). The secretory portion of the glands is drained by the ductal system, composed of nonsecretory columnar and cuboidal epithelium. Reticular connective tissue supports the alveoli and smaller ducts. Bundles of smooth muscle and elastic fibers surround the large ducts. Myoepithelial cells can be found between the alveolar epithelial cells and underlying basement membrane. Myoepithelial cells are immunoreactive for vimentin, CK5/6, CK14, CK17, smooth muscle actin, calponin, p63, and CK10 (Peña et al., 2014; McCourt et al., 2018). The normal histology of mammary gland from immature female dogs and sequential microscopic changes that occur during different stages of the estrous cycle are reviewed elsewhere (Rehm et al., 2007).

Normal Cytology

Low numbers of sloughed secretory epithelial cells, known as foam cells, as well as macrophages and occasional neutrophils on an eosinophilic to basophilic proteinaceous background,

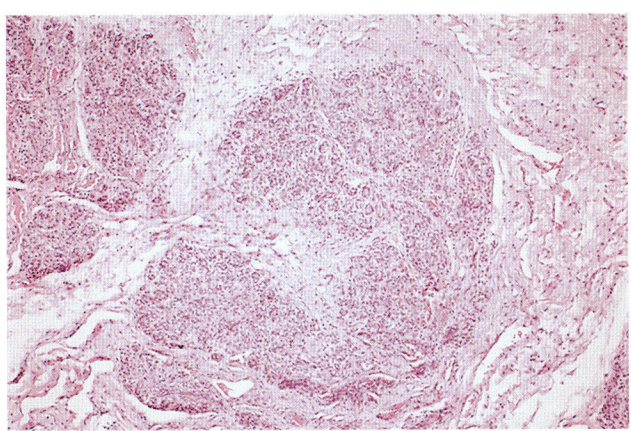

■ **FIGURE 13.1 Normal. Inactive mammary gland. Histology. Dog.** Lobules of glandular tissue are surrounded by abundant interlobular connective tissue. (H&E; LP.)

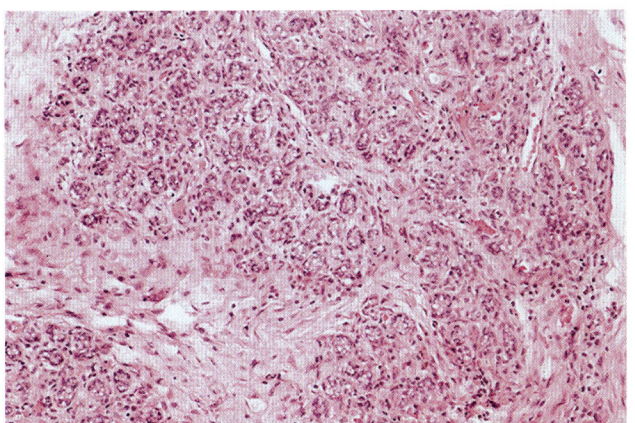

■ **FIGURE 13.2 Normal. Inactive mammary gland. Histology. Dog.** The glandular portion of mammary tissue is composed of alveoli (acini) and intralobular ducts, which are lined by cuboidal to columnar epithelium. The interlobular ducts, composed of nonsecretory columnar and cuboidal epithelium, drain the alveoli. Reticular connective tissue supports the alveoli and smaller ducts. Bundles of smooth muscle and elastic fibers surround the large ducts. (H&E; IP.)

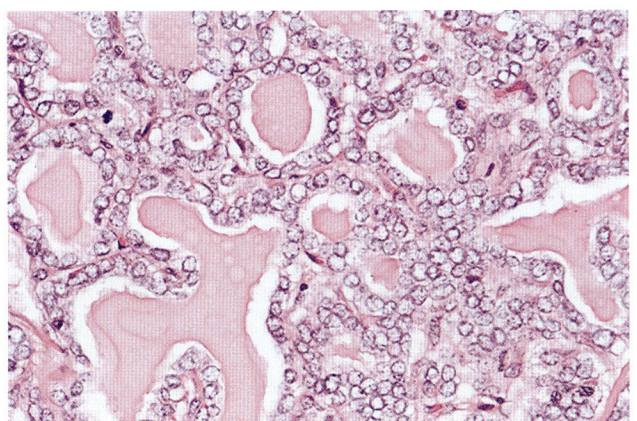

■ **FIGURE 13.3 Normal. Lactational mammary gland. Histology. Dog.** The secretory portion of the gland is well developed, and connective tissue elements are decreased. The mammary alveoli contain bright-pink secretory material. (H&E; HP oil.)

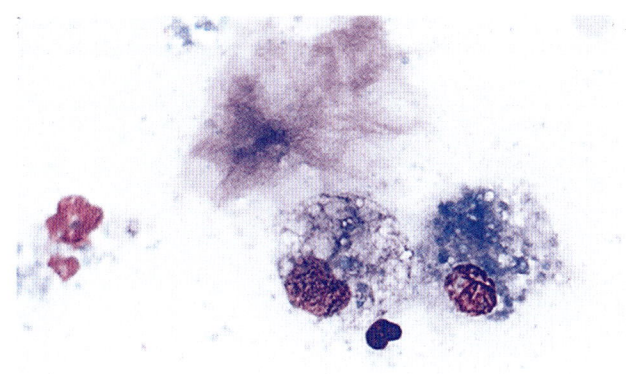

■ **FIGURE 13.4 Foam Cells. Mammary gland aspirate. Cat.** The two foam cells have eccentrically located nuclei, low nucleocytoplasmic ratios, clear and foamy cytoplasmic vacuoles, and basophilic secretory material. The background has a lightly basophilic, proteinaceous appearance consistent with normal mammary aspirates. (Wright-Giemsa; HP oil.)

cytologically characterizes normal mammary secretions. Foam cells are large, individualized cells characterized by round to oval, eccentrically located nuclei and abundant amounts of vacuolated cytoplasm. These cells may also contain amorphous, basophilic secretory material (Fig. 13.4). Foam cells resemble, and can be difficult to distinguish from, foamy macrophages. FNA cytology of normal mammary tissue usually reveals small amounts of blood with no to low numbers of nucleated cells, moderate to large amounts of basophilic proteinaceous material, variously sized and colorless circles (dissolved lipid droplets), and adipocytes. Small sheets and clusters of mammary secretory epithelial cells that are uniform in size and shape may be seen occasionally. Secretory epithelial cells exhibit round, dark nuclei and moderate amounts of basophilic cytoplasm. Acinar formations may be noted. Ductal epithelial cells are characterized by oval, basal nuclei with scant amounts of cytoplasm. Myoepithelial cells may be seen as dark, oval, cell-free nuclei, or spindle-shaped cells.

Mammary Duct Ectasia

Mammary duct ectasia, previously known as mammary cysts, fibrocystic disease, blue-dome cyst, and polycystic mastopathy, is a form of mammary dysplasia in which dilated ducts expand to form cavitary lesions (Box 13.1). Duct ectasia generally occurs in middle-aged to older intact or spayed female dogs, although the disease has been reported in dogs as young as 1 year (Miller et al., 2001). One study found mammary duct ectasia may not be prevented or resolved by ovariohysterectomy and may develop independent of ovarian or exogenous progestogens (Miller et al., 2001). In dogs, rapid growth during estrus and regression during anestrus have been noted. Ovariohysterectomy should be considered when lesions grow and regress in association with the estrous cycle, particularly if multiple glands are involved. Duct ectasia is considered a benign lesion in dogs; however, it has been associated with mammary gland carcinoma (Miller et al., 2001). Duct ectasia is rarely seen in cats (Giménez et al., 2010).

Duct ectasia may present as a well-circumscribed, single cystic nodule or as a flat, rubbery, multinodular mass. The nodules exhibit slow, expansile growth, and the overlying skin may appear

BOX 13.1 Histopathologic Classification of Canine Mammary Gland Tumors

BENIGN MAMMARY GLAND TUMORS

Hyperplasia or Dysplasia
Melanosis of the skin of the teat
Hyperplasia of the teat
Duct ectasia
Lobular hyperplasia (adenosis)
Epitheliosis
Papillomatosis
Gynecomastia

Neoplasms
Duct adenoma
Intraductal papillary adenoma
Adenoma
Fibroadenoma
Complex adenoma[a]
Benign mixed tumor[b]
Myoepithelioma

MALIGNANT MAMMARY GLAND TUMORS

Malignant Epithelial Cells
Carcinoma of the teat
Ductal carcinoma
Intraductal papillary carcinoma
Carcinoma in situ
Carcinoma, tubular
Carcinoma, tubulopapillary
Carcinoma, invasive micropapillary
Carcinoma, solid
Comedocarcinoma
Carcinoma, mucinous
Carcinoma, lipid rich (secretory)
Carcinoma, anaplastic
Carcinoma, spindle cell variant
Carcinoma arising in complex adenoma[a]
Carcinoma arising in benign mixed tumor[b]
Carcinoma, complex type[a]
Carcinoma, mixed type[b]
Carcinoma and malignant myoepithelioma
Malignant myoepithelioma
Squamous cell carcinoma
Adenosquamous carcinoma
Spindle cell carcinoma

Malignant Mesenchymal Cells
Osteosarcoma
Chondrosarcoma
Fibrosarcoma
Hemangiosarcoma

Malignant Epithelial and Mesenchymal Cells
Carcinosarcoma

[a]Complex tumors contain proliferations of mammary epithelial and myoepithelial cells. In complex adenoma, both of these populations are benign. In carcinoma arising in complex adenoma, there is malignant transformation of mammary epithelial cells within complex adenoma. In carcinoma, complex type, the mammary epithelial cells are malignant, but the myoepithelial cells are benign, and there is no identifiable complex adenoma origin.
[b]Mixed tumors are complex tumors with the addition of a benign proliferation of mesenchymal cells, often producing cartilage, bone, or myxoid matrix.
Modified from Goldschmidt M, Peña L, Rasotto R, et al. Classification and grading of canine mammary tumors, *Vet Pathol.* 2011;48:117–131; and Zappulli V, Peña L, Rastottoe R, et al. Mammary tumors. In Kiupel M, ed: *Surgical Pathology of Tumors of Domestic Animals, vol 2.* Washington, DC: Davis-Thompson DVM Foundation; 2019:1–268.

blue, hence the term *blue-dome cyst* (Miller et al., 2001). Histologically, the dilated ducts may be lined by a typical, attenuated, or hyperplastic epithelium, and papillary projections into the duct lumen may be present (Miller et al., 2001). Aspiration of luminal fluid typically yields a green-brown or blood-tinged fluid containing low numbers of foam cells and pigment-laden macrophages. Neutrophils may be increased if inflammation is also present. Cholesterol crystals, which frequently appear as large, rectangular crystalline structures often with a notched corner or less commonly as colorless needle-shapes, may be present as a result of breakdown of exfoliated cell membranes within duct lumens (Fig. 13.5). Epithelial cells derived from the duct lining may be noted, particularly if the lesion has a papillary component. These cells tend to occur in dense sheets and clusters and may display some mild variation in nuclear size and shape.

Duct ectasia may coexist with benign or malignant mammary tumors (Miller et al., 2001). Therefore, fine-needle or tissue biopsies of solid areas of a mass associated with a fluid-filled lesion or other mammary masses are recommended to rule out the presence of concurrent mammary neoplasia.

Mammary Gland Hyperplasia

Hyperplastic and dysplastic lesions of mammary glands include *lobular hyperplasia* (adenosis) and *epitheliosis* (see Box 13.1). These lesions occur in dogs and, less commonly, cats. Mammary hyperplasia is characterized by proliferations of secretory or ductal epithelium or myoepithelial cells resembling the physiologic hyperplasia of pregnancy with some mild histologic atypia. Cytopathologically, these lesions may be difficult to distinguish from each other and from adenomas. Moderate to

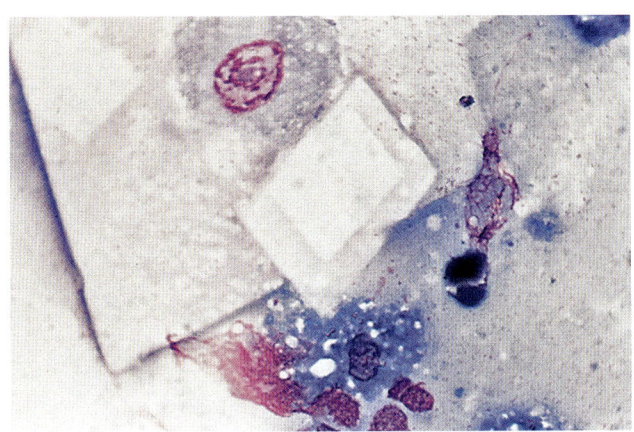

FIGURE 13.5 Duct ectasia. Mammary gland aspirate. Cat. The colorless, rectangular crystals are of varying size. Two foam cells are adjacent to these cholesterol crystals. (Wright-Giemsa; HP oil.)

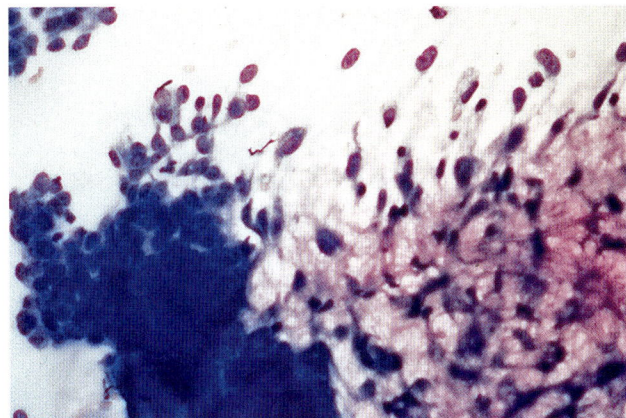

FIGURE 13.6 Fibroadenomatous change. Mammary gland aspirate. Cat. Note the closely associated sheet of epithelial cells *(left)* and aggregate of spindle cells within a pink extracellular matrix *(right)*. The epithelial cells are uniform in size and shape, and the spindle cells display some mild anisokaryosis. (Wright; IP.) (Courtesy Christopher Mesher, Cornell University.)

large numbers of epithelial cells arranged in sheets and clusters can be sampled from hyperplastic mammary tissue. These cells, which are similar in appearance to normal mammary epithelial cells, display round nuclei with fine to lightly stippled chromatin of uniform size and shape and scant to moderate amounts of basophilic cytoplasm. Foam cells and macrophages may also be noted.

Unique to cats is a form of mammary hyperplasia now termed feline *fibroadenomatous change* (formerly termed mammary fibroepithelial hyperplasia) that has been variously identified as feline fibroepithelial hypertrophy, fibroadenomatous hyperplasia, or feline mammary hypertrophy-fibroadenoma complex. Fibroadenomatous change is a clinically benign, common condition affecting estrous-cycling, pregnant, or pseudopregnant female cats usually younger than 2 years (Mesher, 1997). The disorder has also been reported in older intact and neutered cats of either gender (Giménez et al., 2010; Leidinger et al., 2011) mostly after receiving progesterone-containing compounds, such as megestrol acetate or depot medroxyprogesterone acetate. Fibromatous change is considered a form of mammary dysplasia characterized by a rapid, abnormal growth of one or more mammary glands without milk production. The mammary glands may be edematous, painful, ulcerative, and sometimes so large that cats have difficulty walking (Giménez et al., 2010). Systemic signs might include tachycardia, lethargy, and anorexia (Giménez et al., 2010). In contrast to a neoplastic process, there is often bilateral and symmetrical gland enlargement. Fibroadenomatous change is notable for a marked intralobular ductal proliferation identical to that seen during the progesterone-influenced early stages of pregnancy. This typical histologic appearance, along with the occurrence in cycling females or cats administered progesterone and the identification of estrogen and progesterone receptors in these lesions from female and male cats, suggests that both hormones are involved. Fibroadenomatous change usually regresses over time without treatment, although secondary infections may require appropriate antibiotic therapy. Ovariohysterectomy, performed via a flank incision if the glands are greatly enlarged, often results in regression of lesions and prevents future recurrences (Foster, 2017a). However, some cats do not respond to withdrawal of progestogens or ovariectomy and can be treated successfully with the progesterone receptor blocker aglepristone.

The cytopathologic appearance of fibroadenomatous change consists of a very uniform population of cuboidal epithelial cells arranged in thick clusters, sheets, and rows (Figs. 13.6 and 13.7A) (Mesher, 1997). The cuboidal epithelial cells are characterized by dense, round nuclei with small nucleoli and scant amounts of basophilic cytoplasm and minimal atypia (Fig. 13.7B). A mesenchymal population of spindle-shaped cells with narrow oval nuclei, one to two nucleoli, and tapering cytoplasm is also present (see Fig. 13.6). The mesenchymal cells display moderate anisokaryosis and anisocytosis. Moderate amounts of pink extracellular matrix are associated with the mesenchymal cells. These cytopathologic findings correlate with the histologic findings of hyperplastic ductal epithelium (cuboidal epithelial population) and proliferation of edematous stroma (mesenchymal cells with extracellular matrix). Cytopathologic recognition of the characteristic cell types from mammary masses in a cat with appropriate signalment, clinical history, clinical presentation, and ultrasonographic findings can be considered highly suggestive of fibroadenomatous change, thus eliminating the need for mammary gland excision and allowing for appropriate medical or surgical management (Giménez et al., 2010; Leidinger et al., 2011). However, the cytopathologic features of fibroadenomatous change alone cannot be always distinguishable from true benign mammary neoplasms.

Mammary Gland Inflammation and Infection

Inflammation of the mammary glands is referred to as *mastitis* and may present as a focal lesion or involve one or more glands. Mastitis may infrequently occur from hematogenous spread of organisms, nonlactation-associated trauma, fight wounds, or infected neoplasms. *Dirofilaria repens* infection of the mammary gland in bitches (Manuali et al., 2005), mycotic mastitis due to *Blastomyces dermatitidis* in three dogs (Ditmyer and Craig, 2011), and mastitis caused by *Toxoplasma gondii* in a cat (Park et al., 2007) have been reported. Mastitis is most often associated with postparturient lactation. It can also occur during pseudopregnancy and after early

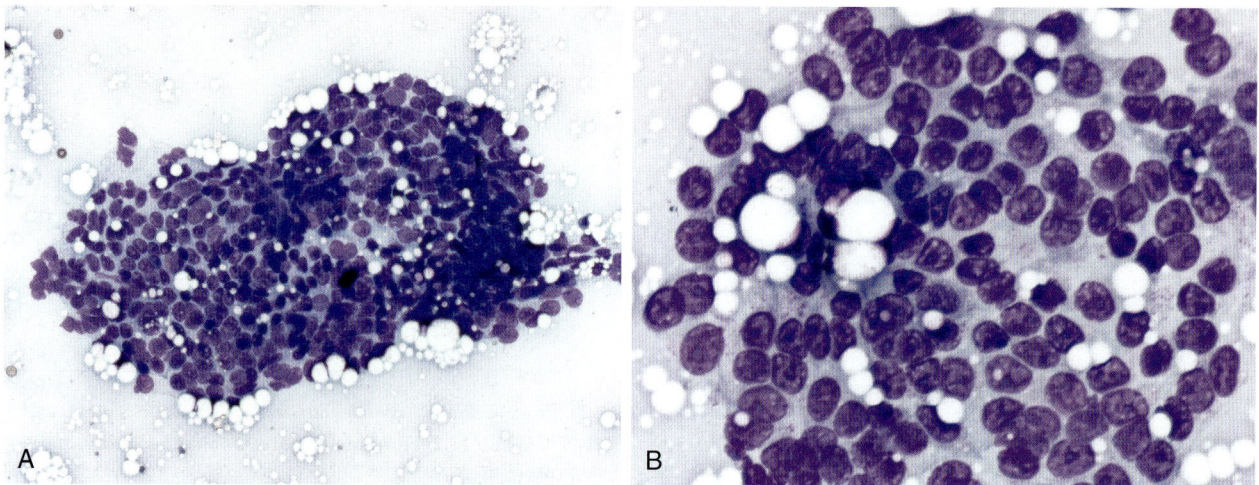

■ **FIGURE 13.7 Fibroadenomatous change. Mammary gland aspirate. Cat.** Same case in A and B. **A,** There is a sheet of uniform epithelial cells with high nucleocytoplasmic ratios and small amounts of light basophilic cytoplasm with indistinct cell borders. The nuclei are often arranged in curved rows, supporting epithelial origin. The light basophilic background contains variably sized, colorless circles, compatible with cell-free lipid that was dissolved during sample fixation. (Wright-Giemsa; IP.) **B,** Epithelial cells display mild anisocytosis and anisokaryosis, smudged chromatin, and a small, round, prominent nucleolus. (Wright-Giemsa; HP oil.) (Courtesy Katie Boes, Virginia Polytechnic Institute and State University.)

weaning of puppies or kittens. It is thought to result from entry of infectious organisms through the teat orifice or damaged overlying skin. Neonatal morbidity or mortality may be the first indication of mastitis. Clinical signs associated with mastitis include swollen, painful glands that result in discomfort while nursing. The glands may become abscessed or gangrenous with necrosis of overlying skin. The bitch or queen may also present with clinical signs of systemic illness such as anorexia, fever, vomiting, or diarrhea. A CBC may reveal an inflammatory leukogram characterized by either an increase in segmented and nonsegmented (band) neutrophils or a degenerative left shift with a predominance of immature neutrophils, especially if gangrenous mastitis is present (Foster, 2017a).

Cytopathologic examination of secretions from inflamed or infected mammary glands is usually diagnostic; however, FNA may be needed for focal lesions. Large numbers of neutrophils are present, which may exhibit degenerative changes of karyolysis and karyorrhexis. Foamy basophilic macrophages, small lymphocytes, and plasma cells may also be seen, particularly with more chronic lesions. Infectious organisms may be seen within neutrophils and, less commonly, macrophages, indicating a septic process. Various bacteria have been incriminated as etiologic agents, such as *Staphylococcus* spp. (Fig. 13.8), *Streptococcus* spp., and *Escherichia coli*. Other types of bacteria, such as *Mycoplasma* spp. and fungi, may also be isolated. Culture and sensitivity of milk, inflamed mammary secretions, or aspirated material are warranted to determine appropriate antibiotic therapy.

The need for antibiotic therapy to treat bacterial mastitis depends on the severity of the lesions. Systemic antibiotic therapy is based on culture and sensitivity results. Abscessed glands should be surgically debrided or drained. Warm, moist topical packs may be used for gangrenous mastitis, and the necrotic tissue can be excised or allowed to slough. Supportive care, including intravenous fluid therapy, may be necessary for the bitch or queen as well as nursing puppies or kittens.

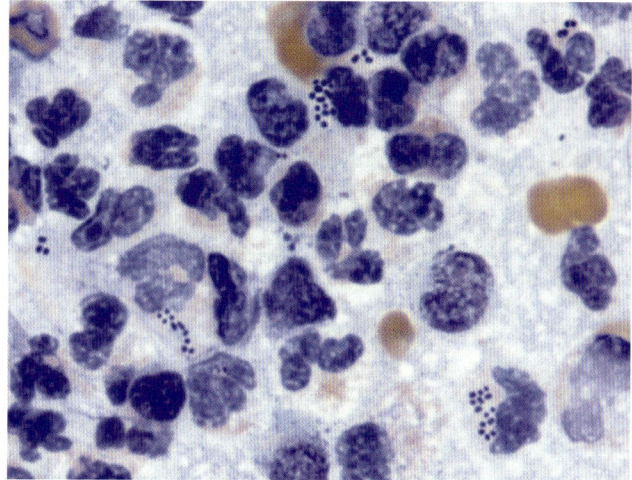

■ **FIGURE 13.8 Mastitis. Milk. Direct smear. Dog.** Specimen of milk from an intact bitch with inflamed mammary gland contains degenerate neutrophils, intracellular and extracellular bacterial cocci, and erythrocytes on a basophilic, foamy, and granular background. Bacterial culture identified a pure growth of *Staphylococcus pseudintermedius*. (Wright-Giemsa; HP oil.) (Courtesy Katie Boes, Virginia Polytechnic Institute and State University.)

In addition, puppies or kittens may require appropriate antibiotic therapy and should be weaned and reared by hand.

Some noninfectious inflammatory conditions of mammary glands have been described. Focal mastitic lesions may leave residual fibrotic nodules consisting of epithelial cell metaplasia, pigment-laden macrophages, nondegenerate neutrophils, small lymphocytes, and plasma cells. Unlike mammary gland tumors (MGTs), fibrotic nodules tend to occur in young dogs, do not increase in size, and are usually associated with a previous history of mastitis.

Mammary Gland Neoplasia

Although histopathology and, more recently, cytopathology have been used to accurately classify mammary lesions as duct ectasia, inflammation, or hyperplasia or neoplasia, determination of the malignant potential of mammary neoplasia can be difficult. Histopathology often shows poor correlation between cellular criteria of malignancy and biologic behavior and prognosis of mammary neoplasms. Although a few studies (Simon et al., 2009; Sontas et al., 2012) have compared cytopathologic evaluation of mammary neoplasms with histopathologic analysis with moderate to good accuracies, limited reports have related biologic behavior with cytopathologic diagnosis (Simon et al., 2009; Dolka et al., 2018). The cytopathologic diagnosis appears to have a good association with the duration of survival, recurrence-free interval, and metastasis-free interval (Simon et al., 2009).

Canine Mammary Gland Tumors

Following skin tumors, mammary neoplasms are the second most common tumor in female dogs and the most commonly seen tumor in intact bitches (Peña et al., 2014; Foster, 2017a). In intact bitches, approximately 50% of MGTs are malignant (Kaszak et al., 2018). MGTs rarely occur in male dogs and are usually benign (Foster, 2017a) with a reported annual incidence of 4 in 100,000, whereas the annual incidence is 207 in 100,000 in female dogs (Saba et al., 2007). Many MGTs reported in male dogs have been associated with small tumor sizes, benign or well-differentiated malignant epithelial tumors, no definitive evidence of metastatic disease at diagnosis, and intense estrogen receptor positivity. The median age for development of canine MGT is 10 to 11 years of age, with rare occurrence in bitches younger than 4 years. Breed tendencies for MGT have been reported with a predisposition in several spaniel breeds, poodles, dachshunds, and other breeds, with a greater prevalence of malignant tumors in large breeds than in small breeds (Kaszak et al., 2018).

Development of MGT appears to have a partial hormonal dependency, as evidenced by the sparing effect of ovariohysterectomy in female dogs and the low incidence in male dogs. Bitches spayed before their first estrous have low mammary cancer risk (0.5%) compared with bitches spayed after one estrous cycle (8% risk) or two or more estrous cycles (26% risk). Although neutering after cancer development has no effect on survival or cause of death, the timing of neutering before mammary carcinoma surgery is prognostic for survival because dogs spayed less than 2 years before tumor surgery survived 45% longer than intact dogs or dogs spayed more than 2 years before tumor surgery (Sorenmo et al., 2013). Estrogen and progesterone receptors have been identified in normal, hyperplastic or dysplastic mammary tissue, and a majority of mammary neoplasms (Peña et al., 2014). Other risk factors for MGT are obesity at age 1 year, a low-fat and low-protein diet, and genetic factors (Kaszak et al., 2018).

Hormone receptor expression, which is a characteristic feature of mature mammary epithelial cells, tends to be decreased or absent in poorly differentiated tumors and metastatic lesions. It is well known that progesterone or synthetic progestin administration increases the incidence of MGT in dogs (Peña et al., 2014). Mechanisms involved in the progesterone-induced MGT include an upregulation of growth hormone production by mammary epithelial cells and a rise in blood levels of insulin-like growth factor (IGF)-I and IGF-II (Sorenmo et al., 2013). Growth hormone and IGF may increase proliferation of susceptible or transformed mammary epithelial cells, resulting in neoplasia.

Molecular targets and biomarkers have been investigated to aid in clinical diagnosis, treatment selection, and prognosis for bitches with MGT, as well to elucidate the pathways of tumorigenesis (Kaszak et al. 2018). A large number of promising molecular targets and biomarkers have been documented. These targets and markers include carcinoembryonic antigen and cancer antigen (CA15.3), cyclooxygenase-2, heat-shock proteins, endothelial growth factor receptor, estrogen and progesterone receptors, human epidermal growth factor receptor 2 (HER-2), breast cancer gene (*BRCA1* and *BRCA2*), *c-erbB-2*, antiapoptotic and proapoptotic proteins, β-catenin, E-cadherin, adenomatous polyposis coli protein (APC), connexin, proliferating cell nuclear tumor protein p53, and Ki-67 (Kaszak et al., 2018). Other promising biomarkers are miRNA, cancer stem cells, and circulating tumor cells (Kaszak et al., 2018).

Clinical behavior and prognosis. Mammary tumors can present as single, firm, well-circumscribed masses to multiple, infiltrative nodules involving one or more glands. In animals with benign mammary tumors, the tumor is small, well circumscribed, and firm on palpation. Clinical findings associated with malignant neoplasms include a tumor diameter greater than 5 cm, recent rapid growth, ill-defined boundaries, infiltration of surrounding tissue, erythema, ulceration, inflammation, and edema (Sorenmo et al., 2013). However, most benign and malignant canine mammary tumors exhibit none of these signs with the exception of dogs with advanced metastatic disease or the clinical syndrome of inflammatory mammary carcinoma (IMC) that typically have systemic signs of illness when they are diagnosed.

The majority of mammary neoplasms occur in the caudal glands, presumably because of the larger amount of glandular tissue present. Multiple MGTs are common, with 50% to 60% of dogs presenting with more than one MGT. Multiple MGTs in a dog are often not of the same histopathologic type and may exhibit differing biologic behaviors. Therefore, a thorough search for additional tumors should be undertaken if a mammary mass is found and separate cytopathologic or histologic analyses should be performed on each MGT.

The ultimate goal of clinical, cytopathologic, and histopathologic evaluation of MGT is to accurately predict the tumor's biologic behavior and therefore the patient's optimal management plan and prognosis. The previous 1999 World Health Organization histologic classification system has been modified by the proposed 2011 canine classification system, which has been found to have prognostic significance (see Box 13.1) (Goldschmidt et al., 2011; Rasotto et al., 2017; Canadas et al., 2019; Zappulli et al., 2019). Prognosis for survival is better for dogs with benign tumors, simple tubular carcinoma, carcinomas arising within benign mixed tumors, complex carcinoma, or mixed carcinomas, and prognosis for survival is worse for dogs with anaplastic carcinoma, carcinosarcoma, solid carcinoma, comedocarcinoma, or adenosquamous carcinoma (Canadas et al., 2019; Rasotto et al., 2017).

Tumor staging and grading. Several histopathologic staging systems for canine mammary carcinomas have been proposed, but the 2013 Peña grading system is most widely used and is prognostic for survival (Peña et al., 2013). The 2013 Peña grading system assesses the tumor's degree of tubular differentiation, amount of nuclear pleomorphism, and mitotic count to determine the histopathologic grade (I, low, well-differentiated; II, intermediate, moderately differentiated; and III, high, poorly differentiated). Another grading system based on the tumor's greatest diameter in millimeters, presence or absence of lymphovascular invasion, and histopathologic lymph nodal stage has also shown to be prognostic for survival (Chocteau et al., 2019a). A recent study applied Robinson's cytopathologic grading system for diagnosis of breast cancer in women to canine mammary tumors and demonstrated 83% agreement between the cytopathologic and histopathologic grading (Dolka et al., 2018).

Histologic classification. Most MGTs are of epithelial origin. In intact bitches, the most common tumor types are tubular adenoma, papillary adenoma, tubular carcinoma (adenocarcinoma), papillary carcinoma, solid carcinoma, complex carcinoma, and carcinosarcoma (Salas et al., 2015). Some tumors contain one cell type (simple tumors), contain both epithelial and myoepithelial tissue (complex tumors), contain areas of cartilage and bone (mixed tumors), or are rarely of entire (sarcoma) or partial (carcinosarcoma) mesenchymal origin (Goldschmidt et al., 2017). Morphologic criteria of malignancy, such as cellular pleomorphism, mitotic activity, and individual grades of anaplasia, are not sufficient criteria for the diagnosis of carcinomas. There are six main histopathologic features that are prognostically significant for mammary tumors: (1) infiltration into skin and soft tissues and metastasis to draining lymph node, (2) intravascular tumor emboli, (3) invasion at the periphery of the mass (peripheral invasion), (4) unique histologic phenotypes, (5) histologic grade, including degree of dysplasia and mitotic rate, and (6) tumor size (Goldschmidt et al., 2017).

Diagnostic accuracy. Accurate and diagnostic exfoliative cytopathology of mammary tumors is difficult. Mesenchymal tumors or tumors with a fibrous or scirrhous component may not exfoliate well, leading to a poorly cellular sample inadequate for diagnosis. Mammary hyperplasia, dysplasia, benign tumors, and well-differentiated carcinomas tend to form a continuum of morphologic appearance, making cytopathologic differentiation of these lesions difficult. Last, the presence of stromal invasion, one of the most important criteria for determining the malignant potential of a mammary neoplasm, cannot be assessed by cytopathology. All of these factors can result in either false-positive or false-negative diagnosis of malignant mammary tumors using cytopathology.

Some studies (Simon et al., 2009; Sontas et al., 2012; Dolka et al., 2018) have examined the accuracy of cytopathology for detecting mammary malignancies and benign lesions compared with histopathologic findings with substantial diagnostic accuracy. Sensitivity and specificity for the diagnosis of malignant tumors and benign lesions are similar between studies, with both ranging from 80% to 90% (Simon et al., 2009; Sontas et al., 2012; Dolka et al., 2018). Cytopathology of canine mammary tumors appears to be a valuable diagnostic tool, although lower accuracy exists when inadequate samples are taken into consideration (Sontas et al., 2012). Limited studies have correlated cytopathologic diagnosis with disease-free intervals or survival times with controversial results (Simon et al., 2009; Dolka et al., 2018). Therefore, the use of cytopathologic criteria to accurately predict the biologic behavior of MGT needs further investigation. Some studies demonstrated that cells in mammary carcinomas had significantly more irregular nuclear shapes than did control epithelial cells or cells in benign epithelial tumors based on differences in fractal dimension and on nuclear diameter and roundness using cytomorphometric analysis (Dolka et al., 2018). These morphometric parameters could help in the preoperative cytopathologic evaluation of canine MGT as demonstrated elsewhere (Simeonov and Simeonova, 2006a, 2006b).

Cytopathology of canine mammary tumors. Cytopathologic examination of mammary tumors frequently reveals a background containing variable amounts of blood, basophilic proteinaceous material, lipid, and foam cells. Aspirates of benign epithelial tumors (adenomas and ductal papillomas) typically reveal moderate to large numbers of epithelial cells arranged in sheets and clusters (Figs. 13.9 and 13.10). These epithelial cells are uniform in appearance with smooth nuclear chromatin and occasionally prominent, single, small, round nucleoli. Occasionally, squamous or apocrine cell differentiation may occur (see Fig. 13.10). Acinar and palisading structures may be seen in samples from adenomas. Papillary and trabecular cell arrangement can be observed in other benign epithelial tumors (Masserdotti, 2006). Benign simple tumors may yield sheets and clusters of uniform-appearing epithelial cells (adenoma) or only myoepithelial cells (myoepithelioma) (Fig. 13.11). In contrast, benign complex tumors comprise a variable number of individual or aggregates of spindle-shaped myoepithelial in addition to epithelial cells (Fig. 13.12). Myoepithelial cells may also appear as oval free nuclei. Examination of benign mixed mammary tumors may reveal the presence of cartilage or bone elements such as osteoblasts, osteoclasts, hematopoietic cells, or bright-pink extracellular material representative of osteoid or chondroid matrix (Fernandes et al., 1998). Benign mixed mammary tumors can be difficult to diagnose using exfoliative cytopathology. For instance, the presence of spindle-shaped cells may not be sufficient for the diagnosis of complex or mixed tumors. Aspirates of mixed tumors also may not reveal all of the cells comprising the tumor. Another case featuring extramedullary hematopoiesis in a benign mixed mammary tumor in a dog contained cortical bone and marrow elements (Grandi et al.,

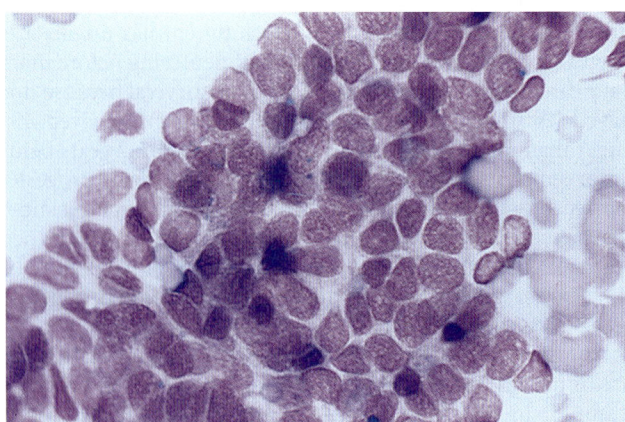

■ **FIGURE 13.9 Mammary adenoma. Mammary gland aspirate. Cat.** Within this sheet of polygonal epithelial cells, individual epithelial cells are of uniform size and shape with a high nucleocytoplasmic ratio and stippled nuclear chromatin. The cytoplasm is lightly basophilic and scant. (Wright-Giemsa; HP oil.)

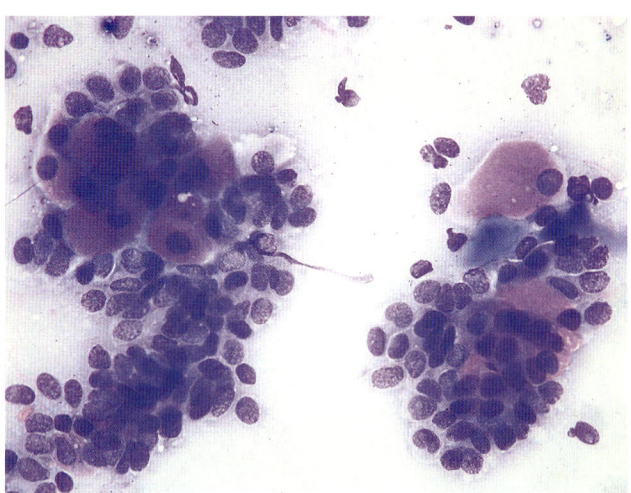

■ **FIGURE 13.10 Apocrine cell differentiation. Mammary adenoma. Mammary nodule aspirate. Dog.** In addition to the uniform population of ductal epithelium, scattered large round eosinophilic cells are admixed in this population. The cells are characterized by an abundant finely granular eosinophilic cytoplasm with a round nucleus with clumped chromatin. These cells resemble apocrine glandular cells, and this neoplasia is a subtype of ductal adenoma. (Wright; HP oil.) (Courtesy Rose Raskin, TDDS, Exeter, UK.)

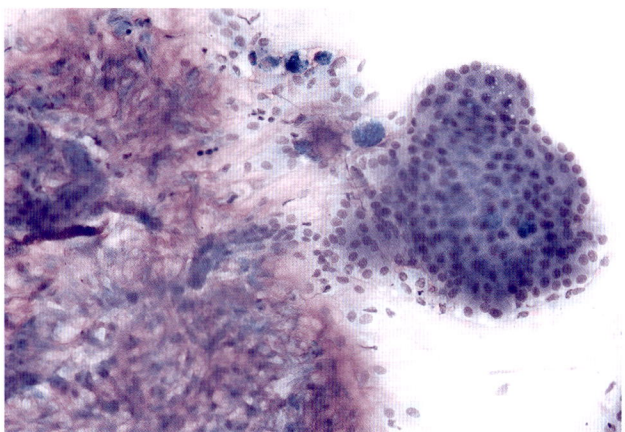

■ **FIGURE 13.12 Myoepithelial and epithelial cells. Complex mammary tumor. Mammary gland aspirate.** Dog. An aggregate of spindle-shaped myoepithelial cells with large amounts of extracellular pink matrix *(left)* is adjacent to a cluster of polygonal epithelial cells *(right)*. Epithelial cells toward the periphery of the cluster are in curved rows, resembling a large acinus. (Wright-Giemsa; IP.)

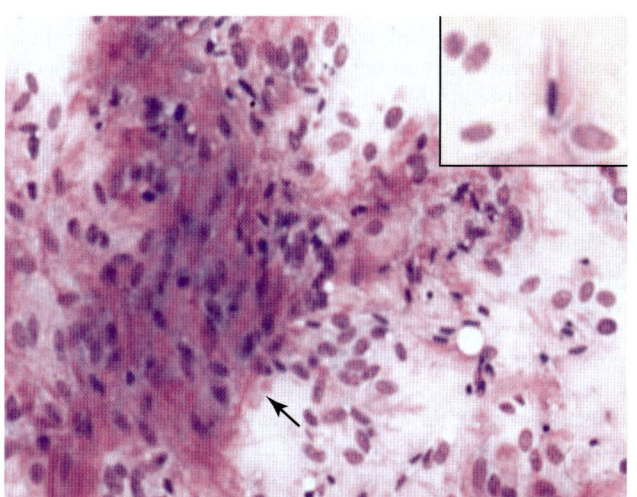

■ **FIGURE 13.11 Myoepithelial cells. Complex mammary tumor. Mammary gland. Fine-needle capillary sampling. Dog.** An aggregate of spindle-shaped myoepithelial cells *(arrow)* associated with an extracellular pink matrix. *Inset:* A benign myoepithelial cell has a small dense eccentric nucleus with fusiform pale cytoplasm. (Giemsa; IP.) (Courtesy Noeme Sousa Rocha, FMVZ-UNESP, Botucatu, Brazil.)

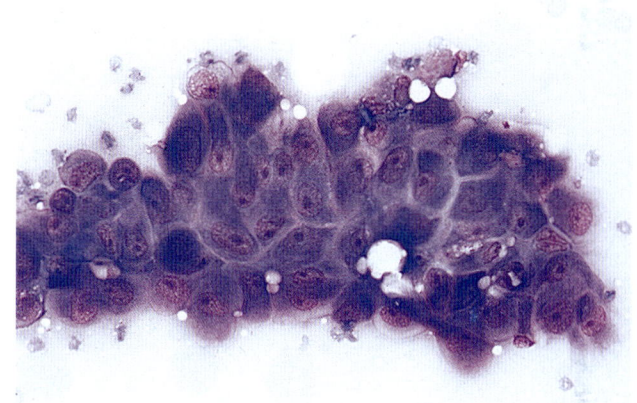

■ **FIGURE 13.13 Mammary carcinoma. Mammary gland aspirate.** Dog. A sheet of epithelial cells displays prominent cell-to-cell junctions. These cells also exhibit moderate anisokaryosis, deeply basophilic cytoplasm, and prominent, large nucleoli. (Wright-Giemsa; HP oil.)

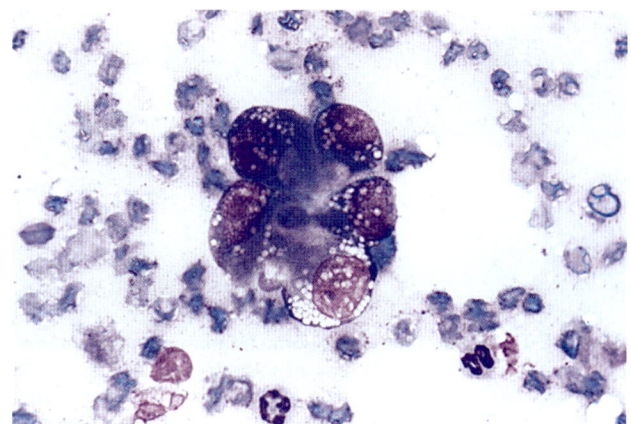

■ **FIGURE 13.14 Mammary carcinoma. Mammary gland aspirate.** Dog. An acinar structure is shown. Note the presence of punctate cytoplasmic vacuoles as well as moderate anisokaryosis and prominent nucleoli. (Wright-Giemsa; HP oil.)

2010). No epithelial cells were noted in the sample. Thus, the multiple differentials included benign or malignant mixed mammary tumor, osseous metaplasia, and osteosarcoma. Histopathology confirmed that the neoplasm was a benign mixed mammary tumor.

Carcinomas are characterized by individualized epithelial cells or epithelial cells arranged in sheets, clusters, acinar formations, papillary arrays, and trabecular arrangements (Figs. 13.13 to 13.17) (Masserdotti, 2006). The epithelial cells are typically

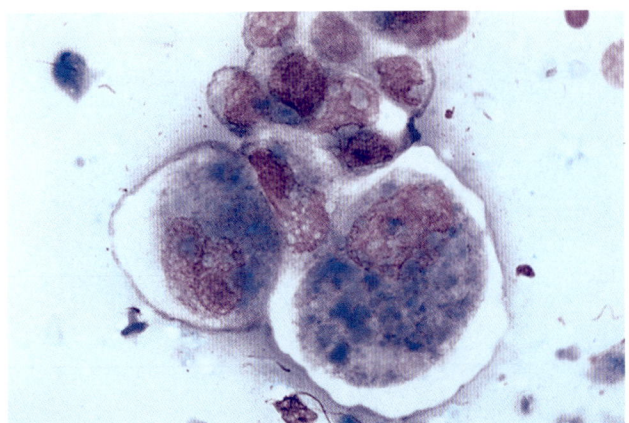

FIGURE 13.15 Mammary carcinoma. Mammary gland aspirate. Dog. Marked anisokaryosis and anisocytosis of the epithelial cells are noted. These epithelial cells contain abundant, foamy, basophilic, secretory material. (Wright-Giemsa; HP oil.)

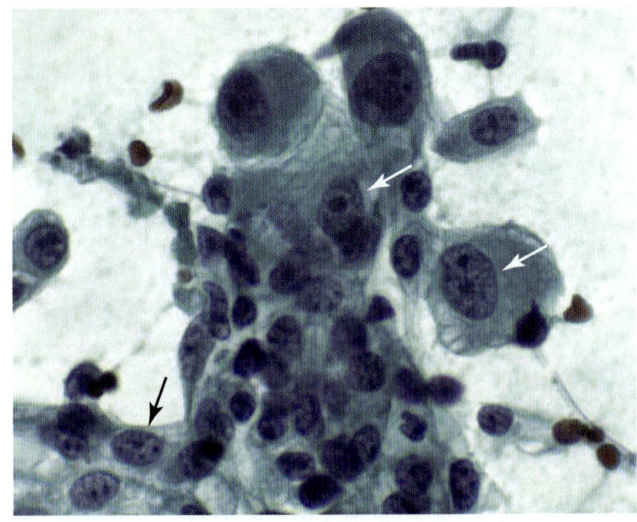

FIGURE 13.17 Mammary carcinoma. Mammary gland. Fine-needle capillary sampling. Dog. Stippled nuclear chromatin with prominent nucleoli within many of the nuclei *(arrows)* are more readily visible in this type of stain. Green color denotes a nonkeratinized cell; a keratinized cell would be orange. (Papanicolaou; HP oil.) (Courtesy Noeme Sousa Rocha, FMVZ-UNESP Botucatu, Brazil.)

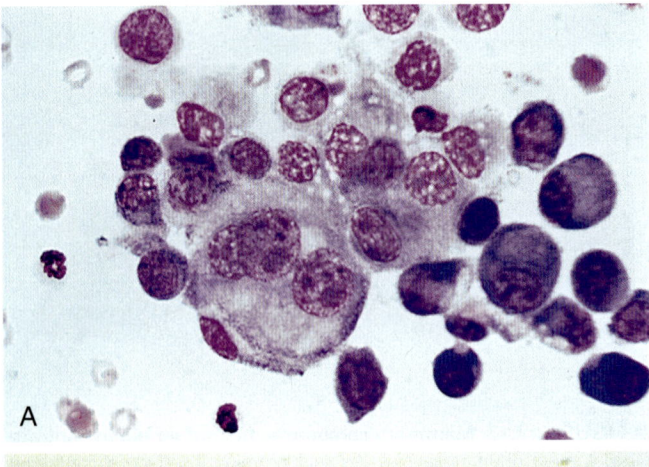

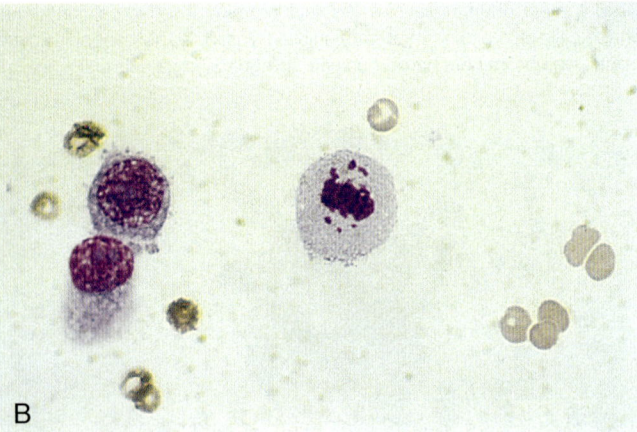

FIGURE 13.16 Mammary carcinoma. Mammary gland aspirate. Dog. Same case in A and B. **A,** Marked anisokaryosis and anisocytosis, prominent nucleoli, coarse chromatin, and binucleation are in neoplastic round cells that also display poor cellular adhesion. (Wright-Giemsa; HP oil.) **B,** Abnormal mitotic figure with lag chromatin. Lag chromatin results from abnormal formation of the mitotic spindle apparatus. Abnormal mitotic figures are considered a criterion of malignancy. (Wright-Giemsa; HP oil.)

round, with round to oval, eccentrically located nuclei and moderate amounts of basophilic cytoplasm that may contain amorphous basophilic secretory product or clear vacuoles (see Fig. 13.14). Some of these vacuoles may appear as punctate vacuoles of variable number or as a diffuse clearing of the cytoplasm that distends the cell and displaces the nucleus peripherally. Criteria of malignancy that may be seen in these cells include increased nucleocytoplasmic ratio (N:C); moderate to marked anisokaryosis; nuclear molding; large, prominent, multiple, or abnormally shaped nucleoli; and binucleation and multinucleation (see Figs. 13.16A and 13.17). Increased mitotic activity and abnormal mitotic figures may be present (see Fig. 13.16B). Ductal carcinomas typically present with sheets and clusters of pleomorphic epithelial cells with high N:C and round, basal nuclei. These cells usually display more than three malignant criteria. Acinar structures, secretory product, and cytoplasmic vacuoles are not characteristic features of ductal carcinomas. Anaplastic carcinomas may present with very large, extremely pleomorphic epithelial cells occurring singly and in small clusters. These cells tend to have bizarre nuclear and nucleolar forms. Multinucleation and abnormal mitotic figures are frequently seen.

Inflammatory mammary carcinoma is a clinical syndrome resulting in local edema, erythema, firmness, pain, and warmth of the mammary glands that mimics mastitis in presentation. These tumors tend to be invasive, aggressive, fast-growing, and highly malignant (Sorenmo et al., 2013). Histopathologically, several types of IMC have been described with invasion of dermal lymphatic vessels by neoplastic cells as the common microscopic feature. The blockage of the superficial lymphatics by tumor cells is responsible for the severe regional edema (de M Souza et al., 2009). The most frequent cytopathologic findings are the presence of anaplastic epithelial cells, singly or in small clusters. Therefore, the cytopathologic findings of highly malignant mammary epithelial cells in association with clinical signs of edema, warmth, pain, and erythema support a clinical diagnosis of IMC. This clinical entity has a guarded prognosis with a short survival time, but medical treatment with piroxicam seems to improve clinical outcome and prolonged survival time (de M Souza et al., 2009).

Squamous cell carcinoma (SCC) of the mammary gland appears cytopathologically similar to those found in other body sites. The malignant squamous cells tend to occur individually or in small sheets. The nuclei may vary from small and pyknotic to large, round, and immature with prominent nucleoli. The N:C is variable, and binucleation may be noted. The cytoplasm of the tumor cells is moderately to deeply basophilic (nonkeratinized) or may have a blue-green color, characteristic of keratinization. Mammary SCC may ulcerate, leading to the presence of inflammatory cells and phagocytized bacteria in the cytopathologic sample.

Fine-needle biopsies of carcinoma arising in complex adenoma, carcinoma arising in benign mixed tumor, complex carcinoma, mixed carcinoma, carcinoma and malignant myoepithelioma, and carcinosarcomas may reveal epithelial and spindle-shaped cells. In these tumors, the spindle-shaped cells are of myoepithelial (complex or mixed tumors) or mesenchymal (carcinosarcoma) cell origin. However, the observance of epithelial and spindle-shaped cells or predominance of one cell type over the other may depend on the area of tumor aspirated (Fig. 13.18). In carcinoma arising in complex adenoma, carcinoma arising in benign mixed tumor, complex carcinomas, and mixed carcinoma, there are malignant epithelial cells and benign-appearing myoepithelial cells, with the mixed types also containing variable amount of osteoid or chondroid matrix. In carcinoma and malignant myoepithelioma and carcinosarcoma, both epithelial and mesenchymal populations should display malignant features.

Mammary sarcomas, such as osteosarcoma, fibrosarcoma, and liposarcoma, are of similar cytopathologic appearance to those found in other body sites. Sarcomas tend to exfoliate poorly, often resulting in samples of low cellularity. Depending on the type of tumor, pink extracellular material or lipid may be present in the background. In general, sarcomas are characterized by spindle-shaped to irregular cells arranged individually

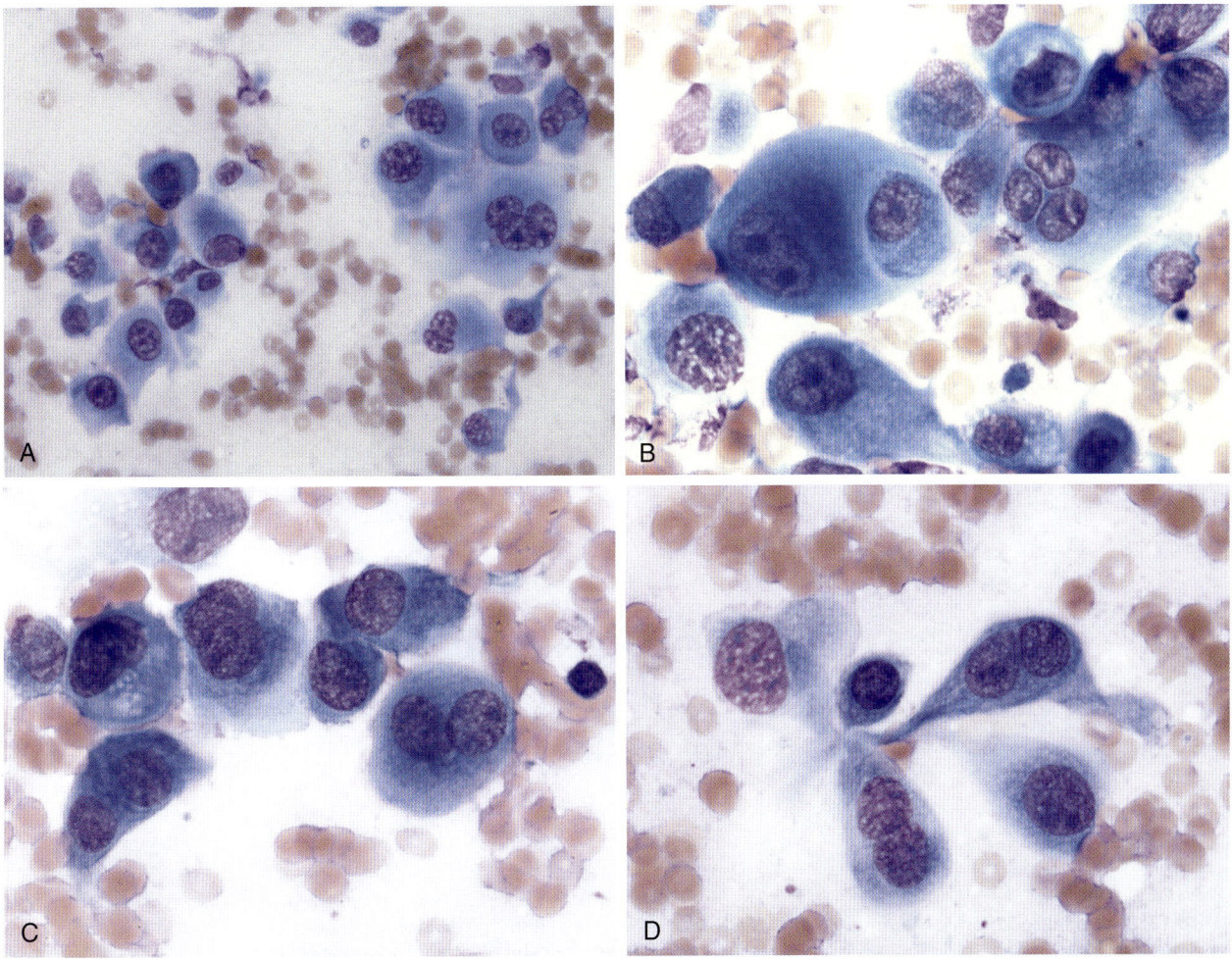

■ **FIGURE 13.18 Mammary carcinoma. Mammary gland aspirate. Dog.** Same case in A to D. Specimen is from a mass (3 cm × 2.5 cm) that exhibited rapid growth and a firm, well-circumscribed, ulcerated appearance that was adherent to underlying tissue. Note the pleomorphic appearance of the malignant epithelial cells, particularly the stellate and spindle forms. Multiple nuclei, prominent and multiple nucleoli, marked anisokaryosis, multinucleation, and nuclear molding are malignant criteria observed. Cytopathologic diagnosis was anaplastic carcinoma, but the histopathologic diagnosis was carcinoma and malignant myoepithelioma. The myoepithelial cell population did not exfoliate within the cytopathologic specimen. Myoepithelial cells may be identified by immunochemistry (calponin, p63, actin, vimentin), but it was not performed in this case. (Wright-Giemsa; HP oil.) (Courtesy Rose Raskin, University of Florida.)

and in aggregates. The cytoplasm of these cells is moderately to deeply basophilic, and the cytoplasmic borders tend to be indistinct. The cells display cytopathologic features of malignancy similar to those described for epithelial neoplasms.

Feline Mammary Gland Tumors

Mammary tumors are the third most common tumor in cats, after hematopoietic neoplasms and skin tumors (Chocteau et al., 2019b). The average age for MGT development in the cat is 11 years (Foster, 2017a). Almost all (99%) of feline MGT occur in intact queens, with rare instance in male cats (Fig. 13.19). Studies of causal factors are limited. Intact animals are at a slightly greater risk, but the effect of spaying is controversial (Foster, 2017a).

Clinical behavior and prognosis. Regular, but not irregular, administration of exogenous progesterone was associated with a significantly increased risk of benign mammary tumors and mammary carcinomas in cats. Hormone receptor analysis has shown that normal feline mammary tissue contains estrogen and progesterone receptors in levels similar to those found in dogs. However, unlike canine MGT but similar to humans, most feline mammary neoplasms express very low levels of estrogen and progesterone receptors, which may be related to the high rate of malignancy found with mammary neoplasia in cats (Chocteau et al., 2019b). Other molecular targets and biomarkers have been investigated to elucidate prognosis, the pathways of tumorigenesis or metastasis such as cyclin A, Cox-2 and HER2, among others (Chocteau et al., 2019b).

In contrast to dogs, the majority of feline MGTs are malignant, with some studies reporting a greater than 85% incidence of malignant neoplasms (Zappulli et al., 2019). Moreover, the majority of feline malignant MGTs are of simple type and epithelial in origin with rare myoepithelial component. Carcinomas (see Fig. 13.19) are the most prevalent malignant MGT followed by sarcomas (Foster, 2017a). Secondary or postsurgical IMC (Millanta et al., 2012) and lipid-rich carcinoma have

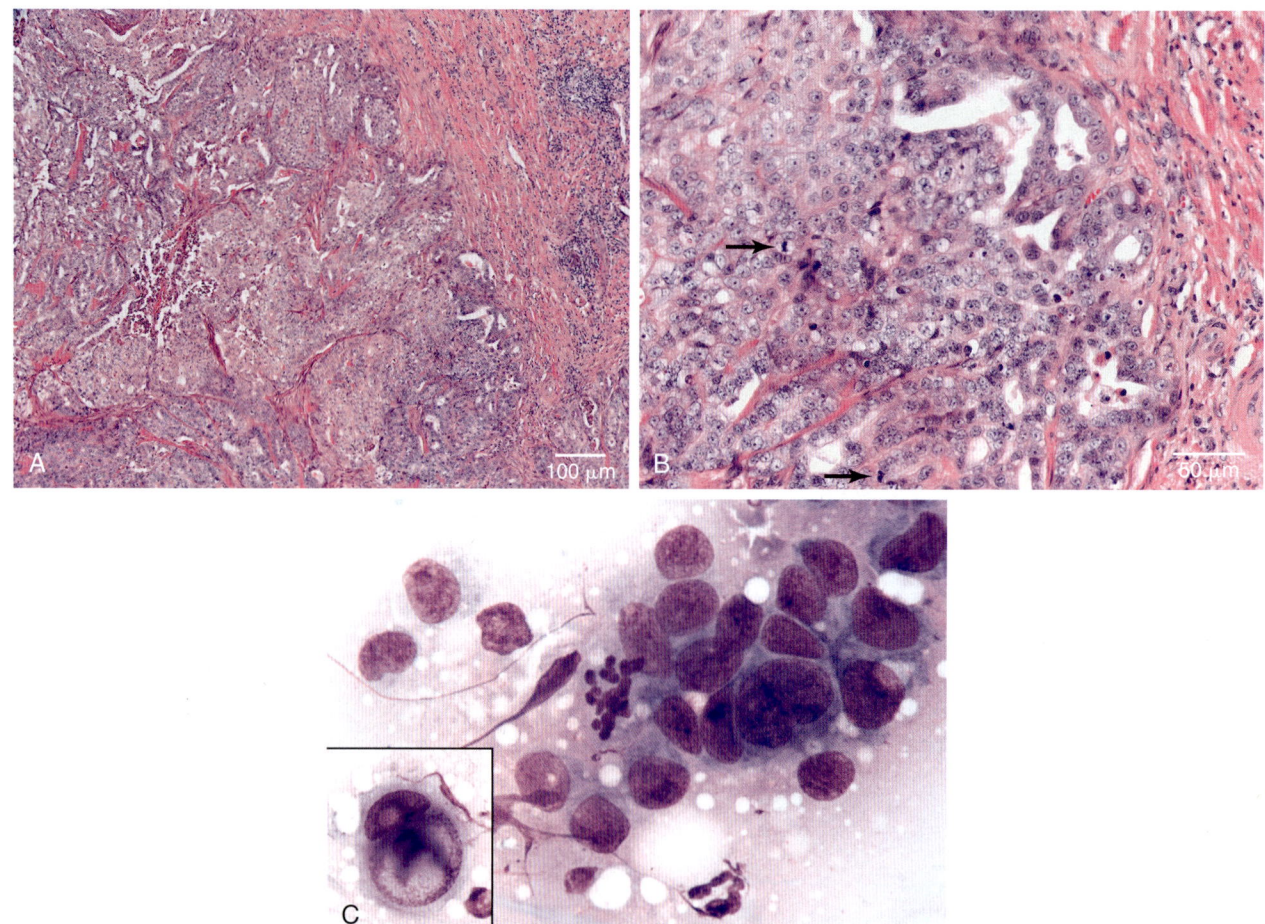

■ **FIGURE 13.19 Ductal carcinoma. Mammary gland. Male cat.** Same case in A to C. **A, Histology.** Loss of normal mammary gland architecture with solid and tubular neoplastic proliferation into surrounding connective tissue. Tubular lumens are slit-like, compatible with ductal origin. The stroma also contains accumulations of small lymphocytes *(upper right).* (H&E; LP.) **B, Histology.** Solid *(left)* and tubular *(center right)* areas of cuboidal to polygonal neoplastic cells infiltrate into the surrounding connective tissue *(right).* Tubules are lined by one to multiple layers of neoplastic cells. Note the two mitotic figures *(arrows)* and conspicuous nucleoli. (H&E; IP.) **C, Cytopathology preparation.** A mitotic figure is in the center and adjacent to epithelial cells arranged in crude acinar formations. Carcinoma cells have high nucleocytoplasmic ratios, multiple and prominent nucleoli, and anisokaryosis. (Romanowsky; HP oil.) *Inset:* A signet ring cell contains a large, granular, cytoplasmic inclusion that peripherally displaces and compresses the nucleus. (Romanowsky; HP oil.) (A–B, Courtesy Frantisek Jelinek, Veterinary Histopathological Laboratory, Prague. C, Courtesy Dita Novakova, Czech Republic.)

been described in cats. Malignant MGTs in cats tend to grow rapidly and metastasize to regional lymph nodes, other mammary glands, lungs, pleura, liver, diaphragm, adrenal glands, and kidneys.

Negative prognostic indicators for survival are the presence of nodal metastasis or lymphovascular invasion, a high histologic grade (grade III), and tumor diameter greater than 3 cm, whereas well-differentiated carcinomas (grade I) have a good prognosis (Foster, 2017a). Median survival times for cats with mammary tumors larger than 3 cm, between 2 and 3 cm, and smaller than 2 cm are 6 months, 2 years, and longer than 3 years, respectively (Foster, 2017a). Thus, early diagnosis and treatment is very important for feline mammary malignancies. A histologic grading system has been validated for feline carcinomas (Mills et al., 2015; Dagher et al., 2019).

Cytopathology of feline mammary tumors. The cytopathologic features of benign and malignant mammary neoplasms in cats (see Fig. 13.19C) are similar to those described in dogs. The reliability of cytopathologic criteria to differentiate between hyperplasia, benign tumors, and malignancies in cats does not appear to have been reported. Given the high rate of mammary malignancy in cats, cytopathologic findings of a benign-appearing population of epithelial cells, particularly in an older cat with no history of progesterone administration, should be treated with some caution. In these cases, samples should be submitted for histopathologic examination to rule out the presence of a malignancy.

Treatment of Mammary Gland Tumors

Treatment considerations should follow clinical and cytopathologic or histopathologic identification of a mammary neoplasm in a dog or a cat. If a malignancy is present, staging the extent of the disease should include three-view thoracic radiographs or computed tomography (CT) or magnetic resonance imaging (MRI) of the lungs and any other potential metastatic sites as well as cytopathologic analysis of regional lymph nodes, suspected metastatic lesions, or body cavity effusions. It has been proposed that treatment guidelines for malignant canine MGT be based on tumor size, histopathologic type, and differentiation (Sorenmo et al., 2013). Surgical excision is the treatment of choice for both canine and feline mammary neoplasms (Giménez et al., 2010). There is limited information regarding the efficacy of adjuvant therapy involving chemotherapeutics, radiation, hormonal therapy, or immune stimulation in canine and feline mammary malignancies and is reviewed elsewhere (Santos and Matos, 2015).

Ovaries

Scarce information is available on ovarian diseases in bitches and queens, but cystic or ovarian tumors are most commonly documented (Arlt and Haimerl, 2016). Cytopathology is a valuable tool for the evaluation of ovarian tumors, as demonstrated by a 94.7% diagnostic agreement between cytopathologic and histopathologic diagnoses of canine ovarian tumors (Bertazzolo et al., 2004). In addition, although oophoritis and ovarian remnant syndrome are rare in dogs and cats (Ball et al., 2010), cytopathologic evaluation might be useful in diagnosis of these disorders.

Collection Techniques

There is little information on ovarian cytopathology collection techniques. Ovarian tissue biopsy for histopathology is performed, and surgical technique is well described elsewhere (Root Kustritz, 2006). Cytopathologic samples can be made by ultrasound-guided percutaneous FNA and could reduce the risk of a tissue biopsy procedure and laparoscopy or exploratory laparotomy in some cases (Bertazzolo et al., 2004).

Normal Anatomy and Histology

The ovary is composed of three broad embryologic origins: (1) the epithelium, (2) the germ cells, and (3) the ovarian stroma, including the sex cords, which together contribute the endocrine apparatus of the ovary (Agnew and MacLachlan, 2017). The epithelium includes the outer layer lining (surface) epithelium of the modified mesothelium, the rete ovarii (remnants of the mesonephric tubules), and in bitches, the subsurface epithelial structures. Each ovary lies within an ovarian bursa, an extension of the mesosalpinx, which is a fold of the peritoneum. Cuboidal epithelium, called germinal epithelium, covers the cortex of the ovary, and a layer of dense connective tissue, the tunica albuginea, is present underneath the epithelium. The canine ovary has small ingrowths of the ovarian surface that are called subsurface epithelial structures. The cortex of the ovary contains follicles, stromal connective tissue, and blood vessels. The ova develop in follicles that are of four types: primordial, primary, secondary, and tertiary. Each developing follicle has the oocyte, multiple layers of granulosa cells, and more peripheral thecal connective tissue cells (Fig. 13.20). Ovulation occurs when the follicle ruptures, releasing the ovum and allowing the space to fill with blood and luteal cells to form the corpus hemorrhagicum and the corpus luteum, respectively. In bitches and queens, cords of epithelial cells called interstitial glands, which are cells of an endocrine type, occur throughout the stroma. A medulla consisting of richly vascularized loose connective tissue, lymphatics, and nerves lies internal to the ovarian cortex. Channels lined by cuboidal epithelium, called *rete ovarii*, are present in this region (Foster, 2017a).

The normal histology of ovaries from immature female dogs and sequential microscopic changes that occur during different stages of the estrous cycle are reviewed elsewhere (Rehm et al., 2007).

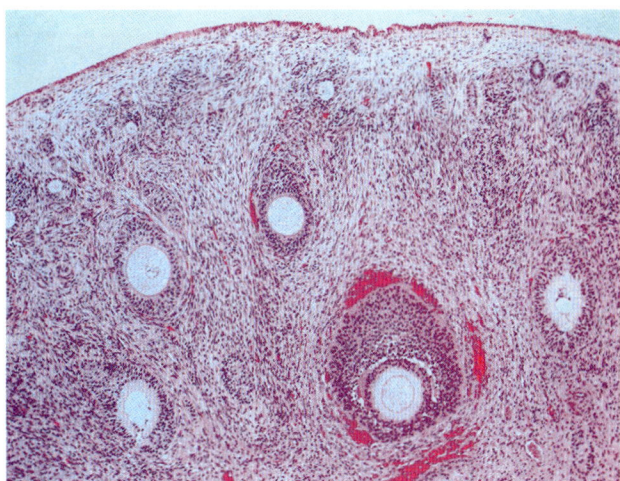

■ **FIGURE 13.20 Normal ovary. Histology. Dog.** Several developing follicles, each with an oocyte surrounded by a layer of granulosa cells, are present within the stroma of the ovarian cortex. The cortex is lined by a simple layer of cuboidal epithelium. (H&E; LP.)

Normal Cytology

Knowledge of specific cytologic features of normal canine ovaries is important for identification of pathologic processes (Piseddu et al., 2012). A detailed cytologic description of aspirates from normal canine ovaries in different stages of estrus with comparison with histologic features is reported elsewhere (Piseddu et al., 2012).

Cytology of normal ovarian tissue usually reveals small amounts of blood with no to moderate numbers of nucleated cells and moderate to large amounts of basophilic, proteinaceous material and clear lipid droplets. Normal ovaries are characterized cytologically by low to moderate numbers of one or more of the following cells based on the stage of the estrous cycle. These cells include adipocytes, individual fibrocytes or fibroblasts, granulosa cells that are uniform in size and shape and are arranged in acinar formations or in small loosely to cohesive aggregates, round cells of unknown origin, rare leukocytes, and luteal cells (Figs. 13.21 to 13.25).

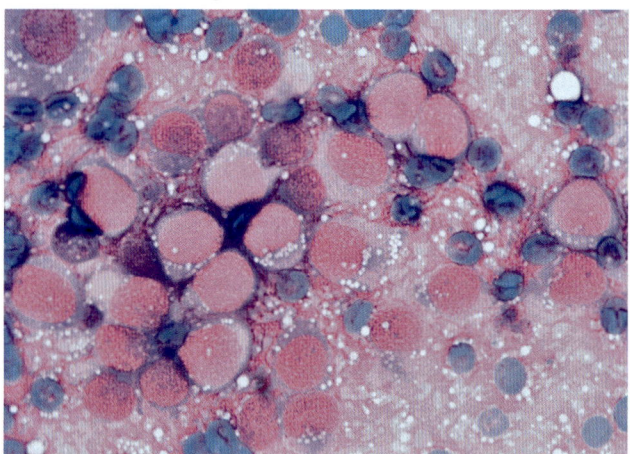

■ **FIGURE 13.23 Normal ovary. Immature cells. Tissue aspirate. Dog.** The immature cells are individualized, round, and 15 to 20 μm in diameter with scant, basophilic, vacuolated cytoplasm. Their nuclei are large and round with reticular chromatin and one to multiple, small, indistinct nucleoli. (Modified Wright; HP oil.) (Courtesy Eleonora Piseddu, IDEXX.)

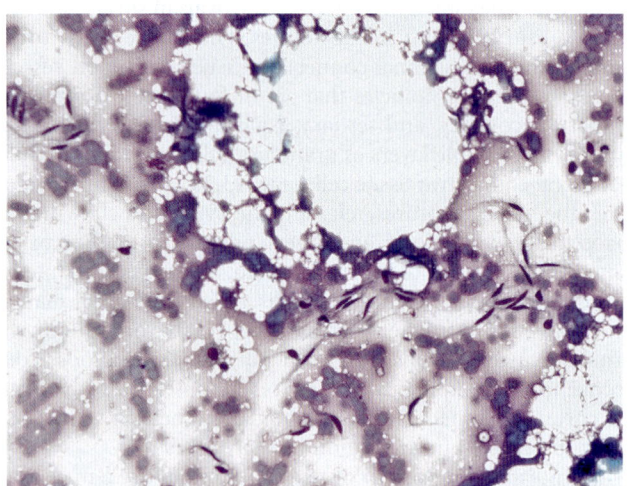

■ **FIGURE 13.21 Normal ovary. Stromal cells. Cytologic preparation. Dog.** The basophilic background contains red blood cells, variable sized lipid droplets, and cellular debris. Numerous fibrocytes and fibroblasts from the stromal area are noted. (May-Grünwald-Giemsa; IP.)

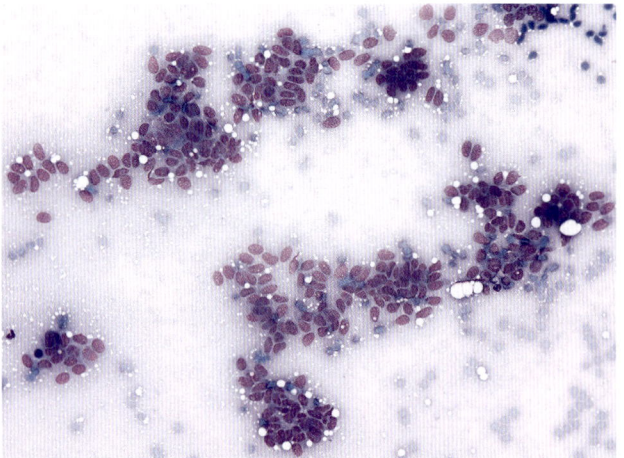

■ **FIGURE 13.22 Normal ovary. Granulosa cells. Tissue aspirate. Dog.** Granulosa cells are uniform in size and shape, and are arranged in small, loose aggregates. (Modified Wright; IP.) (Courtesy Eleonora Piseddu, IDEXX.)

Luteal cells are large cells with low N:C and variable degrees of anisocytosis and anisokaryosis. Cytoplasmic and nuclear features and shapes of luteal cells differed in early (see Fig. 13.24) and late (see Fig. 13.25) diestrus. Anisocytosis and anisokaryosis are increased in early diestrus compared with late diestrus. Luteal cells exfoliated individually or in perivascular arrangements. In early diestrus, most luteal cells are round to polygonal or elongated and have distinct cell borders and mild to moderate anisocytosis and mild anisokaryosis. Nuclei are eccentric round to oval nuclei with finely stippled to reticular chromatin. A variable amount of cytoplasm appears finely granular and amphophilic to deeply basophilic with rarely small to medium-sized intracytoplasmic clear discrete vacuoles (see Fig. 13.24) (Piseddu et al., 2012). In late diestrus, luteal cells are round and frequently have indistinct borders with blebbed margins. The cytoplasm is clear at the periphery and lightly basophilic in the center with numerous small clear discrete vacuoles. Nuclei have the same location and shapes reported for cells in early diestrus but have reticular to coarse chromatin with one to two prominent nucleoli (see Fig. 13.25). Large pale pink dense structures (150–300 μm) are rarely observed extracellularly in late diestrus (Fig. 13.26) and are similar to corpora albicans found in histologic sections (Piseddu et al., 2012). In both early and late diestrus, binucleated cells and leukoemperipolesis are noted frequently (see Figs. 13.24A and 13.25) (Piseddu et al., 2012).

Spindle cells (see Fig. 13.21) and granulosa cells are not associated with any particular estrous stage. Granulosa cells exfoliated in loose to cohesive aggregates, within which palisades and acinar-like arrangements are noted (see Fig. 13.22). The cells are small, 10 to 15 μm in diameter, and round to elongate, sometimes with short cytoplasmic tails. The cytoplasm is scant and basophilic with indistinct borders and, rarely, a few, small, clear vacuoles. Nuclei are oval to round with stippled to finely reticular chromatin and indistinct nucleoli. Granulosa cells frequently are associated with purple amorphous material (Fig. 13.27) (Piseddu et al., 2012). Round immature cells exfoliate individually, and often are mixed with luteal or granulosa

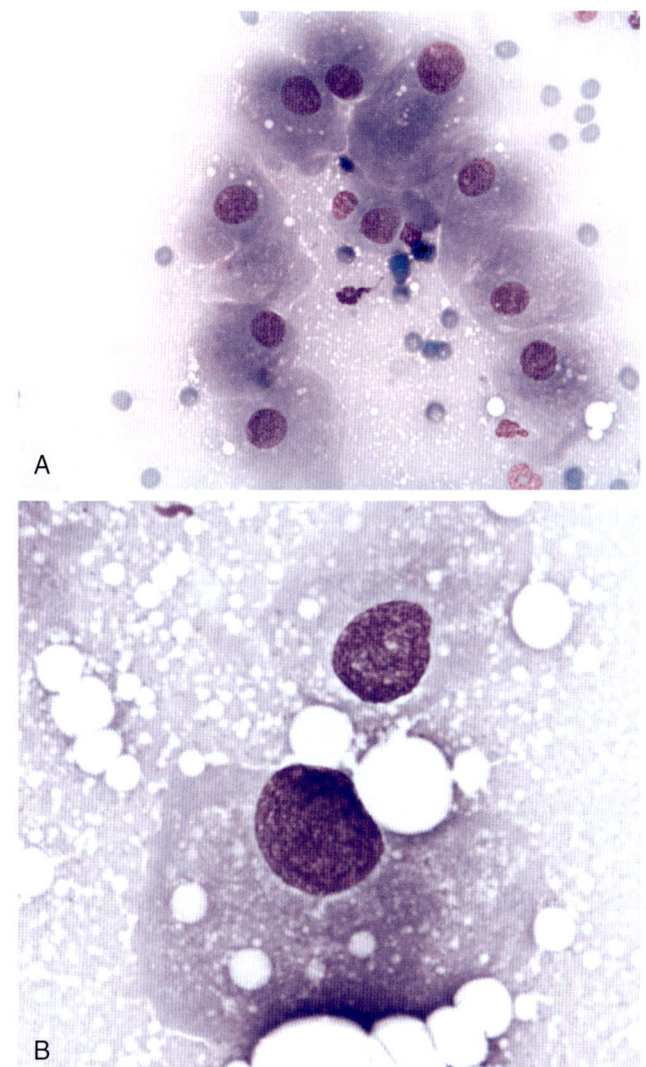

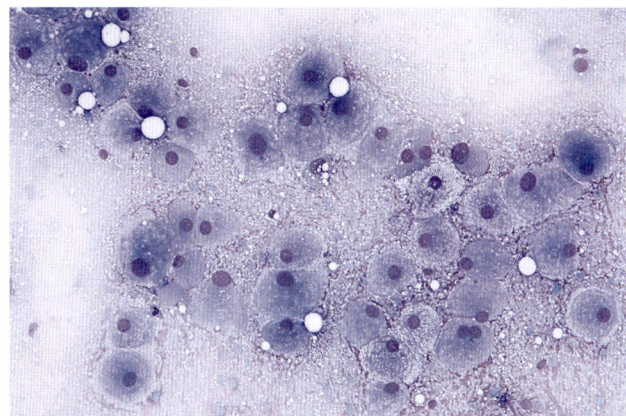

■ **FIGURE 13.25** **Normal ovary (late diestrus). Luteal cells. Tissue aspirate. Dog.** Note many small vacuoles in the background and luteal cells with vacuolated cytoplasm, round and eccentric nuclei, and stippled chromatin. A binucleated cell is also noted. (Modified Wright; IP.) (Courtesy Eleonora Piseddu, IDEXX.)

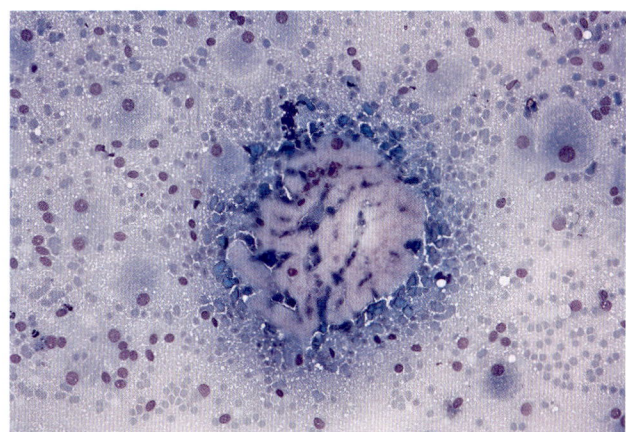

■ **FIGURE 13.26** **Normal ovary (late diestrus). Corpus albicans. Tissue aspirate. Dog.** The pale basophilic background contains variably sized lipid droplets and red blood cells. Freely dispersed luteal cells, erythrocytes, and cell-free nuclei surround a large, pale-pink, dense structure suggestive of a corpus albicans. (Modified Wright; IP.) (Courtesy Eleonora Piseddu, IDEXX.)

■ **FIGURE 13.24** **Normal ovary (early diestrus). Luteal cells. Tissue aspirate. Dog. A,** The pale basophilic background contains variably sized lipid droplets and red blood cells. There are several individual luteal cells characterized by abundant dense basophilic cytoplasm; several, small, colorless, discrete vacuoles; and eccentric, round or oval nuclei. Note the mild to moderate anisokaryosis and mild anisocytosis. (Modified Wright; HP oil.) **B,** Two luteal cells contain abundant pale basophilic cytoplasm, colorless and discrete vacuoles, and eccentric round or oval nuclei. (May-Grünwald-Giemsa; HP oil.) (A, Courtesy Eleonora Piseddu, IDEXX.)

cells. They are medium sized and 15 to 20 μm in diameter with distinct cell borders, high N:C, and scant to moderate amounts of lightly basophilic cytoplasm containing small clear vacuoles. Nuclei are round and usually centrally placed with finely reticular chromatin and often small, multiple, indistinct nucleoli (see Fig. 13.23). These cells are not observed on smears of ovaries in anestrus (Piseddu et al., 2012).

Ovarian Cysts

Cysts in and around the ovary are a common finding during ovariohysterectomy in dogs and cats. There are two types of cysts: intraovarian and paraovarian. Intraovarian cysts include cystic *rete ovarii*, subsurface epithelial structure (dog only), follicular (Fig. 13.28A), lutein, cystic *corporea lutea*, vascular

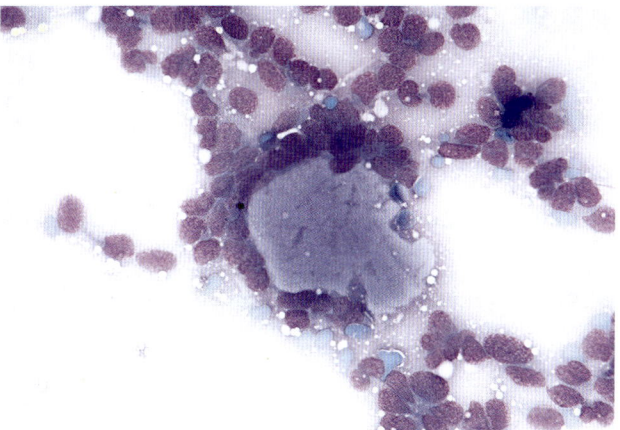

■ **FIGURE 13.27** **Normal ovary. Tissue aspirate. Dog.** Blue-purple amorphous material is surrounded by loose aggregates of partially ruptured granulosa cells. This material is likely mucinous in nature. (Modified Wright; HP oil.) (Courtesy Eleonora Piseddu, IDEXX.)

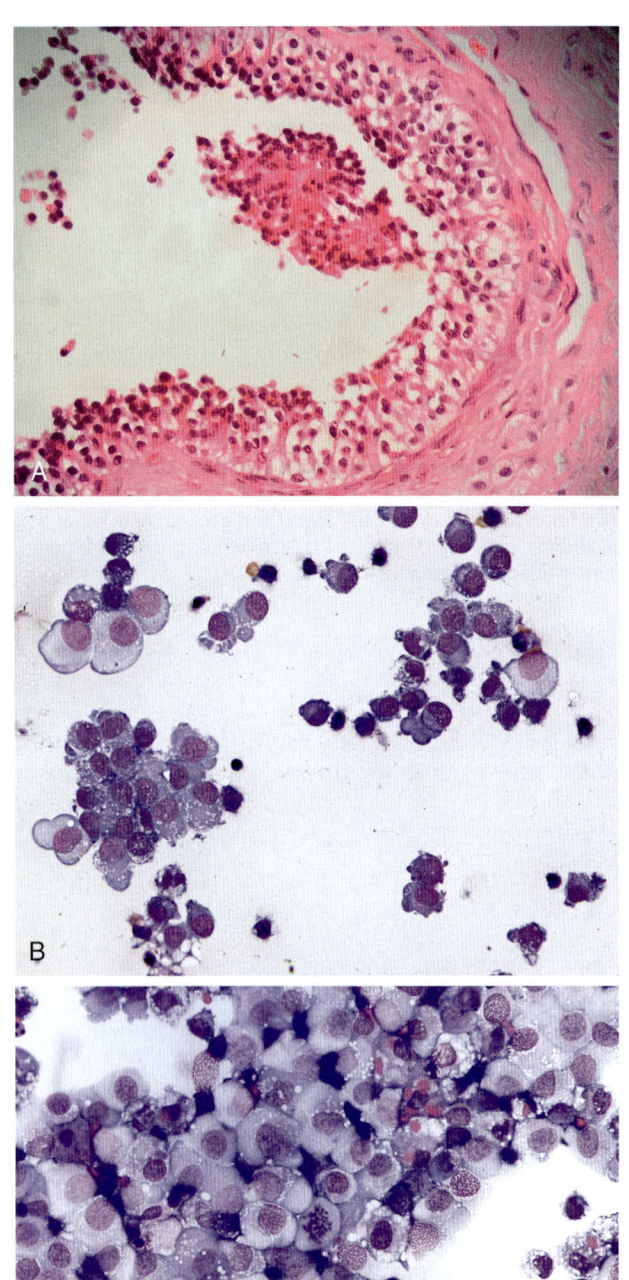

FIGURE 13.28 Ovarian follicular cyst. Dog. Same case in A to C. **A, Tissue section.** The cyst wall is lined by pseudostratified tissue, and the lumen contains sloughed, individualized or adherent lining cells. (H&E; IP.) **B, Cyst fluid aspirate. Direct preparation.** There are individualized or adherent, round cells with variable amounts of basophilic cytoplasm, discrete and colorless vacuoles, and smooth to blebbed cell borders. Their nuclei are round and eccentric with moderate anisokaryosis, stippled chromatin, and small nucleoli. (Modified Wright; HP oil.) **C, Cyst fluid aspirate. Cytocentrifuged preparation.** The same round cells are shown, one of which contains a mitotic figure *(center)*. Scattered erythrophagocytic macrophages and fewer neutrophils are also present. (Modified Wright; HP oil.) (Courtesy Niki Skeldon, Axiom Veterinary Laboratories, Devon, UK.)

hematomas, and adenomatous hyperplasia of the *rete ovarii* (Foster, 2017a; Knauf et al., 2018). General cytopathologic findings are similar to other cysts and are characterized by low nucleated cellularity (e.g., <5000/μL), proteinaceous debris, a variably hemodiluted background with sloughed cells that line the cyst wall, vacuolated macrophages, and evidence of recent and prior hemorrhage (Fig. 13.28B–C). Sloughed granulosa cells may be individualized or in sheets. These cells are round to cuboidal with smooth or blebbed borders; moderate to abundant light basophilic cytoplasm; no or a few discrete, colorless vacuoles; and variably prominent cell borders. Their eccentric nuclei are round to ovoid with coarse chromatin; one to three small, distinct nucleoli; and rare mitotic figures. Anisocytosis and anisokaryosis are moderate with occasional binucleated cells and mitotic figures present (Skeldon et al., 2018).

Ovarian Endometriosis

Endometriosis is ectopic growth of endometrial tissue in extrauterine sites. If the lesion occurs as a well-defined mass, it is termed endometrioma. This condition is common in humans, rare in dogs, and not reported in cats. One case of ovarian endometriosis in a dog described a smooth, flat, hemorrhagic, and thick-walled ovarian cyst on gross examination (Demirel, 2017). Histopathologic examination revealed endometrial lining covering the internal surface of the cyst wall (Demirel, 2017).

Ovarian Inflammation

Oophoritis, or inflammation of the ovary, is rare in domestic animals. Bacterial oophoritis occasionally is found in cats and dogs (Foster, 2017a). The inflammation is around the ovary and within the uterine tube, suggesting that the causative bacteria ascended from the uterus (Foster, 2017a). In cats, feline infectious peritonitis can cause oophoritis.

Ovarian Neoplasia

Tumors of the ovary are uncommon in dogs and cats, accounting for 0.5% to 6.3% of all canine tumors and 0.8% of all feline tumors (McEntee, 2002). The actual frequency of ovarian tumors may be underestimated because ovaries are not routinely sectioned at necropsy and are more commonly examined only if there is a gross lesion. In addition, the low frequency is affected by the fact that many companion animals are neutered at an early age. There are four main categories of ovarian tumors: epithelial, germ cell, sex cord–stromal, and mesenchymal. There are several other miscellaneous neoplastic diseases of the ovaries, including mixed tumors, primary ovarian rhabdomyosarcoma, and metastatic neoplasms, such as lymphoma, carcinoma, and sarcoma (McEntee, 2002). Clinical signs typically occur secondary to a space-occupying mass or to an effusion related to metastasis (Bertazzolo et al., 2012). Clinical signs in dogs with functional tumors secondary to excessive estrogen or progesterone production include signs of persistent estrus, pyometra, and bone marrow toxicity. Ovarian tumors can be an incidental finding at the time of ovariohysterectomy or necropsy.

Epithelial Tumors

Epithelial tumors include papillary adenomas and cystadenomas, papillary adenocarcinoma, cystadenocarcinoma, rete adenomas, and undifferentiated carcinomas (Agnew and MacLachlan, 2017) and account for 40% to 50% of canine ovarian tumors. Fifty percent of malignant epithelial tumors metastasize by implantation or lymphatic or vascular invasion. These tumors occur in older female dogs with a median age of 10 to 12 years (McEntee, 2002). Epithelial tumors are extremely rare in cats.

Papillary adenocarcinoma has been described cytopathologically (Masserdotti, 2006). Cells are arranged in macro- to micropapillary forms, acinar or tubular patterns, in cohesive clusters sometimes tridimensional, and occasionally as single cells (Figs. 13.29 to 13.31). Cells are round to polyhedral with a single oval nucleus. Nuclear chromatin is reticular to coarse. Nucleoli are indistinct to prominent and single or multiple. Mild to marked anisokaryosis and anisocytosis are present. The cytoplasm is scarce to moderate and sometimes contains finely discrete, clear vacuoles. Occasionally, large intracytoplasmic vacuoles or signet ring cells are observed (Bertazzolo et al., 2004; Hori et al., 2006).

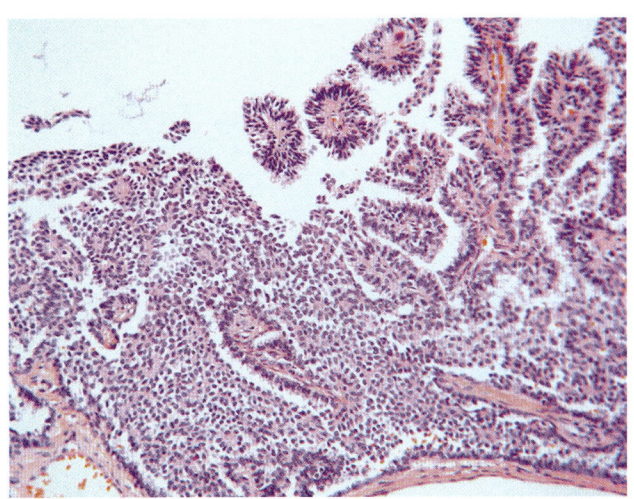

■ **FIGURE 13.31 Ovarian papillary adenocarcinoma. Histology. Dog.** There is dense proliferation of hyperchromic epithelial cells, some of which display acinar and papillary growth formations. (H&E; LP.) (Courtesy Walter Bertazzolo, MyLav Laboratories, Italy.)

Ovarian carcinoma is often not diagnosed until peritoneal or pleural metastases develop, causing malignant neoplastic peritoneal and pleural effusion, with subsequent abdominal distension and dyspnea, respectively (Salgado et al., 2012). Cytopathologic findings of malignant metastatic effusion of this tumor are similar to the findings observed in primary ovarian carcinoma aspirates (Masserdotti, 2006). Numerous large papillary aggregates of cells are present. Acinar arrangements are also seen. Neoplastic cells are monomorphic and show mild cytopathologic atypia (Bertazzolo et al., 2012).

Sex Cord–Stromal Tumors

Sex cord–stromal tumors include granulosa cell tumors (Figs. 13.32 to 13.35), luteomas (also called interstitial gland, lipid, or interstitial cell tumors), thecomas, and Sertoli-Leydig cell tumor. In dogs, granulosa cell tumors account for 50% of ovarian tumors and occur in older bitches with a median age of 10 to 12 years. Some 77% of granulosa cell tumors produce estrogens, progesterone, or both, and up to 20% are malignant. Granulosa cell tumor is the most common sex cord–stromal tumor in older cats, and more than 50% are malignant. Reported metastatic sites include the peritoneum, lumbar lymph nodes, omentum, diaphragm, kidney, pancreas (see Fig. 13.35), spleen, liver, and lungs (McEntee, 2002). Granulosa cell tumors may be confused sometimes with ovarian epithelial tumors, even in histologic preparations. Useful immunohistochemical markers to distinguish these two tumors are cytokeratin 7 and inhibin-α. Ovarian epithelial tumors cells are positive to cytokeratin 7 and negative to inhibin-α, whereas granulosa tumor cells and thecomas are negative to cytokeratin 7 and positive to inhibin-α (Riccardi et al., 2007). Another marker useful to differentiate granulosa cell tumors from ovarian epithelial tumors is Hector Battifora mesothelial epitope-1 (HBME-1). HBME-1 is one of the immunohistochemical markers employed in the diagnosis of ovarian epithelial tumors. Granulosa cells and related tumors are consistently negative for HBME-1 (Banco et al., 2011; Agnew and MacLachlan, 2017).

Cytopathologically, neoplastic granulosa cells are usually in monolayered, loosely cohesive clusters and often have acinar to

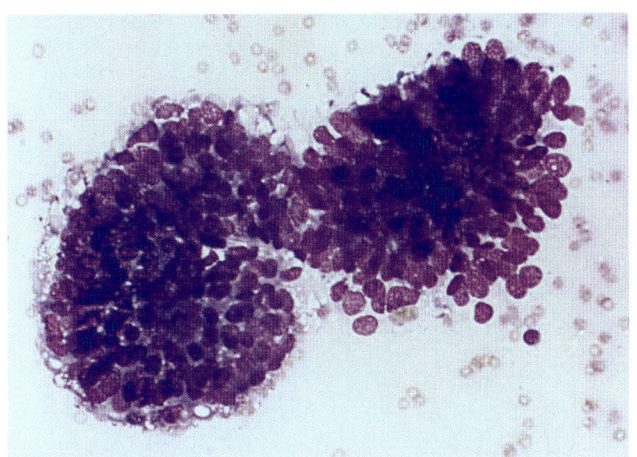

■ **FIGURE 13.29 Ovarian papillary adenocarcinoma. Cytopathologic preparation. Dog.** A cluster of cohesive neoplastic epithelial cells are arranged in a papillary pattern. (May-Grünwald-Giemsa; IP.) (Courtesy Walter Bertazzolo, MyLav Laboratories, Italy.)

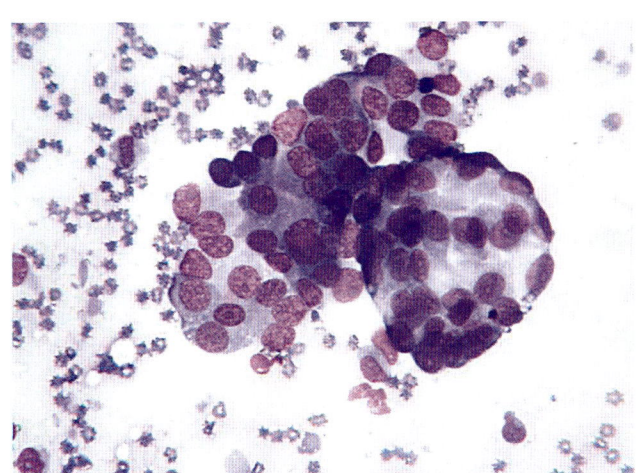

■ **FIGURE 13.30 Ovarian papillary adenocarcinoma. Cytopathologic preparation. Dog.** Shown is a round papillary cluster of cohesive neoplastic epithelial cells known as a cell ball. (May-Grünwald-Giemsa; IP.) (Courtesy Walter Bertazzolo, MyLav Laboratories, Italy.)

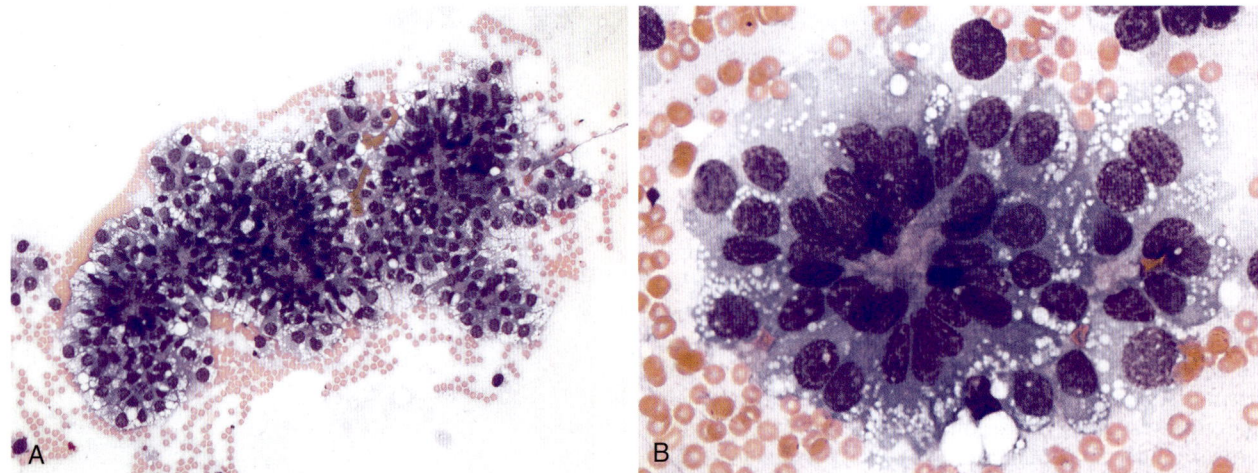

■ **FIGURE 13.32 Granulosa cell tumor. Ovarian mass aspirate. Cat.** Same case in A and B. **A,** A branching, tubule-like structure with granulosa cells is emanating from an eosinophilic, extracellular, mucinous material. (Wright-Giemsa; IP.) **B,** Granulosa cells surround an eosinophilic, mucinous material, forming a small follicle-like structure, termed a Call-Exner body. Individual granulosa cells are irregularly round to columnar with a moderate amount of basophilic cytoplasm, discrete and colorless vacuoles, and indistinct cell borders. Their nuclei are round or compressed with coarse chromatin and a small nucleolus. (Wright-Giemsa; HP oil.) (Courtesy Katie Boes, Virginia Polytechnic Institute and State University.)

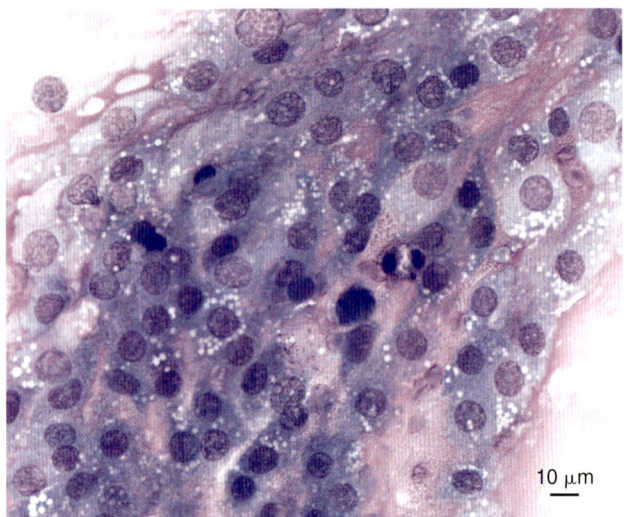

■ **FIGURE 13.33 Granulosa cell tumor. Ovarian mass imprint. Dog.** Presented for evaluation of a mid-abdominal mass that had been steadily growing for 4 months. The patient also had enlarged vulva and mammae. The round to polygonal granulosa cells were immunoreactive to inhibin-alpha and vimentin but negative for cytokeratin 7 (not shown). Cytopathologically, these cells display moderate anisocytosis and anisokaryosis, finely to coarsely stippled chromatin, and variably sized prominent nucleoli. Cells also have abundant basophilic cytoplasm with small clear vacuoles surrounded by abundant brightly eosinophilic material. This material was positive for periodic acid–Schiff and Alcian blue, indicating mucin composition. (Romanowsky; HP oil.) (Courtesy K. Banajee et al., Louisiana State University. Presented at the 2012 ASVCP case review session.)

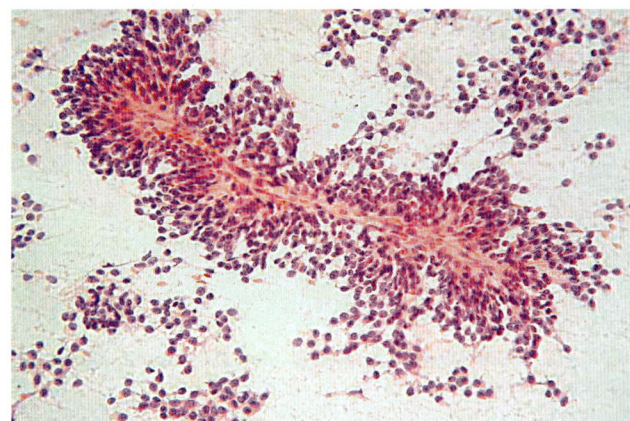

■ **FIGURE 13.34 Granulosa cell tumor. Ovarian mass. Histology. Dog.** A large cluster of granulosa cells appears with a perivascular pattern. (H&E; LP.) (Courtesy Walter Bertazzolo, MyLav Laboratories, Italy.)

tubular pattern (see Fig. 13.32). Granulosa cells sometimes form *Call-Exner* bodies, which are follicle-like structures centered on amorphous, eosinophilic, extracellular, mucinous material (see Fig. 13.32). Capillary-like structures are occasionally evident inside large clusters of cells (see Fig. 13.34). Single cells are round to polyhedral. Nuclei are round to oval with indistinct nucleoli and mild to moderate cellular atypia. The cytoplasm is scarce to moderate with variable amounts of vacuolated cytoplasm (Bertazzolo et al., 2004).

Feline luteomas have been recently cytopathologically described. Large round to oval cells arranged individually or in loose clusters are observed. Nuclei are central to eccentric with granular chromatin with prominent, small, central nucleoli. Anisokaryosis is mild to moderate. Cytoplasm is lightly basophilic with many variably sized clear vacuoles and occasionally small purple granules (Choi et al., 2005).

Germ Cell Tumors

Germ cell tumors include dysgerminoma (counterpart of the testicular seminoma), embryonal carcinoma, teratoma, and teratocarcinoma (Gorman et al., 2010). Dysgerminoma represents a less differentiated tumor than mature teratoma. Germ cell tumors comprise 6% to 20% of canine ovarian neoplasms and 15% to 27% of feline ovarian neoplasms. The median age

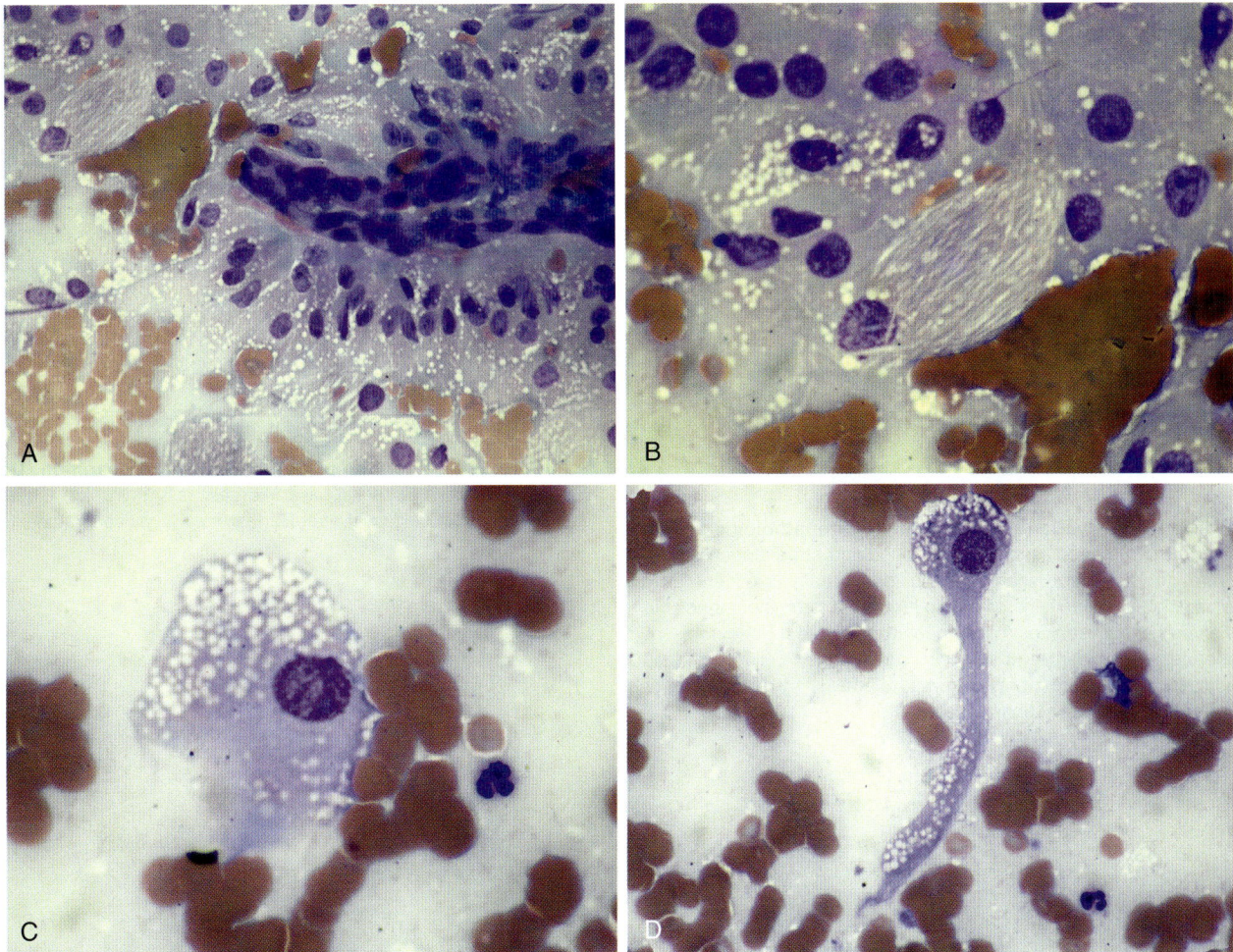

FIGURE 13.35 Metastatic sex cord–stromal neoplasm, presumed granulosa cell tumor. Pancreatic mass aspirate. Female adult neutered dog. Same specimen in A to D. Same case as in Figures 13.44 and 13.52. **A,** Against a background of blood is a large population of cells present in aggregates in association with capillaries. The cells appear elongated with a moderate amount of finely granular basophilic cytoplasm that is poorly demarcated and contains variably sized vacuoles. **B,** The nuclei are uniform, round to oval, with granular chromatin and a single pale nucleolus. One cell appears to contain numerous clear linear crystalline needle-like cytoplasmic inclusions. **C,** A single round to polygonal cell has peripheralized variably sized vacuoles within the lightly basophilic cytoplasm. The round nucleus has granular chromatin with a single prominent pale nucleolus. **D,** An individual elongated cell with indistinct and wispy cytoplasmic borders. The cytoplasm contains numerous small nonstaining vacuoles to two sides of the cell. The nucleus is round with granular chromatin and contains a single prominent nucleolus. (A–D, Wright; HP oil.) (Courtesy Oliver Coldrick, TDDS, Exeter, UK.)

of dogs with dysgerminoma is 10 to 13 years and with teratomas is 4 years. The age of cats that have been reported to have dysgerminomas ranges from 1 to 17 years with a median of 5 years. Metastasis is reported to develop in 10% to 20% of canine dysgerminomas with regional lymph nodes, the liver, the brain, and the kidney as the primary sites. Teratomas are more common in young (<6 months) dogs and rarely documented in cats (Saba and Lawrence, 2013).

Dysgerminomas are seen cytopathologically as a predominant population of markedly pleomorphic, large, round to polygonal cells arranged singly or in loose aggregates. Cells range from 20 to 70 μm in diameter. Nuclei are large and round to oval with chromatin stippled to reticular (Figs. 13.36 and 13.37). Nucleoli are prominent, multiple, and of variable shapes and sizes. Aberrant mitotic figures and bi- or multinucleated cells are commonly noted. Anisocytosis and anisokaryosis are marked. The cytoplasm is scant clear to blue-gray with variably distinct margins. Occasionally, eosinophilic, granular, intracytoplasmic material is noted. Small lymphocytes can be observed (Bertazzolo et al., 2004; Brazzell and Borjesson, 2006).

Cytopathologically, teratomas are characterized by a necrotic background, moderate neutrophilic and macrophagic inflammation, clusters of sebocytes or other mature epithelial cells, abundant keratin debris, and mature keratinocytes (Figs. 13.38 to 13.41) (Bertazzolo et al., 2004). Malignant teratoma or teratocarcinoma is similar cytopathologically to teratoma. However, large, pleomorphic cells with moderate to marked atypia and high mitotic activity are present in malignant teratoma (Gorman et al., 2010).

Surgery remains the mainstay of treatment of ovarian tumors. A complete ovariohysterectomy is recommended. Careful examination of all serosal surfaces and removal with histopathologic biopsy of any lesions suspected for metastatic disease are recommended for staging purposes. Successful

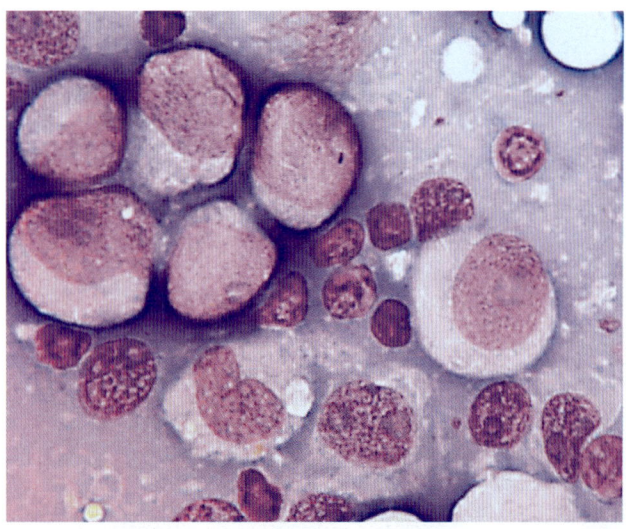

■ **FIGURE 13.36 Ovarian dysgerminoma. Cytopathologic preparation. Dog.** Large neoplastic cells are round and are arranged singly. Nuclei are pleomorphic in shape and located centrally or eccentrically with a stippled to coarse chromatin pattern and prominent nucleoli. Anisokaryosis and anisocytosis are moderate to marked. The cytoplasm is moderate to abundant and pale basophilic. Lysed cells and small lymphocytes are present. (May-Grünwald-Giemsa; HP oil.) (Courtesy Walter Bertazzolo, MyLav Laboratories, Italy.)

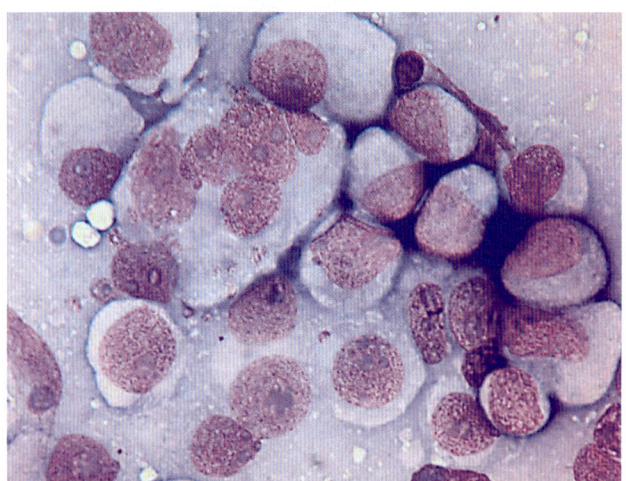

■ **FIGURE 13.37 Ovarian dysgerminoma. Cytopathologic preparation. Dog.** Note the multinucleated cell and marked anisokaryosis and anisocytosis. (May-Grünwald-Giemsa; HP oil.) (Courtesy Walter Bertazzolo, MyLav Laboratories, Italy.)

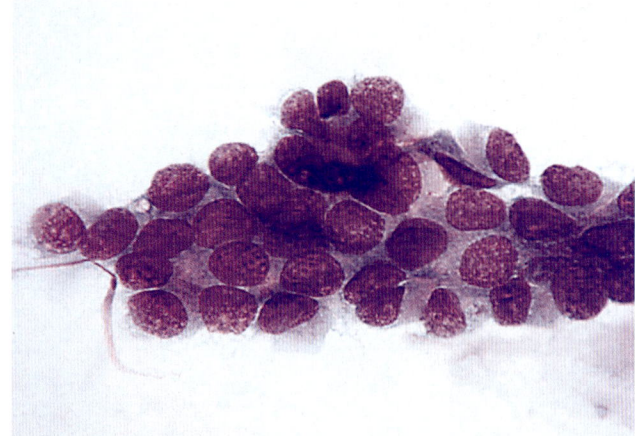

■ **FIGURE 13.38 Teratoma. Cytopathologic preparation. Dog.** A cluster of cohesive epithelial basal-like cells is shown. (May-Grünwald-Giemsa; HP oil.) (Courtesy Walter Bertazzolo, MyLav Laboratories, Italy.)

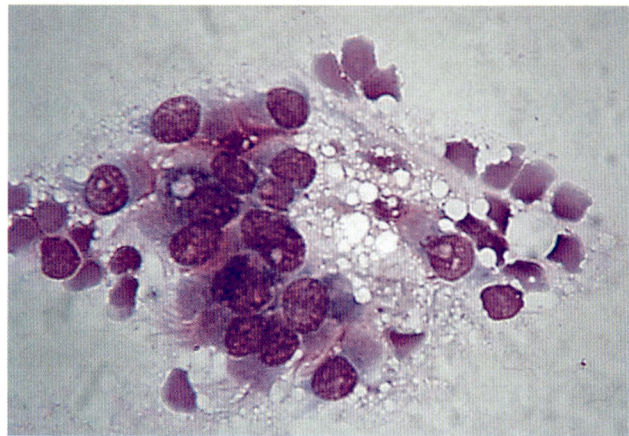

■ **FIGURE 13.39 Teratoma. Cytopathologic preparation. Dog.** Epithelial cells have a basally polarized round to oval nucleus with an eosinophilic, ciliated apical surface suggestive of differentiation toward respiratory epithelium. (May-Grünwald-Giemsa; HP oil.) (Courtesy Walter Bertazzolo, MyLav Laboratories, Italy.)

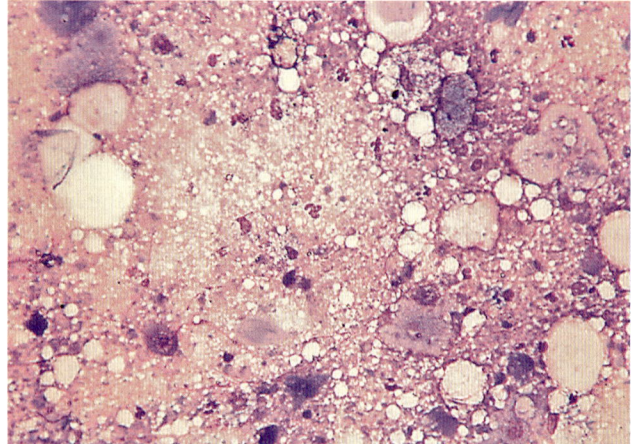

■ **FIGURE 13.40 Teratoma. Cytopathologic preparation. Dog.** Necrotic background, keratin debris, neutrophils, and macrophages are evident. (May-Grünwald-Giemsa; IP.) (Courtesy Walter Bertazzolo, MyLav Laboratories, Italy.)

palliation with chemotherapy has been reported, but no standard recommendations have been established (Saba and Lawrence, 2013).

Uterus

Indications for uterine cytopathology and histopathology include evaluation of degree of cystic endometrial hyperplasia, inflammation, hematometra, inflammatory endometrial polyp, uterine torsion, neoplasia, and prognostic assessment for fertility (Root Kustritz et al., 2006).

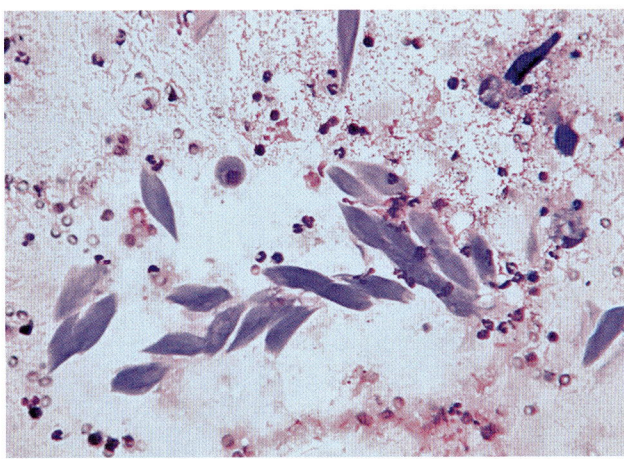

FIGURE 13.41 Teratoma. Cytopathologic preparation. Dog. Note the presence of keratinocytes, keratin debris, neutrophils, and red blood cells. (May-Grünwald-Giemsa; IP.) (Courtesy Walter Bertazzolo, MyLav Laboratories, Italy.)

Collection Techniques

Cells may be collected at the time of hysterotomy or be retrieved transcervically (Root Kustritz, 2006). This latter technique involves visualizing the cervix with a rigid endoscope and passing a catheter through the cervix into the uterus. Samples for microbiology and cytopathology are obtained by the infusion and aspiration of sterile normal saline. This technique allows uterine microbiology and cytology of the bitch throughout the reproductive cycle. Complications include vaginal inflammation, tearing, and endometritis, mainly when samples are taken in anestrus. Another technique is hysteroscopy, performed in anesthetized bitches with a laparoscope and air insufflation of the uterus. Side effects include petechiae or ecchymosis on endometrium.

Normal Anatomy and Histology

Cats and dogs have a bicornuate uterus with uterine horns and a uterine body. The uterine tubes have four regions: the infundibulum, ampulla, isthmus, and uterotubal junction. It is supported by a mesosalpinx. The mesosalpinx of a dog completely surrounds the ovary and has a large amount of fat; a small hole connects the bursa to the abdominal cavity. The infundibulum surrounds the ovary. The wall of the uterus has three layers: outer perimetrium (serosa), middle myometrium, and inner endometrium (mucosa) (Figs. 13.42 and 13.43). The perimetrium is composed of loose connective tissue and covered by peritoneal mesothelium. The myometrium is divided into a thick, inner circular layer and a thin, outer longitudinal layer (see Fig. 13.42A). A richly vascularized and well-innervated *stratum vasculare* usually separates the muscle layers (see Fig. 13.43). The epithelium of the endometrium is simple cuboidal or columnar in bitches and queens, depending on the estrus cycle. Simple, branched endometrial glands extend into the lamina propria (see Fig. 13.42B). The cervix is the structure that separates the external genitalia from the uterus and is an effective barrier from the external environment. The cervix does not have transverse folds and tends to open dorsally (Foster, 2017a). The normal histology of the uterus from immature female dogs and sequential microscopic changes that occur during different stages of the estrous cycle are reviewed elsewhere (Rehm et al., 2007).

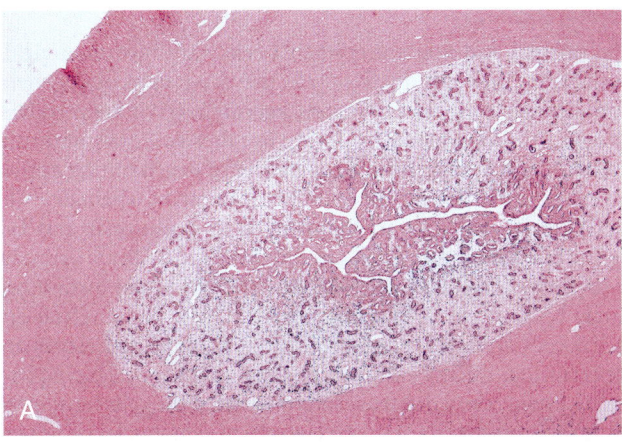
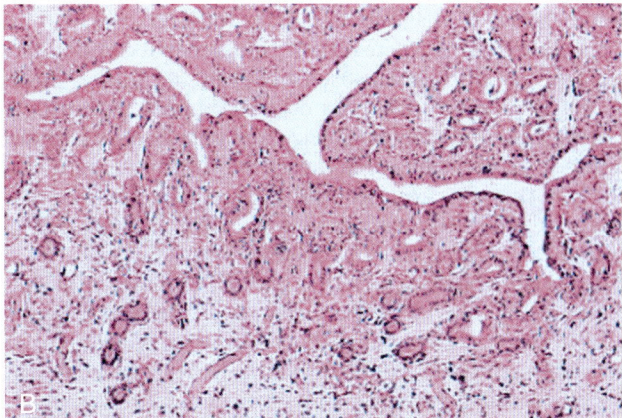

FIGURE 13.42 Normal uterus. Proestrus. Histology. Dog. Same case in A and B. **A,** The dense area surrounding the endometrial glands is the myometrium, which consists of two layers of smooth muscle, the inner circular and outer longitudinal layers. The outermost layer is the perimetrium or mesothelial-lined serosa. (H&E; LP.) **B,** Close magnification of luminal epithelium shows the extension of the uterine glands present of the mucosa into the lamina propria as tubular formations. The inner mucosa or endometrium is lined by cuboidal or columnar epithelium. (H&E; LP.)

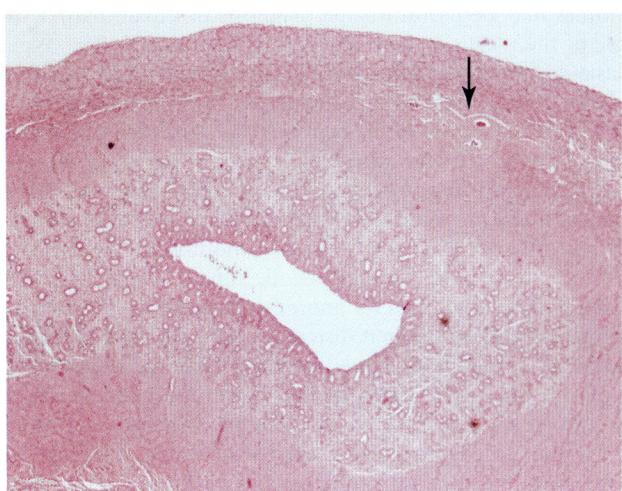

FIGURE 13.43 Normal uterus. Early estrus. Histology. Dog. The mucosal glands and deeper endometrial glands have extended across the lamina propria. *Arrow* indicates a region of prominent blood vessels. (H&E; LP.)

Normal Cytology

The normal endometrial epithelial cells vary morphologically throughout the reproductive cycle; they have signs of degeneration, defined as nuclear pyknosis, karyorrhexis or karyolysis, or cytoplasmic clear vacuoles, during late diestrus, early and mid-anestrus, and postpartum. The number of degenerating epithelial cells decreases with time until late anestrus, when all endometrial epithelial cells are cuboidal to low columnar and lack signs of degeneration. Endometrial epithelial cells are arranged in monolayered sheets, cohesive clusters, and acinar formations. Single cells are less frequently observed. The endometrial epithelial cells are low columnar during proestrus and estrus and are columnar during early diestrus and pregnancy. During proestrus, estrus, early diestrus, and pregnancy, the cells have intact nuclei and uniformly staining cytoplasm. The nuclei of normal endometrial epithelial cells are usually round or oval with fine, stippled chromatin, whereas those of degenerated endometrial cells are often of irregular shape and pyknotic. Neutrophils are the most common leukocytes observed during proestrus, estrus, diestrus, and early pregnancy, and lymphocytes and macrophages are frequently seen during anestrus (Groppetti et al., 2010). Eosinophils are identified in samples collected during proestrus and estrus (Groppetti et al., 2010). Plasma cells are encountered during the late anestrus stage (Groppetti et al., 2010). Erythrocytes are present in variable numbers at all stages of the reproductive cycle. Spermatozoa are observed in samples collected during estrus and early pregnancy in bitches that had their last mating 1 to 3 days previously. Bacteria are commonly observed during proestrus and estrus. Cornified cervical or vaginal cells are present during proestrus and estrus (Groppetti et al., 2010).

Microorganisms are frequently recovered from the uterus during proestrus, estrus, and diestrus but rarely at other stages of the reproductive cycle. The uterine microflora often reflects the vaginal microflora during proestrus, estrus, and diestrus (Maksimović et al., 2012).

Cystic Endometrial Hyperplasia–Pyometra Complex and Metritis

Cytopathologic examination of vaginal discharges or uterus samples may be useful for the diagnosis of inflammatory disease of the uterus in dogs and cats. Cystic endometrial hyperplasia–pyometra complex is a disease that is mainly characterized by progesterone-induced hyperplasia of the endometrium with cystic dilatation of the endometrial glands and inflammation of the uterus with purulent content in the uterine lumen (pyometra), leading to several clinical signs (Hagman, 2018). The common presentation of pyometra involves older, unbred bitches presenting from 4 weeks to 4 months after estrus with mild to severe evidence of systemic illness (Hagman, 2018). Clinical signs may include anorexia, depression, polyuria, or polydipsia and abdominal distention with or without vaginal discharge (open- and closed-cervix pyometra, respectively). Typically, the bitch is afebrile and often has leukocytosis, although leukopenia may occur. Prerenal azotemia commonly accompanies dehydration. This systemic disease may result in death from toxemia, renal disease, and peritonitis. There is an increased risk of pyometra in some breeds (Hagman, 2018).

Cystic endometrial hyperplasia–pyometra complex is considered to be less common in cats, probably because cats are induced ovulators, which limits uterine exposure to progesterone

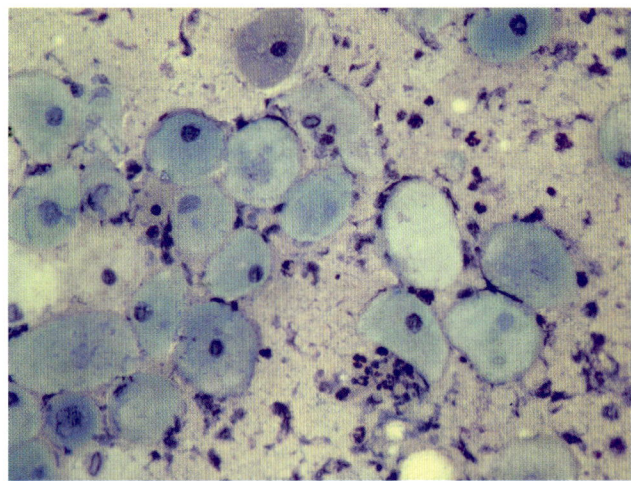

FIGURE 13.44 Uterine inflammation. Uterine stump aspirate. Dog. Same case as in Figures 13.35 and 13.52. The highly cellular preparation contains numerous superficial and anucleate keratinized squamous epithelial cells. Additionally, there are large numbers of poorly preserved neutrophils, and no infectious agents are seen. The squames may be the result of estrogen production by the metastatic tumor. (Modified Wright; HP oil.) (Courtesy Oliver Coldrick, TDDS, Exeter, UK.)

(Hagman, 2018). *Escherichia coli* is the most frequently isolated microorganism in canine and feline pyometras (Hagman, 2018).

Pyometra or uterine stump flushing samples are characterized cytopathologically by a low number of endometrial epithelial cells often with degenerative changes. Subsequent to hyperplasia, the glands become cystic with increased pressure of retained secretion causing the epithelium of the glands to become flattened and simple squamous in type (Agnew and MacLachlan, 2017). Numerous nondegenerate and degenerate neutrophils together with many lymphocytes, macrophages, and plasma cells are also noticed (Fig. 13.44). Intracellular and free bacteria are both abundant (Groppetti et al., 2010).

Treatment of choice for pyometra is ovariohysterectomy with supportive therapy, including appropriate antibiotic administration. The combination of a prolactin inhibitor, prostaglandin, and an antibiotic treatment in bitches with pyometra appears to have been effective in rapid clinical improvement, terminating the luteal phase and promoting uterine evacuation. This combination may be useful not only in bitches that are required for future breeding but also in bitches that have a high anesthetic risk (Hagman, 2018).

Metritis usually follows parturition and is characterized by a systemically ill animal with a malodorous uterine or vaginal discharge. Other causes of metritis can be bacterial, fungal such as aspergillosis, and mating related. Bacterial or nonbacterial metritis is associated with infertility. The treatment of metritis is also ovariohysterectomy if the owner is not interested in further breeding or if severe systemic illness is present. Nursing puppies or kittens should be weaned and hand raised.

Large numbers of neutrophils, many of which are degenerate, characterize the smears prepared from vaginal discharges resulting from open-cervix pyometra or metritis. Bacteria may be seen extracellularly and within the neutrophils. Muscle fibers from decomposing fetuses may rarely be visible in samples from metritis due to pregnancy.

Uterine Neoplasia

Uterine tumors occur infrequently in dogs and cats, accounting for 0.3% to 0.4% of canine and 0.2% to 1.5% of feline tumors. Middle-aged to older animals are most commonly affected (Saba and Lawrence, 2013). In dogs, uterine leiomyomas are most commonly reported, and leiomyosarcomas are comparatively rare. These tumors are of similar cytopathologic appearance to those found in other body sites. Uterine carcinoma, hemangiosarcoma, and lymphoma are rare in dogs (Ko et al., 2013). In cats, both leiomyoma and endometrial adenocarcinoma are reported with similar frequencies (Miller et al., 2003). Other tumors in cats that are less commonly described include leiomyosarcoma, myxoid leiomyosarcoma, endometrial stromal sarcoma, lymphoma, and mixed Mullerian tumor (adenosarcoma) (McEntee, 2002; Miller at al., 2003; Conversy et al., 2017). A complete ovariohysterectomy is recommended, and attempts should be made to remove all tumors and metastatic foci.

Vagina

Examination of exfoliated vaginal cells for staging the estrous cycle is one of the most common uses of cytology in veterinary practice. This technique is easy to perform and can be successfully used to optimize breeding, although some authors suggest that this method should be used with caution to determine the optimal mating period. If used for breeding purposes, serial, and not a single time point, vaginal cytology is recommended. Cytopathologic examination of vaginal mucosal imprints and discharges is also useful for the evaluation of vaginal inflammation and neoplasia of the female reproductive tract (Root Kustritz, 2006).

Collection Techniques

Several techniques have been described for obtaining vaginal cells for cytologic examination. Most commonly, a saline-moistened cotton swab or thin glass rod with a rounded tip is directed craniodorsally into the caudal vagina. The vestibule and clitoral fossa should be avoided because keratinized superficial squamous cells present in these sites may alter cytologic interpretations. When cranial to the urethral orifice, vaginal cells are obtained by gently passing the swab or glass rod over the epithelial lining (Root Kustritz, 2006). In an alternate method of sample collection, a small glass bulb pipette containing sterile saline is passed into the caudal vagina, and cells are obtained by repeatedly flushing and aspirating the saline fluid (Olson et al., 1984). After collection, the exfoliated cells are gently transferred onto a clean microscope slide for staining. In addition, endoscopic vaginoscopy is a useful diagnostic procedure for evaluating the nature and extent of disease in the vestibule and vagina and for obtaining adequate samples for microscopic evaluation (Root Kustritz, 2006).

Although several types of stains have been used for cytologic evaluation of vaginal cells, ones such as methanolic or aqueous Romanowsky stains are most commonly used. These stains are easy to use in a clinical setting and provide good morphologic detail for determining the degree of maturation of the epithelial cells. Papanicolaou or trichrome stains have also been used for estrous cycle staging. These stains impart a distinctive orange staining to the keratin precursors that are abundant in superficial cells. The ratio of orange or eosinophilic cells to noneosinophilic cells, termed the *eosinophilic index*, can be used to assess the degree of maturation of the epithelial cells and subsequently stage the estrous cycle. However, these stains may yield variable staining results, and the need for multiple solutions limits their practical use. Indications for vaginal culture include any disorder of the genitourinary tract associated with vulvar discharge and anterior vaginal culture in proestrus for the diagnosis of uterine infection (Root Kustritz, 2006). The vagina is not sterile, and larger numbers of normal flora are routinely cultured from the caudal vagina than the cranial vagina and during estrus than diestrus or anestrus. However, a larger number of organisms are retrieved from bitches with reproductive tract disease than from normal bitches. It is important to provide a quantitative culture result related to the fact that reproductive tract infection is caused by overgrowth of normal flora.

Normal Anatomy and Histology

The vagina is a musculomembranous canal extending from the uterus to the vulva. The vaginal wall is composed of an inner mucosal layer, a middle smooth muscle layer, and an external coat of connective tissue and peritoneum (cranially) (Foster, 2017a). The mucosal layer consists of stratified squamous epithelium, which undergoes characteristic morphologic changes in association with the estrous cycle. Although the mucosa is typically nonglandular, intraepithelial glands have been observed during estrus in dogs. The vulva is anatomically similar to the caudal vagina. The vulva is composed of the vestibule containing the urethral orifice, clitoral fossa, and labia. The mucosa is lined by stratified squamous epithelium; some keratinized epithelial cells may be found in the vestibule and clitoral fossa. Vestibular glands of the vulva are mucus-secreting compound tubuloacinar glands, which are most notable during estrus and at parturition. These glands are located well within the propria-submucosa with stratified squamous epithelia lining their large ducts (Samuelson, 2007). Histologically, at the base of the clitoris are scattered apocrine glands within the fibrous and adipose tissue of the propria-submucosa (Verin et al., 2018). The normal histology of the vagina from immature female dogs and sequential microscopic changes that occur during different stages of the estrous cycle are reviewed elsewhere (Rehm et al., 2007).

Normal Cytology

Four types of vaginal surface epithelial cells may be identified by exfoliative cytology. In order from the deepest and most immature cells to the most superficial and mature, these cells are basal, parabasal, intermediate, and superficial (Fig. 13.45).

Basal cells are located along the basement membrane and give rise to the other epithelial cell types seen in a vaginal smear. Round nuclei and scant amounts of basophilic cytoplasm characterize these small cells. Because of their deep location, basal cells are rarely seen in vaginal preparations.

Parabasal cells are the smallest of the epithelial cells seen in routine vaginal cytologic samples as basal cells are absent. Parabasal cells have a high N:C, round nuclei of uniform size and shape, and basophilic cytoplasm. Parabasal cells or intermediate cells containing cytoplasmic vacuoles are called *foam cells*; the significance of the vacuoles is unknown (Olson et al., 1984). These cells may be associated with diestrus and anestrus. Large numbers of parabasal cells may be seen in vaginal smears of prepubertal animals and should not be confused with neoplastic cells (Feldman and Nelson, 2004).

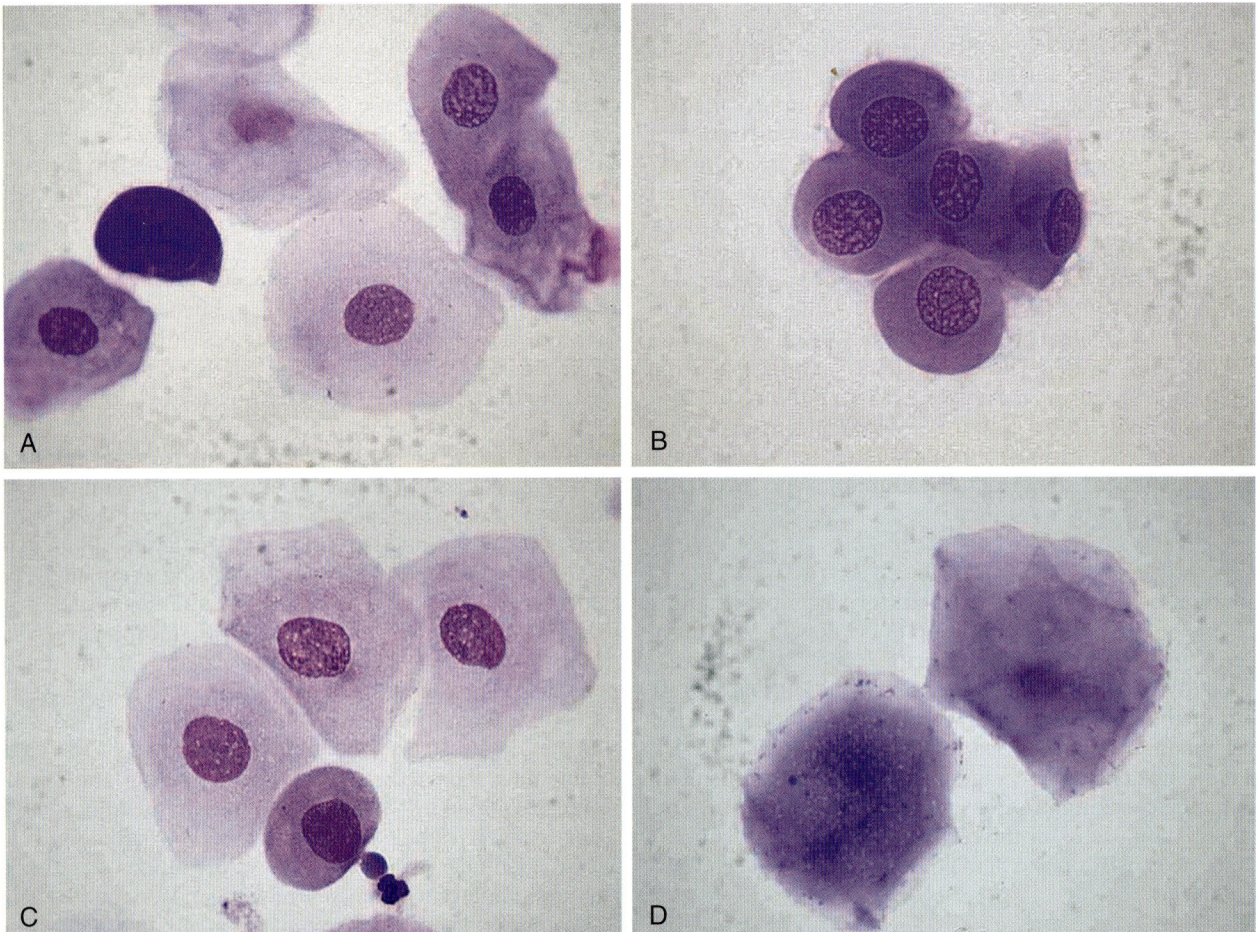

■ **FIGURE 13.45 Vaginal epithelial cells. Vaginal smear. Dog. A,** The small, dense basophilic cell is an immature parabasal cell (basal cell) appearing among several intermediate squamous cells showing varied levels of maturation. **B,** Sheet of parabasal cells with round cell shape and basophilic cytoplasm. **C,** Three large intermediate cells and one parabasal cell. **D,** Anuclear superficial squamous cells. (Wright-Giemsa; HP oil.)

Intermediate cells may vary in size but are generally twice the size of parabasal cells. The N:C is decreased with abundant amounts of blue to blue-green (keratinized) cytoplasm. The cytoplasmic borders are round to irregular and folded. Intermediate cells may also be called *superficial intermediate* or *transitional intermediate cells. Metestrum cells* are large, intermediate vaginal cells that appear to have one or more neutrophils contained within their cytoplasm. These cells are usually seen in diestrus or vaginitis, and such cells are rarely observed in early proestrus (Feldman and Nelson, 2004).

Superficial cells are characterized by small, round to pyknotic nuclei, abundant amounts of light blue to blue-green (keratinized) cytoplasm, and angular to folded cell borders. Some superficial cells contain dark-staining bodies of unknown significance (Olson et al., 1984). As superficial cells age and become degenerate, the nuclei are lost, and the cells become anucleated. Superficial cells with pyknotic nuclei and anucleated superficial cells have the same physiologic significance. Folded, angular cells with pyknotic or absent nuclei are called *anuclear squames* or *anuclear superficial cells* (Feldman and Nelson, 2004).

Staging the Canine Estrous Cycle

Duration, cytologic appearance, and hormonal status of the different stages of canine estrous cycle are described in Table 13.1 and pictorially demonstrated in Figure 13.46. The normal physiology and endocrinology of the estrous cycle of bitches is reviewed elsewhere (Root Kustritz, 2012).

Proestrus. Proestrus (Fig. 13.47) is characterized by rising concentrations of estradiol and low concentrations of progesterone. As the estradiol concentrations increase, the vaginal epithelium proliferates, and red blood cells (RBCs) move via diapedesis through uterine capillaries (Feldman and Nelson, 2004). In early to mid proestrus, neutrophils and a mixture of parabasal, intermediate, and superficial epithelial cells (Olson et al., 1984) characterize the vaginal smear. As proestrus progresses, the neutrophils decrease in number, and superficial epithelial cells begin to predominate.

Estrus. For optimal breeding efficiency, sperm should be present in the female reproductive tract as close to ovulation as possible. Although vaginal cytology has been shown to be a more accurate indicator of estrus (Fig. 13.48) and ovulation than behavioral signs, evidence of vaginal maturation or cornification is not closely associated with ovulation. Maximum cornification of vaginal superficial cells ranges from 6 days before the luteinizing hormone (LH) peak to 3 days after the LH peak (Olson et al., 1984). Because ovulation usually occurs 1 to 2 days after the LH peak, vaginal cytology is not an accurate predictor of ovulation. Ova are viable for up to 2 days postovulation, and sperm may

TABLE 13.1 Duration, Cytologic Appearance, and Hormonal Status of Stages of Canine Estrous Cycle

STAGES AND DURATION OF ESTROUS CYCLE	EPITHELIAL CELLS	NEUTROPHILS	RED BLOOD CELLS	BACTERIA	BACKGROUND	HORMONAL STATUS
Proestrus 9 days; range, 3–21 days						
Early	Mixture of parabasal, intermediate, and few superficial cells	Present	May be abundant or absent; usually present	Present	Granular or dirty appearance; mucus can be present	Follicular development; rise in concentrations of estradiol and low concentrations of progesterone
Late[a]	Mixture of superficial (>80%) and intermediate cells	Few or none	May be abundant or absent; usually present	Present	Clear	
Estrus 9 days; range 3–21 days	>80% superficial and anuclear squames (50%); <5% parabasal or intermediate cells	Absent	Present or absent	Present	Clear	Declining estradiol concentrations with subsequent increase of LH, ovulation, and rising preovulatory progesterone concentration
Diestrus Pregnant bitches: 62–64 days Nonpregnant bitches: 49–79 days	Abrupt decrease in superficial cells and increase in small, intermediate cells	Frequently present (few to many)	May be present but usually none	Present; ingested bacteria within neutrophils may be seen	May contain large amounts of debris	Progesterone rises and then declines over this stage; rapid decline at end (pregnant dogs) or more gradual decline (nonpregnant dogs); progesterone production is supported by LH and prolactin secretion
Anestrus 1–8 months	Predominance of parabasal and intermediate cells; superficial cells absent	Absent or low numbers	Absent	Absent or low numbers	Clear or granular	FSH elevated; LH concentrations increase late in stage after estrogen priming, low concentrations of progesterone

[a]It is not possible to distinguish late proestrus from estrus with vaginal cytology.
FSH, Follicle-stimulating hormone; *LH*, Luteinizing hormone.

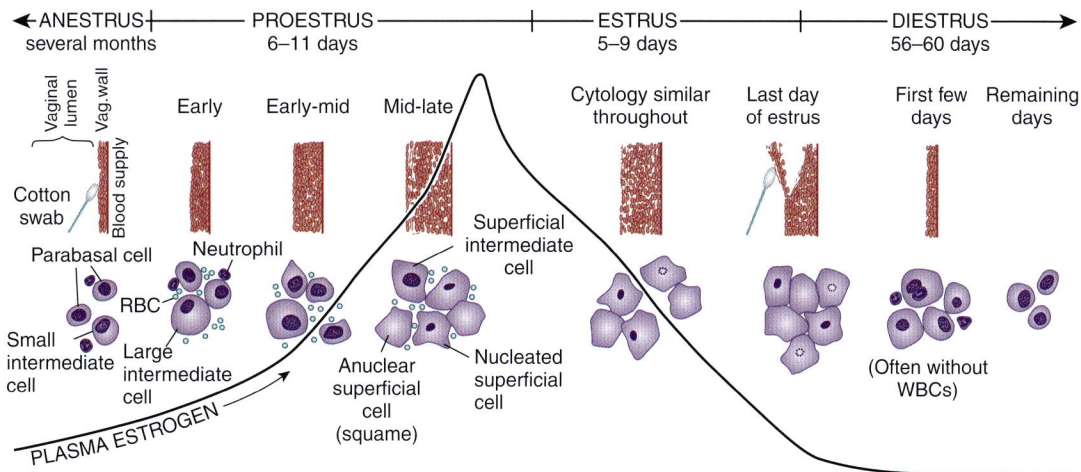

FIGURE 13.46 Changes in vaginal wall thickness, cell cytology, and estrous cycle relative to blood estrogen levels in dogs. *RBC*, Red blood cell; *WBC*, white blood cell. (Modified from Feldman EC, Nelson RW. Ovarian cycle and vaginal cytology. In: Feldman EC, Nelson RW, editors. *Canine and Feline Endocrinology and Reproduction*. 3rd ed. Philadelphia: Elsevier; 2004:755.)

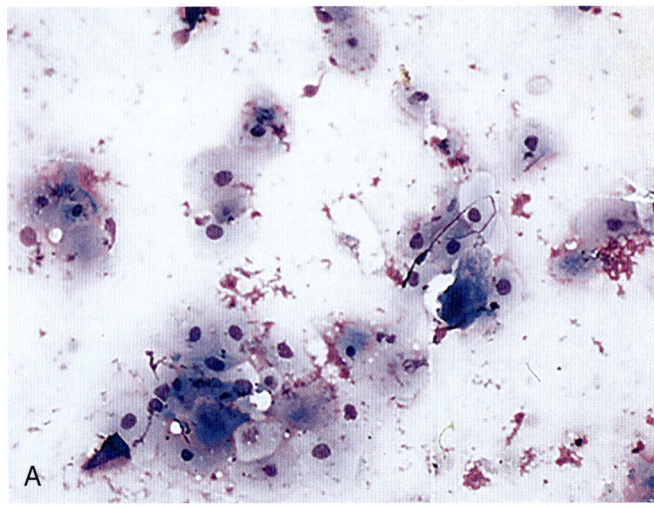

remain viable for up to 4 days within the canine reproductive tract during estrus. Therefore, bitches should be bred every 2 to 3 days during cytologic estrus (>90% superficial cells) for optimal breeding. Use of serum progesterone concentrations in combination with vaginal cytology more accurately indicates the time of ovulation, allowing for even greater breeding efficiency and estimation of the time of expected parturition (Feldman and Nelson, 2004).

Diestrus. Diestrus (Figs. 13.49 and 13.50) is the luteal phase. The decrease of superficial cells at the beginning of diestrus is usually more rapid than the increase of superficial cells occurring at estrus. Neutrophils frequently reappear during diestrus, frequently localized into the cytoplasm of epithelial cells (metestrum cells). Some neutrophils from normal bitches in diestrus contain ingested bacteria. The cytologic appearance of early proestrus and diestrus can be very similar; thus, one

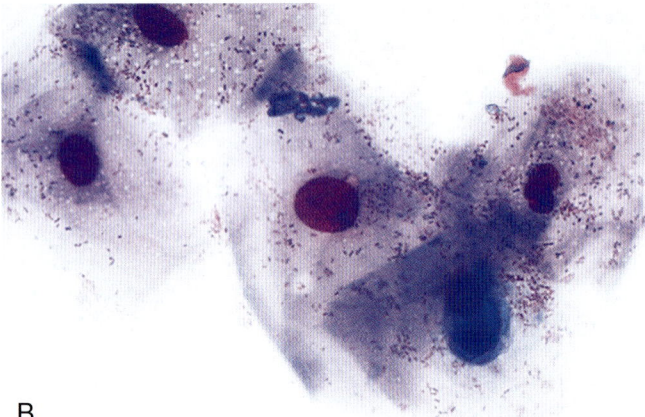

■ **FIGURE 13.47 Late proestrus. Vaginal smear. Dog. A,** Predominantly intermediate epithelial cells with occasional superficial cells. Red blood cells are present. (Wright-Giemsa; HP oil.) **B,** One intermediate and three superficial cells appear with round to pyknotic nuclei and moderately basophilic cytoplasm with angular to folded borders. The cells are associated with large numbers of bacteria. (Wright-Giemsa; HP oil.) (Courtesy Rolf Larsen, University of Florida.)

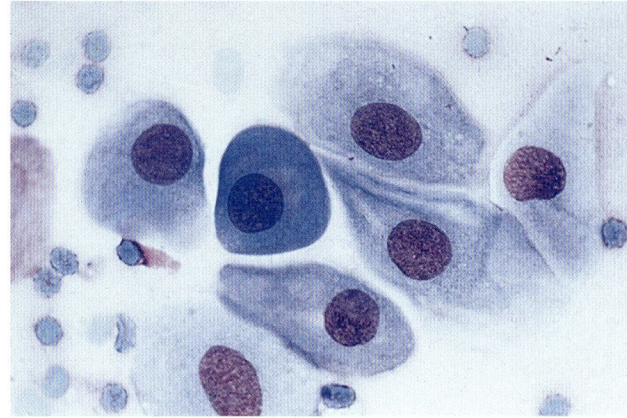

■ **FIGURE 13.49 Diestrus. Vaginal smear. Dog.** Parabasal and intermediate epithelial cells are shown. The two parabasal cells have round nuclei, moderate nucleocytoplasmic ratios, moderately to deeply basophilic cytoplasm, and round cell borders. The intermediate cells are larger with increased amounts of cytoplasm and angular borders. Basophilic staining erythrocytes are present in the background. (Wright-Giemsa; HP oil.) (Courtesy Rolf Larsen, University of Florida.)

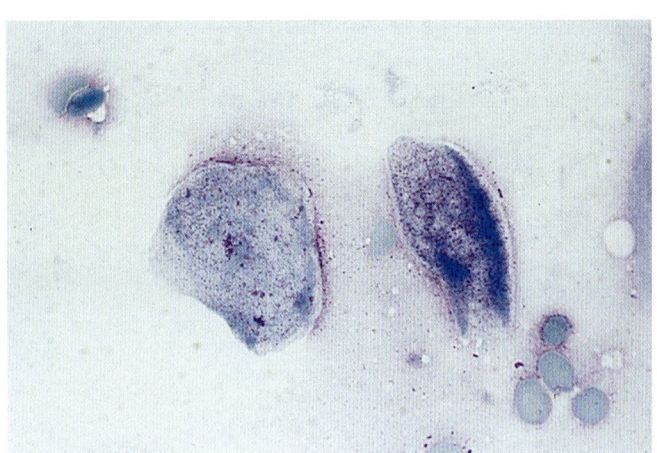

■ **FIGURE 13.48 Estrus. vaginal smear. Dog.** Shown are two anucleated (cornified) superficial epithelial cells and several basophilic staining erythrocytes. (Wright-Giemsa; HP oil.) (Courtesy Rolf Larsen, University of Florida.)

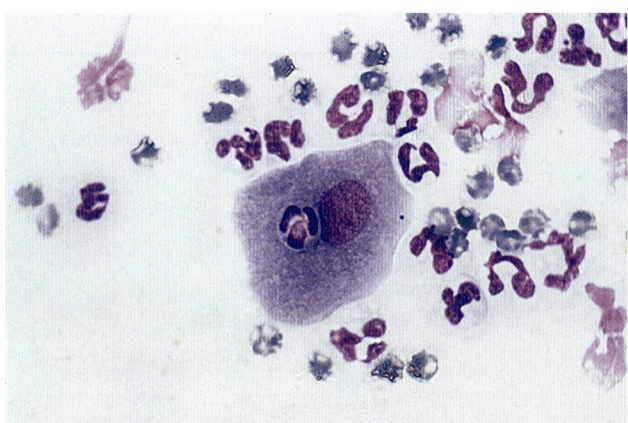

■ **FIGURE 13.50 Diestrus. Vaginal smear. Dog.** Note the large number of neutrophils and erythrocytes in the background. An intermediate epithelial cell containing a neutrophil (metestrus cell) is located in the center. These cells are not specific for diestrus and appear whenever increased numbers of neutrophils are present, including inflammation. (Wright-Giemsa; HP oil.) (Courtesy Rolf Larsen, University of Florida.)

vaginal smear is not adequate for differentiation of these two stages (Olson et al., 1984). When cytologic evidence of diestrus is apparent, breeding is unlikely to be successful.

Anestrus. Anestrus, the period between the end of diestrus and the beginning of the next proestrus, is a time of uterine involution and endometrial repair (Feldman and Nelson, 2004).

Staging the Feline Estrous Cycle

Cats are seasonally polyestrous. Coitus is necessary for ovulation, with successive estrous cycles occurring until ovulation takes place. The average duration of estrus is 8 days (range, 3–16 days) with an intermediate period of 9 days (range, 4–22 days) if ovulation does not occur. In the presence of ovulation without pregnancy, the return to estrus may be delayed for about 45 days (Olson et al., 1984). Vaginal cytology has been shown to accurately predict the various stages of the estrous cycle in cats (Mills et al., 1979). Collection of smears for cytologic evaluation is similar to those described for dogs; collection of feline vaginal samples may rarely result in ovulation.

Changes in feline vaginal cytology during the estrous cycle are similar to those seen in dogs; however, some differences should be noted. RBCs are rarely seen in smears made at any stage of the cycle. Neutrophils are rare in smears from proestrus and are an inconsistent feature of diestrus. Superficial cells are the predominant cell type seen during estrus. In contrast to dogs, superficial cells comprise only 40% to 88% of the epithelial cells seen during feline estrus (Mills et al., 1979). Anucleated cells increase to about 10% of the epithelial population on the first day of estrus, with a maximum average of 40% anucleated cells by the fourth day of estrus. A prominent clearing of the vaginal smear background in association with estrus has been observed. This clearing occurred in 90% of feline estrus smears and was suggested to be a sensitive indicator of estrus in cats (Mills et al., 1979).

Vaginal Inflammation

Inflammatory disease of the vaginal mucosa (vaginitis) is often related to noninfectious factors such as vaginal anomalies, clitoral hypertrophy, retained fetal foreign bodies, neoplasia, or vaginal immaturity ("puppy vaginitis"). Smears for cytopathologic evaluation of inflammation may be obtained from the vaginal mucosa, vaginal discharges, or FNA of vaginal or vulvar masses. Moderate to large numbers of neutrophils characterize acute vaginitis. In addition to neutrophils, lymphocytes and macrophages may be seen in more chronic inflammatory conditions. If an infectious component is involved in the inflammatory process, degenerate neutrophils and phagocytized bacteria may be seen (Figs. 13.51 and 13.52). Less commonly, yeast forms related to fungal infection such as *Malassezia* spp. or hyphal elements as in pythiosis (Fig. 13.53A) may be observed. Cytopathologic specimens may be submitted for silver stains to identify hyphae if mycosis or pythiosis is suspected (Fig. 13.53B).

Treatment of vaginitis should involve identification and correction of any underlying conditions responsible for the inflammation. If sepsis is present, appropriate antibiotic therapy based on culture and sensitivity results should be instituted. Vaginitis can be associated with the presence of epithelial cells displaying atypical cellular features in response to the inflammatory process. In the absence of a tumor, therapy to alleviate the inflammation should eliminate the atypical cells. However, if an observable mass is present or atypical cells remain after appropriate treatment, further tests to rule out the presence of neoplasia should be considered.

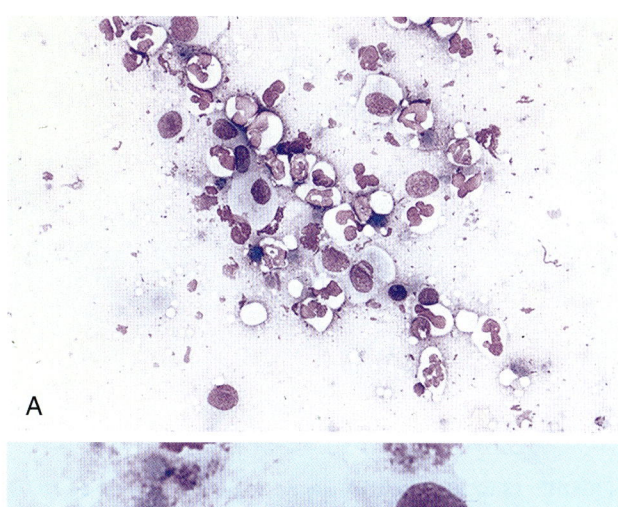
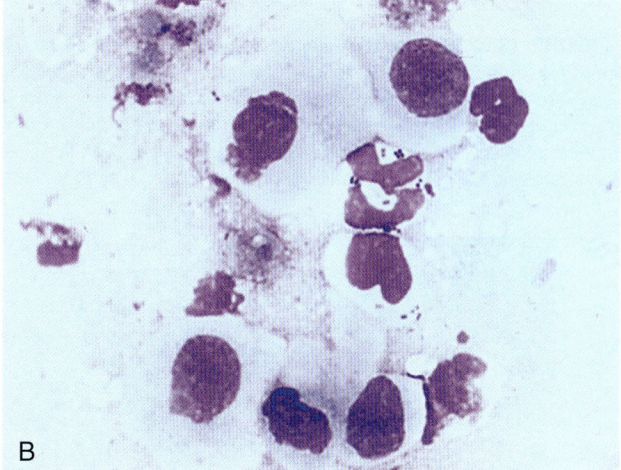

FIGURE 13.51 Suppurative vaginitis. Tissue scraping. Dog. Same case in A and B. **A,** Increased numbers of neutrophils from a vaginal papule. The neutrophils display degenerative nuclear changes of moderate to marked karyolysis. Degenerative changes are typically associated with bacterial infections. A few parabasal and intermediate epithelial cells are also present. (Wright-Giemsa; HP oil.) **B,** Two degenerative neutrophils contain phagocytized bacteria. (Wright-Giemsa; HP oil.)

Vaginal Neoplasia

Vaginal and vulvar tumors are uncommon and tend to occur in older animals (McEntee, 2002). The presenting clinical sign generally is a slow-growing perineal mass. Clinical signs seen less frequently include vulvar bleeding or discharge, an enlarging vulvar mass, dysuria, hematuria, tenesmus, excessive vulvar licking, and dystocia. Leiomyomas, fibroleiomyomas, fibromas, and fibroepithelial polyps (Foster, 2017a) are the most common vaginal neoplasm in dogs and cats. Lipoleiomyomas are also rarely reported (Agnew and MacLachlan, 2017). These benign mesenchymal tumors are characterized by variable numbers of spindle-shaped cells of uniform size and shape arranged individually and in small clumps (Fig. 13.54). The nuclei are typically oval, and scant to moderate amounts of wispy cytoplasm are present. The most common malignant tumor is leiomyosarcoma, and distant metastasis has been reported (McEntee, 2002). Other tumors with malignant potential include transmissible venereal tumors (TVTs), adenocarcinoma, SCC or epidermoid carcinoma, urethral urothelial

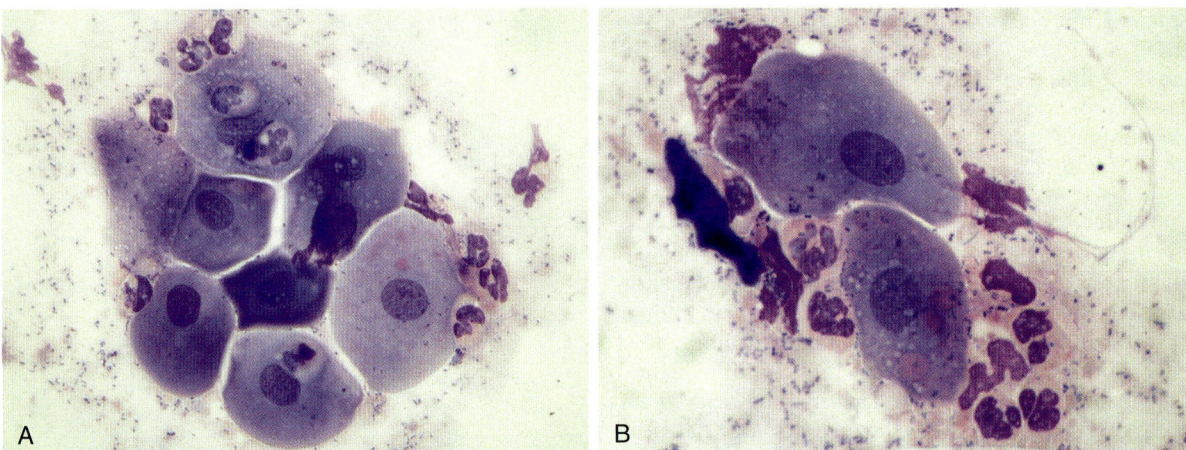

■ **FIGURE 13.52 Suppurative septic vaginitis. Vaginal swab. Dog.** Same specimen A and B. Same case as in Figures 13.35 and 13.44. The patient presented with a persistent vaginal discharge. **A,** Several intermediate to superficial squamous cells, one squame, and one parabasal epithelial cell are present. Numerous karyolytic neutrophils appear around the epithelial cells and several are within these cells (metestrus cells). The background contains many small bacteria. Note the eosinophilic granules within a few squamous cells. (Modified Wright; HP oil.) **B,** Two squamous epithelial cells contain small cytoplasmic vacuoles as well as larger eosinophilic inclusions in one cells that likely represent keratin. Neutrophils are degenerate and karyolytic and often contain short bacilli and cocci. (Modified Wright; HP oil.) (Courtesy Oliver Coldrick, TDDS, Exeter, UK.)

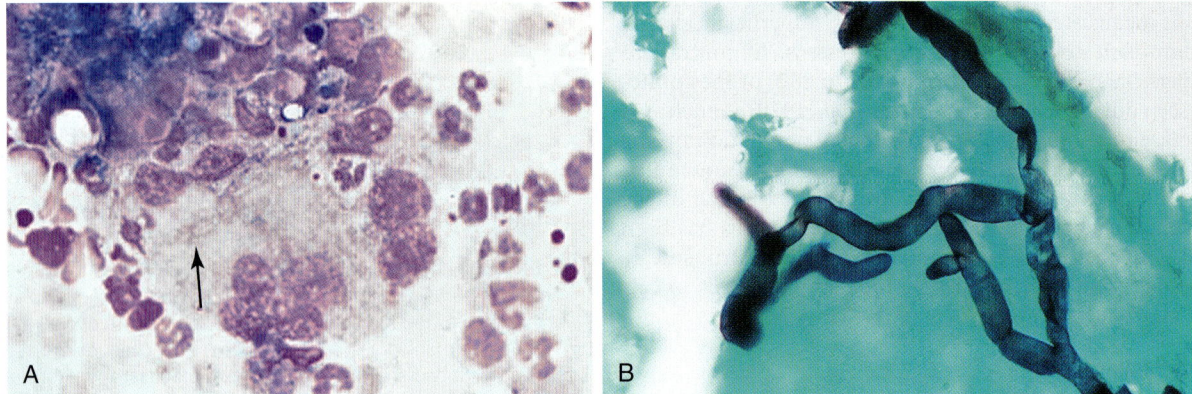

■ **FIGURE 13.53 Pyogranulomatous vaginitis. Pythiosis. Vulvar mass aspirate. Dog.** Same case in A and B. **A,** Large numbers of neutrophils, lower numbers of eosinophils, and a multinucleated macrophage are present. Pale-staining linear structures suspicious for hyphae *(arrow)* are seen within the macrophage. (Wright-Giemsa; HP oil.) **B,** Positive-staining, branching, poorly septate, linear hyphae approximately 6 to 8 μm in width are present. Culture confirmed the presence of *Pythium* spp. (Gomori methenamine silver; HP oil.)

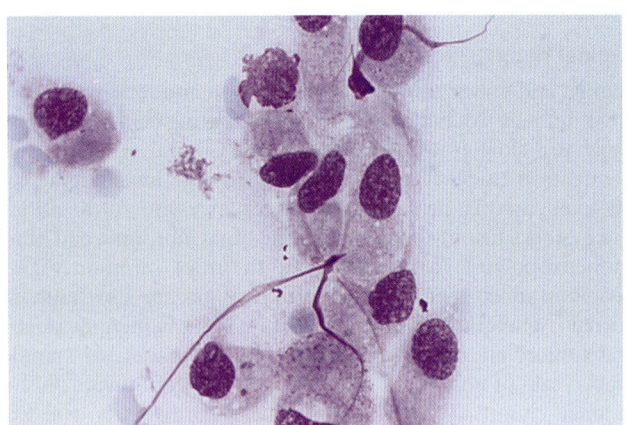

■ **FIGURE 13.54 Vaginal Leiomyoma. Vaginal mass imprint. Dog.** The cells are arranged individually or in small clumps and display round to oval nuclei with coarse nuclear chromatin, moderate nucleocytoplasmic ratios, and inconspicuous nucleoli. The cytoplasm is moderately basophilic and cell borders are indistinct. (Wright-Giemsa; HP oil.)

cell carcinoma (also known as transitional cell carcinoma), osteosarcoma, hemangiosarcoma, rhabdomyosarcoma, lymphoma, and mast cell tumor. The cytopathologic appearance of these tumors is similar to those found in other body sites. One exception is a unique neoplasm recently described by cytopathology (Neihaus et al., 2010; Rout et al., 2016; Verin et al., 2018; Piech et al., 2019). The naked nuclei cytomorphology of the canine clitoral or vulvar adenocarcinoma (Fig. 13.55) appears similar to that of the apocrine gland anal sac adenocarcinoma (AGASACA). Similar to AGASACA, this neoplasm is often associated with secondary hypercalcemia of malignancy and metastasis to regional lymph nodes. Treatment of vaginal tumors usually involves conservative surgical excision combined with ovariohysterectomy, which is usually is curative for benign tumors. In cases of malignant tumors, further evaluation to determine extent of local invasion or metastasis should be performed.

Transmissible venereal tumor may also be diagnosed using cytopathologic examination of vaginal scrapings, swabs, imprints, or aspirates. TVTs are contagious, sexually transmitted tumors

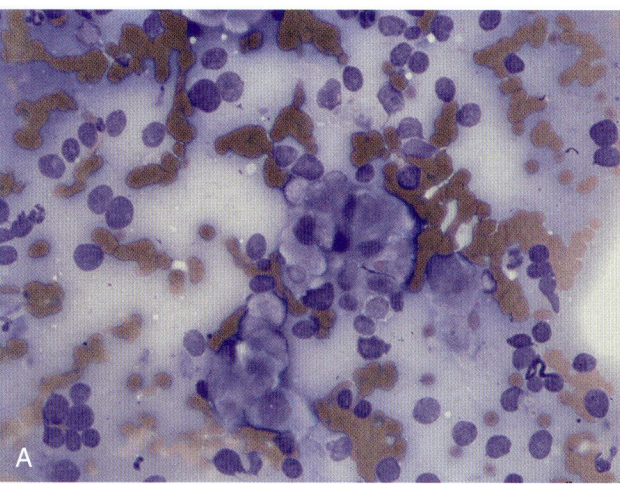 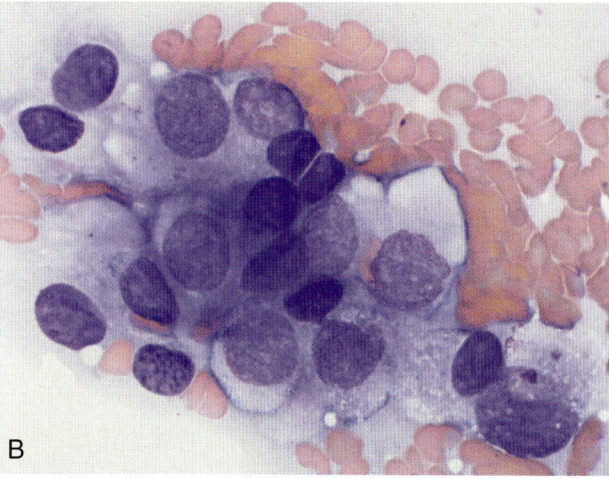

■ **FIGURE 13.55 Adenocarcinoma. Vulvar mass aspirate. Cat.** Same case in A and B. The owner noticed redness of the cat's vulva a few weeks before presentation. There was a mild response to prednisolone; when the drug was stopped, the mass grew larger. At the time of presentation the mass was 1.5 × 2 cm with a necrotic center. **A,** Small aggregates of malignant epithelial cells are present against a background containing many naked nuclei (Wright; HP oil.) **B,** Higher magnification demonstrates the moderate to high nucleocytoplasmic ratios and anisokaryosis of the carcinoma cells. (Modified Wright; HP oil.) (Courtesy Karena Tang, Purdue University.)

occurring in male and female dogs. The tumors may be located in genital areas and extragenital sites such as the rectum, skin, oral and nasal cavities, and eyes (Ganguly et al., 2016). They appear as firm, friable, tan, ulcerated, and nodular or polypoid masses (Fig. 13.56; see also Figs. 3.205 and 3.206). In bitches, TVT may spread directly to the cervix, uterus, and oviducts. Although metastasis is uncommon, TVT can spread to regional lymph nodes, skin, and subcutaneous tissue. Other reported metastatic sites include the lips, oral mucous membranes, eye, bone, musculature, abdominal viscera, lungs, and central nervous system (Park et al., 2006). TVT is suspected to be of histiocytic origin based on positive reactions to lysozyme, alpha-1-antitripsin, vimentin, glial fibrillary acid protein, and a macrophage-specific immunostain and negative reactions to immunostains specific for other cell types, such as cytokeratin, S100, and muscle markers. TVT with intracellular *Leishmania infantum* amastigotes has been documented, which also supports histiocytic origin (Ganguly et al., 2016).

Aspirates of TVT generally yield large numbers of individualized, round cells (Fig. 13.57). The nuclei are round with clumped nuclear chromatin and single or multiple prominent nucleoli. The nuclei are located eccentrically. Moderate amounts of pale-blue cytoplasm frequently contain multiple, punctate vacuoles. Mitotic activity is often high. Inflammation, as indicated by increased numbers of plasma cells, lymphocytes, macrophages, and neutrophils, may be present.

Marginal surgical resection is not considered effective treatment for TVT. The most effective treatments for TVT are chemotherapy and radiation. Single-agent therapy with vincristine has been shown to be very effective for TVT, even in cases of metastatic disease. Doxorubicin is the drug of choice for TVT resistant to vincristine (Ganguly et al., 2016).

MALE REPRODUCTIVE SYSTEM

The focus of this section is the testes, prostate, and semen, including normal anatomy, cytopathology, and histopathology. The lesions discussed involve cystic changes, hyperplasia, metaplasia, inflammation, and neoplasia.

Prostate Gland

Cats have two accessory genital glands: the prostate and bulbourethral glands. Prostatic carcinoma, paraprostatic cysts, prostatic abscess, and prostatic squamous metaplasia are uncommonly reported in cats. Although the prostate gland is present in cats, the vast majority of prostatic disease is reported in dogs. The following discussion of normal and abnormal findings associated with the prostate gland is limited to dogs. Prostatic disorders are common in middle-aged and older male dogs and have been categorized as hyperplasia, cysts, inflammation, squamous metaplasia, and primary or metastatic neoplasia. More than one prostatic disorder may occur simultaneously (Cunto et al., 2019).

The primary presenting clinical findings associated with prostatic disease are signs of systemic febrile illness, lower urinary tract signs (hemorrhagic urethral discharge), abnormalities of defecation, and locomotion problems. Some cases of canine prostatic disease may be present without obvious clinical signs; therefore, palpation of the prostate per rectum should be a part of all physical examination in mature intact and neutered male dogs. Normally, the prostate should be smooth, symmetrical, and nonpainful. Abdominal palpation can be used to evaluate an enlarged prostate that has moved into the abdominal cavity (Cunto et al., 2019). Ancillary diagnostic tests that may be used to evaluate suspected cases of prostatic disease include urinalysis, bacterial culture, and imaging, such as radiography, ultrasonography, elastography, CT, and MRI (Cunto et al., 2019). CBCs and serum biochemical profiles are usually normal in cases of prostatic illness; however, the presence of hemogram and biochemical abnormalities may help in diagnosis. Serum canine prostatic specific esterase (CPSE) may be used as a screening test for prostatic disease because serum CPSE is increased in dogs with prostatic hyperplasia, bacterial prostatitis, or prostatic carcinoma (Alonge et al., 2018). Cytopathology, microbiology, and histopathology may be necessary to classify the type of prostatic disease. Canine prostatic disease is commonly diagnosed using cytopathologic techniques, especially now that ultrasound-guided FNA is widely available. The diagnostic accuracy of

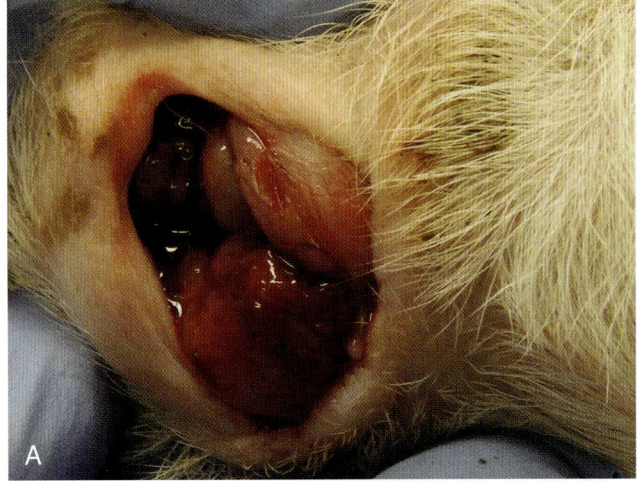
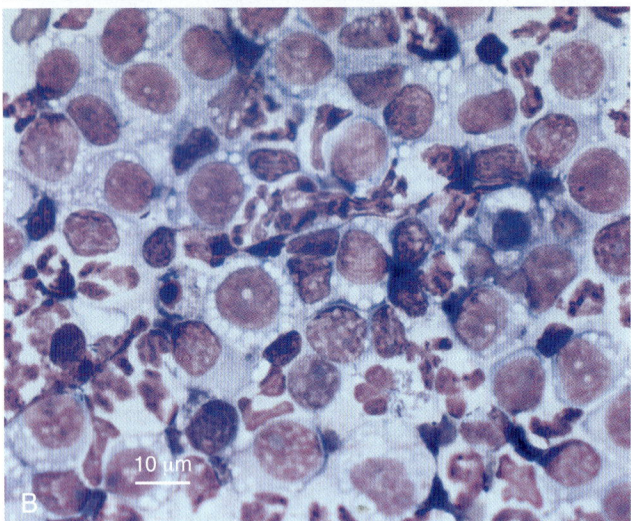
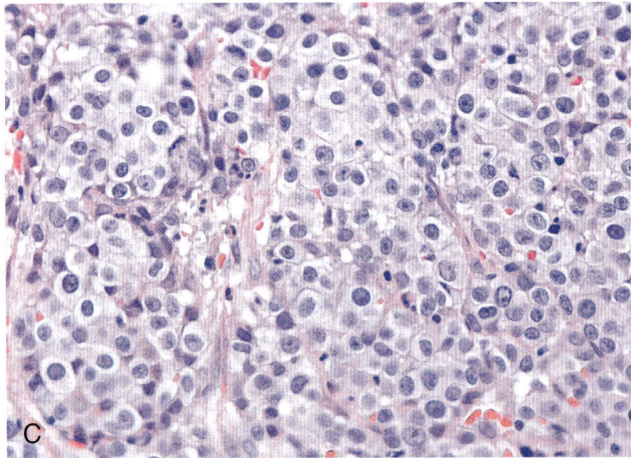

■ **FIGURE 13.56 Transmissible venereal tumor. Vaginal mass. Dog.** Same case in A to C. **A, Macroscopic specimen.** Swelling at the mucocutaneous junction related to multiple hemorrhagic masses. **B, Tissue imprint.** Highly cellular specimen with numerous round cells displaying a round nucleus, prominent nucleolus, and abundant basophilic cytoplasm often containing punctate vacuoles. Inflammatory cells involve degenerative neutrophils with evidence of bacterial sepsis. (Modified Wright; HP oil.) **C, Tissue section.** Dermal proliferation of round cells with prominent nucleoli. Mitotic figures are infrequent. (H&E; IP.) (A, Courtesy Chris Fulkerson, Purdue University. B–C, Courtesy Kristin Fisher, Purdue University.)

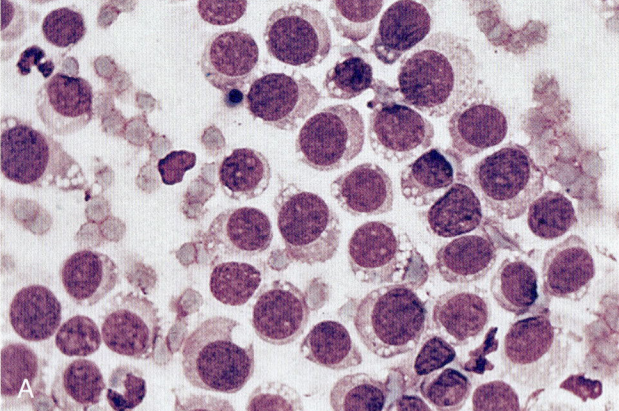
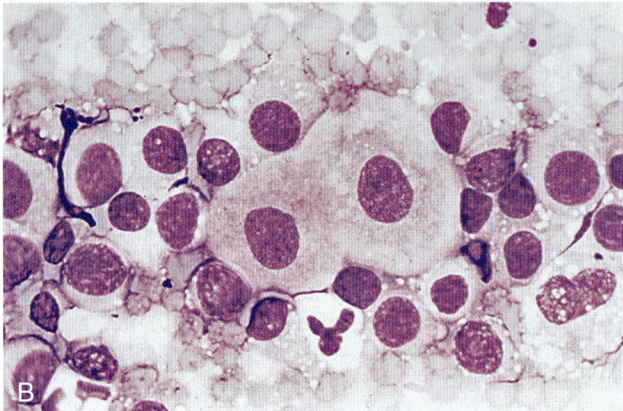

■ **FIGURE 13.57 Transmissible venereal tumor. Vaginal mass imprint. Dog.** Same case in A and B. **A,** Large numbers of round cells have round nuclei, coarse nuclear chromatin, variably prominent nucleoli, and scant to moderate amounts of lightly basophilic cytoplasm. Many of the cells contain punctate cytoplasmic vacuoles, a characteristic feature of this tumor. **B,** Two intermediate epithelial cells *(center)* and individualized tumor cells are shown. Note the larger size and increased amounts of cytoplasm in the epithelial cells compared with the tumor cells. (Wright-Giemsa; HP oil.)

cytopathology in comparison with histopathologic diagnosis is 80% (Powe et al., 2004). In addition, cytopathology is a more sensitive method than histopathology for the detection of bacterial infection. Interestingly, histopathologic terminology standards for the reporting of prostatic epithelial lesions in dogs have been recently described (Palmieri et al., 2019a).

Collection Techniques

Urethral discharge. Sampling of urethral discharge is a simple method to evaluate prostatic abnormalities. If present, urethral discharge is collected by retracting the prepuce, cleaning the glans, and collecting the discharge into a vial or onto a microscope slide for microscopic evaluation. Some samples may also be collected into sterile containers for bacterial culture and colony counts. Concurrent analysis of urine collected by catheterization or cystocentesis should be performed to differentiate between normal urethral flora and cystitis.

Semen collection. A detailed description of canine and feline semen collection is not fully covered in this text, but an in-depth review is available elsewhere (Freshman, 2002; Zambelli and Cunto, 2006). Ejaculate material for the evaluation of prostatic disease can be obtained from intact dogs via manual stimulation; however, collection of semen may not be possible if the dog is inexperienced or in pain. A collection funnel may be used to separate the clear prostatic third fraction of the ejaculate from the sperm-rich first and second fractions. An aliquot for microbiologic analysis should be placed into a sterile culture tube with the remaining fluid retained for cytopathologic evaluation. If inflammation is suspected, the cytopathologic aliquot should be placed into a vial containing ethylenediaminetetraacetic acid (EDTA). Because of the presence of normal bacterial flora in the lower urethra, a quantitative culture should be performed on the ejaculate fluid. In the presence of inflammatory cells, high numbers (>100,000 cfu/mL) of gram-negative or gram-positive bacteria indicates an infectious process (Root Kustritz, 2006). If cytopathologic and microbiologic results are equivocal in regard to prostatic infection versus urethral contamination, a quantitative lower urethral culture to compare with the semen culture results may be useful.

Prostatic massage and wash. Prostatic massage is used primarily to collect prostatic fluid in dogs unable to ejaculate. The simplest method for prostatic massage or wash involves passing a urinary catheter, guided by rectal palpation, to the caudal pole of the prostate. A syringe is attached to the catheter, and fluid is aspirated as the prostate is gently massaged per rectum. A few milliliters of sterile saline may be flushed into the catheter and aspirated to facilitate collection of fluid for analysis. Urinary tract infection (UTI) often accompanies infectious prostatitis, which may confound the results of prostatic massage. For these cases, an alternative massage procedure may be used to determine the source of the infection. The urinary bladder is catheterized, emptied of urine, and flushed with 5 mL of sterile physiologic saline. The fluid from this first flush is collected as the preprostatic massage fraction. The catheter is then retracted to the caudal pole of the prostate. Another 5 mL of sterile physiologic saline is injected through the catheter while the prostate is massaged per rectum. The catheter is then advanced back into the bladder, and all the fluid in the bladder is collected. This fluid is the postprostatic massage fraction, which should be relatively free of urinary contamination (Root Kustritz, 2006; Smith, 2008). Bacterial colony counts and presence or absence of inflammatory cells from the pre- and postprostatic massage fractions can be compared with isolate the source of the infection. Ampicillin, which concentrates in urine but reaches lower concentrations in the prostate owing to its inability to cross the prostatic-lipid barrier, may be administered 1 day before prostatic massage to aid in isolation of the source of infection. In general, prostatic massage should be reserved for evaluation of prostatitis in dogs without UTI or in which the UTI is controlled. It should be noted that cytopathologic preparations obtained by catheterization typically yield a mixed population of urothelial cells (Powe et al., 2004).

Fine-needle biopsy. Fine-needle aspiration or capillary sampling of the prostate gland produce more reliable results and more prostatic cells than prostatic massage, especially with ultrasound guidance. If the gland is enlarged, a transabdominal approach may be used. Transperineal and perirectal approaches have also been described. The method of aspiration of the prostate gland is similar to that used for other tissues. A 22-gauge needle attached to a 13 mL syringe is directed into the gland, and cells, fluid, or both are aspirated. A drop of aspirate material or fluid is placed onto a slide. If necessary, any remaining material may then be submitted for culture.

Historically, the use of FNA in cases of acute prostatitis or abscessation was associated with a risk of peritonitis or seeding the infection or neoplasia along the needle tract. However, there are reports in the veterinary literature documenting FNA for diagnosis or treatment of prostatic disease with no complications (Boland et al., 2003). Ultrasound-guided transabdominal FNA of the prostate is described elsewhere (Root Kustritz, 2006). FNA of the prostate has several advantages over other collection methods. Identification of squamous epithelial cells from a prostatic aspirate allows the diagnosis of squamous metaplasia, whereas the presence of these cells in prostatic massage fluid could be misinterpreted as normal lower urinary tract squamous epithelial cells. Also, the greater cellular detail obtained via FNA increases the confidence of a diagnosis of neoplasia. The primary disadvantage of prostatic FNA is that focal lesions, such as neoplasia, may be missed. However, use of ultrasound to guide the aspirate can lessen this possibility.

Normal Anatomy and Histology

The prostate gland secretes seminal fluid that promotes sperm survival and motility. Normal prostatic fluid is clear and represents the third fraction of the canine ejaculate, although some have suggested that the first fraction may contain some prostatic material. The prostate gland is a glandular, fibromuscular structure surrounding the proximal portion of the male urethra. Before 2 months of age, the prostate is located within the abdominal cavity. After breakdown of the urachal ligament until sexual maturity, the prostate lies in the pelvic canal. With increasing age, the prostate enlarges and moves over the pelvic brim into the abdomen. Bladder distension can also pull the prostate cranially into the abdomen.

The prostate gland is composed of compound tubuloalveolar glands radiating from the urethral opening (Fig. 13.58). The secretory alveoli contain primary and secondary enfoldings of epithelium that project into the alveolar lumen. A fibromuscular stroma surrounds the prostatic ducts, which are lined by cuboidal to columnar epithelium. Urothelial (transitional) epithelium lines the excretory ducts that open onto the urethra (Cunto et al., 2019).

Normal Cytology

The number and type of prostatic cells in cytologic samples from the prostate vary depending on the collection technique. Prostatic epithelial cells obtained via aspiration from normal dogs occur in frequent clusters and are cuboidal to columnar. These cells are uniform in size and shape and contain round to oval nuclei, which may be basilar in columnar cells. Nucleoli are usually small and inconspicuous. The cytoplasm is finely granular or microvesiculated and basophilic. Other cell types that may be seen, particularly from semen samples or prostatic massages, include spermatozoa, squamous epithelial cells, and urothelial (transitional) cells. Spermatozoa stain blue-green with Romanowsky and modified Romanowsky stains and may adhere to other cells. Squamous cells are large with abundant amounts of blue to blue-green (keratinized) cytoplasm. The nuclei of these cells may be round to pyknotic or absent. Cell borders are typically angular to folded. Urothelial (transitional) cells are larger than prostatic epithelial cells and have lighter staining cytoplasm with a lower N:C. Normal ejaculate fluid

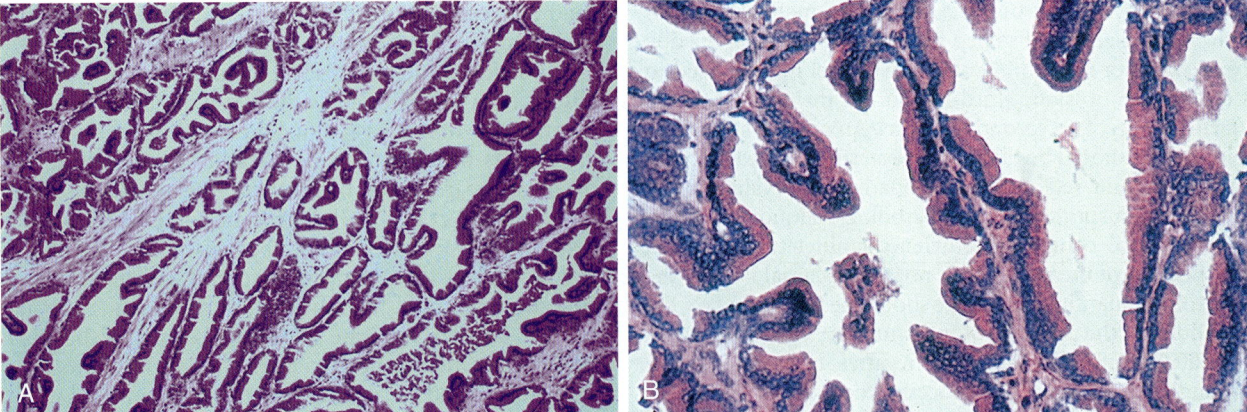

■ **FIGURE 13.58 Normal prostate gland. Histology. Dog.** Same case in A and B. **A,** The tubuloalveolar glands are surrounded by a fibromuscular stroma. Primary and secondary enfoldings of epithelium project into the alveolar lumen. (H&E; L.P.) **B,** Higher magnification shows cuboidal and columnar epithelium line the prostatic lumens and ducts. (H&E; I.P.) (Courtesy Roger Reep and Don Samuelson, University of Florida.)

may contain low numbers of neutrophils and RBCs. Use of excessive amounts of ultrasound gel during ultrasound-guided FNA can result in large amounts of purple, variably sized, granular background debris that may obscure cellular detail. To prevent this artifact, excess gel should be removed before inserting the aspiration needle.

Prostatic Cysts

There are many cysts that develop within and around the prostate. Paraprostatic cysts are those around the prostate, and prostatic cysts are those within the prostate. Prostatic cysts (Fig. 13.59) may occur as multiple, small cysts associated with androgen-dependent prostatic hyperplasia as well as large retention cysts within the prostate tissue. Paraprostatic cysts may become mineralized or result from osseous metaplasia. Except for hyperplasia-associated cysts, prostatic cysts account for 2% to 5% of prostatic abnormalities. Prostatic cavitary lesions containing urine (urinary cysts) due to intraprostatic urethral fistulation have been reported (Bokemeyer et al., 2011). Small cysts may be palpated per rectum as small, fluctuant areas in an asymmetrically enlarged prostate. Large, discrete cysts may be palpated in the caudal abdomen or in the perineal area. Unless the cyst becomes secondarily infected, clinical signs are uncommon. A bloody urethral discharge, dysuria, and tenesmus may be present, owing to increased prostatic size. Recommended treatment is surgical resection, with or without concurrent castration (Cunto et al., 2019). Ultrasound-guided, percutaneous drainage of prostatic cysts appears to be a useful alternative treatment (Boland et al., 2003).

Aspiration of prostatic cysts typically yields variable amounts of serosanguineous to brown fluid (Fig. 13.60; see also Fig. 2.6). Cytopathologic examination of the fluid usually reveals no or few normal-appearing epithelial cells; low to moderate

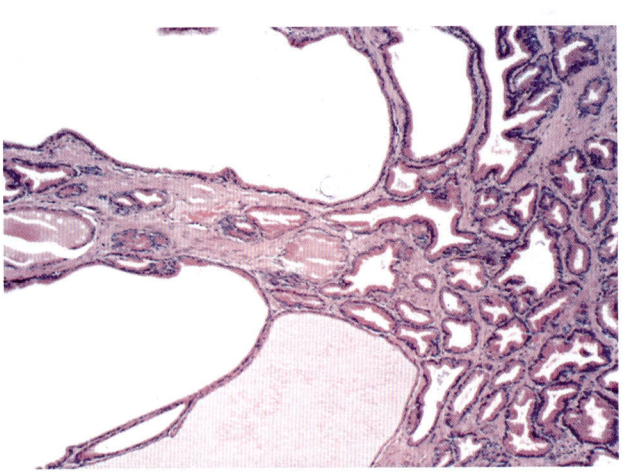

■ **FIGURE 13.59 Prostatic cyst. Histology. Dog.** Cuboidal epithelial cells line large cystic spaces representing dilated ducts. (H&E; L.P.) (Courtesy Rose Raskin, University of Florida.)

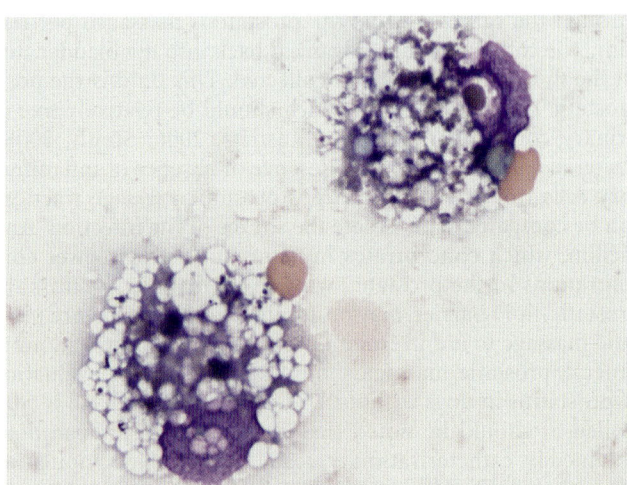

■ **FIGURE 13.60 Prostate cyst. Fluid smear. Dog.** Same case in Figure 2.6. Fluid appeared brown and hazy initially, and postcentrifugation fluid was yellow and clear. Other data included 3 g/dL protein, 3% packed cell volume, and 333 cells/μL. The smears had low cellularity and minimal blood content. Macrophages accounted for more than 95% of nucleated cells and contained abundant dark pigment or blue pigment consistent with hemosiderin as shown, along with cytoplasmic foaminess or vacuolation. Cytopathologic diagnosis was chronic hemorrhage. (Modified Wright; HP oil.) (Courtesy Rose Raskin, Michigan State University.)

numbers of neutrophils, macrophages, and small lymphocytes; and erythrocytes on a lightly proteinaceous background (Boland et al., 2003).

Prostatic Hyperplasia

Prostatic hyperplasia (benign prostatic hyperplasia) is a common finding in older intact male dogs. Prostatic hyperplasia is an increase in gland size and weight related to increases in interstitial tissue and gland lumens. Symmetrical cystic dilation of the glands results from increases in the interstitium and gland lumens. The pathogenesis of prostatic hyperplasia is not completely understood. However, its development is hormonally dependent and requires the presence of functioning testes. Dihydrotestosterone is accepted as a key hormone in stimulating enlargement of the canine prostate by enhancing growth in both stromal and glandular components. Circulating levels of testosterone are often decreased in older male dogs; however, dihydrotestosterone concentrations are often increased in the hyperplastic tissue. Additionally, estrogens appear to act synergistically with androgens in potentiating prostatic hyperplasia and may also act directly on the prostate, resulting in stromal hypertrophy and squamous epithelial metaplasia (Cunto et al., 2019). The treatment of choice for canine prostatic hyperplasia is castration or finasteride administration; finasteride inhibits conversion of testosterone to dihydrotestosterone, causing prostatic involution via apoptosis. Other medical options exist for treating prostatic hyperplasia and are reviewed elsewhere (Cunto et al., 2019).

In dogs, the prostate gland is not fixed, so enlargement occurs in an outward direction, resulting in constipation and tenesmus. Mild hemorrhagic urethral discharge can also be noted. However, clinical signs are often absent in dogs with prostatic hyperplasia. Palpation of the prostate usually reveals a symmetrically enlarged, nonpainful gland; however, an irregular surface is occasionally appreciated (Cunto et al., 2019).

Epithelial cells obtained from a hyperplastic prostate gland are generally arranged in variably sized sheets and clusters in a honeycomb pattern (Fig. 13.61) (Masserdotti, 2006). The cells are uniform in appearance with round nuclei and small, round nucleoli. The N:C is moderate to high, and the cytoplasm is basophilic and finely vesiculated (see Fig. 13.61C). Mild increases in cell size and anisokaryosis may be noted as well as binucleation (see Fig. 13.61B). Cytopathologic and histopathologic samples yielding unremarkable prostatic epithelial cells from a symmetrically enlarged prostate are consistent with a diagnosis of prostatic hyperplasia (Fig. 13.62).

Prostatic Squamous Metaplasia

Squamous metaplasia of the prostatic epithelium may result from chronic irritation, inflammation, or causes of hyperestrogenism, such as Sertoli cell tumors (Powe et al., 2004). Estrogen receptors, which are present on ductal, stromal, and 10% of the prostatic epithelial cells, may mediate this responsiveness. The prostate may be small as a result of decreased concentrations of testosterone or enlarged if cysts or abscesses are present. Cytopathologically, the epithelial cells develop staining and morphologic characteristics of squamous epithelial cells (Fig. 13.63). Treatment for squamous metaplasia is removal of the estrogen source (Cunto et al., 2019).

Prostatic Inflammation

Both acute and chronic infections occur in the canine prostate gland, usually as a result of ascent of normal aerobic urethral

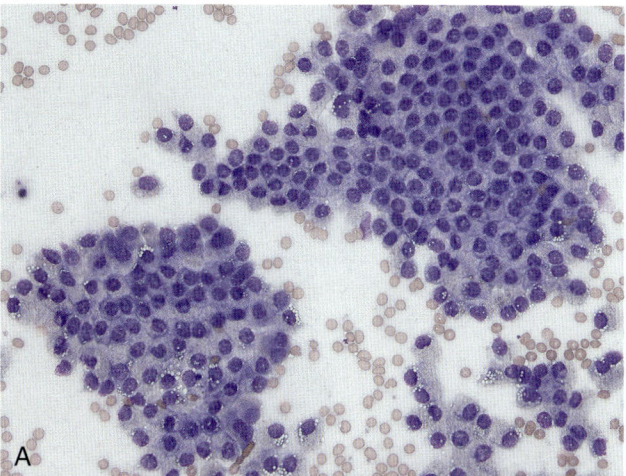
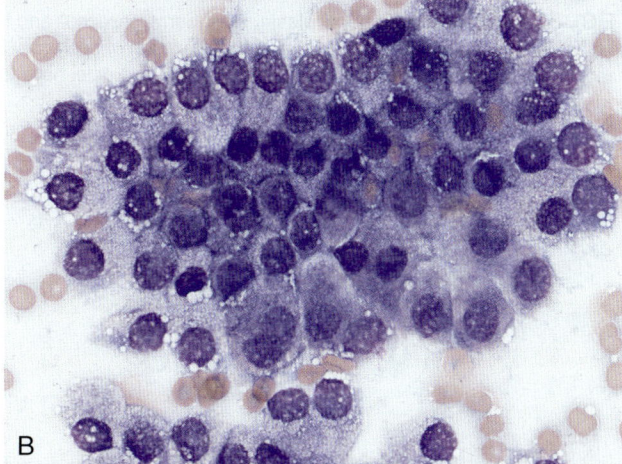
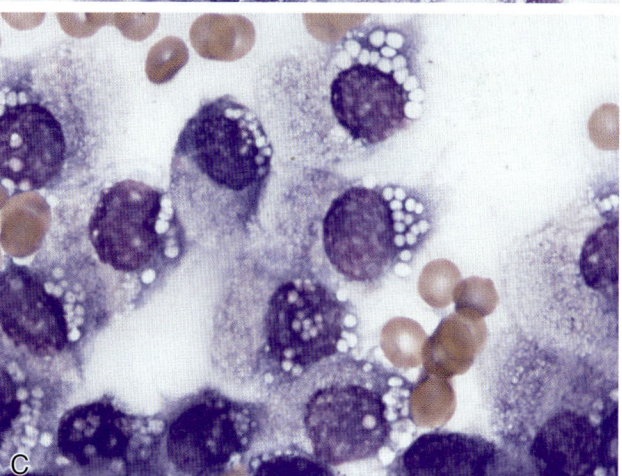

■ **FIGURE 13.61 Prostatic hyperplasia. Prostate mass aspirate. Dog.** Same case in A to C. The patient was presented with a history of dribbling urine for several months. There are both solid and cystic enlargements. This sample is taken from the solid area. **A,** A sheet of prostatic epithelium has uniform cells with high nucleocytoplsamic ratios. (Wright; IP.) **B,** Pavement formation is evident by the cobblestone effect of the cells interlocking with one another. Nucleocytoplasmic ratio appears to vary from high to moderate. (Wright; HP oil.) **C,** Notice the frequent appearance of punctate vacuoles within the cytoplasm. The nuclei are round to ovoid with granular chromatin and small nucleoli. The basophilic cytoplasm is finely granular. (Wright; HP oil.) (Courtesy Rose Raskin, Michigan State University.)

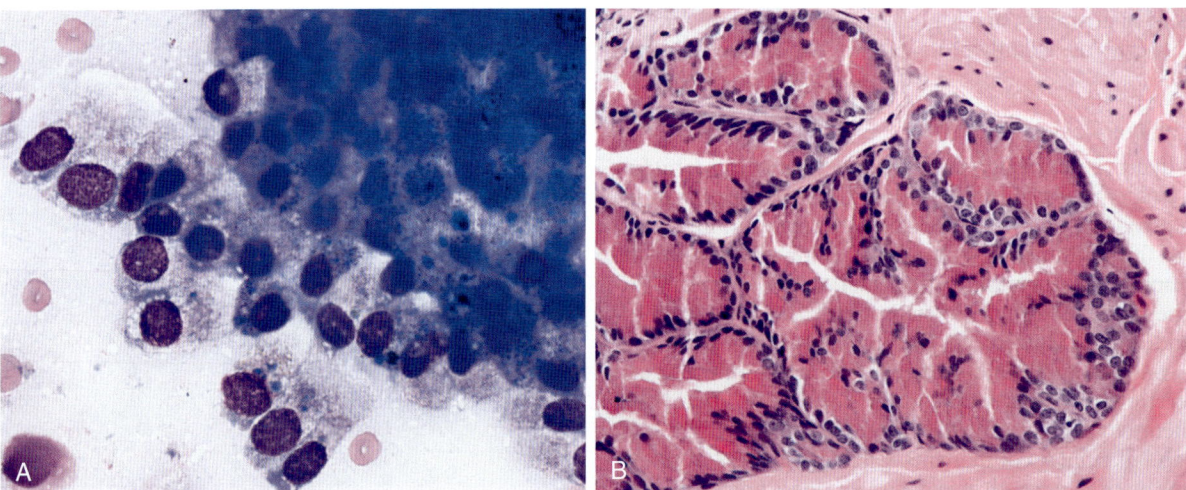

■ **FIGURE 13.62 Prostatic hyperplasia. Dog.** Same case in A and B. **A, Tissue aspirate.** Prostatic epithelial cells are columnar and uniform. Note the granulated appearance of the cells and accumulation of secretory pigment in the cell sheets and clusters. (Wright; HP oil.) **B, Histology.** Minimal anaplastic features characterize hyperplastic epithelium. Nuclei have less nuclear chromatin density than normal but increased prominence of nucleoli. (H&E; IP.) (Courtesy Rose Raskin, Purdue University.)

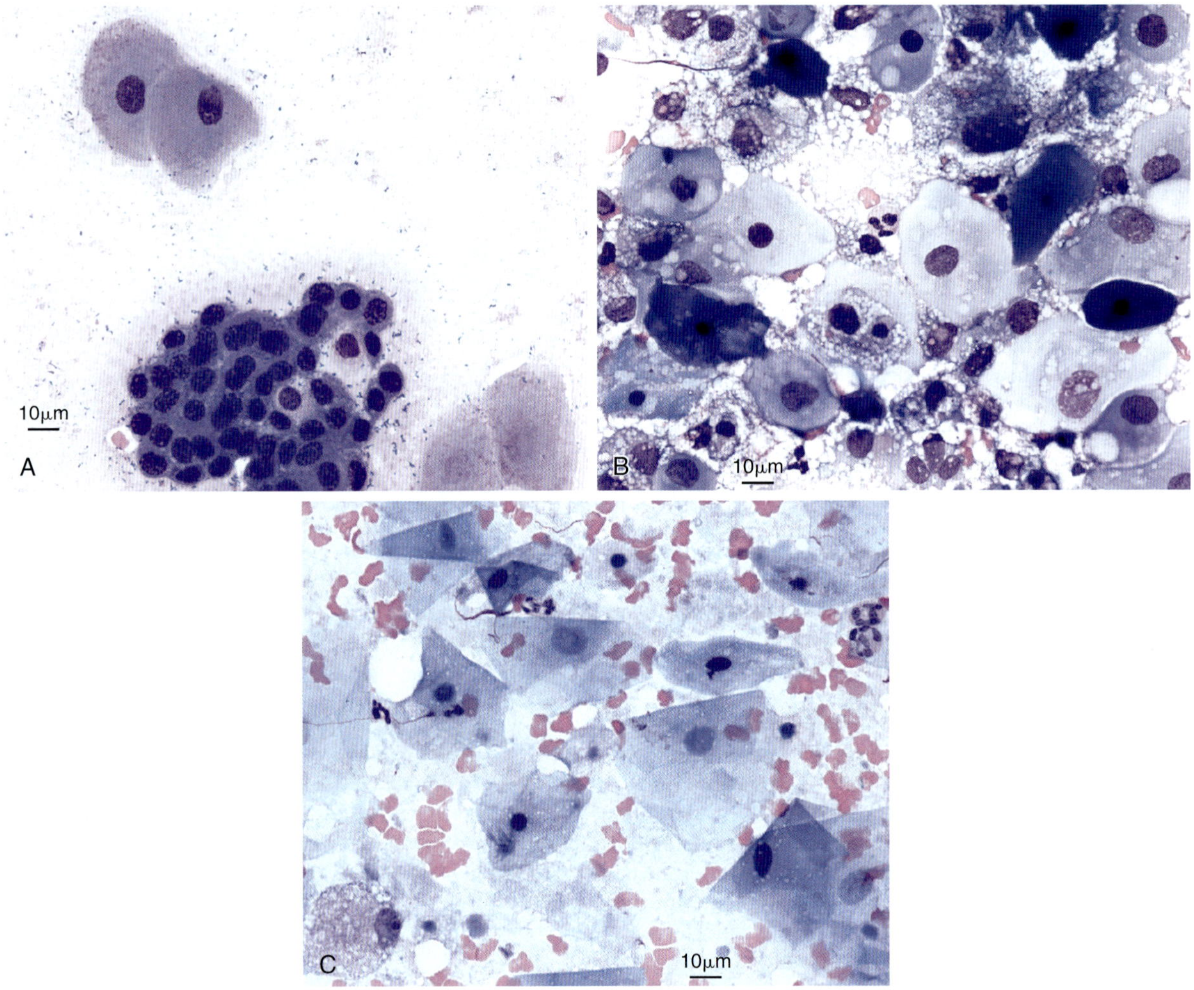

■ **FIGURE 13.63 Squamous metaplasia. Prostate. Dog. A, Wash.** Sheet of hyperplastic epithelium along with several squamous cells, two with small nuclei and two anucleate. The background is dotted by bacteria. Neutrophils (not shown) are mildly increased. (Modified Wright; HP oil.) **B, Tissue aspirate.** Highly cellular specimen with squamous epithelium in various stages of maturation and keratinization. (Modified Wright; HP oil.) **C, Tissue aspirate.** Mild neutrophilic and macrophagic inflammation accompany keratinized superficial squamous cells. (Modified Wright; HP oil.) (Courtesy Rose Raskin, Purdue University.)

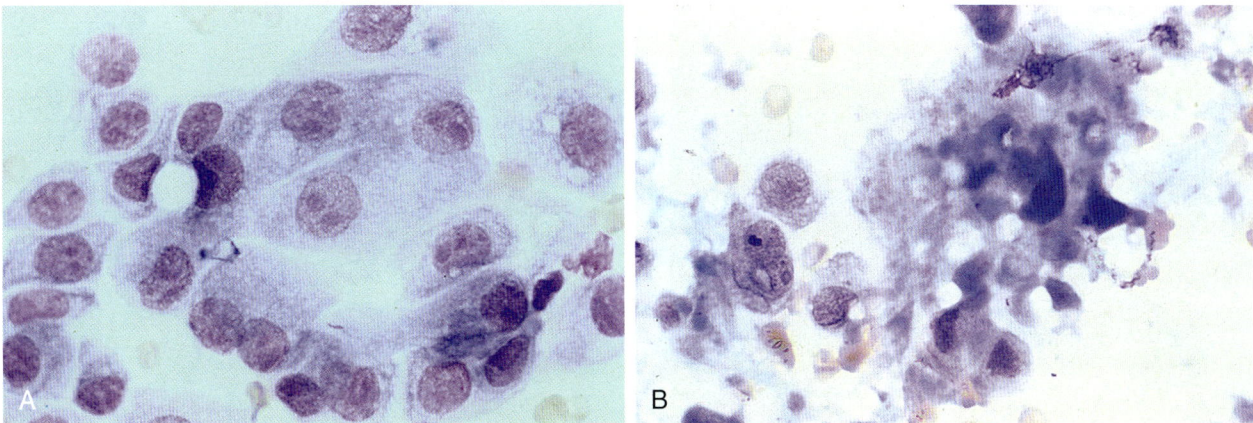

■ **FIGURE 13.69 Prostatic adenocarcinoma. Cytopathologic preparation. Dog.** Same case in A and B. **A,** Neoplastic epithelial cells display prominent, large, multiple nucleoli, coarse nuclear chromatin, moderate anisokaryosis and anisocytosis, variable nucleocytoplasmic ratios, and binucleation. (Wright-Giemsa; HP oil.) **B,** Amorphous basophilic material is compatible with necrosis, which can be found in aspirates of malignant tumors. Cellular features are indistinct. (Wright-Giemsa; HP oil.)

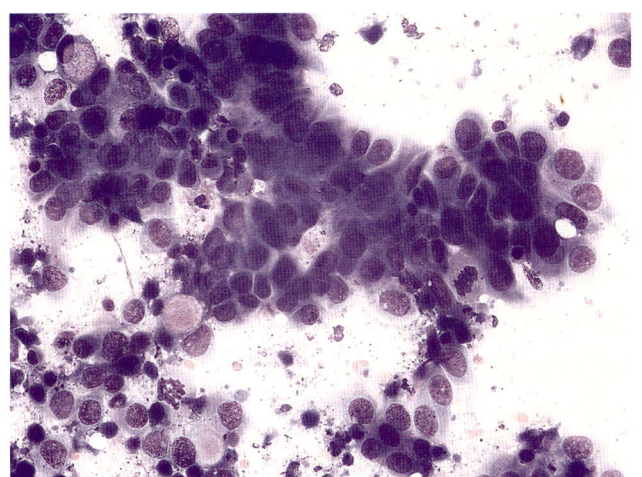

■ **FIGURE 13.70 Prostatic urothelial (transitional cell) carcinoma. cytopathologic preparation. Dog.** A large sheet of epithelial cells with palisading arrays of peripherally located cells. Notice the presence of tailed cytoplasm and of some large cytoplasmic vacuoles. (Wright-Giemsa; HP oil.)

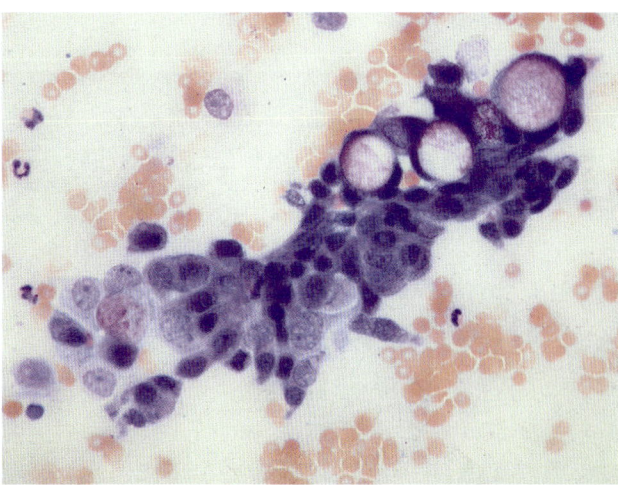

■ **FIGURE 13.71 Prostatic urothelial (transitional cell) carcinoma. Prostate aspirate. Dog.** The patient was noted to have calcification and prostatomegaly on imaging. Several cells show a large eosinophilic granular cytoplasmic vacuole (Melamed-Wolinska body) that displaces the nucleus to the periphery. (Wright; HP oil.) (Courtesy Rose Raskin, TDDS, Exeter, UK.)

carcinoma (Figs. 13.70 to 13.74) can be difficult to distinguish cytopathologically and histopathologically. Some acinar structures may be noted in prostatic adenocarcinoma, which can help to differentiate this neoplasm from urothelial (transitional cell) carcinoma. Moreover, the urothelial (transitional) cells show tailed shapes, and only sporadically exhibit vacuolated cytoplasm as a consequence of glandular metaplasia. The presence of a variably sized magenta-stained cytoplasmic vacuole (Melamed-Wolinska body) is supportive of urothelial origin and may help to distinguish urothelial carcinoma from prostatic adenocarcinoma (Powe et al., 2004). Neoplastic urothelial cells are arranged in discohesive, mostly bidimensional clusters. Nuclei are round to ovoid, with irregularly clumped chromatin, sometimes nucleolated, and show moderate to marked anisokaryosis.

Most canine prostatic carcinomas, mainly urothelial (transitional cell) carcinoma, are locally invasive and metastatic. Metastases are present at necropsy in 80% to 89% of dogs with prostatic carcinoma, and regional lymph nodes and lungs are the most common metastatic sites. Other sites for metastasis are bone, urinary bladder, and mesentery. Bone metastases are most often located in the pelvis, lumbar vertebrae, and femur and can be lytic or proliferative. In untreated dogs, the disease carries a poor prognosis with an expected survival time of less than 2 months (Agnew and MacLachlan, 2017; Cunto et al., 2019). Therapy for prostatic carcinoma is usually palliative and may include prostatectomy or intraoperative radiation (Cunto et al., 2019).

Testes

Unilateral or bilateral testicular enlargement is the primary indication for FNA and cytopathologic evaluation of the testes. Cytopathology is useful for differentiation between inflammatory or neoplastic conditions that cause testicular enlargement

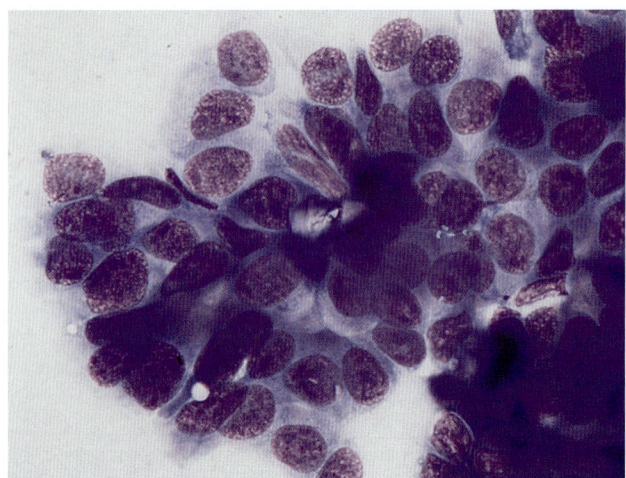

■ **FIGURE 13.72 Prostatic urothelial (transitional cell) carcinoma. Cytopathologic preparation. Dog.** Neoplastic cells have large round to ovoid nuclei, anisokaryosis, and irregular clumped chromatin with prominent multiple nucleoli. (Wright-Giemsa; HP oil.)

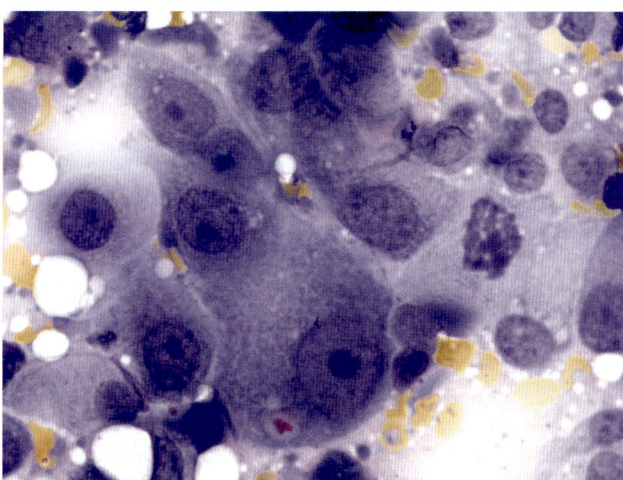

■ **FIGURE 13.74 Prostatic urothelial (transitional cell) carcinoma. Prostate aspirate. Dog.** The patient presented with prostatomegaly. The basophilic background contained some amorphous refractile material suggestive of mineral and a moderate amount of amorphous blue-gray material consistent with necrosis (not shown). Shown here is a cluster of malignant cells and a mitotic figure *(center right)*. Features of malignancy include high and variable nucleocytoplasmic ratio, open chromatin, prominent and irregular nucleoli, and anisokaryosis. The large cell in the center contains a small eosinophilic cytoplasmic inclusion similar to a Melamed-Wolinska body. (Wright-Giemsa; HP oil.) (Courtesy Rose Raskin, University of Florida.)

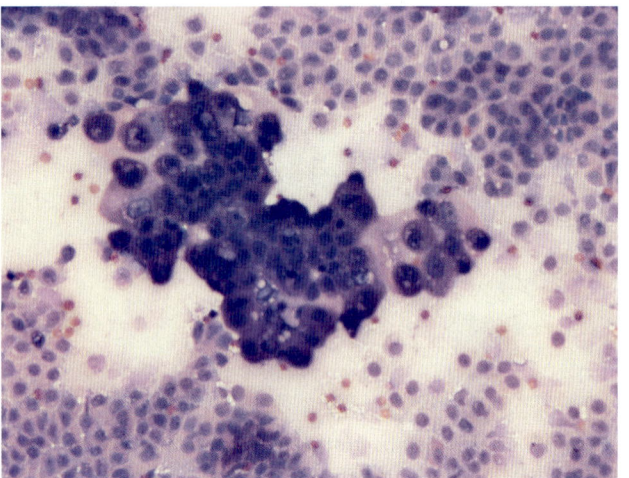

■ **FIGURE 13.73 Prostatic urothelial (transitional cell) carcinoma. Prostatic wash biopsy. Dog.** The patient presented with a history of dribbling urine for 5 months and moderate prostatomegaly. Within a large sheet of uniform hyperplastic, prostatic epithelium are a focal collection and cluster of malignant epithelium. These cells are characterized by moderate anisokaryosis and anisocytosis. The neoplastic cells have abundant pink granular cytoplasm with often perinuclear vacuolation. Nuclei are large and round with coarsely clumped chromatin with one to two prominent nuclei. Binucleation was noted and karyomegaly is common. (Modified Wright; IP.) (Courtesy Rose Raskin, Michigan State University.)

obtain a better cytologic preparation such as atraumatic sampling (FNCS) (Masserdotti et al., 2005). The material should be very lightly smeared when preparing the cell monolayer. Alternatively, gentle touch imprints from available tissue may decrease cellular disruption. Imprints of testicular biopsies should be made rapidly after removal of the tissue to prevent cell degeneration.

Normal Anatomy and Histology

The testes are the site of spermatogenesis in adult animals and exhibit both exocrine and endocrine function. The convoluted seminiferous tubules are lined by some stratified layers of spermatogenic cells, germ cells that are actively involved in spermatogenesis. Sertoli cells or sustentacular cells, which secrete estrogen and provide support for the developing sperm, lie between the germinal cells near the base of the seminiferous tubules (Fig. 13.75). The connective tissue between adjacent tubules contains interstitial (Leydig) cells, which secrete testosterone and are localized near the blood vessels.

Normal Cytology

Normal testicular imprints are highly cellular with a predominance of ruptured cells and streaming nuclear material. When cells rupture, the nuclear chromatin becomes coarse, and nucleoli are prominent. Testicular germinal cells are generally round, with coarse nuclear chromatin, a single large, prominent nucleolus, and moderate amounts of basophilic cytoplasm (Fig. 13.76A and B). The presence of multinucleated cells is possible, as the result of *cytodieresis imperfecta*, a morphologic expression of incomplete separation of germinal cells during subdivision. Mitotic activity is often high. More mature stages of developing sperm are characterized by oval, eosinophilic to pale-staining nuclei, and tails may be noted (Fig. 13.76C and D). Small groups of columnar cells,

as well as classify testicular neoplasia (Masserdotti et al., 2005). Testicular FNA is usually not associated with immediate or long-term adverse effects (Root Kustritz, 2006).

Collection Techniques

Routine FNA with a 20- to 25-gauge needle attached to a 5 to 10 mL syringe is used for cytologic sampling of the testes (Root Kustritz, 2006). Because of the increased fragility of testicular cells, great care should be taken when preparing the slide of aspirated material, and some authors recommend avoiding aspiration to

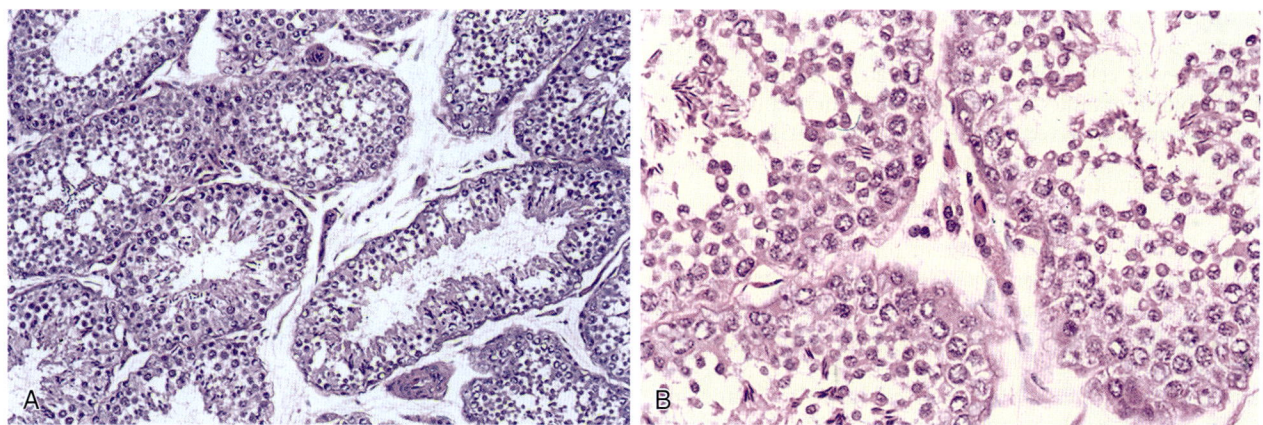

■ **FIGURE 13.75 Normal testes. Histology. Dog.** Same case in A and B. **A,** Multiple seminiferous tubules are surrounded by connective tissue containing low numbers of interstitial cells. (H&E; IP.) **B,** Higher magnification of the seminiferous tubules shows interstitial cells between the tubules. Spermatocytes as well as early and late spermatids are seen within the tubules. Spermatocytes are characterized by round nuclei and coarse nuclear chromatin. During the maturation process, developing sperm move from the periphery of the tubule to the central lumen. Low numbers of Sertoli cells with smooth nuclear chromatin and single, prominent nucleoli are seen at the periphery of the tubules. (H&E; HP oil.)

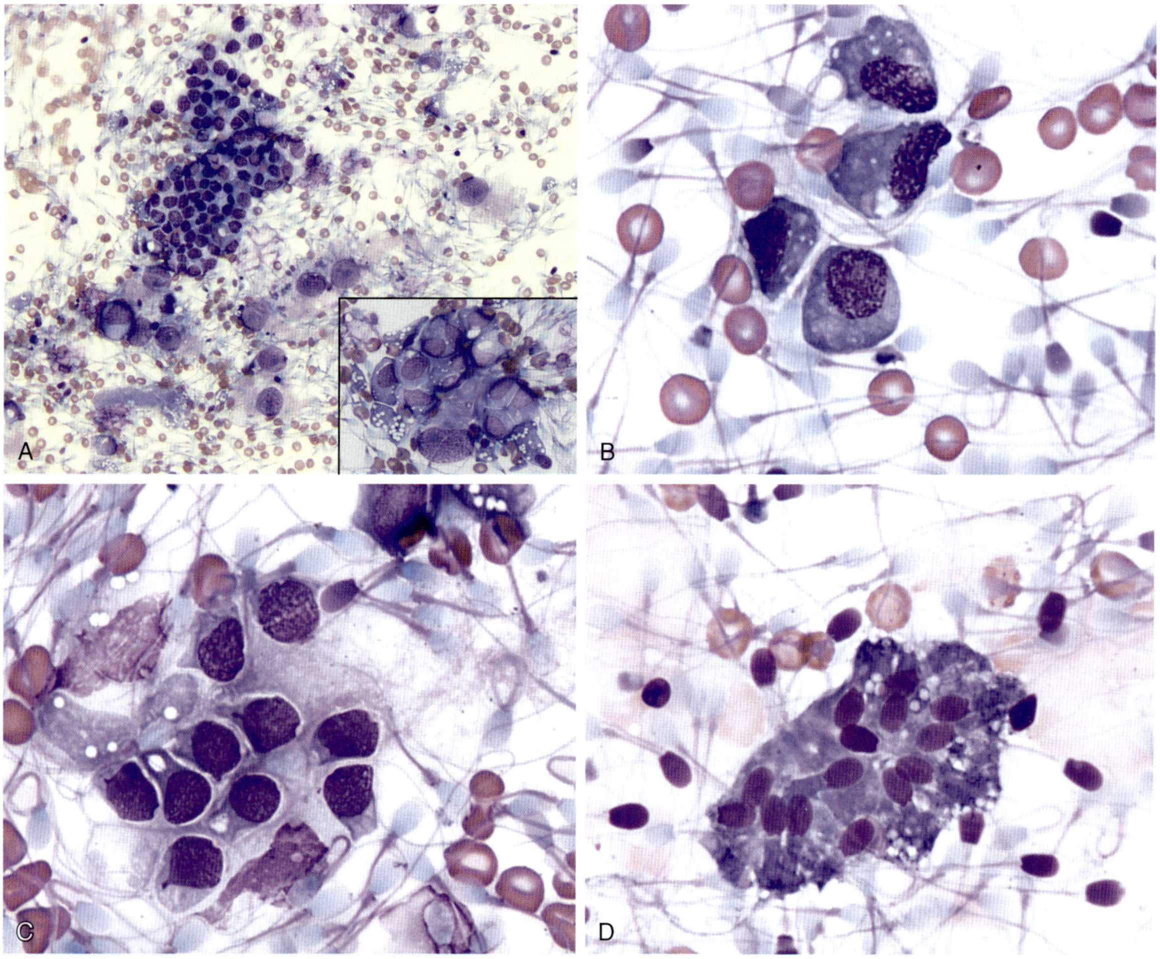

■ **FIGURE 13.76 Normal testes. Testicle aspirate. Dog.** Same case in A and D. **A,** Specimen taken to compare with enlarged opposite diseased testicle. Several ruptured large germinal cells (spermatogonium) with a single prominent nucleolus are scattered in the background along with an aggregate of dense round basophilic spermatocytes. (Wright; IP.) *Inset:* Shown is a collection of large germinal cells with high to moderate nucleocytoplasmic ratios having one or two round to ovoid nuclei. (Wright; HP oil.) **B,** Spermatocytes with coarse chromatin and round to oval nuclei with abundant deeply basophilic and mildly vacuolated cytoplasm. The background contains many intact mature sperm with lightly basophilic heads. (Wright; HP oil.) **C,** Dense spermatocytes with scant lightly basophilic cytoplasm and clumped chromatin represent a step before spermatids. **D,** Elongated spermatids are present as an aggregate, and mature variably basophilic sperm appear in the background. (Wright; HP oil.) (A–D, Courtesy Rose Raskin, Michigan State University.)

with indistinct cytoplasm and large round nuclei as single nucleoli, recognizable as Sertoli cells, can be evident. Scattered stellate or caudate Leydig cells, with microvacuolated cytoplasm, sometimes with bluish granules of lipofuscin pigment and round nuclei, are sometimes observed (Masserdotti et al., 2005).

Testicular Inflammation

In dogs, inflammatory disease of the testes (orchitis) or epididymis (epididymitis) can be due to infection with *B. canis*, *Pseudomonas* spp., *E. coli*, or *Proteus* spp. Intranuclear or intracytoplasmic inclusions may be seen in cases of distemper-associated orchitis. Orchitis and epididymitis may also be due to *B. dermatitidis*, *L. infantum*, *Mycoplasma canis*, or *Rickettsia rickettsii* infection. In cats, orchitis or epididymitis is uncommon, and orchitis has been rarely associated with coronavirus and *Sporothrix schenckii* infections. Acute orchitis is characterized by a predominance of neutrophils, and some of them may exhibit nuclear degenerative changes. Macrophages including multinucleated giant cells and lymphocytes may be seen in chronic inflammation, mycosis (blastomycosis), or protozoonosis (leishmaniosis).

Testicular Neoplasia

In intact male dogs, the testis is the second most common anatomic site for cancer development, and testicular tumors account for approximately 90% of all cancers of male genitalia. The three most common tumors are Leydig cell tumor or interstitial cell tumor (58%), seminoma (23%), and Sertoli cell tumor or sustentacular cell tumor (19%) (Masserdotti et al., 2005), although cases of hemangiomas, teratomas, sarcomas, embryonal carcinomas, gonadoblastomas, lymphomas, and rete testis mucinous carcinomas have been rarely described (Agnew and MacLachlan, 2017). Mixed germ cell–sex cord–stromal tumor with more than one type of testicular tumor is common in dogs (Fig. 13.77). Testicular tumors occur frequently in aged male dogs. Cryptorchid testes have a higher incidence of Sertoli cell tumors and seminomas, with the right testis more frequently being retained and therefore predisposed to tumorigenesis (Agnew and MacLachlan, 2017). Most primary testicular tumors are locally confined, with fewer than 15% undergoing metastasis. In dogs with localized disease, orchiectomy with scrotal ablation remains the treatment of choice and often is curative. Information about appropriate and effective management of metastatic disease is limited, although the use of radiation therapy and chemotherapy has been reported to increase survival time.

Testicular tumors are rare in cats. There are only isolated cases reports of testicular tumors in cats, such as teratoma and interstitial and Sertoli cell tumors (Agnew and MacLachlan, 2017).

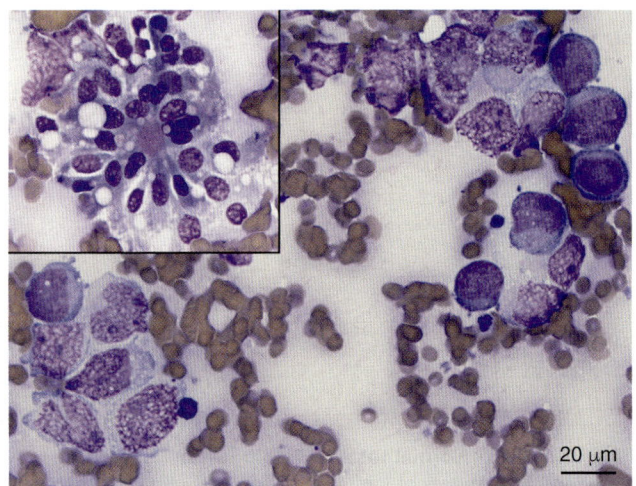

FIGURE 13.77 Mixed germ cell–sex cord stromal tumor. Testicle aspirate. Dog. The same specimen contained two focal cell populations. In some areas, many intact and ruptured large round cells with high nucleocytoplasmic ratio and fine chromatin were present supportive of a germ cell population or seminoma. *Inset:* Aggregate of elongated vacuolated cells with coarse chromatin were present surrounding amorphous eosinophilic material (Call-Exner body) that is consistent with a sex cord–stromal tumor of Sertoli cell origin. (Aqueous Romanowsky; HP oil.) (Courtesy Rose Raskin, Purdue University.)

High sensitivity (95% for seminoma, 88% for Sertoli cell tumor, and 96% for Leydig cell tumor) and specificity (100%) for the cytopathologic diagnosis of canine testicular tumors have been reported compared with histopathologic evaluation. Cytopathologic evaluation permits accurate diagnosis and is useful in the management of the disease (Masserdotti et al., 2005). Expected immunochemical labeling of testicular neoplasms is reviewed elsewhere (Agnew and MacLachlan, 2017) and summarized in Table 13.2.

Seminoma

Seminomas arise from neoplastic transformation of the testicular germ cells. Seminomas most often occur in older animals; boxers, German shepherds, Maltese, and Norwegian elkhounds appear predisposed. Other than testicular enlargement, which may not be readily apparent if the tumor involves a cryptorchid testicle, clinical signs related to seminomas are rare. About 6% to 11% of canine seminomas metastasize, with primary metastatic sites including the inguinal, iliac, and sublumbar lymph nodes and the lungs or abdominal organs (Agnew and MacLachlan, 2017).

Cytopathologic differentiation of seminomas from other testicular tumors may be difficult. Cytopathologic preparations

TABLE 13.2 Immunostaining of Canine Testicular Tumors

TUMORS	VIMENTIN	CYTOKERATIN	GATA-4	INHIBIN-A	MELAN-A	E-CADHERIN	NSE	LH	S-100	C-KIT	DESMIN
Seminoma	±	−	−	±	−	±	±	−	−	+	±
Sertoli cell	+	+	+	+	+	+	+	+	−	±	±
Interstitial cell	+	±	±	+	+	+	−	−	+	±	NA

LH, Luteinizing hormone; *NA*, not available; *NSE*, neuron-specific enolase.
Data from Owston and Ramos-Vara, 2007; Ramos-Vara and Miller, 2009; Yu et al., 2009; Ciaputa et al., 2014; Hohšteter et al., 2014; and Agnew and MacLachlan, 2017.

from seminomas often contain large numbers of lysed cells and free nuclei. These cells are large, discrete, round, and arranged individually or in small aggregates. The nuclei are large and round, sometimes with irregular outlines. Nuclear chromatin is reticular to coarse, and large, prominent nucleoli are common (Fig. 13.78; see also Fig. 13.77). Moderate anisokaryosis and anisocytosis, and frequent binucleation and multinucleation may be present. The cytoplasm is lightly to moderately basophilic with a moderate to high N:C. The presence of clear macrovacuoles in the cytoplasm is rarely noted. Numerous and atypical mitoses are often observed (see Fig. 13.78). Small lymphocytes are frequent and may be focally or multifocally distributed on slides made by tissue imprints (Fig. 13.79). Lacy, granular, eosinophilic material with the appearance of a tigroid or striped background is occasionally seen (Masserdotti et al., 2005).

Sertoli Cell Tumor or Sustentacular Cell Tumor

Sertoli cell tumors are fairly common sex cord stromal tumors in retained testes. Most dogs with Sertoli cell tumors are older than 6 years with a mean age of 9.5 years, although tumors in dogs as young as 3 years have been reported. Miniature schnauzer dogs with persistent Müllerian duct syndrome, Shetland sheepdogs, and collies are overrepresented. About one-third of canine Sertoli cell tumors are associated with excess production of estrogen, although both seminomas and interstitial cell tumors can cause hormonal imbalances. Reductions in the plasma testosterone/estradiol ratio correlate better than increased plasma 17β-estradiol concentrations with clinical signs of feminization, including bilaterally symmetric alopecia and hyperpigmentation, a pendulous prepuce, gynecomastia, galactorrhea, atrophic penis, squamous metaplasia of the prostate, or bone marrow suppression. Metastasis occurs in 10% to 14% of Sertoli cell tumors. Sites of metastasis are primarily iliac lymph nodes and other lymph nodes, the spleen, the liver, and the kidneys (Agnew and MacLachlan, 2017). Sites of extratesticular occurrence of testicular tumors include the skin and may be associated with previous castration procedures, suggesting possible seeding of testicular tissue (Doxsee et al., 2006; Meichner et al., 2016).

Cytopathologically, variable numbers of round to elongate pleomorphic cells with indistinct cytoplasm are common features of Sertoli cell tumors (Figs. 13.80 to 13.82). These cells may occur individually or in small clusters, occasionally forming Call-Exner bodies (see Figs. 13.77 and 13.81) or palisading formation (see Fig. 13.82) (Masserdotti, 2006). Call-Exner bodies are pseudorosette structures characterized by elongated cells surrounding amorphous, eosinophilic, extracellular, dense material (see Figs. 13.77 and 13.81). These structures are also observed in granulosa cell tumors (see Fig. 13.32), which is the ovarian counterpart of Sertoli cell tumors (Masserdotti et al., 2008). Sertoli cell nuclei are generally round to oval with fine nuclear chromatin, and occasionally one to three prominent, large nucleoli are noted. The lightly basophilic cytoplasm may vary from scant to abundant in amount, sometimes with indistinct margins. The presence of moderate-sized to large cytoplasmic vacuoles is typical (see Figs. 13.77, 13.81, and 13.82) (Masserdotti et al., 2005).

Interstitial Cell Tumors

Interstitial cell tumors are very common sex cord–stromal tumors in dogs, but only 16% of these tumors are associated with

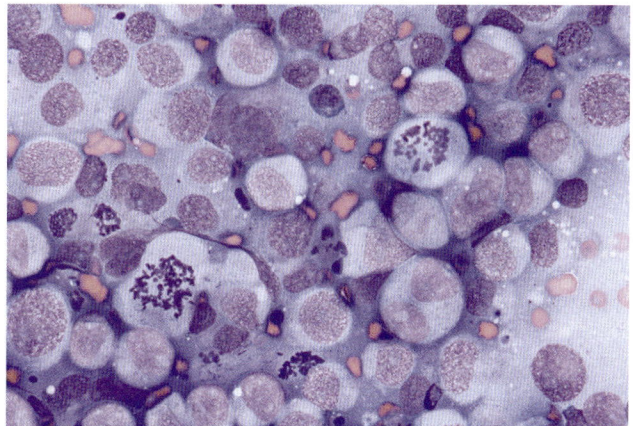

■ **FIGURE 13.78 Seminoma. Testicle aspirate. Dog.** Neoplastic cells appear large with round nuclei, coarse nuclear chromatin, and prominent, large nucleoli. The cytoplasm is lightly basophilic, and some cells contain small numbers of punctate cytoplasmic vacuoles. Two mitotic figures are also evident. (Wright-Giemsa; HP oil.)

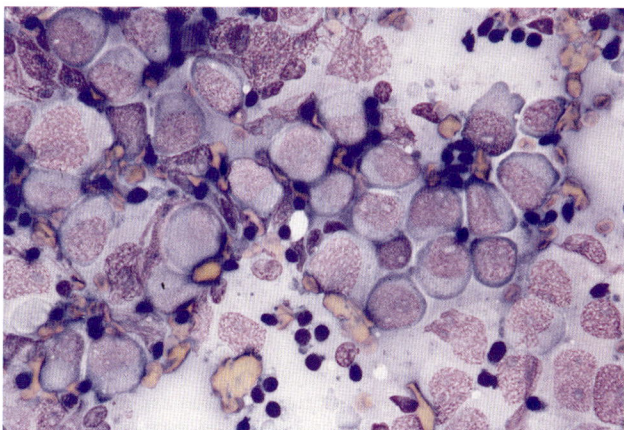

■ **FIGURE 13.79 Seminoma. Testicle aspirate. Dog.** Several round neoplastic, focally disrupted, cells are associated with many small lymphocytes. (Wright-Giemsa; HP oil.)

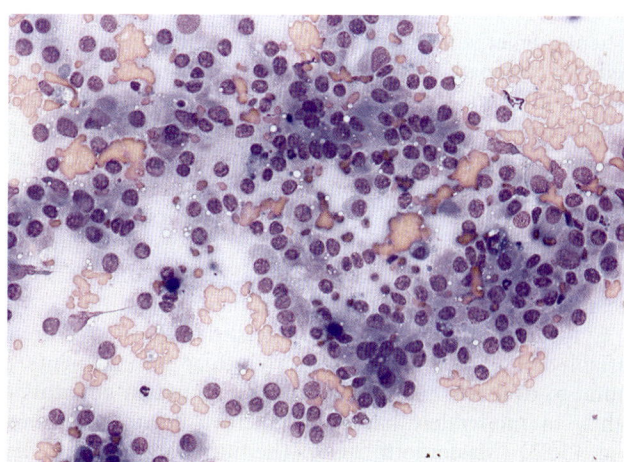

■ **FIGURE 13.80 Sertoli cell tumor. Testicle aspirate. Dog.** The tumor cells are arranged in loose sheets or trabeculae. The cytoplasm is lightly basophilic, and cell borders are often indistinct. Nuclei are round to oval, with slightly coarse nuclear chromatin and moderate nucleocytoplasmic ratios. (Wright-Giemsa; HP oil.)

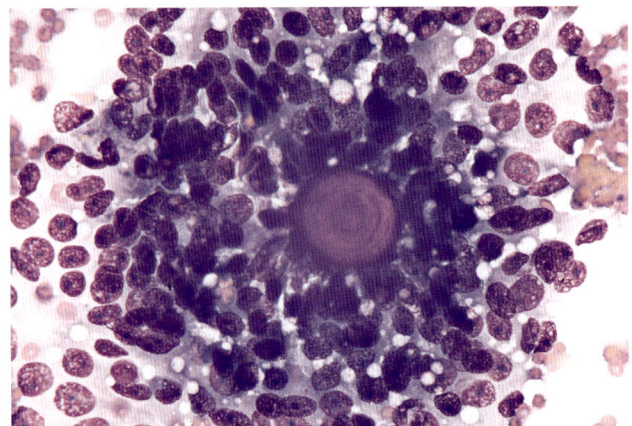

■ **FIGURE 13.81 Sertoli cell tumor. Testicle aspirate. Dog.** A Call-Exner body, a pseudorosette structure characterized by a dense aggregate of cells centered around amorphous eosinophilic extracellular dense material. (Wright-Giemsa; HP oil.)

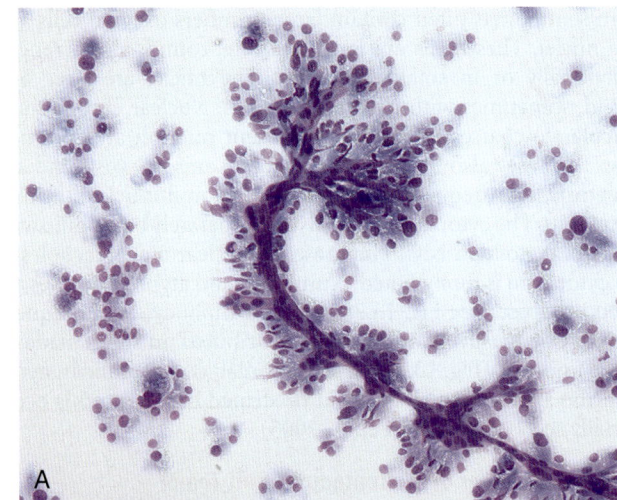

A

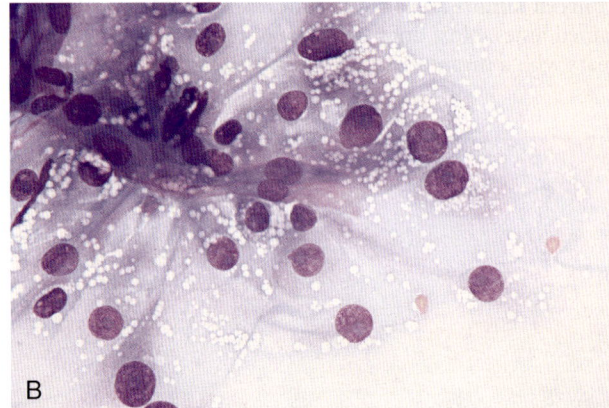

B

■ **FIGURE 13.83 Interstitial cell tumor. Tissue aspirate. Dog.** Same case in A and B. **A,** Perivascular arrangement of interstitial cells is a common finding in this testicular tumor. (Wright-Giemsa; IP.) **B,** Tumor cells display coarse nuclear chromatin, prominent, single nucleoli, and large amounts of moderately basophilic cytoplasm. The nuclei are often located at the periphery of the cell. Small punctate cytoplasmic vacuoles are present in the majority of the cells. (Wright-Giemsa; HP oil.)

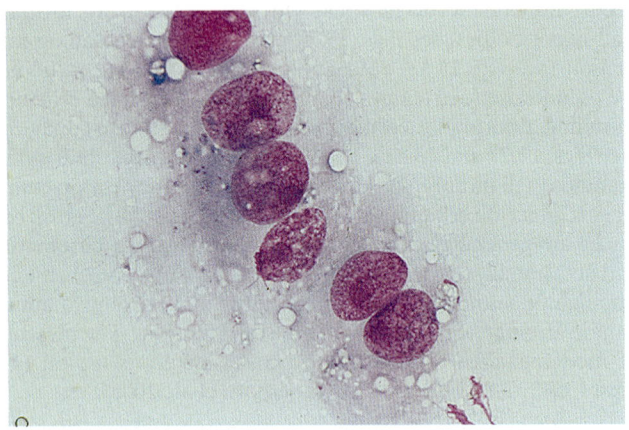

■ **FIGURE 13.82 Sertoli cell tumor. Testicle aspirate. Dog.** A row or palisading array of oval tumor cells is shown. Large cytoplasmic vacuoles are seen in several of the cells. (Wright-Giemsa; HP oil.)

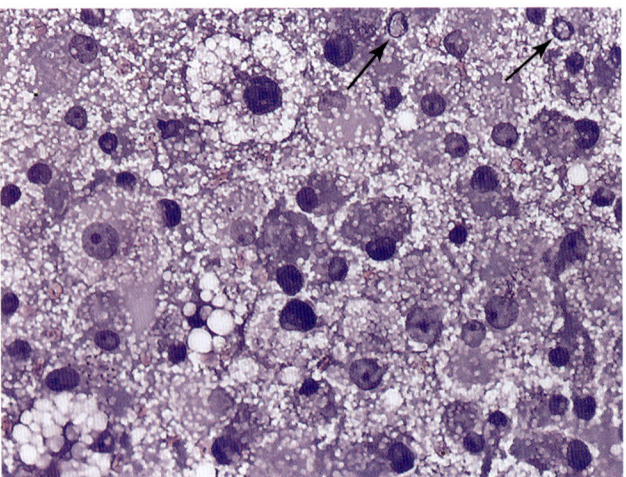

■ **FIGURE 13.84 Interstitial cell tumor. Tissue aspirate. Dog.** Several intact cells are present that have abundant microvacuolated cytoplasm. Note the two nuclei with pseudoinclusions *(arrows)* and the moderate anisokaryosis, which are both common features of interstitial cell tumors. (Wright; HP oil.) (Courtesy Rose Raskin, Purdue University.)

testicular enlargement; therefore, they are infrequently evaluated for cytopathologic analysis (Agnew and MacLachlan, 2017). This tumor is associated with increased production of testosterone and subsequently a high prevalence of prostatic disease and perianal gland neoplasms (McEntee, 2002). Cats with interstitial cell tumors often display tomcat behavior, such as aggression or spraying, or penile barbs (Doxsee et al., 2006). Interstitial tumors may rarely produce estrogen, resulting in myelosuppression and pancytopenia (Suess et al., 1992), and metastasize to the skin (de Lima Nascimento et al., 2019).

Cytopathologic samples from interstitial cell tumors are of variable cellularity. There are perivascular arrangements of round to oval cells that usually contain abundant amounts of lightly to moderately basophilic microvacuolated cytoplasm (Fig. 13.83) (Masserdotti, 2006). The nuclei are round to oval with fine, reticular chromatin and small, prominent nucleoli. The presence of nuclear pseudoinclusions is observed in half of the cases (Fig. 13.84). Moderate to marked anisokaryosis and variable N:C are seen. Numerous small, uniform cytoplasmic clear vacuoles are common (see Figs. 13.83B and 13.84). Dark, irregularly shaped cytoplasmic granules may be present in some cells (Masserdotti et al., 2005).

Semen Abnormalities

A detailed description of canine and feline semen collection and evaluation is not offered in this text, but in-depth reviews are available elsewhere (Freshman, 2002; Zambelli and Cunto, 2006; Axner and Linde Forsberg, 2007; Kolster, 2018). However, the cytopathologist is occasionally presented with seminal material from dogs or cats with infertility or suspected testicular or prostatic disease; thus, the ability to recognize certain abnormalities is useful. Gross evaluation, pH, and light microscopy such as concentration, motility, and morphology are routinely used to evaluate the principal parameters of dog and cat semen. Concentration is usually determined using a counting chamber. Aqueous Romanowsky or methanolic-Romanowsky stains are often used to assess sperm morphology. In high-quality semen, nearly all of the sperm should be of similar morphology. Spermatozoal abnormalities are considered as primary or secondary (Table 13.3). Primary abnormalities occur mostly during defective spermatogenesis and are therefore more serious. Secondary abnormalities may occur during passage through the epididymis (defective maturation) or during collection and preparation of the slide (see Table 13.3). Severe abnormalities include abnormal size or shape of the sperm head or acrosomal cap, proximal or midpiece protoplasmic droplets, and coiled tails (Figs. 13.85 to 13.87). Less severe abnormalities include detached, normal-appearing heads and bent tails (Fig. 13.88A; see also Fig. 13.87). Normal semen samples should have less than

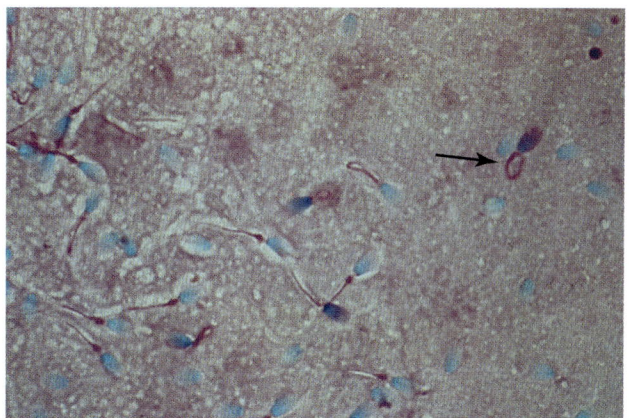

■ **FIGURE 13.86 Primary abnormalities. Semen smear. Dog.** Noninflammatory semen sample from a case of infertility. Against a heavy proteinaceous background, several sperm display tightly coiled tails *(arrow)* and proximal protoplasmic droplets. (Wright; HP oil.) (Courtesy Rose Raskin, University of Florida.)

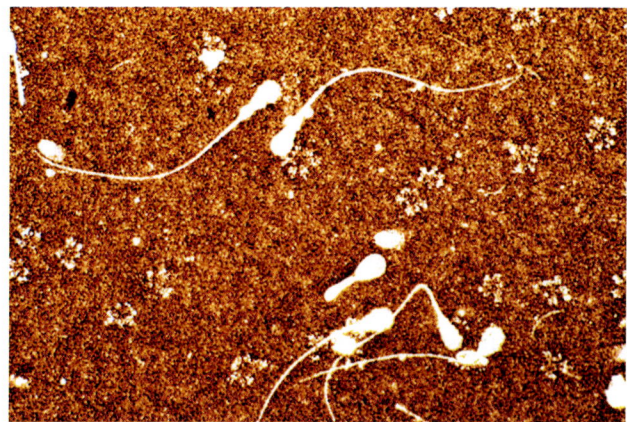

■ **FIGURE 13.87 Primary and secondary abnormalities. Semen smear. Dog.** Noninflammatory semen sample from a case of infertility. Sperm abnormalities include proximal protoplasmic droplets, coiled tails, and bent tails. (India ink; HP oil.) (Courtesy Rose Raskin, University of Florida.)

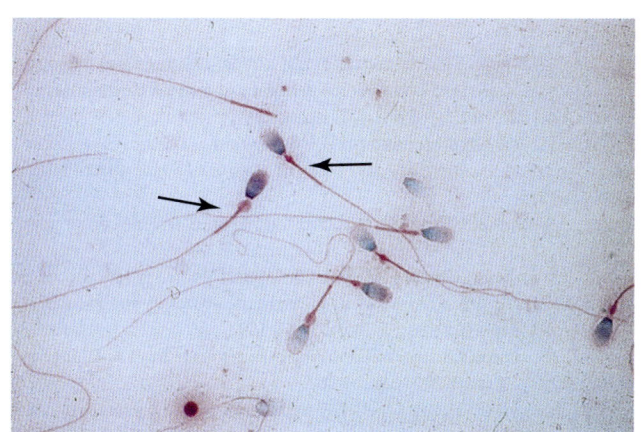

■ **FIGURE 13.85 Primary abnormalities. Semen smear. Dog.** Noninflammatory semen sample from a case of infertility. Sperm have prominent proximal protoplasmic droplets *(arrows)*. (Wright; HP oil.) (Courtesy Rose Raskin, University of Florida.)

10% primary abnormalities and less than 20% secondary abnormalities. Total canine and feline spermatozoal abnormalities should be less than 20% to 30% (Freshman, 2002).

Cytopathology of the sperm-rich and prostatic fractions should be evaluated separately by centrifuge or whole sample (less cellularity). Normal cytology of the sperm-rich fraction contains spermatozoa, white blood cells (WBCs; 2–4/hpf), epithelial cells, bacteria, and RBCs. Increased or degenerate

TABLE 13.3	Canine Spermatozoal Abnormalities	
LOCATION OF ABNORMALITY	**PRIMARY ABNORMALITIES**	**SECONDARY ABNORMALITIES**
Head	Pyriform, tapered, narrow, small (microcephaly), giant (macrocephaly), round, deformed, double heads, nuclear vacuoles	Detached head
Midpiece	Double and swollen midpiece and proximal droplet, pseudodroplet	Distal droplet, bowed midpiece (curved or rounded appearance of midpiece)
Tail	Tightly coiled and double tails	Bent, reverse, and distal coiled tails
Other	Teratoid forms	Released acrosome

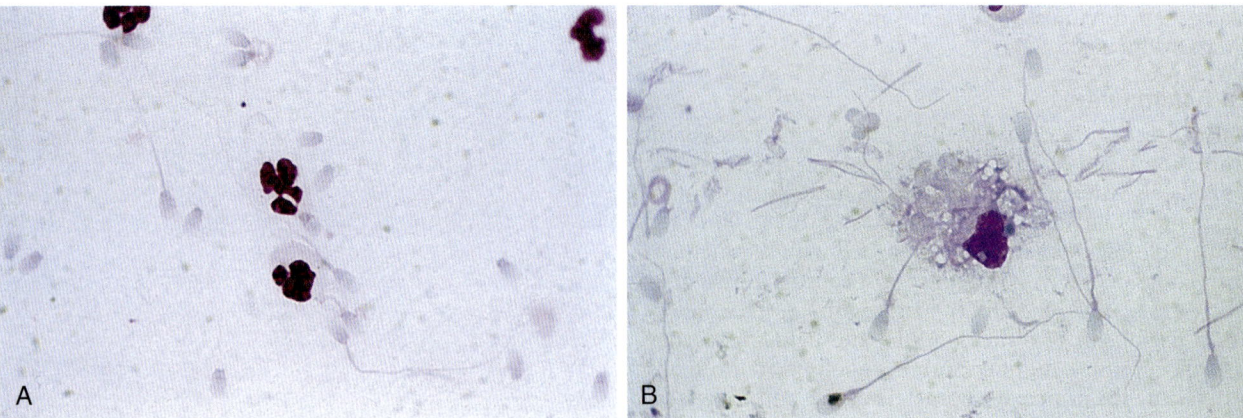

■ **FIGURE 13.88 Inflammation and abnormal sperm. Semen sample. Dog.** Same case in A and B. Ejaculate sample from an animal with intermittent preputial bleeding. **A,** Mildly degenerate neutrophils are present. Several morphologic secondary abnormalities of the sperm (detached heads, bent tails, and coiled tails) are also present. (Wright-Giemsa; HP oil.) **B,** A foamy macrophage and several relatively normal-appearing sperm. (Wright-Giemsa; HP oil.)

neutrophils or macrophages or intracellular bacteria indicate inflammation or infection (see Fig. 13.88). If neutrophils exhibit degenerative changes, a search for infectious organisms should be performed. However, culture of the fluid may be necessary for identification of pathogens related to the fact that 55% of clinically meaningful aerobic, anaerobic, or myoplasmic bacterial growth has noninflammatory seminal fluid cytology (Root Kustritz et al., 2006). Normal cytology of prostatic fluid is characterized by small amounts of epithelial cells, bacteria, and WBCs (2–4/hpf) (Freshman, 2002). Lower urinary tract inflammation and prostatitis should also be considered when inflammatory cells are present in semen. The presence of abnormal prostatic epithelium in the semen sample warrants further evaluation of the prostate gland.

Other miscellaneous tests exist to evaluate semen such as live-dead staining with eosin-nigrosin stains, hypo-osmotic swelling test, and measurement of components of seminal fluid. The most frequently used seminal markers are alkaline phosphatase (ALP) and carnitine. Both components originate from the epididymis in dogs and have the same application as markers of patency of ductal azoospermia. In a semen sample without sperm (azoospermia), measurement of seminal ALP or carnitine activity is essential in determining if the azoospermia is due to problems with libido, testicular failure, or ductal blockage. A low seminal ALP or carnitine activity indicates ductal blockage, whereas a normal seminal ALP or carnitine activity indicates testicular failure (Freshman, 2002; Kolster, 2018).

There are a few limitations of light microscopic methods, such as subjectivity and variability. Recently, several techniques have been described related to the capacity to reach, bind, penetrate, and fertilize an oocyte that may enable a more accurate prediction of the fertilizing capacity of semen sample. Conventional light microscopic semen assessment is being replaced by fluorescent staining techniques, computer-assisted sperm analysis systems, and flow cytometry (Kolster, 2018).

REFERENCES

Agnew DW, MacLachlan NJ. Tumors of the genital systems. In: Meuten DJ, ed. *Tumors in Domestic Animals*. 5th ed. Ames: John Wiley and Sons; 2017:689-722.

Alonge S, Melandri M, Aiudi G, et al. Advances in prostatic diagnostics in dogs: the role of canine prostatic specific esterase in the early diagnosis of prostatic disorders. *Top Companion Anim Med*. 2018;33:105-108.

Arlt SP, Haimerl P. Cystic ovaries and ovarian neoplasia in the female dog: a systematic review. *Reprod Domest Anim*. 2016;51(suppl 1):3-11.

Axner E, Linde Forsberg C. Sperm morphology in the domestic cat, and its relation with fertility: a retrospective study. *Reprod Domest Anim*. 2007; 42:282-291.

Ball RL, Birchard SJ, May LR, et al. Ovarian remnant syndrome in dogs and cats: 21 cases (2000-2007). *J Am Vet Med Assoc*. 2010;236:548-553.

Banco B, Antuofermo E, Borzacchiello G, et al. Canine ovarian tumors: an immunohistochemical study with HBME-1 antibody. *J Vet Diagn Invest*. 2011;23:977-981.

Bertazzolo W, Bonfanti U, Mazzotti S, et al. Cytologic features and diagnostic accuracy of analysis of effusions for detection of ovarian carcinoma in dogs. *Vet Clin Pathol*. 2012;41:127-132.

Bertazzolo W, Dell'Orco M, Bonfanti U, et al. Cytological features of canine ovarian tumours: a retrospective study of 19 cases. *J Small Anim Pract*. 2004;45:539-545.

Bokemeyer J, Peppler C, Thiel C, et al. Prostatic cavitary lesions containing urine in dogs. *J Small Anim Pract*. 2011;52:132-138.

Boland LE, Hardie RJ, Gregory SP, et al. Ultrasound-guided percutaneous drainage as the primary treatment for prostatic abscesses and cysts in dogs. *J Am Anim Hosp Assoc*. 2003;39:151-159.

Brazzell JL, Borjesson DL. Intra-abdominal mass aspirate from an alopecic dog. *Vet Clin Pathol*. 2006;35:259-262.

Bryan JN, Keeler MR, Henry CJ, et al. A population study of neutering status as a risk factor for canine prostate cancer. *Prostate*. 2007;67:1174-1181.

Canadas A, França M, Pereirea C, et al. Canine mammary tumors: comparison of classification and grading methods in a survival study. *Vet Pathol*. 2019; 56:208-219.

Chocteau F, Abadie J, Loussouarn D, et al. Proposal for a histological staging system of mammary carcinomas in dogs and cats. Part 1: canine mammary carcinomas. *Front Vet Sci*. 2019a;6:38.

Chocteau F, Boulay MM, Besnard F, et al. Proposal for a histological staging system of mammary carcinomas in dogs and cats. Part 2: feline mammary carcinomas. *Front Vet Sci*. 2019b6;387.

Choi US, Seo KW, Oh SY, et al. Intra-abdominal mass aspirate from a cat in heat. *Vet Clin Pathol*. 2005;34:275-277.

Ciaputa R, Nowak M, Madej JA, et al. Inhibin-α, E-cadherin, calretinin and Ki-67 antigen in the immunohistochemical evaluation of canine and human testicular neoplasms. *Folia Histochem Cytobiol*. 2014;52(4): 326-334.

Conversy B, Freulon AL, Graille M. Focal uterine T-cell lymphoma in an ovariectomized cat. *J Am Vet Med Assoc*. 2017;251:1059-1063.

Cunto M, Mariani E, Anicito Guido E, et al. Clinical approach to prostatic diseases in the dog. *Reprod Domest Anim.* 2019;54:815-822.

Dagher E, Abadie J, Loussouarn D, et al. Feline invasive mammary carcinomas: prognostic value of histological grading. *Vet Pathol.* 2019;56(5):660-670.

de Lima Nascimento HH, Tochetto C, Lucena RB, et al. Testicular interstitial cell tumor with disseminated cutaneous metastasis in a dog. *Acta Sci Vet.* 2019;47(suppl 1):434.

de M Souza CH, Toledo-Piza E, Amorin R, et al. Inflammatory mammary carcinoma in 12 dogs: clinical features, cyclooxygenase-2 expression, and response to piroxicam treatment. *Can Vet J.* 2009;50:506-510.

Demirel MA. A case of spontaneous abortion related to ovarian endometriosis in a golden retriever dog. *Iran J Vet Res.* 2017;18:63-66.

Ditmyer H, Craig L. Mycotic mastitis in three dogs due to *Blastomyces dermatitidis*. *J Am Anim Hosp Assoc.* 2011;47:356-358.

Dolka I, Czopowicz M, Gruk-Jurka A, et al. Diagnostic efficacy of smear cytology and Robinson's cytological grading of canine mammary tumors with respect to histopathology, cytomorphometry, metastases and overall survival. *PLoS One.* 2018;13:e0191595.

Doxsee AL, Yager JA, Best SJ, et al. Extratesticular interstitial and Sertoli cell tumors in previously neutered dogs and cats: a report of 17 cases. *Can Vet J.* 2006;47:763-766.

Feldman EC, Nelson RW. Ovarian cycle and vaginal cytology. In: Feldman EC, Nelson RW, eds. *Canine and Feline Endocrinology and Reproduction*. St. Louis: Elsevier; 2004:752-775.

Fernandes PJ, Guyer C, Modiano JF. What is your diagnosis? Mammary mass aspirate from a Yorkshire terrier. *Vet Clin Pathol.* 1998;27(79):91.

Foster RA. Female reproductive system and mammae. In: Zachary JF, ed. *Pathologic Basis of Veterinary Disease*. 6th ed. St. Louis: Elsevier; 2017a:1147-1193.

Foster RA. Male reproductive system and mammae. In: Zachary JF, ed. *Pathologic Basis of Veterinary Disease*. 6th ed. St. Louis: Elsevier; 2017b:1194-1222.

Freshman JL. Semen collection and evaluation. *Clin Tech Small Anim Pract.* 2002;17:104-107.

Ganguly B, Das U, Das AK. Canine transmissible venereal tumour: a review. *Vet Comp Oncol.* 2016;14:1-12.

Giménez F, Hecht S, Craig LE, et al. Early detection, aggressive therapy: optimizing the management of feline mammary masses. *J Feline Med Surg.* 2010;12:214-224.

Goldschmidt M, Peña L, Rasotto R, et al. Classification and grading of canine mammary tumors. *Vet Pathol.* 2011;48:117-131.

Goldschmidt MH, Peña L, Zappulli V. Tumors of the mammary gland. In: Meuten DJ, ed: *Tumors in Domestic Animals*. 5th ed. Ames: John Wiley & Sons, Inc; 2017:723-765.

Gorman ME, Bildfell R, Seguin B. What is your diagnosis? Peritoneal fluid from a 1-year-old female German shepherd dog. *Vet Clin Pathol.* 2010;39:393-394.

Grandi F, Colodel MM, Monteiro LN, et al. Extramedullary hematopoiesis in a case of benign mixed mammary tumor in a female dog: cytological and histopathological assessment. *BMC Vet Res.* 2010;6:45.

Groppetti D, Pecile A, Arrighi S, et al. Endometrial cytology and computerized morphometric analysis of epithelial nuclei: a useful tool for reproductive diagnosis in the bitch. *Theriogenology.* 2010;73:927-941.

Hagman R. Pyometra in small animals. *Vet Clin North Am Small Anim Pract.* 2018;48:639-661.

Hohšteter M, Artuković B, Severin K, et al. Canine testicular tumors: two types of seminomas can be differentiated by immunohistochemistry. *BMC Vet Res.* 2014;10:169.

Hori Y, Uechi M, Kanakubo K, et al. Canine ovarian serous papillary adenocarcinoma with neoplastic hypercalcemia. *J Vet Med Sci.* 2006;68:979-982.

Kaszak I, Ruszczak A, Kanafa S, et al. Current biomarkers of canine mammary tumors. *Acta Vet Scand.* 2018;60:66.

Knauf Y, Köhler K, Knauf S, et al. Histological classification of canine ovarian cyst types with reference to medical history. *J Vet Sci.* 2018;19:725-734.

Ko JS, Kim HJ, Han S, Do SH. Primary lymphoma of the uterine horn in a Lhasa Apso dog. *Ir Vet J.* 2013;66:24.

Kolster KA. Evaluation of canine sperm and management of semen disorders. *Vet Clin North Am Small Anim Pract.* 2018;48:533-545.

Leidinger E, Hooijberg E, Sick K, et al. Fibroepithelial hyperplasia in an entire male cat: cytologic and histopathological features. *Tierarztl Prax Ausg K Kleintiere Heimtiere.* 2011;39:198-202.

Maksimović A, Maksimović Z, Filipović S, et al. Vaginal and uterine bacteria of healthy bitches during different stages of their reproductive cycle. *Vet Rec.* 2012;171:375.

Manuali E, Eleni C, Giovannini P, et al. Unusual finding in a nipple discharge of a female dog: dirofilariasis of the breast. *Diagn Cytopathol.* 2005;32:108-109.

Masserdotti C. Architectural patterns in cytology: correlation with histology. *Vet Clin Pathol.* 2006;35:388-396.

Masserdotti C, Bonfanti U, De Lorenzi D, et al. Cytologic features of testicular tumours in dog. *J Vet Med A Physiol Pathol Clin Med.* 2005;52:339-346.

Masserdotti C, De Lorenzi D, Gasparotto L. Cytologic detection of Call-Exner bodies in Sertoli cell tumors from 2 dogs. *Vet Clin Pathol.* 2008;37:112-114.

McCourt MR, Dieterly AM, Mackey PE, et al. Complex mammary carcinoma with metastases to lymph nodes, subcutaneous tissue, and multiple joints in a dog. *Vet Clin Pathol.* 2018;47:477-483.

McEntee MC. Reproductive oncology. *Clin Tech Small Anim Pract.* 2002;17:133-149.

Meichner K, Montgomery SA, Borst LB, et al. Pathology in practice: extratesticular cutaneous Sertoli cell tumor in a dog. *J Am Vet Med Assoc.* 2016;249:1023-1026.

Mesher CI. What is your diagnosis? A 14-month old domestic cat. *Vet Clin Pathol.* 1997;26:4.

Millanta F, Verin R, Asproni P, et al. A case of feline primary inflammatory mammary carcinoma: clinicopathological and immunohistochemical findings. *J Feline Med Surg.* 2012;14:420-423.

Miller MA, Kottler SJ, Cohn LA, et al. Mammary duct ectasia in dogs: 51 cases (1992–1999). *J Am Vet Med Assoc.* 2001;218(8):1303-1307.

Miller MA, Ramos-Vara JA, Dickerson MF, et al. Uterine neoplasia in 13 cats. *J Vet Diagn Invest.* 2003;15:515-522.

Mills JM, Valli VE, Lumsden JH. Cyclical changes of vaginal cytology in the cat. *Can Vet J.* 1979;20:95-101.

Mills SW, Musil KM, Davies JL, et al. Prognostic value of histologic grading for feline mammary carcinoma: a retrospective survival analysis. *Vet Pathol.* 2015;52(2):238-249.

Neihaus SA, Winter JE, Goring RL, et al. Primary clitoral adenocarcinoma with secondary hypercalcemia of malignancy in a dog. *J Am Anim Hosp Assoc.* 2010;46:193-196.

Olson PN, Thrall MA, Wykes PM, et al. Vaginal cytology: part I. A useful tool for staging the canine estrous cycle. *Compend Contin Educ Pract.* 1984;6:288-297.

Owston MA, Ramos-Vara JA. Histologic and immunohistochemical characterization of a testicular mixed germ cell sex cord-stromal tumor and a Leydig cell tumor in a dog. *Vet Pathol.* 2007;44:936-943.

Palmieri C, Foster RA, Grieco V, et al. Histopathological terminology standards for the reporting of prostatic epithelial lesions in dogs. *J Comp Pathol.* 2019a;171:30-37.

Palmieri C, Hood G, Fonseca-Alves CE, et al. An immunohistochemical study of T and B lymphocyte density in prostatic hyperplasia and prostate carcinoma in dogs. *Res Vet Sci.* 2019b;122:189-192.

Park CH, Ikadai H, Yoshida E, et al. Cutaneous toxoplasmosis in a female Japanese cat. *Vet Pathol.* 2007;44:683-687.

Park MS, Kim Y, Kang MS, et al. Disseminated transmissible venereal tumor in a dog. *J Vet Diagn Invest.* 2006;18:130-133.

Peña L, De Andrés PJ, Clemente M, et al. Prognostic value of histological grading in noninflammatory canine mammary carcinomas in a prospective study with two-year follow-up: relationship with clinical and histological characteristics. *Vet Pathol.* 2013;50:94-105.

Peña L, Gama A, Goldschmidt MH, et al. Canine mammary tumors: a review and consensus of standard guidelines on epithelial and myoepithelial phenotype markers, HER2, and hormone receptor assessment using immunohistochemistry. *Vet Pathol.* 2014;51:127-145.

Piech TL, Chu S, Bozynski CC, et al. Pathology in practice: clitoral adenocarcinoma in a dog. *J Am Vet Med Assoc*. 2019;254(10):1167-1170.

Pinto da Cunha N, Ghisleni G, Romussi S, et al. Prostatic sarcomatoid carcinoma in a dog: cytologic and immunohistochemical findings. *Vet Clin Pathol*. 2007;36:368-372.

Piseddu E, Masserdotti C, Milesi C, et al. Cytologic features of normal canine ovaries in different stages of estrus with histologic comparison. *Vet Clin Pathol*. 2012;41:396-404.

Powe JR, Canfield PJ, Martin PA. Evaluation of the cytologic diagnosis of canine prostatic disorders. *Vet Clin Pathol*. 2004;33:150-154.

Ramos-Vara JA, Miller MA. Immunohistochemical evaluation of GATA-4 in canine testicular tumors. *Vet Pathol*. 2009;46:893-896.

Rasotto R, Berlato D, Goldschmidt MH, et al. Prognostic significance of canine mammary tumor histologic subtypes: an observational cohort study of 229 cases. *Vet Pathol*. 2017;54:571-578.

Reed LT, Balog KA, Boes KM, et al. Pathology in practice: granulomatous pneumonia, prostatitis and uveitis with intralesional yeasts consistent with *Blastomyces*. *J Am Vet Med Assoc*. 2010;236:411-413.

Rehm S, Stanislaus DJ, Williams AM. Estrous cycle-dependent histology and review of sex steroid receptor expression in dog reproductive tissues and mammary gland and associated hormone levels. *Birth Defects Res B Dev Reprod Toxicol*. 2007;80:233-245.

Riccardi E, Greco V, Verganti S, et al. Immunohistochemical diagnosis of canine ovarian epithelial and granulosa cell tumors. *J Vet Diagn Invest*. 2007;19:431-435.

Root Kustritz MV. Collection of tissue and culture samples from the canine reproductive tract. *Theriogenology*. 2006;66:567-574.

Root Kustritz MV. Managing the reproductive cycle in the bitch. *Vet Clin North Am Small Anim Pract*. 2012;42:423-437.

Rout ED, Hoon-Hanks LL, Gustafson TL, et al. What is your diagnosis? Clitoral mass in a dog. *Vet Clin Pathol*. 2016;45(1):197-198.

Saba CF, Lawrence JA. Tumors of the female reproductive system. In: Withrow SJ, Vail DM, Page RL, eds. *Withrow & MacEwen's Small Animal Clinical Oncology*. 5th ed. St Louis: Elsevier; 2013:532-537.

Saba CF, Rogers KS, Newman SJ, et al. Mammary gland tumors in male dogs. *J Vet Intern Med*. 2007;21:1056-1059.

Salas Y, Márquez A, Diaz D, et al. Epidemiological study of mammary tumors in female dogs diagnosed during the period 2002-2012: a growing animal health problem. *PLoS One*. 2015;10(5):e0127381.

Salgado BS, Monteiro LN, Grandi F, et al. What is your diagnosis? Ascites fluid from a dog with abdominal distension. *Vet Clin Pathol*. 2012;41:605-606.

Samuelson DA. *Textbook of Veterinary Histology*. St. Louis: Elsevier; 2007: 442-485.

Santos AA, Matos AJ. Advances in the understanding of the clinically relevant genetic pathways and molecular aspects of canine mammary tumours. Part 2: invasion, angiogenesis, metastasis and therapy. *Vet J*. 2015;205:144-153.

Simeonov R, Simeonova G. Computerized morphometry of mean nuclear diameter and nuclear roundness in canine mammary gland tumors on cytologic smears. *Vet Clin Pathol*. 2006a;35:88-90.

Simeonov R, Simeonova G. Fractal dimension of canine mammary gland epithelial tumors on cytologic smears. *Vet Clin Pathol*. 2006b;35:446-448.

Simon D, Schoenrock D, Nolte I, et al. Cytologic examination of fine-needle aspirates from mammary gland tumors in the dog: diagnostic accuracy with comparison to histopathology and association with postoperative outcome. *Vet Clin Pathol*. 2009;38:521-528.

Skeldon N, Spoor M, Klaassen J, et al. What is your diagnosis? Cystic ovarian structure in a dog. *Vet Clin Pathol*. 2018;47:667-669.

Smith J. Canine prostatic disease: a review of anatomy, pathology, diagnosis, and treatment. *Theriogenology*. 2008;70:375-383.

Sontas BH, Yüzbaşıoğlu Öztürk G, Toydemir TF, et al. Fine-needle aspiration biopsy of canine mammary gland tumours: a comparison between cytology and histopathology. *Reprod Domest Anim*. 2012;47:125-130.

Sorenmo KU, Worley DR, Goldschmidt MH. Tumors of the mammary gland. In: Withrow SJ, Vail DM, Page R, eds. *Withrow & MacEwen's Small Animal Clinical Oncology*. 5th ed. St. Louis: Elsevier; 2013:538-556.

Suess Jr RP, Barr SC, Sacre BJ, et al. Bone marrow hypoplasia in a feminized dog with an interstitial cell tumor. *J Am Vet Med Assoc*. 1992;200:1346-1348.

Verin R, Cian F, Stewart J, et al. Canine clitoral carcinoma: a clinical, cytologic, histopathologic, immunohistochemical, and ultrastructural study. *Vet Pathol*. 2018;55(4):501-509.

Yu CH, Hwang DN, Yhee JY, et al. Comparative immunohistochemical characterization of canine seminomas and Sertoli cell tumors. *J Vet Sci*. 2009;10(1):1-7.

Zambelli D, Cunto M. Semen collection in cats: techniques and analysis. *Theriogenology*. 2006;66:159-165.

Zappulli V, Peña L, Rastottoe R, et al. Mammary tumors. In: Kiupel M, ed. *Surgical Pathology of Tumors of Domestic Animals*. Vol 2. Washington, DC: Davis-Thompson DVM Foundation; 2019:1-268.

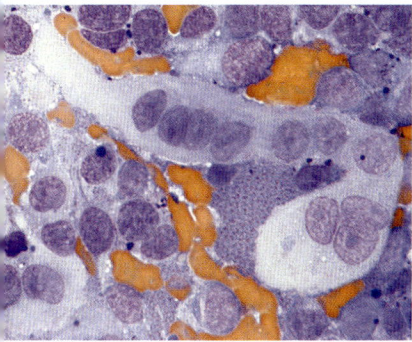

CHAPTER 14

Musculoskeletal System

Anne M. Barger

Lameness is the cardinal clinical sign associated with disease of the musculoskeletal system. Other signs include stiffness, ataxia, weakness, pain, fever, limb and joint swelling, and deformity. Depending on the type of disorder, other organ systems may also be involved, including neurologic, endocrine, urologic, hemolymphatic, digestive, respiratory, and cardiovascular systems; thus, an animal with musculoskeletal disease may present with a variety of problems and signs.

Cytopathology may be a component of the workup in an animal with a suspected musculoskeletal disorder. Materials that may be sampled include synovial fluid as well as fine-needle aspirates of soft tissue masses involving muscle or proliferative or lytic lesions of the bone. Cytopathologic evaluation alone is rarely the sole diagnostic test necessary to completely define a musculoskeletal problem. Other important information includes signalment, history, physical examination, radiographs, complete blood count, and biochemistry. In addition, many lesions will require histopathology for definitive characterization. Some types of muscle, bone, and joint disease cause changes that cannot be detected by cytopathologic methods.

NORMAL JOINT ANATOMY AND SYNOVIAL FLUID PRODUCTION

The articular joints have outer fibrous tissue that attaches to bone enclosing and stabilizing the joint. The innermost tissue is called the synovial membrane (Fig. 14.1). Except for the articular cartilage surface, this thin discontinuous villous membrane covers the inner surface of the joint. The inner surface of this layer may be flat or contain tiny villi. The synovial intimal or lining cells may be up to four cells thick and consist of two cell types, A and B. Type A cells are histiocytes, which remove debris or hemorrhage. Type B are fibroblast-like cells, which are secretory and produce synovial fluid (Carlson and Weisbrode, 2012). Normal synovial fluid is composed of hyaluronic acid, lubricin (a water-soluble glycoprotein), proteinases, and collagenase. Along with lubrication of joint surfaces, the synovial fluid provides oxygen and nutrients to chondrocytes in the articular cartilage and removes their wastes. Below the surface of the membrane are blood and lymph vessels along with variable amounts of adipose tissue (Carlson and Weisbrode, 2012).

SYNOVIAL FLUID EVALUATION

Synovial fluid analysis is a part of the minimum database when assessing an animal for joint disease. It is important to recognize that evaluation of the synovial fluid is only a component of the workup, and the findings must be integrated with other clinical and laboratory findings, including appropriate ancillary diagnostic tests (e.g., culture, serology, antinuclear antibody titer, rheumatoid factor [RF] titer, imaging). Nevertheless, when an animal has suspected joint disease, synovial fluid evaluation is a critical component in determining the cause.

As with other body cavity effusions, a complete fluid analysis is helpful when evaluating synovial fluid. Routine synovial fluid analysis should include evaluation of color, transparency, protein concentration, viscosity, mucin clot test, nucleated cell count, differential, and cytopathologic evaluation. These tests are discussed in further detail later in this chapter. Reference values for synovial fluid from healthy dogs and cats are shown in Box 14.1. If the sample volume is limited, the most important component of analysis is the cytopathology. In that case, a direct smear of a drop of fluid is spread onto a slide and stained for evaluation. Typical results for different kinds of joint disease are shown in Table 14.1.

Sample Collection and Handling

Collection of synovial fluid varies to some degree depending on the joint sampled. Descriptions of approaches to various joints have been described. In general, collection of synovial fluid requires the following materials: 3 to 6 mL syringe, 18- to 22-gauge 1-inch needles, and red-top and lavender-top tubes. The amount of restraint and necessary levels of sedation and anesthesia vary from animal to animal. Enough restraint should be used to minimize struggling during collection. In general, many animals require at least some degree of sedation or anesthesia. Sterile technique is critical when preparing the site and during aspiration. The fur should be clipped and the area of aspiration scrubbed. Care should be taken not to scratch the articular surface during needle insertion. Use the needle alone or attached to a syringe during joint penetration, whichever is easiest for needle insertion. Palpation and slight flexion or hyperextension of the joint help to identify insertion points of the needle. The location of aspiration varies with the joint aspirated. The coxofemoral joint can be aspirated cranioproximal to the trochanter major and slightly ventral and caudal. The stifle should be left at ease or lightly flexed when aspirated. Aspiration can occur medial or lateral to the patellar ligament, midway between the tibia and femur. The tarsocrural joint can be aspirated by hyperextending the joint and inserting the needle lateral or medial to the fibular tarsal bone. To aspirate the shoulder, insert the needle 1 cm distal and slightly caudal to

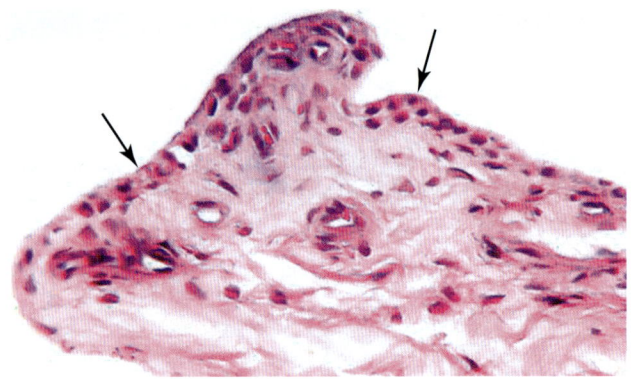

■ **FIGURE 14.1 Synovial membrane. Joint. Histology. Dog.** The normal synovial membrane *(arrows)* consists of an incomplete layer of histiocytes (phagocytic cells) and fibrocytes with subjacent loose fibrous and/or fibrofatty tissue. The joint lumen is at the top of the figure. (H&E; IP.) (From Zachary JF. *Pathologic Basis of Veterinary Disease.* 5th ed. Philadelphia: Elsevier; 2012.)

BOX 14.1 Normal Synovial Fluid Characteristics

Clear to straw colored
Protein <2.5 g/dL (also cited as 1.5–3.0 g/dL)
pH 7 to –7.8
Viscosity: 2 cm in string test
Mucin clot: good (tight clot formation)
Cell count <3000/μL in dogs, <1000/μL in cats
Neutrophils <5%
Mononuclear cells >95% (small: lymphocytes; large: macrophages and fibroblastic synoviocytes)
Quantity: Only a small amount should be present (<0.5 mL in most joints)

---

the acromion process. The elbow should be hyperextended and the needle inserted lateral and alongside the olecranon. The carpal joints can be simply aspirated by flexing the joint and palpating the joint space. The needle should be advanced slowly through the joint capsule into the joint cavity. The amount of fluid withdrawn depends on the size of animal and joint as well as the amount of effusion present. Synovial fluid will be aspirated easily if there is a significant effusion, but a few drops may be obtained from joints without an increase in synovial fluid volume. Before removing the needle from the synovial cavity, the plunger should be released to remove any negative pressure. Normal synovial fluid has a gel-like consistency that should not be mistaken for a clot. The gel-like consistency becomes less viscous when shaken and returns to the original viscosity upon standing; this property is referred to as *thixotropy*. Clotting is likely to occur if there is significant blood contamination, and inflamed joints may form fibrin precipitates or clots. For these reasons, some joint fluid should be put into an ethylenediaminetetraacetic acid (EDTA) tube (lavender-top tube). EDTA interferes with tests such as the mucin clot test and culturing. The synovial fluid should be refrigerated if not being immediately evaluated. For samples that may be cultured based on the cytopathologic findings, the fluid should be put into a red-top tube, left in the sterile syringe, or placed in an aerobic Culturette. There are advocates of putting fluid in blood culture media to improve the chances for bacterial growth. The laboratory should be contacted for their recommendations. In many smaller animals, only one or two drops of joint fluid can be obtained. In these cases, immediate preparation of direct smears is the critical component of sample management (see Chapter 1). Regardless of the amount of fluid collected, it usually is advantageous to make direct smears immediately to best preserve cell morphology. These slides should not be refrigerated before staining.

Appearance and Viscosity

Normal joint fluid is typically present in small amounts (<0.5 mL) and is clear to straw colored (Fig. 14.2). Red-tinged fluid indicates hemorrhage or peripheral blood contamination. True hemorrhage is uniformly discolored throughout aspiration, whereas peripheral blood contamination often occurs at the end of aspiration. This may appear as a red tail or wisp in the fluid. The fluid should be viscous as evidenced by stringiness when suspended between fingertips, touched by an applicator stick, or expelled from the syringe (see Fig. 14.2). The fluid viscosity is related to the concentration and quality of hyaluronic acid. Normal synovial fluid has good viscosity and demonstrates thixotropy (see earlier discussion).

Healthy synovial fluid should be viscous because of the production of mucin. The mucin clot test semiquantitatively

---

TABLE 14.1 Classification of Abnormal Synovial Fluid

	HEMARTHROSIS	NONSUPPURATIVE ARTHROPATHY	SUPPURATIVE ARTHROPATHY
Appearance	Red, cloudy, or xanthochromia	Clear	Cloudy
Protein	Increased	Normal to decreased	Normal to increased
Viscosity	Decreased	Normal to decreased	Normal to decreased
Mucin clot	Normal to poor	Normal to poor	Fair to poor
Cell count	Increased nucleated cells; red blood cells	1000–10,000/μL	5000 to >100,000/μL
Neutrophils	Similar to blood	<10%	>10%–100%
Mononuclear cells	Similar to blood	>90% (both lymphocytes and large mononuclear cells)	10% to <90%
Comments	Erythrophagia or hemosiderin helps confirm hemorrhage	Synoviocytes are present along with macrophages in thick sheets	Septic and nonseptic etiologies; bacteria are rarely observed in infected joints; however, culture is recommended

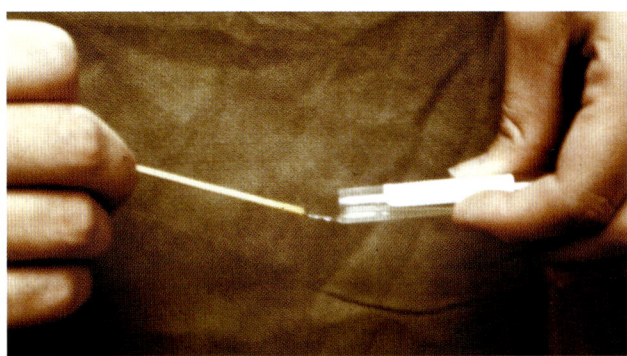

■ **FIGURE 14.2 Synovial fluid viscosity test.** A string of viscous material from normal synovial fluid should measure about 2 cm in length when touched with an applicator stick before it snaps apart. (Courtesy Rose Raskin, University of Florida.)

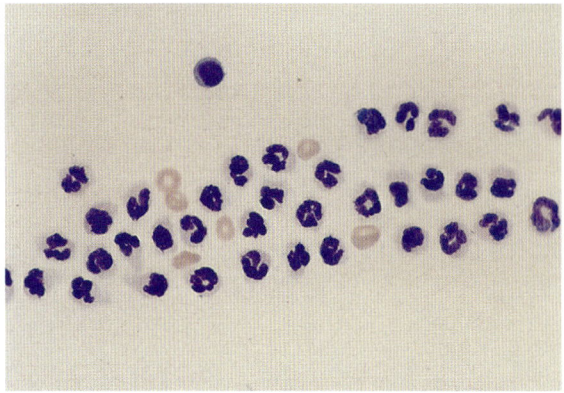

■ **FIGURE 14.4 Synovial fluid windrowing. Fluid aspirate.** The cells in this figure are found in rows, referred to as *windrowing*, which is commonly seen in fluids with increased viscosity or increased protein concentration. Inflamed joints may have decreased viscosity macroscopically but prominent windrowing of cells microscopically. (Wright; HP oil.)

assesses the amount and degree of polymerization of hyaluronic acid in the joint fluid. Because EDTA interferes with this test, heparin can be used if an anticoagulant is required before performing this test. One to two drops of undiluted joint fluid are added to 4 to 8 drops of 2% acetic acid. In a sample with normal hyaluronic acid concentration and quality, a thick, ropy clot will form (Fig. 14.3). As the amount or quality of hyaluronic acid decreases in various forms of joint disease, the mucin clot is less well formed. This test is typically interpreted as good, fair, or poor. Normal joints have good mucin clot results.

The direct smear of the synovial fluid should also be evaluated for the presence of windrowing. In a viscous sample, the cells often line up in rows (Fig. 14.4) or windrows that resemble the arrangement of cut hay. Mucinous material can be identified in the background of the direct smears as eosinophilic granular material (Figs. 14.5 and 14.6) or sometimes as

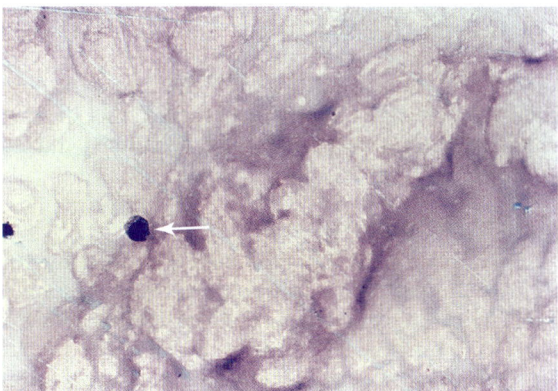

■ **FIGURE 14.5 Synovial fluid granular background. Fluid aspirate.** Normal synovial fluid has low nucleated cell numbers with a thick, granular to ropy background material separating the cells. The granular background is related to the mucin content of the fluid. The low cellularity generally means that fewer than one or two small to medium-sized mononuclear cells are seen on high-power examination *(arrow).* (Wright; IP.)

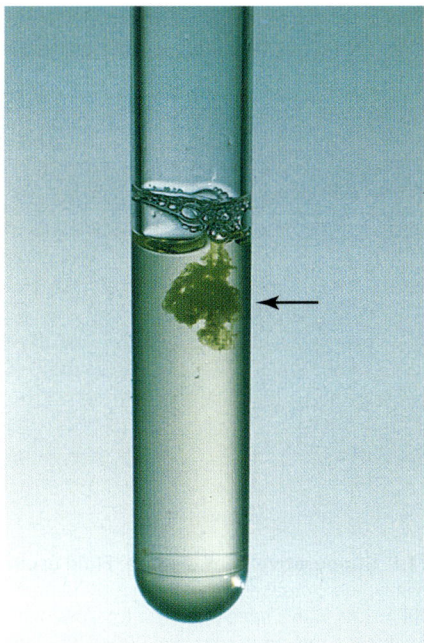

■ **FIGURE 14.3 Synovial fluid mucin clot test.** This sample is from a normal joint. The mucin clot is thick and ropy *(arrow)*, indicating good mucin content and quality. (Courtesy Dr. Sonjia Shelly.)

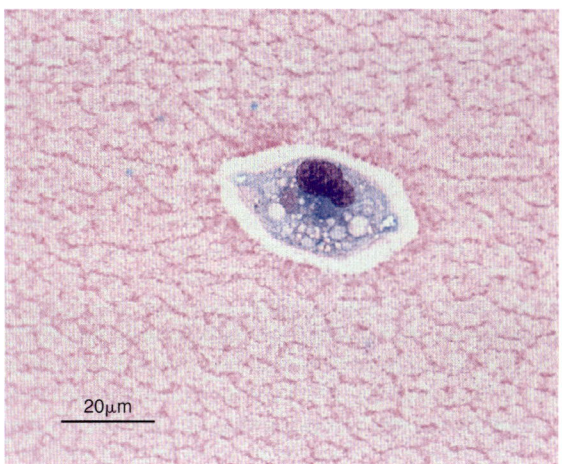

■ **FIGURE 14.6 Synoviocyte against granular background. Fluid aspirate. Dog.** A single synovial cavity-lining cell is present against the normal granular eosinophilic mucin material that is typical of normal synovial fluid. This dog had a degenerative joint condition with normal viscosity. (Wright; HP oil.) (Courtesy Rose Raskin, Purdue University.)

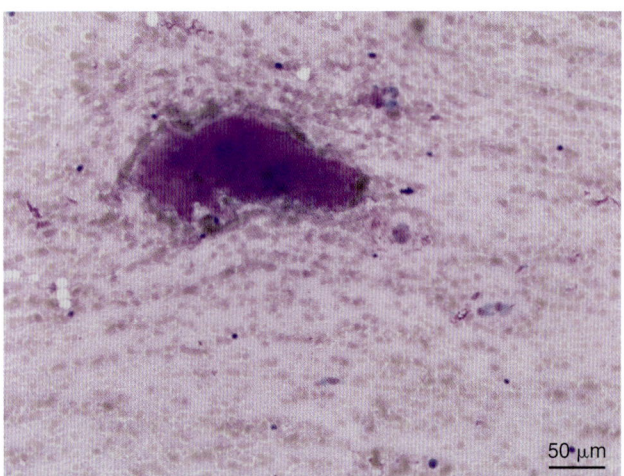

FIGURE 14.7 **Cartilage fragment and windrowing. Stifle joint. synovial fluid. Fluid aspirate. Dog.** Dense magenta staining articular cartilage fragment appears against a background of erythrocyte windrowing. Nucleated cellularity is within normal reference interval. (Wright-Giemsa; IP.) (Courtesy Rose Raskin, University of Florida.)

proteinaceous crescents. Occasional small flecks of magenta amorphous cartilage may be normally aspirated during the procedure (Fig. 14.7).

Cell Counts and Differential

Cell counts and the differential count are done by routine methods. If enough fluid is present, cell counts can be made using a hemocytometer. Some reference laboratories use automated cell counters for cell enumeration. Automated cell counters tend to give a higher cell count than the hemocytometer; however, the difference is not usually great enough to affect the clinical interpretation. The cells may occur in clumps, and accurate assessment of cell numbers may be difficult. In an effort to minimize cell clumping, hyaluronidase can be added to the synovial fluid. Various methods have been described. The easiest procedure is to add a small amount of hyaluronidase powder (amount adherent to an applicator stick) directly into the sample tube, which may result in more accurate cell counts. If only slides are prepared, cell numbers can be roughly estimated by counting the number of cells per low-power field (10×) and multiplying the count by 100 to give an approximate number per microliter. However, estimates from smears are less accurate and tend to be higher than counts from automated counters. Normal joints have low nucleated cell numbers, usually fewer than 3000 cells/μL in dogs and 1000 cells/μL in cats (Pacchiana et al., 2004), although more typically the count is fewer than 500 cells/μL in both species. These counts may vary slightly based on breed, age, body weight, and joint sampled. Consequently, only one to two cells per high-power field (40×) will be observed depending on the thickness of the direct smear (see Fig. 14.5). Gibson et al. (1999) demonstrated the variability in performing these estimates by a group of clinicians on synovial fluid. Cells commonly observed in synovial fluid include lymphocytes, macrophages (*clasmatocytes*), neutrophils, and occasionally synovial lining cells that produce glycosaminoglycans. Neutrophils typically account for less than 5% to 10% of nucleated cells in normal joints. If fluid is obtained, both direct smears and concentrated preparations can be evaluated. If available, a cytocentrifuge is useful in preparing concentrated preparations. Concentrated preparations can also be prepared by centrifuging the fluid, pouring of the supernatant, and resuspending the fluid in one or two drops of supernatant. Smears can then be prepared from this concentrated preparation. Concentrated preparations are useful in synovial fluid, particularly if the cell count is low (<500 cells/μL).

Protein Concentration

Protein concentration is often measured by refractometry, which usually provides a value that is useful for routine clinical classification and interpretation of the synovial fluid. The most accurate measurement of protein requires chemical methods. Normal synovial fluid generally has a low protein concentration (<2.5 g/dL), commonly between 1.5 and 3.0 g/dL (MacWilliams and Friedrichs, 2003) but can be as high as 4.8 g/dL (Fernandez et al., 1983). Protein concentration increases with inflammatory disease, including immune-mediated polyarthritis (Murakami et al., 2015). False increases in protein can occur with EDTA, especially if a short sample is submitted or if the patient has received an intraarticular injection.

Classification of Joint Disease

The primary goal in synovial fluid evaluation is to distinguish suppurative joint disease from nonsuppurative joint disease (see Table 14.1). Other types of joint disease that may be distinguished include hemarthrosis and neoplastic disease. Further defining the disease process, as noted earlier, requires integrating the synovial fluid findings with other historical, physical, and laboratory findings, including imaging techniques. It is important to note that synovial fluid analysis alone rarely differentiates or identifies the specific cause from among the multiple etiologic factors involved in suppurative and nonsuppurative joint diseases.

Suppurative Joint Disease

Suppurative joint disease is characterized by increased numbers of white blood cells, particularly neutrophils, in the joint fluid (Fig. 14.8). Absolute numbers of segmented neutrophils are

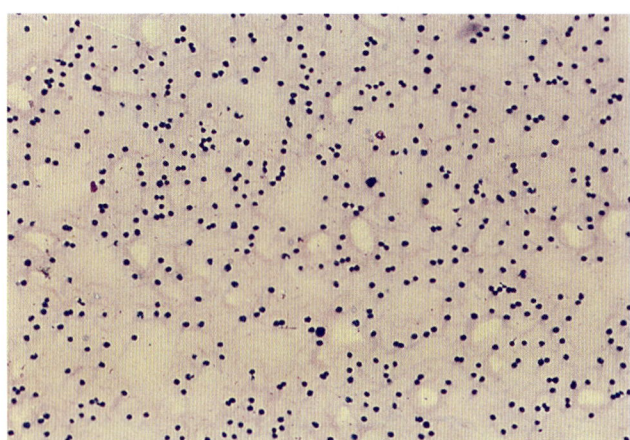

FIGURE 14.8 **Suppurative joint disease. Fluid aspirate.** Inflamed joints have an absolute increase in the number of neutrophils that often exceeds 50,000/μL, as in this specimen. The total cell number occasionally may be within normal limits (i.e., <3000/μL in dogs) in a septic joint, but the neutrophil number will represent more than 70% of the total cell number, emphasizing the need for microscopic examination. (Wright; IP.)

often moderately to markedly increased. However, the inflammatory process appears to wax and wane with time and, if polyarticular, involves other joints with varying intensity. Consequently, repeating joint sampling and, more importantly, sampling multiple joints, even if not clinically affected, has diagnostic value.

> **KEY POINT** Suppurative joint disease has both infectious and noninfectious causes.

Infectious arthritis. Some cases of joint disease are caused by bacteria (Figs. 14.9 and 14.10) or fungal infection (Figs. 14.11 and 14.12). The majority of septic joints have grossly abnormal joint fluid that is cloudy, watery, and often bloody and flocculent (Clements et al., 2005). In general, these joints have very high cell counts often greater than $100 \times 10^3/\mu L$ (Mielke et al., 2018). In most cases, the cells are primarily segmented neutrophils. It is important to evaluate the condition of the neutrophils. Degenerative or karyolytic neutrophils are more commonly observed with septic joints. Degenerate neutrophils have a pale, swollen nucleus with some loss of nuclear segmentation. However, often the majority of the neutrophils appear nondegenerate in septic arthritis. In one study, *Staphylococcus* spp. was the most common bacterial agent isolated in septic joints (Clements et al., 2005). Organisms may gain access to joints either hematogenously or via direct inoculation. In addition, there may be infection elsewhere in the body (e.g., endocarditis) with immune complex deposition in the synovial tissue and resultant nonseptic inflammation in the synovial fluid. Bacterial and fungal arthritis most commonly present with solitary joint involvement but on occasion may involve multiple joints, especially in young animals. Because infectious and noninfectious arthritis can have a similar presentation, it may be advisable to culture inflamed joints, keeping in mind that a negative culture result does not rule out infection because the microorganisms

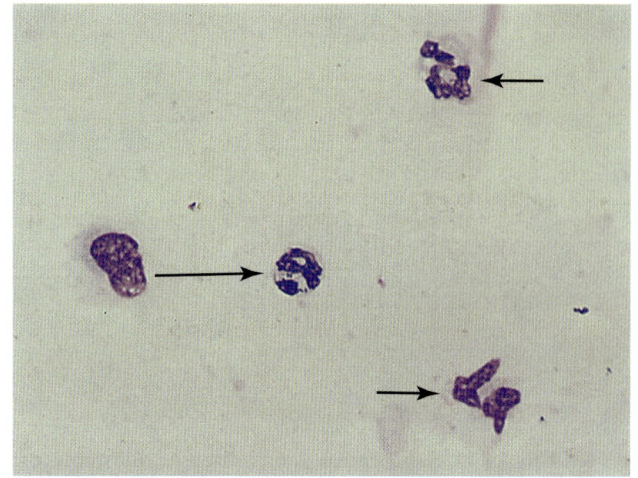

■ **FIGURE 14.9 Suppurative joint disease. Bacterial arthritis. Fluid aspirate.** Bacterial arthritis may be caused by direct inoculation or hematogenous spread. Infected joints typically have high neutrophil counts (>50,000/μL). In this example, the neutrophils display degenerative changes, including nuclear swelling *(short arrows)* and cytoplasmic vacuolization. The presence of degenerative changes strongly supports infection; however, the lack of degenerative changes or observable microorganisms does not rule out the possibility of infection. The bacteria may be located in the joint tissue and not present in the synovial fluid. Rare bacteria were observed after prolonged searching *(long arrow)*. (Wright; HP oil.).

are sometimes limited to the synovial lining tissue. Also, even when bacteria are observed in neutrophils, the synovial fluid may occasionally result in a negative culture. Interestingly, the elbow appears to be predisposed to septic arthritis in dogs with orthopedic surgery at a distant site (Mielke et al., 2018). Other organisms that have been implicated as causative agents of joint disease include mycoplasma; bacterial L-forms; spirochetes (*Borrelia burgdorferi* sensu stricto); protozoa (*Leishmania*

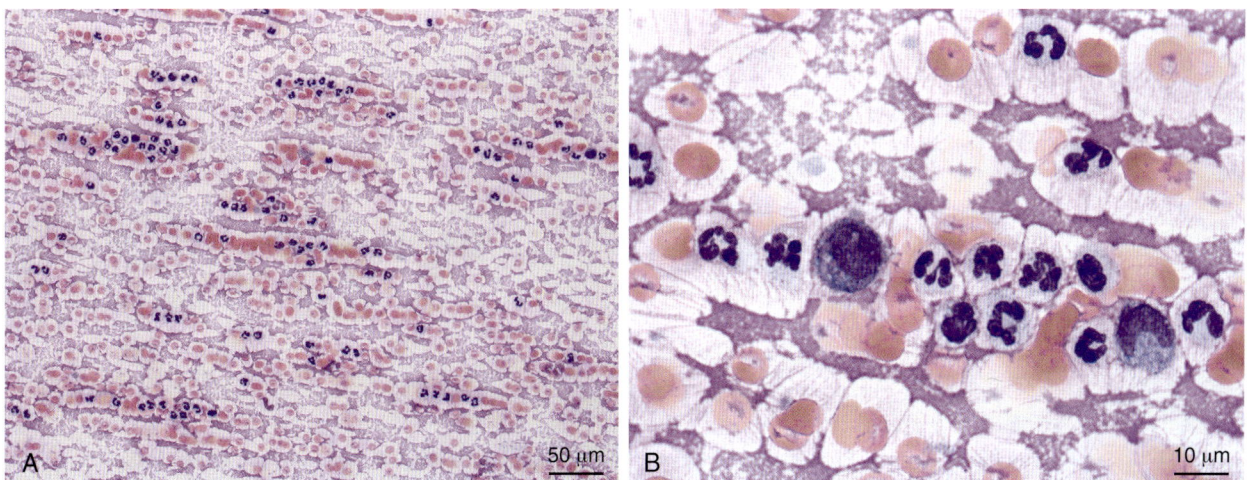

■ **FIGURE 14.10 Suppurative joint disease. Lyme disease. Carpus synovial fluid. Fluid aspirate. Dog.** Same case in A and B. The patient presented with polyarthritis, lethargy, and inappetence. The dog tested positive for Lyme disease on a combination snap test and an ELISA or Lyme quantitative C6 antibody. **A,** Nucleated cell count/μL was estimated to be 188,000 with a leukocyte differential of 99% neutrophils and 1% large mononuclear cells. The specimens contain neutrophils and erythrocytes in windrows. **B,** Nondegenerate neutrophils compose the majority of leukocytes. The background has granular eosinophilic material consistent with synovial fluid mucin. This suppurative reaction is consistent with an immune-mediated response to Lyme disease, a tick-borne disease. (Wright-Giemsa; HP oil.) (Courtesy Rose Raskin, University of Florida.)

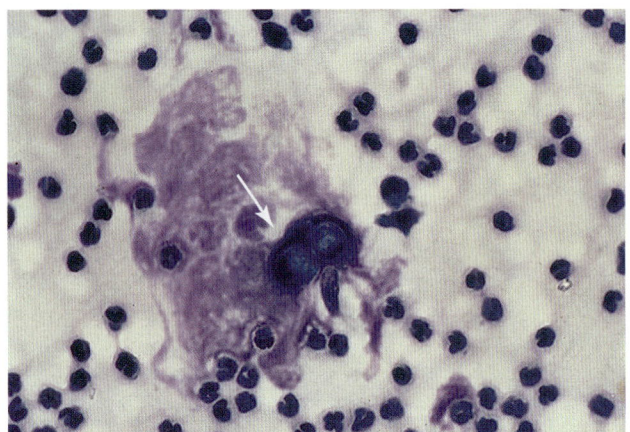

■ **FIGURE 14.11 Suppurative joint disease. Blastomycosis. Synovial fluid. Fluid aspirate.** In addition to bacteria, other types of infectious agents may also involve the joint. This photomicrograph contains numerous neutrophils that are "rounded up" and look like mononuclear cells owing to the thickness of the smear. In the center of the photo, broad-based budding yeasts are found that are consistent with *Blastomyces dermatitidis (arrow)*. Fungal organisms may be present infrequently and are best found on low-power examination. As with bacteria, the lack of observable organisms does not rule out infection. Fungal culture is advisable in suspected cases. (Wright; HP oil.)

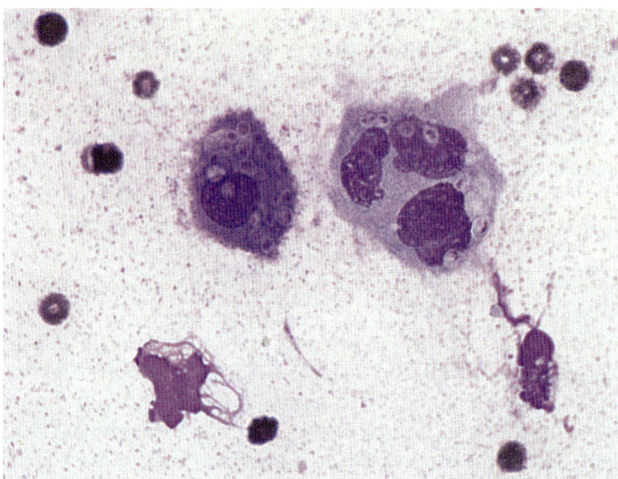

■ **FIGURE 14.12 Suppurative joint disease. Histoplasmosis. Synovial fluid. Fluid aspirate. Cat.** The patient was treated 1 year earlier for histoplasmosis. The fluid had high nucleated cellularity, which consisted primarily of moderately degenerate neutrophils and phagocytic mononuclear cells. Two macrophages contain multiple ovoid yeast organisms, which are approximately 2 to 5 μm with dark interior structures. These organisms are surrounded by a nonstaining clear halo consistent with *Histoplasma capsulatum*. (Wright; HP oil.) (Courtesy Rose Raskin, Kansas State University.)

donovani); viruses (calicivirus, coronavirus); and rickettsia or anaplasma, such as *Ehrlichia canis*, *Ehrlichia ewingii* (Fig. 14.13), *Anaplasma phagocytophilum* (formerly *Ehrlichia equi*), and *Rickettsia rickettsii* (Kornblatt et al., 1985; Santos et al., 2006; Harvey and Raskin, 2004). In one study of *E. ewingii* joint infection cases, in which the diagnosis was confirmed by polymerase chain reaction testing of peripheral blood, nucleated cell counts ranged from 16,000 to 125,000/μL with 63% to 95% neutrophils (Goodman et al., 2003). Interestingly, in a retrospective study of 41 dogs naturally infected with *E. ewingii*, limb or joint pain, often manifesting as polyarthralgia, was the most frequent physical examination finding at presentation (34%) despite polyarthritis per se being reported in only 10% (Qurollo et al., 2019).

> **KEY POINT** Bacterial arthritis often lacks visible evidence of infection; culture of the synovial fluid is therefore recommended.

> **KEY POINT** Limb or joint pain is a frequent finding on physical examination in dogs infected with *E. ewingii*.

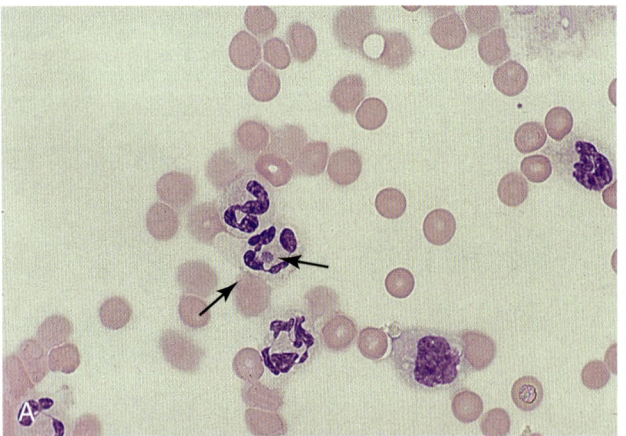
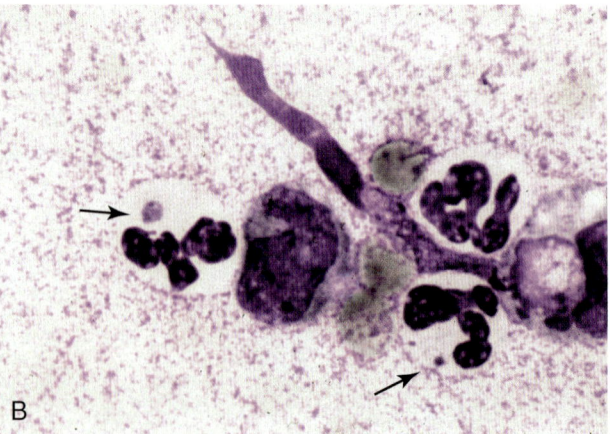

■ **FIGURE 14.13 Suppurative joint disease. Ehrlichiosis. Synovial fluid. Fluid aspirate. Dog. A, Granulocytic ehrlichiosis.** The neutrophil in the center *(arrows)* contains an ehrlichial morula in the cytoplasm. Granulocytic ehrlichiosis may be caused by *Anaplasma phagocytophilum* or *Ehrlichia ewingii*. These organisms may cause joint inflammation as well as a variety of other clinical signs and laboratory problems. It is unusual to find the organisms in clinical samples except for acute infections. Diagnosis is usually based on recognition of clinical signs with appropriate serologic testing. (Wright; HP oil.) **B,** ***E. ewingii*** **joint infection.** Pictured are three neutrophils with intracytoplasmic morulae *(arrows)*. This stifle synovial fluid had an estimated white cell count of higher than 50,000/μL and a predominance of mildly karyolytic neutrophils against an eosinophilic granular background. Diagnosis was confirmed by polymerase chain reaction testing to amplify genus- and species-specific products. (Wright-Giemsa; HP oil.) (Courtesy Rose Raskin, University of Florida.)

> **KEY POINT** Bacterial cultures of synovial fluid are often unrewarding; therefore, sampling of the synovial membrane may be necessary for culture.

Noninfectious arthritis. Many animals with inflamed joints have nonerosive disease (Michels and Carr, 1997). Causes of nonerosive polyarthritis include inflammation secondary to infection or neoplasia at extraarticular sites, breed-specific polyarthritis (e.g., beagle, Chinese Shar-Peis), drug-induced disease, immune-mediated polyarthritis, and systemic lupus erythematosus. As the name implies, polyarthritis typically affects multiple joints but on occasion may present clinically as a solitary affected joint. In addition to Doberman pinschers, miniature schnauzers and Samoyeds are at increased risk of hypersensitivity to sulfonamides with drug-induced suppurative arthritis (Trepanier et al., 2003). Although crystal-induced arthritis (e.g., gout or pseudogout) has been described in animals, it is infrequent in dogs and cats (deHaan and Andreasen, 1992; Forsyth et al., 2007) (Fig. 14.14).

Joints affected by immune-mediated disease often have increased numbers of nondegenerate neutrophils (Meléndez-Lazo et al., 2015). In some cases, increased numbers of lymphocytes and plasma cells may be found (see later discussion). Smaller distal joints are most commonly affected. Diagnosis of immune-mediated disease depends not only on demonstrating joint inflammation but also on ruling out infection via culture, serology, or empiric therapy. Some cases of immune-mediated disease have ragocytes (Fig. 14.15) or lupus erythematosus cells (Fig. 14.16). These are infrequent findings and should not be relied on as an absolute method to diagnose immune-mediated disease.

Erosive arthritis is suggested when lucent cystlike areas in the subchondral bone with narrowing or widening of the joint spaces are found on joint radiographs. Types of erosive arthritis described in animals include rheumatoid arthritis, polyarthritis of greyhounds, and feline chronic progressive polyarthritis (Carr and Michels, 1997; Oohashi et al., 2010). The classic finding is progressive loss of subchondral bone with deformation and destruction of affected joints. Infection or neoplasia may also cause erosive joint disease. Erosive arthritis, as with other types of suppurative joint disease, is characterized by increased numbers of neutrophils in the synovial fluid. Synovial fluid analysis alone cannot distinguish erosive disease from nonerosive disease; therefore, imaging techniques are necessary on animals with inflammatory joint disease. Other clinical features of noninfectious erosive arthritis include morning stiffness, swelling of the same or multiple joints within a 3-month period, symmetric swelling of joints, mononuclear infiltrates observed microscopically in a synovial membrane histopathology, and positive RF titer.

Neoplasia that is adjacent to the joint may induce a secondary suppurative response related to tissue damage and release of cytokines. Nondegenerate neutrophils may predominate in these cases (Fig. 14.17).

Nonsuppurative Joint Disease

Degenerative joint disease (osteoarthritis, osteoarthropathy) is characterized by degeneration of articular cartilage with secondary changes in associated joint structures (Figs. 14.18 and 14.19). The disorder usually occurs secondary to conditions such as osteochondrosis, hip dysplasia, joint instability, chronic bicipital tenosynovitis, and trauma. Changes in the synovial fluid are not as remarkable as seen with suppurative disease. During early degeneration, the joint area appears normal radiographically despite joint swelling. There may be mild cartilage softening related to loss of proteoglycan content and increased water content in the cartilage matrix, which may cause synovial lining reactivity (Fig. 14.20) (Carlson and Weisbrode, 2012). A mild increase in the number of mononuclear cells is the

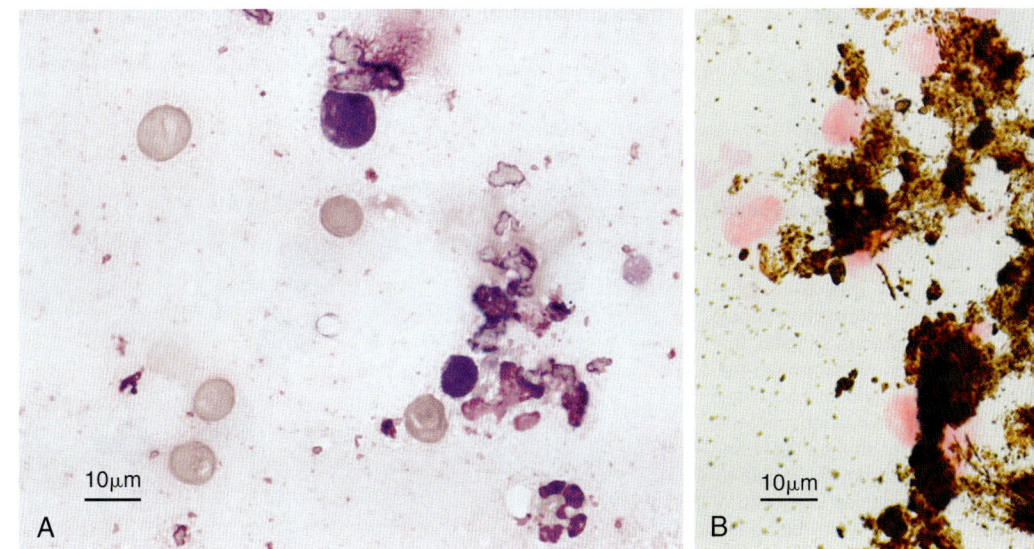
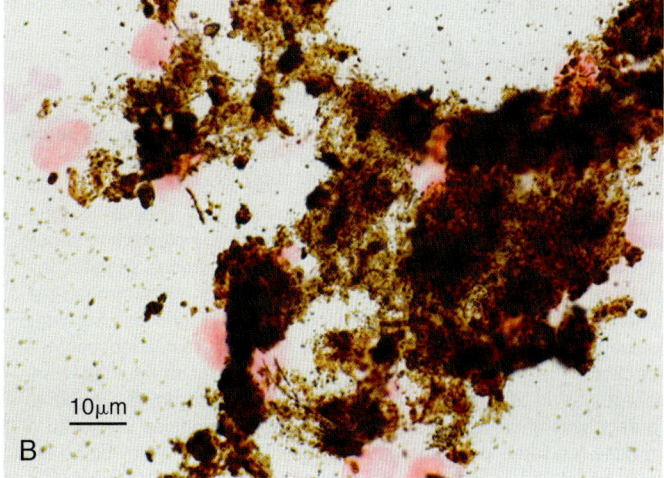

FIGURE 14.14 **Mixed-cell inflammation with calcium deposition. Synovial fluid. Fluid aspirate. Dog.** Same case in A and B. **A,** Neutrophils, mononuclear cells, and several erythrocytes are present within a background containing coarse and fine irregular refractile yellow-green crystalline material. Etiology for the crystal-induced arthropathy is uncertain but may relate to an earlier condition of systemic histoplasmosis. (Wright; HP oil.) **B,** Large collections are present of brown, positive-stained granules confirming calcium composition. Also noted are several inflammatory cells indicated by a nuclear counterstain that is associated with the mineral (Von Kossa; HP oil.) (Courtesy Rose Raskin, Purdue University.)

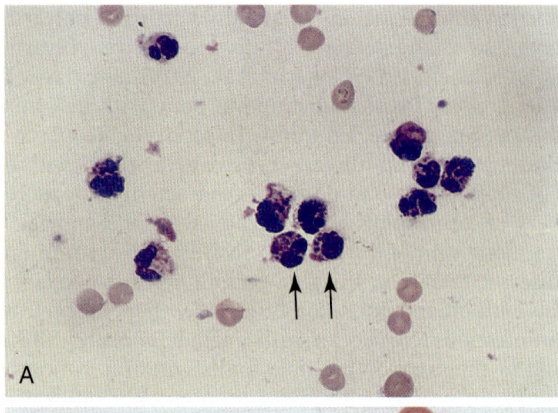
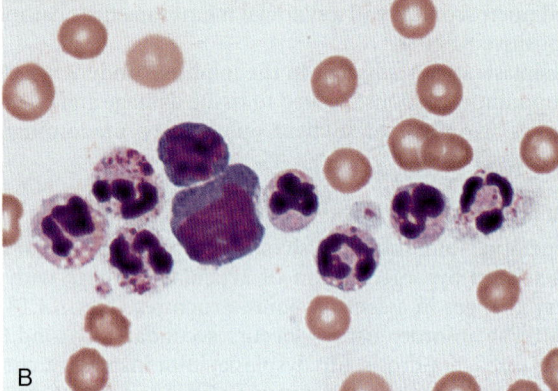
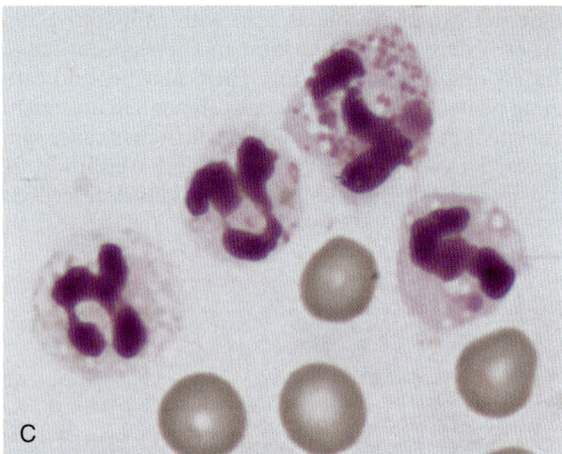

■ **FIGURE 14.15 Suppurative joint disease. Ragocytes. Synovial fluid. Fluid aspirate. Dog.** Same case in A to C. **A,** Ragocytes are phagocytic cells, commonly neutrophils, that contain multiple small, variably sized, purple cytoplasmic inclusions *(arrows)*. They likely represent nuclear remnants or phagocytosed immune complexes and should be distinguished from bacteria or toxicity. Observations suggest that these cells are seen more commonly in association with immune-mediated polyarthropathy but are not considered diagnostic. Serologic evaluation for immune-mediated disease and extraarticular nonbacterial infections such as ehrlichiosis and borreliosis is recommended when polyarthritis is identified. (Wright; HP oil.) **B,** Neutrophils frequently contain several variably sized, dark cytoplasmic granules in a case of immune-mediated polyarthropathy. Stifle fluid had a white blood cell count of 7400/μL, protein of 3.6 g/dL, good mucin clot, 21% nondegenerate neutrophils, 45% small lymphocytes, 34% large mononuclear cells, positive antinuclear antibody titer, and negative rickettsial titers. (Wright; HP oil.) **C,** Higher magnification of affected neutrophils containing fragments of nuclear material. (Wright; HP oil.) (B–C, Courtesy Rose Raskin, Purdue University.)

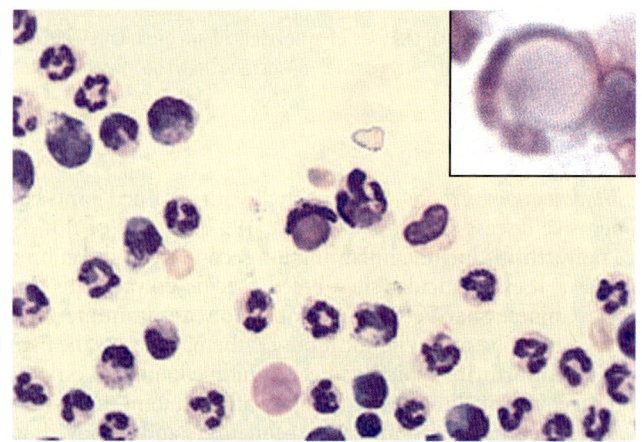

■ **FIGURE 14.16 Suppurative joint disease. Lupus erythematosus cell. Synovial fluid. Fluid aspirate. Dog.** Clinical presentation is shifting leg lameness. The total cell number is moderately increased and composed of predominantly nondegenerate neutrophils with lesser numbers of lymphocytes and monocytes. The neutrophil in the center contains a large, round, homogeneous eosinophilic inclusion in the cytoplasm that displaces the nucleus to the periphery of the cell membrane. This is a lupus erythematosus (LE) cell. The phagocytized material is thought to be nuclear material that has been structurally altered by antinuclear antibody. The homogeneous, light-staining appearance of the material distinguishes it from normal nuclear material. LE cells are rare, but when found, they support the diagnosis of systemic lupus erythematosus. *Inset:* Higher magnification of another LE cell. (Wright; HP oil.) (Courtesy Linda L. Werner. Inset, Courtesy Rose Raskin.)

predominant finding with moderate to chronic degeneration (Stobie et al., 1995). These cells are likely a mixture of macrophages, lymphocytes, and synovial lining cells (Figs. 14.21 to 14.24). Fibroblast-like synovial cell proliferation or fibrosis may occur with chronic degeneration (Fig. 14.25). Cranial cruciate ligament rupture of the stifle (see Fig. 14.24) is associated with nonsuppurative joint disease with synovial fluid composed predominantly of mononuclear cells (large mononuclear cells

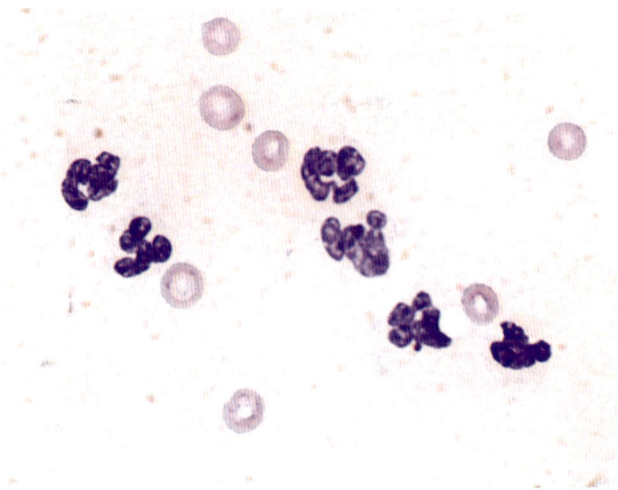

■ **FIGURE 14.17 Suppurative joint disease. Nonseptic inflammation. Synovial fluid. Fluid aspirate.** The fluid contains predominantly well-segmented, nondegenerative neutrophils that resulted secondarily to adjacent neoplasia of the bone. (Wright-Giemsa; HP oil.)

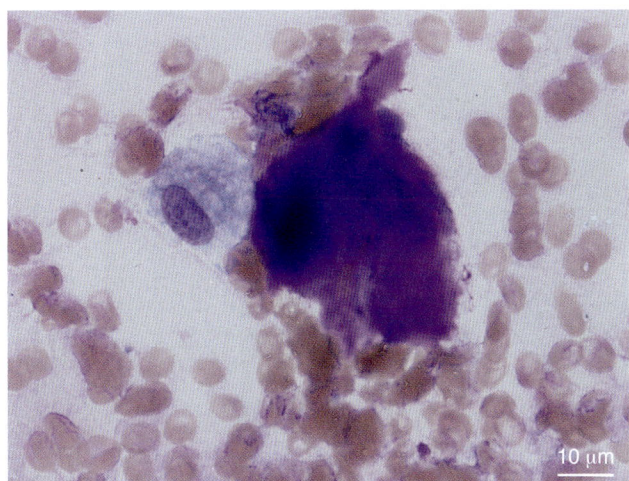

FIGURE 14.18 Nonsuppurative joint disease. Cartilage. Synovial fluid. Fluid aspirate. Dog. Same case as Figure 14.7. The specimen is taken from the stifle joint of a chihuahua with polyarthropathy. The leukocyte estimate of the fluid was 800 to 2000/µL. The leukocyte differential revealed 56% lymphocytes, 38% large mononuclear cells, and 6% neutrophils. In addition to one large mononuclear cell, a large cartilage fragment is present likely related to the small size of the joint region in this dog and its degenerative joint disease. (Wright-Giemsa; HP oil.) (Courtesy Rose Raskin, University of Florida.)

chondrocytes (Camus et al., 2017). The concern is to recognize the variety of reactive changes that occur during joint degeneration and mistake these changes for neoplasia.

Canine rheumatoid arthritis may present with a small mononuclear cell predominance and mildly increased synovial cell counts as well as increased neutrophils, particularly with moderately to markedly increased cell counts over 10,000/µL (MacWilliams and Friedrichs, 2003).

A generalized arthritis with metaphyseal swelling that affects young dogs is recognized as hypertrophic osteodystrophy. Cytologic evaluation of the synovial fluid in one case revealed a low to mildly increased nucleated cell count with 43% nondegenerate neutrophils, 52% large mononuclear cells, and 5% lymphocytes (Hill et al., 2015).

Synovial fluid eosinophilia is a rare idiopathic phenomenon that resembles an immune-mediated response (Christopher and Wallace, 1986; Silverstein et al., 2000; Birckhead et al., 2019). Single or multiple joints were affected in one cat and two dogs, respectively. Lameness in two cases responded to prednisone and one to meclofenamic acid.

Hemarthrosis

If recent trauma has occurred, joint hemorrhage may be detected (Fig. 14.27). True hemorrhage must be distinguished from the much more common artifact of blood contamination. This is best done at the time of sample collection. If hemorrhage has occurred recently, the withdrawn fluid color will appear homogeneously red and cloudy; a yellowish color (xanthochromia) is indicative of prior hemorrhage with resolution. Besides trauma, other causes of hemorrhagic joint fluid include coagulation defects and neoplasia. A congenital coagulation factor deficiency should be considered in a puppy or kitten that presents with repeated episodes of hemarthrosis or with hemarthrosis and a history of minimal trauma. Low numbers of red blood cells can be observed microscopically in normal synovial fluid but should not be present in high enough numbers to

with increased numbers of lymphocytes and plasma cells) along with few neutrophils (Erne et al., 2009). This immune-associated condition may be accompanied by synovial membrane hyperplasia (see Fig. 14.19). In severe cases of degeneration, osteoclasts can be observed, which may suggest erosion of cartilage and exposure of underlying subchondral bone (Fig. 14.26; see also Fig. 14.23B). A case of synovial chondrometaplasia was reported as a sequela of chronic degenerative joint disease in a dog in which cytopathology revealed atypical

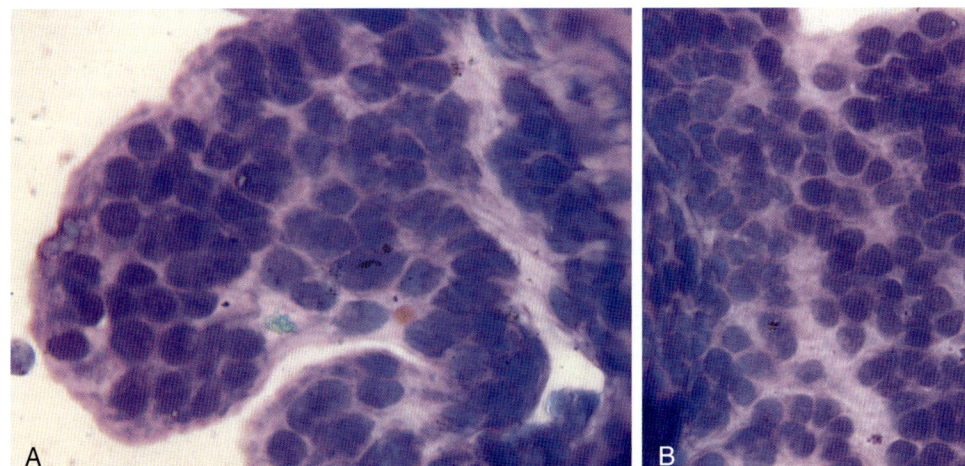

FIGURE 14.19 Nonsuppurative joint disease. Synovial membrane hyperplasia. Elbow synovial fluid. Fluid aspirate. Dog. Same case in A and B. Specimen taken from an 8-month-old Nova Scotia duck tolling retriever with a nucleated cell count within reference interval. Leukocytes are 99% mononuclear within evidence of infection. Also noted is a very large cell aggregate arranged in a papillary formation. The cells have high nucleocytoplasmic ratio, a round central nucleus, and pale eosinophilic wispy cytoplasm. The cells and nuclei appear uniform in size and shape. Within this network of cells are pale eosinophilic ribbons of collagen. The cytopathologic diagnosis is synovial membrane proliferation possibly related to degenerative joint conditions, ligament injuries, or trauma. (Wright; HP oil.) (Courtesy Rose Raskin, University of Bristol, UK.)

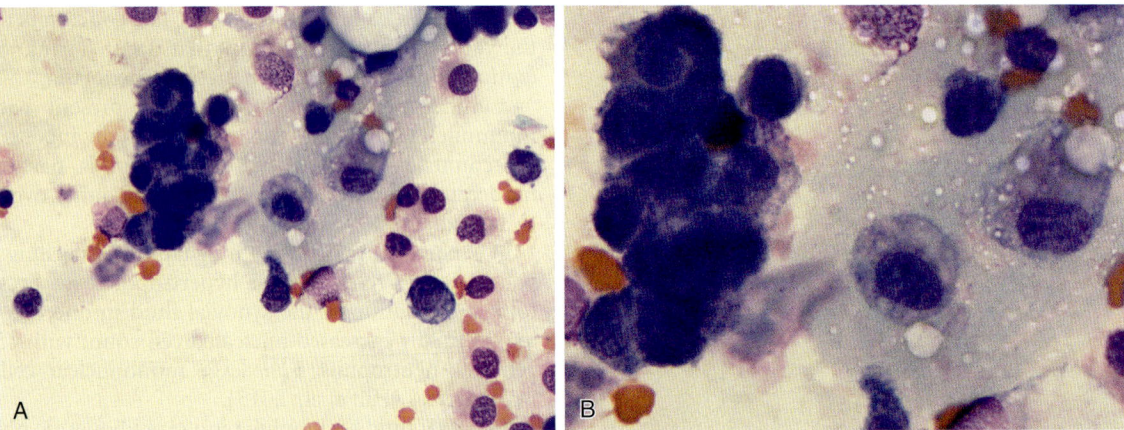

■ **FIGURE 14.20 Reactive synovial tissue. Tibiotarsal joint. Fluid aspirate.** Same case in A and B. Synovial swelling is associated with only this joint. No significant lameness is present, and no radiographic abnormality is noted. The fluid is characterized as pink or slightly hazy before centrifugation and colorless or clear after centrifugation with normal viscosity and a low total solids of less than 2.5 g/dL. The nucleated cell count was also low at 56/μL with 82% large mononuclear cells, 16% lymphocytes, and 2% neutrophils. **A,** A tightly cohesive aggregate of likely synovial lining cells is shown with several mononuclear cells. **B,** Higher magnification of the aggregate reveals the cells contain small amounts of deeply basophilic cytoplasm and a round to oval nucleus with clumped chromatin. The cytoplasmic surface has surface blebbing or villous projections. This synovial membrane reactivity with low cell counts and low protein is consistent with early degenerative joint disease. (Wright; HP oil.) (Courtesy Rose Raskin, Michigan State University.)

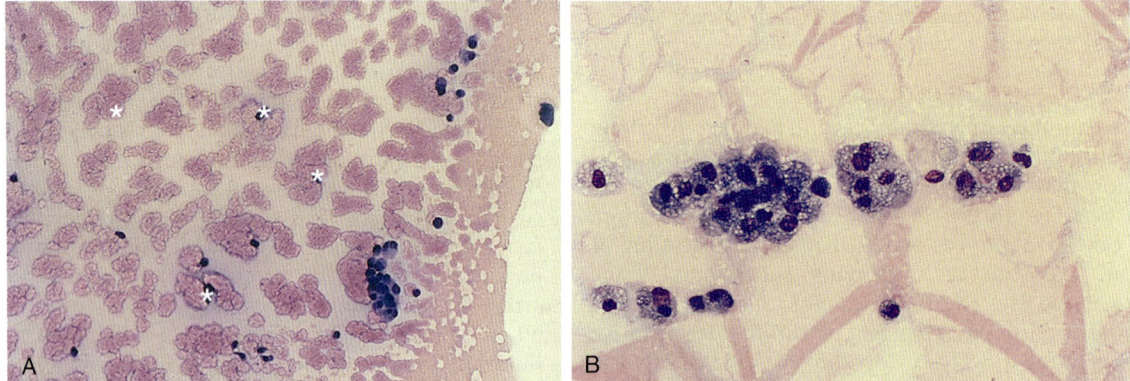

■ **FIGURE 14.21 Nonsuppurative joint disease. Degenerative joint disease. Synovial fluid. Fluid aspirate. Dog.** Same case in A and B. **A,** This sample is from the stifle joint of a large dog with chronic hind limb lameness. Cell numbers appear to be slightly increased but difficult to estimate because of clumping and thickness of the smear. The granular background that includes clumps of mucin *(asterisks)*, resembling erythrocytes, is suggestive of good mucin content. The majority of the cells are mononuclear with some having a macrophage appearance. Further evaluation for underlying disease such as osteochondrosis or meniscal disease is warranted. (Wright; IP.) **B,** Joints with degenerative disease typically have increased numbers of macrophages or phagocytic type A synoviocytes. The cells are usually large and vacuolated and contain numerous pink-staining, cytoplasmic granules. Mucin content may remain good as is evident by the thick pink background. (Wright; HP oil.)

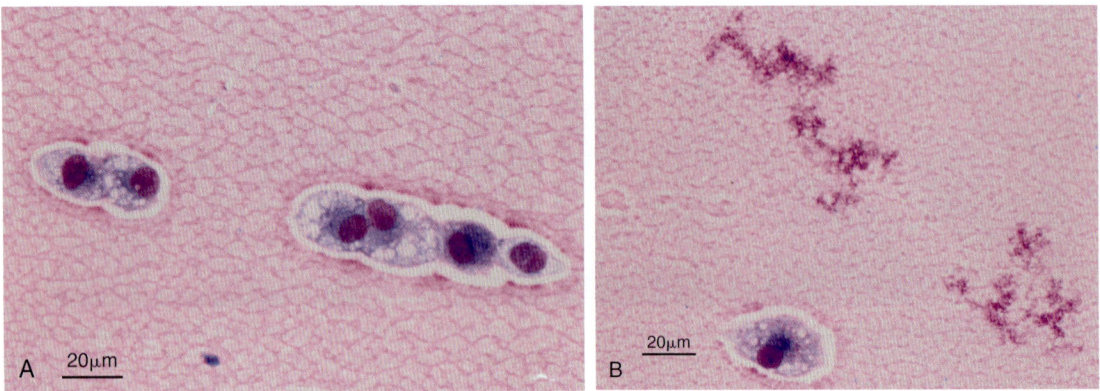

■ **FIGURE 14.22 Nonsuppurative joint disease. Chronic bicipital tenosynovitis. Synovial fluid. Fluid aspirate. Dog.** Same case in A and B. **A,** Windrowing of large mononuclear cells is noted in this shoulder joint fluid specimen with chronic degenerative disease involving the biceps brachii tendon and synovial sheath. It is a common cause of forelimb lameness in adult dogs. (Wright; HP oil.) **B,** A single synoviocyte is shown against the granular background, which contains eosinophilic aggregates of mucin materials likely released from damaged articular surfaces. (Wright, HP oil.) (Courtesy Rose Raskin, Purdue University.)

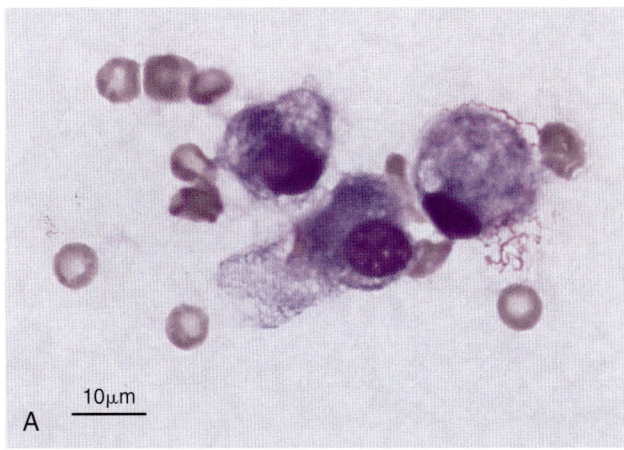

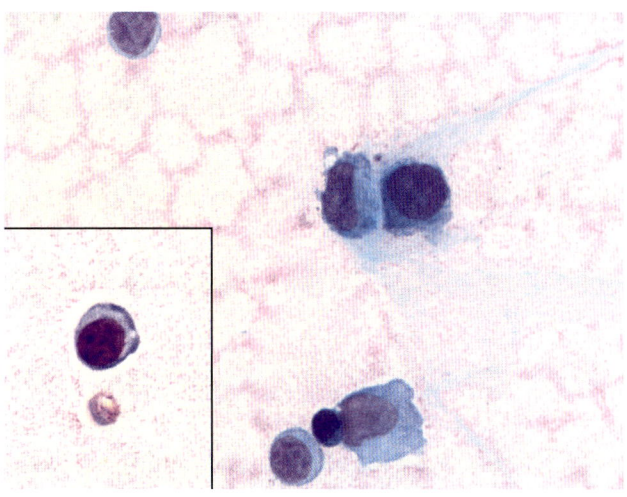

■ **FIGURE 14.24 Nonsuppurative joint disease. Cranial cruciate tear. Synovial fluid. Fluid aspirate. Dog.** Synovial fluid had an estimated cell count of white blood cells of 5000/μL and protein of 4.5 g/dL with normal viscosity in which the cell differential indicated 76% lymphocytes, 15% neutrophils, and 9% large mononuclear cells. Note the plasmacytoid lymphocyte in the *inset* with identical magnification to the other lymphoid cells. (Wright-Giemsa; HP oil.) (Courtesy Rose Raskin, Purdue University.)

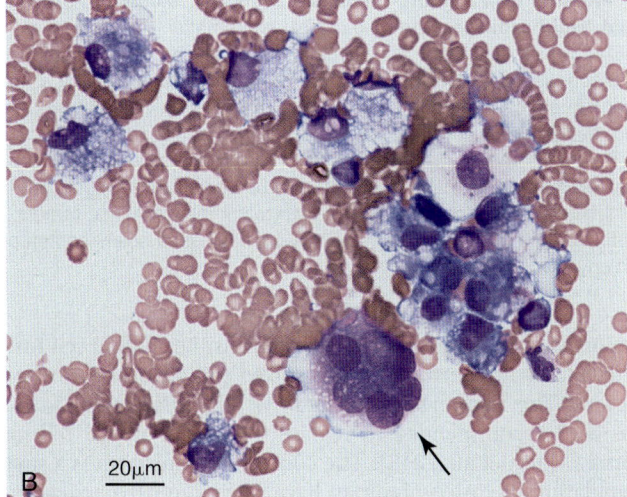

■ **FIGURE 14.23 Nonsuppurative joint disease. Osteoarthritis. Synovial fluid. Fluid aspirate. Dog.** Same case in A and B. **A,** Three individual large mononuclear cells are shown from a direct smear of synovial fluid from a joint with a nonsuppurative degenerative disease. These are consistent with macrophages. (Wright; HP oil.) **B,** *Arrow* indicates a multinucleated osteoclast among the numerous mononuclear cells and erythrocytes. (Wright; HP oil.) (Courtesy Rose Raskin, Purdue University.)

discolor the fluid. Cytopathologically, hemorrhage can be distinguished from peripheral blood contamination by identification of erythrophagia, hemosiderin-laden macrophages, and other red blood cell pigments such as hematoidin. Occasionally, platelets are observed in samples with severe peripheral blood contamination. Care must be taken not to overinterpret erythrophagia because this can occur ex vivo if the sample is not evaluated quickly.

Neoplasia

Normal synovium consists of loose connective tissue containing blood vessels and adipocytes lined by a layer of synoviocytes composed of type A histiocytic and type B fibroblastic cells (see Fig. 14.1). In a study of 35 dogs, the most common synovial

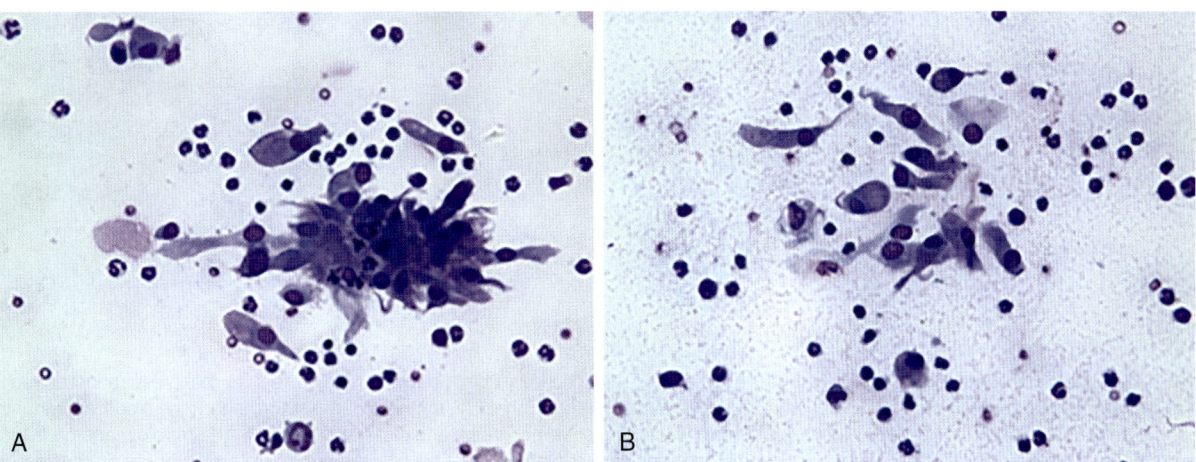

■ **FIGURE 14.25 Fibroblastic proliferation. Carpus synovial fluid. Fluid aspirate. Dog.** Same case in A and B. The patient presented with a swollen carpal joint, and radiographs indicated bony formation. There was a mild to moderate increase in neutrophils along with individual or aggregated mesenchymal cells. These mesenchymal cells may represent reactivity and proliferation of synovial fibroblasts in response to chronic joint disease. (Romanowsky; HP oil.) (Courtesy Ulsoo Choi, South Korea.)

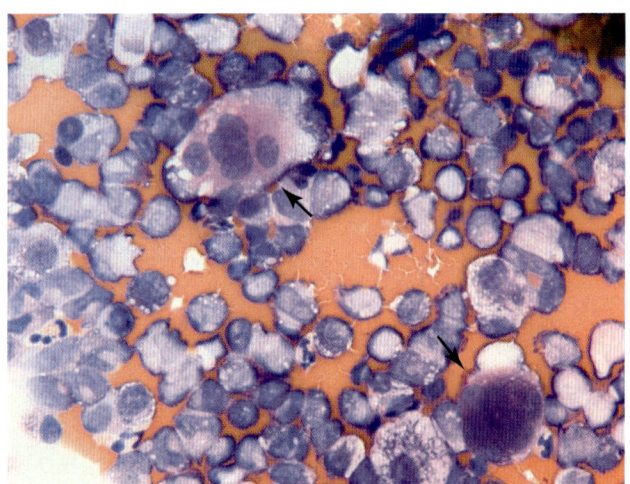

■ **FIGURE 14.26 Nonsuppurative joint disease. Osteoclast. Synovial fluid. Fluid aspirate.** In patients with degenerative joint disease or erosion of cartilage, osteoclasts can be observed *(arrows)*. (Wright; HP oil.)

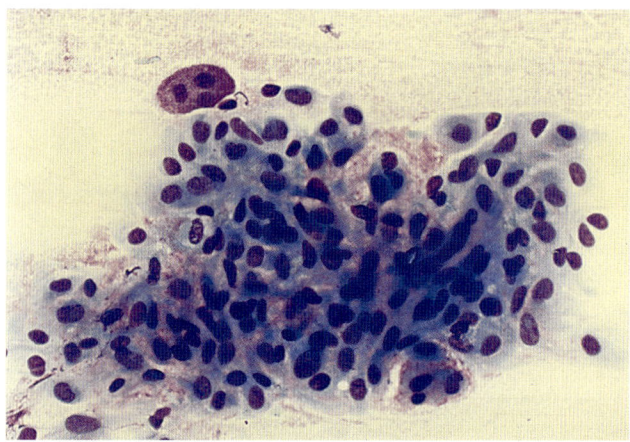

■ **FIGURE 14.28 Joint neoplasia. Synovial sarcoma. Synovial fluid. Fluid aspirate. Dog.** The clinical presentation was lameness localized to a solitary joint. The sample is predominated by large sheets of pleomorphic spindle cells that are sometimes separated by a fine, pink, streaming stroma. The cells display moderate pleomorphism. This joint had an associated soft tissue mass that was ultimately diagnosed as synovial sarcoma. The cells in this photograph display some cytopathologic features of malignancy and may be neoplastic but could potentially be reactive synovial cells. As with many mesenchymal tumors, it is difficult to definitively diagnose malignancy based solely on cytopathology. (Wright; HP oil.)

neoplasm was of histiocytic origin (51%) (Craig et al., 2002), followed by synovial myxomas (17%), synovial sarcomas (14%), and other mixed sarcomas (17%), including anaplastic sarcoma with giant cells (formerly malignant fibrous histiocytoma), fibrosarcoma, chondrosarcoma, and undifferentiated sarcoma. However, in light of recent studies, synovial cell sarcoma is considered a rare tumor in animals (Craig and Thompson, 2017). Immunohistochemical staining was necessary to distinguish between the histologic types of synovial tumors because the prognosis varied greatly among them. A recommended panel of antibodies is suggested to include cytokeratin (AE1/AE3) for synovial cell sarcoma and CD18 for histiocytic sarcoma. Interestingly, normal synovium is negative for cytokeratin (Cazzini et al., 2015). In human medicine, the tumors are called synovial sarcoma, and the detection of a gene translocation is used for diagnosis (Cazzini et al., 2015; Monti et al., 2018). Synovial cell sarcomas may appear most commonly as the spindle cell form (Fig. 14.28) or alternatively as a mixed spindle and epithelioid variant. The term *cytokeratin positive joint–associated sarcoma* has been recommended to replace the term synovial cell sarcoma (Monti et al., 2018). The concern for this term is a small population of osteosarcomas have been reported to express cytokeratin (Nagamine et al., 2015).

Histiocytic sarcomas arise from the antigen-presenting dendritic cells of the synovium layer. These neoplasms are frequently associated with Rottweilers, Bernese mountain dogs, and

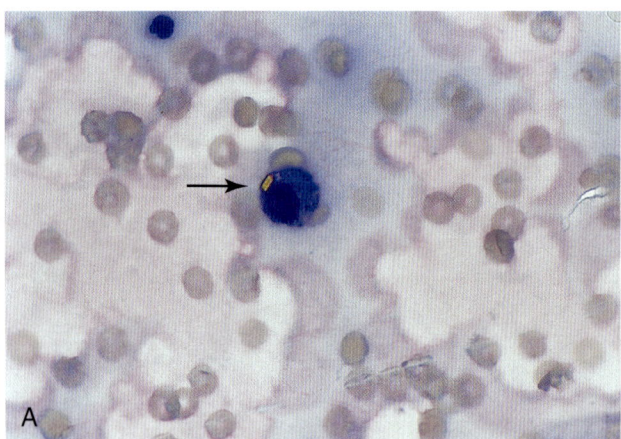
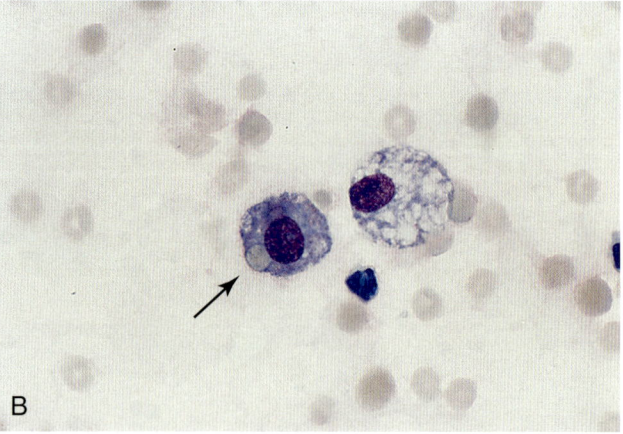

■ **FIGURE 14.27 Hemarthrosis. Synovial fluid. Fluid aspirate.** The small size of canine and feline joints may make aspiration difficult, so it is common to get some degree of blood contamination in most joint specimens. To help distinguish true hemorrhage from blood contamination, the smears should be routinely examined for erythrophagia, hematoidin crystals, hemosiderin, and platelet clumps. **A,** The macrophage contains a small, golden hematoidin crystal *(arrow)*. **B,** The smaller of two macrophages contains a phagocytosed erythrocyte in the lower left area of its cytoplasm *(arrow)*. These findings indicate that there has been previous and active hemorrhage in the joint, respectively. Potential causes of hemarthrosis include trauma, coagulopathy, and neoplasia. Coagulopathies may have evidence of multiple joint involvement and bleeding elsewhere. Abnormal hemostasis is documented by coagulation testing. (Wright; HP oil.)

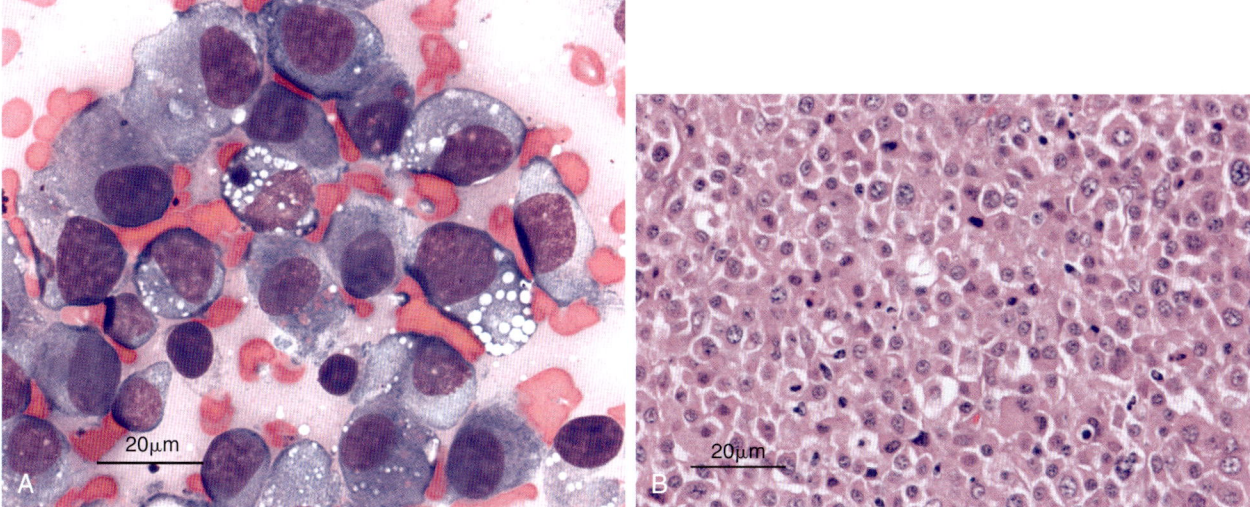

■ **FIGURE 14.29 Joint neoplasia. Histiocytic sarcoma. Periarticular joint tissue. Dog.** Same case in A and B. **A, Tissue aspirate.** A localized soft tissue mass was present around the joint and infiltrated the muscle. The specimen revealed a pleomorphic population of round cells. These cells display malignant features of anisokaryosis, variable nucleocytoplasmic, ratio, coarse chromatin, and prominent nucleoli. The abundant basophilic cytoplasm suggests histiocytic origin, which was confirmed by immunohistochemistry. (Wright; HP oil.) **B, Histology.** Pleomorphic round cell neoplasm was negative for CD3, CD79, and MUM1 (lymphoid) antigens and positive for CD45, CD18, and E-cadherin (leukocyte, histiocytic, and dendritic cell antigens, respectively). (H&E; IP.) (Courtesy Rose Raskin, Purdue University.)

retrievers (Affolter and Moore, 2002; Moore, 2014). Cytopathologically, histiocytic sarcomas display a round cell appearance with anaplastic characteristics, including cellular pleomorphism, multinucleation, anisokaryosis, coarse chromatin, and prominent nucleoli with abundant basophilic cytoplasm (Fig. 14.29). Occasionally, osteosarcoma can penetrate the joint from adjacent bone with osteoblasts appearing in joint fluid (Fig. 14.30).

Another neoplasm occasionally encountered in the joints is metastatic carcinoma. Cases with metastatic neoplastic cells in synovial fluid have been documented arising from the lungs and mammary glands (Meinkoth et al., 1997). A urolithial (transitional) cell carcinoma located in the prostate gland was diagnosed in synovial fluid as the cause of lameness in a dog (Colledge et al., 2013). Cells in the primary site and metastatic sites (carpus and stifle) were immunoreactive to uroplakin-III, a urothelial tissue marker (Fig. 14.31).

Less commonly encountered are multinodular joint masses termed *synovial myxomas*. These produce abundant fluid that

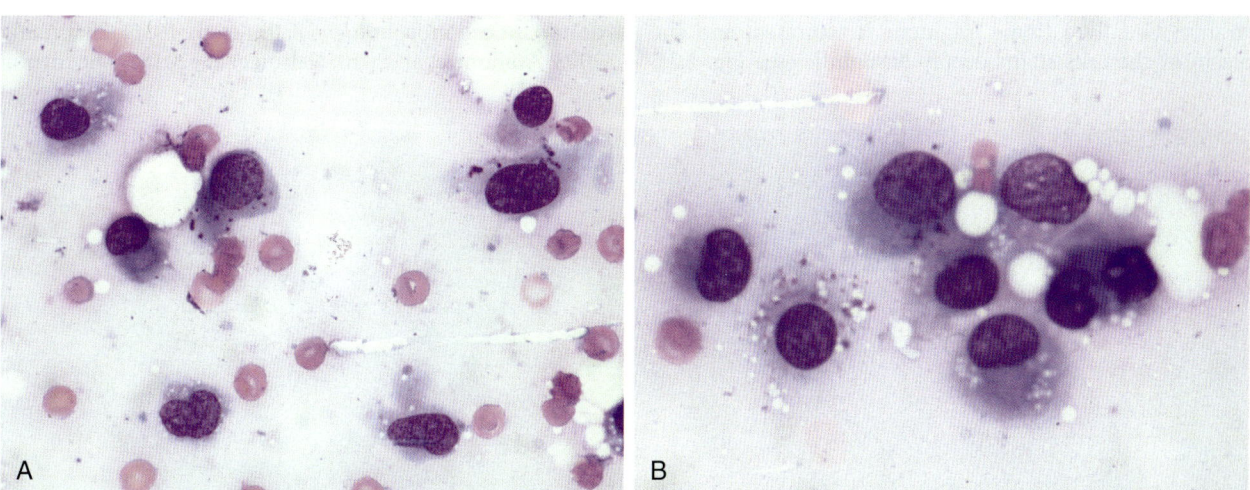

■ **FIGURE 14.30 Joint neoplasia. Osteosarcoma. Stifle synovial fluid. Fluid aspirate. Dog.** Same case in A and B. A palpable soft tissue swelling was caudal to the joint. On radiographs, the stifle shows femoral and tibial changes with areas of osteoproliferation along with lytic bone lesions. The joint fluid has high cellularity consisting of individualized cells with occasional dense aggregates of these cells. Dense eosinophilic matrix material is occasionally noted in the background (not shown). These round to ovoid to occasionally spindle cells are mostly mononuclear and intermediate in size with a round to ovoid nucleus that measures 1.5 to 2 times an erythrocyte diameter. The nuclear chromatin is coarse, and a single nucleolus is noted; however, multiple nucleoli may be seen. The nucleus is often eccentric within the basophilic and vacuolated cytoplasm. Variably sized eosinophilic cytoplasmic granules are noted in many of these cells. Cytopathologic diagnosis is osteosarcoma that is supported by positive alkaline phosphatase staining. (Wright; HP oil.) (Courtesy Rose Raskin, SynLab/TDDS, Exeter, UK.)

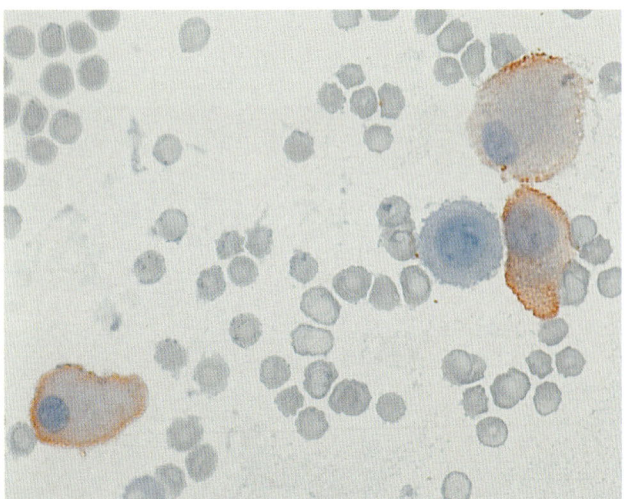

■ **FIGURE 14.31 Joint neoplasia. Metastatic prostatic carcinoma. Synovial fluid. Fluid aspirate. Dog.** Fluid from the carpus revealed individual cells and small clusters of prostatic urothelium. Confirmation of urothelial origin involved using immunocytochemistry. The red cytoplasmic surface staining indicates positive immunoreactivity. (Uroplakin III/AEC; HP oil.) (Courtesy Sarah Colledge, Purdue University.)

has been characterized by vacuolated monocytoid cells consistent with normal-appearing synoviocytes or macrophages in a background of a proteinaceous light pink matrix (Craig and Thompson, 2017).

> **KEY POINT** Sampling of musculoskeletal lesions is similar to that of other mass lesions. Tissue puncture with or without suction and impression smears from tissue are common methods to obtain a sample.

SKELETAL MUSCLE

Normal cytology of skeletal muscle has a characteristic appearance. Usually a tissue fragment is aspirated, and the cytoplasm of the cells stains deeply basophilic (see Fig. 2.1). Often, striations can be visualized by focusing up and down on the cell aggregate. The nuclei are round with a condensed chromatin pattern.

Myositis

Myositis is difficult to diagnose with cytopathology because it may be difficult to associate the inflammatory cells with the myocytes. Necrotizing myopathy appears inflammatory initially, often with neutrophils (Fig. 14.32) but with healing, fibrosis later occurs. Inflammatory cells may involve predominantly neutrophils in acute infections (Fig. 14.33), predominantly eosinophils with insect bite or immune-mediated reactions (Fig. 14.34) or mixed cells, including macrophages and fibroblasts (Fig. 14.35). Diagnosis of myositis and etiology typically requires consideration of history, signalment, and chemistry findings (increased creatine kinase and aspartate transaminase), as well as electromyographic, immunologic, and serologic tests for protozoa. Eosinophilic myositis may be considered an immune-mediated myopathy that is often associated with masticatory muscles. Histopathology is necessary for definitive diagnosis of myositis and degenerative myopathies.

Muscle Neoplasms

Tumors arising from skeletal muscle include rhabdomyoma and rhabdomyosarcoma (Figs. 14.36 to 14.40). These neoplasms are uncommon. On cytopathology, these tumors may appear similar to other mesenchymal tumors. Rhabdomyomas in particular often exfoliate poorly; however, when sufficient cells are obtained, they can be generally classified on cytopathology as a sarcoma. There are three major subclasses of rhabdomyosarcoma based on histologic findings: embryonal, alveolar, and pleomorphic (Caserto, 2013). Botryoid rhabdomyosarcoma is actually a subset of embryonal, but related to its unique location (urinary bladder), it is often considered as a separate subclass (Alleman et al., 1991; Gerber and Rees, 2009). Embryonal subclass is most commonly encountered in dogs and cats with three variants that are distinguished by the predominant cell morphology (Fallin et al., 1995; Chapman et al., 2008; Avallone et al., 2010; Nelson et al., 2018). The myotubular

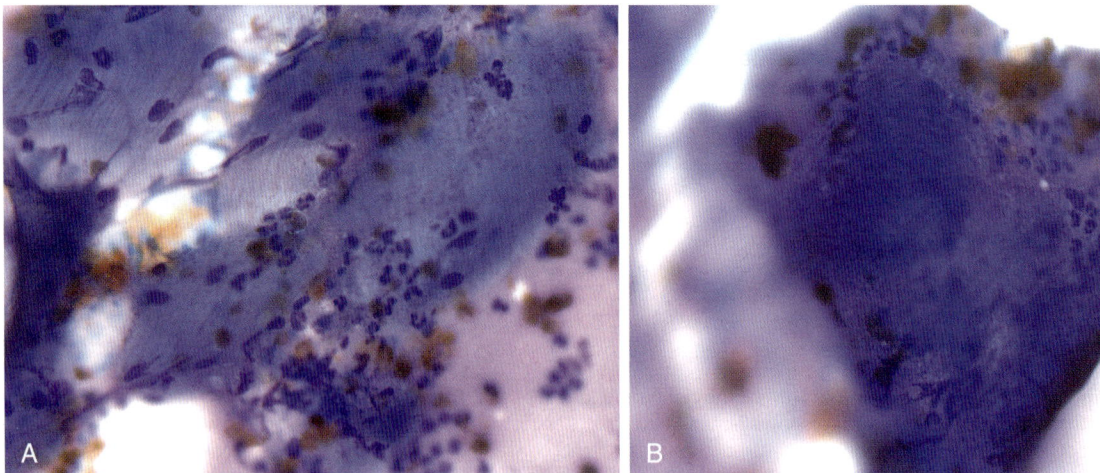

■ **FIGURE 14.32 Necrotizing and neutrophilic myositis. Hind leg, Quadriceps muscle. Tissue aspirate. Dog.** Same case in A and B. Patient presented with severe swelling of the leg with cystic areas and a 5-day history of lethargy and pyrexia. Numerous nondegenerate neutrophils are present within and around granular and poorly striated muscle. Related to the geographic area, season (spring), and clinical signs, strong consideration was given to adder envenomation. (Aqueous Romanowsky; HP oil.) (Courtesy Rose Raskin, University of Bristol, UK.)

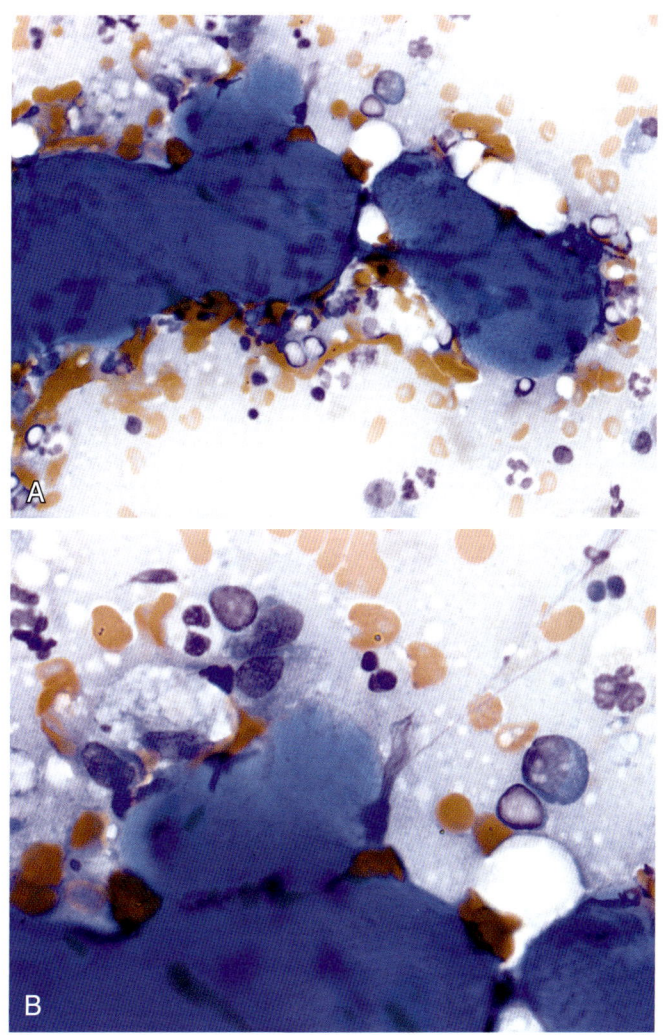

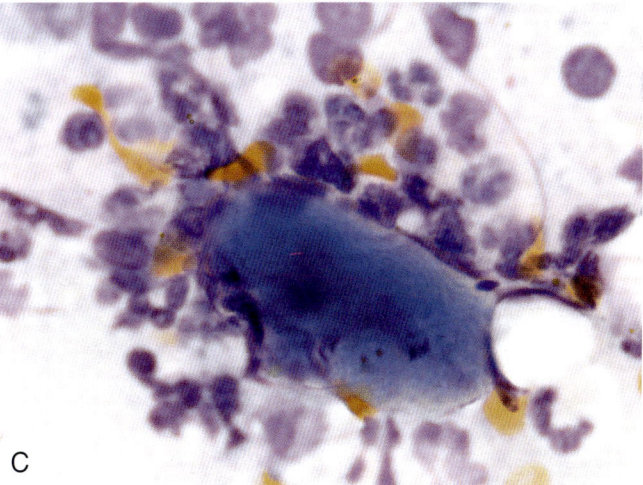

■ **FIGURE 14.33 Neutrophilic myositis. Submandibular region. Tissue aspirate. Dog.** Same case in A to C. Mostly karyolytic neutrophils with lesser numbers of macrophages, lymphocytes, and occasional plasma cells make up the inflammatory population. Suspicious of an infectious etiology related to the clinical response to amoxicillin–clavulanic acid administration. (Wright-Giemsa; HP oil.) (Courtesy Rose Raskin, University of Florida.)

variant is dominated by multinucleated and elongated tubular cells; the rhabdomyoblastic variant is dominated by large round cells with abundant cytoplasm; and the spindle cell variant is dominated by fusiform, elongated cells arranged in streams. It is common to see all three variants together in embryonal rhabdomyosarcomas and hence it is confusing to place in one neoplastic cytomorphologic category. Typically, multinucleated cells are observed with the nuclei arranged in a row consistent with a straplike cell (see Figs. 14.37, 14.38, and 14.40C–D). Rarely, striations are visible within the cytoplasm. The multinucleated cells are formed by the fusion of one or more rhabdomyoblasts, which appear as round cells with high to moderate nucleocytoplasmic ratios. Less common is the alveolar subclass, which may appear in two variants, aggregates or sheets (solid). Cytopathologically, these smears are highly cellular and contain numerous atypical round cells that resemble lymphoid cells with mitotic figures being frequent (Murakami et al., 2010; Snyder and Michael, 2011). The third subclass of rhabdomyosarcomas is pleomorphic with haphazardly arranged plump spindle cells displaying marked anisocytosis and anisokaryosis with bizarre mitotic figures (Caserto, 2013). Although rhabdomyosarcomas often occur in juvenile animals younger than 2 years, the embryonal subclass may be in either juvenile or adults and the pleomorphic is mostly in adults (Caserto, 2013). Specific diagnosis of a rhabdomyoma or rhabdomyosarcoma by cytopathology is sometimes difficult; however, the presence of striations and strap cells can assist with the diagnosis. Histopathology with immunohistochemistry is often necessary for a definitive diagnosis (see Chapter 18). Rhabdomyosarcomas are consistently immunoreactive using antibodies for vimentin, desmin, muscle actin, and src actin, but myoglobin is variable. Both myogenin and MyoD1 have been used to diagnose canine rhabdomyosarcoma but at this time do not appear to help in classification of the subclasses (Caserto, 2013).

BONE

Fine-needle aspiration of bone is becoming a more commonly used technique (Britt et al., 2007; Neihaus et al., 2011). Aspiration of bone is indicated if an osteolytic or osteoproliferative lesion involving cortical lysis or periosteal bone proliferation is observed radiographically. Healthy bone does not exfoliate well; however, inflamed or neoplastic bone exfoliates much more readily. Bone aspiration can be performed with an 18- to 22-gauge needle; if there is considerable lysis, the smaller gauge needle is helpful. Both aspiration and nonsuction penetration techniques can be used to obtain a specimen for cytopathology. Additionally, imprints of tissue obtained for a histopathology can be used for cytopathology. Care must be taken to blot as much blood off the tissue specimen as possible before making the imprints (see Chapter 1). The bone should be sampled in the center of the lesion rather than on the periphery of the lesion, where there may be a transition between normal and abnormal bone.

Normal Bone Anatomy and Cytology

Normal bone consists of mineralized tissue (osteoid) with small cells, osteocytes, enclosed in small lacunae within the osteoid. Osteoblasts appear on the bone surface, produce osteoid, and initiate the mineralization of the matrix. Osteoid appears

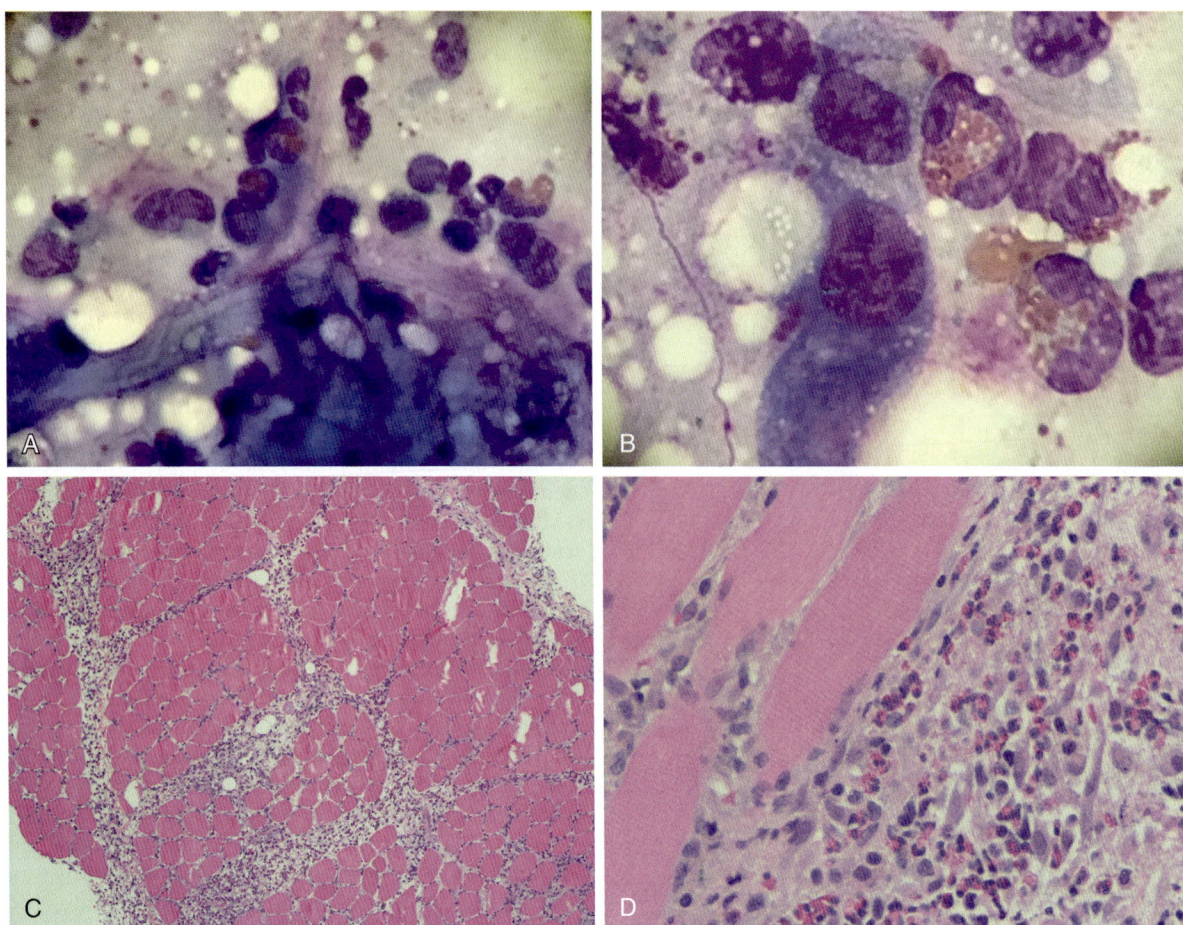

■ **FIGURE 14.34 Eosinophilic myositis. Cervical musculature. Dog.** Same case in A to D. The patient presented with cervical muscle spasms and occasional stumbling. **A, Tissue imprint.** Areas of hyalinized blue skeletal tissue appear along with a predominately eosinophilic with lesser macrophagic and lymphoplasmacytic inflammatory reaction. (Wright-Giemsa; HP oil.) **B, Tissue imprint.** Eosinophils and a fibroblast are prominent in this field. (Wright-Giemsa; HP oil.) **C, Histology.** Numerous eosinophils and fewer macrophages, neutrophils, lymphocytes, and plasma cells admixed with fibrin, and necrotic cellular debris, diffusely, moderately to markedly expand the perimysium and endomysium. Histopathologic diagnosis is myositis, necrotizing, eosinophilic and histiocytic, chronic, diffuse, marked, skeletal muscle. (H&E; LP.) **D. Histology.** Marked eosinophilic infiltrate between muscle fibers. Consideration is given for an immune-mediated myopathy. (H& E; IP.) (Courtesy Rose Raskin, University of Florida.)

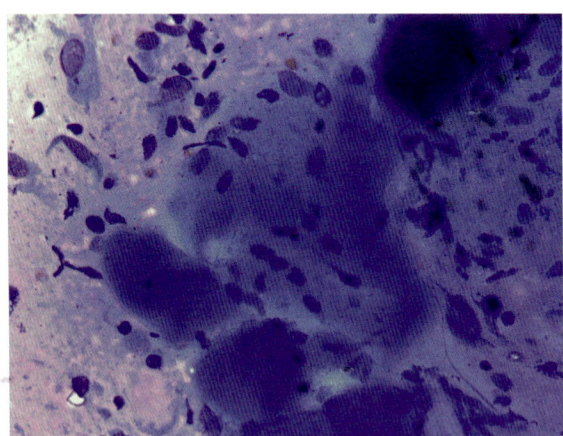

■ **FIGURE 14.35 Mixed cell myositis with fibrosis. Submandibular mass. Tissue aspirate. Dog.** The background consists of blood and bare nuclei from ruptured cells. The large dark blue structures present are consistent with skeletal muscle fragments. Additionally, scattered inflammatory cells and several spindle-shaped cells are identified. (Wright; HP oil.)

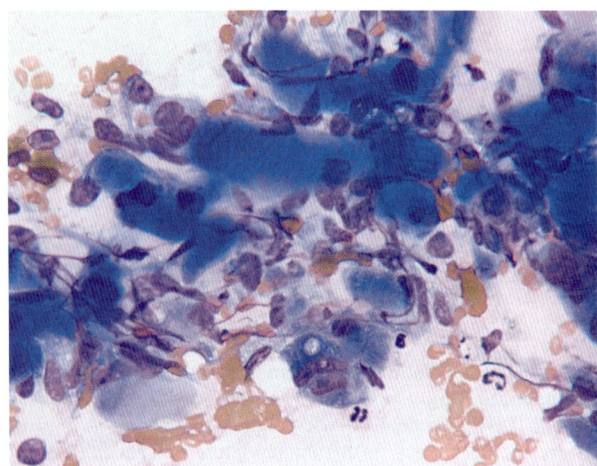

■ **FIGURE 14.36 Rhabdomyosarcoma. Cutaneous mass. Tissue aspirate. Dog.** Cytopathologic specimen from a young mixed-breed dog. A population of neoplastic mesenchymal cells is observed with striations evident within the cytoplasm. The mass was confirmed with histopathology as a rhabdomyosarcoma. (Wright; HP oil.)

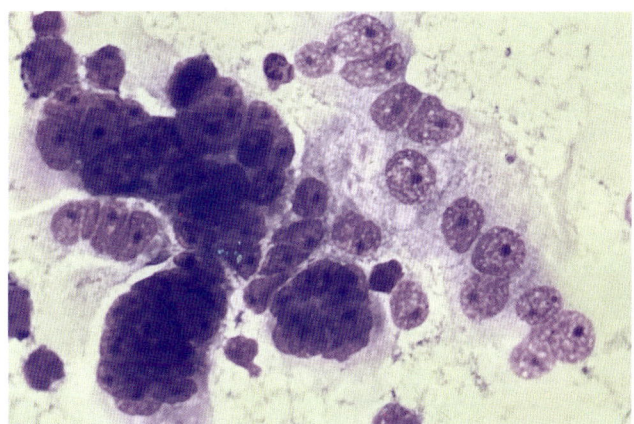

■ **FIGURE 14.37 Rhabdomyosarcoma. Submandibular mass. Tissue aspirate. Dog.** Cytopathologic specimen from a 12-month-old dog with multiple oral and facial masses. Large, multinucleated cells and arrangement of nuclei in rows are present in this histopathologically confirmed case of rhabdomyosarcoma. (Wright-Giemsa; HP oil.) (From Fallin CW, Fox LE, Papendick RE, Christopher MM. What is your diagnosis? A 12-month-old dog with multiple soft tissue masses, Vet Clin Pathol. 1995;24[3]:80.)

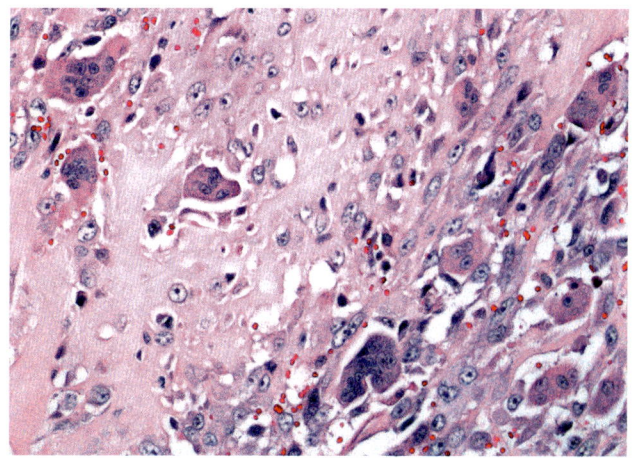

■ **FIGURE 14.39 Rhabdomyosarcoma. Histology. Dog.** Note the many multinucleated cells, some with nuclei in a row. (H&E; IP.) (Courtesy Rose Raskin, University of Florida.)

microscopically as a pink, amorphous, proteinaceous material. On the outer surface of the bone is the periosteum, which consists of fibrous connective tissue. Cytology of normal bone is usually of very low cellularity and may consist of one or two cells per slide or less. The cells that can be seen in healthy bone include osteoblasts, osteoclasts, chondrocytes, hematopoietic precursors, spindle-shaped mesenchymal cells, and periosteal cells (Figs. 14.41 and 14.42). Osteoblasts occur singly or in small groups. Cells are round to triangular and appear plasmacytoid with a small, eccentrically placed nucleus having coarsely stippled chromatin. There may be a perinuclear clearing or Golgi region with few eosinophilic granules in the cytoplasm with indistinct cell borders. Osteoclasts may be occasional and as multinucleated cells, contain multiple uniform nuclei. The cytoplasm is basophilic with a light dusting of eosinophilic granules. These cells are responsible for bone resorption. Chondrocytes are present less commonly unless the specimen is taken near joints or costochondral junctions. They are usually within lacuna as small groups along with cartilaginous fragments. These fragments present as a fibrillar hyaline-like matrix that stains magenta to purple with Romanowsky stains (Akerman et al., 2010).

Reactive Bone and Inflammation

When bone remodeling occurs secondary to trauma, inflammation, or neoplasia, reactive osteoblasts can be observed on cytopathology (Fig. 14.43). These cells are round with deeply basophilic cytoplasm caused by the abundant rough endoplasmic reticulum and mitochondria (Barger, 2017). There is a prominent Golgi apparatus, which appears as a prominent perinuclear clearing. Compared with nonreactive osteoblasts, reactive osteoblasts can exhibit moderate to marked anisocytosis and anisokaryosis and have prominent nucleoli; however, the N:C ratio remains low. It is important not to mistake reactive osteoblasts for neoplastic osteoblasts, which can be challenging cytopathologically and should be interpreted with caution in the absence of inflammation and only minimal criteria of malignancy.

Cytopathology of lytic bone is often very cellular. Processes associated with bone lysis include inflammation, neoplasia, hypertrophic osteopathy, and aneurysmal bone cyst. Osteomyelitis usually consists of suppurative to pyogranulomatous inflammation with varying numbers of neutrophils, macrophages, and multinucleated giant cells depending on the cause of inflammation. Reactive osteoblasts and other mesenchymal cells may also be observed. Osteomyelitis can be caused by bacteria or fungi. Bacterial osteomyelitis can occur secondary to bite wounds, trauma, postsurgical infections, or foreign bodies and less commonly via hematogenous spread. There are many causes of bacterial osteomyelitis; however, organisms commonly associated with osteomyelitis include *Actinomyces* and *Nocardia*. The inflammatory process associated with bacterial osteomyelitis is suppurative rather than pyogranulomatous. It is important to remember when aspirating bone that there is often peripheral blood contamination, and some neutrophils

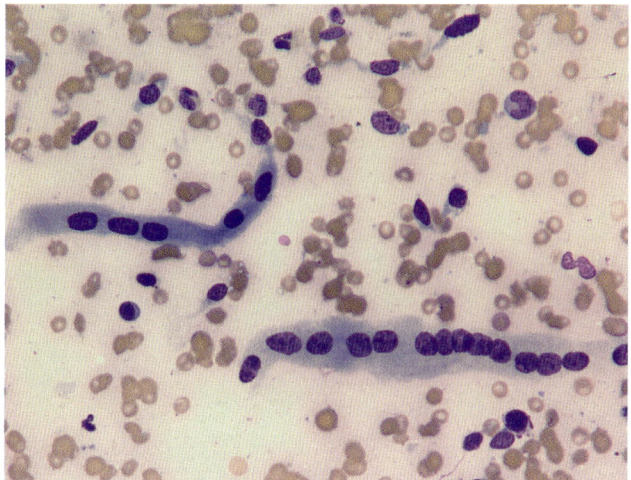

■ **FIGURE 14.38 Rhabdomyosarcoma, myotubular variant. Strap cells. Tissue aspirate.** Two elongated tubular cells are shown. These are formed by the fusion of rhabdomyoblasts. (Romanowsky; HP oil.)

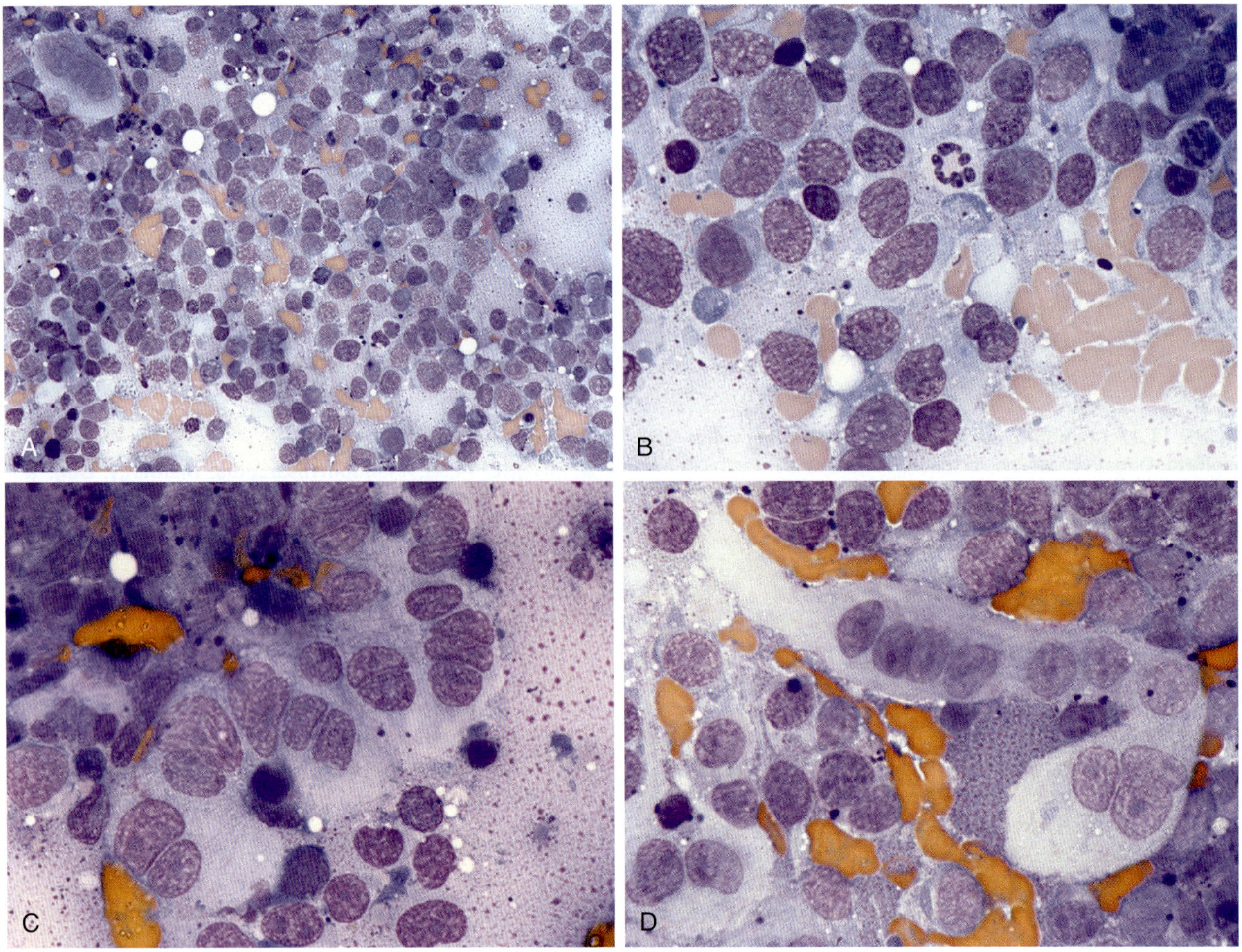

■ **FIGURE 14.40 Embryonal rhabdomyosarcoma. Musculature mass. Tissue aspirate. Dog.** Same case in A to D. Multiple nodular masses in body wall musculature from a 11-month-old bullmastiff. **A,** Highly cellular with mixed cellular morphology. This field is composed of mostly round individualized cells (rhabdomyoblasts) with one multinucleated cell *(upper left)*. (Wright; IP.) **B,** Nuclei are ovoid, round, or polygonal in shape with a stippled chromatin pattern and one to four round to polygonal, prominent nucleoli with moderate anisonucleosis. The nucleocytoplasmic ratio is high. (Wright; HP oil.) **C,** Fusion of rhabdomyoblasts results in a strap cell with multiple often-compressed nuclei. (Wright; HP oil.) **D,** Strap cell with classic myotubular formation. (Wright; HP oil.) (Courtesy Rose Raskin, Kansas State University.)

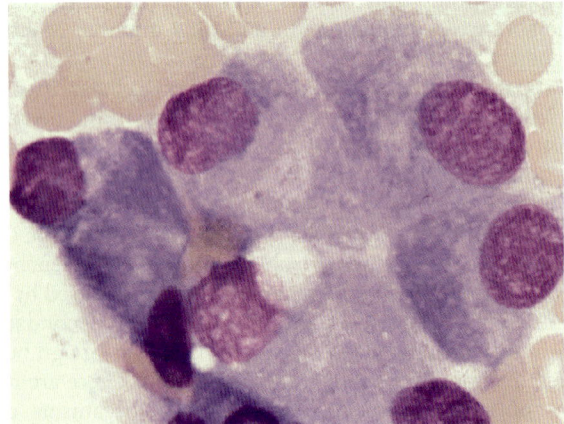

■ **FIGURE 14.41 Normal osteoblasts. Tissue aspirate.** Cells are uniform and oval to triangular with abundant lightly basophilic cytoplasm with pale perinuclear zone. The round to oval eccentrically placed nucleus has coarsely stippled chromatin and small nucleoli. The nucleocytoplasmic ratio is low. (Wright; HP oil.) (Courtesy Purdue Resource Center.)

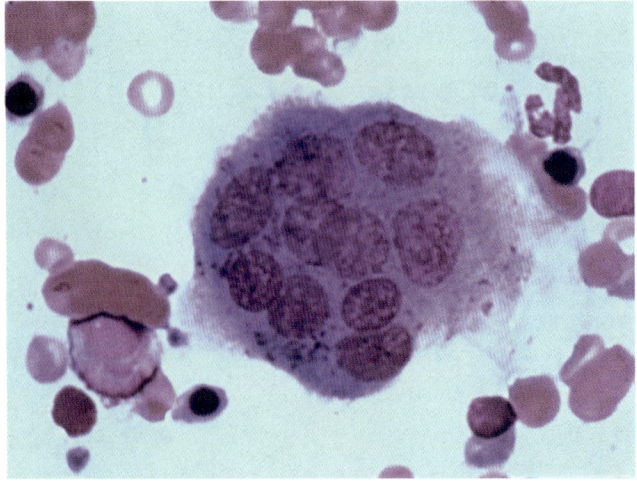

■ **FIGURE 14.42 Normal osteoclast. Tissue aspirate.** A single osteoclast with 10 separate nuclei is shown having a pink-blue granular cytoplasm. (Wright; HP oil.) (Courtesy of Purdue Resource Center.)

CHAPTER 14 *Musculoskeletal System*

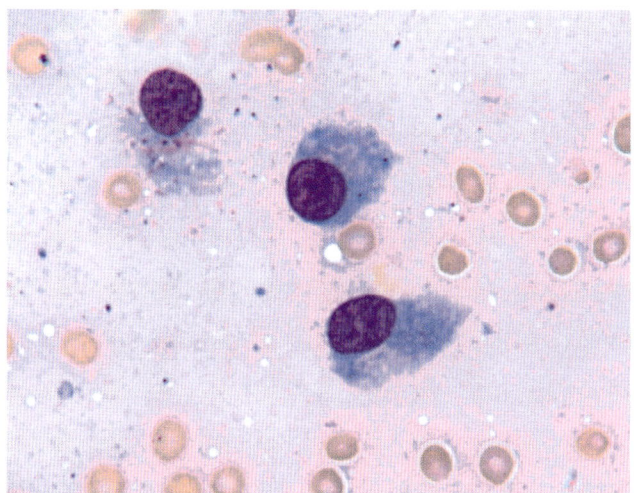

■ **FIGURE 14.43 Reactive osteoblasts. Bone mass. Tissue aspirate. Dog.** Aspirate from a lytic and proliferative lesion in the distal radius. The sample overall is of low cellularity. Pictured are three reactive osteoblasts with mild anisokaryosis and increased cytoplasmic basophilia. These cells commonly have an eccentrically placed nucleus with prominent Golgi apparatus and prominent nucleoli. Care must be taken not to overinterpret reactive osteoblasts for neoplastic cells; contrast with Figures 14.51C and 14.52A. (Wright; HP oil.)

all of the slides. Fungal organisms known to cause osteomyelitis include *Blastomyces dermatitidis* (Fig. 14.44), *Cryptococcus* spp. (Block et al., 2017), *Coccidioides* spp. (Fig. 14.45), *Histoplasma capsulatum* and, less commonly, *Candida* spp., *Aspergillus* spp., *Geomyces* spp. (Erne et al., 2007), *Sporothrix* spp., and *Curvularia* spp. (Fig. 14.46). *Blastomyces* is a round yeast organism with a double-contoured wall and broad-based bud. *Coccidioides* organisms are large (10–100 µm) blue or clear spheres with finely granular protoplasm. *Histoplasma* organisms by comparison are relatively small (2–4 µm), are easily phagocytized by macrophages, and can be observed within the cytoplasm of macrophages. The organisms are round with a thin capsule and crescent-shaped, eccentrically placed, eosinophilic nuclei. Cryptococcal organisms are round with a narrow-based bud and thick, nonstaining with Wright stain, mucoid capsule.

Reactive osteoblasts, osteoclasts, and fibroblasts may be encountered during response to bone fractures from trauma, infection, or neoplasia (Fig. 14.47). Hematopoietic cells (Fig. 14.48) are more commonly encountered in reparative bone lesions (Reinhardt et al., 2005). The healing response is best appreciated in polarized histologic sections where woven bone is laid down, resulting in disorganized collagen instead of normal parallel layers (Carlson and Weisbrode, 2012).

Neoplasia

Bone tumors often cause lysis or proliferation of the bone. They can be categorized as primary bone tumors, tumors of bone marrow, tumors that invade bone, or tumors that are metastatic to bone (Rosol et al., 2003). For osteodestructive lesions caused by primary bone tumors, metastatic carcinoma and non-neoplastic lesions, accuracy was 83% for cytopathology (sensitivity, 83.3%; specificity, 80%) and 82.1% for histology (sensitivity, 72.2%; specificity, 100%). Tumor type was correctly identified on cytopathology and histopathology in 50% and 55.5% of cases, respectively (Sabattini et al., 2017).

Primary bone tumors include osteosarcoma (Figs. 14.49 to 14.55), chondrosarcoma (Figs. 14.56 and 14.57), fibrosarcoma, hemangiosarcoma (Fig. 14.58), and synovial cell sarcoma (Chun,

will be observed secondary to the hemodilution. It may be necessary to evaluate and contrast neutrophil numbers from a hemogram or peripheral blood smear to determine if there are truly increased numbers of neutrophils within the cytopathology sample. Observation of intracellular bacteria is diagnostic for bacterial osteomyelitis. Culture is recommended for all suppurative inflammatory bone aspirates.

Fungal osteomyelitis consists of a pyogranulomatous to suppurative inflammatory process and often consists of neutrophils, macrophages, and multinucleated giant cells. Organisms are not always observed in the aspirate, so it is important to obtain multiple aspirates, three or four if possible, and examine

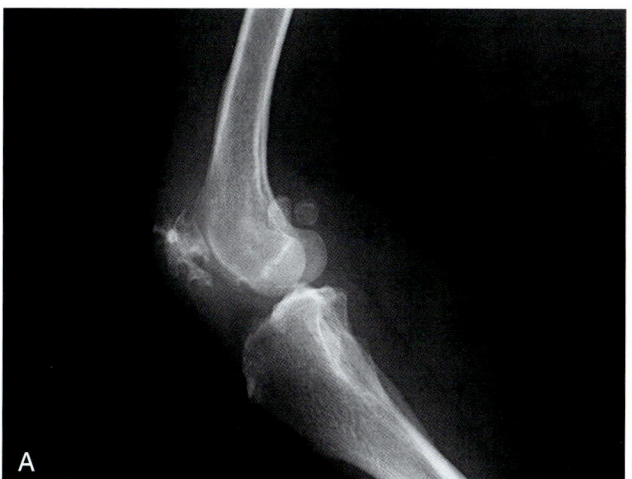 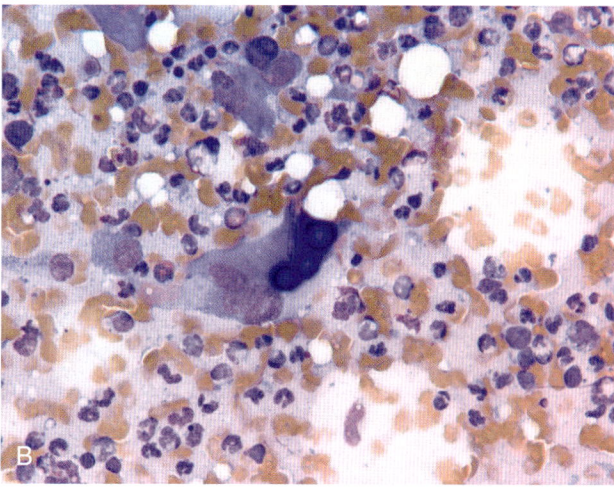

■ **FIGURE 14.44 Blastomycosis. Bone lesion. Dog.** Same case in A and B. **A, Radiograph.** A 3-year-old dog with a history of left hind leg lameness. A lytic lesion is noted in the patella. **B, Tissue aspirate.** The specimen from the lytic lesion is cellular and consists of a mixed inflammatory population predominated by neutrophils. Several fungal yeast organisms, consistent with *Blastomyces dermatitidis,* are observed. (Wright; HP oil.) (A, Courtesy Kristen Odell-Anderson.)

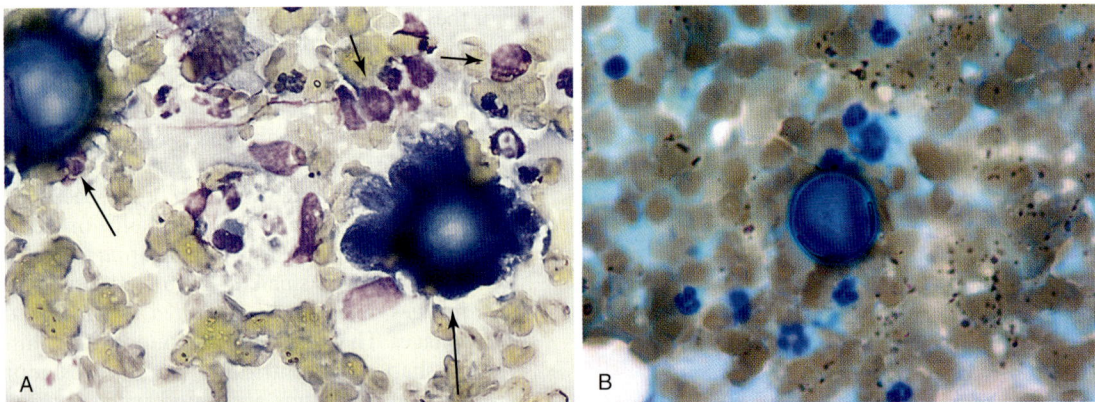

■ **FIGURE 14.45 Coccidioidomycosis. Bone lesion. Tissue aspirate. Dog. A,** Specimen from a lytic lesion in the scapula of a middle-aged dog with pain and lameness of the foreleg. In addition to blood, there is a mixture of inflammatory cells and smudged nuclei *(short arrow)*. Two large, blue, spherical structures are present in this field *(long arrow)*, which are *Coccidioides* spp. spherules. The size of the spherules prevents sharp focusing on both spherules and background cells. When focusing up and down on these spherules, variable numbers of endospores may be seen within. Aspiration of fungal myelitis lesions does not always yield observable organisms (particularly *Coccidioides*); if infection is suspected, culture and appropriate serology are indicated. Relative to the zoonotic potential of some fungal organisms, extreme care should be taken when culturing these lesions. (Wright; HP oil.) **B,** Specimen from a lytic lesion in the proximal humerus of a 4-year-old dog with a history of lameness of the left front leg. The cellularity is low and is markedly hemodiluted, with many red blood cells observed in the background. Few inflammatory cells and one *Coccidioides* spp. spherule are observed. The spherule is filled with many endospores, and occasionally a spherule will rupture, allowing the much smaller endospores to be visualized. It is common to find low numbers of spherules in a bone aspirate. (Wright; HP oil.)

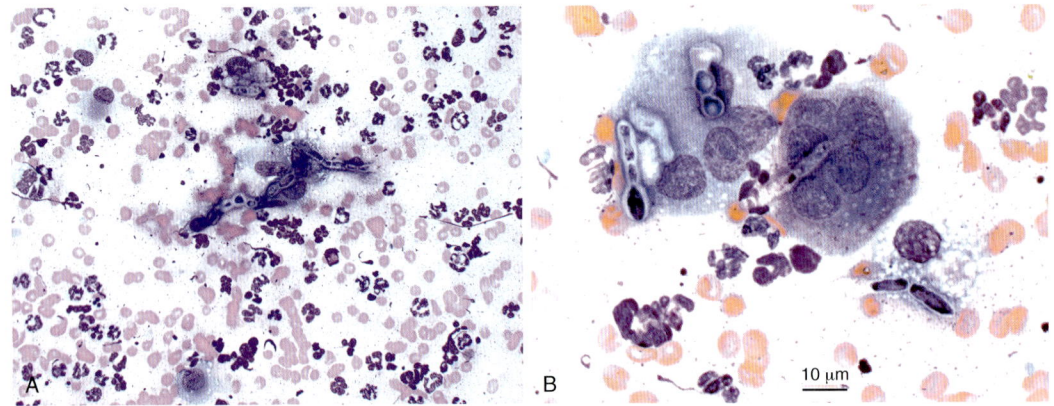

■ **FIGURE 14.46** *Curvularia* **spp. Infection. Osteolytic tarsal bone. Tissue aspirate. Dog.** Same case in A and B. Patient had been treated for a long-standing disseminated phaeohyphomycosis diagnosed by culture as *Curvularia spicifera (Bipolaris spicifera)*. **A,** Highly cellular specimen with numerous neutrophils, both mildly karyolytic and nondegenerate, and several macrophages and giant multinucleated cells. (Wright; HP oil.) **B,** Within macrophages are collections of hyphal structures. These septate hyphae measure approximately 5 μm in width and have swollen bulbous ends. A basophilic internal structure is easily visible. Cytopathologic diagnosis is severe mixed pyogranulomatous (neutrophilic and histiocytic) osteitis with intralesional hyphae. (Wright; HP oil.) (Courtesy Rose Raskin, North Carolina State University.)

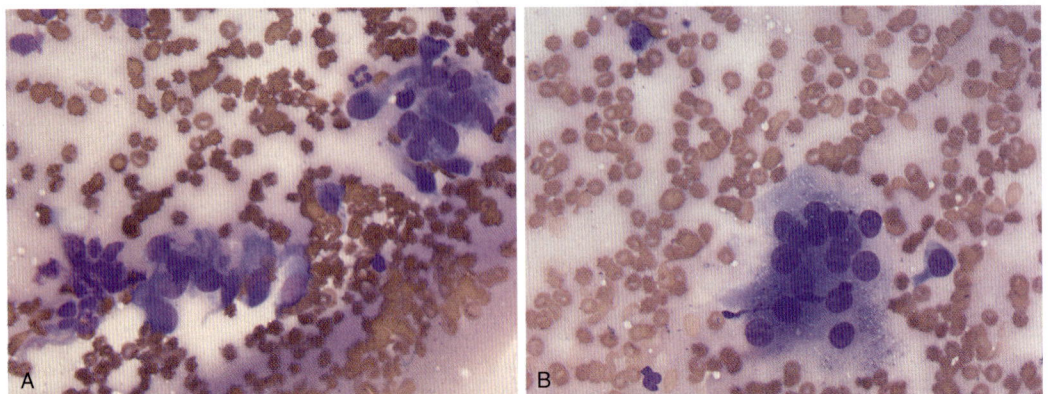

■ **FIGURE 14.47 Osteoclasts and reactive fibrosis. Radius and ulna fracture site. Tissue aspirate. Dog.** Same case in A and B. **A,** Numerous plump fibroblasts are present during bone healing. **B,** Osteoclast is present to assist in bone remodeling. There was no evidence of osteomyelitis or neoplasia. (Wright; HP oil.) (Courtesy Rose Raskin, University of Bristol, UK.)

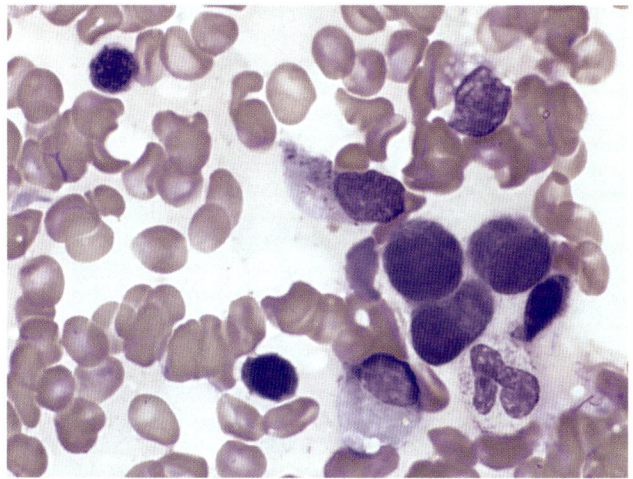

■ **FIGURE 14.48 Reactive osteoblasts and hematopoietic precursors. Humerus. Tissue aspirate.** Three osteoblasts are present having a higher nucleocytoplasmic ratio with deep basophilic cytoplasm. Also present are three erythroid precursors. Reactive bone is more likely to show hematopoietic precursors than osteosarcoma. (Wright; HP oil.) (Courtesy Rose Raskin, Michigan State University.)

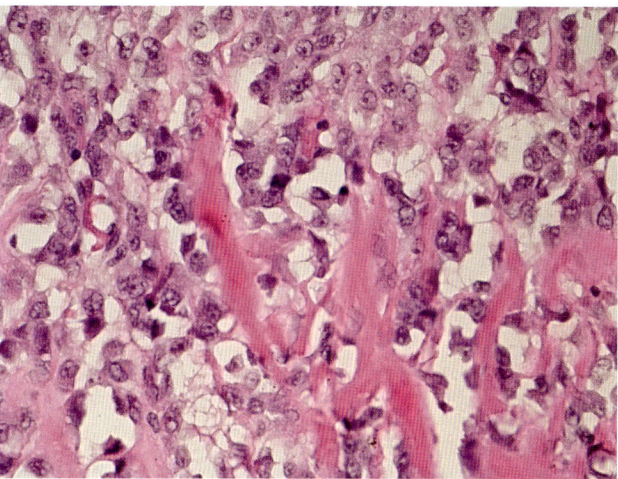

■ **FIGURE 14.50 Osteosarcoma. Histology. Dog.** Classical appearance of sheets of cells with euchromatic nuclei and one or multiple prominent nucleoli. There is scant to moderate pale eosinophilic cytoplasm. Islands and trabeculae of amorphous eosinophilic matrix, interpreted as tumor osteoid, separate the proliferative cells. (H&E; IP.) (Courtesy Rose Raskin, Michigan State University.)

2005). Cytopathologically, these tumors can be difficult to differentiate from one another. General cytopathologic features include round to spindle-shaped cells with basophilic cytoplasm and an eccentrically placed nucleus, with prominent nucleoli (Reinhardt et al., 2005). In one study, several cytopathologic features helped to distinguish histopathologically confirmed osteosarcoma from reparative non-neoplastic bone lesions. (Reinhardt et al., 2005). Cellularity was moderate with frequent necrosis in osteosarcoma but poor to moderate cellularity and minimal necrosis in reparative bone proliferations. Hematopoietic precursor cells occurred frequently in reparative callus material but infrequently in malignant tissue. The nuclei contained one or two nucleoli in callus smears and frequently more than two nucleoli per nucleus in osteosarcoma. In osteosarcoma, the nucleocytoplasmic ratio was significantly increased as a result of an increase in the nuclear diameter and a decrease in the cellular diameter compared with that in dogs with reparative proliferations. Neoplastic osteoblasts showed significantly more criteria of malignancy than reactive osteoblasts, including coarse chromatin, angular nucleoli, thickening of the nuclear membrane, cytoplasmic vacuolization, macronucleosis, aberrant mitoses, and nuclear molding (see Fig. 14.51C). Classical osteosarcomas present with rounded cells and frequent eosinophilic osteoid matrix (see Figs. 14.49B, 14.50, and 14.51). Two variants of osteosarcoma include fibroblastic (see Figs. 14.53 and 14.54) and anaplastic with giant cells (see Fig. 14.55).

Osteosarcoma, hemangiosarcoma, and hemophagocytic histiocytic sarcoma have all been reported to exhibit erythrophagia

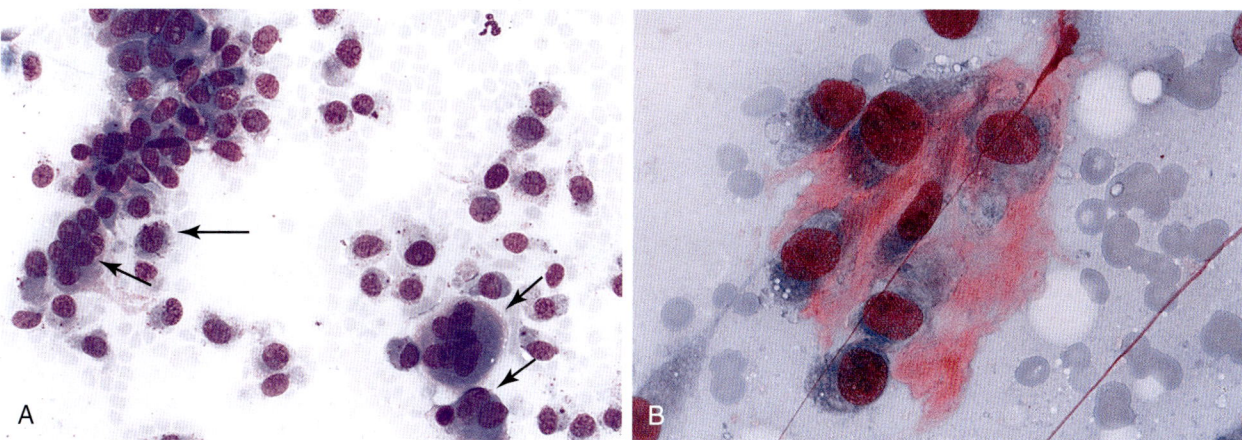

■ **FIGURE 14.49 Osteosarcoma. Tissue aspirate.** Same case in A and B. **A, Cellularity.** Sample taken from a lytic and proliferative lesion of the proximal tibia. The specimen is bloody with high cellularity with a mixture of ellipsoid and multinucleated cells *(short arrows)*. Some areas show thick accumulations of cells *(long arrow)*. (Wright; HP oil.) **B, Eosinophilic background matrix.** Higher magnification of the background demonstrates a group of individualized cells that are presumptively osteoblasts with swirls of a fine, pink extracellular material around them. Note the large cell size by contrasting them to the greenish-stained erythrocytes. This appearance is most consistent with a sarcoma. It is difficult to distinguish by cytopathology different types of sarcoma, and additional tests such as radiography and histopathology are necessary for definitive morphologic diagnosis. Histopathology of this lesion indicated osteosarcoma. (Wright; HP oil.)

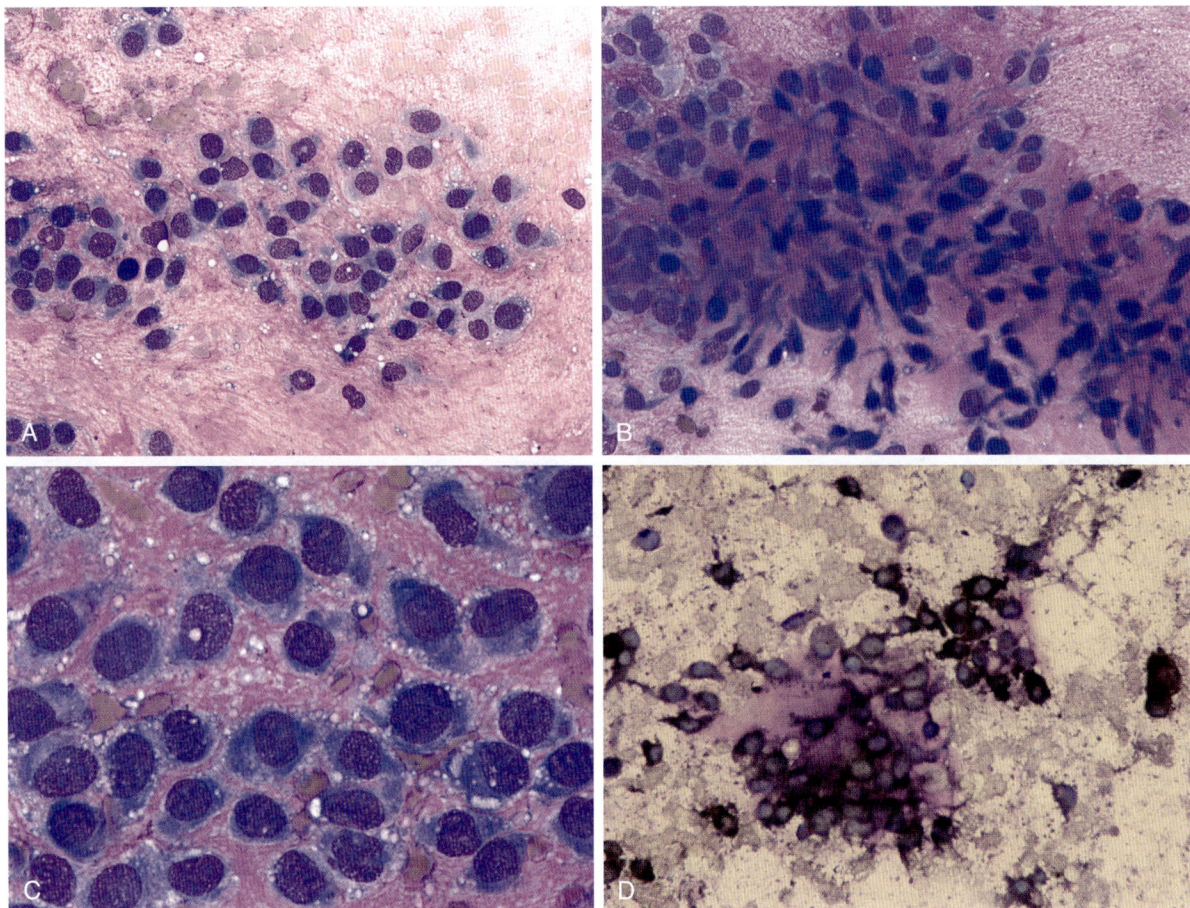

FIGURE 14.51 Osteosarcoma. Humerus. Tissue aspirate. Dog. Same case in A to D. **A,** Highly cellular population of individualized cells with round to oval nuclei and scant basophilic cytoplasm with wispy indistinct cell borders. (Wright; IP.) **B,** Dense eosinophilic matrix is surrounded and admixed with round or spindle cells. (Wright; IP.) **C,** Background stains densely eosinophilic. Cells enmeshed in this matrix have a round or oval nuclei with coarse chromatin and multiple prominent nucleoli. Malignant features involve anisokaryosis, multiple and irregular nucleoli, coarse chromatin, and a high nucleocytoplasmic ratio. Histopathology confirmed cytopathologic diagnosis of osteosarcoma. (Wright; HP oil.) **D,** Black staining reaction supports osteoblast cell origin. Cells are counterstained with a Romanowsky stain to best see the cells. (ALP; IP.) (A–D, Courtesy Rose Raskin, Kansas State University.)

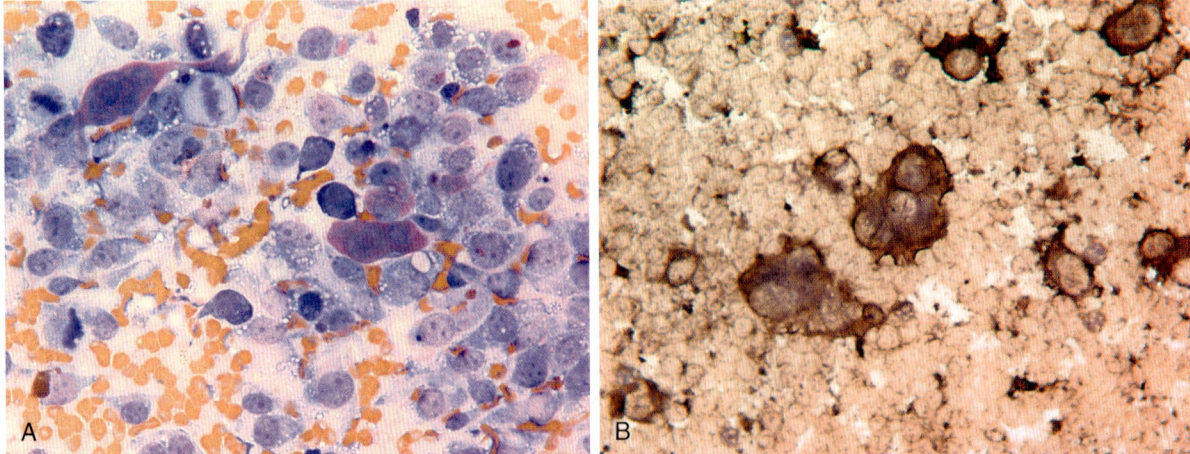

FIGURE 14.52 Osteosarcoma. Bone mass. Dog. Same case in A and B. **A,** Sample from a proliferative and lytic lesion in the proximal humerus of a mixed-breed dog. The sample is cellular and consists of a population of round and spindle-shaped neoplastic cells. Multiple criteria of malignancy are observed, including prominent and multiple nucleoli, anisocytosis and anisokaryosis, and marked variability in the nucleocytoplasmic ratio. Small pools of eosinophilic proteinaceous matrix are identified. The cytopathologic diagnosis is sarcoma. (Wright; HP oil.) **B,** Alkaline phosphatase (ALP) staining of a previously unstained slide demonstrates a strong positive reaction for ALP activity, as indicated by the black staining of the cytoplasm. Diagnosis of osteosarcoma was confirmed with histopathology. (ALP; HP oil.)

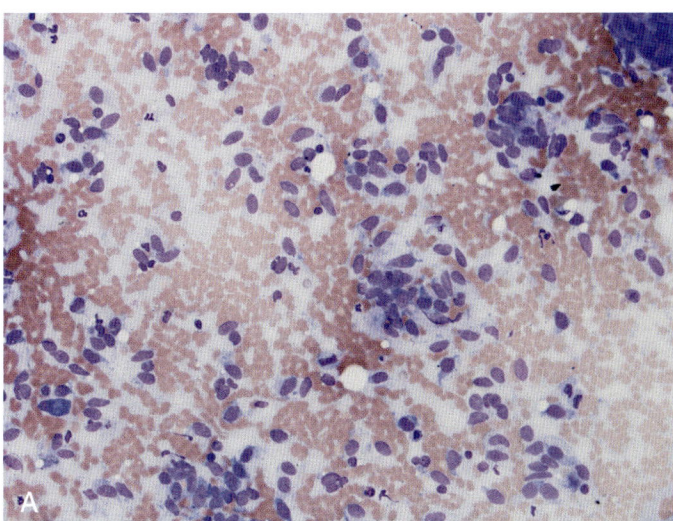
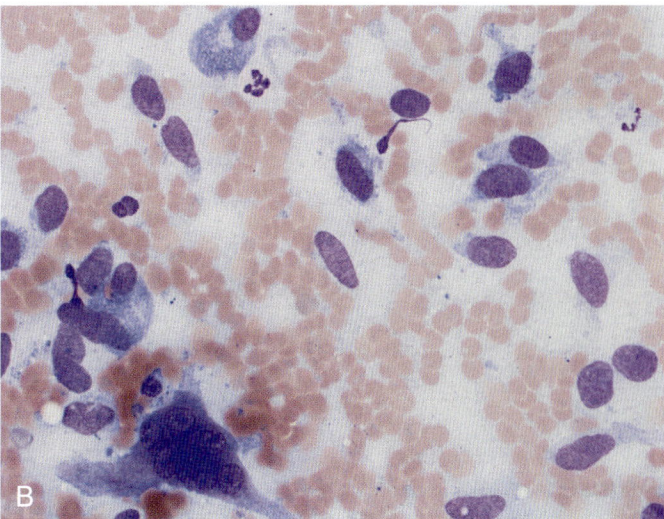

■ **FIGURE 14.53 Osteosarcoma, fibroblastic variant. Scapular mass. Tissue aspirate. Dog.** Same case in A and B. The patient had a 6-month history of an intermittent forelimb lameness. A 6-cm mass was present over the scapula that was painful on palpation. Lysis is seen radiographically. **A,** Highly cellular specimen consisting of spindle cells with fusiform nuclei and wispy pointed basophilic cytoplasmic ends. (Wright-Giemsa; IP.) **B,** Two benign-appearing osteoblasts and one osteoclast are present among the many spindle cells. Cytopathologic diagnosis was sarcoma, possibly fibrosarcoma related to the spindle cell appearance. However, histopathologic diagnosis indicated a fibroblastic osteosarcoma with small islands of osteoid material present. (Wright-Giemsa; HP oil.) (Courtesy Rose Raskin, University of Florida.)

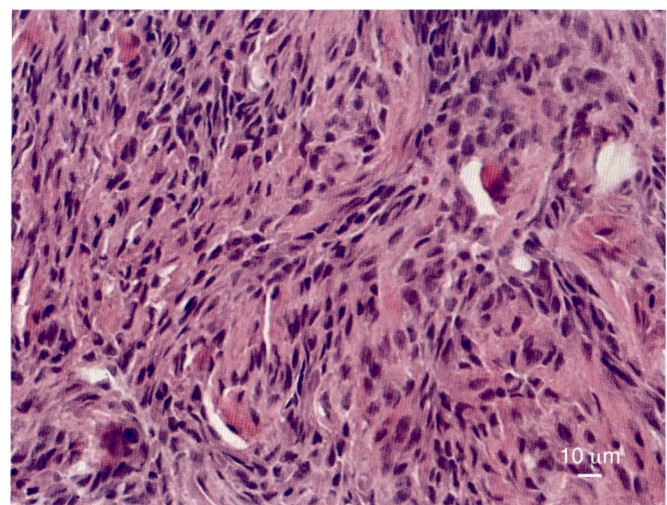

■ **FIGURE 14.54 Osteosarcoma, fibroblastic variant. Histology. Humerus. Dog.** Densely cellular neoplastic mesenchymal cells forming packed interwoven bundles and streams supported by fibrovascular stroma. Scattered throughout are small islands of brightly eosinophilic, amorphous substance (osteoid). Cells are medium to large with indistinct borders and abundant, granular eosinophilic cytoplasm. Nuclei are small to medium, oval to fusiform, with dense chromatin and an occasionally prominent nucleolus. (H&E; IP.) (Courtesy Rose Raskin, Michigan State University.)

(see Fig. 14.58B) (Barger et al., 2012). Osteosarcoma, chondrosarcoma, and fibrosarcoma can have varying amounts of eosinophilic proteinaceous material in the background (see Figs. 14.49B, 14.50, and 14.51). This material can also be observed within the cytoplasm. Osteoid was not detectable in 24% of the osteosarcoma (Reinhardt et al., 2005).

Chondrosarcomas can have a large amount of matrix in the background, which results in understaining of the cells (see Figs. 14.56 and 14.57B and C). Despite these subtle differences, these tumors can be difficult to differentiate by cytopathology, and histopathology is necessary (see Fig. 14.57D). Hemangiosarcoma and telangiectatic osteosarcoma can be difficult to differentiate even with histopathology. Immunohistochemical staining with antibodies against factor VIII–related antigen helps identify hemangiosarcoma of bone more readily (Giuffrida et al., 2017).

Additional cytochemical testing can also be done to improve the sensitivity of cytopathologic diagnosis of osteosarcoma. Staining of the neoplastic cells for alkaline phosphatase (ALP) activity with nitroblue tetrazolium chloride/5-bromo-4-chloro-3-indolyl phosphate toluidine salt (NBT/BCIP) increases the sensitivity and specificity of differentiating osteosarcoma from other mesenchymal tumors (Barger et al., 2005). One limitation of this staining technique is that reactive osteoblasts will stain positive as well, so obvious criteria of malignancy must be observed before this test is performed (see Figs. 14.51C and 14.52A). Grayish-black staining of the cytoplasm (see Figs. 14.5 and 14.52B) indicates positive staining. Previously unstained slides are best used; however, a recent study showed that previously stained slides can be destained and subsequently stained for ALP activity (Ryseff and Bohn, 2012). See Appendix 2 for more procedure details. After staining for ALP activity, cells can be lightly counterstained with a Romanowsky stain to examine the positive cells for the appropriate criteria of malignancy.

> **KEY POINT** Bone tumors can be difficult to distinguish with cytopathology alone; additional stains such as ALP or histopathology may be necessary for definitive diagnosis.

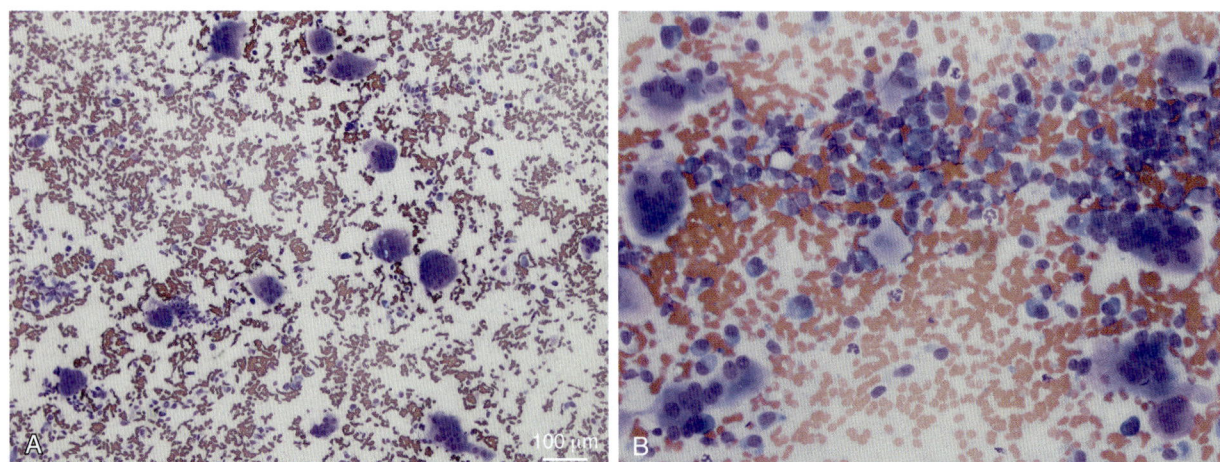

■ **FIGURE 14.55 Osteosarcoma, giant cell variant. Mandibular mass. Tissue aspirate. Dog.** Same case in A and B. Specimen is from a 6 × 8 cm mass on a Boston terrier. **A,** Many large multinucleate giant cells are present against a moderately hemodiluted background. (Wright-Giemsa; LP.) **B,** A highly cellular specimen with many atypical mesenchymal cells is present individually and in loosely associated aggregates in addition to several giant multinucleate cells. Cytopathologic diagnosis was sarcoma, likely anaplastic sarcoma, with giant cells or osteosarcoma. Histopathologic diagnosis confirmed osteosarcoma. (Wright-Giemsa; IP.) (Courtesy Rose Raskin, University of Florida.)

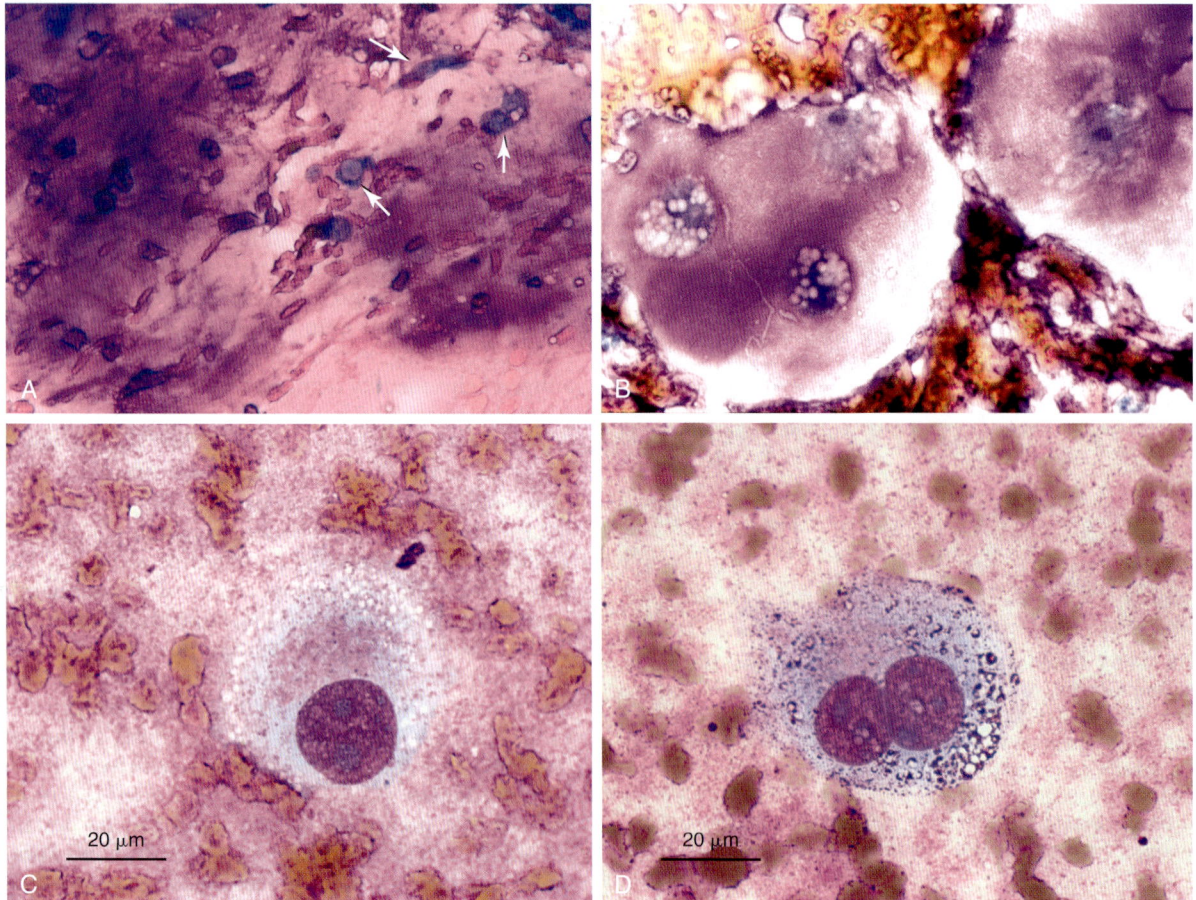

■ **FIGURE 14.56 Chondrosarcoma. Bone lesion. Tissue aspirate. Dog. A,** Aspirate from a lytic bone lesion in the distal radius of a 10-year-old Labrador retriever. The sample is highly cellular. Neoplastic cells *(arrows)* are not stained well because of the abundant amounts of deeply eosinophilic matrix filling the background. The presence of this material is common in bone tumors, particularly chondroma and chondrosarcoma. The cytopathologic diagnosis of this sample is sarcoma, likely chondrosarcoma. Histopathology confirmed the diagnosis of chondrosarcoma. (Wright; HP oil.) **B,** Foamy cytoplasm of the chondrocytes gives the appearance of lacunae within dense, eosinophilic, mucinous material. (Wright; HP oil.) **C,** Note the prominent multiple nucleoli, coarse chromatin clumping, and fine eosinophilic and cytoplasmic granularity in the mononuclear cell. (Wright; HP oil.) **D, Tissue aspirate.** Binucleated cell cytoplasm contains dark-purple cytoplasmic granularity, and the two nuclei have slightly different sizes. (Wright; HP oil.) (B, Courtesy Rick Alleman, University of Florida. C, Courtesy Rose Raskin, Purdue University.)

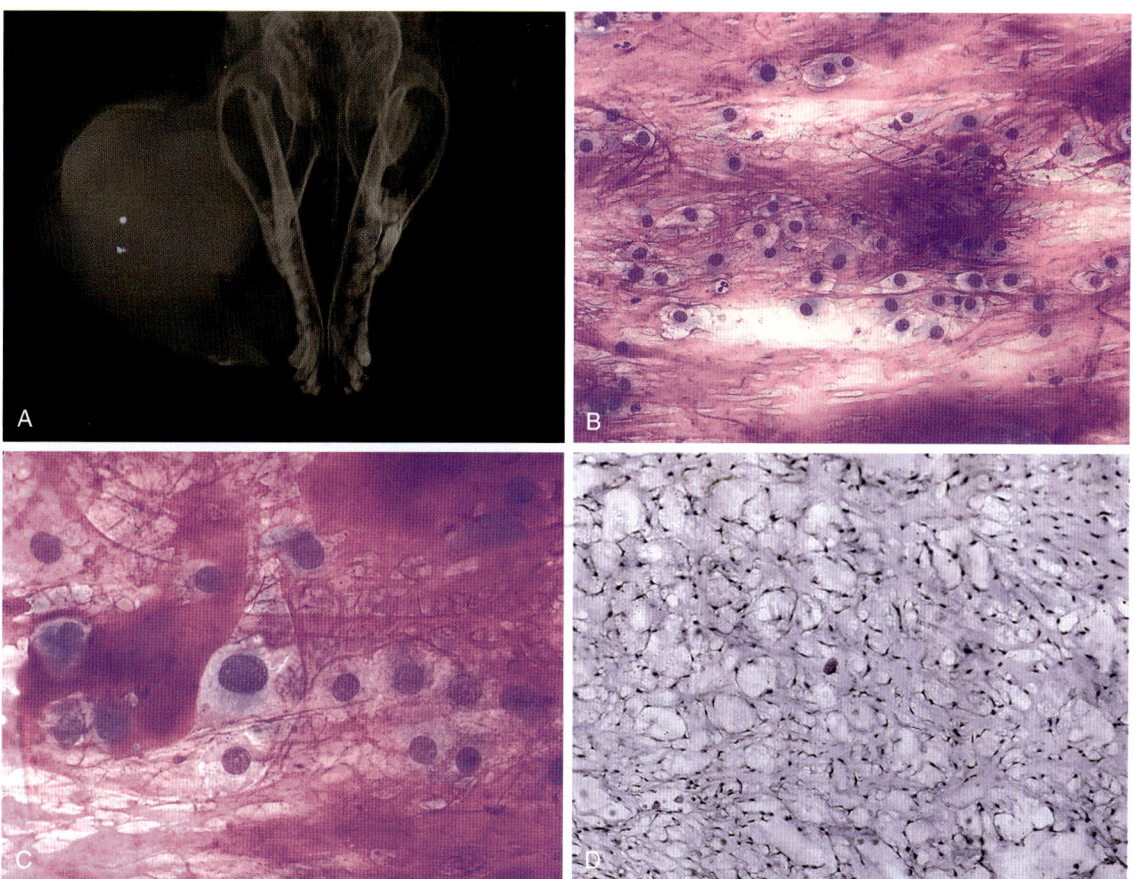

■ **FIGURE 14.57 Chondroid neoplasm. Head mass. Dog.** Same case in A to D. **A, Radiology.** A large homogenous round mass extends from the orbital region without bone lysis. **B, Tissue aspirate.** A dense eosinophilic fibrillary matrix material fills the background. A uniform population of single cells or small cell aggregates arranged in rows is admixed within the matrix. (Romanowsky; HP oil.) **C, Tissue aspirate.** Round cells with abundant pale cytoplasm display moderate anisokaryosis and stippled chromatin. Some cells appear in lacunae within dense deeply eosinophilic matrix. Cytopathologic diagnosis is chondroid neoplasm. (Romanowsky; HP oil.) **D, Histology.** Thin cords of stellate vacuolated chondrocytes are embedded in an abundant, mostly hypovascular, mucinous matrix. Formalin fixation is known to shrink cell nuclei, producing a much smaller nucleocytoplasmic ratio compared with the cytopathologic specimen. Histologic appearance is consistent but not diagnostic for a myxoid chondrosarcoma. (H&E; IP.) (Courtesy of Polly Franco, Brazil.)

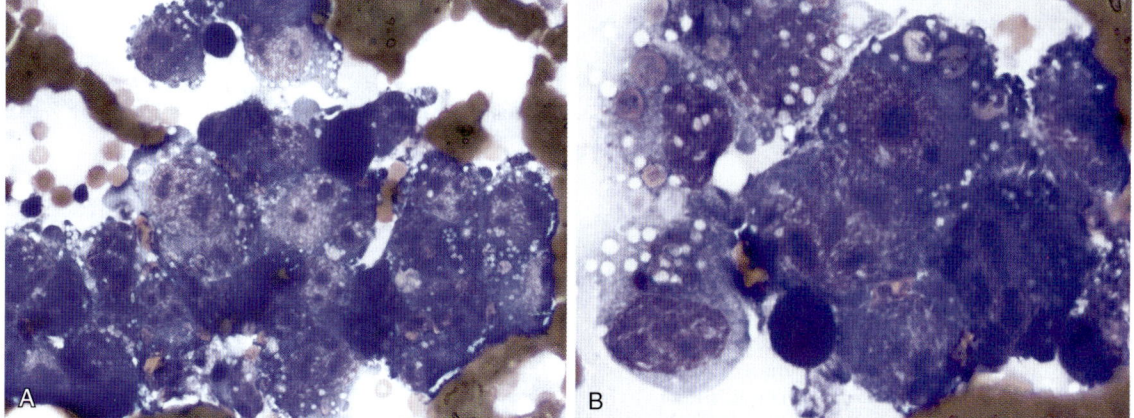

■ **FIGURE 14.58 Hemangiosarcoma. Scapular mass. Tissue aspirate. Dog.** Same case in A and B. Radiographs indicate a destructive bone lesion. Clinically, the scapular swelling was firm. **A,** The specimen is markedly bloody with few large cellular aggregates. Cells display marked anaplastic features, including high to moderate nucleocytoplasmic ratio, coarse chromatin, multiple nucleoli (up to eight), moderate anisokaryosis (3–6 × RBC diameter), and marked anisonucleoliosis. Cells appear irregularly round to stellate when individualized, with frequent surface blebbing. The cytoplasm is dark blue and frequently contains numerous punctate vacuoles. (Wright; HP oil.) **B,** A large percentage of these cells contain erythrocytes within their cytoplasm, as shown here. The cytopathologic diagnosis is hemangiosarcoma. Histopathology was not available to confirm this presumed diagnosis. (Wright; HP oil.) (Courtesy Rose Raskin, Michigan State University.)

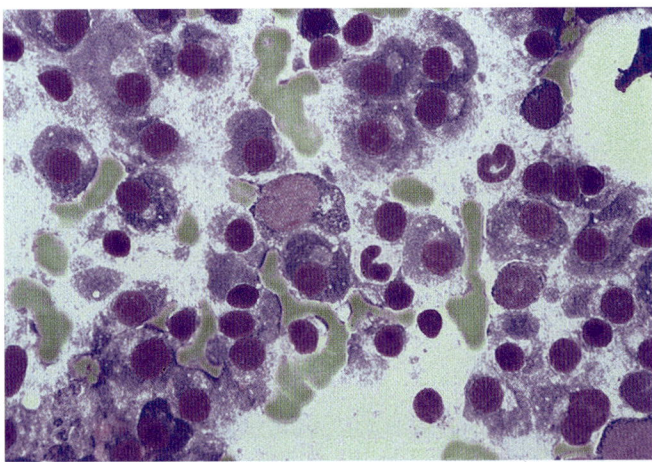

■ **FIGURE 14.59 Multiple myeloma. Bone lesion. Tissue aspirate. Dog.** Sample from a lytic, "punched-out" lesion in a vertebral spinous process of an 8-year-old dog. The specimen is predominated by mildly pleomorphic plasma cells. This finding in combination with the presence of lytic bony lesions is diagnostic for multiple myeloma. (Wright; HP oil.)

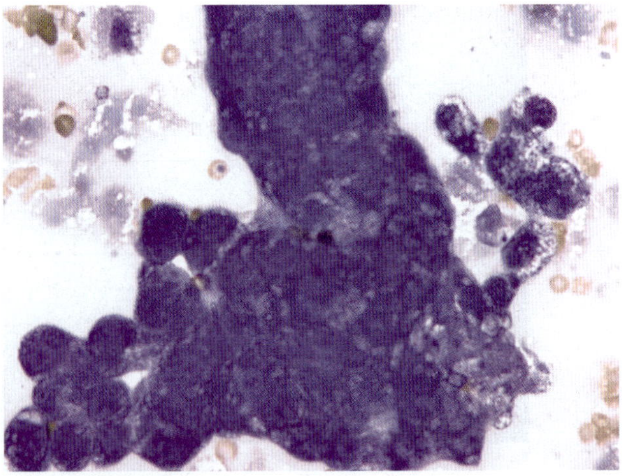

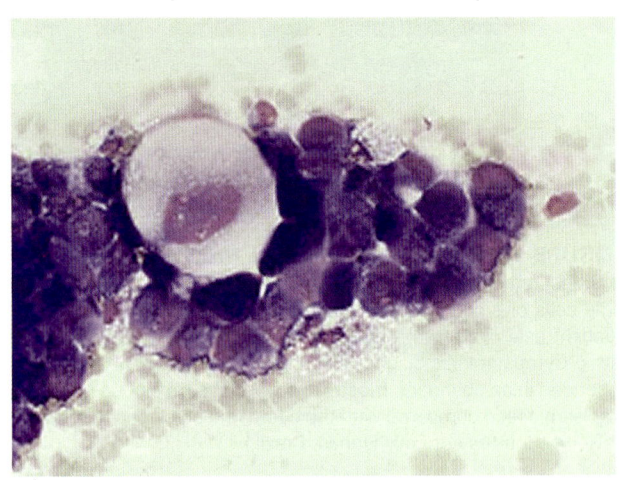

■ **FIGURE 14.60 Metastatic carcinoma. Bone lesion. Tissue aspirate. Dog.** Specimen from a lytic lesion in a vertebral body from a dog with a history of prostatic carcinoma. The cohesive nature of these cells is consistent with carcinoma; in this case, the most likely diagnosis is metastatic prostatic carcinoma. (Wright; HP oil.)

Lymphoma and plasma cell tumors are considered tumors of bone marrow that can result in bone lysis. The morphology of these cells appears similar to that in other tissues (Fig. 14.59). Plasma cell tumors produce a characteristic punched-out radiographic appearance. A combination of diagnostic tests is necessary to diagnose the plasma cell tumor as multiple myeloma. In addition to radiographs and cytopathology, protein electrophoresis of serum and urine plus immunofixation may be diagnostic.

Squamous cell carcinoma is the most common tumor that can invade bone. Usually, the cytopathology reveals neoplastic squamous cells with rare or no osteoblasts. Cytopathologic features of this tumor are similar to those in other locations. Many tumors can metastasize to bone, the common ones being prostatic, lung, and mammary carcinomas (McCourt et al., 2018). Identification of metastatic neoplasms can be difficult because cytopathology is often accompanied by reactive osteoblasts and osteoclasts. However, a second population of cells can often be differentiated from the reactive population. Epithelial neoplasms are usually clustered, but when they metastasize, they may appear more poorly differentiated (Figs. 14.60 and 14.61). Immunostaining may be very helpful for diagnosis.

■ **FIGURE 14.61 Metastatic carcinoma. Joint adjacent to bone lysis. Dog.** This sample is from the stifle joint of a 12-year-old golden retriever. The joint was swollen and painful with evidence of bony lysis. Numerous clusters of pleomorphic cells are present. These cells display marked anisocytosis and anisokaryosis with prominent, irregularly shaped nucleoli. The atypia of the cells is consistent with the diagnosis of metastatic carcinoma. (Wright; HP oil.)

REFERENCES

Affolter VK, Moore PF. Localized and disseminated histiocytic sarcoma of dendritic cell origin in dogs. *Vet Pathol.* 2002;39:74-83.

Akerman M, Domanski HA, Jonsson K. Cytology of normal constituents in bone aspirates and of reactive changes. *Monogr Clin Cytol.* 2010;19:13-17.

Alleman AR, Raskin RE, Uhl EW, et al. What is your diagnosis? Bladder mass from an 11-month-old dog. *Vet Clin Pathol.* 1991;20:44.

Avallone G, Pinto da Cunha N, Palmieri C, et al. Subcutaneous embryonal rhabdomyosarcoma in a dog: cytologic, immunocytochemical, histologic, and ultrastructural features. *Vet Clin Pathol.* 2010;39(4):499-504.

Barger A, Graca R, Bailey K, et al. Utilization of alkaline phosphatase staining to differentiate osteosarcoma from other vimentin positive tumors. *Vet Pathol.* 2005;42:161-165.

Barger AM. Cytology of bone. *Vet Clin North Am Small Anim Pract.* 2017;47: 71-84.

Barger AM, Skowronski MC, MacNeill AL. Cytologic identification of erythrophagocytic neoplasms in the dog. *Vet Clin Pathol.* 2012;41: 587-589.

Birckhead A, Combs M, Croser E, et al. Idiopathic eosinophilic polysynovitis in a dog. *Vet Rec Case Rep.* 2019;7:e000763.

Block K, Battig J. Cryptococcal maxillary osteomyelitis and osteonecrosis in a 18-month-old dog. *J Vet Dent.* 2017;34(2):76-85.

Britt T, Clifford C, Barger A, et al. Diagnosing appendicular osteosarcoma with ultrasound-guided fine-needle aspiration: 36 cases. *J Small Anim Pract.* 2007;48:145-150.

Camus MS, Burnum A, Howerth EW, et al. What is your diagnosis? Digit aspirate from a dog. *Vet Clin Pathol.* 2017;46(4):635-636.

Carlson CS, Weisbrode SE. Bones, joints, tendons, and ligaments. In: Zachary JF, McGavin MD, eds. *Pathologic Basis of Veterinary Disease*. 5th ed. St Louis: Elsevier; 2012:920-971.

Carr AP, Michels G. Identifying noninfectious erosive arthritis in dogs and cats. *Vet Med*. 1997;92:804-810.

Caserto BG. A comparative review of canine and human rhabdomyosarcoma with emphasis on classification and pathogenesis. *Vet Pathol*. 2013;55(5):806-826.

Cazzini P, Frontera-Acevedo K, Garner B, et al. Morphologic, molecular, and ultrastructural characterization of a feline synovial cell sarcoma and derived cell line. *J Vet Diagn Invest*. 2015;27(3):369-376.

Chapman S, Nabity M, Calise D. What is your diagnosis? Lingual mass in a dog. *Vet Clin Pathol*. 2008;37:133-139.

Christopher MM, Wallace LJ. Synovial fluid eosinophilia: a case report in a dog and review of the literature. *Vet Clin Pathol*. 1986;15:25-31.

Chun R. Common malignant musculoskeletal neoplasms of dogs and cats. *Vet Clin North Am Small Anim Pract*. 2005;35:1155-1167.

Clements DN, Owen MR, Mosley JR, et al. Retrospective study of bacterial infective arthritis in 31 dogs. *J Small Anim Pract*. 2005;46:171-176.

Colledge SL, Raskin RE, Messick JB, et al. Multiple joint metastasis of a transitional cell carcinoma in a dog. *Vet Clin Pathol*. 2013;42:216-220.

Craig LE, Julian ME, Ferracone JD. The diagnosis and prognosis of synovial tumors in dogs: 35 cases. *Vet Pathol*. 2002;39:66-73.

Craig LE, Thompson KG. Tumors of joints. In: Meuten DJ, ed. *Tumors in Domestic Animals*. 5th ed. Ames, IA: John Wiley & Sons; 2017:337-355.

deHaan JJ, Andreasen CB. Calcium crystal-associated arthropathy (pseudogout) in a dog. *J Am Anim Hosp Assoc*. 1992;200:943-946.

Erne JB, Goring RL, Kennedy FA, et al. Prevalence of lymphoplasmacytic synovitis in dogs with naturally occurring cranial cruciate ligament rupture. *J Am Vet Med Assoc*. 2009;235:386-390.

Erne JB, Walker MC, Strik N, et al. Systemic infection with *Geomyces* organisms in a dog with lytic bone lesions. *J Am Vet Med Assoc*. 2007;230:537-540.

Fallin CW, Fox LE, Papendick RE, et al. What is your diagnosis? A 12-month-old dog with multiple soft tissue masses. *Vet Clin Pathol*. 1995;24(80):100-101.

Fernandez FR, Grindem CB, Lipowitz AJ, et al. Synovial fluid analysis: preparation of smears for cytologic examination of canine synovial fluid. *J Am Anim Hosp Assoc*. 1983;19:727-734.

Forsyth SF, Thompson KG, Donald JJ. Possible pseudogout in two dogs. *J Small Anim Pract*. 2007;48:174-176.

Gerber K, Rees P. Urinary bladder botryoid rhabdomyosarcoma with widespread metastases in an 8-month-old Labrador cross dog. *J S Afr Vet Assoc*. 2009;80(3):199-203.

Gibson NR, Carmichael S, Li A, et al. Value of direct smears of synovial fluid in the diagnosis of canine joint disease. *Vet Rec*. 1999;144:463-465.

Giuffrida MA, Bacon NJ, Kamstock DA. Use of routine histopathology and factor VIII-related antigen/von Willebrand factor immunohistochemistry to differentiate primary hemangiosarcoma of bone from telangiectatic osteosarcoma in 54 dogs. *Vet Comp Oncol*. 2017;15(4):1232-1239.

Goodman RA, Hawkins EC, Olby NJ, et al. Molecular identification of Ehrlichia ewingii infection in dogs: 15 cases (1997-2001). *J Am Vet Med Assoc*. 2003;222:1102-1107.

Harvey JW, Raskin RE. Polyarthritis in a dog. *NAVC Clinician's Brief*. 2004;2: 37-38.

Hill M, Scudder CJ, Glanemann B, et al. Hypertrophic osteodystrophy in a dog imaged with CT. *Vet Rec Case Rep*. 2015;3:e000155.

Kornblatt AN, Urband PH, Steere AC. Arthritis caused by *Borrelia burgdorferi* in dogs. *J Am Vet Med Assoc*. 1985;186(9):960-964.

MacWilliams PS, Friedrichs KR. Laboratory evaluation and interpretation of synovial fluid. *Vet Clin North Am Small Anim Pract*. 2003;33:153-178.

McCourt MR, Dieterly AM, Mackey PE, et al. Complex mammary carcinoma with metastases to lymph nodes, subcutaneous tissue, and multiple joints in a dog. *Vet Clin Pathol*. 2018;47:477-483.

Meinkoth JH, Rochat MC, Cowell RL. Metastatic carcinoma presenting as hind-limb lameness: diagnosis by synovial fluid cytology. *J Am Anim Hosp Assoc*. 1997;33:325-328.

Meléndez-Lazo A, Fernandez M, Solano-Gallego L, et al. What is your diagnosis? Synovial fluid from a dog. *Vet Clin Pathol*. 2015;44(2):329-330.

Michels GM, Carr AP. Noninfectious nonerosive arthritis in dogs. *Vet Med*. 1997;92:798-803.

Mielke B, Comerford E, English K, et al. Spontaneous septic arthritis of canine elbows: twenty-one cases. *Vet Comp Orthop Traumatol*. 2018;31: 488-493.

Monti P, Barnes D, Adrian AM, et al. Synovial cell sarcoma in a dog: a misnomer—cytologic and histologic findings and review of the literature. *Vet Clin Pathol*. 2018;47:181-185.

Moore PF. A review of histiocytic diseases of dogs and cats. *Vet Pathol*. 2014;51:167-184.

Murakami M, Sakai H, Iwatani N, et al. Cytologic, histologic, and immunohistochemical features of maxillofacial alveolar rhabdomyosarcoma in a juvenile dog. *Vet Clin Pathol*. 2010;39(1):113-118.

Murakami K, Yonezawa T, Matsuki N. Synovial fluid total protein concentration as a possible marker for canine idiopathic polyarthritis. *J Vet Med Sci*. 2015;77(12):1715-1717.

Nagamine E, Hirayama K, Matsuda K, et al. Diversity of histologic patterns and expression of cytoskeletal proteins in canine skeletal osteosarcoma. *Vet Pathol*. 2015;52(5):977-984.

Neihaus SA, Locke JE, Barger AM, et al. A novel method of core aspirate cytology compared to fine-needle aspiration for diagnosing canine osteosarcoma. *J Am Anim Hosp Assoc*. 2011;47:317-323.

Nelson C, Barger A, Roady P. What is your diagnosis? Dermal mass over the ribs with metastasis to lymph nodes in a dog. *Vet Clin Pathol*. 2018;47: 679-681.

Oohashi E, Yamada K, Oohashi M, et al. Chronic progressive polyarthritis in a female cat. *J Vet Med Sci*. 2010;72:511-514.

Pacchiana PD, Gilley RS, Wallace LJ, et al. Absolute and relative cell counts for synovial fluid from clinically normal shoulder and stifle joints in cats. *J Am Vet Med Assoc*. 2004;225:1866-1870.

Qurollo BA, Buch J, Ramaswamy C, et al. Clinicopathological findings in 41 dogs (2008-2018) naturally infected with *Ehrlichia ewingii*. *J Vet Intern Med*. 2019;33(2):618-629.

Reinhardt S, Stockhaus C, Teske E, et al. Assessment of cytological criteria for diagnosing osteosarcoma in dogs. *J Small Anim Pract*. 2005;46:65-70.

Rosol TJ, Tannehill-Gregg SH, LeRoy BE, et al. Animal models of bone metastasis. *Cancer*. 2003;97(suppl 3):748-757.

Ryseff JK, Bohn AA. Detection of alkaline phosphatase in canine cells previously stained with Wright-Giemsa and its utility in differentiating osteosarcoma from other mesenchymal tumors. *Vet Clin Pathol*. 2012; 41:391-395.

Sabattini S, Renzi A, Buracco P, et al. Comparative assessment of the accuracy of cytological and histologic biopsies in the diagnosis of canine bone lesions. *J Vet Intern Med*. 2017;31(3):864-871.

Santos M, Marcos R, Assuncao M, et al. Polyarthritis associated with visceral leishmaniasis in a juvenile dog. *Vet Parasitol*. 2006;141:340-344.

Silverstein DC, Almy FS, Zinkl JG, et al. Idiopathic localized eosinophilic synovitis in a cat. *Vet Clin Pathol*. 2000;29:90-92.

Snyder LA, Michael H. Alveolar rhabdomyosarcoma in a juvenile Labrador retriever: case report and literature review. *J Am Anim Hosp Assoc*. 2011;47(6):443-446.

Stobie D, Wallace LJ, Lipowitz AJ, et al. Chronic bicipital tenosynovitis in dogs: 29 cases (1985-1992). *J Am Vet Med Assoc*. 1995;207:201-207.

Trepanier LA, Danhof R, Toll J, et al. Clinical findings in 40 dogs with hypersensitivity associated with administration of potentiated sulfonamides. *J Vet Intern Med*. 2003;17:647-652.

15 CHAPTER

Nervous System

Davide De Lorenzi and Laura Pintore

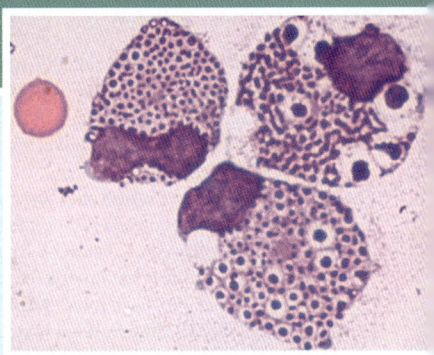

CEREBROSPINAL FLUID

Cerebrospinal fluid (CSF) evaluation is a clinical mainstay in the diagnosis of central nervous system (CNS) disease because it is relatively simple to collect and can provide valuable information. CSF evaluation can identify abnormal changes and, in combination with other tests, yields a specific diagnosis or can contribute to differential diagnoses (Bush et al., 2002; Bohn et al., 2006). Collection of CSF is recommended as a part of the diagnostic investigation of CNS disease of unknown cause when not contraindicated.

The submission of a properly collected specimen is necessary to obtain reliable and accurate information. Proper interpretation of the sample requires knowledge of the clinical presentation, collection site, and specimen handling considerations. The presence of artifacts or contaminants may interfere with an appropriate interpretation unless the conditions surrounding the collection are known.

Cerebrospinal fluid is formed primarily by ultrafiltration and secretion through the ventricular choroid plexuses. Other sites that secrete CSF include the ependymal linings of the ventricles and blood vessels of the subarachnoid spaces and pia mater. The fluid leaves the fourth ventricle and flows caudally, entering the subarachnoid spaces and the central canal of the spinal cord, and is predominantly absorbed from the subarachnoid spaces via veins in the arachnoid and subarachnoid villi that project into subdural venous sinuses (Di Terlizzi and Platt, 2006).

Collection of Cerebrospinal Fluid
Contraindications
Cerebrospinal fluid collection is contraindicated when the CNS signs are associated with known trauma or intoxication, when anesthesia is contraindicated, and when increased intracranial pressure (ICP) is suspected. Increased ICP should be suspected with acute head trauma, active or decompensated hydrocephalus, anisocoria, papilledema, or cerebral edema. Expansive mass lesions and unstable CNS or systemic conditions may result in increased ICP or decreased pressure in the spinal compartment relative to the intracranial compartment. In these situations, herniation of the brain may result in severe compromise of brain function, tetraplegia, stupor or coma, or death. The history, physical and neurologic examinations, and results of imaging studies are critical in determining if these conditions are likely before deciding to collect CSF. If the benefit of obtaining CSF outweighs the risk, the risk of herniation can be reduced by administration of dexamethasone just before induction of anesthesia and by hyperventilation of the patient with oxygen during the procedure. Except in cases in which dexamethasone is administered prophylactically because of suspected increased ICP, CSF collection should predate corticosteroid administration because of potential alteration of CSF composition.

Complications
The risks and benefits of CSF collection should be considered for each individual case. Iatrogenic trauma to the spinal cord or brainstem can occur by the collection needle, but it is minimized by attention to anatomic landmarks and careful collection procedures. Risk of introduction of infectious agents into CNS is minimized by adherence to the basic principles of aseptic technique and correct preparation of the site of collection. Familiarity with the technique is best accomplished by initially practicing on cadavers.

Slight to moderate blood contamination is a common complication of collection associated with penetration of the dorsal vertebral sinuses or small vessels within the meninges; this may complicate interpretation of the fluid analyses and cytopathology but has not been found to be harmful to the patient.

Ketamine should not be used to anesthetize cats for CSF collection because it increases ICP and may induce seizures; gas anesthesia should be used instead.

If three unsuccessful attempts at CSF collection occur, abandonment of the procedure is recommended to decrease the probability of repeated penetration of the spinal cord, which may result in serious complications or death.

Equipment
Clippers, scrub, and alcohol are used to surgically prepare the site of collection. Sterile gloves should be worn during the procedure. A sterile disposable or spinal needle with stylet that can be sterilized is used. A 20- to 22-gauge, 1.5-inch needle with a polypropylene hub is recommended for most cases, although smaller needles may be needed in very small dogs and cats, and longer needles may be needed in large dogs. Several needles should be available because replacement may be needed if the needle is inserted off the midline and enters a venous sinus.

Sterile plain plastic tubes without ethylenediaminetetraacetic acid (EDTA) for CSF collection are generally recommended because leukocytes can adhere to glass, and clotting is rare. It was commonly considered that EDTA may falsely elevate the protein concentration of CSF; however, a recent study demonstrated no difference between plain and EDTA tubes in semiquantitative protein measurement by reagent strips (Koch et al., 2019). Some prefer routine collection into EDTA tubes to avoid clotting secondary to extensive blood contamination. However, such samples probably have limited diagnostic utility. If measurement of glucose is the primary objective, CSF should be collected into a fluoride-oxalate tube, although this may not be necessary if CSF contains few cells and is analyzed rapidly. Collection into red-topped tubes should be avoided when it contains silica for clot activation because the material interferes with cellular detail (Fig. 15.1).

Collection Volume

Approximately 1 mL of CSF per 5 kg of body weight can be collected safely. It may be dangerous to remove more than 1 mL of CSF per 30 seconds, more than 4 to 5 mL of CSF from dogs, more than 0.5 to 1 mL of CSF from adult cats, or more than 10 to 20 drops of CSF from kittens. Approximately 1.0 to 1.5 mL of CSF can usually be collected from cats to avoid meningeal hemorrhage if too much fluid is withdrawn (Rand et al., 1990).

Cerebellomedullary Cistern Collection

Collection at this site is indicated to classify lesions affecting the meninges of the head and neck when the clinical signs involve seizures, generalized incoordination, head tilt, or circling.

Preparation of the site should include clipping of the hair from the head and neck, from the anterior margin of the pinna to the level of the third cervical vertebra, and laterally to the level of the lateral margins of the pinnae. This area should be scrubbed for a sterile procedure (Cellio, 2001).

The animal is positioned in lateral recumbent position with the head and vertebral column positioned at an angle of approximately 90 degrees. Excessive flexion of the neck may result in elevation of ICP and increase the potential for brain herniation or may result in occlusion of the endotracheal tube. The nose should be held or propped so that its long axis is parallel to the table, and it should not be allowed to rotate in either direction. The point of insertion is located on the midline approximately halfway between the external occipital protuberance and the craniodorsal tip of the dorsal spine of C2 (axis) and just rostral to the anterior margins of the wings of C1 (atlas). The needle is inserted at the intersection of a line connecting the anterior borders of the wings of the atlas and a line drawn from the occipital crest to the dorsal border of the axis along the midline. Puncture of the skin first with an 18-gauge needle or a scalpel blade is helpful in overcoming skin resistance in thick-skinned animals and preventing contamination with skin cells or detritus. Alternatively, the skin can be pinched and lifted so that the needle can be safely pushed through the skin with a twisting motion.

The needle should be inserted with the bevel oriented cranially and aimed toward the nose. It should be held perpendicular to the skin surface and then gradually advanced with the stylet in place. Periodically, the needle should be stabilized and the stylet withdrawn to determine if CSF is present. Occasionally, a sudden loss of resistance may be felt as the subarachnoid space is entered, but this may not be recognized in all cases. If the collector suspects that the needle has been inserted too deeply, the stylet may be removed and the needle slowly withdrawn a few millimeters at a time while the collector watches for the appearance of fluid in the hub. If the needle hits bone during insertion, slight redirection of the needle cranially or caudally should be attempted to enter the atlanto-occipital space.

If opening pressure readings are taken, CSF fluid sample is taken by directing the flow of CSF through the manometer using a three-way stopcock. If pressure readings are not taken, CSF may be collected directly from the spinal needle hub by dripping into a test tube or gentle aspiration of drops as they collect at the hub using a syringe. Attachment of a syringe to the needle with aspiration of CSF is not recommended because suction may result in contamination with blood or meningeal cells or obstruction of CSF flow by aspirated meningeal trabeculae. Rarely, if aspiration is necessary, it should be only done by the experienced collector. Passage of the needle through the spinal cord to underlying bone should be avoided at the cerebellomedullary cistern because it may cause damage to the cord or cause blood contamination of the CSF sample. On completion of CSF collection, the needle is smoothly withdrawn. Replacement of the stylet is not necessary.

If the fluid appears bloody at the onset of collection, replacement of the stylet for 30 to 60 seconds may result in clearing of the blood. If the first few drops of CSF are still slightly bloody, they can be collected separately from the following drops, which are often clear. If the rate of flow of CSF is slow, the needle should be rotated slightly to ensure that the tip is not in contact with tissue. The rate of flow also can be increased by compression of the jugular veins, resulting in expansion of the venous sinuses and increased CSF pressure.

Appearance of abundant fresh blood from the collection needle indicates that the point of the needle is most likely off the midline and in a lateral venous sinus. A new approach with a new needle is necessary in this case.

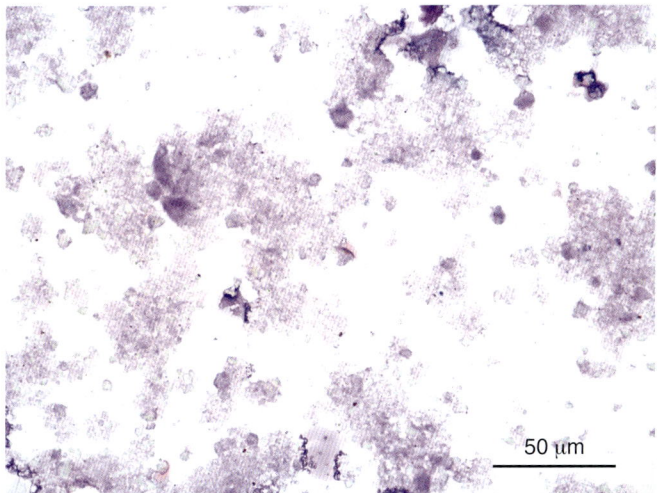

■ **FIGURE 15.1 Collection artifact. Red top tube silica. Cerebrospinal fluid (CSF). Dog.** The background contains refractile crystalline material. The sample had been submitted in a clot-activated red top tube, which may interfere with cytopathologic examination. CSF should be submitted in a red top tube with no additives or an EDTA tube. (Modified Wright; HP oil.) (Courtesy Pierre Deshuillers, Purdue University.)

Lumbar Cistern Collection

Lumbar cistern specimens from L5 to L6 for large breed dogs and L6 to L7 in small breed dogs and cats may be more technically difficult than collection from the cerebellomedullary cistern.

Sometimes no fluid or only a very small amount of blood-contaminated fluid is obtained owing to the small size of the lumbar subarachnoid space. Lumbar puncture is preferred in cases neurolocalized to the thoracolumbar region related to the rostrocaudal flow of CSF; it is therefore more likely to be reflective of the pathology than cerebellomedullary cistern collections (Thomson et al., 1990; Early et al., 2019; Lampe et al., 2020). In a study of 54 dogs with postmortem-confirmed diagnoses, tests of fluid collected from the lumbar cistern were more sensitive for identifying pleocytosis and elevated protein concentrations compared with the fluid from the cerebellomedullary cistern in dogs with spinal cord disease (Early et al., 2019). One study found that the CSF parameter results differed between samples collected concomitantly from the cerebellomedullary and lumbar cisterns in dogs with lesions neurolocalized to the brain or spinal cord, suggesting there may be clinical benefit in collecting and examining fluid from both sites (Lampe et al., 2020).

The dorsal midline is clipped and prepared between the midsacrum and L3, extending laterally to the wings of the ilium. The animal is placed in lateral recumbency, and the back is flexed slightly to open the spaces between the dorsal laminae of the vertebrae. The L5 to L6 or L6 to L7 spaces are most commonly used in dogs because the subarachnoid space rarely extends to the lumbosacral junction. In cats, CSF is frequently collected from the lumbosacral space.

The dorsal spinous process of L7 lies between the wings of the ilia and is usually smaller than that of L6. To collect from the L5 to L6 intervertebral space, the needle is inserted just off the midline at the caudal aspect of the L6 dorsal spinous process and then advanced at an angle cranioventrally and slightly medially to enter the spinal canal between the dorsal laminae of L5 and L6. Misdirection laterally into the paralumbar muscles or underestimation of the length of needle required might result in advancement of the needle to the hub without encountering bone.

Cerebrospinal fluid may be collected from the dorsal subarachnoid space, or the needle may be passed through the nervous structures to the floor of the spinal canal and CSF collected from the ventral subarachnoid space. The stylet is removed, and the needle may be carefully withdrawn a few millimeters to allow for fluid flow. The rate of flow is usually slower than from the cerebellomedullary cistern; it may be increased by jugular compression.

Cerebrospinal Fluid Opening Pressure

Cerebrospinal fluid pressure is measured with a standard spinal fluid manometer as the fluid is collected. Cerebrospinal opening pressure should be measured to confirm a supposed increase in ICP caused by a space-occupying mass or cerebral edema. The normal range is less than 170 mm H_2O and 100 mm H_2O for dogs and cats, respectively (Chrisman, 1992).

Handling of Cerebrospinal Fluid Specimens

Cells lyse rapidly in the low-protein milieu of CSF, so cell counts and cytopathologic preparations of unfixed fluid should be done within 30 to 60 minutes of collection (Fry et al., 2006). The likelihood of misinterpretation caused by sample deterioration depends on the initial protein concentration of the sample and how long the analysis is delayed. For example, if the CSF protein concentration is more than 50 mg/dL, a delay in analysis of less than 12 hours is unlikely to alter final interpretation. Addition of an equal volume of 4% to 10% neutral buffered formalin or 50% to 90% alcohol, depending on availability, is recommended for fixation of specimens that cannot be immediately delivered to a laboratory and processed immediately. Alternatively, the addition of one drop of 10% formalin to 1 to 2 mL of CSF can be used to preserve cells for cell counts and morphologic examination when submitted to a referral laboratory; cell count will be different from unfixed, but the difference is clinically insignificant. Refrigeration helps retard cellular degeneration. Cellular stability can be increased by addition of fresh, frozen, or thawed serum or plasma or by addition of 20% albumin (Bienzle et al., 2000). If a CSF sample is not analyzed within 1 hour from collection, Fry et al. (2006) recommend dividing the fluid into two aliquots, an unadulterated aliquot for total nucleated cell count (TNCC) and protein measurement and an aliquot added with 20% of fetal calf serum (or 10% autologous serum) for differential cell count and morphologic evaluation. For samples of insufficient volume (<0.5 mL total), hetastarch can be added to CSF for routine assays. In the last situation, the dilutional effect of adding a stabilizing agent must be taken into account when calculating results. Hetastarch comes ready to use as 6% hydroxyethyl starch in 0.9% NaCl solution and is then added to CSF 1:1 (vol/vol). Protein and enzyme concentrations in CSF are relatively stable during transit by routine pick-up, overnight postal, and courier delivery. Analyses other than cell counts and cell differentials are best performed on the unadulterated aliquot to ensure no interference. A recent study evaluated cellular morphology preservation using 6% hydroxyethyl starch 130/0.4 in 0.9% sodium chloride (Vetstarch, Abbott Laboratories), finding it does not reduce time-dependent cellular degeneration compared with the saline diluent or serum and is therefore not recommended as a stabilizing agent for canine CSF (Peterson et al., 2020).

Laboratory Analysis of Cerebrospinal Fluid

Usually at least 1 to 2 mL of CSF is available from dogs or cats. The analysis for cell counts requires approximately 0.5 mL (500 μL total or 250 μL for duplicate erythrocyte count and nucleated cell count, respectively). The volume required for chemical protein determination varies depending on the equipment and method used, but it can be expected to be on the order of 200 to 250 μL for large, automated pieces of equipment. Taking these figures into account, approximately 0.25 to 1.25 mL of CSF should be available for cytopathologic evaluation and other tests.

Routine analyses of CSF include the following: macroscopic evaluation, quantitative analysis (erythrocyte count, TNCC, and total protein concentration), and microscopic evaluation, as summarized in Table 15.1. If the volume of CSF is small and all tests are not likely to be obtained, the clinician should rank the tests in order of preference when the specimen is submitted to the laboratory. The most useful diagnostic tests, in decreasing order, are nucleated and erythrocyte counts, sedimentation cytopathology, protein concentration, and cytocentrifuge-sediment cytopathology.

Effect of Blood Contamination

Various formulas have been used to predict the effect of blood contamination on protein concentration and nucleated cell count in CSF (Rand et al., 1990). Subsequent studies have shown that erythrocyte counts in blood contaminated canine

TABLE 15.1 Routine Evaluation of Cerebrospinal Fluid

COMPONENT OF CSF EVALUATION	NORMAL CSF	ABNORMAL CSF	COMMENTS AND NOTES
Macroscopic Evaluation			
Color	Colorless	Pink, red xanthochromic (yellow to yellow-orange); occasional gray to green color may be seen	Compare with tube containing water Red or pink suggests blood; if caused by intact erythrocytes, it will clear with centrifugation Xanthochromia is an indication of previous hemorrhage with accumulation of oxyhemoglobin or methemoglobin from erythrocyte degradation; may occur with hyperbilirubinemia May be graded as slight, moderate, or marked
Clarity	Clear; turbidity absent	Turbid or cloudy—slight, moderate, or marked	Evaluate ability to read printed words through the tube Detectable turbidity corresponds to nucleated cell count >500/µL
Erythrocyte (RBC) count	Zero RBCs is considered normal but frequently present in small numbers	Variable	Standard hemocytometer
Nucleated cell count	Most commonly cited reference intervals: 0–5/µL (dogs) 0–8/µL (cats)	Variable	Standard hemocytometer
Specific gravity	1.004–1.006	Most within reference interval for normal CSF	Of questionable value; only relatively marked increases in total protein result in detectable changes by specific gravity measurement
Total Protein (Microprotein)			
Quantitation	Most commonly cited reference intervals: <25 or <30 mg/dL (cerebellomedullary) or <45 mg/dL (lumbar cistern)	Increased total protein seen in a variety of conditions	Microprotein method and reference values may vary with laboratory; use laboratory-established reference values
Estimation (urine dipstick)	Multistix[a] microprotein concentration: Trace[b] = <30 mg/dL 1+ = 30 mg/dL 2+ = 100 mg/dL 3+ = 300 mg/dL 4+ = >2000 mg/dL	Most sensitive to albumin; detects ranges of protein that are useful for evaluation of most canine and feline CSF specimens; good correlation with standard dye-binding microprotein determinations	
Microscopic Evaluation			

Cell population	Lymphocytes and monocytoid cells predominate; very few mature, nondegenerate neutrophils may be present; a few erythrocytes may be seen	Variable	See other sections for more details of cytopathologic features and specific conditions
			Preparatory techniques for concentrating cells:
			  Cytocentrifuge preparation
			  Membrane filter
			  Sedimentation
			  Chamber

[a]N-Multistix SG, Siemens Medical Solutions.
[b]Trace to 1+ protein on urine dipstick is within normal limits.
CSF, Cerebrospinal fluid; *RBC,* red blood cell.

CSF from dogs with and without neurologic disease poorly correlate with TNCC and protein concentrations and concluded using formulas to correct TNCC and protein concentrations for the number of red blood cell (RBC) in CSF is inappropriate (Hurtt and Smith, 1997; MacNeill et al., 2018). One study did find that blood contamination increased the percentage of neutrophils and the presence of eosinophils; however, finding reactive lymphocytes and activated macrophages was indicative of CNS disease (Doyle and Solano-Gallego, 2009).

The presence of vacuolated basophilic macrophages and reactive lymphocytosis is not significantly affected by blood contamination so it may be useful in identifying dogs with CNS abnormalities even when CSF has a low TNCC.

Although blood contamination may make interpretation of CSF more difficult, red or pink CSF or CSF with a high erythrocyte count should not be discarded as useless because cytopathologic evaluation may detect abnormalities (Chrisman, 1992).

Macroscopic Evaluation

Normal CSF is clear, colorless, and transparent and does not coagulate. Discoloration or cloudiness and degree of change should be recorded as slight, moderate, or marked or graded 1+ to 4+. Turbidity is reported to be detectable if greater than 500 cells/µL or at least 200 leukocytes/µL or 700 erythrocytes/µL are present (Fig. 15.2A) (Fenner, 2000).

Red to pink discoloration may be associated with iatrogenic contamination with blood or pathologic hemorrhage. Erythrophages or siderophages in a rapidly processed CSF specimen with fixative added immediately after collection support pathologic hemorrhage as an underlying cause. Xanthochromia is the yellow to yellow-orange discoloration associated with pathologic hemorrhage caused by trauma, vasculitis, severe inflammation, disc extrusion, or necrotic or erosive neoplasia (Fig. 15.2B). Occasionally, xanthochromia will be seen with leptospirosis, cryptococcosis, toxoplasmosis, ischemic myelopathy, coagulopathy, or hyperbilirubinemia.

Quantitative Analysis

Cell counts. Erythrocyte and nucleated cell counts are often performed using standard hemocytometer techniques. In general, collections from normal animals from the cerebellomedullary cistern have slightly higher numbers of cells and slightly lower protein concentrations than those from the lumbar cistern.

To count nucleated cells, charge both chambers of the hemocytometer with undiluted CSF and place the unit in a humidified Petri dish for 15 minutes to allow cells to adhere to the glass. All nucleated cells are counted in the 10 large squares (four corner squares and one center square on each side) for a TNCC per microliter. Cell counts for erythrocytes are performed similarly.

A study demonstrated a strong positive correlation between the in-house RBC count and TNCC using the Neubauer hemocytometer and those reported by the commercial laboratory (Newton et al., 2017). A study conducted to evaluate the usefulness of an automated cell counter in counting and differentiating cell types from canine CSF determined moderate correlation between this method and a hemocytometer for leukocyte values and excellent correlation for erythrocytes; however, cell differentials were much more variable (Ruotsalo et al., 2008).

Reference intervals for feline CSF erythrocyte counts are reported to range from 0 to 30 cells/µL (Rand et al., 1990). Reference intervals for feline CSF nucleated cell counts are reported to be less than 8 cells/µL (Rand et al., 1990). Reference intervals for canine CSF erythrocyte counts are reported to be zero (Chrisman, 1992). Reference intervals for canine CSF nucleated cell counts are reported to be less than 6 cells/µL for cerebellomedullary cistern and lumbar cistern collections (Chrisman, 1992).

Protein. Reference intervals for the CSF protein concentration may vary slightly with the laboratory and testing method used, but cerebellomedullary CSF protein is usually less than 25 to 30 mg/dL, and lumbar cistern collections are less than 45 mg/dL in dogs and cats (Chrisman, 1992; Fenner, 2000). Microprotein analytic techniques by reference laboratories are used for the measurement protein concentration in CSF. A membrane microconcentrator technique followed by agarose gel electrophoresis was described for measurement of CSF proteins in dogs (Gama et al., 2007).

The refractometer cannot be used for the measurement of protein concentration in the CSF; however, an estimate of CSF protein concentration can be obtained using urine dipsticks (Jacobs et al., 1990). Semiquantitative protein concentration using Multistix (Siemens) are indicated as negative (0 mg/dL), trace (<30 mg/dL), 1+ (30–100 mg/dL), 2+ (100–300 mg/dL), 3+ (300–2000 mg/dL), or 4+ (>2000 mg/dL).

Increased CSF protein concentration may be caused by an alteration in the blood-brain barrier and leakage from plasma

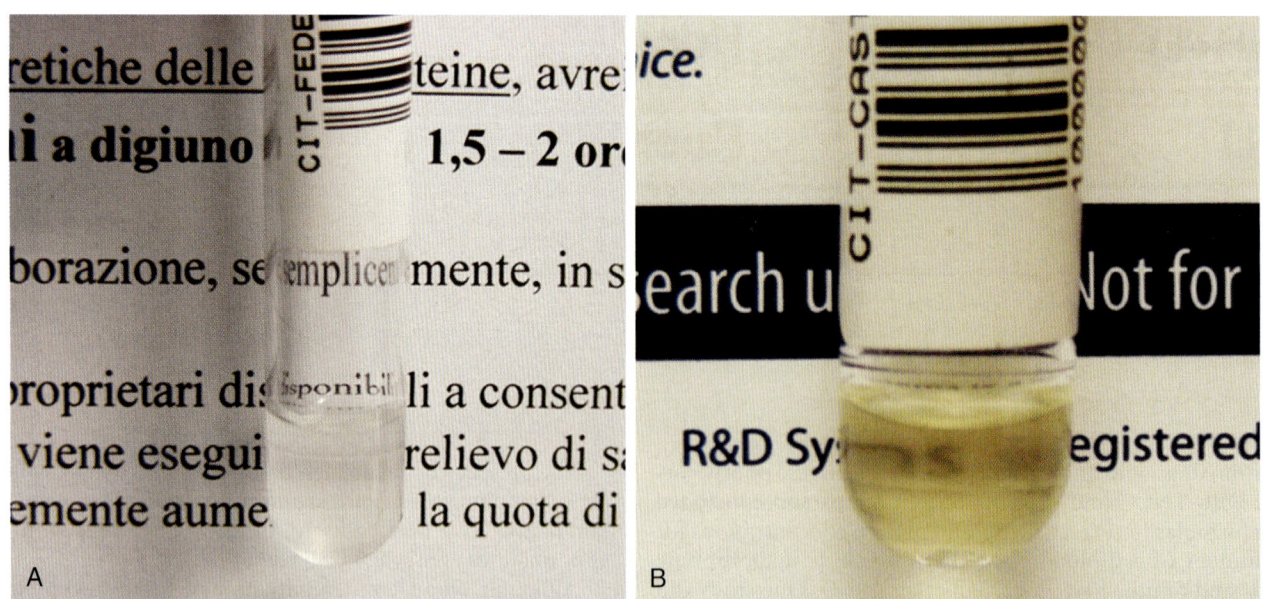

■ **FIGURE 15.2 Clarity testing. Cerebrospinal fluid. Macroscopic. A, Turbid. Dog.** There is marked turbidity or cloudiness against the background of newsprint. This animal had steroid-responsive meningitis with a count of 760 nucleated cells/µL. Turbidity is reported to be detectable if more than 200 leukocytes/µL are present. **B, Xanthochromic. Dog.** The fluid has a yellow-orange discoloration and moderate turbidity from a dog with subarachnoidal hemorrhage of inflammatory origin.

or increased local synthesis. Albumin accounts for 80% to 95% of the protein concentration in normal CSF. Qualitative tests to detect increased globulins in CSF are the Pandy and Nonne-Apelt tests. Use of these tests is limited because of the qualitative nature and absence of specificity regarding underlying cause. Normal CSF contains little if any globulin that can be detected by these methods. Erythrocyte counts in blood-contaminated canine CSF poorly correlate with TNCC and protein concentration. Using formulas to correct TNCC and protein concentration for the number of RBCs in CSF is inappropriate (MacNeill et al., 2018).

Other Tests

Normal CSF glucose is 60% to 80% of the serum or plasma concentration and changes in CSF glucose concentration relative to serum or plasma may take 1 to 3 hours for equilibrium. An increase in the CSF glucose level is not diagnostically important and reflects hyperglycemia within several hours before collection. Decreased CSF glucose concentrations, hypoglycorrhachia, may be associated with bacterial and fungal meningitis, in which microorganisms and polymorphonuclear leukocytes are considered to use glucose. However, in dogs, bacterial meningitis is less common relative to steroid-responsive meningitis-arteritis (SRMA)-associated decreased CSF glucose, a disease in which no infectious cause has been identified. The decreased CSF glucose concentration is attributed to the attendant high numbers of neutrophils in the CSF in that inflammatory disease, which are suggested to have an increased glycolysis, particularly when these cells are active (e.g., phagocytosis, production of oxygen radicals) (Weber et al., 2012). Decreased glucose concentrations also may be associated with diffuse meningeal neoplasia as well as SRMA (Weber et al., 2012). Increased D-dimer concentrations may be considered a diagnostic marker for SRMA in the differential diagnosis of canine neurologic disorders (de la Fuente et al., 2012). A positive bacterial culture of the CSF is essential for confirmation of a bacterial etiology for a decreased CSF glucose concentration.

Although aerobic and anaerobic bacterial cultures are recommended for all CSF samples with neutrophils or when bacteria are identified by cytopathology, culture rarely grows the microorganism. In a series of eight histologically confirmed cases of canine bacterial meningoencephalomyelitis, the CSF culture was positive in only one sample (Radaelli and Platt, 2002). Several factors likely contribute to poor culture performance, including small volume of CSF, organisms mostly confined to the brain parenchyma, organisms are slow growing or require nonstandard culture techniques, and animals have received antibiotic therapy before sampling. *Staphylococcus*, *Streptococcus*, *Klebsiella*, *Escherichia coli*, and *Pasteurella* are aerobic bacteria that may cause CNS infection, whereas *Fusobacterium*, *Bacteroides*, *Peptostreptococcus*, *Clostridium*, and *Eubacterium* are anaerobic species that have been reported.

Other tests recommended by various authors or used in specific situations include electrophoretic determination of albumin and determination of total immunoglobulin levels. In combination with serum albumin and serum immunoglobulin levels, these can be used to calculate the albumin quotient (AQ) and immunoglobulin G (IgG) index. AQ is equal to the CSF albumin divided by serum albumin times 100. AQ greater than 2.35 suggests an altered blood-brain barrier with increased protein concentration in CSF associated with leakage from plasma.

The IgG index is equal to the (CSF IgG/serum IgG) divided by (CSF albumin/serum albumin). An IgG index greater than 0.272 with a normal AQ suggests intrathecal production of IgG. An increased IgG index and increased AQ are suggestive of an altered blood-brain barrier as the source of IgG (Chrisman, 1992).

Alterations in electrophoretic protein fractions have been reported. Dogs with canine distemper have increased gamma globulins, and dogs with granulomatous meningoencephalitis (GME) have increased beta and gamma globulins (Chrisman, 1992).

Using high-resolution protein electrophoresis (paired CSF and serum) in dogs with a variety of neurologic diseases, there was a strong linear correlation between CSF total protein concentration and AQ, suggesting that an increased CSF protein concentration is an indicator of blood-brain barrier dysfunction but not characteristic of a specific disease (Behr et al., 2006). Paired testing of CSF IgA and serum IgA is recommended to confirm the diagnosis of suspected cases of canine SRMA, showing a sensitivity and a specificity of 91% and 78%, respectively (Maiolini et al., 2012).

Detection of specific CSF antibodies and comparison with serum levels may be useful in diagnosis of infectious meningoencephalitides, including infectious canine hepatitis, canine herpesvirus, canine parvovirus, canine parainfluenza virus, canine distemper virus, ehrlichiosis, Rocky Mountain spotted fever, Lyme disease (borreliosis), *Toxoplasma gondii* infection, *Neospora caninum* infection, *Encephalitozoon cuniculi* infection, *Babesia* spp. infection, cryptococcosis (Berthelin et al., 1994), and blastomycosis. In CSF of cats with confirmed feline infectious peritonitis (FIP) involving the CNS, measurement of anticoronavirus IgG is considered of equivocal clinical use (Boettcher et al., 2007). Rising serial titers of serum IgG support active disease. The presence of IgM in serum or CSF is considered more specific than IgG or total immunoglobulin levels in support of active disease (Chrisman, 1992). Vector-transmitted microorganisms in the genera *Ehrlichia*, *Anaplasma*, *Rickettsia*, *Bartonella*, and *Borrelia* spp. have been suspected in dogs with meningoencephalomyelitis. Brain tissue and CSF collected prospectively from dogs with neurological disease and evaluated by broadly reactive polymerase chain reaction (PCR) did not detect pathogen nucleic acids, with one exception, suggesting that microorganisms in the genera *Ehrlichia*, *Anaplasma*, *Rickettsia*, and *Borrelia* spp. are unlikely to be directly associated with canine meningoencephalomyelitis. *Bartonella vinsonii* subsp. *berkhoffii* DNA was amplified from one of six dogs with histopathologically confirmed granulomatous meningoencephalomyelitis (GME) warranting further investigation (Barber et al., 2010).

Cerebrospinal fluid creatine kinase (CK) activity is a useful outcome predictor when combined with CSF myelin basic protein (MBP) concentration and neurologic sign evaluation in dogs with acute thoracolumbar intervertebral disc herniation (IVDH) (Witsberger et al., 2012). The median CSF-CK activity is higher in dogs with thoracolumbar IVDH with unsuccessful outcome (62 U/L) compared with dogs having a successful outcome (20 U/L), a value similar to dogs without thoracolumbar IVDH. The odds of recovery for dogs with thoracolumbar IVDH having CSF-CK activity less than or equal to 38 U/L were greater (35-fold difference) than those dogs having CSF-CK activity higher than 38 U/L. Furthermore, when CSF MBP concentration is higher than 3 ng/mL, there is a sensitivity of 78% and specificity of 76% to predict an unsuccessful outcome of IVDH disease (Levine et al., 2010). The CSF-CK by itself does not appear to be a useful diagnostic marker for neurological diseases (Ferreira, 2016).

Matrix metalloproteinases (MMPs) are proteolytic enzymes secreted as latent enzymes that must be cleaved to become fully active. Among the MMPs, MMP-2 (gelatinase A) and MMP-9 (gelatinase B) are able to digest basal lamina, which can lead to opening of cerebral barriers. MMP-9 expression in the CSF of dogs with IVDH was associated with the severity of neurologic signs and prognosis, suggesting MMP-9 expression after severe spinal cord injury associated with absence of deep pain perception is a predictor of poor prognosis (Nagano et al., 2011). Latent MMP-9 was detected in 9 of 10 dogs with choroid plexus tumors or lymphoma, in a smaller percentage in dogs with meningiomas, gliomas, or pituitary tumors and not in dogs with nonneoplastic neurologic disease (Mariani et al., 2013). Their further diagnostic application of in CNS inflammatory diseases will require combined analyses of their inhibitors and associated cytokine profile (Marangoni et al., 2011).

The CNS lactate is produced via glycolysis by neurons and astrocytes. In dogs, CSF lactate concentration tends to increase in animals with severe cognitive deficit, intracranial disease, and intervertebral disc disease (Witsberger et al., 2012; Caines et al., 2013). Lactate, measured with a commercially available handheld lactate monitor (Nye and Mariani, 2018), was above reference range in 47% of 102 dogs with prospectively and retrospectively diagnosed inflammatory CNS disease subcategorized as SRMA, infectious meningoencephalitis, granulomatous meningoencephalitis, meningoencephalitis of unknown etiology, and necrotizing leukoencephalitis (NLE). There was significant but weak correlations between CSF lactate concentration and TNCC, absolute large mononuclear cell count, absolute small mononuclear cell count, absolute neutrophil cell count, and protein concentration. There was no correlation between CSF lactate concentration and CSF RBC count or association with survival. The results suggest that CSF lactate concentrations could serve as a rapid biomarker of inflammatory CNS disease in dogs (Mariani et al., 2019).

Immunophenotyping of CSF mononuclear cells in healthy dogs examined by flow cytometry was compared with corresponding blood sample (Duque et al., 2002). The mean proportion of CD4+ and CD21+ cells was significantly higher in blood than in CSF, but the mean proportion of CD14+ and CD8α+ cells was not significantly different between blood and CSF. The immunophenotypes of T lymphocytes in CSF in canine visceral leishmaniasis was composed of increased percentages of double negative and double positive T cells, which was similar to the proportions found in the peripheral blood, likely related to inflammation-related alterations of the blood-brain barrier (Grano et al., 2016).

Cellular Evaluation of Cerebrospinal Fluid

The most useful diagnostic tests in decreasing order are nucleated cell and erythrocyte counts, sedimentation cytopathology, protein concentration, and cytocentrifuge cytopathology. When a limited sample volume must be parsed, the sequence of analysis generally recommended is cell counts, protein concentration, and cytopathology. Cytopathology is preferred in cases of suspected GME and lymphoma. Cytopathologic features that may be found in canine and feline CSF are summarized in Table 15.2. Differential diagnoses associated with abnormal CSF findings are summarized in Table 15.3.

Methods of Cytopathologic Preparation

Standardization of the volume used for cytopathologic evaluation may be of benefit in minimizing analytic variation and aid in interpretation (Krimer et al., 2016). Evaluation of multiple preparations or preparations from larger volumes of CSF increases the likelihood of detection of minor abnormalities. Because CSF has low cellularity, a concentration procedure is generally required: cytocentrifugation, sedimentation, or membrane filtration techniques may be used. Cytocentrifugation is commonly available in reference or commercial laboratories; however, it was shown to produce variable numbers of nucleated cells in cytocentrifuge preparations and canine CSF cytocentrifuged cell yield and differential evaluations are imprecise (Krimer et al., 2016).

The membrane filtration technique requires special staining that is not commonly available in practice. Several sedimentation techniques have been described and are suitable for use in practice or commercial or reference laboratories to which rapid submission of CSF specimens is possible. A sample device is demonstrated in Figure 15.3. Sedimentation preparations may be made if a specimen cannot be delivered the same day to the laboratory for cytopathologic processing (Hare et al., 2019). Prepared slides are sent to the laboratory for staining and evaluation.

Cytocentrifuge or sedimentation preparations are air dried and most commonly stained with Romanowsky stains available in commercial or reference laboratories and clinical practice laboratories. Membrane-filtration specimens require wet fixation, and stains appropriate for this method involve Papanicolaou, trichrome, or hematoxylin and eosin (H&E). Wet fixation and these staining methods may also be used on cytocentrifuge or sedimentation preparations and are appropriate for formalin- or alcohol-fixed specimens. Cytocentrifuge or membrane filtration preparatory and staining techniques may vary with laboratory, technical training, and pathologist preference.

A low-cost in-house manual cytocentrifugation using an adapted salad spinner to obtain a cytocentrifuged preparation has been described (Marcos et al., 2016a). The manual cytocentrifuge produced preparations with similar cell yield as the automated cytocentrifuge. The histologic assessment of cell tube blocks (CTBs) from the CSF of a cat was evaluated. Using CTB, cell morphology is comparable to that of cytopathologic preparations, but the cells are smaller because of the formalin and paraffin shrinkage and sectioning (Marcos et al., 2017). One of the main advantages of using the CTB technique on CSF samples could be the possibility of performing immunohistochemical investigations, as well as having the possibility of storing the cellular portion of a liquid material that would otherwise degenerate.

Special stains may be indicated in some cases. Gram stain may be useful for confirmation and identification of categories of bacteria. India ink or new methylene blue preparations have been reported to be helpful in identification of fungal infections, especially *Cryptococcus neoformans*. Special stains used for the identification of *C. neoformans* are Gram, periodic acid–Schiff (PAS), and mucicarmine that specifically stain the mucopolysaccharide capsule. Gomori methenamine silver allows

TABLE 15.2 Cytopathologic Features of Cerebrospinal Fluid in Dogs and Cats

CELL OR FEATURE	DESCRIPTION	SIGNIFICANCE
Lymphocytes	Morphologically similar to those in peripheral blood; 9–15 μm in diameter, scant to moderate, pale basophilic cytoplasm with round to ovoid, slightly indented nucleus	Predominant cell type in normal CSF from healthy dogs; present in normal CSF from healthy cats
Reactive lymphocytes	Morphologically similar to those in peripheral blood; greater amount of cytoplasm and more deeply basophilic cytoplasm than normal lymphocytes; may see prominent perinuclear clear zones and coarse chromatin patterns	Not present in normal CSF from healthy animals but not specific for underlying condition
Monocytoid cells	Large mononuclear cell; 12–15 μm in diameter; moderate amount, pale basophilic, often finely foamy cytoplasm; nuclear shape variable to amoeboid; chromatin pattern open to lacy	Present in CSF from healthy animals in low numbers
Activated monocytoid cells	Morphologically resemble macrophages in many sites; larger than "normal" monocytoid cells (>12–15 μm in diameter); increased amount of cytoplasm that is often paler than normal and possibly vacuolated; nuclei become round to oval and eccentric; chromatin with increased coarseness	Activation associated with irritation, inflammation, or degenerative processes; often phagocytic; reported in cats to be commonly associated with extensive necrosis
Neutrophils	Morphologically similar to those in peripheral blood; polymorphonuclear leukocytes	May be present in low numbers (≤25% of total nucleated cells) in normal CSF from healthy animals
Ependymal lining cells	Uniform, round to cuboidal mononuclear cells; individual cells or in cohesive clusters; eccentric, round nuclei; uniformly granular to coarse chromatin; moderate amount of finely granular cytoplasm	May be present in normal CSF from healthy animals in low numbers; not consistently present in normal or abnormal conditions
Choroid plexus cells	Indistinguishable from ependymal lining cells (as above)	May be present in normal CSF from healthy animals in low numbers; not consistently present in normal or abnormal conditions
Subarachnoid lining cells and leptomeningeal cells	Mononuclear cells with moderate to abundant pale basophilic cytoplasm; round to oval eccentric nuclei; uniform, delicate chromatin pattern; indistinct cytoplasm margins; single or in small clusters	May be present in normal CSF from healthy animals in low numbers; not consistently present in normal or abnormal conditions
Hematopoietic cells	Morphologically similar to those in bone marrow or other locations	Myeloid and erythroid precursors and erythroblastic island reported as contaminants of canine CSF with lumbar collections
Eosinophils	Morphologically similar to those in peripheral blood; polymorphonuclear leukocytes with eosinophilic granules with shape characteristic for species	Occasionally, cells seen in normal CSF from healthy dogs or cats; may be seen as a nonspecific part of an active inflammatory response; also consider parasitic, hypersensitivity, or neoplastic processes (primary or metastatic)
Plasma cells	Morphologically similar to those in other locations; eccentric nuclei with prominent chromatin (clock face pattern); moderately abundant cytoplasm, moderately to deeply basophilic with perinuclear clear zone (Golgi apparatus)	Not present in normal CSF from healthy dogs or cats; may be part of nonspecific reactive or inflammatory process with response to antigenic stimulation
Bacteria	Morphology varies with type, may include cocci, rods of various sizes, coccobacilli, or filamentous forms	Not present in normal CSF from healthy dogs or cats; may be contaminants if collection process or tube are not sterile or if CSF collected close to death; pathologic role likely if suppurative meningitis is present and supported by intracellular location
Neural tissue	Nerve cells morphologically similar to those in nervous tissue; very large cell with prominent nucleolus, abundant cytoplasm, and three to four tentacle-like cytoplasmic processes; neuropil and myelin represented by amorphous, acellular background material	Reported as contaminant in canine CSF associated with accidental puncture of spinal cord; myelin fragments may be associated with demyelination
Paracellular coiled ribbons	Coiled, homogeneous, basophilic material within phagocytic vacuoles	Reported in CSF obtained at postmortem; hypothesized to represent denatured myelin, myelin figures, or myelin fragments
Neoplastic cells	Abnormal cell type or number for location (benign tumors) or atypical features fulfilling criteria for malignancy (malignant tumors); morphology may vary with cell type of origin and degree of differentiation	May be primary or metastatic; presence requires communication with subarachnoid space or ventricles; absence of tumor does not rule out its presence without contribution of cells to CSF
Fungi, yeast, and protozoa	Appearance varies with type; may be primary or opportunistic infections	Characteristic morphology associated with various common pathologic organisms; demonstration of organisms in conjunction with clinical signs and results of other testing increases confidence in diagnosis of fungal or protozoal disease
Mitotic figures	Recognized by characteristic nuclear configurations of cells undergoing mitosis; cell type of origin not identifiable during the mitotic cycle	Rare mitotic figures reported in normal CSF from healthy animals; presence indicates proliferative process, often neoplasia

CSF, Cerebrospinal fluid.

TABLE 15.3 Differential Diagnoses Associated With Cytopathologic Features of Inflammation in Cerebrospinal Fluid

CYTOPATHOLOGIC FEATURES	SPECIAL CONSIDERATIONS OR DIFFERENTIAL DIAGNOSES	COMMENTS
Slight to moderate neutrophilic inflammation; 25%–50% neutrophils, with or without elevated CSF protein, with or without pleocytosis	Bacterial, fungal, protozoal, parasitic, rickettsial, or viral infection	Depends on species, type of infection, focal or diffuse involvement, presence of concurrent necrosis; presence of protozoa, fungi or yeast organisms, or intracellular bacteria confirms diagnosis
	Neoplasia	Depends on type of neoplasm, location, presence of concurrent necrosis; neoplastic cells rarely seen in CSF
	Other noninfectious conditions	Consider traumatic, degenerative, immune mediated, associated with metabolic conditions, ischemia
Marked neutrophilic inflammation (suppurative meningitis)	Bacterial infection	May be focal (abscess) or diffuse (meningoencephalomyelitis); intracellular bacterial confirms diagnosis
Pleocytosis with predominance of neutrophils (>50%), often with increased CSF protein	Severe viral encephalitis	Especially FIP
	Necrotizing vasculitis	May have immune-mediated or infectious basis; Bernese mountain dogs and beagles
	Steroid-responsive meningitis-arteritis	Responsive to glucocorticoids but must rule out infectious causes
	Postmyelography reaction (usually within 24–48 hours)	History of recent, previous myelography
	Neoplasms	Especially meningiomas but may occur with any neoplasm, especially if associated with necrosis
	Trauma	History may be supportive if trauma was observed
	Hemorrhage	History may be supportive; may have traumatic, degenerative, metabolic infectious, neoplastic, or other underlying cause
	Acquired hydrocephalus	May depend on underlying cause of the acquired condition
Mixed-cell inflammation with a variety of cell types (no single cell type predominant)	Often interpreted to represent granulomatous inflammation; consider fungal, protozoal, parasitic, or rickettsial infection	Presence of fungal or protozoal organisms is confirmatory
Mixture of macrophages, lymphocytes, neutrophils, and sometimes plasma cells, with or without elevated CSF protein, with or without pleocytosis	Some idiopathic inflammatory or degenerative diseases	Especially GME
	Inadequately treated chronic bacterial infections or early response to antibacterial treatment	History and previous diagnosis helpful
Nonsuppurative inflammation (mononuclear pleocytosis)	Viral, bacterial, fungal, protozoal, parasitic, or rickettsial infection	Especially non-FIP viral meningoencephalomyelitis in cats and canine distemper infection in dogs
Pleocytosis with predominance of mononuclear cells, especially lymphocytes	Necrotizing encephalitis of small breed dogs	Signalment and lymphocytic predominance helpful in diagnosis, but definitive diagnosis requires histopathology; not responsive to glucocorticoids
	Neoplasia	Neoplastic cells may rarely be seen in CSF
	Noninfectious or degenerative conditions	Consider GME; may require elimination of other possible causes and consideration of multiple factors to arrive at a clinical diagnosis
Eosinophilic inflammation	Parasitic, protozoal, bacterial, viral, fungal, or rickettsial infections	Uncommon manifestation reported with a variety of types of disease
Pleocytosis with predominance of eosinophils	Neoplasia	Occasionally seen with neoplasia
	Hypersensitivity reaction	Consider vaccine reactions or other hypersensitivity components associated with infectious or noninfectious origin
	Inflammatory process	May be seen as part of a nonspecific inflammatory process

CSF, Cerebrospinal fluid; *FIP*, feline infectious peritonitis; *GME*, granulomatous meningoencephalomyelitis.

identification of organisms, but its dark color prevents the visualization of the cellular morphological detail (Marcos et al., 2016b). PAS stain may be used to demonstrate positive intracellular material in dogs with globoid cell leukodystrophy. Luxol fast blue can be used to demonstrate myelin in CSF specimens (Mesher et al., 1996).

Normal Cerebrospinal Fluid

Normal CSF from healthy dogs and cats contains primarily mononuclear cells that are composed of a mixture of lymphocytes and large mononuclear (monocytoid) cells of uncertain origin (Fig. 15.4). Lymphocytes or monocytoid cells are the predominant nucleated cell type in normal canine and feline

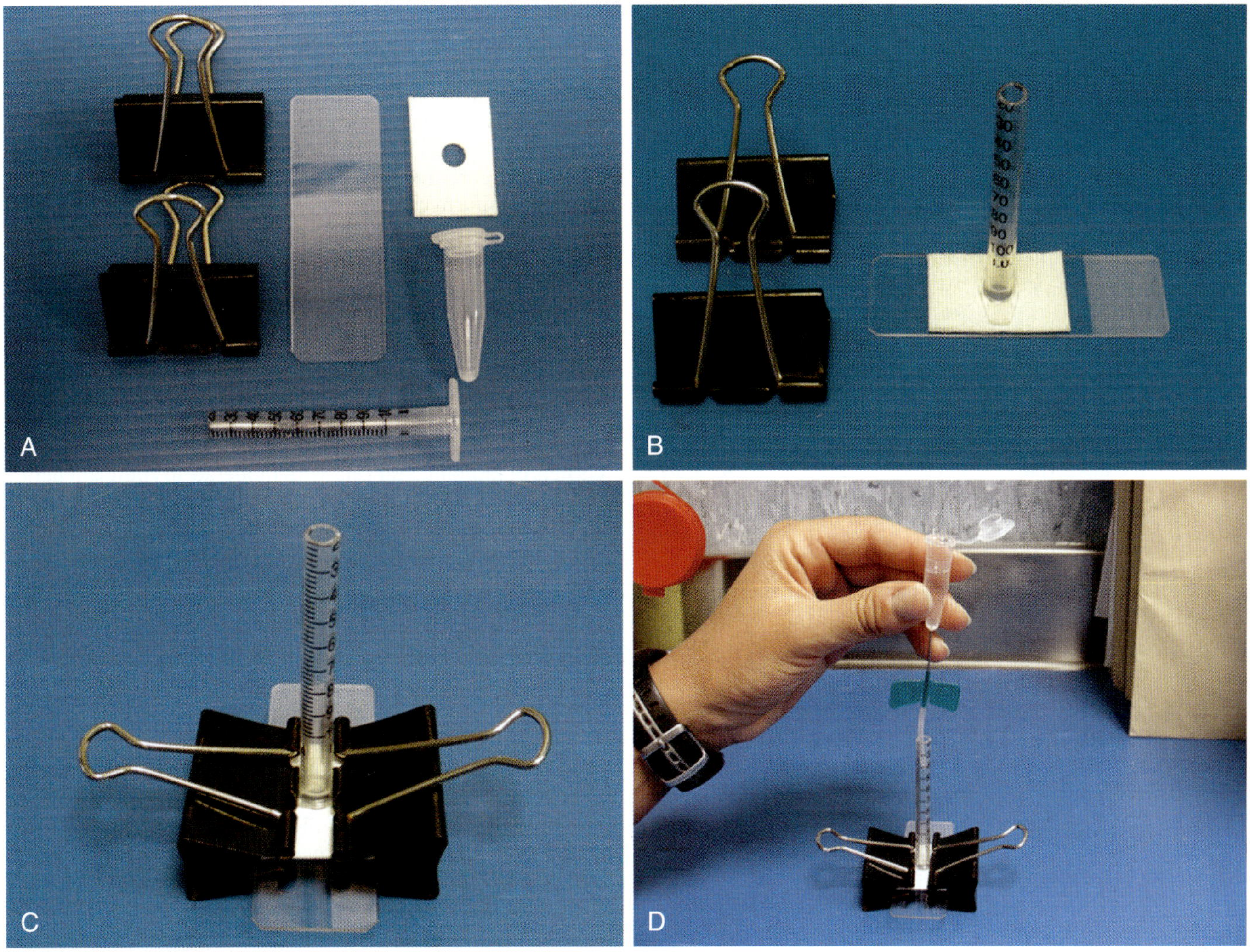

FIGURE 15.3 In-house cerebrospinal fluid (CSF) sedimentation device. A, Unassembled sedimentation device with materials needed: 1 mL modified insulin syringe barrel, filter paper with a hole punched, glass slide, two binder clips, and an Eppendorf tube for CSF collection. **B,** Partially assembled sedimentation device. **C,** Assembled sedimentation device demonstrating the attachment of the binder clips to the barrel flanged portions. **D,** The tube made from the syringe barrel is filled with as little as 100 µL of CSF by transfer pipette or, as the figure demonstrates, using a butterfly needle. The added fluid is allowed to sit undisturbed for 1 hour. Cells concentrate and settle on to the exposed area of the glass slide.

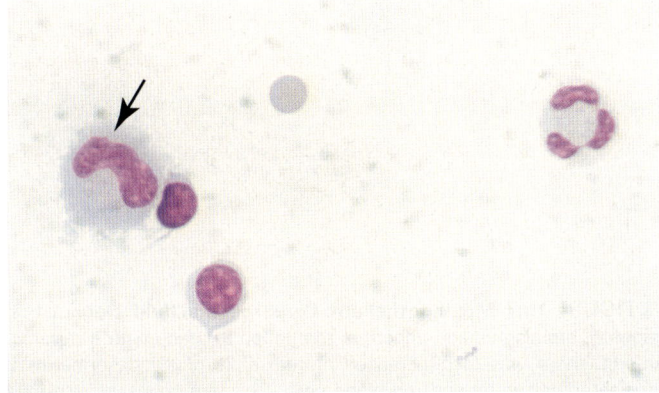

FIGURE 15.4 Normal cerebrospinal fluid cells. Cytocentrifuged preparation. Dog. Two small mononuclear cells (lymphocytes), one large mononuclear (monocytoid) cell *(arrow)*, one nondegenerate neutrophil, and one erythrocyte are present. (Wright-Giemsa; HP oil.)

CSF. Monocytoid cells are the predominant type in normal CSF from healthy cats that make up 69% to 100% of the total nucleated cells; lymphocytes, 0% to 27%; neutrophils, 0% to 9%; macrophages, 0% to 3%; and eosinophils, less than 1% (Rand et al., 1990). Occasional choroid plexus cells, ependymal cells, meningeal lining cells, or mitotic figures may be seen (Fig. 15.5).

Inadvertent Puncture Contaminants

Bone marrow cells have been reported in canine CSF and may be attributed to inadvertent penetration of the bone marrow space during lumbar cistern collections (Christopher, 1992). However, sites of extramedullary hematopoiesis have been described within the interstitium of the choroid plexus at the level of the fourth ventricle in five dogs (Bienzle et al., 1995). Myelin-like material, neurons, and neuropil have been reported as contaminants of canine CSF associated with accidental puncture of the spinal cord during cerebellomedullary cistern collection (Fig. 15.6) (Fallin et al., 1996).

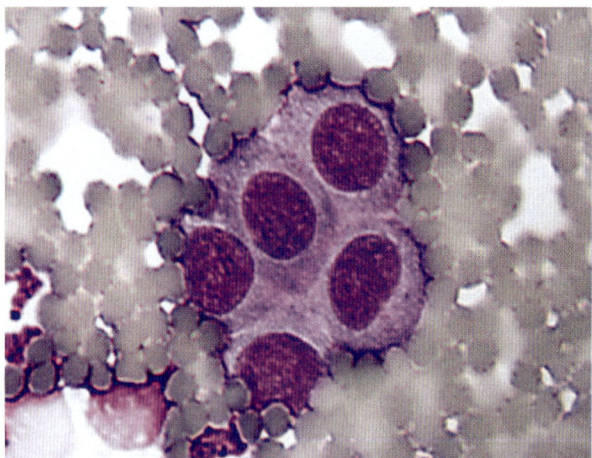

FIGURE 15.5 Normal lining cells. Cerebrospinal fluid. Dog. Both ependymal and choroid plexus cells usually represent an incidental finding in fluid specimens. These cells have no diagnostic importance other than their potential to be mistaken for neoplasia. (Romanowsky; HP oil.)

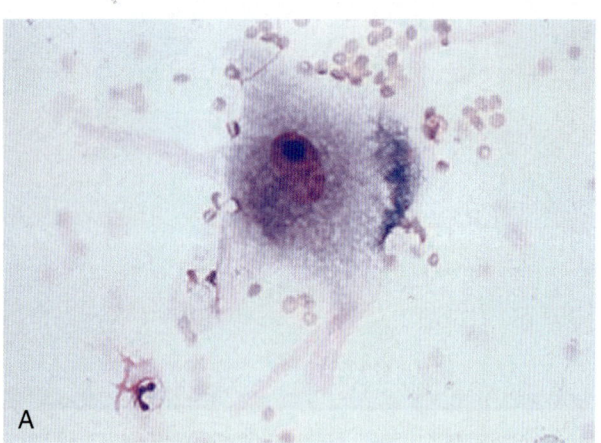

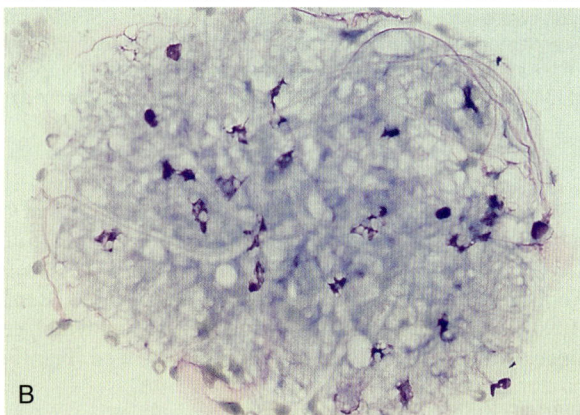

FIGURE 15.6 Nervous tissue. Cerebrospinal fluid. Dog. Same case in A and B. The patient presented with cervical pain. **A, Neuron.** Inadvertent puncture of nervous tissue during collection at the cerebellomedullary cistern demonstrating the large size of the neuron compared with a neutrophil and erythrocytes. Basophilic granular material within the neuronal cell cytoplasm is presumed to be Nissl bodies. (Wright-Giemsa; HP oil.) **B, Neuropil with microglial cells.** The swirling fibrils of nervous tissue are termed *neuropil*. (Wright-Giemsa; HP oil.) (A, From Fallin CW, Raskin RE, Harvey JW. Cytologic identification of neural tissue in the cerebrospinal fluid of two dogs. *Vet Clin Pathol*. 1996;25:127–129. B, Courtesy of Rose Raskin, University of Florida.)

The term *surface epithelium* is used to describe meningeal, choroid plexus, ependymal, and endothelial cells that are found in human CSF. However, because of their fragility, these cells are difficult to identify microscopically with certainty. Ependymal cells, which line the walls of the ventricles, and choroid plexus epithelium, which is continuous with ependymal epithelium, are indistinguishable from one another; they are small uniform cuboidal to columnar cells that are characterized by eccentrically located small, round nuclei, granular to coarse chromatin, and moderate amounts of finely granular cytoplasm (see Fig. 15.5). Three cell types considered to be of canine choroid plexus origin have been described based on Romanowsky staining in which the most prevalent were termed alpha cells (75%) having basophilic granular cytoplasm (Garma-Aviña, 2004). The beta and gamma cells are nongranular or rarely vacuolated, respectively. Leptomeningeal (subarachnoid lining) cells are described as individual or small clusters of mononuclear cells with moderate to abundant lightly basophilic cytoplasm containing round to oval eccentric nuclei with a delicate chromatin pattern (Fig. 15.7). In canine CSF, the presence of occasional surface epithelium cells should be judiciously interpreted as a possible contaminant (Wessmann et al., 2010).

Cerebrospinal Fluid Presentation and Interpretation
Normal Cerebrospinal Fluid Findings in the Presence of Disease

There may be no abnormal CSF cytopathologic findings in cases of idiopathic epilepsy, congenital hydrocephalus, intoxication, metabolic or functional disorders, vertebral disease, or myelomalacia. Most cases of FIP, distemper encephalitis, neoplasia, or GME with neurologic signs have CSF parameters within normal limits. In a series of 17 dogs with neurologic symptoms caused by spinal arachnoid cysts, CSF analysis was

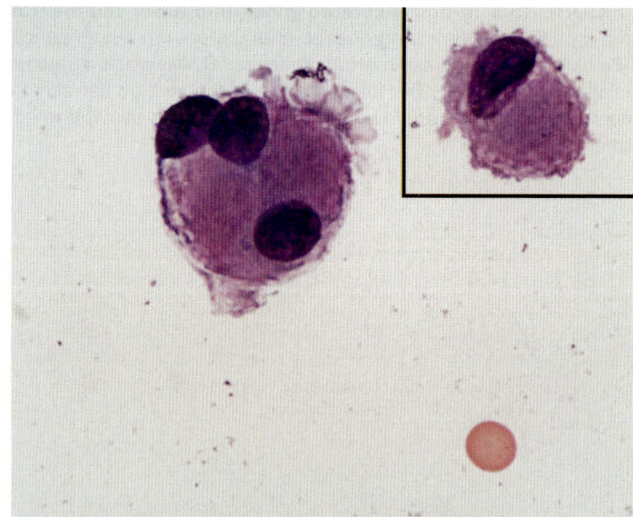

FIGURE 15.7 Meningothelium. Cerebrospinal fluid. Dog. Clinical signs of strabismus and abnormal mentation in a dog with a thalamic infarct. There was mild increased protein (0.28 g/L) and normal total nucleated cell count and red blood cells. Cells are cohesive with mild surface blebbing. *Inset:* One isolated cell has an oval eccentrically placed nucleus with dense clumped chromatin. The cytoplasm is eosinophilic and finely granulated. (Wright; HP oil.) (Courtesy Rose Raskin, Royal Veterinary College, UK.)

unremarkable (Skeen et al., 2003). Absence of cytopathologic abnormality in CSF does not rule out the possibility of neurologic disease.

Protein Abnormalities in Cerebrospinal Fluid

An increase in the protein concentration without an increase in total cells is referred to as *albuminocytologic* or *protein-cytologic dissociation*. The increase in the protein concentration may be associated with an increase in the blood-brain barrier permeability, local necrosis, interruption of normal CSF flow and absorption, or intrathecal globulin production (Chrisman, 1992).

Increases in CSF protein concentration, with or without increases in nucleated cell count or cytopathologic abnormality in CSF, may occur with inflammatory, degenerative, compressive, or neoplastic disease. In a series of 56 cases of canine intracranial meningiomas, increased total protein concentration, in the presence of a normal TNCC, was detected in 16 (30%) dogs (Dickinson et al., 2006). An increase in the protein concentration without an increase in TNCC may occur with neoplasia, ischemic myelopathy, postseizure, fever, intervertebral disc extrusion, degenerative myelopathy, myelomalacia, fibrocartilaginous embolism, or GME (Clemmons, 1991; Gandini et al., 2003). In cats, a marked increase in the protein concentration is supportive of a presumptive diagnosis of FIP (Singh et al., 2005).

In a series of 61 Cavalier King Charles spaniels with Chiari-like malformation, the group with concurrent syringomyelia showed a higher CSF protein concentration (0.26 g/L [0.07–0.42 g/L]) and increases in TNCC and neutrophil percentage compared with dogs without syringomyelia (0.2 g/L [0.12–0.39 g/L]) (Whittaker et al., 2011). The change in dogs with concurrent Chiari-like malformation and syringomyelia was attributed to disruption of the blood–spinal cord barrier.

Increased Cell Type Percentages Without Increased Total Nucleated Cell Counts

Increased percentages of either neutrophils or eosinophils may occur without an increase in the TNCC in a variety of neurologic disorders. If blood contamination is ruled out, increased neutrophil percentages greater than 10% to 20% and eosinophil percentages greater than 1% should be considered unusual. Increased neutrophils may indicate mild or early inflammation or tissue irritation, a lesion that does not contact the meninges or ependymal cells, or previous use of drugs such as glucocorticoids and antibiotics that reduce the inflammatory response. Conditions to consider include degenerative intervertebral disc disease, spinal fractures, cerebrovascular disorders such as infarcts, or compressive disease (e.g., cervical spondylomyelopathy). Increased eosinophils without increased total white blood cell count may occur with parasite migration or protozoal disease.

Pleocytosis

Increases in TNCC of CSF is termed *pleocytosis*, which is further defined by the predominant cell type—that is, neutrophilic, eosinophilic, mononuclear, or mixed cell pleocytosis. Pleocytosis is graded as mild (6–50 cells/µL in dogs and cats), moderate (51–200 cells/µL and 51–1000 cells/µL, in dogs and cats, respectively), or marked (>200 cells/µL and >1000 cells/µL, in dogs and cats, respectively) (Chrisman, 1992; Singh et al., 2005).

Neutrophilic pleocytosis. Neutrophilic pleocytosis has been associated with a wide variety of active inflammatory disorders, including trauma, postmyelographic aseptic meningitis, fibrocartilaginous embolic myelopathy, myelomalacia, hemorrhage, neoplasia, brain infarct, and mycotic and bacterial meningitis (Mariani et al., 2002; Mikszewski et al., 2006). It may be seen with abscesses communicating with the ventricles or subarachnoid space, early viral infections, FIP, Rocky Mountain spotted fever, discospondylitis, acquired hydrocephalus, and necrosis. Marked neutrophilic pleocytosis is most often associated with noninfectious meningoencephalomyelitis such as steroid-responsive meningitis, or necrotizing vasculitis or neoplasia and in bacterial or fungal meningoencephalitis (Fig. 15.8) (Chrisman, 1992; Tipold and Schatzberg, 2010). Infectious agents that may be observed in CSF include *C. neoformans*, *Blastomyces dermatitidis*, *Histoplasma capsulatum*, *N. caninum*, and *Ehrlichia* (Singh et al., 2005; Gaitero et al., 2006). Parasites such as *Toxocara canis*, *Dirofilaria immitis*, *Cuterebra* larva, and *Cysticercus* that may cause neurologic disease have not been reported in CSF cytopathology preparations. The presence of marked neutrophilic pleocytosis or increasing numbers of neutrophils in sequential CSF collections has been reported to be an unfavorable prognostic finding.

The most frequent noninflammatory diseases in cats 7 years or older with progressive neurological signs for more than 4 weeks were neoplasia with a lesser number with ischemic encephalopathy. The CSF protein concentration was slightly increased (<1 g/L; 100 mg/dL) without an increase in the TNCC with infrequent concomitant slight increases in percentage of neutrophils or lymphocytes or both (Rand et al., 1994).

Feline infectious peritonitis, a coronavirus infection, is a common cause of neutrophilic pleocytosis in the cat (Figs. 15.9 and 15.10). The main neurologic signs are depression, tetraparesis, head tilt, nystagmus, and intention tremor (Baroni and Heinold, 1995). It accounted for 44% of 61 feline cases of inflammatory CNS disease (Rand et al., 1994). Marked neutrophilic pleocytosis with counts of more than 100 cells/µL, with neutrophils making up more than 50% of the total, was associated seen with FIP,

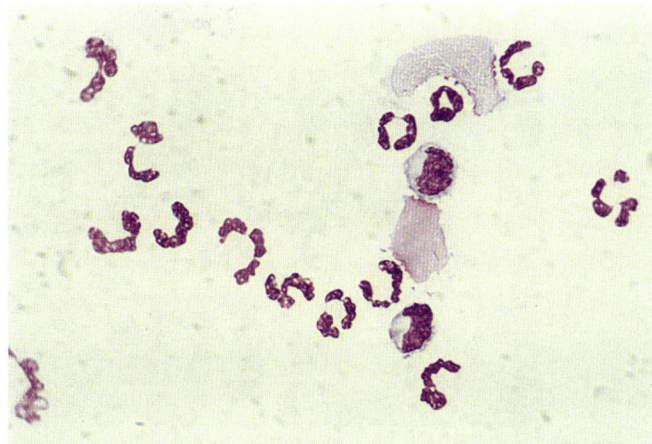

■ **FIGURE 15.8 Neutrophilic pleocytosis. Meningioma. Cerebrospinal fluid. Dog.** Total nucleated cell count was 1018/µL, and the protein concentration was 240 mg/dL with a history of head tilt and hemiplegia related to a cranial meningioma. Nondegenerate neutrophils composed 83% of the cell population. (Wright-Giemsa; HP oil.)

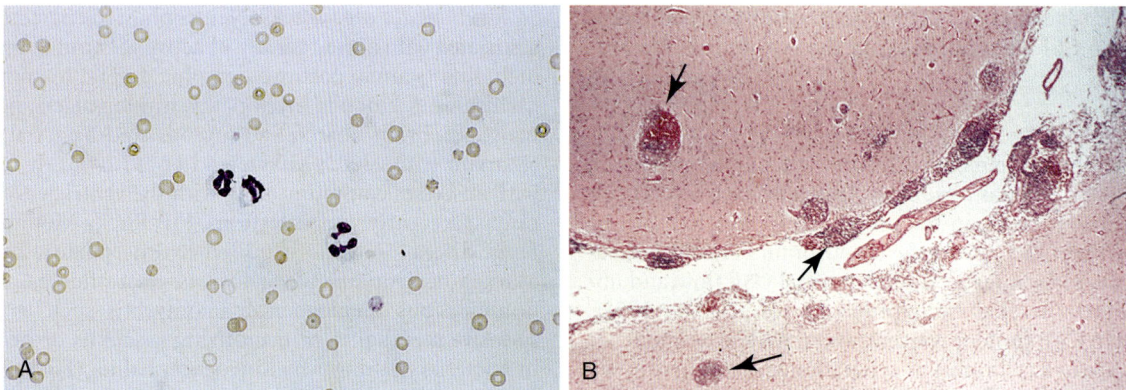

■ **FIGURE 15.9 Neutrophilic pleocytosis. Feline infectious peritonitis (FIP). Cerebrospinal fluid. Cat.** Same case in A and B. **A,** Direct smear made from fluid from a kitten with a 5-day duration of ataxia. A high nucleated cell count supported use of a direct smear to evaluate leukocytes. The case was diagnosed as FIP by positive titer and histologic examination. Numerous erythrocytes and several nondegenerate neutrophils characterize the cells present. Acute hemorrhage was evident but is not demonstrated in this field. (Wright; HP oil.) **B,** Section of midbrain and third ventricle demonstrating multifocal neutrophilic perivascular infiltrates *(arrows)* in a cat with FIP. The proximity of the infiltrates to the ventricle contributed to the neutrophilic pleocytosis. (H&E; LP.)

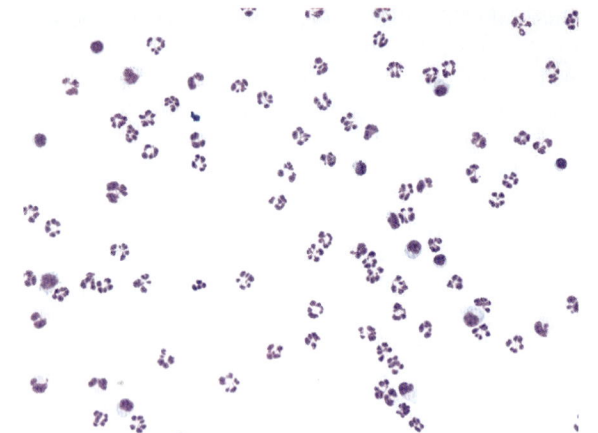

■ **FIGURE 15.10 Neutrophilic pleocytosis. Feline infectious peritonitis. Cerebrospinal fluid. Cat.** There is a mixed population with predominant nondegenerate segmented neutrophils with low numbers of small and intermediate lymphocytes. (MGG, HP oil.)

along with increased CSF protein concentration (usually >200 mg/dL). The study results indicated a high probability of FIP if a cat is younger than 4 years with multifocal neurologic signs referable to the cerebellum or brainstem, a protracted course of illness, and CSF protein concentration greater than 200 mg/dL. Later in the course of the disease, a mixed cellular population may be found with large mononuclear cells and lymphocytes present to a significant degree (Fig. 15.11). Similar results were found in a series of 11 cats with FIP (Singh et al., 2005). The study results indicated that the CSF characterized as suppurative in seven cats, mixed cell types in one, and primarily mononuclear in three. Five cats had marked elevations in the CSF TNCC (>1000 cells/µL), three had moderate elevations (51–1000 calls/µL), and two had mild elevations (6–50 cells/µL). A CSF titer of 1:640 or higher is supportive of a presumptive diagnosis of FIP (Soma et al., 2018). Immunocytochemical staining of feline coronavirus antigen (FCoV) within macrophages of CSF is a highly sensitive test for antemortem diagnosis of neurologic FIP but with low specificity. Immunocytochemical staining of FCoV

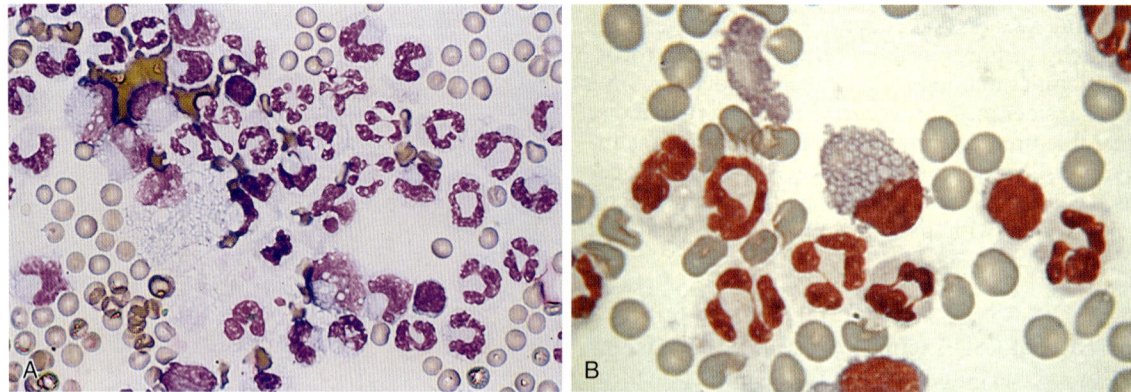

■ **FIGURE 15.11 Mixed cell pleocytosis with neutrophilic predominance. Feline infectious peritonitis (FIP). Cerebrospinal fluid. Cat. A,** Increased numbers of large mononuclear cells consistent with macrophages were present in a cat with fever, high titers for FIP, and histopathologic support of FIP at necropsy. The duration of disease was several months, accounting for the more mononuclear response than the case in Figure 15.9. (Wright-Giemsa; HP oil.) **B,** Chronicity of infection with FIP is suggested by the presence of plasma cells indicated by the Mott cell *(center).* Nondegenerate cells and erythrocytes are also seen. Plasma cells are not seen in cerebrospinal fluid of healthy animals. (MGG; HP oil.)
(A, Courtesy Rick Alleman, University of Florida.)

could be helpful to discover preneurologic stages of CNS FIP but cannot be recommended as a diagnostic test for FIP (Gruendl et al., 2017). Real-time reverse transcriptase polymerase chain reaction (real-time RT-PCR) detecting FCoV RNA in CSF of cats showed a moderate sensitivity (42.1%) and excellent specificity, indicating that is a reliable tool for diagnosing FIP (Doenges et al., 2016).

Non-FIP viral meningoencephalitis was considered most likely in cats younger than 3 years of age with progressive neurologic disease and focal neurologic signs referable to the thalamocortex (Rand et al., 1994). The TNCC was less than 50 cells/µL, and the CSF protein concentration was less than 100 mg/dL. The study results indicated that non-FIP viral meningoencephalitis had a favorable prognosis for recovery.

Steroid-responsive suppurative meningitis-arteritis occurs in young to middle-aged dogs that present with signs of fever, cervical pain, hyperesthesia, and paresis. Pleocytosis is often greater than 500 cells/µL with greater than 75% nondegenerate neutrophils if glucocorticoids have not been recently administered (Fig. 15.12) (Chrisman, 1992). Bacteria are not observed or cultured, and improvement is often seen within 72 hours after glucocorticoid administration; the long-term prognosis is favorable. The finding of IgG and IgA in the CSF was attributed to intrathecal synthesis and suggested the humoral response was primary rather than the result of a generalized immune complex disease (Tipold et al., 1995). In a series of 12 cases of aseptic suppurative meningitis in juvenile boxers, of which 10 of the dogs exhibited the acute form of the disease, the TNCC was greater than 100 cells/µL, with the percentage of neutrophils ranging from 72% to 100% (Behr and Cauzinille, 2006). The CSF from two other dogs with a more clinically chronic disease had a mixed pleocytosis with a percentage of neutrophils of approximately 60%. An abnormal cell count of mixed cell population or mononuclear cells in CSF are seen in the protracted form, and monitoring of CSF cell count in dogs with this condition seems to be a sensitive indicator of success of treatment (Cizinauskas et al., 2000).

Necrotizing vasculitis is a syndrome of aseptic suppurative meningitis in young Bernese mountain dogs involving the leptomeningeal arteries. Animals present with severe cervical pain and neurologic deficits. The CSF TNCC is generally greater than 1000 cells/µL, with nondegenerate neutrophils predominating. A similar condition has been reported in beagles and Welsh springer spaniels (Caswell and Nykamp, 2003). Clinical improvement occurred with corticosteroid administration.

Bacterial meningoencephalitis (Fig. 15.13) is suspected if more than 75% neutrophils are present in CSF regardless of the total cell count. Bacteremia is usually the cause with septic emboli to the brain as a result. Untreated cases often produce marked pleocytosis with greater than 1000 cells/µL. Intracellular location of bacteria and accompanying inflammation are particularly important in eliminating the possibility of bacterial contamination associated with nonsterile collection technique or nonsterile collection tubes. Neutrophils show mild to severe

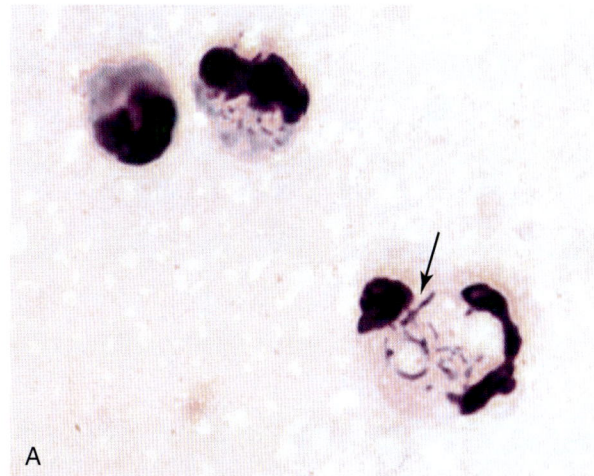

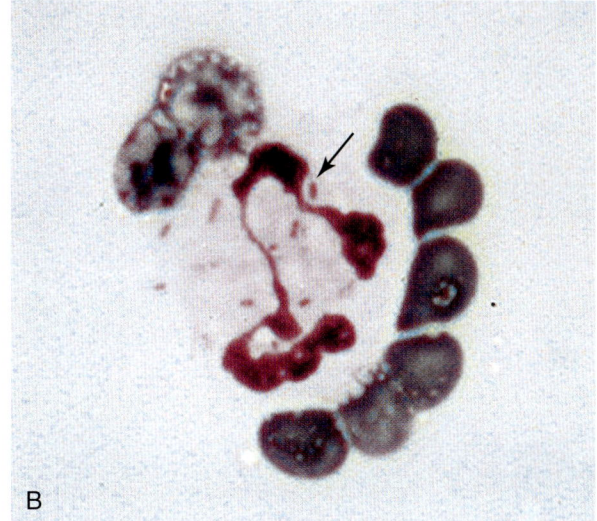

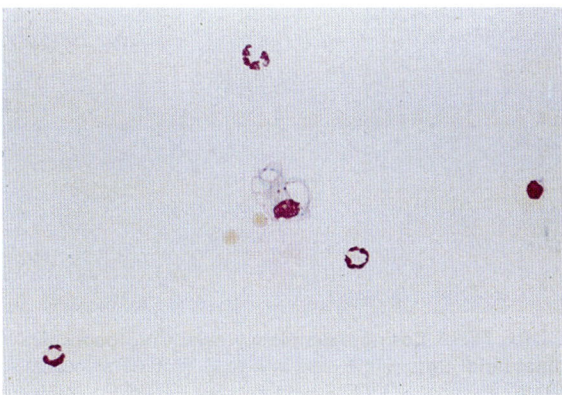

■ **FIGURE 15.12 Neutrophilic pleocytosis. Steroid-responsive meningitis. Cerebrospinal fluid. Dog.** Generalized nonseptic inflammatory response in a 1-year-old dog exhibiting fever and cervical, thoracic, and lumbar pain. Total nucleated cell count was 106/µL with protein concentration of 41 mg/dL and red blood cells of 3700/µL. Three nondegenerate neutrophils, one large mononuclear cell, and one lymphocyte are present. Multiple joints were similarly affected in this case. Immune-mediated corticosteroid-responsive meningitis was suspected. (Wright-Giemsa; HP oil.)

■ **FIGURE 15.13 Neutrophilic pleocytosis. Bacterial infection. Cerebrospinal fluid (CSF). Cat. A,** Direct smear of cloudy CSF indicates increased cellularity with many degenerate neutrophils present. Associated with the karyolytic neutrophils shown are intracellular, small, rod-shaped bacteria *(arrow)* cultured as *Enterobacter* spp. (Wright; HP oil.) **B, Septic meningoencephalitis.** Several rod bacteria *(arrow)* are present within the cytoplasm of the neutrophil. Several erythrocytes surround the inflammatory cell. (MGG; HP oil.)

karyolysis. Identification of bacteria in CSF cytopathology and by culture is rare because of the small sample size. Bacteria were identified by using CSF cytopathology in 62 of 109 (57%) adult humans, zero of 14 (0%) dogs, and two of five (40%) cats with confirmed bacterial CNS infection (Messer et al., 2006). Other causes of neutrophilic pleocytosis, especially SRMA, need to be ruled out by signalment before a presumptive diagnosis of bacterial CSF infection is made, a relatively rare occurrence.

Eosinophilic pleocytosis. Eosinophilic pleocytosis (usually >10% TNCC) has been associated with parasites, hypersensitivity, toxoplasmosis, neosporosis, *C. neoformans* infection, migrating internal parasites (e.g., *Baylisascaris procyonis* or *Angiostrongylus cantonensis*), *Prototheca* spp., canine distemper virus infection, and rabies (Chrisman, 1992; Windsor et al., 2009; Galgut et al., 2010; Gupta et al., 2011; Lane et al., 2012; Lunn et al., 2012) (Figs. 15.14 to 15.16). Eosinophilic

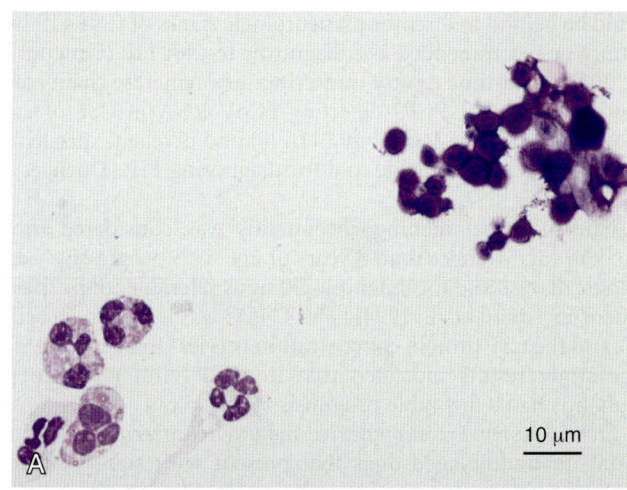

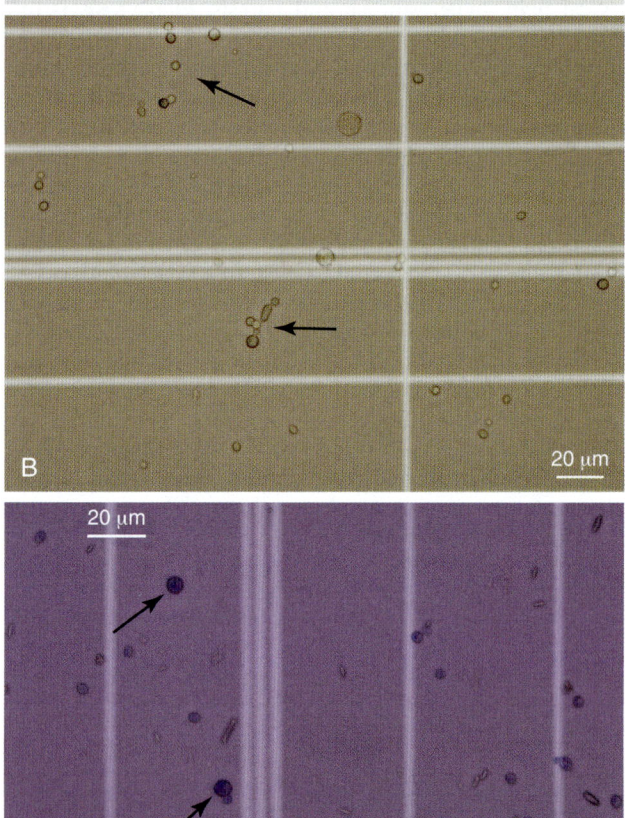

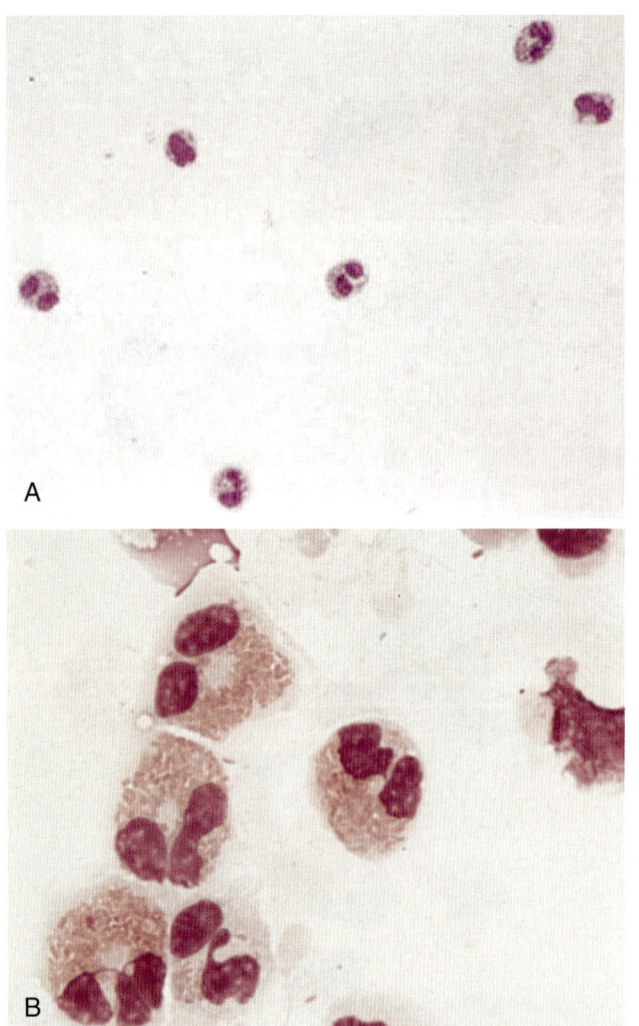

■ **FIGURE 15.14 Eosinophilic pleocytosis. Toxoplasmosis. Cisternal cerebrospinal fluid. A, Dog.** This acutely paraparetic animal with upper motor neuron dysfunction to the rear legs was diagnosed as having toxoplasmosis by serum titer. Total nucleated cell count was 124/μL with a high normal protein. Eosinophils accounted for 98% of the cell population. Peripheral eosinophilia was not present. (Wright-Giemsa; HP oil.) **B, Cat.** Note the predominance of typical bilobate eosinophils in the cerebrospinal fluid from this case of toxoplasmosis confirmed by polymerase chain reaction of cerebrospinal fluid. (MGG; HP oil.)

■ **FIGURE 15.15 Eosinophilic pleocytosis. Cryptococcosis. Cerebrospinal fluid. Dog.** Same case in A to C. Marked pleocytosis (total nucleated cell count, 7300/μL), erythrocytes (5500/μL), and increased microprotein (61 mg/dL). Cell differential indicated 46% eosinophils, 33% neutrophils, 11% large mononuclear cells, and 10% lymphocytes. **A, Cytocentrifuged preparation.** Group of round refractile yeasts appear in the *upper right* with a mixed granulocyte response at the *lower left*. (Wright-Giemsa; HP oil.) **B, Unstained wet mount.** Yeast are recognized on the unstained hemocytometer *(arrows)*. (Unstained; IP.) **C, Stained wet mount.** Three round yeast nuclei *(arrows)* are easily appreciated with staining. (NMB; IP.) (A–C, Courtesy Jere Stern, University of Florida.)

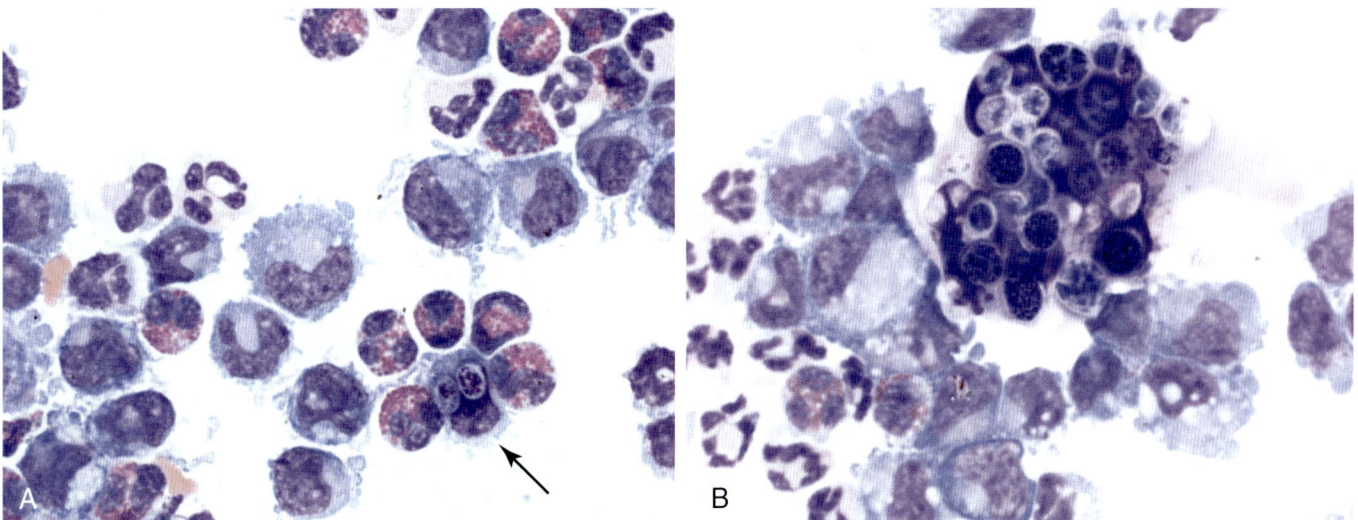

■ **FIGURE 15.16 Eosinophilic pleocytosis. Prototheosis. Cerebrospinal fluid (CSF). Dog.** Same case in A and B. The patient had clinical signs of ataxia and proprioceptive deficits. Brain magnetic resonance imaging revealed a lesion on one side of the pons and medulla extending dorsally to the fourth ventricle. CSF revealed 2000/μL total nucleated cell count and 1898 mg/dL total protein. The marked pleocytosis consisted of 65% eosinophils, 25% nondegenerate neutrophils, and 10% small lymphocytes and large mononuclear cells. **A,** Mixed cell population with large mononuclear cells with two round to ovoid *Prototheca* organisms *(arrow).* (Wright-Giemsa; HP oil.) **B,** Large group of single spherical and dividing forms of extracellular organisms. (Wright-Giemsa; HP oil.) (Courtesy Mary Leissinger, Louisiana State University.)

pleocytosis associated with *Angiostrongylus vasorum* infection may persist several weeks following treatment and negative fecal Baermann test result (Alcoverro et al., 2019). Pleocytosis composed of a predominance of eosinophils and monocytes was associated with a coinfection of *N. caninum* and *Ehrlichia canis*. Intracytoplasmic inclusions consistent with *E. canis* morulae were observed within eosinophils and intracytoplasmic tachyzoites consistent with *N. caninum* were observed within mononuclear cells (Aroch et al., 2018).

Eosinophilic pleocytosis was reported in a cat associated with T-cell spinal lymphoma (Bray et al., 2016).

Eosinophilic pleocytosis without a defined underlying etiopathogenesis is termed *idiopathic eosinophilic meningoencephalomyelitis* or *eosinophilic meningoencephalitis of unknown etiology* and is often associated with large breed dogs (Windsor et al., 2009; Olivier et al., 2010; Cardy and Cornelis, 2018). Steroid-responsive meningoencephalitis with a predominance of eosinophils has been described in dogs and cats (Chrisman, 1992) (Fig. 15.17). Finding more than 80% eosinophils with mild to marked pleocytosis present and finding no evidence of protozoal, parasitic, or fungal infection usually supports the diagnosis. In the canine study, golden retrievers were overrepresented, which may suggest a breed predisposition to this condition (Fig. 15.18). Animals usually respond to glucocorticoid therapy with dramatic decreases in cell numbers and changes in differential percentages. An allergic or type I hypersensitivity reaction is suspected in some cases.

Mononuclear pleocytosis. Mononuclear pleocytosis of CSF usually presents with increased lymphocytes in viral, protozoal, or fungal infection; uremia; intoxication; vaccine reaction; meningoencephalomyelitis of unknown etiology (MUE); and discospondylitis. Furthermore, it may be seen with necrotizing encephalitis, steroid-responsive meningoencephalomyelitis, ehrlichiosis, or treated bacterial meningoencephalitis (Tipold and Schatzberg, 2010). However, monocytoid and

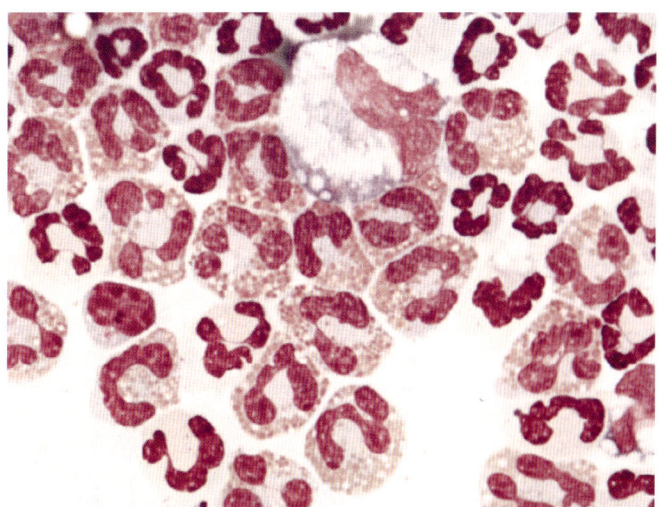

■ **FIGURE 15.17 Eosinophilic pleocytosis. Eosinophilic meningoencephalitis of unknown etiology. Cerebrospinal fluid. Dog.** Total nucleated cell count was 125/μL, and 85% were eosinophils. Several nondegenerate neutrophils and a large, foamy macrophage are also present. (MGG; HP oil.)

macrophage cells may also predominate in these conditions and most commonly with cryptococcosis (Figs. 15.19 and 15.20). Mononuclear pleocytosis was noted in two cats with cuterebriasis (Glass et al., 1998) and in another cat with cerebral cholesterol granuloma (Fluhemann et al., 2006).

The appearance of CSF macrophages containing vacuoles and pink-purple amorphous granular material in a young cat with mononuclear pleocytosis, increased protein concentration, seizures, incoordination, and tremors indicated the presence of a lysosomal storage disease (GM_2-gangliosidosis) (Johnsrude et al.,

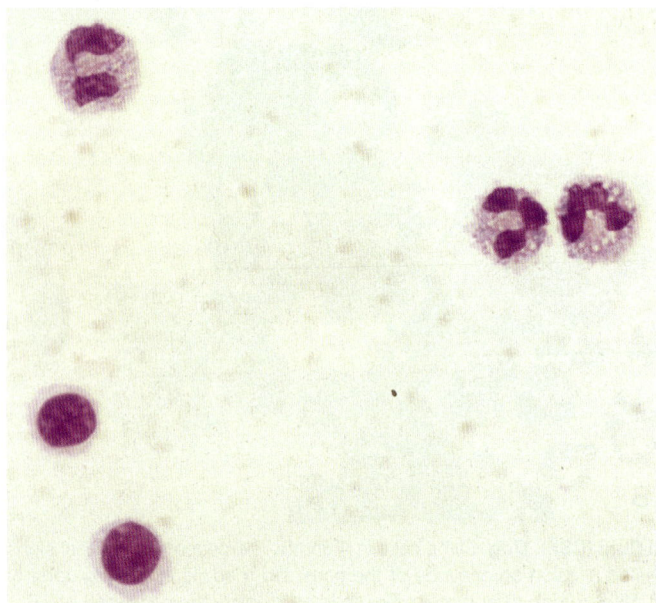

■ **FIGURE 15.18 Eosinophilic pleocytosis. Eosinophilic meningoencephalitis of unknown etiology. Cerebrospinal fluid. Dog.** This sample is from a golden retriever with a total nucleated cell count of 43/μL and protein of 77 mg/dL. The cell differential was 43% eosinophils, 50% lymphocytes, and 7% large mononuclear phagocytes. Three eosinophils and two small lymphocytes are shown. This condition is often associated with this breed. (Wright-Giemsa; HP oil.)

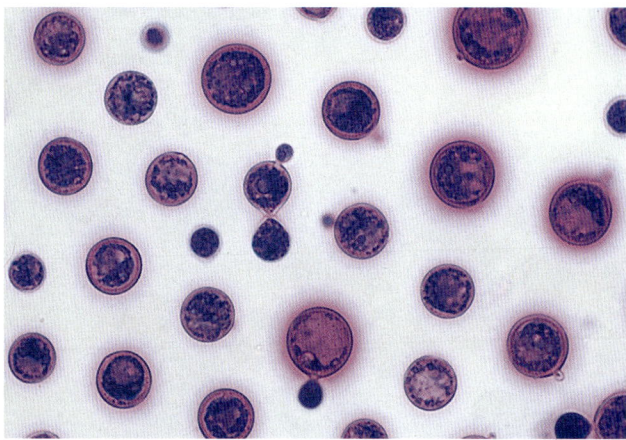

■ **FIGURE 15.20 Cryptococcosis. Cerebrospinal fluid. Dog.** These spherical organisms display frequent budding. (NMB; HP oil.) (Courtesy Rick Alleman, University of Florida.)

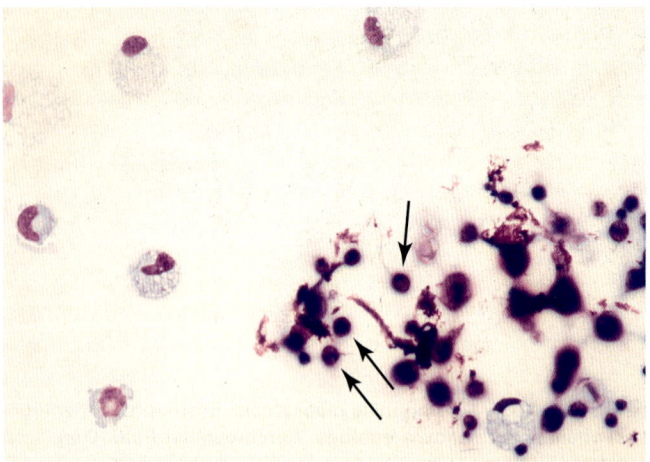

■ **FIGURE 15.19 Mononuclear pleocytosis. Cryptococcosis. Cerebrospinal fluid. Dog.** Clusters of basophilic-staining extracellular yeast measuring approximately 10 to 20 μm in diameter are present. Three yeast structures *(arrows)* have well-defined cell walls that surround a single nucleus along with cytoplasmic organelles. The fluid contained a total nucleated cell count of 60/μL of which 85% were mononuclear phagocytes. Several mononuclear cells have abundant foamy to vacuolated pale cytoplasm and are classified as reactive mononuclear cells. (Wright-Giemsa; HP oil.)

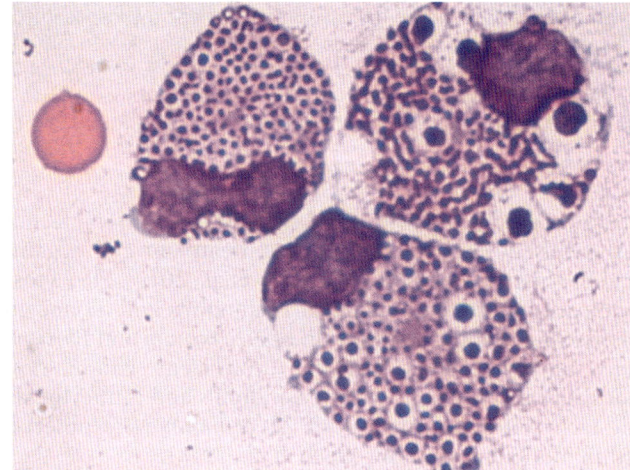

■ **FIGURE 15.21 Lysosomal storage disease. GM_2-gangliosidosis. Cerebrospinal fluid (CSF). Cat.** A 5-month-old kitten presented with a history of seizures, incoordination, and tremors since birth. Neuroanatomic localization suggested diffuse cerebral and cerebellar disease. CSF analysis indicated a mononuclear pleocytosis with total nucleated cell count of 88/μL, red blood cells of 196/μL, and a mildly increased protein (30 mg/dL). The cell differential was primarily macrophages. An enzyme assay determined the condition as a GM_2-gangliosidosis (β hexosaminidase B deficiency). Note the large mononuclear cells contain prominent, purple or vacuolar inclusions consistent with lysosomal storage material. (Wright-Giemsa; HP oil.) (Courtesy Rose Raskin, University of Florida.)

1996) (Fig. 15.21). Another type of lysosomal storage disease with a similar cytopathologic appearance occurred in a young dog with neuronal ceroid lipofuscinosis (Gardini et al., 2019).

The most frequent noninflammatory neurologic diseases of CNS in cats are neoplasia and ischemic encephalopathy, which usually present with an increased CSF protein concentration and slight lymphocytic pleocytosis or normal TNCC (Rand et al., 1994). Hemorrhagic conditions may be accompanied by a mononuclear pleocytosis composed of foamy macrophages (Fig. 15.22). Compressive conditions such as Chiari-like caudal occipital malformation syndrome with syringomyelia may occur in small breeds with a lymphocytic pleocytosis (Fig. 15.23).

Meningoencephalitis of unknown etiology or *unknown origin* is an umbrella term for a heterogeneous group of inflammatory, noninfectious, and presumed autoimmune inflammatory CNS diseases that affect young to middle-aged dogs. It includes primarily cerebellar syndrome (idiopathic cerebellitis or generalized tremor syndrome), eosinophilic meningoencephalitis, and encephalitides defined histopathologically as necrotizing or granulomatous that are diagnosed clinically by a combination of magnetic resonance imaging (MRI) and CSF findings and negative infectious disease test results (Talarico and Schatzberg, 2010; Coates and Jeffery, 2014; Cornelis et al., 2019; Stafford et al., 2019). Specific disease entities included under MUE are GME and two variants of necrotizing encephalitis that affect small breed dogs such as pugs, Maltese, Yorkshire terriers, chihuahuas, shih tzus, Pekinese, and French bulldogs. One variant is necrotizing meningoencephalitis (NME), which was previously termed *pug encephalitis*. Histologically, inflammation is marked, nonsuppurative, and associated with marked gliosis of the cerebral cortex involving the meninges and perivascular spaces. A second variant is NLE involving Yorkshire terriers and other toy breeds, which involves the white matter of the cerebrum. Histologically, there is marked nonsuppurative inflammation accompanied by gliosis, cavitation, edema, and gitter cell infiltration (Uchida et al., 2016).

A validated assay was used to detect antibodies to 6 neuronal cell surface proteins associated with autoimmune encephalitis in human in the CSF of dogs clinically diagnosed with inflammatory and noninflammatory CNS disease. Anti-N-methyl-D-aspartate receptor (NMDAR1) antibodies were detected in a cohort of three dogs. The dogs responded to treatment for MUE, suggesting that defining antigenic targets associated with encephalitis in dogs might allow diagnostic categorization of MUE antemortem (Stafford et al., 2019). Pugs have an autoantibody against astrocytes by indirect immunofluorescence assay, suggesting an immune-mediated etiopathogenesis (Uchida et al., 1999).

The dogs are usually younger than 4 years; present frequently with seizures, depression, and ataxia; and do not respond to glucocorticoids. Brainstem signs are more likely with NLE than NME that progresses quickly to become fatal or leading to euthanasia (Tipold et al., 1993; Stalis et al., 1995; Uchida et al., 1999; Timmann et al., 2007). The CSF has mild to moderate pleocytosis, generally greater than 200 cells/µL composed of predominantly lymphocytes, CSF protein concentration often greater than 50 mg/dL, and negative for an infectious cause (e.g., distemper and herpesviruses) (Figs. 15.24 and 15.25). A young

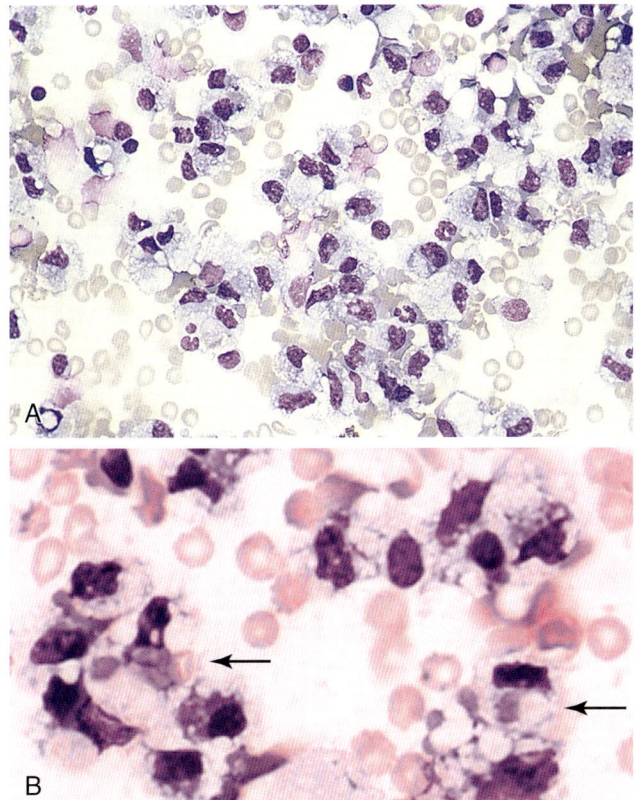

■ **FIGURE 15.22 Acute hemorrhage with mononuclear pleocytosis. Cerebrospinal fluid. Dog.** Same case in A and B. **A,** There was a history of seizures and dementia. Total nucleated cell count was 190/µL with 91% mononuclear phagocytes and protein 72 mg/dL. (Wright-Giemsa; HP oil.) **B,** Several vacuolated, phagocytic macrophages with engulfed erythrocytes *(arrows)* are shown. (Wright-Giemsa; HP oil.)

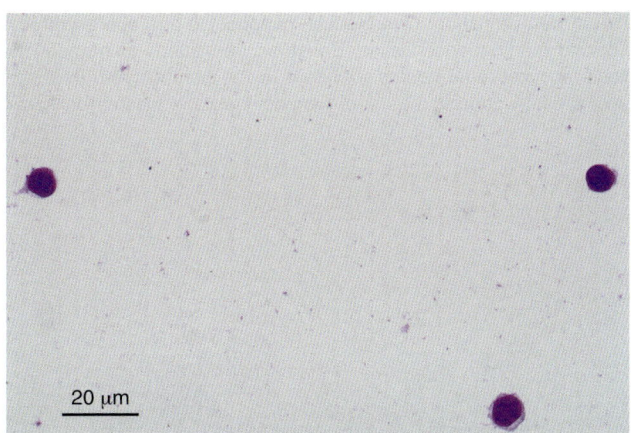

■ **FIGURE 15.23 Lymphocytic pleocytosis. Chiari-like malformation with syringohydromyelia. Cerebrospinal fluid. Dog.** This toy fox terrier presented with progressive head tilt and vestibular ataxia. Cerebrospinal fluid indicated a mild pleocytosis (total nucleated cell count, 9/µL) and normal protein. Lymphocytes accounted for 74%, and the remainder were mononuclear phagocytes. Further testing by magnetic resonance imaging confirmed a caudal occipital malformation syndrome, cerebellar vermis foramen magnum herniation, and cranial cervical syringohydromyelia. The lymphocytes are small with scant cytoplasm and dense chromatin clumping. (Wright-Giemsa; HP oil.) (Courtesy Jere Stern, University of Florida.)

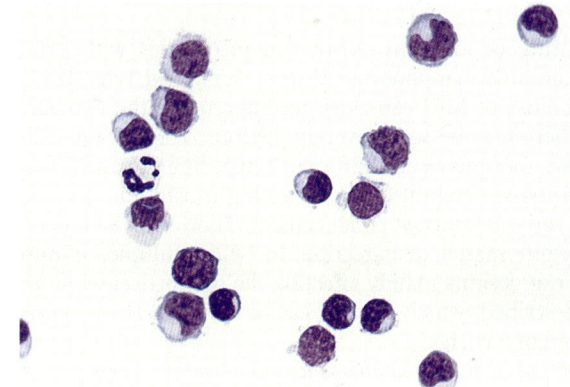

■ **FIGURE 15.24 Lymphocytic pleocytosis. Necrotizing encephalitis. Cerebrospinal fluid (CSF). Dog.** Previously termed *pug encephalitis*, this condition is present in a variety of small breed dogs. This CSF is characterized by pleocytosis (265 cells/µL) with 87% lymphocytes. Lymphocytes are small to medium size with normal morphology. (Wright-Giemsa; HP oil.)

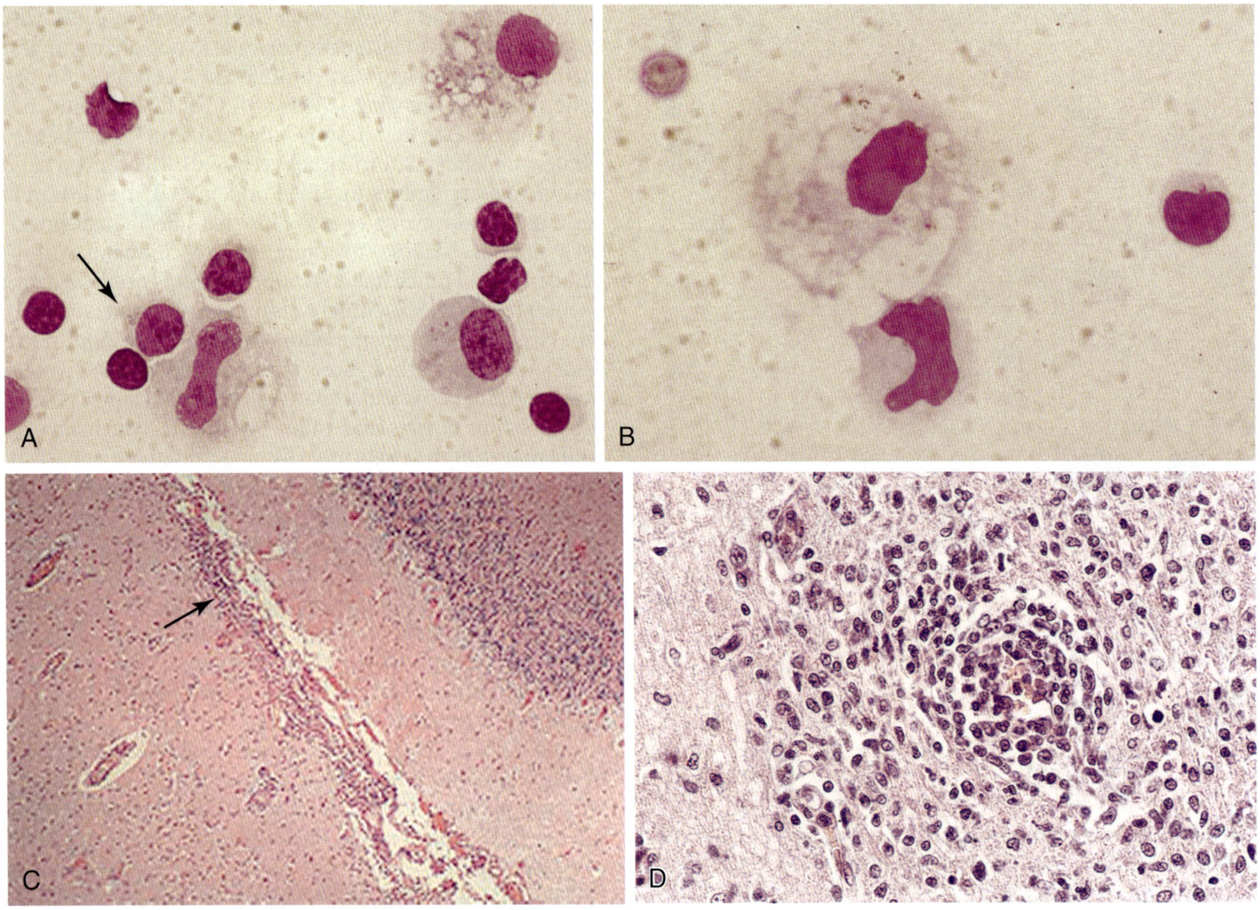

■ **FIGURE 15.25 Lymphocytic pleocytosis. Necrotizing encephalitis. Dog.** Same case in A to D. A 6-year-old Maltese presented with acute seizures unresponsive to glucocorticoids and anticonvulsants. **A, Cerebrospinal fluid (CSF).** Total nucleated cell count was 430/μL with 82% lymphocytes, 11% large mononuclear cells, and 7% nondegenerate neutrophils and 3+ protein on the urine chemistry reagent test strip (dipstick). Shown are many lymphocytes, one of which is a granular lymphocyte *(arrow)*, and three large mononuclear cells demonstrating various nuclear shapes and vacuolated, granular cytoplasm. (Wright-Giemsa; HP oil.) **B, CSF.** Mononuclear pleocytosis is evident in this field with two large mononuclear cells; one of them displays marked cytoplasmic vacuolization suggestive of demyelination. One granular lymphocyte and one erythrocyte are also present. (Wright-Giemsa; HP oil.) **C, Histology.** Nonsuppurative necrotizing meningoencephalitis. Dense accumulations of mononuclear cells along the meninges *(arrow)* extend into the parenchyma. There are gliosis and neuronal necrosis evident in the parenchyma. (H&E; LP.) **D, Histology.** Severe, focally extensive, perivascular meningoencephalitis. Cells present consist mostly of lymphocytes and plasma cells, with smaller numbers of large mononuclear phagocytes. (H&E; HP oil.)

miniature poodle with NME had pleocytosis with primarily large granular lymphocytes (Garma-Aviña and Tyler, 1999).

The use of MRI can assist to differentiate the two variants, but there may be some overlap. Lesions of NME typically appear as asymmetric, multifocal T2 hyperintense and T1 iso- to hypointense cerebral lesions affecting mostly the gray matter, with variable contrast enhancement. There may be loss of gray and white matter demarcation. In NLE, multiple, asymmetric forebrain lesions mainly affecting the subcortical white matter are described, which may be cavitary, with relative sparing of the cerebral cortex.

Granulomatous meningoencephalomyelitis (Figs. 15.26 to 15.28) is a noninfectious inflammatory disease of CNS in primarily young to middle-aged female dogs, primarily toy and terrier breeds (Sorjonen, 1990; Munana and Luttgen, 1998). Clinical signs include fever, ataxia, tetraparesis, cervical hyperesthesia, and seizures. Lesions are histologically found in both white and gray matter of the brain and predominantly the white

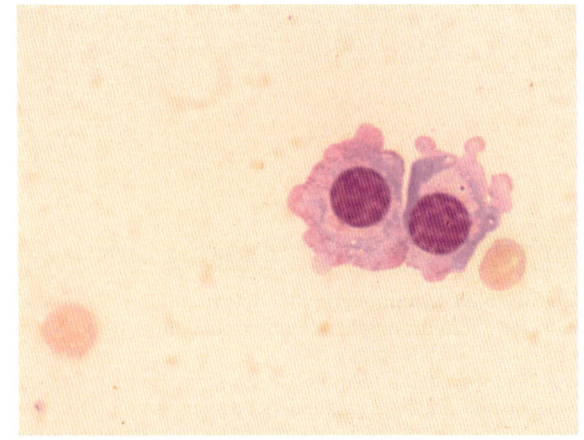

■ **FIGURE 15.26 Flaming plasma cells. Granulomatous meningoencephalitis. Cerebrospinal fluid. Dog.** High-normal nucleated cell count and protein (361 mg/dL) in a suspected case of granulomatous meningoencephalomyelitis. *Flaming* is a descriptive term for the red-pink periphery of the cytoplasm but has no diagnostic meaning. (Wright-Giemsa; HP oil.)

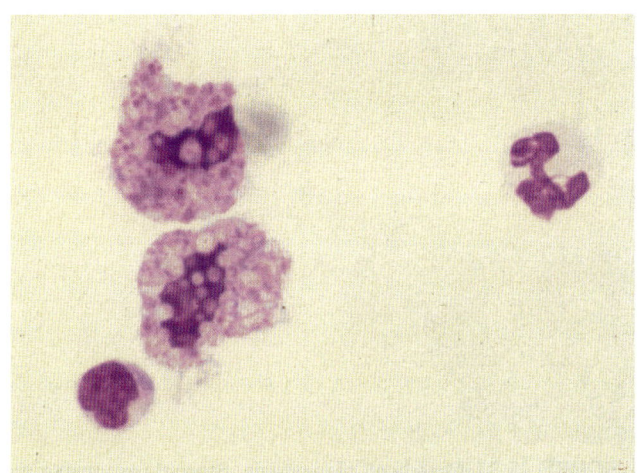

FIGURE 15.27 Granular large mononuclear phagocytes. Granulomatous meningoencephalitis. Cerebrospinal fluid. Dog. Granulated and vacuolated phagocytic mononuclear cells in a case of suspected granulomatous meningoencephalomyelitis. One neutrophil and one lymphocyte are also observed. (Wright-Giemsa; HP oil.) (Courtesy Rick Alleman, University of Florida.)

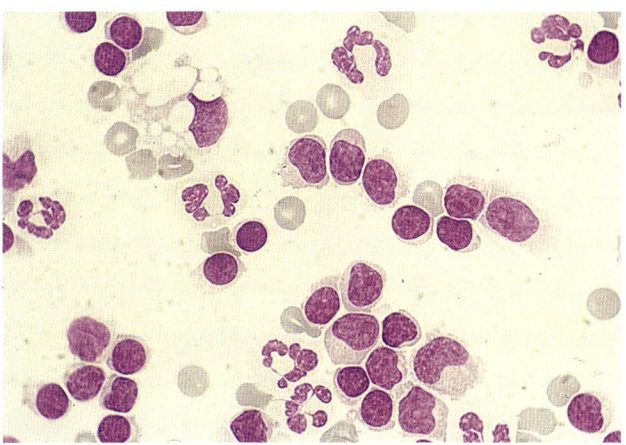

FIGURE 15.28 Mixed-cell pleocytosis. Granulomatous meningoencephalitis. Cerebrospinal fluid. Dog. A young dog presented with neck pain. There are numerous small and medium-sized lymphocytes (70%), fewer numbers of nondegenerate neutrophils (18%), and large mononuclear cells (12%), one of which contains large cytoplasmic vacuoles. Total nucleated cell count was 208 cells/μL, and protein concentration was 256 mg/dL. The dog died 5 days later of unknown cause. Histopathology indicated moderate to marked, multifocal, nonsuppurative meningoencephalitis and mild, multifocal vacuolization of axons and neuronal necrosis. (Wright-Giemsa; HP oil.)

matter of the caudal brainstem and spinal cord and characterized by the accumulation of lymphocytes and macrophages with epithelioid morphology, forming granulomas around blood vessels (Uchida et al., 2016). The CSF has variable cytopathology ranging from a mild to moderate lymphocytic, mixed cell pleocytosis to neutrophilic predominance (Chrisman, 1992). Nucleated cell counts had a median of 250 cells/μL (range, 0–11,840) with the majority having counts greater than 100 cells/μL (Munana and Luttgen, 1998). In this same study, dogs with multifocal signs all had pleocytosis, whereas some of the dogs with focal signs had normal cell counts. The predominant cell type was lymphocytic (52%), monocytic (21%), neutrophilic (10%), and mixed cell (17%). The CSF protein concentration is variably increased with a mean value of 256 mg/dL (range, 13–1119) (Bailey and Higgins, 1986). Electrophoretic separation of CSF proteins in GME has shown increases in the alpha and beta globulin fractions, whereas these fractions are generally decreased in canine distemper, which can be diagnosed by antibody titers or enzyme-linked immunosorbent assay performed on CSF (Sorjonen, 1990; Chrisman, 1992). Prognosis is generally better for GME for long-term survival than the necrotizing encephalitis variants with immunosuppressant therapy.

Canine viral infections such as canine distemper infection and rabies infection each present with CSF that exhibits a lymphocytic pleocytosis (Figs. 15.29 and 15.30). Cell counts may be

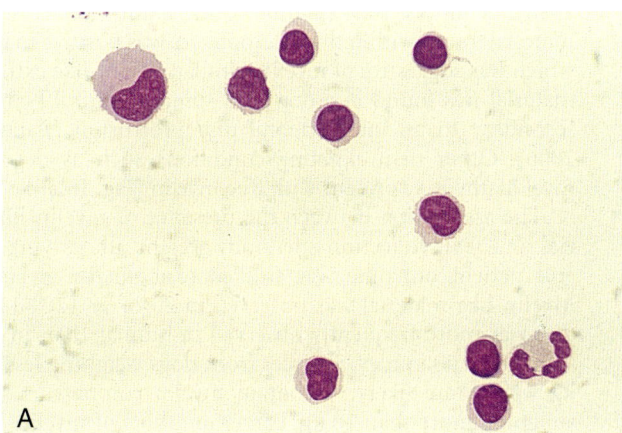
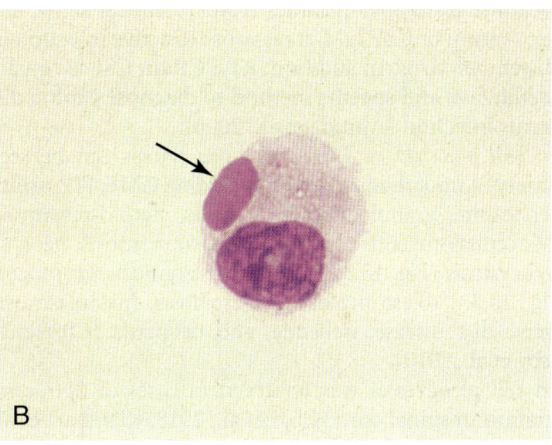

FIGURE 15.29 Canine distemper infection. Cerebrospinal fluid (CSF). Dogs. A, Lymphocytic pleocytosis. Pleocytosis (292 cells/μL) with 72% lymphocytes and protein concentration of 126 mg/dL from a cerebellomedullary cistern sample in a dog with acute ataxia and head tilt. The CSF distemper titer was positive, suggesting a distemper-related encephalopathy, which clinically responded within 6 months using glucocorticoid therapy. Shown are numerous small lymphocytes, one neutrophil, and one large mononuclear cell. (Wright-Giemsa; HP oil.) **B, Distemper inclusion.** Example of an eosinophilic inclusion in a large mononuclear cell *(arrow)* that represents viral proteins from a dog diagnosed with canine distemper. (Wright-Giemsa; HP oil.) (B, From Alleman AR, Christopher MM, Steiner DA, et al. Identification of intracytoplasmic inclusion bodies in mononuclear cells from the cerebrospinal fluid of a dog with canine distemper. *Vet Pathol.* 1992;29:84–85.)

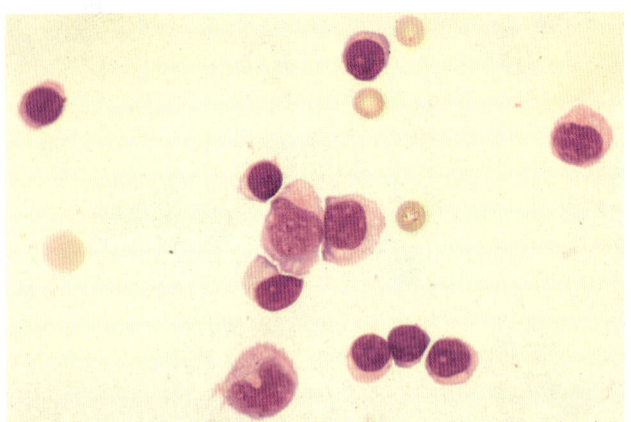

■ **FIGURE 15.30 Lymphocytic pleocytosis. Rabies infection. Cerebrospinal fluid (CSF). Dog.** A 6-month-old stray dog presented with weakness on one hind leg that progressed over the course of 1 week to bilateral forelimb paresis and later seizures. The initial clinical presentation of a leg bite wound that progressed with neurologic deficits and the cytopathology of the CSF warranted euthanasia. Subsequently, a diagnosis of rabies was made. If infectious agents are suspected, gloves and a facial mask must be worn when handling diagnostic specimens, and cytocentrifugation must be covered to prevent aerosolization. Note the predominance of small lymphocytes in addition to two large mononuclear cells. Total nucleated cell count was 1140 cells/μL with a protein concentration 366 mg/dL. (Wright-Giemsa; HP oil.) (Courtesy Rose Raskin, University of Florida.)

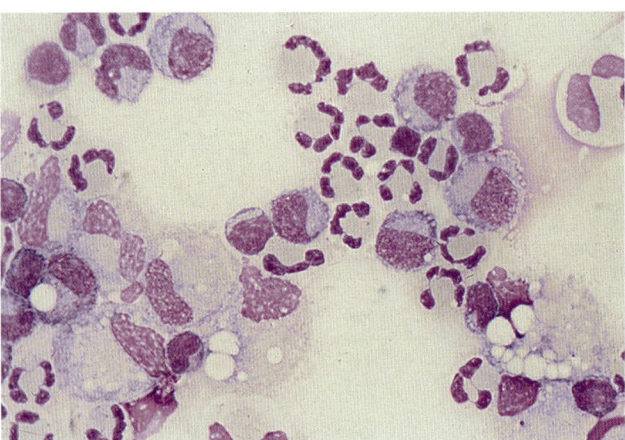

■ **FIGURE 15.31 Mixed-cell pleocytosis. Steroid-responsive meningoencephalitis. Cerebrospinal fluid. Dog.** This sample is from an adult female cairn terrier with a 4-month history of neck pain and muscle spasms that were responsive to glucocorticoids. Mononuclear phagocytes (52%) were mostly reactive as indicated by a foamy or vacuolated cytoplasm and phagocytized granular debris. Neutrophils made up 35% and lymphocytes 13% of the total cell population. (Wright-Giemsa; HP oil.)

variable, ranging from normal to greater than 50 cells/μL, and lymphocytes represent the greater than 60% of the TNCC. The CSF associated with distemper had increases in macrophages, protein concentration, and gamma-globulin fraction by electrophoretic separation and the presence of cellular inclusions (Abate et al., 1998). A 7-month-old dog with PCR-confirmed viral distemper had marked CSF pleocytosis (554 cells/μL) composed of 70% lymphocytes, 25% neutrophils, and 5% monocytes with no increase in the protein concentration (Amude et al., 2006). Evidence used for the presumptive diagnosis of canine distemper includes history, clinical signs, and evidence of serum or CSF IgM in response to active infection by canine distemper virus. In addition, RT-PCR on CSF is considered a useful, fast, and specific method to diagnose canine distemper virus infection (Amude et al., 2006).

Mixed cell pleocytosis. Mixed cell pleocytosis can be seen with a variety of underlying diseases, including GME, FIP, canine distemper, canine granulocytic ehrlichiosis, steroid-responsive meningoencephalomyelitis (Fig. 15.31), toxoplasmosis, neosporosis, sarcocystosis (Fig. 15.32), encephalitozoonosis, cryptococcosis (Fig. 15.33), blastomycosis, aspergillosis, histoplasmosis, degenerative disc disease, ischemia, and neoplasia (Chrisman, 1992; Bisby et al., 2010).

Mixed cell pleocytosis was observed in cases of *Spirocerca lupi* migration in spinal cord (Chai et al., 2018; Klainbart et al., 2018). In one case, variably basophilic staining *Spirocerca lupi* elliptical ova were present in cytocentrifuged CSF (Klainbart et al., 2018).

Neural Tissue Injury Findings

In addition to blood contamination encountered during collection, the presence of erythrocytes in a cytopathologic preparation may result from cranial or spinal hemorrhage. Macrophages with phagocytized erythrocytes may be seen in cases of acute spinal cord injury such as IVDH, neoplasia, inflammation, or degenerative conditions (Fig. 15.34). Chronic hemorrhage is indicated by the presence of hemosiderin-laden macrophage or hematoidin crystals (Fig. 15.35). Tissue damage with necrosis induces macrophage removal of dead cells and leukophagocytosis (Fig. 15.36).

Homogeneous ribbons of basophilic material hypothesized to represent degenerated myelin because myelin figures or myelin fragments have been reported in a postmortem collection of CSF from a dog (Figs. 15.37 and 15.38) (Fallin et al., 1996). Spinal cord infarction with diffuse myelomalacia in a dog resulted in the presence of foamy macrophages in CSF (Mesher et al., 1996). Luxol fast blue staining of the amorphous eosinophilic material found within the macrophages was positive in this case, which was suggestive of myelin. Similar myelin-like extracellular material was found in a dog with spinal subdural hemorrhage secondary to an intervertebral disc protrusion (Bauer et al., 2006). Other demyelinating conditions such as degenerative myelopathy may present with free myelin (Fig. 15.39).

The association between the presence of myelin-like material and CSF collection site, body weight, underlying disease, and patient outcome was studied (Zabolotzky et al., 2010). Myelin-like material was observed in 20 of 98 (20%) samples and was more frequently observed in lumbar than in cerebellomedullary samples. Samples from dogs weighing less than 10 kg were more likely to contain myelin compared with dogs weighing more than 10 kg. Larger amounts of myelin-like material were observed in CSF from dogs with intervertebral disc disease compared with other diseases. These results suggest that the presence of extracellular myelin-like material in canine CSF samples may be encountered as an artifact of collection technique.

Spinal injury with myelomalacia caused by fibrocartilaginous embolism was described clinically in five cats; neutrophilic

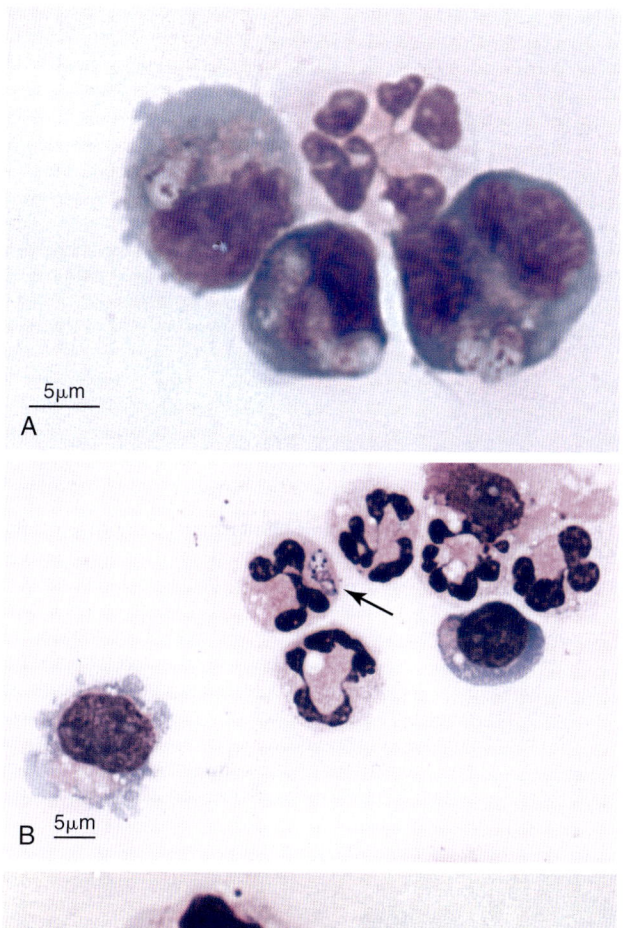

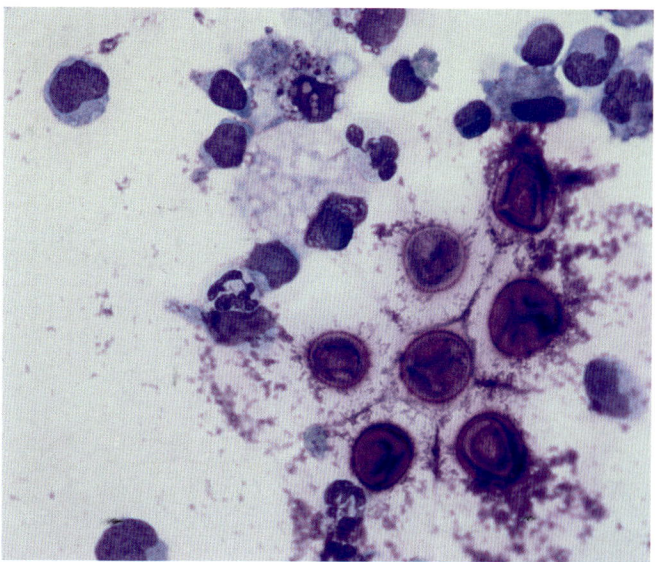

■ **FIGURE 15.33 Mixed cell pleocytosis. Cryptococcosis. Cerebrospinal fluid. Dog.** There are moderate pleocytosis (total nucleated cell count, 158/μL), increased erythrocytes (29/μL), and microprotein (221 mg/dL). The predominant cells were macrophages with lower numbers of neutrophils and lymphocytes. Shown are seven magenta round yeast organisms with a wide, poorly staining capsule measuring 15–20 μm surrounding the prominent cell wall. In the *top center* are two eosinophils with the remainder of cells shown being mixed mononuclear cells and neutrophils. (Modified Wright; HP oil.) (Courtesy Rose Raskin, Kansas State University.)

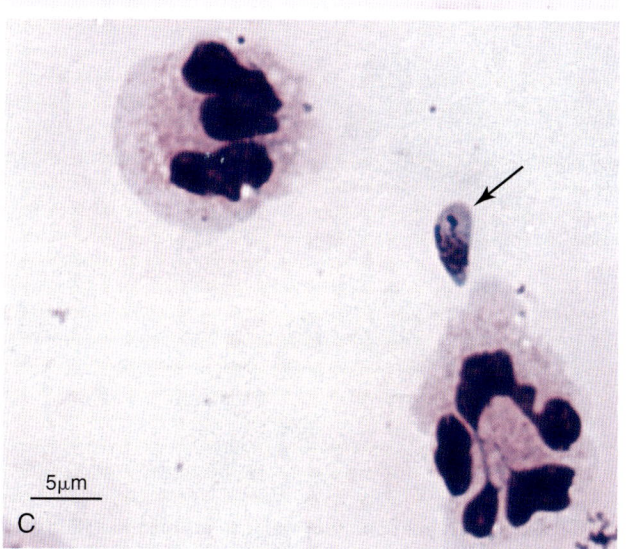

■ **FIGURE 15.32 Mixed cell pleocytosis. *Sarcocystis* spp. infection. Cisternal cerebrospinal fluid. Cat.** Same case in A to C. A 5-month-old cat presented with paraparesis and pain upon palpation of the spine. **A,** *Sarcocystis* spp. merozoites are observed within the cytoplasm of three large mononuclear cells. Polymerase chain reaction and gene sequencing established the specific diagnosis. (Wright; HP oil.) **B,** There is a *Sarcocystis* merozoite within a neutrophil *(arrow)*. Neutrophils appear mostly nondegenerate and account for 80% of the total nucleated cell population, along with 11% lymphocytes and 9% large mononuclear cells. The cytocentrifuge preparation was highly cellular but insufficient fluid did not allow an accurate cell count. (Wright; HP oil.) **C,** An extracellular, pear-shaped merozoite *(arrow)* measures approximately 2–3 × 5 μm (Wright; HP oil.) (A–C, Courtesy Rose Raskin, Purdue University.)

pleocytosis was detected in three of them (Mikszewski et al., 2006). In 16 cats diagnosed with ischemic myelopathy by MRI and evaluated by CSF examination, three had neutrophilic pleocytosis, and eight had increased CSF protein concentration (Theobald et al., 2013). The presence of neutrophilic pleocytosis did not have an adverse effect on clinical outcome.

Pleocytosis (>5 cells/μL) was present in 51% of dogs, including 23% with cervical IVDH and 61% with thoracolumbar IVDH. Moderate or marked inflammation (>20 cells/μL) was identified in the CSF of 51% of dogs with thoracolumbar IVDH and neutrophilic pleocytosis was observed most frequently. A predominance of lymphocytes was significantly more common in dogs examined after 7 days from onset of signs (Windsor et al., 2008). In dogs with intervertebral disc disease that presented without deep pain sensation and did not regain ambulation, there were greater than 13% macrophages in the lumbar CSF, suggesting that the percentage of CSF macrophages can be used as a prognostic indicator for regaining ambulation in dogs that have lost deep pain sensation (Srugo et al., 2011).

Neural Cystic and Neoplastic Lesion Findings in Cerebrospinal Fluid

Rare developmental defects have been demonstrated mainly in young dogs associated with squamous epithelial lined cysts that occur within the fourth ventricle, cerebellopontine angle and fourth ventricle, cerebellum, brainstem, and vertebral canal (Lipitz et al., 2011). They are thought to arise from entrapment of ectodermal cells in the neural tube during

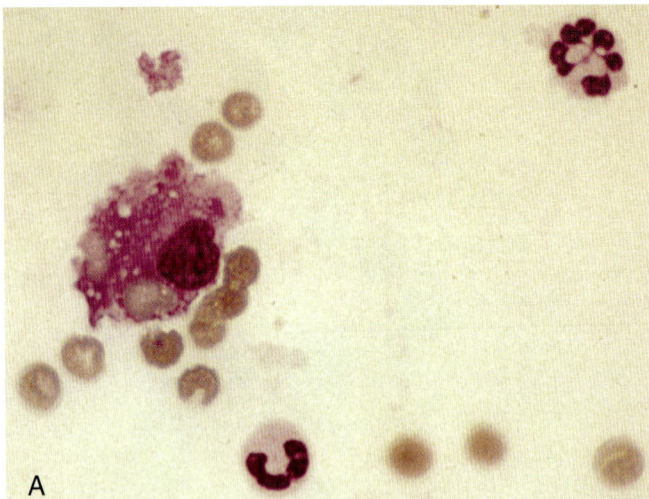
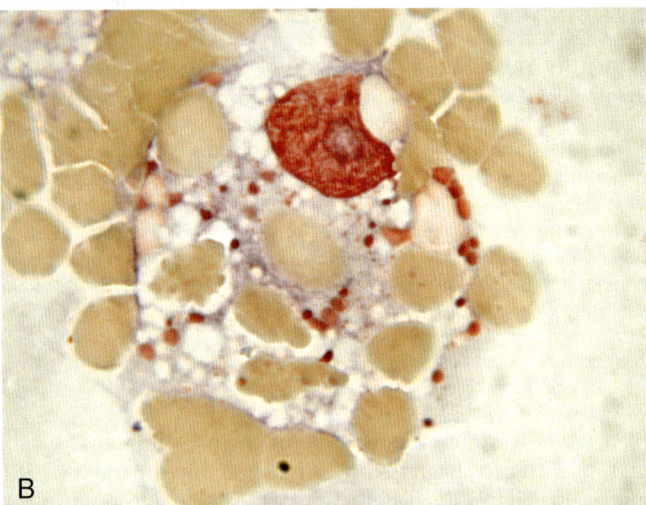

■ **FIGURE 15.34 Erythrophagocytosis. Cerebrospinal fluid. Dogs.
A,** This lumbar site collection was bloody with a total nucleated cell count of 84/µL, red blood cell count of 7000/µL, and protein concentration of 104 mg/dL. A car-related injury caused a thoracic spinal fracture that contributed to the acute hemorrhage exhibited in this example. Vacuolated (foamy) and basophilic macrophages are present; one has phagocytized neutrophil *(upper right)*. (Wright-Giemsa; HP oil.) **B,** Erythrophagocytosis; a macrophage has phagocytized erythrocytes. (MGG; HP oil.) (A, Courtesy Rick Alleman, University of Florida.)

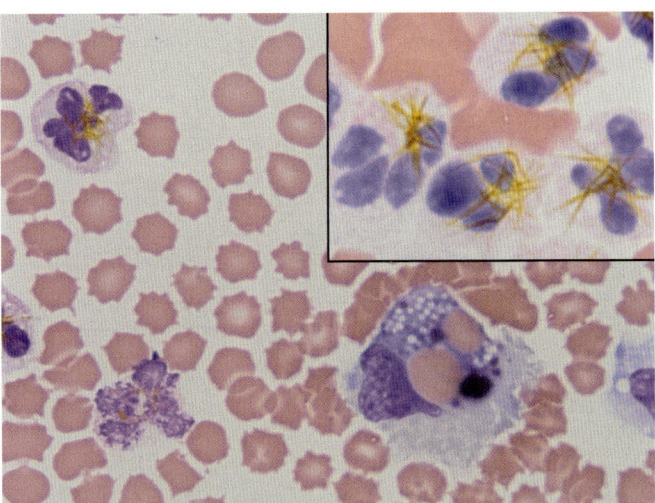

■ **FIGURE 15.35 Acute and chronic hemorrhage. Cerebrospinal fluid (CSF). Dog.** A 2-month-old Irish setter presented with a history of seizures. The CSF was red and cloudy, with increased cell counts (red blood cell count, 220,000/µL; total nucleated cell count, 1100/µL) and increased microprotein (1930 mg/dL). The cell differential indicated nearly equal numbers of neutrophils and macrophages. A brain mass was determined from computed tomography. A macrophage contains engulfed erythrocytes and hemosiderin suggesting both acute and chronic hemorrhage, respectively. *Inset:* Several neutrophils contain yellow needle-like crystals consistent with bilirubin or heme degradation without iron (hematoidin). (Modified Wright; HP oil.) (Courtesy Matt Williams, Mississippi State University.)

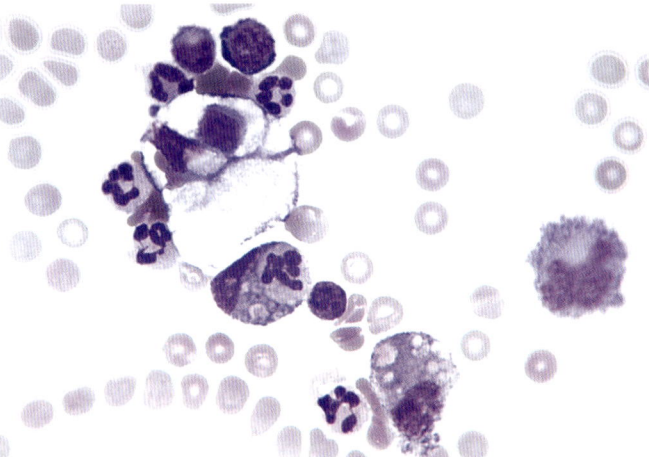

■ **FIGURE 15.36 Leukophagocytosis. Cerebrospinal fluid. Dog.** The response to tissue injury may be increased numbers of nondegenerate neutrophils, one of which was phagocytized by a macrophage. (MGG; HP oil.)

embryologic development or from trauma of repeated spinal taps. The cyst material, and occasionally CSF, contains numerous mature squamous epithelium, consistent with an epidermoid cyst (Fig. 15.40). Spinal arachnoid cysts, also referred to as meningeal cysts and leptomeningeal cysts, have been reported as an uncommon cause of neurologic deficits in dogs and cats and are generally related to a normal CSF analysis (Galloway et al., 1999).

With neoplasia, the protein concentration is often increased with only occasional neoplastic cells observed in CSF. This depends on the location of the mass with its proximity to the ventricle, its involvement with the meninges, or its communication with the subarachnoid space in order to have access to CSF. A mixed cell pleocytosis was the most common cytopathologic finding in CSF collected from 51 dogs with primary intracranial neoplasia; neoplastic cells were detected in only two dogs with CNS lymphoma (Snyder et al., 2006). Similarly, in 28 cats with intracranial neoplasia, a definitive diagnosis of lymphoma was made in only one cat in which lymphoid blast cells were detected in CSF (Troxel et al., 2003).

In a series of 56 dogs with confirmed intracranial meningioma, pleocytosis was detected in cisternal CSF in 27% of dogs,

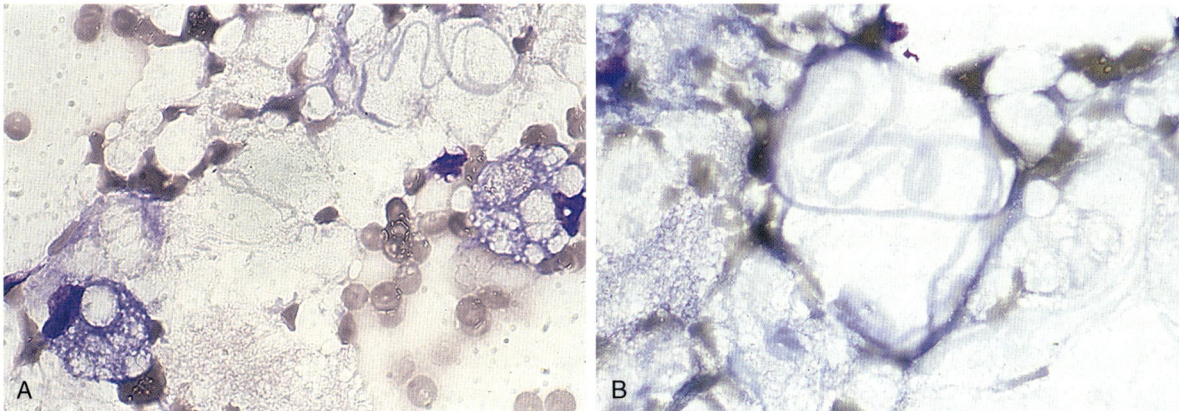

■ **FIGURE 15.37 Myelomalacia. Cerebrospinal fluid (CSF). Dog.** Same case in A and B. The dog presented with acute paraplegic and absent deep pain related to a disc protrusion at L1–L2. Myelogram confirmed dorsal spinal compression from T11 to L1. A cerebellomedullary cistern sample was taken 4 days after surgery at the time of euthanasia. **A,** Two macrophages *(arrows)* with large lipid-filled cytoplasmic vacuoles and basophilic ribbons of material extracellularly. Necropsy confirmed a necrotic spinal cord at T11–L1. (Wright-Giemsa; HP oil.) **B, Myelin figures. CSF.** Basophilic ribbonlike structures likely represent phospholipids, derived from damaged cytomembranes. (Wright-Giemsa; HP oil.)

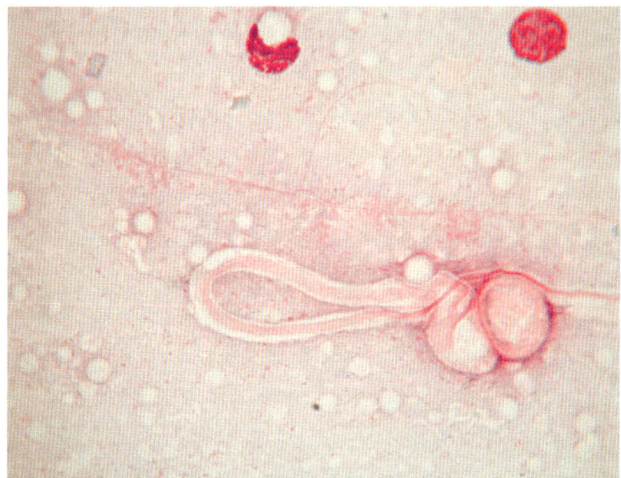

■ **FIGURE 15.38 Myelin ribbon. Lumbar cerebrospinal fluid. Dog.** An eosinophilic ribbonlike structure is present along with two mononuclear cells. It likely represents phospholipids derived from damaged membranes. (MGG; HP oil.)

with a predominance of neutrophils detected only in 19% of dogs (Dickinson et al., 2006). Although TNCC was generally less than 5/μL, total protein concentration was mild to moderately increased with a median result of 52 mg/dL. They concluded in particular that neutrophilic pleocytosis may not be detected in CSF samples from dogs with meningiomas located within the middle or rostral portion of the cranial fossae. Rarely, the presence of neoplastic or proliferative meningeal cell clumps may be encountered (Figs. 15.41 and 15.42).

The presence of mitotic cells in CSF is unusual and often indicates a proliferative population such as a neoplasm. The presence of immature lymphocytes is diagnostic for the presence of CNS lymphoma (Figs. 15.43 to 15.47) (Seo et al., 2011). The use of immunocytochemistry can assist to determine the immunophenotype of suspected lymphoma cases (see Fig. 15.45).

A recent study examined neuroanatomic patterns in primary or secondary canine nervous system lymphoma. The presence of neoplastic cells in the CSF was noted only in tumors in which histologic examination showed meningeal or

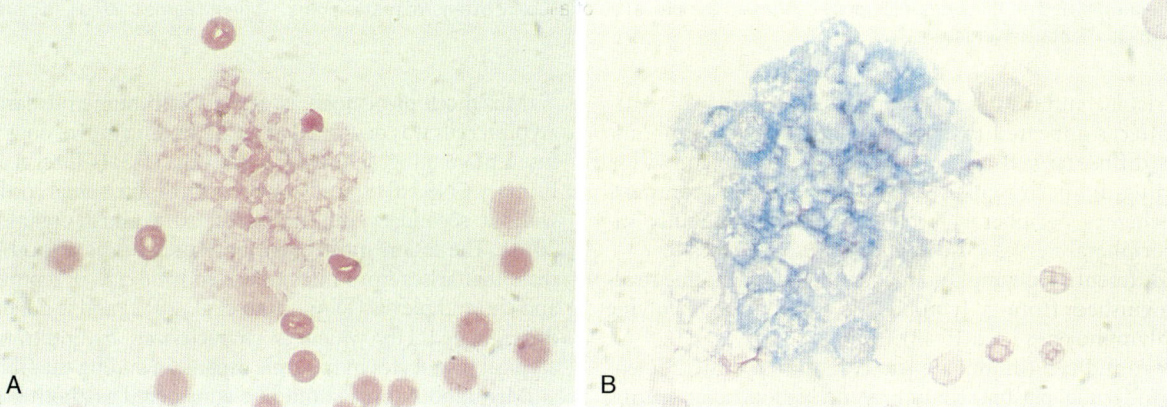

■ **FIGURE 15.39 Myelin. Cerebrospinal fluid. Dog.** Same case in A and B. Mixed-breed dog with a history of degenerative myelopathy with normal total nucleated cell count and increased protein concentration (62 mg/dL). **A,** Collections of pale eosinophilic foamy material are shown extracellularly suspected to be myelin. (Wright-Giemsa; HP oil.) **B,** Extracellular material stained positive for myelin. Demyelination was suspected. (Luxol fast blue; HP oil.)

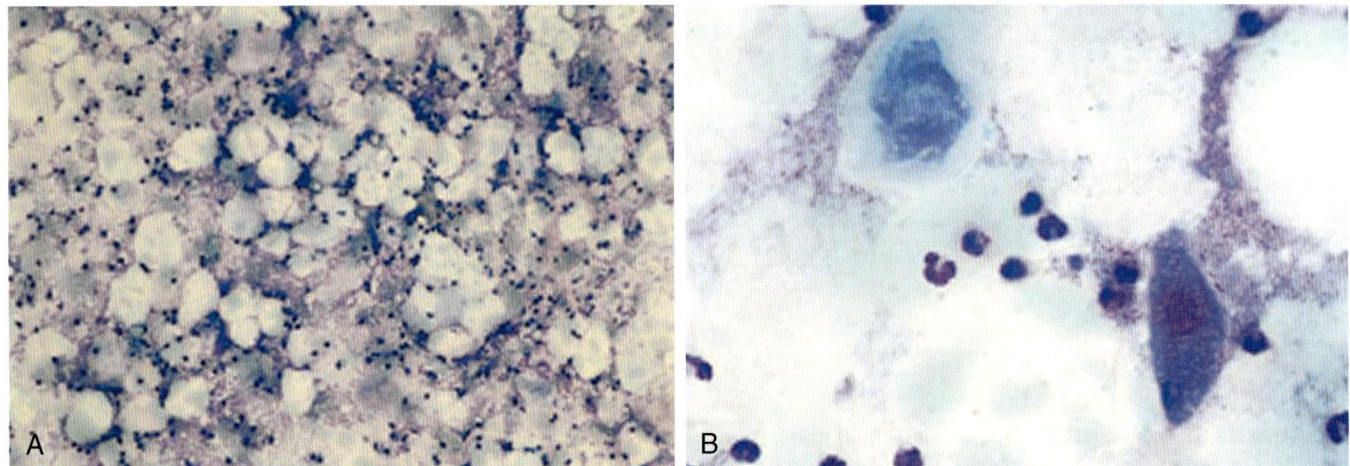

■ **FIGURE 15.40 Epidermoid cyst. Cerebrospinal fluid. Dog.** Same case in A and B. This dog had a 3-month duration of seizures. **A,** Direct smear of creamy, opaque fluid with a total nucleated cell count of 80,000/μL taken from the cerebellomedullary cistern. Numerous large, blue-green cells are evident at low magnification. (Romanowsky-type stain; IP.) **B,** Keratinized squamous epithelial cell *(upper left)* and intermediate squamous epithelial cell *(lower right)* along with numerous nondegenerate neutrophils. (Romanowsky-type stain; HP oil.) (Courtesy Joseph Spano.)

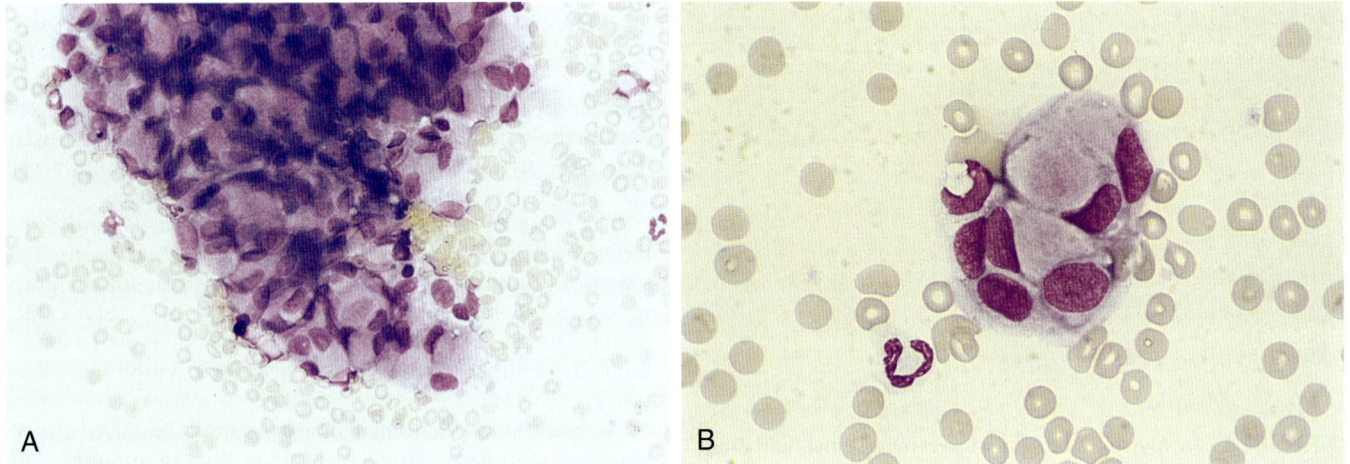

■ **FIGURE 15.41 Meningothelial meningioma. Cerebrospinal fluid. Dog.** Same case in A and B. **A,** Large dense clump of cohesive cells in a sample taken from the cerebellomedullary cistern of a dog with a spinal cord lesion in the C1–C2 region that presented with weakness. (Wright-Giemsa; HP oil.) **B,** Higher magnification of the cell clusters showing plump cells with oval to round eccentric nuclei with occasional prominent nucleoli and surrounded by variably abundant granular that may contain eosinophilic secretory material; the large size is illustrated by comparison with the neutrophil and erythrocytes. Necropsy confirmed the presence of a locally extensive meningioma. (Wright-Giemsa; HP oil.) (Courtesy Rose Raskin, Michigan State University.)

periventricular infiltration of neoplastic lymphocytes. Anatomic patterns appeared to correlate with specific lymphoma subtypes: diffuse large B-cell lymphoma tended to occur within the meningeal, perivascular, and periventricular compartments, whereas peripheral T-cell lymphoma frequently involved peripheral nerves (Sisò et al., 2017).

Well-differentiated lymphoid malignancies may not be readily distinguished from a lymphocytic pleocytosis involving granular lymphocytes (Fig. 15.48).

Other round cell tumors are less common and include encephalic and spinal plasma cell tumors and histiocytic-appearing neoplasms that may be difficult to distinguish from GME (Figs. 15.49 and 15.50) (Sheppard et al., 1997; Greenberg et al., 2004; Zimmerman et al., 2006; Tzipory et al., 2009; Stowe et al., 2012).

Mixed cell pleocytosis associated with numerous large round atypical cells was described as a CSF finding in two dogs with diffuse leptomeningeal histiocytic sarcoma (HS) (Cluzel et al., 2016). Primary CNS HS typically involves the brain, spinal cord, or both without secondary infiltration of extracranial organs (Moore, 2014). The lesion most commonly presents as a focal subdural mass that arises from interstitial dendritic cells of leptomeninges and choroid plexus (D'Agostino et al., 2012) and is different from disseminated HS, which is characterized by infiltration with atypical histiocytes in multiple organs, including the CNS.

Medulloblastoma should be considered as another differential diagnosis for atypical round cells in CSF of young dogs (Thompson et al., 2003). Rarely, individualized cells from choroid plexus papillomas are found in CSF as large round cells (see discussion later under Neoplasms of Neuroepithelial Cells).

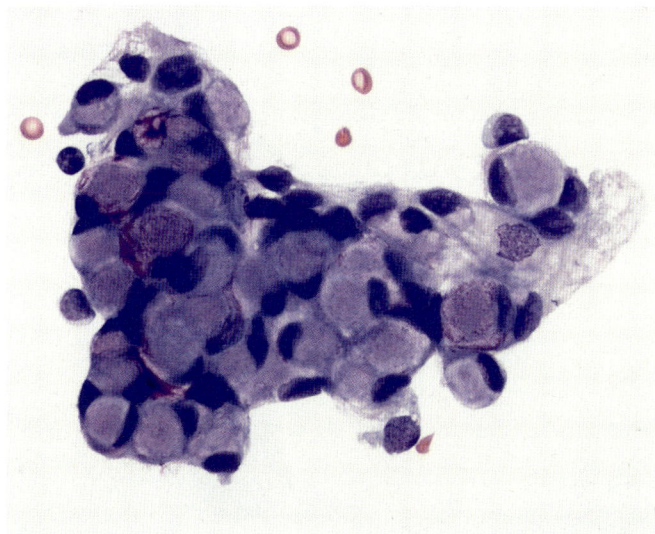

■ **FIGURE 15.42 Meningothelial proliferation. Cerebrospinal fluid (CSF). Dog.** An 11-year-old Staffordshire bull terrier presented with rapidly progressive bilateral blindness. Magnetic resonance imaging revealed multifocal extraaxial intracranial lesions, most severe in the cerebellum and brainstem. CSF showed increased microprotein (41 mg/dL) with normal total nucleated cell count and mildly increased red blood cell count (74/μL) consistent with an albuminocytologic dissociation. The only cytopathologic abnormality was the presence of a large cohesive aggregate of approximately 28 cells. These cells have an abundant granular cytoplasm that displaces the nucleus to the side. These cells strongly resemble meningothelium; meningioma or meningioangiomatosis was suspected but not confirmed. (Modified Wright; HP oil.) (Courtesy Rose Raskin, Michigan State University.)

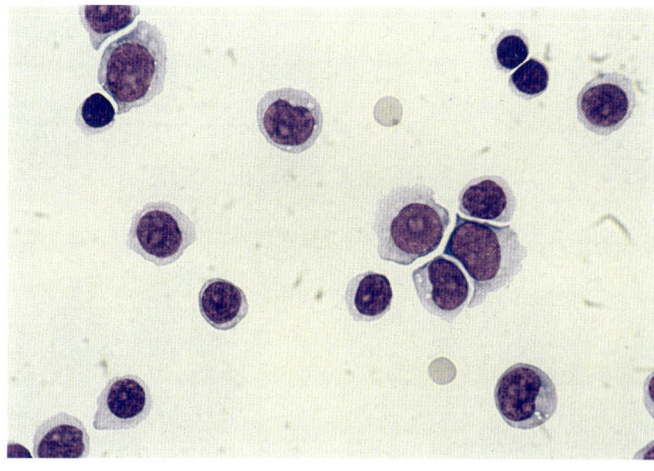

■ **FIGURE 15.44 Mononuclear pleocytosis. Lymphoma. Cerebrospinal fluid. Dog.** Clinical signs were a head tilt and ataxia of 3 months' duration. Increased protein concentration (170 mg/dL) and pleocytosis (1417/μL) were present in the clear fluid from the cerebellomedullary site. A mixed population of small, well-differentiated lymphocytes and large lymphoid blast cells that often contain a single prominent nucleolus; the cytopathologic diagnosis was lymphoma. (Wright-Giemsa; HP oil.)

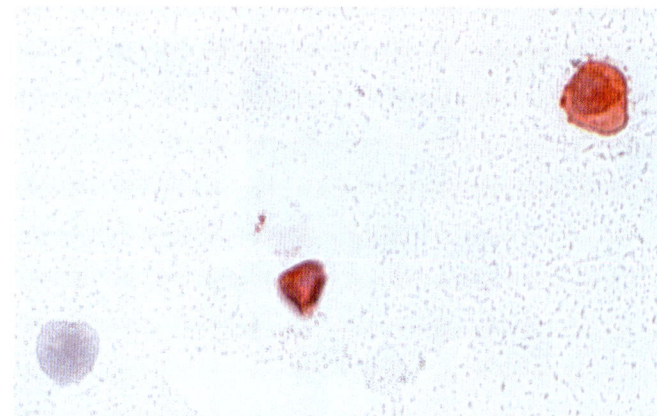

■ **FIGURE 15.45 Mononuclear pleocytosis. B-cell lymphoma. Cerebrospinal fluid (CSF). Dog.** Clinical signs suggested pituitary origin related to nonresponsive pupils, absent menace response, and polyuria and polydipsia. Increased protein (74 mg/dL) and pleocytosis (41 cells/μL) were present in the clear CSF. A sellar tumor was detected on magnetic resonance imaging. The large mononuclear cells were predominantly immunoreactive to CD20 antibody. Shown are three cells of which two are immunoreactive *(red)* and one is negative *(blue)*. (CD20/AEC; HP oil.) (Courtesy Rose Raskin, Purdue University.)

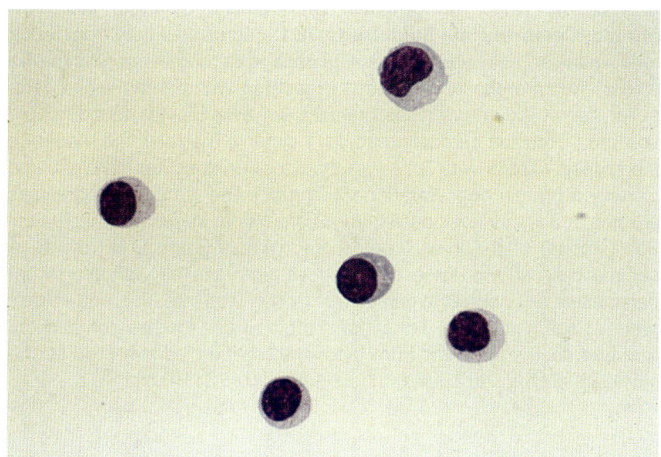

■ **FIGURE 15.43 Mononuclear pleocytosis. Lymphoma. Cerebrospinal fluid (CSF). Cat.** The cat had hindlimb paresis, urinary and fecal incontinence, and flaccid anal tone and tail. Cerebellomedullary collected CSF has a total nucleated cell count of 60/μL with 80% lymphocytes and a protein concentration of 140 mg/dL. Intermediate-sized lymphocytes predominate in the field shown. Myelogram revealed a lumbar spinal cord mass that was cytopathologically diagnosed as large cell lymphoma. (Wright-Giemsa; HP oil.) (Courtesy Rick Alleman, University of Florida.)

Finding metastatic carcinoma cells in CSF (Fig. 15.51) is the gold standard for the diagnosis of leptomeningeal carcinomatosis in humans. Patients with extensive meningeal involvement are more likely to have positive CSF cytopathology results (66%) than those with only focal involvement of the leptomeninges (38%). In three cases of canine leptomeningeal carcinomatosis, neoplastic cells were detected in CSF (Stampley et al., 1986; Pumarola and Balash, 1996; Behling-Kelly et al., 2010). In a case of meningeal carcinomatosis and spinal cord infiltration

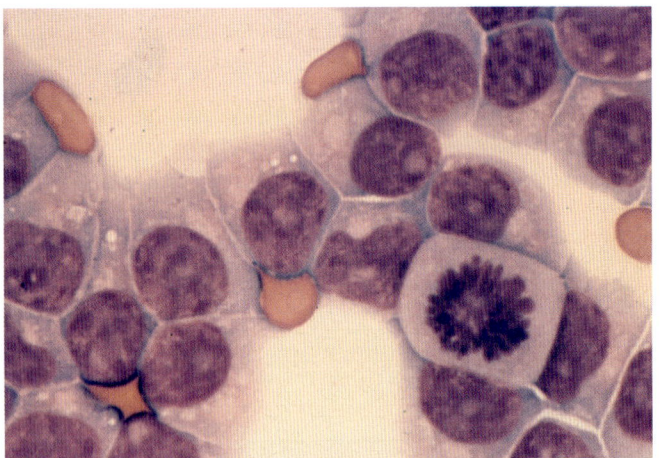

■ **FIGURE 15.46 Mononuclear pleocytosis. Lymphoma. Cerebrospinal fluid (CSF). Dog.** A cream-colored CSF was withdrawn from the cerebellomedullary cistern of a dog with vestibular deficits. The fluid had marked pleocytosis (total nucleated cell count, 109,400/μL) and increased protein concentration of 220 mg/dL. There is a monomorphic population of large lymphoid blast cells with a prominent single nucleolus making up 92% of the total nucleated cell count. A normal appearing mitotic figure is present. (Wright; HP oil.) (Courtesy Rose Raskin, Michigan State University.)

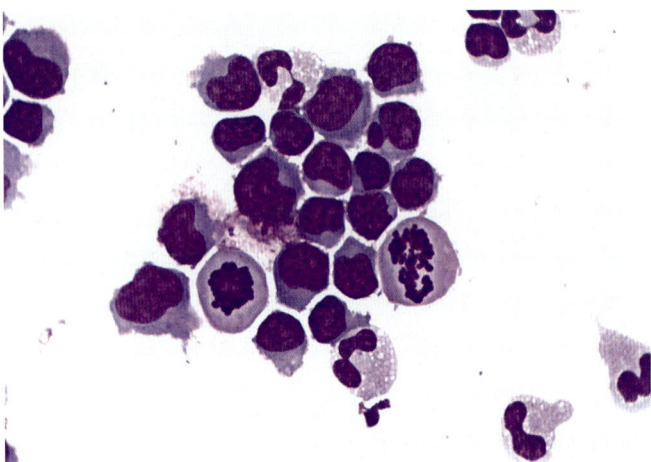

■ **FIGURE 15.47 Mononuclear pleocytosis. Lymphoma. Cerebrospinal fluid. Dog.** This fluid had a near monomorphic population of neoplastic lymphoid cells with indented nucleus, prominent Golgi zone, and frequent mitotic figures, one of which that appears abnormal. Several neutrophils are noted, which can be used for cell size comparison. (MGG; HP oil.)

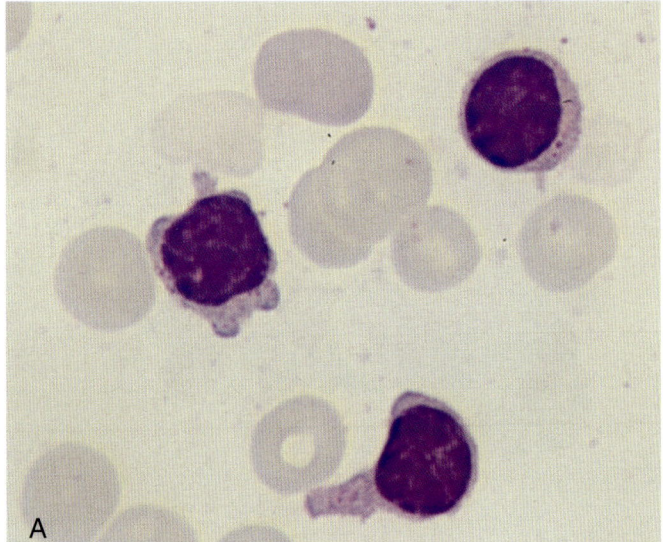

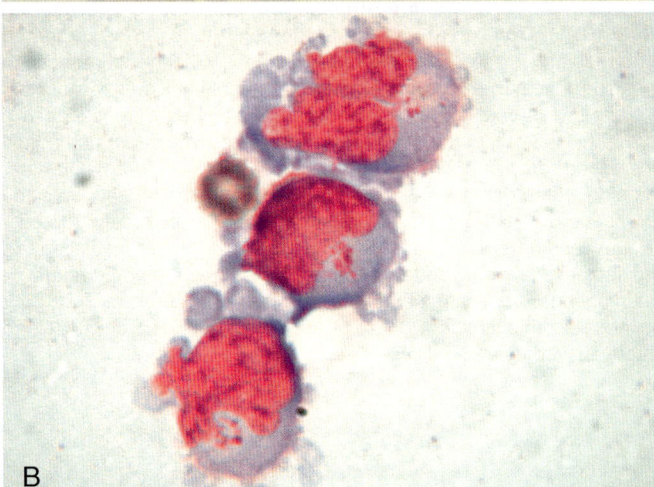

■ **FIGURE 15.48 Mononuclear pleocytosis. Granular cell lymphoma. Cerebrospinal fluid. Dogs. A,** Cerebrospinal fluid from a dog with granular cell lymphocyte leukemia that originated within the spleen. Two months later, the dog presented with dementia and cerebellar signs. Shown are three granular cell lymphocytes found in fluid collected from the cerebellomedullary cistern. The fluid had moderate pleocytosis (32/μL) with 91% lymphocytes, erythrocytes (520/μL), and increased protein concentration (69 mg/dL). The lymphocyte granules are fine and lightly eosinophilic (most prominent in cytoplasmic projection [uropod] of the lower center cell). (Wright-Giemsa; HP oil.) **B,** A second case shows three granular cell lymphocytes with prominent paranuclear eosinophilic granules from a dog with intestinal and splenic granular cell lymphoma. Note the red blood cell for size comparison. Some artifact is apparent from cytocentrifugation, as indicated by the surface blebbing and nuclear incontinence. (MGG; HP oil.)

caused by a pulmonary adenocarcinoma in a cat, CSF examination showed lymphocytic pleocytosis but no neoplastic cells (Posporis et al., 2017).

CYTOPATHOLOGY OF NERVOUS SYSTEM TISSUE

Collection and Preparation of Nervous System Tissues

When an intracranial or spinal mass is suspected, the veterinary neurologist often relies on imaging such as computed tomography (CT) and MRI to identify the lesion. Even if imaging can give some information about the location, the size, and the relationship to other surrounding structures, very often the differential diagnosis for the mass found on imaging includes an inflammatory (sterile or septic) lesion or benign and malignant tumor.

Each disease has a different prognosis and requires different therapies; therefore, a definitive diagnosis needs to be sought, but this can be achieved only by histologic examination. Intraoperative cytopathology has been successfully applied in veterinary

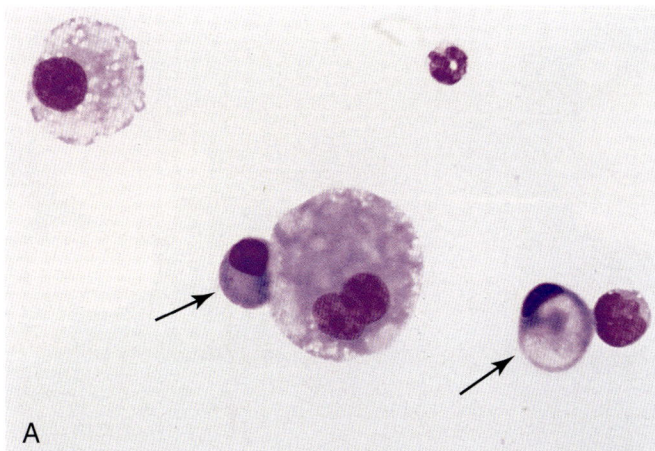

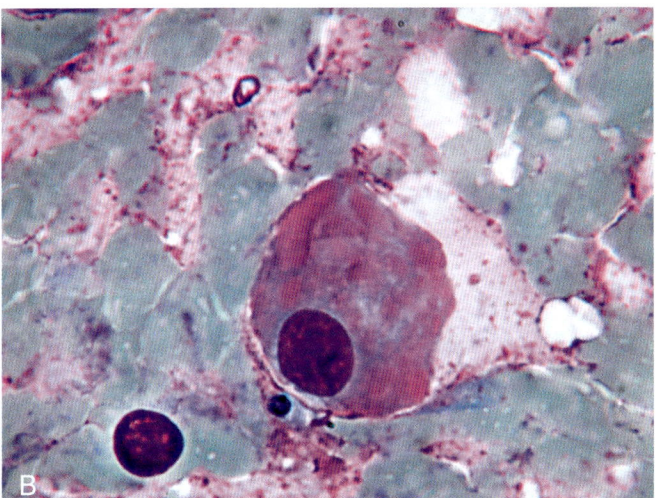

FIGURE 15.49 Plasma cell tumor. Cerebrospinal fluid. Dogs. A, Plasma cell tumor. Two large foamy, granular macrophages and two atypical plasmacytoid cells *(arrows)* are shown from the spinal fluid with marked mononuclear pleocytosis (27,600/μL) and increased protein concentration (>2000 mg/dL). A primary encephalic plasma cell tumor involving the brainstem was diagnosed at necropsy with diagnostic support by electron microscopy and immunocytochemistry. (Wright-Giemsa; HP oil.) **B, Spinal plasmacytoma. Lumbar cerebrospinal fluid.** A large atypical plasma cell with pink and blue cytoplasm is shown against a proteinaceous background with numerous erythrocytes. Compare the size of this neoplastic cell with the small lymphocyte on the lower left. (MGG; HP oil.)

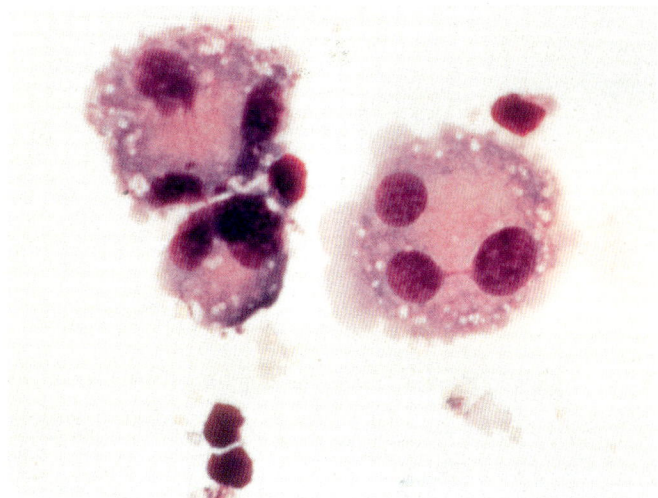

FIGURE 15.50 Histiocytic tumor. Cerebrospinal fluid. Dog. A tumor of unknown origin in the area of the thalamus produced clinical signs of pain initially and later tetraparesis. The fluid had mild pleocytosis (21/μL) composed of 59% large mononuclear cells and 37% lymphocytes with an increased protein concentration (70 mg/dL). The pleomorphism of the large mononuclear cells with vacuolation along with many giant, multinucleated forms suggested a histiocytic neoplasm rather than an inflammatory disease, but a definitive diagnosis was not available. (Wright; HP oil.)

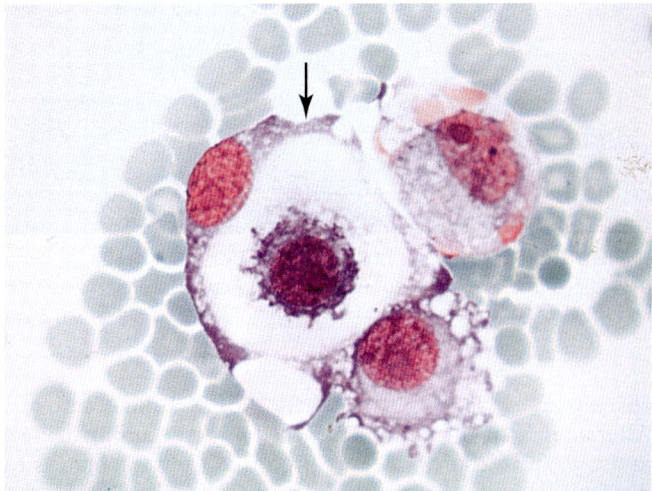

FIGURE 15.51 Metastatic mammary adenocarcinoma. Cerebrospinal fluid (CSF). Dog. The dog underwent surgery for a malignant mammary tumor. Six months after surgery, the dog presented with seizures and ataxia. The CSF sample was hemorrhagic and highly cellular, with the presence of a gigantic signet ring cell *(arrow)* that contains another neoplastic cell (cell within a cell). Contrast cell sizes to erythrocytes in the background. (MGG; HP oil.)

medicine (Vernau et al., 2001). Using this technique, the accuracy between cytopathology and histopathology was examined, and the results found a satisfactory cytopathologic diagnosis obtained in more than 90% of examined cases (De Lorenzi et al., 2006). Elective employment of smear cytopathology is based on several considerations: it is very simple and quick to perform, it requires few materials and equipment, and the specimens can be prepared directly in the operating or adjacent room. Small pieces of tissue can be examined, and smear preparation can be repeated several times with different portions of the same specimens. Various fast-staining techniques can be used. Smear preparations appear to be of greater diagnostic value, with fewer nondiagnostic specimens, compared with touch preparations (Long et al., 2002).

Stereotactic CT-guided brain biopsy can be considered as a valued technique in the neurologic workup of patients with brain diseases, and an early cytopathologic assessment is considered important even during conventional intracranial and spinal surgery (Moissonnier et al., 2002). The methods allow tissue sampling from a precise point for histologic or microbiologic assay, aspiration of a cystic structure or

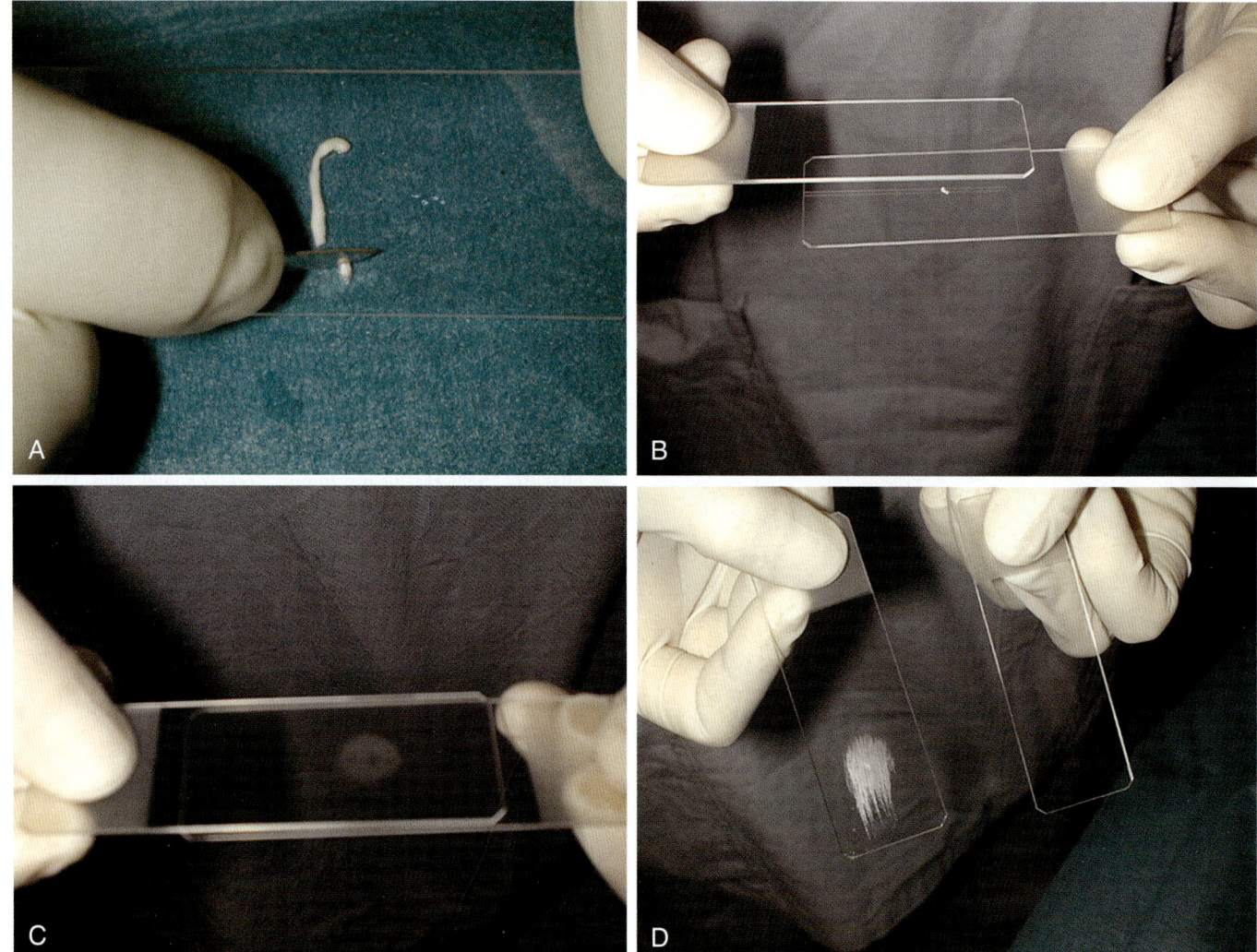

■ **FIGURE 15.52 Squash prep technique for brain tissue. A,** A portion of brain tissue biopsy for the smear. **B,** Place the small fragment near the frosted end of a standard glass slide. **C,** Apply pressure using a second slide, maintain compression, and then slide the top slide over the held bottom slide. **D,** The tissue is smeared onto the slide, resulting in an oval preparation.

abscess cavity, as well as installation of treatment systems. After anesthesia, the animal is placed in a restraining device, and x, y, and z coordinates are produced from CT images to precisely identify the area of interest. The biopsy needle for cutting or aspiration is then introduced into the calculated area of tissue via a hole previously burred into the cranium. The smear preparation technique for tissue is demonstrated in Figure 15.52.

Cytology of Normal Nervous System Tissues

Central nervous system cells have two main origins: neuroectoderm and mesenchyme. Whereas neurons and glial cells (astrocytes, oligodendrocytes, Schwann cells, ependymal cells, and choroid plexus cells) are of neuroectodermal origin, meningeal cells and microglia are of mesenchymal origin.

Cytology of Normal Nervous System Cells

Normal cerebral tissue is an easy-to-smear tissue of low cellular density. In general, the gray matter contains neurons and a few nonmyelinated fibers, whereas the white matter displays myelinated axonal fibers. Specific cells and cellular material are described next.

Neuropil. *Neuropil* is the term used to define the dense network of fine glial processes, neuronal processes (axons and dendrites), and fibrils in the gray matter of CNS (Fig. 15.53). The neuropil is particularly prominent with May-Grünwald-Giemsa (MGG) staining, in which it appears blue-purple. The characteristic and almost distinctive blue staining and foaminess shown by normal neuropil is particularly important to recognize because it is rarely, if ever, present in tumors and in most lesions.

Neurons. Neurons are the principal components of the nervous system. More than any other cell, neurons vary in size from location to location. Most neurons are very large cells, measuring up to 40 µm in diameter, but their size can vary from 5 µm (granular layer of the cerebellum) to 100 µm (motor cortex) (Figs. 15.54 and 15.55; see also Fig. 15.6A). Despite this variation in size, neurons share a common morphologic feature in both dogs and cats—an angulated shape with multiple and branching cytoplasmic processes composed of dendrites and a single axon.

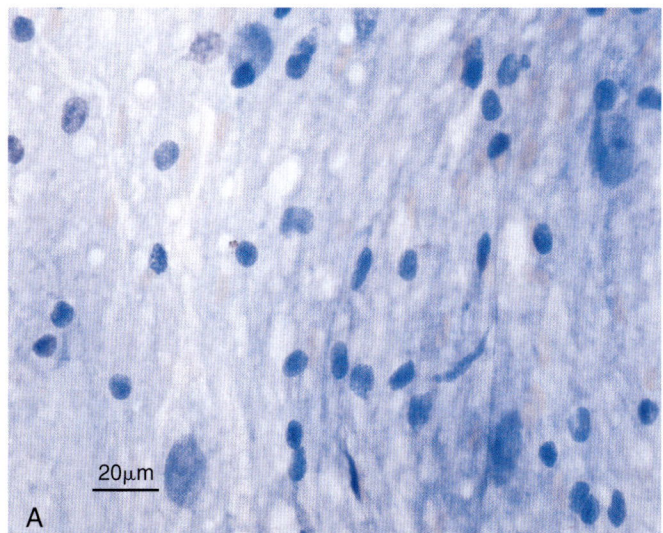

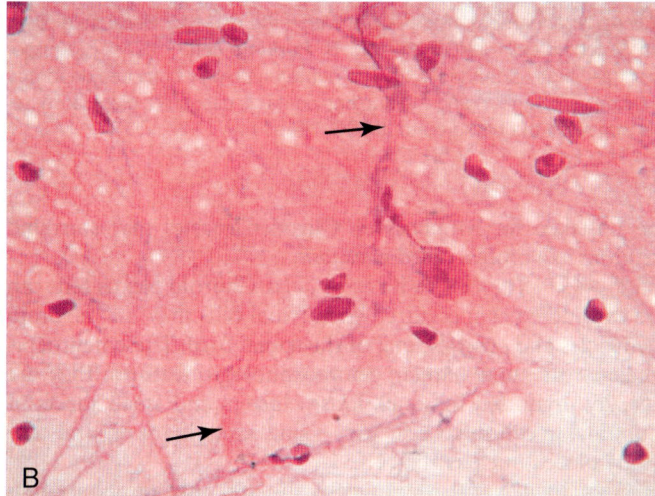

■ **FIGURE 15.53 Neuropil. A, Brain cortex aspirate. Dog.** Inadvertent puncture of cerebral cortex during aspiration of the sinus cavity demonstrates the vacuolated foamy and amorphous basophilic appearance of neuronal and glial processes of the gray matter. (Wright; HP oil.) **B, Normal brain cortex. Squash preparation. Cat.** A neuron (large nucleus with prominent nucleolus) and several hyperchromatic glial cell nuclei within a meshwork of fibrillary processes known as neuropil. Blood vessels *(arrows)* are present within the neuropil. (MGG; HP oil.) (A, Courtesy Rose Raskin, Purdue University.)

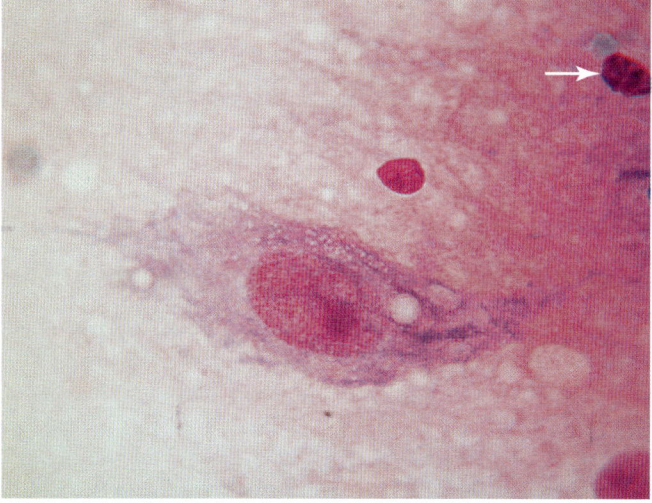

■ **FIGURE 15.54 Neuron. Normal brain cortex. Squash preparation. Cat.** A neuron with a prominent nucleolus is shown. Neurons are huge and vary in size and shape depending on location. Common morphologic features shared by most neurons include a single, centrally placed nucleus with prominent nucleolus and angulated indistinct cytoplasmic borders with wispy basophilic, granular cytoplasm that represents rough endoplasmic reticulum (Nissl substance). Small hyperchromatic glial cell nuclei are noted in the background *(arrow)*. (MGG; HP oil.)

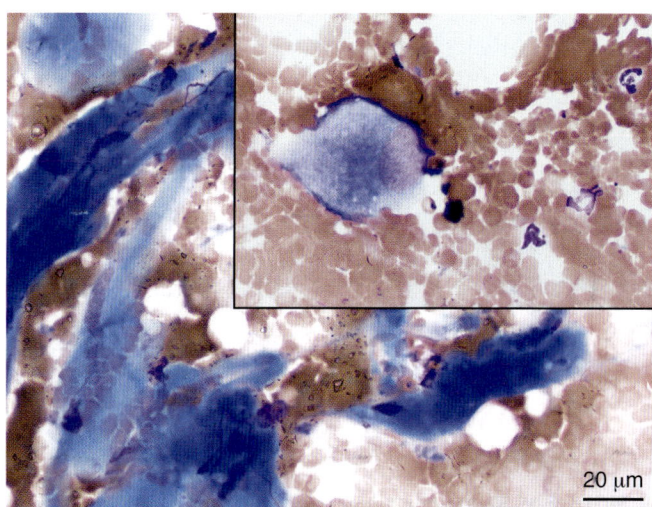

■ **FIGURE 15.55 Neuron. Myenteric nerve plexus. Intestinal aspirate. Dog.** History of vomiting prompted an ultrasound-guided aspirate biopsy of the proximal duodenum. The background contains many basophilic fibers of smooth muscle origin with blood contamination. (Wright-Giemsa; HP oil.) *Inset:* A large neuron, approximately 50 μm in length, was present in an adjacent area to the smooth muscle fibers. Compare its size with the neutrophils in the field. This combination of neuronal tissue within the intestinal wall is consistent with a myenteric nerve plexus and is of no diagnostic significance. (Wright-Giemsa; HP oil.) (Courtesy Rose Raskin, University of Florida.)

The real number of extensions of these specialized structures cannot be evaluated by MGG stain because special stains are needed for this purpose. All neurons have a very large, centrally placed nucleus and frequently a single, prominent nucleolus. The cytoplasm is usually abundant and granular because of the presence of Nissl substance—the rough endoplasmic reticulum often so abundant as to obscure the nucleus. In some areas of the brain, the cytoplasm may contain melanin pigments (neuromelanin) and microvacuoles (neuromediators). Smears from the cerebellar cortex have a highly characteristic appearance because the cellularity is usually higher than in the brain cortex, with sheets of small, hyperchromatic granular cells (Fig. 15.56A) from the inner, granular layer that are occasionally sprinkled between large Purkinje cells (Fig. 15.56B).

Astrocytes. Astrocytes have a supportive function to neurons and are distributed throughout the nervous system. The cells appear as small, oval, naked nuclei that measure between 7 and

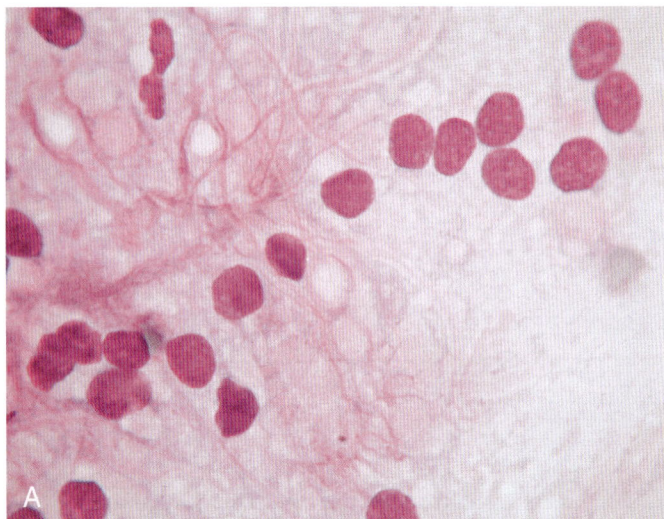 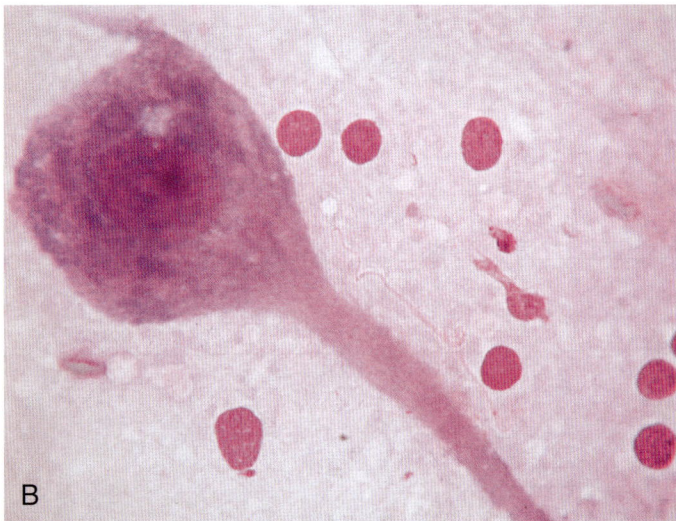

■ **FIGURE 15.56 Cerebellar cortex. Squash preparation. Dog. A, Granular cells.** Several small hyperchromatic neuron nuclei are shown from the inner granular layer of the cerebellar cortex. Note the hypercellularity and linear arrangement of the nuclei within the neuropil. Because of their small size and near absence of cytoplasm, these cells can be confused with lymphoid cells. (MGG; HP oil.) **B, Purkinje cell.** Present is a large, distinctive, flask-shaped neuron with single, central nucleus and characteristic single, large, extended axon. The numerous highly branched dendrites for this cell are usually not evident using the May-Grünwald-Giemsa stain. The cytoplasm surrounding the nucleus contains basophilic granular material known as Nissl bodies or substance. Several hyperchromatic granular cells appear in the background. (MGG; HP oil.)

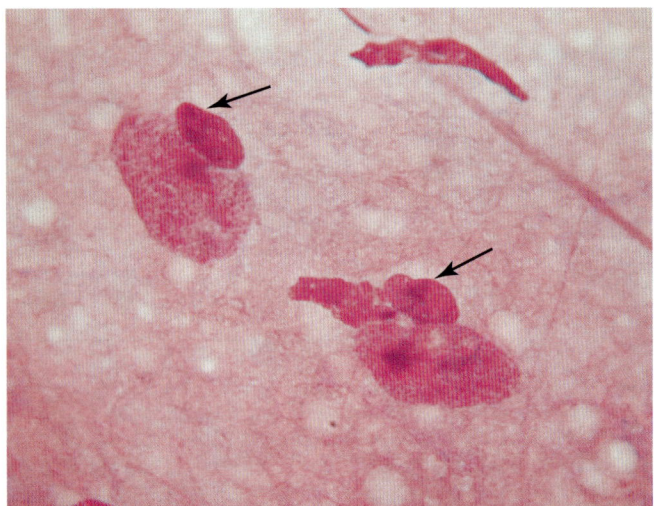

■ **FIGURE 15.57 Normal astrocytes. Squash preparation. Dog.** In May-Grünwald-Giemsa stained samples, astrocytes appear as small, oval, naked nuclei that measure between 7 and 10 μm *(arrows)* surrounded by neuropil. (MGG; HP oil.)

10 μm, surrounded by neuropil (Fig. 15.57). In response to neural tissue injury in the brain and spinal cord, there is a proliferation and hypertrophy of the resident neuroglial cells, which include the astrocyte, a supporting cell with branched cellular projections (Fig. 15.58). The characteristic star-shaped appearance of astrocytes may rarely be demonstrated with Romanowsky stain (Fig. 15.59).

Oligodendrocytes. These are the myelin-forming cells of the CNS. In smears, their nuclei are smaller (5–7 μm) and rounder than astrocytes and, like astrocytes, their cytoplasm is not well defined (Fig. 15.60). Because of their size and shape, oligodendrocytes can be mistaken for lymphocytes. Oligodendrocytes may surround neurons in a process called *satellitosis*.

Ependymal and choroid plexus cells. Choroid plexus cells can be considered as specialized ependymal cells that line the brain ventricles and central canal of the spinal cord. These neuroepithelial cells show similar cytomorphologic features: they are usually organized in small, loose clusters and small sheets of cuboidal to columnar cells with a single, small, round, and centrally placed nucleus (Fig. 15.61).

Meningeal cells. Meningeal cells are only rarely seen or recognized in brain smears. The cells are usually organized in sheets or in loose clusters, showing a rather pleomorphic storiform pattern. Cell borders are poorly defined, and the nuclear shape ranges from round to oval to elongate (Fig. 15.62). Occasionally, cells are organized in pseudoacinar structures mimicking a glandular origin, which is more common in meningiomas, but can also be identified in normal meningeal tissue.

Microglia. These neuroglial cells are derived from bone marrow elements, likely macrophages that have specific phagocytic functions. They have small and elongated nuclei, giving them the name *rod cells*. In many smears from brain cortex, microglia are localized in perivascular areas. When reactive, they show lipophagocytosis, filling the cytoplasm with well-defined vacuoles, producing a foamy appearance (Fig. 15.63).

Cytopathology of Abnormal Nervous System Tissues

An accuracy value of 92.8% was obtained with the cytopathologic evaluation of nervous system lesions from 42 cases in dogs and cats, in which changes were initially classified as nonneoplastic or neoplastic (De Lorenzi et al., 2006). The non-neoplastic group consisted of tissues derived from inflammation, cyst, granuloma, or scar lesion, whereas the neoplastic group included lesions of neuroepithelial origin (neural, glial, and ependymal-choroidal proliferations) or of

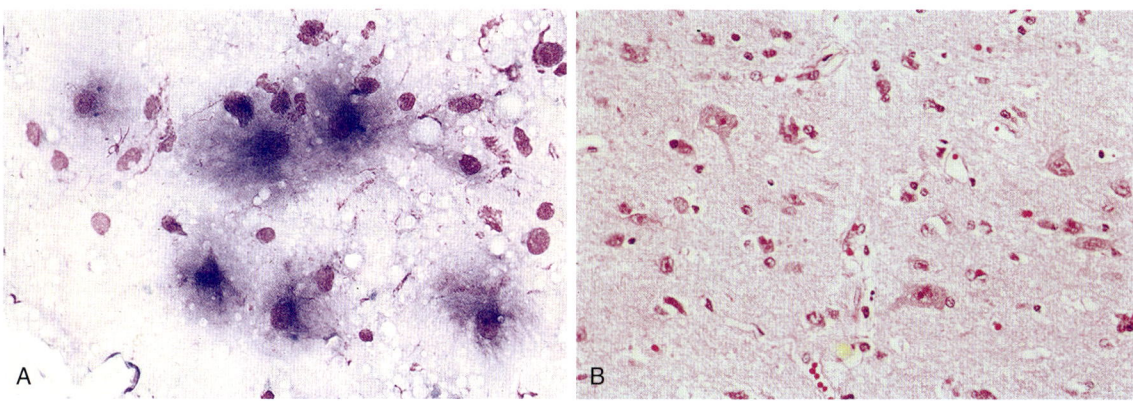

■ **FIGURE 15.58 Astrocytosis. Brain. Cat.** Same case in A and B. **A, Aspirate biopsy.** Six large cells with a wispy basophilic cytoplasm are evident in this aspirate from a cat with a 14-day progression of dementia and head pressing. Nuclei are round to oval with a single small prominent nucleolus, and the nucleocytoplasmic ratio is mildly increased. (Wright-Giemsa; HP oil.) **B, Histology.** Magnetic resonance imaging revealed an intracranial mass. Tissue biopsy revealed normal gray matter with hypertrophied astrocytes, which is a nonspecific reaction. (H&E; HP oil.)

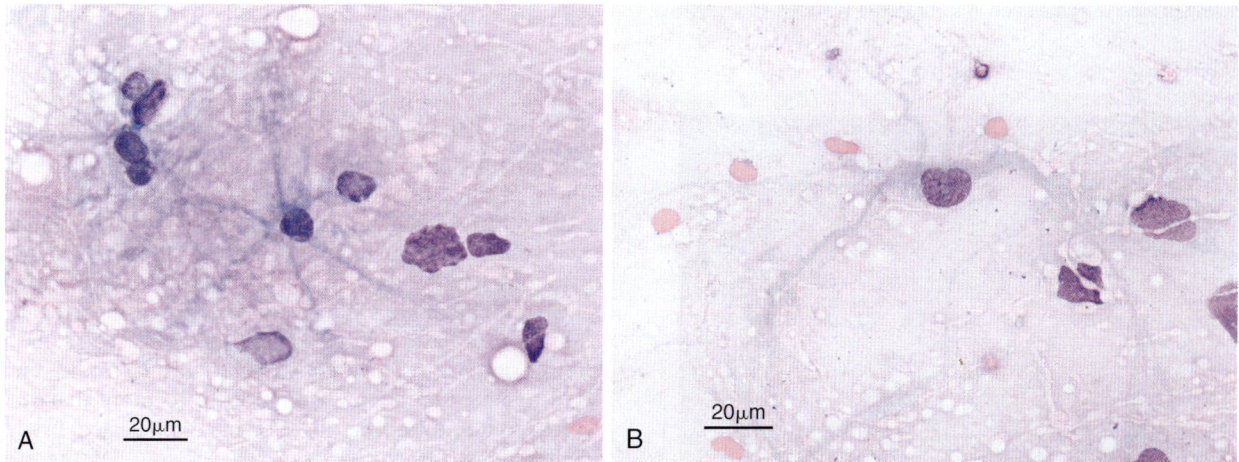

■ **FIGURE 15.59 Astrocytosis. Brain tissue imprint. Dog.** Same case in A and B. **A,** Injury from an adjacent oligodendroglioma (not shown) resulted in astrocyte response. The center cell demonstrates a characteristic star appearance with a small dense nucleus and streaming fibrillar cytoplasm. (Wright; HP oil.) **B,** Single astrocyte with long extensions of cytoplasm. (Wright; HP oil.) (Courtesy Rose Raskin, Purdue University.)

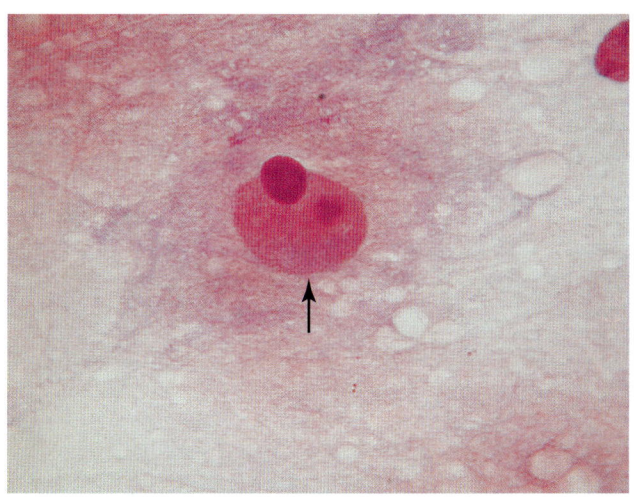

■ **FIGURE 15.60 Oligodendrocyte. Normal brain cortex. Squash preparation. Dog.** In May-Grünwald-Giemsa stained smears, the oligodendrocyte looks like a round, naked nucleus (arrow) that often surrounds neurons in a process called satellitosis. (MGG; HP oil.)

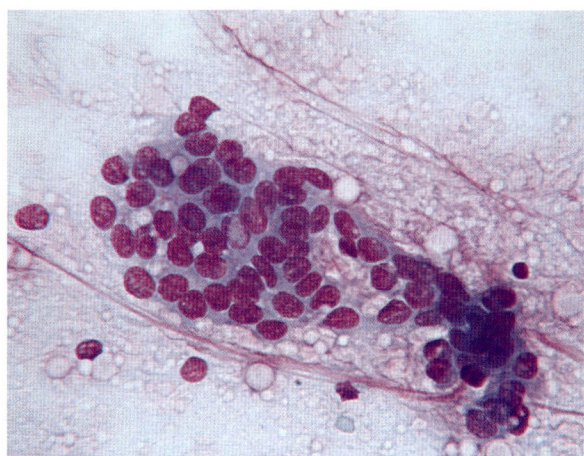

■ **FIGURE 15.61 Normal choroid cells. Squash preparation. Dog.** Cohesive cluster of cuboidal to columnar cells have a uniform nuclear appearance and high nucleocytoplasmic ratio. The single small, round, and centrally placed nuclei are arranged occasionally in a palisade or linear arrangement. Choroid cells are indistinguishable from ependymal cells by cytopathology. (MGG; HP oil.)

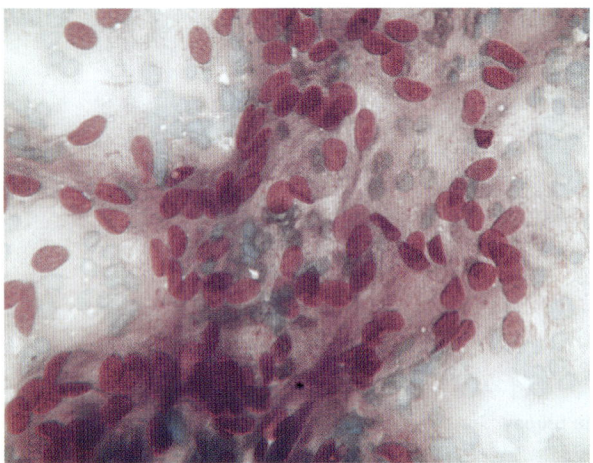

■ **FIGURE 15.62 Normal meningeal cells. Squash preparation. Dog.** The dense collection of oval nuclei is surrounded by eosinophilic streaming, wispy cytoplasm. This appearance is more common in meningiomas, but it can also be seen in samples from normal brain. (MGG; HP oil.)

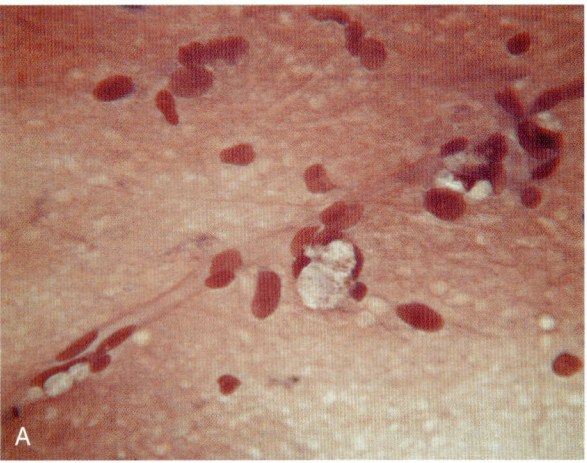

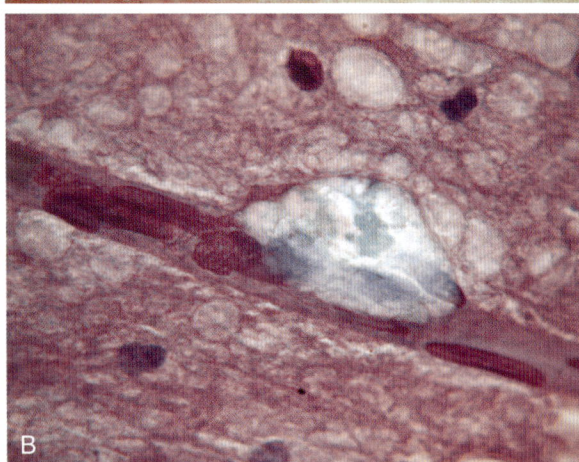

■ **FIGURE 15.63 Microglial cells. Normal brain cortex. Squash preparation. A, Dog.** A perivascular microglial cells *(center)* has plump abundant vacuolated cytoplasm. The background contains other glial cells along with neural fibrils. (MGG; HP oil.) **B, Cat.** A single plump vacuolated, lipid-filled microglial cell is noted adjacent to a blood vessel. When reactive, these macrophage-derived cells undergo lipophagocytosis. (MGG; HP oil.)

non-neuroepithelial origin, divided further into epithelial, mesenchymal, and round cell tumors.

Cytopathologic features suggesting a neuroepithelial origin include highly cellular smears related to the soft texture of the specimen, fine fibrillar background, perivascular arrangement with processes approaching the vascular lumen, round nuclei with finely stippled chromatin, and endothelial cell proliferation. Cytopathologic features of non-neuroepithelial lesions can vary considerably because of the extreme heterogeneous morphology of these groups. Nevertheless, the presence of cohesive cellular clusters or epithelial sheets; tightly packed spindle cells; whorls; large, round cells with prominent nucleoli and discernible cytoplasm; and numerous inflammatory cells suggests consideration of non-neuroepithelial tumors. The distinction between neuroepithelial and non-neuroepithelial depends to a large extent on pattern recognition (an advantage of histopathology) and individual cell morphology. Therefore, overlapping of morphologic features for the differentiation of neoplastic and non-neoplastic lesions and the primitive tumor heterogeneity is a limitation of cytopathology. The cytopathologic features of 93 primary brain tumors in dogs and cats have been described (Vernau et al., 2001).

Inflammatory Conditions of the Central Nervous System

Inflammatory lesions of CNS can mimic neoplastic proliferation clinically and radiographically. Cytopathology can be a useful tool in distinguishing tumor from an inflammatory or reactive lesion. Romanowsky stain can effectively stain many infectious agents. For example, a space-occupying lesion in the temporal lobe of an adult cat was diagnosed by cytopathology as brain toxoplasmosis (Falzone et al., 2008). The squash prep showed intense reactive gliosis surrounding round, encapsulated tissue cysts ranging from 15 μm to more than 100 μm, which contained numerous elongated nucleated bradyzoites identified as *Toxoplasma* spp. (Fig. 15.64). Of the systemic fungi, CNS infections have occurred with *Coccidioides* spp., *Blastomyces dermatitidis* (Fig. 15.65), *H. capsulatum*, and *C. neoformans*, but only *C. neoformans* has a particular affinity for the CNS (Miller and Zachary, 2017).

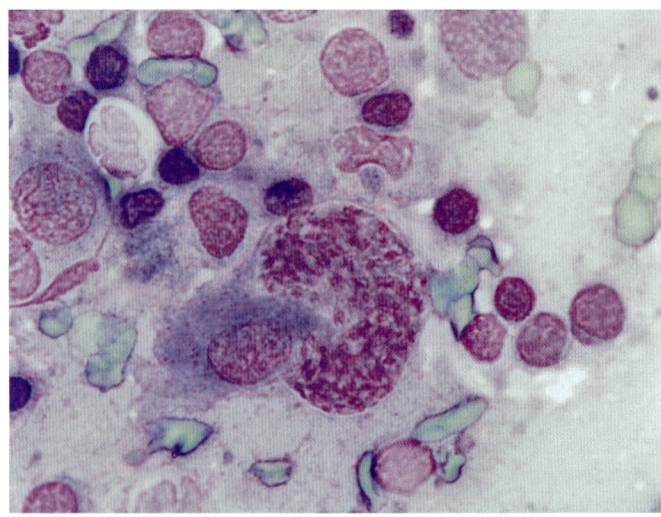

■ **FIGURE 15.64 Toxoplasmosis tissue cyst. Brain mass. Squash preparation. Cat.** A round, encapsulated structure (tissue cyst) is filled with nucleated bradyzoites of *Toxoplasma* spp. (MGG; HP oil.)

Neoplasms of the Meninges and Nerve Sheaths

Meningioma. Non-neuroepithelial tumors that arise from the arachnoid meningeal layer are termed *meningiomas* (Table 15.4), the most common intracranial tumor in dogs and cats. In cats, approximately 60% of primary CNS tumors are meningiomas. Meningiomas have a statistically higher incidence in golden retrievers and boxers (Higgins et al., 2017). The tumors are derived from leptomeningocytes that associate with neural crest tissue and have both epithelial and fibroblastic ultrastructural characteristics. As a result, these tumors have several variant forms (Montoliu et al., 2006), which are found both in cervical and lumbar regions of the spinal cord (15%) as well as intracranially (82%) and within the retrobulbar region (<3%) (Zimmerman et al., 2000; Higgins et al., 2017). Spinal cord meningiomas are mostly extramedullary (Fig. 15.66), but few reports note the radiographic presentation of them as intramedullary (Hopkins et al., 1995). Meningiomas are negative for the immunomarker glial fibrillary acid protein (GFAP), synaptophysin, and PAS but may be positive for acid mucopolysaccharides or mucins (Raskin, 1984; Barnhart et al., 2002). Histologically, some of the variant types include meningothelial, transitional, fibrous (fibroblastic), psammomatous, angiomatous (vascular), microcystic, or secretory (Higgins et al., 2017). Surgical removal is often the treatment of choice.

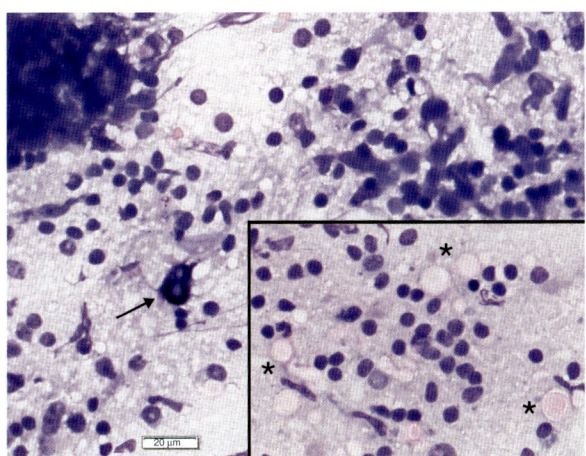

■ **FIGURE 15.65 Blastomycosis. Brain imprint. Dog.** A young dog presented with head tilt and ataxia. Magnetic resonance imaging revealed a contrast-enhancing mass within the ventral rostral cerebellum. **Cerebrospinal fluid** had increased protein (46 mg/dL) and total nucleated cell count (31/μL) with mixed-cell pleocytosis (suppurative, mononuclear) without evidence of a cause. At necropsy, the brain granuloma revealed yeast organisms; one is shown *(arrow)* among glial cells. (Wright; HP oil.) *Inset:* In addition to gliosis, several collections of eosinophilic myelin are present *(asterisks)*. (Wright; HP oil.) (Courtesy Rose Raskin, Purdue University.)

TABLE 15.4 Nervous System Tumors on Cytopathology and Their Diagnostic Immunomarkers[a]

TUMORS	POSITIVE IMMUNOREACTIVE	NEGATIVE IMMUNOREACTIVE
Meningeal Origin		
Meningioma	VIM, CK, E-cadherin	GFAP
Granular cell tumor	Ubiquitin	GFAP, CD18, Iba1, leukocyte markers
Melanoma	Melan A, S-100	
Nerve Sheath Origin		
Peripheral nerve sheath tumors	VIM, laminin, Olig-2; CNPase	
Schwannoma	GFAP +/−	Claudin-1
Neurofibrosarcoma	Claudin-1 +/−	GFAP
Neuroepithelial Origin		
Gliomas		
Oligodendroglioma	GFAP, Olig-2	CK
Astrocytoma	GFAP, Olig-2, EGFR, VIM, nestin	CK
Ependymoma	CK (AE1/AE3), GFAP	S-100, leukocyte markers
Choroid plexus tumors (papilloma, carcinoma)	VIM, GFAP, CK (AE1/AE3), laminin	
Primitive Neuroectodermal Tumors		
Medulloblastoma	SYN, GFAP, NeuN, MAP-2, SMI 31, TNF	CK (AE1/AE3)
Neuroblastoma	NeuN	
Hematopoietic Origin		
Lymphoma	CD3, CD20, CD79a, PAX5	CK
Plasma cell tumor	MUM1	CK
Histiocytic sarcoma	CD1a, CD11c, CD18	CK
Extramedullary (Renal) Origin		
Nephroblastoma	WT1, VIM, CK	GFAP, SYN, NeuN

[a]Higgins et al., 2017.

CK, Cytokeratin; *CNPase*, cyclic nucleotide phosphodiesterase; *EGFR*, epidermal growth factor receptor; *GFAP*, glial fibrillary acid protein; *MAP-2*, microtubule-associated protein; *MUM1*, multiple myeloma 1; *NeuN*, neuron-specific nuclear protein; *Olig2*, oligodendrocyte transcription factor 2; *PDGFR*, platelet-derived growth factor receptor; *SMI 31*, phosphorylated neurofilaments; *SYN*, synaptophysin; *TNF*, triple neurofilament; *VIM*, vimentin; *WT1*, Wilms tumor 1.

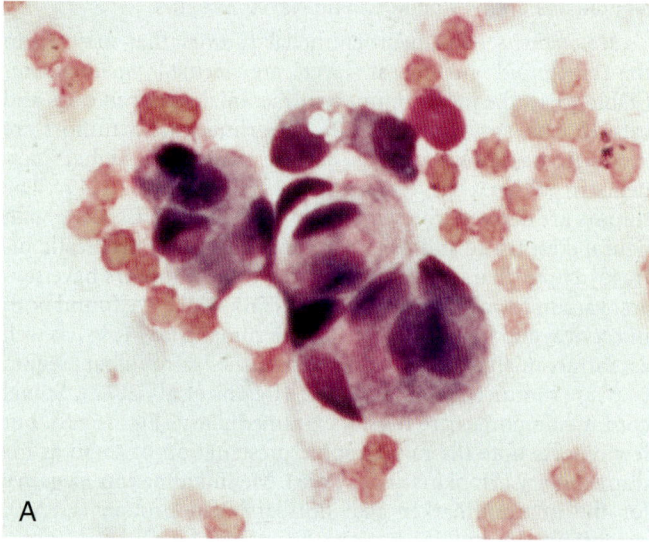
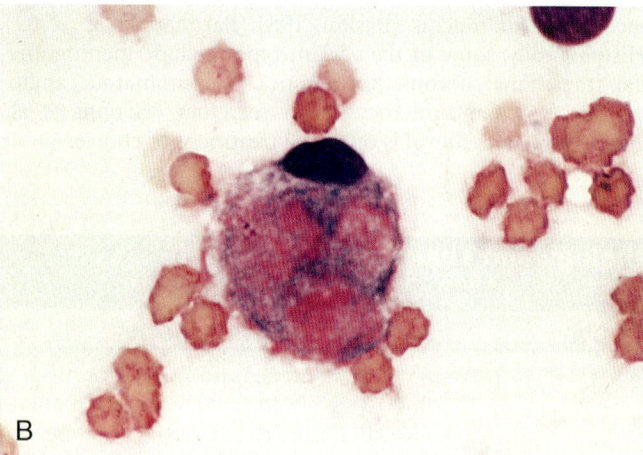

■ **FIGURE 15.66 Meningothelial meningioma. Spinal cord mass imprint. Dog.** Same case in A and B. **A,** A dog presented with a 2-year history of neck pain and front leg paresis. Imaging revealed an extradural mass compressing the spinal cord that was confirmed at surgery and necropsy. **A,** Cytopathologic features demonstrate cohesive ball formation with an epithelial-like appearance. (Wright; IP.) **B,** Individual meningeal cell with histiocytic appearance. The cytoplasm is abundant with eosinophilic secretory material that was positive for acid mucopolysaccharides. (Wright; HP oil.) (Courtesy Rose Raskin, Michigan State University.)

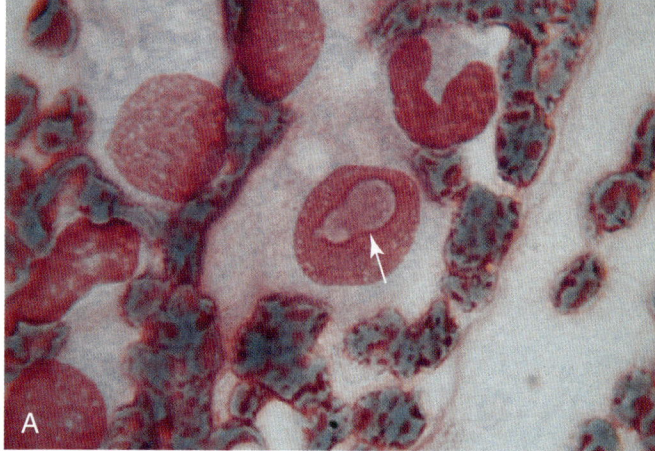
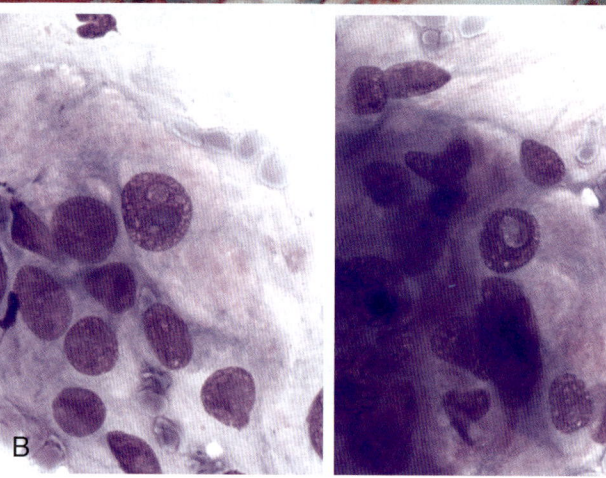

■ **FIGURE 15.67 Meningioma with nuclear inclusion. Squash preparation from surgical biopsy. Dog. A,** A single meningothelial cell contains an intranuclear inclusion *(arrow)* that is thought to represent cytoplasmic evagination. Cytoplasmic evagination may be commonly encountered in meningiomas of meningothelial origin. (MGG; HP oil.) **B,** Another canine case showing two additional presentations of cytoplasmic evaginations. (MGG; HP oil.)

According to Bailey and Higgins (1986), meningiomas are associated with a high prevalence of pleocytosis (nucleated cell counts >50/µL), with a predominance of neutrophils that is attributed to a response to tumor necrosis. In contrast, pleocytosis was detected in only 27% of 56 dogs with intracranial meningioma, and a neutrophil predominance was observed in only 19% of dogs. It is possible that the incidence of the tumor necrosis was less in their study. Myelography, MRI, and CT are imaging tools used currently to identify tumors of the brain and spinal cord. Fine-needle aspirations, crush preparations (Moissonnier et al., 2002; De Lorenzi et al., 2006), and incisional cutting needles (Platt et al., 2002) have been used to obtain cytopathologic and histopathologic specimens. The cytopathologic features of meningiomas have been discussed in several reports (Hopkins et al., 1995; Zimmerman et al., 2000).

Crush preparations from wet-fixed, rapid H&E-stained meningiomas from 44 dogs and seven cats were evaluated (Vernau et al., 2001). At low magnification, tumor cells were broken up into many clusters or cohesive cell aggregates, as well as separated into individual cells. Meningioma cells had round to slightly elongate, uniform-sized nuclei with a small, prominent nucleolus, diffusely coarse chromatin, and a well-defined nuclear border. Rarely, there were intranuclear cytoplasmic evaginations, but these were plentiful in some individual tumor cells of the meningothelial subtype (Fig. 15.67). More elongated cells sometimes had a central bar or fold through the longitudinal axis of their nucleus. There were variable amounts of eosinophilic, granular, wispy to solid cytoplasm that appeared round to elongate, often with a polar location. Mitotic figures were extremely rare. Some tumors had marked cellular anaplasia or nuclear atypia. Neutrophils were usually found in tumors that had histologic foci of necrosis and focal accumulations. A common cytopathologic appearance is meningothelial (also known as endotheliomatous or syncytial meningioma) (Figs. 15.66 to 15.68). Psammoma bodies appear as dense, dark-staining

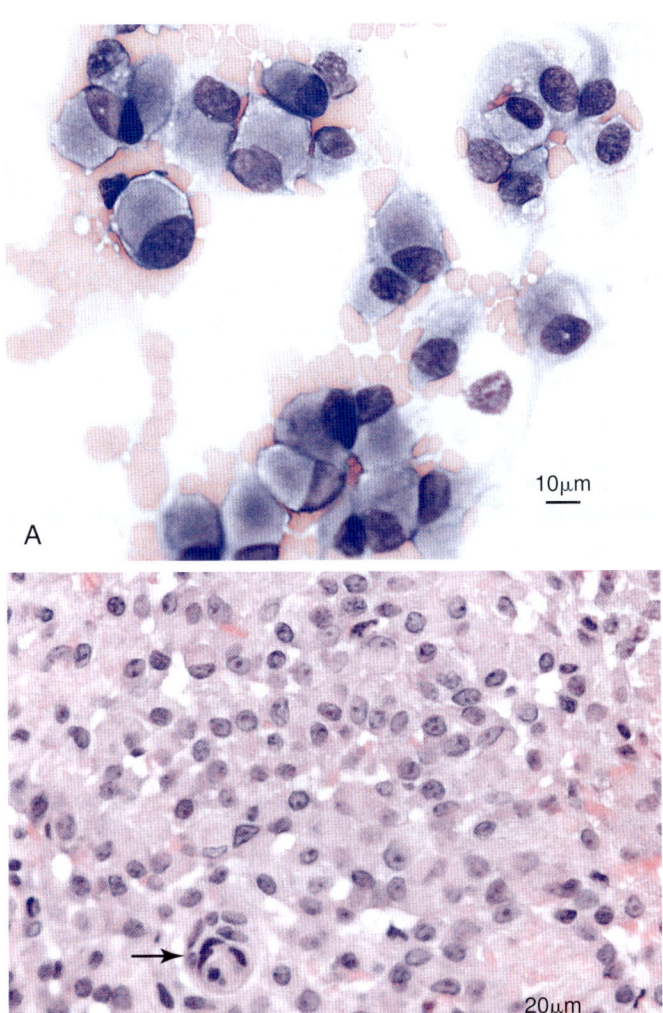

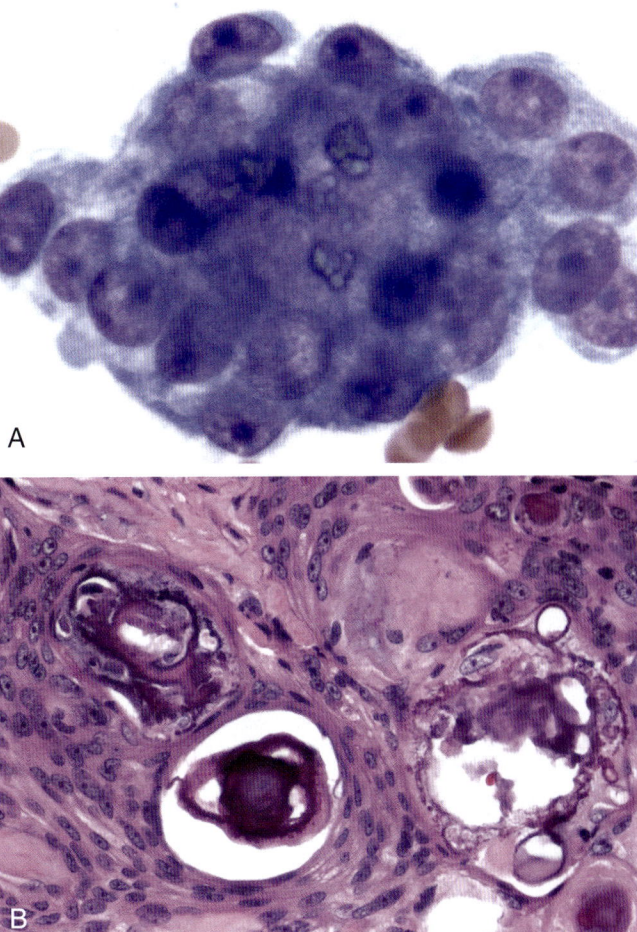

■ **FIGURE 15.68** **Meningothelial meningioma. Brain mass imprint. Dog.** Same case in A and B. The patient's history included head bobbing and exaggerated placing response of the right foreleg. A lesion was suspected clinically within the right cerebellum. The total nucleated cell count was 1/μL with a mildly increased protein concentration (46 mg/dL). **A,** The nucleated cells are large, having abundant granular basophilic cytoplasm with an eccentric nucleus and demonstrate mild anisocytosis and anisokaryosis. The cells have both an epithelial-like appearance suggestive of an epithelial neoplasm. (Wright; HP oil.) **B, Histologic section.** A meningothelial meningioma was diagnosed with histopathology. There is a psammoma body (laminar, circular collection of calcium believed to form from degradation of necrotic tissue that has no diagnostic meaning) *(arrow)* along with a sheetlike appearance of the majority of the cells. Meningiomas is one of several tumor types in which psammoma bodies can be found. Meningothelial cells wrap around small blood vessels. (H&E; HP oil.) (Courtesy Kristin Nunez-Fisher, Purdue University.)

■ **FIGURE 15.69** **Meningioma. Psammoma bodies. Brain mass. Dog.** Same case in A and B. Clinical signs were seizures, ataxia, abnormal behavior, and weakness. Neurologic examination localized the lesion to the forebrain, and magnetic resonance imaging identified a large mass in the left olfactory or frontal lobe. **A, Surgical biopsy imprint.** A cluster of spindle neoplastic cells with small circular refractile mineralized concretions. These concretions are likely small amounts of material from psammoma bodies. (Wright-Giemsa; HP oil.) **B, Histology.** Note the dense mineralized psammoma bodies within the meningioma. (H&E; IP.) (Courtesy Brenda Yamamoto et al., The Ohio State University. Presented at the 2005 ASVCP case review session.)

structures that composed of calcium phosphate from mitochondria or phospholipid membrane vesicles from dying cells (Fig. 15.69). Cholesterol crystals may also be found from cell membranes remnants. Meningiomas often appear with a spindle cell appearance and psammomatous histologic appearance (Figs. 15.70 to 15.72).

Perivascular whorling around blood vessels with a predominance of dilated vessels is an uncommon pattern termed *angiomatous* (Fig. 15.73) (Higgins et al., 2017). Less frequently, tumors with a sarcomatous appearance and high mitotic count are malignant and may have a disseminated nature (Higgins et al., 2017).

Granular cell tumor. Another tumor associated with the meninges is the granular cell tumor, an uncommon tumor of animals and humans that occurs within or outside the nervous system. The cell of origin is unclear, but the morphologic appearance is thought to be the result of the accumulation of lysosomes, as demonstrated by electron microscopy (Sharkey et al., 2004; Levitin et al., 2019), that reflects metabolic derangements in the cell. The cytopathologic features include large, round cells with eccentric nuclei and cytoplasm distended by many variably stained eosinophilic granules (Fig. 15.74). Cells stain strongly positive for PAS as well as for the immunomarker ubiquitin (see Table 15.4). Other staining reactions for these

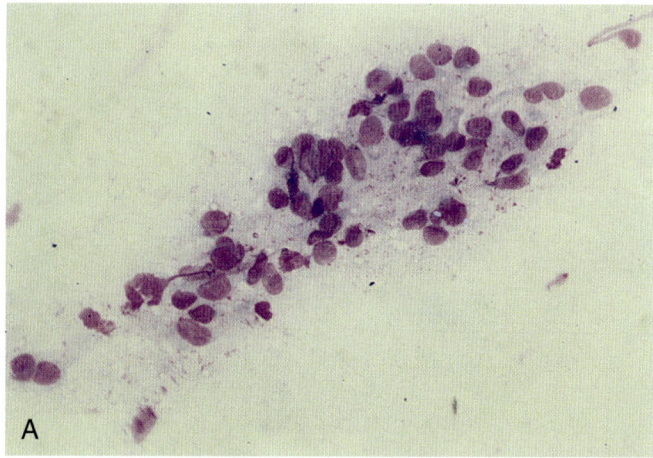
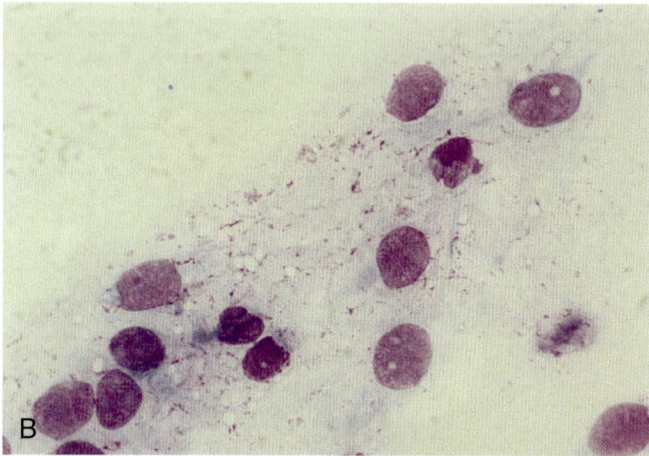
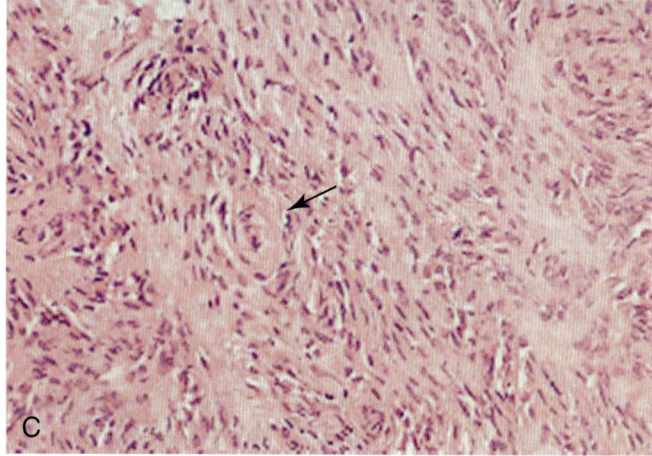

■ **FIGURE 15.70 Meningioma. Spindle pattern. Dog.** Same case in A to C. **A–B, Tissue imprint. A,** Progressive quadriparesis was associated with an intramedullary lesion observed with magnetic resonance imaging. Large cellular aggregates of mesenchymal-appearing cells are shown against a pink, finely granular background. (Wright-Giemsa; HP oil.) **B,** Higher magnification of a meningioma demonstrating the round to oval nucleus with finely granular chromatin, small nucleoli, and lightly basophilic cytoplasm that forms wispy tails. A finely granular eosinophilic material surrounds the cells and is seen within the cytoplasm as well. (Wright-Giemsa; HP oil.) **C, Tissue section.** Interweaving bundles of spindle cells are prominent with dense collagenous bands separating the cells. A small psammoma body is present (arrow). (H&E; IP.)

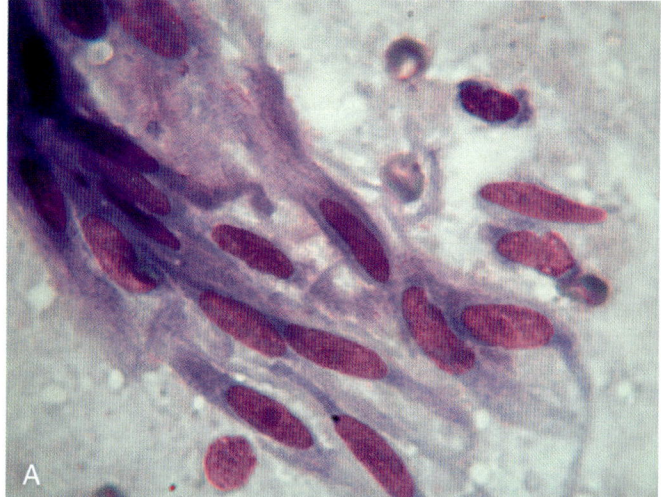
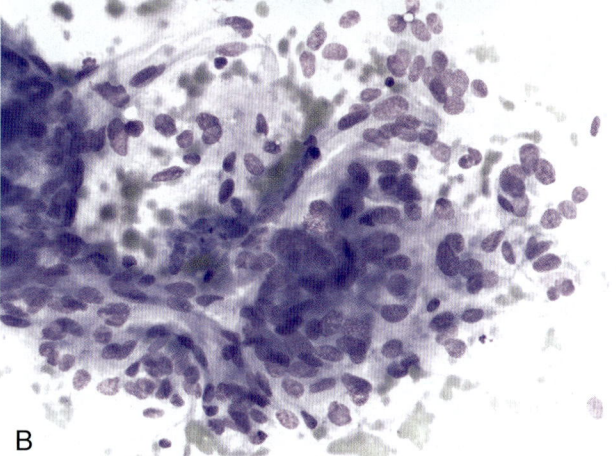

■ **FIGURE 15.71 Meningioma. Spindle pattern. Squash preparation from surgical biopsy. Dogs. A,** Spindle-like tumor cells are arranged in a storiform pattern. These elongate cells with oval nuclei have a single small but prominent nucleolus and moderately coarse chromatin. The cytoplasm is basophilic with wispy, pointed ends. (MGG; HP oil.) **B,** Spindle cells are present as aggregates or balls of cells. (MGG; HP oil.)

cells include a variably positive reaction for S-100, α-1-antichymotrypsin, α-1-antitrypsin, and vimentin as well as a negative reaction for GFAP, pancytokeratins, and markers for subpopulations of lymphocytes and macrophages (Higgins et al., 2001; Sharkey et al., 2004).

Peripheral nerve sheath tumor. Peripheral nerve sheath tumors (PNSTs) may be encountered in cytopathologic preparations (see Table 15.4). These are most often associated with peripheral nerve roots and include those of the neural crest–derived Schwann cell that assists in myelination as well as fibroblastic connective tissue cells that surround nerve bundles. A cytopathologic distinction among benign PNST (schwannoma and neurofibroma) can be difficult or impossible (Figs. 15.75 and 15.76A). Benign schwannomas and neurofibromas can show cytopathologic features of atypia so that differentiation between benign and malignant PNST is problematic even for the experienced, and histopathologic examination is required (Figs. 15.76B and 15.77).

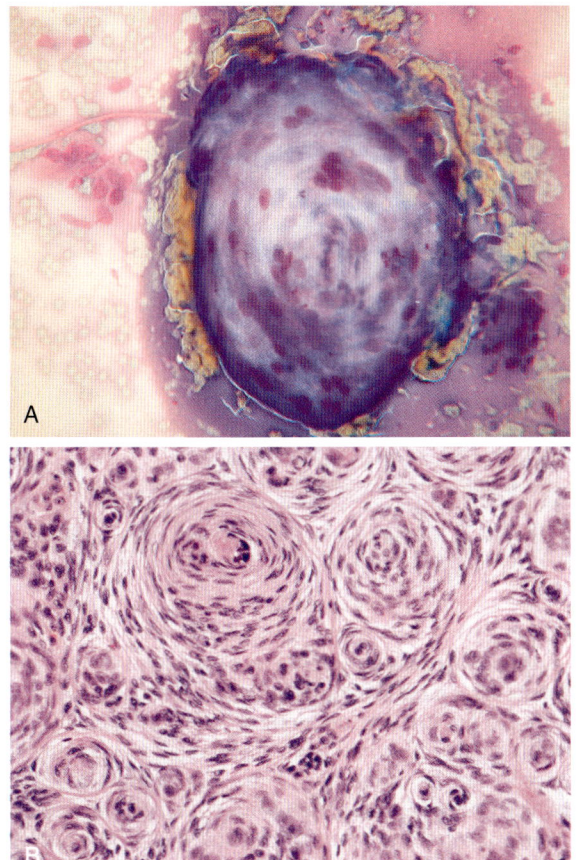

■ **FIGURE 15.72 Meningioma. Psammomatous pattern. Cerebrum. Cat.** Same case in A and B. **A, Squash preparation from surgical biopsy.** A cohesive aggregate of meningeal cells are present in a distinctive whorl formation characteristic of a psammomatous meningioma. Nuclei are round to slightly elongated, and the cell border is poorly defined. (MGG; IP.) **B, Histology.** Frequent island and whorl patterns of neoplastic meningeal spindyloid cells are a significant feature of the psammomatous pattern. (H&E; IP.)

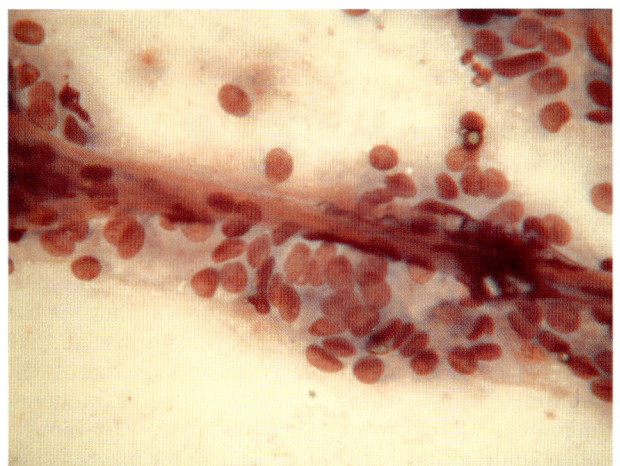

■ **FIGURE 15.73 Meningioma. Perivascular pattern. Squash preparation from surgical biopsy. Dog.** The spindle-shaped cells are strongly associated with an eosinophilic linear capillary blood vessel. This pattern may be found in the angiomatous pattern composed of a predominance of blood vessels. (MGG; HP oil.)

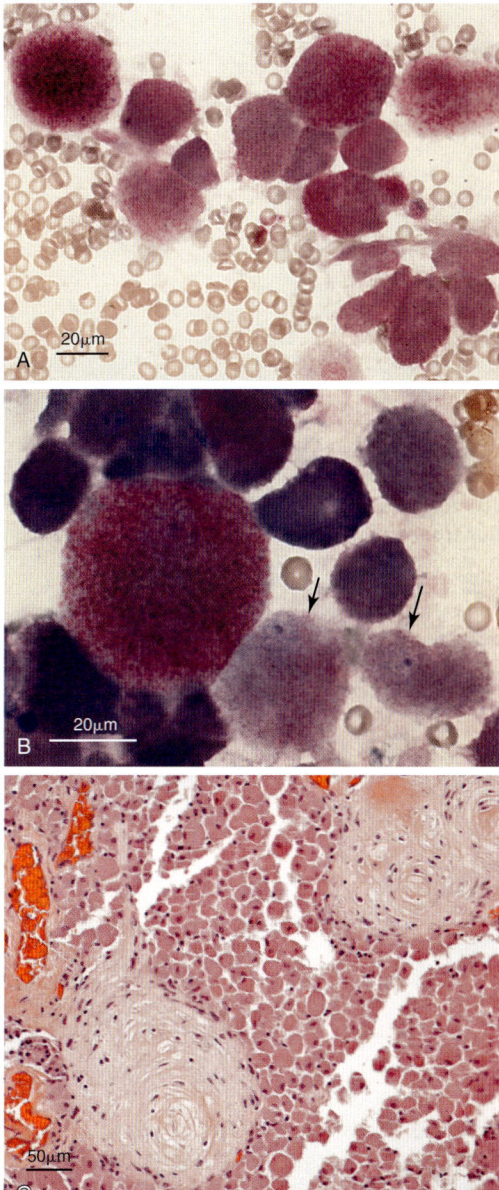

■ **FIGURE 15.74 Granular cell tumor. Brain. Dog.** Same case in A to C. This 10-year-old golden retriever became aggressive and developed seizures 2 months preceding the detection of a cerebral tumor by magnetic resonance imaging. **A, Tissue imprint.** A group of huge pleomorphic oval to round granular cells are present with variable degrees of cytoplasmic granularity. One granular cell with sparse granules permits the observation of a small round nucleus (bottom center). (Wright-Giemsa; HP oil.) **B, Tissue imprint.** One cell measuring approximately 50 μm contains numerous pink-purple, coarse granules in the cytoplasm believed to be the result of the accumulation of lysosomes as demonstrated by electron microscopy, not to be confused with a mast cell. Note two poorly granular adjacent cells with small round nuclei and single small nucleoli (arrows). (Wright-Giemsa; HP oil.) **C, Tissue section.** The meningeal tumor was comprised of two tumor cell types: a psammomatous meningioma with characteristic pattern of islands of tumor cell whorls and interspaced are granular cell tumor cells. The histogenesis of the granular cell tumor is unclear and may be variable. The cells are periodic acid–Schiff positive with diastase-resistant granules and are immunohistochemically negative for muscle markers and positive for either neuron-specific enolase, S-100, or both. (H&E; IP.) (Courtesy Rose Raskin, University of Florida.)

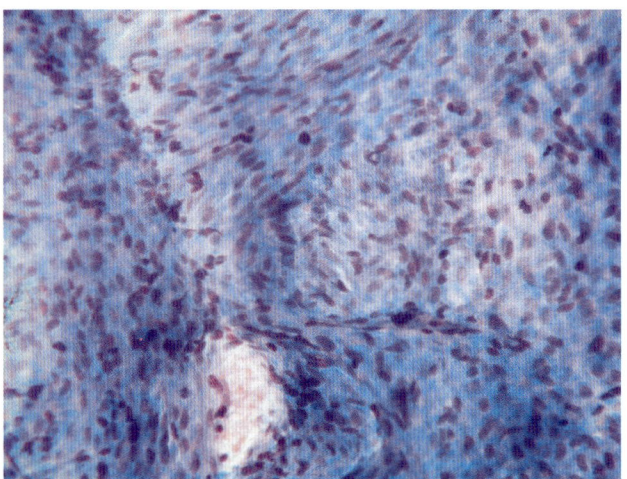

■ **FIGURE 15.75 Peripheral nerve sheath tumor (PNST). Squash preparation from surgical biopsy. Dog.** A dense collection of pleomorphic, elongated cells with oval nuclei is organized in a storiform pattern with focal palisade arrangement. Distinction between schwannoma and neurofibroma is not possible by cytopathology. PNST can be more easily diagnosed if a neoplasm with these cytomorphologic features is associated with a peripheral nerve root. (MGG; IP.)

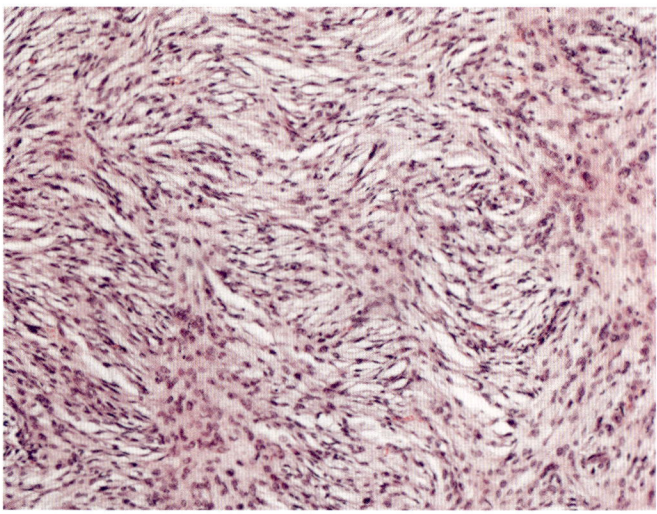

■ **FIGURE 15.77 Benign nerve sheath tumor. Tissue section. Dog.** A dense weave pattern of neoplastic cells. (H&E; HP oil.)

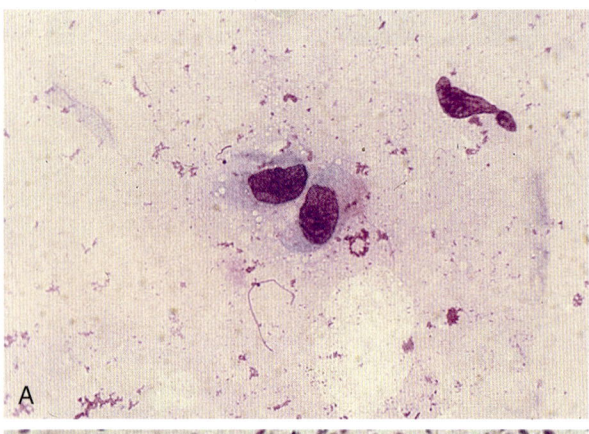

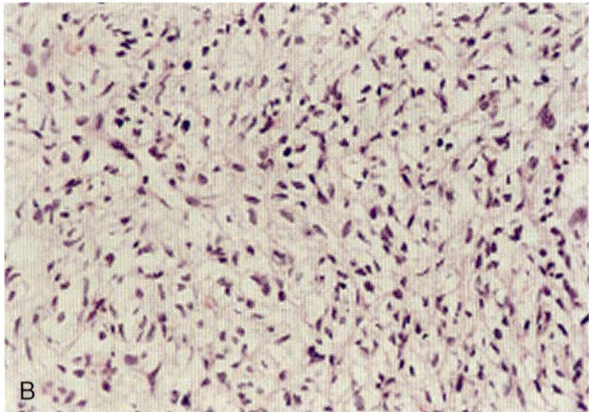

■ **FIGURE 15.76 Benign nerve sheath tumor.** Same case in A and B. **Dog.** Clinical presentation included tetraparesis, ataxia, cervical pain, and Horner syndrome. A compressive extradural lesion was found in the spinal canal at the nerve root region of C2–C3. **A, Tissue imprint.** Two intact plump spindle cells demonstrate minimal anaplastic features. (Wright-Giemsa; HP oil.) **B, Tissue section.** Neoplastic mesenchymal cells with eosinophilic fibrillary cell borders are arranged loosely within a fibroblastic stroma. (H&E; HP oil.)

A diagnosis of suspect PNST can be made in the presence of neoplasms associated with a peripheral nerve root, showing cytopathologic features of moderate to high cellularity. The cells are mainly grouped in thick fragments even if smaller clusters or single cells can be present and are characteristically spindle shaped with elongated nuclei and inconspicuous nucleoli.

An unusual cytopathologic presentation of PNST from the forelimb of one cat was described (Tremblay et al., 2005). The cells revealed a pleomorphic population of individual round cells resembling histiocytes or plasma cells with round, central to eccentric nuclei; basophilic cytoplasm; numerous mitotic figures; and large, multinucleated cells.

Benign nerve sheath tumors are shown in Figures 15.75 to 15.77. Malignant nerve sheath tumors may be locally extensive and recur more often. The histologic distinction between malignant fibroblasts and malignant Schwann cells is not readily discernible without immunohistochemistry and electron microscopy (see Table 15.4). A confirmed neurofibrosarcoma case confirmed by histopathology is shown in Figure 15.78. See Figs. 3.143 to 3.146 for more examples of nerve sheath tumors and schwannomas.

Neoplasms of Neuroepithelial Cells

Gliomas are neoplasms of specific neuroglial cells that include oligodendrocytes and astrocytes, which are immunoreactive to GFAP (see Table 15.4). Tumors from these cells most often produce a normal CSF related to their deep parenchymal location.

Oligodendroglioma. One report of oligodendrogliomas in cats described their cytopathologic features as they appeared in cytocentrifuge preparations of CSF (Dickinson et al., 2000). Cells were large with nuclei four to six times the size of RBCs. Nuclei were eccentric within a densely basophilic, moderately abundant cytoplasm. An imprint from the surgery biopsy of an oligodendroglioma presenting as a brain mass is shown Figure 15.79. Normally, these cells are responsible for myelination of neurons in the CNS and appear as small cells with condensed chromatin. Tumors on histopathology often demonstrate a unique honeycomb appearance and increased proliferation of blood vessels (Figs. 15.79D and 15.80).

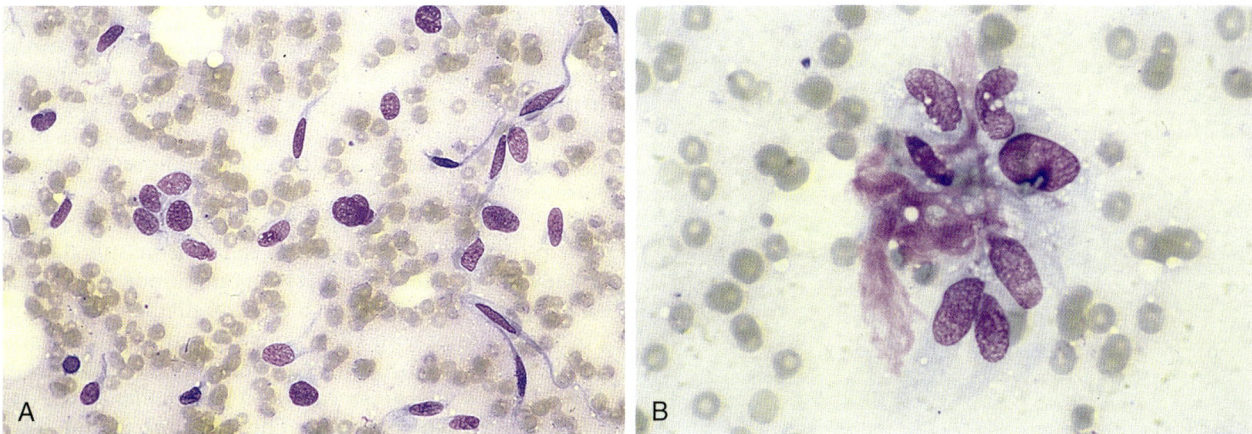

■ **FIGURE 15.78 Malignant nerve sheath tumor. Tissue imprint. Dog.** Same case in A and B. Clinical presentation included paraparesis that progressed to tetraparesis. A mass within the spinal canal at the C2–C3 nerve root was resected but recurred 2 months later. **A,** Spindle cells predominate with two populations present. Some cells have elongated fusiform nuclei, and others have plump round to oval nuclei. The cytoplasm forms tails more distinct on the more elongated cells. (Wright-Giemsa; HP oil.) **B,** Aggregate of neoplastic cells with associated amorphous eosinophilic collagenous stroma. Cells have oval nuclei with coarse chromatin, small distinct nucleoli, and vacuolated scant pale blue cytoplasm. Histopathologic diagnosis was neurofibrosarcoma. Malignancy cannot be determined by cytopathology. (Wright-Giemsa; HP oil.)

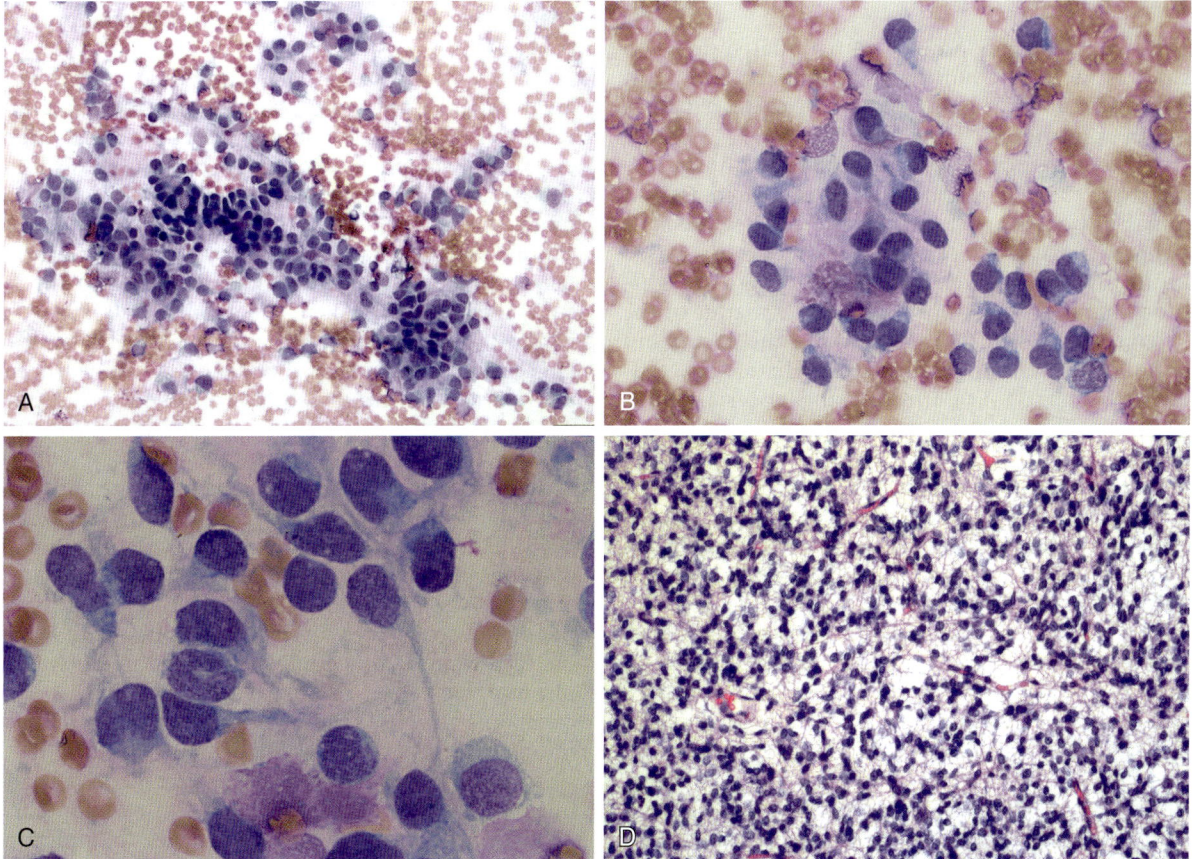

■ **FIGURE 15.79 Oligodendroglioma. Brain.** Same case in A to D. **Dog.** Clinical signs were seizures that began clustering in this 2-year-old dog. Magnetic resonance imaging indicated a 1.1 × 1.2 × 1.3 cm mass in the left frontal lobe, and the cerebrospinal fluid revealed no abnormalities. Surgical biopsy resulted in mass imprints and a histopathology specimen. **A–C, Cytopathologic preparations. A,** Dense aggregates and loose individualized cells produce a highly cellular specimen. (Wright-Giemsa; IP.) **B,** Individualized cells are enmeshed in an eosinophilic wispy matrix. (Wright-Giemsa; HP oil.) **C,** Round to ovoid nuclei have scant to moderate amounts of wispy basophilic cytoplasmic extensions. Chromatin is finely stippled with indiscernible nucleoli. (Wright-Giemsa; HP oil.) **D,** Individualized hyperchromic nuclei surrounded by clear spaces and fine wispy matrix along with linear arrays of capillaries. (H&E; IP.) (A–D, Courtesy Rose Raskin, University of Florida.)

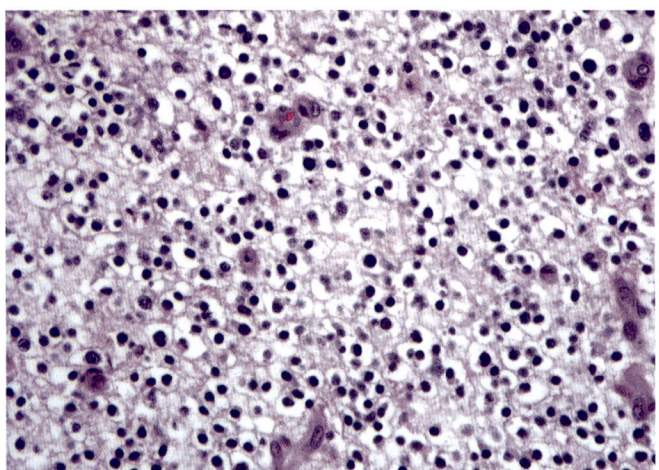

FIGURE 15.80 Oligodendroglioma. Brain. Tissue section. Classic histopathology with hyperchromic round cells with a perinuclear halo producing a honeycomb appearance. Cross-sections of capillaries are visible along with an eosinophilic wispy intercellular matrix. (H&E; IP.) (Courtesy Rose Raskin, University of Florida.)

Astrocytoma. Astrocytes provide nutritional support to neurons, act as metabolic buffers or detoxifiers, and assist in repair and scar formation. They have been described as histiocytic in appearance (Fernandez et al., 1997). An example of reactive astrocytes was described previously (see Figs. 15.57 to 15.59). There may be an increased risk of astrocytomas in boxers and Boston terriers. They are subdivided into two distinct morphological subgroups based on an infiltrative versus well-circumscribed growth pattern. Astrocytomas arise mainly within white matter of the cerebral hemispheres, and they can invade the cortex but generally not into the ventricular system. Histologic grading of astrocytomas (I–IV) involves the criteria of increased cell density, nuclear atypia, and mitotic count (Higgins et al., 2017).

Astrocytomas examined by crush preparation or aspirate biopsy preserve the cytoplasmic features of an eccentrically placed nucleus within a moderately abundant basophilic cytoplasm with prominent nucleoli (Fig. 15.81A–C). High mitotic activity is associated with a grade III or IV (Fig. 15.81D). GFAP is a marker used to distinguish astrocytes (Hostetter et al., 2018) from other neuroglial and meningeal cells but it may sometimes yield a positive reaction in neuroepithelial tumors, such as ependymoma and choroid plexus tumor (Fernandez et al., 1997), and meningeal tumors (Montoliu et al., 2006).

Recent articles in veterinary medicine have evaluated the expression of immunohistochemical markers (see Table 15.4) to classify cerebral and spinal cord canine gliomas (Higgins et al., 2017; Rissi et al., 2017; Kishimoto et al., 2018). A simplified classification scheme of canine glioma based on histopathology and immunohistochemistry results was carried out in a large comprehensive review to collect clinical outcome and molecular data in a defined way (Koehler et al., 2018). The immunohistochemical panel proposed includes GFAP for astrocytic neoplasms with some limitations, Olig2, which may not reliably differentiate between astrocytic and oligodendrocytic lineage; CNPase, a myelinating enzyme specific to oligodendrocytes and Schwann cells; and Ki67, a marker of proliferation (growth fraction rate) even if its use as prognostic indicator of cerebral high-grade gliomas is still debated (Stoyanov et al., 2017).

Ependymoma. The ependymal cells line the ventricular system of the brain and central canal of the spinal cord. The ependymoma (see Table 15.4) is a rare tumor (Fig. 15.82). An anaplastic ependymoma in a dog was diagnosed from partial positive staining with GFAP and vimentin but a negative reaction with S-100, CD3, and cytokeratin (Fernandez et al., 1997). In a study of 18 cats with ventricular and extraventricular ependymal tumors, clinical signs included altered behavior, seizures, circling, abnormal gait, generalized discomfort, and poor condition (Woolford et al., 2013). These cats had intraventricular masses that often arose from the lining of the lateral or third ventricles. On histopathology, perivascular pseudorosettes were observed in all of the ependymomas; however, true rosettes with a core of cell processes were less common. Some tumors had areas of necrosis, mineralization, cholesterol clefts, or hemorrhage. Most feline ependymomas reacted to GFAP immunostaining (Woolford et al., 2013).

Choroid plexus tumor. The choroid plexus cells represent a highly vascular portion of the pia mater that projects into the ventricles of the brain and is thought to secrete CSF. Positive cytokeratin staining is expected in choroid plexus tumors (see Table 15.4). A cytopathologic example of a choroid plexus tumor is shown as an imprint of the tumor mass (Fig. 15.83). The choroid plexus tumors were associated with increased CSF protein concentration and increased CSF nucleated cell count in a study (Bailey and Higgins, 1986; Lipsitz et al., 1999). These cells within the CSF appear similar to mesothelial cells, having a large, round nucleus with abundant, well-defined, deeply basophilic cytoplasm having surface projections (Fig. 15.83C). A papillary appearance with epithelial features can be seen in cytopathologic preparations of choroid plexus papilloma (see Fig. 15.83A). Two choroid plexus carcinomas were misdiagnosed by cytopathology as choroid plexus papillomas (De Lorenzi et al., 2006). Both of these tumors occurred within a ventricular site and consisted of large, pedunculated, friable masses that presented as well-formed papillary structures, usually showing a fine fibrovascular core covered by uniform cuboidal or columnar epithelium having minimal cytologic atypia with moderate pleomorphism (Fig. 15.84A). The final histologic diagnosis of carcinoma was based on the presence of single-cell infiltration into the fibrovascular cores, suggesting that a definitive diagnosis of choroid plexus carcinoma can be made only after thorough histologic examination of the resected specimen (Fig. 15.84B). MRI and CSF analysis were helpful in determining a difference between choroid plexus papilloma and choroid plexus carcinoma (Westworth et al., 2008). In this study, golden retrievers were overrepresented compared with the hospital population, and median CSF protein concentration in carcinomas was 108 mg/dL (range, 27–380 mg/dL), which was significantly higher compared with papillomas, whose median was 34 mg/dL (range, 32–80 mg/dL).

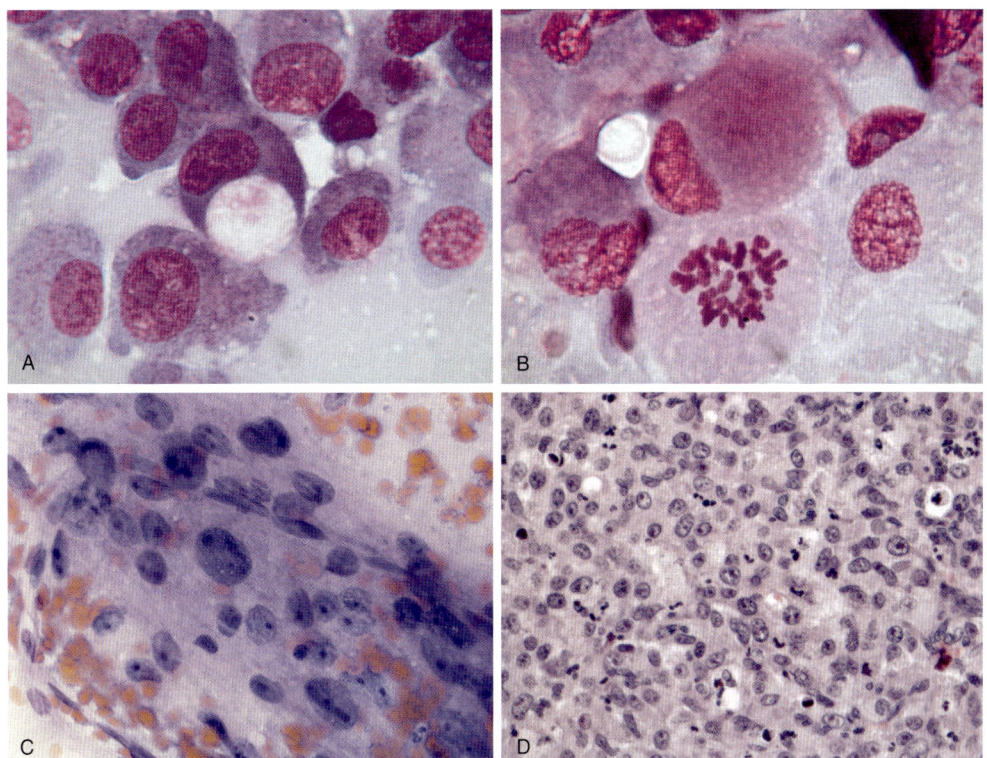

■ **FIGURE 15.81 Astrocytoma. A, Brain. Squash preparation. Dog.** Pleomorphic cells are individualized, having an eccentrically placed nucleus with prominent nucleoli and moderately abundant, deeply basophilic cytoplasm, giving them a plasma cell–like appearance. One cell appears to contain a vacuole. (MGG; HP oil.) **B, Spinal mass. Squash preparation from surgical biopsy. Cat.** This intradural spinal mass is composed of large cells with an eccentrically placed nucleus and abundant pink, granular cytoplasm, giving the appearance of a histiocytic cell; a mitotic figure is observed. A positive immunohistochemical stain for glial fibrillary acid protein was determined that confirmed the astrocytic origin. (MGG; HP oil.) **C, Brain mass. Intraoperative aspirate specimen. Dog.** History of head tilt, circling, ataxia, and change in mentation. Magnetic resonance imaging revealed a circular mass within the caudal fossa. The mass was approximately 17 × 21 × 15 mm in diameter. Diffuse, strongly positive cytoplasmic staining with glial fibrillary acid protein and negative immunoreactivity for synaptophysin supported the diagnosis on histopathology. The predominant cell was a pleomorphic cell population that formed clumps and loose clusters around small blood vessels, appearing as a linear array. Cells borders of the neoplastic cells were indistinct with moderate to abundant, slightly granular, amphophilic cytoplasm. Nuclei were round to oval with stippled chromatin and prominent nucleoli. These cells exhibited marked anisokaryosis with often abnormally shaped nucleoli. (Modified Wright; HP oil.) **D, Spinal mass. Tissue section. Cat.** Medium-grade astrocytoma (anaplastic astrocytoma) with astrocytic neoplastic population characterized by high cellularity and pleomorphism, marked nuclear atypia, and several mitotic figures. (H&E; IP.) (C, Courtesy Shannon Hostetter, Iowa State University.)

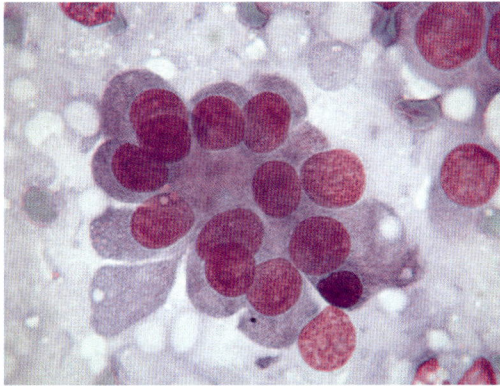

■ **FIGURE 15.82 Ependymoma. Spinal mass. Squash preparation from surgical biopsy. Dog.** These monomorphic cuboidal cells are arranged in a tight cluster with a true rosette pattern. There are mild anisokaryosis and occasional prominent nucleoli. Nuclei are round with uniform chromatin features. Cytoplasm is scant to moderately abundant and pink-blue with fine granularity giving them a plasma cell–like appearance. (MGG; HP oil.)

A potential diagnostic pitfall among tumors of different neuroectodermal and non-neuroectodermal origin can arise with ependymal or choroid plexus tumors and metastasis from well-differentiated adenocarcinomas. In fact, these two categories of neoplasms can share some analogous cytomorphologic findings such as epithelioid aspects with cohesive glandlike fragments, round to polygonal cellular shape, and well-defined cytoplasm with distinct margins and round nuclei often with evident nucleoli. Additional information, such as the age of the patient, the precise location within the brain or spinal cord, and a complete clinical history, especially the presence of a known primary tumor, may be critical in making the correct diagnosis.

Extramedullary Tumors

Cytopathologic features of a canine nephroblastoma (see Table 15.4) involving the thoracolumbar spinal nerves have been described in two young dogs (Neel and Dean, 2000; De Lorenzi et al., 2007). The pseudorosette formation and cytokeratin reactivity help to differentiate the nephroblastoma from tumors of neuroepithelial origin.

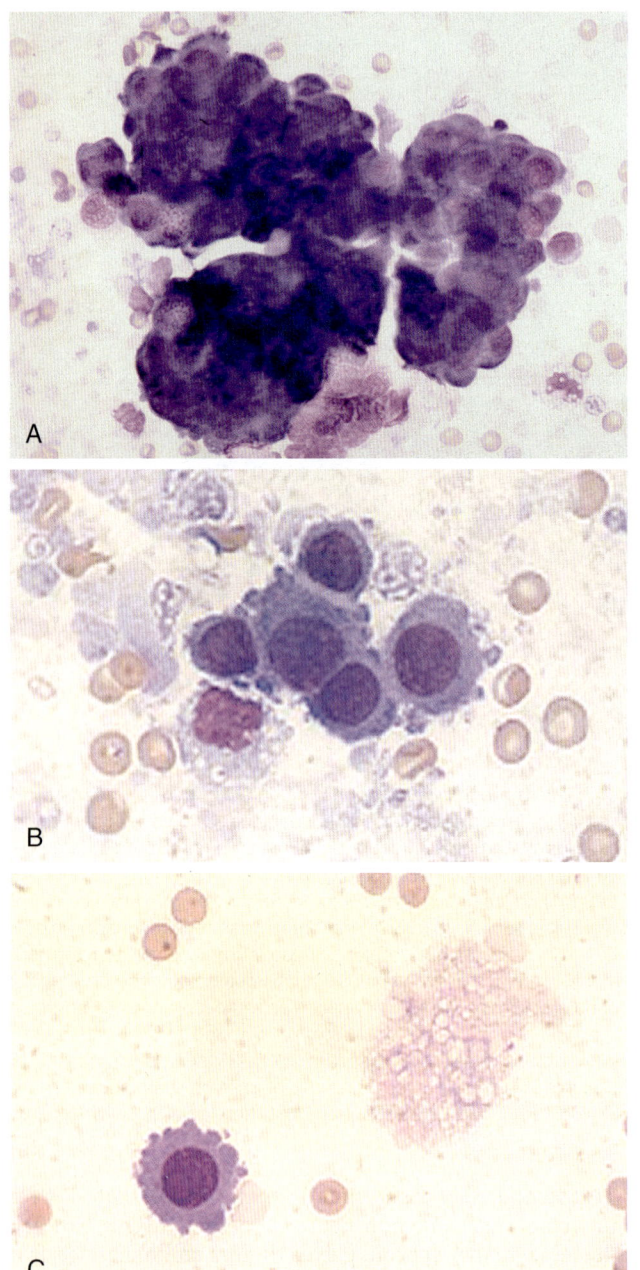

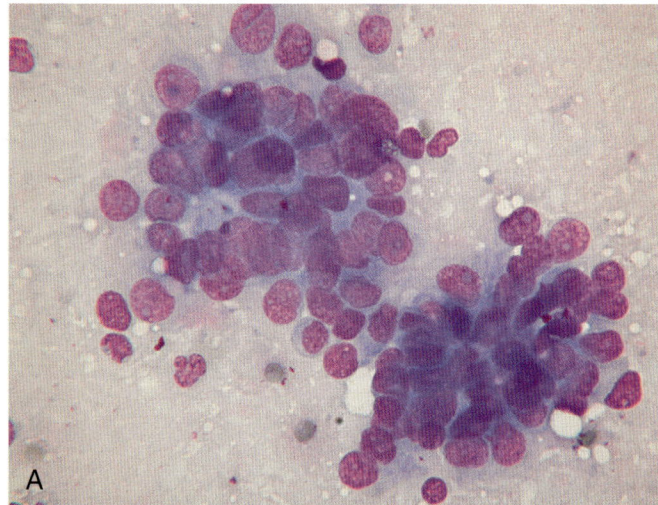

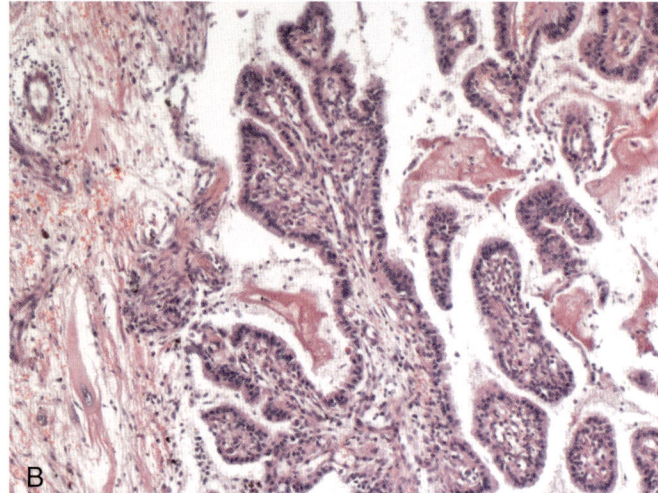

■ **FIGURE 15.84 Choroid plexus carcinoma. Dog.** Same case in A and B. **A, Squash preparation.** Cells are grouped in tight clusters with an acinar-like appearance. There are moderate anisokaryosis, prominent nucleoli, coarse chromatin, and a high nucleocytoplasmic ratio. These cytomorphologic features suggest a carcinoma that has metastasized from well-differentiated tumor cells. (MGG; HP oil.) **B, Tissue section.** Papillary figures are characterized by cuboidal to columnar neoplastic neuroepithelial cells of one or more layers in thickness. The adjacent subependymal brain tissue is affected by severe edema and glial reaction. (H&E; LP.)

■ **FIGURE 15.83 Choroid plexus papilloma. Dog.** Same case in A to C. Seizure, dementia, ataxia, and tetraparesis were clinical signs present in this dog in which magnetic resonance imaging revealed a ventricular mass. **A–B, Ventricular mass imprint. A,** The sample was highly cellular with large, densely clustered cohesive cells with scant to moderately abundant, deeply basophilic cytoplasm. Contrast tumor cell size with the erythrocytes. (Wright-Giemsa; HP oil.) **B,** Higher magnification demonstrating the tight cohesion between cells. The nucleocytoplasmic ratio is high. The nucleus is round with finely granular chromatin and large prominent nucleoli. The cytoplasm is basophilic and finely granular. (Wright-Giemsa; HP oil.) **C, Cerebrospinal fluid specimen.** The fluid had increased protein concentration (98 mg/dL) and a normal total nucleated cell count. One neoplastic cell was present in two cytocentrifuge preparations. The nucleus is very large and round with dispersed chromatin and a single prominent nucleolus. The cytoplasm is dark blue with smooth surface projections. To the right of the cell is granular, pink-gray, vacuolated material with an indistinct irregular border, consistent with myelin, suggesting a degenerative process. (Wright-Giemsa; HP oil.)

REFERENCES

Abate O, Bollo E, Lotti D, et al. Cytological, immunocytochemical and biochemical cerebrospinal fluid investigations in selected central nervous system disorder of dogs. *J Vet Med Series B*. 1998;45:73-85.

Alcoverro E, Bersan E, Sanchez-Masianet D, et al. Eosinophilic cerebrospinal fluid pleocytosis associated with neural *Angiostrongylus vasorum* infection in a dog. *Vet Clin Pathol*. 2019;48(1):78-82.

Amude AM, Alfieri AA, Balarin MRS, et al. Cerebrospinal fluid from a 7-month-old dog with seizure-like episodes. *Vet Clin Pathol*. 2006;35:119-122.

Aroch I, Baneth G, Salant H, et al. *Neospora caninum* and *Ehrlichia canis* co-infection in a dog with meningoencephalitis. *Vet Clin Pathol*. 2018;7: 289-293.

Bailey CS, Higgins RJ. Characteristics of cerebrospinal fluid associated with canine granulomatous meningoencephalomyelitis: a retrospective study. *J Am Vet Med Assoc*. 1986;88:418-421.

Barber RM, Li Q, Diniz PPVP, et al. Evaluation of brain tissue or cerebrospinal fluid with broadly reactive polymerase chain reaction for *Ehrlichia*, *Anaplasma*, spotted fever group *Rickettsia*, *Bartonella*, and *Borrelia* species in canine neurological diseases (109 cases). *J Vet Intern Med*. 2010;4(2):372-378.

Barnhart KF, Wojcieszyn J, Storts RW. Immunohistochemical staining patterns of canine meningiomas and correlation with published immunophenotypes. *Vet Pathol*. 2002;9(3):311-321.

Baroni M, Heinold Y. A review of the clinical diagnosis of feline infectious peritonitis viral meningoencephalitis. *Prog Vet Neurol*. 1995;6:88-94.

Bauer NB, Basset H, O'Neill EJ, et al. Cerebrospinal fluid from a 6-year-old dog with severe neck pain. *Vet Clin Pathol*. 2006;35:123-125.

Behling-Kelly E, Petersen S, Muthuswamy A, et al. Neoplastic pleocytosis in a dog with metastatic mammary carcinoma and meningeal carcinomatosis. *Vet Clin Pathol*. 2010;39(2):247-252.

Behr S, Cauzinille L. Aseptic suppurative meningitis in juvenile boxer dogs: retrospective study of 12 cases. *J Am Anim Hosp Assoc*. 2006;42:277-282.

Behr S, Trumel C, Cauzinille L, et al. High resolution protein electrophoresis of 100 paired canine cerebrospinal fluid and serum. *J Vet Intern Med*. 2006;20:657-662.

Berthelin CF, Legendre AM, Bailey CS, et al. Cryptococcosis of the nervous system in dogs, part 2: diagnosis, treatment, monitoring, and prognosis. *Prog Vet Neurol*. 1994;5:136-145.

Bienzle D, Kwiecien JM, Parent JM. Extramedullary hematopoiesis in the choroid plexus of five dogs. *Vet Pathol*. 1995;32:437-440.

Bienzle D, McDonnell JJ, Stanton JB. Analysis of cerebrospinal fluid from dogs and cats after 24 and 48 hours of storage. *J Am Vet Med Assoc*. 2000;216:1761-1764.

Bisby TM, Holman PJ, Pitoc GA, et al. *Sarcocystis* sp. encephalomyelitis in a cat. *Vet Clin Pathol*. 2010;39:105-112.

Boettcher IC, Steinberg T, Matiasek K. Use of anti-coronavirus antibody testing of cerebrospinal fluid for diagnosis of feline infectious peritonitis involving the central nervous system. *J Am Vet Med Assoc*. 2007;230:199-206.

Bohn AA, Willis TB, West CL, et al. Cerebrospinal fluid analysis and magnetic resonance imaging in the diagnosis of neurologic disease in dogs: a retrospective study. *Vet Clin Pathol*. 2006;35:315-320.

Bray KY, Muñana K, Meichner K, et al. Eosinophilic meningomyelitis associated with T-cell lymphoma in a cat. *Vet Clin Pathol*. 2016;45(4):698-702.

Bush WW, Barr C, Darrin EW, et al. Results of cerebrospinal fluid analysis, neurological examination findings, and age at the onset of seizures as predictors for results of magnetic resonance imaging of the brain in dogs examined because of seizures: 115 cases (1992-2000). *J Am Vet Med Assoc*. 2002;220:781-784.

Caines D, Sinclair M, Wood D, et al. Evaluation of cerebrospinal fluid lactate and plasma lactate concentrations in anesthetized dogs with and without intracranial disease. *Can J Vet Res*. 2013;77:297-302.

Cardy TJA, Cornelis I. Clinical presentation and magnetic resonance imaging findings in 11 dogs with eosinophilic meningoencephalitis of unknown etiology. *J Small Anim Pract*. 2018;59:422-431.

Caswell JL, Nykamp SG. Intradural vasculitis and hemorrhage in full sibling Welsh springer spaniels. *Can Vet J*. 2003;44:137-139.

Cellio BC. Collecting, processing, and preparing cerebrospinal fluid in dogs and cats. *Compend Contin Educ Pract Vet*. 2001;23:786-794.

Chai O, Yas E, Brenner O, et al. Clinical characteristics of *Spirocerca lupi* migration in the spinal cord. *Vet Parasitol*. 2018;253:16-21.

Chrisman CL. Cerebrospinal fluid analysis. *Vet Clin North Am Small Anim Pract*. 1992;22:781-810.

Christopher MM. Bone marrow contamination of canine cerebrospinal fluid. *Vet Clin Pathol*. 1992;21:95-98.

Cizinauskas S, Jaggy A, Tipold A. Long-term treatment of dogs with steroid-responsive meningitis-arteritis: clinical, laboratory and therapeutic results. *J Small Anim Pract*. 2000;41:295-301.

Clemmons RM. Therapeutic considerations for degenerative myelopathy of German shepherds. *Proceedings of the 9th ACVIM Forum*. New Orleans: 1991:773-775.

Cluzel C, Aboulmali AA, Dugas S, et al. Diffuse leptomeningeal histiocytic sarcoma in the cerebrospinal fluid of 2 dogs. *Vet Clin Pathol*. 2016;45(1):184-190.

Coates JR, Jeffery ND. Perspectives on meningoencephalitis of unknown origin. *Vet Clin North Am Small Anim Pract*. 2014;44:1157-1185.

Cornelis I, Van Hama L, Gielen I, et al. Clinical presentation, diagnostic findings, prognostic factors, treatment and outcome in dogs with meningoencephalomyelitis of unknown origin: a review. *Vet J*. 2019;244:37-44.

D'Agostino PM, Gottfried-Blackmore A, Anandasabapathy N, et al. Brain dendritic cells: biology and pathology. *Acta Neuropathol*. 2012;124:599-614.

de la Fuente C, Monreal L, Cerón J, et al. Fibrinolytic activity in cerebrospinal fluid of dogs with different neurological disorders. *J Vet Intern Med*. 2012;26(6):1365-1373.

De Lorenzi D, Baroni M, Mandara MT. A true "triphasic" pattern: thoracolumbar spinal tumor in a young dog. *Vet Clin Pathol*. 2007;36:200-203.

De Lorenzi D, Mandara MT, Tranquillo M, et al. Squash-prep cytology in the diagnosis of canine and feline nervous system lesions: a study of 42 cases. *Vet Clin Pathol*. 2006;35:208-214.

Dickinson PJ, Keel MK, Higgins RJ, et al. Clinical and pathologic features of oligodendrogliomas in two cats. *Vet Pathol*. 2000;37:160-167.

Dickinson PJ, Sturges BK, Kass PH, et al. Characteristics of cisternal cerebrospinal fluid associated with intracranial meningiomas in dogs: 56 cases (1985-2004). *J Am Vet Med Assoc*. 2006;228:564-567.

Di Terlizzi R, Platt S. The function, composition and analysis of cerebrospinal fluid in companion animals: part I—function and composition. *Vet J*. 2006;172:422-431.

Doenges SJ, Weber K, Dorsch R, et al. Detection of feline coronavirus in cerebrospinal fluid for diagnosis of feline infectious peritonitis in cats with and without neurological signs. *J Feline Med Surg*. 2016;8(2):104-109.

Doyle C, Solano-Gallego L. Cytologic interpretation of canine cerebrospinal fluid samples with low total nucleated cell concentration, with and without blood contamination. *Vet Clin Pathol*. 2009;38(3):392-396.

Duque C, Parent J, Bienzle D. The immunophenotype of blood and cerebrospinal fluid mononuclear cells in dogs. *J Vet Intern Med*. 2002;16:714-719.

Early PJ, Munana KJ, Olby NR, et al. Comparison of cerebrospinal fluid parameters from the cerebellomedullary and lumbar cisterns in 54 dogs. *Can Vet J*. 2019;60(8):885-888.

Fallin CW, Raskin RE, Harvey JW. Cytologic identification of neural tissue in the cerebrospinal fluid of two dogs. *Vet Clin Pathol*. 1996;25:127-129.

Falzone C, Baroni M, De Lorenzi D, et al. *Toxoplasma gondii* brain granuloma in a cat: diagnosis using cytology from an intraoperative sample and sequential magnetic resonance imaging. *J Small Anim Pract*. 2008;49:95-99.

Fenner WR. Diseases of the brain. In: Ettinger SJ, Feldman EC, eds. *Textbook of Veterinary Internal Medicine*. 5th ed. Philadelphia: WB Saunders; 2000:552-602.

Fernandez FR, Grindem CB, Brown TT, et al. Cytologic and histologic features of a poorly differentiated glioma in a dog. *Vet Clin Pathol*. 1997;26:182-186.

Ferreira A. Diagnostic value of creatine kinase activity in canine cerebrospinal fluid. *Can Vet J*. 2016;57(10):1081-1086.

Fluhemann G, Konar M, Jaggy A, et al. Cerebral cholesterol granuloma in a cat. *J Vet Intern Med*. 2006;20:1241-1244.

Fry MM, Vernau W, Kass PH, et al. Effects of time, initial composition, and stabilizing agents on the results of canine cerebrospinal fluid analysis. *Vet Clin Pathol*. 2006;35:72-77.

Gaitero L, Anor S, Montoliu P, et al. Detection of *Neospora caninum* tachyzoites in canine cerebrospinal fluid. *J Vet Intern Med*. 2006;20:410-414.

Galgut BI, Janardhan KS, Grondin TM, et al. Detection of *Neospora caninum* tachyzoites in cerebrospinal fluid of a dog following prednisone and cyclosporine therapy. *Vet Clin Pathol*. 2010;39(3):386-390.

Galloway AM, Curtis NC, Sommerlad SF, et al. Correlative imaging findings in seven dogs and one cat with spinal arachnoid cyst. *Vet Radiol Ultrasound*. 1999;40:445-452.

Gama FGV, Santana AE, de Campos Filho E, et al. Agarose gel electrophoresis of cerebrospinal fluid proteins of dogs after sample concentration using a membrane microconcentrator technique. *Vet Clin Pathol*. 2007;36:85-88.

Gandini G, Cizinauskas S, Lang J, et al. Fibrocartilaginous embolism in 75 dogs: clinical findings and factors influencing the recovery rate. *J Small Anim Pract*. 2003;44(2):76-80.

Gardini A, de Brot S, Cherubini GB. Pathology in practice: neuronal ceroid lipofuscinosis in a Jack Russell terrier. *J Am Vet Med Assoc*. 2019;254(3):359-362.

Garma-Aviña A. Cytology of the normal and abnormal choroid plexi in selected domestic mammals, wildlife species, and man. *J Vet Diagn Invest*. 2004;16:283-292.

Garma-Aviña A, Tyler JW. Large granular lymphocyte pleocytosis in the cerebrospinal fluid of a dog with necrotizing meningoencephalitis. *J Comp Pathol*. 1999;121:83-87.

Glass EN, Cornetta AM, deLahunta A, et al. Clinical and clinicopathologic features in 11 cats with *Cuterebra* larvae myiasis of the central nervous system. *J Vet Intern Med*. 1998;12:365-368.

Grano FG, Dos S. Silva JE, et al. T lymphocyte immunophenotypes in the cerebrospinal fluid of dogs with visceral leishmaniasis. *Vet Parasitol*. 2016;232:12-20.

Greenberg MJ, Schatzberg SJ, deLahunta A, et al. Intracerebral plasma cell tumor in a cat: a case report and literature review. *J Vet Intern Med*. 2004;18:581-585.

Gruendl S, Matiasek K, Matiasek L, et al. Diagnostic utility of cerebrospinal fluid immunocytochemistry for diagnosis of feline infectious peritonitis manifesting in the central nervous system. *J Feline Med Surg*. 2017;9(6):576-585.

Gupta A, Gumber S, Bauer RW, et al. What is your diagnosis? Cerebrospinal fluid from a dog [Protothecosis]. *Vet Clin Pathol*. 2011;40(1):105-106.

Hare C, Sanchini L, Worrall C, et al. Rapid in-house method of CSF analysis utilising sedimentation direct from the spinal needle. *J Small Anim Pract*. 2019;60:486-492.

Higgins RJ, Bollen AW, Dickinson PJ, et al. Tumors of the nervous system. In: Meuten DJ, ed. *Tumors in Domestic Animals*. 5th ed. Ames: John Wiley and Sons; 2017:834-891.

Higgins RJ, LeCouteur RA, Vernau KM, et al. Granular cell tumor of the canine central nervous system: two cases. *Vet Pathol*. 2001;38:620-627.

Hopkins AL, Garner M, Ackerman N, et al. Spinal meningeal sarcoma in a Rottweiler puppy. *J Small Anim Pract*. 1995;36:183-186.

Hostetter SJ, Hu HZ, Haynes JS. What is your diagnosis? Caudal fossa mass from a dog. *Vet Clin Pathol*. 2018;47:322-323.

Hurtt AE, Smith MO. Effects of iatrogenic blood contamination of results of cerebrospinal fluid analysis in clinically normal dogs and dogs with neurologic disease. *J Am Vet Med Assoc*. 1997;211:866-867.

Jacobs RM, Cochrane SM, Lumsden JH, et al. Relationship of cerebrospinal fluid protein concentration determined by dye-binding and urinary dipstick methodologies. *Can Vet J*. 1990;31:587-588.

Johnsrude JD, Alleman AR, Schumacher J, et al. Cytologic findings in cerebrospinal fluid from two animals with GM_2-gangliosidosis. *Vet Clin Pathol*. 1996;25:80-83.

Kishimoto TE, Uchida K, Thongtharb A, et al. Expression of oligodendrocyte precursor cell markers in canine oligodendrogliomas. *Vet Pathol*. 2018;55(5):634-644.

Klainbart S, Chai O, Vaturi R, et al. Nematode eggs observed in cytology of cerebrospinal fluid diagnostic for intramedullary *Spirocerca lupi* spinal cord migration. *Vet Clin Pathol*. 2018;47(1):138-141.

Koch BC, Daniels LO, Thomsen LT, et al. Collection of cerebrospinal fluid into EDTA versus plain tubes does not affect the standard analysis in dogs. *Acta Vet Scand*. 2019;61:23.

Koehler JW, Miller AD, Miller CR, et al. A revised diagnostic classification of canine glioma: towards validation of the canine glioma patient as a naturally occurring preclinical model for human glioma. *J Neuropathol Exp Neurol*. 2018;77(11):1039-1054.

Krimer PM, Haley AC, Harvey SB, et al. Evaluation of cytospin precision in low cellularity canine cerebrospinal fluid. *J Vet Diagn Invest*. 2016;28(2):158-164.

Lampe, R, Foss KD, Vitale S, et al. Comparison of cerebellomedullary and lumbar cerebrospinal fluid analysis in dogs with neurological disease. *J Vet Intern Med*. 2020;34(2):838-843.

Lane LV, Meinkoth JH, Brunker J, et al. Disseminated protothecosis diagnosed by evaluation of CSF in a dog. *Vet Clin Pathol*. 2012;41(1):147-152.

Levine GJ, Levine JM, Witsberger TH, et al. Cerebrospinal fluid myelin basic protein as a prognostic biomarker in dogs with thoracolumbar intervertebral disk herniation. *J Vet Intern Med*. 2010;24:890-896.

Levitin HA, Foss KD, Hague DW, et al. The utility of intraoperative impression smear cytology of intracranial granular cell tumors: three cases. *Vet Clin Pathol*. 2019;48:282-286.

Lipitz L, Rylander H, Pinkerton ME. Intramedullary epidermoid cyst in the thoracic spine of a dog. *J Am Anim Hosp Assoc*. 2011;47:e145-e149.

Lipsitz D, Levitski RE, Chauvet AE. Magnetic resonance imaging of a choroid plexus carcinoma and meningeal carcinomatosis in a dog. *Vet Radiol Ultrasound*. 1999;40:246-250.

Long SN, Anderson TJ, Long FHA, et al. Evaluation of rapid staining techniques for cytologic diagnosis of intracranial lesions. *Am J Vet Res*. 2002;3:381-386.

Lunn JA, Lee R, Smaller J, et al. Twenty two cases of canine neural angiostrongylosis in eastern Australia (2002-2005) and a review of the literature. *Parasit Vectors*. 2012;5:70.

MacNeill AL, Andre BG, Zingale Y, et al. The effects of iatrogenic blood contamination on total nucleated cell counts and protein concentrations in canine cerebrospinal fluid. *Vet Clin Pathol*. 2018;47(3):464-470.

Maiolini A, Carlson R, Schwartz M, et al. Determination of immunoglobulin A concentrations in the serum and cerebrospinal fluid of dogs: an estimation of its diagnostic value in canine steroid-responsive meningitis–arteritis. *Vet J*. 2012;191(2):219-224.

Marangoni NR, Melo GD, Moraes OC, et al. Levels of matrix metalloproteinase-2 and metalloproteinase-9 in the cerebrospinal fluid of dogs with visceral leishmaniasis. *Parasite Immunol*. 2011;33(6):330-334.

Marcos R, Malhao F, Santos J, et al. The cryptic Cryptococcus. *Vet Clin Pathol*. 2016b;45(4):532-533.

Marcos R, Santos M, Marrinhas C, et al. Cell tube block: a new technique to produce cell blocks from fluid cytology samples. *Vet Clin Pathol*. 2017;46(1):195-201.

Marcos R, Santos M, Marrinhas C, et al. Cytocentrifuge preparation in veterinary cytology: a quick, simple, and affordable manual method to concentrate low cellularity fluids. *Vet Clin Pathol*. 2016a;45(4):725-731.

Mariani CL, Boozer LB, Braxton AM, et al. Evaluation of matrix metalloproteinase-2 and -9 in the cerebrospinal fluid of dogs with intracranial tumors. *Am J Vet Res*. 2013;74(1):122-129.

Mariani CL, Nye CJ, Tokarz DA, et al. Cerebrospinal fluid lactate in dogs with inflammatory central nervous system disorders. *J Vet Intern Med*. 2019;33:2701-2708.

Mariani CL, Platt SR, Scase TJ, et al. Cerebral phaeohyphomycosis caused by *Cladosporum* spp. in two domestic shorthair cats. *J Am Anim Hosp Assoc*. 2002;38:225-230.

Mesher CI, Blue JT, Guffroy MRG, et al. Intracellular myelin in cerebrospinal fluid from a dog with myelomalacia. *Vet Clin Pathol*. 1996;25:124-126.

Messer JS, Kegge SJ, Cooper ES, et al. Meningoencephalomyelitis caused by *Pasteurella multocida* in a cat. *J Vet Intern Med*. 2006;20:1033-1036.

Mikszewski JS, Van Winkle TJ, Troxel MT. Fibrocartilaginous embolic myelopathy in five cats. *J Am Anim Hosp Assoc*. 2006;42:226-233.

Miller AD, Zachary JF. Nervous system. In: Zachary JF, ed. *Pathologic Basis of Veterinary Disease*. 6th ed. St Louis: Elsevier; 2017;805-907.

Moissonnier P, Blot S, Devauchelle P, et al. Stereotactic CT-guided brain biopsy in the dog. *J Small Anim Pract*. 2002;43:115-123.

Montoliu P, Añor S, Vidal E, et al. Histological and immunohistochemical study of 30 cases of canine meningioma. *J Comp Pathol*. 2006;135:200-207.

Moore PF. A review of histiocytic diseases of dogs and cats. *Vet Pathol*. 2014;51(1):167-184.

Munana KR, Luttgen PJ. Prognostic factors for dogs with granulomatous meningoencephalomyelitis: 42 cases (1982-1996). *J Am Vet Med Assoc*. 1998;212:1902-1906.

Nagano S, Kim SH, Tokunaga S, et al. Matrix metalloprotease-9 activity in the cerebrospinal fluid and spinal injury severity in dogs with intervertebral disc herniation. *Res Vet Sci*. 2011;91(3):482-485.

Neel J, Dean GA. A mass in the spinal column of a dog (nephroblastoma). *Vet Clin Pathol.* 2000;29:87-89.

Newton PL, Fry DR, Best MP. Comparison of direct in-house cerebrospinal fluid cytology with commercial pathology results in dogs. *J Small Anim Pract.* 2017;58(12):694-702.

Nye CJ, Mariani CL. Validation of a portable monitor for assessment of cerebrospinal fluid lactate in dogs. *Vet Clin Pathol.* 2018;47(1):108-114.

Olivier AK, Parkes JD, Flaherty HA, et al. Idiopathic eosinophilic meningoencephalomyelitis in a Rottweiler dog. *J Vet Diagn Invest.* 2010;22:646-648.

Peterson LN, Christian JA, Bentley RT, et al. Evaluation of the hydroxyethyl starch stabilizing agent, Vetstarch, in the preservation of canine cerebrospinal fluid samples. *Vet Clin Pathol.* 2020;49:95-99.

Platt SR, Alleman AR, Lanz OI, et al. Comparison of fine-needle aspiration and surgical-tissue biopsy in the diagnosis of canine brain tumors. *Vet Surg.* 2002;31:65-69.

Posporis C, Grau-Roma L, Travetti O, et al. Meningeal carcinomatosis and spinal cord infiltration caused by a locally invasive pulmonary adenocarcinoma in a cat. *JFMS Open Rep.* 2017;3(2):2055116917742812.

Pumarola M, Balash M. Meningeal carcinomatosis in a dog. *Vet Rec.* 1996;25:523-524.

Radaelli ST, Platt SR. Bacterial meningoencephalomyelitis in dogs: a retrospective study of 23 cases (1990-1999). *J Vet Intern Med.* 2002;16:159-163.

Rand JS, Parent J, Jacobs R, et al. Reference intervals for feline cerebrospinal fluid: cell counts and cytological features. *Am J Vet Res.* 1990;51:1044-1048.

Rand JS, Parent J, Percy D, et al. Clinical, cerebrospinal fluid and histological data from thirty-four cats with primary noninflammatory disease of the central nervous system. *Can Vet J.* 1994;35:174-181.

Raskin RE. An atypical spinal meningioma in a dog. *Vet Pathol.* 1984;21:538-540.

Rissi DR, Barber R, Burnum A, et al. Canine spinal cord glioma. *J Vet Diagn Invest.* 2017;29(1):126-132.

Ruotsalo K, Poma R, da Costa RC, et al. Evaluation of the ADVIA 120 for analysis of canine cerebrospinal fluid. *Vet Clin Pathol.* 2008;37:242-248.

Seo KW, Choi US, Lee JB, et al. Central nervous system relapses in 3 dogs with B-cell lymphoma. *Can Vet J.* 2011;52(7):778-783.

Sharkey LC, McDonnell JJ, Alroy J. Cytology of a mass on the meningeal surface of the left brain in a dog. *Vet Clin Pathol.* 2004;33:111-114.

Sheppard BJ, Chrisman CL, Newell SM, et al. Primary encephalic plasma cell tumor in a dog. *Vet Pathol.* 1997;34:621-627.

Singh M, Foster DJ, Child J, et al. Inflammatory cerebrospinal fluid analysis in cats: clinical diagnosis and outcome. *J Feline Med Surg.* 2005;7:77-93.

Sisò S, Marco-Salazar P, Moore PF, et al. Canine nervous system lymphoma subtypes display characteristic neuroanatomical patterns. *Vet Pathol.* 2017;54(1):53-60.

Skeen TM, Olby NJ, Munana KR, et al. Spinal arachnoid cysts in 17 dogs. *J Am Anim Hosp Assoc.* 2003;39:271-282.

Snyder JM, Shofer FS, Van Winkle TJ, et al. Canine intracranial primary neoplasia: 173 cases (1986-2003). *J Vet Intern Med.* 2006;20:669-765.

Soma T, Saito N, Kawaguchi M, et al. Feline coronavirus antibody titer in cerebrospinal fluid from cats with neurological signs. *J Vet Med Sci.* 2018;80(1):59-62.

Sorjonen DC. Clinical and histopathological features of granulomatous meningoencephalomyelitis in dogs. *J Am Anim Hosp Assoc.* 1990;26:141-147.

Stafford EG, Kortum A, Castel AC, et al. Presence of cerebrospinal fluid antibodies associated with autoimmune encephalitis of humans in dogs with neurologic disease. *J Vet Intern Med.* 2019;33(5):2175-2182.

Stalis IH, Chadwick B, Dayrell-Hart B, et al. Necrotizing meningoencephalitis of Maltese dogs. *Vet Pathol.* 1995;32:230-235.

Stampley AR, Swaynev DE, Prasse KW. Meningeal carcinomatosis secondary to a colonic signet-ring cell carcinoma in a dog. *J Am Anim Hosp Assoc.* 1986;23:655-658.

Stowe DM, Escobar C, Neel JA. What is your diagnosis? Cerebrospinal fluid from a dog (histiocytic sarcoma). *Vet Clin Pathol.* 2012;41(3):429-430.

Stoyanov GS, Dzhenkov DL, Kitanova M, et al. Correlation between Ki-67 index, World Health Organization grade and patient survival in glial tumors with astrocytic differentiation. *Cureus.* 2017;9(6):e1396.

Srugo I, Aroch I, Christopher MM, et al. Association of cerebrospinal fluid analysis findings with clinical signs and outcome in acute nonambulatory thoracolumbar disc disease in dogs. *J Vet Intern Med.* 2011;25:846-855.

Talarico, LR, Schatzberg, SJ. Idiopathic granulomatous and necrotising inflammatory disorders of the canine central nervous system: a review and future perspectives. *J Small Anim Pract.* 2010;51:138-149.

Theobald A, Volk HA, Dennis R, et al. Clinical outcome in 19 cats with clinical and magnetic resonance imaging diagnosis of ischaemic myelopathy (2000-2011). *J Fel Med Surg.* 2013;15:132-141.

Thompson CA, Russell KE, Levine JM, et al. Cerebrospinal fluid from a dog with neurologic collapse. *Vet Clin Pathol.* 2003;32:143-146.

Thomson CE, Kornegay JN, Stevens JB. Analysis of cerebrospinal fluid from the cerebellomedullary and lumbar cisterns of dogs with focal neurologic disease: 145 cases (1985-1987). *J Am Vet Med Assoc.* 1990;196:1841-1844.

Timmann D, Konar M, Howard J, et al. Necrotizing encephalitis in a French bulldog. *J Small Anim Pract.* 2007;48:339-342.

Tipold A, Fatzer R, Jaggy A, et al. Necrotizing encephalitis in Yorkshire terriers. *J Small Anim Pract.* 1993;34:623-628.

Tipold A, Schatzberg SJ. An update on steroid responsive meningitis-arteritis. *J Small Anim Pract.* 2010;51:150-154.

Tipold A, Vandevelde M, Zurbriggen A. Neuroimmunological studies in steroid-responsive meningitis-arteritis in dogs. *Res Vet Sci.* 1995;58:103-108.

Tremblay N, Lanevschi A, Doré M, et al. Of all the nerve! A subcutaneous forelimb mass in a cat. *Vet Clin Pathol.* 2005;34:417-420.

Troxel MT, Vite CH, Van Winkle TJ, et al. Feline intracranial neoplasia: review of 160 cases (1985-2001). *J Vet Intern Med.* 2003;17:850-859.

Tzipory L, Vernau KM, Sturges BK, et al. Antemortem diagnosis of localized central nervous system histiocytic sarcoma in 2 dogs. *J Vet Intern Med.* 2009;23:369-374.

Uchida K, Hasegawa T, Ikeda M, et al. Detection of an autoantibody from pug dogs with necrotizing encephalitis (pug dog encephalitis). *Vet Pathol.* 1999;36:301-307.

Uchida K, Park E, Tsuboi M, et al. Pathological and immunological features of canine necrotising meningoencephalitis and granulomatous meningoencephalitis. *Vet J.* 2016;213:72-77.

Vernau KM, Higgins RJ, Bollen AW, et al. Primary canine and feline nervous system tumours: intraoperative diagnosis using the smear technique. *Vet Pathol.* 2001;38:47-57.

Weber J, Maiolini A, Tipold A. Untersuchungen zu erniedrigten glukosewertenim liquor cerebrospinalis des hundes [Evaluation of decreased glucose levels in the cerebrospinal fluid of dogs]. *Tierarztl Prax Ausg K Kleintiere Heimtiere.* 2012;40(5):325-332.

Wessmann A, Volk HA, Chandler K, et al. Significance of surface epithelial cells in canine cerebrospinal fluid and relationship to central nervous system disease. *Vet Clin Pathol.* 2010;39:358-364.

Westworth DR, Dickinson PJ, Vernau W, et al. Choroid plexus tumors in 56 dogs (1985–2007). *J Vet Intern Med.* 2008;22:1157-1165.

Whittaker DE, English K, McGonnell IM, et al. Evaluation of cerebrospinal fluid in Cavalier King Charles Spaniel dogs diagnosed with Chiari-like malformation with or without concurrent syringomyelia. *J Vet Diagn Invest.* 2011;23:302-307.

Windsor RC, Sturges BK, Vernau KM, et al. Cerebrospinal fluid eosinophilia in dogs. *J Vet Intern Med.* 2009;23(2):275-281.

Windsor RC, Vernau KM, Sturges BK, et al. Lumbar cerebrospinal fluid in dogs with type I intervertebral disc herniation. *J Vet Intern Med.* 2008;22:954-960.

Witsberger TH, Levine JM, Geoffrey T, et al. Associations between cerebrospinal fluid biomarkers and long-term neurologic outcome in dogs with acute intervertebral disk herniation. *J Am Vet Med Assoc.* 2012;240(5):555-562.

Woolford L, de Lahunta A, Baiker K, et al. Ventricular and extraventricular ependymal tumors in 18 cats. *Vet Pathol.* 2013;50(2):243-251.

Zabolotzky SM, Vernau KM, Kass PH, et al. Prevalence and significance of extracellular myelin-like material in canine cerebrospinal fluid. *Vet Clin Pathol.* 2010;39(1):90-95.

Zimmerman K, Almy F, Carter L, et al. Cerebrospinal fluid from a 10-year-old dog with a single seizure episode. *Vet Clin Pathol.* 2006;35:127-131.

Zimmerman KL, Bender HS, Boon GD, et al. A comparison of the cytologic and histologic features of meningiomas in four dogs. *Vet Clin Pathol.* 2000;29:29-34.

16 CHAPTER

Eyes and Ears

Pierre L. Deshuillers and Rose E. Raskin

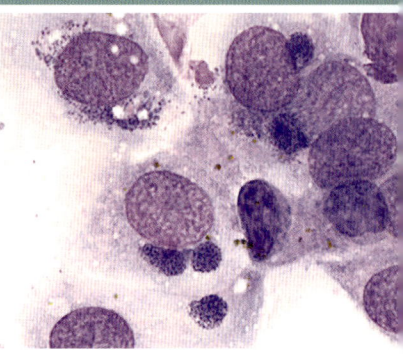

EYE AND ORBITAL STRUCTURES

Cytopathologic examination of the eye and surrounding structures is frequently helpful in determining the general categories of pathology before performing more invasive or expensive procedures. The following cytodiagnostic categories apply to the various anatomic sites of the eye. It should be noted that more than one presentation might occur in a specimen at a time.

General Cytodiagnostic Groups for Ocular Cytopathology
- Normal
- Cyst or hyperplasia
- Inflammation
- Neoplasia
- Response to tissue injury

Sample Collection and Preparation
Aspiration of focal and diffuse lesions is recommended for the lesions of the eyelid, eye, and other associated structures. Exudate material, duct washings, and aspirate material can be used as specimens of the nasolacrimal apparatus. Specialized collection techniques are discussed under the areas sampled by these methods.

EYELIDS

Normal Anatomy and Histology
The dorsal and ventral eyelids are thin extensions of facial skin that meet at the lateral and medial margins called canthi. Two to four rows of lashes are found on the upper eyelid at the free margin in dogs, whereas cats have only one row of cilia (Samuelson, 1999). The rostral surface (outermost layer) resembles typical skin, with keratinized squamous epithelium and numerous hair follicles that lie in close association with sebaceous and modified sweat glands (Fig. 16.1). Striated muscle fibers course through the deeper layers. The caudal surface or innermost layer is the palpebral conjunctiva and is lined by pseudostratified squamous to columnar epithelium that may contain goblet cells. Near the margins of both eyelids deep to the palpebral conjunctiva are the Meibomian or tarsal glands (see Fig. 16.1). These modified sebaceous glands lie adjacent to the palpebral conjunctiva and empty into a duct that opens onto the palpebral surface near the junction between keratinized and nonkeratinized squamous epithelium. These secretions contribute to the lipid component of the tear film along with the goblet cell secretions.

Inflammation
Blepharitis refers to inflammatory conditions of the eyelid. On cytopathology, the predominant cell type categorizes the inflammation. Neutrophilic or purulent blepharitis most often involves bacteria such as *Staphylococcus* and *Streptococcus* spp.; however, immune-mediated disease or foreign body reactions may result in purulent inflammation. Eosinophilic inflammation should be considered for allergic reactions, some autoimmune conditions, parasitic migration (*Cuterebra* spp.), and conditions associated with collagen degeneration. Dermatophytosis or other fungal infections may be associated with granulomatous inflammation containing macrophages alone or mixed with other cell types.

Chalazion, or meibomian adenitis, refers to the granuloma formed from a foreign body reaction to the sebaceous secretion product of the Meibomian glands. It is often associated with Meibomian gland neoplasms such as adenomas or epitheliomas, which can cause blockages. In this situation, numerous foamy macrophages, few giant cells, neutrophils, lymphocytes, amorphous debris, sebaceous epithelium, or basal cells are present (Black et al., 2018). In both histopathology and cytopathology, polarization demonstrates birefringent needle-shaped phagocytized sebum within macrophages (Fig. 16.2). *Hordeolum* refers to a suppurative lesion resulting from infection of the eyelash follicles or Zeis, Moll, or Meibomian glands. Contrary to chalazion, hordeolum is characterized by the presence of septic suppurative inflammation.

Neoplasia
Diffuse neoplasms of the eyelids involve squamous cell carcinoma (SCC; especially in cats), sarcoma, mast cell tumor, and lymphoma. Focal presentations (Fig. 16.3) may involve sebaceous gland adenoma or adenocarcinoma (canine), papilloma (canine), mast cell tumor, benign and malignant melanoma, SCC, hemangioma, hemangiosarcoma, cutaneous basilar epithelial neoplasm, histiocytoma (Fig. 16.4), and other histiocytic neoplasms. Benign tumors predominate in dogs (Krehbiel and Langham, 1975; Roberts et al., 1986), whereas malignant neoplasms are more frequent in cats. In cats, these tumors are often locally invasive but rarely metastasize (Newkirk and Rohrbach, 2009). In dogs and cats, malignant neoplasms, such as apocrine sweat gland tumors, can invade the globe and extensively damage the eye (Hirai et al., 1997).

CHAPTER 16 Eyes and Ears

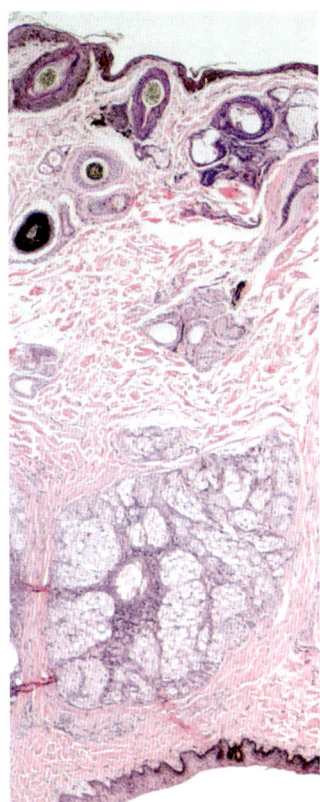

FIGURE 16.1 Eyelid. Histology. Dog. The top outermost layer resembles typical skin with keratinized squamous epithelium, hair follicles, and associated sebaceous and sweat glands. The innermost layer (palpebral conjunctiva) is lined by a pseudostratified squamous to columnar epithelium. Note the large sebaceous gland lobules (meibomian gland) adjacent to the palpebral conjunctiva. (H&E; LP).

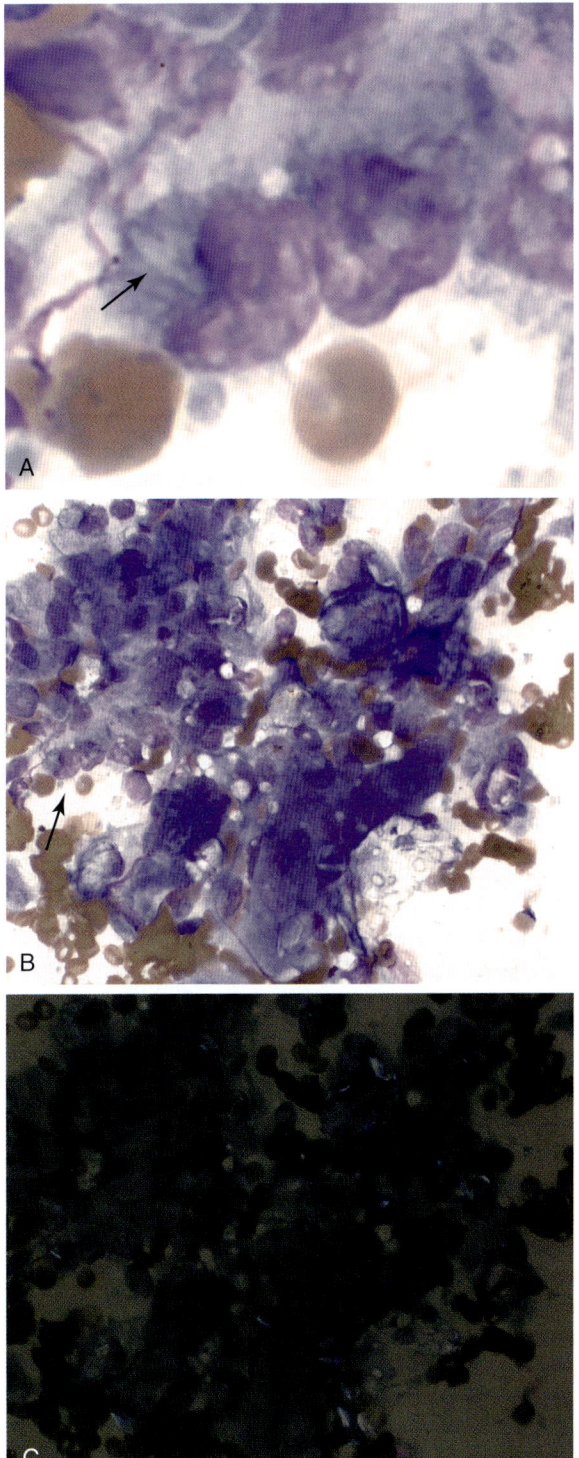

FIGURE 16.2 Macrophagic adenitis. Eyelid mass aspirate. Dog. Same case in A to C. **A,** High magnification of two macrophages, one of which contains a pale linear structure *(arrow)*. (Wright-Giemsa; HP oil.) **B,** Overview of field displaying macrophagic inflammation secondary to meibomian epithelioma (not shown). Note the location of the same two macrophages shown in part A *(arrow)*. (Wright-Giemsa; HP oil.) **C,** Polarization of the same field as shown in part B demonstrating bright birefringent needle-shaped sebum-containing structures throughout the specimen. Note the location of the macrophage, demonstrating birefringence of the linear structure shown in part A. (Polarized Wright-Giemsa; HP oil.) (A–C, Courtesy Laura Black and Mary Leissinger, University of Florida.)

CONJUNCTIVAE

Normal Anatomy and Histology

The palpebral conjunctiva is lined by a pseudostratified epithelium (see Fig. 16.1) with increasing numbers of goblet cells from the eyelid margin to the fornix. The *fornix* is the blind sac created at the junction of the palpebral and bulbar conjunctivae that is lined by stratified cuboidal to columnar epithelium containing many goblet cells. The palpebral conjunctiva is continuous with the bulbar conjunctiva, which reflects onto the globe and joins the corneal epithelium. The bulbar conjunctiva consists of sheets of stratified nonkeratinized squamous epithelium. The substantia propria of the conjunctiva is composed of two layers, a superficial layer, which in dogs and cats contains lymphatic follicles and glands, and a deep fibrous layer. The nerves and vessels of the conjunctiva are in the fibrous layer (Samuelson, 1999). There are no significant numbers of inflammatory cells; however, mucosa-associated lymphoid tissue (MALT) is located below the squamous layer of the palpebral conjunctiva near the fornix, where goblet cells are absent.

Sample Collection From the Conjunctiva

The thinner conjunctival tissue requires scraping with a blunt instrument such as an ophthalmic spatula or soft brush (Fig. 16.5). The use of a brush was shown to reduce

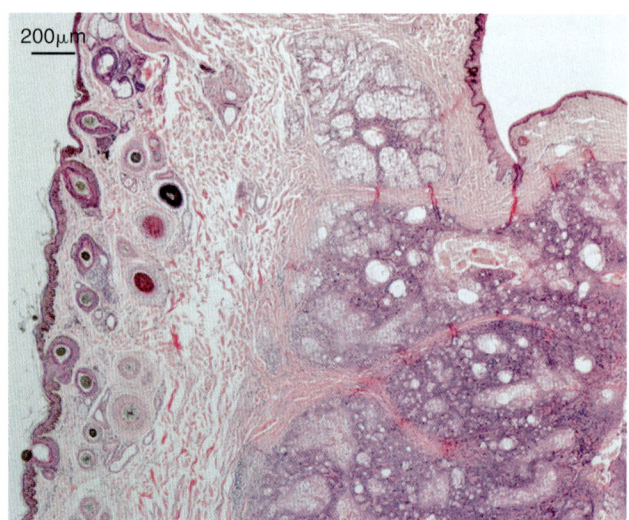

■ **FIGURE 16.3 Sebaceous epithelioma. Eyelid mass. Histopathology. Dog.** Focal adenomatous change is demonstrated within the sebaceous lobules. The mass is encapsulated with proliferation of adnexal epithelium. (H&E; LP.)

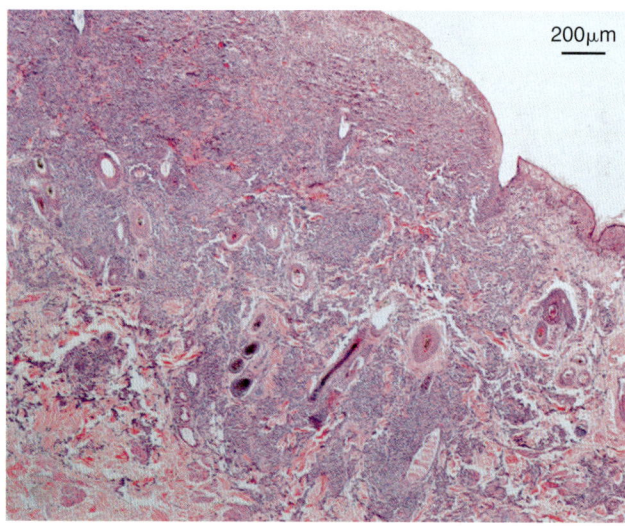

■ **FIGURE 16.4 Histiocytoma. Eyelid mass. Histopathology. Dog.** The dermis is densely populated with round cells in this neoplasm that presents with a top-heavy appearance of the tumor's growth pattern. (H&E; LP.)

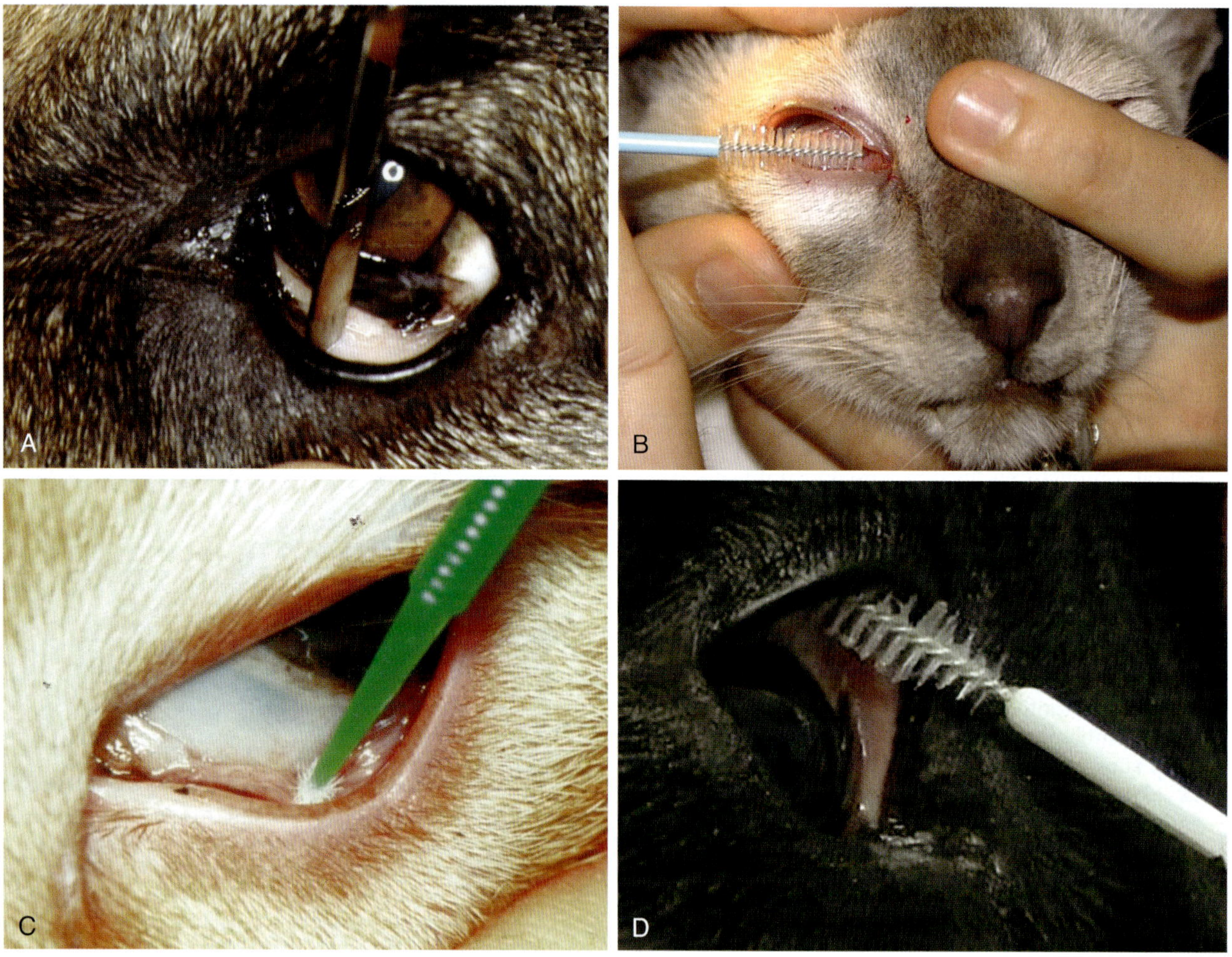

■ **FIGURE 16.5 Conjunctival sampling techniques. A, Dog. Kimura spatula.** The palpebral surface of the nictitating membrane is sampled. **B, Cat. Cytobrush.** Notice the animal handling and collection method. **C, Nylon bristle brush.** Collection of lower palpebral conjunctiva. **D, Dog. Cytobrush.** Collection of upper palpebral conjunctiva. (A, Courtesy Alain Regnier, Ecole Nationale Vétérinaire de Toulouse, France. B, Courtesy Thomas Dulaurent, Centre Hospitalier Vétérinaire Saint-Martin, France. C, From Greene CE. *Infectious Diseases of the Dog And Cat.* 4th ed. Elsevier; 2012. D, Courtesy Jean-Yves Douet, Ecole Nationale Vétérinaire de Toulouse, France.)

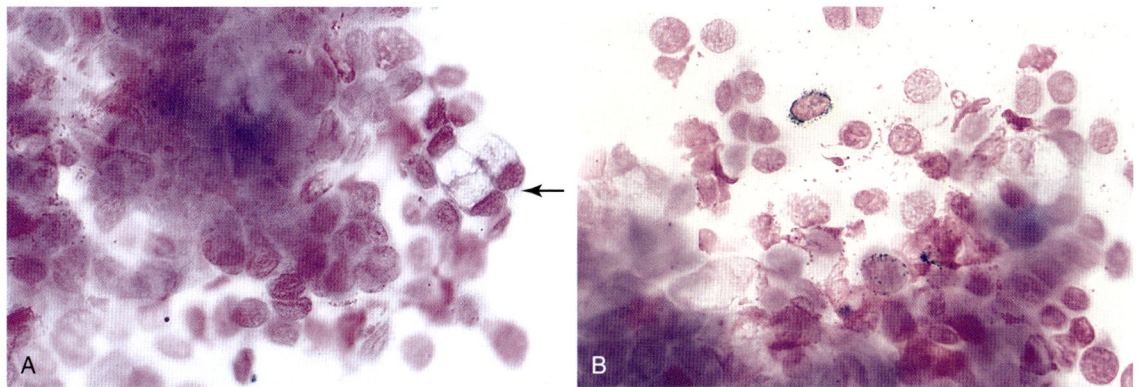

■ **FIGURE 16.6 Hyperplastic epithelium. Conjunctival scraping. Cat.** Same case in A and B. **A, Goblet cell hyperplasia.** Chronic conjunctival disease in this animal resulted in increased numbers of goblet cells. Two are shown *(arrow)* characterized by a columnar shape, basal nucleus, and pale foamy cytoplasm. (Wright-Giemsa; HP oil.) **B, Pigmentation and hyperplastic epithelium.** Two cells are present with abundant fine black-green cytoplasmic granules. Also note the hyperplastic epithelium with increased nucleocytoplasmic ratio. (Wright-Giemsa; HP oil.)

cellular clumping of samples and provide less cellular distortion (Willis et al., 1997). Impressions can be a good alternative for the bulbar conjunctiva (Eördögh et al., 2015); however, cytopathologic details may be more difficult to evaluate compared with brush samples (Perazzi et al., 2017).

Normal Cytology and Artifacts

Bulbar conjunctiva consists of mostly intermediate and superficial squamous epithelium with less than 1% goblet cells as detected by impression cytology (Bolzan et al., 2005). Goblet cells appear as distended, polarized cells with a basal nucleus. Their cytoplasm may contain clear vacuoles or red-blue granules. Mucus, from goblet cells, is common on cytologic specimens, appearing as lightly basophilic amorphous strands. Small and intermediate-sized lymphocytes from MALT may be present.

Hyperplasia

Conditions such as keratoconjunctivitis sicca, vitamin A deficiency, chronic disease, and trauma from mechanical irritants result in increased cell numbers, sometimes with evidence of metaplasia. These specimens contain many keratinized epithelial cells and goblet cells (Fig. 16.6A) (Murphy, 1988). Increased pigmentation of the epithelium may also occur such that the cytoplasm contains numerous fine, black-green melanin granules (Fig. 16.6B).

Inflammation

The predominant cell type present characterizes conjunctivitis. Neutrophilic conjunctivitis may be associated with infectious agents such as bacteria and viruses or noninfectious causes. A bacterial origin should be suspected if degenerative changes are present. With viruses such as feline herpesvirus-1 (FHV-1) and chronic canine distemper virus, nondegenerate neutrophils predominate (Fig. 16.7). However, in FHV-1 infections, a mixed inflammation including eosinophils is often noted along with the presence of binucleated and multinucleated epithelial cells along with dysplastic changes (Volopich et al., 2005; Hillström et al., 2012) (Fig. 16.8). Eosinophils are associated with FHV-1 infection, and their presence supports confirmatory testing (Fig. 16.9) (Volopich et al., 2005; Hillström et al., 2012).

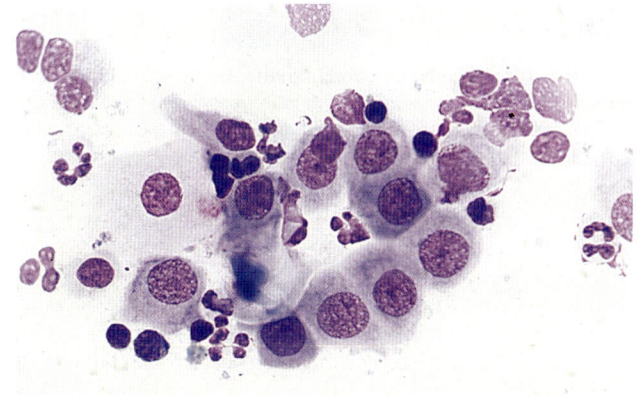

■ **FIGURE 16.7 Suppurative conjunctivitis. Conjunctival scraping. Cat.** The bulbar conjunctiva is hyperplastic with many nondegenerate neutrophils and few lymphocytes in this young cat with chronic conjunctivitis. Infection with feline herpesvirus was suspected. (Aqueous Romanowsky; HP oil.)

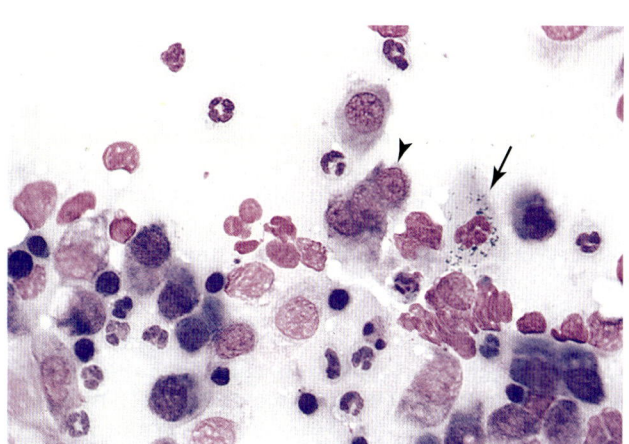

■ **FIGURE 16.8 Herpesvirus infection with suppurative conjunctivitis. Conjunctival scraping. Cat.** Many nondegenerate neutrophils are present along with reactive epithelium, including multinucleation *(arrowhead)*. This case was confirmed previously for herpesvirus infection by polymerase chain reaction. One pigmented epithelial cell *(arrow)* is also noted. (Wright-Giemsa; HP oil.)

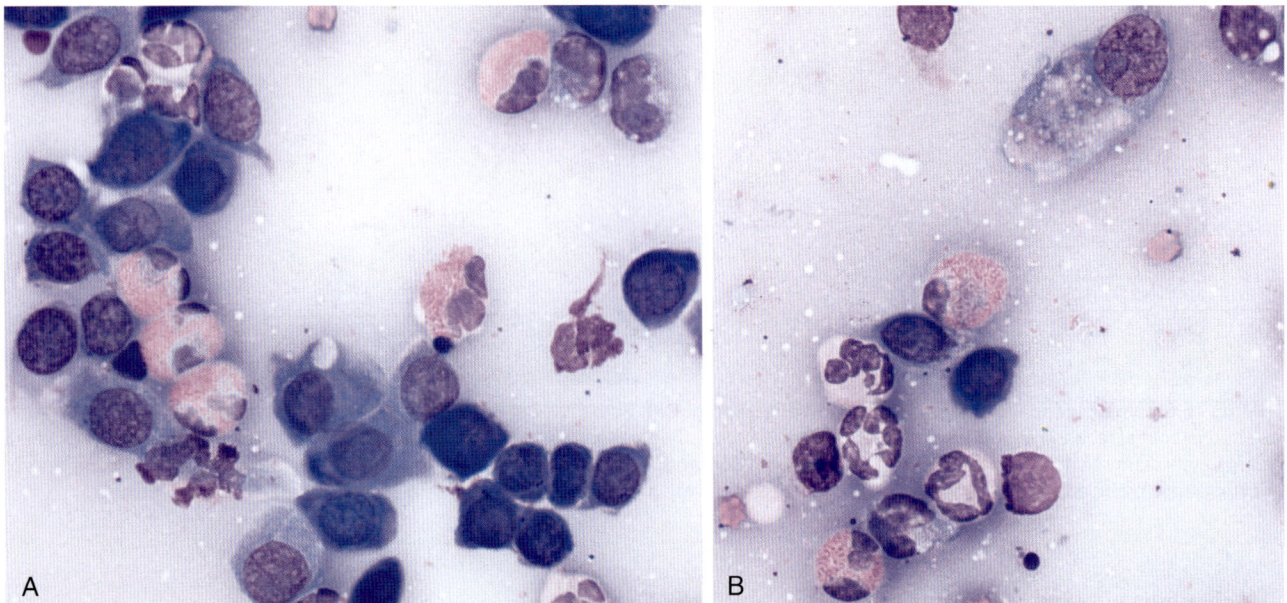

■ **FIGURE 16.9 Mixed cell conjunctivitis. Conjunctival brushing. Cat.** Same case in A and B. **A,** Eosinophils predominate in the inflammatory response of this suspected herpesvirus infection with hypersensitivity in an adult cat. The small, deeply basophilic cells are the basal epithelium. Clinical signs exhibited were sneezing, tearing, blepharospasms, chemosis, and hyperemia. (Wright; HP oil.) **B,** In this field, nondegenerate neutrophils predominate in addition to the notable increase in eosinophils. A goblet cell *(upper right)* is present with columnar shape and pale foamy cytoplasm. (Wright; HP oil.)

Intranuclear viral inclusions in FHV-1 infection are occasionally encountered in conjunctival smears (Volopich et al., 2005) but are more readily seen in histologic sections (Fig. 16.10). Confirmation of the infection requires a polymerase chain reaction (PCR) test, which has greater sensitivity for detection of the virus than other tests (Stiles et al., 1997). Canine distemper inclusions appear pink with methanolic Romanowsky stains (Fig. 16.11) and purple with aqueous Romanowsky stains (Henderson et al., 2015). In addition to cytopathology, methods such as direct immunofluorescence assay and immunohistochemistry for the canine distemper virus nucleoprotein in conjunctival smears and tissues, respectively, are available to support the diagnosis (Gonzales-Viera et al., 2018).

Other infectious causes include feline chlamydiosis caused by the bacterial agent *Chlamydia felis* (basionym: *Chlamydophila felis*) spp. (Nunes and Gomes, 2014). The organism presents initially as variably sized discrete basophilic to bright magenta bodies that attach to the epithelial cells within the first 2 weeks of infection. These small elementary bodies measure 0.2 to 0.6 μm (Figs. 16.12 and 16.13A) and are taken into the cytoplasm, where they divide and differentiate into a large (0.5–1.5 μm) membrane-bound reticulate body (Figs. 16.13B and 16.14). The cycle continues as the reticulate body condenses into multiple elementary bodies that are released upon cell lysis to infect new cells (Fig. 16.14C–D) (Sykes, 2014). Chlamydial infection was identified in 7% to 12% of conjunctival samples from cats with conjunctivitis by positive PCR for *C. felis* (von Bomhard et al., 2003; Low et al., 2007; Hillström et al., 2012). *C. felis* inclusions are more easily identified early in the course of the disease, whereas they may disappear with chronicity. In one study, all eight cats with conjunctivitis

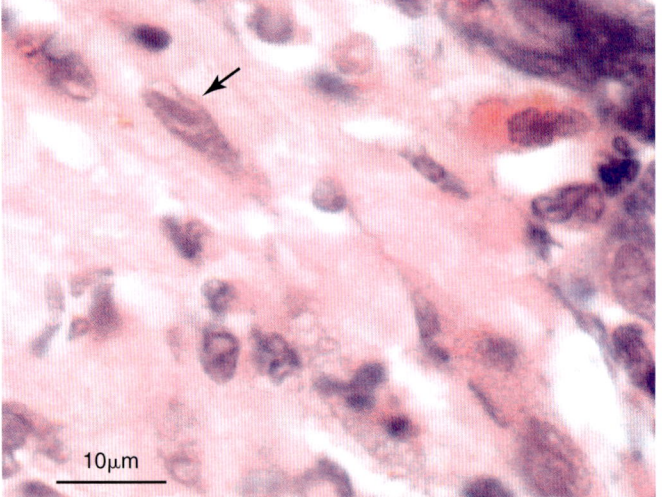

■ **FIGURE 16.10 Neutrophilic and eosinophilic keratoconjunctivitis. Herpesvirus infection. Tissue section. Cat.** Large irregular eosinophilic intranuclear inclusion *(arrow)* within an epithelial cell. (H&E; HP oil.)

that tested PCR positive for *Chlamydia* had cytopathologic evidence of the disease (Hillström et al., 2012). In another study of 226 conjunctival samples, 39% were positive for non–*C. felis* chlamydial DNA, identified as *Neochlamydia hartmannella,* in cytopathologic samples with eosinophilic inflammation (von Bomhard et al., 2003).

Infection with feline *Mycoplasma* spp. presents as small basophilic granules similar to the elementary bodies of chlamydial infections except that they are adherent to the surface

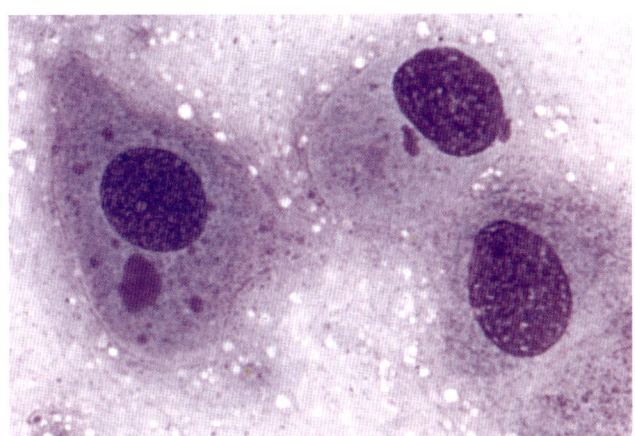

■ **FIGURE 16.11 Canine distemper viral inclusions. Conjunctiva. Cytopathologic preparation. Dog.** Variably sized pink cytoplasmic inclusions are present in two of the three conjunctival cells. (Aqueous Romanowsky; HP oil.) (Courtesy Catherine Trumel, Ecole Nationale Vétérinaire de Toulouse, France.)

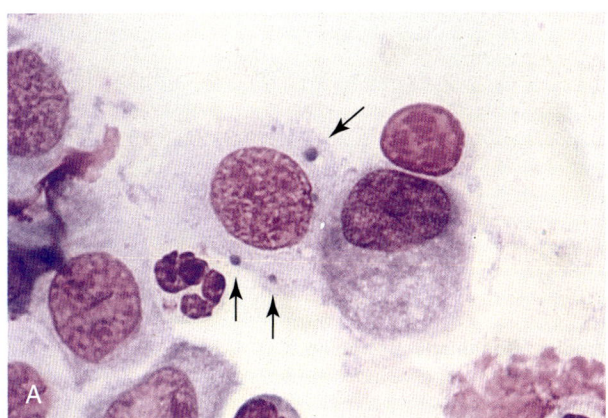

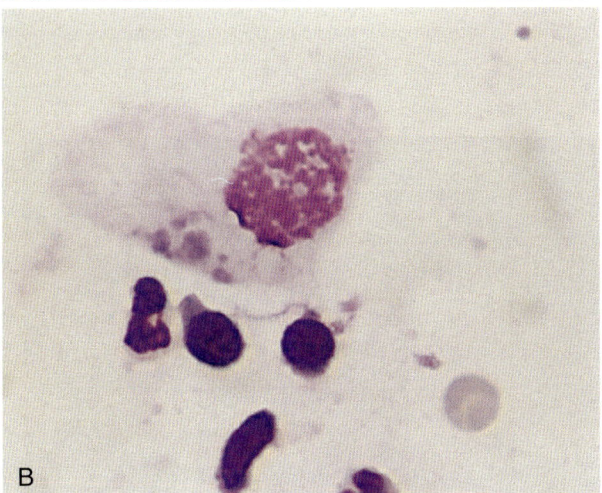

■ **FIGURE 16.12 Chlamydiosis with elementary bodies. Conjunctival scraping. Cat.** Same case in A and B. **A,** Three small basophilic inclusions *(arrows)* are present in the cytoplasm of one epithelial cell of this 10-month-old kitten. (Wright-Giemsa; HP oil.) **B,** Degenerating epithelial cell contains several small basophilic granular elementary bodies. A second cat in the house as well as the owner had conjunctivitis. Nondegenerate neutrophils and small lymphocytes are also present in this sample. (Wright-Giemsa; HP oil.)

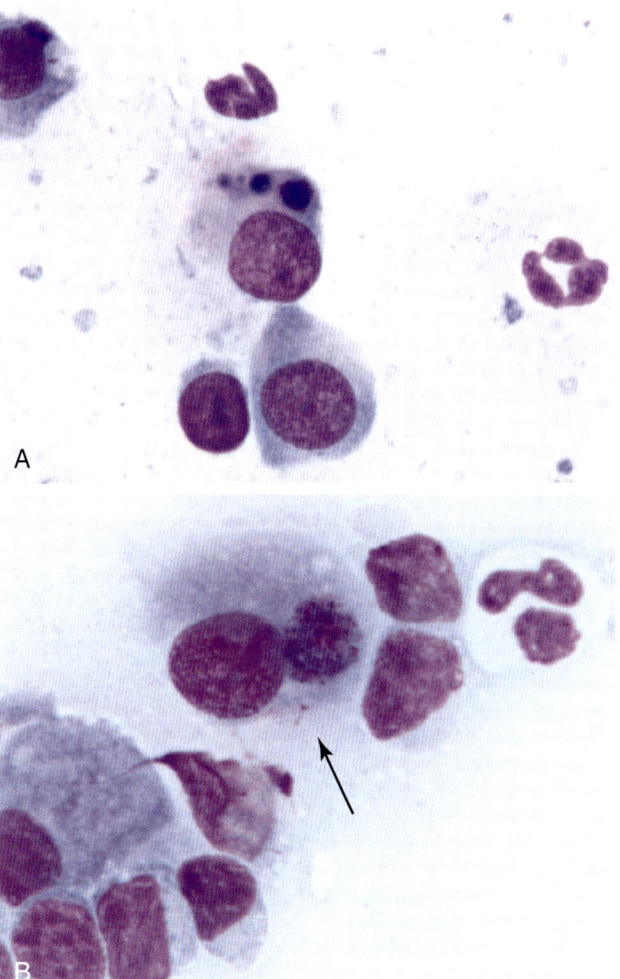

■ **FIGURE 16.13 Chlamydiosis with elementary and reticulate bodies. Conjunctival scraping. Cat.** Same case in A and B. **A,** Several variably sized basophilic and magenta inclusions appear in the cytoplasm of an acutely ill animal. Two neutrophils and a lymphocyte are present. (Wright; HP oil.) **B,** The epithelial cell *(arrow)* contains a large (~10 µm) paranuclear inclusion containing numerous small elementary bodies. Small and intermediate lymphocytes are frequent. (Modified Wright; HP oil.) (Courtesy Pierre Deshuillers, Purdue University.)

membrane (Fig. 16.15). One study from Belgium indicated that mycoplasmal infection had an incidence of 25% in cats with conjunctivitis (Haesebrouck et al., 1991), but the prevalence was lower in other studies (Low et al., 2007; Hillström et al., 2012). *Mycoplasma felis* is considered resident bacteria in young cats but may become more pathogenic in association with FHV-1 or *C. felis* infection. (Sykes, 2014). Cytopathology is of limited use for the detection of *M. felis* in conjunctival samples given the high number of false negative results (Hillström et al., 2012).

Ocular leishmaniasis is identified most commonly in the conjunctiva and limbus region (Peña et al., 2008). Other sites in order of frequency were the ciliary body, iris, cornea, sclera and iridocorneal angle, choroid, and optic nerve sheath. Organisms may appear in uveal specimens as well. Leishmaniasis commonly causes a granulomatous inflammation with the

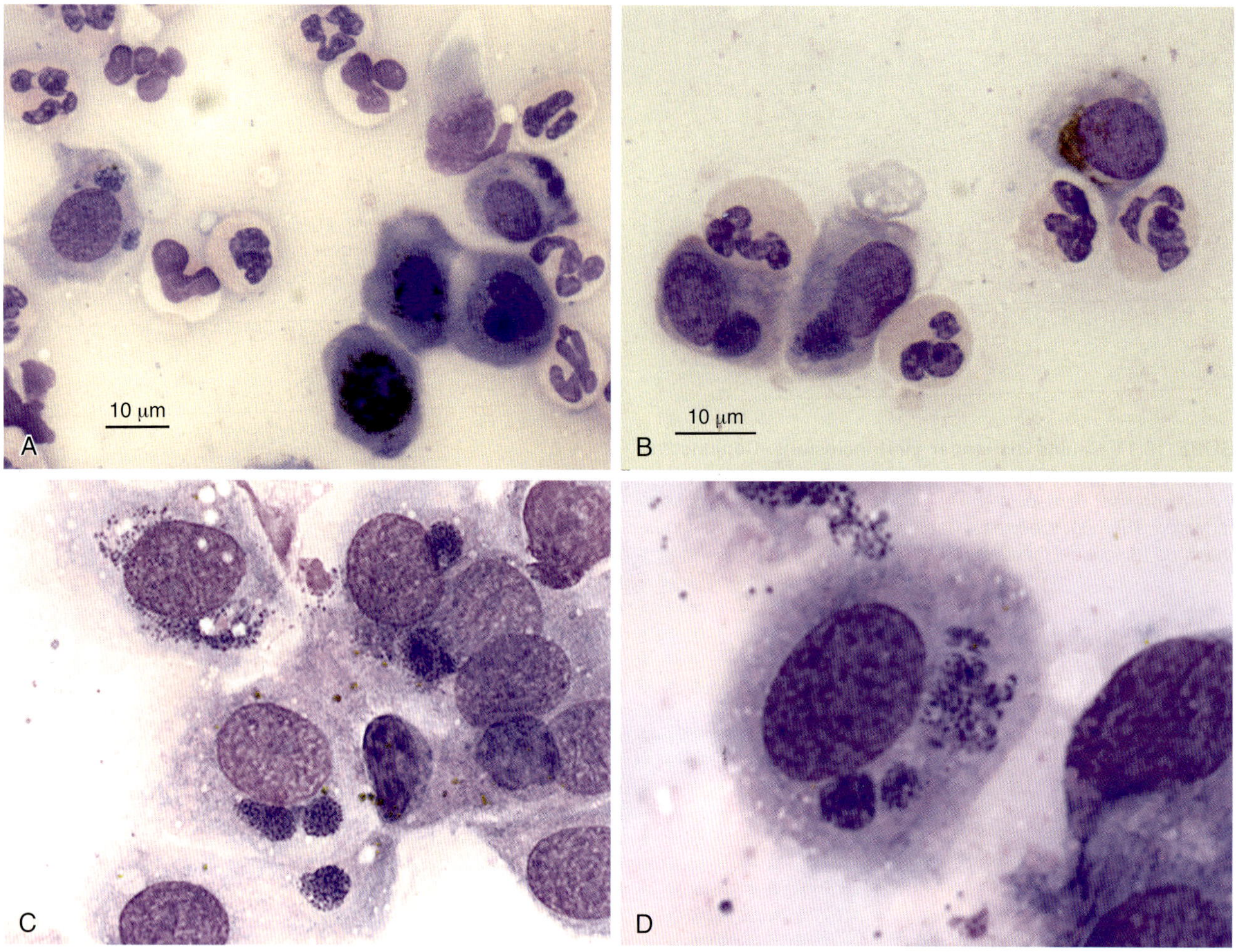

FIGURE 16.14 Chlamydiosis with reticulate and infective elementary bodies. Conjunctival scraping. Cat. Same case in A to D. **A,** An epithelial cell *(middle right)* contains multiple elementary bodies at the cell's periphery, and one cell *(middle left)* contains granular paranuclear reticulate bodies. Three epithelial cells at *lower right* contain black melanin granules. **B,** Two epithelial cells *(left)* contain a single large granular reticulate body. Note the golden melanin granules in the epithelial cell *(right)*. **C,** Multiple cells contain large granular reticulate bodies, and one cell *(upper left)* contains dispersed infective elementary bodies. **D,** One epithelial cells contains large granular reticulate bodies and infective elementary bodies that are loose in the cytoplasm. (A–D, Modified Wright; HP oil.)

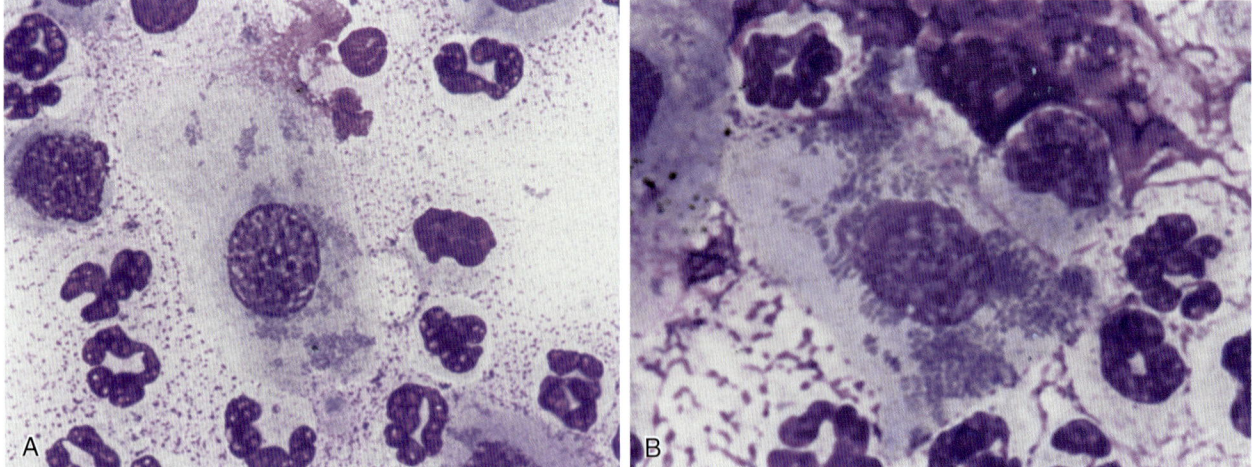

FIGURE 16.15 Mycoplasmosis. Conjunctival scraping. Dog. Same case in A and B. **A,** Numerous small gray bacteria in small aggregates are associated with the epithelial cell. Nondegenerate neutrophils are frequent. (May-Grunwald Giemsa; HP oil.) **B,** Note the numerous organisms over the cytoplasm and nucleus. These granules are adherent to the surface membrane and extend into the background. (May-Grunwald Giemsa; HP oil.) (Courtesy Catherine Trumel, Ecole Nationale Vétérinaire de Toulouse, France.)

CHAPTER 16 Eyes and Ears

the conjunctiva (Fig. 16.18A). This may result in proliferation or hyperplasia of the epithelium (see Fig. 16.18B).

Neoplasia

Epithelium is frequently atypical and hyperplastic as a result of severe inflammation; therefore, neoplasia may be difficult to diagnose confidently. Neoplasms involving the conjunctival include SCC, papilloma (Beckwith-Cohen et al., 2015) melanoma, lymphoma, hemangiosarcoma, and mast cell tumor. In dogs, the majority of conjunctival mast cell tumors presented as Patnaik grade I or II in one study (Fife et al., 2011) (Fig. 16.19). An uncommon location of transmissible venereal tumor is the conjunctivae of the upper and lower eyelids (Boscos et al., 1998).

Miscellaneous Findings

Dark blue to blue-black, sharply demarcated, 0.3 to 2.5 μm bodies scattered throughout the cytoplasm of squamous epithelium have been attributed to ophthalmic ointment use, particularly those containing Neosporin (bacitracin zinc, neomycin sulfate, and polymyxin B sulfate) (Fig. 16.20) (Streeten and Streeten, 1985; Young, 2006). Larger bodies could be found in a paranuclear location. Ultrastructurally, these inclusions consist of a variety of dense bodies and phagolysosomal vacuoles containing complex lipids, supporting epithelial cell injury (Streeten and Streeten, 1985).

NICTITATING MEMBRANE

Normal Histology and Cytology

The third eyelid, or nictitating membrane, is a large fold of conjunctiva protruding from the medial canthus. It contains a T-shaped cartilaginous plate surrounded by glandular epithelium that is serous in the cat and seromucoid in dogs (Samuelson, 1999). The palpebral and bulbar surfaces are covered by nonkeratinized stratified squamous epithelium.

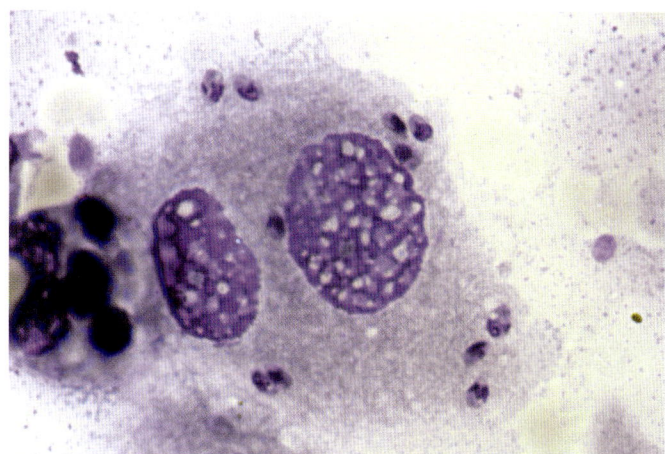

FIGURE 16.16 Leishmaniasis. Conjunctival scraping. Dog. Numerous amastigotes are associated with a degenerating cell, which may be a macrophage or a conjunctival cell on which free organisms are laying. To the left of this cell is a macrophage containing debris or hemosiderin. The organisms have a round nucleus and rod-shaped kinetoplast. Ocular leishmaniasis occurs in decreasing order in the conjunctiva and limbus, ciliary body, iris, cornea, sclera and iridocorneal angle, choroid, and optic nerve sheath. (May-Grunwald Giemsa; HP oil.) (Courtesy Catherine Trumel, Ecole Nationale Vétérinaire de Toulouse, France.)

organism in the characteristic amastigote form having a rod-shaped kinetoplast and round nucleus (Fig. 16.16).

Noninfectious causes include allergic conjunctivitis, canine keratoconjunctivitis sicca, and feline lipogranulomatous conjunctivitis. Allergic conjunctivitis in cats may result in eosinophilic and mastocytic inflammation (Fig. 16.17). (Beckwith-Cohen et al., 2017). Lymphocytes and plasma cells have been associated with allergic conditions but may also occur with early canine distemper infection, and chronic inflammation of

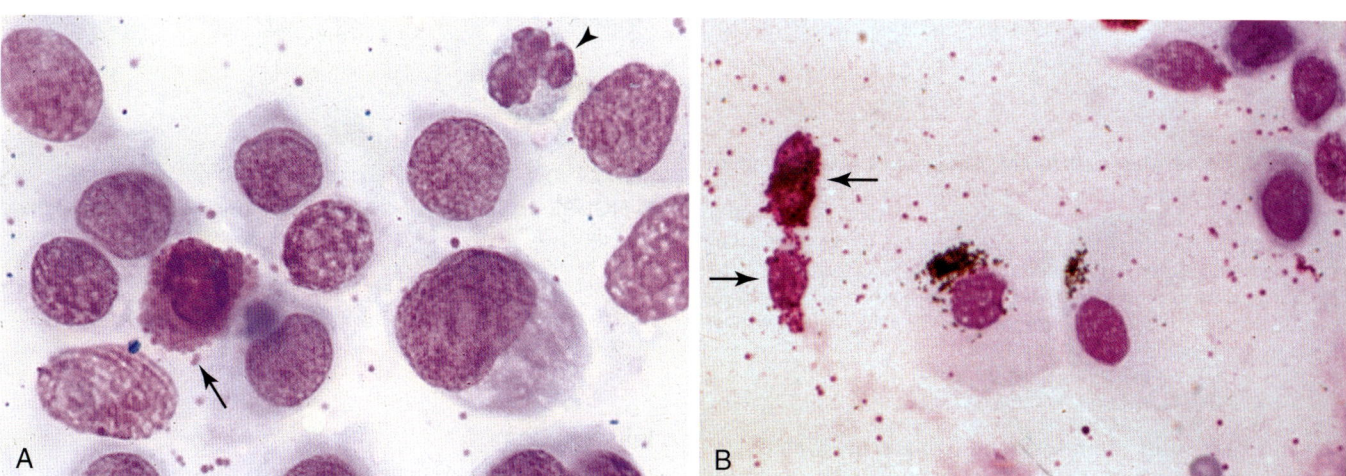

FIGURE 16.17 Eosinophilic conjunctivitis. Conjunctival scraping. Cat. Same case in A and B. **A,** Bilateral conjunctivitis is present in this animal. A lightly stained eosinophil *(arrowhead)* is shown along with a mast cell *(arrow).* Note the mast cell granules in the background. This response occurred with a suspected hypersensitivity reaction of noninfectious causes. (Wright-Giemsa; HP oil.) **B,** Many mast cell granules are free in the background. Two mast cells *(arrows)* and two pigmented epithelial cells are present in the center. The mast cells may be so numerous as to cause concern for a mast cell tumor. (Wright-Giemsa; HP oil.)

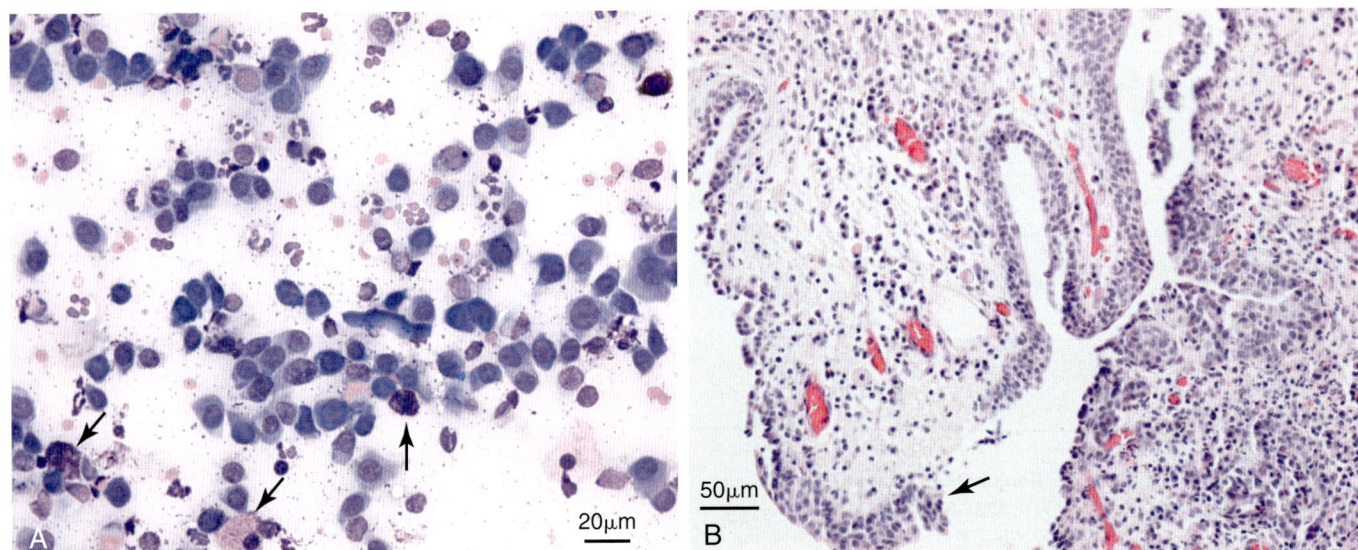

■ **FIGURE 16.18 Mixed cell conjunctivitis with epithelial hyperplasia. Cat.** Same case in A and B. **A, Conjunctival swab.** Chronic inflammation of the conjunctiva present for 4 months has been nonresponsive to medications. The patient now has nodular proliferations on the upper and lower eyelids. Inflammatory cells include approximately 60% neutrophils, 15% mast cells, 10% eosinophils, 5% plasma cells, and 4% lymphocytes against a loose background of mast cell granules. Three mast cells are indicated *(arrows)*. The conjunctival epithelium demonstrates increased cytoplasmic basophilia, increased nucleocytoplasmic ratio, and pleomorphism of cell shape. (Wright; IP.) **B, Tissue section.** The tissue is edematous indicated by increased spacing between cells within the submucosa, well vascularized with a predominance of segmented and mononuclear inflammatory cells. The expanded epithelium is polypoid and lined by stratified squamous epithelium *(arrow)*. (H&E; LP.)

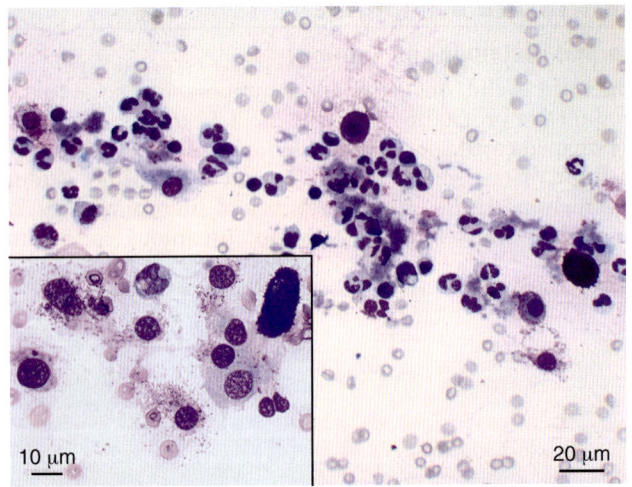

■ **FIGURE 16.19 Mast cell tumor. Conjunctiva. Mass aspirate. Dog.** There are frequent well-granulated and poorly granulated mast cells along with occasional eosinophils. Small numbers of neutrophils, lymphocytes, and macrophages are present. *Inset*: Many granules are in the background from ruptured mast cells. Anisocytosis and aniso-karyosis is mild to moderate. Histopathology confirmed a low-grade mast cell tumor. (Aqueous Romanowsky; HP oil.) (Courtesy Rose Raskin, North Carolina State University.)

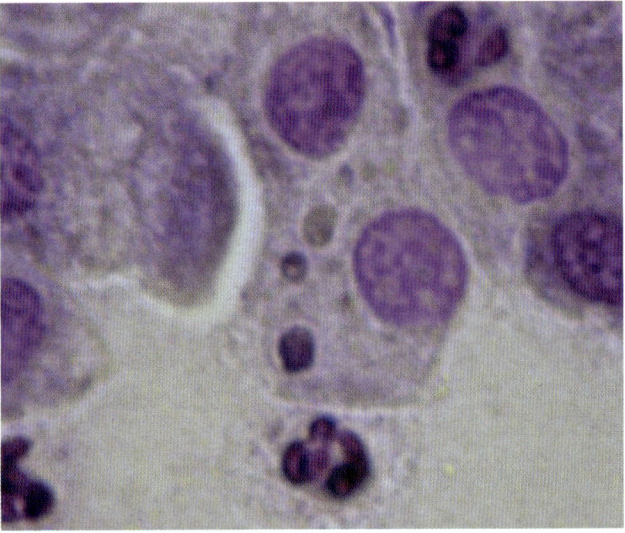

■ **FIGURE 16.20 "Blue body" ointment inclusions. Conjunctiva.** Four irregularly sized, shaped, and colored cytoplasmic inclusions were associated with ophthalmic ointment administration. It may resemble chlamydial elementary bodies, so history is important to determine the cause of these inclusions. (Courtesy Jean Stiles, Purdue University.)

The free margin of the membrane is pigmented, and cytologically, fine green-black melanin granules can be found within the epithelium. Numerous variably sized lymphoid aggregates with overlying epithelium having microvilli or microfolds (M cells) on the apical surface are associated with the bulbar surface of the nictitating membrane (Giuliano et al., 2002). The stroma also contains fibrous connective tissue.

Inflammation

With follicular conjunctivitis, there is a mixed population of lymphoid cells that resembles a hyperplastic lymph node (Fig. 16.21). Plasma cell infiltrates (plasmacytic conjunctivitis or plasmoma) have been seen in German shepherds. These thickened depigmenting lesions are composed of numerous well-differentiated plasma cells.

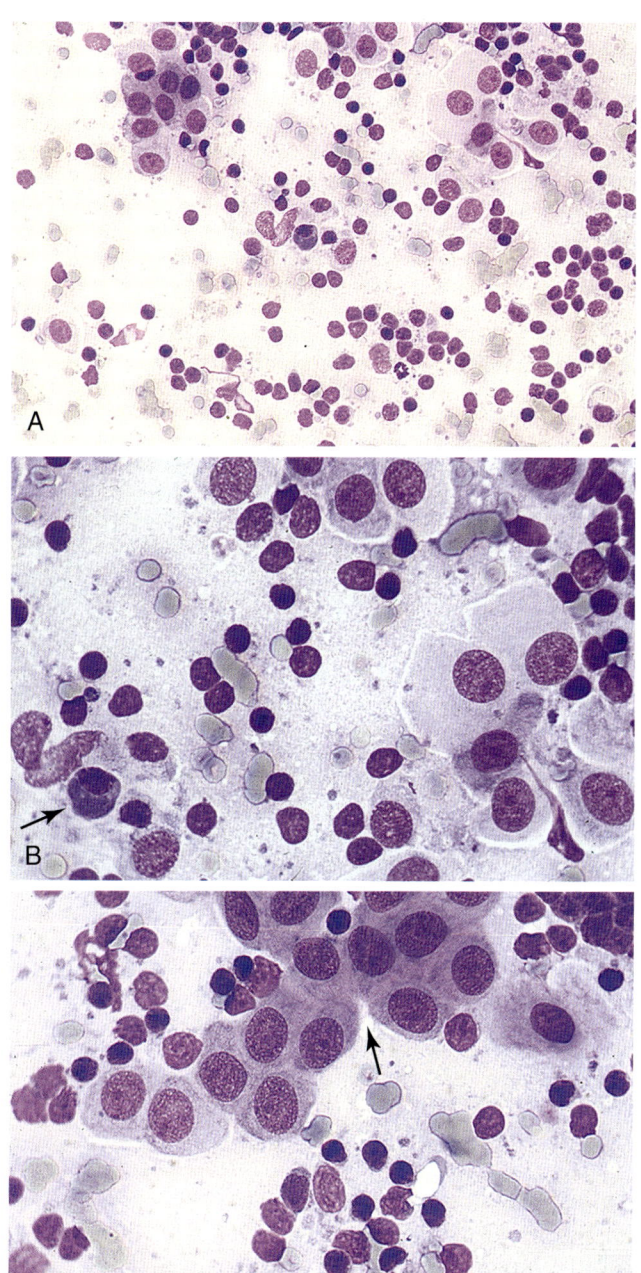

FIGURE 16.21 Follicular hyperplasia. Nictitating membrane. Cat. Same case in A to C. **A,** Numerous small lymphocytes predominant. **B,** Higher magnification to demonstrate the presence of a plasma cell *(arrow)* and several intermediate lymphocytes in addition to the small lymphocytes. **C,** Reactive epithelium *(arrow)* accompanies the lymphoplasmacytic population. (Aqueous Romanowsky; HP oil.)

Neoplasia

Tumors of the nictitating membrane are similar to those seen in the conjunctivae. In one retrospective study, adenocarcinomas was the most common neoplasm of the third eyelid followed by adenomas and SCCs in dogs and cats (Dees et al., 2016); however, papillomas and malignant melanomas are also common. SCC of the nictitating membrane is considered an extension from the eyelid. SCCs appear similar to those found in the skin often with nonseptic purulent inflammation (Fig. 16.22). Dogs and cats most commonly present with hemangiosarcoma and hemangioma within the nonpigmented epithelium of the nictitating membrane compared with the conjunctivae. Exposure to ultraviolet light is suspected to be a risk factor for these endothelial neoplasms (Pirie and Dubielzig, 2006; Pirie et al., 2006).

SCLERA

Normal Histology and Cytology

The sclera is a fibrous covering of the globe that merges with the peripheral cornea and bulbar conjunctiva at the limbus, where it is pigmented. Pigment is found in all layers of the limbus except the superficial squamous cells. The underlying stroma contains dense collagen fibers, elastic fibers, fibrocytes, melanocytes, and blood vessels. Aspirates may be poorly cellular, with mostly collagen present and occasional melanocytes.

Inflammation

A tan-pink raised mass may appear at the corneoscleral limbus as a small tag or an inflamed focal area. *Nodular granulomatous episclerokeratoconjunctivitis* or proliferative keratoconjunctivitis is a dome-shaped lesion that arises from the subconjunctiva or episclera (Figs. 16.23 and 16.24). This disease is recognized in several breeds, especially in rough collies, and is suspected to be immune mediated. Cytopathologically, it is composed of variable numbers of epithelioid or dendritic-appearing histiocytes with many lymphocytes and occasional neutrophils (see Fig. 16.24). Fibroblasts are commonly noted; hence, this has been also termed *nodular fasciitis*. Melanocytes may be seen.

Onchocerciasis should be a differential consideration in cases of canine episcleral nodules or periorbital swelling, particularly in dogs from the southern and western United States as well as Europe (Grácio et al., 2015). These granulomas contain the adult worm along with a variable number of eosinophils (Zarfoss et al., 2005).

Neoplasia

Neoplasms present in the sclera include melanoma, mast cell tumor, lymphoma, and sarcoma.

CORNEA

Normal Histology and Cytology

The surface of the cornea is composed of nonkeratinized stratified squamous epithelium (Fig. 16.25A). Below this surface is a thick layer of parallel bundles of collagenous stroma (Fig. 16.25B) with infrequent intermixed fibrocytes, called *keratocytes*. Deeper to the stroma is a basement membrane, termed *Descemet membrane*, composed of fine collagen fibrils. The deepest layer consists of a single layer of flattened endothelium. Cytologically, basal and intermediate squamous epithelial cells that normally lack pigmentation predominate in scrapings.

Inflammation

Infectious keratitis involves bacterial and fungal agents. Bacterial agents such as *Pseudomonas* sp., *Streptococcus* spp., and *Staphylococcus* spp. produce suppurative responses with degenerative neutrophils. Fungal agents commonly isolated in mycotic keratitis are *Aspergillus* sp., *Fusarium* spp., and *Candida* spp. (Fig. 16.26). These infections produce mostly neutrophilic

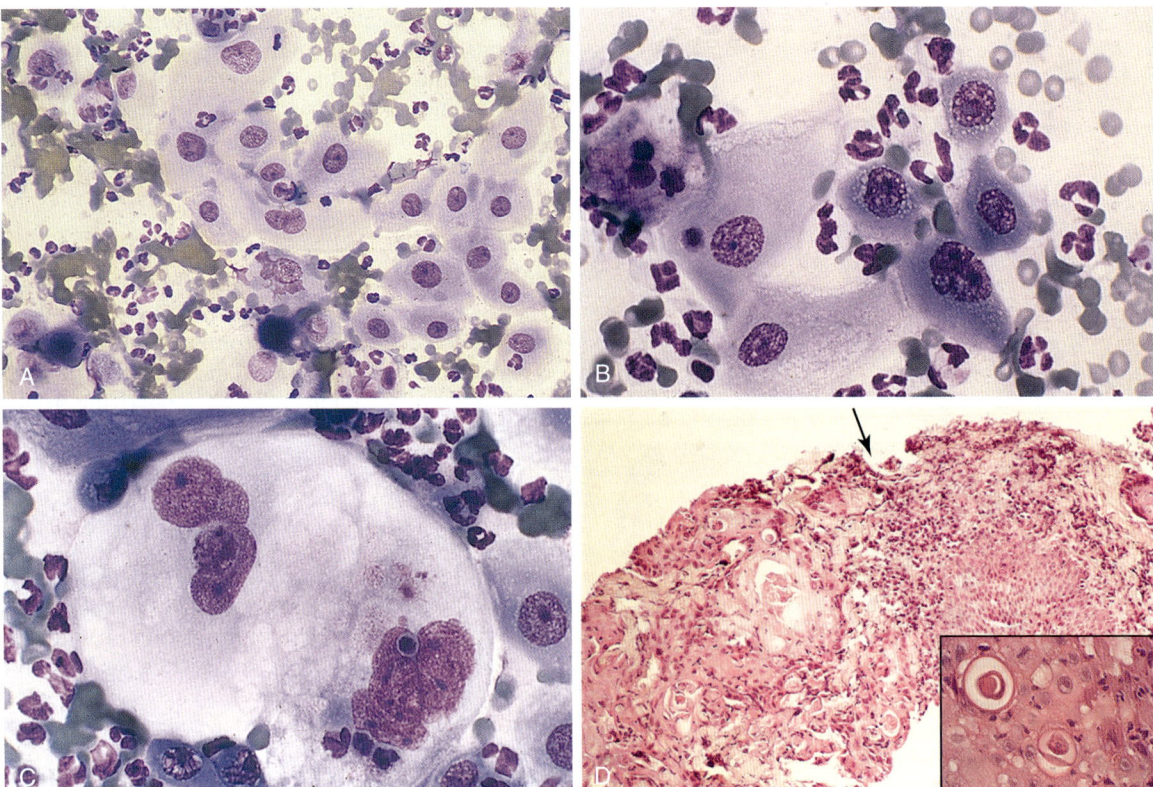

■ **FIGURE 16.22 Squamous cell carcinoma. Nictitating membrane. Cat.** Same case in A to D. **A,** Several weeks' duration of erythema and edema along with proliferative lesions on the conjunctiva and third eyelid were present in this 14-year-old cat. Sheets of epithelium appear with some features of malignancy, including anisokaryosis, multinucleation, variable nucleocytoplasmic ratio, and coarse chromatin. Many nondegenerate neutrophils are noted without evidence of sepsis. (Aqueous Romanowsky; HP oil.) **B,** In addition to the previously mentioned malignant features, there is perinuclear vacuolation, a feature often associated with malignant squamous epithelium. The presence of severe suppurative inflammation likely accounts for some of the dysplastic changes in the epithelium. (Aqueous Romanowsky; HP oil.) **C,** Two giant epithelial cells with multiple nuclei contrast in size to the adjacent neutrophils. The presence of very bizarre morphologic changes and the absence of sepsis further support the malignant, not dysplastic, nature of the epithelium. (Aqueous Romanowsky; HP oil.) **D,** Section taken from the junction between the palpebral conjunctiva on the left and the nictitating membrane on the right. Note the marked disorganization of the mucous membrane and dermis at their junction *(arrow)*. This tumor is thought to originate from the eyelid with extension to the nictitating membrane. (H&E; IP.) *Inset:* Two keratin pearls that are often associated with malignant squamous epithelium appear in the center and help to identify the neoplasm. (H&E; HP oil.)

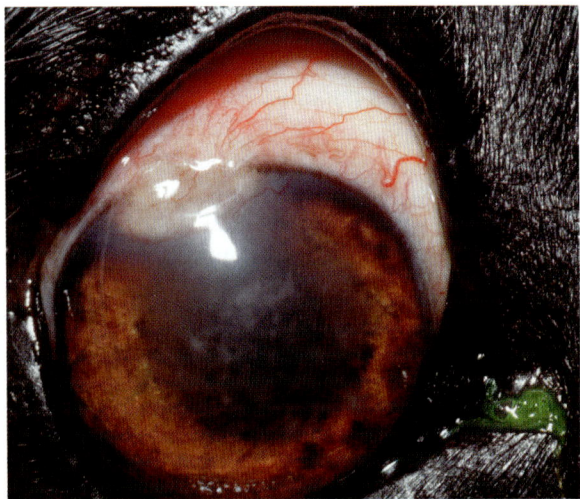

■ **FIGURE 16.23 Nodular granulomatous episcleritis. Dog. A,** The globe has a tan slightly raised tissue extending from the sclera into the corneal stroma. (From Maggs DJ, Miller PE, Ofri R. *Slatter's Fundamentals of Veterinary Ophthalmology.* 5th ed. Elsevier; 2013.)

infiltration, but macrophages are common with occasional eosinophils. Hyphal elements are best seen with stains such as Grocott-Gomori methenamine silver. Samples should be obtained from deep within the lesion or at its edge. When used together with microbial culture, cytopathologic evaluation of scrapings from corneal ulcers results in a maximal identification of infectious ulcerative keratitis (Massa et al., 1999; Nevile et al., 2016). Scott and Carter (2014) found several predisposing factors for fungal keratitis, including underlying endocrinopathy, preexisting corneal disease, intraocular surgery, or prolonged use of either topical antibiotics or corticosteroids at the time of initial examination. Neutrophilic inflammation may accompany corneal ulceration along with emperipolesis and squamous dysplasia (Fig. 16.27). *Capnocytophaga* keratitis is a severe, rapidly progressive corneal infection in dogs that is associated with corneal ulceration with a relatively poor prognosis (Ledbetter et al., 2018). On cytopathology, severe neutrophilic inflammation was present with long, thin, gram-negative rods in some dogs.

Eosinophilic keratitis is a raised, opaque, fleshy pink mass with white granular surface; it is seen in cats (O'Connell et al.,

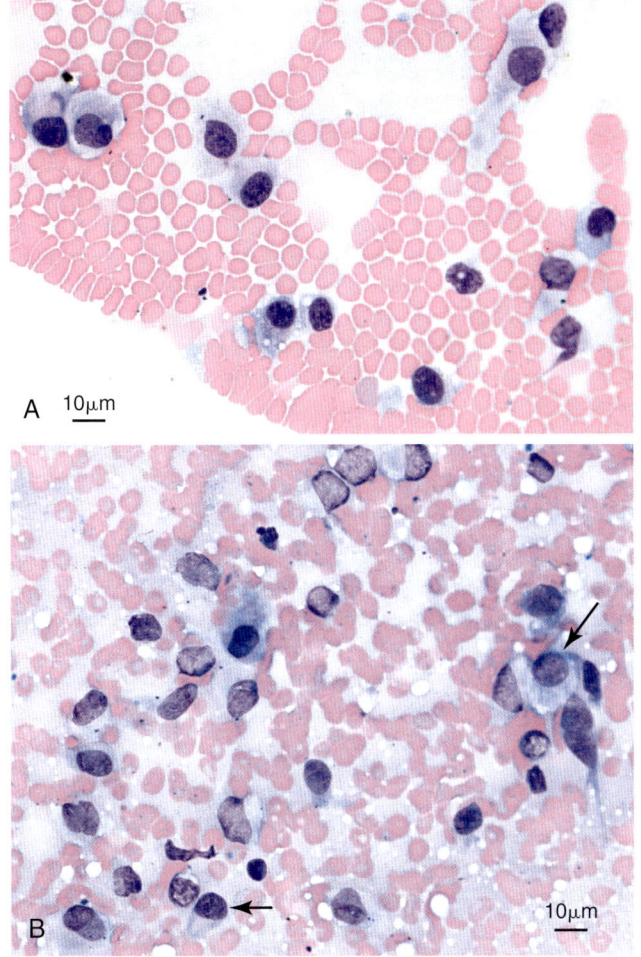

■ **FIGURE 16.24 Nodular granulomatous episcleritis (NGE). Scleral mass imprint. Dog.** Same case in A and B. **A,** This Yorkshire terrier presented with a 10 × 10 × 4 mm nodule in the ventral sclera. A large population of epithelioid macrophages make up the majority of inflammatory cells present. (Wright; HP oil.) **B,** A mixed population of small and intermediate lymphocytes along with plasma cells *(arrows)* is also present and suggest an immune response. Histologic examination was consistent with NGE. (Wright; HP oil.)

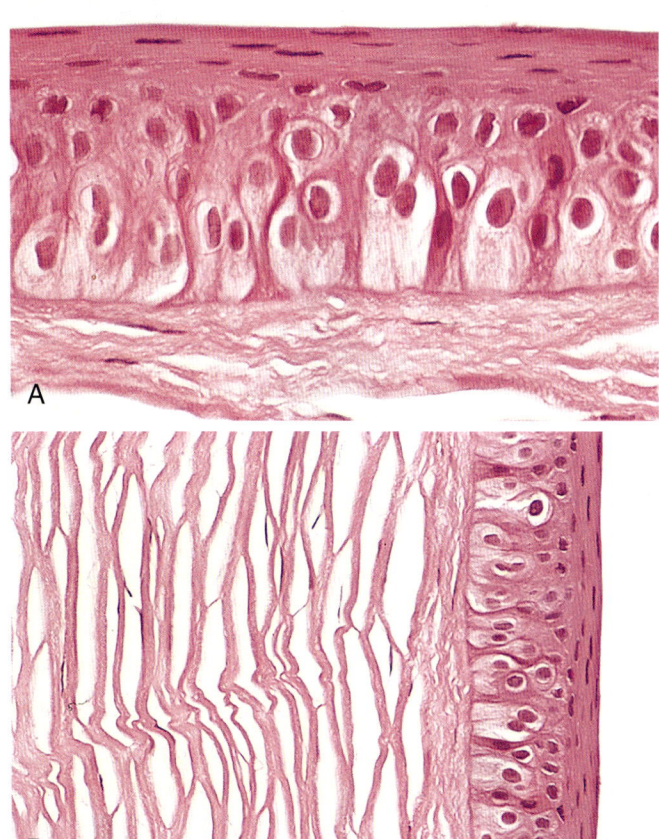

■ **FIGURE 16.25 Normal cornea. Histology. Dog. A,** The outer surface is composed of nonkeratinized stratified squamous epithelium. (H&E; HP oil.) **B,** Below the surface epithelium is a thick layer of parallel bundles of collagenous stroma. (H&E; HP oil.)

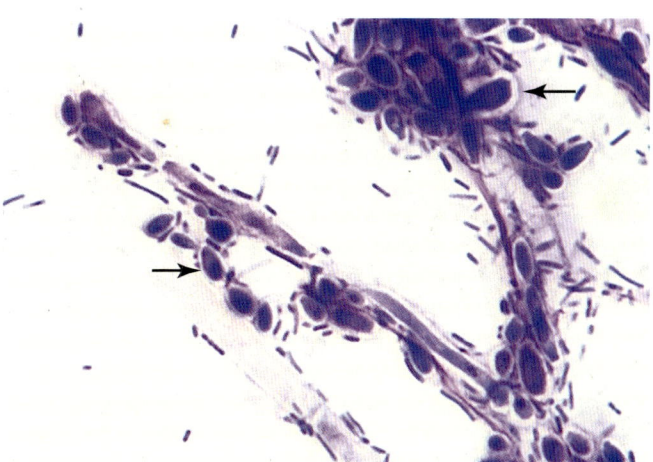

■ **FIGURE 16.26 Mycotic keratitis. Corneal scraping. Dog.** There is a 1-week history of raised white punctate masses on the cornea. Against the background of extracellular rod-shaped bacteria are hyphal elements and many yeast forms *(arrows)*. Infection with *Candida* spp. was suspected. Neutrophils were present in other fields of the specimen. (Aqueous Romanowsky; HP oil.)

2017). The surface scrapings are composed of squamous epithelium; cellular debris, including eosinophil granules; and numerous mast cells with lower numbers of intact eosinophils (Fig. 16.28A). Deeper scrapings contain predominantly eosinophils and lymphoid cells (Figs. 16.28B and 16.29) (Dean and Meunier, 2013). The histopathology and cytopathology are well described in an article by Prasse and Winston (1996). In a study involving detection of FHV-1 infection, there was a significant association between viral presence and epithelial keratitis (Volopich et al., 2005). In another study of eosinophilic keratitis, 76% cases had detectable FHV-1 DNA by PCR analysis, suggesting that the virus may play a role in the pathogenesis of some cases (Nasisse et al., 1998). Treatment usually involves topical corticosteroids with possible cyclosporine administration (O'Connell et al., 2017).

Pannus, or chronic superficial keratitis, is a chronic immune-mediated keratoconjunctivitis. Although common in German shepherds, greyhounds, Belgian Tervuren, or Belgian

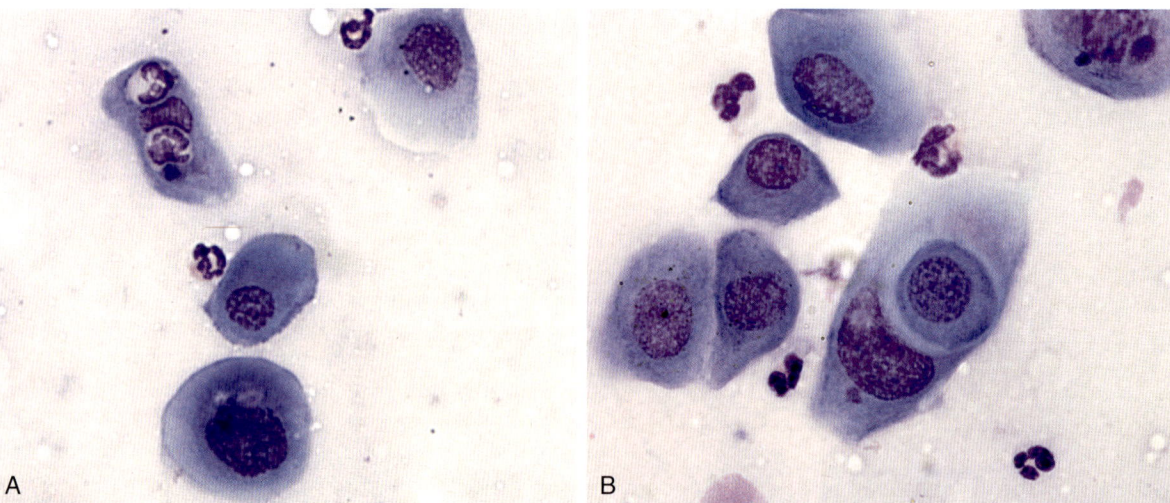

■ **FIGURE 16.27 Epithelial dysplasia and emperipolesis, corneal ulcer with inflammation. Corneal scraping. Dog.** Same case in A and B. **A,** This patient had chronic corneal ulceration attributed to distichiasis and currently has anterior uveitis from a cataract. Mild bacterial sepsis was noted (not shown). The epithelium displays moderate to marked anisocytosis and anisokaryosis with hyalinized or keratinized cytoplasm. Two neutrophils are present within the cytoplasm (emperipolesis) related to the moderate inflammation. **B,** Note the homotypic cell cannibalism or cell-in-cell occurrence. This feature should signal concern for neoplasia because this cell interaction is most often attributed to malignancy, but confirmation of neoplasia was lacking in this case. (Wright-Giemsa; HP oil.) (Courtesy Rose Raskin, University of Florida.)

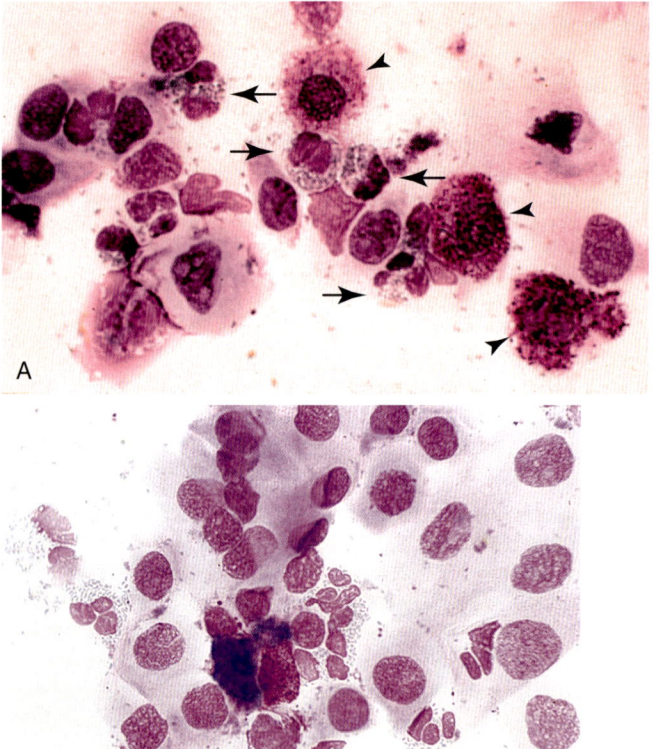

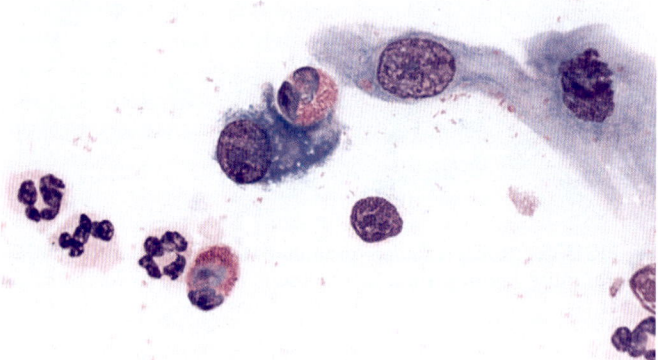

■ **FIGURE 16.29 Eosinophilic keratitis. Corneal brushing. Cat.** This sample is taken from an adult cat with a raised white proliferative lesion of 2 months' duration. Reactive squamous epithelium is shown along with a mixed population of nondegenerate neutrophils and eosinophils. Rod-shaped eosinophil granules produce the stippled background. (Wright-Giemsa; HP oil.)

■ **FIGURE 16.28 Eosinophilic keratitis. Corneal scraping. Cat.** Same case in A and B. **A,** There was a gritty, white proliferative mass at the lateral limbus of this animal with recurrent keratitis. Note the mixture of eosinophils *(arrows)* and many mast cells *(arrowheads)* along with corneal epithelium. Surface granular material often contains high numbers of mast cells in addition to eosinophils. (Wright-Giemsa; HP oil.) **B,** This sample was likely taken from deeper into the cornea because it contains many more eosinophils than mast cells admixed among numerous pale-staining epithelial cells. (Wright-Giemsa; HP oil.)

Malinois, other breeds may also be affected, especially with high exposure to ultraviolet radiation. It initially appears at the limbus as a red, vascularized lesion that progresses centrally, becoming fleshlike and later pigmented and scarred. Initially, it appears cytopathologically as mixed inflammation with plasma cells, lymphocytes, macrophages, and neutrophils.

Response to Tissue Injury

Noninflammatory opaque corneal lesions may result from disease. Corneal degeneration with lipid deposits is seen on histopathology as cholesterol clefts within the stroma in animals with systemic metabolic disease, in particular hyperlipidemia (Wilcock and Njaa, 2015). Cytopathologically, only normal epithelium is seen or rarely cholesterol crystals. This should be contrasted with corneal dystrophy, the most common cause of lipid or mineral deposition in the canine cornea related to a genetic defect in keratocyte metabolism that leads to an accumulation of lipids within corneal fibroblasts.

The deposition of calcium salts is associated with corneal stromal edema and tissue injury or hypercalcemia and appears as a granular plaque. Cytopathology reveals nonstaining crystalline material, which often stains positive for calcium using the von Kossa stain.

Corneal epithelial cysts are an uncommon sequela to corneal injury with surface keratinocytes collected within the stroma producing a raised white to tan mass. Cytopathology resembles that of follicular cyst in the skin (Choi et al., 2010).

Neoplasia

Squamous cell carcinoma, papilloma, melanoma, and sarcoma are the predominant tumor types, although tumors of the cornea are rare.

IRIS, CILIARY BODY, AND AQUEOUS HUMOR

Normal Anatomy and Histology

The iris and ciliary body are termed the *anterior uvea*. The uvea is highly vascular and often pigmented (Fig. 16.30). The anterior border layer contains a single layer of fibroblasts with several underlying layers of melanocytes (Samuelson, 1999). These melanocytes in dogs and cats contain rod to oval brown melanin granules. The iris stroma consists of fine collagenous fibers along with blood vessels and nerves. Unstriated muscle fibers within the stroma help to dilate the iris. The posterior iridal surface is covered by pigmented epithelium that is continuous with the ciliary body. The main portion of the ciliary body consists of smooth muscle along with vascular sinuses and heavily pigmented epithelium at the surface, containing large, round melanin granules. As an extension of the choroid layer, the ciliary body provides nutrients and removes wastes for the cornea and lens through the formation of the aqueous humor. Aqueous humor is a clear fluid that originates from the vascular sinuses within the folds and processes of the posterior portion of the ciliary body. The fluid flows from the posterior chamber of the anterior compartment through the pupil and into the anterior chamber toward the filtration angle. Excess fluid is removed at the iridocorneal angle through a vascular meshwork.

Sample Collection and Preparation of the Anterior Uvea Specimens

When a uveal mass is present, aspiration may be accomplished through the anterior chamber using a 25-gauge or smaller needle. When aqueous humor is cloudy, cytopathologic evaluation of the fluid may help diagnose the presence of infectious agents or neoplasms. Aspiration of the uvea is seldom performed when no mass is present; therefore, cytopathology of aqueous humor may be a good alternative (Linn-Pearl et al., 2015).

Fine-needle aspiration biopsy of fluid in the anterior chamber is conducted under anesthesia using a 25-gauge or smaller needle by entering at the limbus through the bulbar conjunctiva; it is termed *aqueocentesis* (Figs. 16.31 and 16.32). A small

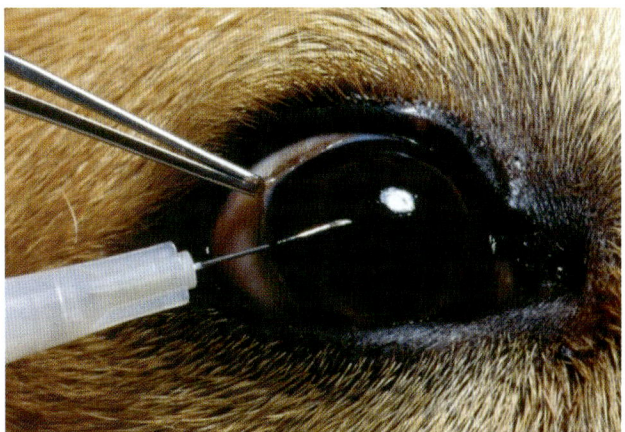

■ **FIGURE 16.31 Aqueocentesis. Cadaver. Dog.** The proper location for sampling is demonstrated on this cadaver. A 27- to 30-gauge needle enters at the limbus, avoiding the iris and corneal endothelium. (From Greene CE. *Infectious Diseases of the Dog and Cat.* 4th ed. Elsevier; 2012.)

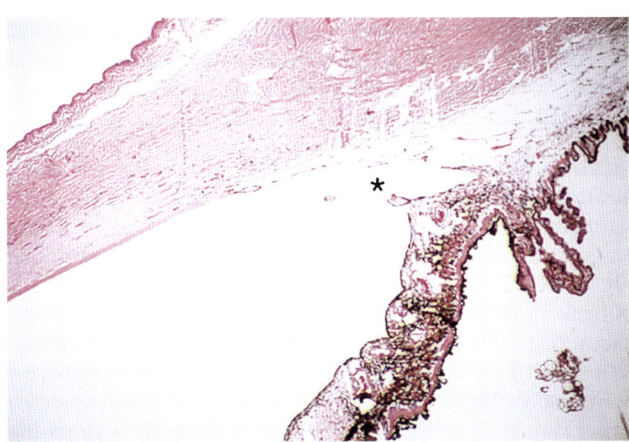

■ **FIGURE 16.30 Normal anterior uvea. Dog.** Present in this view is the cornea near the limbus where the iris and ciliary body attach at the iridocorneal angle *(asterisk)*. Portions of both the anterior and posterior chambers of the anterior humor compartment are shown. (H&E; LP.)

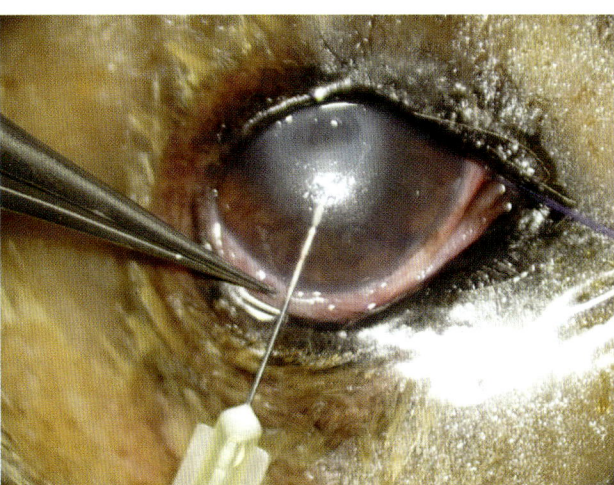

■ **FIGURE 16.32 Aqueocentesis. Clinical case. Dog.** Collection of fluid from the anterior chamber. The procedure is intended for patients with diseased eyes. (Courtesy Thomas Dulaurent, Centre Hospitalier Vétérinaire Saint-Martin, France.)

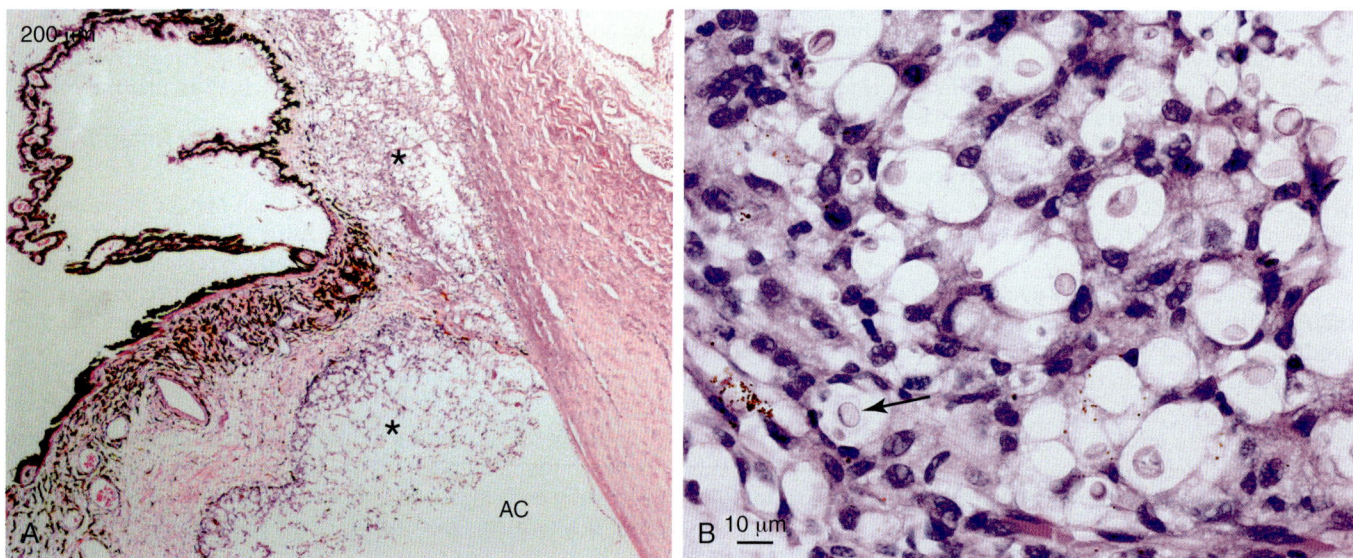

■ **FIGURE 16.33 Pyogranulomatous iridocyclitis. Cryptococcosis. Tissue section. Dog.** Same case in A and B. **A, Tissue section.** A mixed population of neutrophils and macrophages infiltrates *(asterisks)* the iris and ciliary body. The reaction extends into the anterior chamber (AC). (H&E; LP.) **B,** Closer magnification of the numerous yeast, one of which displays budding *(arrow)*. Note the colorless capsules, which mimic epithelial cells. (H&E; HP oil.)

amount of fluid is removed without anticoagulant and processed immediately. A direct cell count using a hemocytometer is performed followed by sedimentation of the fluid for smear or cytocentrifuge preparation. Additional fluid is used to measure total protein by a microprotein technique.

Normal Cytology and Artifacts

Cytologically, the low-protein fluid is clear, colorless, and acellular with only occasional free rod to oval melanin granules or melanin-containing cells. Normal aqueous humor in dogs has a mean direct cell count of 8.2/μL (range, 0–37) and mean protein of 36.4 mg/dL (range, 21–65). Normal aqueous humor in the cat has a mean direct cell count of 2.2/μL (range, 0–15) and mean protein of 43.7 mg/dL (range, 22–75) (Hazel et al., 1985).

Inflammation

Uveal inflammation is typically evaluated from aqueous humor. Anterior uveitis most often produces a neutrophilic infiltrate with infectious causes such as bacteria or from a penetrating injury. Mixed neutrophilic and macrophagic inflammation may occur with fungal infections such as coccidioidomycosis, blastomycosis, cryptococcosis (Fig. 16.33), and histoplasmosis. Feline infectious peritonitis may also produce an anterior uveitis with pyogranulomatous iridocyclitis (Fig. 16.34). An amplification of the infectious agent's nucleic acid can be performed on aqueous humor and may prove useful; however, information regarding the utility of reverse transcription PCR for the feline coronavirus is still lacking (Wiggans et al., 2014; Tasker, 2018). Mononuclear uveitis may occur in the presence of hemorrhage.

Other infectious conditions associated with granulomatous or lymphoplasmacytic uveitis include protothecosis, toxoplasmosis, leishmaniasis (see Fig. 16.16), and canine adenovirus 1 infection (Peña et al., 2008; Di Pietro et al., 2016). Canine monocytic ehrlichiosis has been associated with an anterior uveitis (Komnenou et al., 2007).

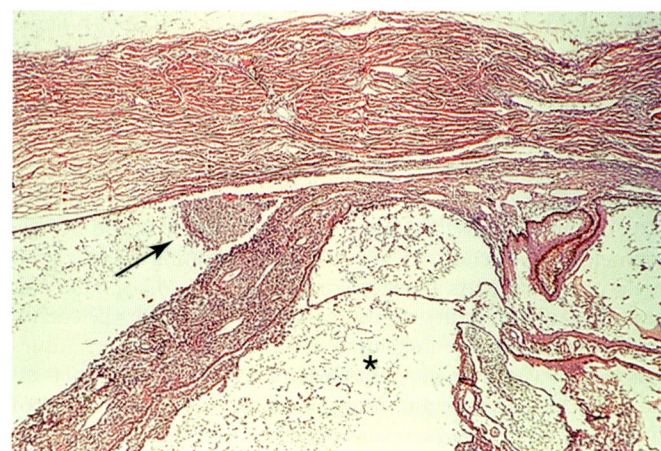

■ **FIGURE 16.34 Pyogranulomatous iridocyclitis. Feline infectious peritonitis. Tissue section. Cat.** Note the presence of an anterior uveitis with accumulation of inflammatory cells in the iridocorneal angle *(arrow)* and in the junction between the iris and ciliary body *(asterisk)* in this animal with confirmed feline infectious peritonitis. (H&E; LP.)

Lens-induced uveitis may produce a lymphoplasmacytic infiltration consistent with immune reactivity to lens proteins. Glaucoma may induce damage to the iris with release of melanin granules and a resulting anterior uveitis from tissue damage (Fig. 16.35). Evidence of damage to the ciliary body or iris can result in frequent rod to round melanin granules engulfed by macrophages (Fig. 16.36). Regardless of the primary cause of uveitis, with time, the predominant cell type may become mononuclear (see Fig. 16.36).

Hemorrhage

Hyphema may present as acute or chronic hemorrhage. Acute hemorrhage may be indicated by the presence of erythrophagocytosis by macrophages. Platelets may be present if ongoing

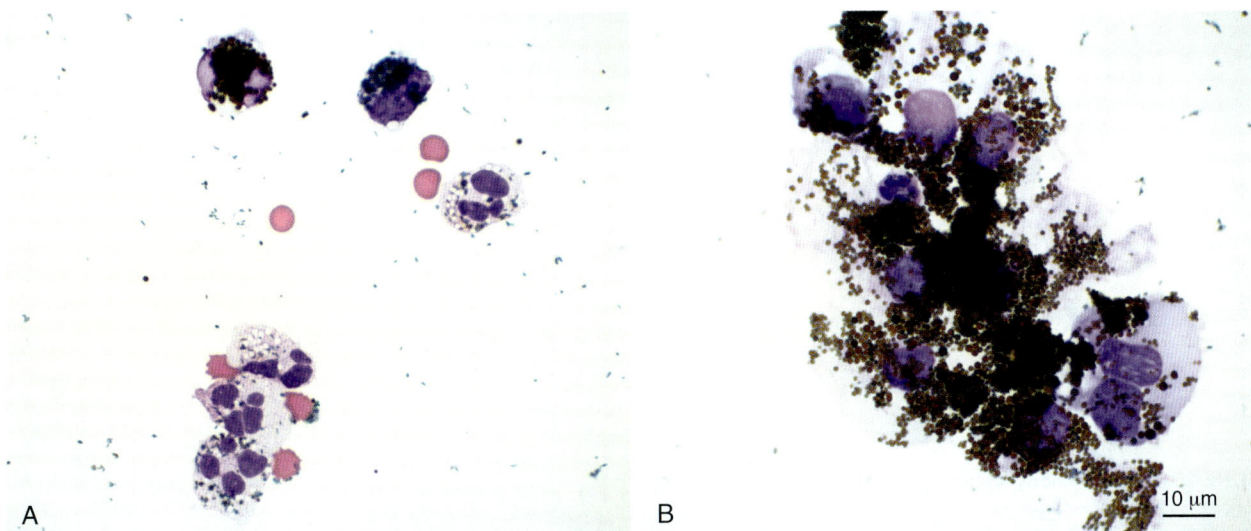

■ **FIGURE 16.35 Glaucoma-induced anterior uveitis. Aqueous humor aspirate. Cytocentrifuged smear. Dog.** Same case in A and B. **A,** The anterior chamber appeared yellow-brown and cloudy. Many neutrophils contain blue-green rod-shaped iris melanin granules. One cell in the upper left contains round, brown melanin granules. **B,** A raft of pigmented epithelium containing round brown melanin granules is present. Enucleation was performed, and histopathology revealed goniodysgenesis (pectinate ligament dysplasia) that likely produced secondary glaucoma, retinal atrophy, and loss of the posterior iris epithelium with pigment dispersion. Neutrophilic uveitis is secondary to iridal and retinal damage. (Modified Wright; HP oil.) (Courtesy Priscila Beatriz Da Silva Serpa, Purdue University.)

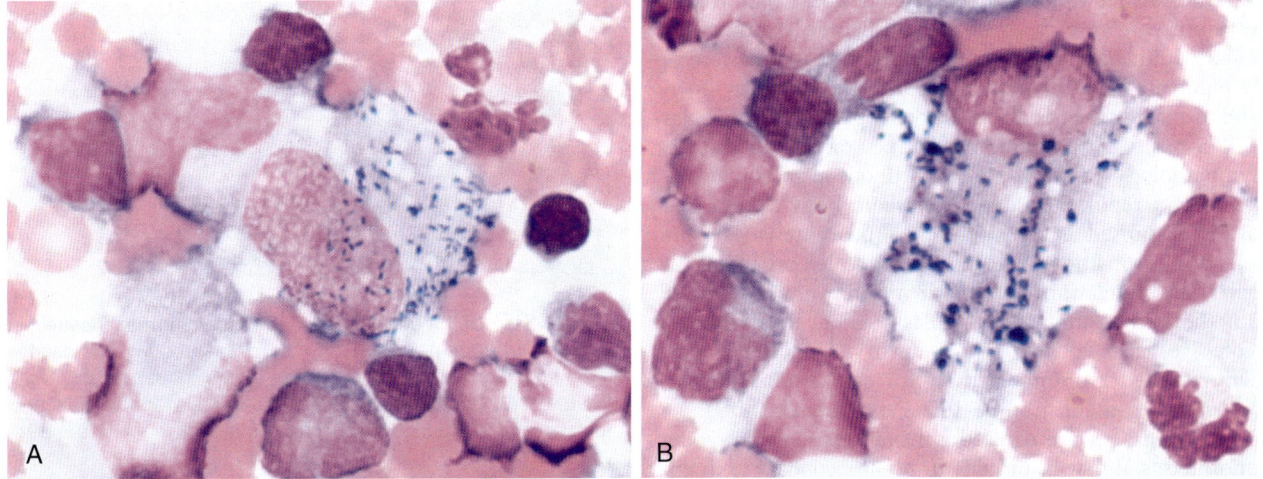

■ **FIGURE 16.36 Mixed mononuclear inflammation. Aqueous humor aspirate. Dog.** Same case in A and B. **A,** Variably sized lymphocytes and macrophages predominate in this case of chronic anterior uveitis with secondary glaucoma. One macrophage contains numerous rod-shaped melanin granules, typical of the anterior iris. (Wright-Giemsa; HP oil.) **B,** Small and intermediate lymphocytes predominate in this field. One macrophage contains both rod and round shapes of melanin granules, consistent with those of the iris and ciliary body. (Wright-Giemsa; HP oil.)

hemorrhage is occurring, but the presence of platelets alone may indicate blood contamination only. Chronic hemorrhage is indicated by the presence of hemosiderin-laden macrophages.

Uveal Hematopoiesis

Studies of six young cats with early life ocular disease (collapse of the globe, corneal perforation with protrusion of the anterior uvea) detected hematopoiesis by histomorphology in three cases. Erythroid and white cell precursors along with occasional megakaryocytes were present in the anterior and posterior uvea (Jacobi and Dubielzig, 2008). Aspirates of damaged eyes in these cases would be expected to demonstrate the extramedullary hematopoiesis.

Neoplasia

Nodular melanomas are the most common primary intraocular tumor in dogs and develop from the iris, ciliary body, and choroid (Labelle and Labelle, 2013). Metastases are infrequent. Diffuse melanomas are common in cats and affect the iris and ciliary body. Distant metastasis spread is relatively frequent. In both nodular and diffuse melanomas, neoplastic cells are variably shaped from plump polygonal to spindle to epithelioid with variable amounts of melanin. Cytopathologic features of mitotic index, nuclear size and pleomorphism, and degree of pigmentation are helpful for prognostic purposes in dogs but not in cats. The presence of anisokaryosis, variable nucleocytoplasmic

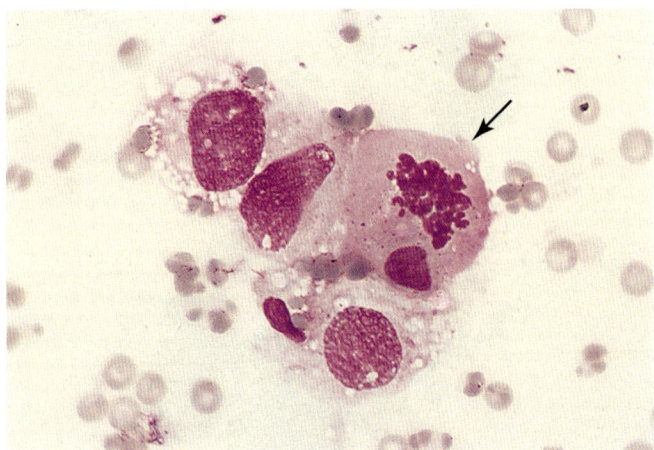

FIGURE 16.37 Ciliary body adenocarcinoma. Iris mass aspirate. Dog. Shown is a tight cluster of epithelial cells with a high nucleocytoplasmic ratio, coarse chromatin, anisokaryosis, and a mitotic figure *(arrow)*. The cytoplasm is foamy with numerous discrete vacuoles. (Wright-Giemsa; HP oil.)

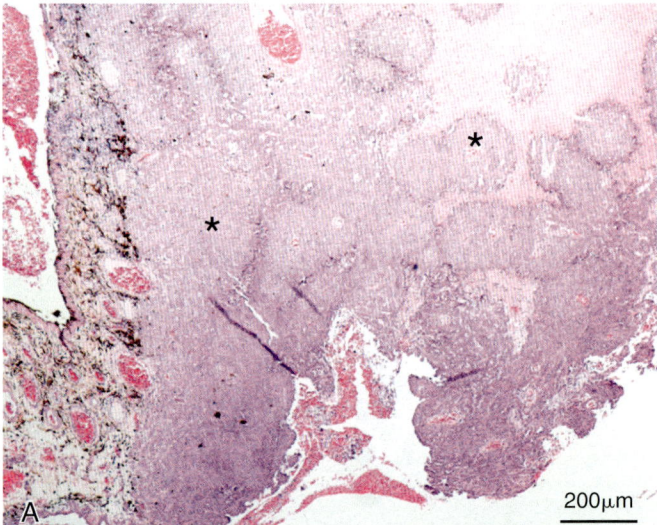
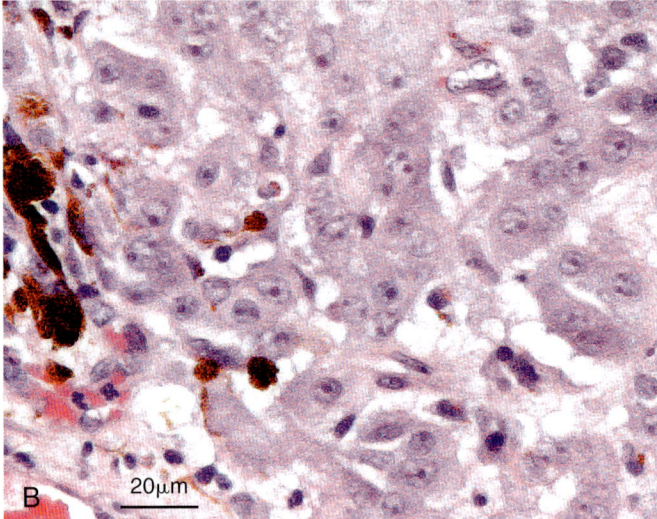

FIGURE 16.38 Ciliary body adenocarcinoma. Tissue section. Dog. Same case in A and B. **A,** The pigmented iris is expanded by a poorly pigmented densely cellular epithelial population *(asterisks)*. (H&E; LP.) **B,** Prominent nucleoli, anisokaryosis, and variable nucleocytoplasmic ratio characterize the malignant epithelium. (H&E; IP.)

ratio (N:C), and prominent nucleoli should help distinguish malignant melanocytes from melanophages.

Ciliary neoplasms such as iridociliary adenoma (Petterino et al., 2014) and adenocarcinoma are the second most common primary intraocular tumors in dogs (Figs. 16.37 and 16.38). These tumors are rare in cats. On ophthalmic examination, iridociliary epithelial neoplasms may appear as a pink, tan, or lightly pigmented masses protruding into the pupillary aperture and displacing the iris. Iridociliary neoplasms often display thick, PAS-positive basement membranes on histopathology and cytopathology may note pink amorphous intracellular material. A recent report of a dog with ciliary body adenocarcinoma was diagnosed as carcinoma by aqueocentesis (Ferreira et al., 2019). Cytopathology in this case revealed an anaplastic epithelial cell population along with melanin granules noted in both the background and cytoplasm of the macrophages and cohesive cells. Immunohistochemistry from the excised eye demonstrated immunoreactivity for cytokeratin, neuron-specific enolase, vimentin, and S-100 (Ferreira et al., 2019).

Lymphoma has been recognized as the most frequent intraocular tumor in cats. It may be primary or occur secondary to multicentric disease. Primary uveal lymphomas may be more frequent in dogs (Lanza et al., 2018). Lymphoma occurs as a diffuse or nodular iris lesion that may be aspirated (Fig. 16.39A). Cytopathologic changes are similar to lymphoid neoplasms in other sites (Fig. 16.39B and C). Metastatic tumors rarely exfoliate with the exception of lymphoma, and aqueocentesis is often diagnostic (Linn-Pearl et al., 2015) (Fig. 16.40). Diffuse large B-cell lymphoma was the most common subtype (53%), followed by peripheral T-cell lymphoma (27%) in a study of 163 cats (Musciano et al., 2020). In that study, primary ocular lymphoma made up the majority of cases (64%), with the remainder being secondary multicentric involvement, and the survival rate was significantly higher in the primary presentation than the systemic form.

RETINA

Normal Histology and Cytology

The retina is composed of 10 classic layers: inner limiting membrane, nerve fiber layer, ganglion cell layer, inner plexiform layer, inner nuclear layer, outer plexiform layer, outer nuclear layer, outer limiting membrane, rod and cone layer, and retinal pigment epithelium (Figs. 16.41 to 16.43A). The outer nuclear layer in cats and dogs contains nuclei associated with mostly rod photoreceptors. These nuclei are small, round, and dense, with a very distinctive appearance having divided dark heterochromatin with one or more cleavages of pale euchromatin (Knoll, 1990; Tvedten and Hillström, 2013) (Fig. 16.43B–D). The retinal pigment epithelium is continuous with the outer layer of the ciliary body and is highly pigmented except in the region of the tapetum lucidum. Melanin within the pigmented retinal epithelial cells appears as lanceolate or elongated (Fig. 16.44). External to the retina and closely adherent to the retinal pigment epithelium is the choroid, also termed the *posterior uvea*, which is mostly composed of large, round, brown to black melanin granules (see Figs. 16.41, 16.42, and 16.44). The outermost area is the sclera composed of fibrous connective tissue (see Fig. 16.41)

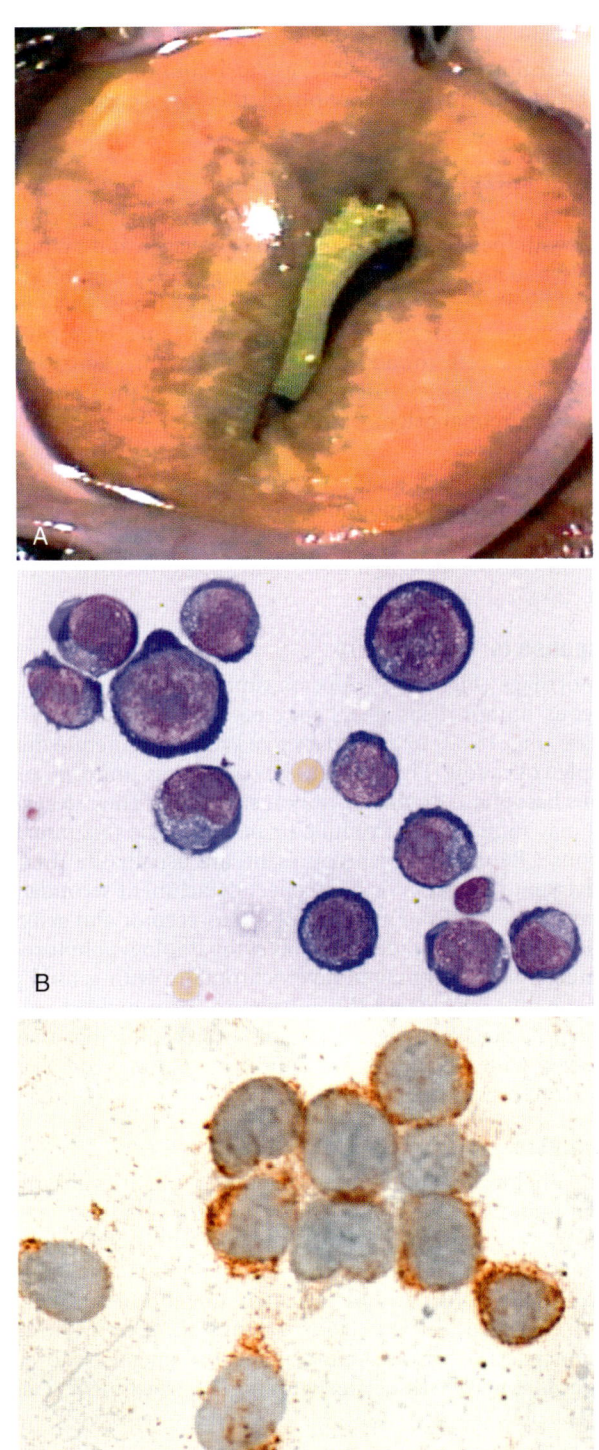

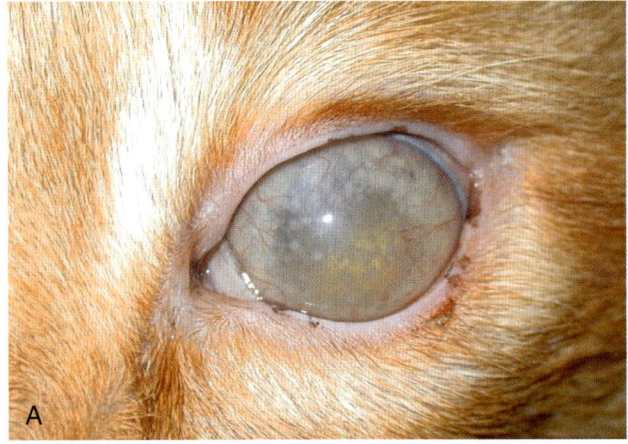

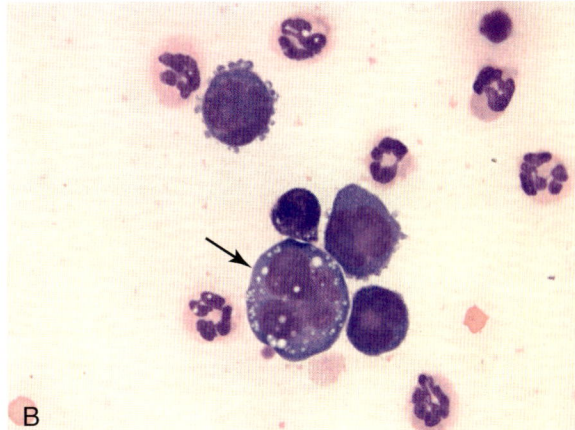

■ **FIGURE 16.40 Lymphoma with neutrophilic uveitis. Cat.** Same case in A and B. **A, Macroscopic.** Cloudiness with flocculent material within the aqueous chamber. Consideration is given for both inflammation and neoplasia. **B, Aqueous humor aspirate.** In addition to nondegenerate neutrophils, several large (4 × RBC diameter) basophilic mononuclear neoplastic lymphocytes are present. One multinucleated cell *(arrow)* is also noted. (Wright; HP oil.) (A, Courtesy Jean Stiles, Purdue University.)

■ **FIGURE 16.39 Lymphoma. Iris mass. Cat.** Same case in A to C. **A, Macroscopic.** Severe thickening and neovascularization of the entire iris. The anterior chamber is very shallow, and the pupil is narrowed by the thickened iris. The nictitans is swollen and the conjunctiva chemotic. **B, Mass imprint.** Large, deeply basophilic round cells are present. Compared with an erythrocyte and small lymphocyte *(lower right)*, these cells measure up to 25 μm in diameter. Notice the RBC size of the nucleolus in several of the cells. Lymphoma is the most frequent intraocular tumor in cats. (Wright-Giemsa; HP oil.) **C, Immunocytochemistry.** Neoplastic round cell population reactive to a B-cell marker. (anti-BLA.36/AEC; HP oil.) (A, Courtesy Maria Kallberg, University of Florida.)

Response to Tissue Injury

Retinal components can be accidentally collected during retrobulbar mass aspiration biopsy, producing retinal hemorrhage (Roth and Sisson, 1999; Tvedten et al., 2013). Retinal detachment may produce a subretinal cavity that contains only normal retinal cells, as demonstrated in one feline case (Knoll, 1990). Ultrasound examination can assist in determining the presence of vitreous debris consistent with retinal detachment. Cytopathologically, intact retinal epithelium along with evidence of acute or chronic hemorrhage with mild neutrophilic inflammation may suggest detachment (Fig. 16.45).

CHOROID AND VITREOUS BODY

Sample Collection of Vitreous Humor

Vitreous humor is likely formed by the nonpigmented epithelium of the ciliary body. In dogs and cats, the vitreous humor is dense in the center of the chamber and fluid at the periphery. Vitreocentesis may be attempted under general anesthesia using

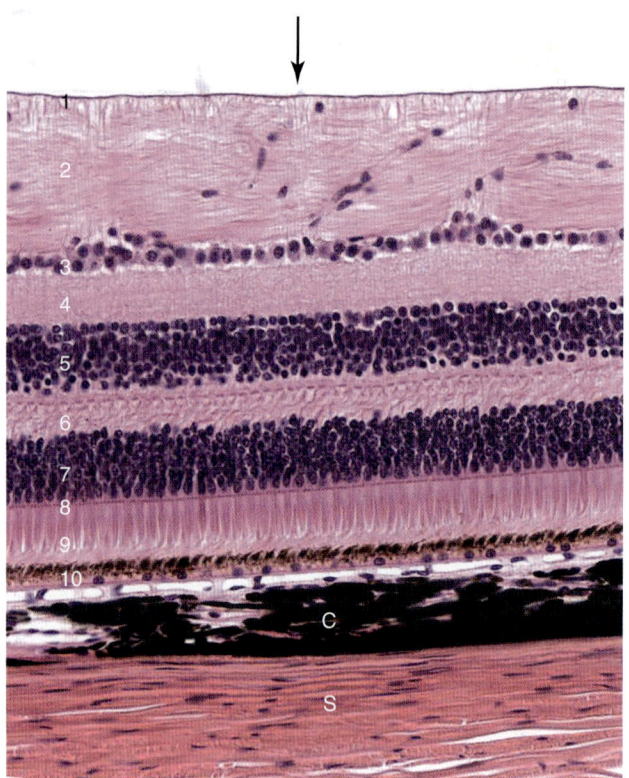

FIGURE 16.41 Normal retina. Dog. Light passes through the vitreous humor *(arrow)* to the retina. The retina is composed of 10 classic layers: *(1)* inner limiting membrane, *(2)* nerve fiber layer, *(3)* ganglion cell layer, *(4)* inner plexiform layer, *(5)* inner nuclear layer, *(6)* outer plexiform layer, *(7)* outer nuclear layer, *(8)* outer limiting membrane, *(9)* rod and cone layer, and *(10)* retinal pigment epithelium. Behind the retina are the vascular choroid (C) and external fibrous sclera (S). (H&E; LP.) (Courtesy Harold Tvedten, Swedish University of the Agricultural Sciences, Sweden.)

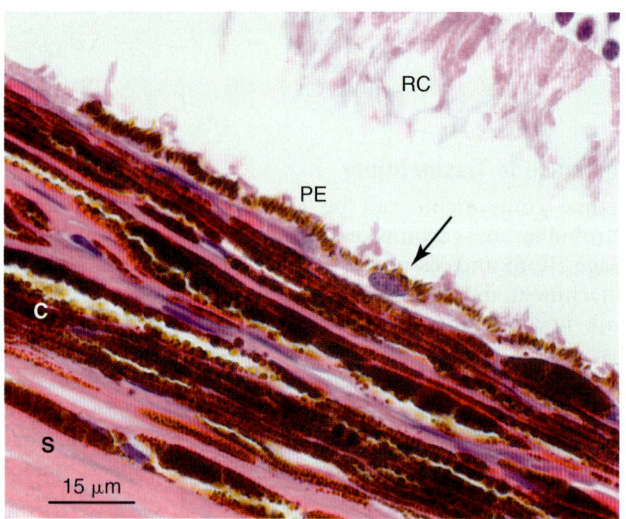

FIGURE 16.42 Normal retina. Dog. High magnification of the outer retinal layers, choroid (C), and external sclera (S). The most external retinal layer is the pigmented epithelium (PE) that contains a palisading row of lanceolate melanin granules in addition to their nucleus *(arrow)*. The artifactually displaced rod and cone layer (RC) normally lies adjacent to the pigmented epithelial layer of the retina. The choroid layer contains numerous round brown granules. (H&E; HP oil.)

a 23-gauge or smaller needle to extract 0.2 to 0.5 mL of fluid from a region 6 to 8 mm caudal to the limbus toward the center of the eye to avoid disruption of the lens (Figs. 16.46 and 16.47).

Normal Vitreous Fluid Cytology

The fluid is a transparent gel-like material that is primarily water with the remainder composed of collagen and hyaluronic acid (Samuelson, 1999). It is acellular except for hyalocytes, a type of histiocyte, plus rare fibrocytes and glial cells. In addition to hyalocytes, fibrocytes and glial cells make up a small portion of the vitreal cells found in the fluid. Occasional lanceolate or caraway seed–shaped melanin granules may be present that are likely from retinal origin.

Inflammation

Infectious causes of endophthalmitis include bacteria, aspergillosis (Gelatt et al., 1991) (Fig. 16.48), blastomycosis (Fig. 16.49), cryptococcosis, histoplasmosis, and prototheosis (Stenner et al., 2007) (Fig. 16.50).

Response to Tissue Injury

Hemorrhage (Fig. 16.51) appears similar to that found in the aqueous humor. Lens fibers may be seen with primary lens disease (Fig. 16.52) or secondary to accidental puncture during sample collection (Fig. 16.53). They appear as uniform amorphous basophilic strands or ribbon structures. Their degeneration may induce a neutrophilic or macrophagic inflammatory response. Retinal cells, when present, are usually the result of inadvertent aspiration or may reflect detachment secondary to disease (e.g., uveitis or glaucoma). Photoreceptor and ganglion cells have been rarely identified on cytopathology; photoreceptor nuclei have marginated heterochromatin with central pale euchromatin, producing the appearance of a divided or segmented nucleus (see Fig. 16.43C). Photoreceptor rods may be observed with retinal disease, appearing as long, rod-shaped, gray structures (see Fig. 16.43B–C).

Neoplasia

Cytopathology rarely discovers neoplasia, but it is diagnostic when found. Feline ocular posttraumatic sarcomas are the second most common intraocular neoplasm in cat. They are thought to arise from lens epithelium when disrupted (trauma, surgery, and so on) and often invade the choroid. (Dubielzig et al., 1990; Zeiss et al., 2003; Grahn et al., 2006). Choroidal melanocytic neoplasms appear as focal pigmented subretinal masses that may be associated with retinal detachment (Labelle and Labelle, 2013).

ORBITAL CAVITY

Sample Collection

The orbit has bony borders and contains vascular and nervous structures as well as lacrimal and salivary glands that are best avoided by imaging-guided biopsies (Boydell, 1991; Cirla et al., 2016). The most direct routes by fine-needle aspiration biopsy are through the lateral and medial canthi, dorsal to the lacrimal bone, or between the mandibular coronoid process and the temporal bone. Specimens were diagnostic in the majority of cases with rare cases of inadvertent retina aspiration (Roth and Sisson, 1999; Tvedten et al., 2013).

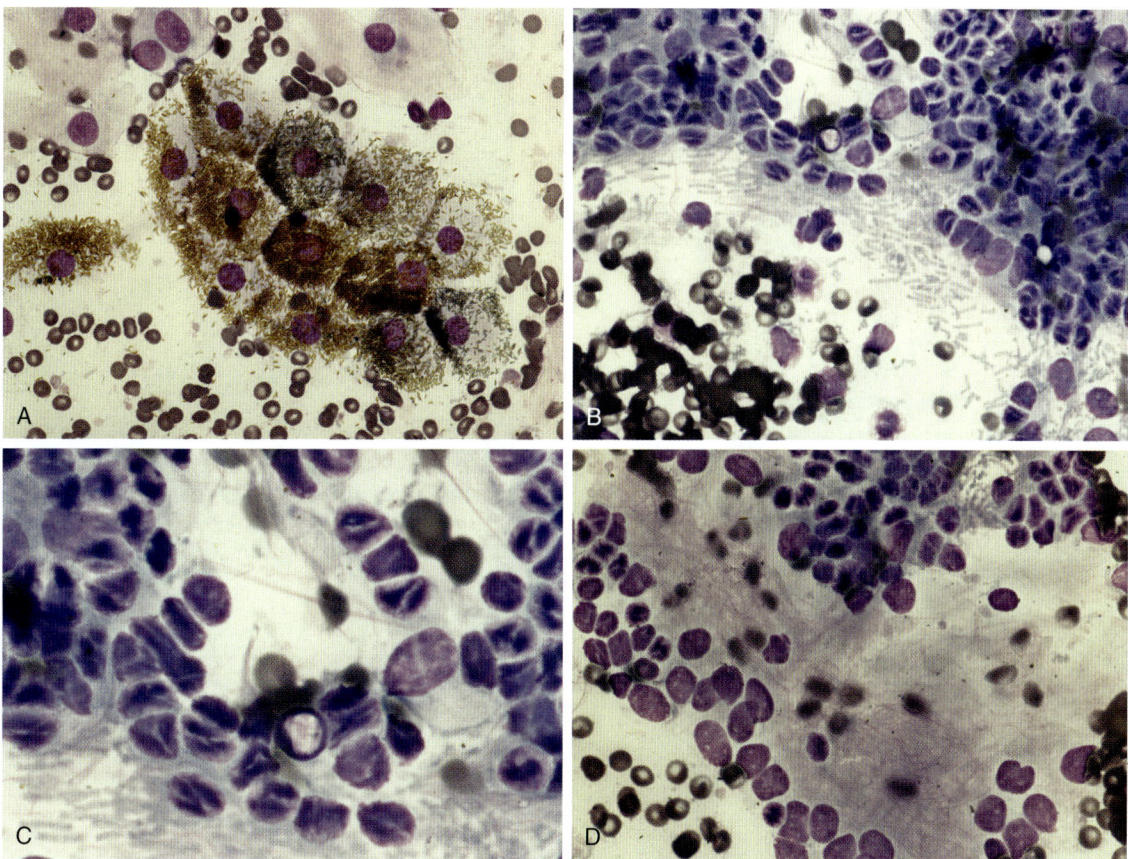

■ **FIGURE 16.43 Normal retina. Aspirate biopsy. Dog.** Same case in A to D. **A,** A monolayer of pigmented epithelium contains numerous lanceolate brown melanin granules and a single round, centrally located nucleus. **B,** A collection of outer nuclear layer cells are present in the upper half along with numerous long gray rods from the rod and cone layer that lie directly below and intermixed among the nuclei. **C,** A higher magnification of the outer nuclear layer cells and rod photoreceptors. Notice the characteristic appearance of the outer nuclear layer cells with margination of the chromatin creating a pale slit so the nuclei appear segmented. **D,** The outer nuclear layer with rods appears in the upper portion of the image with a pink fibrillar region below them representative of the nerve fibers from the outer plexiform layer. Below this layer is a row of large round nuclei with fine chromatin from the inner nuclear layer. (A–D, Hemacolor stain; HP oil.) (Courtesy Harold Tvedten, Swedish University of the Agricultural Sciences, Sweden.)

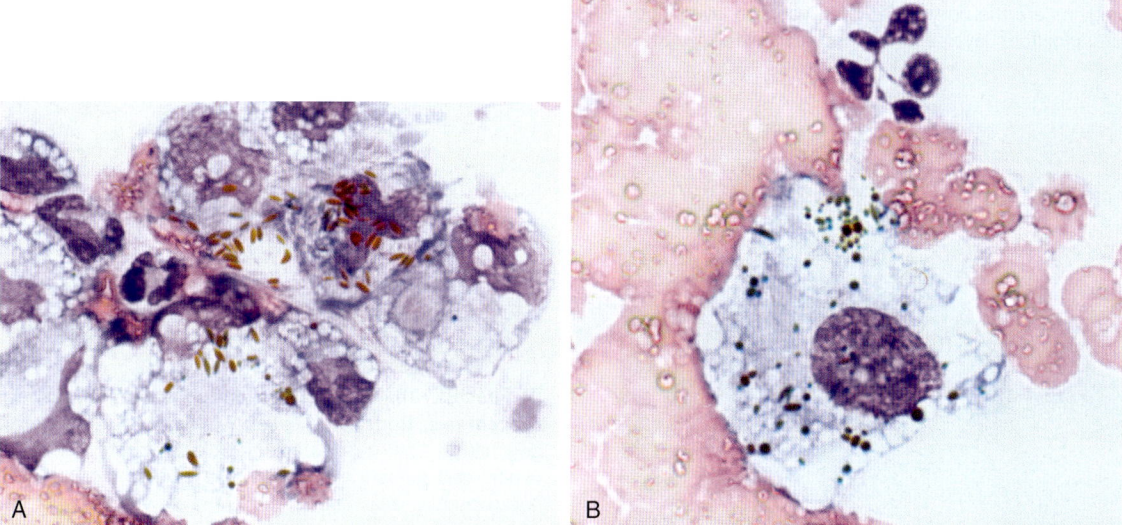

■ **FIGURE 16.44 Melanin granules in vitreous humor. Vitreocentesis. Dog.** Same case in A and B. **A, Retinal melanin granules.** Characteristic lanceolate or caraway seed–shaped melanin granules from the pigmented retinal epithelium are present within macrophages. (Wright-Giemsa; HP oil.) **B, Uveal melanin granules.** The choroid layer adjacent to the retina contains numerous large round brown-black granules as shown within the macrophage. Few lanceolate retinal melanin granules are also present. (Wright-Giemsa; HP oil.)

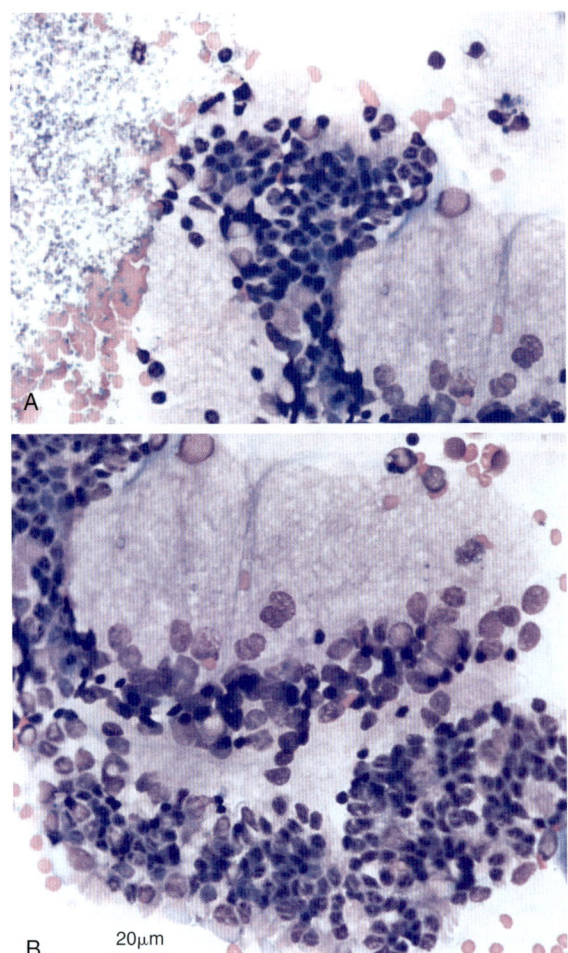

■ **FIGURE 16.45 Retinal detachment. Vitreocentesis. Dog.** Same case in A and B. **A,** Visual impairment was noted for several months. Ocular ultrasound detected vitreous debris. Cytocentrifuged preparation produced a mixture of retinal pigment granules (upper left), dense round retinal cells, and pale neural fibers. (Wright; IP.) **B,** Higher magnification demonstrates the various retinal layers. From top to bottom, the most visible regions are the nerve fiber layer, ganglion layer, inner nuclear layer, outer plexiform layer, and outer nuclear layer. (Wright; IP.)

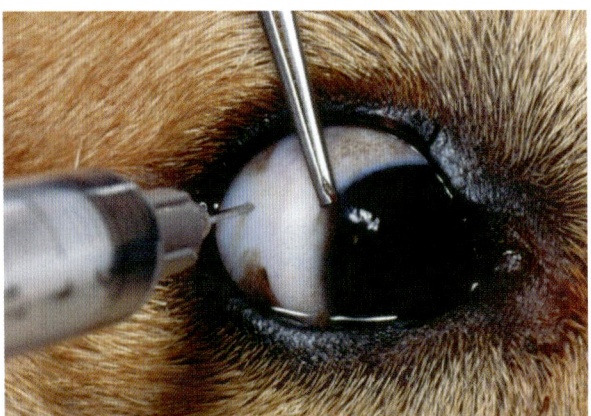

■ **FIGURE 16.46 Vitreocentesis. Cadaver. Dog.** A 22- to 25-gauge needle enters 6 mm posterior to the limbus, directed posterior and toward the center of the globe. (From Greene CE. *Infectious Diseases of the Dog And Cat.* 4th ed. Elsevier; 2012.)

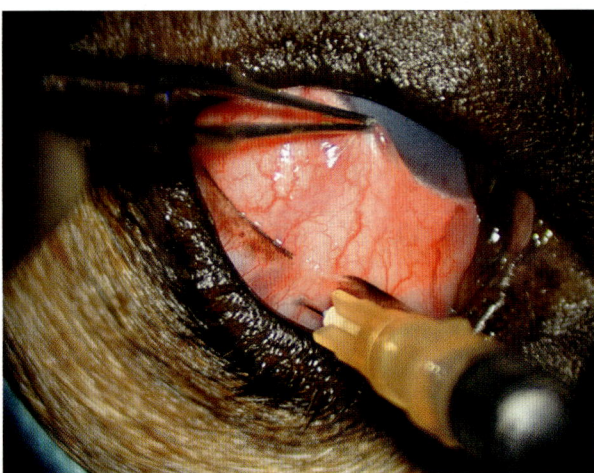

■ **FIGURE 16.47 Vitreocentesis. Clinical case. Dog.** Collection of vitreous fluid. The procedure is intended for patients with diseased eyes. (Courtesy Thomas Dulaurent, Centre Hospitalier Vétérinaire Saint-Martin, France.)

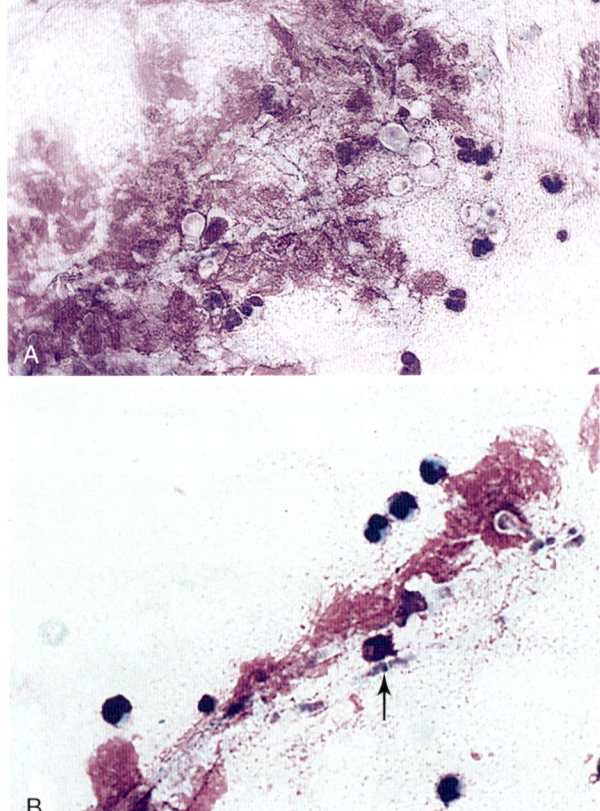

■ **FIGURE 16.48 Infectious endophthalmitis. Aspergillosis. Vitreocentesis. Dog.** Same case in A and B. **A,** This German shepherd dog had a history of paraplegia related to discospondylitis. Bilateral uveitis was present along with other systemic signs of infection. The background is eosinophilic and granular with degenerate neutrophils. Against this proteinaceous material are the clear-staining hyphae and round spores of this fungal agent, which were cultured and identified as *Aspergillus terreus*. (Wright-Giemsa; HP oil.) **B,** Hyphae are barely visible *(arrow)* against the light background. Aspergillosis is a common cause of infectious endophthalmitis. (Wright-Giemsa; HP oil.)

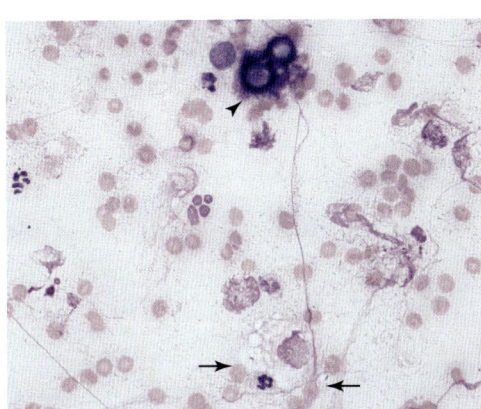

■ **FIGURE 16.49 Infectious endophthalmitis. Blastomycosis. Vitreocentesis. Dog.** Two blue-stained round yeast forms *(arrowhead)* are present along with numerous degenerate neutrophils against a background of many erythrocytes and nuclear debris. One macrophage is vacuolated and phagocytized a lanceolate retinal melanin granule *(arrow)*. Another granule is noted in the background *(arrow)*. (Wright; HP oil.)

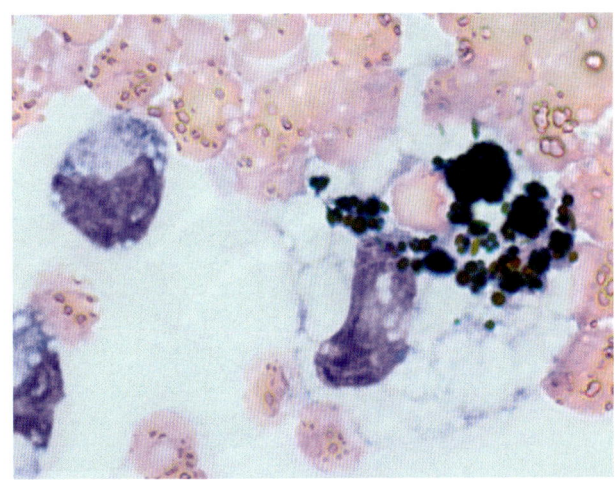

■ **FIGURE 16.51 Acute hemorrhage with uveal melanin granules. Vitreous humor aspirate. Dog.** Same case as in Figure 16.44. A macrophage is shown that has engulfed an erythrocyte as well as clumps of large round brown to black melanin granules consistent with the choroid layer. (Wright-Giemsa; HP oil.)

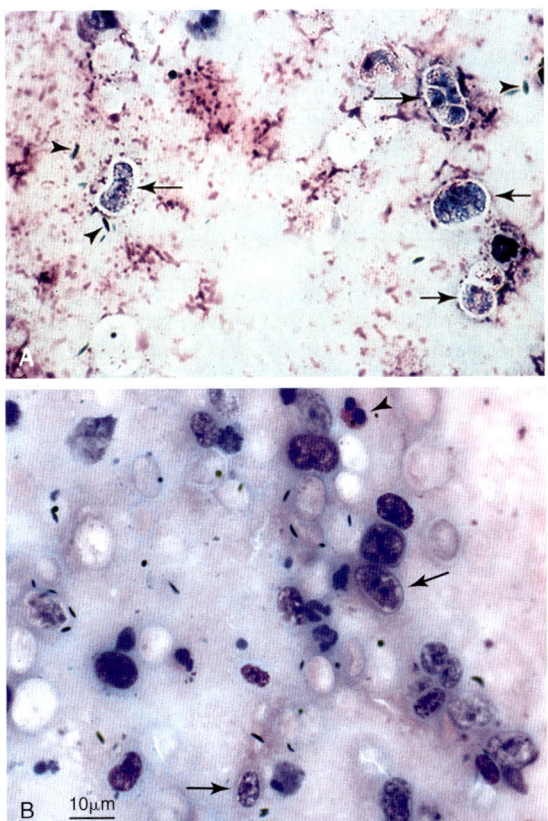

■ **FIGURE 16.50 Protothecosis. Vitreocentesis. Dog. A,** Shown present against the eosinophilic granular vitreal material are four sporulating forms *(arrows)* indicating two sporangia containing 2 to 4 sporangiospores and two free sporangiospores without internal divisions of *Prototheca zopfii*. Also present in the background are several lanceolate melanin granules typical of the retina melanocytes *(arrowheads)*. (Wright-Giemsa; HP oil.) **B,** Fluid contained numerous spherical to oval variably basophilic sporangiospores *(arrows)* having a thin clear wall. Organisms were approximately 3 to 9 μm in diameter by 3 to 10 μm in length with a cell wall (~0.5–1.0 μm thick). A mild inflammatory response consisted mostly of moderately to severely degenerate neutrophils. One eosinophil *(arrowhead)* along with scattered lanceolate melanin granules are also noted in this field. (A, Courtesy Eric Schultze, University of Tennessee. B, Courtesy Heather Flaherty et al., Michigan State University. Presented at the 2004 ASVCP case review session.)

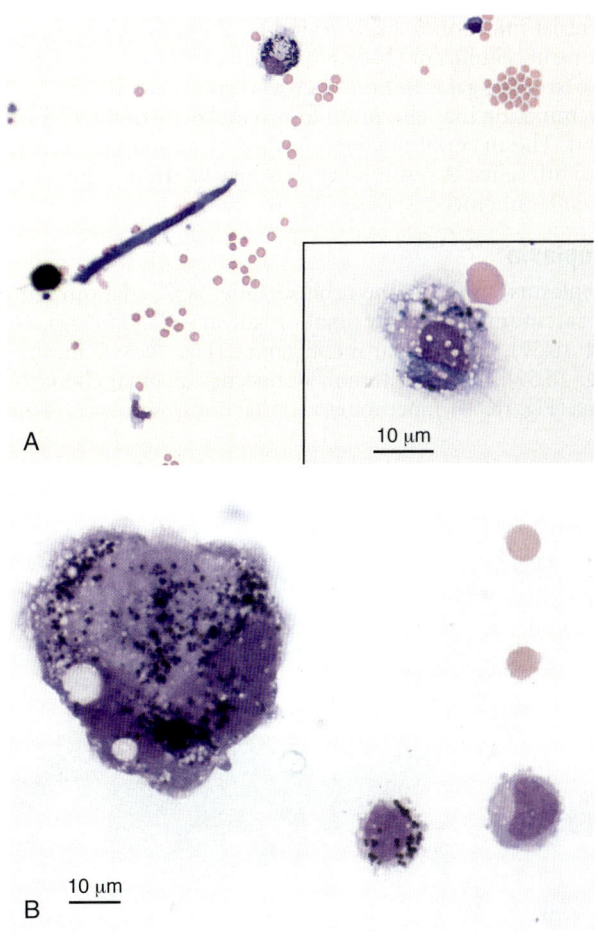

■ **FIGURE 16.52 Lens damage with macrophagic inflammation. Vitreocentesis. Dog.** Same case in A and B. **A,** A single basophilic lens fiber and a mononuclear inflammatory reaction. A macrophage *(top center)* contains lanceolate melanin granules (Modified Wright; IP.) Two lymphocytes are present. *Inset:* A macrophage contains round melanin granules and a short piece of phagocytized lens fiber. (Modified Wright; HP oil.) **B,** One multinucleated and two mononucleated macrophages are present with phagocytized melanin granules. (Modified Wright; HP oil.)

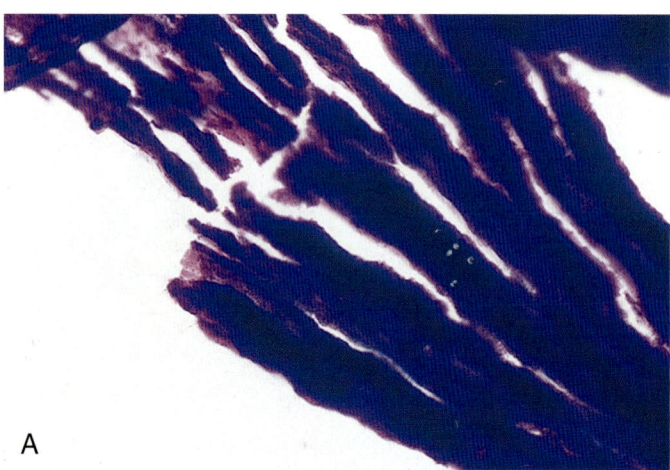
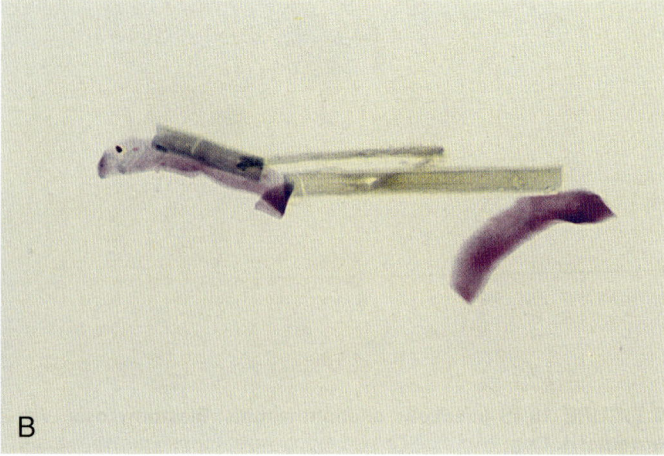

■ **FIGURE 16.53 Inadvertent lens puncture. Vitreocentesis. Dog.** Same case in A and B. **A,** Dark basophilic-staining lens fibers appear in parallel fashion. A mononuclear infiltrate of small lymphocytes (not shown) was present in low numbers in the vitreous humor. The presence of the lens fibers was the result of inadvertent puncture of the lens. (Wright-Giemsa; HP oil.) **B,** Isolated lightly basophilic lens fibers are recognized by the rectangular sharp outlines and ribbon-like appearance. (Wright-Giemsa; HP oil.)

Inflammation

Bacterial infection is likely to induce a purulent response, resulting in cellulitis or abscess formation. Periorbital masses may arise from fungal infections such as cryptococcosis (Fig. 16.54). Inflammation may also result from a mucocele of the zygomatic gland. The material obtained is often clear and viscid, consistent with saliva. A resulting abscess may be sterile with a mixed cell inflammatory response (Fig. 16.55).

Neoplasia

Neoplasms involving the orbit include: SCC, adenoma or adenocarcinoma of the lacrimal or salivary glands (Figs. 16.56 and 16.57), lymphoma, meningioma (Fig. 16.58), melanoma (Fig. 16.59), mast cell tumor, histiocytic sarcoma, chondrosarcoma (Fig. 16.60), hibernoma, and rhabdomyosarcoma (Hendrix et al., 2000; Armour et al., 2011; Tvedten and Hollström, 2013; Cirla et al., 2016; Scott et al., 2016; Piccione and Dial, 2020). The classification of feline intraocular neoplasms by histochemistry and immunohistochemistry was reviewed (Grahn et al., 2006). Histiocytic sarcoma must be considered in the differential diagnosis of dogs with intraocular masses, especially in Rottweilers and retriever breeds. It may be distinguished from melanoma by finding CD18-positive cells and no reactivity using Melan-A. The ocular manifestation of histiocytic sarcoma arises from the systemic form of the disease (Naranjo et al., 2007). An uncommon benign neoplasm of the orbit is *hibernoma* (Ravi et al., 2014),

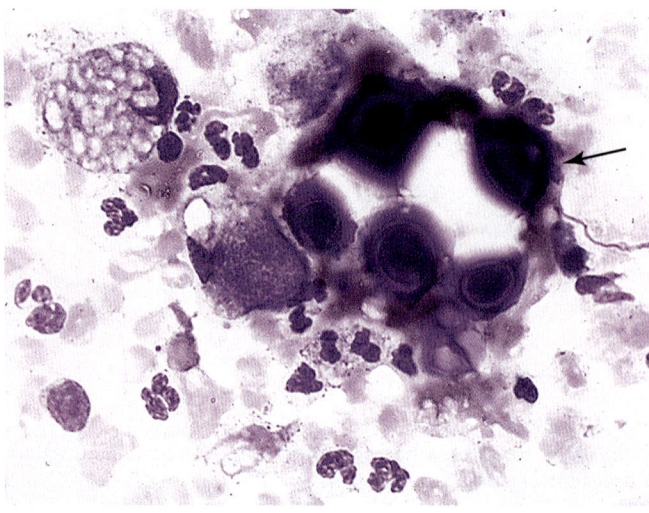

■ **FIGURE 16.54 Cryptococcosis. Tissue aspirate of periorbital mass. Dog.** This animal presented with protuberance of the frontal bone and blindness. Pyogranulomatous reaction occurred in response to the dark spherical yeast forms *(arrow)* of *Cryptococcus neoformans*. (Wright-Giemsa; HP oil.)

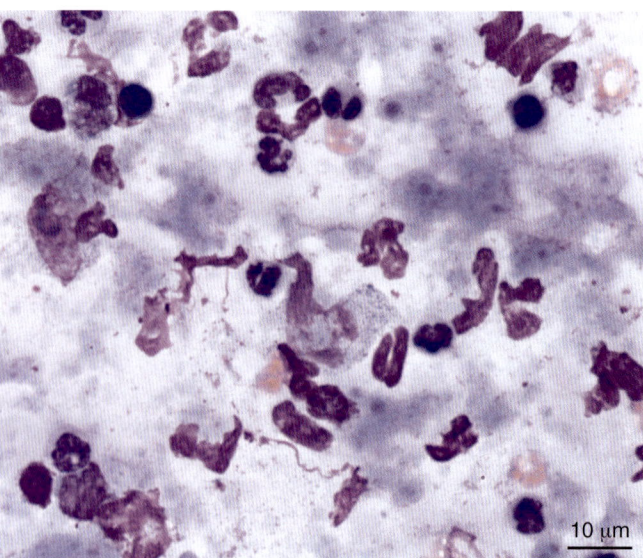

■ **FIGURE 16.55 Retrobulbar salivary gland abscess. Tissue aspirate. Dog.** The patient presented with inflamed and erythematous eyelids and resistance to opening the mouth. Ultrasound-guided aspirate biopsy of periorbital swelling taken revealed moderate neutrophilic inflammation with evidence of gray-blue mucus and occasional epithelium (not shown). Previous antibiotic administration may have precluded finding infectious agents. (Wright-Giemsa; HP oil.) (Courtesy Rose Raskin, University of Florida.)

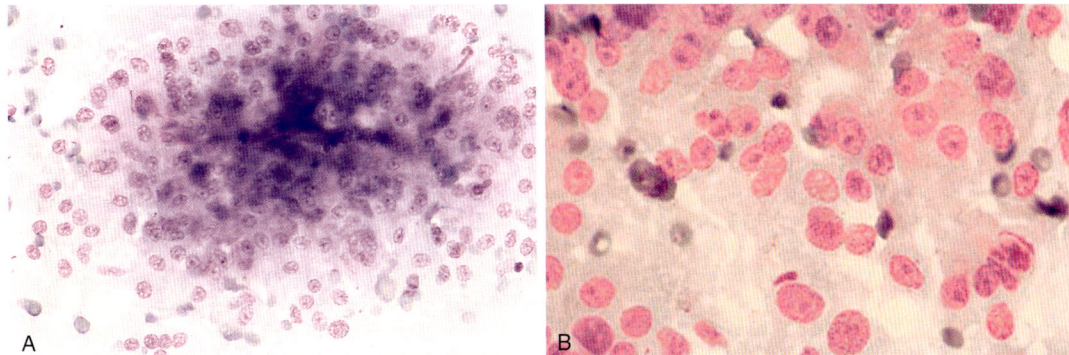

■ **FIGURE 16.56 Salivary and lacrimal gland adenocarcinoma. Tissue aspirate of retrobulbar mass. Dog.** Same case in A and B. **A,** Dense cluster of a monomorphic population of epithelial cells having high nucleocytoplasmic (N:C) ratios and anisokaryosis. The exact origin was not clear on histopathology. It produced minor degenerative changes to the retina but did not invade the globe. (Wright-Giemsa; HP oil.) **B,** Higher magnification demonstrates an acinus *(upper right)* and the foamy secretory appearance of the cytoplasm. Several nuclear features of malignancy are present, including a high N:C ratio, anisokaryosis, coarse chromatin, prominent nucleoli, and multinucleation. (Wright-Giemsa; HP oil.)

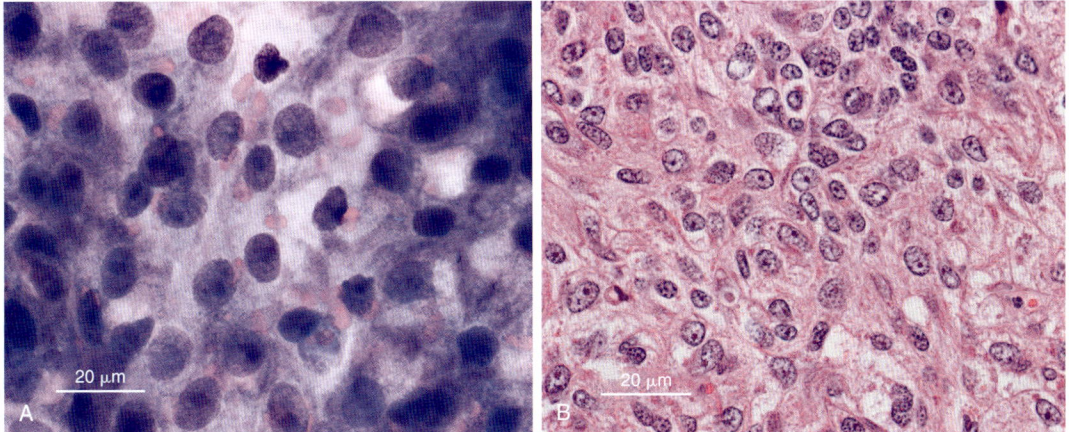

■ **FIGURE 16.57 Retrobulbar salivary and lacrimal carcinoma. Cat.** Same case in A and B. **A, Tissue aspirate.** A monomorphic cluster of small to medium epithelial cells is present. Each cell has a single round to oval nucleus set in a moderate amount of wispy, blue to grey cytoplasm with indistinct margins. The nuclei exhibit a finely stippled chromatin pattern and often contain one or two prominent round to slightly angular nucleoli. Slight anisokaryosis and anisocytosis are noted. Nucleocytoplasmic (N:C) ratios are only slightly increased. The minimal anaplastic features suggest a low-grade carcinoma on cytopathology. (Wright; HP oil.) **B, Tissue section.** Mild to moderate anisokaryosis, moderate N:C ratio, and low numbers of mitotic figures (not shown) confirm a low-grade neoplasia. Cell clusters with junctions that were confirmed by electron microscopy support the epithelial origin. The pale or foamy or vacuolar appearance of the cytoplasm suggests a secretory or glandular product. Top considerations include salivary or lacrimal origin or, less likely, nasal epithelium. (H&E; HP oil.)

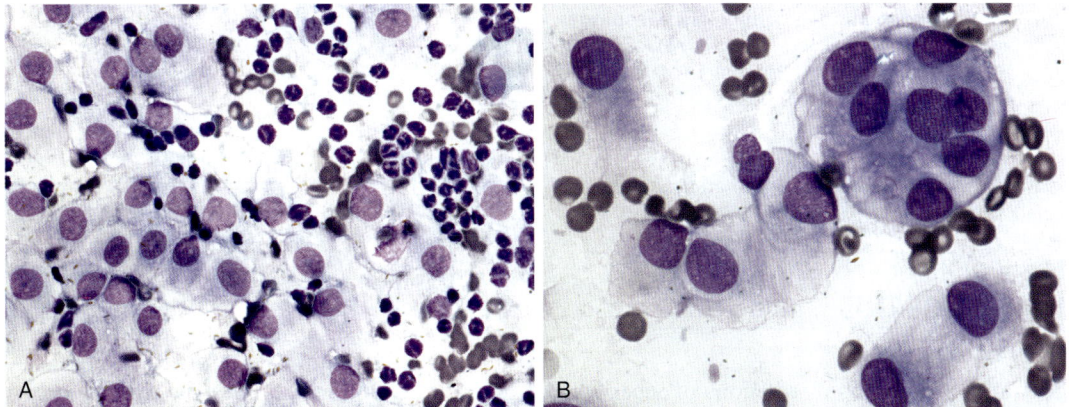

■ **FIGURE 16.58 Periorbital meningioma. Tissue aspirate. Dog.** Same case in A and B. **A,** Meningioma growing around the optical nerve was composed of cells with moderate to large amounts of lightly basophilic cytoplasm. Indistinct cell borders suggested mesenchymal cytomorphology. Nuclei displayed mild anisokaryosis, a uniform chromatin pattern, and small nucleoli, suggesting a benign tumor. Nuclei were about 1.5 to 2.5 times an erythrocyte in diameter. Collections of outer nuclear retinal cells are visible at *upper right*. (Hemacolor stain; HP oil.) **B,** One aggregate of meningioma cells are arranged in a ball with other cells appearing individualized with indistinct cell borders. (Hemacolor stain; HP oil.) (Courtesy Harold Tvedten, Swedish University of the Agricultural Sciences, Sweden.)

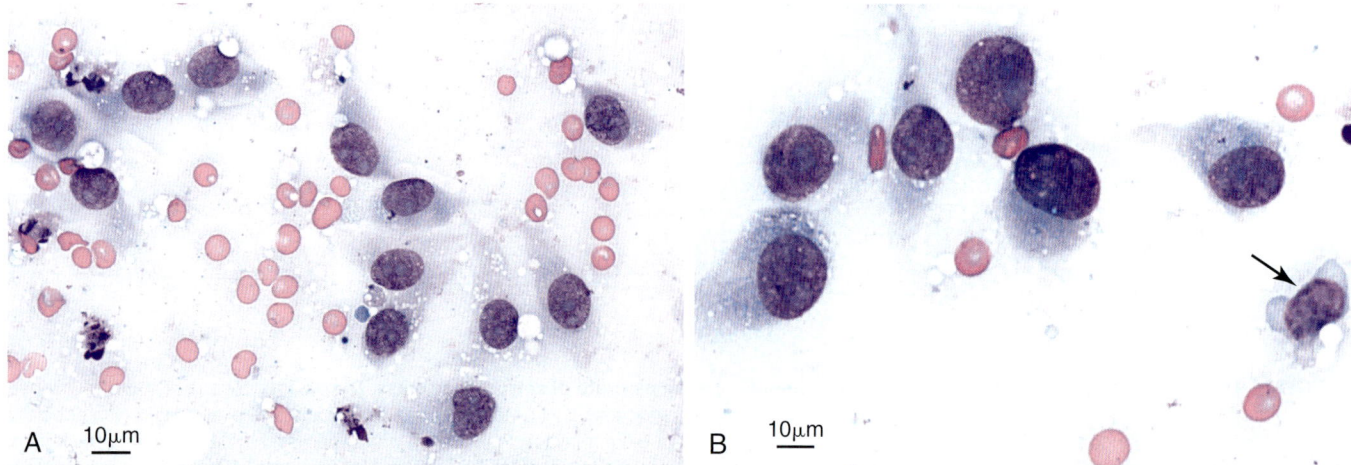

■ **FIGURE 16.59 Retrobulbar melanoma. Tissue aspirate. Dog.** Same case in A and B. **A,** The patient was treated for an incompletely excised oral melanoma 1 year earlier. This retrobulbar mass is composed of a uniform population of individualized cells having spindle to oval shapes. (Wright; HP oil.) **B,** Higher magnification demonstrates moderately basophilic amelanotic cytoplasm with tail extensions and round to oval nuclei with multiple prominent nucleoli. One lymphocyte is present *(arrow)* for size comparison. (Wright; HP oil.)

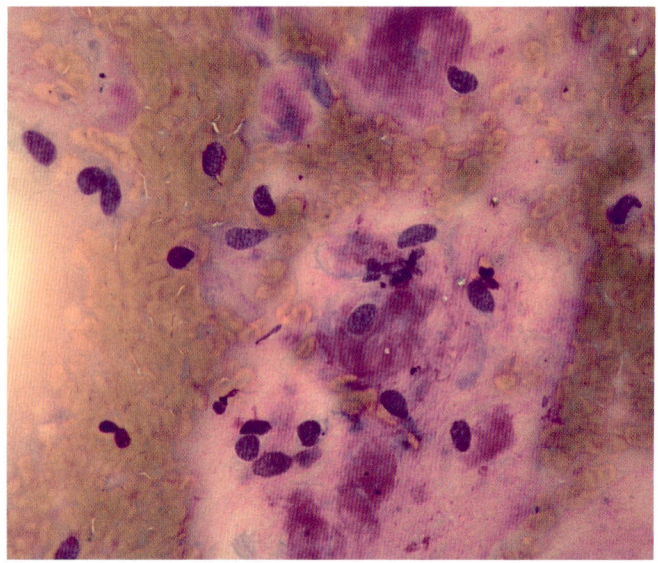

■ **FIGURE 16.60 Retrobulbar chondrosarcoma. Tissue aspirate. Dog.** Moderate numbers of mesenchymal cells with oval nuclei display mild anisokaryosis. Abundant magenta, fibrillar matrix material surrounds these cells. (Modified Wright; HP oil.) (Courtesy Rose Raskin, TDDS, Synlab, Exeter, UK.)

which on cytopathology contains finely granulated and highly vacuolated fat cells with many small droplets, consistent with brown fat.

NASOLACRIMAL APPARATUS

Normal Histology and Cytology

Tears are formed in part by the lipid secretions of sebaceous glands, such as the meibomian glands, by mucin from conjunctival goblet cells, and by seromucoid secretions from the gland of the nictitating membrane. However, tears are formed predominantly by aqueous fluid from the lacrimal gland located dorsolateral to the globe. The lacrimal gland is composed of serous gland epithelium in cats but is seromucoid in dogs. Ducts are lined by flattened, cuboidal epithelium.

Inflammation

Inflammation of the lacrimal sac, or *dacryocystitis*, is frequently bacterial in origin with neutrophilic exudates that may obstruct the ducts.

Cyst

In dogs and cats, a cyst may arise within the duct of the lacrimal gland that is termed *dacryops*. On cytopathology, smears contain serous or seromucoid material of low cellularity. The cyst contents may be mixed with few neutrophils and macrophages (Ota et al., 2009; Zemljič et al., 2011; Delgado, 2013) (Fig. 16.61).

OTIC CYTOPATHOLOGY

Cytopathology of the ear is a frequently used tool in clinical practice to manage ear conditions and determine an underlying cause. The ear involves the pinna, external ear canal, middle ear, and inner ear (Fig. 16.62). Although most areas of the ear are examined, the inner ear being contained within bone is not clinically examined by cytopathology.

EXTERNAL EAR AND PINNA

Normal Anatomy and Histology

The external ear is composed of the pinna or auricle and the external ear canal or auditory acoustic meatus. There are many muscles in and around the pinna, which act to move the ear in specific directions. The pinna functions to collect, focus, and direct sound down the funnel-shaped external acoustic meatus to the tympanic membrane. The *external acoustic meatus* is a conical opening made up of elastic cartilage and bone (Njaa, 2017). The vertical ear canal in dogs extends about 1 inch before forming the horizontal ear canal. The skin of the pinna (Fig. 16.63) contains apocrine sweat glands, sebaceous glands, and hair follicles, and the external acoustic meatus is lined by

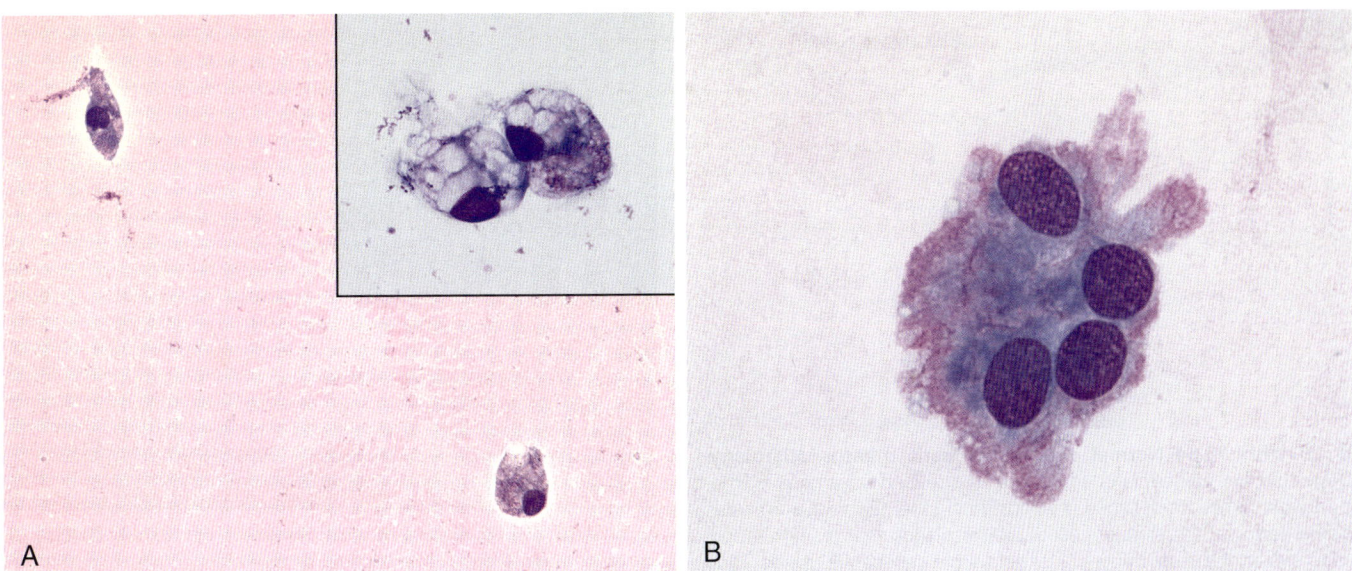

FIGURE 16.61 Lacrimal gland dacryops. Fluid aspirate. Dog. Same case in A and B. **A,** Swelling on the side of the head revealed a fluid with low nucleated cellularity against a lightly eosinophilic background. Nucleated cells consist primarily of individualized mononuclear cells. The cyst arises as a swelling within the lacrimal gland duct. (Modified Wright; IP) *Inset:* Two vacuolated mononuclear cells with pink granulated and foamy cytoplasm. (Modified Wright; HP oil.) **B,** An aggregate of four lacrimal ductular cells appears with associated pink matrix. (Modified Wright; HP oil.) (Courtesy Rose Raskin, Kansas State University.)

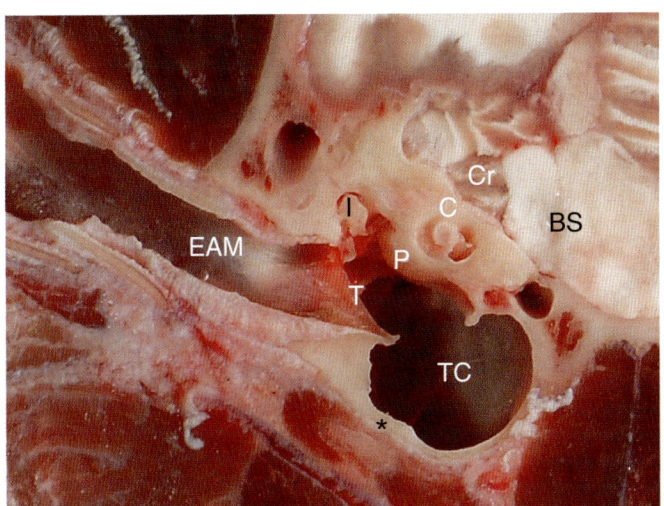

FIGURE 16.62 Cross section of the head through the normal right ear. Rostral aspect. Dog. The horizontal canal portion of the external ear canal or external acoustic meatus (EAM) is shown that ends at the tympanic membrane (T), which has been torn off. The middle ear consists of the tympanic cavity (TC), which is surrounded by a thin bone *(asterisk)*. The promontory (P) portion of the temporal bone demarcates the medial portion of the tympanic cavity. The three ossicles also located in the middle ear with one present, the incus (I). The auditory tube is indicated *(arrowhead)*. One portion of the inner ear enclosed by bone is visible, the cochlea (C). BS, Brainstem; Cr, cerebellar cortex. (Courtesy Bradley Njaa, Kansas State University.)

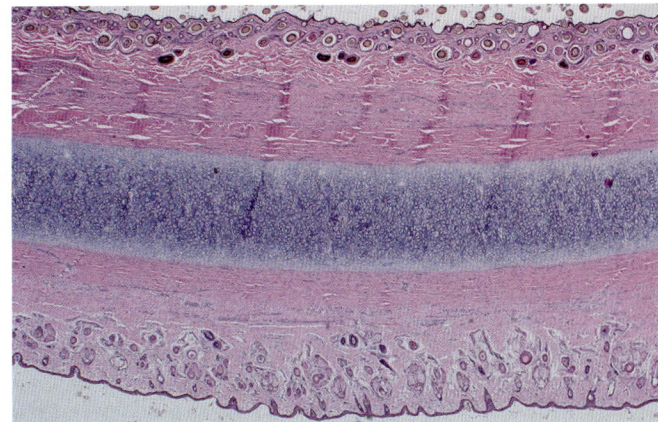

FIGURE 16.63 Normal pinna. Histology. Dog. The convex side is at the top containing numerous hair follicles and a denser adnexal region than the less haired concave bottom side. Cartilage is present as structural support in the auricle. (H&E; LP.) (Courtesy Bradley Njaa, Kansas State University.)

thin epidermis of stratified squamous epithelium and thin dermis that contains similar sebaceous glands, fewer hair follicles, and many more ceruminous glands (Fig. 16.64). Ceruminous glands are simple coiled tubular glands that resemble apocrine sweat glands located in the deeper dermis below the sebaceous glands. The secretory portion of the ceruminous glands is lined with high columnar cells, whereas the tubular part is lined by a single row of flattened cells. Cerumen is a clear emulsion that coats the ear canal composed of sloughed keratinized squamous epithelial cells and secretions from the sebaceous and ceruminous glands.

Sample Collection and Preparation

Historically, sample collection of ear swabs used heat fixation to ensure good-quality smears. This debate has been addressed in two separate reports that show that samples taken as swabs for ear cytopathology do not need heat fixation (Toma et al., 2006; Griffin et al., 2007). Specimens should be evaluated for the

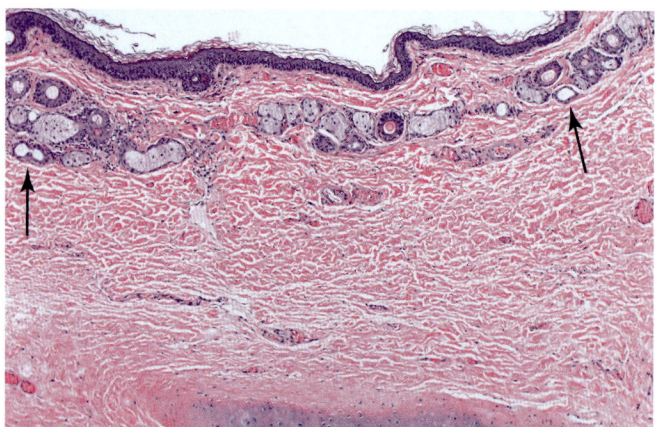

FIGURE 16.64 Normal external acoustic meatus. Histology. Dog. The thin epidermis is composed of stratified squamous epithelium with numerous sebaceous glands within the dermis. Ceruminous glands *(arrows)* are simple, coiled, tubular glands that resemble apocrine sweat glands and appear just below the sebaceous glands. Their ducts open either into hair follicles or directly to the epidermal surface. (H&E; LP.) (Courtesy Bradley Njaa, Kansas State University.)

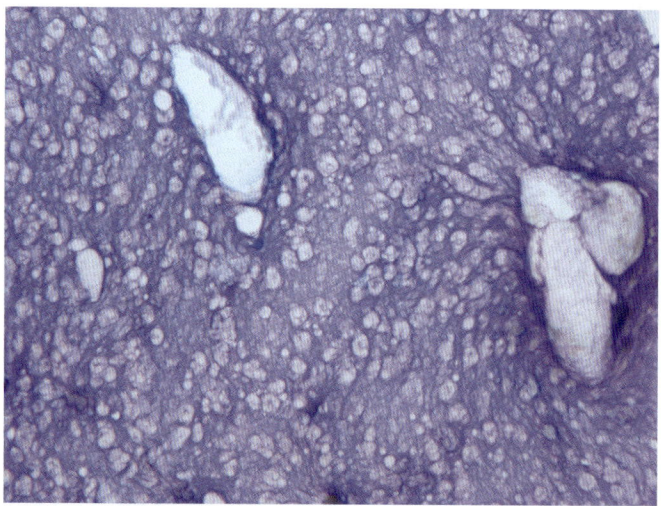

FIGURE 16.65 Otic ointment. External ear canal. Discharge biopsy smear. Dog. A low number of pale-staining keratinocytes appears within an abundant lipid mucin material. This gel medication stains pink-purple and contains variably sized colorless foamy lipid-like droplets. Clinical history indicated recent use of Osurnia (florfenicol terbinafine betamethasone acetate). (Modified Wright; HP oil.) (Courtesy Rose Raskin, University of Bristol, UK.)

presence, numbers, and characteristics of nonhematopoietic cells and leukocytes as well as microbiologic or parasitic agents (bacteria, yeast, arthropods) (Angus, 2004).

It is recommended to take aspirate biopsies of external ear masses, which in cats showed good association with the histopathology (De Lorenzi et al., 2005).

Normal Cytology and Artifacts

In a study of the normal vertical ear canal, yeasts, were detected in 96% of the dogs and 83% of the cats. Gram-positive cocci were found in 42% of the dogs and 71% of the cats, but rods were not seen in either species (Tater et al., 2003). Organisms cultured from the external ears of dogs without ear disease include *Staphylococcus* spp., *Bacillus* spp., yeast, *Escherichia coli*, *Corynebacterium* spp., *Streptococci* spp., and *Micrococcus* spp. (Cole, 2009). In a study of normal ears, the average number of yeast per 10/hpf (400× magnification) was 2.6 in dogs and 3.3 in cats with a median value for each species of fewer than 0.3 yeast per high power field (Tater et al., 2003).

Nucleated keratinocytes are observed in canine and feline ear canals and should not be mistaken for a pathological process. The presence of topical medication may appear as oily discharges that contain occasional keratinocytes against a background of foamy basophilic material (Fig. 16.65).

Inflammation

Many of the inflammatory lesions found elsewhere on the body may occur on the outer side of the pinna, including parasitic dermatitis (demodex), pyoderma (coccoid bacteria) (Fig. 16.66), mycotic dermatitis (Fig. 16.67), or protozoanosis (e.g., leishmaniasis) (Fig. 16.68).

Mycobacteriosis, including canine leproid granuloma (CLG), is an uncommon condition that appears mostly in Australia with fewer cases in North America (Kastl et al., 2020), South America, Africa, and Europe. The etiologic agent is a nontuberculous mycobacterial species that is difficult to grow in culture. The disease is self-limiting, resolving spontaneously within 6 months, and up to 86% of CLG lesions resolve

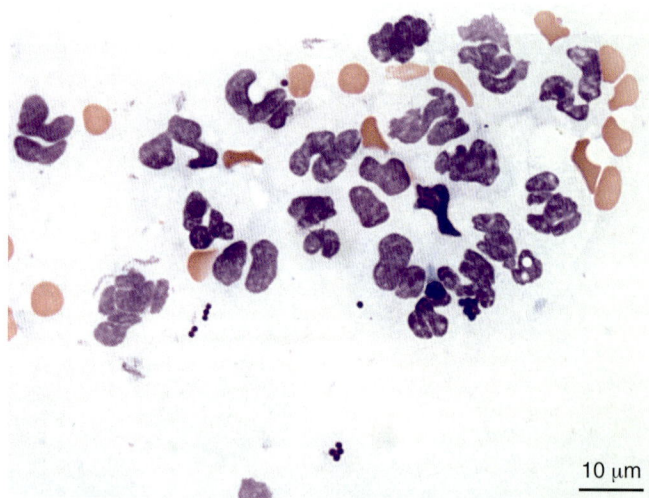

FIGURE 16.66 Otitis externa. Bacterial infection. Discharge biopsy smear. Cat. Many karyolytic (degenerate) neutrophils with extracellular and occasional intracellular large coccoid bacteria. There was concurrent yeast infection in other areas (not shown). (Wright-Giemsa; HP oil.) (Courtesy Rose Raskin, University of Florida.)

spontaneously within 1 to 3 months without medical or surgical intervention (Kastl et al., 2020). Short-haired breeds such as boxers and boxer-cross dogs and German shepherds are predisposed. Single to multiple, firm, painless nodules appear often on the head or pinna (Fig. 16.69A). The inflammation involves macrophages and varies with neutrophils, lymphocytes, and plasma cells (Fig. 16.69B). Diagnosis involves use of Fite or Ziehl-Neelsen acid-fast stains (Fig. 16.69C) with specific identification by PCR testing.

Macroscopically, otitis externa may include discharge from the ear (otorrhea), hemorrhage from the ear (otorrhagia),

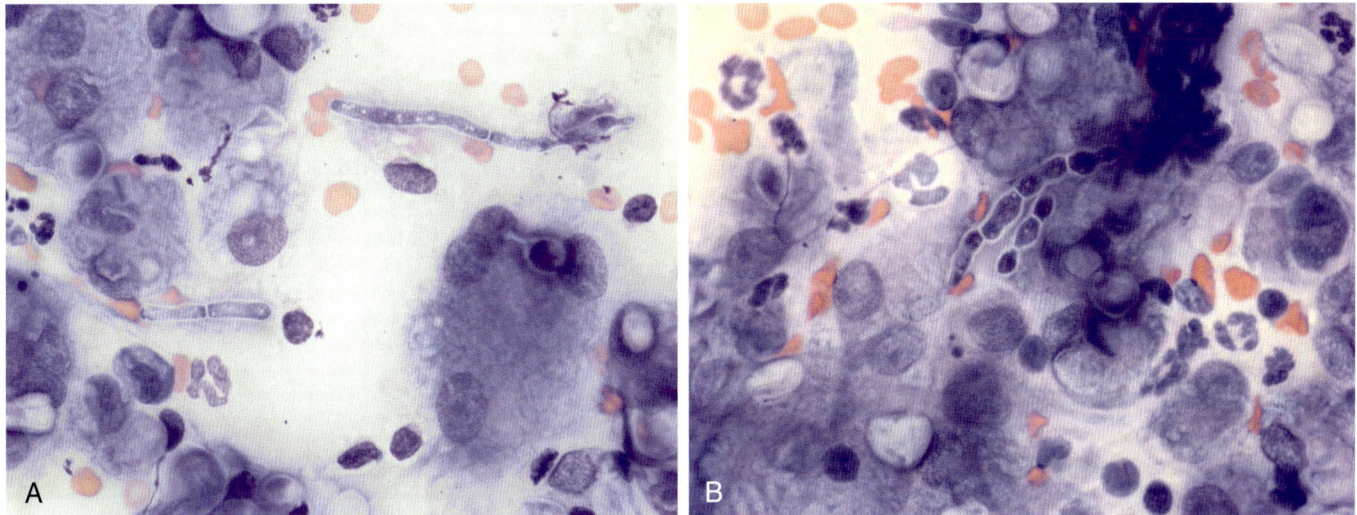

■ **FIGURE 16.67 Otitis externa. Fungal infection. Mass biopsy smear. Cat.** Same case in A and B. **A,** Many macrophages with fewer neutrophils surround and phagocytize septate fungal hyphae. **B,** Swollen septate hyphae with globose conidia consistent with an opportunistic fungal agent. (Modified Wright; HP oil.) (Courtesy Robert Lukacs, TDDS, Synlab, Exeter, UK.)

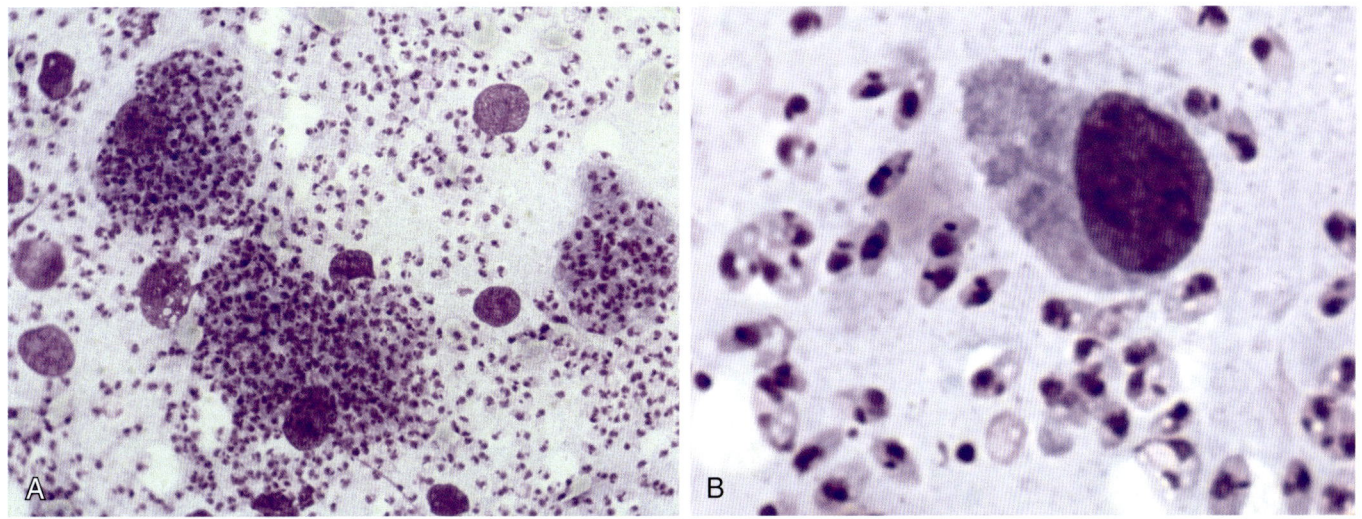

■ **FIGURE 16.68 Leishmaniasis. Granulomatous inflammation. Pinna nodule. Aspirate biopsy. Cat.** Same case in A and B. Multiple soft round nodules are present on the ear surface. The largest measured 5 to 7 mm was evaluated. **A,** The majority of nucleated cells were macrophages, several of which are intact or partially ruptured against a background of numerous free amastigotes. (Aqueous Romanowsky; HP oil.) **B,** One intact macrophage is present along with amastigotes that measure 0.5 to 2.0 μm. The amastigote has pale oval cytoplasm containing a round, dense, purple nucleus with a single short dark rod-shaped kinetoplast. (Aqueous Romanowsky; HP oil.) (Glass slide material courtesy of Ruanna Gossett et al., Texas A&M University. Presented at the 1991 ASVCP case review session.)

and pain elicited when palpating the ear (Njaa, 2017). Otitis externa results in epidermal and follicular hyperplasia, dermal inflammation, reduced activity of sebaceous glands, and dilated ceruminous glands (Cole, 2009) (Fig. 16.70). The adnexa transforms from an initially dominant sebaceous gland population to an overabundance of ceruminous glands that tend to be large, ectatic, and infiltrated by inflammatory cells. The overlying epidermis is typically both hyperplastic and hyperkeratotic and may be eroded or ulcerated (Njaa, 2017).

Typically, the ear infection is minimally inflamed with *Malassezia* yeast organisms adhered to squamous epithelium (Figs. 16.71 to 16.73). Brown cerumen had more yeasts per high-power field than clear or white cerumen (Tater et al., 2003)

Inflammatory polyps originating from the middle ear may extend through the tympanic membrane into the external ear canal, causing otorrhea and head shaking and occasionally presenting as a visible mass obstructing the external ear canal (Sula, 2012). Inflammatory polyps in one study were accurately diagnosed by cytologic examination and were easily distinguished from neoplasia (De Lorenzi et al., 2005). Cytopathologic specimens were highly cellular, containing a mixed, inflammatory cell population predominately composed of neutrophils, macrophages, and lymphocytes, with a lower component of plasma

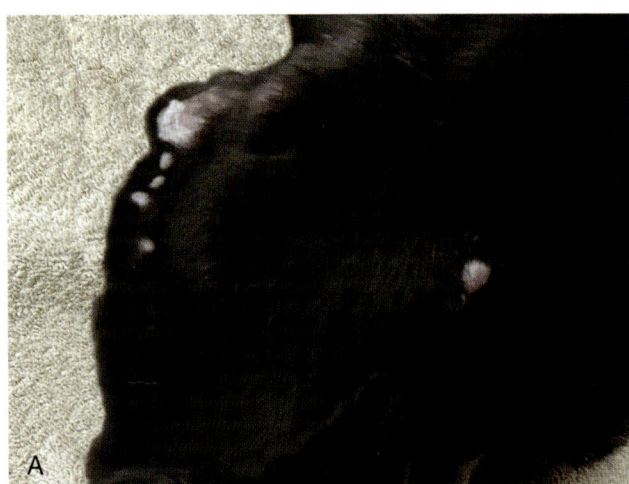

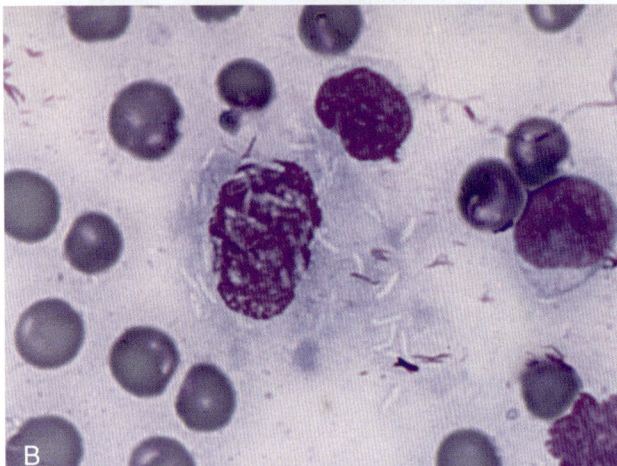

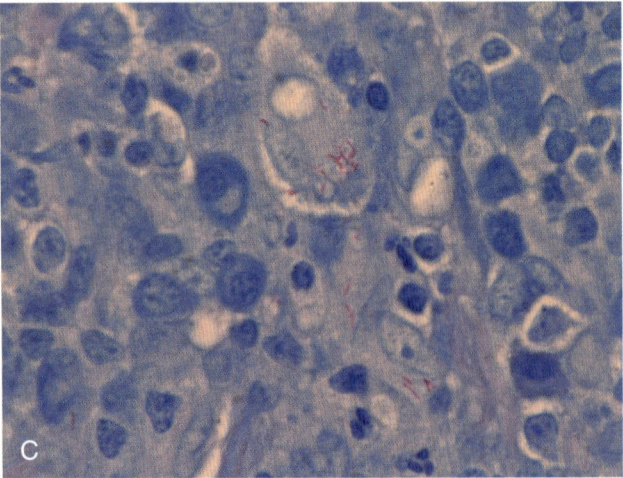

■ **FIGURE 16.69 Canine leproid granuloma. Pinna. Dog.** Same case in A to C. **A, Macroscopic nodules.** Right pinna of a 5-year-old boxer cross. Multiple focal to coalescing, firm, alopecic dermal masses 0.5 to 1.5 cm in diameter appear at the base and margins. **B, Nodule aspirate.** A lymphocyte is present along with a macrophage that contains many negatively stained, 2 to 5 μm long bacilli confirmed by molecular testing as *Mycobacterium* spp. (Modified Wright stain; HP oil.) **C, Histopathology.** Mixed inflammatory response with neutrophils, lymphocytes, plasma cells, and macrophages. Two macrophages contain several positively stained bacilli. (Ziehl-Neelsen; HP oil.) (A, Courtesy Becky Rankin, Abilene Animal Hospital, Kansas. B–C, Courtesy Rose Raskin, Kansas State University.)

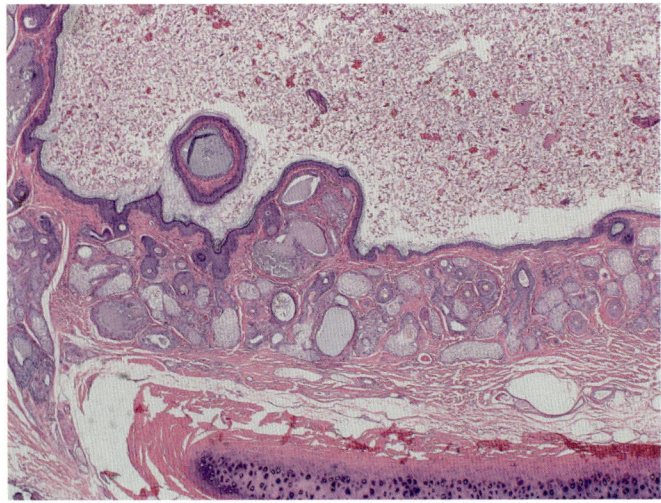

■ **FIGURE 16.70 Chronic otitis externa with adnexal hyperplasia. External acoustic meatus. Histopathology. Dog.** The ear canal is filled with cellular debris at the top with hyperplastic and hyperkeratotic epidermis below it. The superficial dermis consists of abundant and prominent sebaceous glands associated with hair follicles. Smaller, ectatic, tubular ceruminous glands located in the deeper layers of dermis contain variably basophilic secretions. (H&E; LP.) (Courtesy Bradley Njaa, Kansas State University.)

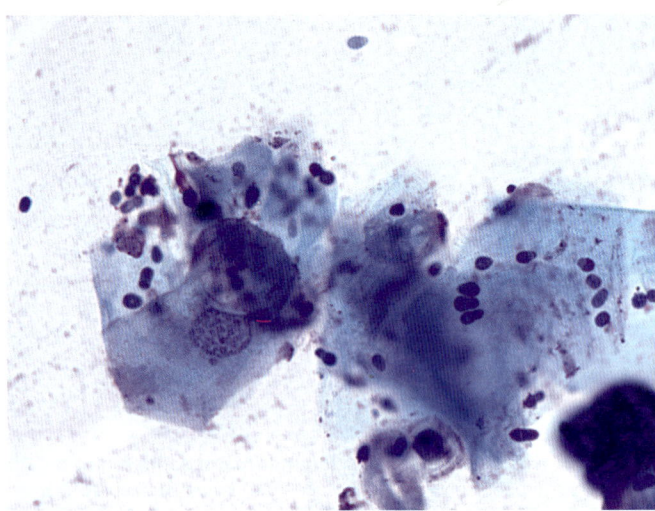

■ **FIGURE 16.71 Chronic otitis externa.** *Malassezia pachydermatis.* **Ear swab. Dog.** Sheets of large, angular keratinized squamous epithelial cells have adherent budding, dark blue to purple yeast. Most keratinocytes are anucleate, but one keratinocyte contains a karyolytic nucleus. Inflammatory cells are not present, but the number of yeast organisms exceeds 5/hpf. (Modified Wright stain; HP oil.) (Courtesy Rose Raskin, Kansas State University.)

cells. Variable numbers of multinucleated giant cells were present along with reactive fibroplasia. Epithelial cells resembled squamous or secretory cells.

Pemphigus foliaceus is the most common autoimmune skin disease in dogs and cats. Drugs, chronic disease, and spontaneous causes have been associated with their occurrence. Grossly, lesions appear as erythematous macules that progress to white or yellow pustules and finally to crusts (Fig. 16.74A). The head and feet are preferred sites, although the ears, trunk, and neck

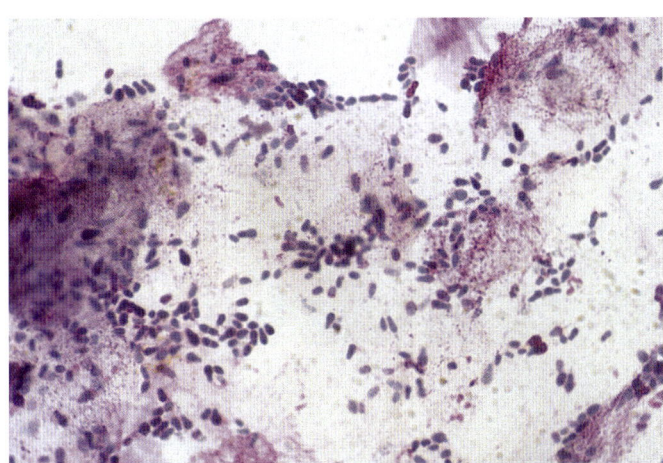

FIGURE 16.72 *Malassezia pachydermatis* infection. Ear swab. **Dog.** Numerous bottle-shaped budding basophilic yeast without an inflammatory response. (Aqueous Romanowsky; HP oil.)

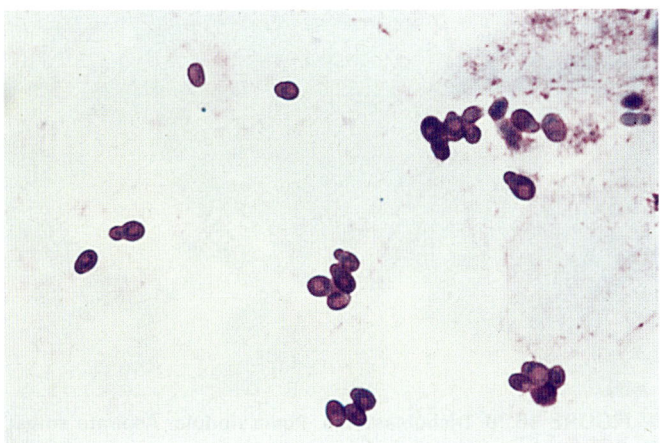

FIGURE 16.73 *Malassezia pachydermatis* infection. Ear swab. **Dog.** High magnification of characteristic shoeprint morphology of the broad-based budding yeast associated with chronic otitis externa. (Aqueous Romanowsky; HP oil.)

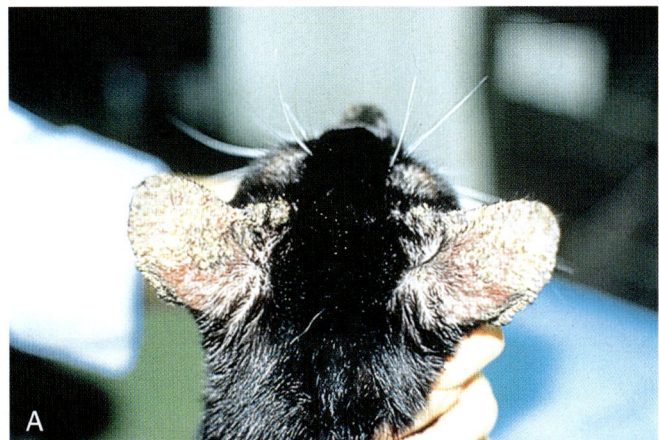

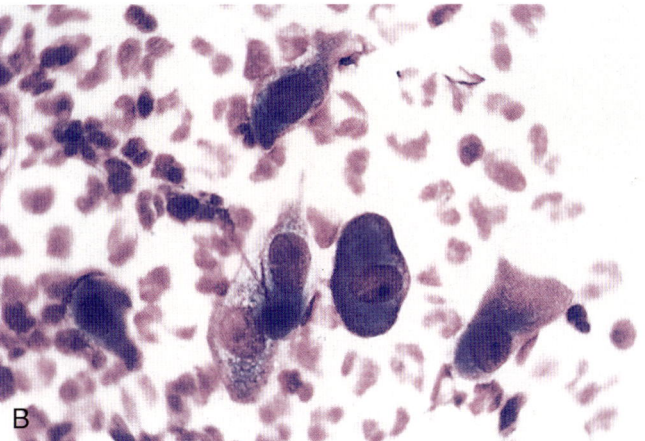

FIGURE 16.74 Pemphigus foliaceous. Cat. **A**, Macroscopic view. Crusty and erythematous lesions on the ear pinnae. **B**, Microscopic view. Acantholytic cells. Pustule aspirate. Cat. Densely stained individualized keratinocytes from a skin pustule on an animal with pemphigus foliaceous. These cells are often associated with immune-mediated skin diseases. Numerous neutrophils, mostly nondegenerate, are present. (Wright-Giemsa; HP oil.) (A, Courtesy Janet Wojciechowski, University of Florida.)

are often affected in cats. Direct imprint of the underside of a crust or aspiration of a pustule reveals nondegenerate neutrophils and *acantholytic cells* appearing as intensely stained individualized oval keratinocytes (Fig. 16.74B).

Response to Tissue Injury

Irritation within the ear canal causes the animal to shake their head vigorously that may produce an aural hematoma with a swollen pinna. Aspiration will yield erythrocytes with evidence of macrophagic inflammation.

Proliferative and necrotizing otitis externa is a distinctive condition of 2-month-old to 5-year-old cats (Sula, 2012). On the concave surface of the pinna, dark brown to black, proliferative, plaque-like coalescing lesions extend into and obstruct the vertical ear canal. Thick exudate and secondary bacterial or yeast otitis externa occur concurrently. The condition appears to arise from T cell–mediated apoptosis of keratinocytes and may undergo spontaneous regression. Cytopathology is expected to reveal keratinocytes, neutrophilic or mixed cell inflammation, and likely infectious agents (yeast, bacteria). Treatment involves use of a T-cell inhibitor of keratinocyte apoptosis (topical tacrolimus).

Non-neoplastic Tumors

Feline ceruminous cystomatosis appears as multiple dark gray to blue to black nodules aggregated along the concave surface of the auricle. They arise from a cystic dilation and hyperplasia of ceruminous glands and are filled with dark inspissated cerumen, which grossly resemble melanoma or vascular tumors.

See the discussion under Middle Ear for keratinized cysts that extend into the external ear.

Neoplasia

Sebaceous gland tumors, histiocytomas, plasmacytomas, and mast cell tumors (Fig. 16.75) are the most common types of aural neoplasms in dogs. Neoplastic transformation of adnexal structures is the most common neoplasia of the external ear canal in dogs and cats. Trichoblastomas are encountered in both dogs and cats (Fig. 16.76). SCC is common in cats as well.

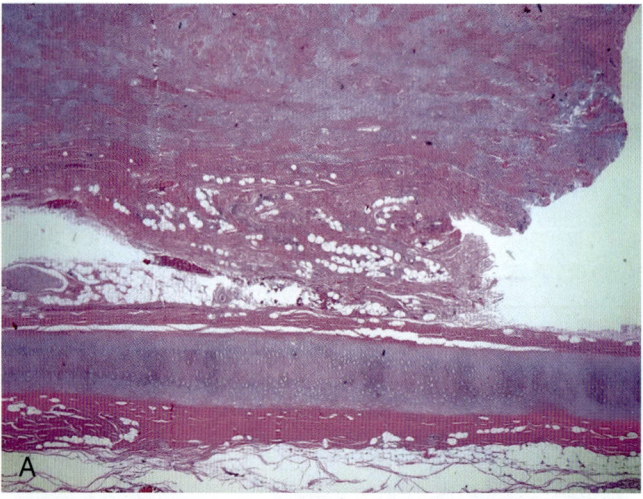
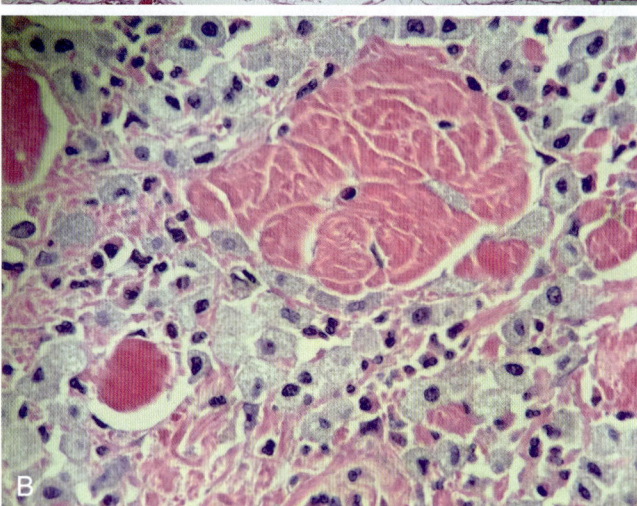
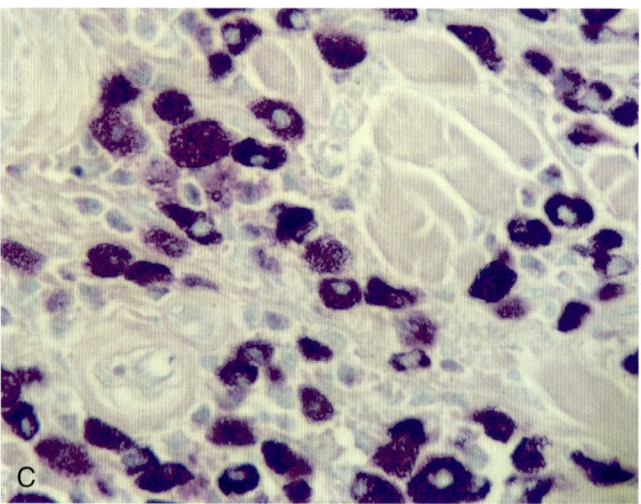

■ **FIGURE 16.75 Mast cell tumor. Pinna nodule. Histopathology.** Same case in A to C. **A,** Multiple to coalescing dermal infiltration of pale-staining neoplastic cells without encapsulation or distinct borders. (H&E; LP.) **B,** Pale-staining neoplastic cells infiltrated around and between muscle fibers. Neoplastic cells are individualized with abundant finely granular cytoplasm, a round nucleus, and mild anisokaryosis. (H&E; IP.) **C,** Prominent dark-purple staining of cytoplasmic granules identifies the round cells as mast cells. Lack of multinucleation, mitotic activity, and anisokaryosis support a low-grade tumor. (Giemsa; HP oil.) (Courtesy Rose Raskin, University of Florida.)

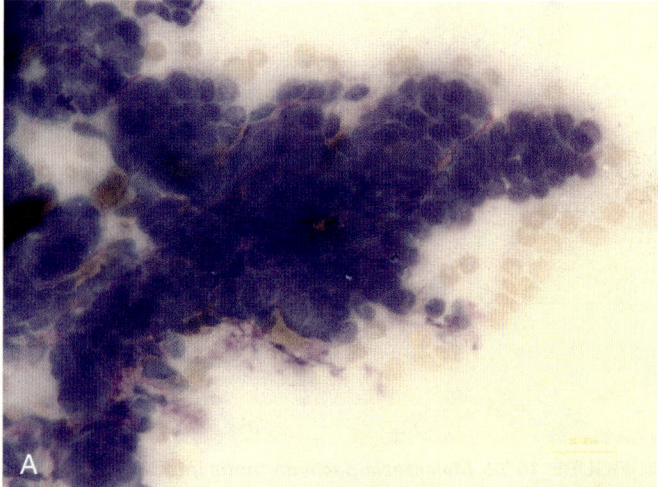
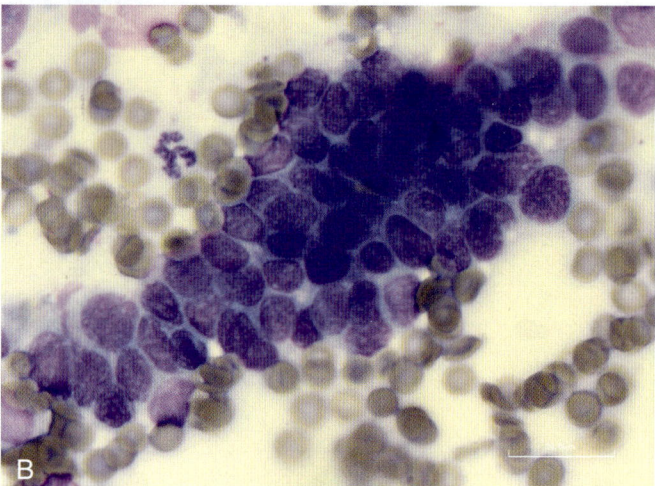

■ **FIGURE 16.76 Trichoblastoma. Pinna nodule. Aspirate smear. Dog.** Same case in A and B. **A,** A fast-growing pink mass revealed a population of tightly clustered epithelial cells with papillary projections. (Wright-Giemsa; HP oil.) **B,** One cluster of mildly atypical dense, tightly cohesive epithelial cells. Some of the epithelial cells are admixed with a small amount of bright-pink extracellular matrix. The small cells are cuboidal to polygonal with a scant amount of pale basophilic cytoplasm and high nucleocytoplasmic ratio. The round to oval nucleus has stippled chromatin and no discernible nucleolus. The pattern suggests a cutaneous basilar epithelial neoplasm of germinal hair origin. (Wright-Giemsa; HP oil.) (Courtesy Rose Raskin, University of Florida.)

Although aspiration cytopathology of external ear masses of cats was sufficiently accurate for distinguishing inflammatory polyps from neoplasia, distinction between benign and malignant ceruminous neoplasms was best determined by histopathology (De Lorenzi et al., 2005).

Canine cutaneous histiocytoma appears on the pinna as a raised ulcerated lesion. Cytopathologically, it is similar to that found elsewhere on the skin (see Chapter 3). Because these masses typically regress within 3 months, cytopathologic diagnosis may be confusing with massive lymphocytic infiltration and only occasional histiocytes (Fig. 16.77).

The majority of feline (85%) and canine (60%) aural neoplasms are malignant. Of these, ceruminous gland adenocarcinoma (Figs. 16.78 to 16.80A–B) is the most common neoplasms

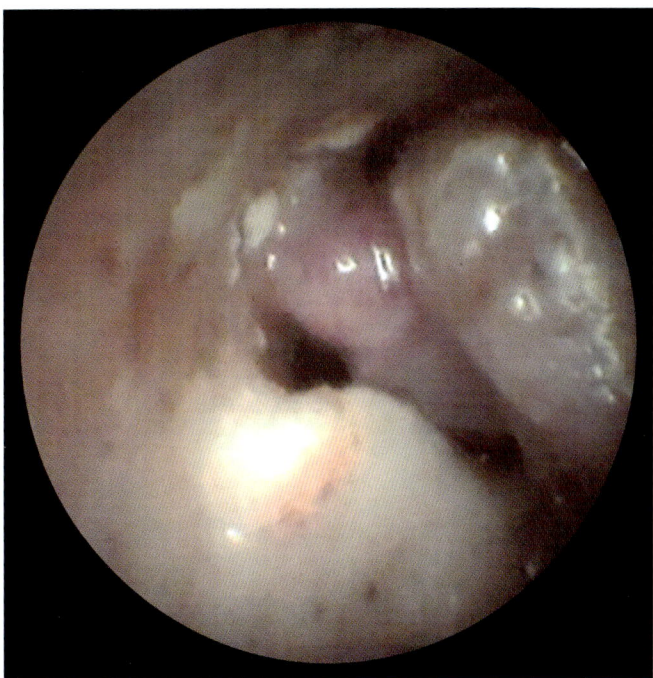

FIGURE 16.78 Ceruminous gland adenocarcinoma. External ear canal mass. Otoscopic view. Cat. A pink mass is visible in the center of the canal. (Courtesy Lisa Akucewich, University of Florida.)

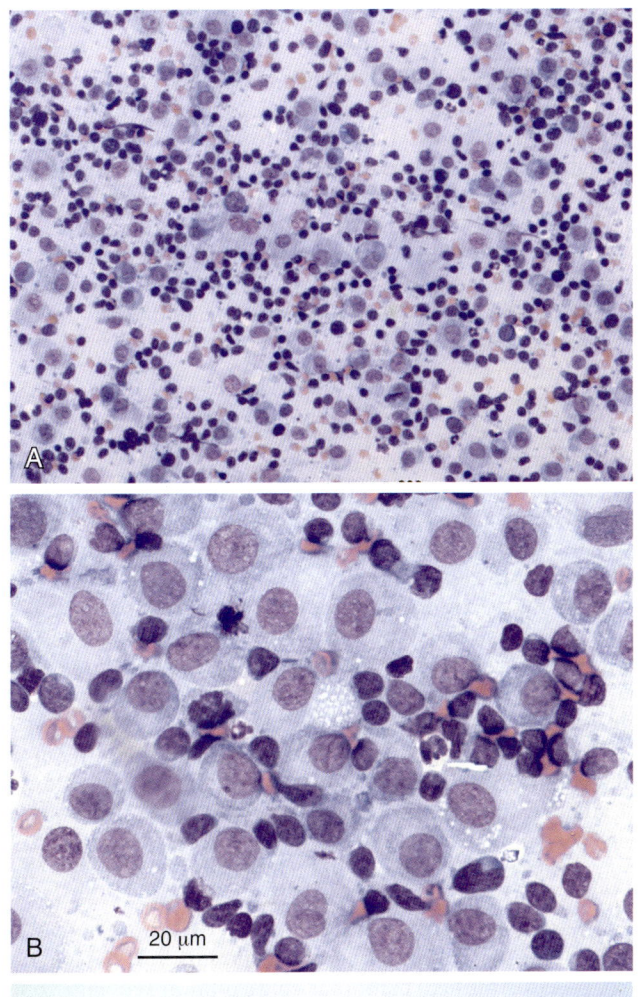

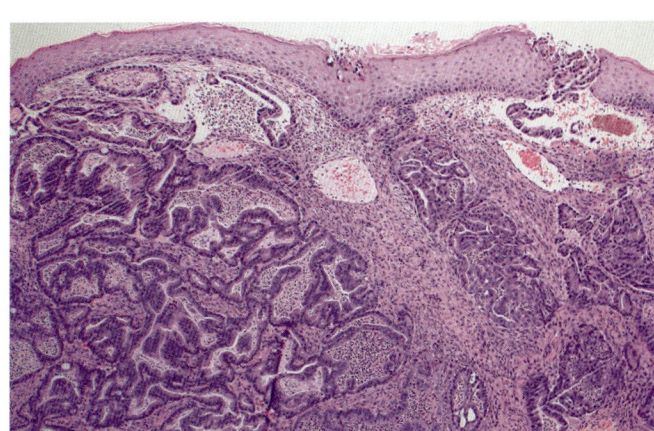

FIGURE 16.79 Ceruminous gland adenocarcinoma. External ear canal mass. Histopathology. Cat. The epidermal surface is broken in three areas by expansion of a tubular gland neoplasm originating from the ceruminous glands in the superficial dermis. There are inflammatory cells throughout the dermis. (H&E; LP.) (Courtesy Bradley Njaa, Kansas State University.)

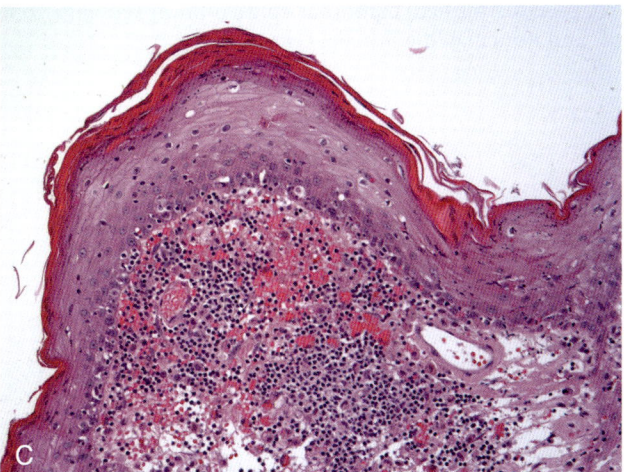

FIGURE 16.77 Regressing histiocytoma. Pinna mass. Dog. Same case in A to C. **A, Mass aspirate.** The nucleated cells are a mixed cell population. (Wright-Giemsa; IP.) **B, Mass aspirate.** Many small lymphocytes are intermixed between fewer large mononuclear cells having abundant lightly basophilic cytoplasm and round to ovoid paracentral nucleus. (Wright-Giemsa; HP oil.) **C, Histopathology.** A dense population of cells, predominantly small lymphocytes, is concentrated within the superficial dermis and basal layers of the epidermis. The high numbers of lymphocytes can be misleading but are typical during regression of histiocytomas. (H&E; LP.) (A–C, Courtesy Rose Raskin, University of Florida.)

diagnosed in the external acoustic meatus of both dogs and cats (Njaa, 2017). Middle-aged to older animals are generally affected. Cytopathology reveals tight clusters of epithelial cells with high N:C ratios, anisokaryosis, coarse chromatin, prominent nucleoli, and black variably sized cytoplasmic granules (Fig. 16.80C).

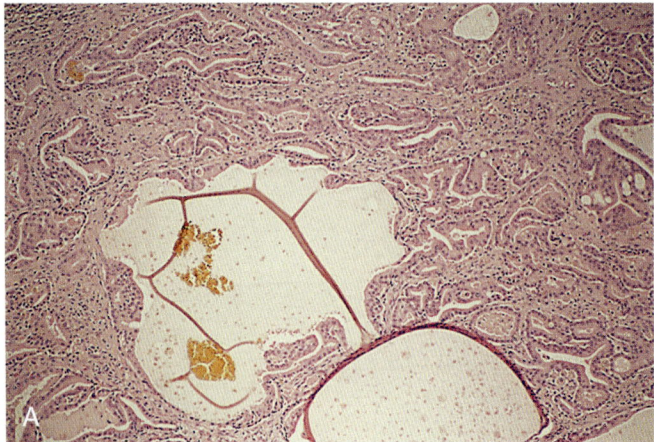
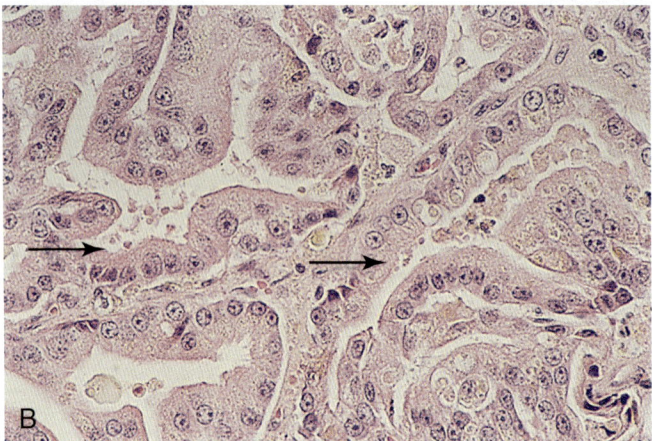
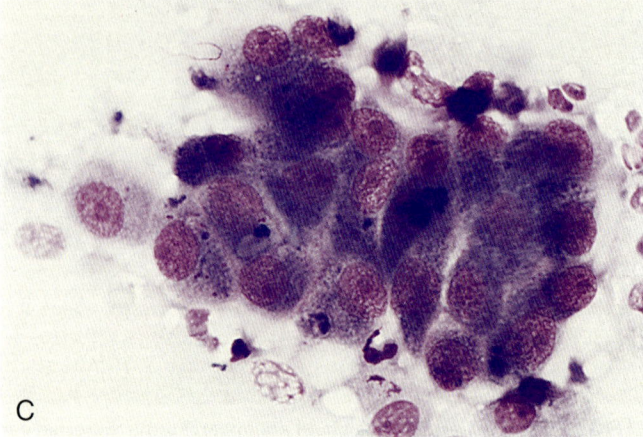

■ **FIGURE 16.80 Ceruminous gland adenocarcinoma. External ear canal mass. Cat.** Same case in A to C. **A, Histopathology.** Neoplastic proliferation of tubular and acinar glandular epithelium with ectasis or dilated areas containing brown sebum. (H&E; LP.) **B, Histopathology.** Malignant changes are noted by anisokaryosis, vesicular nuclei, prominent nucleoli, and marked anisocytosis of tubular epithelium. The apocrine function of these cells is indicated by the eosinophilic droplets at the apical surface *(arrows).* (H&E; HP oil.) **C, Mass imprint.** Tight clusters of epithelium demonstrate increased nucleocytoplasmic ratio, prominent single nucleoli, coarse chromatin, anisokaryosis, and anisocytosis. Note the intracytoplasmic presence of black globular secretory material in some cells, which when finely dispersed in other cells resembles melanin pigment. (Aqueous Romanowsky; HP oil.)

MIDDLE EAR

Normal Anatomy and Histology

Sound waves travel via the external ear to the tympanic membrane, where sound is transferred from the attached malleus through the other middle ear ossicles (incus and stapes) to produce movement of endolymph within the cochlea of the inner ear. The ossicles lie within the tympanic cavity, an air-filled region whose air pressure is stabilized from the auditory tube that lies between the tympanic cavity and the nasopharynx. The middle ear begins with the tympanic membrane; includes the ossicles, tympanic cavity, and auditory tube; and ends at the vestibular oval window of the cochlea.

The tympanic membrane (Fig. 16.81) is a thin, three-layered membrane in which the manubrium of the malleus is embedded. The majority of the area is transparent and composed of an outer layer of keratinizing squamous epithelium; a middle layer of thin, variably vascularized fibrous connective tissue; and an inner layer of very low cuboidal to nonkeratinizing squamous epithelium.

An air-filled compartment, the tympanic cavity (see Fig. 16.81) is surrounded by bone that is separated from the external ear by the tympanic membrane and communicates with the pharynx via the auditory tube (Eustachian tube). The *mucoperiosteum* represents a fused mucosa and periosteum lining the surface of bony structures of the middle ear. In cats and dogs, the lining epithelium varies, depending on the location. Dorsally, close to the auditory tube opening, the mucoperiosteum contains mostly ciliated columnar cells mixed with goblet cells and basal cells contiguous with the nasopharyngeal mucosae (Fig. 16.82) (Njaa, 2017).

The auditory tube (see Fig. 16.81) is derived from endoderm and reflects the nasopharyngeal cell population, namely ciliated, pseudostratified, columnar epithelium mixed with goblet cells and nonciliated epithelial cells.

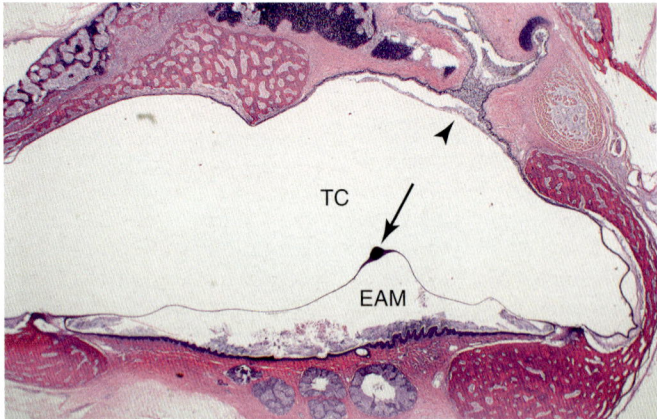

■ **FIGURE 16.81 Normal middle ear. Histology. Cat.** The large central cavity (TC) is the tympanic cavity that lies between the auditory tube *(arrowhead)* and tympanic membrane *(arrow).* A small section of the external acoustic meatus (EAM) or ear canal contains sloughed squamous epithelium. Within the dermis of the ear canal are sebaceous glands with ducts to the surface. The dark area on the tympanic membrane indicated by the *arrow* is the malleus, an ossicle firmly attached to the membrane. (H&E; LP.) (Courtesy Bradley Njaa, Kansas State University.)

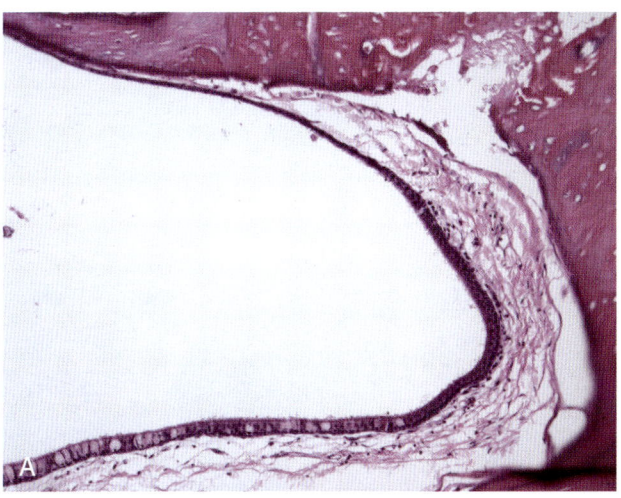 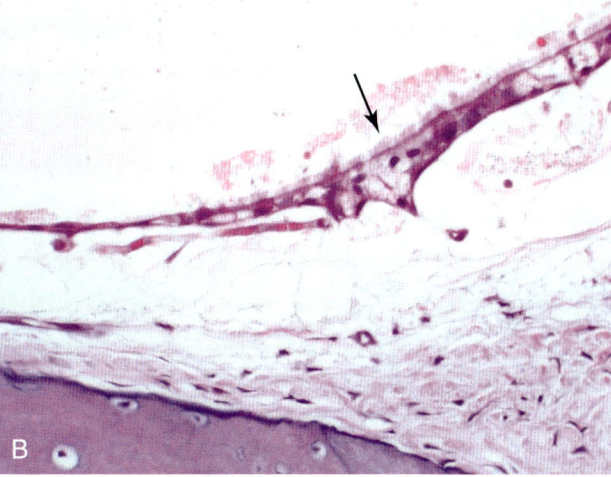

FIGURE 16.82 Normal middle ear. Mucoperiosteum. Histology. Cat. Same case in A and B. **A,** Lining cells of the middle ear vary in size with those closest to the auditory tube and nasopharynx having ciliated columnar epithelium with intermixed pale-staining goblet cells *(bottom)*, while farther away, the cells become cuboidal and flattened *(top)*. (H&E; LP.) **B,** Higher magnification of the ciliated columnar cells *(arrow)*, which fuse with the underlying periosteum of the bone to form the mucoperiosteum. (H&E; HP oil.) (Courtesy Bradley Njaa, Kansas State University.)

The ossicles are composed of calcified cartilaginous matrix interwoven with lesser lamellar bone (Sula et al., 2014).

Sample Collection and Preparation

A bulging tympanic membrane or abnormal scan from computed tomography or magnetic resonance imaging (MRI) supports the presence of disease within the middle ear. Masses may be removed or sampled through ventral bulla osteotomy, whereas fluid samples for cytopathology or microbiologic testing are obtained by piercing the tympanic membrane (myringotomy) or via the auditory tube from the nasopharynx.

Normal Cytology and Artifacts

The middle ear is mostly air filled with few nucleated cells present. If found, these are ciliated cuboidal to columnar epithelium from the mucoperiosteum and auditory tube and few nonkeratinized squamous cells from the tympanic membrane.

Inflammation

Middle ear infections are common in small animal veterinary patients. Predisposing factors in dogs include infections, tumors, and allergies. In cats, tumors and chronic upper respiratory disease are responsible (Fig. 16.83). Otitis externa, if chronic, may extend into the middle ear. Infections from the nasopharynx may also extend into the middle ear. Acute inflammation of the middle ear may result in rapid expansion of the mucoperiosteum by edema, congestion, and acute inflammatory cells. Chronic otitis media may produce a granulomatous inflammatory response with cholesterol crystal accumulation (see Fig. 16.83)

Primary secretory otitis media (PSOM) is associated with Cavalier King Charles spaniels, boxers, and other brachycephalic breeds. MRI reveals material within the tympanic bulla that has been described macroscopically as white to yellow, opaque, and viscous; this condition has been called "glue ear." Cytopathology of PSOM material reveals few to many mature keratinocytes against a background of basophilic to lavender, amorphous, mucin-like material that stains positive with Alcian blue and periodic acid–Schiff. There may be no evidence of inflammatory cells or infection (Fig. 16.84) (Weinstein et al., 2016).

Non-neoplastic Tumors

Inflammatory polyps arise from the mucosal lining of the middle ear, auditory tube, or nasopharynx and are the most commonly reported external ear canal mass in cats. Chronic inflammation results in mucoperiosteal expansion by mononuclear inflammatory cells and granulation tissue (Njaa, 2017). Cytopathology through imprint biopsy may display low cuboidal and tall columnar cells with abundant pale basophilic cytoplasm, a basally located oval nucleus, finely stippled chromatin, and rarely a small nucleolus (see Fig. 16.83D and 5.13A–D). The apical side of these cells often has abundant brightly eosinophilic cilia. Small lymphocytes and nondegenerate neutrophils are admixed with the epithelial cells. Brightly eosinophilic amorphous extracellular matrix or amphophilic, streaming, mucous material may appear in the background (Wong and Jaffe, 2018). On histopathology, these masses have a core of proliferative fibrovascular stroma lined superficially by simple to pseudostratified squamous nonkeratinized epithelium. Aggregates of lymphocytes and plasma cells are scattered throughout the mass. Surgical treatment often involves a ventral bulla osteotomy with middle ear involvement.

Tympanokeratoma (formerly referred to as aural cholesteatoma or aural keratinizing cyst) is a non-neoplastic, cystic structure composed of a central cavity of keratin debris often with cholesterol surrounded by keratinizing, stratified squamous epithelium that originates from the tympanic membrane (Njaa, 2017). Macroscopically, the cyst has a layered, pearly appearance owing to the abundant laminated keratin. Cytopathologically, the lesions resemble follicular cysts of the skin with abundant anucleate, keratinized squamous epithelial cells, mixed cell inflammation, and evidence of fibroplasia (Newman et al., 2015). In middle-aged to older dogs, these are considered acquired

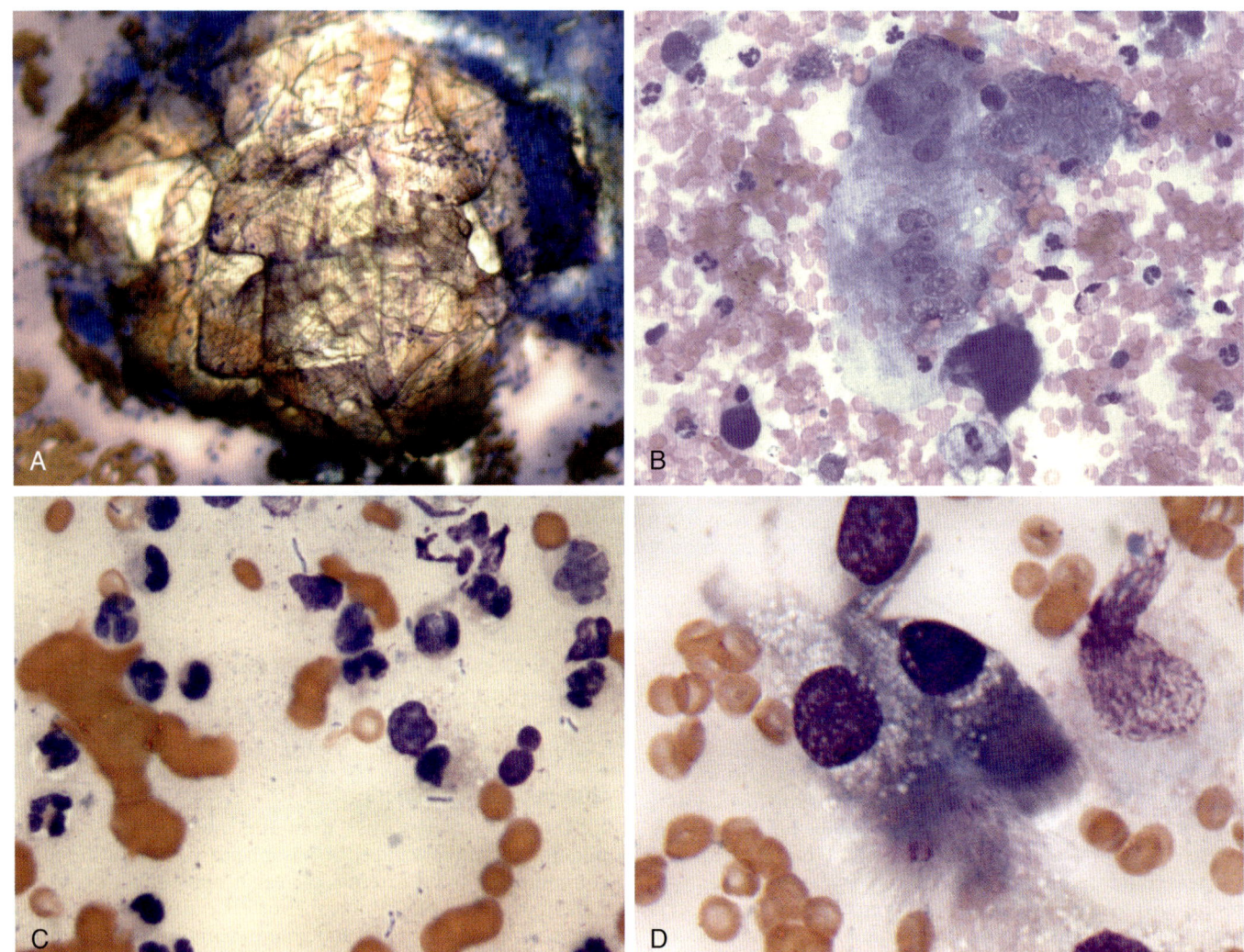

■ **FIGURE 16.83 Bilateral chronic otitis media. Mixed neutrophilic and macrophagic inflammation with bacterial infection. Myringotomy specimens. Cat.** Same case in A to D. The cat had a chronic respiratory infection and was displaying vestibular signs. Magnetic resonance imaging indicated bilateral involvement and both ears showed similar pathologic findings. **A,** Large accumulations of cholesterol crystals are present in both ears. (Modified Wright; LP.) **B,** Several multinucleated giant cells are mixed with neutrophils and macrophages likely in response to cholesterol deposits. (Modified Wright; HP oil.) **C,** Large numbers of mildly to moderately degenerate (karyolytic) neutrophils are present with a monotypic population of extracellular rod bacteria typical of the oral cavity. (Modified Wright; HP oil.) **D,** Two ciliated columnar epithelium cells are shown that likely represent the mucoperiosteal lining cells. The round nucleus is located basally, opposite to the cilia on the apical surface. The basophilic cytoplasm displays mild foaminess. (Modified Wright; HP oil.) (Courtesy Rose Raskin, University of Bristol, UK.)

entities, secondary to migration or invagination of stratified squamous epithelium from the external ear canal. They are most commonly found in the middle ear and can result in enlargement of the tympanic bulla, as well as bony lysis of bullae, but can extend into the external ear canal. A similar expansive mass to the tympanokeratoma that is associated with chronic otitis media and otitis externa is granulomatous inflammation with granulation tissue laden with cholesterol (cholesterol clefts on histopathology) (Njaa, 2017).

Neoplasia

Neoplasms occur rarely in the middle ear. SCCs are diagnosed most frequently in cats, whereas carcinomas of undetermined origin more commonly occur in dogs (Njaa, 2017). Neoplasms may originate within the middle ear or arise in the external ear canal and penetrate through the tympanic membrane into the tympanic cavity. Lymphoma within the bulla has been reported to occur in cats. One case of angiocentric or angioinvasive T-cell lymphoma within the tympanic bulla and nasopharynx was documented in a young adult cat by cytopathology and histopathology (Santagostino et al., 2015). Neoplastic cells expressed CD3, feline leukemia virus p27, and gp70 antigens. Since disseminated lymphoma was present in this case, it is uncertain whether the ear involvement was primary.

INNER EAR

Normal Anatomy and Histology

Sound waves arrive at the oval window via the stapes and produce inward fluid waves within the perilymph of the cochlea, located in the petrous portion of the temporal bone. A round window membrane also in the cochlea acts as a pressure relief

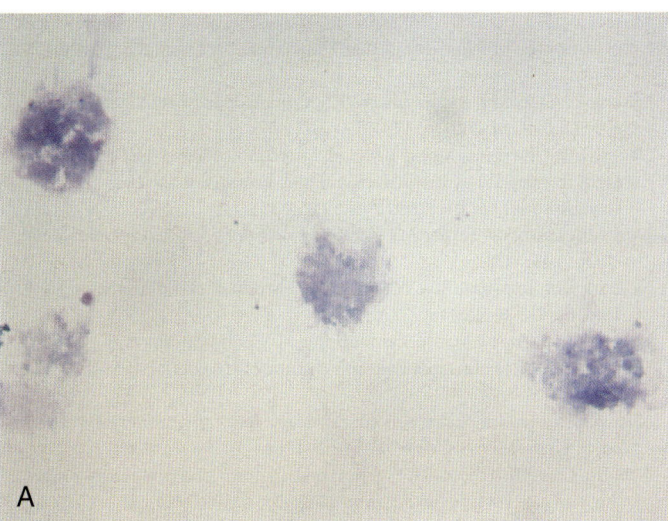 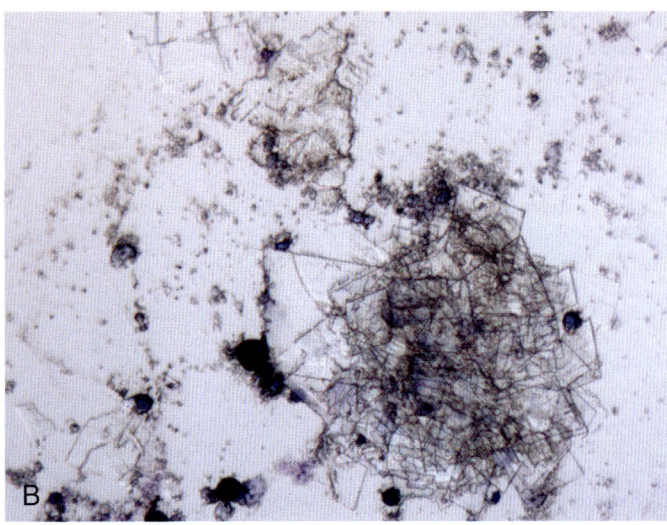

FIGURE 16.84 Primary secretory otitis media. Myringotomy specimens. Dog. Same case in A and B. This boxer presented with vestibular signs. Magnetic resonance imaging of the head showed contrast enhancement of a facial nerve with fluid present in both middle ears. Bilateral myringotomy removed brown, thick, and gelatinous fluid. **A,** The background contains deposits of lightly basophilic granular material. Not shown, but also present, are highly vacuolated macrophages. **B,** Focally noted are dense collections of cholesterol crystals within the granular deposits. (Modified Wright; HP oil.) (Courtesy Rose Raskin, University of Bristol, UK.)

port for the perilymph wave movement. Perilymph is an extracellular fluid similar in electrolyte composition to cerebrospinal fluid. Between the perilymph in the outer portion of the cochlea and endolymph in the inner cochlear duct is a membrane. Endolymph resembles intracellular fluid with a higher potassium and low sodium concentrations than perilymph. The cochlear duct is filled with endolymph, and within the cochlear portion of the membranous labyrinth duct is the spiral organ with specialized neurosensory epithelium (hair cells) that convert the fluid waves into action potentials that are transmitted to the brainstem and auditory cortex, resulting in hearing (Njaa et al., 2012). Because the inner ear is enclosed within bone, it is rarely accessed for cytopathology.

Inflammation

Otitis interna results from extension of otitis media. Microscopically, the inflammatory infiltrate is similar to that affecting the middle ear, namely neutrophils, macrophages, lymphocytes, and plasma cells. The most plausible portal of entry is through the membranous covering of the cochlear round window (Njaa, 2017).

REFERENCES

Angus JC. Otic cytology in health and disease. *Vet Clin North Am Small Anim Pract.* 2004;34:411-424.

Armour MD, Broome M, Dell'Anna G, et al. A review of orbital and intracranial magnetic resonance imaging in 79 canine and 13 feline patients (2004-2010). *Vet Ophthalmol.* 2011;14:215-226.

Beckwith-Cohen B, Dubielzig RR, Maggs DJ, et al. Feline epitheliotropic mastocytic conjunctivitis in 15 cats. *Vet Pathol.* 2017;54:141-146.

Beckwith-Cohen B, Teixeira LBC, Ramos-Vera JA, et al. Squamous papillomas of the conjunctiva in dogs: a condition not associated with papillomavirus infection. *Vet Pathol.* 2015;52:676-680.

Black LJ, da Costa Martins B, Plummer CE, et al. What is your diagnosis? Eyelid mass in a dog. *Vet Clin Pathol.* 2018;47:157-159.

Bolzan AA, Brunelli ATJ, Castro MB, et al. Conjunctival impression cytology in dogs. *Vet Ophthalmol.* 2005;8:401-405.

Boscos CM, Ververidis HN, Tondis DK, et al. Ocular involvement of transmissible venereal tumor in a dog. *Vet Ophthalmol.* 1998;1:167-170.

Boydell P. Fine needle aspiration biopsy in the diagnosis of exophthalmos. *J Sm Anim Pract.* 1991;32:542-546.

Choi US, Labelle P, Kim S, et al. Successful treatment of an unusually large corneal epithelial inclusion cyst using equine amniotic membrane in a dog. *Vet Ophthalmol.* 2010;13:122-125.

Cirla A, Rondena M, Bertolini G. Automated tru-cut imaging-guided core needle biopsy canine orbital neoplasia. A prospective feasibility study. *Open Vet J.* 2016;6:114-120.

Cole LK. Anatomy and physiology of the canine ear. *Vet Dermatol.* 2009;20:412-421.

Dean E, Meunier V. Feline eosinophilic keratoconjunctivitis: a retrospective study of 45 cases (56 eyes). *J Feline Med Surg.* 2013;15:661-666.

Dees DD, Schobert CS, Dubielzig RR, et al. Third eyelid gland neoplasms of dogs and cats: a retrospective histopathologic study of 145 cases. *Vet Ophthalmol.* 2016;19:138-143.

Delgado E. Dacryops of the lacrimal gland in a dog. *Vet Ophthalmol.* 2013;16:153-158.

De Lorenzi D, Bonfanti U, Masserdotti C, et al. Fine-needle biopsy of external ear canal masses in the cat: cytologic results and histologic correlations in 27 cases. *Vet Clin Pathol.* 2005;34(2):100-105.

Di Pietro SD, Bosco VRF, Crinò C, et al. Prevalence, type, and prognosis of ocular lesions in shelter and owned client dogs naturally infected by *Leishmania infantum*. *Vet World.* 2016;9(6):633-637.

Dubielzig RR, Everitt J, Shadduck JA, et al. Clinical and morphologic features of post-traumatic ocular sarcoma in cats. *Vet Pathol.* 1990;27:62-67.

Eördögh R, Schwendenwein I, Tichy A, et al. Impression cytology: a novel sampling technique for cytology of the feline eye. *Vet Ophthalmol.* 2015;18:276-284.

Ferreira H, Scurrell E, Bass J, et al. What is your diagnosis? Aqueous humor from a dog. *Vet Clin Pathol.* 2019;48(3):484-486.

Fife M, Blocker T, Fife T, et al. Canine conjunctival mast cell tumors: a retrospective study. *Vet Ophthalmol.* 2011;14:153-160.

Gelatt KN, Chrisman CL, Samuelson DA, et al. Ocular and systemic aspergillosis in a dog. *J Am Anim Hosp Assoc.* 1991;27:427-431.

Giuliano EA, Moore CP, Phillips TE. Morphological evidence of M cells in healthy canine conjunctiva-associated lymphoid tissue. *Graefe's Arch Clin Exp Ophthalmol.* 2002;240:220-226.

Gonzales-Viera O, Casey K, Keel MK. What is your diagnosis? Conjunctival smear in a dog. *Vet Clin Pathol.* 2018;47:509-510.

Grácio AJS, Richter J, Kommenou AT, et al. Onchocerciasis caused by *Onchocerca lupi*: an emerging zoonotic infection. Systematic review. *Parasitol Res.* 2015;114:2401-2413.

Grahn BH, Peiffer RL, Cullen CL, et al. Classification of feline intraocular neoplasms based on morphology, histochemical staining, and immunohistochemical labeling. *Vet Ophthalmol.* 2006;9:395-403.

Griffin JS, Scott DW, Erb HN. *Malassezia* otitis externa in the dog: the effect of heat-fixing otic exudate for cytological analysis. *J Vet Med A.* 2007;54:424-427.

Haesebrouck F, Devriese LA, van Rijssen B, et al. Incidence and significance of isolation of *Mycoplasma felis* from conjunctival swabs of cats. *Vet Microbiol.* 1991;26:95-101.

Hazel SJ, Thrall MAH, Severin GA, et al. Laboratory evaluation of aqueous humor in the healthy dog, cat, horse, and cow. *Am J Vet Res.* 1985;46:657-659.

Henderson SE, Clark ES, Stromberg PC, et al. Pathology in practice: canine distemper virus infection in a puppy. *J Am Vet Med Assoc.* 2015;247(12):1375-1377.

Hendrix DV, Gelatt KN. Diagnosis, treatment and outcome of orbital neoplasia in dogs: a retrospective study of 44 cases. *J Small Anim Pract.* 2000;41:105-108.

Hillström A, Tvedten H, Källberg M, et al. Evaluation of cytologic findings in feline conjunctivitis. *Vet Clin Pathol.* 2012;41:283-290.

Hirai T, Mubarak M, Kimura T, et al. Apocrine gland tumor of the eyelid in a dog. *Vet Pathol.* 1997;34:232-234.

Jacobi S, Dubielzig RR. Feline early life ocular disease. *Vet Ophthalmol.* 2008;11:166-169.

Kastl B, Peddireddi L, Rankin B, et al. Pathology in practice. *J Am Vet Med Assoc.* 2020;256(12):1331-1334.

Knoll JS. What is your diagnosis? *Vet Clin Pathol.* 1990;19:32-34.

Komnenou AA, Mylonakis ME, Kouti V, et al. Ocular manifestations of natural canine monocytic ehrlichiosis (*Ehrlichia canis*): a retrospective study of 90 cases. *Vet Ophthalmol.* 2007;10:137-142.

Krehbiel JD, Langham RF. Eyelid neoplasm of dogs. *Am J Vet Res.* 1975;36:115-119.

Labelle AL, Labelle P. Canine ocular neoplasia: a review. *Vet Ophthalmol.* 2013;16:3-14.

Lanza MR, Musciano AR, Dubielzig RD, et al. Clinical and pathological classification of canine intraocular lymphoma. *Vet Ophthalmol.* 2018;21:167-173.

Ledbetter EC, Franklin-Guild RJ, Edelmann ML. *Capnocytophaga* keratitis in dogs: clinical, histopathologic, and microbiologic features of seven cases. *Vet Ophthalmol.* 2018;21(6):638-645.

Linn-Pearl RN, Powell RM, Newman HA, et al. Validity of aqueocentesis as a component of anterior uveitis investigation in dogs and cats. *Vet Ophthalmol.* 2015;18:326-334.

Low HC, Powell CC, Veir JK, et al. Prevalence of feline herpesvirus 1, *Chlamydophila felis*, and *Mycoplasma* spp. DNA in conjunctival cells collected from cats with and without conjunctivitis. *Am J Vet Res.* 2007;68:643-648.

Massa KL, Murphy CJ, Hartmann FA, et al. Usefulness of aerobic microbial culture and cytologic evaluation of corneal specimens in the diagnosis of infectious ulcerative keratitis in animals. *J Am Vet Med Assoc.* 1999;215:1671-1674.

Murphy JM. Exfoliative cytologic examination as an aid in diagnosing ocular diseases in the dog and cat. *Semin Vet Med Surg (Small Anim).* 1988;3:10-14.

Musciano AR, Lanza MR, Dubielzig RR, et al. Clinical and histopathological classification of feline intraocular lymphoma. *Vet Ophthalmol.* 2020;23:77-89.

Naranjo C, Dubielzig RR, Friedrichs KR. Canine ocular histiocytic sarcoma. *Vet Ophthalmol.* 2007;10:179-185.

Nasisse MP, Glover TL, Moore CP, et al. Detection of feline herpesvirus 1 DNA in corneas of cats with eosinophilic keratitis or corneal sequestration. *Am J Vet Res.* 1998;59:856-858.

Nevile JC, Hurn SD, Turner AG. Keratomycosis in five dogs. *Vet Ophthalmol.* 2016;19:432-438.

Newkirk KM, Rohrbach BW. A retrospective study of eyelid tumors in 43 cats. *Vet Pathol.* 2009;46:916-927.

Newman AW, Estey CM, McDonough S, et al. Cholesteatoma and meningoencephalitis in a dog with chronic otitis externa. *Vet Clin Pathol.* 2015;44:157-163.

Njaa BL. The ear. In: Zachary JF, ed: *Pathologic Basis of Veterinary Disease.* 6th ed. St Louis, MO: Elsevier; 2017:1223-1264.

Njaa BL, Cole LK, Tabacca N. Practical otic anatomy and physiology of the dog and cat. *Vet Clin Small Anim.* 2012;42(6):1109-1126.

Nunes A, Gomes JP. Evolution, phylogeny, and molecular epidemiology of *Chlamydia. Infect Genet Evol.* 2014;23:49-64.

O'Connell KE, Bruce CJ, Cazzini P. Pathology in practice. Eosinophilic keratitis in a cat. *J Am Vet Med Assoc.* 2017;251(2):165-167.

Ota J, Pearce JW, Fihn MJ, et al. Dacryops (lacrimal cyst) in three young labradors retrievers. *J Am Anim Hosp Assoc.* 2009;45:191-196.

Peña MT, Naranjo C, Klauss G, et al. Histopathological features of ocular leishmaniosis in the dog. *J Comp Pathol.* 2008;138(1):32-39.

Perazzi A, Bonsembiante F, Gelain M, et al. Cytology of the healthy canine and feline ocular surface: comparison between cytobrush and impression technique. *Vet Clin Pathol.* 2017;46:164-171.

Petterino C, Bjomson S, Hayes S. What is your diagnosis? An intraocular mass in a dog. *Vet Clin Pathol.* 2014;43:289-290.

Piccione J, Dial SM. Cytologic appearance of hibernoma in two dogs. *Vet Clin Pathol.* 2020;49(1):125-129.

Pirie CG, Dubielzig RR. Feline conjunctival hemangioma and hemangiosarcoma: a retrospective of eight cases (1993-2004). *Vet Ophthalmol.* 2006;9:227-231.

Pirie CG, Knollinger AM, Thomas CB, et al. Canine conjunctival hemangioma and hemangiosarcoma: a retrospective evaluation of 108 cases (1989-2004). *Vet Ophthalmol.* 2006;9:215-226.

Prasse KW, Winston SM. Cytology and histopathology of feline eosinophilic keratitis. *Vet Comp Opthalmol.* 1996;6:74-81.

Ravi M, Schobert CS, Kiupel M, et al. Clinical, morphologic, and immunohistochemical features of canine orbital hibernomas. *Vet Pathol.* 2014;51:563-568.

Roberts SM, Severin GA, Lavach JD. Prevalence and treatment of palpebral neoplasms in the dog: 200 cases (1975-1983). *J Am Vet Med Assoc.* 1986;189:1355-1359.

Roth L, Sisson A. Aspirate of a mass posterior to the eye. *Vet Clin Pathol.* 1999;28:89-90.

Samuelson DA. Ophthalmic anatomy. In: Gelatt KN, ed. *Veterinary Ophthalmology.* 13th ed. Philadelphia: Lippincott Williams & Wilkins; 1999:31-150.

Santagostino SF, Mortellaro CM, Buchholz J, et al. Primary angiocentric/angioinvasive T-cell lymphoma of the tympanic bulla in a feline leukaemia virus-positive cat. *JFMS Open Rep.* 2015;1:2055116915593966. doi:10.1177/2055116915593966.

Scott EM, Carter RT. Canine keratomycosis in 11 dogs: a case series (2000-2011). *J Am Anim Hosp Assoc.* 2014;50:112-118.

Scott EM, Teixeira LBC, Flanders DJ, et al. Canine orbital rhabdomyosarcoma: a report of 18 cases. *Vet Ophthalmol.* 2016;19:130-137.

Stenner VJ, Mackay B, King T, et al. Protothecosis in 17 Australian dogs and a review of the canine literature. *Med Mycol.* 2007;45:249-266.

Stiles J, McDermott M, Bigsby D, et al. Use of nested polymerase chain reaction to identify feline herpesvirus in ocular tissue from clinically normal cats and cats with corneal sequestra or conjunctivitis. *Am J Vet Res.* 1997;58:338-342.

Streeten BW, Streeten EA. "Blue body" epithelial cell inclusions in conjunctivitis. *Ophthalmol*. 1985;92:575-579.

Sula MM. Tumors and tumorlike lesions of dog and cat ears. *Vet Clin Small Anim*. 2012;42(6):1161-1178.

Sula MM, Njaa BL, Payton ME. Histologic characterization of the cat middle ear: in sickness and in health. *Vet Pathol*. 2014;51(5):951-967.

Sykes JE. Chlamydial infections; mycoplasma infections. In: Sykes JE, ed. *Canine and Feline Infectious Diseases*. 1st ed. St. Louis: Elsevier; 2014:326-333, 382-389.

Tasker S. Diagnosis of feline infectious peritonitis. Update on evidence supporting available tests. *J Feline Med Surg*. 2018;20:228-243.

Tater KC, Scott DW, Miller WH Jr, et al. The cytology of the external ear canal in the normal dog and cat. *J Vet Med A Physiol Pathol Clin Med*. 2003;50(7):370-374.

Toma S, Cornegliani L, Persico P, et al. Comparison of 4 fixation and staining methods for the cytologic evaluation of ear canals with clinical evidence of ceruminous otitis externa. *Vet Clin Pathol*. 2006;35:194-198.

Tvedten H, Hillström A. Cytologic appearance of retinal cells included in a fine-needle aspirate of a meningioma around the optic nerve of a dog. *Vet Clin Pathol*. 2013;42:234-237.

Volopich S, Benetka V, Schwendenwein I, et al. Cytologic findings, and feline herpesvirus DNA and *Chlamydophila felis* antigen detection rates in normal cats and cats with conjunctival and corneal lesions. *Vet Ophthalmol*. 2005;8:25-32.

von Bomhard W, Polkinghorne A, Lu ZH, et al. Detection of novel chlamydiae in cats with ocular disease. *Am J Vet Res*. 2003;64:1421-1428.

Weinstein NM, Boes KM, Mauldin E, et al. What is your diagnosis? Middle ear material from a dog. *Vet Clin Pathol*. 2016;45:195-196.

Wiggans KT, Vernau W, Lappin MR, et al. Diagnostic utility of aqueocentesis and aqueous humor analysis in dogs and cats with anterior uveitis. *Vet Ophthalmol*. 2014;17:212-220.

Wilcock BP, Njaa BL. Special senses. In: Maxie MG, ed. *Jubb, Kennedy, and Palmer's Pathology of Domestic Animals*. 6th ed. St. Louis: Elsevier; 2016:407-508.

Willis M, Bounous DI, Hirsh S, et al. Conjunctival brush cytology: evaluation of a new cytological collection technique in dogs and cats with a comparison to conjunctival scraping. *Vet Comp Ophthalmol*. 1997;7:74-81.

Wong VM, Jaffe MH. Pathology in practice. *J Am Vet Med Assoc*. 2018;252(3):297-299.

Young KM. Laboratory medicine: yesterday today tomorrow (Eye on the cytoplasm). *Vet Clin Pathol*. 2006;35:141.

Zarfoss MK, Dubielzig RR, Eberhard ML, et al. Canine ocular onchocerciasis in the United States: two new cases and a review of the literature. *Vet Ophthalmol*. 2005;8:51-57.

Zeiss CJ, Johnson EM, Dubielzig RR. Feline intraocular tumors may arise from transformation of lens epithelium. *Vet Pathol*. 2003;40:355-362.

Zemljič T, Matheis FL, Venzin C, et al. Orbito-nasal cyst in a young European short-haired cat. *Vet Ophthalmol*. 2011;14:122-129.

17 CHAPTER

Endocrine and Neuroendocrine Systems

Ul-Soo Choi and Tara Arndt

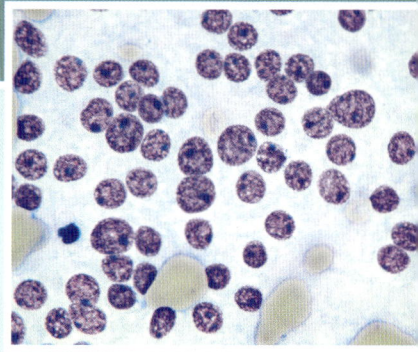

The endocrine system consists of the thyroid, parathyroid, adrenal cortex, and pancreatic islet cells. These highly integrated and vascularized glands have sinusoids that are closely associated with secretory parenchymal cells, from which hormones are produced. The neuroendocrine system involves paraganglionic cells, which synthesize and secrete catecholamines and other regulatory peptides. The neuroendocrine cells of the adrenal medulla and extra-adrenal sites are derived from neuroectoderm. The extra-adrenal paraganglionic cells include the aortic and carotid bodies, which have chemoreceptor activity in blood gas regulation. Embryologically, neuroendocrine cells are present in gastrointestinal (GI) tissue, the tracheobronchial tree, and the liver (Hamilton et al., 1999).

Conditions involving the endocrine and neuroendocrine systems may involve hyperplasia, hypoplasia, inflammation, and neoplasia, with the latter condition of most interest to cytopathologists (Table 17.1).

Cytopathology preparations from endocrine system tumors are often highly cellular, with the exception of aspirates from some thyroid tumors, which are often blood contaminated with low nucleated cellularity. Neuroendocrine neoplasms may arise from chemoreceptor organs, giving rise to both adenomas and adenocarcinomas. These tumors arise from the neuroendocrine cells in the nasal cavity, lung, liver, skin, or GI tract and are generally termed *carcinoids*. Endocrine gland– and neuroendocrine cell–derived tumors share characteristic cytopathologic features, including naked or free nuclei embedded in a background of pale cytoplasm with few distinct cytoplasmic borders resulting from the fragile nature of these cells. These cytopathologic features can mimic poorly prepared samples from other tissues, where cell lysis occurs when excessive pressure is applied to the slides during sample preparation. In the latter case, cell damage such as nuclear lysis and nuclear streaming will also be evident (Fig. 17.1).

Although neuroendocrine tumors share common cytomorphologic characteristics, they can often be distinguished from each other by the location of the lesion and other distinctive cytopathologic features. Identification of the tissue of origin is important to aid prediction of biologic behavior because these tumors often have a relatively bland cytopathologic appearance and lack cytopathologic criteria for malignancy. If criteria of malignancy are present, neuroendocrine tumors are more likely to metastasize or locally invade surrounding structures. Thus, tissue of origin and identification and knowledge of the malignant potential of the specific neoplasms in different species are critical for prognosticating tumors of endocrine and neuroendocrine origin and are particularly important when evaluating thyroid tumors, which are the most commonly encountered endocrine system tumor.

> **KEY POINT** The presence of numerous intact free or naked nuclei aids in the identification of the endocrine or neuroendocrine origin tumors; however, it can be difficult to predict biologic behavior based on cytopathologic findings alone because aggressive tumors may lack characteristics of cytopathologic malignancy.

THYROID GLAND

The thyroid is composed of variably sized follicles lined by simple epithelium. Squamous to low cuboidal epithelium is found in the resting stage, and cuboidal to columnar epithelium is found in the active stage (Fig. 17.2). The follicular colloid contains thyroglobulin, from which thyroid hormone is produced. Follicles are separated by parafollicular cells, which are found within the delicate fibrous septa along with an abundant vascular supply. Active follicles have small vacuoles adjacent to the epithelium that are recognized as endocytosis of thyroglobulin.

Non-neoplastic Thyroid Diseases

Non-neoplastic thyroid diseases include lymphocytic thyroiditis, follicular atrophy, nodular hyperplasia (goiter), and thyroid cysts (Fig. 17.3 and Table 17.2) with lymphocytic thyroiditis and follicular atrophy making up the majority of causes of hypothyroidism in dogs (La Perle, 2013). In cases of suspected thyroiditis or follicular atrophy, measurement of serum tetraiodothyronine (T_4) and/or a thyroglobulin autoantibody titer biopsy and histologic assessment should be considered before fine-needle aspiration (FNA) cytopathology because of the inherent challenges of aspirating these poorly exfoliating lesions. According to recent literature on histologic evaluation of lymphocytic thyroiditis, varying numbers of lymphocytes, plasma cells, macrophages, and thyroid epithelial cells with or without colloid will be exfoliated (La Perle, 2013). In atrophic lesions, small numbers of thyroid epithelial cells and spindle cells may be found in the smears with or without colloid.

Lymphocytic thyroiditis and follicular atrophy are clinically identified infrequently versus nodular hyperplasia, which can be frequently encountered in clinical settings because more than 98% of hyperthyroid cats develop thyroid hyperplasia and adenoma (Mooney and Peterson, 2004).

TABLE 17.1 Pathology of the Endocrine and Neuroendocrine Systems

TISSUE OF ORIGIN	LOCATION	PATHOLOGY
Thyroid	Neck or ectopic	**Non-neoplastic** Lymphocytic thyroiditis Follicular atrophy Nodular hyperplasia (goiter) Cysts **Neoplastic** Follicular adenoma or adenocarcinoma Thyroid C-cell adenoma or carcinoma
Parathyroid	Neck	**Non-neoplastic** Parathyroid cyst Lymphocytic parathyroiditis Parathyroid gland hyperplasia Cysts **Neoplastic** Parathyroid adenoma Parathyroid carcinoma
Pancreatic endocrine (islet cell)[a]	Pancreas	**Neoplastic** Glucagonoma (α islet cell) Insulinoma (β islet cell) Gastrin-secreting islet cell tumor (non-β islet cell) Somatostatinoma (δ islet cell) PPoma (pancreatic polypeptide–secreting cell) Others: vasoactive intestinal peptide adenoma
Adrenal cortex	Adrenal gland	**Non-neoplastic** Adrenalitis Adrenocortical hyperplasia Idiopathic adrenocortical atrophy **Neoplastic** Adrenocortical adenoma or adenocarcinoma
Adrenal medulla	Adrenal gland	**Neoplastic** Pheochromocytoma (paraganglia, chromaffin cell) Neuroblastoma Ganglioneuroma
Chemoreceptor (paraganglia, nonchromaffin cell)	Aortic body, carotid body, other areas	**Neoplastic** Aortic body tumor Carotid body tumor Chemodectoma
Other neuroendocrine	Gastrointestinal tract, liver, lung, nasal cavity	**Neoplastic** Carcinoid (Well-differentiated benign, well-differentiated or poorly differentiated malignant)
	Retroperitoneum, para-aorta	Extra-adrenal paraganglia, (chromaffin cell)
	Skin, oral cavity	**Neoplastic** Merkel cell tumor or carcinoma

[a]Endocrine pancreas discussed fully in Chapter 8.

Cytopathologic differentiation of benign lesions such as hyperplasia and adenoma and well-differentiated carcinoma can be difficult based on cytomorphologic features alone because of the often-bland cytopathologic appearance and lack of distinguishing features. Regular-appearing thyroid epithelial cells along with extracellular eosinophilic material (colloid) should be expected in fine-needle aspirate cytopathologic smears of thyroid glands, regardless of benign or malignant state.

Thyroid cysts include thyroglossal duct cysts, cystadenomas, and thyroid carcinomas that are encountered in hyperthyroid and euthyroid cats with benign and malignant thyroid tumors. Clinically, thyroid cysts can be subclinical or cause signs of dysphagia, regurgitation, cough, and laryngeal paralysis by compression of surrounding structures (Miller et al., 2017). One cat had a large ventral neck mass containing approximately 60 mL of clear fluid. The fluid was reported as an acellular transudate with no observed infectious organisms. The cyst fluid T_4

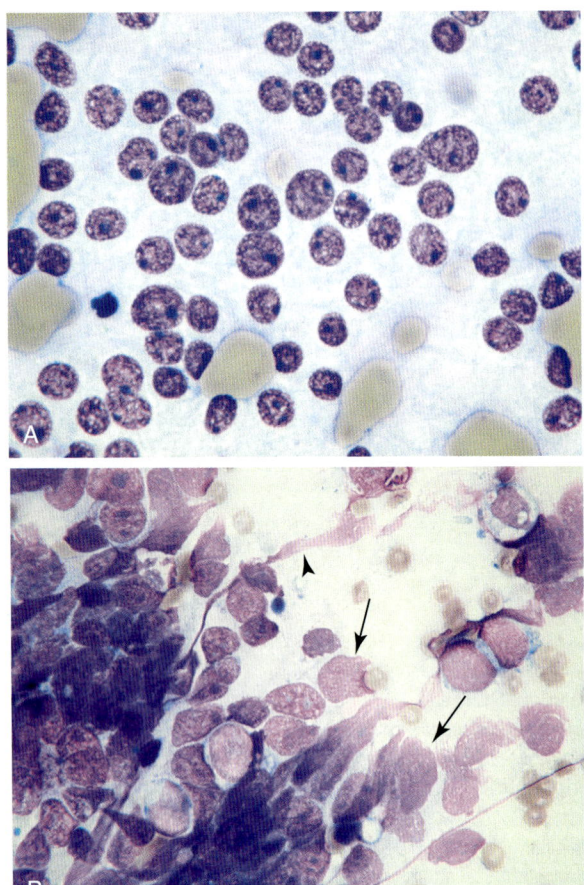

■ **FIGURE 17.1 Naked nuclei versus lysed cell nuclei. A,** Numerous freely scattered and intact naked nuclei are embedded in a background of pale, basophilic cytoplasm, typical of neuroendocrine cell origin. This case is of a chemodectoma. (Aqueous Romanowsky; HP oil.) **B,** Free nuclei caused by cell lysis *(arrows)* and nuclear material streaming *(arrowhead)* are indicative of excess pressure applied at the time of sample preparation. (Wright-Giemsa; HP oil.) (A, From Choi US. *Practical Guide to Diagnostic Cytology of the Dog and Cat.* OKVET; 2012.)

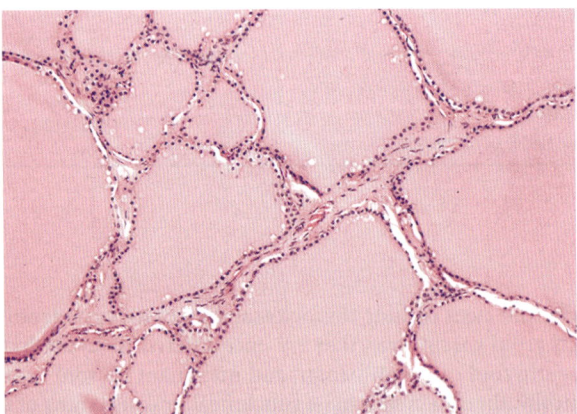

■ **FIGURE 17.2 Normal active thyroid gland. Histology. Cat.** Variably sized thyroid follicles contain homogeneous eosinophilic colloid lined by uniform cuboidal epithelium. Vacuoles are present adjacent to the epithelium, indicating active endocytosis of thyroglobulin. Parafollicular cells present between the follicles produce calcitonin. (H&E; IP.) (Courtesy Rose Raskin, University of Florida.)

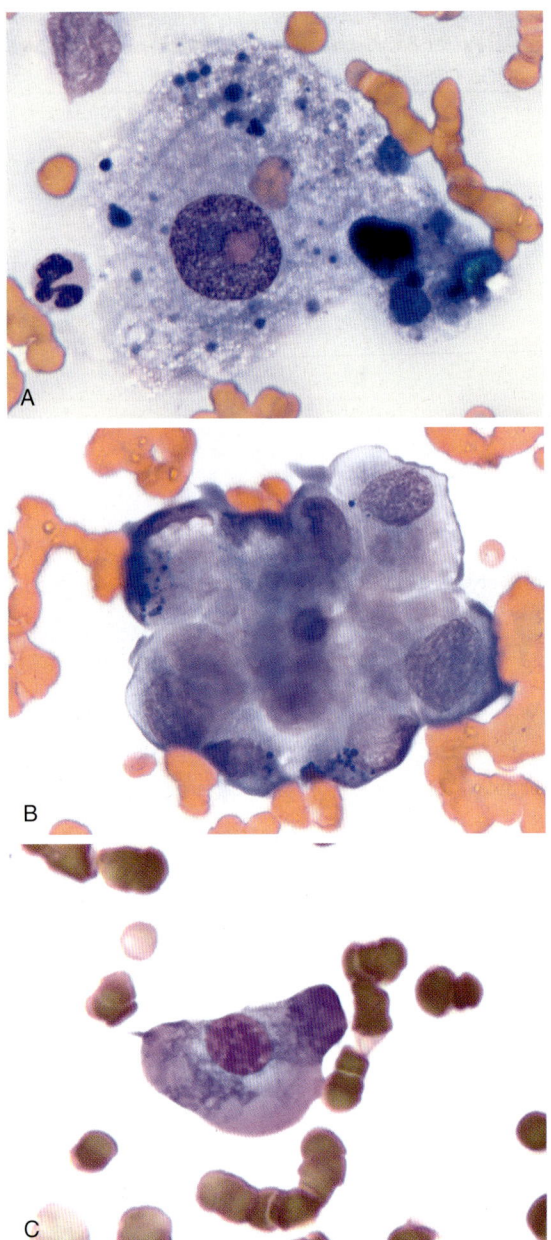

■ **FIGURE 17.3 Thyroid cyst. Tissue aspirate. Cat.** This cervical mass was present for 3 months with hemorrhage only found on an initial cytopathologic biopsy. Computed tomography revealed a 3.2 × 1.6 cm mixed soft tissue and fluid attenuating mass around one thyroid lobe. **A, Hemorrhage.** The fluid was poorly cellular with moderate to marked hemodilution with few macrophages displaying acute (erythrophagocytosis) and chronic hemorrhage (hemosiderin granules). (Modified Wright; HP oil.) **B, Thyroid epithelial cell cluster.** Single cohesive cluster of small to medium-sized round to angular cells with a central, round to ovoid nucleus that measured approximately three times red blood cell (RBC) diameter and having stippled chromatin with occasional prominent single nucleolus. Low amounts of basophilic cytoplasm containing pink amorphous material are present. These cells exhibited minimal atypia with mild anisocytosis and anisokaryosis. (Modified Wright; HP oil.) **C, Thyroid epithelial cell.** One round to angular cell with a central to paracentral round to ovoid nucleus that measured three times RBC diameter having clumped chromatin. There is an abundant amount of basophilic cytoplasm containing pink homogenous material (presumed colloid). Also present in the fluid were low numbers of fibroblasts (not shown). (Modified Wright; HP oil.) (Courtesy Rose Raskin, Michigan State University.)

CHAPTER 17 Endocrine and Neuroendocrine Systems

TABLE 17.2 Features of Non-neoplastic Lesions in the Thyroid Gland of Dogs and Cats

PATHOLOGY	CYTOPATHOLOGY	CLINICAL COMMENTS
Lymphocytic thyroiditis	Lymphocytes, plasma cells, macrophages, and thyroid epithelial cells ± colloid	Common in canine hypothyroidism, with decreased serum T_4 concentration ± increased thyroglobulin autoantibody titer
Follicular atrophy	Well-differentiated thyroid epithelial cells ± adipose connective tissue cells ± colloid	Most common in canine hypothyroidism
Nodular hyperplasia (goiter)	Common to see thyroid epithelial cells ± colloid	Most common in hyperthyroid cats with elevated levels of serum T_4 and T_3
Thyroid cysts	Clear to brown turbid fluid with low cellularity Hemorrhagic, mononuclear predominance, ± thyroid epithelium with colloid	Euthyroid or hyperthyroid Variably sized ventral neck masses Most common in cats Should distinguish from parathyroid cyst by hormonal analysis

T_3, Triiodothyronine; T_4, tetraiodothyronine.

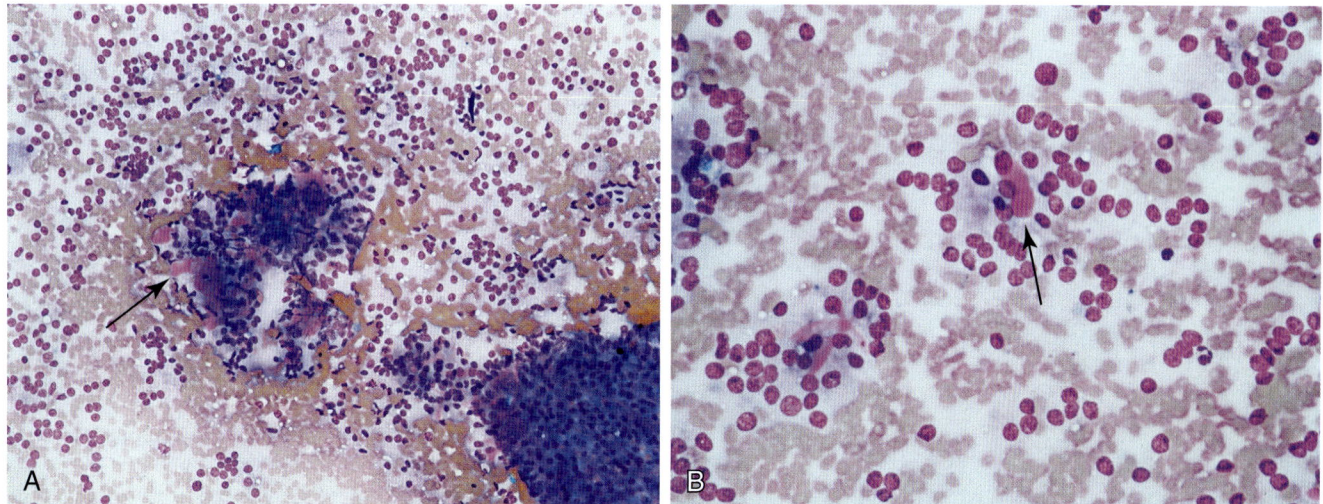

■ **FIGURE 17.4 Thyroid follicular carcinoma. Neck mass. Tissue aspirate. Dog.** Same case in A and B. **A**, Subcutaneous mass located on the neck consists of sheets and clusters with high numbers of free cell nuclei and variably intact epithelial cells having poorly defined cytoplasmic borders. Extracellular eosinophilic material *(arrow)* is colloid. (Aqueous Romanowsky; IP.) **B**, Higher magnification showing dense extracellular colloid *(arrow)* associated with numerous naked nuclei. (Aqueous Romanowsky; IP.) (B, Courtesy Choi US. *Practical Guide to Diagnostic Cytology of the Dog and Cat*. OKVET; 2012.)

concentration was within reference range, which was similar to the serum concentration (Giles et al., 2007). Histopathology revealed that the cyst was supported by fibrous connective tissue lined by a single layer of cuboidal thyroid epithelium. Within the stroma, numerous colloid-filled follicles were lined by attenuated epithelium; the diagnosis was thyroglossal duct cyst. Others report smaller structures with a brown, cloudy appearance with high protein content, approximately 1000 nucleated cells/µL consisting primarily of lymphocytes and macrophages, similar to a hematoma or seroma (Phillips et al., 2003). Furthermore, analysis of cystic fluid of total thyroxine and parathormone may help distinguish the origin of the mass (Phillips et al., 2003)

Thyroid Tumors in Dogs and Cats

Thyroid tumors occur most frequently in dogs, cats, horses, and guinea pigs (Rosol and Meuten, 2017). They often present clinically as subcutaneous masses located on the neck, usually lateral to the trachea (Figs. 17.4 to 17.13), at or near the thoracic

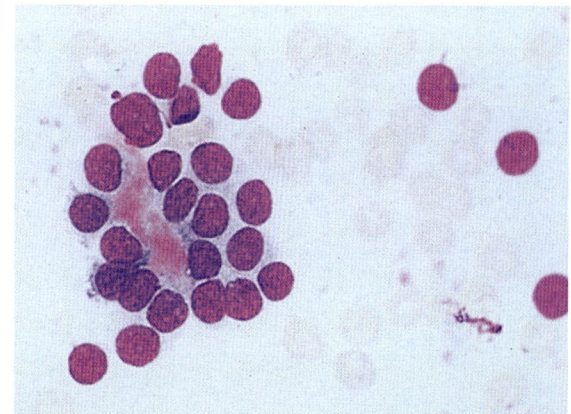

■ **FIGURE 17.5 Thyroid follicular carcinoma. Neck mass. Tissue aspirate.** A cluster of cells with pale cytoplasm and poorly defined cytoplasmic borders. Nuclei are fairly uniform with only mild anisokaryosis. A small amount of amorphous eosinophilic material or colloid can be seen within the cluster of cells. (Wright-Giemsa; HP oil.)

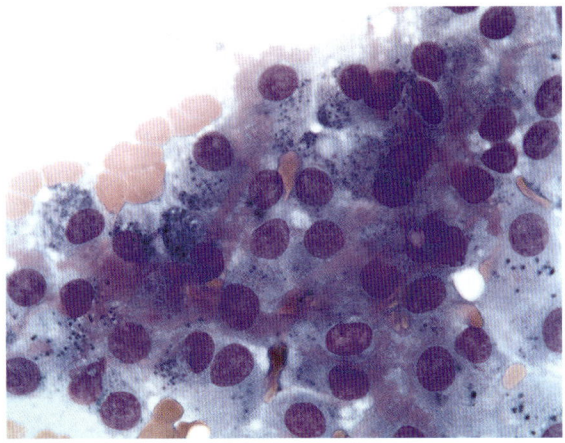

■ **FIGURE 17.6 Thyroid adenocarcinoma. Subcutaneous neck mass. Tissue aspirate. Dog.** The cytoplasm of the cells has poorly defined borders, and pink colloid is observed within and around cell clusters. The dark, cytoplasmic pigment seen throughout the cluster is believed to be tyrosine granules. The nuclei display mild anisokaryosis. (Wright-Giemsa; HP oil.)

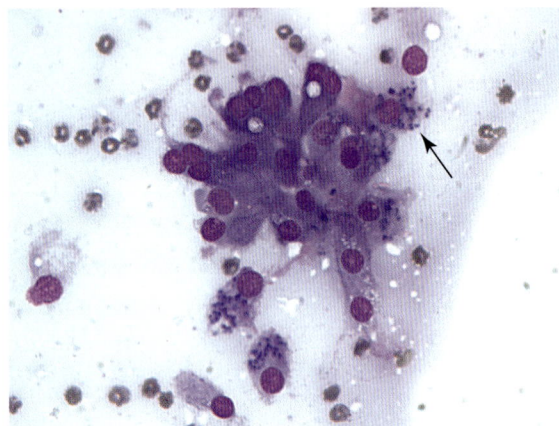

■ **FIGURE 17.7 Thyroid adenocarcinoma. Neck mass. Dog.** The *arrow* indicates pigmented granules considered to be tyrosine. (Wright-Giemsa; HP oil.)

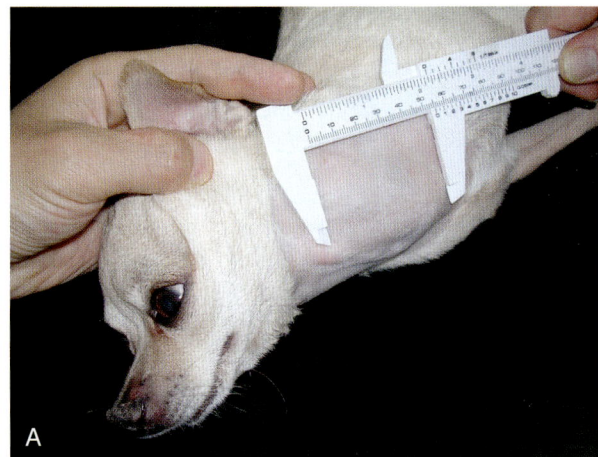

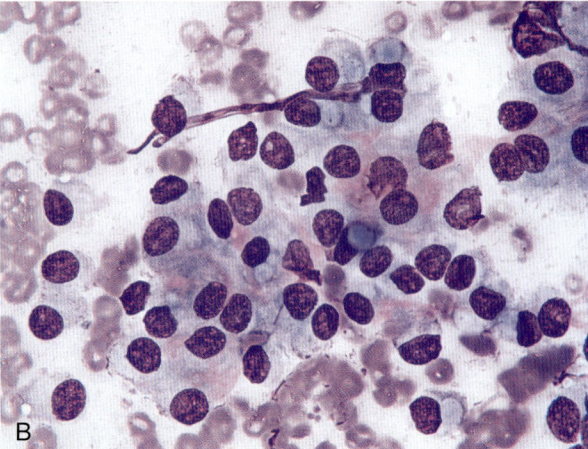

■ **FIGURE 17.8 Thyroid follicular cell adenocarcinoma. Neck mass. Dog.** Same case in A and B. **A, Clinical view.** Firm, cervical mass had grown to 5 cm over 19 months with no reported change in appetite or behavior. **B, Tissue aspirate.** Cells have pale cytoplasm with poorly defined cytoplasmic borders. Nuclei are fairly uniform with only mild anisokaryosis. A small amount of amorphous eosinophilic material (colloid) can be seen between cells. The case was confirmed as follicular cell adenocarcinoma on histopathology. (Aqueous Romanowsky; HP oil.)

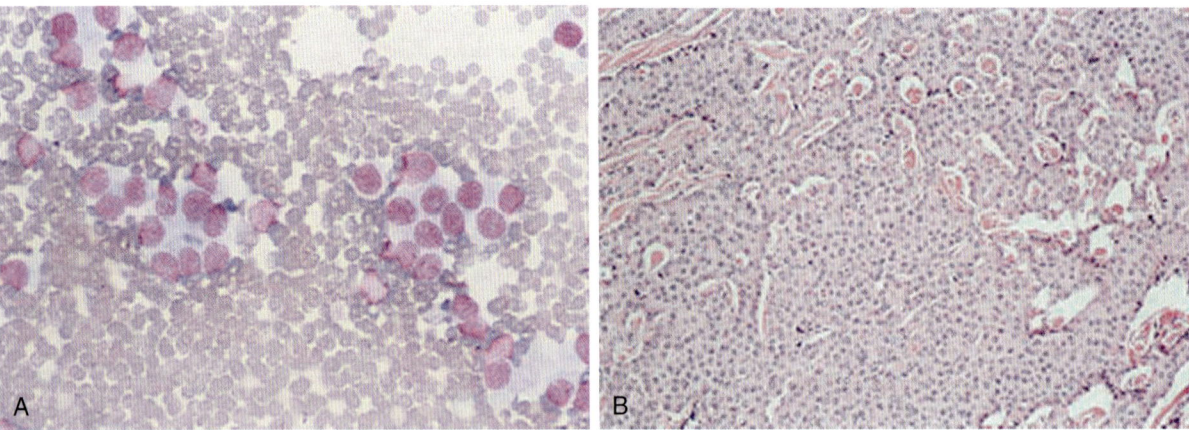

■ **FIGURE 17.9 Thyroid adenocarcinoma. Neck mass. Dog.** Same case in A and B. **A, Tissue aspirate.** This animal had an intermittent honking cough. On physical examination, there was a 2 to 3 cm firm, round, moveable mass lateral to the trachea at the mid neck. Present are groups of loosely adherent cells appearing as naked nuclei against a blood-contaminated background. (Wright-Giemsa; HP oil.) **B, Histology.** Variably sized compact nests and diffuse sheets of neoplastic cells efface the gland, leaving normal thyroid gland with small follicles at the periphery. (H&E; IP.) (Courtesy Rose Raskin, University of Florida.)

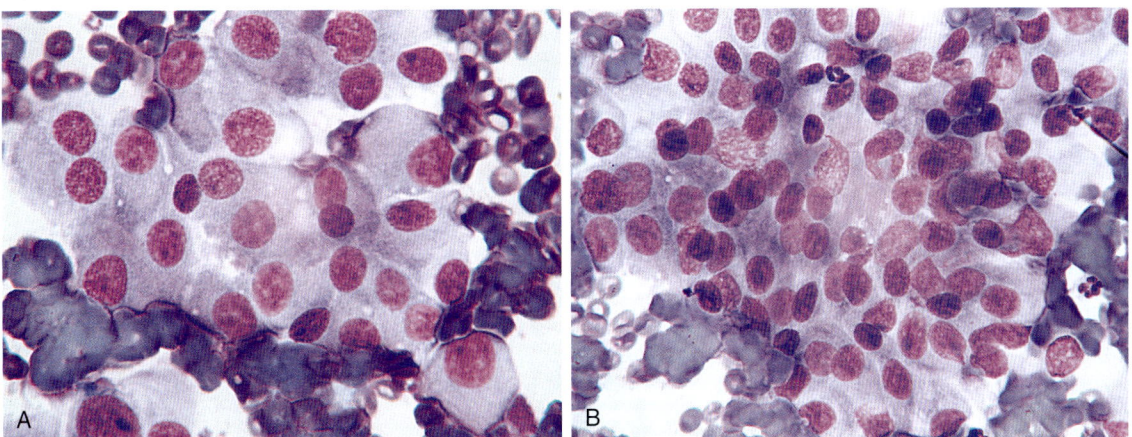

■ **FIGURE 17.10 Thyroid medullary carcinoma. Dog.** Same case in A and B. **A,** Note the distinct cell borders, giving a more cohesive epithelial cytomorphologic appearance compared with follicular carcinoma, which has a naked nuclei cytomorphology. Criteria of malignancy included mild to moderate anisokaryosis, binucleation, and prominent nucleoli. The case was histologically confirmed as thyroid medullary carcinoma with immunoreactivity to calcitonin. (Hemacolor; HP oil.) **B,** This cluster of cells has indistinct cytoplasmic borders. (Hemacolor; HP oil.) (Courtesy Walter Bertazzolo, Italy.)

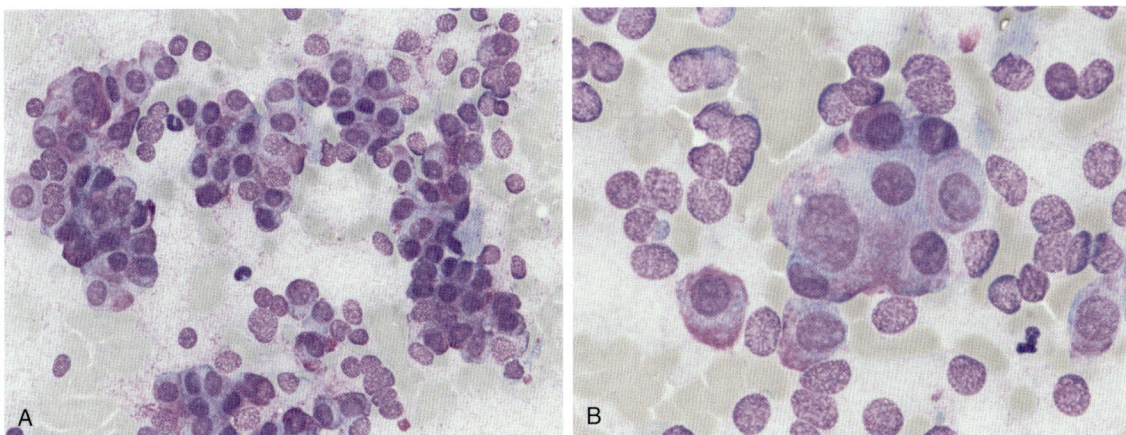

■ **FIGURE 17.11 Thyroid medullary carcinoma. Dog.** Same case in A and B. **A,** A trabecular pattern of epithelial cell clusters contains numerous intracytoplasmic azurophilic granules and scattered numerous granules appear in the background. (Wright-Giemsa; IP.) **B,** Higher magnification of a small cluster of epithelial cells and numerous naked nuclei that contain distinctive azurophilic cytoplasmic granules. (Wright-Giemsa; HP oil.) (Courtesy Jean-Sebastien Latouche, IDEXX Laboratories.)

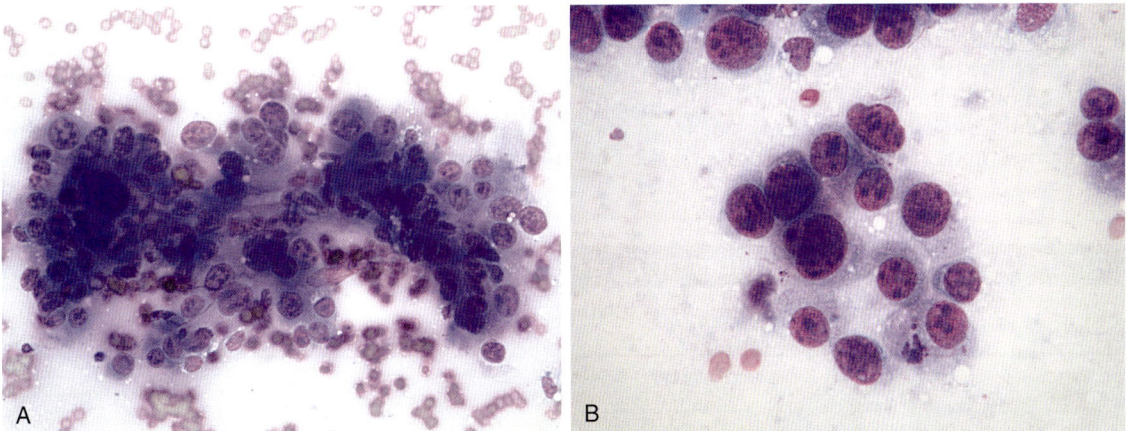

■ **FIGURE 17.12 Poorly differentiated thyroid carcinoma. Dog.** Same case in A and B. **A,** This specimen is taken from a recurrent cervical mass. Present are numerous criteria of malignancy that include anisocytosis, anisokaryosis, anisonucleosis, satellite nuclei, and nuclear crowding and molding. (Aqueous Romanowsky; IP.) **B,** Higher magnification of loosely clustered cells, displaying prominent nucleoli and irregular nuclear shapes. The mass was confirmed on histopathology as an undifferentiated carcinoma. (Aqueous Romanowsky; HP oil.) (A, From Choi US. *Practical Guide to Diagnostic Cytology of the Dog and Cat.* OKVET; 2012.)

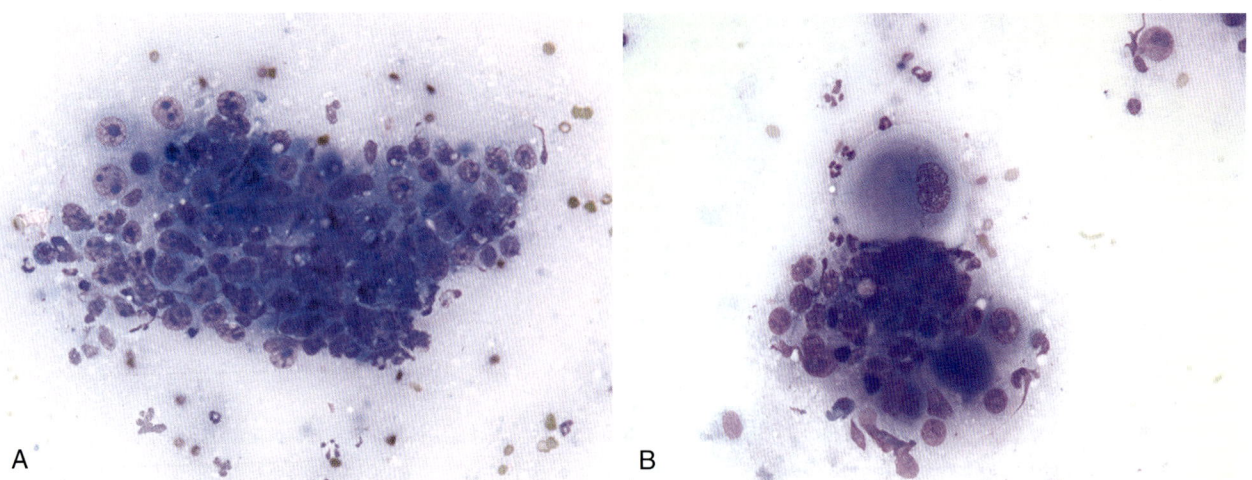

■ **FIGURE 17.13** **Poorly differentiated thyroid carcinoma with squamoid features. Dog.** Same case in A and B. **A,** Single loose cluster of epithelial cells with indistinct cellular margins shows prominent nucleoli with rare macro nucleolus. (Wright-Giemsa; IP.) **B,** Several squamous cells with prominent malignant features were admixed within a cluster of epithelial cells. Note the nuclear molding in a binucleated squamous cell. This case was histologically confirmed as poorly differentiated thyroid carcinoma (squamoid cell type). (Wright-Giemsa; HP oil.)

inlet. Ectopic thyroid tumors may occasionally be found in the cranial thoracic cavity, at the base of the heart or even in the oral cavity at the base of the tongue (Lantz and Salisbury, 1989). There is marked species variability in the biologic behavior of thyroid tumors, and only the most frequently reported features of these lesions are described in this chapter as they relate to dogs and cats (Table 17.3).

Canine Thyroid Tumors

Thyroid tumors represent 1.1% to 3.8% of all canine tumors (Lunn and Page, 2013). No sex predilection has been established; however, a breed predilection has been suggested for Siberian huskies, beagles, and golden retrievers. A recent review indicates that 90% of thyroid tumors identified clinically in dogs are carcinomas (Lunn and Page, 2013), including thyroid follicular carcinoma arising from the follicular epithelium and, less commonly, medullary carcinoma from parafollicular or C-cell origin (Bertazzolo et al., 2003; Barber, 2007). The biologic behavior of canine thyroid tumors is well characterized. Thyroid adenocarcinomas are invasive and can metastasize if given sufficient time. The prognosis and the potential for metastasis may depend on tumor size, and in one study, 14% of dogs with tumor volumes less than 20 mL had evidence of metastasis, whereas a metastatic rate of 74% to 100% was seen in dogs with tumor volumes between 21 and 100 mL (Leav et al., 1976). The earliest and most frequent site of metastasis is the lungs often following local expansion into the larynx, resulting from invasion of tumor cells into the thyroid or jugular vein (Rosol and Meuten, 2017). When possible, surgical resection is the treatment of choice; however, carcinomas are rapidly invasive and may involve vital structures such as the jugular vein, carotid artery, and esophagus. In dogs, hypersecretion of thyroid hormones in association with a thyroid tumor (functional tumor) is of low occurrence and may involve only 10% of cases (Lunn and Page, 2013). Medullary carcinomas are known to be more encapsulated and less invasive than thyroid follicular carcinoma and carry a more favorable prognosis (Carver et al., 1995; Barber, 2007).

Cytopathologic preparations from thyroid tumors, particularly carcinomas, may be hemodilute and contain a large amount of blood contamination. Tumor cells from thyroid follicular carcinoma are exfoliated in clusters or sheets of epithelial cells mixed with variable numbers of free or naked nuclei scattered in the background (see Fig. 17.4), of which the latter may be more prominent in thyroid follicular carcinoma than in medullary carcinoma (Bertazzolo et al., 2003). Aggregates of epithelial cells usually have indistinct cytoplasmic borders and appear as intact free nuclei embedded in a

TABLE 17.3	Cytopathologic Features of Thyroid Tumors	
THYROID TUMOR	**FOLLICULAR ADENOMA, FOLLICULAR ADENOCARCINOMA**	**MEDULLARY OR C-CELL ADENOMA OR CARCINOMA**
Cytopathology	Naked nuclei morphology ± epithelial cell clusters and cytoplasmic blue to black pigment ± colloid Blood contamination is common	Naked nuclei morphology ± epithelial cell clusters ± colloid ± cytoplasmic granules (azurophilic) Blood contamination is common
Clinical comments	Dogs: ~90%–95% are malignant carcinoma; nonfunctional Cats: mostly adenoma; functional; ±cystic	<10% of thyroid tumors in dogs and cats
Immunochemical markers	Thyroglobulin	Calcitonin

background of pale-blue cytoplasm (see Figs. 17.4 and 17.5), with few cells having distinct cytoplasmic borders. Dark blue to black pigment, thought to represent tyrosine-containing granules, can be identified in the cytoplasm of intact epithelial cells (see Figs. 17.6 and 17.7). Extracellular amorphous pink material (colloid) may be associated with some clusters (see Figs. 17.4 and 17.5). Colloid and pigmented granules, along with the naked nuclei appearance of the cells, are helpful to identify the tissue as thyroid in origin. Other findings may include low numbers of macrophages laden with distinct cytoplasmic vacuoles and blue green granules (hemosiderin), indicating recent hemorrhage and red cell turnover.

The nuclei of most neoplastic cells are round to oval with minimal anaplastic features. Most thyroid tumors, even adenocarcinomas, are usually composed of a relatively uniform cell population displaying few, if any, criteria of malignancy (see Figs. 17.4 to 17.9). There may be mild to moderate anisokaryosis (see Fig. 17.8B), and small, indistinct nucleoli are occasionally observed. As previously mentioned, approximately 90% to 95% of clinically apparent canine thyroid tumors are adenocarcinomas and should be considered a probable carcinoma until histopathologic confirmation is obtained.

In thyroid medullary carcinoma or C-cell thyroid carcinoma, cytopathologic features are similar to those in thyroid follicular carcinoma except that neoplastic cells may exfoliate more in clusters and aggregates, and naked nuclei may not be present (see Fig. 17.10). Amorphous pink material or colloid can be seen in the absence of blue-black granules (tyrosine), which has been used as a differentiating feature from thyroid follicular carcinoma. Definitive diagnosis as medullary carcinoma requires histopathology and immunohistochemistry (Bertazzolo et al., 2003). Azurophilic granules can be seen in a low number of tumor cells in thyroid medullary carcinomas (see Fig. 17.11), which may represent cytoplasmic calcitonin (Kini, 2008).

Poorly differentiated thyroid carcinoma are composed of numerous anaplastic tumor cells showing prominent malignant criteria (see Fig. 17.12). Some neoplastic cells may display a squamous differentiation in a rare anaplastic thyroid carcinoma with squamoid subtype (see Fig. 17.13). In a rare thyroid carcinosarcoma case, there were two distinct cell populations, both epithelial and mesenchymal origin, with numerous criteria of malignancy (Fernandez et al., 2008).

Feline Thyroid Tumors

Feline thyroid tumors have similar cytomorphologic features to those of dogs. Unlike dogs, the vast majority of feline thyroid tumors are benign adenomas, occasionally referred to as adenomatous hyperplasia (Figs. 17.14 and 17.15). Bilateral thyroid gland involvement is present in about 70% of feline cases, and functional adenocarcinomas occur in only 1% to 3% of cats presenting with clinical signs of hyperthyroidism (Lunn and Page, 2013). In cats, a uniform population of nuclei with no criteria for malignancy generally indicates a benign lesion. It is not possible to differentiate between adenomas and adenocarcinomas based on cytopathology alone; histologic evaluation of capsular or lymphatic invasion is often required for this characterization (Rosol and Meuten, 2017).

Unlike in dogs, most feline thyroid adenomas are functional and actively secrete thyroid hormones. Adenomas are usually well encapsulated and often have an excellent prognosis with

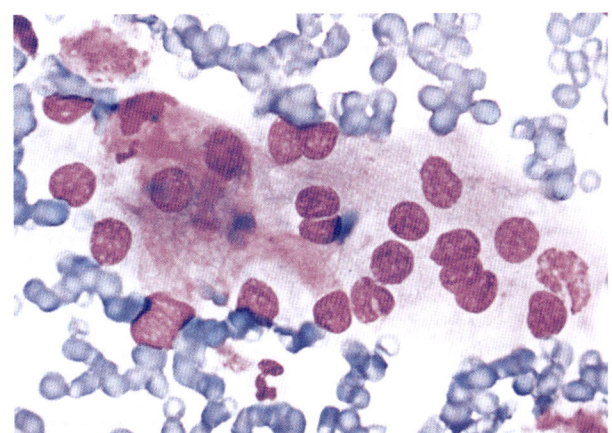

■ **FIGURE 17.14 Thyroid adenoma with colloid. Subcutaneous neck mass. Tissue aspirate. Cat.** The cytoplasm of the cells has poorly defined borders, and amorphous pink material (colloid) is observed within the cluster. The nuclei are uniform consistent with adenoma or adenomatous hyperplasia. (Wright-Giemsa; HP oil.)

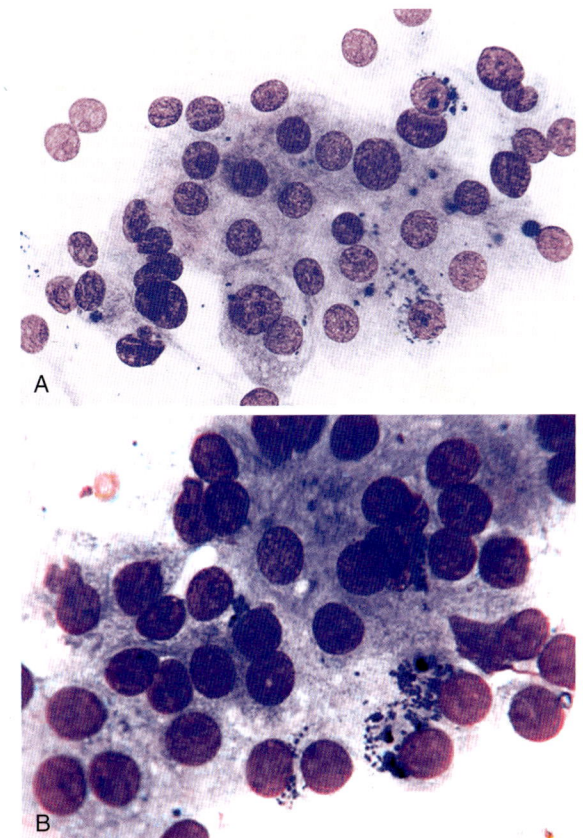

■ **FIGURE 17.15 Thyroid adenoma with tyrosine. Neck mass. Tissue aspirate.** Same case in A and B. **Cat. A,** Clinical hyperthyroidism of 3-year duration. The cat was treated 3 months earlier with radioactive iodine and now presented with reoccurrence of hyperthyroidism. Several binucleated forms are present along with black granular cytoplasmic inclusions thought to represent tyrosine granules. A moderate degree of anisocytosis and anisokaryosis is noted that may relate to the relapse and radiation therapy. (Wright-Giemsa; HP oil.) **B,** Several binucleated forms appear to be present along with black granular cytoplasmic inclusions, likely tyrosine. (Wright-Giemsa; HP oil.) (Courtesy Rose Raskin and Rick Alleman, University of Florida.)

complete surgical removal. After bilateral thyroidectomy, the patient must be monitored for signs of hypothyroidism and hypocalcemia resulting from inadvertent removal of the parathyroid glands (Lunn and Page, 2013). Adenocarcinomas are locally invasive and often metastasize to regional lymph nodes, with metastatic disease reported in up to 70% of cats with adenocarcinomas (Lunn and Page, 2013).

Alternative treatment to surgical removal may consist of antithyroid drugs, which are not generally cytotoxic but do reduce the metabolic effects of thyrotoxicosis. Radiotherapy with iodine-131 is another alternate treatment used to reduce the size of the neoplasm, especially for cats with hyperfunctional ectopic thyroid tissue.

> **KEY POINT** Iatrogenic blood contamination is common in FNA cytopathology of thyroid tumors. Free naked nuclei and amorphous extracellular eosinophilic material (colloid) and cytoplasmic blue to black pigment (probable tyrosine) are key cytomorphologic features.

PARATHYROID GLANDS

Reported pathologic changes of the feline and canine parathyroid gland are listed in Table 17.4. Most animal species have paired parathyroid glands located in the cranial cervical area. External and internal parathyroid glands are found in dogs and cats, in which the predominant cells are secretory chief cells. In histology sections, chief cells are cuboidal or polyhedral epithelial cells with lightly eosinophilic cytoplasm; however, cytopathologic preparations may contain free nuclei embedded in a background of lightly basophilic cytoplasm with indistinct borders (Diaconu et al., 2008).

Non-neoplastic Parathyroid Disease

Parathyroid cysts within the glandular parenchyma or near the glands in the mediastinum occur frequently in dogs and occasionally in cats and can occasionally be large enough to be seen macroscopically (Swainson et al., 2000; Rosol and Meuten, 2017). Cytopathologic evaluation of parathyroid cysts is considered similar to that described for branchial cysts (see Chapter 4) with a reported description of clear, acellular fluid with few proteinaceous strands (Swainson et al., 2000). Histologically, the cysts are lined by cuboidal to columnar, often ciliated, and epithelial cells filled with densely eosinophilic proteinaceous material (Swainson et al., 2000). Another report noted a small fluid-filled mass with an anechoic center. Only 1 to 2 mL of a clear fluid was aspirated. Fluid parathormone concentration was four times the serum concentration and 25 times the reference interval. The clinical significance of cystic parathyroid lesions in veterinary species is unknown but is likely subclinical (Swainson et al., 2000; Barber, 2004).

Lymphocytic parathyroiditis, attributed to an immune-mediated mechanism, is one cause of hyperparathyroidism. Histologically, lesions have been described to contain lymphocytes, plasma cells, fibroblasts, neocapillaries, and varying number of chief cells (La Perle, 2013). Cytopathologic smears may yield chief cells and inflammatory cells associated with immune-mediated disease, including lymphocytes and plasma cells. In dogs, idiopathic hyperparathyroidism is usually caused by lymphocytic parathyroiditis.

Parathyroid gland hyperplasia can be seen in dogs with hypercalcemia either primary or compensatory to chronic renal disease and nutritional imbalances (DeVries et al., 1993; Rosol and Meuten, 2017). Palpable, enlarged parathyroid glands may be clinically palpated, and surgical removal can be curative with normalization of serum calcium levels in cases of primary parathyroid gland hyperplasia (DeVries et al., 1993). On histopathology, these lesions have been described as adenomatous hyperplasia. On cytopathology, free nuclei embedded in the background of lightly basophilic cytoplasm with indistinct cellular borders are often observed, and differentiation between hyperplasia and parathyroid adenoma is not possible on cytopathologic specimens alone (Diaconu et al., 2008).

Parathyroid Gland Tumors

Parathyroid tumors are uncommon neoplasms in domestic animals with most reported in dogs and cats (Kallet et al., 1991; Berger and Feldman, 1987; DeVries et al., 1993; den Hertog et al., 1997). Generally, these tumors are recognized in older animals, dogs older than 7 years, and cats older than 8 years, with a potential breed predisposition in keeshonds (Berger and Feldman, 1987).

The most frequently reported parathyroid tumor is the adenoma of the parathyroid chief cells. Parathyroid carcinomas are rare and have been reported in older dogs and cats (Kallet et al., 1991; Marquez et al., 1995; den Hertog et al., 1997; Ramaiah et al., 2001). Cytopathologic evaluations have been described as useful for diagnosis and are usually performed on

TABLE 17.4 Pathology of the Parathyroid Gland in Dogs and Cats

PATHOLOGY	CYTOPATHOLOGY	CLINICAL COMMENTS
Non-neoplastic		
Parathyroid cyst	Epithelial cells and eosinophilic proteinaceous material	May cause hypercalcemia; measure cyst fluid parathormone level to help distinguish from thyroid cysts
Lymphocytic parathyroiditis	Lymphocytes, plasma cells, and chief cells	Hypoparathyroidism in dogs
Hyperplasia, primary or compensatory	Naked nuclei embedded in the background of lightly basophilic cytoplasm	Hypercalcemia
Neoplastic		
Parathyroid adenoma or carcinoma of parathyroid chief cells	Naked nuclei ± needle-like eosinophilic cytoplasmic inclusions	Rare carcinoma Hypercalcemia and relevant clinical signs

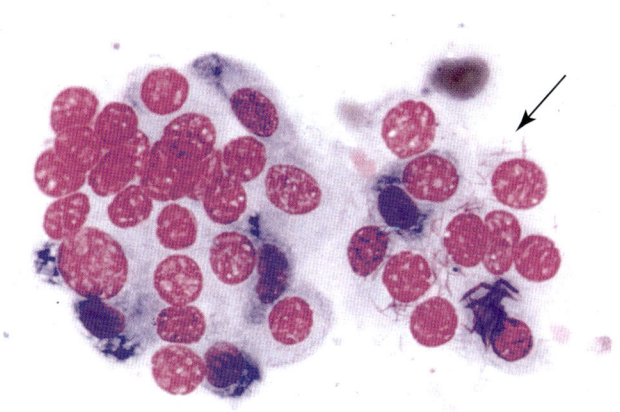

FIGURE 17.16 Adenocarcinoma. Parathyroid. Subcutaneous neck mass. Tissue imprint. Dog. The animal had persistent hypercalcemia and increased serum parathormone concentration. The cytoplasm of the cell cluster is pale blue with indistinct cytoplasmic borders and pale eosinophilic needle-like inclusions of unknown significance *(arrow)*. Some intact cells contain black needle intracytoplasmic structures. Nuclei are dense with a high nucleocytoplasmic ratio and moderate anisokaryosis. (Wright-Giemsa; HP oil.) (Courtesy Shashi Ramaiah, University of Florida.)

surgically excised tissue imprints because of the small size of the tumors and difficulty in aspirating them (Ramaiah et al., 2001). However, in one report, four of seven cats with primary hyperparathyroidism had palpable cervical masses (Kallet et al., 1991).

Chief cells aspirated from parathyroid adenomas have a typical naked nuclei appearance on cytopathologic preparations. Cells appear as free nuclei in a lightly basophilic background of cytoplasm. In addition, some parathyroid tumors contain needle-like, eosinophilic cytoplasmic inclusions of unknown composition (Fig. 17.16). Nuclei are round to oval and relatively uniform in size and shape. Parathyroid adenocarcinomas are typically larger than adenomas; however, they may appear similar cytopathologically. The diagnosis of adenocarcinoma is made when there is histologic or gross evidence of capsular invasion into surrounding structures or metastasis to regional lymph node(s) or lungs (Rosol and Meuten, 2017).

Because parathyroid tumors, especially adenomas, are often not palpable, the presurgical diagnosis frequently relies on recognition of clinical signs and characteristic laboratory findings. The vast majority of parathyroid tumors actively secrete excess parathormone, and most cases are presented for clinical signs associated with increased hormonal activity. Commonly reported abnormalities include hypercalcemia, most common finding, polydipsia and polyuria, muscle wasting, skeletal abnormalities, and urinary bladder calculi (DeVries et al., 1993; Marquez et al., 1995; Lunn and Page, 2013).

Surgical exploration of the cervical area is warranted if laboratory and clinical findings establish a diagnosis of primary hyperparathyroidism. Parathyroid adenomas are well encapsulated and can often be surgically removed by blunt dissection. Patients must be monitored closely for the rapid development of postsurgical hypocalcemia (Lunn and Page, 2013). The long-term prognosis for patients with parathyroid adenomas is good.

EXTRA-ADRENAL PARAGANGLIOMAS

Paragangliomas are tumors of neuroendocrine cells with components of the sympathetic or parasympathetic nervous systems. *Paraganglioma* is the preferred terminology when they occur in areas other than adrenal medulla (i.e., aortic body, carotid body, or elsewhere in the body). Chromaffin paragangliomas arising within adrenal medulla are termed *pheochromocytoma*. Most chromaffin extra-adrenal paraganglionic cells in the retroperitoneum of dogs occur in the mid-retroperitoneum ventral and lateral to the abdominal aorta, with smaller aggregates distributed around the origin of the caudal mesenteric artery (likely organ of Zuckerkandl) and adrenal glands (Ilha and Styer, 2013). Pheochromocytomas and extra-adrenal paragangliomas of sympathetic origin are usually composed of chromaffin cells (staining positive with chromium salts), which have secretory granules containing norepinephrine, epinephrine, or both.

Chemodectomas

Chemoreceptor tumors are generally referred to as chemodectomas or nonchromaffin paragangliomas. Paragangliomas from aortic and carotid body are also called according to their location, aortic body or heart base tumors, and carotid body tumors, respectively. Aortic and carotid body tumors typically develop from the parasympathetic nervous system and are usually negative for chromaffin cells (nonchromaffin paragangliomas) (Shaw et al., 2010; Rosol and Meuten, 2017).

Chemodectomas are uncommon tumors of dogs and have rarely been reported in cats (Tillson et al., 1994; Ware and Hopper, 1999; Caruso et al., 2002; Hardcastle et al., 2013). Most dogs affected are between 10 and 15 years of age, and there is a higher incidence of these tumors in brachycephalic breeds, particularly boxers and Boston terriers (Rosol and Meuten, 2017). The majority (80%–90%) of chemodectomas reported in animals originated from the aortic bodies; however, there are rare reports of carotid body tumors in dogs (Obradovich et al., 1992) (Table 17.5).

TABLE 17.5 Location and Clinical Aspects of Chemoreceptor Tumors		
CHEMORECEPTOR TUMORS	**LOCATION**	**CLINICAL ASPECTS**
Aortic body tumor or heart base tumor	Within the pericardial sac at or near the base of the heart	Nonfunctional; space-occupying effects (pericardial effusion, right-sided congestive heart failure)
Carotid body tumor	In the neck, near the angle of the jaw, at the carotid bifurcation	Nonfunctional; space-occupying effects (dyspnea, esophageal disease, compression of the carotid artery)

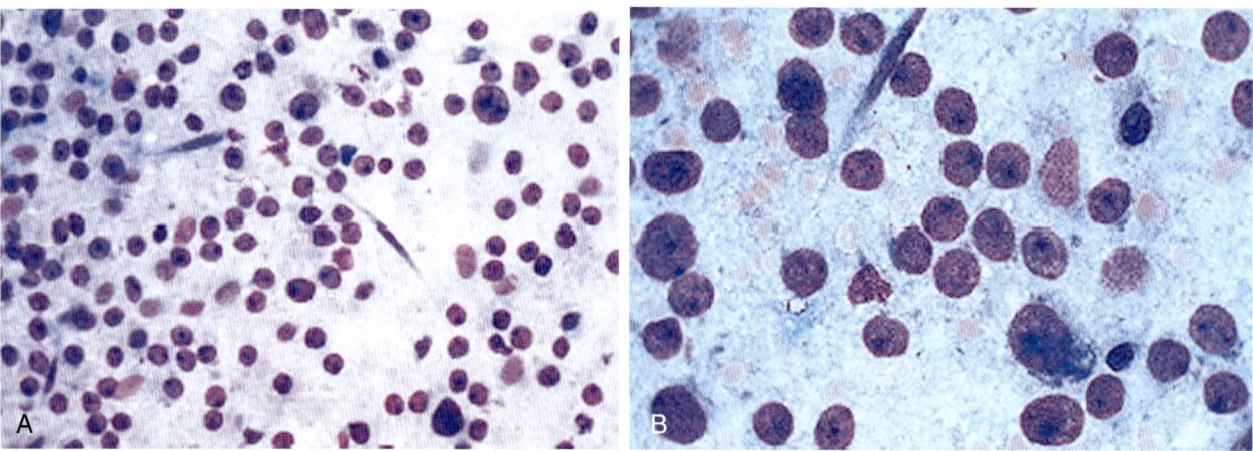

FIGURE 17.17 Aortic body tumor (chemodectoma). Thoracic mass. Tissue aspirate. Dog. Same case in A and B. **A,** The mass was located in the thoracic cavity just dorsal to the base of the heart. Cytopathology is composed of free nuclei with moderate anisokaryosis and prominent nucleolus in a background of lightly basophilic, granular free cytoplasm from the ruptured cells. Two spindle-shaped cells are considered to be of stromal origin. (Wright-Giemsa; HP oil.) **B,** Higher magnification of tumor cells with moderate anisokaryosis and prominent nucleoli in a sea of lightly basophilic, granular free cytoplasm. A stromal cell located in the upper center. (Wright-Giemsa; HP oil.)

Aortic Body Tumor

The aortic body tumor generally occurs as a single mass within the pericardial sac at or near the base of the heart (Rosol and Meuten, 2017). Presenting clinical signs are usually those associated with cardiac decompensation, particularly right heart failure resulting from significant pericardial effusion. Cytopathologic evaluation of this pericardial effusion rarely identifies tumor cells. Reactive mesothelium often associated with the fluid may be mistaken for neoplastic cells in dogs (see Chapter 6). Unlike pericardial fluid, ultrasound-guided fine-needle aspirates taken directly from the lesions are usually very cellular and often diagnostically rewarding. Care must be taken when performing this procedure because of the close association of aortic body tumors with atria and major vessels.

Aspirates and imprints taken from aortic body tumors are usually cellular. The typical naked nuclei appearance with free nuclei in a background of cytoplasm is a prominent feature (Fig. 17.17A). Nuclei are round with clumped chromatin and usually contain a single, prominent nucleolus, typical of neuroendocrine cell tumors (Fig. 17.17B). Both benign and malignant forms occur, and anaplastic features of anisokaryosis and multiple, variable nucleoli are not reliable indicators of the malignant potential. Both adenomas and adenocarcinomas can have scattered areas of the tumor that contain larger, more pleomorphic cells and bizarrely shaped giant cells (Rosol and Meuten, 2017). Carcinomas are identified by invasion into the surrounding capsule, blood vessels, lymphatics, or adjacent structures (Rosol and Meuten, 2017). Aortic body tumors may be difficult to distinguish from ectopic thyroid tumors, which may appear on cytopathology similar and may on occasion occur in the same area. The identification of colloid or cytoplasmic blue-green pigment granules (tyrosine) can help to identify the tissue as thyroid origin (Boes et al., 2010).

Most aortic body tumors in dogs are benign adenomas (Rosol and Meuten, 2017). They are usually well encapsulated and are slow growing with low metastatic potential; however, they can be expansive lesions and with potential to compress the atria or vena cava. Surgical resection is the treatment of choice for adenomas; however, long-term success is limited because complete resection is difficult to achieve because of the close association of these neoplasms with major vessels. Malignant forms or carcinomas are invasive and may spread locally to veins, lymphatics, or myocardium (Zimmerman et al., 2000; Rosol and Meuten, 2017). When distant metastasis occurs, it is usually to the lung or liver, but any number of organs may be involved. The prognosis for cats with chemodectomas may be worse because of the frequent invasive nature of the tumor in this species (Tillson et al., 1994).

Carotid Body Tumor

Carotid body tumors are rare neoplasms that are located in the neck, near the angle of the jaw, at the bifurcation of the common carotid artery (Rosol and Meuten, 2017). Carotid body tumors appear similar on cytopathology to aortic body tumors (Fig. 17.18A). The location of carotid body tumors also necessitates differentiation from thyroid tumors. Identification of colloid or pigment granules would help to identify tissue as thyroid origin. Although case reports are limited, these tumors are more likely to be malignant than are aortic body tumors, and they are characterized by local tissue invasion and a tendency to metastasize to multiple sites in the body (Fig. 17.18B) (Obradovich et al., 1992; Rosol and Meuten, 2017). Metastasis usually occurs late in the course of the disease, primarily to the liver, mediastinum, brain, heart, and lungs. Early surgical excision is the treatment of choice, and the role of chemotherapy in the treatment of these tumors has not been evaluated (Obradovich et al., 1992).

> **KEY POINT** Chemodectoma should be differentiated from ectopic (heart base) or cervical thyroid tumor, which shares similar cytopathologic features, including naked nuclei. The presence of colloid or cytoplasmic blue-green pigment granules (tyrosine) may be helpful to identify thyroid origin. Histologic and immunohistochemical evaluation is often necessary for confirmation.

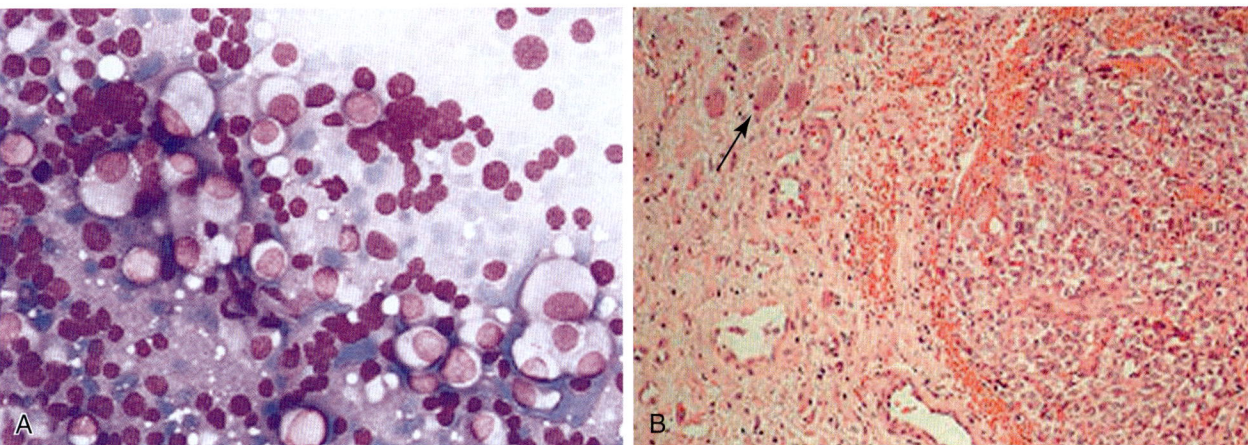

■ **FIGURE 17.18 Carotid body tumor (chemodectoma). Cervical mass. Dog.** Same case in A and B. The animal presented with a head tilt. Magnetic resonance imaging indicated the presence of the mass in the neck region near the tympanic bulla. **A, Surgical excision imprint.** There are numerous free nuclei with a small number of intact cells with variably abundant clear cytoplasm showing marked anisocytosis and anisokaryosis. (Wright-Giemsa; HP oil.) **B, Histology.** This section contains dense sheets of neoplastic cells *(right)* adjacent to fibrovascular stroma *(left)* and nerve cell bodies *(arrow)*. Tumor emboli were observed in blood vessels (not shown), demonstrating the invasive nature of the tumor. (H&E; IP.) (Courtesy Rose Raskin, University of Florida.)

ADRENAL GLAND

The adrenal glands consist of two morphologically and functionally distinct parts, the cortex and medulla. The adrenal cortex originates from the cells of the coelomic epithelium of mesoderm, and the cells of the adrenal medulla are derived from ectoderm of the neural crest, becoming paraganglion cells and chromaffin cells. The adrenal cortex comprises three layers: the zona glomerulosa (outer zone), zona fasciculata (middle zone), and zona reticularis (inner zone), secreting mineralocorticoid hormones, glucocorticoid hormones, and sex hormones, respectively. Of the three layers, approximately 80% involves the zona fasciculata, 15% the zona glomerulosa, and 5% the zona reticularis. Normal adrenal cortex cells are cohesive and have an abundant amount of vacuolated cytoplasm, whereas adrenal medulla cells have a smaller volume of cytoplasm and appear as naked nuclei or individualized cells. Using these cytopathologic features, there is a high accuracy in determining the cortical or medullary origin of adrenal tumors; however, cytopathology was not sufficient in evaluating the malignancy of the tumors (Bertazzolo et al., 2014).

Enlargement of the adrenal gland may arise from either the cortex or medulla. Enlargements originating within the cortex often result in the excessive production of corticosteroids and the clinical condition of hyperadrenocorticism. Tumors of the adrenal medulla cause the paroxysmal release of catecholamines, primarily norepinephrine (Table 17.6). Reported pathologies of the adrenal gland are listed in Table 17.7.

TABLE 17.6 Comparison of Features for Medullary and Cortical Adrenal Tumors

	ADRENAL MEDULLA	ADRENAL CORTEX
Tumors	Pheochromocytoma (common) Neuroblastoma (rare) Ganglioneuroma (rare)	Adenoma or adenocarcinoma
Cytopathology	*Pheochromocytoma:* Naked nuclei Indistinct nucleoli High nucleocytoplasmic ratio Occasional faint basophilic granules Pale blue cytoplasm	Intact cells, singly or in clusters ± prominent nucleoli Low nucleocytoplasmic ratio Numerous lipid vacuoles Basophilic cytoplasm 6 extramedullary hematopoiesis
Blood tests	*Pheochromocytoma:* Plasma metanephrine and normetanephrine measurement	ACTH stimulation test Low-dose dexamethasone suppression test High-dose dexamethasone suppression test Serum aldosterone
Clinical comments	Clinical signs associated with catecholamine secretion	Hyperadrenocorticism

ACTH, Adrenocorticotropic hormone.

Tumors of the Adrenal Medulla

The most common tumor of the adrenal medulla is *pheochromocytoma*, also called chromaffin paraganglioma or chromaffin cell tumor. Rarely, other tumors, such as neuroblastomas and ganglioneuromas, may arise from the primitive neuroectodermal cells in this area (Rosol and Meuten, 2017). Neuroblastomas are often seen in very young animals, resulting in large intraabdominal masses, which often metastasize to peritoneal surfaces. Ganglioneuromas are small benign tumors in the adrenal medulla.

Pheochromocytoma

Pheochromocytomas are tumors of the chromaffin cells of the adrenal medulla (Figs. 17.19 to 17.22). They occur most frequently in middle-aged to older dogs, with no apparent gender

TABLE 17.7 Pathology of the Adrenal Gland

TISSUE OF ORIGIN	PATHOLOGY
Adrenal cortex	**Non-neoplastic**
	Adrenalitis
	Adrenocortical hyperplasia
	Idiopathic adrenocortical atrophy
	Neoplastic
	Adrenocortical adenoma/adenocarcinoma
Adrenal medulla	**Neoplastic**
	Pheochromocytoma (paraganglia, chromaffin cell)
	Neuroblastoma
	Ganglioneuroma

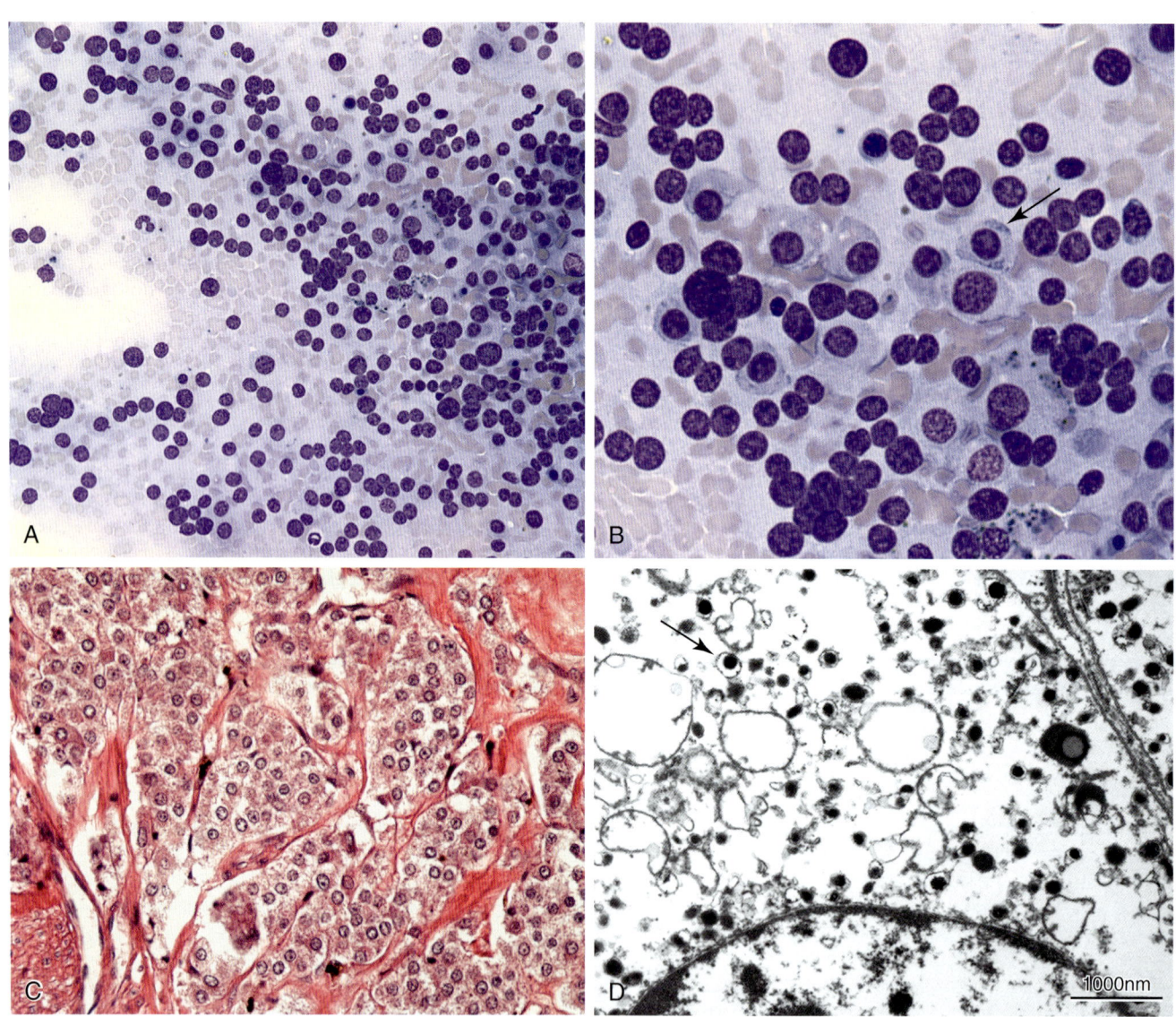

■ **FIGURE 17.19 Pheochromocytoma. Adrenal mass. Dog.** Same case in A to D. **A, Tissue aspirate.** Highly cellular preparation composed predominantly by free nuclei with moderate to marked anisokaryosis in a background of red blood cells. (Aqueous Romanowsky, IP.) **B, Tissue aspirate.** Higher magnification demonstrating few intact cells with distinct cytoplasmic borders and faint basophilic granules in some cells *(arrow)*. The adrenal mass invaded the caudal vena cava, and the dog was hypertensive. (Aqueous Romanowsky; HP oil.) **C, Tissue section.** Neoplastic cells were arranged in sheets subdivided into cords and packets by thin fibrovascular trabeculae. (H&E, IP.) **D, Electron microscopy.** Cytoplasmic dense core granules have a wide submembranous space, which is consistent with norepinephrine granules *(arrow)*. Urine metanephrine excretion was increased (56.0 mg/day; control dog, 10.4 mg/day). (From Choi US. *Practical Guide to Diagnostic Cytology of the Dog and Cat.* OKVET; 2012.)

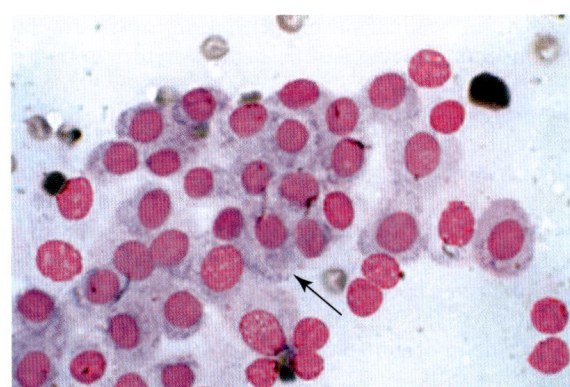

■ **FIGURE 17.20 Pheochromocytoma. Adrenal gland mass. Tissue aspirate. Dog.** Cluster of cells with round nuclei surrounded by moderately abundant lightly basophilic cytoplasm with fine, basophilic granules *(arrow)*. Their relatively benign appearance is misleading because there was local invasion into the caudal vena cava detected by ultrasound, and a pheochromocytoma was confirmed histologically after surgical excision of the tumor. (Wright-Giemsa; HP oil.)

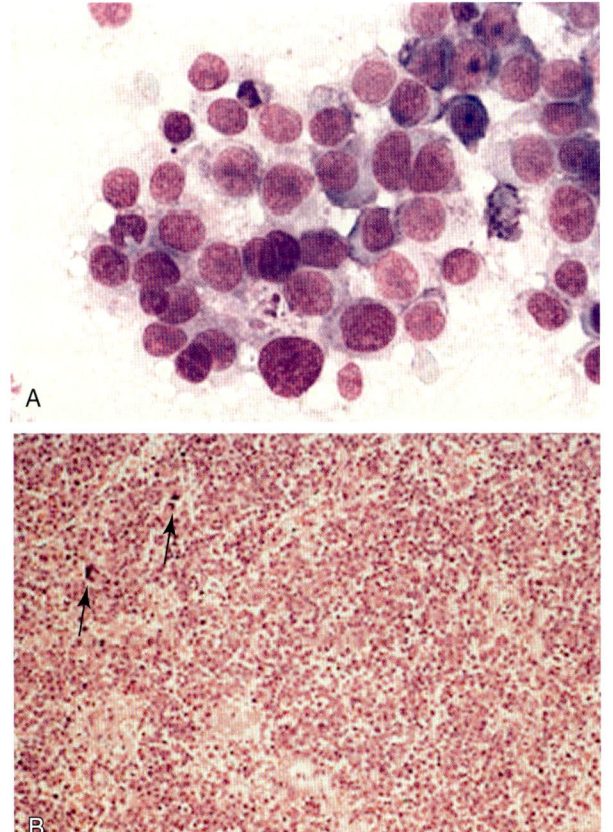

■ **FIGURE 17.21 Pheochromocytoma. Abdominal mass. Dog.** This animal presented with cervical and thoracic pain that progressed rapidly to paraparesis. A myelogram revealed an epidural mass at L1 to L2, and ultrasound examination indicated an abdominal mass. Same case in A and B. **A, Tissue aspirate.** Cluster of loosely adherent cells with a round to oval nucleus with stippled chromatin surrounded by minimal to moderate lightly basophilic cytoplasm demonstrating moderate to marked anisocytosis, anisokaryosis, variable nucleocytoplasmic ratios, and prominent nucleoli. (Wright-Giemsa; HP oil.) **B, Histology.** The mass is composed of pleomorphic neoplastic cells arranged in a dense lobular formation separated by fibrovascular septa. *Arrows* denote two multinucleate cells. (H&E; IP.) (Courtesy Rose Raskin, University of Florida.)

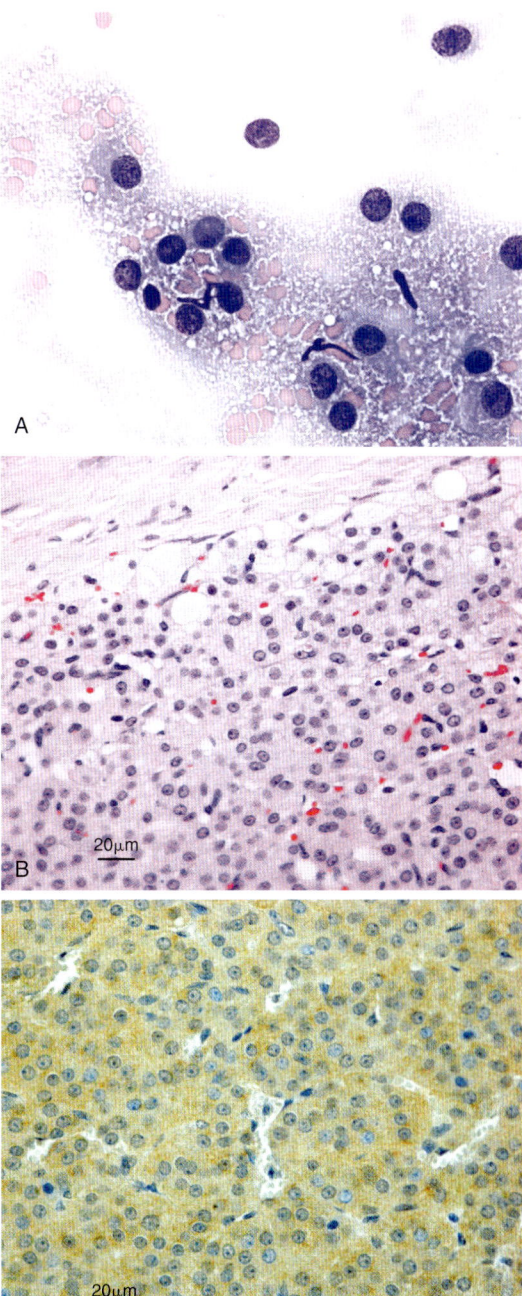

■ **FIGURE 17.22 Pheochromocytoma. Abdominal mass. Cat.** The patient was presented on emergency with anorexia and vomiting. A 2.2 cm anechoic nodule in midcranial abdomen was evaluated. Same case in A to C. **A, Tissue aspirate.** There is low cellularity composed of free round nuclei and cells with round nuclei surrounded by mildly basophilic cytoplasm in a granular basophilic sea of free cytoplasm. (Wright; HP oil.) **B, Histology.** Tissue section from adrenalectomy demonstrating neoplastic tissue that extends focally into the adrenal capsule. The polyhedral cells are arranged in packets that are separated by fine fibrovascular septa. The neoplastic cells have a round nucleus, mild anisokaryosis, distinct nucleolus, and abundant faintly granular eosinophilic cytoplasm with distinct cell borders. (H&E; IP.) **C, Immunohistochemistry.** Tissue section demonstrating moderately strong immunoreactivity to synaptophysin, confirming a neuroendocrine origin and ruling out adrenocortical neoplasia. The diagnosis of pheochromocytoma was confirmed by immunohistochemical detection of synaptophysin and PGP 9.5 in the neoplastic cells of the adrenal gland. (Synaptophysin/diaminobenzidine; IP.) (Courtesy Kristin Fisher, Purdue University.)

or breed predilection, and are rarely reported in cats (Barthez et al., 1997). Clinical evidence of this tumor is usually seen on release of large amounts of catecholamines from the neoplasm. However, clinical signs are varied and vague, and in one study, 57% of the cases were diagnosed as incidental findings (Barthez et al., 1997). Two cases of pheochromocytoma in dogs presented with paraparesis related to the invasion into the spinal canal (Platt et al., 1998). In addition, a large number of patients with pheochromocytomas have concurrent diseases, including other neoplasms originating from other tissues (Bouayad et al., 1987; Barthez et al., 1997). Concurrent pituitary adenomas or adrenocortical tumors resulted in some dogs with pheochromocytomas having concurrent hyperadrenocorticism. Consequently, the clinical signs may be a combination of those attributable to the release of catecholamines and those caused by concomitant disease. Measurement of plasma free metanephrines and normetanephrine (catecholamine metabolites) or urine catecholamine and their metabolites to urine creatinine ratio has been shown to be highly sensitive and specific for the detection of pheochromocytoma and can be used for their diagnosis (Quante et al., 2010; Gostelow et al., 2013).

Abdominal ultrasonography is able to detect adrenal pheochromocytomas in approximately 50% of the cases (Barthez et al., 1997). In these situations, ultrasound-guided FNA may be used to make a more definitive diagnosis. Care must be taken during the sampling procedure because manipulation of the affected adrenal gland could cause the paroxysmal release of catecholamines, resulting in hypertension, tachycardia, or arrhythmias. In addition, many of these lesions are closely associated with the caudal vena cava and may invade this vessel; however, this is not specific for pheochromocytoma because adrenocortical tumors can also show invasion (Kyles et al., 2003). Differentiating between adrenocortical tumors and pheochromocytomas requires cytopathologic evaluation of the lesion or diagnostic tests for hyperadrenocorticism such as adrenocorticotropic hormone (ACTH) stimulation test or low-dose dexamethasone suppression test (Bertazzolo et al., 2014).

The cytopathologic appearance of pheochromocytomas is typical of other neuroendocrine tumors. Much of the cytopathologic preparation may appear as the familiar naked nuclei against a background of pale basophilic cytoplasm; however, intact cells are usually identified in most carefully prepared specimens (see Fig. 17.19B). The cytoplasm of the cells is lightly basophilic to amphophilic with faint granules sometimes visible using Romanowsky-type stains (see Figs. 17.19B and 17.20). Nuclei are round to oval, and a single, small nucleolus may occasionally be observed. Both benign and malignant forms of the tumor exist. Nuclear features of malignancy are unreliable in predicting the biologic behavior of the lesion because even small tumors with well-differentiated cells have been reported to metastasize or invade surrounding structures, but the presence of nuclear criteria of malignancy strongly suggests a high potential for local invasion or metastasis (Bouayad et al., 1987; Rosol and Meuten, 2017) (see Fig. 17.21).

Pheochromocytomas may be recognized clinically on the release of large quantities of catecholamines, primarily norepinephrine, which often results in a variety of clinical signs related to the cardiovascular system and nervous system. Immunocytochemical stains (see Chapter 18) such as chromogranin A and synaptophysin on cytopathologic specimens may be used to support the diagnosis of a medullary tumor (Bilek et al., 2008) (see Fig. 17.22). Although not routinely performed, ultrastructural studies of pheochromocytomas are helpful to demonstrate the cytoplasmic neurosecretory granules (see Fig. 17.19D).

The prognosis for patients is guarded to poor because 50% or more of these tumors are nonresectable because of early invasion of the venous system and distant metastasis via the caudal vena cava at the time of diagnosis (Bouayad et al., 1987; Barthez et al., 1997; Rosol and Meuten, 2017). Complete surgical excision does offer long-term survival in some cases. Several reports indicate a greater than 50% frequency of concurrent neoplasia of patients with pheochromocytomas, many of which are endocrine in origin (Bouayad et al., 1987; von Dehn et al., 1995; Barthez et al., 1997). The concurrent finding of pituitary adenoma or adrenocortical neoplasia resulted in a significant number of dogs with pheochromocytomas having concurrent hyperadrenocorticism (von Dehn et al., 1995; Barthez et al., 1997). Notably, in bulls and humans, pheochromocytomas are associated with a condition termed *multiple endocrine neoplasia*, which can include concurrent adrenal pheochromocytoma, thyroid C-cell carcinoma, and pituitary chromophobe adenomas (Rosol and Meuten, 2017).

Non-neoplastic Adrenocortical Disease

Infectious adrenalitis can occur in dogs and cats by bacteria in the course of bacterial septicemia, fungi (occasionally by *Histoplasma capsulatum, Coccidioides immitis,* and *Cryptococcus neoformans*), or protozoa (*Toxoplasma gondii*). Inflammation is usually suppurative or granulomatous accompanied by necrosis, which can be a cause of hypoadrenocorticism (La Perle, 2013). Cytopathologic specimens can be obtained by ultrasound-guided FNA, and the diagnosis of adrenalitis can be made based on the presence of inflammatory cells and specific infectious organisms, which can be aided by either culture or molecular assay, such as polymerase chain reaction.

Adrenocortical atrophy can occur bilaterally in young adult dogs (La Perle, 2013). The precise pathogenesis of hypoadrenocorticism is unknown but is most likely immune mediated. Atrophy of the adrenal cortex (specifically the zona fasciculata and zona reticularis) can be caused by the destruction of the pituitary gland, which is under ACTH control, with no apparent electrolyte abnormalities. In contrast, idiopathic atrophy of adrenal cortex is characterized by severe atrophy of all three layers of the cortex initiated by early focal infiltration of lymphocytes and plasma cells (La Perle, 2013). Hypoadrenocorticism can be diagnosed by unresponsiveness to ACTH stimulation test.

Adrenocortical hyperplasia can occur as nodular hyperplasia or diffuse cortical hyperplasia in dogs and cats (La Perle, 2013). Hyperplastic nodules are usually multiple and bilateral, involving any of the three zones of the adrenal cortex. Diffuse cortical hyperplasia results in bilateral enlargement of the adrenal cortices. Hypertrophy and hyperplasia of cells of the zona fasciculata and reticularis can occur in response to an autonomous hypersecretion of ACTH by a pituitary gland adenoma (>80% of Cushing disease cases). Cytopathologic evaluation of ultrasound-guided FNA of the hyperplastic lesion is performed occasionally to rule in or rule out hyperplasia, tumor, or inflammation. Cytopathologic preparations reveal naked nuclei and some intact cells with a moderate to abundant amount of pale cytoplasm laden with lipoid vacuoles, which can also punctuate the background. However, cytopathology, and occasionally histopathology, cannot differentiate between hyperplasia, adenoma, and well-differentiated adenocarcinoma. Functional hyperplasia can be demonstrated with an ACTH stimulation test or dexamethasone suppression test.

Adrenocortical Tumors

Hyperadrenocorticism is a common endocrinopathy in dogs and is rarely identified in cats. In dogs, the condition is most often the result of a pituitary tumor; however, between 15% and 20% of the cases are associated with adrenocortical neoplasia (Fig. 17.23) (Lunn and Page, 2013). In 89 reported cases of dogs with adrenocortical tumors, adenocarcinomas were diagnosed in 53 dogs, and adenomas were found in 36 (Scavelli et al., 1986; Penninck et al., 1988; Reusch and Feldman, 1991). The mean age was approximately 11 years (range, 5–16 years), with no significant breed or sex predilection. Both adrenocortical adenomas and adenocarcinomas have rarely been reported in cats (Nelson et al., 1988; Jones et al., 1992).

Patients with adrenocortical tumors usually present with clinical and laboratory signs of hyperadrenocorticism. After a diagnosis of hyperadrenocorticism is made, discriminatory tests such as the high-dose dexamethasone suppression test, measurement of endogenous ACTH concentrations, and abdominal ultrasonography should be used to distinguish pituitary-dependent hyperadrenocorticism (PDH) from adrenal tumors. In contrast to PDH, which causes bilateral adrenal enlargement, an adrenal tumor typically causes enlargement of one adrenal gland and atrophy of the contralateral adrenal gland. In one study, abdominal ultrasonography detected 18 of 25 dogs (72%) with adrenal tumors (Reusch and Feldman, 1991). In this situation, an ultrasound-guided FNA of the affected adrenal gland can be performed for cytopathologic evaluation of the lesion.

Cytopathologic specimens taken from adrenocortical adenomas contain cells resembling normal secretory cells from the zona fasciculata or zona reticularis. Preparations are typical of other endocrine tumors with most cells appearing as naked nuclei in a background of abundant free cytoplasm. The cytoplasm is moderately basophilic and often contains distinct clear, lipid vacuoles (Figs. 17.23 and 17.24). Nuclei of adenomas are round and uniform in size and may contain a prominent, often singular nucleolus. Focal areas of hematopoiesis, adipocytes, and mineral deposits may be found in some cortical adenomas (Figs. 17.23B and 17.25) (Rosol and Meuten, 2017). The presence of hematopoietic precursors from erythroid, granulocytic, and megakaryocytic lines along with adipose tissue suggests another adrenal cortical neoplasm, namely myelolipoma (see Chapter 4) (Tursi et al., 2005; de Swarte et al., 2019). This is typically a benign adrenal neoplasm that is rarely encountered in dogs but may occur alone or in combination with adrenocortical adenoma or adrenocortical hyperplasia (de Swarte et al., 2019).

It should be noted that cells aspirated from adrenal glands that are hyperplastic, as seen in dogs with PDH, and cells from adrenal adenomas are cytopathologically indistinguishable. Therefore, cytopathology cannot be used as a tool to distinguish between PDH and hyperadrenocorticism associated with adrenal tumors.

Tumor cells from adrenocortical adenocarcinomas may be more pleomorphic than those from adenomas (Rosol and Meuten, 2017). Two cases of aldosterone-producing adrenocortical carcinoma in cats have been described by cytopathology

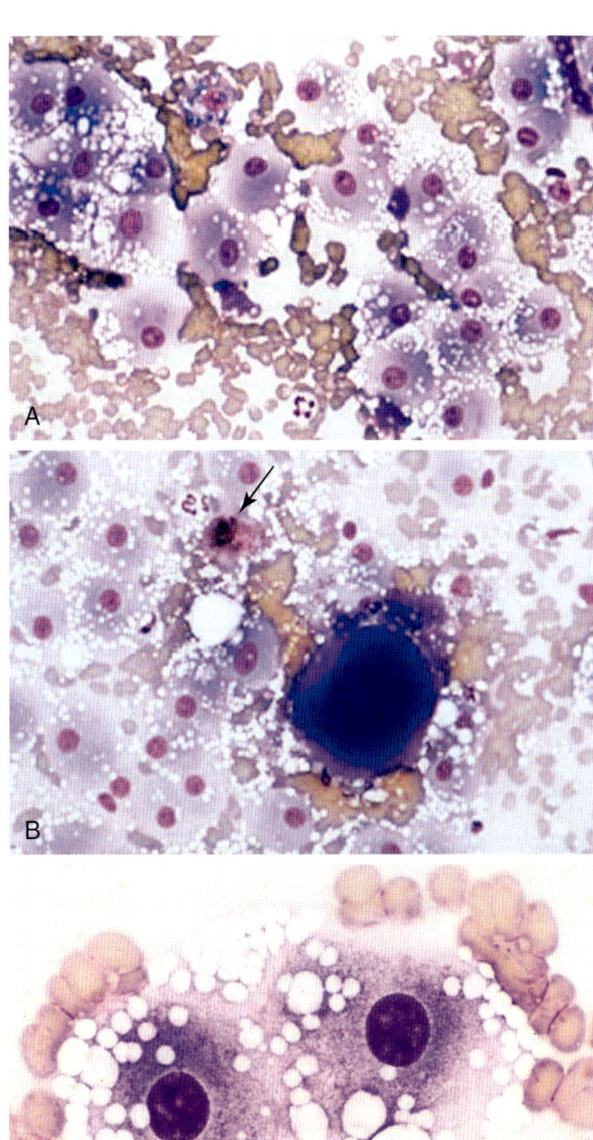

■ **FIGURE 17.23 Adrenocortical adenoma. Adrenal mass. Tissue aspirate. Dog.** The patient was presented with clinical signs of hyperadrenocorticism. The specimen was obtained via ultrasound guidance from a single nodule off the cranial pole of the adrenal gland. Same case in A to C. **A,** Loosely adherent cells and sheet of uniform cells with small round nucleus surrounded by abundant, amphophilic cytoplasm containing numerous punctate vacuoles. Cells have poorly defined cytoplasmic borders. (Wright-Giemsa; HP oil.) **B,** A large, dark, basophilic-staining megakaryocyte *(center)* indicates the presence of extramedullary hematopoiesis that is sometimes seen in adrenocortical tumors. A macrophage contains dark blue-black, variably sized granules consistent with hemosiderin indicative of prior intratumor hemorrhage *(arrow)*. (Wright-Giemsa; HP oil.) **C,** Two adrenocortical cells with centrally located, round nuclei having prominent nucleoli are surrounded by abundant granular amphophilic cytoplasm, which contains variably sized punctate vacuoles suggestive of secretory function, and that appear predominantly along the cell periphery. (Wright-Giemsa; HP oil.) (A–B, Courtesy Peter Fernandes, University of Florida. C, Courtesy Rose Raskin, University of Florida.)

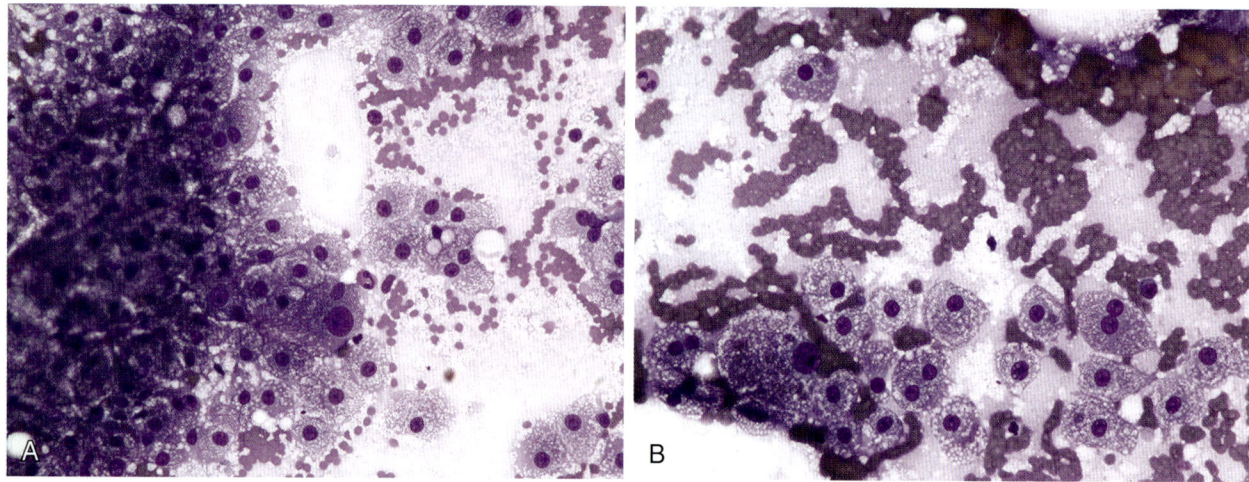

■ **FIGURE 17.24 Adrenal mass. Tissue aspirate. Cat.** Same case in A and B. **A–B,** The cat presented with polyuria and polydipsia, increased appetite, and bilateral alopecia at the pelvic region. Only the right adrenal gland was enlarged (3 cm in diameter). Ultrasound-guided collection from the enlarged right adrenal mass is shown. A large cluster of uniform epithelial cells has numerous distinct small cytoplasmic vacuoles along with a low number of individualized cells. Note the rare gigantic nuclei with distinct nucleoli and occasional binucleation. (Wright-Giemsa; IP.)

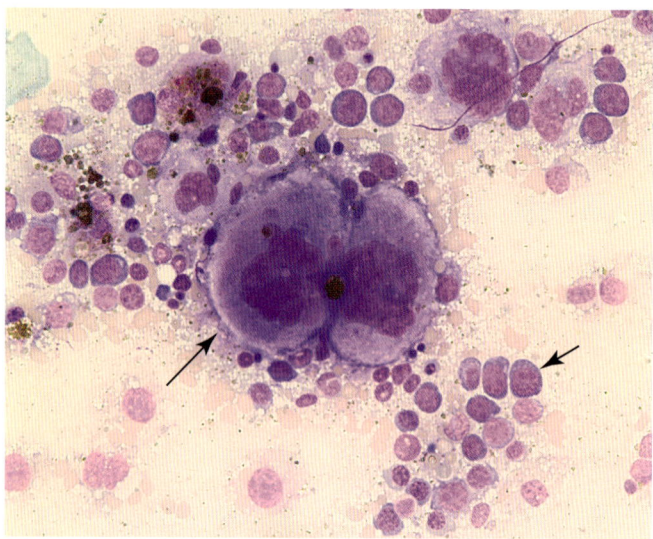

■ **FIGURE 17.25 Extramedullary hematopoiesis. Adrenal mass. Dog.** Two megakaryocytes *(long arrow)* and one of multiple erythroblasts *(short arrow)* that are indicative of extramedullary hematopoiesis, a common observation in an adrenocortical adenoma. Left of center are multiple aggregates of yellow-gold, variably sized crystals consistent with hematoidin along with a clump of dark blue-black granules consistent with hemosiderin indicative of prior intratumor hemorrhage. (Wright-Giemsa; HP oil.)

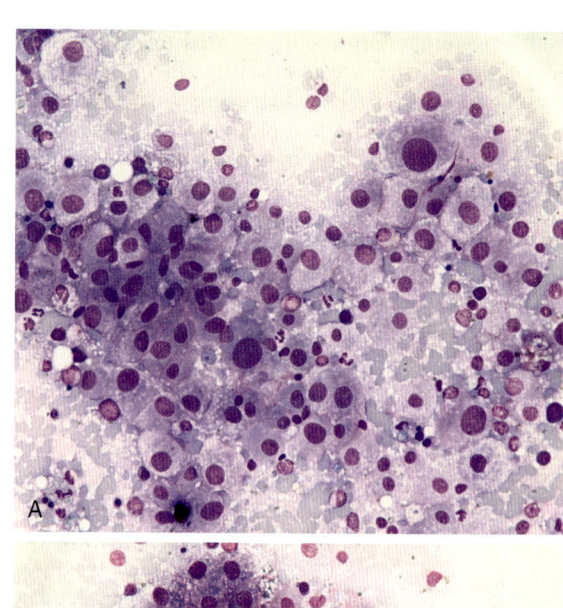

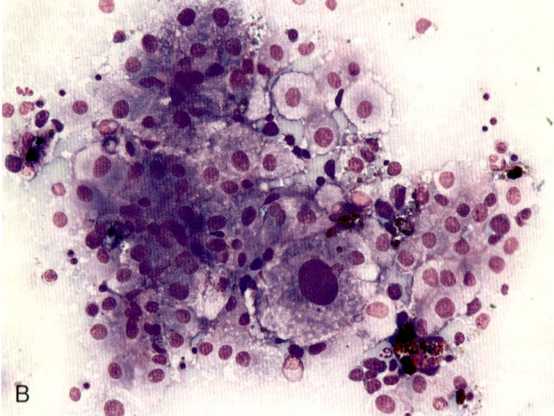

■ **FIGURE 17.26 Adrenocortical adenocarcinoma. Dog.** Same case in A and B. **A–B,** Loosely adherent cells with centrally located round nucleus surrounded by abundant amphophilic to lightly basophilic cytoplasm. Criteria of malignancy include karyomegaly, nuclear crowding increased nucleocytoplasmic ratio, binucleation, and anisokaryosis. The irregular clumps of black-colored material is consistent with hemosiderin suggestive of prior intratumor hemorrhage. (Wright-Giemsa; HP oil.)

(Renschler and Dean, 2009; Attipa et al., 2018). Adenocarcinomas may display features of anaplasia, including anisokaryosis and multiple nucleoli (Figs. 17.26 and 17.27). However, because some adenocarcinomas may contain well-differentiated cells, histologic evaluation for invasion of capsule, adjacent structures, or vessels is the preferred method of distinction between adenomas and adenocarcinomas. If the cytopathologic criteria of malignancy are fulfilled, a diagnosis of adenocarcinoma can reliably be made; however, in the absence of such criteria, caution should be used in making an interpretation based on cytomorphologic features alone.

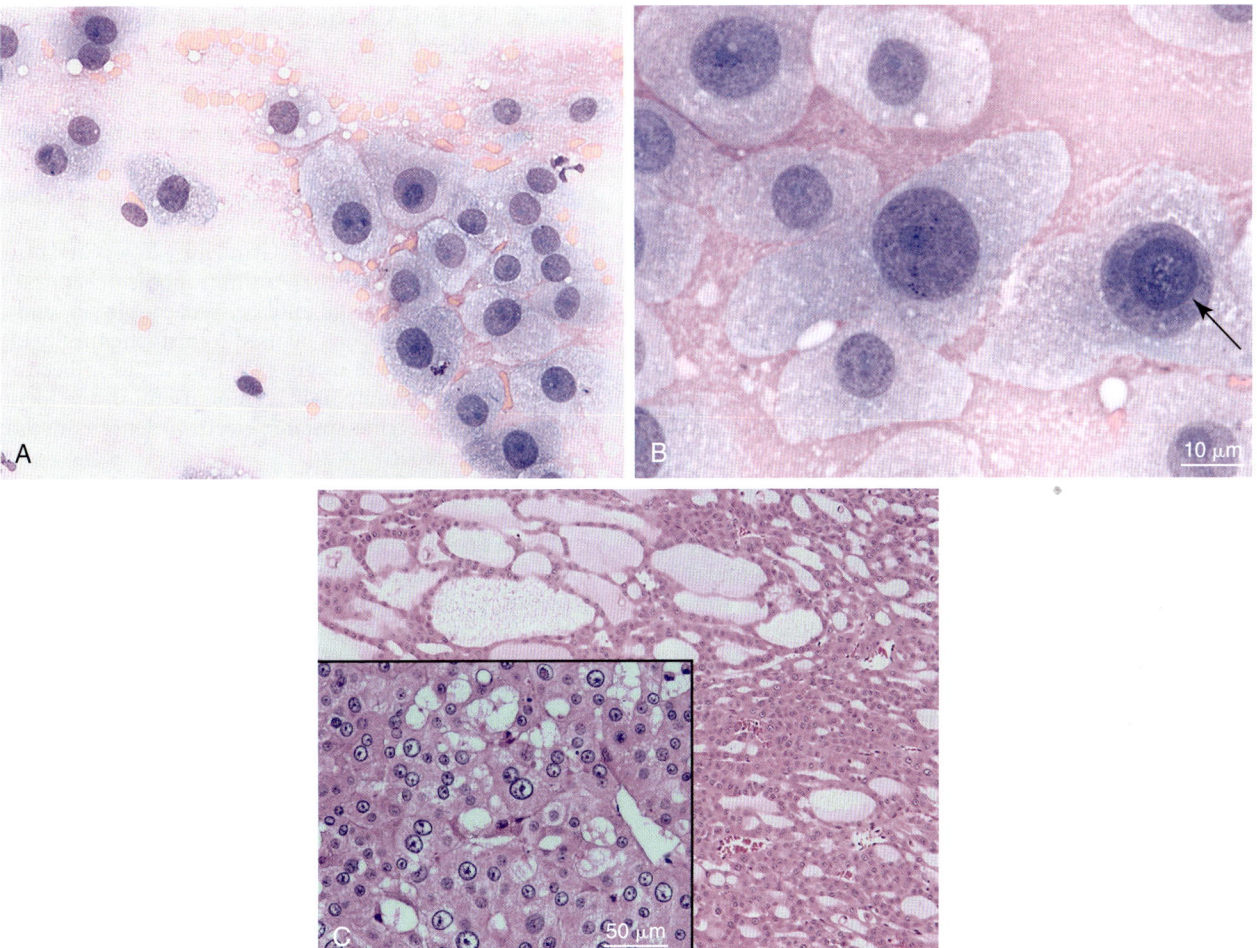

FIGURE 17.27 Aldosterone-producing adrenocortical carcinoma with myxoid differentiation. Adrenal mass. Cat. Same case in A to C. **A, Tissue imprint.** Individualized and loosely adherent cells with round nuclei having finely stippled chromatin and one or two small, variably prominent nucleoli are present within an eosinophilic material. Cells had moderate amounts of pale basophilic to amphophilic, finely granular cytoplasm, which often contained low numbers of small cytoplasmic vacuoles. Cytologic criteria of malignancy included moderate to rarely marked anisocytosis and anisokaryosis (10–25 μm) and occasional binucleation. (Modified Wright; IP.) **B, Tissue imprint.** Marked anisocytosis and anisokaryosis are prominent against an eosinophilic mucinous background. Note anisonucleosis, including one marked macronucleolus *(arrow)*. Presurgical analyses revealed a marked increase in serum aldosterone concentration, a mildly decreased basal cortisol concentration, and a normal total thyroxine concentration compared with reference intervals, consistent with a diagnosis of feline primary hyperaldosteronism. (Modified Wright; HP oil.) **C, Histology.** The neoplasm has a mixed multilobular and cystic arrangement. The cystic spaces were later identified to contain epithelial mucins. (H&E; LP.) *Inset:* Neoplastic cells are mildly pleomorphic with abundant eosinophilic cytoplasm that contains a single round to oval nucleus, with open chromatin and one to two nucleoli. Anisokaryosis and anisocytosis are moderate. A cell with intranuclear cytoplasmic invagination is seen at the top, not to be confused with a viral inclusion or macronucleolus. Immunohistochemistry (not shown) demonstrated immunoreactivity to cytochrome P450 aldosterone synthase. (H&E; IP.) (Courtesy Charalampos Attipa, Royal Veterinary College, UK.)

Adenomas of the zona fasciculata or zona reticularis are usually small and do not metastasize. Surgical resection is treatment of choice for adenomas; however, operative and postoperative complications involving the removal of the gland are frequently seen. Approximately half of dogs with adrenocortical adenocarcinomas have gross evidence of local invasion into the caudal vena cava or renal artery, or distant metastasis, primarily to the liver, lung, or kidney (Scavelli et al., 1986). Surgical resection of adenocarcinomas is difficult and, as with adrenal adenomas, the incidence of postoperative complications is high (Scavelli et al., 1986). Treatment of adenocarcinomas with mitotane and trilostane appears to be beneficial when surgery is a poor option (Lunn and Page, 2013).

CARCINOIDS

Carcinoids are rare tumors arising from disseminated neuroendocrine cells in various organs. These cells are found dispersed in the GI tract, endocrine pancreas, biliary tract, respiratory tract, thymus, thyroid, urogenital tract, and skin (Klopel, 2007). These lesions were first described as "karzinoide" by Oberndorfer in 1907, referring to intestinal tumors that appeared to behave in a more indolent nature than the typical intestinal adenocarcinoma (Kulke and Mayer, 1999). Carcinoids have also been referred to as APUD (amine precursor uptake and decarboxylation) tumors, or apudomas because these neuroendocrine cells are able to synthesize, secrete, and metabolize biologically active amines. At present, these tumors are classified as well-differentiated neuroendocrine tumors (benign) and well-differentiated to poorly differentiated neuroendocrine carcinomas (malignant) (Klopel, 2007).

In dogs and cats, the most common location for carcinoids is in the GI tract (Albers et al., 1998; Sako et al., 2003). Other locations include the nasal cavity (Sako et al., 2005), pharynx (Patnaik et al., 2002), lung (Fig. 17.28) (Saegusa et al., 1994; Ferreira et al., 2005; Choi et al., 2008), liver (Patnaik et al., 1981, 2005a), gallbladder (Morrell et al., 2002), and skin (Konno et al., 1998; Joiner et al., 2010). In cats, carcinoid tumors have been reported in the liver and gallbladder (Patnaik et al., 2005b), stomach (Rossmeisl et al., 2002), intestines (Slawienski et al., 1997), esophagus (Patnaik et al., 1990), tracheobronchus (Rossi et al., 2007), and skin (Patnaik et al., 2001). There appears to be no apparent sex or breed predilection. Carcinoids have been reported in animals ranging from 4 months to 18 years of age, but most were reported in animals older than 7 years (Table 17.8).

Animals with carcinoids can have a variety of clinical findings, or in some cases, benign carcinoids have been found incidentally in the lungs or intestines of clinically healthy animals during physical examination or imaging studies (Sykes and Cooper, 1982; Choi et al., 2008). Clinical signs generally reflect the anatomic location of the lesion. Gallbladder tumors can cause icterus or hematemesis (Morrell et al., 2002). In one report, a cat with a 5-month history of vomiting was found with a stomach carcinoid (Rossmeisl et al., 2002).

Although neuroendocrine tumor cells may have granules containing various bioactive amines such as serotonin, histamine, substance P, kallikrein, and corticotropin, there are no known reports indicating that the release of these bioactive amines causes the development of clinical symptoms in humans or animals with benign carcinoids. In cases of malignant carcinoids, clinical signs can be attributed to the release of bioactive amines. In humans, carcinoids can result in what is known as *carcinoid syndrome*, a clinical syndrome consisting of diarrhea, erythema, asthenia, organomegaly, and right-sided congestive heart failure (Kulke and Mayer, 1999). These are attributed to synthesis, release, and delayed hepatic metabolism of 5-HT (hydroxytryptamine, serotonin) and tachykinins by tumor cells. In these cases, measurement of serum or urine 5-HT concentration can be used as a screening test. However, unlike in humans, most dogs and cats with malignant lesions have clinical signs related to advanced stages of tumor growth and metastasis, not the release of biologically active substances. In one case, a dog with a jejunal carcinoid presented with a 4-month history of anemia, fatigue, anorexia, vomiting, intermittent diarrhea, and intestinal bleeding (Sako et al., 2003). In this animal, the concentration of serum 5-HT was approximately 10 times the reference range. There have also been rare reports of hypercortisolism in dogs with carcinoids (Churcher, 1999).

Carcinoids have a typical neuroendocrine cytomorphology with naked nuclei embedded in a background of pale cytoplasm (see Fig. 17.28C). A small number of round or polygonal intact cells with a moderate to abundant amount of weakly basophilic cytoplasm may also be identified (sese Fig. 17.28D). The nuclei are round to polygonal with fine chromatin and occasional nucleoli. Cells from some carcinoids may contain fine, pale basophilic intracytoplasmic granules (see Fig. 17.28E). The cytopathologic appearance of carcinoids is similar regardless of anatomic location. A recent report of a neuroendocrine carcinoma *(Merkel cell tumor)* developing in the skin of a dog yielded aspirates with numerous naked nuclei and intact round to polygonal cells with moderate amounts of pale basophilic cytoplasm (see Chapter 3) (Joiner et al., 2010). These tumors may be grossly and on cytopathology appear similar to cutaneous lymphoma or histiocytoma, and special procedures (immunohistochemistry or electron microscopy) may be necessary to confirm the tissue of origin (Grimelius, 2004; Gil da Costa et al., 2009; Joiner et al., 2010). An immunohistochemical panel containing neuron-specific enolase, synaptophysin, and chromogranin A antibodies can be used to histochemically identify cells of neuroendocrine origin (see Fig. 17.28F). Electron microscopy, not commonly used, can be useful in the identification of neuroendocrine-specific, electron-dense core granules (Patnaik et al., 2005b).

As with other neuroendocrine tumors, the biologic behavior of carcinoids is difficult to predict on the basis of cell morphology. Most of the reported neuroendocrine tumors, especially those of hepatic and intestinal origin, were malignant with poor prognosis. In all of the 26 reported cases of hepatic carcinoids in dogs, the animals were either euthanized or died because the tumors were diffuse, involving all liver lobes, or had evidence of metastatic disease at the time of diagnosis (Patnaik et al., 1981, 2005a; Churcher, 1999). In cats with hepatic carcinoids, most of the animals were euthanized during or soon after surgical exploration because of either metastatic disease or diffuse involvement of liver lobes (Patnaik et al., 2005b). In animals with GI carcinoids, including those with lesions in the esophagus, stomach, and intestinal tract, 10 of 12 canine cases and 4 of 5 feline cases had evidence of either local or distant metastasis at the time of presentation. These animals frequently presented with severe clinical signs of intestinal hemorrhage, vomiting, or both. There are few reports of carcinoid tumors at sites other than liver and GI, and in these, tumor behavior was variable (Saegusa et al., 1994; Konno et al., 1998; Patnaik et al., 2001; Choi et al., 2008). In benign tumors, surgical removal is the treatment of choice. There are no known reports of successful chemotherapeutic management of malignant carcinoids. One locally invasive, cutaneous neuroendocrine tumor was successfully treated with radiation therapy, and the animal remained in complete remission for 18 months (Whiteley and Leininger, 1987).

SUMMARY

Lesions involving endocrine glands and neuroendocrine tissues are a varied group of conditions that may arise from a number of specialized organs. Even so, these lesions share cytomorphologic features, including the appearance of naked nuclei within a background of lightly basophilic cytoplasm and indistinct cellular borders. In addition, as a group, it is difficult to predict the biologic behavior of these lesions based solely on the presence or absence of abnormal cytomorphologic features. The potential biologic behavior should be evaluated based on the specific tumor type and the species involved, along with histologic or clinical evidence of invasion of adjacent tissues. Endocrine and neuroendocrine cytopathology often have shared cytomorphologic features, necessitating further consideration of organ sampled, relevant clinical signs, clinical pathology results, or imaging findings for a definitive diagnosis.

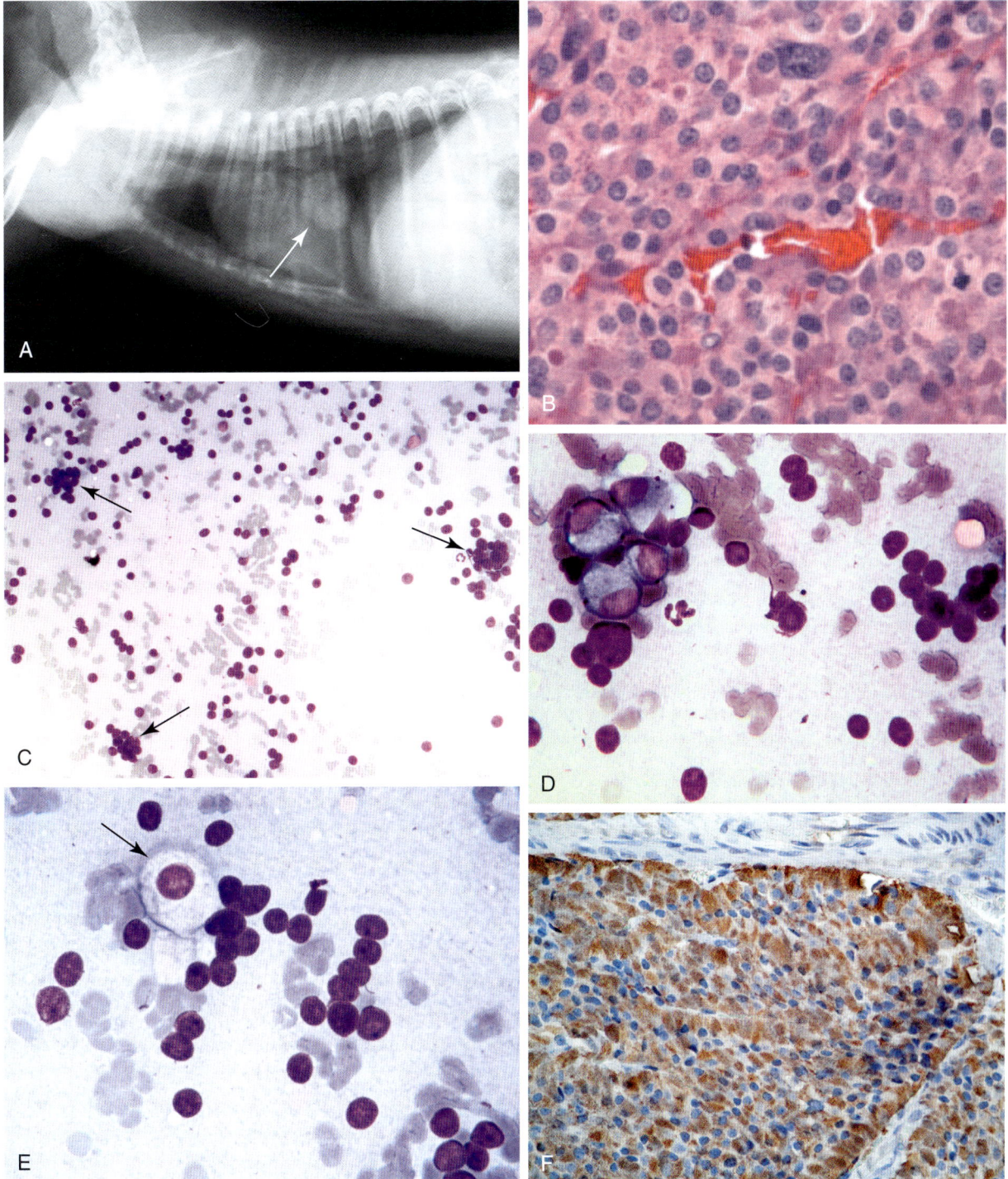

■ **FIGURE 17.28 Carcinoid. Lung mass. Dog.** Same case in A to F. **A,** Thoracic radiograph showing incidental mass *(arrow)* in a caudal lung lobe of an 11-year-old neutered male Yorkshire terrier. **B, Histology.** Packets of round to polygonal cells with round nuclei surrounded by abundant eosinophilic granular cytoplasm, interlaced by a rich capillary network histologically characterized the carcinoid neoplasm. (H&E; IP.) **C, Tissue aspirate.** Free nuclei embedded in a background of lightly basophilic cytoplasm from ruptured cells predominate with scattered aggregates of free nuclei *(arrows).* (Wright-Giemsa; IP.) **D, Tissue aspirate.** Naked nuclei are seen as a prominent feature with intact cells comprised of an oval eccentric nucleus surrounded by a moderate to abundant amount of mildly basophilic cytoplasm *(upper left).* The neutrophil, used for comparison, denotes the relatively large size of the neoplastic cells. (Wright-Giemsa; HP oil.) **E, Tissue aspirate.** An intact cell has faint basophilic granules sprinkled in the cytoplasm *(arrow).* (Wright-Giemsa; HP oil.) **F, Immunohistochemistry.** Strong cytoplasmic immunoreactivity demonstrates expression of chromogranin A, a member of the granin family of neuroendocrine secretory proteins located in secretory vesicles of neurons, neuroendocrine cells, and endocrine cells and is an indicator of neoplasms of those cell types. (Chromogranin A antibody/diaminobenzidine/hematoxylin; IP.) (B, From Choi US, Alleman AR, Choi J, et al. Cytologic and immunohistochemical characterization of a lung carcinoid in a dog with comparisons to human typical carcinoid. *Vet Clin Pathol* 2008;37:249-252; E, From Choi US. *Practical Guide to Diagnostic Cytology of the Dog and Cat.* OKVET; 2012.)

TABLE 17.8 Location of Carcinoids in Dogs and Cats

LOCATION	SPECIES	REPORTED SITES OF CARCINOIDS
Gastrointestinal tract	Dogs	Oral cavity, stomach, intestine, liver, gallbladder
	Cats	Liver, gallbladder, stomach, intestines, esophagus
Respiratory tract	Dogs	Nasal cavity, pharynx, lung
	Cats	Tracheobronchus
Skin	Dogs and cats	Dermis

REFERENCES

Albers TM, Alroy J, McDonnell JJ, et al. A poorly differentiated gastric carcinoid in a dog. *J Vet Diagn Invest.* 1998;10:116-118.

Attipa C, Beck S, Lipscomb V, et al. Aldosterone-producing adrenocortical carcinoma with myxoid differentiation in a cat. *Vet Clin Pathol.* 2018;47:660-664.

Barber LG. Thyroid tumors in dogs and cats. *Vet Clin North Am Small Anim Pract.* 2007;37:755-773.

Barber PJ. Investigation of hypercalcemia and hypocalcemia. In: Mooney CT, Peterson ME, eds. *BSAVA Manual of Canine and Feline Endocrinology.* 3rd ed. Gloucester, UK: BSAVA Publications; 2004:26-32.

Barthez PY, Marks SL, Woo J, et al. Pheochromocytoma in dogs: 61 cases (1984-1995). *J Vet Intern Med.* 1997;11:272-278.

Berger B, Feldman EC. Primary hyperparathyroidism in dogs: 21 cases (1976-1986). *J Am Vet Med Assoc.* 1987;191:350-356.

Bertazzolo W, Didier M, Gelain ME, et al. Accuracy of cytology in distinguishing adrenocortical tumors from pheochromocytoma in companion animals. *Vet Clin Pathol.* 2014;43:453-459.

Bertazzolo W, Giudice C, Dell'Orco M, et al. Paratracheal cervical mass in a dog. *Vet Clin Pathol.* 2003;32:209-212.

Bilek R, Safarik L, Ciprova V, et al. Chromogranin A, a member of neuroendocrine secretory proteins as a selective marker for laboratory diagnosis of pheochromocytoma. *Physiol Res.* 2008;57(suppl 1):S171-S179.

Boes K, Messick J, Green H, et al. What is your diagnosis? Impression smear from an intracardiac mass in a dog. *Vet Clin Pathol.* 2010;39:119-120.

Bouayad H, Feeney DA, Caywood DD, et al. Pheochromocytoma in dogs: 13 cases (1980-1985). *J Am Vet Med Assoc.* 1987;191:1610-1615.

Caruso KJ, Cowell RL, Upton ML, et al. Intrathoracic mass in a cat [chemodectoma]. *Vet Clin Pathol.* 2002;31:193-195.

Carver JR, Kapatkin A, Patnaik AK. A comparison of medullary thyroid carcinoma and thyroid adenocarcinoma in dogs: a retrospective study of 38 cases. *Vet Surg.* 1995;24:315-319.

Choi US, Alleman AR, Choi J, et al. Cytologic and immunohistochemical characterization of a lung carcinoid in a dog with comparisons to human typical carcinoid. *Vet Clin Pathol.* 2008;37:249-252.

Churcher RK. Hepatic carcinoid, hypercortisolism and hypokalaemia in a dog. *Aust Vet J.* 1999;77(10):641-645.

den Hertog E, Goossens MM, van-der-Linde-Sipman JS, et al. Primary hyperparathyroidism in two cats. *Vet Q.* 1997;19:81-84.

de Swarte M, Hecht S, Lane MB. What is your diagnosis? (Adrenal myelolipoma). *J Am Vet Med Assoc.* 2019;255(5):525-527.

DeVries SE, Feldman EC, Nelson RW, et al. Primary parathyroid gland hyperplasia in dogs: six cases (1982-1991). *J Am Vet Med Assoc.* 1993;202:1132-1136.

Diaconu IV, Bucur EO, Tihulca CR. Histopathological and histochemical aspects in a case of dog hyperparathyroidism. *Lucrări Stiintifice Medicină Veterinară.* 2008;41:608-618.

Fernandez NJ, Clark EG, Larson VS. What is your diagnosis? Ventral neck mass in a dog. *Vet Clin Pathol.* 2008;37:447-451.

Ferreira AJA, Peleteiro MC, Correia JHD, et al. Small-cell carcinoma of the lung resembling a brachial plexus tumour. *J Small Anim Pract.* 2005;46:286-290.

Gil da Costa RM, Rema A, Pires MA, et al. Two canine Merkel cell tumours: immunoexpression of c-KIT, E-cadherin, β-catenin and S100 protein. *Vet Dermatol.* 2009;21:198-201.

Giles JT, Rochat MC, Snider TA. Surgical management of a thyroglossal duct cyst in a cat. *J Am Vet Med Assoc.* 2007;230:686-689.

Gostelow R, Bridger N, Syme HM. Plasma-free metanephrine and free normetanephrine measurement for the diagnosis of pheochromocytoma in dogs. *J Vet Intern Med.* 2013;27:83-90.

Grimelius L. Silver stains demonstrating neuroendocrine cells. *Biotech Histochem.* 2004;79(1):37-44.

Hamilton SR, Farber JL, Rubin E. Neoplasms. In: Rubin E, Farber JL, eds. *Pathology.* 3rd ed. Philadelphia: Lippincott-Raven; 1999:720-721.

Hardcastle MK, Meyer J, McSporran KD. Pathology in practice. *J Am Vet Med Assoc.* 2013;242:175-177.

Ilha MRS, Styer EL. Extra-adrenal retroperitoneal paraganglioma in a dog. *J Vet Diagn Invest.* 2013;25(6):803-806.

Joiner KS, Smith AN, Henderson RA, et al. Multicentric cutaneous neuroendocrine (Merkel cell) carcinoma in a dog. *Vet Pathol.* 2010;47(6): 1090-1094.

Jones CA, Refsal KR, Stevens BJ, et al. Adrenocortical adenocarcinoma in a cat. *J Am Anim Hosp Assoc.* 1992;28:59-62.

Kallet AJ, Richter KP, Feldman EC, et al. Primary hyperparathyroidism in cats: seven cases (1984-1989). *J Am Vet Med Assoc.* 1991;199:1767-1771.

Kini SR. Medullary carcinoma. In: Kini SR, ed. *Thyroid Cytopathology.* Philadelphia: Lippincott Williams & Wilkins; 2008:272-273.

Klopel G. Tumour biology and histopathology of neuroendocrine tumours. *Best Pract Res Clin Endocrinol Metab.* 2007;21(1):15-31.

Konno A, Nagata M, Nanko H. Immunohistochemical diagnosis of a Merkel cell tumor in a dog. *Vet Pathol.* 1998;35(6):538-540.

Kulke MH, Mayer RJ. Carcinoid tumors. *N Engl J Med.* 1999;340:858-868.

Kyles AE, Feldman EC, De Cock HE, et al. Surgical management of adrenal gland tumors with and without associated tumor thrombi in dogs: 40 cases (1994-2001). *J Am Vet Med Assoc.* 2003;223:654-662.

La Perle KMD. Endocrine system. In: Zachary JF, McGavin MD, eds. *Pathologic Basis of Veterinary Disease.* 4th ed. St. Louis: Mosby; 2013:660-697.

Lantz GC, Salisbury SK. Surgical excision of ectopic thyroid carcinoma involving the base of the tongue in dogs: three cases (1980-1987). *J Am Vet Med Assoc.* 1989;195:1606-1608.

Leav I, Schillert AL, Rijnberk A, et al. Adenomas and adenocarcinomas of the canine and feline thyroid. *Am J Pathol.* 1976;83:61-93.

Lunn KF, Page RL. Tumors of the endocrine system. In: Withrow SJ, Vail DM, Page RL, eds. *Withrow & MacEwen's Small Animal Clinical Oncology.* 5th ed. St. Louis: Elsevier-Saunders; 2013:504-523.

Marquez GA, Klausner JS, Osborne CA. Calcium oxalate urolithiasis in a cat with a functional parathyroid adenocarcinoma. *J Am Vet Med Assoc.* 1995;206:817-819.

Miller ML, Peterson ME, Randolph JF, et al. Thyroid cysts in cats: a retrospective study of 40 cases. *J Vet Intern Med.* 2017;31:723-729.

Mooney CT, Peterson ME. Feline hyperthyroidism. In: Mooney CT, Peterson ME, eds. *BSAVA Manual of Canine and Feline Endocrinology.* 3rd ed. Gloucester, UK: BSAVA Publications; 2004:95-110.

Morrell CN, Volk MV, Mankowski JL. A carcinoid tumor in the gallbladder of a dog. *Vet Pathol.* 2002;39(6):756-758.

Nelson RW, Feldman EC, Smith MC. Hyperadrenocorticism in cats: seven cases (1978-1987). *J Am Vet Med Assoc.* 1988;193:245-250.

Obradovich JE, Withrow SJ, Powers BE, et al. Carotid body tumors in the dog: eleven cases (1978-1988). *J Vet Intern Med.* 1992;6:96-101.

Patnaik AK, Lieberman PH, Hurvitz AI, et al. Canine hepatic carcinoids. *Vet Pathol.* 1981;18(4):445-453.

Patnaik AK, Erlandson RA, Lieberman PH, et al. Extra-adrenal pheochromocytoma (paraganglioma) in a cat. *J Am Vet Med Assoc.* 1990;197:104-106.

Patnaik AK, Erlandson RA, Lieberman PH. Esophageal neuroendocrine carcinoma in a cat. *Vet Pathol.* 1990;27(2):128-130.

Patnaik AK, Post GS, Erlandson RA. Clinicopathologic and electron microscopic study of cutaneous neuroendocrine (Merkel cell) carcinoma in a cat with comparisons to human and canine tumors. *Vet Pathol.* 2001;38(5):553-556.

Patnaik AK, Ludwig LL, Erlandson RA. Neuroendocrine carcinoma of the nasopharynx in a dog. *Vet Pathol.* 2002;39(4):496-500.

Patnaik AK, Newman SJ, Scase T, et al. Canine hepatic neuroendocrine carcinoma: an immunohistochemical and electron microscopic study. *Vet Pathol.* 2005a;42(2):140-146.

Patnaik AK, Lieberman PH, Erlandson RA, et al. Hepatobiliary neuroendocrine carcinoma in cats: a clinicopathologic, immunohistochemical, and ultrastructural study of 17 cases. *Vet Pathol.* 2005b;42(3):331-337.

Penninck DG, Feldman EC, Nyland TG. Radiographic features of canine hyperadrenocorticism caused by autonomously functioning adrenocortical tumors: 23 cases (1978-1986). *J Am Vet Med Assoc.* 1988;192:1604-1608.

Phillips DE, Radlinski MG, Fischer JR, et al. Cystic thyroid and parathyroid lesions in cats. *J Am Anim Hosp Assoc.* 2003;39:349-354.

Platt SR, Sheppard BJ, Graham J, et al. Pheochromocytoma in the vertebral canal of two dogs. *J Am Anim Hosp Assoc.* 1998;34:365-371.

Quante S, Boretti FS, Kook PH, et al. Urinary catecholamine and metanephrine to creatinine ratios in dog with hyperadrenocorticism or pheochromocytoma and in healthy dogs. *J Vet Intern Med.* 2010;24:1093-1097.

Ramaiah SK, Alleman AR, Hanel R, et al. A mass in the ventral neck of a hypercalcemic dog. *Vet Clin Pathol.* 2001;30:177-179.

Reusch CE, Feldman EC. Canine hyperadrenocorticism due to adrenocortical neoplasia. *J Vet Intern Med.* 1991;5:3-10.

Renschler JS, Dean GA. What is your diagnosis? Abdominal mass aspirate in a cat with an increased Na:K ratio. *Vet Clin Pathol.* 2009;38(1):69-72.

Rosol TJ, Meuten DJ. Tumors of the endocrine glands. In: Meuten DJ, ed. *Tumors in Domestic Animals.* 5th ed. Ames, IA: Wiley-Blackwell; 2017:766-833.

Rossi G, Magi GE, Tarantino C, et al. Tracheobronchial neuroendocrine carcinoma in a cat. *J Comp Pathol.* 2007;137(2-3):165-168.

Rossmeisl JH Jr, Forrester SD, Robertson JL, et al. Chronic vomiting associated with a gastric carcinoid in a cat. *J Am Anim Hosp Assoc.* 2002;38(1):61-66.

Saegusa S, Yamamura H, Morita T, et al. Pulmonary neuroendocrine carcinoma in a four-month-old dog. *J Comp Pathol.* 1994;111(4):439-443.

Sako T, Shimoyama Y, Akihara Y, et al. Neuroendocrine carcinoma in the nasal cavity of ten dogs. *J Comp Pathol.* 2005;133:155-163.

Sako T, Uchida E, Okamoto M, et al. Immunohistochemical evaluation of a malignant intestinal carcinoid in a dog. *Vet Pathol.* 2003;40(2):212-215.

Scavelli TD, Peterson ME, Matthiesen DT. Results of surgical treatment of hyperadrenocorticism caused by adrenocortical neoplasia in the dog: 25 cases (1980-1984). *J Am Vet Med Assoc.* 1986;189:1360-1364.

Shaw TE, Harkin KR, Nietfeld J, et al. Aortic body tumor in full-sibling English bulldogs. *J Am Anim Hosp Assoc.* 2010;46:366-370.

Slawienski MJ, Mauldin GE, Mauldin GN, et al. Malignant colonic neoplasia in cats: 46 cases (1990-1996). *J Am Vet Med Assoc.* 1997;211(7):878-881.

Swainson SW, Nelson L, Niyo Y, et al. Radiographic diagnosis: mediastinal parathyroid cyst in a cat. *Vet Radiol Ultrasound.* 2000;41:41-43.

Sykes GP, Cooper BJ. Canine intestinal carcinoids. *Vet Pathol.* 1982;19(2):120-131.

Tillson DM, Fingland RB, Andrews GA. Chemodectoma in a cat. *J Am Anim Hosp Assoc.* 1994;30:586-590.

Tursi M, Iussich S, Prunotto M, et al. Adrenal myelolipoma in a dog. *Vet Pathol.* 2005;42(2):232-235.

von Dehn BJ, Nelson RW, Feldman EC, et al. Pheochromocytoma and hyperadrenocorticism in dogs: six cases (1982-1992). *J Am Vet Med Assoc.* 1995;207:322-324.

Ware WA, Hopper DL. Cardiac tumors in dogs: 1982-1995. *J Vet Int Med.* 1999;13:95-103.

Whiteley LO, Leininger JR. Neuroendocrine (Merkel) cell tumors of the canine oral cavity. *Vet Pathol.* 1987;24:570-572.

Zimmerman KL, Rossmeisl JH, Thorn CE, et al. Mediastinal mass in a dog with syncope and abdominal distension. *Vet Clin Pathol.* 2000;29:19-21.

18 CHAPTER

Advanced Diagnostic Techniques

José A. Ramos-Vara and Maria Elena Gelain

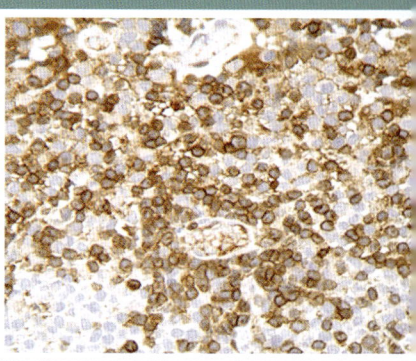

IMMUNODIAGNOSIS

The detection of antigens by immunologic and chemical reactions in tissue sections, immunohistochemistry (IHC), or immunocytochemistry (ICC) in cytopathologic preparations has become one of the most commonly used ancillary morphologic techniques in diagnostic pathology. The advantages of IHC and ICC are as follows: (1) They do not require the use of expensive equipment. (2) Both prospective and retrospective studies can be done on a variety of samples. (3) Antigen detection by IHC can be correlated with histomorphology and its cellular location detected by ICC. (4) Stained slides can be stored for many months. (5) Routine processing of samples is usually acceptable for these techniques. Both IHC and ICC are practical in the characterization of poorly differentiated neoplasms, differentiation of primary from metastatic tumors, and determination of sites of origin of metastatic lesions, and prognostic assessments. IHC and ICC methods, if properly applied and interpreted, increase diagnostic accuracy in pathology. Technical aspects of ICC, interpretation of results, and pitfalls are reviewed in this chapter. An algorithmic approach to the diagnosis of tumors, the diagnosis of metastatic disease, and the use of antibodies as prognostic markers are also presented.

Antibodies

Immunocytochemistry demonstrates antigens in cell preps by incubating them with specific antibodies and demonstrating the immunologic reaction with a histochemical (enzyme-substrate) reaction to produce a colored (visible) reaction (Ramos-Vara and Miller, 2014). Polyclonal or monoclonal antibodies can be used. Polyclonal antibodies are usually raised in rabbits and have higher affinity but lower specificity than monoclonal antibodies (Kim et al., 2016). Cross-reactivity (defined as recognition of unrelated antigens) is more common with polyclonal antibodies. Key in the use of polyclonal antibodies in diagnostic IHC and ICC is their degree of purification. (Examples of commercially available antibodies include whole serum antibodies, antibodies purified by precipitation of immunoglobulins [Igs], and Igs purified by affinity chromatography.) Monoclonal antibodies, produced in mice using the hybridoma technology, recognize a single epitope (a 4- to 8-amino acid chain in a protein) and therefore are highly specific and have constant characteristics among different batches of antibody. Selection of a particular antibody is determined by published information or the experience of other laboratories. Nanoantibodies are antibodies that only contain heavy chains. Their advantages include smaller size, which makes them able to recognize epitopes hidden to conventional IgGs; high affinity; and very stable to high temperatures and a wide range of pH (Wong et al., 2018). In addition, they can be genetically engineered. There are no guarantees that an antibody that recognizes an antigen in one species will do so in another species; only testing will determine if this is the case. Needless to say, the large number of species from which samples can be obtained is one of the biggest challenges that a veterinary pathologist must face in immunodiagnostics.

For technical aspects of IHC and ICC and detailed protocols, readers are referred to more recent reviews (Polak and Van Noorden, 2003; Ramos-Vara, 2013; Ramos-Vara and Miller, 2014; Anonymous, 2017) and Appendix 2 of this book. Table 18.1 includes a selection of antibodies used at Purdue University College of Veterinary Medicine Animal Disease Diagnostic Laboratory and Clinical Pathology Laboratory for infectious and neoplastic diseases of dogs and cats as well as others validated elsewhere. Immunohistochemical protocols can be divided into three stages: (1) pretreatment procedures; (2) incubation of the primary antibody, secondary, and tertiary reagents; and (3) visualization of the immunologic reaction.

Processing of Cytopathologic Samples

Immunocytochemistry can be performed on most types of cytopathologic samples, including cytocentrifuge and smear preparations, tissue imprints, cell blocks, cell cultures, liquid-based monolayer preparations, and previously Romanowsky-stained slides (Ramos-Vara et at., 2016; Raskin et al., 2019). Cytocentrifuge and smear preparations are used when the sample volume is small. The advantage of cytocentrifuge preparations is better preservation of cytomorphology. Aspirate or imprint smears give reproducible results with nuclear markers but may be less suitable for cytoplasmic and membrane markers because of the high background produced by cell damage during slide preparation (Skoog and Tani, 2011). To offset this concern, aspirates may be placed in a normal saline solution first followed by preparation of a cytocentrifuge specimen, which will clear away background blood and noncellular proteins, lipids, and carbohydrates. The use of pretreated slides to promote cell adhesion may reduce loss of cells over the course of the ICC procedure (Dupré and Courtade-Saidi, 2012) but would not be necessary if specimens are left to completely dry overnight before staining, which aids in adhesion.

Cell or tube blocks are helpful for cytopathologic specimens, particularly when cells are numerous (Zanoni et al., 2012; Ramos-Vara, 2013; Marcos et al., 2017; Heinrich et al., 2019). See

TABLE 18.1 Selected Antigen Markers, Sources, Tissue Controls, and Uses for Selected Antibodies Used in Dogs and Cats

ANTIGEN[a]	SPECIES REACTIVITY[b]	CLONE/CATALOG NUMBER	VENDOR	TISSUE CONTROL (CELL LOCALIZATION)	USES
Actin muscle	Dogs	HHF35	Dako	Skeletal muscle and heart (cyto)	Muscle neoplasms
Actin sarcomeric	Dogs	Alpha-Sr-1	Dako	Skeletal muscle and heart (cyto)	Striated muscle tumors
Actin smooth muscle	Dogs	1A4	Dako	Stomach/intestine (cyto)	Smooth muscle tumors
Adenovirus (blend)	Dogs	20/11 and 2/6	Millipore-Sigma	Infected tissue (nuclear)	Infection
Amylin (IAPP)	Cats and dogs	R10/99	Bio-Rad	Pancreas (extracellular)	Pancreatic islet amyloid
Aspergillus	Cats and dogs	Mab-WF-AF-1	Dako	Infected tissue	Infected tissue
Bcl-2 oncoprotein	Cats only	NCL-bcl-2	Novocastra	Lymphoid tissue (cyto)	Lymphoid tumors
B-lymphocyte antigen (BLA.36)	Cats and dogs	A27-42	Dako	Lymph node, spleen (memb)	B-cell, histiocytic tumors
CD1a (IHC)	Cats and dogs	O10	Dako	Thymus (memb)	Cortical thymocytes, Langerhans cells, T-cell lymphoblastic lymphoma
CD1a (ICC)	Cats only	FE1.5F4	UCD	Hematolymphatic (memb)	Dendritic cells, feline progressive histiocytosis
CD1a (ICC, IHC, FC)	Dogs only	CA13.9H11	UCD	Hematolymphatic (memb)	Dendritic cell tumors, reactive or systemic histiocytosis
CD1c (ICC)	Cats	FE5.5C1	UCD	Hematolymphatic (memb)	Dendritic cells, feline progressive histiocytosis
CD3 (ICC, FC)	Dogs only	CA17.2A12	Bio-Rad	Lymph node, spleen (memb)	T-cell lymphoma
CD3 epsilon (ICC, IHC)	Cats and dogs	CD3-12 / A0452	Bio-Rad / Dako	Lymph node, spleen (cyto, memb)	T-cell lymphoma
CD4 (ICC, FC)	Cats	FE1.7B12, sVpg34	UCD, Bio-Rad	Hematopoietic (memb)	T-cell neoplasia
CD4 (ICC, FC)	Dogs	CA13.1E4, YKIX302.9	Bio-Rad	Hematopoietic (memb)	T-cell neoplasia, reactive or systemic histiocytosis
CD5 (ICC, FC)	Dog / Cats	YKIX322.3 / FE1.1B11	Bio-Rad / Bio-Rad	Spleen (memb)	T-cell lymphocytes
CD8α (ICC, FC)	Dogs	YCATE55.9 / CA9.JD3	Bio-Rad / Bio-Rad	Spleen (memb)	T-cell lymphocytes
CD8α (ICC, FC)	Cats	FE1.10E9	Bio-Rad	Spleen (memb)	T-cell lymphocytes
CD8β (ICC, FC)	Dogs	CA15.4G2	Bio-Rad	Spleen (memb)	T-cell lymphocytes
CD10 (CALLA antigen)	Dogs	56C6	Abcam	Kidney (cyto, memb)	Renal, stromal tumors
CD11b (ICC, FC)	Cats and dogs	CA16.3E10	Bio-Rad	Spleen (memb)	Granulocytes, monocytes, macrophages
CD11c (ICC, FC)	Dogs	CA11.6A1	Bio-Rad	Spleen (memb)	Granulocytes, monocytes, dendritic cells
CD11d (IHC)	Dogs only	CA18.3C6	UCD	Spleen (memb)	Lymphoid, histiocytic tumors
CD11d (ICC, FC)	Cats and dogs	CA11.8H2	Bio-Rad	Spleen, bone marrow (memb)	Lymphoid, histiocytic tumors
CD14 (ICC, IHC)	Cats and dogs	TÜK4	Dako	Hematopoietic (memb)	Monocytes, macrophages
CD18 (IHC)	Cats only	FE3.9F2	UCD	Spleen (memb)	Leukocytic tumors
CD18 (IHC)	Dogs only	CA16.3C10	UCD	Spleen, lymph node (memb)	Leukocytic tumors
CD18 (ICC, FC)	Cats and dogs	CA1.4E9	Bio-Rad	Spleen, lymph node (memb)	Leukocytic tumors
CD20 (ICC, IHC)	Cats and dogs	RB-9013 / PA5-16701 (FC)	Thermo-Fisher Scientific	Spleen, lymph node (memb)	B-cell tumors
CD21 (ICC, FC)	Cats and dogs	CA2.1D6	Bio-Rad	Lymph node (memb)	B-cell tumors
CD31 (IHC, ICC, FC)	Cats and dogs	JC70A/M0823	Dako	Skin, other (memb)	Vascular endothelial and megakaryocytic tumors
CD34 (ICC, IHC, FC)	Dogs (cats)	1H6	Bio-Rad	Hematopoietic (memb)	Hematopoietic stem cells, vascular neoplasms
CD41/61 (ICC, FC)	Cats and dogs	CO.35E4	Thermo-Fisher Scientific (Invitrogen)	Bone marrow (memb)	Megakaryocytes, platelets

Continued

TABLE 18.1 Selected Antigen Markers, Sources, Tissue Controls, and Uses for Selected Antibodies Used in Dogs and Cats—cont'd

ANTIGEN[a]	SPECIES REACTIVITY[b]	CLONE/CATALOG NUMBER	VENDOR	TISSUE CONTROL (CELL LOCALIZATION)	USES
CD45 (FC, ICC)	Dogs only	CA12.10C12 (IHC) YKIX716.13	Bio-Rad	Spleen, lymph node (memb)	Leukocytic tumors
CD45RA (IHC, ICC, FC)	Dogs only	CA21.4B3	UCD	Lymphoid tissue (memb)	Lymphoid tumors
CD71 [transferrin receptor] (ICC, FC)	Cats	Ber-T9	Dako	Bone marrow (memb)	Erythroid precursors
CD71 (IHC)	Cats	EPR4012	Abcam	Bone marrow (memb, cyto)	Erythroid precursors
CD79a (IHC, ICC)	Cats and dogs	HM57	Bio-Rad	Lymph node, spleen (memb)	B-cell lymphoma
CD90 [Thy-1]	Dogs Dogs	CA1.4G8 (ICC, FC, IHC) YKIX337.217 (FC)	UCD Bio-Rad	Spleen (memb)	Interstitial dendritic cells, reactive or systemic histiocytosis, T-lymphocytes
CD117 (*c-kit* protein)	Dogs and cats	A4502	Dako	Mast cell tumor (memb, cyto)	Mast cell tumor, GIST, melanoma
CD163 (macrophage scavenger receptor)	Dogs and cats	AM-3K	TransGenic	Spleen (memb)	Histiocytic (phagocytic) sarcoma
CD204 (macrophage scavenger receptor)	Dogs	SRA-E5/sc-166184	Santa Cruz	Spleen (memb, cyto)	Histiocytic (phagocytic) sarcoma
Calcitonin	Cats and dogs	A0576	Dako	Thyroid (cyto)	C-cell (medullary) tumors
Calponin	Cats and dogs	CALP, h-CP	Dako, Sigma	Small intestine, stomach (cyto)	Smooth muscle, myofibroblastic and myoepithelial tumors
Calprotectin (myeloid/histiocytic antigen) (IHC, ICC)	Cats and dogs	MAC 387	Dako, Bio-Rad	Spleen, liver (cyto)	Macrophages, myeloid cells
Calretinin	Cats and dogs	DC8/18.0211 Calret 1/M7245	Thermo-Fisher Scientific Dako	Kidney (cyto, nuclear)	Renal tubules, nerve tissue, adrenocortical tumors, mesothelioma
Canine distemper virus	Dogs	CDV-NP	VMRD	Infected tissue (nuclear, cyto)	Infection
Carcinoembryonic antigen	Dogs	A0115	Dako	Intestine (cyto)	Epithelial tumors
Chromogranin A	Cats and dogs	LK2H10	Thermo Scientific	Pancreas (cyto)	Neuroendocrine marker
Claudin 1	Cats and dogs	Ab15098	Abcam	Epidermis (memb)	Epithelial neoplasms, meningioma
CNPase (myelin enzyme)	Dogs	SMI-91	BioLegend	Nerve (cyto)	Peripheral nerve sheath tumors (Schwann cells), oligodendrogliomas
Coronavirus	Cats and dogs	FIPV3-70	CMI	Infected tissue (cyto)	Infection
COX-1	Cats and dogs	160108	Cayman Chemical	Normal urinary bladder (cyto, nuclear)	Normal urothelium, endothelium
COX-2	Cats and dogs	/160116	Cayman Chemical	Urothelial carcinoma (cyto)	Carcinomas
Cytokeratin 5	Dogs	XM26	Vector	Mammary gland, skin (cyto)	Myoepithelium, epithelial basal cells, mesothelium
Cytokeratin 7	Cats and dogs	OV-TL 12/30	Dako	Skin, urinary bladder, biliary epithelium (cyto)	Glandular epithelium neoplasms
Cytokeratins 8/18	Dogs	5D3	Novocastra	Liver, stomach (cyto)	Glandular epithelium neoplasms
Cytokeratins AE1-AE3 (ICC, IHC)	Cats and dogs	AE1 and AE3	Dako	Skin (cyto)	General epithelial cell marker
Cytokeratins Pan	Dogs	MNF116	Dako	Glandular or squamous epithelium (cyto)	General epithelial cell marker
Cytokeratins HMW	Dogs	34βE12	Dako	Skin (cyto)	Squamous epithelium, mesothelium
Desmin	Dogs	D33	Dako	Skin, stomach, intestine (cyto)	Muscle tumors
E-Cadherin	Dogs Cats	36 4A2C7	BD Transduction Zymed	Skin (memb)	Langerhans cells, epithelial neoplasms, canine histiocytoma, meningioma
Estrogen receptor alpha	Cats and dogs	CC4-5	Novocastra	Uterus (nuclear)	Estrogen receptor–expressing tumors

TABLE 18.1 Selected Antigen Markers, Sources, Tissue Controls, and Uses for Selected Antibodies Used in Dogs and Cats—cont'd

ANTIGEN[a]	SPECIES REACTIVITY[b]	CLONE/CATALOG NUMBER	VENDOR	TISSUE CONTROL (CELL LOCALIZATION)	USES
Factor VIII–related antigen (vWF) (IHC, ICC)	Cats and dogs	A0082	Dako	Skin, other (cyto)	Vascular endothelial and megakaryocytic tumors
Feline calicivirus	Cats	S1-9	CMI	Infected tissue (cyto)	Infection
Feline herpesvirus 1	Cats	FHV5	CMI	Infected tissue (nuclear, cyto)	Infection
Feline leukemia virus	Cats	C11D8-2C1	CMI	Infected tissue	Infection
Francisella tularensis	Cats and dogs	240939	Becton Dickinson	Infected tissue	Infected tissue
Gastrin	Cats and dogs	A0568	Dako	Stomach (cyto)	Gastrin-producing tumors
GATA-3	Dogs	CM 405	Biocare	Urinary bladder (nuclear)	Urothelial carcinoma
GATA-4	Dogs	sc-1237	Santa Cruz	Testis (nuclear)	Sex cord–stromal tumors
Glial fibrillary acidic protein	Dogs	Z0334	Dako	Brain (cyto)	Neural (glial) tumors
Glucagon	Cats and dogs	A0565	Dako	Pancreas (cyto)	Glucagon-producing tumors
Glut 1	Dogs	A3536	Dako	Peripheral nerve (cyto)	Peripheral nerves, stromal cells, kidney
Glycophorin A [CD235a] (ICC, FC, IHC)	Cats	JC159	Dako	Bone marrow (memb)	Erythroid leukemia
Granzyme B (IHC)	Cats and dogs	E2580	Spring Bioscience	Spleen (focal cyto granules)	Cytotoxic T-lymphocytes, natural killer cells
Hepatocyte marker-1 (Hep Par 1)	Cats and dogs	OCH1E5	Dako	Liver (cyto)	Hepatocellular tumors
Iba1	Cats and dogs	CP290	Biocare	Microglia, histiocytes (memb)	Hematopoietic neoplasia; nervous tissue
Ig kappa chains	Dogs	A0191	Dako	Lymph node (cyto, memb)	Plasmacytomas, B-cell lymphoma
Ig lambda chains	Dog	A0193	Dako	Lymph node (cyto, memb)	Plasmacytomas, B-cell lymphoma
Immunoglobulin M	Cats and dogs	CM7	CMI	Lymph node (cyto, memb)	Lymphoid tumors
Inhibin-alpha	Dogs	R1	Bio-Rad	Testicle, Sertoli cell tumor (cyto)	Sex cord–stromal and adrenal cortical tumors
Insulin	Dogs	Z006	Zymed	Pancreas (cyto)	Insulin-producing tumors
Ki-67	Dogs	7B11	Zymed	Lymphoma (nuclear)	Cell proliferation marker
	Cats and dogs	MIB-1	Dako		
Laminin	Cats and dogs	Z0097	Dako	Skin/kidney (extracellular)	Perivascular wall tumors and basement membrane
Leptospira	Dogs	—	NVSL	Infected tissue (cyto)	Infection
Lysozyme (ICC, IHC)	Dogs and cats	A0099	Dako	Liver, spleen (cyto)	Histiocytes (macrophages)
LYVE-1	Cats and dogs	Ab33682	Abcam	Small intestine (cyto)	Lymphatic endothelial tumors
Melan-A (ICC, IHC)	Cats and dogs	A103	Dako	Melanoma (cyto)	Melanocytic neoplasms, steroid-producing tumors
Melanocytic antigen (IHC, ICC)	Dogs	PNL2/sc-59306	Santa Cruz	Melanoma (cyto)	Melanocytic neoplasms
MHC II	Cats	42.3	UCD	Hematopoietic (memb)	Macrophage, dendritic lineage
MHC II (HLA-DR) (ICC, IHC)	Dogs	TAL.1B5	Dako	Histiocytoma, LN (memb)	Antigen-presenting cells, lymphocytes
Microphthalmia transcription factor	Dogs	C5	Abcam	Melanoma (nuclear)	Melanocytic neoplasms
Myeloperoxidase (IHC, ICC)	Dogs	CA25.10A6	UCD	Bone marrow (cyto)	Granulocytic leukemia
	Cats and dogs	CA25.7G1	UCD		
MUM1 protein (IHC, ICC)	Cats and dogs	MUM1p	Dako	Plasma cells (nuclear)	Plasmacytomas, myelomas, some B-cell tumors, some histiocytomas
MyoD1	Dogs	5.8A	Dako	Rhabdomyosarcoma (nuclear)	Rhabdomyosarcoma
Myosin smooth muscle	Cats and dogs	SMMS-1	Dako	Intestine (cyto)	Smooth muscle tumors
Neospora caninum	Dogs	210-70-NC	VMRD	Infected tissue (cyto)	Infection
Nerve growth factor receptor	Cats and dogs	NGFR5	Santa Cruz, Life Technologies	Nerve (memb)	Nerves
Neurofilament-2	Dogs	SMI-31	BioLegend	Brain (cyto)	Neoplastic cells of neural origin

Continued

TABLE 18.1 Selected Antigen Markers, Sources, Tissue Controls, and Uses for Selected Antibodies Used in Dogs and Cats—cont'd

ANTIGEN[a]	SPECIES REACTIVITY[b]	CLONE/CATALOG NUMBER	VENDOR	TISSUE CONTROL (CELL LOCALIZATION)	USES
Neuron-specific enolase	Dogs	BBS/NC/VI-H14	Dako	Pancreas (cyto)	Neuroendocrine marker
OCT-3/4	Dogs	C-10/sc-279	Santa Cruz	Mast cell tumor (nuclear)	Germ cells, stem cells
Olig-2	Dogs	AB9610	EMD Millipore	Cerebrum (nuclear)	Oligodendrogliomas
p63	Dogs	4A4	EMD Millipore	Skin, mammary gland (nuclear)	Myoepithelium, epithelial basal cells, urothelial tumors
Papilloma virus	Dogs	BPV-1/18+CAM	Abcam	Infected tissue (nuclear)	Infection
Parathyroid hormone	Cats and dogs	A1/70/ab14493	Abcam	Parathyroid (cyto)	Parathyroid neoplasms
Parvovirus	Dog	A3B10	VMRD	Infected tissue (nuclear, cyto)	Infection
Pax5 (ICC, IHC)	Cats and dogs	DAK-Pax5 24/Pax5	Dako BD Biosciences	Lymph node (nuclear)	B-cell lymphoma
Pax8	Dogs	BC12	Biocare Medical	Kidney (nuclear)	Renal, thyroid follicular tumors
Progesterone receptor	Dogs	SP2	Thermo Scientific	Uterus (nuclear)	Progesterone receptor expressing tumors
Proliferating cell nuclear antigen (PCNA)	Cats and dogs	PC10	Dako, Bio-Rad	Lymphoma, lymph node (nuclear)	Proliferation marker
Prostatic specific antigen	Dogs	A0562	Dako	Prostate (cyto)	Prostatic carcinoma
Protein gene product 9.5	Cats and dogs	Z5116	Dako	Adrenal gland (cyto)	Neuroendocrine marker
Prox-1	Cats and dogs	11-002	AngioBio	Lymph node (nuclear)	Lymphatic endothelium neoplasms
S-100 protein	Cats and dogs	Z0311	Dako	Nerve, brain (cyto, nuclear)	Neural marker, neuroendocrine tumors
Somatostatin	Dogs	A0566	Dako	Pancreas (cyto)	Pancreatic islet tumors, some carcinoids
Synaptophysin	Dogs	SP11	Thermo Scientific	Pancreas (cyto)	Neuroendocrine cells and their tumors
Thyroglobulin	Cats and dogs	12G9/ab1983	Abcam	Thyroid (cyto)	Thyroglobulin-producing tumors
Thyroid transcription factor-1	Dog	8G7G3/1	Dako	Lung, thyroid (nuclear)	Lung and thyroid neoplasms
Tryptase (ICC, IHC)	Cats and dogs	AA1	Bio-Rad	Mast cell tumor (cyto)	Mast cell tumors
Tyrosinase	Cats and dogs	SPM360	Abcam	Melanoma (cyto)	Melanocytic tumors
Uroplakin II	Dogs	BC21	Biocare Medicare	Urinary bladder (cyto, memb)	Urothelial carcinoma
Uroplakin III (IHC, ICC)	Dogs	AU1	Fitzgerald	Urinary bladder (cyto, memb)	Urothelial carcinoma
Vimentin (ICC, IHC)	Cats and dogs	SP20, V9	Spring Bioscience, Dako	Skin, stomach (cyto)	Mesenchymal tumor marker
WT1 (ICC, IHC)	Cats and dogs	6F-H2	Dako	Mesothelium (nuclear)	Mesothelioma, nephroblastoma, ovarian carcinoma

[a]The antigen markers listed are indicated for IHC use unless other methods are indicated.
[b]Known species reactivity is listed; dogs or cats only indicates both species were tested but only one is reactive.
CMI, Custom Monoclonals International; *CNPase*, 2′,3′-cyclic nucleotide-3′phosphodiesterase; *cyto*, cytoplasmic reactivity; *Dako*, owned by Agilent Technologies; *FC*, flow cytometry; *GIST*, gastrointestinal stromal tumor; *HMW*, high molecular weight; *ICC*, immunocytochemistry; *IHC*, immunohistochemistry (paraffin embedded); *LN*, lymph node; *LYVE-1*, lymphatic vessel endothelial receptor 1; *memb*, surface membrane reactivity; *NVSL*, National Veterinary Services Laboratories; *UCD*, University of California–Davis; *WSU*, Washington State University (Monoclonal Antibody Laboratory); *WT1*, Wilms tumor 1.

Appendix 5 for more detail about specimen preparation with these techniques. Cell or tube blocks are processed similar to histopathology specimens, so IHC methods can be used without adaptive modifications. In addition, multiple sections can be produced from a single block, so multiple markers can be evaluated in the same cell population. However, cell blocks can alter cytopathologic detail through fixative-induced cell shrinkage and cause variation in cellularity depending on the lesion sampled by aspiration biopsy, the cellularity of aspirate needle rinses, the sampling effectiveness during dedicated aspiration for the cell block, and postprocedural handling of the needle rinse specimen. Importantly, because cell blocks are fixed in formaldehyde-containing solutions, sections from cell blocks need to undergo additional time for antigen retrieval (AR) procedures and are not able to use some antibodies intended for lymphocyte subset identification. Cell blocks are preferred for nuclear antigens (e.g., Ki-67, p53, proliferating cell nuclear antigen [PCNA]), whereas air-dried cytocentrifuge preparations are preferred for the detection of surface antigens (e.g., leukocytic antigens). Liquid-based cytology using ThinPrep preparations enhances retrieval of cells from small samples with preservation of cellular detail and, theoretically, a reduction of background because of less blood, mucin, and proteinaceous material in the sample (Dupré and Courtade-Saidi, 2012). ThinPrep preparations are less suitable than cell blocks for detection of nuclear antigens (Gong et al., 2003). A more detailed discussion of the pros and cons of different cytopathologic preparation methods is available (Fowler and Lachar, 2008).

Under certain circumstances, ICC may be performed on previously stained Romanowsky or Papanicolaou slides when that is the only available specimen and produces similar results to that of unstained slides (Raskin et al., 2019). The ICC staining does not require destaining of the routine stain (Raskin et al., 2019). However, there are some technical drawbacks to using previously stained slides: possible loss of cells from the slide, cell disruption (affecting mostly ICC of membranous and cytoplasmic markers), and signal reduction for some markers. In cases in which only a slide is available and the area containing cells is large, multiple markers can be tested simultaneously, using wax pens to separate specimens (Raskin et al., 2019). Alternatively, the sample can be divided following tissue-transfer techniques (Stone and Gan, 2014). Cell transfer techniques allow the evaluation of multiple markers when few slides are available for ICC. If cell transfer from previously stained cytopathologic smears is anticipated, nonadhesive treated slides are recommended.

Storage of air-dried preparations for up to 2 weeks at 2°C to 8°C before ICC does not appear to reduce their antigenicity (Fetsch and Abati, 2004). Samples are placed in a plastic microscope slide box and then into a zip-lock plastic bag containing desiccant. Samples should equilibrate to room temperature before the bag is opened to avoid cell rupture. However, acetone-fixed slides kept refrigerated may retain their antigenicity for 4 to 5 months (Raskin et al., 2019). If longer storage is needed, slides should be kept at −70°C. Guidelines from the American Society for Veterinary Clinical Pathology provide additional specimen handling advice regarding ICC (Arnold et al., 2019).

Fixation and Antigen Retrieval

Approximately 85% of antigens fixed in formalin require some type of AR to optimize the immunoreaction (Ramos-Vara et al., 2016). The need for AR and choice of AR method depend not only on the antigen examined but also on the antibody used (Ramos-Vara and Miller, 2014; Kim et al., 2016). Polyclonal antibodies are more likely to detect antigens than monoclonal antibodies in the absence of AR (Ramos-Vara et al., 2016). Although AR allows detection of multiple antigens, background staining or antigen detection in unusual locations due to harsh AR methods is common and can affect diagnostic interpretation. In addition to conformational changes in the structure of proteins, fixation produces major changes in the electrostatic charge of proteins (antigens), which is critical for the initial attraction between antigens and antibodies. Therefore, recovery of the electrostatic charges lost during formalin fixation has been proposed as another mechanism of AR for many (but not all) proteins. In other words, it appears that more than one mechanism may be involved in the lack of recognition of antigens by antibodies after fixation in cross-linking fixatives. The two more common AR procedures for formalin-fixed, paraffin-embedded (FFPE) tissue sections include protease-induced AR (proteolytic enzymes, e.g., pronase, trypsin, proteinase K) and heat-induced AR (immersion of slides in buffer at high temperature). Each antibody may react differently to AR; therefore, it is necessary to test several methods when optimizing the immunochemistry procedure. In general, heat-induced epitope retrieval (HIER) procedures appear to produce optimal results in a wide variety of antibodies (Denda et al., 2012; Ramos-Vara et al., 2014; Raskin et al., 2019).

As mentioned earlier, fixation and tissue processing may modify the three-dimensional structure of proteins (antigens), which can render them undetectable by specific antibodies. This fact is better understood if we remember that, in general, an immunologic reaction between antigen and antibody depends on the conformation of the former (Hayat, 2002). One challenge of ICC is to develop AR methods that reverse the changes produced by fixation. AR is particularly necessary when tissues are fixed in cross-linking fixatives. A main difference between IHC and ICC is the type of fixation. Contrary to the situation in histopathology and IHC in which 10% formalin is the universal fixative, there is no standard fixative for cytopathologic specimens. In general, the type of fixation is determined by the antigens to be tested (Skoog and Tani, 2011). Slides are either wet fixed or air dried and fixed immediately before ICC is performed (Dabbs, 2002; Valli et al., 2009; Raskin et al., 2019).

For nuclear antigens, fixation of air-dried specimens in buffered 4% to 10% formalin alone or followed by methanol-acetone produces excellent results (Skoog and Tani, 2011). For membrane and cytoplasmic antigens, the type of fixation is not as critical as for nuclear antigens; a variety of fixatives, including formalin followed by ethanol, a 1:1 mixture of methanol-absolute ethanol, or fixation in −20°C acetone produces good results (Skoog and Tani, 2011). Extra caution is needed when using acetone alone as a fixative for ICC to detect small peptides. Acetone solubilizes cell membranes, leading to diffusion of small peptides out of cells and false-negative results (Van der Loos, 2007). However, using an initial fixation with ethanol followed by acetone appeared to minimize loss of cellular peptides and provide good staining (Raskin et al., 2019). Antigens such as S-100 protein, Hep Par 1, hormone receptors, and gross cystic fluid protein 15 are leached by alcohol fixatives, producing false-negative results (Dabbs, 2002; Chivukula and Dabbs, 2010). One laboratory proposes these guidelines: (1) samples should be fixed immediately before the ICC procedure, and (2) for leukocyte and nuclear markers, fix slides with 95% ethanol for 10 minutes followed by fixation with cold acetone for 15 minutes and air dry before AR if performed (Raskin et al., 2019). In general, leukocyte markers are best performed after acetone fixation.

Antigen retrieval is necessary in many instances even if formalin fixation is not used, especially if the slides have been previously stained with a Romanowsky stain (Dorfelt et al., 2019; Raskin et al., 2019). Unfortunately, the wide range of fixation procedures makes standardization of AR procedures among laboratories very difficult; each laboratory must optimize the procedure for each antigen. Whereas citrate buffer (pH, 6.0) with HIER is best for most leukocyte markers, a Tris-buffer (pH, 9.0) with HIER was useful for routine tissue markers (Raskin et al., 2019). Guidelines about AR and suggested antibody concentration are often provided by the manufacturers of the antibodies and should be used as starting points for validation trials.

Enzymatic AR is much less commonly used than HIER in ICC (Zhang et al., 2012). When the amount of cytopathologic specimen is limited, the same slide can often be tested for a second marker if the first test result is negative (Ramos-Vara et al., 2016).

> **KEY POINT** When using heat-based AR, the slides are placed in a buffer that is heated. The type of heating device is not critical, although commercially available sophisticated units, microwave ovens, or an inexpensive rice steamer can produce similar results in many cases.

Immunochemical Reaction

The immunochemical reaction can be divided into an immunologic (antigen-antibody) reaction followed by its demonstration with a histochemical (colored) reaction. The sensitivity of the immunochemical reaction is mostly the result of the detection method used (Ramos-Vara, 2013; Ramos-Vara and Miller, 2014). The two main enzymes used in IHC are peroxidase and alkaline phosphatase. Peroxidase is probably the most commonly used, but in some cases, particularly with heavily pigmented samples or samples rich in endogenous peroxidase, alkaline phosphatase is an excellent alternative. Current ICC methods can be divided into avidin-biotin or non–avidin-biotin systems. After incubation with the primary antibody, a secondary antibody specific for the primary antibody (secondary reagent) is added. For avidin-biotin systems, the secondary reagent is biotinylated. For avidin-biotin methods, a tertiary reagent labeled with avidin molecules and an enzyme (peroxidase or alkaline phosphatase) is needed (Ramos-Vara et al., 2014). The most common non–avidin-biotin method is based on polymer technology. The polymers contain many molecules of secondary antibodies and enzyme. Polymer methods are usually two-step methods; however, supersensitive polymer methods consist of three steps, which are similar to avidin-biotin methods. Polymer-based methods have fewer steps, do not have endogenous avidin-biotin background problems, and are usually more sensitive (Ramos-Vara and Miller, 2014). Detection of multiple antigens in the same tissue section is also possible. Issues to keep in mind in double or multiple immunostaining is the compatibility of AR among antigens to be detected, the type of primary antibodies (polyclonal or monoclonal), cellular localization of antigens, and the color of chromogens used (Ramos-Vara and Miller, 2014).

Protocols

Immunocytochemical methods parallel those of IHC (Ramos-Vara and Miller, 2014; Anonymous, 2017; Raskin et al., 2019). There are several steps before the incubation of the primary antibody (e.g., endogenous peroxidase block, nonspecific binding block, avidin-biotin block, AR). After the primary antibody incubation, a secondary, and sometimes a tertiary, reagent is necessary to demonstrate the immune reaction. The peroxidase block is necessary when using immunoperoxidase techniques with blood-rich smears; the usual method is with 3% H_2O_2 in deionized water. There is no rule to determine a priori whether AR is needed or which method is optimal. The approach to standardize ICC is similar to that for IHC.

Visualization of the Immunologic Reaction

The addition of a substrate for the enzyme used plus a chromogen will produce a colored reaction if there is binding of antibodies to tissue antigens. For immunoperoxidase methods, the most common chromogen is 3,3′-diaminobenzidine tetrahydrochloride hydrate (DAB), which produces a brown deposit. Another common chromogen is 3-amino-9-ethylcarbazole (AEC). For alkaline phosphatase, Fast Blue and Fast Red are common chromogens. The use of a chromogen needs to be coordinated with the counterstaining and coverslipping methods.

Interpretation of Immunohistochemistry and Immunocytochemistry

Immunochemistry is an ancillary method and therefore needs to be interpreted in conjunction with clinicopathologic data, including cytopathologic and histopathologic findings, if available. Specific knowledge of the right staining pattern of a given marker is extremely important to determine whether the staining is significant or not. As stressed in a later section on immunohistochemical diagnosis of metastatic tumors, very few, if any, antibodies are truly specific for a single cell type. The interpretation of IHC and ICC reactions is based on the expected antibody "personality profile" (see later) and the infidelity of tumor-specific markers (e.g., reactivity in T cells with B-cell markers) (Yaziji and Barry, 2006). The simultaneous presence of an antigen in more than one cellular compartment is possible in neoplastic cells but usually results from diffusion of proteins caused by cellular damage during processing. An antigen detected in an unusual location must be interpreted with caution and indicated in the immunohistochemical report. Antibodies used in IHC may or may not work in ICC and vice versa, the latter especially related to lymphocyte subset markers, which work only in ICC and not IHC.

The interpretation of an immunohistochemical or immunocytochemical reaction requires a definition of positive or negative staining. This is a controversial issue, so only guidelines will be given. Some markers are expected to be present in most cells in a tumor (e.g., cytokeratins [CKs] in a carcinoma), whereas the detection of other markers (e.g., uroplakin III in urothelial cell carcinoma) in only a small group of cells is considered a positive result. As recommended in human pathology, a statement in the report indicating the intensity of the staining and the percentage of positive tumor cells would be more informative than merely a positive or negative result (Höinghaus et al., 2008). The lack of expression of a particular antigen may be as significant as its presence in prognostication (e.g., absence of expression of progesterone receptor is linked to poor outcome in human breast cancer; lack of bcl-6 expression combined with MUM1 expression in cutaneous large B-cell lymphoma is linked to short survival) (Bardou et al., 2003; Sundram et al., 2005). In human pathology IHC antibodies are classified as class I devices by the Food and Drug Administration, meaning that antibodies are considered special stains as adjuncts to conventional histopathologic diagnostic examination (Rhodes, 2005). In other words, with some exceptions, IHC is not a standalone technique. Results must be interpreted by the pathologist in the context of the disease. Some IHC tests (e.g., assays for ER, PR, HER2/neu) are considered class II devices with potential predictive or prognostic value. Similarly, in veterinary medicine, immunohistochemical results are part of the pathology report and should be interpreted by the pathologist (Ramos-Vara et al., 2008).

Interpretation of ICC may be more challenging than that of IHC because of the difficulty in obtaining positive and negative control samples treated in a similar way to the test sample and the additional difficulty of distinguishing normal from neoplastic cells. With the general lack of clear guidelines in this regard, each laboratory should document and state in the ICC report what is interpreted as a positive result. Interpretation of ICC tests should be done in conjunction with a standard cytologic stain (e.g., Wright-Giemsa, Romanowsky, Papanicolaou) and in concert with the clinicopathologic correlations.

Standardization and Validation of an Immunochemical Test

Like any other ancillary technique, IHC needs to be standardized and validated. *Optimization* (standardization) of a new antibody or test is the process of serially testing and modifying components of the procedure (e.g., fixation, AR, antibody dilution, detection system, incubation time) with the aim of producing a consistent, high-quality assay. The reader is advised to standardize every antibody used in his or her laboratory despite the existence of published protocols, to ensure optimal results. In our IHC laboratory, every new antibody is tested following a standard protocol that includes three pretreatments—no AR, AR with a proteolytic enzyme (e.g., proteinase K), and HIER (e.g., citrate buffer, pH of 6.0)—and four twofold dilutions of the primary antibody (Ramos-Vara and Miller, 2014). With this standard protocol, the total number of slides initially processed for each antibody is 15, including a negative reagent control for each pretreatment. A similar process has been reported for ICC (Raskin et al., 2019). The positive control section used in standardization (and later in a diagnostic setting) is one in which the antigen in question has been detected with a different method for infectious diseases (e.g., virus isolation) and its cellular location is known; for tumor markers, it is a specific neoplasm with expected reactivity for that antibody. A negative control section (containing cells known by independent methods to lack the antigen in question) also should be included. Usually, the same tissue block used for the positive control is used for the negative reagent control.

Incubation of the primary antibody is done at room temperature; its duration varies from 30 minutes to 2 hours. Overnight incubations (usually at 4°C) may be beneficial in reducing the background staining or increasing the dilution of the primary antibody. Based on the results of this initial procedure, the optimal AR method and dilution of the primary antibody are selected as the slide with the best signal (specific staining)-to-noise (background staining) ratio. If staining is nonspecific or suboptimal, other AR methods and dilutions should be tested. Keep in mind that some antibodies raised against human antigens may not be reactive in animal tissues. For standardization, tissue samples are processed in the same way as the diagnostic samples that eventually will be tested.

Test validation in ICC follows standardization; however, because it is time consuming and expensive, it is seldom done in veterinary medicine. Validation of a test examines technical aspects such as the effects of prolonged fixation but focuses more on the ability of the antibody to be used as a marker of a specific cell, tumor, or infectious agent. Antibodies used as tumor markers need to be tested against tumors that may be difficult to distinguish from the one in question (tumors with similar phenotype, e.g., round cell tumors) with routine stains and tumors present in the same location or organ (Ramos-Vara and Miller, 2007). Validation should also include evaluation of staining differences among different tumors, staining differences within tumors—particularly when different phenotypes are present (e.g., spindle and epithelioid melanomas staining differences with Melan-A)—and differences between primary and metastatic tumors. Validation is critical given the relative immunologic promiscuity (recognition of more than one cell type or tumor) of most antibodies. Finally, standardization and validation of an immunochemical procedure must be done in each species examined (Bricker et al., 2012). Because of the large resources needed to perform in-house validation studies in veterinary medicine, it is acceptable to use the information provided by other researchers or reported in the literature to validate a test.

Limitations of Immunochemical Methods

Although IHC and ICC have largely displaced electron microscopy as the ancillary technique of choice in diagnostic pathology, they have some limitations. One of the main problems is the lack of standardization and quality control among laboratories, particularly in regard to AR. Interpretation of immunostaining is also subjective (wide range of interobserver interpretations), and a degree of knowledge of ICC and the antibodies used is required to interpret the results correctly. What constitutes a positive result (percentage of positive cells needed, intensity of the reaction) is still controversial, but it is a critical issue for therapeutic decisions in oncology. Some tumors do not express specific markers beyond the generic ones, which makes testing with multiple markers expensive and unrewarding. Neoplastic cells upregulate and downregulate gene expression, resulting in the lack of expression of expected antigens or the expression of new antigens. All these issues are perhaps more serious in veterinary medicine, in which the degree of sophistication and use of ICC techniques is not as advanced as in human pathology and are exacerbated by interspecies differences in antigen expression and detection.

An alternative to a slightly longer enzyme-based ICC procedure on smears requires a special fluorescent microscope to examine antibodies against multiple tissue markers (Sawa et al., 2018). However, this study noted problems with nonspecific background staining and weak immunostaining. One report successfully used multiplex fluorescent immunocytochemical staining using antibodies against CK and vimentin for a dog with pulmonary carcinoma (Moore et al., 2016).

Troubleshooting
General Lack of Staining

The most common cause of lack of staining in the test and control samples is improper procedure (including fixation, AR, antibody concentration, and improper counterstain) (Dabbs, 2002). A systematic approach to the entire procedure is necessary to determine the cause of staining failure.

Weak Staining

In this context, weak staining applies to both the positive (tissue) control and the test sample and may be the result of too much buffer left after a rinsing step, excessive antibody dilution, inadequate AR, insufficient incubation time, or improper storage of reagents such as buffers, antibodies, and substrates. If weak staining only affects the test sample, it might be the result of loss of epitopes in the tissue or overfixation.

Background Staining, False-Positive Staining, and False-Negative Staining

There are multiple causes of background staining. A common one is inadequate blocking of serum proteins. Other causes of false-positive staining are necrotic tissue, crushed cells, improper fixation, incomplete blocking of endogenous peroxidase or endogenous biotin, spurious staining of cells that have phagocytized other cells, and high concentration of the primary antibody. Thick samples tend to trap reagents and produce background staining. Carcinoma cells in fluids often express vimentin and lose their immunoreactivity for CKs; antigens shed into effusion fluid can be absorbed onto the surfaces of other cells present in the same fluid. Some antigens in cytopathologic samples such as factor VIII-rAg and Igs may diffuse into the surrounding tissue, contributing to incorrect interpretation of immunostaining (Ramos-Vara and Miller, 2014). To avoid overstaining because of the concentration of the primary antibody, retitration of primary antibodies on cytopathologic preparations is recommended. Other causes of background staining are included elsewhere (Ramos-Vara et al., 2016). When using detection kits that recognize primary antibodies made in the same species than the tissue or cell examined, extensive background in both positive and negative controls is observed because of the presence of endogenous Igs recognized by the secondary antibody. A similar problem is observed with rabbit monoclonal antibodies tested on rabbit tissues or mouse monoclonal antibodies tested on mouse tissues. Special detection procedures are commercially available to avoid this background staining. Figures 18.1 to 18.15 show examples of inappropriate methods, materials, nonspecific staining, and interpretation.

False-positive reactions may reflect endogenous biotin if an avidin or biotin blocking step is not performed. The vitamin biotin is found in tissues such as the liver, kidney, adrenal cortex, pancreas, thyroid and parathyroid, and adipose tissue (Fetsch and Abati, 2004). When using CD79a (HM-57 clone), it is not unusual to see diffuse cytoplasmic staining that is considered a nonspecific reaction (see Fig. 18.7).

Other causes of false-negative staining are improper fixation, inadequate antibody titration, insufficient AR, or cell damage during slide preparation (Chivukula and Dabbs, 2010).

Although not an example of nonspecific background staining, it is very important in ICC to distinguish positive staining in normal or reactive cells from that in neoplastic cells. This distinction can be challenging when the number of reactive cells is higher than that of the neoplastic cells (e.g., T cell–rich B-cell lymphoma). An overwhelming positively stained reactive lymphoid cell population may overshadow the negatively stained Langerhans cells in regressing histiocytomas, leading to a false-positive interpretation of lymphoid neoplasia (see Fig. 18.15).

Use of Controls

The use of positive and negative controls is well established and is standard for human and veterinary IHC procedures (Ramos-Vara et al., 2008; Ramos-Vara et al., 2016). Positive and negative controls for ICC must be performed with each test sample using a comparably fixed cytopathology sample (Arnold et al., 2019). In one review of the human ICC literature, only 13% of publications listed positive and negative controls processed identical to the samples; 54% did not mention the use of controls or processed controls separately (Colasacco et al., 2010).

Cytopathologic control preparations fixed in acetone will lose antigenicity after 4 to 5 months even if wrapped in aluminum foil and refrigerated; control samples fixed in formalin retain their antigenicity indefinitely (Raskin et al., 2019; Valli et al., 2009). The production of cytopathologic controls from organs (e.g., lymph node, liver) is described elsewhere (Valli et al., 2009). The ideal positive cell control should demonstrate immunoreactivity

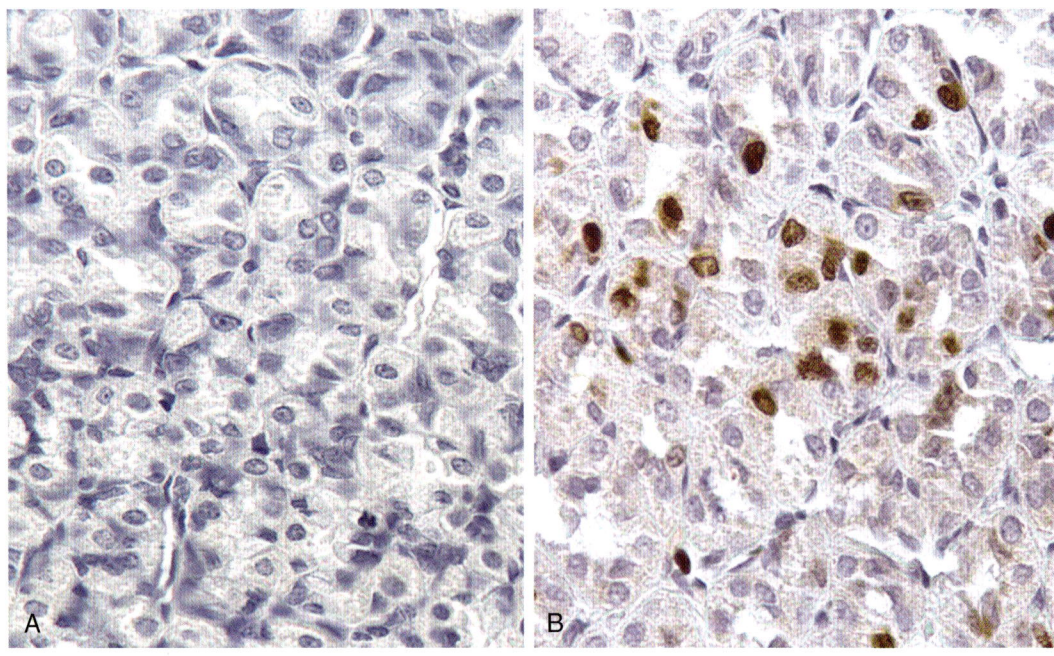

FIGURE 18.1 Troubleshooting in immunohistochemistry. Aged tissue. Same case in A and B. **A,** Tissue section cut several weeks before immunohistochemical testing shows no staining for Ki67 as a result of tissue section aging. (HP; Anti-Ki67/DAB.) **B,** Compare the same tissue section when cut fresh and immunohistochemistry is performed, which shows Ki67 nuclear staining in several cells. (IP; Anti-Ki67/DAB) (Courtesy Kim Maratea, Purdue University.)

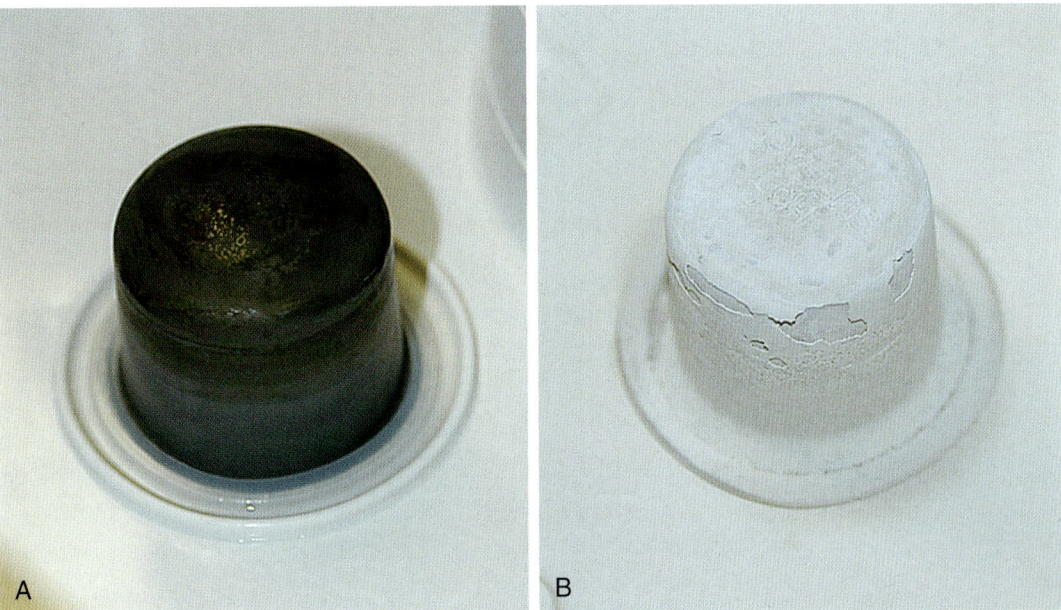

■ **FIGURE 18.2 Troubleshooting in immunohistochemistry.** **Temperature fluctuation.** Same equipment in A and B. **A,** A clean heating unit of a steamer used for antigen retrieval is shown, which helps avoid fluctuations in the incubation temperature. **B,** Note the buildup of salt deposits in the steamer heating unit.

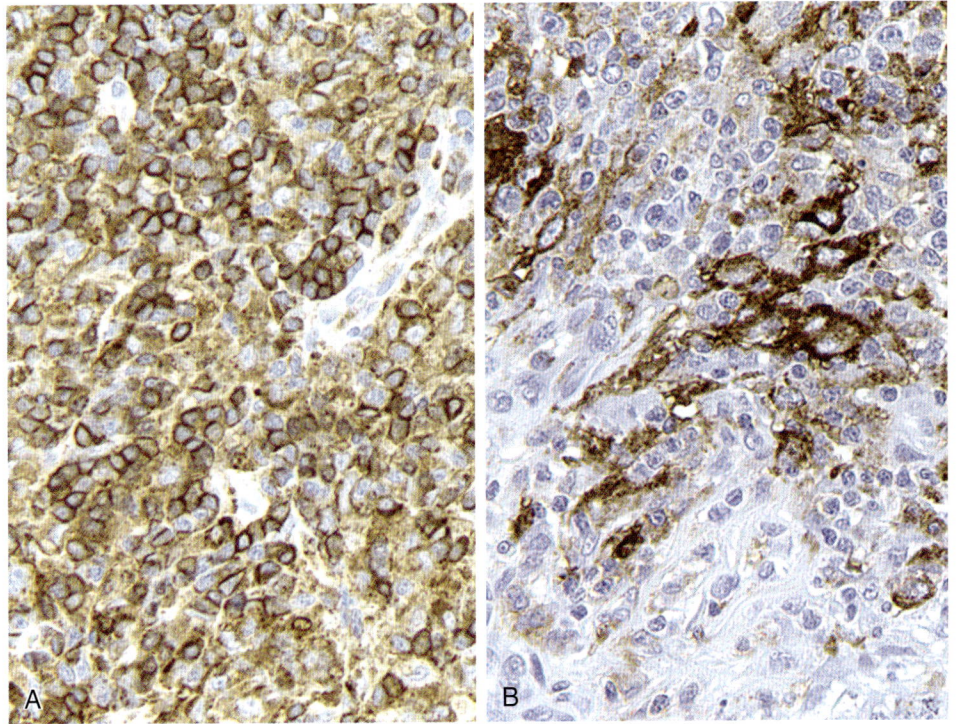

■ **FIGURE 18.3 Troubleshooting in immunohistochemistry.** **Antigen retrieval.** **Skin mass section.** Same tissue in A and B. **A,** Antigen retrieval (HIER with citrate) demonstrates major histocompatibility II–positive cells that include lymphocytes and histiocytes in a case of regressing canine cutaneous histiocytoma. (IP; anti-MHCII/DAB.) **B,** Note only dendritic (Langerhans) cells are demonstrated when not using antigen retrieval. (IP; anti-MHCII/DAB.)

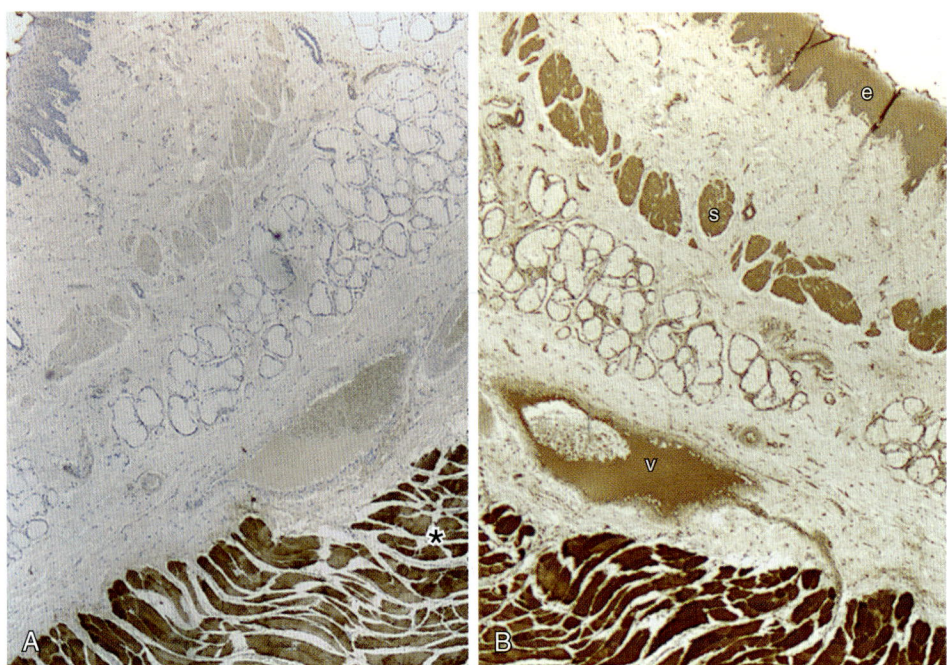

■ **FIGURE 18.4 Troubleshooting in immunohistochemistry. Nonspecific staining. Esophagus section.** Same tissue in A and B. **A,** Myoglobin is only detected in striated muscle *(asterisk)* of the esophagus when no antigen retrieval is used (IP; anti-myoglobin/DAB.) **B,** Nonspecific staining caused by antigen retrieval with proteinase K in blood vessels (v), smooth muscle (s), and mucosal epithelium (e).

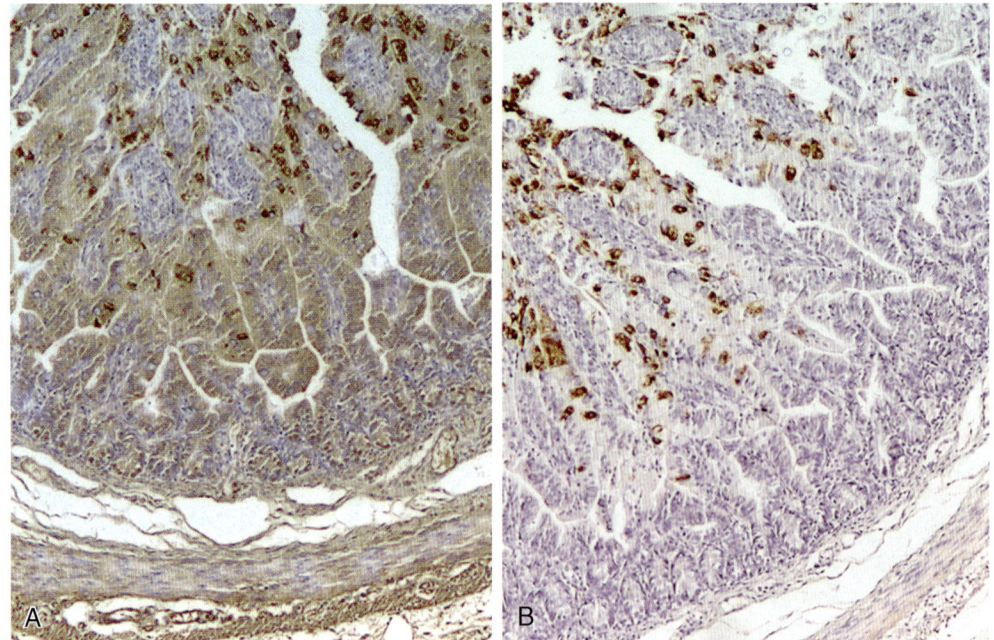

■ **FIGURE 18.5 Troubleshooting in immunohistochemistry. Antibody concentration. Intestine section.** Same case in A and B. **A,** The primary antibody is too concentrated and nonspecifically reacts with many cells. (LP; anti-rotavirus A/DAB.) **B,** Optimal dilution of the primary antibody shows reactivity for anti–rotavirus A only in infected cells of this section of small intestine. (IP; anti-rotavirus A/DAB.)

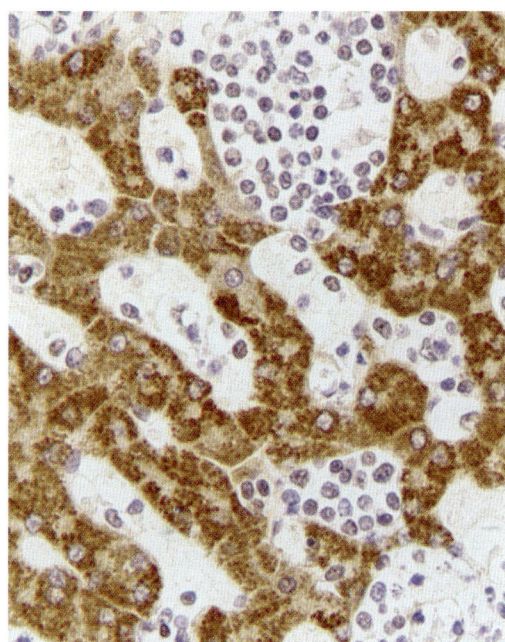

■ **FIGURE 18.6 Troubleshooting in immunohistochemistry. Inappropriate tissue reaction. Liver section.** Strong staining of hepatocytes with antibody to CD79a, a B-cell marker. (IP; anti-CD79a/DAB.)

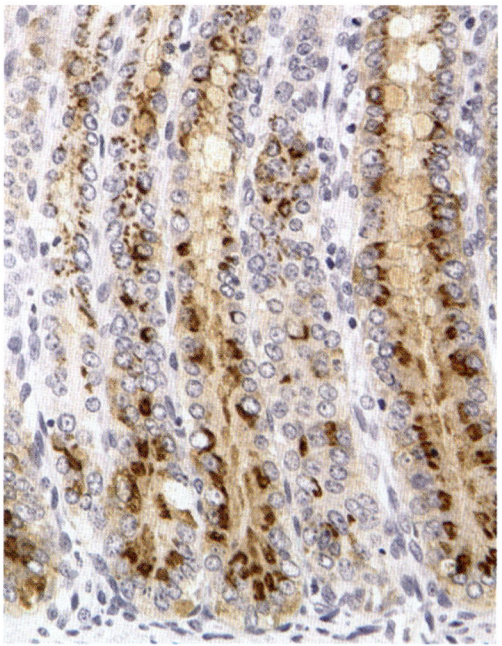

■ **FIGURE 18.8 Troubleshooting in immunohistochemistry. Atypical stain reaction. Intestine section.** The majority of epithelial cells in this section of small intestine have strong supranuclear staining with anti–rotavirus A, which was considered nonspecific. Similar staining (supranuclear) has been observed in different mucosal epithelia with other monoclonal antibodies targeting infectious agents. (IP; anti-rotavirus A/DAB.)

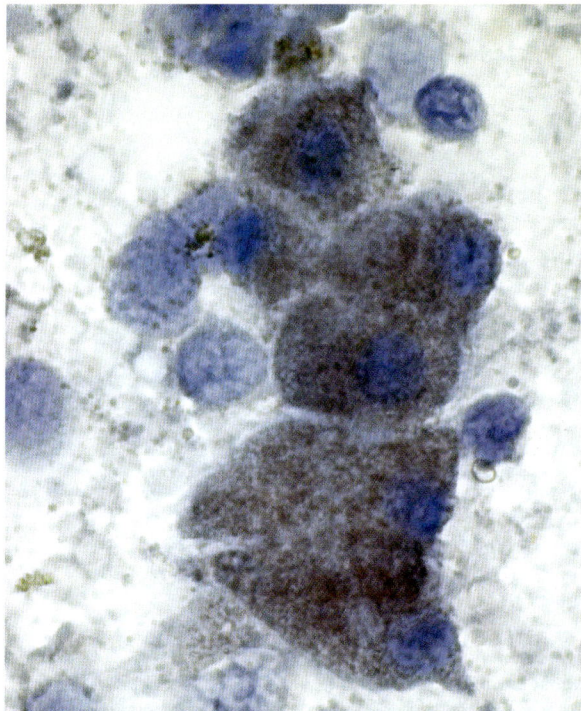

■ **FIGURE 18.7 Troubleshooting in immunocytochemistry. Inappropriate tissue reaction. Liver aspirate.** Diffuse cytoplasmic staining of hepatocytes by a lymphocyte marker. With avidin-biotin staining methods, tissues containing the vitamin biotin, such as the liver, stain positive. (IP oil; anti-CD79a/AEC.) (Courtesy Rose Raskin, Purdue University.)

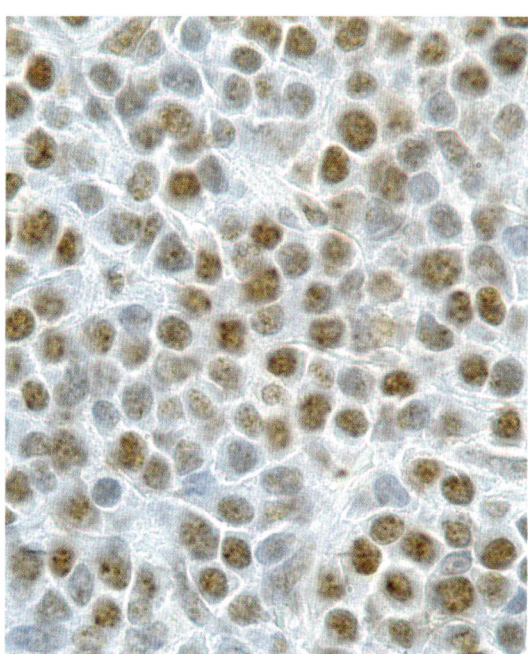

■ **FIGURE 18.9 Troubleshooting in immunohistochemistry. Atypical stain reaction. Lymphoid tissue section.** Sometimes CD79a antibody produces strong nuclear staining in lymphocytes without demonstrable cytoplasmic staining. This pattern of staining is considered nondiagnostic. (IP; anti-CD79a/DAB.)

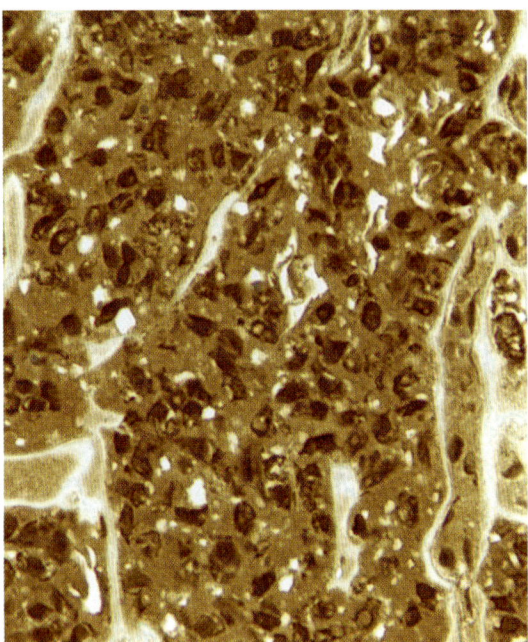

■ **FIGURE 18.10 Troubleshooting in immunohistochemistry. Autolyzed tissue. Parathyroid section.** Autolyzed tissues may show abnormal location of some proteins. Parathyroid gland shows strong nuclear and cytoplasmic staining for cytokeratins. (IP; anti-CK/DAB.)

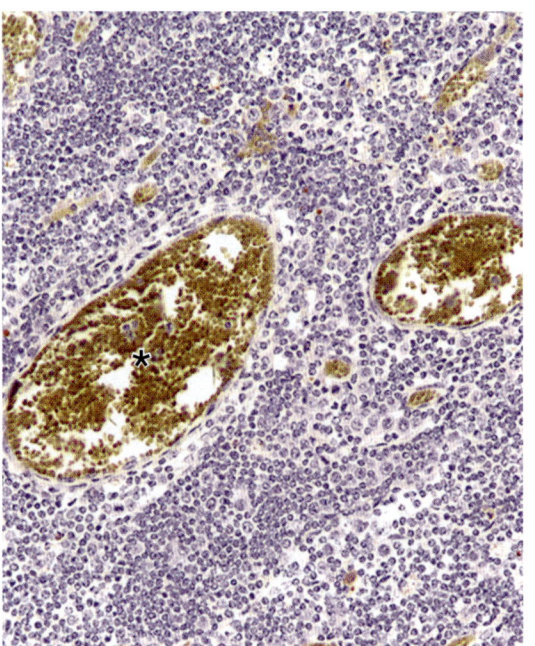

■ **FIGURE 18.12 Troubleshooting in immunohistochemistry. Endogenous peroxidase. Lymphoid tissue section.** This tissue was not pretreated with hydrogen peroxide to remove endogenous peroxidase activity. Red blood cells *(asterisk)* contain abundant endogenous peroxidase activity. (IP; unspecified antibody/DAB.)

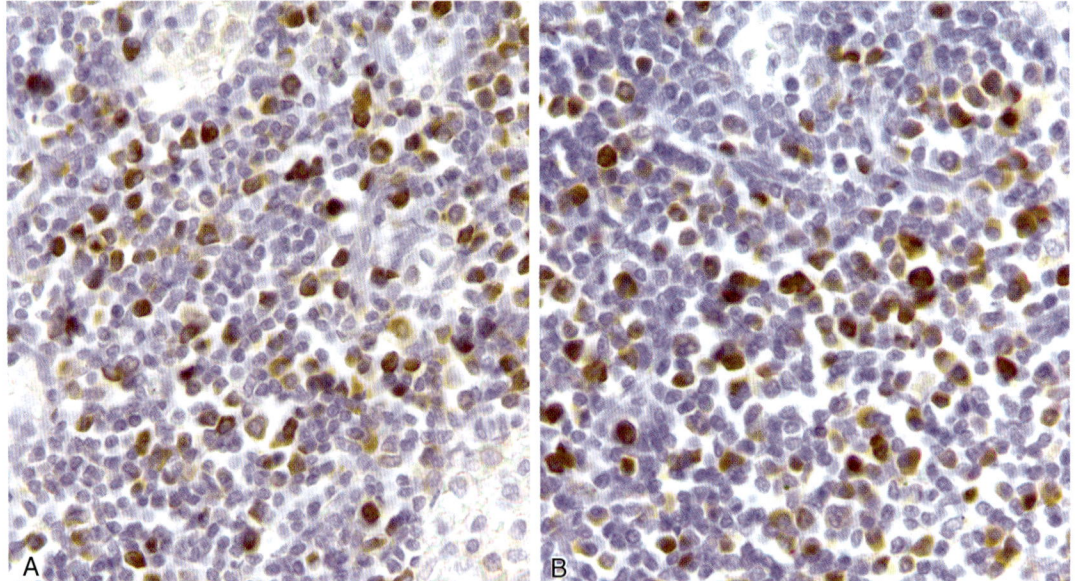

■ **FIGURE 18.11 Troubleshooting in immunohistochemistry. Immunoglobulins. Lymph node section.** Same case in A and B. **A,** Strong cytoplasmic staining with a primary antibody for natural killer cells. (IP; anti-NK/DAB.) **B,** A similar strong cytoplasmic reaction; however, the primary antibody is replaced with nonimmune serum. Use of negative reagent control section helps to demonstrate positive nonspecific staining by numerous plasma cells. These results are interpreted as binding of the secondary antibody to immunoglobulin-producing cells (plasma cells). (IP; nonimmune serum/DAB.)

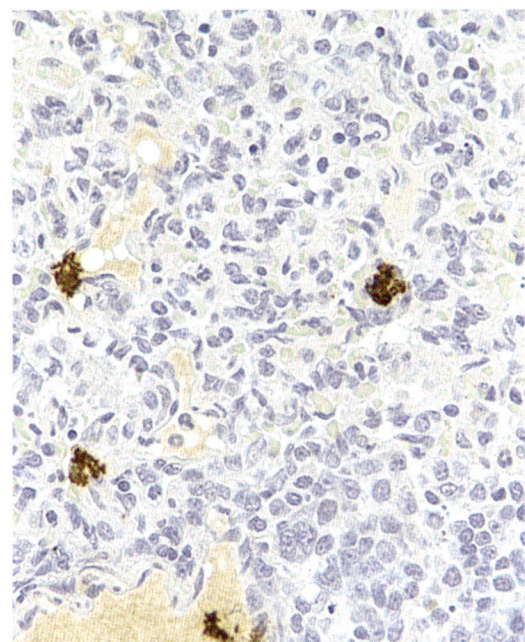

■ **FIGURE 18.13 Troubleshooting in immunohistochemistry. Chromogen precipitate. Tissue section.** Nonspecific DAB precipitate can mimic true staining. (IP; unspecified antibody/DAB.)

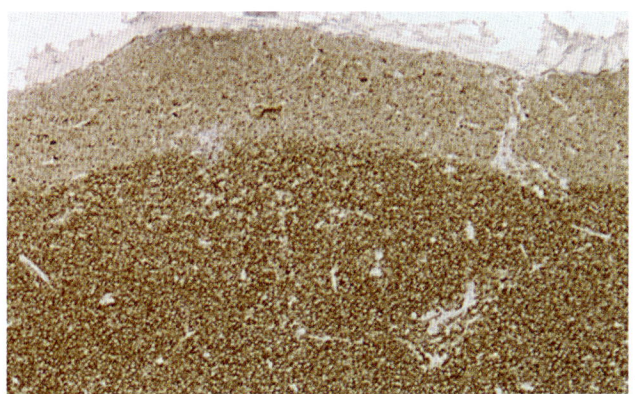

■ **FIGURE 18.14 Troubleshooting in immunohistochemistry. Improper incubation. Lymphoma tissue section.** The border of the section is less stained than the center because of loss (evaporation) of reagents during prolonged incubation (IP; anti-CD3/DAB.)

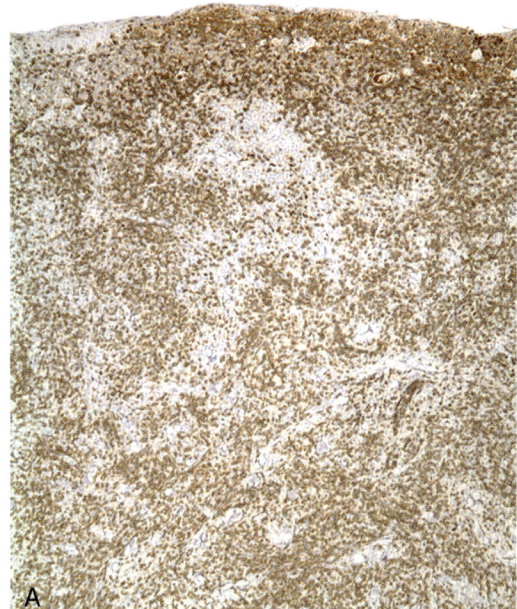

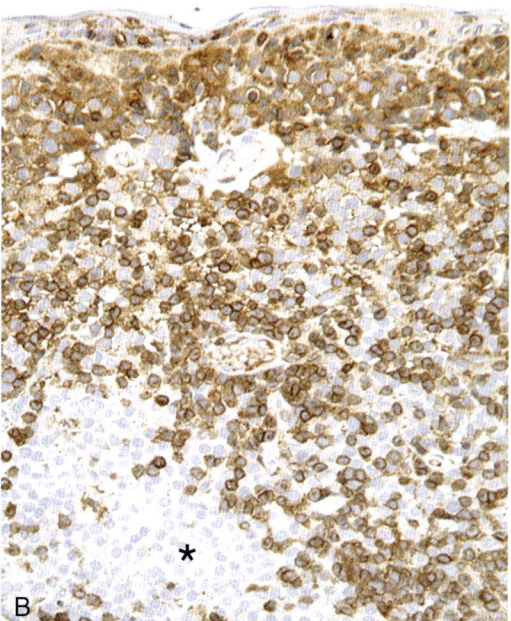

■ **FIGURE 18.15 Troubleshooting in immunohistochemistry. Skin mass section. False interpretation.** Same case in A and B. **A,** Low magnification of a case of regressing cutaneous histiocytoma demonstrates the more abundant positive reactive lymphocytes than neoplastic Langerhans cells. (IP; anti-CD3/DAB.) **B,** Higher magnification showing Langerhans cells that are unstained *(asterisk)*. (IP; anti-CD3/DAB.)

that is weak in some places and strong in others. A negative reagent control is also necessary for each antibody tested (Fig. 18.16). For the negative reagent control, either an irrelevant antibody, nonimmune serum from the same species as the primary antibody (and ideally the same Ig isotype for monoclonal antibodies), or Tris-buffered saline replaces the primary antibody (Fetsch and Abati, 2004; Raskin et al., 2019). The slide with the negative reagent control should be processed in an identical manner as the slide with the primary antibody. The negative control slide is used to assess nonspecific staining that is not the result of specific antigen-antibody binding (see Fig. 18.11). If only one slide is available, it may be used divided into test and negative reagent controls using a commercial hydrophobic barrier pen or by using cell transfer technique (Stone and Gan, 2014; Raskin et al., 2019). In some instances, a slide negative for one marker can be used to test a second marker. See the Appendix 2 for further information regarding these techniques.

Panel Markers for Diagnostic Immunocytochemistry and Immunohistochemistry of Tumors

The goal of diagnostic ICC is to maximize sensitivity without compromising specificity of results. A typical approach is to cover the main tumor types with antibody panels that include CKs (carcinoma), vimentin (sarcoma), S-100 (melanomas or

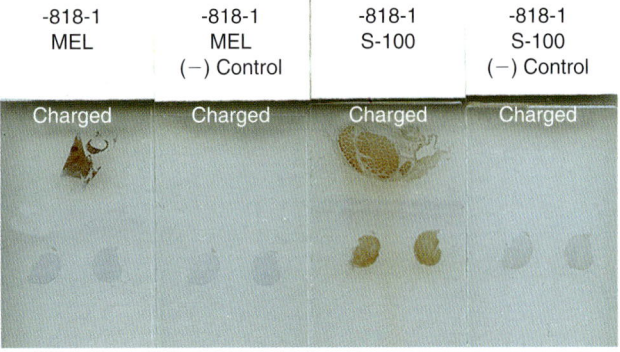

FIGURE 18.16 Troubleshooting in immunohistochemistry. Proper use of controls. Four slides show the results for the two markers, Melan-A and S-100. Each marker has two tissue sections on two slides. One slide is incubated with each primary antibody (slides labeled as MEL and S-100), and one slide each has the primary antibody replaced with nonimmune serum or immunoglobulins (slides labeled as (−) Control). It is advisable to add a known positive control to the same slide that contains the test tissue section (in this case, the positive control is the brown-stained tissue in the upper half of the slides). This case was positive for S-100 and negative for Melan-A (test tissues are in the lower half of the slides).

peripheral nerve sheath tumors), and CD18 (leukocytic neoplasms). To achieve maximum sensitivity, the use of "redundant" antibodies for a given antigen is recommended—in other words, the use of several antibodies that should label the same cell type. Table 18.2 lists cell markers and their use in the immunochemical diagnosis of tumors, with emphasis on organ systems. In human pathology, the following expanded panel has been proposed: pancytokeratin (carcinomas), CD45 and CD43 (lymphomas), S-100 and Melan-A or gp 100 (melanomas), and vimentin and collagen IV (sarcoma) (Yaziji and Barry, 2006). Some of these markers are not available or not reactive in animal tissues, so alternatives need to be found. After other clinicopathologic data have been examined, judicious use of antibodies is the best approach: it will reduce both the cost of testing and the need to explain unexpected reactions to the client. After a particular tumor group has been identified (e.g., sarcoma), more specific markers to determine the type of tumor are used. This approach is based on algorithms. Figure 18.17 shows a basic algorithm to characterize tumors frequently found in domestic species. This algorithmic approach is borrowed from the human experience; unfortunately, many markers currently used in human pathology are not reactive in animal tissues, or their reactivity is different. The lack of predictive behavior (percentage of positive cases of a tumor with a particular antibody) is one of the most difficult barriers to overcome in veterinary diagnostic ICC. Many antibodies with diagnostic or prognostic significance in human pathology await validation in similar tumors of animals.

Antibody personality profile (APP) is a concept introduced by Yaziji and Barry (2006). An APPF is defined by:
- Location of expected signal (e.g., CKs are exclusively cytoplasmic, S-100 protein and calretinin are cytoplasmic and nuclear; CD45, CD11 are in the cell membrane; and laminin, collagen IV are found only in the interstitium)
- Antibody pattern (S-100 produces a homogeneous signal; CKs, a filamentous signal; chromogranin A and Melan-A, a granular signal)

TABLE 18.2 Markers Used for the Differential Diagnosis of Major Tumor Categories

TUMOR TISSUE	MARKERS
Adrenal	Cortex: Melan-A, inhibin-alpha, calretinin Medulla: PGP 9.5, chromogranins, synaptophysin
Endocrine tumors (generic)	Chromogranin A, synaptophysin, PGP 9.5, neuron-specific enolase (NSE), S100
Epithelial vs mesenchymal	Cytokeratins (epithelial), vimentin (mesenchymal), E-cadherin (epithelium), claudin-1 (epithelial), p63 (basal cells, myoepithelium)
Leukocytic	CD45 (panleukocytic); CD18 (with emphasis in histiocytic cells); CD11d (macrophages, some splenic T cells); CD90, E-cadherin (Langerhans cells); lysozyme (histiocytes); calprotectin, CD163, CD204 (histiocytes, myeloid cells); Iba1 (histiocytes, dendritic cells, Langerhans cells)
Liver	Hep Par 1 (hepatocytes), cytokeratin 7 (bile duct epithelium)
Lymphoid	CD3 (T-cell), CD79a and CD20 (B-cell), CD45 and CD18 (panleukocytic), MUM1 (plasma cells), Pax5 (B-cell)
Mast cell tumors	CD117, tryptase, OCT3/4
Melanocytic tumors	Melan-A, melanocytic marker PNL2, NSE, S100
Muscle differentiation	Actin muscle (all muscle), actin sarcomeric (striated muscle), calponin (smooth muscle, myofibroblast, myoepithelium), desmin (all muscle), smooth muscle actin (smooth muscle)
Neurogenic tumors	S100 (neurons, glial cells), neurofilament (neurons); GFAP, Olig-2, CNPase (glial cells); glut1, nerve growth factor receptor (perineural cells)
Pancreas (endocrine)	Chromogranin A, glucagon, gastrin, insulin, somatostatin, synaptophysin, PGP 9.5
Squamous vs adenocarcinoma	Squamous cell carcinoma (CK5, p63); adenocarcinoma (CK7, CK8/18)
Testis and ovary	Sex cord–stromal tumors (inhibin-α, NSE); germ-cell tumors (calretinin, KIT, Oct3/4, PGP 9.5)
Thyroid	Thyroglobulin (follicular cells), calcitonin (medulla, C cells), TTF1 and Pax8 (follicles and medulla)
Urinary tumors	Uroplakins II and III, GATA-3, cytokeratin 7, COX-2, COX-1, p63
Vascular tumors (endothelium)	Factor VIII–related antigen, CD31, CD34 (blood and lymphatic endothelium); LYVE-1 and Prox-1 (lymphatic endothelium)

- Antibody-characteristic pattern across tissues and tumors (thyroid transcription factor-1 [TTF-1] stains most neoplastic cells in a pulmonary carcinoma; uroplakin III stains only a small percentage of tumor cells).

Knowledge of the profile facilitates accurate interpretation of immunohistochemical results. Keep in mind that APP may vary among animal species (Ramos-Vara et al., 2000; Ramos-Vara et al., 2002b).

Immunochemical Diagnosis of Anaplastic or Metastatic Tumors

The number of antibodies available for diagnostic purposes has increased exponentially in the past few years. This gives

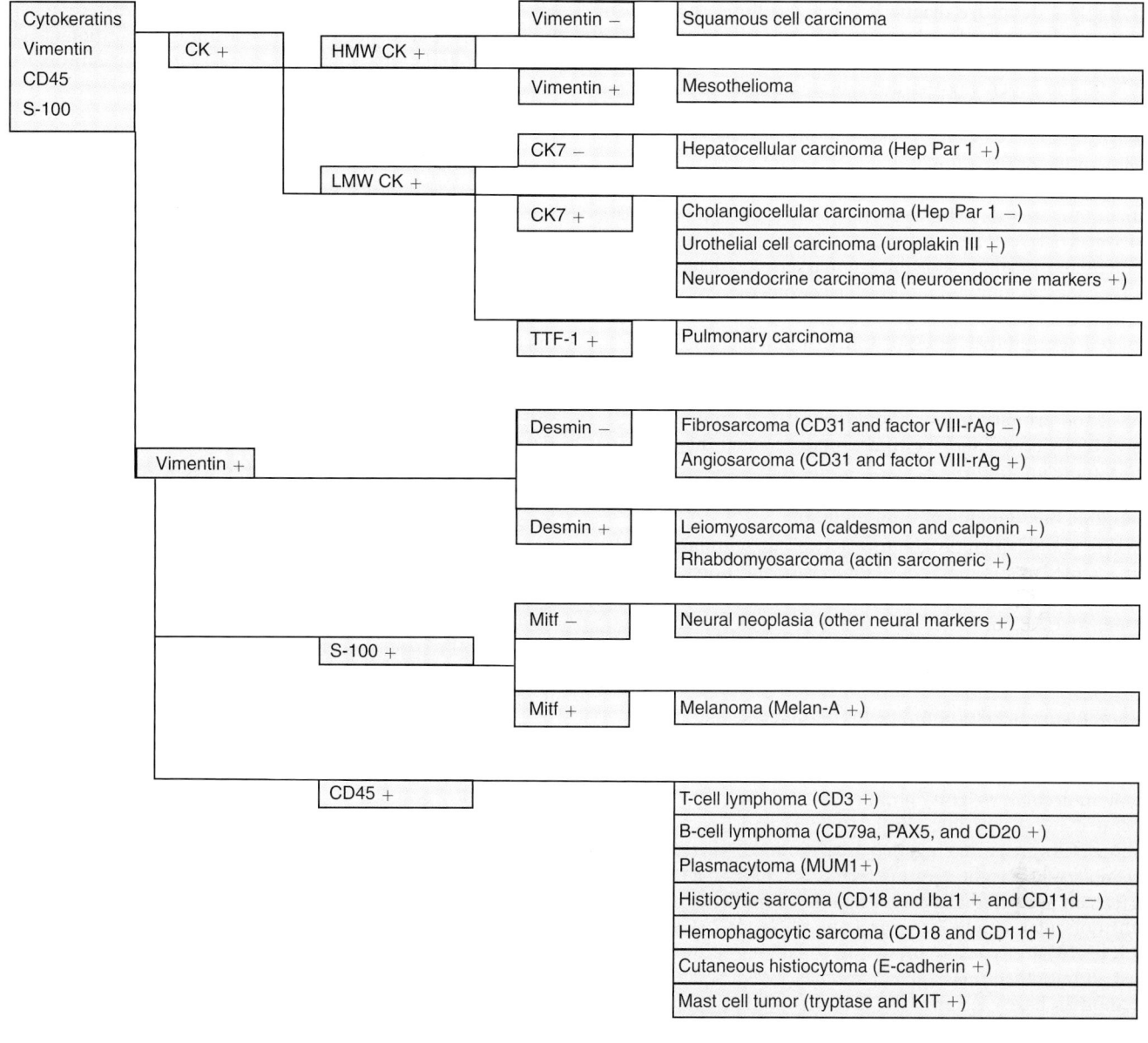

■ **FIGURE 18.17 Simplified algorithmic approach for canine tumor diagnosis using immunochemistry.** Cytokeratins, vimentin, CD45, and S-100 provide the starting point to help distinguish several carcinomas, sarcomas, neural tumors, and hematopoietic neoplasms from each other.

diagnosticians more opportunities to make a definitive diagnosis—or get more confused. Keep in mind that regardless of the number of markers used to characterize a particular tumor, the gold standard before attempting IHC should be hematoxylin and eosin (H&E) and for ICC the standard staining for cytopathology. A careful examination of H&E-stained slides will reduce the number of markers needed to arrive to a definitive diagnosis.

Even after that, it is uncommon to make a definitive diagnosis with only one marker because expression (or lack of thereof) of proteins in tumor cells may differ from that in the normal cell counterpart. Upregulation and downregulation of gene expression and the proteins codified by such genes is common in neoplastic cells. The use of tumor marker panels in the diagnosis of metastatic disease is key to improving the chances of arriving at a definitive diagnosis. An algorithmic approach to human carcinomas of unknown primary has been reported (Stelow and Yaziji, 2018). Considering the relatively low cost of IHC and the expenses of treating some tumors, clinicians are keen to get a definitive answer from the pathologist. A treatment tailored to a specific tumor will more likely improve the quality of life of the animal.

Modified proposed series of steps to characterize a metastatic tumor are listed (Bhargava and Dabbs, 2010; Ramos-Vara and Borst, 2017). The steps are (1) determine the cell line of differentiation using major lineage markers; (2) determine the CK type for carcinomas and possible coexpression of vimentin; and (3) determine if there is expression of cell-specific products, cell-specific structures, or transcription factors unique to specific cell types. The main difference with the algorithmic approach for a metastatic tumor is that without knowing the location of the primary tumor, the differential diagnosis includes more tumor types, and the tumor marker panel therefore includes more antibodies.

Determine the Cell Line of Differentiation

Markers should include keratins as well as lymphoid, melanoma, and sarcoma markers (Ramos-Vara and Borst, 2017). A basic panel of markers for small animals is pancytokeratins (clones AE1/AE3 or MNF 116), CD45 or CD18 (panleukocytic markers), Melan-A or PNL2 (melanocytic differentiation), and vimentin (mesenchymal differentiation).

Determine the Cytokeratin Type for Carcinomas and Coexpression of Vimentin

Cytokeratins comprise approximately 20 polypeptides with different molecular weights, numbered 1 through 20. They are separated by charge into acidic (type I) and basic (type II) keratins. CKs are paired together as acidic and basic types. Most low-molecular-weight keratins (e.g., CK7, CK8, CK18, CK20) are present in all epithelia except squamous epithelium, whereas high-molecular-weight keratins (e.g., CK1, CK2, CK3, CK4, CK9, CK10) are typically present in squamous epithelium. Almost all mesotheliomas and carcinomas, except squamous cell carcinomas, have CK8 and CK18. The coordinate expression of CK7 and CK20 is one criterion to classify carcinomas in human pathology. This approach has proven very useful in metastatic carcinomas of undetermined origin. Coordinate expression of CK7 and CK20 in feline and canine carcinomas has been reported (Espinosa de los Monteros et al., 1999). Results for CK7 were similar to those in humans, but major differences were observed for CK20 between both animal species. CK5 is a useful marker of myoepithelial differentiation in glandular tumors as well as for squamous epithelium and mesothelial cells. Although CKs are the typical marker of epithelial differentiation, they can be detected in mesenchymal tumors (melanoma, leiomyosarcoma, gastrointestinal stromal tumors, liposarcoma, meningioma, and angiosarcoma) but usually in only a few cells as opposed to the diffuse and strong staining of carcinomas and sarcomatoid carcinomas (Dabbs, 2006). Coexpression of intermediate filaments has been reported in certain human fetal and adult tissues.

Some carcinomas frequently express vimentin, particularly endometrial carcinoma, renal cell carcinoma, salivary gland carcinoma, spindle cell carcinoma, and thyroid follicular carcinoma. In a few cases, coexpression of CK and vimentin is observed in colorectal, mammary, prostatic, and ovarian carcinomas. ICC performed on synovial fluid preparations from a stifle joint and carpal joint and on prostate gland smears from a dog with metastatic urothelial cell carcinoma demonstrated reactivity to CK and uroplakin III, confirming that the neoplastic population in the joint fluid and prostate was both epithelial and urothelial in origin (Colledge et al., 2013). In this same case, there was coexpression of vimentin with CK on the metastatic tumor cells in the joints, suggesting epithelial to mesenchymal transition, which contributed to metastasis.

Expression of Cell-Specific Products

This group of markers includes proteins or glycoproteins produced by a few cell types. The exact function of some of these proteins is unknown.

Specific Immunomarkers

Every year, numerous scientific papers report the characterization of "novel" markers (antibodies) that are extremely specific for particular human cells or tumors. Most eventually are relegated to use in combination with other antibodies (as part of a tumor panel). This section presents some markers that are useful in the characterization of specific animal tumors.

Thyroid Transcription Factor-1

Thyroid transcription factor-1, a nuclear transcription factor, is frequently expressed in thyroid tumors (more common in follicular but also present in medullary tumors) and pulmonary tumors (Ramos-Vara et al., 2002a; Ramos-Vara et al., 2005). Other tumors, including mesotheliomas, are usually negative.

Hepatocyte Paraffin 1

Hepatocyte paraffin 1 (Hep Par 1) is consistently detected in hepatocytes and their tumors, with no staining of biliary epithelium, which makes it a good choice to distinguish these tumors, particularly when used in conjunction with CK7 (Ramos-Vara et al., 2001b). However, some intestinal, and probably pancreatic, tumors can be positive (Ramos-Vara and Miller, 2002).

Melan-A and PNL2

Melan-A and PNL2 are two of the most specific and sensitive markers of melanomas in dogs (less sensitive in feline melanomas) and certainly more specific than other classic markers such as S-100 and neuron-specific enolase (Ramos-Vara et al., 2000; Ramos-Vara et al., 2002b). It should be noted that many steroid-producing tumors from the adrenal cortex, testis, and ovary show strong reactivity for Melan-A (Ramos-Vara et al., 2001a). Protein gene product 9.5 (PGP9.5) is present in neurons, nerve fibers, and many neuroendocrine tumors; however, some canine lymphomas can express this protein as well (Ramos-Vara and Miller, 2007).

Uroplakin III

Uroplakin III, a major component of the asymmetric unit of the urothelium, is expressed in most canine urothelial carcinomas, and in conjunction with CK7, the number of urothelial carcinomas detected approaches 100% (Ramos-Vara et al., 2003). Uroplakin III has not been detected in nonurothelial normal or neoplastic tissues of dogs except in some prostatic carcinomas (Lai et al., 2008), which makes this marker extremely specific.

Calretinin

A marker widely used in human pathology to discriminate mesothelioma from carcinoma is calretinin. However, attempts to use it in canine mesotheliomas with a variety of antibodies have been equivocal. The use of both CKs and vimentin (usually coexpressed in mesotheliomas) is probably the best approach to distinguish mesothelioma from pulmonary carcinoma in animals (Sato et al., 2005; Vural et al., 2007).

Calponin A

Calponin A, smooth muscle–specific protein, has been evaluated along with p63 in canine mammary tumors (Łopuszyński et al., 2019). The study indicated p63 was more sensitive and specific than p63 for myoepithelial cells in mammary tumors. A list of markers used in veterinary pathology is included in Ramos-Vara and Borst (2017).

Antibodies as Prognostic Markers in Veterinary Oncology

Immunohistochemistry in oncology is useful as a tool to determine tumor prognosis or disease outcome. This is a topic of intense investigation in human pathology and not without controversy. Prognostic markers are currently under investigation for some animal tumors. Briefly discussed below are proliferation markers, telomerase activity, and KIT stem cell factor.

Proliferation and Cell Cycle Markers

This group includes Ki67, PCNA, and cyclins and in general indicates the proportion of proliferating or cycling cells in a given tumor; these markers correlate well with mitotic index. Malignant tumors generally have more proliferating cells than benign tumors, with some exceptions. Lymphomas, mammary tumors, melanocytic tumors, and mast cell tumors are probably the tumors in domestic species in which these markers have been studied the most extensively (Zuccari et al., 2004; Ishikawa et al., 2006; Carvalho et al., 2016). In mast cell tumors, there is good correlation between decreased survival time and Ki67 index and between the histochemical detection of argyrophilic nuclear organizing regions (AgNORs), which determine the rate of cellular proliferation (generation time), and decreased disease-free interval (Webster et al., 2007). Both AgNORs and Ki67 scores are considered useful prognostic markers for canine mast cell tumors, with Ki67 score used to divide Patnaik grade 2 mast cell tumors into two groups showing markedly different actual survival times study (Scase et al., 2006). PCNA score did not correlate with differences in patients with survival times of several types of tumors (Webster et al., 2007). The detection of cyclins in animal tumors has not been fully evaluated, but one study indicated prognostic significance in canine oral melanoma (Zamboni et al., 2020).

Telomerase

Telomeres are portions of repetitive DNA that protect chromosomes from degradation and loss of essential genes (Pang and Argyle, 2010). With each cell division, telomeres progressively shorten in all somatic cells until cells undergo replicative senescence or apoptosis. Telomerase is a ribonucleoprotein enzyme complex that synthesizes telomere DNA. In normal cells, telomerase is detected in male germ cells, activated lymphocytes, lens tissue, and stem cell populations but not in somatic cells. In human cancer, telomerase activity is detected in 85% to 90% of cases, and in dogs more than 90% of tumors examined have telomerase activity (Kow et al., 2006). Telomerase expression in dogs is significantly associated with tumor proliferation (Ki67 labeling index) or tumor grade (Long et al., 2006). Immunohistochemical detection of telomerase could be useful as a prognostic marker and tool to determine the therapeutic approach to cancer, but supportive evidence is still lacking (Argyle and Nasir, 2003).

KIT

The KIT protein, a tyrosine kinase receptor product of the *c-kit* proto-oncogene, is expressed in numerous tissues and cells, including mast cells and mast cell tumors. Immunohistochemical staining patterns of KIT in canine mast cell tumors have been used as a prognostic tool (Kiupel et al., 2004). In a normal mast cell, KIT is localized in the cell membrane; localization within the cytoplasm in mast cell tumors has been linked to increased rate of local recurrence, decreased survival rate, and increased tumor grade (Reguera et al., 2000). Additionally, paranuclear and cytoplasmic patterns in cytopathologic specimens stained with CD117 antibodies generally matched with the presence of the *c-kit* mutation in canine mast cell tumors (Sailasuta et al., 2014).

> **KEY POINT** Immunohistochemistry and ICC are a useful complementary adjunct to histopathology and cytopathology, and immunologic-stained preparations for the characterization of canine and feline neoplasia.

ELECTRON MICROSCOPY

Ultrastructural examination of tissues and cells is a relatively common ancillary method used in diagnostic cytopathology and histopathology. If the markers of ICC are structural or secretory proteins specific for a cell or tissue, then the markers of electron microscopy (EM) are subcellular structures such as organelles or matrix constituents. EM has contributed in great measure to an understanding of the structural features of normal and pathologic tissues. Although its use has declined in the last decade and partially replaced by other techniques, e.g., IHC, EM is still a very valuable tool to reach a definitive diagnosis in some difficult cases, particularly in peripheral nerve sheath tumors, some synovial sarcomas, pleomorphic sarcomas, and mesotheliomas (Dardick and Herrera, 1998; Mackay, 2007). New ultrastructural methods applied to biologic specimens have expanded the use of EM in pathology (Cheville and Staskos, 2014). Both EM and ICC should be used in a complementary fashion based on the type of diagnostic problem. As an ancillary technique, EM raises the level of confidence in diagnoses based on light microscopy.

Pros and Cons of Electron Microscopy
Advantages

- It is the only method to examine the fine detail of tissues and cells (organelles, inclusions, pigments, extracellular matrix).
- There is a wealth of information on ultrastructural pathology in the literature of the past 40-plus years.
- Although not optimal, formalin-fixed (and even paraffin-embedded) tissues can be used.
- It can identify infectious agents not previously reported (and therefore without specific antibodies or genetic probes).

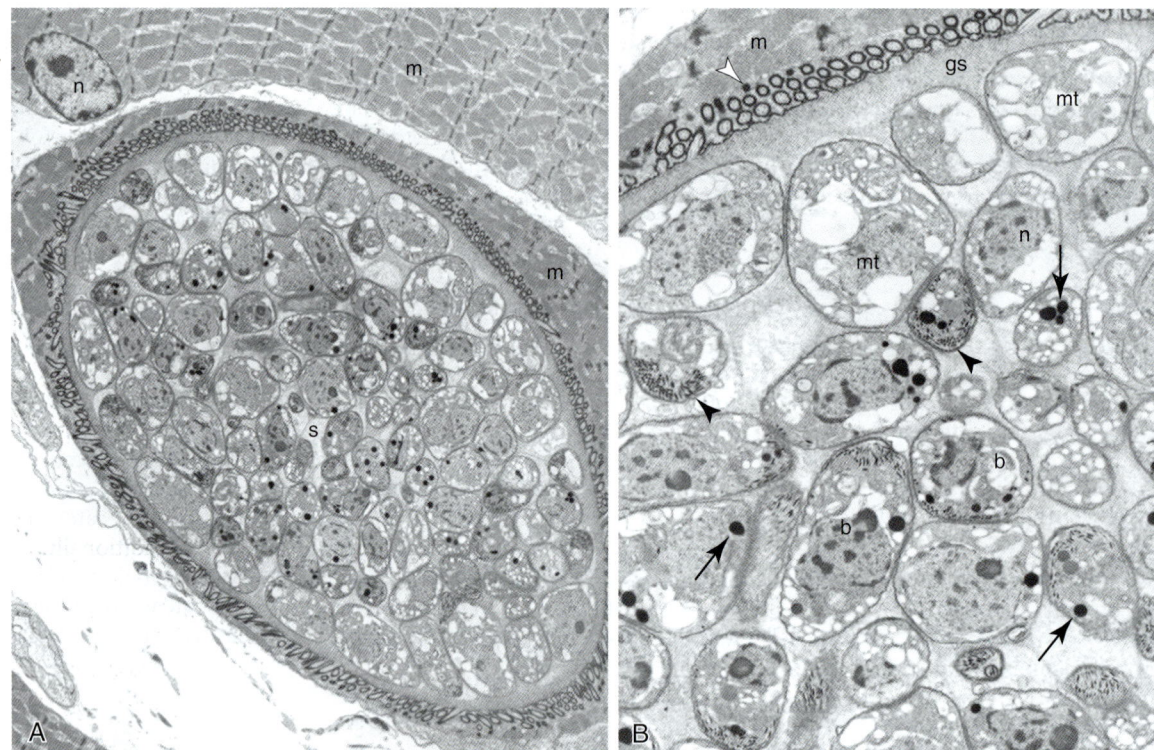

■ **FIGURE 18.18** Ultrastructure of microorganisms. *Sarcocystis*. Skeletal muscle. Mink. Same case in A and B. **A,** *Sarcocystis* cyst (s) within a skeletal muscle cell (m) along with its nucleus (n). **B,** Higher magnification of the *Sarcocystis* cyst reveals metrocytes (mt), bradyzoites (b), and ground substance (gs) surrounded by the cyst wall *(white arrowhead)*. Typical structures of coccidian parasites are micronemes *(arrowheads)* and rhoptries *(arrows)*. Skeletal muscle (m) contains the cyst. Note the nucleus (n) of a bradyzoite.

- Many microorganisms are more resistant to autolysis than eukaryotic cells (and therefore warrant ultrastructural examination in suboptimally preserved tissues) (Figs. 18.18 to 18.26).
- For some tumors, it is the most reliable method for diagnosis (Figs. 18.27 to 18.29).
- For certain lesions (e.g., glomerular disease), it is still the gold standard method (Fig. 18.30).
- Immunologic assays can be performed on EM samples.
- EM complements IHC and ICC.
- Cellular structures are nearly identical among animal species at the ultrastructural level. In contrast, IHC or ICC is often unable to demonstrate a particular antigen in a new species due to lack of interspecies cross-reactivity.

Disadvantages
- Sample preparation is rather tedious.
- Optimal preparation is only achieved with special fixation.
- Pathologic changes are sometimes difficult to distinguish from autolysis or processing artifacts.
- Sampling may not be representative because of small sample size (an important limiting factor for heterogeneous lesions); pitfalls include the presence of necrotic, normal, or stromal tissue.
- Overall, it is more expensive than IHC.
- It requires expensive equipment and highly skilled technicians.
- Examination of samples is very tedious.
- Dwindling numbers of pathologists have extensive experience and interest in ultrastructural pathology.

Basics of Electron Microscopy
Fundamentals
The principle on which the transmission electron microscope operates is similar to that of the light microscope (i.e., lenses are used to magnify images). The main difference used to produce images is in the type of radiation, which for EM is electrons, and the means to focus, which for EM is electromagnetic lenses. The resolving power of an electron microscope is around 0.2 nm or less, much higher than that obtained with a photonic microscope (200 nm) or with a fluorescence microscope (100 nm) (Ramos-Vara et al., 2016). Processing a sample for EM is basically similar to that for light microscopy, paraffin-embedded samples, but the reagents used are different.

Fixation
The speed of fixation is critical in EM to avoid changes caused by autolysis. For routine EM, glutaraldehyde is the gold standard, with secondary fixation in osmium tetroxide. These two fixatives are complementary: glutaraldehyde stabilizes proteins, and osmium tetroxide stabilizes lipids. Glutaraldehyde has a slower diffusion rate than formaldehyde, and very small samples (~ 1 mm^3) are required for optimal fixation. Formaldehyde is not an optimal fixative, but in diagnostic pathology, it is the most commonly used primary fixative for EM, particularly when ultrastructural studies are not considered initially in the diagnostic workup. Because of the impurities of commercially available formaldehyde solutions (e.g., formic acid, methanol), ultrastructural preservation is compromised. Tissues fixed in paraformaldehyde (an aldehyde from which formaldehyde is

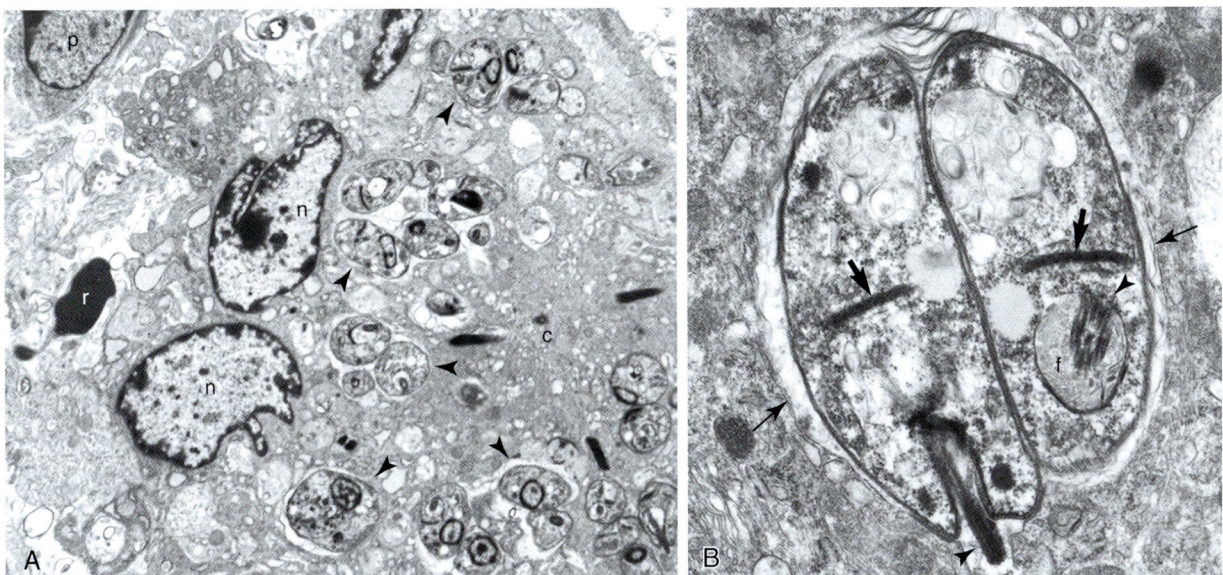

■ **FIGURE 18.19 Ultrastructure of microorganisms.** *Leishmania.* **Dermis. Horse.** Same case in A and B. **A,** *Leishmania* amastigotes *(arrowheads)* appear within a multinucleate giant cell. Note the nucleus (n) and cytoplasm (c) of this cell. A red blood cell (r) and plasma cell nucleus (p) are partially visible. **B,** Higher magnification of two *Leishmania* amastigotes showing the kinetoplast *(thick arrows)*, flagellum *(arrowhead)*, and flagellar pocket within the parasitophorous vacuole *(thin arrows)*.

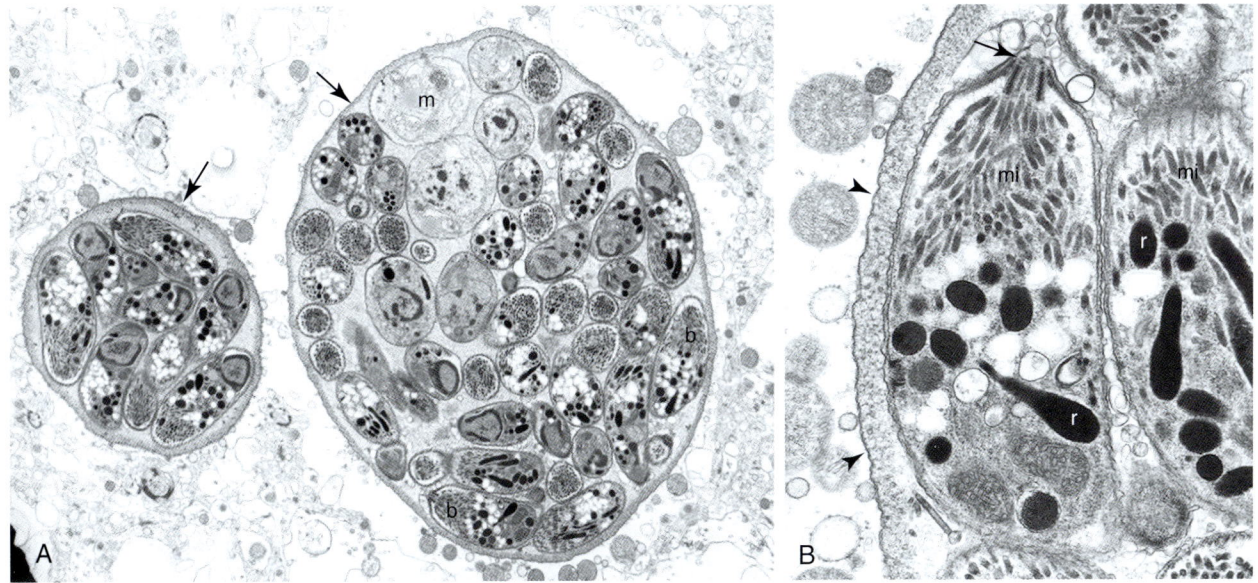

■ **FIGURE 18.20 Ultrastructure of microorganisms.** *Toxoplasma.* **Brain. Cat.** Same case in A and B. **A,** Two *Toxoplasma gondii* cysts *(arrows)* contain numerous bradyzoites (b) and fewer immature merozoites (m). **B,** *Toxoplasma* bradyzoites with conoid *(arrow)*, micronemes (mi) and rhoptries (r) surrounded by a cyst wall *(arrowheads)*.

produced) are more amenable to immunoelectron microscopy than those fixed in glutaraldehyde.

Processing of Fixed Samples

Fixed samples are dehydrated and embedded in a liquid resin that polymerizes to produce a hard block that is cut using special glass or diamond knives in an ultramicrotome. Epoxy resins are the standard embedding material, but for special procedures (e.g., immunoelectron microscopy) acrylic resins, such as Lowicryl and LR White resins, are preferred (Ramos-Vara et al., 2016). For cell suspensions obtained by aspiration, samples are pre-embedded in a protein medium (e.g., agar, bovine serum albumin). Pelleted cytopathologic specimens can be prepared by low-speed centrifugation of the cell suspension followed by removal of the supernatant and replacement with the fixative. Semi-thin sections (0.5–1.0 μm) are first cut to localize the most appropriate portion of the sample to section at an approximate thickness of 60 to 90 nm (silver to straw-colored ultrathin sections). Routine sections are usually stained with uranyl acetate and lead citrate (osmium fixative will also stain

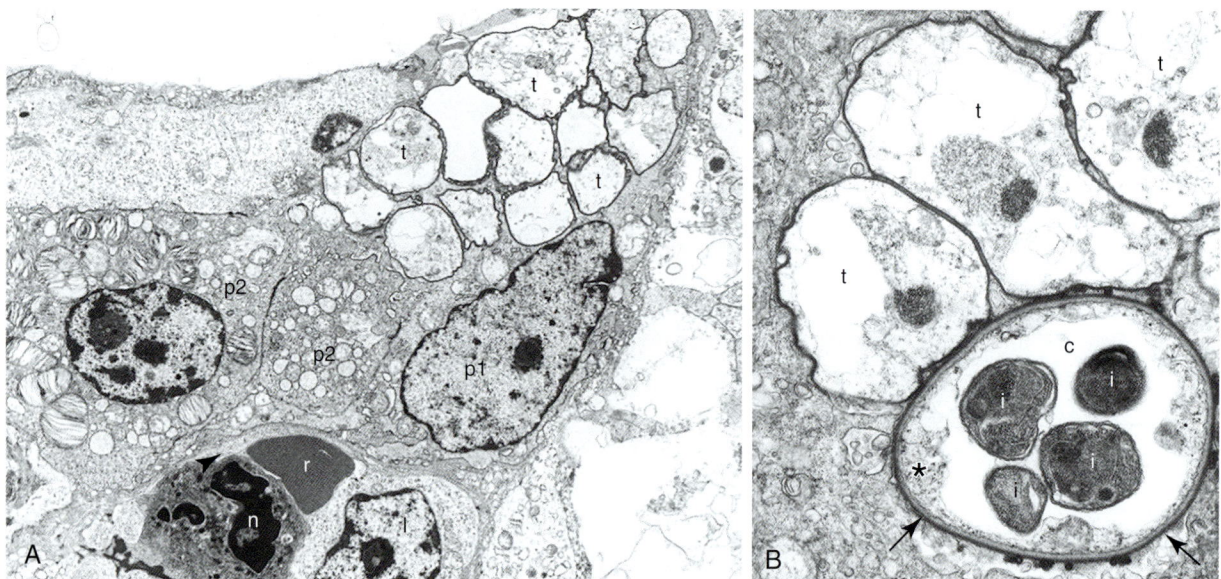

■ **FIGURE 18.21 Ultrastructure of microorganisms. *Pneumocystis*. Lung. Pig.** Same case in A and B. **A,** Numerous *Pneumocystis carinii* trophozoites (t) on the alveolar surface. Note the type 1 (p1) and type 2 (p2) pneumocytes, red blood cell (r), neutrophil (n), and lymphocyte (l). **B,** Three trophozoites (t) and one cyst (c) form. Note the cyst has a thick cell wall *(arrows)*, a rudimentary cytoplasm *(asterisk)*, and four intracystic bodies (i).

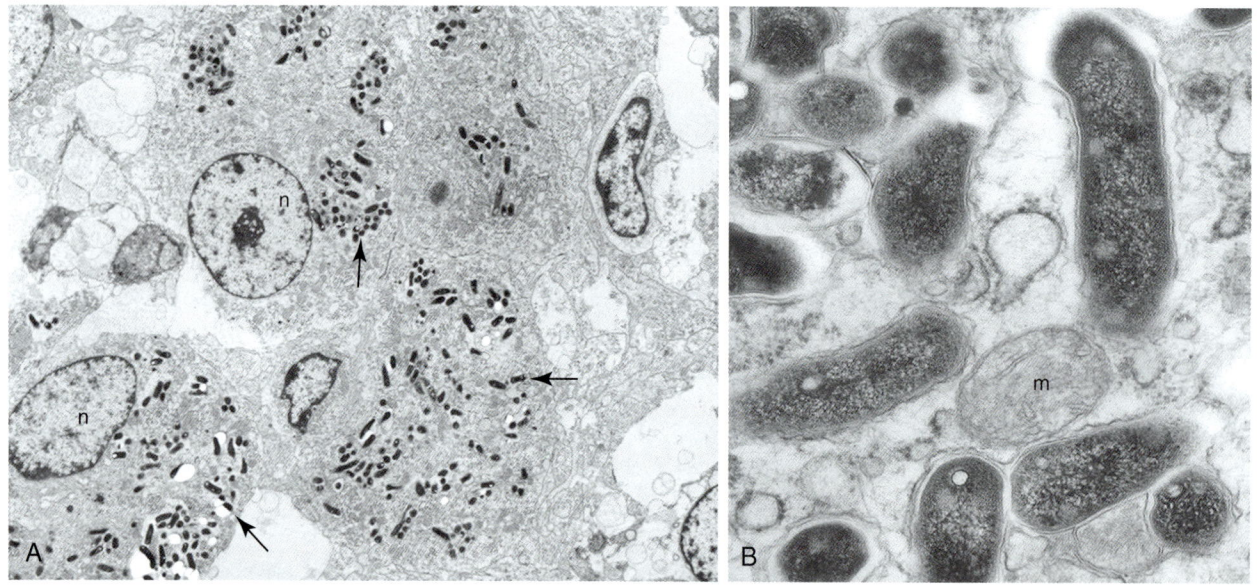

■ **FIGURE 18.22 Ultrastructure of microorganisms. *Mycobacterium*. Intestine. Goat.** Same case in A and B. **A,** Present within epithelioid macrophages are *Mycobacterium avium* subsp. *paratuberculosis* bacteria *(arrows)*. Note the nucleus (n) of the macrophages. **B,** Higher magnification of mycobacterial organisms, indicating a mitochondrion (m).

membranes and lipid vacuoles). FFPE tissues can be used when no other sample is available. Keep in mind that the degree of preservation of organelles and membranes in FFPE samples may be severely compromised.

Approach to Diagnostic Ultrastructural Pathology

Sample selection and interpretation of electron micrographs is heavily biased by the clinical history and light microscopy findings. After examination of FFPE tissues under light microscope, differential diagnoses are made, and additional ancillary techniques (e.g., EM, IHC) are requested for further characterization of that lesion. After examining a lesion by light microscopy, the pathologist will determine which features to seek at the ultrastructural level. During the ultrastructural examination, an experienced observer may find additional, unexpected features that prompt reconsideration of the original diagnosis. Formalin fixation or delayed fixation will probably create artifacts that may render the sample unsuitable for thorough ultrastructural evaluation but still be adequate to detect specific features (e.g., viral particles, parasites, inclusions, crystals).

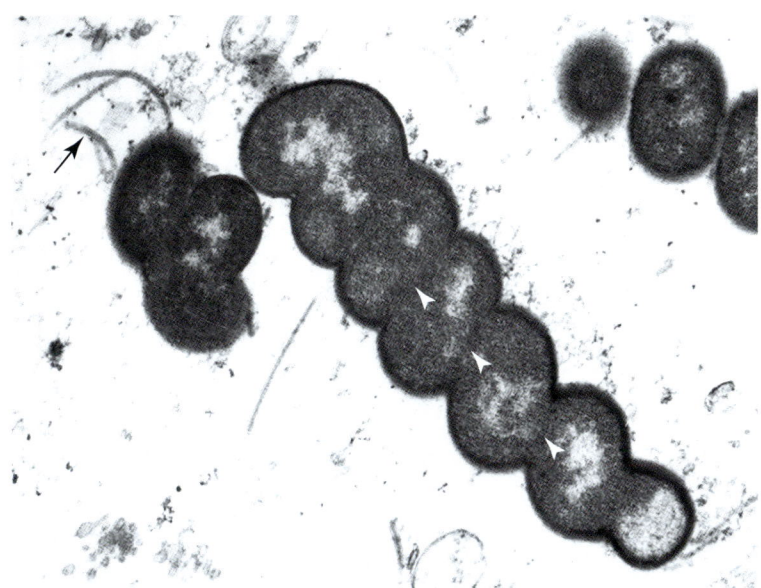

■ **FIGURE 18.23** **Ultrastructure of microorganisms.** *Helicobacter.* **Stomach. Pig.** Bacteria identified as *Helicobacter* sp. have a flagella *(arrow)* and periplasmic filaments *(arrowheads in white).*

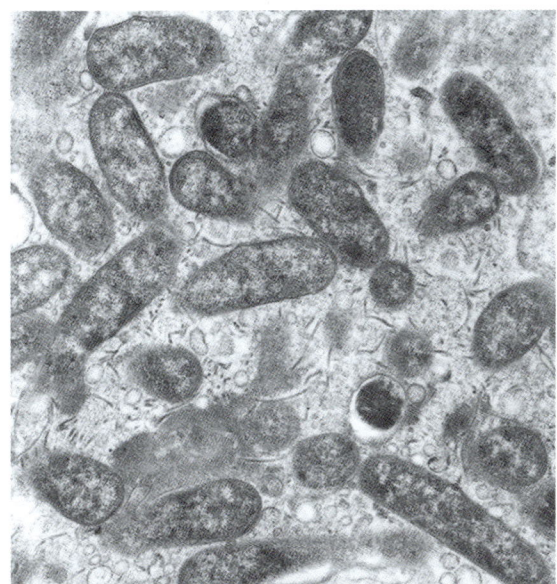

■ **FIGURE 18.24** **Ultrastructure of microorganisms.** *Campylobacter-like bacteria.* **Stomach. Dog.** Numerous flagella are observed in this field.

Buffered formaldehyde (pH of ~7.4) will reduce the loss of cellular components and tissue shrinkage.

In case of a conflict of interpretation between light microscopy and EM, reevaluation of findings is mandatory. As a rule, if discrepancies persist, light microscopy findings should prevail due to the far greater amount of tissue examined. However, the current specialization of pathology makes the use of multiple ancillary techniques (EM, IHC, polymerase chain reaction [PCR]) common in difficult cases and careful evaluation of all results must be made before establishing a final diagnosis. Malignancy cannot be determined on ultrastructural grounds.

Establishment of a malignant phenotype is in the realm of light microscopy and tumor biologic behavior, supported in very specific cases by immunohistochemical and molecular tests. Tables 18.3 and 18.4 are intended to give readers a general approach to the ultrastructural characterization of common tumors.

There are excellent atlases on ultrastructural pathology available (Dvorak and Monahan-Earley, 1992; Erlandson, 1994; Eyden, 1996; Ghadially, 1998; Dickersin, 2000).

> **KEY POINT** A sequential, orderly approach to the ultrastructural study of tumors involves the following: topographic cellular relationships, external lamina, cell contours, intercellular junctions; cytoplasmic granules, filaments, vacuoles, and vesicles; type and distribution of organelles; nuclear and nucleolar morphology; and stroma.

HISTOCHEMICAL STAINS

Stains used in histopathology and cytopathology bind tissues and cells by a chemical reaction. Histochemical stains remain important techniques in the characterization of numerous lesions and tissues. Before the advent of IHC and molecular techniques, histochemical stains were the main tool to characterize lesions beyond HE stain. The majority of laboratories are capable of doing these stains with the same equipment available for routine histopathology.

Advantages of Histochemical Stains

- They are easy and usually quick to produce.
- Most have standard and very reproducible protocols.
- Currently, numerous histochemical stains can be purchased as kits and used in automatic stainers.
- They have been extensively validated, and numerous variations to original protocols have been produced to improve their quality.

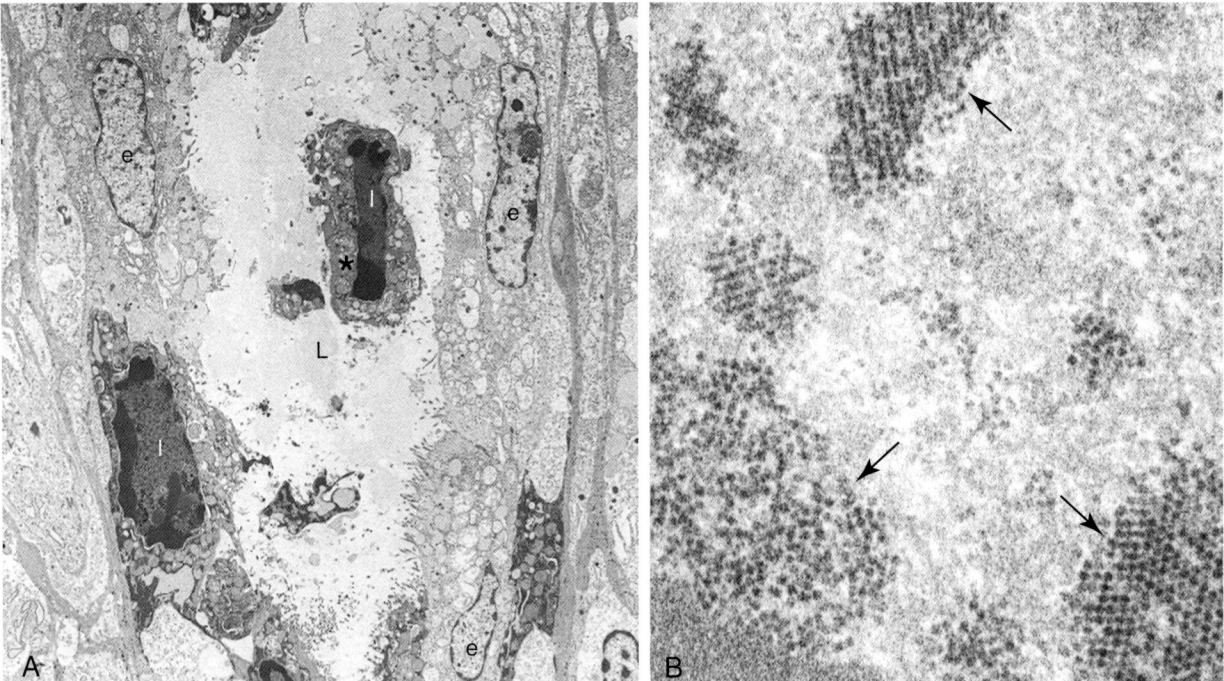

■ **FIGURE 18.25 Ultrastructure of microorganisms. Panleukopenia viral inclusions. Intestine. Cat.** Same case in A and B. **A,** Shown is an intestinal crypt lined by epithelial cells (e). Two epithelial cells, one free *(asterisk)* in the crypt lumen (L), have pyknotic nuclei and intranuclear feline panleukopenia viral inclusions (I). **B,** Higher magnification of feline panleukopenia viral particles forming distinct arrays *(arrows)*.

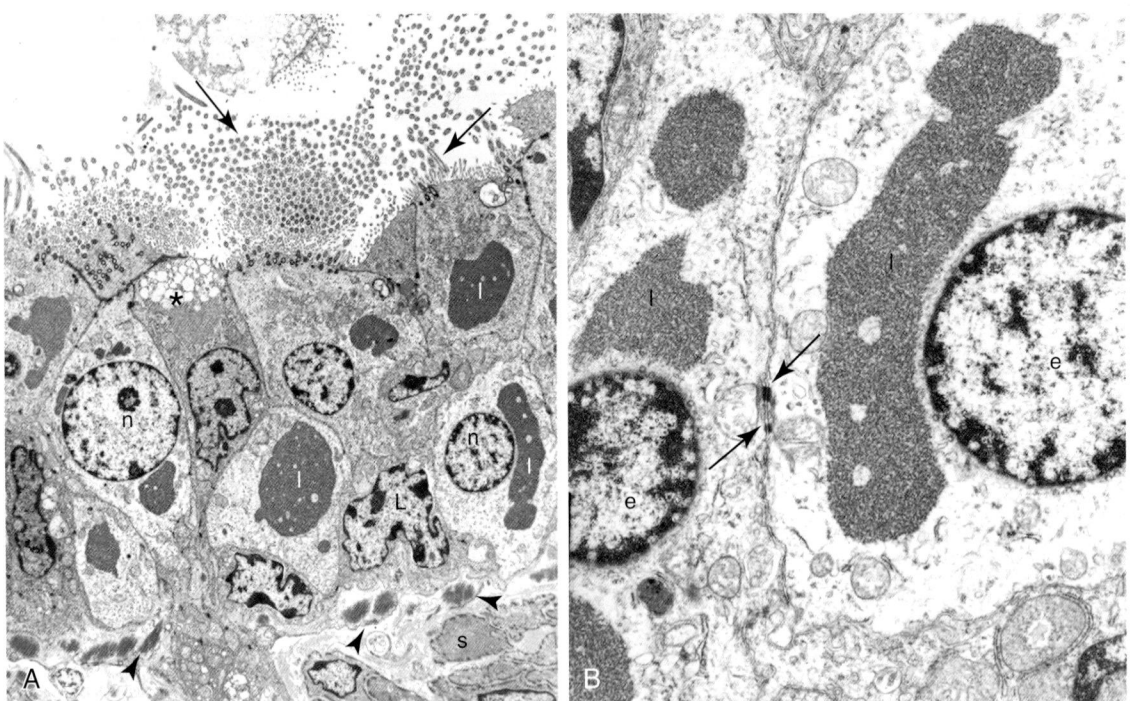

■ **FIGURE 18.26 Ultrastructure of microorganisms. Distemper viral inclusions. Lung. Mink.** Same case in A and B. **A,** Bronchiole with numerous ciliated cells that contain intracytoplasmic distemper viral inclusions (I). Note the nucleus (n) of the epithelial cells, many cilia *(arrows)*, mucus cell *(asterisk)*, basement membrane with collagen bundles *(arrowheads)*, and a smooth muscle cell (s). **B,** Higher magnification of bronchiole demonstrating distemper viral inclusions (I). Note the intercellular junctions *(arrows)* between two infected epithelial cells and the nuclei of the two epithelial cells (e).

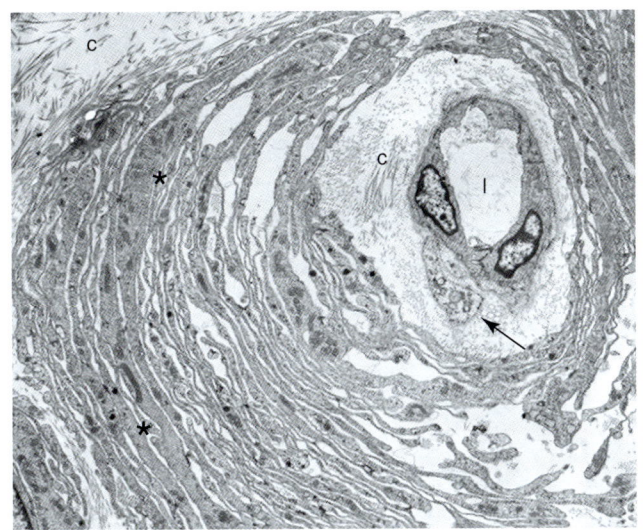

■ **FIGURE 18.27 Ultrastructure of mesenchymal neoplasia. Perivascular wall tumor. Skin. Dog.** Shown is a capillary vessel lumen (l) that is lined by endothelial cells, a pericyte *(arrow)*, and collagen fibers (c). Neoplastic pericytes *(asterisks)* form multiple layers around the vessel.

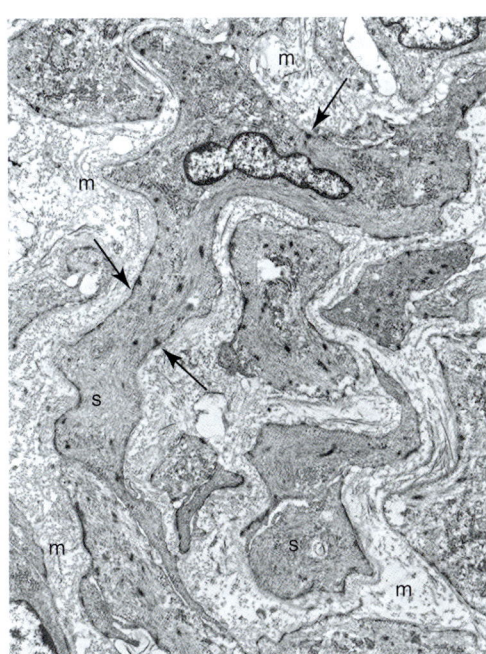

■ **FIGURE 18.28 Ultrastructure of mesenchymal neoplasia. Leiomyosarcoma. Intestine. Dog.** Spindle-shaped neoplastic cells (s) show characteristic subplasmalemmal and cytoplasmic densities *(arrows)* of smooth muscle cells. Note the extracellular matrix (m).

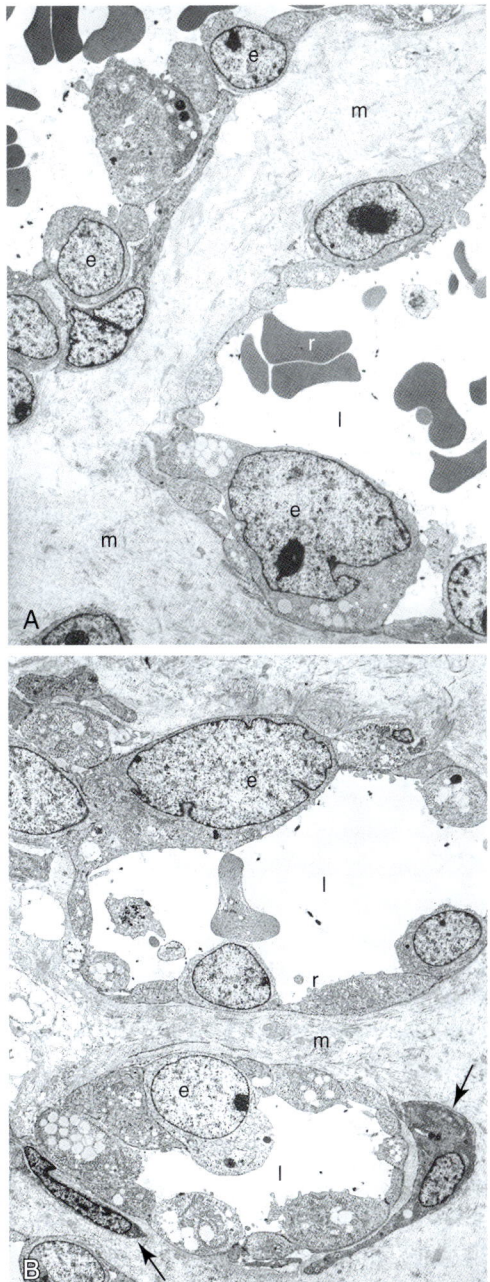

■ **FIGURE 18.29 Ultrastructure of mesenchymal neoplasia. Hemangiosarcoma. Skin. Dog.** Same case in A and B. **A,** Low magnification. **B,** High magnification. The neoplastic capillary vessel lumens (l) are lined by atypical endothelial cells (e) that have a large nucleus with abundant euchromatin and a prominent nucleolus. Also present are red blood cells (r), extracellular matrix (m), and pericytes *(arrows)*.

- They are relatively inexpensive.
- They detect substances to which there are no commercial antibodies to be detected by IHC.

Disadvantages of Histochemical Stains
- Some stains are somewhat unpredictable.
- Because of the nature of the histochemical reaction, large chemical groups rather than a small number of amino acids encompassing an epitope of an antigen as in IHC or short sequences of nucleic acids (molecular techniques) are detected; in other words, they are less specific than IHC or molecular techniques.

Staining Principles
Numerous factors contribute to dye–tissue affinities. They include (1) solvent-solvent interactions (e.g., hydrophobic bonding between enzymes and their substrates), (2) stain-stain

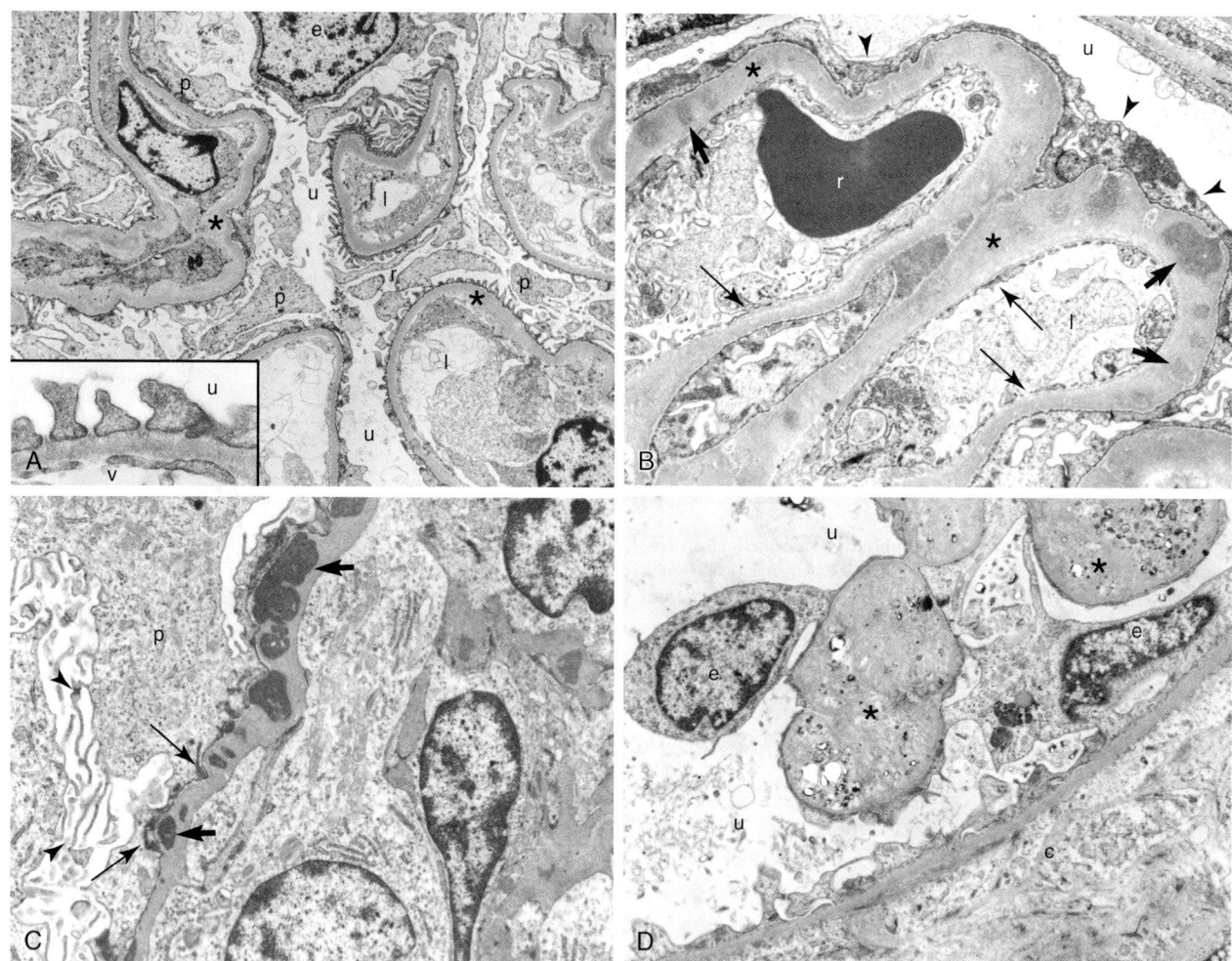

■ **FIGURE 18.30 Ultrastructure of normal kidney and glomerular disease. A, Normal glomerulus. Horse.** Shown is the urinary space (u) with basement membrane *(asterisks)* lined by podocyte processes (p). Note that foot processes of podocytes are distributed evenly over the surface of the basement membrane. Lumen of capillary (l) is shown. *Inset*: Higher magnification of the filtration unit of the glomerulus showing the urinary side (u) versus the vascular side (v). **B, Membranous glomerulonephritis. Cat.** Shown is irregular thickening of the basement membrane *(asterisks)* of the glomerulus from multiple immune-complex electron-dense deposits *(large arrows)*. Note the fused foot processes of podocytes *(arrowheads)*. Lumen of a capillary vessel (l) is surrounded by a fenestrated lining *(small arrows)*. Also shown is a red blood cell (r) and the urinary space (u). **C, Membranous glomerulonephritis. Dog.** Demonstrated is an irregular thickening of the basement membrane that contains multiple immune-complex electron-dense deposits *(long arrows)* with some in a subepithelial location *(short arrows)*. Note microvilli *(arrowheads)* on the surface of a podocyte (p). **D, Glomerulocystic kidney disease. Dog.** The parietal epithelium (e) is hypertrophic and distorted, containing abundant, mildly electron-dense material *(asterisks)*. The associated Bowman capsule (c) is expanded by extracellular matrix and surrounds the urinary space (u).

interactions (e.g., metachromatic staining with basic dyes, silver impregnation), and (3) reagent-tissue interactions. The latter involves Coulombic attractions (e.g., acid and basic dyes), Van der Waals forces (e.g., detection of large molecules such as elastic fibers), hydrogen bonding (e.g., staining of polysaccharides by carminic acid from nonaqueous solutions), or covalent bonding (e.g., nuclear detection by the Feulgen reaction, PAS stain) (Horobin, 2013).

Histochemical stains are used mainly to demonstrate specific chemical groups characteristic of a substance (e.g., glycogen, myelin) (Fig. 18.31 and Table 18.5) and to demonstrate the general morphology of microorganisms (e.g., fungi, bacteria) (Figs. 18.32 and 18.33; Table 18.6). There are excellent books regarding special stains and other aspects of histotechnology (Prophet et al., 1992; Carson and Cappellano, 2015; Suvarna et al., 2018).

FLOW CYTOMETRY

Although cytomorphology alone is often sufficient for cell identification, in many instances, more objective or detailed identification is needed to provide diagnostic or prognostic information. Flow cytometry (FC) is a valuable and readily available tool that allows the analysis of individual cells as they pass in front of a laser as a single cell suspension. The light absorbance and scatter properties of the cells can provide information about cell size and internal complexity or granularity, respectively, and the use of specific antibodies allows the quantification of both intracellular and surface-expressed components. The most widely used clinical application involves incubating cells with fluorescent-labeled antibodies directed at surface antigens to determine the frequency of cells that express the given molecule as well as the relative expression levels on

TABLE 18.3 Organelle Approach to Tumor Diagnosis

ORGANELLE	FEATURES	TUMORS
Basal lamina	50 to 100 nm-thick, moderately dense layer following the contours of the cell membrane	Epithelium, mesothelium, meningothelium, granulosa cell, Sertoli cell, muscle, nerve sheath, adipose, and endothelial tumors (Not present in hematopoietic cells, fibroblasts, neurons, chondrocytes, osteoblasts, or myofibroblasts)
Extracellular matrix	*Collagen:* cross-striated periodicity of 50 nm, 50 to 100 nm thick	Numerous epithelial and mesenchymal tumors
	Elastin: amorphous, moderately dense component and 10 to 12 nm tubular filaments in different arrangements	Chondrosarcoma; variable in mesenchymal tumors
	Proteoglycans: poorly stained, amorphous with occasional granular to filamentous structures	
Fibronexus	Cell-to-matrix structure composed of fibronectin filaments in the extracellular space and subplasmalemmal plaques with intracellular smooth muscle myofilaments	Myofibroblastic tumors
		Not present in smooth muscle tumors and fibrosarcomas
	Difficult to observe in formalin-fixed tissues	
Filaments, intermediate	~10 nm thick; located in cytoplasmic matrix	Carcinomas, neuroendocrine tumors, melanomas, sarcomas
	Noncytokeratin: vimentin, desmin, neurofilaments, glial filaments; impossible to distinguish them by EM; variable amounts; between organelles, forming bands of spheroidal masses	Squamous, basal cell, mesothelioma, endocrine, ameloblastoma, synovial, and epithelioid sarcomas
	Cytokeratins: tonofibril (bundles of cytokeratin filaments); loosely organized (nonsquamous epithelium, e.g., mesothelium) or high electron density (squamous and basal cell epithelium).	Myoepithelium (along with myofilaments)
Filament, smooth muscle	5 to 7 nm (actin) and 15 nm (myosin) thick with dense bodies and attachment plaques	Leiomyosarcoma, hemangiopericytoma, myoepithelium, myofibroblast
Filaments, striated muscle	Variable degree of differentiation (organization) of sarcomeric myofilaments (actin, myosin)	Rhabdomyosarcoma, rhabdomyoma
Glycogen	Small, pale to dense particles (30 nm) or rosettes (100–200 nm); empty areas of cytoplasm caused by extraction during processing	Muscle and liver tumors; variable amount in many carcinomas and sarcomas
Golgi apparatus	Packaging and biochemically altering proteins produced in RER; stacks of membranes	No specific tumor types
Intercellular junctions	*Desmosomes:* uniform width of 20–30 nm with intermediate linear density, subcytoplasmic membrane plaques, and tonofilaments	Many epithelial and mesenchymal tumors
	Gap junctions: closely apposed membranes (2-nm space) without associated filaments or dense material	
Lipid	Not membrane bound with amorphous to lamellar, variably dense matrix	Abundant in steroidogenic tumors, adipose tumors, sebaceous carcinoma, renal cell carcinoma
	Membrane bound if in lysosomes	
Lysosomes, primary	Small (100–300 nm), rounded, or oval, single-membrane–bound granules. Dense, homogeneous, granular matrix; crystalline core in eosinophil granules	Myeloid sarcomas, histiocytic sarcomas, follicular thyroid carcinoma, endocrine and steroidogenic tumors, granular cell tumors
Lysosomes, secondary	Variably sized, single-membrane–bound organelles with remnants of digested material	Granular cell tumor; myeloid leukemias, histiocytic sarcoma, prostatic and neuroendocrine tumors
Melanosomes	Rod-shaped or elliptical, 200- to 600-nm, single-membrane granules	Melanoma, melanocytic schwannoma
Melanosome, compound	Aggregates of melanosomes within secondary lysosomes; variable stages of digestion	Keratinocytes, macrophages, fibroblasts
Microtubules	Long, cytoplasmic, 25 nm diameter tubules	Abundant in neuronal and neuroendocrine tumors
Mitochondria	Rounded, ovoid, rod-shaped, elongated, branched, annular (1000 nm width); two limiting membranes and intermediate clear space; cristae represent infoldings of inner membrane; tubular or tubulovesicular cristae in cells with lipid and SER indicate steroidogenic phenotype (liver, adrenal cortex, Leydig, and ovarian cells)	Abundant in oncocytomas, hepatocellular tumors, renal cell carcinoma, steroid and muscle tumors
Mucin granules	Single limiting membrane granules with flocculent, filamentous, reticulate, or homogeneous matrix with no halo	Mucinous carcinomas
Neuroendocrine granules	Location: below plasma membrane, within basal cytoplasm and cell processes Size: typically 200–400 nm, with range from 60 to 1000 nm Center: very dense matrix (core) separated from the membrane by clear halo	Neuroendocrine, paraneuronal, neuronal tumors
	Small granules (80–150 nm)	Retinoblastoma, neuroblastoma, Merkel cell tumor
	Large granules (1000 nm)	Pituitary gland tumors
	Norepinephrine granules: eccentric cores	Pheochromocytomas, paragangliomas
	Biphasic (rounded and rod-shaped profile) granules	Abdominal and urogenital neuroendocrine tumors
	Crystal-like granules and sometimes multiple cores	Insulinoma

Continued

TABLE 18.3 Organelle Approach to Tumor Diagnosis—cont'd

ORGANELLE	FEATURES	TUMORS
Nucleus	Nuclear irregularities are common in neoplastic cells; artifact of sectioning with contained portions of cytoplasm (pseudoinclusions or nuclear pockets)	Multiple tumor types; nonspecific features, osteoclast-like giant cell tumors
	Multilobation: multiple nuclear profiles connected by thin bridges	Myeloid leukemia, large B-cell lymphoma
	Multinuclearity: nuclear profiles not joined	
RER	Common; active protein synthesis (immunoglobulins, matrix, neuroendocrine, lysosomes)	Fibrosarcoma, plasmacytoma, osteosarcoma
SER	Common in cells rich in lipid, glycogen, or steroid metabolism	Sex cord–stromal tumors, hepatocellular tumors
Serous/zymogen granules	Large (≤1000 nm), single membrane bound with a dense to pale matrix and no halo	Serous carcinomas (e.g., salivary, pancreatic)
Synaptic vesicles	40- to 80-nm, membrane-bound structures with clear interiors	Differentiated neuronal tumors

EM, Electron microscopy; *RER*, rough endoplasmic reticulum; *SER*, smooth endoplasmic reticulum.

TABLE 18.4 Common Ultrastructural Features of Tumors

TUMOR TYPE	CELLULAR FEATURES	EXTRACELLULAR MATRIX
Adenocarcinoma	Microvilli, lumens, junctional complexes, secretory granules, Golgi apparatus, ER, cilia[a]	Basal lamina
Carcinoid or islet cell tumors	Insular arrangement of cells	Basal lamina surrounding cell clusters, collagen
	Intercellular junctions (e.g., desmosomes)	
	Numerous dense-core granules (variable size and morphology depending on tumor type)	
	Variable intermediate filaments	
C-cell carcinoma of thyroid	Dense-core granules	Basal lamina surrounding cell clusters, collagen
	Variable number of organelles (Golgi apparatus, RER, mitochondria)	
Chondrosarcoma	Scalloped or villous-like cell surface	Variable; collagen, glycoprotein, glycosaminoglycans
	Abundant and dilated RER	
	Large Golgi apparatus	
	Abundant glycogen	
	Variable intermediate filaments	
Fibrosarcoma	Abundant RER	No basal lamina; abundant collagen
	Cytoplasmic filaments	
	Golgi apparatus	
	Filopodia[a]	
Gastrointestinal stromal tumor	Lack of distinct nuclear/cytoplasmic features or morphology similar to smooth, fibroblastic, or nerve cells	Basal lamina[a]; collagen
Glomus tumor	Epithelioid cells	Basal lamina; collagen
	Many mitochondria	
	Thin filaments	
	Dense bodies	
	Pinocytotic vesicles	
Granular cell tumor	Tightly apposed cells	Basal lamina around groups of cells
	Numerous cytoplasmic, membrane-bound, variable electron-dense granules (secondary lysosomes)	
Hemangiopericytoma	Palisading arrangement around capillaries	Abundant basal lamina and matrix
	Focal attachments and intercellular junctions	
	Pinocytotic vesicles	
	Intermediate filaments	
	Variable number of mitochondria, RER	
Hemangiosarcoma	Prominent junctional complexes	Basal lamina
	Villous-like projections on the luminal aspect	
	Pinocytotic vesicles	
	Intermediate cytoplasmic filaments	
	Free ribosomes	
	Some mitochondria and RER	

TABLE 18.4 Common Ultrastructural Features of Tumors—cont'd

TUMOR TYPE	CELLULAR FEATURES	EXTRACELLULAR MATRIX
Histiocytic sarcoma	Variably sized and shaped nuclei Numerous cytoplasmic organelles (lysosomes, mitochondria, Golgi apparatus, lipid droplets)[a] Phagocytosed red blood cells or leukocytes[a]	No basal lamina
Langerhans histiocytosis	Large, irregularly shaped nucleus Numerous organelles (mitochondria, free ribosomes, RER, primary lysosomes) Filopodia Absence of secondary lysosomes	No basal lamina
Leiomyosarcoma	Thin (6 nm) filaments and dense bodies among filaments within cytoplasm and subjacent to plasmalemma Pinocytotic vesicles Little RER Round-ended nuclei Contraction indentations of nuclei	Basal lamina
Leydig cell tumor	Lipid droplets Abundant SER Mitochondria with tubular cristae Microvilli on cell surface Canalicular-like spaces between cells	Partial basal lamina
Liposarcoma	Lipid droplets Pinocytotic vesicles Glycogen[a] Intermediate filaments Mitochondria[a] Golgi apparatus[a] SER and RER[a]	Basal lamina
Lymphoma	Many free ribosomes or polyribosomes No intercellular junctions Smooth, indented, or convoluted nuclear membrane	No basal lamina
Mast cell tumor	Round, indented nucleus Numerous membrane-bound cytoplasmic granules of variable density Filopodia	No basal lamina; collagen
Meningioma	Long, interdigitating cellular processes Numerous intermediate filaments Numerous intercellular junctions (e.g., desmosomes) Variable number of organelles Glycogen[a]	Basal lamina[b]
Mesothelioma	Numerous long microvilli Intercellular junctions Filaments Tonofibrils Glycogen Intracytoplasmic lumens Lack of mucinous granules and glycocalyx	Basal lamina
Myofibroblastic sarcoma	Spindle shape Prominent RER Some thin (6 nm) and peripherally located filaments with focal densities Fibronexus junction[a]	No basal lamina; abundant matrix with collagen, proteoglycans, and glycosaminoglycans; fibronectin
Osteosarcoma	Scalloped or villous-like cell surface Abundant and dilated RER Large Golgi apparatus Abundant glycogen	Hydroxyapatite deposits on collagen fibers (osteoid)[a]
Paraganglioma	Clusters of cells Round, dense-core granules Prominent Golgi apparatus Interweaving cytoplasmic processes Paranuclear filaments[a] Sustentacular (Schwann-like) cells with filaments at the periphery of cell clusters	Basal lamina surrounding cell clusters

Continued

TABLE 18.4 Common Ultrastructural Features of Tumors—cont'd

TUMOR TYPE	CELLULAR FEATURES	EXTRACELLULAR MATRIX
Parathyroid carcinoma	Islands of cells Intercellular junctions Interdigitation of lateral membranes Dense-core secretory granules Variable glycogen and cell organelles (RER, mitochondria, Golgi) Occasional clusters of oncocytic cells	Basal lamina surrounding cell clusters
Perineuroma	Whorls of slender cells with bipolar cytoplasmic processes Pinocytotic vesicles Scant organelles	Discontinuous basal lamina; collagen
Pheochromocytoma	Clusters of polygonal cells Large, pleomorphic, dense-core granules (sometimes clear or partially filled) Prominent Golgi apparatus No significant number of sustentacular cells	Basal lamina surrounding cell clusters, many small blood vessels
Plasmacytoma	Abundant RER Membrane-bound dense bodies[a] Intercellular junctions[a] Eccentric nucleus Paranuclear area with Golgi apparatus, centriole, mitochondria	No basal lamina, amyloid[a]
Rhabdomyosarcoma	Thick (15 nm) myosin filaments Z-band formations Sarcomeres Thin (6 nm) filaments Glycogen Mitochondria[a]	Incomplete basal lamina, collagen
Schwannoma	Long intertwining processes Variable number of mitochondria, RER, lysosomes Intermediate filaments	Basal lamina, collagen in matrix
Seminoma	Closely appositioned, round to polygonal cells Intercellular junctions Large, euchromatic nucleus Prominent nucleoli Abundant glycogen Variable number of organelles; mainly free ribosomes	Basal lamina[a]
Sertoli cell tumor	Polygonal cells Intercellular junctions Indented nuclei Junctional complexes Interdigitating lateral cell membranes Abundant SER Lipid droplets Mitochondria with tubular cristae Secondary lysosomes	Basal lamina, collagenous matrix
Squamous cell carcinoma	Desmosomes Keratohyalin granules Tonofibrils	Basal lamina

[a]Feature not present in all tumors or cells.
[b]Feature rarely observed.
ER, Endoplasmic reticulum; *RER*, rough endoplasmic reticulum; *SER*, smooth endoplasmic reticulum.

individual cells. Because antibodies can be labeled with a variety of fluorochromes that have different excitation and emission wavelengths, the expression of several surface molecules can be detected simultaneously. The major advantage of FC is that it allows the rapid and objective identification of large numbers of cells. Clinically, it is most commonly used for the analysis of hematopoietic cells to characterize lymphoma and various forms of leukemia and quantify cells in cases of suspected immunologic disorders.

The information provided in this chapter focuses on methods of cell preparation, antibodies, and data analysis for veterinary species. *Practical Flow Cytometry*, 4th ed, by Howard Shapiro is an extremely thorough text to which all readers should turn for detailed information about virtually any aspect of FC, including methodology, instrumentation, and data analysis. This e-book has been made available at no charge by Beckman Coulter and can be accessed through the website beckman.com/resources/reading-material/ebooks/practical-flow-cytometry.

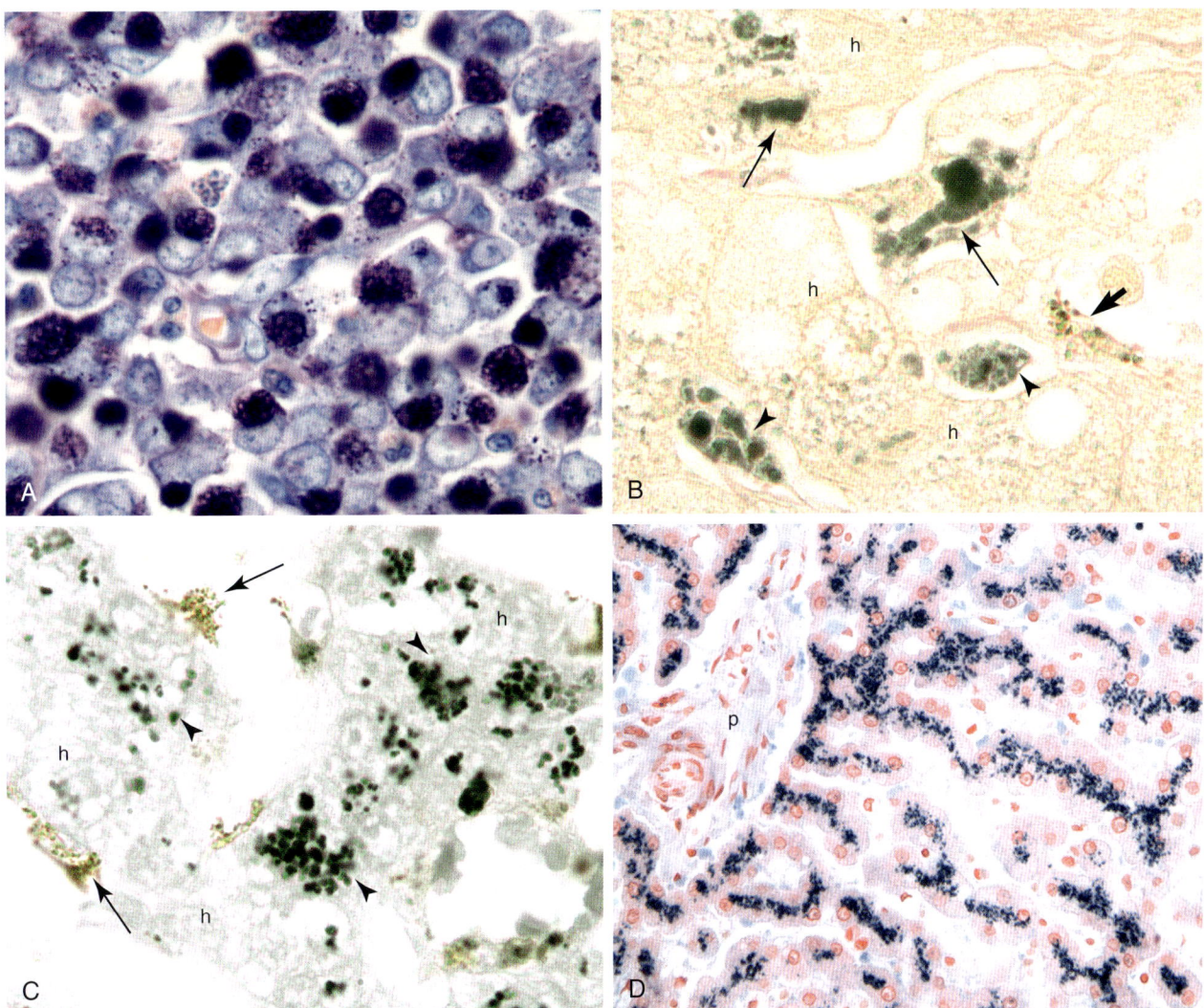

■ **FIGURE 18.31 Detection of granules and pigments by histochemical stains. A, Giemsa stain. Mast cell tumor. Skin. Dog.** Cells are filled with numerous dense metachromatic granules *(purple)* characteristic of mast cells. **B, Hall stain. Liver. Dog.** The green pigment present within bile canaliculi *(short arrows)* and Kupffer cells *(arrowheads)* is bile. Hemosiderin *(long arrow)* is not stained but is apparent because of its refractile nature. Hepatocytes (h) are noted. **C, Rubeanic acid stain. Liver. Dog.** This stain reveals copper granules *(arrowheads)* within hepatocytes (h). Kupffer cells with hemosiderin granules *(arrows)* are shown. **D, Perl's stain for iron. Liver. Dog.** Iron pigment appears blue within hepatocytes. The portal area (p) is shown.

Methodology

Sample Collection

To analyze a sample with FC, the cells must be in suspension and free of any clumping or debris. Anticoagulated whole-blood or cavity effusions can generally be submitted directly to an FC facility for analysis. Aspirates from solid tissue can be resuspended in media with serum. In university or laboratory settings, tissue culture media such as RPMI or DMEM, buffered with HEPES and supplemented with 5% to 10% fetal bovine serum is ideal. However, in the clinic setting, 0.9% saline can be used, and 10% serum from the patient or another animal of the same species can be added. Because a minimum of 10,000 cells is needed for each antibody combination, several tissue aspirates are needed for a complete analysis. One way to ensure a good yield of cells is to expel the aspirate into the saline-serum suspension and rinse the hub of the needle in the suspension. The suspension fluid should appear slightly cloudy rather than clear for best cell yield. If samples are to be shipped, they must be shipped overnight with a cold pack. Cian et al. (2014) determined some benefit in using Cyto-Chex BCT tubes (Streck) for cell stabilization of whole blood for immunophenotyping when shipping specimens to remote laboratories. However, CD45 and CD3 expression in normal dog blood was significantly decreased after 3 days.

Preanalytical variables. The increasing popularity of FC in veterinary medicine for the diagnosis of leukemia and lymphoma both in dogs and cats has led to an increasing number of samples being processed by specialized laboratories. However, the correct evaluation of preanalytical variables is fundamental to ensure to obtain a sample suitable for the analysis and to increase the diagnostic utility of this technique. The quality of samples could be influenced by several factors related to the animal, the operator, or the type of sample. Poor cellularity and

TABLE 18.5 Histochemical Stains for Intracellular and Extracellular Substances

STAIN OR METHOD	SUBSTANCE OR STRUCTURE	COLOR
Acid phosphatase	Prostate	Black
Alcian blue	Sialomucins, hyaluronic acid, sulfated mucosubstances	Blue
Alizarin red S	Calcium	Orange-red
Best's carmine	Glycogen	Deep red
Bielschowsky silver stain	Axons	Black
Congo red	Amyloid	Orange-red[a]
Cresyl violet	Nissl substance	Violet
Dunn-Thompson	Hemoglobin	Emerald green
Feulgen	DNA	Red-purple
Fontana-Masson	Melanin	Black
Gordon and Sweets reticulin fiber	Reticulin fibers	Black
Grimelius	Argyrophilic granules	Black
Hall's method	Biliverdin, bilirubin	Green
Jones silver methenamine	Basement membranes	Black
Kinyoun (modified Ziehl-Neelsen)	Lipofuscin	Red
Luxol fast blue	Myelin	Blue
Mallory's PTAH	Muscle, fibrin, glial processes	Dark blue
Masson's trichrome	Muscle, collagen	Muscle: red Collagen: blue
Mayer's mucicarmine	Mucin, hyaluronic acid, chondroitin sulfate	Rose to red
Methyl green pyronin	Nucleic acids	DNA: green-blue RNA: red
Oil red O	Fat	Orange–bright red
Periodic acid–Schiff (PAS)	Glycogen, mucin	Red
Prussian blue	Ferric iron	Blue
Rhodanine	Copper	Red
Rubeanic acid	Copper	Green-black
Schmorl's reaction	Melanin, lipofuscin, bile	Dark blue
Sudan black B	Fat	Black
Toluidine blue	Mast cells	Purple
Verhöeff's stain	Elastic fibers	Black
von Kossa stain	Calcium	Black

[a]Apple-green birefringence with polarized light.

the presence of necrotic debris can make a sample unsuitable for processing (Comazzi et al., 2018). To avoid the first limitation, some authors suggest the use of 21-gauge needles, especially in cats in which smaller needles could disrupt cells and large needles could increase the hemodilution in samples and be more traumatic for surrounding tissues (Martini et al., 2018). In any case, it is not advisable to sample the centers of very large neoplastic lymph nodes because of the more likely presence of necrosis. Another preanalytical variable is the technical skill of the operator, which affects the likelihood of obtaining diagnostic samples. Other possible preanalytical factors such as signalment, shipping procedures, and sampling site seem not to affect the quality of samples (Comazzi et al., 2018; Martini et al., 2018).

Laboratory Preparation of Sample

The preparation of cells for FC varies widely among laboratories (Vernau and Moore, 1999; Lana et al., 2006b; Villiers et al., 2006; Gelain et al., 2008), and there is no consensus about the best method. Most commonly, the first step in cell preparation is to remove the red blood cells (RBCs) by lysis in a hypotonic solution. An alternative method is to prepare the cells by differential density centrifugation through a solution such as Histopaque. Neutrophils, RBCs, and platelets will pass through the solution, whereas mononuclear cells will remain on top of the Histopaque layer. Although this technique concentrates the mononuclear cells considerably, it is possible that cells of interest may pass through the density gradient and be lost from the analysis. Therefore, this method is not recommended for diagnostic assays.

For analysis of antigens expressed on the cell surface, such as CD4 and CD8, cells are incubated with antibodies to cell surface markers in a buffer such as phosphate-buffered saline with added protein (bovine serum albumin or fetal bovine serum). Primary antibodies are either unlabeled or have been directly conjugated to fluorescent molecules. Directly conjugated antibodies can be visualized immediately after staining, and they greatly facilitate the use of multiple markers simultaneously. Cells stained with unlabeled antibodies are subject to a second staining reaction using fluorescent-labeled antibody that recognizes Ig of the species of the primary antibody (e.g., goat anti-mouse IgG for a mouse primary antibody). In general, only a single unconjugated antibody can be used in a staining reaction, preventing the simultaneous quantification of multiple markers on individual cells. It is important to include negative

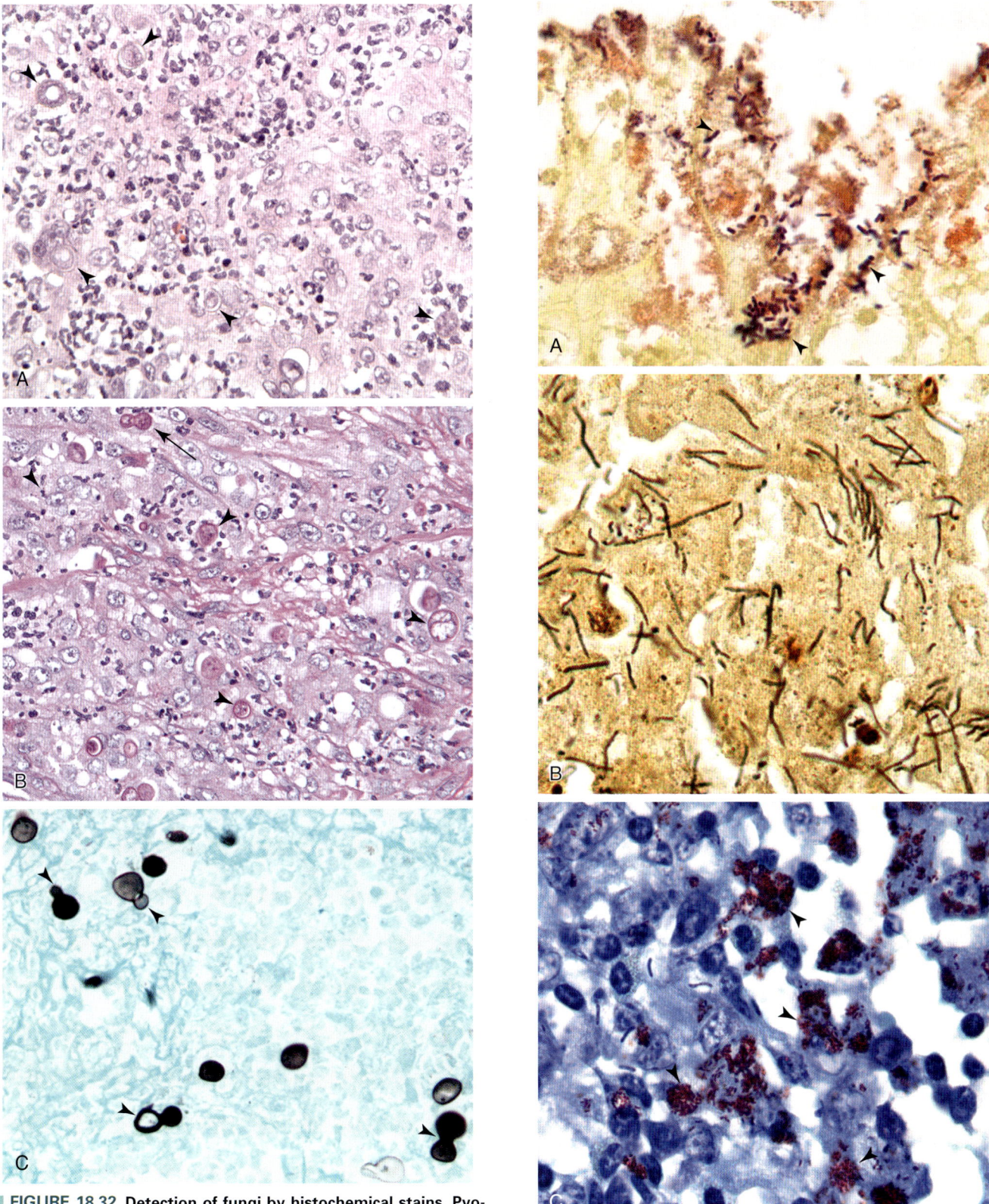

FIGURE 18.32 Detection of fungi by histochemical stains. Pyogranulomatous dermatitis. Skin. Dog. Blastomycosis. Same case in A to C. **A,** Cellular detail of the inflammatory reaction is excellent but detection of yeasts *(arrowheads)* is difficult. (H&E.) **B,** Improved detection of yeasts due to staining cell walls magenta *(arrowheads)*. Note the broad-based budding formation *(arrow)*. (PAS.) **C,** Excellent yeast morphology, but detail of the inflammatory process is poor. Numerous broad-based budding yeasts are observed *(arrowheads)*. (Grocott methenamine silver stain.)

FIGURE 18.33 Detection of bacteria by histochemical stains. A, Gram stain. Intestine. Dog. Stain depicts many gram-positive bacterial rods *(arrowheads)*. **B, Warthin-Starry stain. Liver. Horse.** This staining method is excellent to detect *Clostridium piliforme* because of the high contrast with the background. **C, Ziehl-Neelsen stain. Skin. Dog.** Acid-fast mycobacterial organisms *(arrowheads)* stain bright red. Note the presence of unstained bacilli.

TABLE 18.6 Histochemical Stains for Microorganisms

STAIN	MICROORGANISM
Giemsa	Metachromatic granules; good stain for protozoa and some bacteria
Gram	Standard staining for bacteria
Grocott methenamine silver	Fungi, oomycetes, *Pneumocystis*
Jimenez	Chlamydiae
Macchiavello	Chlamydiae
Mucicarmine	Capsule of *Cryptococcus*
Periodic acid–Schiff	Fungi
Steiner and Steiner silver	Numerous bacteria, including *Helicobacter* (good contrast between the black staining of the bacteria and the background)
Toluidine blue	Metachromatic granules
Wade-Fite	Acid-fast bacteria, including mycobacteria, *Nocardia*
Warthin-Starry	Similar uses to Steiner stain
Ziehl-Neelsen	Acid-fast bacteria; *Nocardia* is difficult to detect

TABLE 18.7 Antibody Panels of the Most Common Clones Used for Characterization of Canine and Feline Leukocytes by Flow Cytometry

CELL TYPE	ANTIGEN	CLONE	SPECIES REACTIVITY
Dogs			
T cells	CD3	CA17.2A12	Dogs
T-cell subset/neutrophils	CD4	YKIX302.9/CA13.1E4	Dogs
T cells	CD5	YKIX322.3	Dogs
T-cell subset	CD8α	YCAT 55.9/CA9.JD3	Dogs
T-cell subset	CD8β	CA15.4G2	Dogs
Most leukocytes	CD11/18	YKIX490.6.4	Dogs
Monocytes or neutrophils	CD14	TUK4/UCHM1[a]	Humans
Neutrophils or monocytes	CD11b	CA163E10	Dogs
Splenic lymphocytes or macrophages	CD11d	CA11.8H2	Dogs
Most leukocytes	CD18	CA1.4E9	Dogs
B cells	CD21	CA2.1D6/B-ly4	Dogs and humans
Precursors	CD34	1H6	Dogs
All leukocytes	CD45	YKIX716.13/CA12.10C12	Dogs
Histiocytes	CD90	CA1.4G8	Dogs
Mast cells, precursors	CD117	ACK45	Mice and dogs
Histiocytes	MHC II	YKIX334.2/CA2.1C12	Dogs
T-cell subset	TCR αβ	CA15.8G7	Dogs
T-cell subset	TCR γδ	CA20.6A3	Dogs
Cats			
T-cell subset	CD4	Vpg39	Cats
T cells	CD5	FE1.1B11/f43	Cats
T-cell subset	CD8α/β	Vpg9	Cat
Splenic lymphocytes and macrophages	CD11d	CA11.8H2	Cats and dogs
Most leukocytes	CD11/18	YKIX490.6.4	Cats and dogs
Monocytes	CD14	TUK4[a]	Cat
B cells	CD21	CA2.1D6/LB21	Dogs and humans
All leukocytes	CD18	CA1.4E9	Cats and dogs
All leukocytes	CD44	IM7	Mice, cats, and dogs

[a]TUK4 does not appear to stain neutrophils, but UCHM1 may weakly stain granulocytes.

control samples for each diagnostic sample. Controls consist of cells left unstained and cells stained with an antibody of the same isotype that should not specifically bind to any antigens on the cells of interest. The unstained cells enable the operator to correct for autofluorescence, and the fluorescent intensity of the irrelevant antibody reaction can be used to determine the level of background staining.

Laboratories use a variety of different antibodies in different combinations for immunophenotyping. Table 18.7 lists a basic panel for lymphoma and various leukemias in dogs and cats, but most laboratories use additional antibodies, chosen based on the experience and training of the personnel (Burkhard and Bienzle, 2013). The largest supplier of directly conjugated antibodies for use in routine veterinary FC is Bio-Rad (www.bio-rad-antibodies.com), and the majority of clones listed in Table 18.7 are available through this company. Other suppliers, such as Bio-Techne brand (www.bio-techne.com), B-D Biosciences (www.bdbiosciences.com), and Southern Biotech (www.southernbiotech.com, cats only) have fewer antibodies. See Table 18.1 for suppliers of specific antibodies used in IHC and ICC.

The cells are washed after the final staining reaction and then can either be fixed in paraformaldehyde for later analysis or analyzed immediately without fixation. If cells are analyzed immediately, they can be additionally stained with a number of different dyes that will determine the viability of the cells; therefore, it is possible to make data analysis only on live cells. This technique is extremely useful because dead cells tend to bind antibodies nonspecifically. In addition, cell death changes the size and scatter properties of cells, and there are at least two studies demonstrating that size is prognostic in cases of B-cell leukemia (Williams et al., 2008) and B-cell lymphoma (Rao et al., 2011).

In addition to surface molecules, several useful antigens are located within the cytoplasm. For example, most human T-cell acute lymphoblastic leukemias (ALLs) lack surface expression of CD3 but have cytoplasmic expression of CD3 (Szczepanski et al., 2006). The CD3 reagent commonly used for IHC in dogs can also be used for FC (Wilkerson et al., 2005) and could be included in a panel used to phenotype acute leukemia. The monocyte and granulocyte lineage markers myeloperoxidase (MPO) and MAC387 (calprotectin) are also cytoplasmic and can be useful for analyzing acute myeloid leukemia (AML) (Villiers et al., 2006). Similarly, CD79a and Pax5, B-cell lineage antigens, can be used to establish a B-cell origin neoplasm when B-cell antigens are not expressed on the cell surface. To expose these cytoplasmic and nuclear molecules, respectively, cell membranes must be permeabilized before staining using commercial kits (e.g., Fix & Perm from Life Technologies).

Flow Instruments

Since the 1960s, different flow cytometers were produced by different manufacturers, among which Beckman Coulter, BD Biosciences, and Sysmex-Partec are the largest and longest operating ones. Each of these companies manufactures flow cytometers that range from small instruments designed for use in individual laboratories with minimal automation to large automated analyzers. More recently, additional machines such as Guava (Luminex Corporation) and Attune (Life Technologies) have entered the market.

Flow cytometers are highly complex instruments that record information about each individual cell in your cell suspension. To accomplish this, cells are focused in a fluid stream that passes in front of one or more lasers. The way that the cell scatters light is recorded by detectors, as is the level of fluorescence exhibited by each cell, which in turns reflects the level of antigen expression for the antigen detected by the fluorescent-labeled antibody.

Data Analysis

The most important aspect of FC is data analysis, which begins with the examination of the light scatter properties of the cells. As cells pass in front of the laser, they scatter the light, and detectors record the amount of forward- and side-scattered light. The total amount of forward-scattered light detected depends on cell surface area or size, whereas the amount of side-scattered light indicates cellular complexity or granularity. Figure 18.34 demonstrates a typical scatter plot from canine peripheral blood, in which each dot represents an individual cell placed relative to the amount of forward and side scatter recorded as it passes in front of the laser. Light scatter properties allow the identification of lymphocyte, monocyte, and neutrophil populations.

Although there is no consensus on analysis methods in veterinary medicine, in general, the first step of an analysis is to "gate" different populations of cells based on their scatter properties. As shown in Figure 18.34, lymphocytes have lower forward and side scatter, whereas neutrophils have higher forward and side scatter, with monocytes falling in between.

The next step is to determine the percentage of cells within each population that expresses the markers of interest by looking at the fluorescence profile of each population. The fluorochromes used to label antibodies are excited by the laser and emit light over a narrow range of wavelengths, which can be

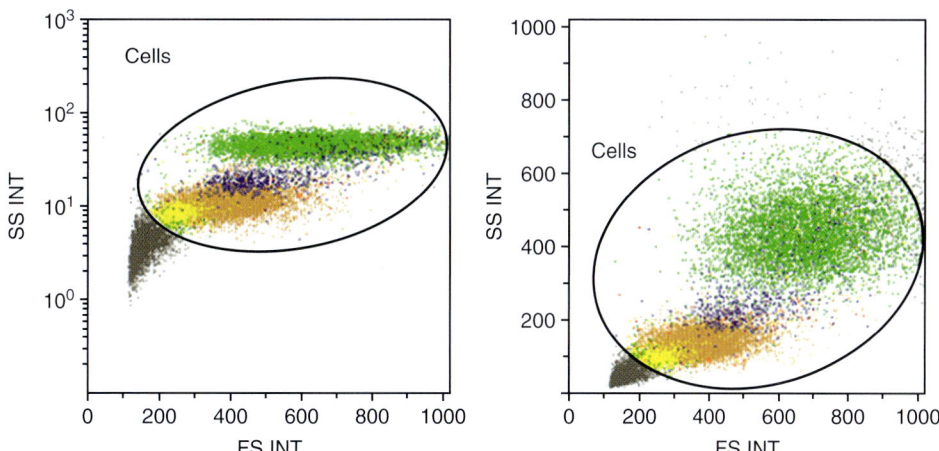

■ **FIGURE 18.34 Light scatter properties of canine peripheral blood by flow cytometry.** Forward (x-axis) and side scatter (y-axis) of peripheral blood showing individual neutrophils *(green)*, monocytes *(blue)*, and lymphocytes *(yellow and beige)*. These two plots represent the same sample graphed using the log value of the side scatter *(left panel)* and the linear value *(right panel)*. Either method can be used. Forward scatter is roughly equivalent to size or surface area, whereas side scatter indicates cytoplasmic complexity. *FS INT,* forward scatter intensity; *SS INT,* side scatter intensity.

detected by the flow cytometer. Different fluorochromes have distinct peak emission wavelengths, so antibodies conjugated to several different fluorochromes can be used simultaneously in one staining reaction. The amount of fluorescent signal detected is proportional to the number of fluorochrome molecules on the cell. The data can then be displayed as a single parameter in the form of a histogram or two parameters displayed simultaneously as a dot plot (Fig. 18.35). Two-parameter dot plots allow individual events or cells to be displayed so that the relative fluorescence for two individual markers can be examined simultaneously.

Electronic gating of different populations allows the user to determine the percentage of cells in each population that are positive for a given molecule (Figs. 18.35 and 18.36). The percentage of positive cells is usually determined by first analyzing the isotype control and setting gates based on this control. The percentage of positive cells is determined by the number of cells that fall above the gate set by the negative control. Although the isotype control is used as a guideline, it is generally accepted that there is some flexibility in the placement of gates to include logical populations of cells. For example, there are two discrete populations of cells corresponding to B and T cells, but it is clear that there is a population of T cells that coexpresses the B-cell antigen CD21 (see Fig. 18.35C). Therefore, the gates were redrawn to reflect this observation, resulting in a more accurate T-cell count (see Fig. 18.35D).

Electronic gating can also allow the user to focus on a particular population of interest. A lymph node from a dog with B-cell lymphoma is illustrated (see Fig. 18.36). When the whole node is analyzed, it appears that 59% of the cells are B cells (see Fig. 18.36B). More important, however, it is clear that the B cells fall almost exclusively into a discrete population of large cells. When these cells are specifically examined, almost 90% are B cells (see Fig. 18.36D). Such a homogeneous expansion of large cells can be considered diagnostic for B-cell lymphoma. It should be noted that although the diagnosis in this case is unambiguous, consistent guidelines have not yet been established in the literature, making a definitive diagnosis of neoplasia. In addition, the definition of cutoff values to define a cell population positive for a specific antigen is still discussed, and it could be variable based on tissue and antigen analyzed. Thus, this technique retains some subjectivity in data interpretation.

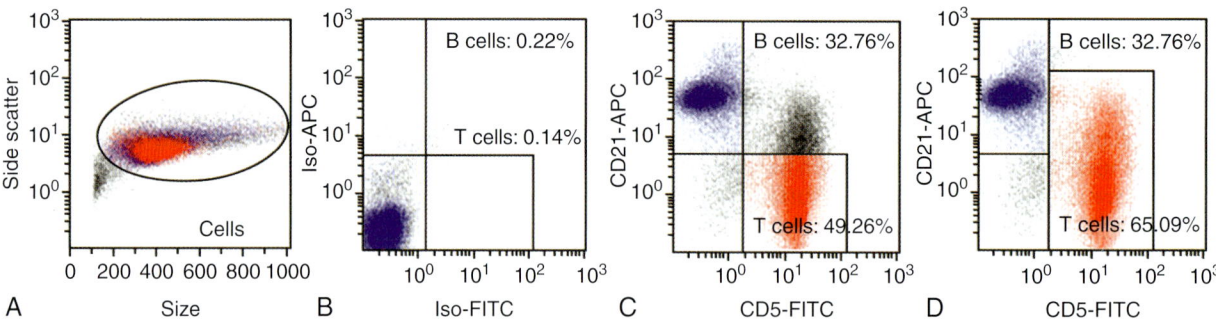

■ **FIGURE 18.35 Flow cytometry. Examining cell surface proteins. Reactive lymph node. Dog.** Same sample in A to D. **A,** Shown is the forward and side scatter histogram of lymph node cells. **B,** The two axes in this panel show the staining with isotype (Iso) control antibodies, antibodies that should not bind specifically to canine lymphocytes but are conjugated with the fluorochromes used for specific staining. APC is the dye allophycocyanin, and FITC is fluorescein isothiocyanate. Two rectangular gates are drawn so that less than 1% of the cells fall within either gate (four quadrants could also be used instead of rectangular gates). **C,** Specific staining for CD5 (T-cell antigen) and CD21 (B-cell antigen) is shown in this panel with the gates drawn as guided by the isotype controls. It is clear, however, that a population of the CD5+ cells is co-expressing CD21, so the gate must be adjusted. **D,** The adjusted gate reflects the true T-cell population. The percentage of T cells in this sample was further verified as being 65% using an anti-CD3 antibody.

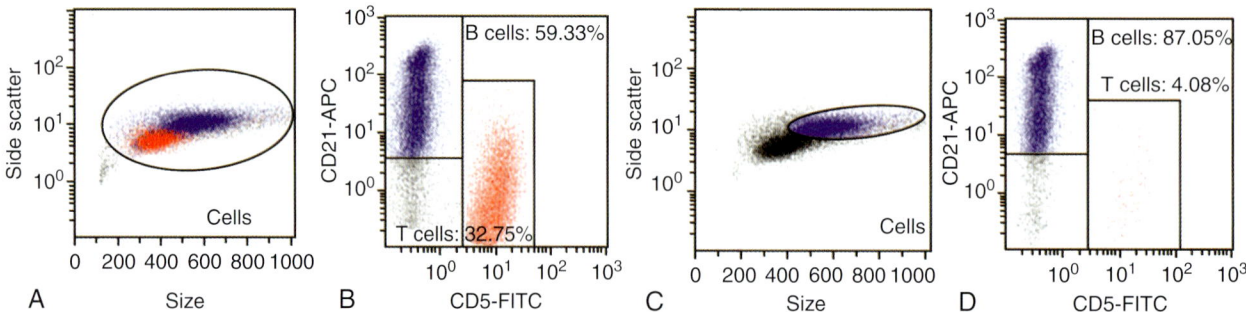

■ **FIGURE 18.36 Flow cytometry. Gating a population of interest. B-cell lymphoma. Lymph node. Dog.** Same case in A to D. **A,** Forward and side scatter histograms detect two discrete cell populations. **B,** B- and T-cell populations are identified and electronically colored so that the cells expressing CD21 are blue and those expressing CD5 are red. Using this backgating technique, the large cells appear to be almost exclusively B cells. **C,** The suspicion that the large cells are B cells is confirmed when only the large cells are examined. **D,** Within the large cell population, almost 90% of the cells are B cells, a finding that can be considered diagnostic for B-cell lymphoma. *APC,* Allophycocyanin; *FITC,* fluorescein isothiocyanate.

Reporting Flow Cytometry Data

All laboratories report FC data differently mainly because a widely accepted standardization on reporting FC data is still lacking in veterinary medicine (Meichner et al., 2020). In Europe, the European Canine Lymphoma Network publishes consensus recommendations trying to standardize the report among institutions and countries (Comazzi et al., 2017). The final target users of FC data are usually clinicians who are interested in defining the immunophenotype or the subtype of hematopoietic neoplasia to establish the prognosis, determine therapy, and monitor the outcome. One study aimed to determine inter-investigator agreement on the interpretation of flow cytometer results from split samples analyzed in different laboratories (Meichner et al., 2020). Although overall agreement was strong in that lymphoproliferations were readily recognized, it appeared the identification of the categories of hematolymphatic neoplasia was variable, concluding a need for more standardization of FC.

Generally, both the percentage of positive cells and the cell count are reported. In peripheral blood analysis, the most useful information is the absolute number of a lymphocyte subset in peripheral blood per microliter. When only percentages are reported, it may be difficult to distinguish the relative loss of one population because of expansion of another population. Although normal values have been published (Byrne et al., 2000), preparation methods differ so widely between laboratories that each one should generate its own normal values.

For other samples, percentages of lymphocyte subsets are reported usually after gating on the relevant population by size. For example, in lymph node aspirates from dogs with lymphoma, the neoplastic lymphocytes are usually large (see Fig. 18.36). Therefore, the percentage of each lymphocyte subset is determined after gating on the large cells. However, this approach has some limitations, including the percentages directly related to the gating strategies (e.g., identify relevant population based on CD45 vs side scatter rather than only on scatter properties), and the controls used to set the cutoff values. Reporting only the percentage of positive cells is not useful to distinguish normal versus neoplastic cells because it does not provide information on antigen coexpression (Comazzi et al., 2017).

Reporting the quantitative expression for some antigens may provide information on maturation stage, aberrancy, or prognosis (Rao et al., 2011). These data are usually reported as dim or bright, even if these definitions are quite subjective and poorly standardized among laboratories. In addition, the presence of a specific aberrant pattern could be useful to identify specific lymphoma subtypes (Martini et al., 2015), detect neoplastic cells in blood or bone marrow, and detect minimal residual disease (MRD). This additional information, as well as a descriptive interpretation of the whole FC analysis, could be included in the report as the description. Other information more related to technical aspects, such as the gating strategies and eventually some plot images, should be added only if the report is sent to clinical pathologists or flow cytometrists. In summary, a flow cytometric report should contain, besides the patient identification and the type of sample analyzed, the percentage of positive cells, a descriptive section, and the diagnosis and interpretation plus any possible comments or references (Comazzi et al., 2017).

Uses for Flow Cytometry
Reactive Versus Neoplastic Lymphocytosis

A lymphoproliferative disorder can often be diagnosed based on the cytopathologic appearance of the cells if the cells exhibit clear criteria of malignancy. Furthermore, when the lymphocytes exhibit a mature phenotype but the lymphocyte count is greater than 30,000 cells/μL, the diagnosis of a lymphoproliferative disorder can be made with certainty because survival is significantly different from cases with lower counts (Williams et al., 2008).

When a dog has lymphocytosis of less than 30,000 cells/μL composed of small mature lymphocytes and no other clinical signs that would point to a diagnosis, FC can be used to distinguish chronic lymphocytic leukemia (CLL) from non-neoplastic causes of lymphocytosis. As a rule of thumb, expansion of a single lymphocyte subtype (CD4 T cells, CD8 T cells, or B cells) would be considered most consistent with neoplasia (except for *Ehrlichia canis* infection as noted later).

Veterinary clinical pathologists have not yet come to an agreement about the criteria for making the distinction between reactive and neoplastic lymphocytosis. For example, canine peripheral blood typically has 300 B cells/μL. Would a B-cell count of 3000 cells/μL in the context of a total lymphocyte count of 6000 cells/μL be considered diagnostic for B-cell neoplasia? Most likely the answer is yes, but definitive studies confirming this assumption with clinical follow-up and clonality assays are lacking. Criteria to determine breed distribution and clinical characteristics of B-cell chronic lymphocytic leukemia (B-CLL) in one study used a lymphocyte count greater than 5000 cells/μL and a percentage of small CD21+ lymphocytes (calculated as the number of CD21+ cells divided by the total B and T cells) of more than 60% (Bromberek et al., 2016).

In addition to homogeneous expansion of a single lymphocyte subset, the presence of cells with aberrant antigen expression (i.e., loss of expression of antigens that should be found on normal lymphocytes or expression of antigens not found on normal lymphocytes) can be considered diagnostic for malignancy (Gelain et al., 2008). For example, the loss of CD45 expression is a consistent feature of small clear cell, or T-zone, lymphoma (Seelig et al., 2014; Martini et al., 2015). Even in the absence of a significantly expanded uniform population of lymphocytes, the presence of a small number of aberrant cells can point to neoplasia. Similarly, normal peripheral blood contains virtually no cells expressing the stem cell antigen CD34. The finding of even a minor population of CD34+ cells in peripheral blood points to a diagnosis of hematopoietic neoplasia.

Other less common differentials for small, mature lymphocytosis in dogs include hypoadrenocorticism, thymoma, and *E. canis* infection. When cases of thymoma involve lymphocytosis, the lymphocytosis is usually characterized by an expansion of CD4 T cells, CD8 T cells, and sometimes T cells that express neither cell surface protein (Batlivala et al., 2010). *E. canis* infection, on the other hand, almost exclusively causes the expansion of CD8 T cells that are described as having azurophilic cytoplasmic granules (Weiser et al., 1991; McDonough and Moore, 2000; Heeb et al., 2003). These CD8 T cells do not exhibit aberrant antigen expression, an observation that can help distinguish them from neoplastic T cells, which can exhibit loss or gain of a variety of T cell–associated antigens.

Prognostic Significance of Immunophenotype

Lymphoma. Studies of canine multicentric lymphoma have consistently demonstrated that immunophenotype (B vs. T) provides prognostically useful information in conjunction with clinical stage (Teske et al., 1994; Ruslander et al., 1997). T-cell lymphomas typically have a worse prognosis than B-cell lymphomas, especially in extranodal sites such as the skin or liver. It is important to note, however, that there are histologic subtypes of T-cell lymphoma that have a good prognosis and histologic subtypes of B-cell lymphoma that have a poor prognosis (Ponce et al., 2004; Valli et al., 2006). In human medicine, surface markers have been identified to help distinguish between some histologic subtypes of lymphoma via FC. T-cell lymphomas (CD4+, CD45+) that express low levels of class II major histocompatibility complex (MHC) consistently had a poor prognosis (Avery et al., 2014). T-zone lymphoma can be definitively diagnosed by FC often with a lack of CD45 antigen (Seelig et al., 2014; Martini et al., 2015). T-zone lymphoma, unlike lymphoblastic T-cell lymphoma, is indolent, with very long median survival (Flood-Knapik et al., 2013). Thus, simply distinguishing B- from T-cell lymphoma gives only an incomplete prognostic picture.

Other testing, such as FC or histopathology assessed by an experienced hematopathologist, is important for providing accurate prognosis. Some prognostic information is aided by flow cytometric evaluation of proliferation markers such as Ki67 or the fraction of cells in S-phase. The percentage of Ki67-positive cells in lymph node aspiration biopsies helped differentiate high- from low-grade lymphoma with 96.3% sensitivity and 100% specificity using 12.2% positive cells as the cut-off value (Poggi et al., 2015). The same authors have demonstrated its prognostic value in high-grade B-cell lymphomas (Poggi et al., 2017). FC can also be used to assess the DNA content: during cell cycle, the DNA content of cells varies, increasing in S-phase until duplication. Thus, using DNA fluorescent dyes, the cell distribution in the different phases could be easily detected. In canine lymphomas, S-phase fraction discriminated between low- and high-grade lymphomas and strongly correlated with Ki67 expression (Miniscalco et al., 2018).

The evaluation of peripheral blood and bone marrow involvement is crucially important to establish the stage V, one of the most important prognostic factors. Even if bone marrow evaluation is not usually required in absence of peripheral cytopenias, blood abnormalities are not always predictive of marrow involvement in large B-cell lymphomas (Martini et al., 2015). However, in veterinary medicine, there are no standardized methods to assess lymphoma infiltration. Recently, FC has been reported to have good analytical precision and accuracy (CV <10%) in the quantification of large CD45 and CD21-positive cells in blood and bone marrow of dogs with high-grade B-cell lymphoma when cut-offs of 0.56% and 2.45% were proposed to define positive blood and bone marrow, respectively (Riondato et al., 2016).

Also in cats, flow cytometric analysis of lymph node aspirates in conjunction with cytopathologic examination is recommended for the diagnosis of lymphoma. One study was successful in evaluating cells from body cavity fluids, intestines, spleen, and mesenteric lymph nodes to identify lymphoma involving internal organs and distinguish neoplasia from lymphoid reactivity (Guzera et al., 2016).

Peripheral lymphocytosis. The question of how to classify leukemia remains unresolved in veterinary medicine. In humans, a disease characterized by circulating small mature B lymphocytes is called chronic lymphocytic leukemia/small cell lymphoma (CLL/SCL); it is not clinically or prognostically relevant to distinguish leukemia from lymphoma. One group of pathologists adopted this convention for lymphoproliferative disease of mature B cells in their study (Vezzali et al., 2010). Forty percent of dogs with small B-cell expansion also had lymphadenopathy (Williams et al., 2008). As a group, these cases have a median survival time of greater than 1000 days and behave like CLL, but it is not clear if all these cases can be classified as CLL/SCL because the lymph nodes are often not evaluated by surgical biopsy. In a study of more than 46% of dogs with lymphadenopathy, splenomegaly, hepatomegaly, or mediastinal mass, B-CLL could not be differentiated from B-cell small cell lymphoma because of the absence of histologic examination of involved organs (Bromberek et al., 2016).

Canine T-cell CLLs are more common than B-cell CLLs in dogs (Workman and Vernau, 2003), and they usually have a longer survival time (Comazzi et al., 2011). It should be noted that dogs with T-zone lymphoma often show peripheral blood involvement at presentation (Seelig et al., 2014; Martini et al., 2016). The unique phenotype with lost expression of the pan-leukocyte antigen CD45 helps differentiate leukemic involvement of T-zone lymphoma compared to other types of T-cell CLL.

Lymphocytosis composed of small mature T cells is not confined to the T-zone phenotype. CD8 T-cell lymphocytosis is common, and when the lymphocyte count is less than 30,000 cells/μL, the disease behaves like CLL (Williams et al., 2008). Lymphocytosis involving CD4 T cells is uncommon, but these diseases can also, in some cases, exhibit an indolent course.

Very little is known about leukemia in cats, but one study demonstrated that the most common form of feline CLL involves CD4+ lymphocytes and has a median survival time of 15 months (Campbell et al., 2012). A more aggressive form of leukemia is associated with intestinal lymphoma, typically of CD8+ lymphocytes, consistent with granular lymphocytes. The maximum survival time in these cases was 84 days (Roccabianca et al., 2006).

Classification of Acute Leukemia

Acute leukemia, diagnosed by cellular morphology, has long been known to have a poor prognosis. Cytopathologic differentiation between ALL and AML is often not possible because of shared cytopathologic features of malignancy. FC can be extremely useful in these cases, although few reports have been published correlating morphologic characteristics with immunophenotype. The use of anticanine CD34, a marker generally found on precursor leukocytes, is useful in objectively identifying cases of acute leukemia. CD34 is most likely expressed on both ALL and AML (Workman and Vernau, 2003; Villiers et al., 2006). Often CD34+ cells in acute leukemia lack MHC II expression. The presence of CD5 expression and CD14 could help in the diagnosis of ALL and AML, respectively (Rout and Avery, 2017). Despite this fact, a significantly shortened survival time in dogs with increased numbers of circulating CD34+ cells has been documented (Williams et al., 2008). Recently, an increased expression of CD117 and CD44 has been reported in acute leukemia, suggesting the use of these two markers as an additional aid in the diagnosis of acute leukemia (Giantin et al., 2013; Gelain et al., 2014).

Cytoplasmic staining of acute leukemias may be more useful than surface staining because human T-cell ALLs express CD3 only in their cytoplasm (Szczepanski et al., 2006). Acute B-cell leukemias may also express only cytoplasmic antigens associated with their lineage, such as CD79a. Leukemias expressing either of these antigens can be classified as lymphoid. Cells expressing surface antigens such as CD14 or CD11b are classified as myeloid. Intracellular staining with an antibody to myeloperoxidase or using the antibody MAC387 may provide further confirmation of the myeloid origin of these cells. There is an excellent study correlating AML subclassification (AML-M1, M4, and M5) with immunophenotype using a variety of markers (Villiers et al., 2006). Several studies have evaluated canine acute leukemia and chronic lymphoid leukemia by immunophenotyping using FC to consider hematologic abnormalities, epidemiologic considerations, and prognostic factors (Adam et al., 2009; Tasca et al., 2009; Novacco et al., 2016).

Diagnosis of Mediastinal Masses

A particularly useful application of FC involves distinguishing lymphoma from thymoma in cases of lymphocyte-rich mediastinal masses in dogs or cats (Lana et al., 2006b; Lara-Garcia et al., 2008). The neoplastic cell type in thymoma is the thymic epithelial cell, which directs differentiation of normal T cells. During differentiation in the thymus, T cells pass through a stage in which they coexpress CD4 and CD8. The thymus is the only place such cells are produced, so their presence in a mediastinal mass of adult dogs or cats can be considered diagnostic for thymoma (Fig. 18.37). After the CD4+ CD8+ stage of development but before exiting the thymus, T cells downregulate one of these antigens. Thus, the number of circulating T cells can be increased in cases of thymoma, but rarely do double-positive cells escape a thymoma and appear in the blood (Deshuillers et al., 2015). By contrast, lymphomas involving the mediastinum are generally T cell but express only one or neither of the subset markers CD4 or CD8. The cells in mediastinal lymphoma are invariably large, whereas the lymphocytes in thymoma are small. Therefore, FC can usually distinguish between these two entities. Because making this distinction determines whether a patient will have chemotherapy or surgery, this is a particularly important use for this assay.

Flow Cytometry in Mast Cell Tumors

Mast cell tumors are some of the most common skin tumors in dogs and readily exfoliative. These features make canine mast cell tumor a good candidate for flow cytometric analysis. Common features for the neoplastic mast cell phenotype include the expression of common antigen (CD45, CD18, CD44) and CD117 (Sulce et al., 2018). The majority of cases were also IgE and CD11b positive. Different from human mastocytosis, CD25 was expressed in only one case. As well as in lymphoma, the definition of a multicolor approach to identify mast cell phenotype could be used to detect neoplastic infiltration on lymph nodes, the spleen, and the liver, making more accurate the diagnosis of metastases.

LYMPHOCYTE CLONALITY TESTING

In human medicine, determination of clonality by detecting clonally rearranged antigen receptor genes is often the test of choice if routine cytopathology, histopathology, and immunophenotyping are not able to provide a definitive diagnosis of lymphoid malignancy (Swerdlow, 2003). Clonality testing is based on the observation that lymphocytes mount a diverse response to antigens, whether they are derived from the environment (e.g., allergens), from pathogens, or from self (autoantigens). By contrast, malignant lymphocytes are homogeneous, arising from a single transformed cell. Normal lymphocyte differentiation depends on the process of antigen receptor rearrangement; therefore, all mature lymphocytes have antigen receptor genes that have undergone VJ or VDJ rearrangement. Ig genes are rearranged in B lymphocytes and

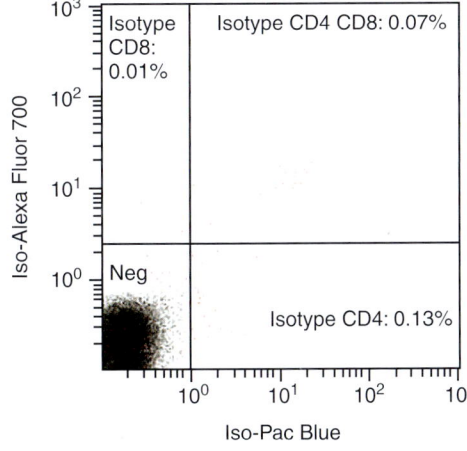
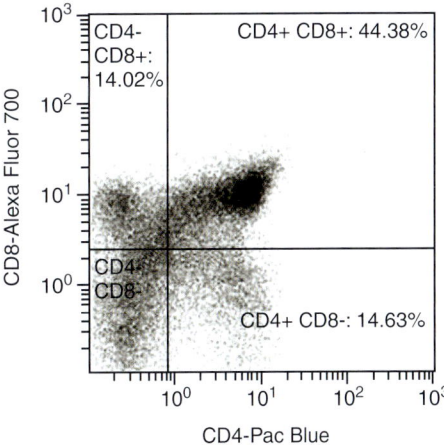

■ **FIGURE 18.37 Flow cytometry. Thymoma. Mediastinal mass cells. Dog.** Both panels show fluorescence of the small lymphocyte population, gated based on forward and side scatter (not shown). *Left,* Isotype control showing placement of quadrants. *Right,* CD4 and CD8 fluorescence, showing that 51% of the cells coexpress CD4 and CD8 *(upper right quadrant).* Note the presence of cells that express only CD4 or CD8. These cells represent the stage of thymic differentiation following the double-positive (CD4+CD8+) stage, when one or the other of the two markers has been downregulated. These single-positive cells exit the thymus into the blood. Double-positive T cells generally do not exit the thymus and are only rarely found in circulation in cases of thymoma.

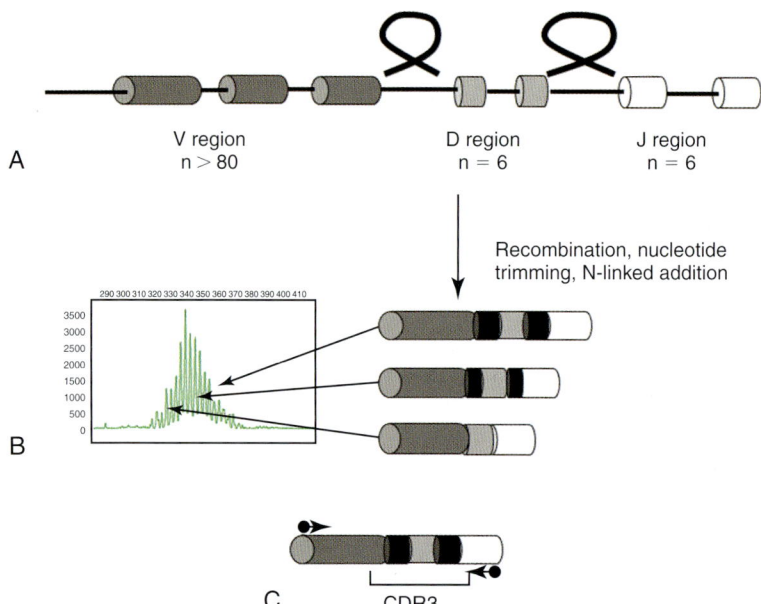

FIGURE 18.38 Immunoglobulin gene rearrangement. A, One V region gene (of ~80 in the canine genome) recombines with a randomly selected D region gene (6 in the canine genome) and a J region gene (6 in the canine genome), looping out the intervening DNA. **B,** During this process, nucleotides are added *(black bars)* between genes, which generate length and sequence diversity in the complementarity determining region 3 (CDR3). Differentially sized DNA can be separated by capillary electrophoresis and will appear as a ladder representing different populations of B cells (shown at *left*). **C,** Primers with homology to the conserved framework regions of V and J regions *(arrows)* will amplify polymerase chain reaction products of different sizes when DNA is derived from different lymphocytes. Primers are located outside the hypervariable CDR3 region to detect as many different V and J genes as possible.

T-cell receptor (TCR) genes α/β and/or γ/δ in T lymphocytes (Jung and Alt, 2004). During this process (Fig. 18.38), nucleotides are trimmed or added between genes as they recombine, resulting in significant length and sequence heterogeneity, particularly within the complementarity determining region 3 (CDR3). Further diversity within B-cell Ig genes is created by somatic hypermutation during antigen-driven B-cell activation. The end result of this differentiation is a diverse population of lymphocytes with virtually limitless antigen specificity and a large variety of CDR3 sequences and lengths. Lymphocytes derived from the same clone have CDR3 regions of the same length and sequence.

Because all lymphomas, lymphocytic leukemias, and myelomas are clonal expansions of lymphocytes, an assay that uses polymerase chain reaction for antigen receptor rearrangement (PARR) was developed to amplify the variable regions of Ig genes and TCR genes to detect the presence of a clonal lymphocyte population. In one study, the assay detected clonally rearranged antigen receptor genes in 91% of the 77 dogs with lymphoid malignancy (Burnett et al., 2003). Gene rearrangement was appropriate for the immunophenotype (Ig gene rearrangement in B-cell leukemias and TCR gene rearrangement in T-cell leukemias). Potential applications of this assay include (1) the diagnosis of lymphoma or leukemia in tissue samples, fluid smears, aspirate biopsies, bone marrow specimens, and peripheral blood; (2) the staging of lymphoma; and (3) the detection of residual disease after chemotherapy (Burnett et al., 2003).

In another study for discrimination of lymphoma versus nonlymphoma, a revised PARR protocol, referred to as ePARR, was performed on fresh-frozen tissue, FFPE tissue, FC pellets, and aspirate biopsies (Ehrhart et al., 2019). Assay performance was determined for FFPE from 56 dogs (18 B-cell lymphoma, 24 T-cell lymphoma, and 14 nonlymphomas), 80 frozen FC pellets (66 B-cell lymphoma, 14 T-cell lymphoma, 0 non-lymphoma), and 41 air-dried aspirate slides (23 lymphoma, 18 nonlymphoma). The assay had 92% and 92% sensitivity and specificity on FFPE with 92% accuracy, 85% sensitivity from FC pellets (nonlymphoma was not evaluated to calculate specificity) with 85% accuracy, and 100% and 100% sensitivity and specificity for aspirate biopsy with 100% accuracy. The results indicate effective interpretation and application of PARR assays in multiple sample types (Ehrhart et al., 2019).

The term PARR is used to distinguish it from other types of PCR assays and other methods of determining clonality. It was coined by Keller et al. (2004) and is not used when referring to the same assay performed by human diagnostic laboratories. Additional means of determining clonality in human medicine include the amplification of *BCL1-IGH* and *BCL2-IGH* genes because the chromosomal translocation that brings the BCL and IGH loci together is relatively common in human B-cell lymphomas (van Dongen et al., 2003).

Methodology
Sample Collection
The principle behind this assay has been described in detail (Workman and Vernau, 2003; Avery and Avery, 2004). The steps to carry out a clonality assay begin with DNA extraction from tissue. Virtually any type of tissue can be used as a source of DNA, including blood, cavity fluids, aspirates, cerebrospinal fluid, stained or unstained cytopathology preps, and tissue in paraffin blocks. The latter is the least desirable because formalin fixation degrades DNA and can result in both more false negatives and false positives. Archival samples, including old cytopathology slides, can be used as a source of material for retrospective analysis.

DNA Amplification

Primers that hybridize to the conserved portions of V and J region genes of Ig and TCR genes are then used to amplify DNA in a PCR reaction. Although TCRs can be either α/β or γ/δ, primers recognizing TCRγ are typically used. Because there are fewer TCRγ genes, fewer primers are needed to detect the majority of malignancies, and TCRγ is rearranged before TCRβ, so it will be clonal even if the malignancy ultimately expresses TCRα/β. In human medicine, primers recognizing TCRγ, TCRβ, and TCRδ, as well as VJ, DJ, and BCL-IgH rearrangements are used to detect clonality (van Dongen et al., 2003).

Amplification of a positive control gene is an important part of the clonality assay. Almost any gene can be used. The goal of amplification is to verify that there is sufficient DNA of adequate quality to be able to interpret the results. In the absence of a positive control, a negative result may not reflect the lack of clonally expanded lymphocytes; it may rather indicate that a sample has no good amplifiable DNA.

Data Analysis

Analysis of these PCR products can be carried out using a variety of methods designed to evaluate the size of the products and in some cases the sequence heterogeneity. Although the original description of clonality assays in both human and veterinary medicine involved the use of polyacrylamide gels to separate PCR products by size, these methods have largely been replaced by capillary gel electrophoresis, which can give better resolution to the size of the products and provide results that are more consistent. Agarose gel electrophoresis is never appropriate for the analysis of PARR assays because even high-resolution agarose gels have insufficient resolution.

The presence of one or more single-sized PCR products indicates a clonal population of lymphocytes. Although it might be hypothesized that at most two PCR products would be seen in a malignancy (one rearrangement on each chromosome), in practice, particularly for TCR rearrangements, more than two rearrangements can be seen (Kisseberth et al., 2007). A comprehensive study of the maximum number of clonally rearranged antigen receptors that can be found in a single malignancy has not been carried out, so the cutoff between a "clonal" population and an "oligoclonal" population is not yet clear. One recommendation suggests that multiple single-sized PCR products appearing oligoclonal should be termed "clonal" (Keller and Moore, 2012). The presence of variably sized products suggests a polyclonal population of lymphocytes. There are examples of the PARR assay carried out on a reactive lymph node, a case of B-cell lymphoma, and a case of T-cell leukemia (Fig. 18.39).

There are no guidelines in veterinary medicine for how positive and negative results are reported. A convention used in the laboratory at the College of Veterinary Medicine and Biomedical Sciences at Colorado State University is to call a result positive (clonal) if the clonal peak is three times the height of the baseline, in accordance with published human studies (Miyata-Takata et al., 2014). Regardless of the method chosen, the laboratory running the test should be able to report sensitivity and specificity of their assay using the method of result calling they have chosen. The laboratory should be able to carry out the assay in such a way that their results are objective and can stand alone. Specificity can be a difficult value to establish. The presence of a clonally rearranged antigen receptor gene in the absence of confirmation of lymphoproliferative disease by histopathology or cytopathology is not necessarily a false-positive result. Because of the assay's sensitivity, clonality testing can detect neoplasia before it is evident by other means. Some presentations of lymphoma, such as T-zone lymphoma, are often diagnosed as lymphoid hyperplasia in the early stages. Thus, the only way to properly evaluate the specificity of the clonality assay is to assess the results in patients with good clinical follow-up for 6 months to 1 year to determine if a positive result indicates early-stage disease.

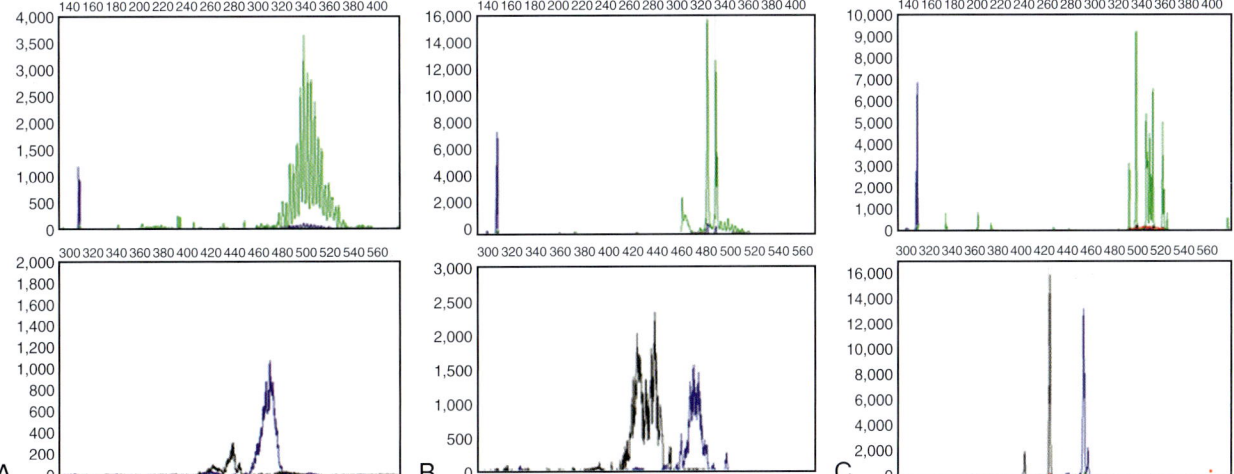

■ **FIGURE 18.39 Results of the polymerase chain reaction for antigen receptor rearrangement assay.** For all three cases, the *top panel* shows amplification of immunoglobulin genes (green) and a positive control gene (left side spike). The *bottom panel* shows amplification of T-cell receptor genes using two different primer pairs (blue and black), which results in slightly different-sized products. The size of the product (number of bases) is depicted on the *x*-axis, and the fluorescence intensity of the product is depicted on the *y*-axis. **A, Lymph node from a dog with reactive lymphoid hyperplasia secondary to dermatitis.** Note that both upper and lower panels contain large amounts of different-sized products. **B, Lymph node from a dog with B-cell lymphoma.** Note the limited spikes of product in the upper panel and numerous products in the lower panel. **C, Peripheral blood from a dog with T-cell leukemia.** Note that although there are multiple immunoglobulin gene products, the number of products is lower than shown in case A. This result reflects the fact that the peripheral blood of this patient contained very few B cells.

In a clinical setting, the interpretation of clonality assay results must be done in the light of clinical data, cytopathologic or histopathologic pattern, and immunophenotype. In fact, the possibility of a polyclonal result in the presence of neoplasia (false-negative results), a clonal result without evidence of neoplasia (false-positive results), or the presence of pseudoclonal results (one or more nonreproducible peaks), or nonspecific products should be considered when interpreting results.

The reasons for a negative PARR assay in a case of lymphoma confirmed by histopathology or cytopathology might include:
- The malignancy uses a V or J gene to which the primers do not hybridize
- Somatic hypermutation in cases of B-cell lymphoma or leukemia that altered the sequence to which the primers hybridize
- A polyclonal background if the samples contained a significant population of non-neoplastic lymphocytes that provide a background noise that obscures the clonal peak
- The malignancy is natural killer in origin and therefore does not contain a rearranged antigen receptor gene
- The malignancy is from an early precursor cell that has not yet rearranged the antigen receptor genes
- The malignancy has lost the chromosome carrying the antigen receptor genes

In some cases, clonal populations are detected in patients without lymphoproliferative disease. Such a "false-positive" rate differs among laboratories and may have a variety of causes. One of the most well recognized is clonal expansions in response to specific antigenic stimulation such as in *E. canis* and *Leishmania infantum* infections. It should also be considered the possibility of unspecific amplification when the clonal peak falls outside the range of the expected molecular size. This situation could be due to low target DNA concentration, but in any case, sequencing of the PCR product should be considered to avoid false-positive results. A review of PARR concepts and its pitfalls and limitations was well covered by Keller et al. (2016).

Sensitivity and specificity of PARR assays can be variable among laboratories, ranging from 72% to 100% and from 96% to 110%, respectively (Ehrhart et al., 2019). Diagnostic accuracy varies between laboratories because of sample type, DNA extraction and amplification protocols used, set of primers, and interpretation of the results. Thus, harmonization in procedures for clonality test in veterinary medicine is lacking and clearly needed.

Uses for Clonality Testing
Diagnosis of Lymphoma and Leukemia
Clonality testing is now routinely available for dogs and cats. Studies have demonstrated the presence of clonally rearranged TCR genes in canine malignancies (Dreitz et al., 1999; Fivenson et al., 1994; Vernau and Moore, 1999; Burnett et al., 2003).

The most common application of this technique is in cases in which cytopathology or histopathology is ambiguous. The assay can detect a malignant clone in a nonlymphoid organ that makes up as little as 0.1% of the tissue, but in lymphoid tissues, it requires a minimum of 10% of DNA to detect a single clone (Burnett et al., 2003). Thus, it can be useful in early cases of lymphoma or leukemia but depends on the tissue being used. Stained or unstained cytopathology slides or cells freshly aspirated into ethylenediaminetetraacetic acid (EDTA) tubes are the best samples for this purpose. Interpretation of the results varies depending on the sensitivity and specificity of the assay in each laboratory offering the test.

It is not advisable to use rearrangement to establish the phenotype of a lymphoma because the presence of double or aberrant rearrangements is often reported (Keller et al., 2016) as well as clonal rearrangements in dogs with AML (Stokol et al., 2017). Thus, clonality assessment could be used to confirm the diagnosis of neoplasia, but it is not useful for distinguishing between T- and B-cell neoplasms or between AML, ALL, or lymphoma with peripheral blood involvement.

Staging Lymphoma and Monitoring Disease
Because the PARR assay is more sensitive than visual examination of cells, it can detect neoplastic cells in the peripheral blood when they are not detected by cytopathology (Keller et al., 2004). Approximately 75% of stage III lymphomas, which have no visually detectable circulating neoplastic cells, will have a PARR+ result in the peripheral blood (Lana et al., 2006a). The presence of these cells does not appear to correlate with a worse outcome; therefore, clinical staging remains the most useful predictor of prognosis.

Clonal Relationships Between Tumors and Detection of Minimal Residual Disease
The sequence of the CDR3 region that is amplified during the PCR process is unique to each lymphocyte clone. Therefore, this sequence can be used to establish the relationship between neoplastic cells that arise in different organs, at different times, or have a dramatically different morphologic appearance. For example, the relationship between *Helicobacter pylori* infection and human gastric lymphoma was established by showing that the B-cell lymphoma in a patient with a history of *Helicobacter* infection had the same CDR3 sequence as clones found in reactive gastritis tissue biopsy specimens obtained several years earlier (Zucca et al., 1998).

The unique CDR3 sequence can be used to determine if two tumors with morphologically different phenotypes are related. Two human patients with two distinct forms of lymphoma occurring simultaneously were reported (Bräuninger et al., 1999). Both patients had classic Hodgkin's lymphoma, but one also had a follicular lymphoma, and the other had a T-cell–rich B-cell lymphoma. The CDR3 sequence of the Ig gene in the Reed-Sternberg cells of the Hodgkin's lymphoma was identical to the CDR3 sequence of the other form of B-cell lymphoma in both patients. This finding indicates that a single clone can evolve into dramatically different morphologic phenotypes. A similar study in a dog treated for classical non-Hodgkin's B-cell lymphoma and then developed multiple myeloma was reported (Burnett et al., 2004). By sequencing the CDR3 regions of both tumors, it was shown that the B cells from the lymphoma and plasma cells from the multiple myeloma had the same clonal origin.

Because CDR3 uniquely identifies an individual B cell, a primer that binds to this region can be used to selectively amplify DNA from a single tumor, as distinct from amplifying DNA from all B cells in a sample. Detection of neoplastic cells is considerably more sensitive using this method, and such an assay has been used to detect MRD in the blood of human patients treated for a variety of lymphoid malignancies. The technique was shown to demonstrate the reappearance of clonal B cells in the blood of dogs treated for B-cell lymphoma before clinical relapse (Yamazaki et al., 2008).

Both FC and PARR are promising techniques for detecting MRD in canine lymphoma. A study of dogs affected with diffuse large B-cell lymphoma (DLBCL) that compared results in lymph node, peripheral blood, and bone marrow samples reported that PARR was more sensitive than FC in predicting time to remission, whereas the combination of PARR and FC was more sensitive than either technique alone in predicting lymphoma-specific survival using peripheral blood samples. The results suggest that immunologic and molecular techniques should be used in combination when monitoring for MRD in canine DLBCL (Aresu et al., 2014).

However, MRD detection with PARR is complex and requires both sequencing the Ig gene involved in the malignancy and creating tumor-specific standard curves to be used in the quantification. Therefore, it is unlikely to be applied to routine monitoring in its current form, but it may be useful when false-negative results of FC are suspected or in a research setting. MRD detection will likely be replaced by next-generation sequencing. In the latter method, all the Ig or TCR genes within a particular sample are sequenced and quantified. This method will allow investigators to directly count the number of tumor cells in a sample.

Clonality Assays in Cats

The sequences of TCRγ and Ig genes from cats have been published and were used for clonality assays in cases of visceral B-cell lymphoma and intestinal T-cell lymphoma (Moore et al., 2005; Werner et al., 2005; Mochizuki et al., 2012). One study found that 79% of cases of intestinal T-cell lymphoma and 50% of B-cell lymphomas could be identified using clonality assays (Moore et al., 2012). Other studies reported a diagnostic sensitivity and specificity of 70% and 90%, respectively, with a diagnostic accuracy of 77% (Hammer et al., 2017).

Perhaps the most important use of the clonality assay in cats is to distinguish neoplastic from non-neoplastic lymphocytic infiltrates when clinicians are trying to distinguish intestinal lymphoma from severe inflammatory bowel disease (IBD). The available data clearly show that full-thickness intestinal tissue biopsy is by far the most useful diagnostic procedure for making this distinction. Only full-thickness biopsies allow the pathologist to assess the extent to which neoplastic cells have infiltrated (mucosal vs transmural) and the size of the neoplastic cells. Both of these features, together with immunophenotype, are prognostic in feline intestinal lymphoma (Moore et al., 2012). The inclusion of clonality assay in the diagnostic procedures to differentiate lymphoma from IBD may be useful. However, recently, some authors reported a high frequency of clonal rearrangements, both with and without a polyclonal background, in cats that did not reveal signs of lymphoma at the follow-up examination (Marsilio et al., 2019). Thus, because of the variable specificity, the PARR results had to be evaluated in the light of all the clinical, histopathologic, and immunophenotypic results.

DETECTION OF TRANSLOCATIONS, CHROMOSOMAL ABERRATIONS, AND GENE MUTATIONS

Translocations

Lymphoma and leukemia are frequently associated with translocations because the process of recombining antigen receptor genes leaves lymphocytes susceptible to mistakes in recombination. Most translocations found in human leukemia and lymphoma involve the Ig heavy chain gene locus. For example, t(11;14) juxtaposes the locus encoding cyclin D1 on chromosome 11 to an Ig-enhancer sequence on chromosome 14. This translocation, which results in the overexpression of cyclin D1, is found in virtually all cases of mantle cell lymphoma (Campo, 2003). Detection of the translocation by PCR or the overexpressed protein by IHC can be used to confirm the diagnosis of mantle cell lymphoma in histologically ambiguous cases. A consortium of European researchers found that the combined use of clonality determination through antigen receptor rearrangements together with detection of this and other translocations by PCR resulted in detection of a clonal population in 95% of human cases of confirmed lymphoid malignancies (van Krieken et al., 2003).

Two translocations that might be targets of future diagnostic testing for canine lymphoma are the IgH-myc translocation in B-cell lymphoma and the BCR-ABL translocation in acute and chronic canine myeloid leukemia (Breen and Modiano, 2008; Culver et al., 2013). IgH-myc is commonly found in aggressive human B-cell lymphomas. The BCR-ABL translocation is found in approximately 95% of human CML cases. Routine detection of this translocation in dogs by any number of methods would be a useful way of distinguishing CML from inflammatory conditions. It is likely that testing for these and other rearrangements will be commercially available in veterinary medicine in the near future.

Chromosomal Aberrations

Chromosomal aberrations in the form of increased or decreased chromosome copy number have been described in multiple different histologic subtypes of lymphoma (Thomas et al., 2011). These investigators used array comparative genomic hybridization, a technique that allows the detection of copy number changes (deletions or duplications) on whole chromosomes or portions of chromosomes throughout the entire canine genome. Although this technique is not currently available as a clinical tool, further studies will likely lead to the discovery of targeted PCR and IHC or FC-based assays that can be used for detecting malignant lymphocytes in ambiguous cases and subclassifying malignancies into discrete prognostic and therapeutic groups.

Gene Mutations

Detection of mutations in oncogenes is a mainstay in the characterization of human malignancies for diagnosis, prognosis, and therapy. For example, mutations in the *FLT3* gene (FMS-like tyrosine kinase 3) result in constitutive activation of this tyrosine kinase receptor. The presence of such mutations is prognostic in human AML (Kayser and Levis, 2014) and can help guide therapy with the appropriate tyrosine kinase inhibitors. Similar *FLT3* mutations have been described in canine ALL (Suter et al., 2011). Although detection of these mutations is not a standard diagnostic test, the methodology is straightforward and could be readily adopted for routine use after there are data to show that the presence of the mutation has prognostic or therapeutic significance.

A similar type of mutation is now commonly detected in canine mast cell tumors. The *c-kit* gene, which encodes the receptor for stem cell factor, is a receptor tyrosine kinase. When a portion of the gene that is adjacent to the cell membrane is duplicated (called an internal tandem duplication), the result is

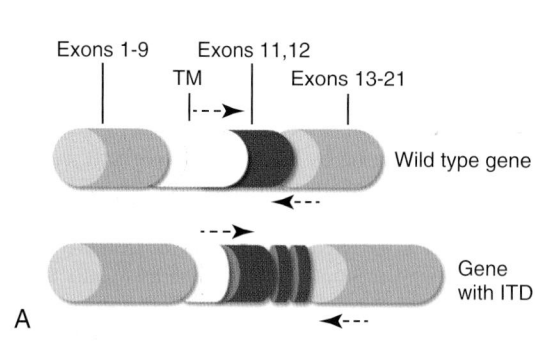
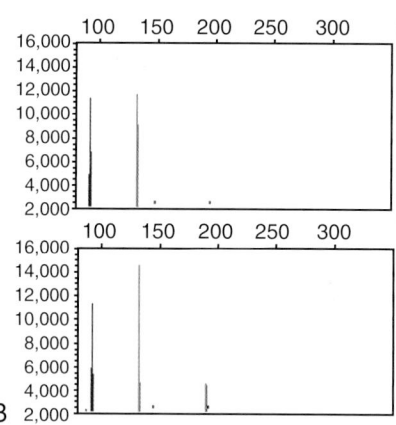

■ **FIGURE 18.40** Assessment of *c-kit* mutation status in canine mast cell tumors. **A,** Diagram of the *c-kit* gene demonstrating where the most common mutation is found (internal tandem duplication of exon 11). The portion of the protein encoded by exons 1 to 9 is found on the cell surface, and the portion encoded by exons 11 to 21 is found in the cytoplasm. The second most common site of internal tandem duplication is exon 8 (not shown). *ITD,* internal tandem duplication; *TM,* transmembrane region. **B,** Amplification of exons 8 and 11 by polymerase chain reaction (PCR). In this example, both exons are amplified in the same PCR reaction, with primers conjugated to different fluorochromes. The top graph shows amplification of wild type exon 8 (blue) and exon 11 (green). The bottom graph shows wild type exons 8 and 11, as well as an internal tandem duplication of exon 11 (~190 bases).

constitutive activation of the receptor. After the initial description of this mutation, a comprehensive analysis of mast cell tumors found that although the most common mutation is seen in exon 11, an internal tandem duplication in exon 8 and point mutations in exons 9 and 17 are also found (Letard et al., 2008). *C-kit* mutations are diagnosed by a PCR assay that amplifies the region of the gene where the mutation is commonly found (Fig. 18.40). The internal tandem duplication in exon 11 creates a larger PCR product of variable size (most commonly between three and 45 additional bases; Letard et al., 2008). The internal tandem duplication in exon 8 is always the same, an addition of 12 bases. Thus, detection of both of these mutations is straightforward. An internal control for this assay is the presence of the wild-type PCR product—almost all samples contain non–tumor-derived DNA, which would contain wild-type *c-kit*. In addition, presumably, the mast cells themselves have one wild-type *c-kit* gene. The assay can be performed on tissue biopsies or aspirate biopsies, and mast cells must comprise at least 10% of the total cell numbers. Mast cell tumors with mutated *c-kit* gene are associated with higher grade, more aggressive behavior and a worse clinical outcome (Webster et al., 2007), but *c-kit* mutation status seems not be predictive of the response to therapy. In a prospective, randomized study, the outcome of dogs was not related to the presence of the *c-kit* mutation in dogs treated with *c-kit* inhibitors as well as with vinblastine (Weishaar et al., 2018).

REFERENCES

Adam F, Villiers E, Watson S, et al. Clinical pathological and epidemiological assessment of morphologically and immunologically confirmed canine leukaemia. *Vet Comp Oncol.* 2009;7:181-195.

Anonymous. *Immunocytochemistry (ICC) Handbook.* Centennial, CO: Novus Biologicals; 2017. Available at: https://www.novusbio.com/support/immunocytochemistry-icc-handbook.

Aresu L, Aricò A, Ferraresso S, et al. Minimal residual disease detection by flow cytometry and PARR in lymph node, peripheral blood and bone marrow, following treatment of dogs with diffuse large B-cell lymphoma. *Vet J.* 2014;200:318-324.

Argyle DJ, Nasir L. Telomerase: a potential diagnostic and therapeutic tool in canine oncology. *Vet Pathol.* 2003;40:1-7.

Arnold JE, Camus MS, Freeman KP, et al. ASVCP guidelines: principles of quality assurance and standards for veterinary clinical pathology (version 3.0). *Vet Clin Pathol.* 2019;48:542-618.

Avery PR, Avery AC. Molecular methods to distinguish reactive and neoplastic lymphocyte expansions and their importance in transitional neoplastic states. *Vet Clin Pathol.* 2004;33:196-207.

Avery PR, Burton J, Bromberek JL, et al. Flow cytometric characterization and clinical outcome of CD4+ T-cell lymphoma in dogs: 67 cases. *J Vet Intern Med.* 2014;28:538-546.

Bardou VJ, Arpino G, Elledge RM, et al. Progesterone receptor status significantly improves outcome prediction over estrogen receptor status alone for adjuvant endocrine therapy in two large breast cancer databases. *J Clin Oncol.* 2003;21:1973-1979.

Batlivala TP, Bacon NJ, Avery AC, et al. Paraneoplastic T cell lymphocytosis associated with a thymoma in a dog. *J Small Anim Pract.* 2010;51:491-494.

Bhargava R, Dabbs DJ. Immunohistology of metastatic carcinomas of unknown primary. In: Dabbs DJ, ed. *Diagnostic Immunohistochemistry. Theranostic and Genomic Applications.* 3rd ed. Philadelphia: Saunders; 2010:206-255.

Bräuninger A, Hansmann ML, Strickler JG, et al. Identification of common germinal-center B-cell precursors in two patients with both Hodgkin's disease and non-Hodgkin's lymphoma. *N Engl J Med.* 1999;340:1239-1247.

Breen M, Modiano JF. Evolutionarily conserved cytogenetic changes in hematological malignancies of dogs and humans–man and his best friend share more than companionship. *Chromosome Res.* 2008;16:145-154.

Bricker NK, Raskin RE, Densmore CL. Cytochemical and immunocytochemical characterization of blood cells and immunohistochemical analysis of spleen cells from 2 species of frog, *Rana (Aquarana) catesbeiana* and *Xenopus laevis. Vet Clin Pathol.* 2012;41:353-361.

Bromberek JL, Rout ED, Agnew MR, et al. Breed distribution and clinical characteristics of B cell chronic lymphocytic leukemia in dogs. *J Vet Intern Med.* 2016;30:215-222.

Burkhard MJ, Bienzle D. Making sense of lymphoma diagnostics in small animal patients. *Vet Clin Small Anim.* 2013;43:1331-1347.

Burnett RC, Vernau W, Modiano JF, et al. Diagnosis of canine lymphoid neoplasia using clonal rearrangements of antigen receptor genes. *Vet Pathol.* 2003;40(1):32-41.

Burnett RC, Blake MK, Thompson LJ, et al. Evolution of a B-cell lymphoma to multiple myeloma after chemotherapy. *J Vet Intern Med.* 2004;18:768-771.

Byrne KM, Kim HW, Chew BP, et al. A standardized gating technique for the generation of flow cytometry data for normal canine and normal feline blood lymphocytes. *Vet Immunol Immunopathol.* 2000;73:167-182.

Campbell MW, Hess PR, Williams LE. Chronic lymphocytic leukaemia in the cat: 18 cases (2000-2010). *Vet Comp Oncol.* 2012;11:256-264.

Campo E. Genetic and molecular genetic studies in the diagnosis of B-cell lymphomas I: mantle cell lymphoma, follicular lymphoma, and Burkitt's lymphoma. *Human Pathol.* 2003;34:330-335.

Carson FL, Cappellano CH. *Histotechnology: A Self-Instructional Text.* 4th ed. Chicago: American Society for Clinical Pathology; 2015.

Carvalho MI, Pires I, Prada J, et al. Ki-67 and PCNA expression in canine mammary tumors and adjacent nonneoplastic mammary glands: prognostic impact by a multivariate survival analysis. *Vet Pathol.* 2016;53(6):1138-1146.

Cheville NF, Stasko J. Techniques in electron microscopy of animal tissue. *Vet Pathol.* 2014;51:28-41.

Chivukula M, Dabbs DJ. Immunocytology. In: Dabbs DJ, ed. *Diagnostic Immunocytochemistry.* 3rd ed. New York: Churchill Livingstone; 2010: 890-918.

Cian F, Guzera M, Frost S, et al. Stability of immunophenotypic lymphoid markers in fixed canine peripheral blood for flow cytometric analysis. *Vet Clin Pathol.* 2014;43:101-108.

Colasacco C, Mount S, Leiman G. Documentation of immunocytochemistry controls in the cytopathologic literature: a meta-analysis of 100 journal articles. *Diagn Cytopathol.* 2010;39:245-250.

Colledge SL, Raskin RE, Messick JB, et al. Multiple joint metastasis of a transitional cell carcinoma in a dog. *Vet Clin Pathol.* 2013;42(2):216-220.

Comazzi S, Avery PR, Garden OA, et al. European canine lymphoma network consensus recommendations for reporting flow cytometry in canine hematopoietic neoplasms. *Cytometry B Clin Cytom.* 2017;92:411-419.

Comazzi S, Cozzi M, Bernardi S, et al. Effects of pre-analytical variables on flow cytometric diagnosis of canine lymphoma: a retrospective study (2009-2015). *Vet J.* 2018;232:65-69.

Comazzi S, Gelain ME, Martini V, et al. Immunophenotype predicts survival time in dogs with chronic lymphocytic leukemia. *J Vet Intern Med.* 2011;25:100-106.

Culver S, Ito D, Borst L, et al. Molecular characterization of canine BCR-ABL-positive chronic myelomonocytic leukemia before and after chemotherapy. *Vet Clin Pathol.* 2013;42(3):314-322.

Dabbs DJ. Immunocytology. In: Dabbs DJ, ed. *Diagnostic Immunohistochemistry.* New York: Churchill Livingstone; 2002:625-639.

Dabbs DJ. Immunohistology of metastatic carcinoma of unknown primary. In: Dabbs DJ, ed. *Diagnostic Immunohistochemistry.* 2nd ed. New York: Churchill Livingstone; 2006.

Dardick I, Herrera GA. Diagnostic electron microscopy of neoplasms. *Hum Pathol.* 1998;29:1335-1338.

Denda T, Kamoshida S, Kawamura J, et al. Optimal antigen retrieval for ethanol-fixed cytologic smears. *Cancer Cytopathol.* 2012;120:167-176.

Deshuillers PL, Santos AP, Raskin RE. First report of circulating double positive CD4/CD8 T lymphocytes in a cat with thymoma. *Vet Clin Pathol.* 2015;44(4):E1-E18.

Dickersin GR, ed. *Diagnostic Electron Microscopy: A Text/Atlas.* 2nd ed. New York: Springer; 2000.

Dorfelt S, Matiasek LA, Felten S, et al. Antigens under cover: the preservation and demasking of selected antigens for successful poststaining immunocytochemistry of effusion, brain smears, and lymph node aspirates. *Vet Clin Pathol.* 2019;48(suppl 1):98-107.

Dreitz MJ, Ogilvie G, Sim GK. Rearranged T lymphocyte antigen receptor genes as markers of malignant T cells. *Vet Immunol Immuopathol.* 1999;69:113-119.

Dupré MP, Courtade-Saidi M. Immunocytochemistry as an adjunct to diagnostic cytology. *Ann Pathol.* 2012;32:433-437.

Dvorak AM, Monahan-Earley RA, eds. *Diagnostic Ultrastructural Pathology I.* Boca Raton: CRC Press; 1992.

Ehrhart EJ, Wong S, Richter K, et al. Polymerase chain reaction for antigen receptor rearrangement: benchmarking performance of a lymphoid clonality assay in diverse canine sample types. *J Vet Intern Med.* 2019; 33(3):1392-1402.

Erlandson RA, ed. *Diagnostic Transmission Electron Microscopy of Tumors.* New York: Raven Press; 1994.

Espinosa de los Monteros A, Fernández A, Millán MY, et al. Coordinate expression of cytokeratins 7 and 20 in feline and canine carcinomas. *Vet Pathol.* 1999;36(3):179-190.

Eyden B, ed. *Organelles in Tumor Diagnosis: An Ultrastructural Atlas.* New York: Igaku Shoin; 1996.

Fetsch PA, Abati A. Ancillary techniques in cytopathology. In: Atkinson BF, ed. *Atlas of Diagnostic Cytopathology.* 2nd ed. Philadelphia: Saunders; 2004:747-775.

Fivenson DP, Saed GM, Beck ER, et al. T-cell receptor gene rearrangement in canine mycosis fungoides: further support for a canine model of cutaneous T cell lymphoma. *J Invest Dermatol.* 1994;102:227-230.

Flood-Knapik KE, Durham AC, Gregor TP, et al. Clinical, histopathological and immunohistochemical characterization of canine indolent lymphoma. *Vet Comp Oncol.* 2013;11:272-286.

Fowler LJ, Lachar WA. Application of immunohistochemistry to cytology. *Arch Pathol Lab Med.* 2008;132:373-383.

Gelain ME, Martini V, Giantin M, et al. CD44 in canine leukemia: analysis of mRNA and protein expression in peripheral blood. *Vet Immunol Immunopathol.* 2014;159:91-96.

Gelain ME, Mazzilli M, Riondato F, et al. Aberrant phenotypes and quantitative antigen expression in different subtypes of canine lymphoma by flow cytometry. *Vet Immunol Immunopathol.* 2008;121:179-188.

Ghadially FN, ed. *Diagnostic Ultrastructural Pathology: A Self-Evaluation and Self-Teaching Manual.* 2nd ed. Boston: Butterworth-Heinemann; 1998.

Giantin M, Aresu L, Aricò A, et al. Evaluation of tyrosine-kinase receptor c-kit mutations, mRNA and protein expression in canine lymphoma: might c-kit represent a therapeutic target. *Vet Immunol Immunopathol.* 2013;154:153-159.

Gong Y, Sun X, Michael CW, et al. Immunocytochemistry of serous effusion specimens: a comparison of ThinPrep vs. cell block. *Diagn Cytopathol.* 2003;28:1-5.

Guzera M, Cian F, Leo C, et al. The use of flow cytometry for immunophenotyping lymphoproliferative disorders in cats: a retrospective study of 19 cases. *Vet Comp Oncol.* 2016;14(suppl 1):40-51.

Hammer SE, Groiss S, Fuchs-Baumgartinger A, et al. Characterization of a PCR-based lymphocyte clonality assay as a complementary tool for the diagnosis of feline lymphoma. *Vet Comp Oncol.* 2017;15:1354-1369.

Hayat MA. Factors affecting antigen retrieval. In: Hayat MA, ed. *Microscopy, Immunohisto-chemistry, and Antigen Retrieval Methods for Light and Electron Microscopy.* New York: Kluwer Academic; 2002:53-69.

Heeb HL, Wilkerson MJ, Chun R, et al. Large granular lymphocytosis, lymphocyte subset inversion, thrombocytopenia, dysproteinemia, and positive Ehrlichia serology in a dog. *J Am Anim Hosp Assoc.* 2003;39:379-384.

Heinrich DA, Avery AC, Henson MS, et al. Cytology and the cell block method in diagnostic characterization of canine lymphadenopathy and in the immunophenotyping of nodal lymphoma. *Vet Comp Oncol.* 2019;17(3):365-375.

Höinghaus R, Hewicker-Trautwein M, Mischke R. Immunocytochemical differentiation of canine mesenchymal tumors in cytologic imprint preparations. *Vet Clin Pathol.* 2008;37:104-111.

Horobin RW. How histological stains work. In: Suvarna K, Layton C, Bancroft JD, eds. *Bancroft's Theory and Practice of Histological Techniques.* 7th ed. Edinburgh: Churchill Livingstone; 2013:157-172.

Ishikawa K, Sakai H, Hosoi M, et al. Evaluation of cell proliferation in canine tumors by the bromodeoxyuridine labeling method, immunostaining of Ki-67 antigen and proliferating cell nuclear antigen. *J Toxicol Pathol.* 2006; 19:123-127.

Jung D, Alt FW. Unraveling V(D)J recombination; insights into gene regulation. *Cell.* 2004;116:299-311.

Kayser S, Levis MJ. FLT3 tyrosine kinase inhibitors in acute myeloid leukemia: clinical implications and limitations. *Leuk Lymphoma.* 2014;55:243-255.

Keller RL, Avery AC, Burnett RC, et al. Detection of neoplastic lymphocytes in peripheral blood of dogs with lymphoma by polymerase chain reaction for antigen receptor gene rearrangement. *Vet Clin Pathol.* 2004;33: 145-149.

Keller SM, Moore PF. A novel clonality assay for the assessment of canine T cell proliferations. *Vet Immunol Immunopathol.* 2012;145:410-419.

Keller SM, Vernau W, Moore PF. Clonality testing in veterinary medicine: a review with diagnostic guidelines. *Vet Pathol.* 2016;53:711-725.

Kim SW, Roh J, Park CS. Immunohistochemistry for pathologists: protocols, pitfalls, and tips. *J Pathol Translat Med.* 2016;50:411-418.

Kisseberth WC, Nadella WV, Breen M, et al. A novel canine lymphoma cell line: a translational and comparative model for lymphoma research. *Leuk Res.* 2007;31:1709-1720.

Kiupel M, Webster JD, Kaneene JB, et al. The use of KIT and tryptase expression patterns as prognostic tools for canine cutaneous mast cell tumors. *Vet Pathol.* 2004;41:371-377.

Kow K, Bailey SM, Williams ES, et al. Telomerase activity in canine osteosarcoma. *Vet Comp Oncol.* 2006;4:184-187.

Lai C-L, van den Ham R, van Leenders G, et al. Histopathological and immunohistochemical characterization of canine prostate cancer. *Prostate.* 2008;68:477-488.

Lana SE, Jackson TL, Burnett RC, et al. Utility of polymerase chain reaction for analysis of antigen receptor rearrangement in staging and predicting prognosis in dogs with lymphoma. *J Vet Intern Med.* 2006a;20:329-334.

Lana S, Plaza S, Hampe K, et al. Diagnosis of mediastinal masses in dogs by flow cytometry. *J Vet Intern Med.* 2006b;20:1161-1165.

Lara-Garcia A, Wellman M, Burkhard MJ, et al. Cervical thymoma originating in ectopic thymic tissue in a cat. *Vet Clin Pathol.* 2008;37:397-402.

Letard S, Yang Y, Hanssens K, et al. Gain-of-function mutations in the extracellular domain of KIT are common in canine mast cell tumors. *Mol Cancer Res.* 2008;6:1137-1345.

Long S, Argyle DJ, Nixon C, et al. Telomerase reverse transcriptase (TERT) expression and proliferation in canine brain tumors. *Neuropathol Appl Neurobiol.* 2006;32:662-673.

Łopuszyński W, Szczubiał M, Millán Y, et al. Immunohistochemical expression of p63 protein and calponin in canine mammary tumours. *Res Vet Sci.* 2019;123:232-238.

Mackay B. Electron microscopy in tumor diagnosis. In: Fletcher CDM, ed. *Diagnostic Histopathology of Tumors.* 3rd ed. New York: Churchill Livingstone; 2007:1831-1859.

Marcos R, Santos M, Marrinhas C, et al. Cell tube block: a new technique to produce cell blocks from fluid cytology samples. *Vet Clin Pathol.* 2017;46(1):195-201.

Marsilio S, Ackermann MR, Lidbury JA, et al. Results of histopathology, immunohistochemistry, and molecular clonality testing of small intestinal biopsy specimens from clinically healthy client-owned cats. *J Vet Intern Med.* 2019;33:551-558.

Martini V, Bernardi S, Marelli P, et al. Flow cytometry for feline lymphoma: a retrospective study regarding pre-analytical factors possibly affecting the quality of samples. *J Feline Med Surg.* 2018;20:494-501.

Martini V, Poggi A, Riondato F, et al. Flow-cytometric detection of phenotypic aberrancies in canine small clear cell lymphoma. *Vet Comp Oncol.* 2015;13: 281-287.

Martini V, Marconato L, Poggi A, et al. Canine small clear cell/T-zone lymphoma: clinical presentation and outcome in a retrospective case series. *Vet Comp Oncol.* 2016;14(suppl 1):117-126.

McDonough SP, Moore PF. Clinical, hematologic, and immunophenotypic characterization of canine large granular lymphocytosis. *Vet Pathol.* 2000;37:637-646.

Meichner K, Stokol T, Tarigo J, et al. Multicenter flow cytometry proficiency testing of canine blood and lymph node samples. *Vet Clin Pathol.* 2020;49:249-257.

Miniscalco B, Poggi A, Martini V, et al. Flow cytometric characterization of S-phase fraction and ploidy in lymph node aspirates from dogs with lymphoma. *J Comp Pathol.* 2018;161:34-42.

Miyata-Takata T, Takata K, Yamanouchi S, et al. Detection of T-cell receptor gamma gene rearrangement in paraffin-embedded T or natural killer/T-cell lymphoma samples using the BIOMED-2 protocol. *Leuk Lymphoma.* 2014;55:2161-2164.

Mochizuki H, Nakamura K, Sato H, et al. GeneScan analysis to detect clonality of T-cell receptor gamma gene rearrangement in feline lymphoid neoplasms. *Vet Immunol Immunopathol.* 2012;145:402-409.

Moore AR, Coffey E, Leavell SE, et al. Canine bicavitary carcinomatosis with transient needle tract metastasis diagnosed by multiplex immunocytochemistry. *Vet Clin Pathol.* 2016;45:495-500.

Moore PF, Rodriguez-Bertos A, Kass PH. Feline gastrointestinal lymphoma: mucosal architecture, immunophenotype, and molecular clonality. *Vet Pathol.* 2012;49:658-668.

Moore PF, Woo JC, Vernau W, et al. Characterization of feline T cell receptor gamma (TCRG) variable region genes for the molecular diagnosis of feline intestinal T cell lymphoma. *Vet Immunol Immunopathol.* 2005;106:167-178.

Novacco M, Comazzi S, Marconato L, et al. Prognostic factors in canine acute leukaemias: a retrospective study. *Vet Comp Oncol.* 2016;14: 409-416.

Pang LY, Argyle D. Cancer stem cells and telomerase as potential biomarkers in veterinary oncology. *Vet J.* 2010;185:15-22.

Poggi A, Miniscalco B, Morello E, et al. Flow cytometric evaluation of Ki67 for the determination of malignancy grade in canine lymphoma. *Vet Comp Oncol.* 2015;13:475-480.

Poggi A, Miniscalco B, Morello E, et al. Prognostic significance of Ki67 evaluated by flow cytometry in dogs with high-grade B-cell lymphoma. *Vet Comp Oncol.* 2017;15:431-440.

Polak JM, Van Noorden S. *Introduction to Immunocytochemistry.* 3rd ed. Oxford: Garland Science/BIOS Scientific Publishers; 2003.

Ponce F, Magnol JP, Ledieu D, et al. Prognostic significance of morphological subtypes in canine malignant lymphomas during chemotherapy. *Vet J.* 2004;167:158-166.

Prophet EB, Mills B, Arrington JB, et al., eds. *AFIP Laboratory Methods in Histotechnology.* Washington DC: American Registry of Pathology; 1992.

Ramos-Vara JA. Immunohistochemical methods. In: Howard GC, Kaser MR, eds. *Making and Using Antibodies: A Practical Handbook.* 2nd ed. Boca Raton: CRC Press; 2013:303-341.

Ramos-Vara JA, Avery PR, Avery AV. Advanced diagnostic techniques. In: Raskin RE, Meyer DJ, eds. *Canine and Feline Cytology: A Color Atlas and Interpretation Guide.* 3rd ed. St. Louis: Elsevier; 2016:453-494.

Ramos-Vara JA, Beissenherz ME, Miller MA, et al. Immunoreactivity of A103, an antibody to Melan-A, in canine steroid-producing tissues and their tumors. *J Vet Diagn Invest.* 2001a;13:328-332.

Ramos-Vara JA, Beissenherz ME, Miller MA, et al. Retrospective study of 338 canine oral melanomas with clinical, histologic, and immunohistochemical review of 129 cases. *Vet Pathol.* 2000;37:597-608.

Ramos-Vara JA, Borst LB. Immunohistochemistry: fundamentals and applications. In: Meuten DJ, ed. *Tumors in Domestic Animals.* 5th ed. Ames, IA: Wiley Blackwell; 2017:44-87.

Ramos-Vara JA, Frank CB, DuSold D, et al. Immunohistochemical expression of melanocytic antigen PNL2, Melan A, S100 and PGP 9.5 in equine melanocytic neoplasms. *Vet Pathol.* 2014;51:161-166.

Ramos-Vara JA, Kiupel M, Baszler T, et al. Suggested guidelines for immunohistochemical techniques in veterinary diagnostic laboratories. *J Vet Diagn Invest.* 2008;20:393-413.

Ramos-Vara JA, Miller MA. Immunohistochemical characterization of canine intestinal epithelial and mesenchymal tumors with a monoclonal antibody to hepatocyte paraffin 1 (Hep Par 1). *Histochem J.* 2002;34:397-401.

Ramos-Vara JA, Miller MA. Immunohistochemical detection of protein gene product 9.5 (PGP 9.5) in canine epitheliotropic T-cell lymphoma (mycosis fungoides). *Vet Pathol.* 2007;44:74-79.

Ramos-Vara JA, Miller MA. When tissue antigens and antibodies get along: revisiting the technical aspects of immunohistochemistry—the red, brown, and blue technique. *Vet Pathol.* 2014;51:42-87.

Ramos-Vara JA, Miller MA, Boucher M, et al. Immunohistochemical detection of uroplakin III, cytokeratin 7, and cytokeratin 20 in canine urothelial tumors. *Vet Pathol.* 2003;40:55-62.

Ramos-Vara JA, Miller MA, Johnson GC. Immunohistochemical characterization of canine hyperplastic hepatic lesions and hepatocellular and biliary neoplasms with monoclonal antibody hepatocyte paraffin 1 and a monoclonal antibody to cytokeratin 7. *Vet Pathol.* 2001b;38:636-643.

Ramos-Vara JA, Miller MA, Johnson GC, et al. Immunohistochemical detection of thyroid transcription factor-1, thyroglobulin, and calcitonin in canine normal, hyperplastic, and neoplastic thyroid gland. *Vet Pathol.* 2002a;39:480-487.

Ramos-Vara JA, Miller MA, Johnson GC, et al. Melan A and S100 protein immunohistochemistry in feline melanomas: 48 cases. *Vet Pathol.* 2002b;39: 127-132.

Ramos-Vara JA, Miller MA, Johnson GC. Usefulness of thyroid transcription factor-1 immunohistochemical staining in the differential diagnosis of primary pulmonary tumors of dogs. *Vet Pathol.* 2005;42:315-320.

Rao S, Lana S, Eickhoff J, et al. Class II major histocompatibility complex expression and cell size independently predict survival in canine B-cell lymphoma. *J Vet Intern Med.* 2011;25:1097-1105.

Raskin RE, Vickers J, Ward JG, et al. Optimized immunocytochemistry using leukocyte and tissue markers on Romanowsky-stained slides from dogs and cats. *Vet Clin Pathol.* 2019;48:88-97.

Reguera MJ, Rabanal RM, Puigdemont A, et al. Canine mast cell tumors express stem cell factor receptor. *Am J Dermatopathol.* 2000;22:49-54.

Rhodes A. Quality assurance of immunocytochemistry and molecular morphology. In: Hacker GW, Tubbs RR, eds. *Molecular Morphology in Human Tissues: Techniques and Applications.* Boca Raton: CRC Press; 2005:275-293.

Riondato F, Miniscalco B, Poggi A, et al. Analytical and diagnostic validation of a flow cytometric strategy to quantify blood and marrow infiltration in dogs with large B-cell lymphoma. *Cytometry B Clin Cytom.* 2016;90:525-530.

Roccabianca P, Vernau W, Caniatti M, et al. Feline large granular lymphocyte (LGL) lymphoma with secondary leukemia: primary intestinal origin with predominance of a CD3/CD8aa phenotype. *Vet Pathol.* 2006;43:15-28.

Rout ED, Avery PR. Lymphoid neoplasia: correlations between morphology and flow cytometry. *Vet Clin North Am Small Anim Pract.* 2017;47:53-70.

Ruslander DA, Gebhard DH, Tompkins MB, et al. Immunophenotypic characterization of canine lymphoproliferative disorders. *In Vivo.* 1997;11:169-172.

Sailasuta A, Ketpun D, Piyaviriyakul P, et al. The relevance of CD117-immunocytochemistry staining patterns to mutational exon-11 in c-kit detected by PCR from fine-needle aspirated canine mast cell tumor cells. *Vet Med Int.* 2014;2014:787498. doi:10.1155/2014/787498.

Sato T, Miyoshi T, Shibuya H, et al. Peritoneal biphasic mesothelioma in a dog. *J Vet Med A.* 2005;52:22-25.

Sawa M, Yabuki A, Kohyama M, et al. Rapid multiple immunofluorescent staining for the simultaneous detection of cytokeratin and vimentin in the cytology of canine tumors. *Vet Clin Pathol.* 2018;47:326-332.

Scase TJ, Edwards D, Miller J, et al. Canine mast cell tumors: correlation of apoptosis and proliferation markers with prognosis. *J Vet Intern Med.* 2006;20:151-158.

Seelig DM, Avery P, Webb T, et al. Canine T-zone lymphoma: unique immunophenotypic features, outcome, and population characteristics. *J Vet Intern Med.* 2014;28:878-886.

Shapiro H. *Practical Flow Cytometry,* 4th ed. Hoboken, NJ: John Wiley & Sons; 2003.

Skoog L, Tani E. Immunocytochemistry: an indispensable technique in routine cytology. *Cytopathology.* 2011;22:215-229.

Stelow EB, Yazjii H. Immunohistochemistry, carcinomas of unknown primary, and incidence rates. *Semin Diagn Pathol.* 2018;35:143-152.

Stokol T, Nickerson GA, Shuman M, et al. Dogs with acute myeloid leukemia have clonal rearrangements in T and B cell receptors. *Front Vet Sci.* 2017;4:76.

Stone BM, Gan D. Application of the tissue transfer technique in veterinary cytopathology. *Vet Clin Pathol.* 2014;43:295-302.

Sulce M, Marconato L, Martano M, et al. Utility of flow cytometry in canine primary cutaneous and matched nodal mast cell tumor. *Vet J.* 2018;242:15-23.

Sundram U, Kim Y, Mraz-Gernhard S, et al. Expression of the bcl-6 and MUM1/IRF4 proteins correlate with overall and disease-specific survival in patients with primary cutaneous large B-cell lymphoma: a tissue microarray study. *J Clin Pathol.* 2005;32:227-234.

Suter SE, Small GW, Seiser EL, et al. FLT3 mutations in canine acute lymphocytic leukemia. *BMC Cancer.* 2011;11:38.

Suvarna SK, Layton C, Bancroft JD. *Bancroft's Theory and Practice of Histological Techniques.* 8th ed. Philadelphia: Elsevier; 2018.

Swerdlow SH. Genetic and molecular genetic studies in the diagnosis of atypical lymphoid hyperplasia versus lymphoma. *Human Pathol.* 2003;34:346-351.

Szczepanski T, van der Velden VHJ, Van Dongen JJ. Flow-cytometric immunophenotyping of normal and malignant lymphocytes. *Clin Chem Lab Med.* 2006;44:775-796.

Tasca S, Carli E, Caldin M, et al. Hematologic abnormalities and flow cytometric immunophenotyping results in dogs with hematopoietic neoplasia: 210 cases (2002–2006). *Vet Clin Pathol.* 2009;38:2-12.

Teske E, van heerde P, Rutteman GR, et al. Pronostic factors for treatment of malignant lymphoma in dogs. *J Am Vet Med Assoc.* 1994;205:1722-1728.

Thomas R, Seiser EL, Motsinger-Reif A, et al. Refining tumor-associated aneuploidy through 'genomic recoding' of recurrent DNA copy number aberrations in 150 canine non-Hodgkin lymphomas. *Leuk Lymphoma.* 2011;52:1321-1335.

Valli V, Peters E, Williams C, et al. Optimizing methods in immunocytochemistry: one laboratory's experience. *Vet Clin Pathol.* 2009;38:261-269.

Valli VE, Vernau W, de Lorimier L-P, et al. Canine indolent nodular lymphoma. *Vet Pathol.* 2006;43:241-256.

Van der Loos CM. A focus on fixation. *Biotech Histochem.* 2007;82:141-154.

van Dongen JJ, Langerak AW, Bruggemann M, et al. Design and standardization of PCR primers and protocols for detection of clonal immunoglobulin and T-cell receptor gene recombinations in suspect lymphoproliferations: report of the BIOMED-2 Concerted Action BMH4-CT98-3936. *Leukemia.* 2003;17:2257-2317.

van Krieken JH, Langerak AW, San Miguel JF, et al. Clonality analysis for antigen receptor genes: preliminary results from the Biomed-2 Concerted Action PL 96-3936. *Human Pathol.* 2003;34:359-361.

Vernau W, Moore PF. An immunophenotypic study of canine leukemias and preliminary assessment of clonality by polymerase chain reaction. *Vet Immunol Immunopathol.* 1999;69:145-164.

Vezzali E, Parodi AL, Marcato PS, et al. Histopathologic classification of 171 cases of canine and feline non-Hodgkin lymphoma according to the WHO. *Vet Comp Oncol.* 2010;8:38-49.

Villiers E, Baines S, Law AM, et al. Identification of acute myeloid leukemia in dogs using flow cytometry with myeloperoxidase, MAC387, and a canine neutrophil-specific antibody. *Vet Clin Pathol.* 2006;35:55-71.

Vural SA, Ozyldilz Z, Ozsoy SY. Pleural mesothelioma in a nine-month-old dog. *Irish Vet J.* 2007;60:30-33.

Webster JD, Yuzbasiyan-Gurkan V, Miller RA, et al. Cellular proliferation in canine cutaneous mast cell tumors: associations with c-KIT and its role in prognostication. *Vet Pathol.* 2007;44:298-308.

Weiser MG, Thrall MA, Fulton R, et al. Granular lymphocytosis and hyperproteinemia in dogs with chronic ehrlichiosis. *J Am Anim Hosp Assoc.* 1991;27:84-88.

Weishaar KM, Ehrhart EJ, Avery AC, et al. c-Kit mutation and localization status as response predictors in mast cell tumors in dogs treated with prednisone and toceranib or vinblastine. *J Vet Intern Med.* 2018;32:394-405.

Werner JA, Woo JC, Vernau W, et al. Characterization of feline immunoglobulin heavy chain variable region genes for the molecular diagnosis of B-cell neoplasia. *Vet Pathol.* 2005;42:596-607.

Wilkerson MJ, Dolce K, Koopman T, et al. Lineage differentiation of canine lymphoma/leukemias and aberrant expression of CD molecules. *Vet Immunol Immunopathol.* 2005;106:179-196.

Williams MJ, Avery AC, Lana SE, et al. Canine lymphoproliferative disease characterized by lymphocytosis: immunophenotypic markers of prognosis. *J Vet Intern Med.* 2008;22:596-601.

Wong A, Sykora C, Rogers L, et al. Modified nanoantibodies increase sensitivity in avidin-biotin immunohistochemistry. *Appl Immunohistochem Mol Morphol.* 2018;26:682-688.

Workman HC, Vernau W. Chronic lymphocytic leukemia in dogs and cats: the veterinary perspective. *Vet Clin North Am Sm Anim Pract.* 2003;33:1379-1399.

Yamazaki J, Baba K, Goto-Koshino Y, et al. Quantitative assessment of minimal residual disease (MRD) in canine lymphoma by using real-time polymerase chain reaction. *Vet Immunol Immunopathol.* 2008;126:321-331.

Yaziji H, Barry T. Diagnostic immunohistochemistry: what can go wrong? *Adv Anat Pathol.* 2006;13:238-246.

Zamboni C, Brocca G, Ferraresso S, et al. Cyclin D1 immunohistochemical expression and somatic mutations in canine oral melanoma. *Vet Comp Oncol.* 2020;18:231-238.

Zanoni DS, Grandi F, Cagnini DQ, et al. Agarose cell block technique as a complementary method in the diagnosis of fungal osteomyelitis in a dog. *Open Vet J.* 2012;2(1):19-22.

Zhang Z, Zhao L, Guo H, et al. Diagnostic significance of immunocytochemistry on fine needle aspiration biopsies processed by thin-layer cytology. *Diagn Cytopathol.* 2012;240:1071-1076.

Zucca E, Bertoni F, Roggero E, et al. Molecular analysis of the progression from *Helicobacter pylori*-associated chronic gastritis to mucosa-associated lymphoid-tissue lymphoma of the stomach. *N Engl J Med.* 1998;338:804-810.

Zuccari DA, Santana AE, Cury PM, et al. Immunocytochemical study of Ki-67 as a prognostic marker in canine mammary neoplasia. *Vet Clin Pathol.* 2004;33:23-28.

APPENDIX 1

Microscope and Telecytopathology Basics

Rose E. Raskin

MICROSCOPE BASICS

Parts of the Microscope

Overview of Microscope Parts

The locations of major control parts of the microscope are illustrated in Figure A1.1, along with a closer view of the substage condenser and its aperture diaphragm in Figure A1.2. This section highlights a few important considerations regarding microscopes and their proper usage.

Lens Objectives

The microscopist should be able to optimize resolution and color correctness to best view and record images. This involves an understanding about chromatic and spherical aberration (color and lens curvature errors) plus field curvature (flatness of field). *Chromatic aberration* is caused by a lens having a different refractive index for each wavelength of light so the rays do not focus in one location, thus producing blurring of colors. *Spherical aberration* is produced by the lens curvature that results in a refraction of light at the periphery. To overcome these aberrations, additional lenses are added to the objective. The increased number of internal lenses influences the quality and cost of the objective lens. The least expensive is *achromat*, which has minimal chromatic and spherical aberration correction and is best intended for black and white photography. A better lens relative to correction but higher in cost is Fluorite or semiapochromat. These lenses correct for several colors and are adequate for color photography. The finest type of lens objective for color correction bringing red, blue, and green into one focal point is *Apochromat*, which is the most expensive. Each of the objectives can also be corrected for the field of view so that it is in focus from center to periphery. This will avoid the fuzzy rim at the outer edge of the field seen with inexpensive lenses. Lenses that correct for field curvature are termed *Plan*, so the best combination for an objective is *Plan Apochromat*. See Table A1.1 on lens corrections relative to aberrations and curvature.

Each objective is labeled with its specifications on the outside of the barrel (Fig. A1.3). Listed are the manufacturer, magnification (10×, 20×, etc.), optimum tube length and working distance (in millimeters), coverslip thickness, suggested immersion medium, color coding, numerical aperture (NA), and any specialized designations.

The tube length for the objective is that designed to produce optimum images (usually 160 mm or the Greek infinity symbol [∞]), whereas the working distance is the amount of space between the front lens of the objective and the surface of the cover glass or specimen. The parfocal distance is the length between the objective mounting position and the surface of the coverslip; if it is equal for all objectives, there is no need for coarse focus adjustment when switching objectives. The thickness of cover glass (coverslip) protecting the specimen is suggested for each objective to correct for spherical aberration (usually 0.17 mm or size #1.5 cover glass). If oil is designed for use with the objective, OIL, OEL (oil between lens and specimen), or HI (homogeneous immersion) will be engraved on the objective along with a black color band below the objective magnification color band (e.g., white for 100×, light blue for 50×, green for 20×, yellow for 10×).

If the objective carries no designation of higher aberration correction, one can usually assume it is achromatic. More highly corrected objectives are inscribed as **Apochromat** or **Apo**, **Plan** or **UPLAN** (Olympus), **FL** or **Fluor**, and so on. In addition to those mentioned earlier, some commonly engraved specialized objective designations include **Corr** (correction collar), **I** or **Iris** (adjustable NA with iris diaphragm) (Fig. A1.4). Other designations include **DIC** (differential interference contrast), **M** (metallographic, no coverslip), **D** (darkfield), **H** (used with heating stage), **ICS** (infinity corrected system [Zeiss]), and **UIS** (universal infinity system [Olympus]), **N** or **NPL** (normal field of view plan), **Ultrafluar** (fluorite objective), and **CF** or **CFI** (chrome-free; chrome-free infinity [Nikon]) (see Figs. A1.3 and A1.4).

Optimizing Microscope Usage
Köhler Illumination

Proper Köhler illumination technique is recommended for best image resolution. The microscope must have a field diaphragm and a variable aperture diaphragm for the substage condenser. The goal is to focus on the diaphragm opening of the substage condenser. See Box A1.1 for the step-by-step procedure. Each objective should be adjusted using both field and substage diaphragms for best image resolution; however, setting the high-dry in this fashion initially allows all objectives to be used in a routine fashion.

Use of Cover Glasses (Coverslips)

Not all size #1.5 cover glasses are manufactured to this specification, and some specimens may have media of variable refractive index between them and the cover glass. Therefore, compensation for abnormal distance can be performed by mechanically adjusting the tube length of the microscope or by use on some lens objectives with coverslip correction collars that change the spacing between internal lenses (see Appendix Fig. 1.4A).

The image may focus poorly at high-dry magnifications (40×, 60×) without a coverslip. A loosely applied coverslip

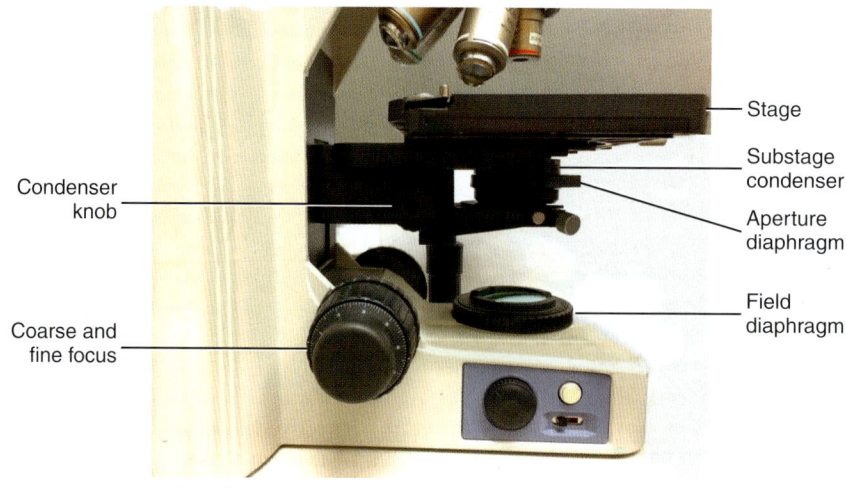

FIGURE A1.1 Major controls for image resolution.

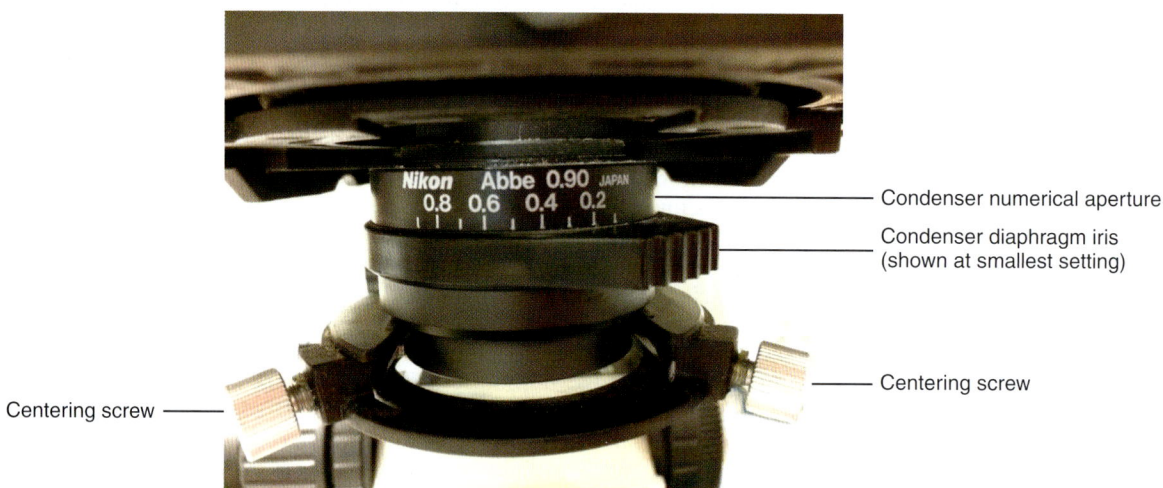

FIGURE A1.2 Substage condenser.

TABLE A1.1	Color Aberrations and Flatness of Field Corrections Relative to Objective Lens Types		
	LENS CORRECTIONS		
OBJECTIVE LENS TYPES	SPHERICAL ABERRATION	CHROMATIC ABERRATION	FIELD CURVATURE
Achromat	One color	Two colors	No
Plan Achromat	One color	Two colors	Yes
Fluorite	Two or three colors	Two or three colors	No
Plan Fluorite	Three or four colors	Two to four colors	Yes
Plan Apochromat	Three or four colors	Four or five colors	Yes

over a stained specimen may improve image resolution. Plastic coverslips should be avoided unless the high-dry objective is designed to work with them. Plastic coverslips are only suggested for routine wet-mount fecal or urine examinations.

Numerical Aperture and Resolution

Numerical aperture refers to the area for light rays to pass through the specimen for viewing in the eyepieces. There is a NA for the substage condenser as well as a NA for the lens objective that must be optimized for adequate viewing and good resolution. The NA typically increases with higher magnifications and may vary from 0.04 for low-power objectives to 1.3 or 1.4 for high-power oil-immersion apochromatic objectives. It is best for the NA of the objective to be equal or greater than the NA of the condenser lens in order to gather the most light. The higher the NA of the total system, the better the resolution.

APPENDIX 1 *Microscope and Telecytopathology Basics*

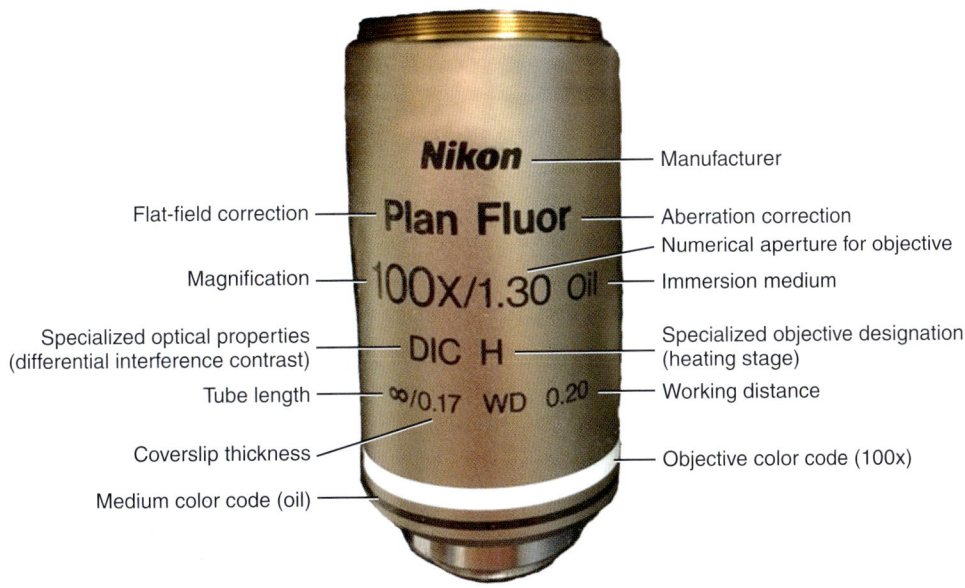

FIGURE A1.3 Parts of the lens objective.

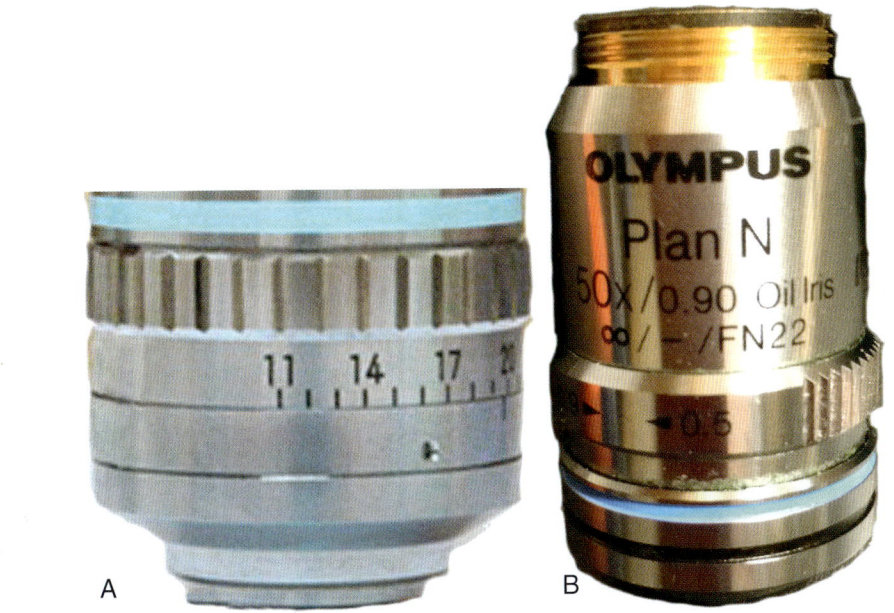

FIGURE A1.4 Special objective adjustment rings. **A,** Cover glass correction collar (0.11–0.22 mm) or 11 to 22. **B,** Numerical aperture iris (shown as 0.9 ▶ ◀ 0.5).

BOX A1.1 Procedure for Köhler Illumination

1. Turn on the microscope and fully open both the field diaphragm and the substage condenser diaphragm shown in Fig. A1.5A.
2. With the 10× objective in place, focus on the specimen on the slide. Close the field diaphragm down most of the way. Using the condenser knob, raise or lower the substage condenser to focus on the image of the field diaphragm, which should appear as a polygon (Fig. A1.5B).
3. If the image is not centered (Fig. A1.5B), use the centering screws to adjust the image (Fig. A1.5C).
4. When centered, open the field diaphragm until the polygon edges just touch the outside with the blue or darker rim visible along the edges (Fig. A1.5D). Then open the diaphragm a little further so these edges just disappear from view.
5. Remove an eyepiece and look down the tube of the microscope to see the full circle (Fig. A1.6A). Adjust the substage condenser diaphragm so that it is two-thirds to three-quarters open (Fig. A1.6B). This provides the best compromise of resolution and contrast.

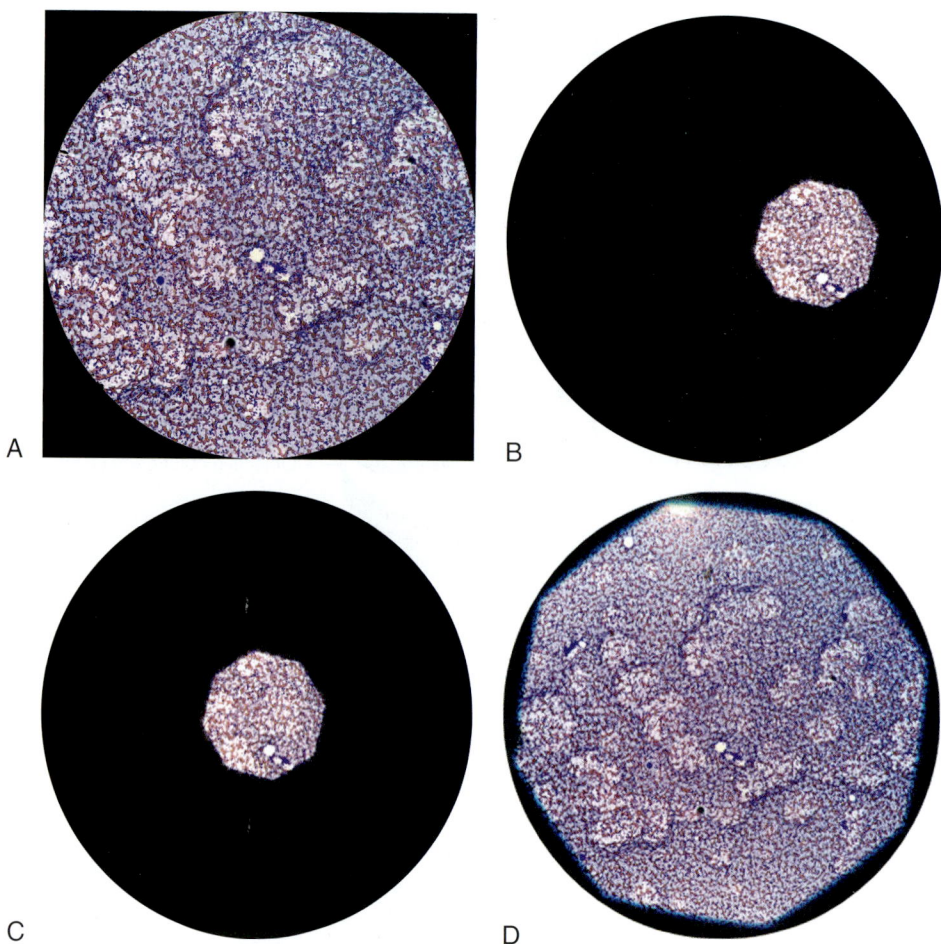

FIGURE A1.5 Köhler illumination procedure using a condenser. **A,** Focus on the specimen using the 10×objective. **B,** Focus the diaphragm condenser aperture to produce a sharply edged polygon. **C,** Use the centering screws to place the polygon in the center of the field of view. **D,** Open the field diaphragm until the polygon edges just disappear from view.

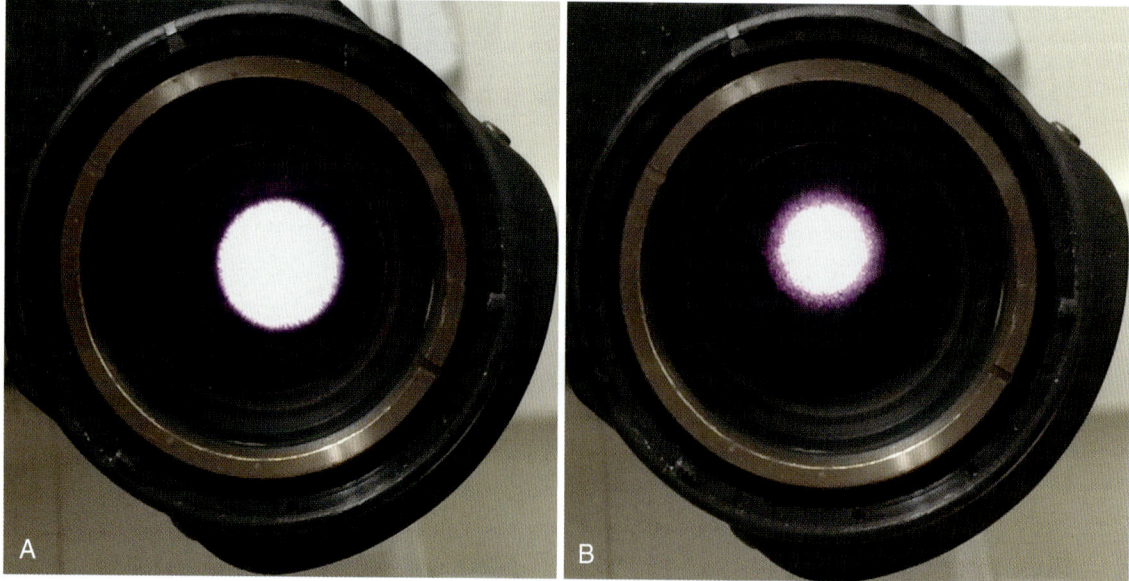

FIGURE A1.6 Köhler illumination procedure continued using an eyepiece. Contrast adjustment by removing eyepiece and noting the field of view. **A,** Fully open. **B,** Reduced light at 75% by dialing down the condenser diaphragm numerical aperture to improve contrast and resolution.

Higher values of the NA allow increasingly oblique rays to enter the objective front lens, which help resolve the image, particularly for brightfield microscopy. Living cells and other transparent, unstained specimens are often difficult to observe under traditional brightfield illumination using the full aperture and resolution of the microscope objective and condenser system. In these cases, reducing the NA by use of an iris diaphragm is possible on some objectives (see Fig. A1.4B).

Resolution is defined as the smallest distance between two points on a specimen that can be discerned as separate. This ability to collect light can be influenced by the refractive index of the medium (e.g., air, oil) between the front lens of the objective and the specimen cover glass, a value that ranges from 1.00 for air to 1.51 for some immersion oils. To obtain the best resolution, check the NA on the objective; then dial the substage condenser NA (see Fig. A1.2) to the proper numerical opening or open completely when the objective NA is higher than available on the condenser. This produces a similar effect to step 4 in Box A1.1.

VERNIER SCALE USAGE

Located on the microscope stage are two scales placed both horizontally and vertically on many microscopes (Fig. A1.7A). These scales may be used to measure distances in millimeters or record areas on a glass slide for later viewing using the same microscope. The larger main scale indicates the whole millimeter number, and the secondary smaller Vernier scale represents one tenth of a millimeter. First note the whole number on the main scale using the 0 from the smaller scale; then look on both scales where the lines match up. That will be the second digit. See the example in Figure A1.7B. Using the vertical and horizontal scales helps to relocate an area of interest at a later time.

SMARTPHONE TELECYTOPATHOLOGY BASICS

Manual Technique

With a little practice, one can take diagnostic images for telecytopathology referral or archiving personal cases using a smartphone as the sole method. An example of the technique can be viewed online at www.youtube.com/watch?v=cfd9ViHBlR4. Selected views are captured in Figure A1.8 for reference of the technique. Briefly, the phone is held horizontally at the edges, allowing free use of a finger (e.g., thumb) to capture the image. The smartphone is held in the hand, which steadies the unit by touching one eyepiece while holding the camera's lens over the other eyepiece. The image is centered and is allowed to fill the eyepiece circle or the rectangular field. The image can be focused by touching the screen just before it is captured.

Over-the-Eyepiece Holders

The use of a camera holder allows sharper images as well as video recording of specimens such as parasite movement or specimen scanning. There are several inexpensive models of microscope camera phone holders or adapters on the market. One of the most current popular models is Snapzoom (www.snapzooms.com; Fig. A1.9A), which is compatible with any smartphone up to 3.67 inches (93 mm) wide and 0.79 inches

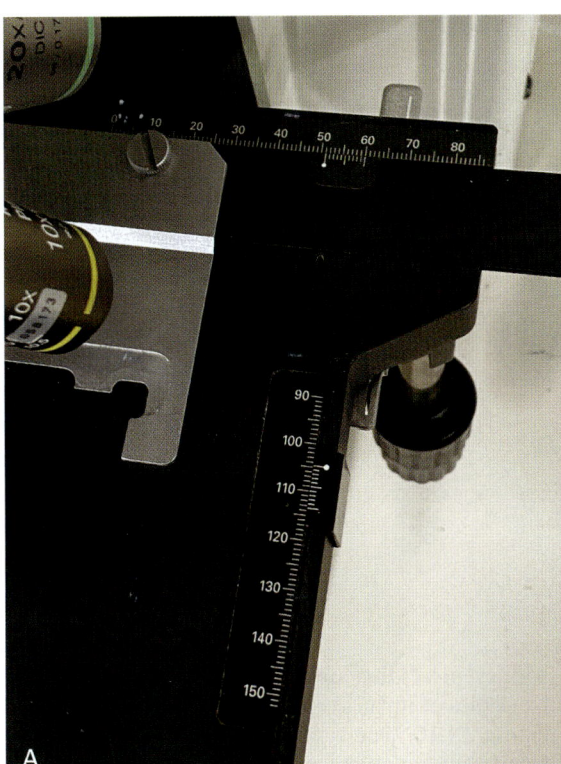
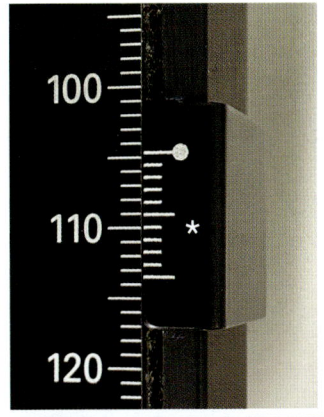
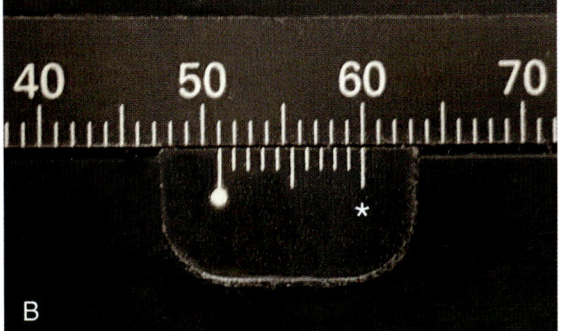

■ **FIGURE A1.7** Microscope stage Vernier scale. **A,** Horizontal and vertical markers are placed on the stage to help record a region of future interest using coordinates or measure of an area. **B,** Close-up on the two sliding scales measured in millimeters. The first digit is the site of the starting closed circle on the small scale. Preceded by a decimal point, the second digit is the mark where lines from both scales align, indicated by a star. The two examples shown are 104.6 mm *(top)* and 51.0 mm *(bottom)*, which represent the coordinates in part A.

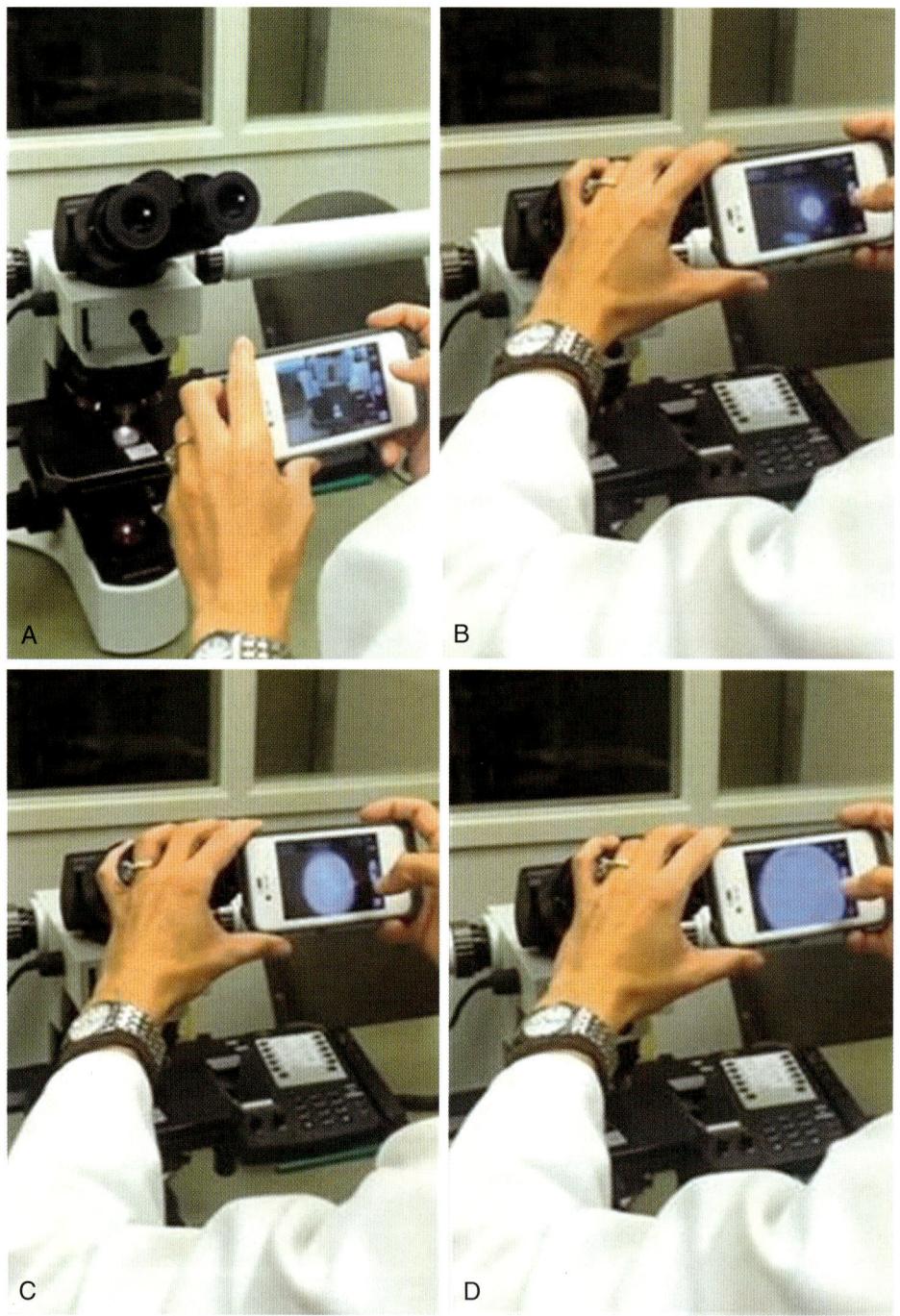

■ **FIGURE A1.8 A–D,** Manual image capture with a smartphone for microscope images. (From Morrison A. Smartphone microscopic photography—the Morrison technique: free hand, no adapter. http://youtu.be/cfd9ViHBIR4.)

(23 mm) thick, with or without a case. The eyepiece jaw accepts an outside diameter between 0.91 and 2.17 inches (23 and 55 mm) wide, and a minimum 1 inch (25 mm) in height. Another is a more restrictive adapter designed only for iPhones. Magnifi (www.arcturuslabs.com; Fig. A1.9B) is designed to work with eyepieces that are 1 to 1.5 inches in diameter (25–38 mm). Examples of images captured using a smartphone are shown in Figure A1.10. One report highlights the advantages of several smartphone adapters and recommends the two mentioned here (Roy et al., 2014).

APPENDIX 1 *Microscope and Telecytopathology Basics*

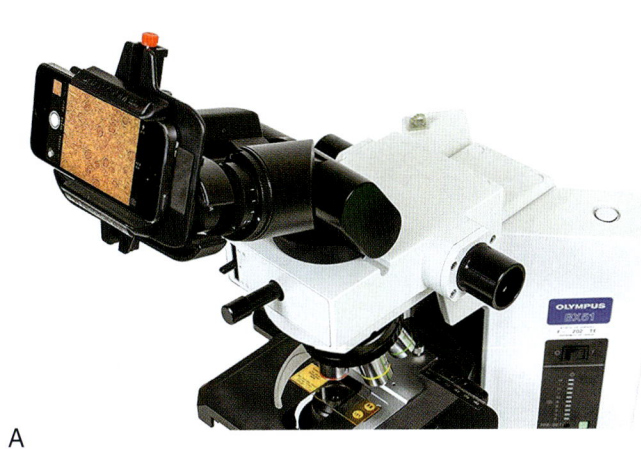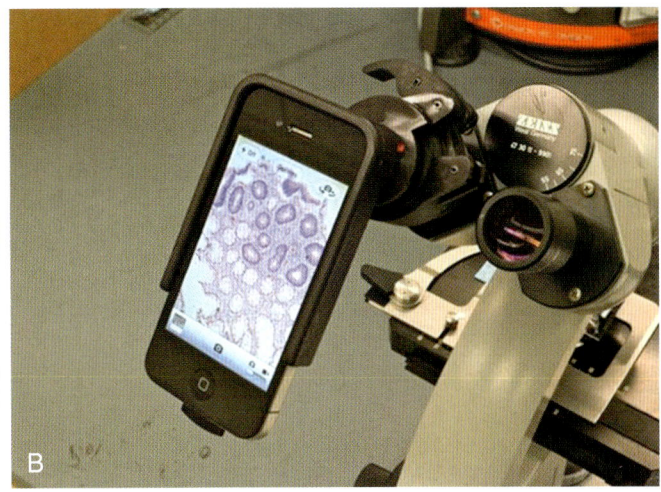

■ **FIGURE A1.9** Two examples of over-the-eyepiece smartphone holders for photomicroscopy. **A,** Snapzoom. **B,** Magnifi 2.

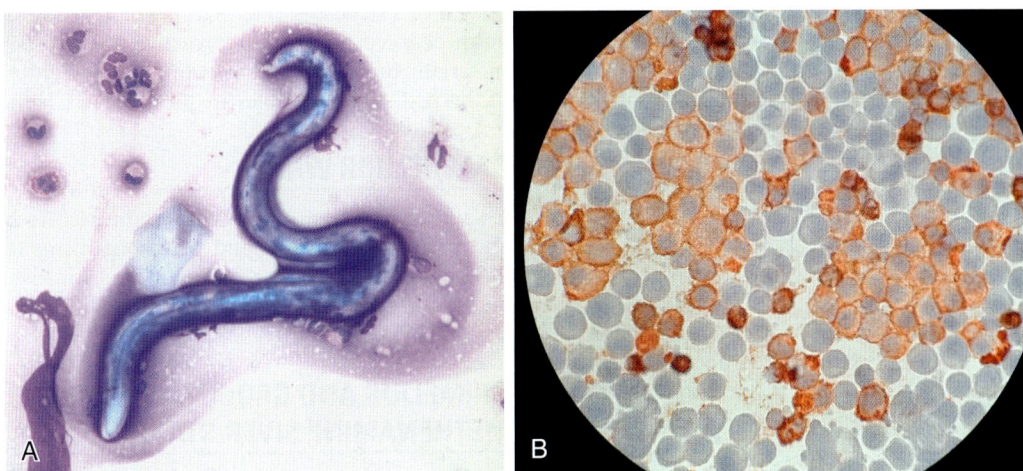

■ **FIGURE A1.10** Two examples of telecytopathology using an iPhone 6SP. **A,** Full-screen view of a feline lungworm larva. (Romanowsky; HP oil.) **B,** Tube view of a canine B-cell lymphoma. (Immunocytochemistry; HP oil.)

REFERENCE

Roy S, Pantanowitz L, Amin M, et al. Smartphone adapters for digital photomicrography. *J Pathol Inform.* 2014;5:24. Available at: www.jpathinformatics.org/text.asp?2014/5/1/24/137728.

APPENDIX 2

Selected Stains and Protocols

Rose E. Raskin

ACID-ALCOHOL

Histochemical stains may be used on unstained or Romanowsky-stained cytology slides (Marcos et al., 2009). It may be helpful or necessary to remove the previous stain before restaining with stains such as periodic acid–Schiff (PAS) or Grocott methenamine silver, both of which may be used to reveal fungal organisms. An overnight methanol soak will accomplish this goal; however, another procedure is a brief exposure to acid-alcohol.

Materials
70% ethyl alcohol: 0.99 mL
Concentrated hydrochloric acid: 1 mL

Protocol
The slide is rapidly dipped two or three times into the acid-alcohol mixture to decolorize the Romanowsky staining followed by washing with running tap water to stop the reaction. For thick specimens, consider destaining slides using 5% acid-alcohol from 1 to 15 minutes.

ALKALINE PHOSPHATASE

Materials
BCIP/NBT Phosphatase Substrate (Cat. #: 5420-0038, 100 mL) comes as a solution of 5-bromo-4-chloro-3-indolyl phosphate (BCIP) at a concentration of 0.21 g/L and nitroblue tetrazolium (NBT) at a concentration of 0.42 g/L in an organic base/Tris buffer. This product is available through KPL (www.seracare.com).

The reaction product is deposited at the site where the hydrolysis of (BCIP/NBT) by alkaline phosphatase occurs. This is best used on unfixed, unstained slides; however, previously Romanowsky-stained slides may be used (Ryseff and Bohn, 2012). Light counterstaining for unstained slides with a Romanowsky stain assists in examination of the positive cells.

Protocol
Warm the solution to room temperature before use. For previously examined slides, remove oil with xylene and rinse briefly with saline buffer. Positive controls consist of hepatic tissue or equine neutrophils.
1. Flood slide or immerse in solution.
2. Incubate for 3 to 5 minutes for unstained slides or approximately 1 hour for previously stained slides.
3. Rinse with distilled water to stop the reaction.
4. Air dry.

Reaction
An intense purple to black granularity within the cytoplasm of osteoblasts, chondroblasts, and rare other cells but not macrophages or osteoclasts (Fig. A2.1). The reaction does not distinguish between malignant or reactive osteoblasts. See images for metastatic tumor cell visualization in the previous (third) edition of this text. More examples are provided in Chapter 14.

CALCOFLUOR WHITE

This is a fluorescent microscopy stain used to highlight chitin and cellulose in animal and plant organisms (Collicutt et al., 2015). It is often used for fungal or parasitic visualization. Algal and yeast cell walls appear as blue-white round to elliptical shapes (Fig. A2.2).

GRIMELIUS AND GROCOTT-GOMORI METHENAMINE SIVER STAINS

Methenamine silver stains help to reveal fungal and algal organisms (see Fig. A2.2A). The Grimelius silver method visualizes argyrophilic granules in neurosecretory tumors (Fig. A2.3).

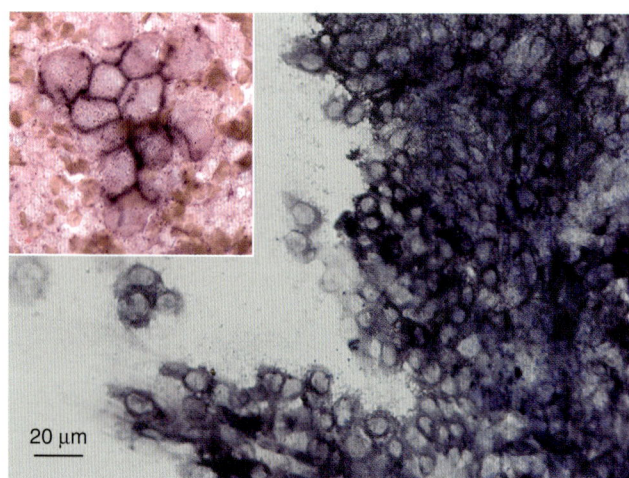

■ **FIGURE A2.1 Alkaline phosphatase. Osteosarcoma. Nasal dorsum aspirate. Dog.** Staining displays black positive aggregates in neoplastic cells. (BCIP/NBT/Romanowsky; IP.) *Inset:* Positive control using a liver specimen demonstrates the intrahepatic canalicular system. (BCIP/NBT; HP oil.)

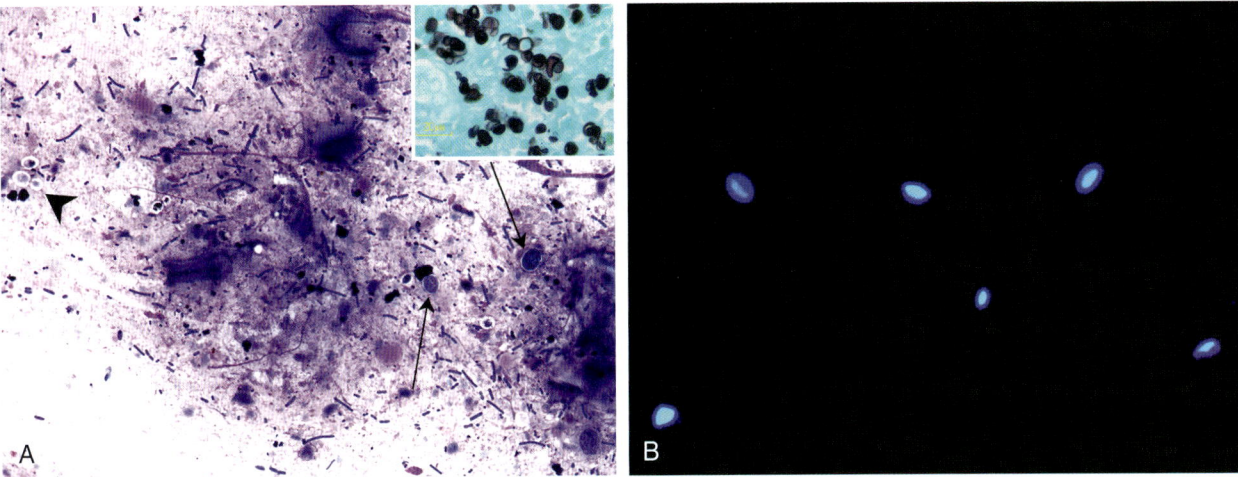

■ **FIGURE A2.2** *Prototheca zopfii*. **Rectal scrape. Dog.** Same case in A and B. **A,** There is a mixed bacterial population in the background along with few yeast *(arrowhead)* and algae *(arrows)*. (Modified Wright; IP.) *Inset:* Histopathologic section of rectum demonstrates positive reaction with a silver stain. (GMS; IP.) **B,** Blue-white reaction to cell walls of yeast and algae (Calcofluor white; IP.) (A, Courtesy Yvonne Wikander; Inset, Courtesy Jonathon Sego. B, Courtesy Kaori Knights, Kansas State University.)

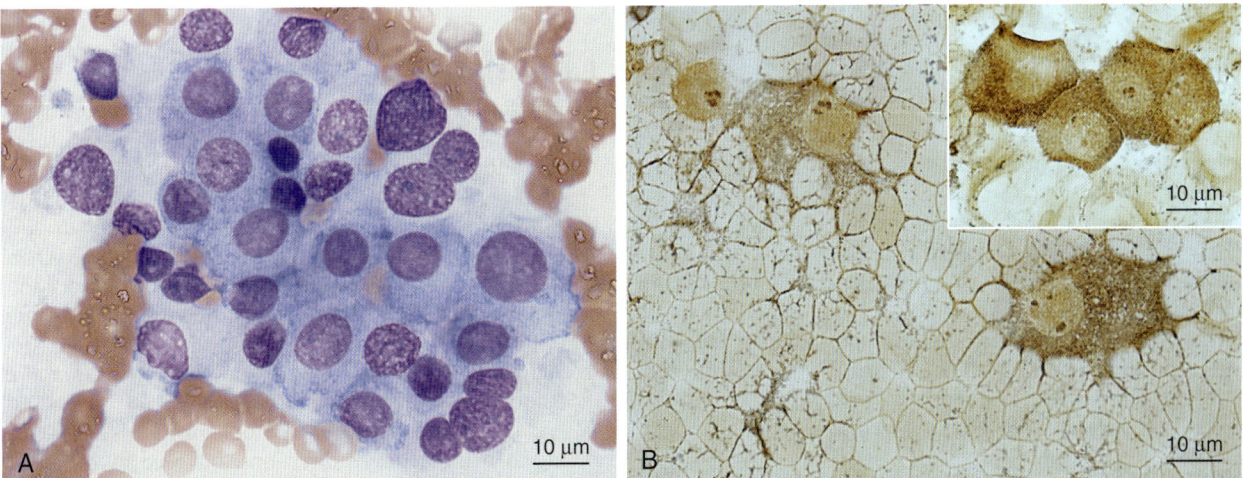

■ **FIGURE A2.3** Neuroendocrine neoplasm. **Caudoventral peritoneal cavity mass. Tissue aspirate. Dog.** Same case in A and B. **A,** A well-defined, slightly lobular, hypoechoic nodule yielded cell clusters with lightly granular cytoplasm, suggestive of a pheochromocytoma. (Wright-Giemsa; HP oil.) **B,** Positive staining to cytoplasmic granules. Note the nucleolar argyrophilic organizing regions as multiple prominent nucleoli. (Grimelius silver; HP oil.) *Inset:* Additional cluster of positive cells. (Grimelius silver; HP oil.)

MUCINS AND GLYCOGEN STAINS

Mucins are high-molecular-weight, heavily glycosylated proteins (glycoconjugates). Depending on the site in the body, they may be composed of acid mucins or neutral mucins. The acid type carry a negative charge while the neutral type have no charge. Stains such as mucicarmine react with the capsule of *Cryptococcus* spp. to detect acid mucins. Alcian blue (AB) at pH 2.5 detects all acid mucins, but some will not stain at pH 1.0. PAS detects glycogen, glycoproteins, carbohydrates, and mucins, including neutral mucins. Mucins can be distinguished when stained first blue with AB and then red with PAS. In addition, PAS with diastase digestion is used to differentiate glycogen from mucins. Two slides are used; one untreated slide is placed in water, while a second slide is treated with diastase. After the treatment step, both slides are stained for PAS. Diastase removes glycogen, and PAS only stains positive if mucins are present.

OIL RED O

For general localization of fats, this stain is followed by a nuclear counterstain. It is best used on unstained smears and frozen sections. Its use may assist in the diagnosis of lipid-containing neoplasms (Masserdotti et al., 2006).

Materials

Oil Red O (ORO) stock solution is prepared by reconstituting Sigma-Aldrich (Cat # O0625) 60 mg with 20 mL of 100% isopropanol and leaving it undisturbed for 20 minutes. This is stable for 1 year. The working solution involves three parts ORO stock solution and two parts distilled water. Allow the mixture to sit for 10 minutes, filter through Whatman No. 1 filter paper, and use within 2 hours.

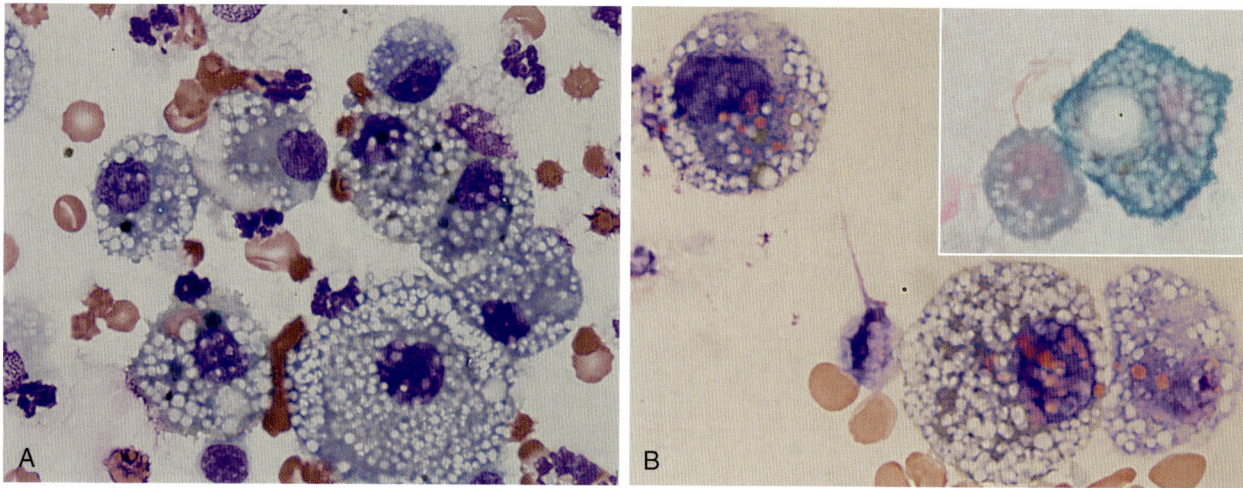

■ **FIGURE A2.4 Lipid pneumonia. Bronchoalveolar wash specimen. Dog.** Same case in A and B. **A,** Mixed leukocyte population composed of neutrophils, macrophages, lymphocytes, and eosinophils. Macrophages display erythrophagia and contain blue-black granules and numerous punctate colorless vacuoles. (Wright-Giemsa; HP oil.) **B,** Red-stained vacuoles support the presence of phagocytized lipid. (Oil Red O/Giemsa; HP oil.) *Inset:* Hemosiderin is identified by the presence of blue intervacuolar material. (Prussian blue/red counterstain; HP oil.) (Courtesy Jacqueline Dolan, University of Florida.)

Protocol

1. Apply the fresh ORO working solution to the unstained cytopathologic specimen smear.
2. Incubate for 5 to 10 minutes.
3. Rinse with water.
4. Dip in counterstain, such as hematoxylin, for 1 minute.
5. Air dry and mount (e.g., Cytoseal) with coverslip. If examining without a coverslip, do not add oil as it will dilute the stain reaction.

Alternatively, for wet examination, add an equal amount of Oil Red O and new methylene blue on the slide, mix and let settle for a short while, and then apply a coverslip and drain excess fluid on a paper towel before viewing.

Reaction

Fat staining appears pale orange (Fig. A2.4), whereas free unincorporated dye forms dark orange globules.

IMMUNOCYTOCHEMISTRY

A more complete description of the stain procedure is found in Chapter 18. In the previous third edition, a complete protocol is given for the streptavidin–horseradish peroxidase method. Next is a brief description of a polymer methodology, which is considered the most advanced. The procedure may be applied to unstained and Romanowsky-stained slides (Raskin et al., 2019).

Protocol

1. Antigen retrieval involves citrate buffer pH6 for CD3ε, CD20, and Pax5 and Tris/EDTA pH9 for cytokeratin, vimentin, and Melan-A at 95°C for 25 minutes in a decloaking chamber (Biocare).
2. After peroxidase and casein protein blocking, primary antibodies are incubated for 30 minutes within a moistened chamber.
3. Negative controls for each specimen lack the primary antibody, and positive controls must be run concurrently to ensure valid results.
4. Signal amplification involves a polymer secondary antibody (Biocare) with horseradish peroxidase.
5. A chromogen such as 3,3′ diaminobenzidine is applied according to manufacturer's directions, followed by a hematoxylin counterstain (40 seconds).

REFERENCES

Collicutt N, Camus M, Dill J. Fluorescent fungus and foliage. *Vet Clin Pathol.* 2015;44(1):6-7.

Marcos R, Santos M, Santos N, et al. Use of destained cytology slides for the application of routine special stains. *Vet Clin Pathol.* 2009;38(1):94-102.

Masserdotti C, Bonfanti U, De Lorenzi D, et al. Use of Oil Red O stain in the cytologic diagnosis of canine liposarcoma. *Vet Clin Pathol.* 2006;35(1):37-41.

Raskin RE, Vickers J, Ward JG, et al. Optimized immunocytochemistry using leukocyte and tissue markers on Romanowsky-stained slides from dogs and cats. *Vet Clin Pathol.* 2019;48:88-97.

Ryseff JK, Bohn AA. Detection of alkaline phosphatase in canine cells previously stained with Wright–Giemsa and its utility in differentiating osteosarcoma from other mesenchymal tumors. *Vet Clin Pathol.* 2012;41(3):391-395.

APPENDIX 3

Peculiar Findings and Polarizing Materials

Rose E. Raskin

SPECIMEN ACQUISITION AND PROCESSING

Sometimes it is difficult to differentiate artifact from a pathologic or diagnostic finding. The following examples illustrate some of the more common materials or structures associated with cytologic specimens that may be puzzling or distracting. In some cases, artifacts are induced by specimen collection into inappropriate tubes (see Fig. 15.1), processing (see Fig. 2.18B), rough handling (Fig. A3.1A), presence of ultrasound gel (see Fig. 4.112), precipitate formation from methanolic Romanowsky stain (Fig. A3.1B), and talc or cornstarch granules from surgical gloves (Fig. A3.1C). Fingerprints are typically located at the slide edges (Fig. A3.1D) with numerous anucleate squames or keratin bars. A circular area on the slide containing mature squamous epithelial cells often with a mixed bacterial

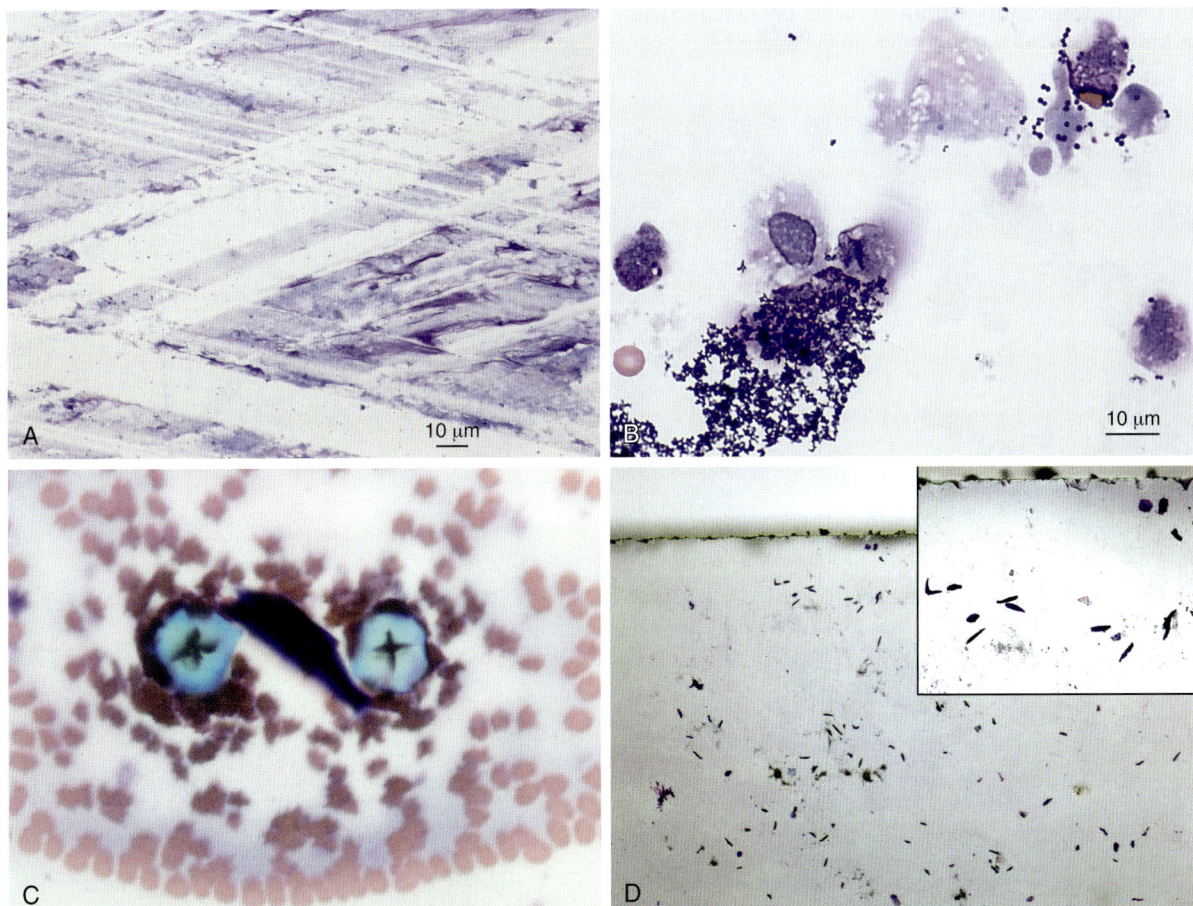

■ **FIGURE A3.1 Artifacts from sample acquisition and processing. A, Scratches.** Linear clear streaks in the stained background typically arise from slides contacting other slides during staining or accidental wiping of the slide. (Romanowsky, HP oil.) **B, Stain precipitate and bacteria. Dog.** The lower left dark granular material represents residue following methanolic Romanowsky staining. Compare a similar granularity and color with coccoid bacteria in the upper right. (Romanowsky, HP oil.) **C, Cornstarch granules. Cat.** This foreign material is characterized by the cross mark in the center of the crystal cell. (Modified Wright; HP oil.) **D, Fingerprint keratin bars.** Near the glass slide edges are numerous individualized squamous epithelial cells represented by dense, dark keratin bars. These surface epithelial cells related to excessive handling of the slide may confuse the diagnosis if they appear within the center of the slide and specimen. (Aqueous Romanowsky; LP.) *Inset:* Higher magnification focused on the squames. (Aqueous Romanowsky; IP.)

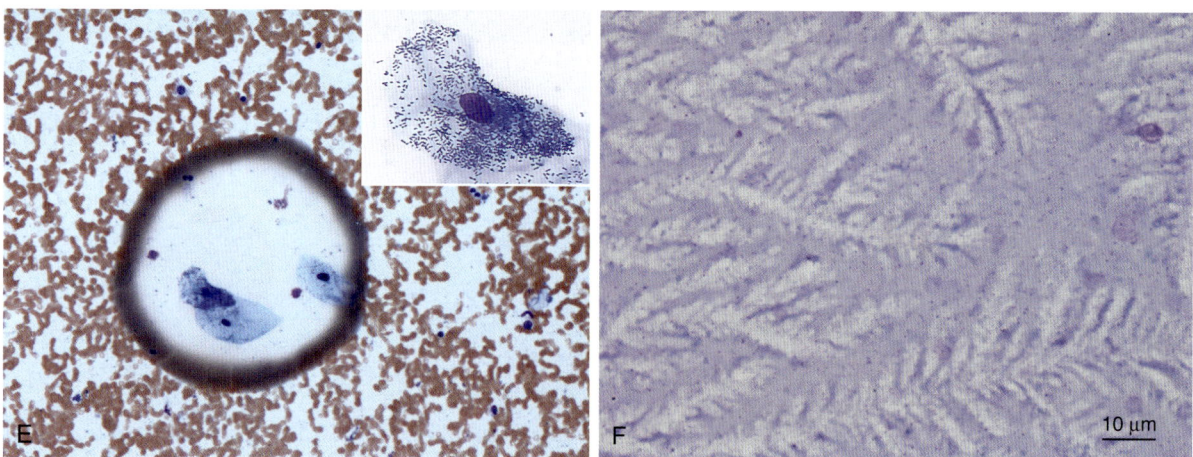

FIGURE A3.1, cont'd E, Saliva droplet. A circular area appears unrelated to adjacent areas. (Wright-Giemsa; IP.) *Inset:* Within the circle are superficial squamous epithelial cells covered with a mixed bacterial population. (Wright-Giemsa; HP oil.) **F, Ferning.** A crystallization artifact during drying of sodium chloride on mucus. (Wright-Giemsa; HP oil.)

population on or around the cells (Fig. A3.1E) suggests saliva droplets originating from the patient or collector. A drying artifact of material collected may produce fernlike patterns related to crystallization of sodium chloride on mucus. This pattern is known as arborization or ferning (Fig. A3.1F).

Plant pollen or spores are often green or brown and are often found in areas with easy access to the environment, including slide surfaces (Fig. A3.2). These should be considered as contaminants under most circumstances. Table A3.1 indicates additional extracellular examples.

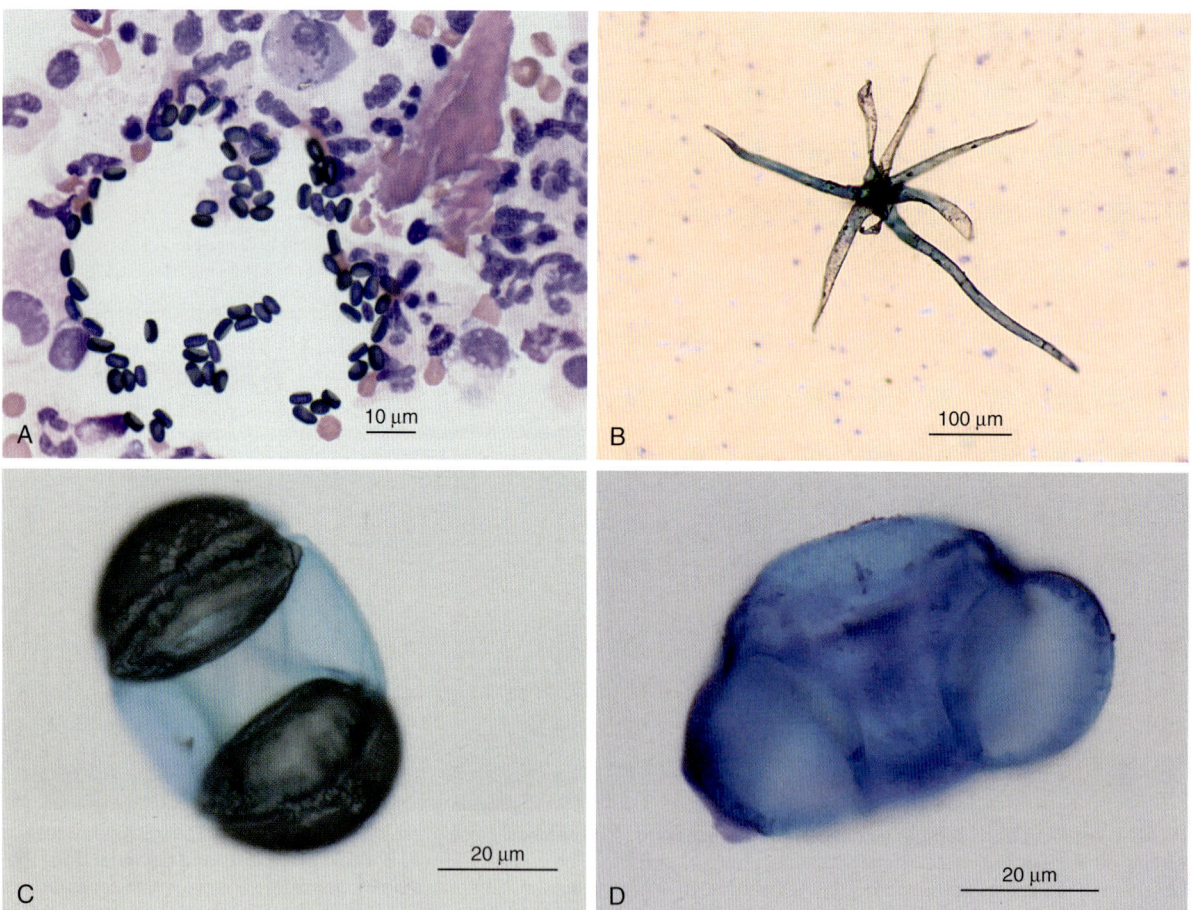

FIGURE A3.2 Plant materials. A, Pollen grains. Urine cytospin preparation. Dog. An aggregate of blue-green ovoid spores is found in voided urine. Although there is an inflammatory process occurring, these extracellular structures are considered to be contaminants. (Modified Wright; HP oil.) **B, Trichome. Spleen aspirate. Dog.** These green-brown stellate plant hairs are found on oak leaves and often contaminant specimens. (Wright-Giemsa; HP oil.) **C–D, Pine pollen at various development stages and staining.** (C, Aqueous Romanowsky; HP oil. D, Methanolic Romanowsky; HP oil.)

APPENDIX 3 Peculiar Findings and Polarizing Materials

TABLE A3.1 Peculiar Findings Based on Cytopathologic Characteristics

EXTRACELLULAR AND CRYSTALLINE MATERIALS	LINEAR FORMATIONS	BASOPHILIC STRUCTURES	EOSINOPHILIC SECRETIONS
Lymphoglandular bodies (see Fig. 2.22)	Nuclear streaming (see Fig. 2.23)	White bile (see Figs. 6.37 and A3.5C)	Medical lubricant (see Fig. 4.112)
Pollen (see Figs. 12.54 and A3.2)	Collagen (see Figs. 2.25A and 3.188)	Necrosis (see Fig. 2.30)	Synovial/IVD MPS (see Figs. 14.5 and A3.6B)
Hemoglobin crystals (see Fig. A3.3E–F)	Cotton fiber (see Figs. 12.53 and A3.4D)	Hemosiderin (see Figs. 4.45A and 5.47)	Osteoid (see Figs. 7.21 and 14.49B)
Talc or cornstarch crystals (see Figs. 12.52 and A3.1C)	Hair (see Fig. A3.4B)	Melanin (see Figs. 3.164C and 16.44A–B)	Amyloid (see Figs. 9.33 and A3.6A)
Mineral crystals (see Figs. 3.212 and 14.14)	Capillaries (see Figs. 3.148A and 4.116B)	Tyrosine granules (see Fig. 17.15A–B)	Thyroid colloid (see Fig. 17.5)
Muscle fragments (see Fig. 2.1)	Curschmann spiral (see Figs. 3.29 and 5.44)	Mammary secretion (see Fig. 13.4)	Call-Exner body (see Fig. 13.81)
Parasite fragments (Fig. A3.7)	Lens fibers (see Fig. 16.53)	Blastomycosis yeast (see Fig. 16.49)	Vaccine adjuvant (see Fig. 3.12B)
Diatoms (see Fig. 5.55)	Gamna-Gandy bodies (see Figs. 4.46 and 4.132)	Sperm (see Fig. 6.40)	Splendore-Hoeppli phenomenon (see Fig. 3.222)

IVD, Intervertebral disk; *MPS*, mucopolysaccharides.

CRYSTALLINE STRUCTURES

Background material often reflects degenerative changes such as dystrophic calcification (Fig. A3.3A) or urate crystals in tissues (Fig. A3.3B). When viewed against a proteinaceous background, crystals such as cholesterol present in a rectangular shape commonly but also as needles and clefts (Figs. A3.3C–D). Slow specimen drying may result in the formation of hemoglobin crystals as bars or as needles (termed *acicular*; Fig. A3.3E–F). Table A3.1 indicates additional crystal examples.

LINEAR SHAPES

Linear shapes can be confusing within samples. Although commonly associated with respiratory specimens, Curschmann's spirals (Fig. A3.4A) represent inspissated mucus and have been seen rarely in dermal lesions. Capillaries lined by endothelium that occasionally contain erythrocytes are common with lymphoid organs and other highly vascularized tissues (Fig. A3.4B–C). Organic or synthetic fibers may resemble hyphae or hair shafts but are distinguished by a refractile or colored feature (Fig. A3.4D). In contrast, fungal hyphae may appear pigmented or nonpigmented (Fig. A3.4E) with uniform width and sometimes distinctive septation or presence of a fruiting body (Fig. A3.4F). Table A3.1 indicates additional linear shape examples.

BASOPHILIC MATERIALS

The background may contain regular or irregularly shaped materials that stain basophilic. The sulfur granule seen grossly in actinomycosis in which mats of bacterial filaments appear as amorphous

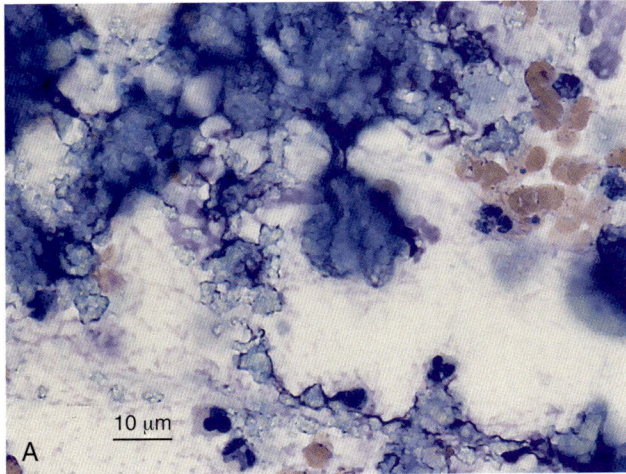 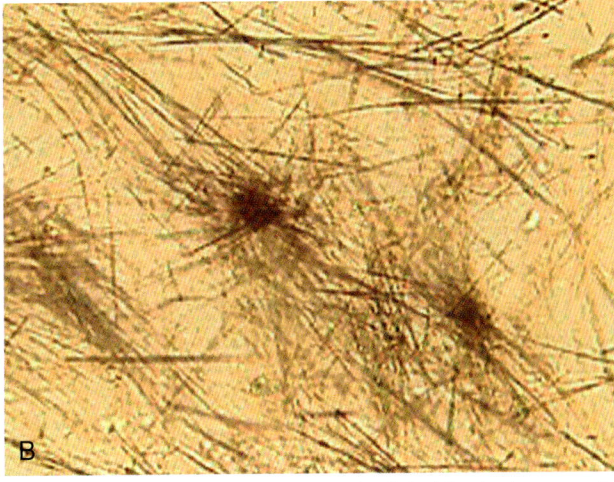

■ **FIGURE A3.3 Crystals. A, Calcium mineralization. Lung aspirate. Cat.** Refractile crystalline material stains light blue in the area of tissue necrosis. (Modified Wright; HP oil.) **B, Urate crystals. Joint aspirate. Tortoise.** Gout arthritis is noted by the presence of long thin needle-like crystals. (Unstained; HP oil.)

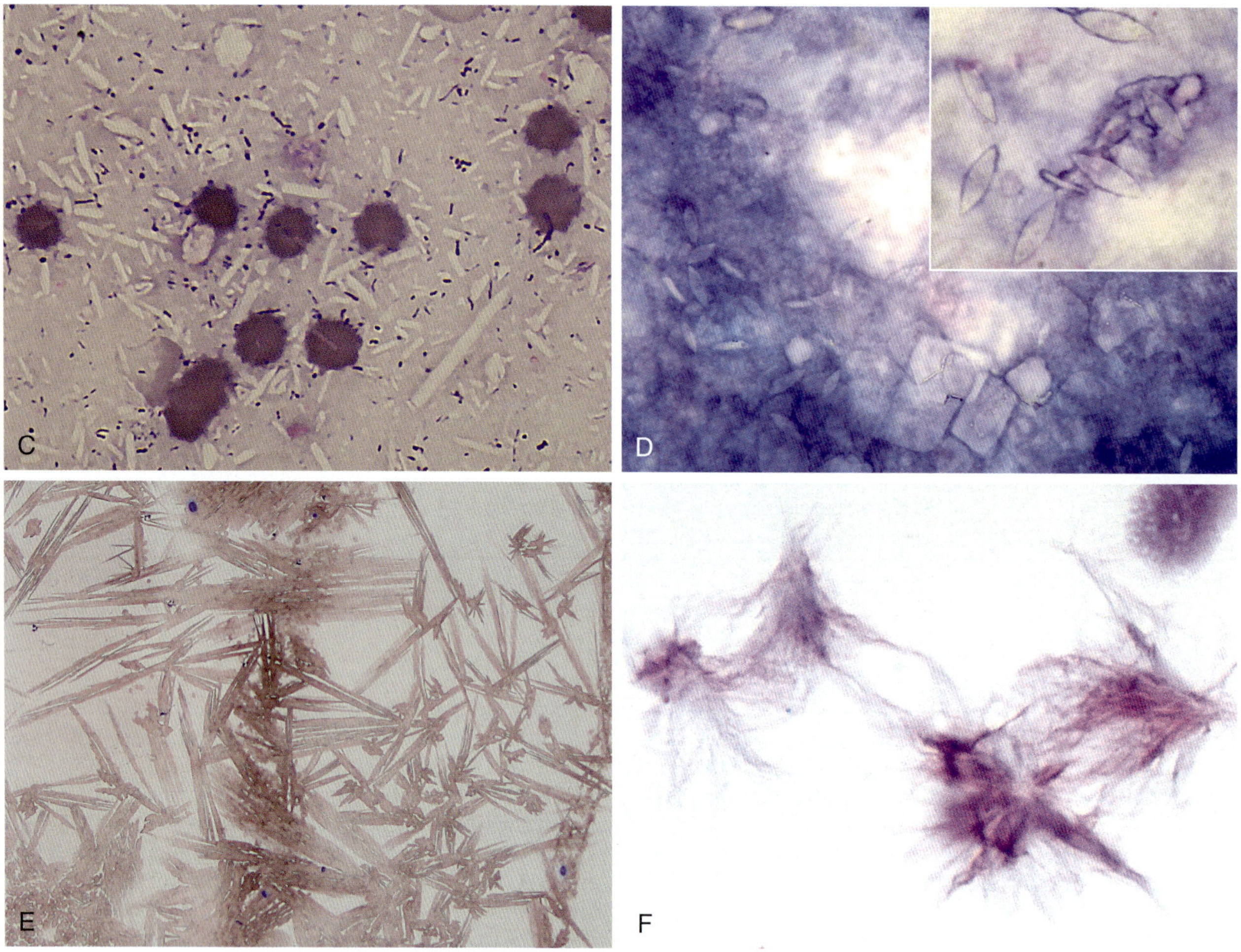

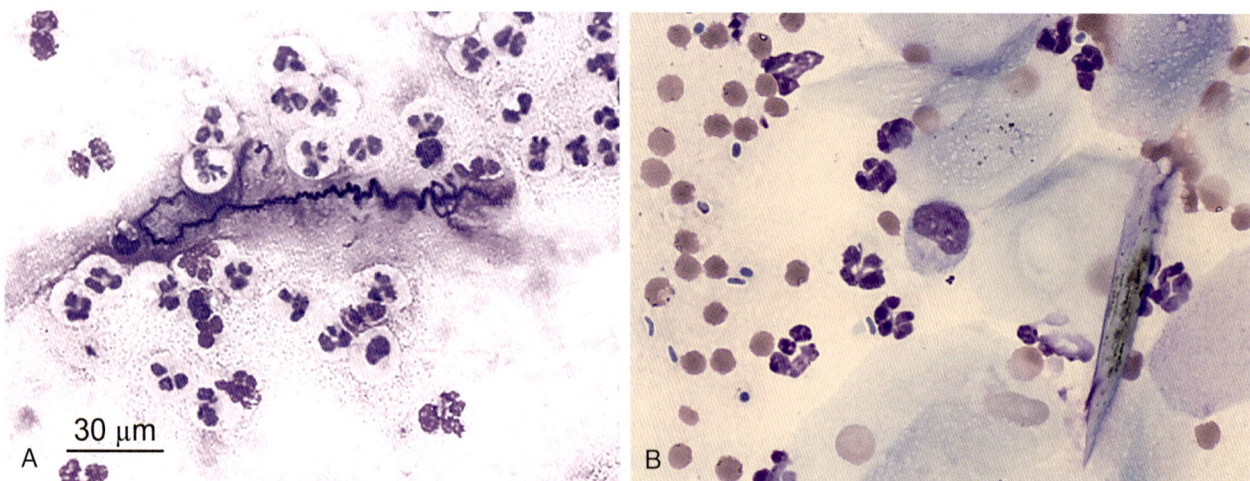

■ **FIGURE A3.3, cont'd C, Cholesterol needle crystals. Perianal mass aspirate. Dog.** The background contains numerous linear streaks of various lengths and widths having sharp sides. It is likely the result of tissue damage with release of cell membrane lipids. (Modified Wright; HP oil.) **D, Cholesterol rectangles and clefts. Dog.** Present in the sample of tissue damage are typical rectangular shapes with corner notch. (Modified Wright; HP oil.) *Inset:* Higher magnification to show additional cholesterol crystals in an elliptical cleft shape. (Modified Wright; HP oil.) **E, Hemoglobin crystals. Dog.** Numerous pale pink, needle-like crystals that may arise from slow drying of a highly blood-contaminated sample. (Modified Wright; HP oil.) **F, Hemoglobin crystals, acicular habit. Dog.** This form of hemoglobin crystal has thin needle- or hairlike projections and was present in a splenic specimen. (Wright-Giemsa; HP oil.)

■ **FIGURE A3.4 Linear structures. A, Curschmann's spiral. Skin aspirate. Dog.** Long linear corkscrew strand is indicative of inspissated mucus that may be found in sites other than the respiratory tract. (Modified Wright; HP oil.) **B, Hair. Tissue imprint. Dog.** Squamous epithelium, remnant hair shaft, and mostly neutrophilic inflammation are present along with moderate numbers of arthrospores in this case of dermatophytosis. These basophilic, oval to elongate structures have a thin, clear capsule and measure 2 to 3 μm in width by 2 to 5 μm in length. (Modified Wright; HP oil.)

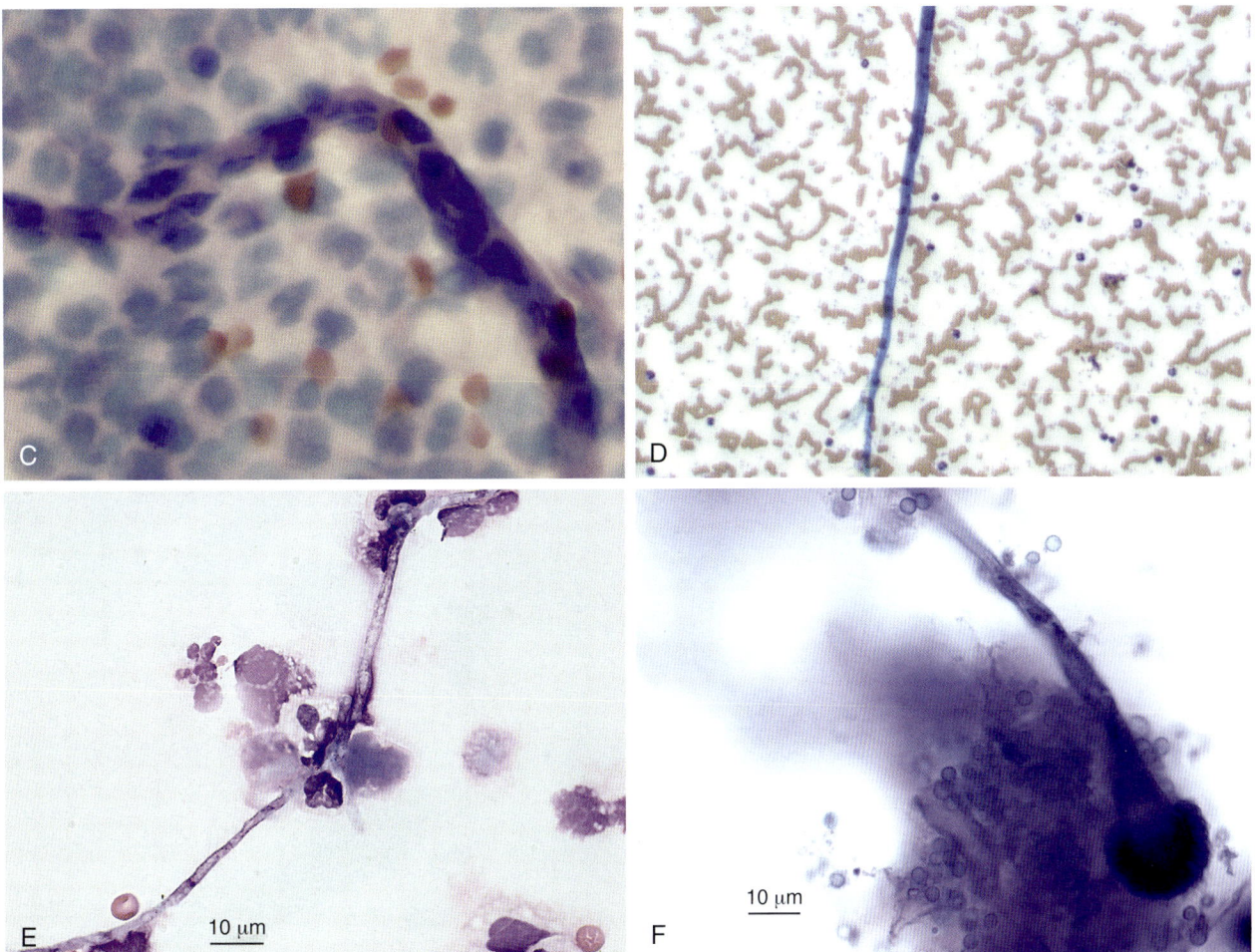

■ **FIGURE A3.4, cont'd C, Blood vessel. Nasal aspirate. Cat.** Note the curving pattern and red cells within the capillary that are covered by endothelial cells. (Modified Wright; IP and HP oil.) **D, Synthetic fiber. Blood. Cat.** The blue transparent thread found on the top red cells as a contaminant structure. The variable width and color are helpful features. (Modified Wright; HP oil.) **E, Fungal hyphal segment. Urine. Dog.** Degenerate neutrophils surround the structure, which is septate. (Modified Wright; HP oil.) **F, *Aspergillus* fruiting body with conidia. Nasal plaque imprint. Dog.** The swollen part of the conidiophore, termed the vesicle, is covered by a dense cap or phialides from which small round conidia arise, each measuring 3 μm in diameter. (New methylene blue; HP oil.)

junk-like material until closely examined (Fig. A3.5A–B). Always examine this material, especially around the periphery, to find the typical beaded filamentous bacteria. In addition to the yellow bile material found within the abdominal cavity upon rupture of the biliary ducts, amorphous mucus of various sizes and shapes appears pale blue within cells or extracellularly (Fig. A3.5C). Large deeply basophilic, thick fibers may indicate skeletal muscle tissue (Fig. A3.5D). Upon close inspection of the muscle tissue, one often observes surface nuclei along with cross-striations. Table A3.1 provides additional basophilic examples.

EOSINOPHILIC MATERIALS

Materials that contain amyloid or mucopolysaccharides will stain brightly pink and appear amorphous or fibrillar (Fig. A3.6). Table A3.1 provides additional eosinophilic examples.

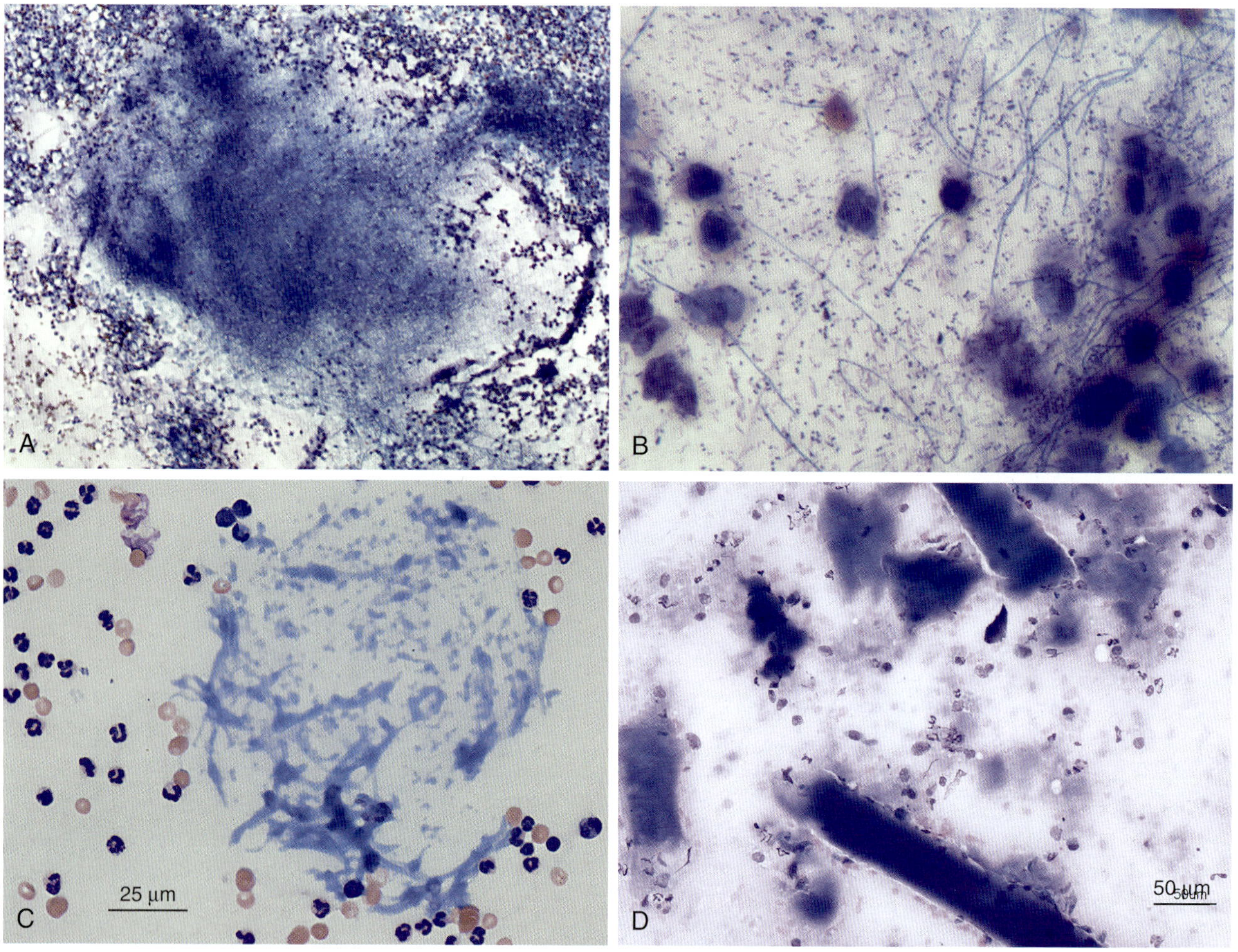

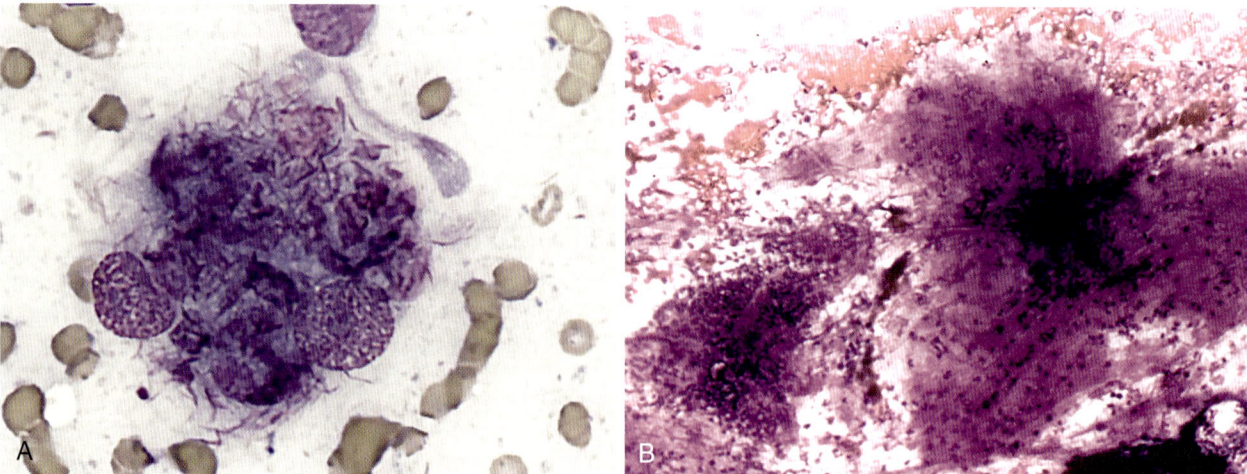

■ **FIGURE A3.5 Basophilic materials. A and B, Actinomycosis. Nasal imprint. Cat.** Low and higher magnification of bacterial mats and purulent inflammation. Bacteria are rarely found in areas away from the large mats of bacteria (not shown). However, just adjacent to the basophilic granular masses are numerous thin beaded filamentous bacteria. (Modified Wright; LP and HP oil.) **C, Bilious effusion. Abdominal fluid smear. Dog.** The background contains abundant strands and amorphous blue-green mucus material appearing as a large lake. This is consistent with white bile or mucus released from a rupture in the biliary tree. (Modified Wright; HP oil.) **D, Muscle fragments. Tissue aspirate. Dog.** The presence of deeply basophilic rectangular pieces suggests skeletal muscle. Confirmation is performed at higher magnification to see cross-striations (see Fig. 2.1). (Modified Wright; IP.)

■ **FIGURE A3.6 Eosinophilic materials. A, Amyloid. Splenic aspirate. Cat.** A single macrophage is surrounded by eosinophilic strands and many similar fibrils are present within the macrophage. (Romanowsky; HP oil.) **B, Intervertebral disk material. Tissue aspirate. Dog.** This specimen consists of a magenta amorphous mucopolysaccharide-containing substance with blood contamination. (Wright-Giemsa; LP). (A, Courtesy Sharon Dial, University of Arizona.)

APPENDIX 3 Peculiar Findings and Polarizing Materials 681

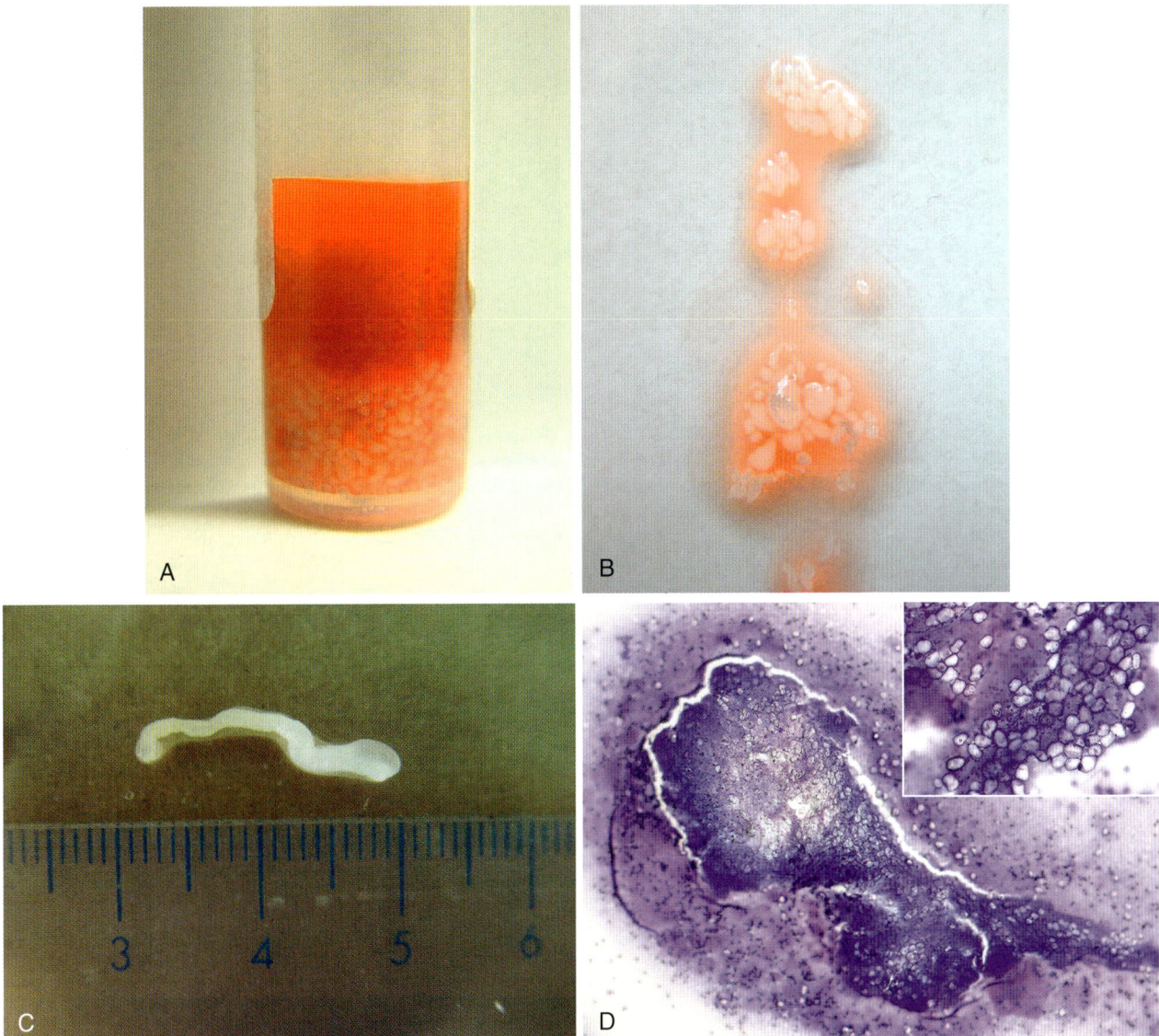

■ **FIGURE A3.7 Canine cestodiasis.** Sequenced as *Mesocestoides corti*. **A, Peritoneal effusion**. Macroscopic appearance of abdominal fluid from the dog with *Mesocestoides* sp. infection. Note the pink to red color, moderately turbid fluid, and numerous white flecks settled at the bottom of the tube. **B, Parasite segments.** Gross appearance of white flat flecks presented throughout abdominal fluid. Several 1 to 4 mm white flecks are visible on the slide. **C, Cestode.** Occasional white flecks are up 1 to 2 cm in length, nonsegmented with thickened head and a long tail. Canine cestodiasis. It was identified by molecular sequencing as *M. corti*. **D,** Segment displaying mucinous background and basophilic segments. (Modified Wright; IP.) *Inset:* Numerous calcareous corpuscles (mineralized refractile structure characterized by concentric rings) are supportive of cestodes. (Modified Wright; HP oil.) (Courtesy Eleonora Piseddu, Padua, Italy.)

POLARIZING MATERIALS

See Table A3.2.

APPENDIX TABLE 3.2 Selected Materials That Polarize

CRYSTALS	LINEAR FORMATIONS	BIOLOGIC MACROMOLECULES
Urate (see Figs. 12.22 and 12.25)	Synthetic suture (Fig. A3.8)	Collagen (Figs. A3.9 and A3.10)
Oxalate (see Figs. 11.12 and 12.29)	Cotton fiber (gossypiboma) (see Fig. 6.41)	Amyloid (see Fig. 9.33C)
Bile microspheroliths (see Fig. 9.37)	Hair shafts (Fig. A3.11)	Ultrasound lubricant gel (Fig. A3.12)
Cornstarch or silica (Fig. A3.13)	Wood (cellulose)	Sebum (see Fig. 16.2)

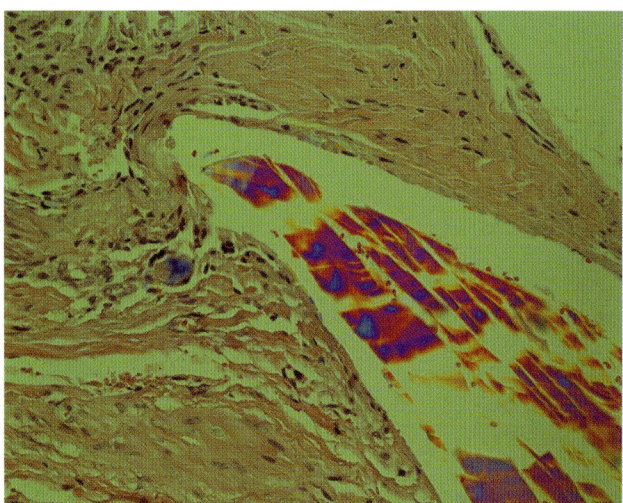

■ FIGURE A3.8 **Suture material. Tissue section. Polarized.** Remnant suture material in the urinary bladder of a dog shows colorful birefringence when polarized. (H&E; IP.)

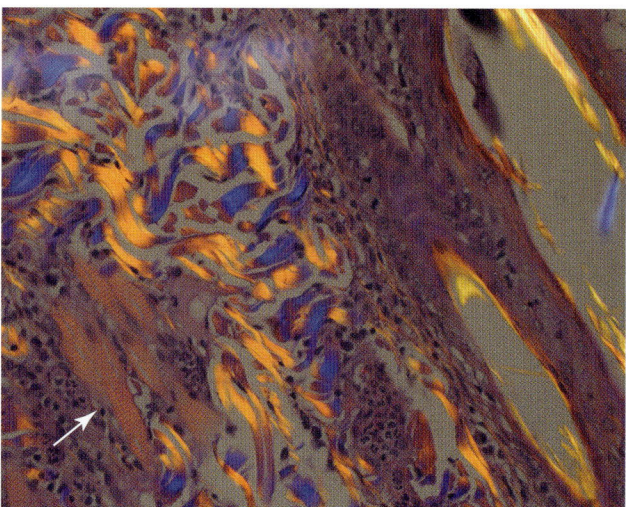

■ FIGURE A3.9 **Collagen fibers. Tissue section. Polarized.** Note that skeletal muscle *(arrow)* does not polarize while the collagen birefringence in this skin specimen from a dog. (H&E; IP.)

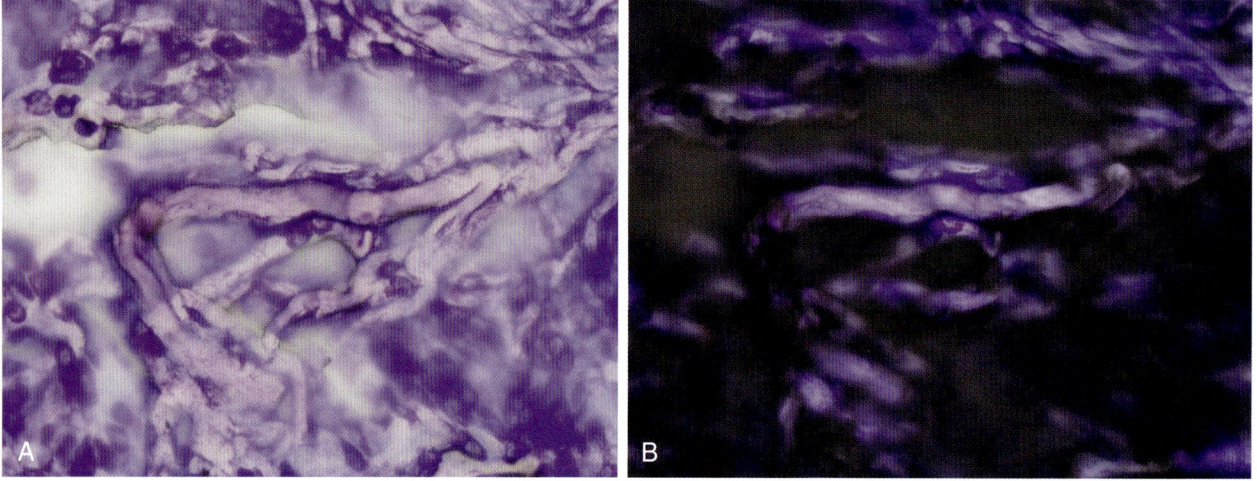

■ FIGURE A3.10 **Collagen fibers. Mast cell tumor. Skin mass aspirate. Dog.** Same case in A and B. **A,** Dense collagen strands are present along with several mast cells. (Modified Wright; IP.) **B,** Pink-white birefringence is noted in the collagen when polarized. (Modified Wright/Polarized; IP.) (Courtesy Yvonne Wikander and Nora Springer, Kansas State University.)

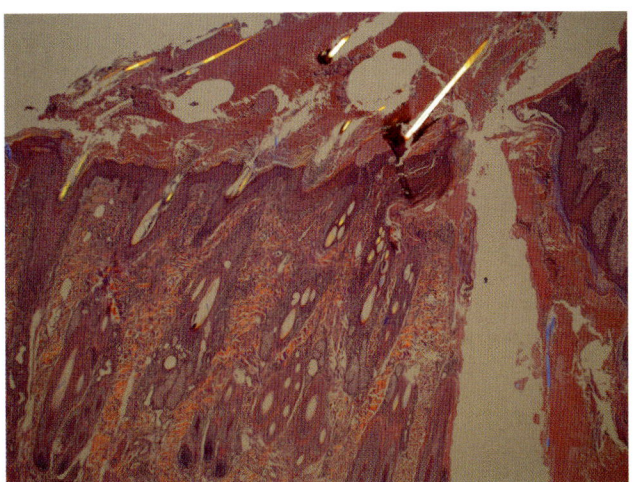

■ **FIGURE A3.11 Hair shafts. Tissue section. Polarized.** Note the multiple hairs that display a bright white-yellow birefringence. (H&E; IP.)

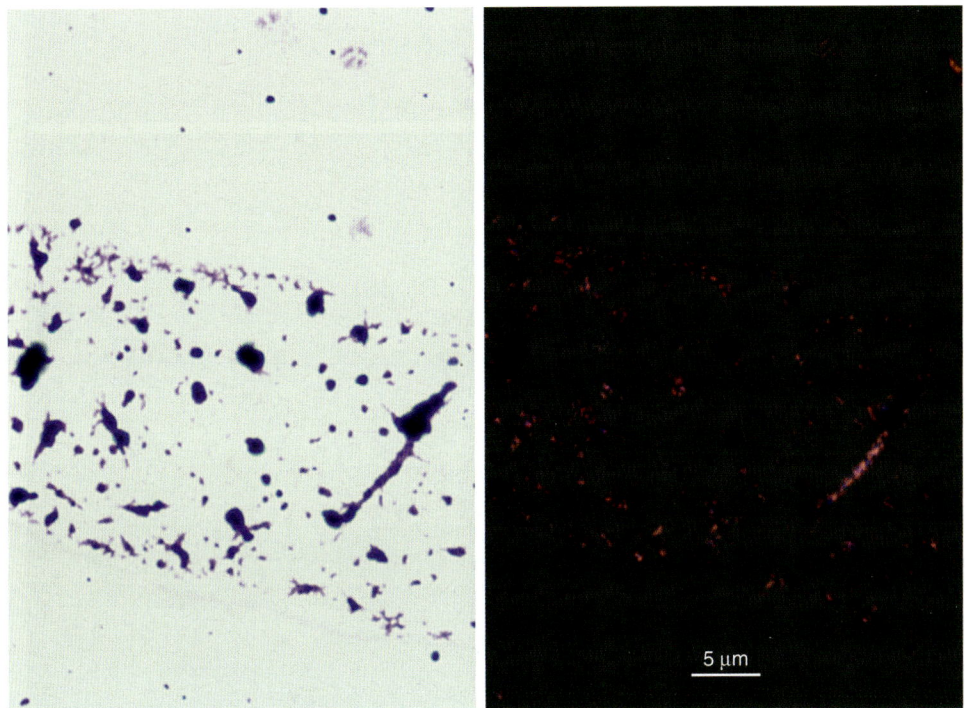

■ **FIGURE A3.12 Ultrasound coupling gel. Imprint. Polarized.** This is a direct smear of the gel on the slide. Note the polarized right panel displays a bright red birefringence compared with the unstained left panel. (Wright-Giemsa; HP oil.) (Courtesy Jere Stern, University of Florida.)

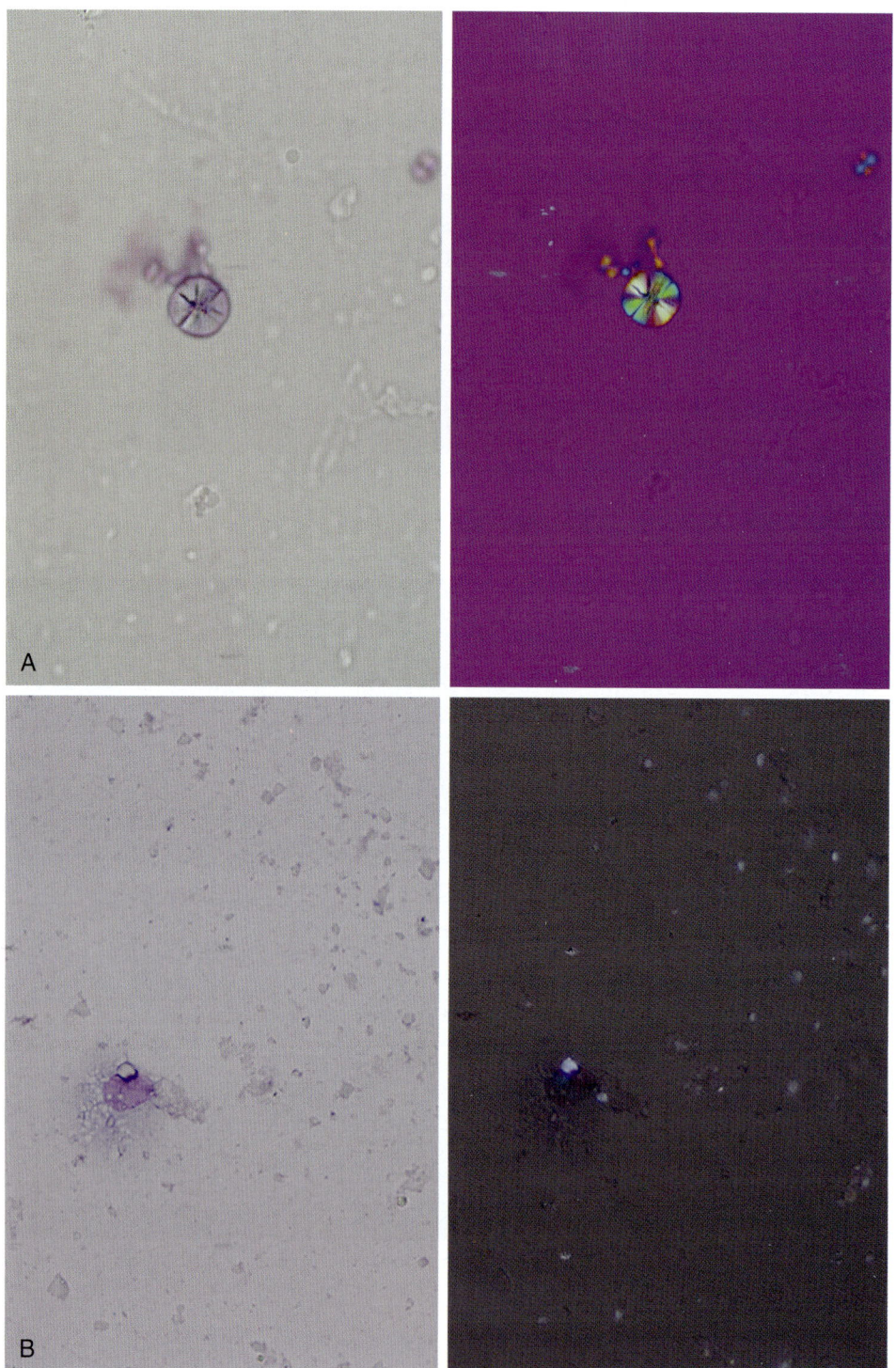

■ **FIGURE A3.13 A, Cornstarch powder. Polarized.** Unknown sample contaminated with glove powder demonstrates birefringence in the polarized *right panel*. The *left panel* is not polarized. (Romanowsky; HP oil.) **B, Red top silica. Polarized.** Tail cyst fluid, placed in a red top tube used for clot activation, is contaminated with silica, which demonstrates polarized fragments *(right panel)* in the background and within a macrophage. The *left panel* is not polarized. (Wright-Giemsa; HP oil.) (B, Courtesy Jere Stern, University of Florida.)

APPENDIX 4

Mitotic Figures and Chromatin Patterns

Rose E. Raskin

Mitotic figures from normal cytology may be recognized in several phases, including prophase, metaphase, anaphase, telophase, and cytokinesis (Fig. A4.1).

In histopathology, mitotic figures are best appreciated as the metaphase and telophase steps (Fig. A4.2). On cytopathology, malignant specimens may contain abnormal mitotic figures (Fig. A4.3) with irregularly dispersed or bridging chromatin, lag chromatin, or tri- or multipolar division (Tvedten, 2009).

Nuclear chromatin patterns are described as stippled as demonstrated in Figure A4.4A–C and as clumped in Figure A4.4D–F. The nucleus may be positioned in the cytoplasm centrally, paracentrally (near the center, as in Fig. A4.4B), or eccentrically (as in Fig. A4.4E). Chromocenter is a densely staining nuclear body associated with chromatin (Fig. A4.4F). The nucleoli (Fig. A4.4B–C) form centrally to the associated chromatin and stains pale to medium blue with Romanowsky owing to RNA content compared with the purple DNA content of the nucleus.

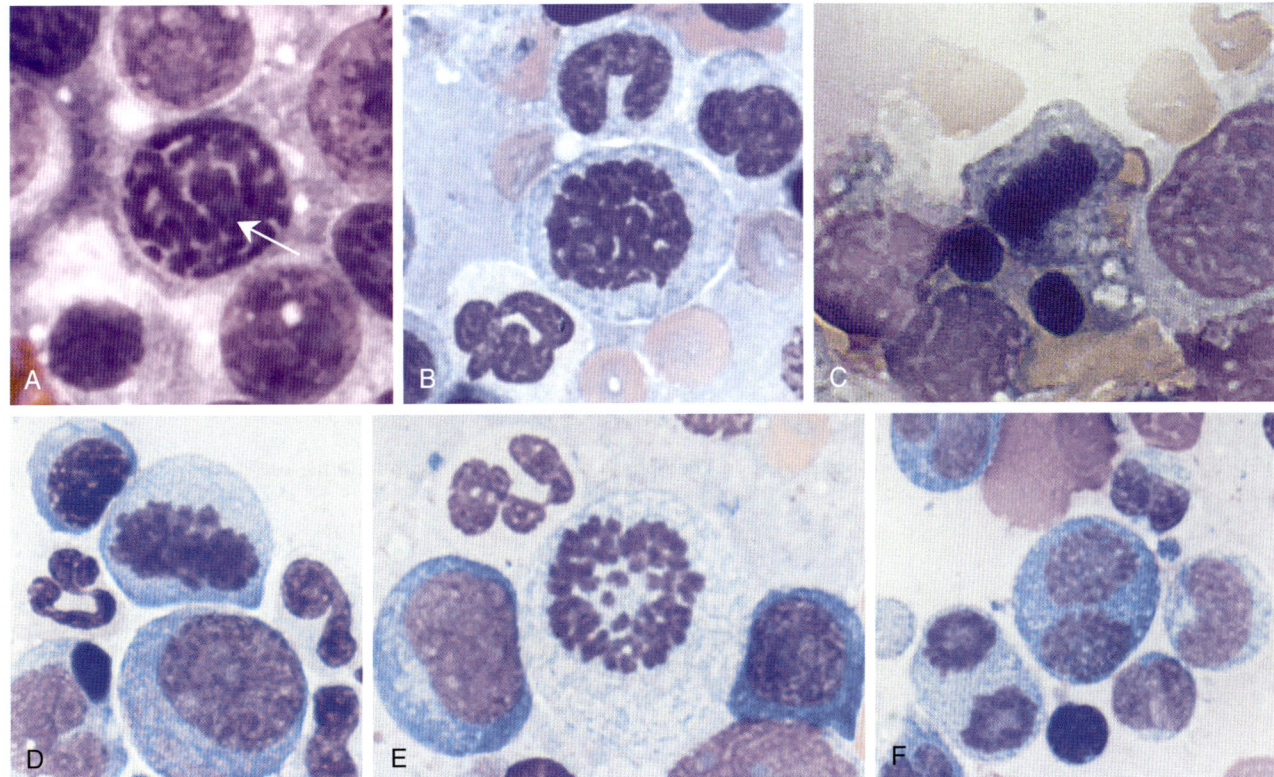

■ **FIGURE A4.1 Normal mitotic figures. Dog. A, Early prophase.** Chromatin condenses into chromosomes, and occasionally a nucleolus *(arrow)* remains. **B, Prophase.** The nucleolus disappears, leaving the coarse clumps of chromosomes. **C** and **D, Metaphase.** The chromosome clumps line up at the equator. **E, Metaphase.** The chromosomes form a ring when viewed head on to the plate, or perpendicular as in parts C and D. Note the even distribution around the circle. **F, Anaphase and binucleated prophase.** The cell in the lower left displays anaphase with two groups of chromosomes pulled apart. The center cell is binucleated cell, and both nuclei are undergoing prophase.

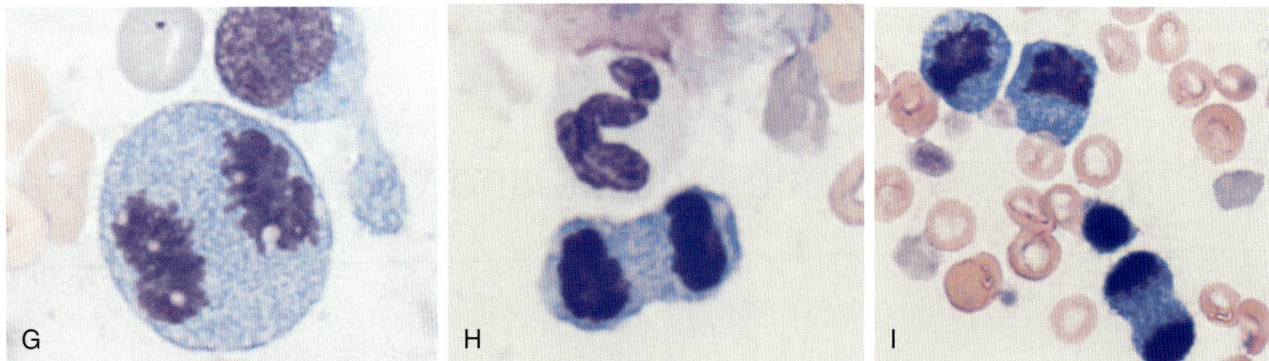

■ **FIGURE A4.1, cont'd G, Anaphase.** The two sets of chromosomes are pulled to opposite poles of the mitotic spindle. **H, Telophase.** After condensation of the chromosomes, there is the beginning of a division in the cytoplasm. **I, Telophase and cytokinesis.** The bottom cell is in telophase as it begins to divide, and the top two cells have just formed from complete division of the cytoplasm, creating two daughter cells. Part A is from a dog with transmissible venereal tumor. (Weight-Giemsa; HP oil.) Parts B–I are from a canine bone marrow aspirate. (Aqueous Romanowsky; HP oil.) (A, Courtesy Mary White, Midwestern University.)

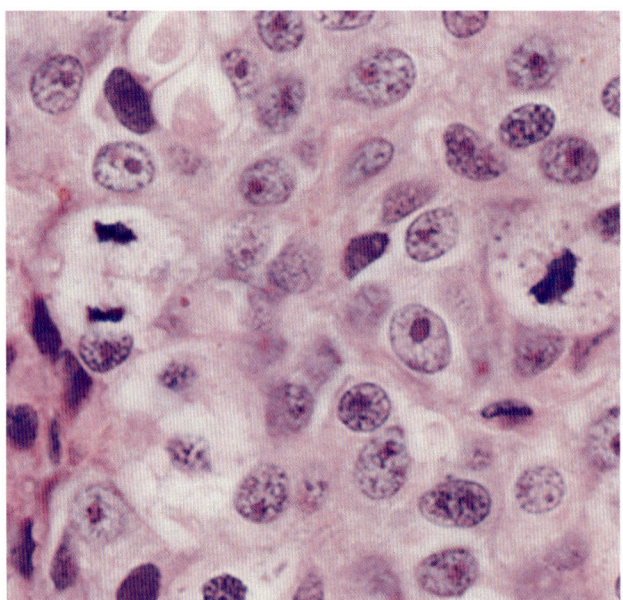

■ **FIGURE A4.2 Normal mitosis. Melanoma tissue section. Metaphase and telophase. Dog.** Note the cell in metaphase at the 3 o'clock position and the cell in telophase at the 9 o'clock position. (HE; HP oil.)

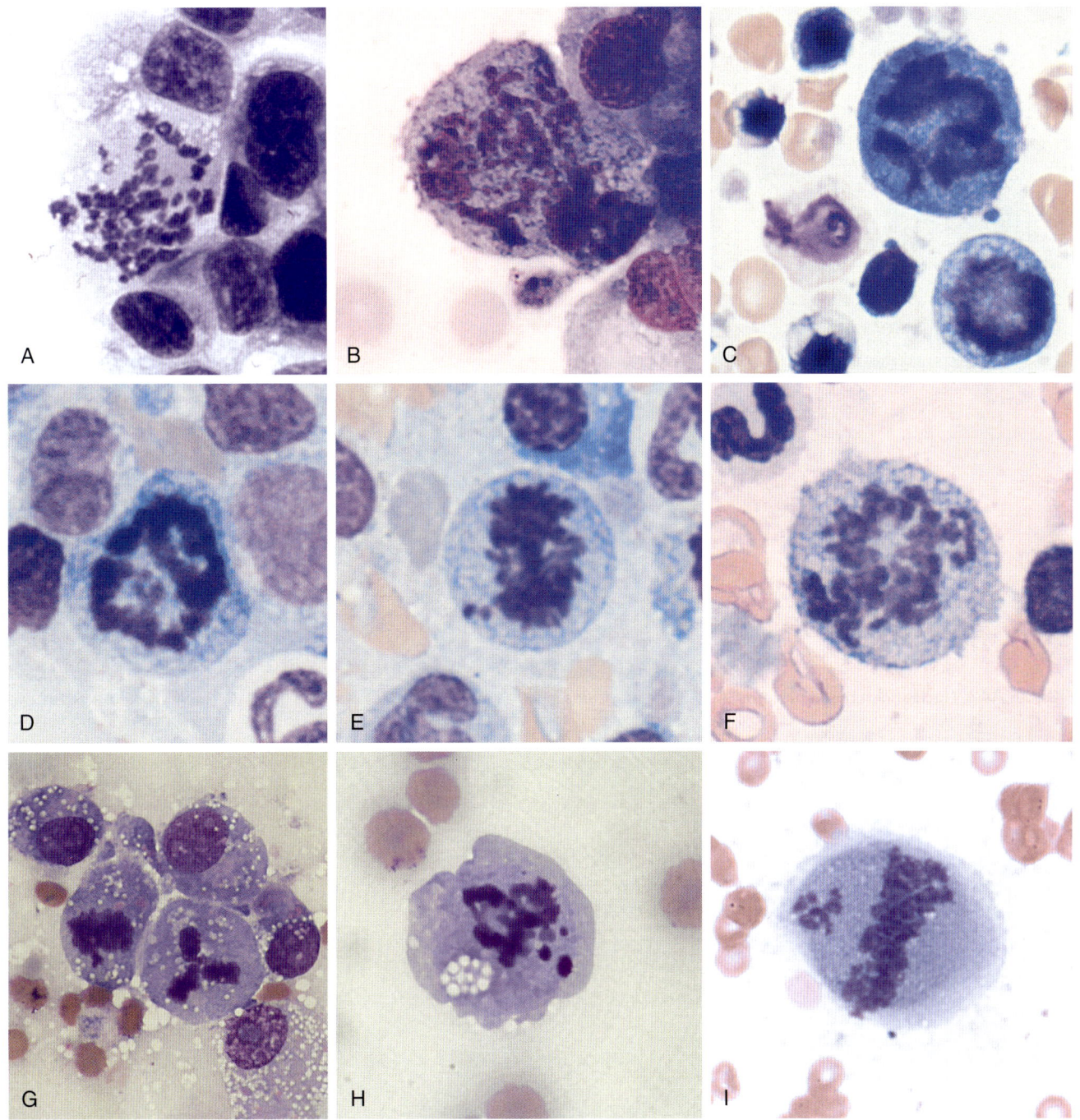

■ **FIGURE A4.3 Abnormal mitosis. Tissue aspirates. Dog. A–I,** Multiple views of abnormal mitotic figures with uneven distribution of chromatin **(C–F)**. Chromosomal fragments are dispersed irregularly with one or more isolated from the rest, termed *lag chromatin* **(A, E, G–I)**. Tripolar **(G)** and multipolar mitosis **(B and H)** are noted. Increased mitotic activity does not necessarily indicate pathology, but abnormal mitotic division supports malignancy. (Methanolic Romanowsky; HP oil.)

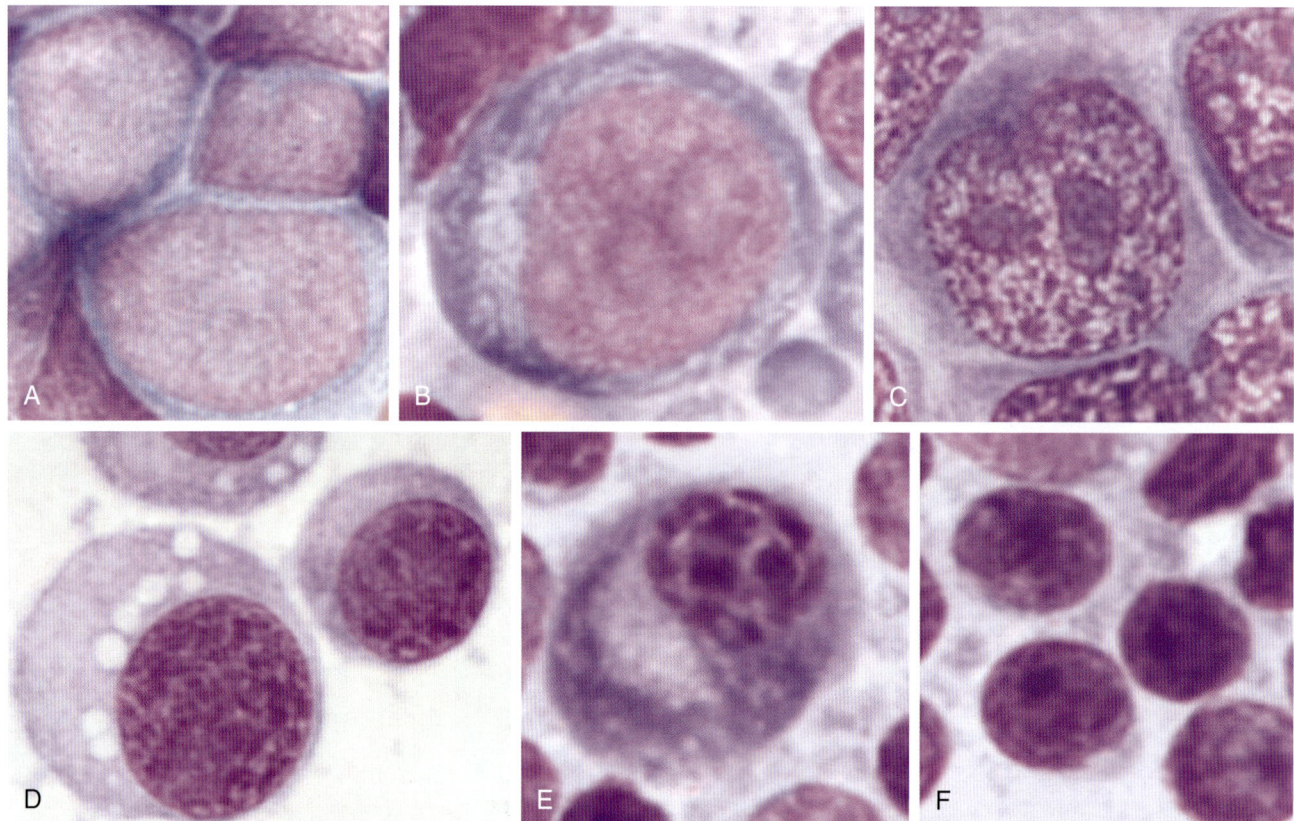

■ **FIGURE A4.4 Nuclear chromatin patterns. A–F,** Chromatin is described as stippled **(A–C)** or clumped **(D–F)**. **A,** *Finely stippled*, smooth, evenly or uniformly distributed chromatin. **B,** *Stippled*, lacy, finely reticular, uniform thin strands of chromatin. **C,** *Coarsely stippled*, open (euchromatin) with uneven clumped (heterochromatin). **D,** *Finely or loosely clumped*, unevenly dispersed with small aggregates. **E,** *Coarsely clumped* with blocks or large uneven dense aggregates. **F,** *Tightly clumped*, smudged, or condensed chromatin. (Romanowsky; HP oil.) (Courtesy Khush Banajee, Louisiana State University.)

REFERENCE

Tvedten H. Atypical mitoses: morphology and classification. *Vet Clin Pathol*. 2009;38:418-420.

APPENDIX 5

Advanced Collection and Preparation Techniques

Rose E. Raskin

CELL BLOCK

The main advantage of the cell block technique is retention of architectural patterns, such as acinar, pavement, honeycomb, papillary, and perivascular, for tissue aspirate biopsies. The technique applied to tissue and fluid materials can be used for diagnostic and ancillary tests such as immunohistochemistry and histochemical stains. The differences in preparation depend on the liquid medium used to rinse the aspirate biopsy material out of the needle and hub, the fixative, and the method used to form a clot or pellet for the cell block to be processed by histopathology. One technique involves rinsing and fixing the aspirate biopsy material in 70% ethanol in 0.6-mL Eppendorf tubes followed by centrifugation at 2800 g for 10 minutes (Zanoni et al., 2012). The supernatant is removed and 2% liquid agarose is added. The tube is recentrifuged at 2800 g for 10 minutes to obtain a solid pellet, which can be embedded in paraffin and routinely processed as a histopathologic specimen. A second method involves needle rinses with saline followed by clotting the sample with plasma and thrombin or if bloody, adding no clot enhancer. The pellet is then fixed with formalin. An alternate method uses HistoGel or Gelfoam to embed specimens followed by formalin fixation (Joiner and Spangler, 2012; Wallace et al., 2015). Last, another technique uses formalin needle rinses into a polymer-lined tube called a collodion bag to help form the pellet (Balassanian et al., 2016). Furthermore, a commercial embedding system (the Shandon Cytoblock Cell Block Preparation System) is available that requires longer incubation with a nonformalin fixative in a proprietary unit for a cytocentrifuge.

One study compared two cell block methods using a suspension of cells aspirated from canine lymph nodes (Fernandes et al., 2016). This suspension was divided for comparison between a fixed sediment method using Bouin's solution and an agar method using agarose in formalin. Pellets from the two methods were evaluated for morphology and immunohistochemistry. The fixed sediment method produced more highly cellular and aggregated groups compared to the agar method.

A modification for small-volume fluid specimens such as cerebrospinal fluid, cystic fluid, body cavity effusions, bronchoalveolar lavage, urine, and blood involves centrifugation of the sample within a microhematocrit tube. Adding a drop of density gradient media (e.g., Percoll) helps to separate the specimen from the clay sealant. The tube is then broken at the liquid-solid interface and fixed in 10% formalin for 24 hours. The plug is removed and embedded in paraffin for histopathology diagnostic and ancillary tests (Marcos et al., 2017).

CELL TRANSFER

Cell transfer of archived cytologic smears previously stained by an aqueous Romanowsky method is demonstrated in Figure A5.1. This method (Stone and Gan, 2014) allows for a variety of additional diagnostic tests such as special histochemical stains, immunocytochemical staining, and molecular testing for infectious agents. Transfer of cells was found to be easier when archived slides had been previously coverslipped. Staining of media-coated sections requires removal of the hardened Pertex by soaking in xylene for 20 to 30 minutes. Each slide is then briefly dried in a 55°C oven to ensure optimal adhesion of the cells to the slides. Routine coverslipping is performed before microscopic examination.

REFERENCES

Balassanian R, Wool GD, Ono JC, et al. A superior method for cell block preparation for fine-needle aspiration biopsies. *Cancer Cytopathol*. 2016; 124(7):508–518.

Fernandes NC, Guerra JM, Réssio RA, et al. Liquid-based cytology and cell block immunocytochemistry in veterinary medicine: comparison with standard cytology for the evaluation of canine lymphoid samples. *Vet Comp Oncol*. 2016;14:107–116.

Joiner KS, Spangler EA. Evaluation of HistoGel-embedded specimens for use in veterinary diagnostic pathology. *J Vet Diagn Invest*. 2012;24:710–715.

Marcos R, Santos M, Marrinhas C, et al. Cell tube block: a new technique to produce cell blocks from fluid cytology samples. *Vet Clin Pathol*. 2017;46(1):195–201.

Stone BM, Gan D. Application of the tissue transfer technique in veterinary cytopathology. *Vet Clin Pathol*. 2014;43(2):295–302.

Wallace KA, Goldschmidt MH, Patel RT. Converting fluid-based cytologic specimens to histologic specimens for immunohistochemistry. *Vet Clin Pathol*. 2015;44(2):303–309.

Zanoni DS, Grandi F, Rocha NS. Agarose cell block technique as a complementary method in the diagnosis of fungal osteomyelitis in a dog. *Vet Clin Pathol*. 2012;41:307–308.

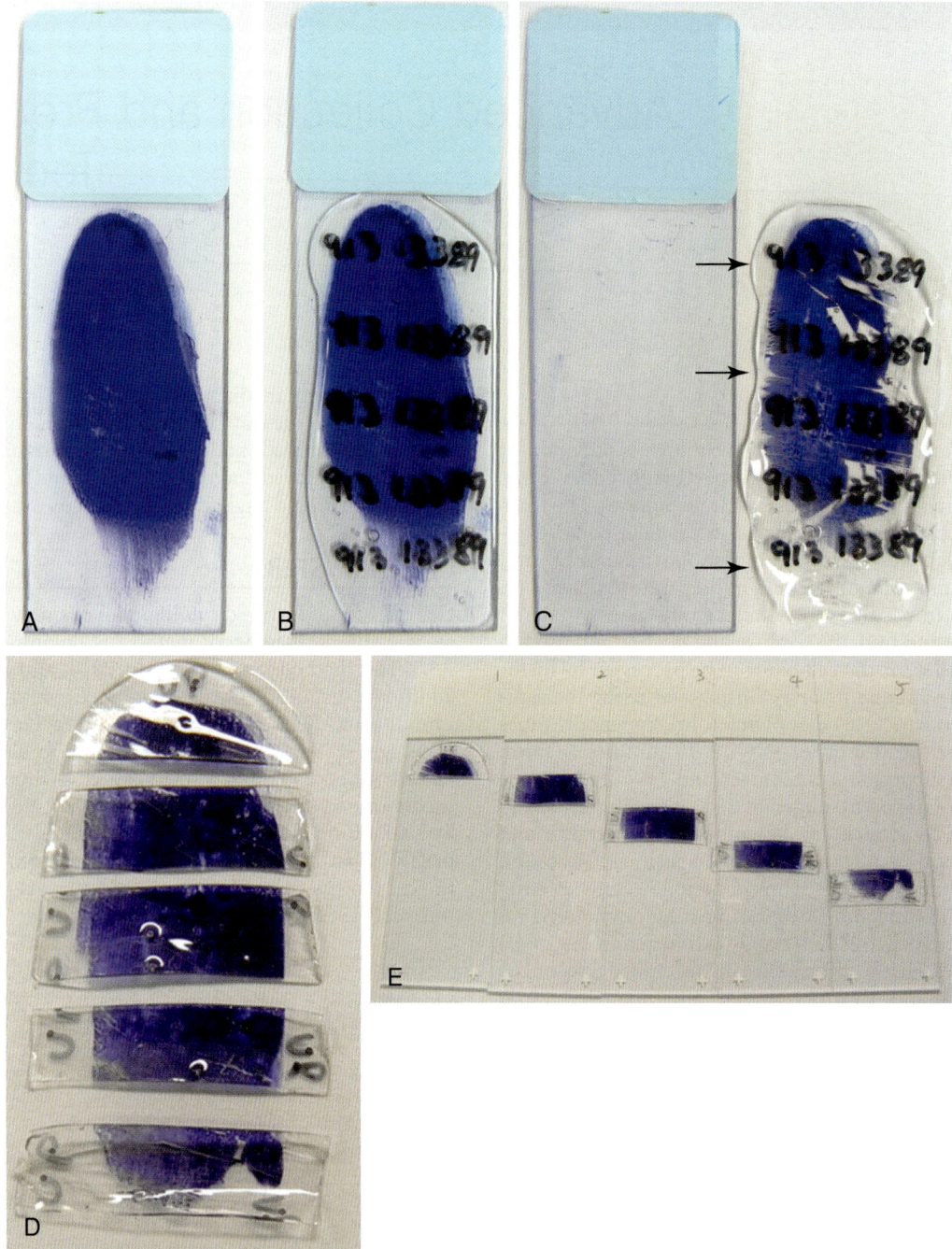

FIGURE A5.1 Cell transfer method. Lymph node aspirate from a dog. A, Archived aqueous Romanowsky coverslipped slide. **B,** Coverslip removal by xylene immersion followed by coating of cytologic material with rapid mounting medium (e.g., Pertex). The slides are then baked in an oven at 55°C for 3 hours until the media hardens. The up direction is labeled on the strip where separate sections will be created. **C,** Pertex and attached cells are removed by scraping the surface of the slide and simultaneously lifting the cell-containing hardened media from the slide using a disposable microtome blade. **D,** The hardened Pertex layer is cut into multiple sections. **E,** The individual pieces are pressed firmly onto positively charged slides that are baked in an oven at 55°C for 1 hour. Slides are stored at room temperature until processed further. (Courtesy Brett Stone, Australia.)

APPENDIX 6

Composing Pathology Reports

Katie M. Boes

The pathology report is the primary form of communication between the pathologist and referring veterinarian. It contains information to aid in interpretation and traceability of the sample—the pathologist's observations, diagnosis, and comments (Figs. A6.1 to A6.4):
- *Referring veterinarian:* name, contact information
- *Client:* name, contact information
- *Patient:* name, species, breed, sex, age, clinical history
- *Sample:* unique laboratory identification number, submission date and time, collection method, source, type, ± fluid characteristics
- *Pathologist contributions:* cytopathologic or histopathologic description, cytologic or morphologic diagnosis, comments
- *Pathologist information:* name, signature, credentials
- *Laboratory:* name, contact information
- *Report information:* issuing date and time, priority status

CYTOPATHOLOGY REPORT

Cytopathologic Description

The description contains the cytopathologist's observations of the microscopic features of the sample, with an emphasis on features that aid in the sample's diagnosis.
1. **Sample quality.** Describe the diagnostic quality of the sample, commenting on the quantity of intact and lysed cells, thickness of preparation, and contaminants such as blood or ultrasound gel.
   Example: There is an extensive monolayer of intact nucleated cells with rare lysed cells and minimal hemodilution, representing an excellent diagnostic sample.
   Example: There are rare droplets containing thick blood and protein that compress the interspersed nucleated cells and obscure their cellular detail, warranting a nondiagnostic sample.
2. **Specimen overview.** Describe the low magnification (e.g., 4× to 10× objective) diagnostic elements in the sample. This includes listing the types and proportions of cells, infectious agents, and noncellular structures that are present; the arrangement of the cells relative to each other (Masserdotti, 2006) or relative noncellular structures; and the background description.
3. **Diagnosis-focused description.** Describe the intermediate to high magnification (e.g., 20× to 100× objective) features of the cells or structures listed in the overview that aid in interpretation of the sample; normal cells and structures are not further described. Descriptions may include one or more of the four categories listed below.
   - *Infectious inflammation:* Describe the characteristics of the agent that aid in identification, such as size, shape, staining characteristics, presence of cellular structures, and location within host cells (see Appendix 8).
   - *Noninfectious inflammation:* If not already included in the overview sentence, further describe structures that could be inciting the inflammation, such as adjuvant or other foreign-body material.
   - *Proliferation (hyperplasia, metaplasia, dysplasia, neoplasia):* Describe the morphology of the proliferating cells, such as cell size, prominence of cell borders, cytoplasmic staining quality and features, nuclear and nucleolar size and shape, nucleus location within the cytoplasm, and chromatin pattern that aid in cell origin identification (see Chapter 2). List and quantify criteria of malignancy (see Chapter 2).
   - *Degenerative or metabolic changes:* Describe cellular changes of degeneration (e.g., cytoplasmic vacuolization, cell swelling, karyolysis), necrosis (e.g., hypereosinophilic cytoplasm, cell shrinkage, karyorrhexis, pyknosis), and cytoplasmic accumulations (e.g., vacuoles or granules suggestive of glycogen or lipid, copper, lipofuscin, hemosiderin). Include the affected cell type, the relative amount of cells affected, and the severity of the change. Follow the description with a parenthetical interpretive phrase (see Fig. A6.2).
4. **Negative findings.** State what was not observed, such as inflammation, infectious agents, or neoplastic cells. This sentence is helpful if a specific etiology is suggested by the clinician.

Cytopathologic Diagnosis (Interpretation)

The cytopathologic diagnosis (interpretation) is a short phrase that summarizes the important aspects of the sample with the intention of conveying a concise medical communication to the submitting clinician. Potential information to include are the cellularity (if the low cellularity hinders interpretation), the certainty of the interpretation, and the key features of the description. The cytopathologic diagnosis is similar to a histopathologic diagnosis except the lack of tissue architecture may preclude statements on lesion origin, distribution, or severity. For example, a lesion interpreted by histopathology as, "lung, moderate, multifocal, pyogranulomatous pneumonia with intralesional broad-based budding yeast" may be interpreted as "pyogranulomatous inflammation with broad-based budding yeast" on cytopathology.

Example: Low cellularity; nondiagnostic
Example: Carcinoma, probable squamous cell carcinoma
Example: Mixed neutrophilic and macrophagic inflammation without evidence of sepsis
Example: Reactive lymphoid hyperplasia
Example: Hepatocytes, moderate microvesicular vacuolar change

Veterinary Laboratory Services
Cytologyville, Virginia, USA
(800) XXX-XXXX

Patient Name:	Molly	**Veterinarian:**	Doctor, Good
Patient ID:	143852	**Clinic Name:**	Great Veterinary Clinic
Patient Owner:	McOwner, Morose	**Clinic Phone:**	(800) XXX-XXXX
Species:	Canine	**Sample ID:**	C20-02193
Breed:	Labrador Retriever	**Received Date:**	01/16/2020 12:00PM
Sex:	SF	**Issued Date:**	01/16/2020 12:30PM
Age:	11 Years	**Priority:**	STAT

Final Cytopathology Report

Clinical history: Acute lethargy, vomiting, abdominal distension

Sample collection method–source: Centesis–peritoneal fluid

Sample type: 1 purple top tube, 1 red top tube (hold for culture)

Color (pre-centrifugation):	Tan	TNCC:	110,000 /μL
Color (post-centrifugation):	Yellow	RBC:	150,000 /μL
Clarity (pre-centrifugation):	Flocculent	Protein:	3.2 g/dL
Clarity (post-centrifugation):	Cloudy		

Cytopathologic description: Direct preparations are evaluated that contain a monolayer of intact nucleated cells, and is of good diagnostic quality. There are many erythrocytes and inflammatory cells (80% neutrophils, 19% macrophages, 1% lymphocytes, and rare eosinophils) that are freely dispersed or aggregated around large fragments of skeletal muscle, hair, amorphous debris, or keratinocytes (digesta). The neutrophils display moderate nuclear swelling and loss of segmentation (degeneration), and frequently contain phagocytized bacterial bacilli and cocci of various morphologies. The macrophages contain deeply basophilic and foamy cytoplasm, phagocytized erythrocytes, green-brown granular material (hemosiderin), brown globular material (digesta), or 3 μm x 6 μm, oval, narrow-based budding yeast with 1 μm-thick, refractive walls. There is no evidence of neoplasia.

Cytopathologic diagnosis: Septic mixed cell exudate with digesta, bacteria, yeast, and mild hemorrhage.

Case comments: This sample is compatible with septic peritonitis secondary to gastrointestinal rupture, which warrants emergency surgery and has a guarded to poor prognosis. Potential causes of gastrointestinal rupture in dogs include dehiscence of a prior surgical site, perforating foreign body, perforating neoplasm, or less likely, external trauma.

Electronically signed by
Katie Boes, DVM, MS, Diplomate ACVP
01/16/2020 at 12:30 PM

End of report (final)

FIGURE A6.1 Example cytopathology report for a metabolic condition in a fluid.

Case Comments

The case comments contain information that helps the clinician decide the next course of action. If the cytopathologic diagnosis was definitive for a disease condition, then the comments may contain information about the condition's clinical behavior, management, or prognosis. If the cytopathologic diagnosis was not definitive, then the comments could list differential diagnoses, the relative probability of certainty for the listed differential diagnoses, and recommended diagnostic testing.

HISTOPATHOLOGY REPORT

Histopathologic Description: Neoplasms

1. **Name the organ or tissue.** This is a word or phrase followed by a colon.
2. **Subgross morphology.** Note the neoplasm's size, tissue location, demarcation with non-neoplastic tissue (e.g., unencapsulated, encapsulated, well-delineated, poorly delineated), effect on pre-existing tissue (e.g., effacing or replacing, elevating, compressing, separating), cell shape (e.g., round, polygonal, elongate), cellular arrangement (e.g., sheets, cords, trabeculae, whorls), cellular density, and type and amount of supporting stroma. If complete excision was attempted, include the amount and type of non-neoplastic tissue between the neoplasm and cut border.
3. **Cellular morphology.** Describe the cellular and nuclear characteristics of the proliferating cells that aid in identification of the cell origin, which may include the cell size, prominence of cell borders, cytoplasmic staining quality and features, nuclear and nucleolar size, nucleus shape, nucleus location within the cytoplasm, and chromatin pattern.

> **Veterinary Laboratory Services**
> Cytologyville, Virginia, USA
> (800) XXX-XXXX
>
> | | | | |
> |---|---|---|---|
> | **Patient Name:** Max | | **Veterinarian:** | Doctor, Good |
> | **Patient ID:** 154365 | | **Clinic Name:** | Great Veterinary Clinic |
> | **Patient Owner:** Daddy, Doggie | | **Clinic Phone:** | (800) XXX-XXXX |
> | **Species:** Canine | | **Sample ID:** | C20-02192 |
> | **Breed:** Boxer | | **Received Date:** | 01/16/2020 11:00AM |
> | **Sex:** MN | | **Issued Date:** | 01/16/2020 1:30PM |
> | **Age:** 6 years | | **Priority:** | Routine |
>
> ### Final Cytopathology Report
>
> **Clinical history:** 2x3 cm skin mass on left rear thigh, freely movable, first noticed this week by groomer
>
> **Sample collection method–source:** Aspirate biopsy–Skin mass
>
> **Sample type:** 1 previously stained slide, 3 unstained slides
>
> **Cytopathologic description:** There is an extensive monolayer of intact nucleated cells with rare lysed cells and minimal hemodilution, representing an excellent diagnostic sample. There are many individualized neoplastic round cells, frequent eosinophils and plump fusiform cells (fibroblasts) emanating from an eosinophilic fibrillar matrix (collagen), and occasional nondegenerate neutrophils on a background containing many cell-free coarse purple granules. The round cells measure 20-30 μm in diameter, and contain a moderate amount of basophilic cytoplasm with discrete cell borders and many coarse purple granules. Their nuclei are round, central, 10-15 μm in diameter, partially obscured by cytoplasmic granules, and display coarse chromatin. Nucleoli, binucleation, and mitotic figures are not observed. There is no evidence of infection.
>
> **Cytopathologic diagnosis:** Mast cell tumor
>
> **Case comments:** All canine cutaneous/subcutaneous mast cell tumors should be treated as potentially malignant. Wide surgical excision with subsequent histopathology is advised if there is no current evidence of metastasis to regional lymph nodes or visceral organs. Histopathology is required for definitive tumor grading, but if this tumor is located within the cutis (versus subcutis), then the cytologic features are most compatible with a low-grade canine cutaneous mast cell tumor, based on the two-tiered grading system. Mast cell tumors may release histamine and other bioactive substances, which may result in local edema and hemorrhage, as well as gastric ulceration. Investigation into gastrointestinal hemorrhage or administration of gastroprotectants should be considered.
>
> Electronically signed by
> *Katie Boes, DVM, MS, Diplomate ACVP*
> 01/16/2020 at 1:30 PM
>
> End of report (final)

■ **FIGURE A6.2** Example cytopathology report for a proliferative and noninfectious inflammatory mass.

4. **Criteria of malignancy.** List the type and degree of cellular criteria of malignancy, such as anisocytosis, anisokaryosis, nuclear pleomorphism, binucleation, multinucleation, presence and morphology of nucleoli, and presence and amount of hemorrhage or necrosis within the neoplasm. The mitotic count is provided as the number of mitotic figures over 2.37 mm^2 (~ten 40× objective fields) of the most densely cellular areas of the neoplasm free from necrosis, hemorrhage, cysts, and other disturbances in tumor homogeneity (Meuten et al., 2016). Note vascular invasion as present or not observed.
5. **Secondary changes.** Describe tissue and cellular abnormalities secondary to the presence of a tumor, such as degeneration, necrosis, hemorrhage, inflammation, or mineralization.

Histopathologic Description: Non-neoplastic

1. **Name the organ.** This is a word or phrase followed by a colon.
2. **Subgross morphology.** Describe the architectural disturbances of the tissue section, including the disturbance's location, distribution, shape, and size. State how the disturbance affects the preexisting tissue (e.g., disrupting, replacing, elevating, compressing, separating).
3. **Diagnosis-focused description.**
   - *Infectious inflammatory lesions:* List and quantify all the inflammatory cells that are present, using their specific names (e.g., lymphocytes instead of mononuclear cells). State the location and quantity of the causative agent and

Histopathologic description: Skin, footpad: Numerous inflammatory cells multifocally infiltrate the dermis and superficial hypodermis and obscure normal architecture by surrounding and separating dermal collagen bundles and hypodermal adipose tissue. The inflammatory infiltrate consists of numerous plasma cells and fewer small lymphocytes and neutrophils. Many of the plasma cells contain globular, eosinophilic, intracytoplasmic vacuoles (Mott cells containing Russell bodies). Collagen fibers are separated by clear spaces (edema); ectatic lymphatics (edema) contain a few small lymphocytes and plasma cells. The overlying epidermis is diffusely thickened (acanthosis) with increased intercellular clear spaces (spongiosis).

Morphologic diagnosis: Skin, footpad: Pododermatitis, plasmacytic, diffuse, marked.

Case comments: The patient's signalment (cat), historical lesion distribution (multiple foot pads), and histopathologic findings are compatible with feline plasma cell pododermatitis. Feline plasma cell pododermatitis is an idiopathic immune-mediated disease, and immunosuppressive therapy should be considered. Some cats develop immune-mediated glomerulosclerosis or renal amyloidosis, which warrants monitoring of renal health (e.g., serum chemistry and urinalysis).

FIGURE A6.3 Example abbreviated histopathologic report for a noninfectious inflammatory lesion.

Histopathologic description: Mucosa and submucosa. The submucosa contains a 2.0 cm x 2.0 cm, nonencapsulated, well-demarcated, densely cellular mass that elevates the overlying mucosa, compresses the surrounding submucosal collagen, and is composed of sheets and cords of neoplastic round cells with scant intervening stroma. The individual cells have well-defined cytoplasmic borders and moderate amounts of eosinophilic cytoplasm; many cells have a hyaline appearance to the cytoplasm or a prominent Golgi zone, and some have peripheralization and lateral compression of the nucleus. Nuclei are round or ovoid, with clumped chromatin and one to multiple variably prominent nucleoli. Anisokaryosis, anisocytosis, and nuclear pleomorphism are generally moderate, with scattered karyomegalic cells that often have bizarre nuclear morphology. Binucleate cells are present in moderate numbers, with fewer multinucleated cells. There are 18 mitotic figures over 2.37 mm^2 (ten 400X fields). Surgical margins contain 0.2 cm – 0.4 cm of nonneoplastic submucosa. Within the mass, there is mild focal hemorrhage; neoplastic cells adjacent to this region often contain golden-brown cytoplasmic granules (hemosiderin). The epithelium overlying the mass is multifocally spongiotic, eroded, or ulcerated, and the underlying submucosa contains dilated lymphatics and mild hemorrhage.

Morphologic diagnosis: Mucosa, plasmacytoma.

Case comments: Canine oral plasmacytomas tend to be benign, and complete surgical excision is expected to be curative. Surgical excision appears complete in this case. Oral plasmacytomas may rarely represent the malignant plasma cell tumor variant, multiple myeloma. Therefore, measurement of the serum globulins concentration is recommended as a screening test for multiple myeloma.

FIGURE A6.4 Example abbreviated histopathologic report for a neoplastic lesion.

describe the agent's characteristics that aid in identification (see Cytopathologic Description).
- *Noninfectious inflammatory lesions:* List and quantify all the inflammatory cells that are present, using their specific names. If not already described in the subgross sentence, describe structures that could be inciting the inflammation (e.g., vaccine adjuvant, ruptured hair follicles) or could implicate a specific condition (e.g., vasculitis, acantholytic keratinocytes, "tombstoning").
- *Proliferative lesions (hyperplasia, metaplasia, dysplasia):* These descriptions are similar to describing a neoplasm (see Histopathologic Description: Neoplasms). Emphasize the cellular characteristics of the proliferating cells that aid in identification of the cell origin and interpretation as hyperplastic, metaplastic, or dysplastic growth.
- *Degenerative or metabolic lesions:* Describe the type, severity, and distribution of cellular attenuation, loss, degeneration, necrosis, and cytoplasmic accumulations. Follow descriptions by a parenthetical interpretive phrase when appropriate.
4. **Secondary changes.** Describe tissue and cellular abnormalities secondary to the presence of inflammation or mass effect, such as degenerative or hyperplastic changes in adjacent tissue.

Histopathologic (Morphologic) Diagnosis

Neoplastic morphologic diagnoses state the organ or tissue name and neoplasm's name. Non-neoplastic morphologic diagnoses list the organ or tissue name, lesion, inflammation type or duration, distribution, and severity followed by significant findings that support the diagnosis.

Example: Haired skin: mast cell tumor.
Example: Lymph node: Lymphadenitis, granulomatous and necrotizing, diffuse, severe, with lymphocyte loss and intracellular rickettsiae, etiology consistent with *Neorickettsia helminthoeca*.

Case Comments

Case comments in a histopathology report are similar to those in a cytopathology report. Notable differences are that the histopathologic tumor grade and extent of surgical margins should be provided when appropriate.

REFERENCES

Masserdotti C. Architectural patterns in cytology: correlation with histology. *Vet Clin Pathol.* 2006;35:388-396.

Meuten DJ, Moore FM, George JW. Mitotic count and the field of view area: time to standardize. *Vet Pathol.* 2016;53:7-9.

7 APPENDIX

Specialized Diagnostic Testing Sites

Rose E. Raskin

The list presented in Table A7.1 not complete to all sources but is known to be accurate as of November 2021. Please contact the laboratory before any submission for test availability, cost, turnaround time, and specimen requirements.

TABLE A7.1 Tests, Submission Materials, and Selected Laboratories Available for Specimen Submission

TEST	SUBMISSION MATERIALS	LABORATORY
C-Kit mutation PCR analysis for mast cell tumor or gastrointestinal stromal tumor	Canine aspirates/imprints (stained or unstained) of mast cell tumors or formalin-fixed tissues, paraffin blocks	**K9/Feline Oncology Diagnostic Lab** Research Bldg., Rm. #330C 1060 William Moore Drive Raleigh NC 27607 (919) 513-1925 cvmoncodiagnosticlab@ncsu.edu cvm.ncsu.edu/research/labs/clinical-sciences/k9feline-oncology-diagnostic/
	Canine and feline: paraffin block, formalin fixed tissue, fresh tissue, or minimum of six unstained, positively charged slides	**Michigan State University** Veterinary Diagnostic Laboratory 4125 Beaumont Road Lansing, MI 48910-8104 (517) 353-1683 cvm.msu.edu/vdl/laboratory-sections/anatomic-surgical-pathology/biopsy-service/detecting-c-kit-mutations
Echinococcus multilocularis, *Echinococcus granulosus*, and *Taenia* spp.: PCR panel	Liver tissue (preferred) and abdominal fluid, cyst or cyst fluid	**University of Guelph** Animal Health Laboratory Laboratory Services Division Box 3612 Guelph, Ontario N1H 6R8 ahlmolec@uoguelph.ca uoguelph.ca/ahl/services/echinococcus-multilocularis-e-granulosus-and-taenia-spp-pcr-panel
Endocrine testing	Serum	**Michigan State University** Veterinary Diagnostic Laboratory 4125 Beaumont Road Lansing, MI 48910-8104 (517) 353-1683 cvm.msu.edu/vdl/laboratory-sections/endocrinology
Flow cytometry	EDTA whole blood, bone marrow aspirate in EDTA, tissue aspirates in saline, effusion fluid or CSF in EDTA	**North Carolina State University** CVM Diagnostic Laboratory Services Clinical Pathology & Immunology Lab 1060 William Moore Dr, Rm. C269 Raleigh, NC 27607 (919) 513-6363 or (919) 513-6550 ncstateimmunology@ncsu.edu cvm.ncsu.edu/research/labs/population-health-pathobiology/clinical-pathology/

TABLE A7.1 Tests, Submission Materials, and Selected Laboratories Available for Specimen Submission—cont'd

TEST	SUBMISSION MATERIALS	LABORATORY
	Tissue aspirates in saline and serum, effusion fluid in EDTA and red tube (if low protein, add serum)	**Colorado State University** Clinical Immunology/Veterinary Diagnostic Laboratory 2450 Gilette Drive Fort Collins, CO 80526 (970) 491-1170 csu-cvmbs.colostate.edu/academics/mip/ci-lab/
	Contact laboratory	**Kansas State University** Veterinary Diagnostic Laboratory Clinical Immunology/Immunophenotyping 1800 Denison Avenue, Mosier D117 Manhattan, KS 66506 (866) 512-5650 ksvdl.org/laboratories/clinical-immunology/
Fungi, organism ID PCR with sequencing	Contact laboratory	**University of Tennessee** College of Veterinary Medicine Bacteriology/Mycology Laboratory 2407 River Drive, Room C121 Knoxville, TN 37996-4543 (865) 974-5639 vetmed.tennessee.edu/vmc/dls/Bacteriology/
Fungi, systemic quantitative antigen EIA (*Blastomyces, Coccidioides, Histoplasma*)	Specimen: urine, serum, plasma, CSF: BAL Anticoagulant: heparin, EDTA: NaCit Volume: Serum/plasma 1.2 mL, CSF 0.8 mL, urine and BAL 0.5 mL	**MiraVista Veterinary Diagnostics** 4705 Decatur Boulevard Indianapolis, IN 46241 (888) 841-8387 MiraVistaVets.com
Genetic testing for metabolic disease	Urine, serum, EDTA blood; contact laboratory	**University of Pennsylvania** PennGen Laboratories School of Veterinary Medicine 3900 Delancey Street Philadelphia, PA 19104 (215) 573-7545 PennGen@lists.upenn.edu vet.upenn.edu/research/academic-departments/clinical-sciences-advanced-medicine/research-labs-centers/penngen/penngen-tests
Heterobilharzia PCR test for canine schistosomiasis	Fresh fecal sample	**Texas A&M University** College of Veterinary Medicine & Biomedical Sciences Gastrointestinal Laboratory College Station, TX 77843-4474 (979) 862-2861 vetmed.tamu.edu/gilab/service/assays/heterobilharzia-americana
Immunochemistry	Formalin-fixed tissues, paraffin block, cell suspension for ICC	**Michigan State University** Veterinary Diagnostic Laboratory 4125 Beaumont Road Lansing, MI 48910-8104 (517) 353-1683 cvm.msu.edu/vdl/laboratory-sections/anatomic-surgical-pathology/immunohistochemistry
	Formalin-fixed tissues, paraffin block, unstained slides	**Purdue University** Animal Disease Diagnostic Laboratory 406 S University Street West Lafayette, IN 47907-2065 (765) 494-7440 vet.purdue.edu/addl/tests/fees.php?id=283

Continued

TABLE A7.1 Tests, Submission Materials, and Selected Laboratories Available for Specimen Submission—cont'd

TEST	SUBMISSION MATERIALS	LABORATORY
	IHC/ICC, contact laboratory	**University of California** VMTH–Histology Lab 1 Garrod Drive Davis, CA 95616 530-752-3901 vetmed.ucdavis.edu/hospital/support-services/lab-services/anatomic-pathology-service
	ICC; four air-dried unstained smears	**Colorado State University** Clinical Immunology/Veterinary Diagnostic Laboratory Veterinary Diagnostic Laboratory 2450 Gilette Drive Fort Collins, CO 80526 (970) 491-1170 csu-cvmbs.colostate.edu/academics/mip/ci-lab
In situ hybridization for selected infectious agents	Tissue (formalin fixed paraffin embedded)	**Michigan State University** Veterinary Diagnostic Laboratory 4125 Beaumont Road Lansing, MI 48910-8104 (517) 353-1683 cvm.msu.edu/vdl/laboratory-sections/anatomic-surgical-pathology/in-situ-hybridization
Oomycete testing	Serum for serology; minimum 100 µL; contact laboratory	**Auburn University** Pythium Laboratory Department of Pathobiology 158 Greene Hall Auburn, AL 36849-5519 (334) 844-2694 bargepc@auburn.edu vetmed.auburn.edu/academic-departments/dept-of-pathobiology/diagnostic-services/
PARR/PCR for antigen receptor rearrangements (clonality testing for lymphoma)	EDTA whole blood, bone marrow, and tissue aspirates in EDTA or placed on slides, effusions, or CSF in EDTA or cytocentrifuged onto slides, noncoverslipped glass slides (stained or unstained)	**Colorado State University** Clinical Immunology/ Veterinary Diagnostic Laboratory 2450 Gilette Drive Fort Collins, CO 80526 (970) 491-1170 csu-cvmbs.colostate.edu/academics/mip/ci-lab/Pages/default.aspx **North Carolina State University** College of Veterinary Medicine K9/Feline Oncology Diagnostic Lab 1060 William Moore Drive Research Building, Room #330C Raleigh NC 27607 (919) 513-1925 cvmoncodiagnosticlab@ncsu.edu cvm.ncsu.edu/research/labs/clinical-sciences/k9feline-oncology-diagnostic/ **SYNLAB VPG Exeter (formerly TDDS)** Unit 1B, Exeter Science Park Babbage Way Clyst Honiton Exeter, EX5 2FN, United Kingdom 01392 247914 vpg.exeter@synlab.co.uk vet.synlab.co.uk/

TABLE A7.1 Tests, Submission Materials, and Selected Laboratories Available for Specimen Submission—cont'd

TEST	SUBMISSION MATERIALS	LABORATORY
PCR (infectious agents)	Contact each laboratory	**University of Guelph** Animal Health Laboratory Laboratory Services Division Box 3612 Guelph, Ontario, Canada N1H 6R8 ahlmolec@uoguelph.ca uoguelph.ca/ahl/ahl-laboratory-sections **North Carolina University** Vector Borne Disease Diagnostic Lab Room 462A 1060 William Moore Drive Raleigh, NC 27607 (919) 513-8279 ncstatevectorborne@ncsu.edu cvm.ncsu.edu/research/labs/clinical-sciences/vector-borne-disease/ **SYNLAB VPG Exeter (formerly TDDS)** Unit 1B, Exeter Science Park Babbage Way Clyst Honiton Exeter, EX5 2FN, United Kingdom 01392 247914 vpg.exeter@synlab.co.uk vet.synlab.co.uk/
Urine BRAF mutation detection assay for urothelial carcinoma (canine, feline)	Urine	**Sentinel Biomedical/Antech Diagnostics** antechdiagnostics.com/laboratory-diagnostics/molecular-diagnostics/cadet-braf-plus

BAL, Bronchoalveolar fluid; *CSF*, cerebrospinal fluid; *EDTA*, ethylenediaminetetraacetic acid; *EIA*, enzyme immunoassay; *ICC*, immunocytochemistry; *IHC*, immunohistochemistry; *PARR*, polymerase chain reaction for antigen receptor rearrangement; *PCR*, polymerase chain reaction.

8 APPENDIX

Quick Reference for Morphologic Features of Microorganisms

Katie M. Boes

OVERVIEW

Microorganisms are identified based on a combination of the clinical history, lesion location, and the agent's cytologic characteristics. Size is particularly helpful in initial categorization as a bacterium, fungus or fungus-like organism, protozoan, or multicellular parasite (Fig. A8.1).

Viruses

Viral inclusions are often round, homogenous, and intranuclear or intracytoplasmic (Fig. A8.2). Distemper viral inclusions are more easily observed using aqueous Romanowsky stains.

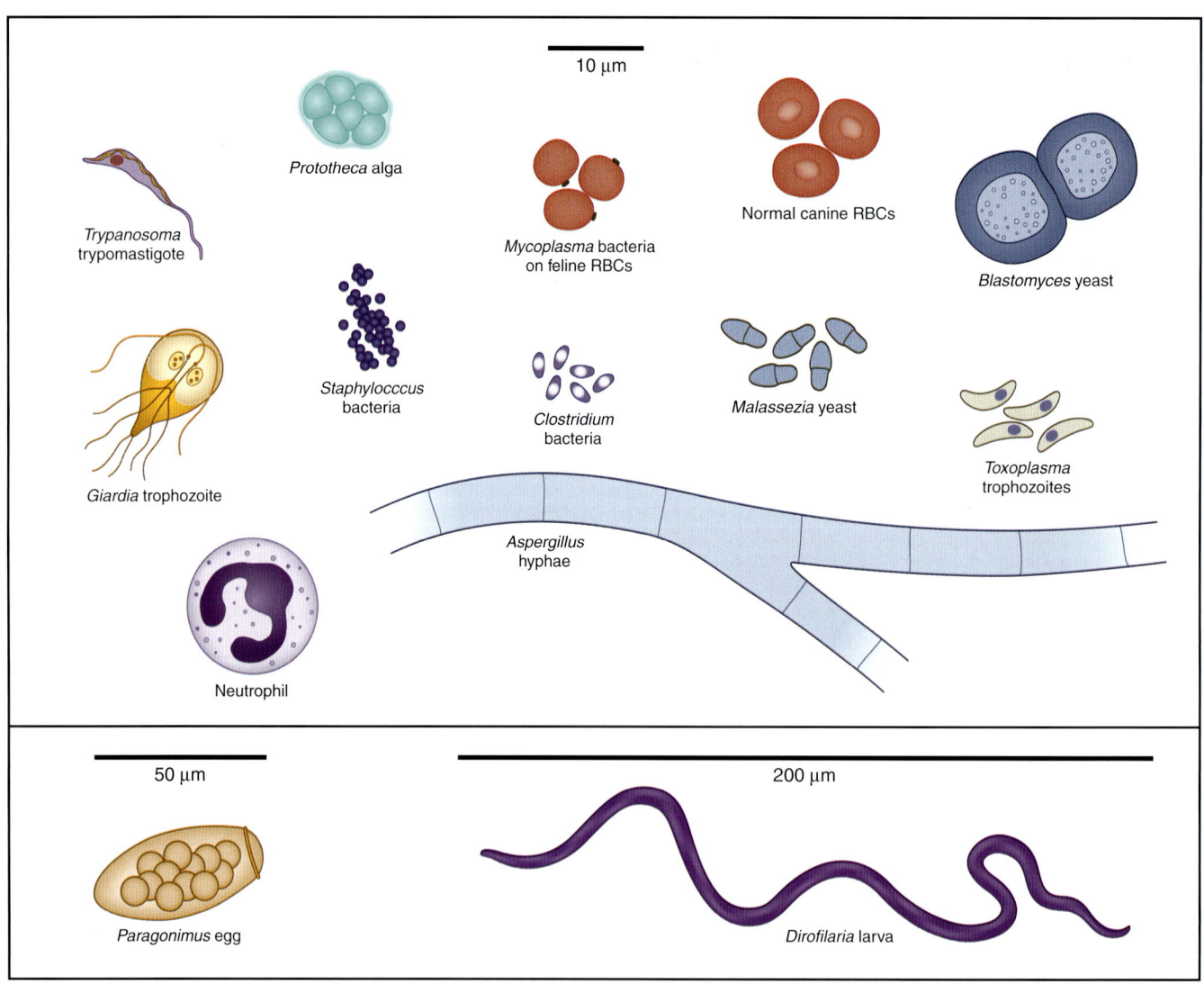

FIGURE A8.1 Relative sizes of microorganisms. *RBC,* Red blood cell.

APPENDIX 8 *Quick Reference for Morphologic Features of Microorganisms*

Viruses

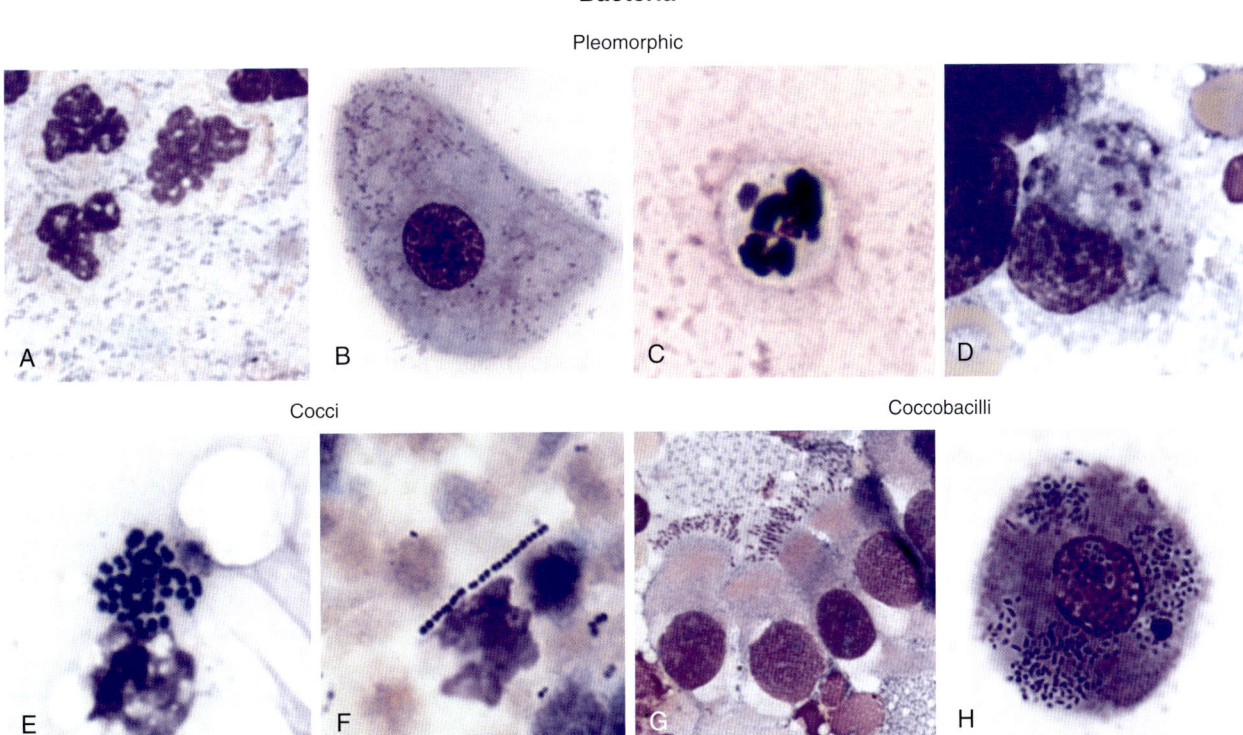

■ **FIGURE A8.2 Cytology of viruses. Canine distemper virus inclusions.** Intracytoplasmic viral inclusions are in hematopoietic cells and epithelial cells. **A,** Lymphocyte. **B,** Neutrophil. **C,** Urothelial cell. (A and C, Aqueous Romanowsky; B, Wright-Giemsa; HP oil.) **D, Canine adenovirus-1 inclusions.** A poorly preserved, binucleated hepatocyte contains one intranuclear viral inclusion in each nucleus. (Modified Wright, HP oil.) (C, Courtesy Thomas Cecere, Virginia Tech.)

Bacteria

Common features of bacteria are their relatively small size compared with most other infectious agents and their lack of a nucleus and unapparent or thin cell wall (Fig. A8.3). Some bacteria, such as *Mycoplasma* spp., *Ureaplasma* spp., *Bordetella bronchiseptica*, and *Simonsiella* spp., live on the surface of epithelial cells, but most bacteria are seen phagocytized by neutrophils. Some bacteria, such as *Neorickettsia helminthoeca*, *Rhodococcus equi*, and *Mycobacterium* spp., preferentially live within macrophages.

Algae, Fungi, and Oomycetes

Common features of algae, fungi, and oomycetes are the presence of a nucleus and a cell wall, which is a 1 μm thick,

Bacteria

■ **FIGURE A8.3 Cytology of bacteria. A,** *Mycoplasma* **spp. Canine infectious respiratory disease.** Numerous small *Mycoplasma* spp. appear within the background mucus of bronchoalveolar lavage fluid. (Wright-Giemsa; HP oil.) **B,** *Ureaplasma* **spp.** Small bacteria colonize the surface of a canine urothelial cell from prostatic wash fluid. (Wright-Giemsa; HP oil.) **C,** *Ehrlichia ewingii.* **Canine granulocytic ehrlichiosis.** Synovial fluid shows neutrophilic inflammation and an *E. ewingii* morula in the upper left cytoplasm of a neutrophil. (Wright-Giemsa; HP oil.) **D,** *Neorickettsia helminthoeca.* **Salmon poisoning disease.** A macrophage contains cytoplasmic *N. helminthoeca* morulae inclusions. (Wright-Giemsa; HP oil.) **E,** *Staphylococcus* **spp.** There is a grapelike cluster of cocci from a pyoderma. (Wright-Giemsa; HP oil.) **F,** *Streptococcus* **spp.** Lymphadenitis with chains of cocci are admixed with necrotic cells. (Wright-Giemsa; HP oil.) **G,** *Bordetella bronchiseptica.* **Canine infectious tracheobronchitis (kennel cough).** Bacteria colonize the cilia of four respiratory epithelial cells in transtracheal wash fluid. (Wright-Giemsa; HP oil.) **H,** *Rhodococcus equi.* **Rhodococcal pleuropneumonia.** Pleural fluid from a dyspneic cat shows intrahistiocytic coccobacilli. (Wright-Giemsa; HP oil.)

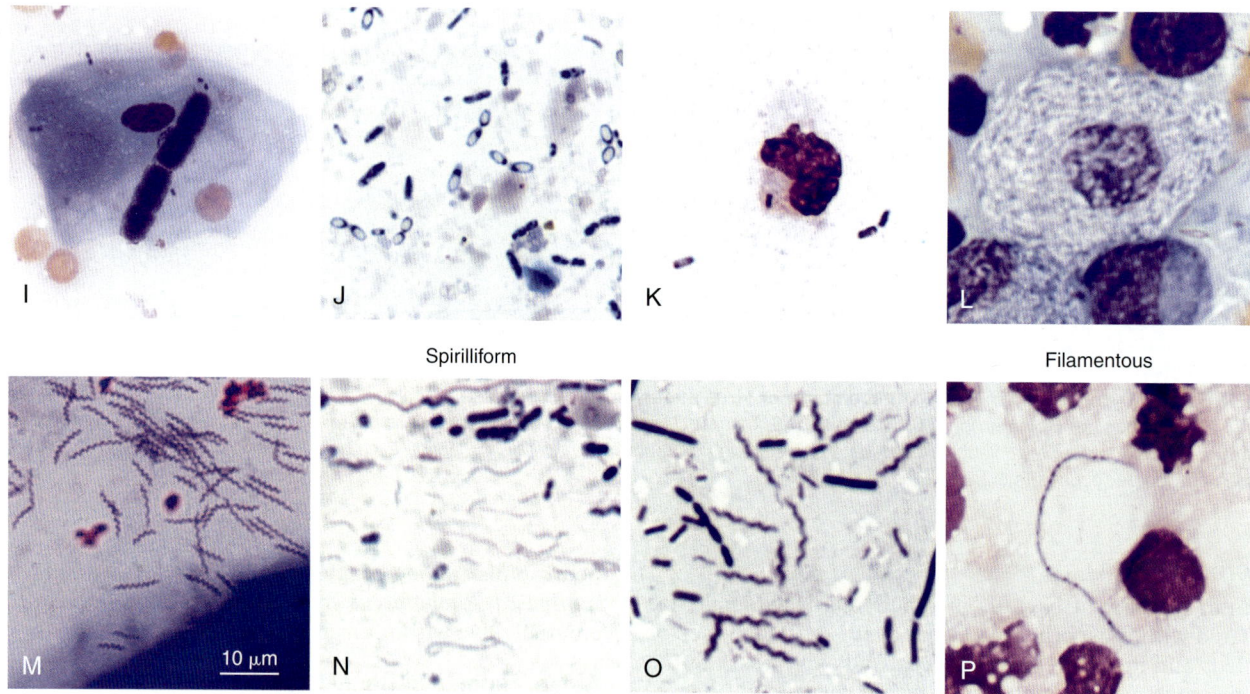

■ **FIGURE A8.3, cont'd** **I**, *Conchiformibius* (basionym: *Simonsiella*) **spp. Oral flora.** A squamous epithelial cell is colonized by longitudinally dividing bacilli. (Wright-Giemsa; HP oil.) **J,** *Clostridium perfringens.* **Clostridial enterotoxicosis.** A fecal smear shows many spore-forming bacilli in a dog with diarrhea. (Wright-Giemsa; HP oil.) **K,** *Escherichia coli.* **Colibacillosis.** *E. coli* bacilli in a peritoneal exudate from a septicemic dog. (Wright-Giemsa; HP oil.) **L,** *Mycobacterium avium.* **Systemic mycobacteriosis.** A splenic aspirate from a dog shows nonstaining, intrahistiocytic *M. avium* bacilli. (Wright-Giemsa; HP oil.) **M,** *Helicobacter*-**like bacteria.** A touch imprint shows spirochetes from the stomach. (Wright; HP oil.) **N,** *Campylobacter* **spp.** Small, thin, curved bacteria in a fecal smear from a dog with diarrhea. (Wright-Giemsa; HP oil.) **O,** *Treponema*-**like bacteria.** Large, thick, spiral-shaped bacteria are in a fecal smear from a dog with diarrhea. Smaller *Campylobacter* spp. bacteria are also present. (Wright-Giemsa; HP oil.) **P, Actinomycete. Pyothorax.** A long, thin, beaded filamentous bacterium is shown. (Wright-Giemsa; HP oil.) (D, Courtesy Austin Viall et al., Oregon State University. Presented at the 2012 ASVCP case review session.)

nonstaining, refractive structure surrounding the cell membrane (Fig. A8.4). These organisms are identified based on their structures of growth (e.g., yeast, hyphae) and reproduction (e.g., budding, fruiting bodies).

Protozoa

Protozoa are unicellular parasites with a wide size range (Fig. A8.5). Kinetoplastids have a characteristic, large mitochondrion, termed a *kinetoplast*. In their mammalian hosts, *Leishmania* spp. and *Trypanosoma* spp. have nonflagellated stages, termed *amastigotes*. Flagellated blood stages, termed *trypomastigotes*, may also be seen in trypanosomiasis. Depending on the agent, multiple life stages may be present in infections with metamonads and amoebas (trophozoites and cysts) or apicomplexans (tachyzoites, schizonts containing merozoites, cysts containing bradyzoites, and gamonts).

Multicellular Parasites: Helminths

This group includes tissue stages of trematodes, cestodes, and nematodes (Fig. A8.6). Ova may have one operculum (*Paragonimus* spp.) or two opercula (*Eucoleus* spp., *Pearsonema* spp.) or contain morulae or larvae (*Aelurostrongylus* spp.). Cestode larvae contain calcareous corpuscles. Nematode larvae are identified by their size and head and tail morphology.

APPENDIX 8 *Quick Reference for Morphologic Features of Microorganisms*

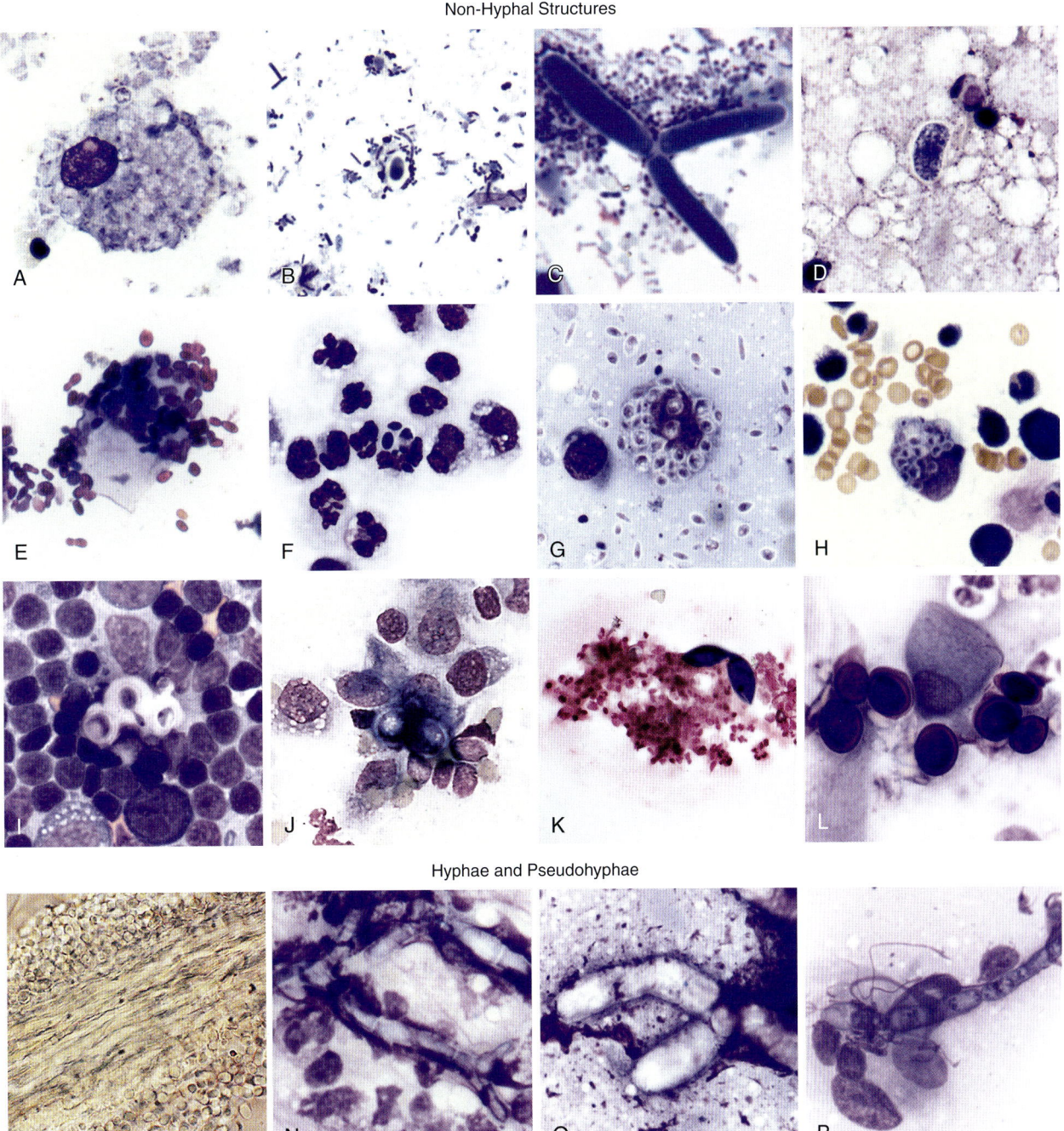

■ **FIGURE A8.4** Cytology of fungi and fungal-like organisms. **A,** *Pneumocystis* **spp.** Bronchoalveolar fluid from a dog contains intrahistiocytic and extracellular trophozoites and cysts. (Wright-Giemsa; HP oil.) **B–C, Intestinal yeast flora. B,** An incidental yeast is in a fecal smear from a dog. (Wright-Giemsa; HP oil.) **C,** *Cyniclomyces guttulatus*. Budding yeast in a fecal smear from a dog. (Wright-Giemsa; HP oil.) **D,** *Prototheca* **spp.** *Prototheca* spp. algae is in a fecal smear from a dog. (Wright-Giemsa; HP oil.) **E,** *Malassezia pachydermatis*. This overgrowth is from a broad-based budding yeast that colonized the surface of a squamous epithelial cell. (Wright-Giemsa; HP oil.) **F,** *Candida* **spp.** Narrow-based buddying yeast are phagocytized by a leukocyte in peritoneal fluid from a dog. (Wright; HP oil.) **G,** *Sporothrix schenckii*. Sporotrichosis. Oval to elongate *Sporothrix* yeast are within a macrophage and the background. (Wright-Giemsa; HP oil.) **H,** *Histoplasma capsulatum*. Intrahistiocytic, oval yeasts are in a bone marrow aspirate from a cat with pancytopenia. (Wright-Giemsa; HP oil.) **I,** *Cryptococcus* **spp.** A lymph node aspirate shows narrow-based budding yeast surrounded by a thick, nonstaining capsule. (Wright-Giemsa; HP oil.) **J,** *Blastomyces dermatitidis*. This deeply basophilic yeast displays broad-based buddying. (Wright-Giemsa; HP oil.) **K,** *Coccidioides immitis*. A ruptured spherule releases many endospores. (Aqueous Romanowsky; HP oil.) **L,** *Rhinosporidium seeberi*. Sporangia from this aquatic protistan parasite surround a nonciliated, columnar, respiratory epithelial cell. (Wright; HP oil.) **M, Dermatophytes.** A keratin-cleared hair pluck shows central hyphae surrounded by arthrospores. (Unstained; HP oil.) **N,** *Aspergillus* **spp.** Hyphae show parallel cell walls, regular septation, and dichotomous branching from a nasal specimen. (Wright-Giemsa; HP oil.) **O, Oomycete.** Hyphae of *Pythium* spp. and *Lagenidium* spp. are nonstaining and poorly septate with rounded ends. (Wright-Giemsa; HP oil.) **P, Pigmented fungi. Phaeohyphomycosis.** A poorly pigmented fungus shows a transition from a pseudohyphae with budlike indentations to a true hypha without indentations. (Wright-Giemsa; HP oil.) (A, Courtesy Catherine Shoemake and Angela Royal, University of Missouri. Presented at the 2018 ASVCP case review session. L, Courtesy Sara Hill et al., University of Minnesota. Presented at the 2008 ASVCP case review session.)

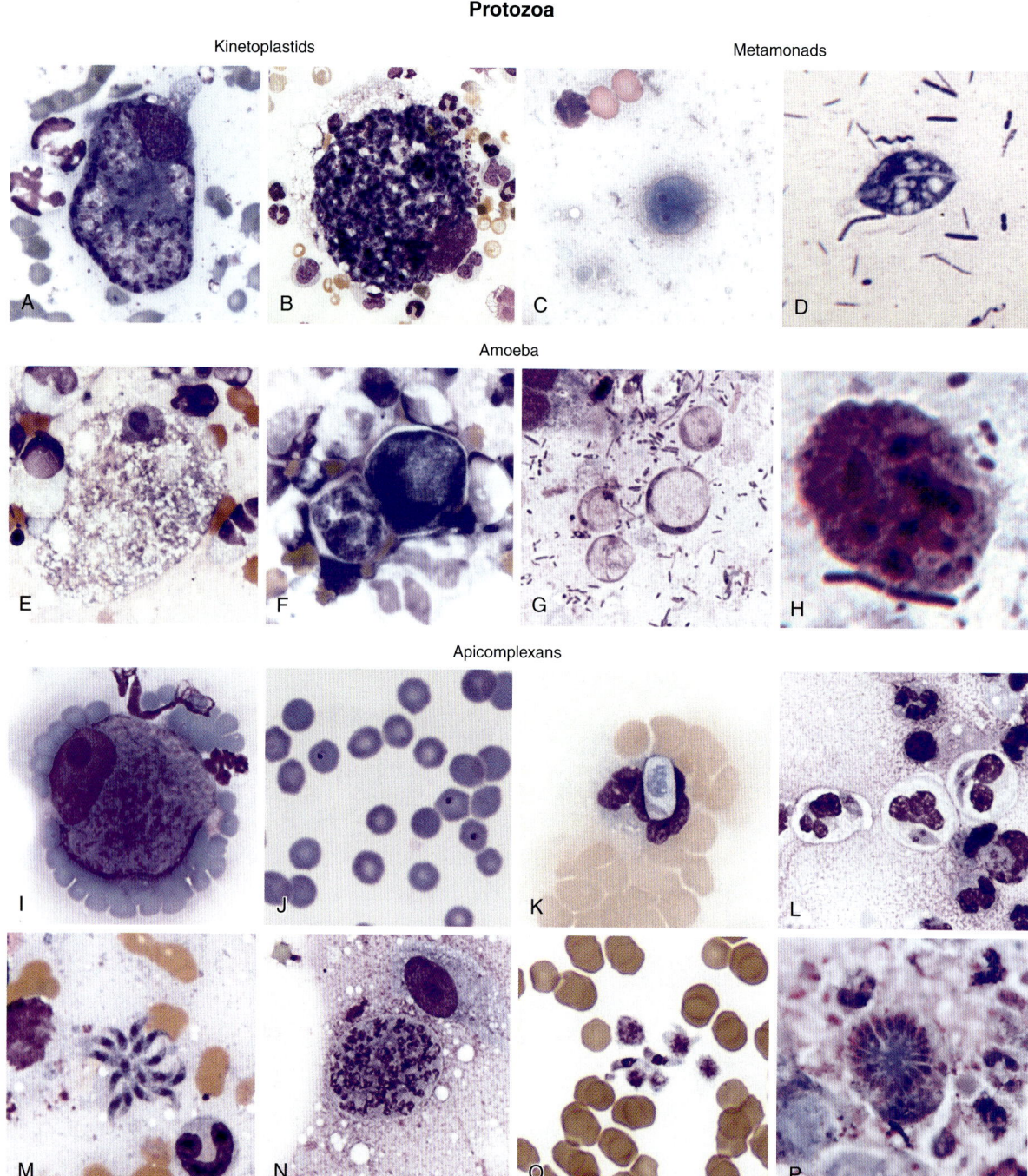

■ **FIGURE A8.5 Cytology of protozoa. A,** *Leishmania* **spp. Cutaneous leishmaniasis.** A macrophage contains many amastigotes characterized by an elongate kinetoplast perpendicular to the protozoan nucleus. (Wright-Giemsa; HP oil.) **B,** *Trypanosoma cruzi.* **Chagas disease.** (Wright; HP oil.) A macrophage contains many amastigotes similar to those of *Leishmania* spp. (Wright-Giemsa; HP oil.) **C,** *Giardia* **spp.** A trophozoite is pear shaped with two nuclei, a central axostyle, and flagella. (Modified Wright; HP oil.) **D,** *Tritrichomonas* **spp.** The trophozoite is football-shaped with one nucleus, a central axostyle, flagella, and an undulating membrane. (Wright-Giemsa; HP oil.) **E–F,** *Acanthamoeba* **spp. E, Trophozoite.** The trophozoite has abundant foamy cytoplasm, a round nucleus, and prominent nucleolus. (Modified Wright; HP oil.) **F, Cyst.** Two cysts have granular, basophilic cytoplasm, a round nucleus (more apparent in the left cyst), and nonstaining, undulating walls. (Modified Wright; HP oil.) **G,** *Blastocystis* **spp.** cysts have one to multiple peripheral nuclei. (Aqueous Romanowsky; HP oil.) **H,** *Entamoeba histolytica.* A trophozoite is present in the feces of a dog with diarrhea. (Wright-Giemsa; HP oil.) **I–J,** *Cytauxzoon felis.* **I, Schizont.** A macrophage contains a merozoite-laden schizont, which peripherally displaces the macrophage nucleus. (Aqueous Romanowsky; HP oil.) **J, Trophozoites.** Erythrocytes contain signet-ring-shaped piroplasms. (Aqueous Romanowsky; HP oil.) **K,** *Hepatozoon canis.* A neutrophil contains a clear oblong gamont. (Wright-Giemsa; HP oil.) **L,** *Neospora caninum.* The neutrophils contain banana-shaped trophozoites. (Wright-Giemsa; HP oil.) **M–N,** *Toxoplasma gondii.* **M,** Trophozoites are presumably released from a ruptured schizont. (Wright-Giemsa; HP oil.) **N,** Cyst contains many bradyzoites. (Wright-Giemsa; HP oil.) **O–P,** *Sarcocystis* **spp. O, Trophozoites.** Two banana-shaped trophozoites are surrounded by six platelets. (Wright-Giemsa; HP oil.) **P, Schizont.** Schizont shows radially arranged merozoites. (Wright; HP oil.) (G, Courtesy Craig Thompson, Purdue University. H, Courtesy Rick Alleman, University of Florida. L, Courtesy Tara Holmberg et al., University of California, Davis. O, Courtesy Nina Zitzer et al., The Ohio State University. P, Courtesy Charlotte Hollinger et al., Michigan State University.)

Helminths

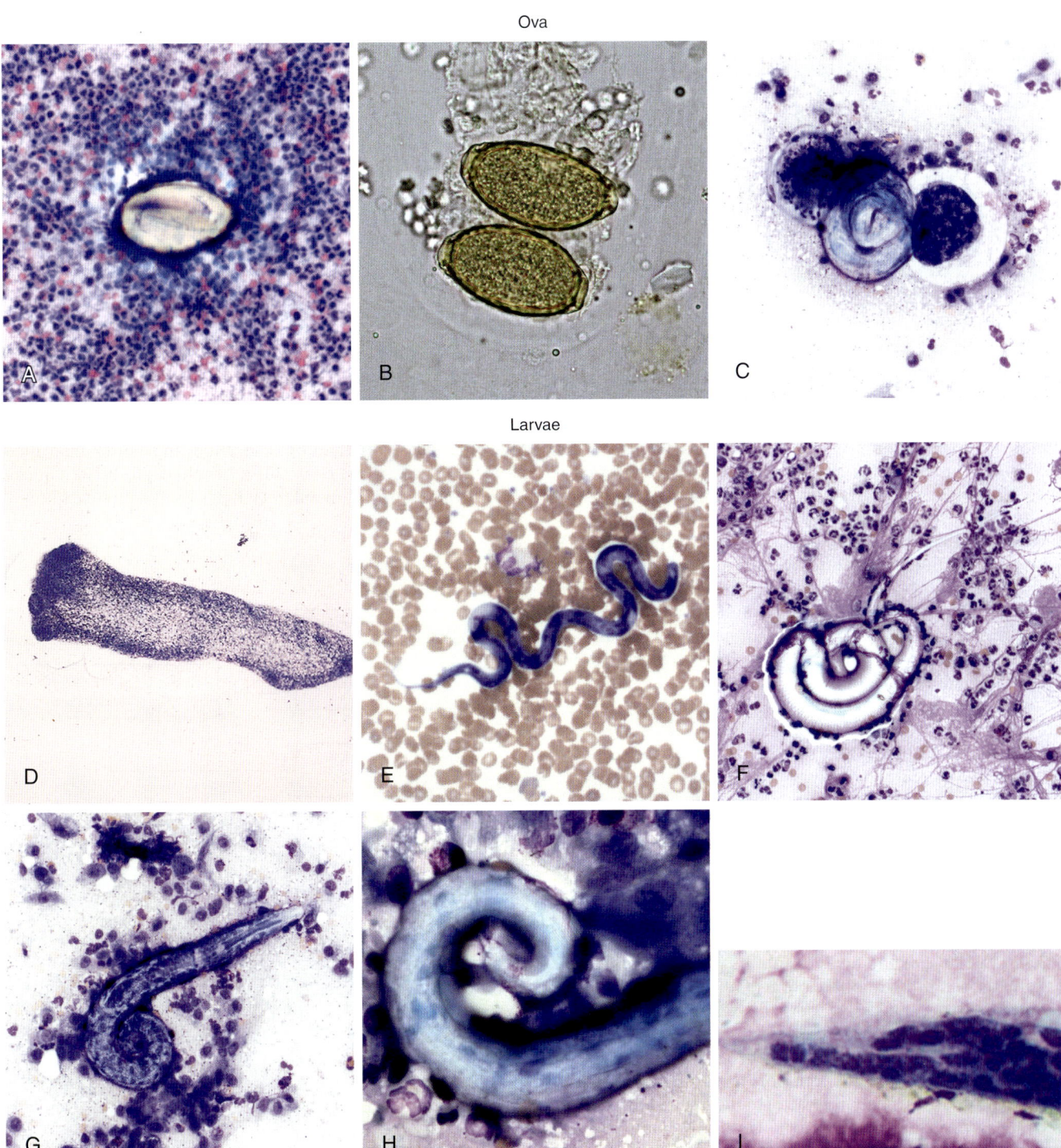

■ **FIGURE A8.6 Cytology of helminths. A**, *Paragonimus kellicotti*. **Ovum**. Eggs of this and other flukes are yellow-brown with a single operculum. (Wright-Giemsa, IP.) **B**, *Pearsonema plica* (basionym *Capillaria plica*). **Ova**. Two eggs are asymmetrically bioperculated in a urine wet mount from a dog. Eggs of other capillarid nematodes, such as *Eucoleus* spp., appear similar. (Wright-Giemsa, HP oil.) **C**, *Aelurostrongylus abstrusus*. **Ova**. There are three nematode eggs in various stages of development, progressing from left (early morula) to right (late morula) to middle (larvated). Larvated eggs hatch into larvae (see part G). (Wright-Giemsa, HP oil.) **D**, *Mesocestoides* spp. **Larva**. Cytologic sampling and processing often ruptures the larvae, resulting in fragments of loose parenchymatous matrix with interspersed calcareous corpuscles. (Aqueous Romanowsky, LP.) **E**, *Dirofilaria immitis*. **Heartworm disease. Microfilaria**. Hemodilute solid tissue aspirates from dogs with heartworm disease may contain larvae. (Wright-Giemsa, HP oil.) **F**, *Dracunculus insignis*. **Larva**. Larvae have long tapered tails and may be sampled from skin lesions, which also contain the adult, female nematode. (Modified Wright, IP.) **G–H**, *Aelurostrongylus abstrusus*. **G, Larva**. Larvae of respiratory helminths are often curled, obscuring tail morphology. (Wright-Giemsa, IP.) **H, Larva tail**. Note the kinked tail morphology. (Wright-Giemsa, HP oil.) **I**, *Crenosoma vulpis* **larva tail**. The tail is smooth and tapered. (Wright-Giemsa, HP oil.) (A, Courtesy Linda Berent et al., University of Illinois. D, Courtesy Jocelyn Johnsrude, IDEXX. F, Courtesy Helen Michael and Leslie Sharkey, University of Minnesota.)

9 APPENDIX

Quality Management Recommendations for Veterinary Diagnostic Cytopathology Services

Bente Flatland

This appendix summarizes recommendations from published human (Chandra et al., 2009; Kocjan et al., 2009; Path2Quality, 2013; Clinical and Laboratory Standards Institute [CLSI], 2014; Nakhleh et al., 2016) and American Society for Veterinary Clinical Pathology (Gunn-Christie et al., 2012; Arnold et al., 2019) guidelines regarding quality assurance for diagnostic cytopathology and makes additional suggestions tailored to veterinary diagnostic laboratories. In this appendix, *sample* denotes material submitted to the laboratory for testing. *Specimen* denotes the portion of submitted sample undergoing examination. Sample and specimen may be the same (e.g., tissue aspirate biopsy smear) or different (e.g., buffy coat smear made from submitted whole blood). Fluid samples, in particular, may yield more than one specimen type (e.g., direct smear, cytocentrifuged preparation, cell block).

Laboratories should consider the cytopathology service's path of workflow and implement policies, standard operating procedures (SOPs), and quality monitoring for processes at each workflow step. A generic workflow path is given in Figure A9.1, and additional examples are published (Path2Quality, 2013; CLSI, 2014). Laboratory work areas should be uncluttered and free of unnecessary distractions that could adversely impact personnel concentration and lead to errors. Written policies and SOPs should govern the various cytopathology service components and should be easily accessible and familiar to all relevant laboratory personnel (including residents in training) (Arnold et al., 2019). Policies and SOPs should be identified by date or version number, with prompt removal of old versions when new versions are issued. Suggested topics for veterinary cytopathology service policies and SOPs are given in Tables A9.1 and A9.2.

In the veterinary setting, involvement of laboratory personnel in sample acquisition and transport to the laboratory is not typical, and most preanalytical factors affecting cytopathology specimens are outside the laboratory's control. Laboratories can facilitate submission of good-quality specimens by providing specimen preparation and handling instructions for use by laboratory clients and by having clearly stated policies governing sample rejection. On laboratory websites, frequently asked questions (FAQs) can be used to address common preanalytical errors, and laboratory "fact sheets" can be used to help clients better understand test indications and limitations. If issued separately from a catalogue of laboratory tests and services, instructions and fact sheets should be clearly identified by a version number and date, with prompt removal of old versions when new versions are issued. Additionally, laboratory submission forms should be designed to capture information that minimizes error (e.g., require two unique patient identifiers and sample acquisition date) and facilitates the pathologist's diagnostic interpretation (e.g., require patient demographic information, sample anatomic location, and a brief clinical history) (Gunn-Christie et al., 2012; Arnold et al., 2019). On electronic forms, use of mandatory fields can facilitate capture of key information.

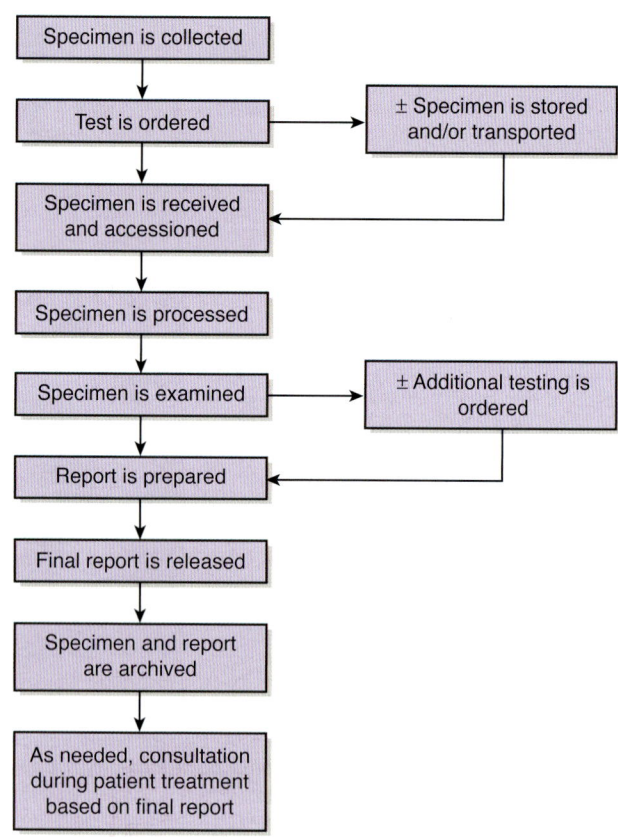

■ **FIGURE A9.1** Workflow path. Example cytopathology service workflow path, adapted from Clinical and Laboratory Standards Institute (CLSI) guideline GP23 (CLSI, 2014). Workflow mapping facilitates quality management by dividing cytopathology processes into component parts for which policies and standard operating procedures can be developed separately.

TABLE A9.1 List of Suggested Content for Veterinary Cytopathology Service Policies and Procedures

TESTING PHASE	SUGGESTED TOPICS
Preanalytical	• Sample handling and transport, including biosafety requirements and considerations for potentially hazardous samples (e.g., risk of zoonotic infection) • Test ordering process (TATs, priority designations,[a] required patient information, required specimen information) • Criteria for acceptable and unacceptable samples • Sample accessioning process • Specimen preparation (e.g., smear types, concentration, drying and fixation) • Labeling process, including for routine vs. potentially hazardous samples or specimens • Staining process, including routine staining and any special stains offered by the laboratory

Analytical	• Total nucleated cell counting (indications, methods)
	• Total protein measurement (indications, methods)
	• Pathologist's workflow (how and where are specimens conveyed to pathologist, how priority designations[a] are communicated to pathologist)
	• Reporting, including policies for:
	  • Paper vs. electronic reports
	  • Preliminary, finalized, addendum, and revised reports and how they are communicated to laboratory clients
	  • Contacting submitting clinicians regarding priority submissions
	  • Handling of reports for routine diagnostic specimens vs. research specimens (if applicable)
	  • Verification of report release
	• Specialized and follow-up tests, if offered by the laboratory (e.g., cell blocks, flow cytometry, PARR testing)

Postanalytical	• Archiving (physical specimens, reports), including criteria for routine diagnostic samples or reports vs. research (if applicable)[b] • Policy in the event of nondiagnostic samples • Handling of consultations and second opinion requests • Second reviews of diagnoses made (type of reviews, procedures) • Accounting and billing procedures, and verification of correct billing

[a]*Priority designations* refer to samples requiring faster processing than typical turnaround time (TAT), e.g., "STAT" samples or other urgent priorities, as defined by the laboratory.
[b]Applicable laws and regulations concerning archiving of veterinary laboratory samples should be followed. If none exist regarding laboratory samples specifically, a suggestion is to follow applicable laws and regulations concerning archiving of veterinary medical records.
PARR, Polymerase chain reaction for antigen gene receptor rearrangements.

TABLE A9.2 Suggested Standard Operating Procedures (SOPs) for Diagnostic Cytopathology Services

TOPIC AREA	SOP FOR PREPARATION AND ANALYSIS OF
General	Tissue aspirates Potentially biohazardous or zoonotic samples
Fluid samples	Cavity effusions Cerebrospinal fluid Respiratory lavages (BAL, TW) Synovial fluid
Other (as applicable)	Buffy coat Cell block Cytochemical stains (one SOP per stain type) Immunocytochemical stains (one SOP per stain type) Flow cytometry Protein electrophoresis

BAL, Bronchoalveolar lavage; *TW*, tracheal wash.

In human medicine, use of "rapid onsite evaluation" (ROSE) may be used to screen cytopathologic specimens at the time of sample acquisition, before laboratory submission. ROSE can be performed by pathologists or nonpathologists (e.g., specially trained medical technologists) (Kocjan et al., 2009). Systematic literature review and meta-analysis have shown that ROSE can improve adequacy of cytopathology specimens (defined as whether a sample provides sufficient material for diagnosis) in human medicine by 12% on average, although exact improvement varies by tissue type (Schmidt et al., 2013). In the author's experience, consistent or formalized ROSE is uncommon in veterinary medicine; screening of specimen adequacy, if performed, is typically done by the clinician(s) obtaining the cytopathologic sample. It seems likely that the proportion of inadequate and nondiagnostic specimens could be reduced by selective adoption of ROSE in veterinary cytopathology. Laboratories considering the incidence of nondiagnostic specimens to be unacceptably high should consider procedures and outreach to laboratory clients to improve specimen screening and quality at the time of sampling.

Cytologic samples are potential biohazards, and local biosafety rules and precautions should be followed during all phases of cytologic testing. Use of secondary containers (additionally containing absorbent material, as appropriate) during transport of primary sample containers to the laboratory is strongly recommended. Exposure to formalin and its fumes should be avoided during acquisition and handling of cytopathology samples because these may adversely affect sample quality (Gunn-Christie et al., 2012; Arnold et al., 2019).

For cytopathology of fluid samples, use of a worksheet to document sample preparation and ancillary measurements (e.g., total protein, hemocytometer counts, biochemical measurements) is recommended, particularly if multiple laboratory staff are involved in sample processing. An example worksheet is given in Figure A9.2. If total nucleated cell counts or biochemical quantities are measured, copies of instrument printouts should be appended to the relevant fluid processing worksheet and cytopathology submission form. Where applicable, hematology analyzer scattergrams and numeric data should be examined as part of the cytopathologic evaluation (Pinto da Cunha et al., 2009; Giordano et al., 2015). Also where applicable (e.g., hemorrhagic effusions, blood-contaminated specimens), correlation of cytopathologic data and concurrent hematologic data should be performed if it can facilitate cytopathologic interpretation.

Clinical Pathology Laboratory Fluid Cytology Sample Worksheet Version #   **Cytology Accession #**

Specimen type:
- ☐ BAL
- ☐ CSF
- ☐ Pericardial
- ☐ Peritoneal (abdominal)
- ☐ Pleural (thoracic)
- ☐ Synovial
- ☐ TTW
- ☐ Other (specify): _____

Fluid submitted in:
- ☐ EDTA
  - EDTA tube less than ½ full: ☐ No ☐ Yes
- ☐ Conical plastic tube
- ☐ Clot tube (plastic)
- ☐ Clot tube (glass)
- ☐ Other (specify): _____

 # Slides received:
_____ Unstained
_____ Previously stained

 # Slides prepared by laboratory:
_____ Direct smears
_____ Smears restained
_____ Cytospin preps
_____ Sediment smears
_____ Squash preps
_____ Imprints

Fluid color:
- ☐ Colorless
- ☐ Straw-colored
- ☐ Yellow
- ☐ Blood-tinged (light red)
- ☐ Grossly bloody (looks like blood)
- ☐ White, milky (lipemic, lactescent)
- ☐ Pink, milky (lipemic, lactescent)
- ☐ Red-brown
- ☐ Brown
- ☐ Tan
- ☐ Light green

Comments about fluid (if needed):

Fluid clarity:
- ☐ Clear
- ☐ Hazy
- ☐ Cloudy
- ☐ Opaque
- ☐ Flocculent material
- ☐ Clot in tube

Fluid Analysis (peritoneal, pleural, pericardial, synovial):

Total protein (g/dL, refractometry): _____
Performed using ☐ unaltered fluid ☐ supernatant
DO NOT PERFORM IF FLUID/SUPERNATANT LIPEMIC (MILKY).

TNCC ($\times 10^3/\mu L$): _____
DO NOT PERFORM IF FLUID CLOTTED.

RBC ($\times 10^6/\mu L$): _____
DO NOT PERFORM IF FLUID CLOTTED.

CSF Total protein (mg/dL, dye-binding): _____

CSF TNCC (#/μL): Average of both chambers _____
Chamber 1: _____ ; _____ × _____ = _____
           (squares) (#cells) (factor) (cells/uL)
Chamber 2: _____ ; _____ × _____ = _____
           (squares) (#cells) (factor) (cells/uL)

CSF RBC (#/μL): Average of both chambers _____
Chamber 1: _____ ; _____ × _____ = _____
           (squares) (#cells) (factor) (cells/uL)
Chamber 2: _____ ; _____ × _____ = _____
           (squares) (#cells) (factor) (cells/uL)

Chemistries (if applicable):

Sample	Bilirubin (mg/dL)	Creat (mg/dL)	K+ (mmol/L)	TG (mg/dL)	Other (specify)
FLUID					
PLASMA					

Technologist Initials:
_____

■ **FIGURE A9.2** Example fluid sample processing worksheet for veterinary cytopathology services. The purposes of this worksheet are to document and reduce errors during fluid specimen preparation, particularly when multiple personnel are involved. *BAL*, Broncheoalveolar fluid; *Creat*, creatinine; *CSF*, cerebrospinal fluid; *EDTA*, ethylenediaminetetraacetic acid; *RBC*, red blood cell; *TG*, triglycerides; *TTW*, tracheal wash.

Specimen descriptions should clearly support the morphologic diagnosis. Explanatory and interpretive comments should be clear and cite supporting scientific literature as needed. Suggestions for further testing should be made if applicable and appropriate. Although cytopathology reports should include descriptions of sample inadequacies and limitations (CLSI, 2014), language should be neutral and avoid accusatory, inflammatory, or judgmental statements that risk damaging the relationship between the submitting veterinarian and pet owner if an owner reviews the cytopathology report.

It has been shown that clinical pathologists use modifiers expressing disease probability and diagnostic certainty differently and that variable interpretation of the pathologist's diagnostic certainty by clinicians impacts patient management (Christopher and Hotz, 2004; Christopher et al., 2010). In one study, clinicians considered the interpretive comment the most important part of a cytopathology report (Christopher et al., 2008). Pathologists in a given laboratory should discuss and reach consensus regarding use of diagnostic probability modifiers in their reporting. Pathologists and laboratory staff should be available to clinicians to answer questions and provide consultation as needed (Christopher et al., 2008; Gunn-Christie et al., 2012).

Reducing errors is important for patient safety, and published quality guidelines in human medicine suggest use of "patient safety" checklists to accompany each cytopathology sample (Path2Quality, 2013; CLSI, 2014). Safety checklists could be included in the veterinary cytopathology workflow path and relevant SOPs. A proposed safety checklist, modified from the list provided in CLSI GP23-A2, is given in Figure A9.3. Known or suspected errors in sample preparation, diagnosis, and reporting should be investigated, and efficacy of corrective actions should be confirmed. Categorization and logging of errors over time is encouraged because data can be used for personnel training (e.g., to correct systematic errors in sample preparation or interpretation) and outreach to laboratory clients (e.g., to correct recurring pre-analytical errors). Suggested cytopathology service quality metrics are given in Box A9.1.

Equipment supporting cytopathologic services (e.g., hematology instruments, chemistry analyzers, automated stainers, cytocentrifuges) should be properly maintained with regular quality control. Validation procedures (e.g., of staining characteristics or automated data) should be performed to verify that instruments perform as intended using the cytology specimen types evaluated by the laboratory (Gunn-Christie et al., 2012).

Random error (imprecision) in routine diagnostic cytopathology is most relevant to total nucleated cell counting (TNCC) performed as part of fluid analysis. Automated TNCC of effusions is typically performed using hematology instruments, and TNCC of cerebrospinal fluid and respiratory lavage specimens may be performed using a manual counting chamber (e.g., Neubauer hemocytometer). Quality control of these methods is beyond the scope of this appendix and interested readers should consult other resources (Flatland and Vap, 2012; Vap et al., 2012; Nabity et al., 2018). Automated TNCC should be verified using slide review. Because cytopathologic specimens often include nonleukocytes that are not accurately enumerated by automated methods (e.g., mesothelial cells, activated macrophages, neoplastic cells), manual nucleated cell differential counting should be performed when relevant. Manual cell differential counting is imprecise, and enumeration of 500 cells is recommended if differential percentages are critical to the diagnostic interpretation (De Lorenzi et al., 2009; Path2Quality, 2013).

Both "second reviews" (periodic revisiting of selected cytopathologic diagnoses, specimen types, or portions of the caseload by pathologists within a single laboratory) and correlation of cytologic and corresponding histologic diagnoses can help assess accuracy of cytopathologic diagnoses. In human anatomic pathology, second reviews have been shown to lower diagnostic error rates (Nakhleh et al., 2016). Academic veterinary medical centers may engage in second reviews organically as part of rounds and review of cases used for teaching. Laboratories are encouraged to formalize periodic second reviews and to monitor the outcome over time to facilitate dialogue among pathologists within the laboratory and to identify areas for improvement (e.g., reaching consensus on discordant interpretations, standardization of terminology, standardization of expressions of diagnostic probability). When review of individual cases alters diagnostic interpretation, particularly in a way that has potential to impact patient management, revised cytopathology reports should be issued and clinicians notified in a timely manner. Formalized second reviews (and the outcome thereof) should be governed by written policies and procedures and viewed as learning opportunities (i.e., not punitive).

An important limitation of cytologic–histologic comparisons is sampling bias of the respective cytologic and histologic procedures. (Is the lesion homogenous, and did cytologic and histologic procedures sample the same area within the lesion?) Additional possible sources of disagreement include discordant interpretations by the cytopathologist and histopathologist and interobserver variability in interpretation or reporting of diagnostic certainty (Christopher and Hotz, 2004; Christopher et al., 2010; CLSI, 2014). For diagnosis of malignancy, a correlaion rate (CR) for cytologic-histologic comparisons can be calculated using the formula

$$CR(\%) = \frac{CHA}{CHA + CHD} \times 100$$

in which *CHA* refers to cytologic-histologic agreement (follow-up histopathology is positive for malignancy) and *CHD* refers to cytologic-histologic disagreement (follow-up histopathology is negative for malignancy) (CLSI, 2014). Monitoring cytologic-histologic disagreement rates per cytopathologist should only be undertaken using adequate data and rigorous statistical analysis, with the intent being education and improvement of skills (not punitive action) (CLSI, 2014). Similar to second reviews, academic veterinary medical centers may engage in cytologic-histologic comparisons organically as part of rounds and review of cases used for teaching. Laboratories are encouraged to maintain and periodically review an index of corresponding cytologic and histologic diagnoses, such that discordant cytologic and histologic diagnoses (per time period, per lesion type, or per caseload portion) are identified and leveraged to help improve cytopathology services.

Telepathology and digitization of cytologic images (whole-slide imaging [WSI]) are becoming increasingly common, and readers using WSI systems should consult relevant guidelines from human and veterinary medicine for comprehensive recommendations regarding equipment, implementation, and validation (Pantanowitz et al., 2013; García-Rojo, 2016; Bonsembiante et al., 2019). Considerations for digitization of cytopathology images include technical aspects (e.g., hardware and software specifications) and information technology aspects (e.g., image size and compression, file formats, network architecture) (García-Rojo, 2016; Bertram

#	Step	Status	Notification Outcome, Explanation, or Notes	Initials
Cytopathology Service Patient Safety Checklist Version #			**Cytology accession #**	
Pre-Analytical (Laboratory Staff)				
1	Sample type appropriate for test ordered	☐ Yes ☐ No ☐ If no, clinician notified	☐ New sample ☐ Order revised ☐ Order canceled	
2	Sample condition acceptable (e.g., appropriate container[s], label type)	☐ Yes ☐ No ☐ If no, clinician notified	☐ New sample ☐ Condition modified ☐ Sample rejected	
2	Sample patient information matches order and submission form	☐ Yes ☐ No ☐ If no, clinician notified	☐ Information corrected ☐ Sample rejected	
3	Submission form properly completed	☐ Yes ☐ No ☐ If no, clinician notified	☐ Missing information obtained ☐ Sample rejected	
4	Sample priority recorded and communicated to pathologist if urgent	☐ Routine ☐ STAT ☐ Other priority	If STAT or urgent, time of pathologist notification: _____ a.m. ☐ _____ p.m ☐	
Analytical (Pathologist)				
5	Number of slides or specimens matches submission form and/or fluids worksheet	☐ Yes ☐ No ☐ If no, lab staff notified	☐ Error investigated, corrected ☐ Sample rejected	
6	Slide/specimen label matches submission form (check both patient identification and laboratory accession number)	☐ Yes ☐ No ☐ If no, lab staff notified	☐ Error investigated, corrected ☐ Sample rejected	
7	Specimen limitations documented in the report	☐ Yes ☐ No	If no, explanation:	
8	If electronic reporting, release of finalized report is verified	☐ Yes ☐ No		
Post-Analytical (Laboratory Staff ± Pathologist)				
9	Specimen archived	☐ Yes ☐ No	If no, explanation:	
10	Accession paperwork (submission form, worksheets, instrument printouts, report copy) archived	☐ Yes ☐ No	If no, explanation:	
11	Additional testing ordered	☐ Special stain(s) ☐ ICC ☐ Flow cytometry ☐ PARR ☐ Cell block ☐ Other (specify)	Specify special stain(s) or other:	
12	Release of additional test result(s) is verified (if applicable)	☐ Yes ☐ No ☐ Not applicable	If no (and additional tests were ordered), explanation:	

FIGURE A9.3 Patient safety checklist. Proposed patient safety checklist for cytopathology services, adapted from Clinical and Laboratory Standards Institute (CLSI) guideline GP23 (CLSI, 2014). The purpose of this checklist is to help prevent errors during processing, examination, and reporting of cytopathology specimens. The checklist is intended to accompany the cytopathology submission form and to be used by both laboratory staff and the attending pathologist(s). *ICC*, Immunocytochemistry; *PARR*, polymerase chain reaction for antigen receptor rearrangement.

BOX A9.1 Suggested Quality Metrics for Veterinary Cytopathology Services[a]

- Turn-around times (routine, priority)
- Proportion of delayed cytopathology reports (vs. timeframe guaranteed by laboratory)
- Number test ordering errors per time period
- Number accessioning errors per time period
- Number labeling errors per time period
- Performance in EQA program testing events (e.g., vs. appropriate peer group)
- Regular "second reviews" of selected cytopathologic diagnoses, with documentation of results
- Proportion of inadequate specimens per sample type *or* proportion of nondiagnostic specimens per caseload
- Proportion of revised cytopathology reports
- Proportion of cytologic diagnoses with discordant histologic diagnoses
- Proportion of second opinion requests by laboratory clients

[a]The intent of using suggested metrics should be improvement of services and staff and pathologist skills, not punitive treatment of involved personnel.

EQA, External quality assessment program (a.k.a. proficiency testing program).

BOX A9.2 Recommendations for Whole Slide Imaging (WSI) System Validation[a]

- Validation study conditions should closely mimic real-world conditions under which equipment will be used.
- Validation should include all the components of the WSI system (slide scanner, computer hardware, computer software, viewing monitors, computer network).
- Revalidation should be carried out if any significant change is made to one or more components of the WSI system.
- A pathologist adequately trained to use the WSI system must be involved with the validation process.
- The validation process should include at least 60 specimens for each application of the system to be validated. The specimens used should reflect the spectrum and complexity of specimens and diagnoses likely to be encountered as part of the laboratory's routine caseload.
- The validation study should establish intraobserver variability for agreement of diagnoses made using digital vs. glass slides.
- Either random or nonrandom order can be used to evaluate digital vs. glass slides during the validation process.
- A wash-out period of at least 2 weeks should occur between evaluation of digital vs. glass slides during the validation process.
- The validation process should include verification that all material present on a glass slide to be scanned is also present in the resulting digital image.
- WSI validation procedures and personnel training should be documented.

[a]Validation should consider intended clinical use of the equipment, specimen type(s), and the setting in which equipment will be used. The goal of validation is to document that equipment will perform as needed for *each* intended diagnostic purpose.

Modified from Pantanowitz L, Sinard JH, Henricks WH, et al. Validating whole slide imaging for diagnostic purposes in pathology. Guideline from the College of American Pathologists Pathology and Laboratory Quality Center. *Arch Pathol Lab Med*. 2013;137:1710–1722.

and Klopfleisch, 2017). As for any laboratory equipment, validation of WSI systems is needed to ensure quality, and recommendations from the College of American Pathologists are given in Box A9.2. Cytopathology reports should include that a WSI system was used during the diagnostic evaluation.

REFERENCES

Arnold JE, Camus MS, Freeman KP, et al. ASVCP guidelines: principles of quality assurance and standards for veterinary clinical pathology (version 3.0). *Vet Clin Pathol*. 2019;48:542-618.

Bertram CA, Klopfleisch R. The pathologist 2.0: an update on digital pathology in veterinary medicine. *Vet Pathol*. 2017;54(5):756-766.

Bonsembiante F, Bonfanti U, Cian F, et al. Diagnostic validation of a whole-slide imaging scanner in cytological samples: diagnostic accuracy and comparison with light microscopy. *Vet Pathol*. 2019;56:429-434.

Chandra A, Cross P, Denton K, et al. The BSCC code of practice—exfoliative cytopathology (excluding gynaecological cytopathology). *Cytopathology*. 2009;20:211-223.

Christopher MM, Hotz CS. Cytologic diagnosis: expression of probability by clinical pathologists. *Vet Clin Pathol*. 2004;33(2):84-95.

Christopher MM, Hotz CS, Shelly SM, et al. Use of cytology as a diagnostic method in veterinary practice and assessment of communication between veterinary practitioners and veterinary clinical pathologists. *J Am Vet Med Assoc*. 2008;232(5):747-754.

Christopher MM, Hotz CS, Shelly SM, et al. Interpretation by clinicians of probability expressions in cytology reports and effect on clinical decision-making. *J Vet Intern Med*. 2010;24:496-503.

Clinical and Laboratory Standards Institute. *Non-gynecological cytology specimens: preexamination, examination, and postexamination processes; Approved guideline.* CLSI document GP23-A2. (2nd ed.). Wayne, PA: Clinical and Laboratory Standards Institute; 2014.

De Lorenzi D, Masserdotti C, Bertoncello D, et al. Differential cell counts in canine cytocentrifuged bronchoalveolar lavage fluid: a study on reliable enumeration of each cell type. *Vet Clin Pathol*. 2009;38(4):532-536.

Flatland B, Vap LM. Quality management recommendations for automated and manual in-house hematology of domestic animals. *Vet Clin North Am Small Anim Pract*. 2012;42(1):11-22.

García-Rojo M. International clinical guidelines for the adoption of digital pathology: a review of technical aspects. *Pathobiology*. 2016;83:99-109.

Giordano A, Stranieri A, Rossi G, et al. High diagnostic efficacy of the Sysmex XT2000iV delta total nucleated cells on effusions for feline infectious peritonitis. *Vet Clin Pathol*. 2015;44(2):295-302.

Gunn-Christie RG, Flatland B, Friedrichs KR, et al. ASVCP quality assurance guidelines: control of pre-analytical, analytical, and post-analytical factors for urinalysis, cytology, and clinical chemistry in veterinary laboratories. *Vet Clin Pathol*. 2012;41(1):18-26.

Kocjan G, Chandra A, Cross P, et al. BSCC code of practice—fine needle aspiration cytology. *Cytopathology*. 2009;20:283-296.

Nabity MB, Harr KE, Camus MS, et al. ASVCP guidelines: allowable total error hematology. *Vet Clin Pathol*. 2018;47(1):9-21.

Nakhleh RE, Nosé V, Colasacco C, et al. Interpretive diagnostic error reduction in surgical pathology and cytology. Guideline from the College of American Pathologists Pathology and Laboratory Quality Center and the Association of Directors of Anatomic and Surgical Pathology. *Arch Pathol Lab Med*. 2016;140:29-40.

Pantanowitz L, Sinard JH, Henricks WH, et al. Validating whole slide imaging for diagnostic purposes in pathology. Guideline from the College of American Pathologists Pathology and Laboratory Quality Center. *Arch Pathol Lab Med*. 2013;137:1710-1722.

Path2Quality. *Standards2Quality: guidelines for quality management in pathology professional practices: version 2*. Ontario, ON: Partnership of the OMA Section on Laboratory Medicine and the Ontario Association of Pathologists; 2013.

Pinto da Cunha N, Giordano A, Caniatti M, et al. Analytical validation of the Sysmex XT2000iV for cell counts in canine and feline effusions and concordance with cytologic diagnosis. *Vet Clin Pathol*. 2009;38(2):230-241.

Schmidt RL, Witt BL, Lopez-Calderon LE, et al. The influence of rapid on-site evaluation on the adequacy rate of fine-needle aspiration cytology. *Am J Clin Pathol*. 2013;139:300-308.

Vap LM, Harr KE, Arnold JE, et al. ASVCP quality assurance guidelines: control of pre-analytical and analytical factors for hematology for mammalian and non-mammalian species, hemostasis, and cross-matching in veterinary laboratories. *Vet Clin Pathol*. 2012;41(1):8-17.

INDEX

Entries with a *b* indicate box, *f* indicate figure, and *t* indicate table.

A

Abdominal fluid, collection of, 242
Abscess
  bacterial, 45–46, 45f
  pancreatic, 329–330, 330f
Acanthamoeba spp. infection, 224, 225f
Acantholytic cells, in pemphigus foliaceus, 42, 42f, 43f
Acanthoma, infundibular keratinizing, 73b, 75f
Acetone, as fixative, 623
Achromat, 665
Acid-alcohol, 672
Acinar cells, 322
Acinar pattern, 29, 30f
Acral lick dermatitis, 35, 35b, 38f
Actinomycosis, 46–47, 46f, 47b, 47f
Actinomycotic pyoabdomen, 254
Actinomycotic pyothorax, 264–266, 265f
Acute pancreatitis, 327–329, 328f, 329b
Adenocarcinoma, 8f, 596
  adrenocortical, 612f
  anal sac, 78–79, 79b, 79f
  apocrine gland anal sac, 78–79, 82b
  ciliary body, 574f
  endometrial, 461
  intestinal, 315f
  mammary, canine, 446
  nasal, 193–194, 195f
  neoplastic effusion from, 273–274, 273f, 274f, 275f
  pancreatic, 331f, 332f, 333f
  papillary, ovarian, 455, 455f
  prostatic, 473–474
  salivary gland, 299f, 300f, 581f
  thyroid gland, 600f, 602
Adenoma, 596
  adrenocortical, 611f
  apocrine duct, 80f, 81f, 82f
  hepatic, 354–355
  mammary, 446f
  pancreatic, 331
  parathyroid, 605
  perianal gland, 76–78, 77f, 78b, 78f, 79f
  renal, 403–404, 403f, 404f
  sebaceous, 73–74, 74b, 75f, 77f
  thyroid, 596–597, 603–604, 603f
  of zona fasciculata, 613
  of zona reticularis, 613
Adipocytes
  in lipoma, 92f
  mesenteric, 347f
Adrenal cortex, 597t, 607
Adrenal gland, 607–613, 607t, 608t
Adrenal medulla, tumors of, 597t, 607t, 608–610, 608t
Adrenocortical adenomas, 611f
Adrenocortical atrophy, 610
Adrenocortical disease, nonneoplastic, 610–611
Adrenocortical tumors, 611–613, 611f, 612f, 613f
Advanced collection and preparation techniques, 689

Advanced diagnostic techniques, 618–664
  for detection of translocations, chromosomal aberrations, and gene mutations, 659–660, 660f
  electron microscopy, 635–639
  flow cytometry, 642–655, 650t, 651f
  immunodiagnosis, 618–635
    immunocytochemistry, 624–625
  PCR for antigen receptor rearrangements, 655–656, 656f, 657f
  special histochemical stains, 639–642, 647f
AEC. *see* 3-Amino-9-ethyl carbazole
Aelurostrongylus abstrusus infection, 224, 225f
Air-drying, 623
Albumin
  as blocking agent, 637–638
  in cerebrospinal fluid, 516–517
Albuminocytologic dissociation, 523
Algae, 701–702, 703f
Algal infection, nasal, 191, 222
Alkaline phosphatase (ALP), 624, 672, 672f
  in liver disease, 354–355
Allergic rhinitis, 186, 187f
ALP. *see* Alkaline phosphatase
Alternaria spp. infection, nasal, 191
Amastigotes, 702
  in leishmaniasis, 57–59, 59f
Amebiasis, infectious causes of, 224
Amelanotic melanoma, 23–25, 27f
3-Amino-9-ethyl carbazole (AEC), 624
Ammonium biurate crystals, 433f
Amylase, in body cavity fluids, 283t
Amyloid, in plasmacytoma, 111f
Amyloidosis, hepatic, 353–354, 354f
Anal sac adenocarcinoma, 78–79, 79b, 79f
Anaplastic carcinoma
  of lung, 232f
  of mammary gland, 447–448
  nasal, 193–194, 195f
Anaplastic sarcoma with giant cells, 91–92, 91f, 92b
Anaplastic tumor, immunochemical diagnosis of, 632–634
  cell line of differentiation, determination of, 634
  cell-specific products and, expression of, 634
    specific immunomarkers of, 634–635
  cytokeratin type, determination of, 634
  vimentin and, co-expression of, 634
Anesthesia, in collection of cerebrospinal fluid, 512
Anestrus, canine, 463t, 465
Angiosarcoma, 93–95, 94f, 95b
Angiostrongylus vasorum infection, 227f, 228, 228f
Anisocytosis, 25f
Anisokaryosis, 25f
Antibodies
  in immunodiagnostics, interpretation of, 624–625
  in immunohistochemistry, 618, 619–622t
  for immunophenotyping, 650–651, 650t

Antibodies *(Continued)*
  as prognostic markers in veterinary oncology, 635
    KIT protein, 635, 635b
    proliferation/cell cycle markers in, 635
    telomerase in, 635
  "redundant," 631–632
Antibody personality profile (APF), 632
Antigen(s)
  detection of, 618
  fixation of, 623
  flow cytometry of, 642–646
  in formalin-fixed, paraffin-embedded (FFPE) tissues, 623
  in immunohistochemistry, 618
  as markers, in immunodiagnostics, 619–622t
  retrieval, in immunohistochemistry, 623–624, 624b
Antigen receptor rearrangements, PARR/PCR for, 696–699t
Aortic body tumor, 606, 606f
APF. *see* Antibody personality profile
Apochromat, 665
Apocrine cyst, 63, 63b, 63f
Apocrine gland adenocarcinoma, of anal sac, 78–79, 79b, 79f
Apocrine gland anal sac adenocarcinoma, 78–79, 80f, 82b
  spindle cell variant, 80f
Aqueocentesis, 571–572, 571f
Aqueous humor, 571–574
Argyrophilic nuclear organizing regions (AgNORs), 635
Argyrophilic nucleolar organizing regions (AgNOR), in lymphoma, 141
Array comparative genomic hybridization, 659
Arthropathy, synovial fluid and, 486t
Arthropod bite reaction, 37, 37b, 40f
Arthrospores, in dermatophytosis, 53–54, 54f
Artifacts, cytologic, thymus, 173, 174f
Ascites
  chylous, 257–259
  parasitic, 263
Aspergillosis, 255f
Aspergillus spp. infection, nasal, 189, 189t, 190f
Astrocytes, tumors from, 550
Astrocytomas, 552, 553f
Avidin-biotin activity, 624

B

Bacteria, 701, 701–702f
Bacterial cystitis, 417f
Bacterial flora, normal, in dry-mount fecal cytology, 379f
Bacterial infections, 216–219
  in nasal cavity, 188–189, 188f
Barium crystals, 260f
Basal cells, of vagina, 461
Basilar cell tumor, 70
Basilar epithelial neoplasms, cutaneous, 70–71, 70f, 71b, 71f

713

Basophilic inclusion, conjunctival, 563f
Basophilic materials, 677–679, 677t, 680f
Basosquamous carcinoma, 69–70, 70f
B-cell chronic lymphocytic leukemia/lymphoma, 143f
BCIP/NBT phosphatase substrate, 672
Benign prostatic hyperplasia (BPH), 471, 471f, 472f
Bicavitary effusions, 279, 283f
Bile
    in hepatocytes, 349, 350t, 351f
    infection of, 361–362, 363f, 364f, 365f
    normal cytology and artifacts of, 341, 342f, 343f
    sampling of, 339–340
Biliary epithelium, 340–341, 341f, 342f
Biliary neoplasia, 365–368, 366f, 367f
Biliary sludge, 355–356, 356f
Bilious effusion, 259–261, 261f, 262f
Bilirubin
    in body cavity fluids, 283t
    in urinary sediment, 426t, 429f
Biopsy
    of lymph nodes
        cytopathologic considerations, 124b, 126b
        indications for, 125, 126t
    splenic
        artifacts on, 158f, 159f
        aspirate, 157, 157b, 158f, 161f, 162f
        indications for, 156–157
    thymic, 171–178
Bladder
    anatomy and histology of, normal, 406–407
    inflammatory disorders of, 407–408, 408f
    neoplasia of, 408–411
    normal cytology and artifacts of, 407, 407f
    specimen collection from, 407
Blastocystosis, dry-mount fecal cytology in, 394f
Blastomyces dermatitidis infection, 312f
    in lung, 219–220
    in respiratory tract, 189t
Blastomycosis, 221f, 254f, 545f
    cutaneous lesions from, 50–51, 51f
    in joint, 490f
    osteomyelitis from, 503f
Blepharitis, 558
Blue-dome cyst, 441–442
B-lymphoblastic leukemia/lymphoma, 143f, 144–145, 145f
Body cavity fluids, 242–286
    abdominal, collection of, 242
    ancillary tests in, 279, 283t
    bilious, 259–261, 261f
    chylous, 257–259
    eosinophilic, 253
    exudate as, 248–250, 249f
    in feline infectious peritonitis, 250–252, 250f, 251f, 252b
    hemorrhagic, 257, 258f
    hyperplasia and, 247
    lymphoid cells in, 246, 246f
    macrophages in, 246f
    mesothelial cells in, 245, 245f
    mesothelioma in, 274–278, 276f, 277f
    modified transudate as, 246f, 247
    neoplastic, 244f, 272–279, 273f, 274f, 275f, 276f, 277f, 278f, 279f, 280f, 281f, 282f
    neutrophils in, 246, 246f

Body cavity fluids *(Continued)*
    nocardial/actinomycotic and, 265–266
    normal cytology in, 245–246
    nucleated cell differential, 245
    organ rupture in, 250
    parasitic ascites, 263
    pericardial, 269–272, 271f
        collection of, 242–243
    peritoneal, collection of, 242
    peritoneal effusions in, 250–263
    physical characteristics of, 243, 243f
    pleural, collection of, 242
    protein quantitation for, 243, 243b
    red blood cell in, 244–245, 245b
    sample, handling of, 243–245, 243f
    slide examination for, 8f
    slide preparation of, 243, 243b
    total nucleated cell count and, 244–245, 245b
    transudate as, 246f, 247–248, 248f
    uroperitoneum, 261–263, 262f
    vessel rupture in, 250
Bone, 499–510
    fine-needle aspiration of, 499
    histology of, 503
    lytic, cytopathology of, 501–503
    squamous cell carcinoma of, 510, 510f
    tumors of, 503, 504f, 505f, 506f, 507b, 507f, 508f
Bone marrow, tumors of, 503
BPH. *see* Benign prostatic hyperplasia
Brain, herniation of, cerebrospinal fluid collection and, 512
Branchial cleft, 173, 175f
Brick bodies, 341–343
Bronchi, 204–237
    anatomy of, 204
    collection techniques for, 204–207
    cytology of, 207–209, 207b, 207f, 207t, 208f
Bronchial brushing, 206
Bronchitis
    bacterial, 216, 216f
    chronic, 210, 215
    viral, 215
Bronchoalveolar lavage, 205–206, 205f
Bronchogenic carcinoma, 229f
Bronchoscopy, for bronchoalveolar lavage, 205
Buffy coat technique, 9, 9f
Butterfly needle, 3f

C

Calcinosis circumscripta, 117, 117f, 118f, 288
Calcinosis cutis, 117, 117f
Calcium carbonate crystals, 426t, 434f
Calcium hydrogen phosphate dihydrate crystals, 426t, 430f
Calcium oxalate crystals, in renal tubules, 399, 400f
Calcium oxalate dihydrate crystals, 426t, 428f
Calcium oxalate monohydrate crystals, 426t, 428f, 429f
Calcium phosphate crystals, 426t, 430f
Calcofluor white, 672, 673f
Calponin A, as marker, 635
Calretinin, as marker, 635
Campylobacteriosis, dry-mount fecal cytology in, 389f
Candida peritonitis, 255, 255f

Candida spp. infection, gastric, 310
Candidiasis, dry-mount fecal cytology in, 383f
Canine cestodiasis, 681f
Canine cutaneous Langerhans cell histiocytosis, 101
Canine distemper infection, 531–532, 531f
    cerebrospinal fluid analysis for, 517
Canine schistosomiasis, heterobilharzia PCR test for, 696–699t
Cannibalism, 32
Carcinoid syndrome, 614
Carcinoids, 596, 613–614, 615f, 616t
    hepatic, 368, 368f, 369f
Carcinoma(s)
    choroid plexus, 552–553, 554f
    endocrine, 115–116, 115f
    hepatocellular, 354–355, 365f, 366f
    laryngeal, 201, 201f
    of lung, 228–237, 229f, 231f
        squamous cell, 230–231, 232f
    mammary, 447f, 448f
    metastatic, 231f
        of bone, 510f
        in cerebrospinal fluid, 537–538, 539f
    nasal, 195f
        anaplastic, 193–194, 195f
        squamous cell, 193–194, 196f
        transitional, 196, 196f
    neoplastic effusion from, 273–274, 273f, 274f, 275f
    renal, 403–404, 403f, 404f
    sebaceous, 76, 76b, 77f
    thyroid
        follicular, 599f
        medullary, 601f, 602
        poorly-differentiated, 601f, 602f, 603
    urothelial, 408–411, 410f
    uterine, 461
Carcinosarcoma, of mammary gland, 446
Carotid body tumors, 606, 606b, 607f
Carpal joints, sample collection from, 485–486
Carprofen, liver injury from, 349f
Case comments
    in cytopathology report, 692
    in histopathology report, 695
Catheterization, urethral, traumatic, for bladder specimen, 407
Cavitational lesion, large, 339
Cell block
    advanced collection and preparation techniques of, 689
    for immunocytochemistry, 618–623
Cell line of differentiation, 634
Cell smears, for immunocytochemistry, 625
Cell transfer, advanced collection and preparation techniques of, 689, 690f
Cellular cast, in urinary sediment, 423f
Cellular infiltrate, 15–22, 17f, 18f, 19f
Cellular morphology, of neoplasm, 692
Cellulitis
    clostridial, 46, 46f
    Rhodococcus equi, 46
Central nervous system
    astrocytes in, 541–542, 542f, 543f
    cells of, 540–542
    choroid plexus cells in, 542, 543f
    ependymal cells in, 542, 543f

Central nervous system (Continued)
  extramedullary tumors of, 553
  lymphoma in, 534, 537f, 538f
  meningeal cells in, 542, 544f
  microglia in, 542, 544f
  neoplasia of, 534
  neurons in, 540–541, 541f, 542f
  neuropil in, 540, 541f
  oligodendrocytes in, 542, 543f
  tissues of
    collection and cytologic preparation of, 538–540, 540f
    cytopathology of, 538–553
    normal cytology of, 540–542
    pathologic, cytology of, 542–553
  tumors of, 545t
Centroacinar cells, 322
Cerebellar cortex, neurons in, 540, 542f
Cerebellomedullary cistern, cerebrospinal fluid collection from, 513
Cerebrospinal fluid (CSF), 512–538
  albumin in, 516–517
  basophilic ribbon material in, 532
  blood contamination of, 512
    effect of, 514–515
  cell counts in, 516
  cellular evaluation of, 518–522, 519t, 520t
    preparation for, 518–520, 521f
  collection of, 512–514
    in cerebellomedullary cistern, 513
    complications of, 512
    contraindications to, 512
    equipment for, 512–513, 513f
    in lumbar cistern, 513–514
    volume of, 513
  cystic findings in, neural, 533–538, 536f, 537f, 538f, 539f
  cytocentrifugation of, 518
  cytopathologic features of, 519t, 520t
  discoloration of, 515t, 516
  enzymes in, 518
  eosinophils in, 523
  erythrophagocytosis in, 20f
  in feline infectious peritonitis, 523, 524f
  formalin for fixation of, 514
  formation of, 512
  glucose in, 517
  immunoglobulin G in, 517
  laboratory analysis of, 514–518, 515t
  lesion findings in, neoplastic, 533–538, 536f, 537f, 538f, 539f
  macrophages in, 520–521
    in differential diagnoses, 520t
  macroscopic evaluation of, 516, 516f
  myelin in, 532, 535f
  neural tissue injury findings in, 532–533, 534f, 535f
  neutrophils in, 523
  normal, 520–521, 521f, 522f
    in presence of disease, 522–523
  opening pressure, 514
  pleocytosis of, 523–532
    eosinophilic, 526–527, 526f, 527f, 528f
    lymphocytic, 529f, 530f
    mixed cell, 532, 532f, 533f
    mononuclear, 527–532, 528f, 529f, 530f, 531f, 532f
    neutrophilic, 523–526, 523f, 524f, 525f

Cerebrospinal fluid (Continued)
  presentation and interpretation of, 522–538
  protein in, 515t, 516–517
    abnormalities in, 523
  puncture contaminants in, 521–522, 522f
  quantitative analysis of, 516–517
  refrigeration of, 514
  sedimentation preparation of, 518, 521f
  specific gravity of, 515t
  specimen of
    handling of, 514
    management of, 9
  stains for, 518–520
  turbidity of, 516, 516f
  xanthochromia of, 516, 516f
Ceroid, in hepatocytes, 350t, 352
Cestodiasis
  nodular, 263, 264f
  peritoneal, 256, 257f
Chalazion, 558
Chemodectomas, 605–606, 605t, 606f
Chemoreceptor, 597t
  tumors, 605, 605t
Chlamydiosis, conjunctival, 563f, 564f
Cholangiocellular carcinoma, 367f
Cholangiohepatitis, neutrophilic, 359f
Cholangitis, suppurative, 360f
Cholesterol, in body cavity fluids, 283t
Cholesterol crystals, 21, 22f, 247, 247f
  in epidermal cysts, 61–62
  in mammary cyst, 441–442, 443f
Chondrosarcoma
  of bone, 507, 508f, 509f
  nasal, 196–197, 197f
Choroid plexus cells, 542, 543f
Choroid plexus tumors, 545t, 552–553, 554f
Chromatic aberration, 665
Chromatin
  in neoplasia, 25f
  patterns, 685
Chromocenter, 685
Chromogens, for immunohistochemistry, 624
Chromogranin A, 632
Chronic lymphocytic leukemia/small cell lymphoma (CLL/SCL), 654
Chronic pancreatitis, 329, 329b, 329f
Chronic sinusitis, 187, 187f
Chyloabdomen (chylous ascites), 257–259, 324
Chylopericardium, 272
Chylothorax, 267, 267f, 268f
Chylous ascites. see Chyloabdomen
Chylous effusion, 18f, 19f, 267, 267f
Ciliary body, 571–574
  adenocarcinoma of, 574
C-kit gene, mutation in, 659–660, 660f
C-Kit mutation PCR analysis, for mast cell tumor, 696–699t
Clear cell adnexal carcinoma, 82, 82f
Clonality assays, in cats, 659
Clonality testing, 655–659, 656f
Clostridium infection, cutaneous, 46, 46f
Clostridium perfringens infection
  colitis as, dry-mount fecal cytology in, 388–389, 389f
  colonic, 315–316, 316f
Coccidioides immitis infection
  in lung, 220, 221f
  in respiratory tract, 189t

Coccidioidomycosis, 221f, 255f
  cutaneous lesions from, 51–52, 51f, 52f, 53f
  osteomyelitis from, 504f
Colitis
  clostridial, 316f
    dry-mount fecal cytology in, 389f
  eosinophilic, 308f
  lymphocytic, 317f
  neutrophilic, 315–316, 316f
Collagen, 20–21, 21f
Collagenolysis, 22f
Colon, 315–318
  Clostridium perfringens infection of, 315–316, 316f
  Cyniclomyces guttulatus infection of, 303, 304f
  epithelial cells of, 315f, 316f
  Histoplasma capsulatum infection of, 316–317, 318f
  hyperplasia of, 315, 316f
  inflammation of, 315–317, 316f, 317f, 318f
  lymphoma of, 317, 318f
  neoplasia of, 317–318, 318f, 319f
  normal cytology of, 315, 315f
  plasmacytoma of, 317, 319f
  Trichuris vulpis infection of, 315–316
Compression (spread) preparation, 3–5, 5b, 4f, 5f
Compression (squash) preparation, 4b
Conjunctivae, 559–565, 559f
  basophilic inclusion of, 563f
  hyperplasia of, 561, 561f
  inflammation of, 561–565, 561f, 562f, 563f, 564f, 565f, 566f
  miscellaneous findings of, 565, 566f
  neoplasia of, 565, 566f
  normal cytology and artifacts of, 561
  normal histology and anatomy of, 559
  sample collection from, 559–561, 560f
Conjunctivitis, 561–562
  eosinophilic, 565f
  follicular, 566, 567f
  mixed cell, 562f
    with epithelial hyperplasia, 566f
  suppurative, 561f
Copper, in hepatocytes, 350–352, 350t, 352f, 353f
Cornea, 567–571
  inflammation of, 567–570, 569f, 570f
  neoplasia of, 571
  normal histology and cytology of, 567, 569f
  response to tissue injury, 570–571
Cortical adrenal tumors, 607t
Corticosteroids, hepatopathy with, 349f
Cotton fibers, in urinary sediment, 437f
Cotton swab biopsy technique, 6, 7f
Cover glasses (coverslips), use of, 665–666
Coxofemoral joint, sample collection from, 485–486
Creatinine, in body cavity fluids, 283t
Crenosoma vulpis infection, 226–228, 227f
Cryptococcosis, 220, 254f
  cutaneous lesions from, 52–53, 53f
  dry-mount fecal cytology in, 394f
  periorbital, 580f
Cryptococcus neoformans infection, nasal, 189t
Cryptococcus spp. infection, nasal, 190–191, 191f, 221f
Crystalline structures, polarizing materials, 677, 677–678f, 677t

Crystals
  ammonium biurate, 426t, 433f
  barium, 260f
  calcium carbonate, 426t, 434f
  calcium hydrogen phosphate dihydrate, 426t, 430f
  calcium oxalate, in renal tubules, 399, 400f
  calcium oxalate dihydrate, 426t, 428f
  calcium oxalate monohydrate, 426t, 428f, 429f
  calcium phosphate, 426t, 430f
  cholesterol, 21, 22f, 247, 247f
    in mammary cyst, 441–442, 443f
  cystine, 426t, 430f
  hematoidin, 19–20, 20f, 118, 119f
  magnesium ammonium phosphate, 426t
  radiopaque contrast dye, 437f
  sodium urate, 426t, 427f
  struvite, 432f
  sulfonamide, 426t, 430f, 431f
  tyrosine, 426t
  uric acid, 426t, 427f, 428f
CSF. see Cerebrospinal fluid
Culture, of cerebrospinal fluid, 517
Curschmann's spirals, 46, 46f, 211, 213f
Cutaneous extraskeletal osteosarcoma, 98
Cutaneous metastatic carcinomas, 82–83
Cutaneous metastatic sarcomas, 87
Cuterebriasis, 61f
Cyclins, in veterinary oncology, 635
Cyniclomyces guttulatus
  in dry-mount fecal cytology, 379, 380f
  infection, colonic, 303, 304f
Cyst(s)
  apocrine, 63, 63b, 63f
  dermoid, 62–63, 63b
  epidermoid, 533–534, 536f
  laryngeal, 200
  leptomeningeal, 533–534
  mammary, 441
  meningeal, 533–534
  nailbed, 62f
  ovarian, 453–454
  prostatic, 16f, 470–471, 470f
  renal, 402, 402f
  spinal arachnoid, 533–534
Cystadenoma, hepatic, 365–366, 366f
Cystic endometrial hyperplasia-pyometra complex, 460
Cystic lesions, of pancreas, 324, 325f
Cystitis, polypoid, 407–408
Cysts, of oral cavity, 288
Cytauxzoonosis, macrophagic splenitis in, 158–161, 161f, 162f
Cytauxzoonosis schizont, hepatic, 362f
Cytocentrifugation, of cerebrospinal fluid, 518
Cytocentrifuge, 9
Cytodiagnostic groups, 15, 15b
  for lymphoid organ cytopathology, 124
Cytokeratin, 634
Cytologic artifacts, thymus, 173
Cytologic interpretations, general categories of, 15–34, 15b
  cellular infiltrate as, 15–22, 17f, 18f, 19f
  common cell relationships, 29–32
    cell-in-cell, 31–32, 33f
    cell-to-cell, 29–31
  cystic mass as, 15
  hyperplastic tissue as, 15, 16f

Cytologic interpretations, general categories of *(Continued)*
  inflammation as, 15–22, 17f, 18f, 19f
  neoplasia as, 22–28, 23f, 24f, 24t, 25f, 26b, 26f, 26t, 27b, 28f
  normal tissue as, 15, 16f
Cytologic samples, 707
Cytology kit, contents of, 2b
Cytopathologic description, 691
Cytopathologic diagnosis (interpretation), 691
Cytopathology report, 691–692, 692f, 693f

D

Dacryocystitis, 582
Dacryops, 582
Degenerative joint disease, 491–493, 492f
Degenerative lesions
  cytopathology report for, 691
  histopathology report for, 694
Demodicosis, 59, 60f
Dendritic cell histiocytosis, progressive, feline, 101, 101b, 102f
Dermatitis, acral lick, 35, 35b, 38f
Dermatophilosis, 47, 48f
Dermatophytosis, 53–55, 54f, 55f
Dermis, 35, 36f
Dermoid cyst, 62–63, 63b
Desmosomes, 27f
Diagnosis-focused description
  in cytopathology report, 691
  in histopathology report, 693–694
Diagnostic imaging, sample collection guided by, 1–3, 3b
3, 3'-Diaminobenzidine tetrahydrochloride hydrate (DAB), 624
Diestrus, canine, 453f, 463t, 464–465, 464f
Diff-Quik (RAL Diagnostics), 12f, 11–12
Diffuse large B-cell lymphoma (DLBCL), 145–147, 146f, 147f, 148f
  anaplastic variant of, 165f
Dirofilaria immitis
  infection from, pulmonary eosinophilic granulomatosis and, 212
  in urinary sediment, 436f
Dirofilaria repens infection, mammary gland, 443–444
Dirofilariasis, 59, 60f, 158f
Distemper viral inclusions, 700, 701f
DLBCL. see Diffuse large B-cell lymphoma
DNA
  amplification of, 657
  extraction of, for PARR, 655–656
Doxorubicin, for mammary gland neoplasia, 467
Dracunculiasis, 59, 60f
Dry-mount fecal cytology
  cell types in, 386–394, 386f, 387f, 388f
  evaluation of, systematic method of, guidelines for, 377b
  microbial pathogens in, potential, 387–394, 388f, 389f, 390b, 390f, 391f, 392f, 393f, 394f, 395f
  microscopic findings in
    abnormal, 381–383, 382f, 383b, 383f
    normal or incidental, 379–381, 379f, 380f, 381b, 381f
  sample in
    collection of, 377–378, 377b, 378b, 378f
    processing of, 377–378, 377b, 378b, 378f

Duodenum, 309f
Dysgerminoma, ovarian, 456–457
Dysplasia, 200
  of lung, 213
  nasal, 185, 186f
Dysplastic squamous epithelium, 67–68

E

Ears, 558–595
"Edge of the cliff syndrome," 8, 8f
Effusions
  body cavity fluid, classification of, 244f, 247
  in feline infectious peritonitis, 250–252, 250f, 251f, 252b
Ehrlichia canis infection, 653
Ehrlichiosis, granulocytic, in joint, 490f
Electron microscopy, 635–639
  advantages of, 635–636, 636f, 637f, 638f, 639f, 640f, 641f, 642f
  basics of, 636–638
    fixation in, 636–637
    and fixed samples, processing of, 637–638
    fundamentals, 636
  and diagnostic ultrastructural pathology, approach to, 638–639, 639b, 643–644t, 644–646t
  of mesenchymal neoplasia, 641f
  of microorganisms, 636f, 637f, 638f, 639f, 640f
    disadvantages of, 636
  of normal kidney and glomerular disease, 642f
Electronic gating, 652, 652f
Emperipolesis, 31, 32f, 67–68, 68f
Endocrine cells, 322
Endocrine pancreas, 322–338
  histology of, 322, 323f
  normal anatomy of, 322, 323f
Endocrine system, 596–617, 596b, 597t, 598f
  tumors, 596
Endocrine testing, 696–699t
Endometriosis, ovarian, 454
Endophthalmitis, infectious, 578f, 579f
Endothelial venules, of lymph nodes, 125f, 129
Endotracheal tube, for bronchoalveolar lavage, 205
Enolase, neuron-specific, 634
Entamoebiasis, dry-mount fecal cytology in, 393f
Enteritis
  eosinophilic, 313f
  lymphocytic, 313f
  neutrophilic, 310f, 311f
Entosis, 32
Enzymes, in cerebrospinal fluid analysis, 518
Eosinophilia, in lung, 211
Eosinophilic effusion, 253
Eosinophilic exudates, 253, 253f
Eosinophilic hypersensitivity dermatitis, 38–42, 42b
Eosinophilic index, of vagina, 461
Eosinophilic lesions, 19, 19f
Eosinophilic materials, 679, 680f
Eosinophils
  in cerebrospinal fluid, 519t, 520–521
    increased percentages of, 523
  tracheal, 207–209, 208f
Ependymal cells, 542, 543f
Ependymoma, 545t, 552, 553f
Epidermal inclusion cysts, 61–62

Epidermis, 36f
Epidermoid cysts, 61–62, 533–534, 536f
Epithelial cells
　biliary, 340–341, 341f, 342f
　in dry-mount fecal cytology, 379–381, 381f, 386, 386f
Epithelial hyperplasia, 200
Epithelial neoplasia/neoplasms, 23, 23f, 24f, 26b
　of nasal cavity, 193–196, 194t
　odontogenic, 291, 294f
Epithelial tumors, ovarian, 454–455, 455f
Epithelioid macrophages, 18, 19f
Epithelioma, sebaceous, 74, 74b, 76f, 77f
Epithelium, dysplastic squamous, 67–68, 68f
Epulis, 291, 294f
Erosive arthritis, 491
Erythrocyte engulfment, 33f
Erythrocytes
　body cavity fluids in, 244
　in cerebrospinal fluid
　　effect of, 514
　　in neural tissue injury, 532, 534f
Erythroid precursors, splenic, 170, 172f
Erythrophagocytosis, 19–20, 20f
Escherichia coli infection, of prostate gland, 444
Esophageal perforation, 268–269, 270f
Esophagitis, 300f
　reflux, 297–298
Esophagus, 296–301
　inflammation of, 297–300, 300f
　leiomyosarcoma of, 300–301, 301f
　neoplasia of, 300–301, 301f
　normal cytology of, 296–297
Estrous cycle
　canine, 462–465, 463f, 463t, 464f
　feline, 465
Estrus, canine, 462–464, 463t, 464f
Ethylene glycol toxicosis, renal tubules in, 400f, 401f
Eucoleus aerophilus infection
　in lung, 225, 226t
　nasal, 225
Eurytrema procyonis, 330
Exocrine pancreas, 322–338
　histology of, 322, 323f
　normal anatomy of, 322, 323f
External acoustic meatus, 582–583
External ear, 582–589
　inflammation of, 584–587, 584f, 585f, 586f, 587f
　neoplasia of, 587–589, 588f, 589f, 590f
　nonneoplastic tumors of, 587
　normal anatomy and histology of, 582–583, 583f, 584f
　normal cytology and artifacts of, 584, 584f
　response to tissue injury of, 587
　sample collection and preparation of, 583–584
Extra-adrenal paragangliomas, 605–606
Extramedullary hematopoiesis, 324
Extramedullary tumors, of central nervous system, 553
Exudates, 248–250, 249f
　eosinophilic, 253, 253f
　nonseptic, 249f, 250–253, 264
　pericardial, 270–271
　postoperative, 252, 252f
　septic, 249f, 253–256, 253f, 264–266

Eyelids, 558
　inflammation of, 558, 559f
　neoplasia of, 558, 560f
　normal anatomy of, 558, 559f
　normal histology of, 558, 559f
Eyes, 558–595

F

Fasciitis, nodular, of sclera, 567
Fatty liver, 343–344
FCG. see Feline chronic gingivostomatitis
Fecal cytopathology, 377–396
Feces, 316–317
Feline chronic gingivostomatitis (FCG), 287–288
Feline fibroadenomatous change, 443, 444f
Feline herpesvirus infection, conjunctival, 561–562
Feline immunodeficiency virus infection, lymphadenopathy in, 131
Feline infectious peritonitis (FIP), 358, 523, 524f
　cerebrospinal fluid analysis for, 517
　effusions in, 250–252, 250f, 251f, 252b
　hepatic inflammation in, 358, 361f
Feline leukemia virus, 131
Feline plasmacytic pododermatitis, 44–45, 45f
Fibrocystic disease, mammary, 441
Fibroepithelial polyp, 408
Fibroma, 83–84, 84b, 84f
Fibroplasia, responsive, 117, 118f, 119f
Fibrosarcoma, 85–86, 85f, 86b
　of bone, 503–505
　keloidal, 83–84, 86f
　laryngeal, 201–203, 202f
　oral cavity, 292
Fibrosis, 21, 23f
　in panniculitis, 37–38
Filaroides hirthi infection, 225–226, 226t
Fine-needle aspiration (FNA)
　of bone, 499
　of kidney, 397
　of prostate gland, 469
　in prostatitis, 469
　of testes, 475–476
Fine-needle aspiration biopsy (FNAB)
　of liver, 339
　of lymph node, 2f
　of nasal cavity, 184
　transthoracic, 206–207
　ultrasound-guided, 1–2, 3f
　　biopsy guidance in, 2
　　complications of, 2–3, 4b
　　equipment for, 2, 3f
　　technique for, 2, 3f
Fine-needle capillary sampling, 1
FIP. see Feline infectious peritonitis
Fixation
　in electron microscopy, 636–637
　with formalin, 623
　in immunohistochemistry, 623–624, 624b
Flow cytometry, 642–655, 696–699t
　antibody panels for characterization of canine and feline leukocytes by, 650t
　cytometers in, 651
　examining cell surface proteins by, 652f
　light scatter properties of canine peripheral blood by, 651f
　methodology of, 647–653
　　data analysis of, 651–652, 651f, 652f

Flow cytometry *(Continued)*
　　laboratory preparation of sample in, 648–651, 650t
　　reporting data from, 653
　　sample collection in, 647–648
　uses for, 653–655
　　in classification of acute leukemia, 654–655
　　in diagnosis of mediastinal masses, 655, 655f
　　immunophenotype, prognostic significance of, 654
　　reactive *versus* neoplastic lymphocytosis, 653
Fluid sample processing worksheet, 707–708, 708f
Fluid samples, 706
Fluids, management of, 6–9, 9b, 7f, 8f, 9f, 10f
Fluorochromes, 651–652
FNA. see Fine-needle aspiration
FNAB. see Fine-needle aspiration biopsy
Foam cells
　of mammary glands, 440–441, 441f
　of vagina, 461
Follicular neoplasms, differentiated, 71–73
Foreign body(ies)
　nasal, 186
　reaction, 35b, 36–37, 37b, 39f, 40f
　　in suppurative inflammation of lung, 211f
Formaldehyde, as fixative, in electron microscopy, 636–637
Formalin
　in cerebrospinal fluid handling, 514
　as fixative, for immunohistochemistry, 623
Fungal infections
　localized opportunistic, 49–50, 50f
　nasal, 189–191, 189t
　systemic, cutaneous lesions from, 50–53
Fungi, 701–702, 703f

G

Gallbladder, normal, 339, 343f
Gallbladder mucoceles, 355–356, 356f
Ganglion cyst, 63–64, 63f
Gastrin-secreting tumor, 335f
Gastritis
　candidiasis, 305f
　lymphocytic, 303f, 304f
　neutrophilic, 304f
Gastrointestinal cytopathology, 301
Gastrointestinal perforation, 259, 260f
Gastrointestinal stromal tumor (GIST), metastatic, 374f
Genetic testing, for metabolic disease, 696–699t
Germinal epithelial neoplasms, cutaneous, 70–71
Giant cell tumor, of bone, of sinonasal cavity, 199, 199f
Giant cells
　anaplastic sarcoma with, 91–92, 92b, 92f
　multinucleate, 18, 19f
Giardiasis, 310, 312f
　dry-mount fecal cytology in, 392f
GIST. see Gastrointestinal stromal tumor
Gliomas, 545t, 550
Glomerulus
　cytology of, normal, 398–399, 400f
　normal, 397, 398f
Glomus tumor, 116–117, 116f
Glucose
　in body cavity fluids, 283t
　in cerebrospinal fluid analysis, 517

Glutaraldehyde, as fixative, in electron microscopy, 636–637
Glycogen stains, 673
Goblet cells, 322
  tracheal, 207, 208f
Gossypiboma (textiloma), 263, 264f
Granular cast, in urinary sediment, 424f
Granular cell lymphoma, cerebrospinal fluid in, 538f
Granular cell tumor(s)
  laryngeal, 203t
  of meninges, 545t, 547–548, 549f
  oral cavity, 292, 296f
Granulation tissue, 117, 118f
Granuloma
  eosinophilic, 38–39, 41f, 42f
  lick, 35, 35b, 38f
Granulomatosis
  eosinophilic, pulmonary, 212
  lymphomatoid, in lung, 234–237, 235f
Granulomatous laryngitis, 200
Granulomatous meningoencephalitis, 517, 530–531, 530f, 531f
Granulosa cell tumor, ovarian, 455
Grimelius and Grocott-Gomori Methenamine Siver stain, 672, 673f

H

Hair follicle tumors, 71–72, 71b, 73f
Hassall's corpuscles, 171–172, 174f
HE staining, 632–634
Heat-induced epitope retrieval (HIER), 623
Helminths, 702, 705f
Hemangioma, 93, 93b, 93f
Hemangiopericytoma, canine, 87–91, 90f, 91b
Hemangiosarcoma, 23–25, 27f, 93–95, 94f, 95b
  of bone, 503–505, 509f
  of spleen, 166, 169f
Hemarthrosis, 493–495, 496f
  synovial fluid and, 486t
Hematoidin crystals, 19–20, 20f, 118, 119f
Hematoma, 64, 65f, 66f, 118
Hematopoiesis, extramedullary, 155, 157f
  hepatic, 352–353, 354f
  splenic, 170–171, 172f, 173f
Hematuria, 418f
Hemolymphatic neoplasia, 197–198
  of lung, 232–237, 234f
Hemolymphatic system, 124–181
Hemopericardium, 271, 272f
Hemoperitoneum (hemoabdomen), 257, 258f
Hemorrhage
  acute, 19–20
  chronic, 19–20, 20f
  erythrophagocytosis in, 19–20, 20f
  hematoidin crystals in, 19–20, 20f
  of iris, 572–573
  pulmonary, 213–214, 214f
Hemorrhagic effusion, 257, 258f
Hemosiderin, 19–20
  in hepatocytes, 348, 349–350, 350t, 351f
Hemosiderosis, hyperplastic spleen and, 158, 159f
Hemostasis, abnormal, as contraindication to fine-needle aspiration biopsy of liver, 339
Hemothorax, 266
Hepatic cell death, 356–357, 357f, 358f
Hepatic fibrosis, 356–357, 357f, 358f
Hepatitis, 359f
Hepatobiliary system, 339–376
Hepatocyte paraffin 1 (Hep Par 1), 634
Hepatocytes
  cytoplasmic rarefaction of, 345–347, 348f
  glycogen accumulation by, 345–347, 348f, 349f
  hydropic (ballooning) degeneration of, 345–347, 349f
  in lung aspirate, 233f, 236f
  in normal liver, 340, 340f
  pigments in, 348, 350t
  "signet ring" appearance of, 345f
Herpesvirus infection, conjunctival, 561f
Heterobilharzia PCR test, for canine schistosomiasis, 696–699t
HIER. see Heat-induced epitope retrieval
Histiocytic lesions, 17–18, 18f
Histiocytic sarcoma, 101, 101b, 102f, 103f
  of lung, 210f, 233–234
  nasal, 198
  of spleen, 171f
  in synovial fluid, 496–497
Histiocytoma
  canine, 98–100, 100b, 100f, 101f
  fibrous, malignant, 91–92, 92b, 92f
Histiocytosis
  dendritic cell, progressive, feline, 101, 101b, 102f
  malignant, hepatic, 372f
  reactive, 103, 103b, 104f
Histopathologic (morphologic) diagnosis, 694
Histopathology report, 692–695, 694f
Histoplasma capsulatum infection, 189, 189t
  in lung, 220, 221f
Histoplasmosis, 221f, 254f
  cutaneous lesions from, 53, 54f
  in joint, 490f
  macrophagic splenitis in, 158–161, 161f
  systemic, peritoneal effusion in, 254
Hodgkin-like lymphoma, 149–150, 150f, 151f
Honeycomb pattern, 29, 29f, 30f
Hyaline cast, in urinary sediment, 422f
Hyalohyphomycosis, 359f
Hydropic degeneration, 15
Hygroma, 118, 119f
Hyperadrenocorticism, 611
Hypergastrinemia, 334–335
Hyperplasia, 15, 16f
  adrenocortical, 610–611
  conjunctival, 561, 561f
  hepatic, 345, 354–355, 355f
  intestinal, 303
  of lung, 213
  of lymph node, 127–131, 128f, 129f, 130f, 131f, 132f
  lymphoid
    of larynx, reactive, 200
    nasal, 197
  mammary, 442–443, 443f
  nasal, 185, 186f
  of nictitating membrane, 567f
  of oral cavity, 287
  of parathyroid gland, 604
  prostatic, 471, 471f, 472f
  of salivary gland, 292–293
  sebaceous, nodular, 64, 64b, 64f, 65f
  splenic, 158, 159f
Hyperplastic pancreatic nodule, 326f
  of exocrine pancreas, 326f
Hyphema, 572–573

I

ID PCR with sequencing, 696–699t
Image resolution, major controls for, 666f
Immune-mediated disease, joints affected by, 491
Immunochemistry, 696–699t
Immunocytochemistry, 624–625, 674
  interpretation of, 624–625
  methods of, 625
  positive and negative controls for, 626
Immunodiagnosis, 618–635
  of anaplastic or metastatic tumors, 632–634
  and antibodies as prognostic markers, 635
  immunocytochemistry, 624–625
  troubleshooting in, 625–631, 626f, 627f, 628f, 629f, 630f, 631f
  use of controls in, 632f
Immunoglobulins
  CDR3 sequence of, 658
  in cerebrospinal fluid, 517
  gene, rearrangement of, 655–656, 657f
  nonspecific binding of, 624
Immunohistochemistry
  antibodies in, 618, 619–622t
  antigen retrieval, 623–624, 624b
  fixation in, 623–624, 624b
  immunochemical reaction, 624
  interpretation of, 624–625
  limitations of, 625
  protocols for, 619–622t, 624
    pretreatment procedures, 618
  sample processing in, 618–623
  standardization and validation of, 625
  test validation in, 625
  troubleshooting in, 625–631, 626f, 627f, 628f, 629f, 630f, 631f
    for background staining, 625–626, 626f, 627f, 628f, 629f, 630f, 631f
    for false-negative staining, 625–626, 626f, 627f, 628f, 629f, 630f, 631f
    for false-positive staining, 625–626, 626f, 627f, 628f, 629f, 630f, 631f
    for lack of staining, 625
    use of controls in, 626–631, 632f
    for weak staining, 625
  of tumors, panel markers for, 631–632, 632t, 633f
  visualization of the immunologic reaction, 624
Immunophenotype
  antibodies for, 650–651, 650t
  prognostic significance of, 654
    in lymphoma, 654
    in peripheral lymphocytosis, 654
In situ hybridization, for selected infectious agents, 696–699t
Inadvertent lens puncture, 580f
Incubation, in immunohistochemistry, 625
Infections
  bacterial, in nasal cavity, 188–189, 188f
  canine distemper, 531–532, 531f
    cerebrospinal fluid analysis for, 517
  feline herpesvirus, conjunctival, 561–562
  feline immunodeficiency virus, lymphadenopathy in, 131

Infections *(Continued)*
  hepatic, 357–362
  mycotic, 312f
  rabies, 531–532, 532f
Infectious inflammation
  cytopathology report for, 691
  histopathology report for, 693–694
Infectious inflammatory disorders, 200
Infertility, male, 481, 481f
Inflammation, 15–22, 17f, 18f, 19f
  of bone, 501–503
  colonic, 315–317, 316f, 317f, 318f
  conjunctival, 561–565, 561f, 562f, 563f, 564f, 565f, 566f
  corneal, 567–570, 569f, 570f
  eosinophilic, 19f
    in dry-mount fecal cytology, 386
    eyelid, 558
    nasal, 184
  of external ear and pinna, 584–587, 584f, 585f, 586f, 587f
  of eyelid, 558, 559f
  gastric, 303–306, 304f, 305f
  hepatic, 352–353, 359f, 361f, 362f
  intestine, 309–310, 310f, 311f, 312f, 313f, 314f
  of joint, 489–491, 490b, 491b
  of lymph node, 131
  mammary gland, 443–444
  of nictitating membrane, 567f
  of oral cavity, 287–288, 288f, 289f, 290f, 291f
  ovarian, 454
  prostatic, 471–473
    fine-needle aspiration in, 468–469
  pyogranulomatous, 18, 19f
  of salivary gland, 293–294, 298f, 299f
  of skeletal muscle, 498
  of skin
    infectious, 45–59
    noninfectious, 35–45
  splenic, 158–161
  testicular, 478
  uterine, 460f
  vaginal, 465, 465f, 466f
Inflammatory disease
  bowel
    clonality assay for, 659
    lymphoplasmacytic, microscopic findings in, 384–385
  nasal
    eosinophilic, 184
    noninfectious, 186–187
Inflammatory effusions, 249
Inflammatory pseudotumours, 408, 409f
Infundibular cyst, 61–62, 61f, 62b, 62f
Inner ear, 592–593
Insect bite reaction, 37, 40f
Insulinoma (-cell tumor), 333f, 334f
Integumentary system, 35–123
  normal histology of, 35
Intercalated ducts, 322
Interlobular ducts, 322
Intermediate cells, of vagina, 462
Interstitial cell tumors, of testes, 479–481, 480f
Intestine, 307–315
  adenocarcinoma of, 315f
  epithelial cells of, 307f, 309f
  hyperplasia of, 309

Intestine *(Continued)*
  inflammation of, 309–310, 310f, 311f, 312f, 313f, 314f
  lymphoma, 314f
  mucosal cells of, 308f
  neoplasia of, 310–315, 314f, 315f
  normal cytology of, 307–308, 307f, 308f, 309f
Intracranial pressure, increased, as contraindication to CSF collection, 512
Iridocyclitis, pyogranulomatous, 572, 572f
Iris, 571–574
  hemorrhage of, 572–573
  inflammation of, 572, 572f, 573f
  lymphoma of, 575f
  neoplasia of, 573–574, 574f, 575f
  normal histology and cytology of, 571, 571f
  uveal hematopoiesis, 573
Islet cell carcinoma, 334f
Islet cell tumor, 333
  metastatic, 156f

J

Joints
  classification of disease of, 488–498, 489b
  degenerative disease of, 491–493, 492f
  hemarthrosis of, 493–495, 496f
  infectious arthritis of, 489–491, 489f, 490b, 490f, 491b
  noninfectious arthritis of, 491, 491f, 492f
  sample collection from, 485–486

K

Karyolysis, 15, 17f
Karyorrhexis, 15–17, 17f, 18f
Keratin bars, 35
Keratin pearl, in squamous cell carcinoma, 67–68, 69f
Keratinocytes, 35
Keratitis
  eosinophilic, 568–569, 570f
  infectious, 567–568
  mycotic, 567–568, 569f
Keratoacanthoma, 73, 73b
Kerion, in dermatophytosis, 53–54, 54f
Ketamine, in collection of cerebrospinal fluid, 512
Ki-67
  antigen, in lymphoma, 141
  in veterinary oncology, 635
Kidneys
  anatomy and histology of, normal, 397, 398f
  crystals in, 399–401, 400f, 401f, 402f
  cysts of, 402, 402f
  cytology of, normal, 398–399, 399f, 400f
  infectious inflammatory disorders of, 401–402, 402f
  neoplasia of, 402–406
  noninfectious inflammatory disorders, 399–401
  specialized collection techniques for, 397–398, 397b
Kiel classification, of lymphoma, 140
Kinetoplast, 702
Kinetoplastids, 702
KIT protein, as marker, in veterinary oncology, 635, 635b
Köhler illumination, 665, 667b, 668f

L

Lactate, in body cavity fluids, 283t
Laryngitis, granulomatous, 200
Laryngoscopy, 199
Larynx, 199–204
  carcinoma of, 201, 201f
  cellular responses to injury, 199–200
  cysts of, 200
  cytologic features of, 199
  fibrosarcoma of, 201–203, 202f
  granular cell tumor of, 203t
  histologic features of, 199
  lymphoma of, 203, 203f
  mucoceles of, 200
  neoplasia of, 200–204
    mesenchymal, 201–203, 202f
  normal anatomy of, 199
  oncocytoma of, 203–204, 203t
  plasmacytoma of, 203
  reactive lymphoid hyperplasia of, 200
  rhabdomyoma of, 201–203, 202f, 203t
  sample collection from, 199
  squamous cell carcinoma of, 200–201, 200f
Leiomyoma, 461
  vaginal, 465–466, 466f
Leiomyosarcoma
  esophageal, 300–301, 301f
  hepatic, 373f
Leishmania infection, nasal, 193
Leishmaniasis, 57–59, 59f
  macrophagic splenitis in, 158–161, 162f
Lens damage, with macrophagic inflammation, 579f
Lens fibers, in vitreous humor, 576
Lens objectives, 665, 666t
  parts of, 667f
Leptomeningeal carcinomatosis, cerebrospinal fluid in, 537–538
Leptomeningeal cells, 522
Leptomeningeal cysts, 533–534
Leukemia
  acute, classification of, flow cytometry and, 654–655
  diagnosis of, PARR and, 658
  granular lymphocytic, of spleen, 165, 167f
  granulocytic, metastasis to lymph nodes, 152–153
  lymphoblastic, 139
  lymphocytic, chronic, of B-cell origin, 143f
  myeloid, acute, 368, 372f
  translocations and, 659
Leukocytes
  fecal, in dry-mount fecal cytology, 383–385, 383f, 384f, 385b, 385f
  globule, intestinal, 307
Lignin test, performing, for sulfonamides in urine, 431b
Linear shapes, polarizing materials, 677, 677t, 678–679f
Linguatula serrata infection, nasal, 193
Lipase, in body cavity fluids, 283t
Lipid
  droplets of, in urinary sediment, 416, 417f
  in lipoma, 92, 92f
Lipid pneumonia, 215, 215f
Lipid storage diseases, hepatic changes in, 347f

Lipidosis, hepatic, 344–345, 345f
Lipofuscin, in hepatocytes, 348, 350t
Lipoma, 92, 92b, 92f
Liposarcoma, 92–93, 93b, 93f
Liver
    accidental aspiration of, 233f
    in acute myeloid leukemia, 368, 372f
    adenoma of, 354–355
    amyloidosis of, 353–354, 354f
    carcinoid of, 368, 368f, 369f
    carcinoma of, 354–355
    carprofen and, 349f
    cell of, 340
    cystic lesions of, 352, 354f
    cytoplasmic changes in, 343–347, 345f, 346f, 347b, 347f, 348f, 349f, 350f
    cytoplasmic rarefaction of, 345–347, 348f
    extramedullary hematopoiesis of, 352–353, 354f
    fatty, 343–344
    hydropic (ballooning) degeneration of, 345–347, 349f
    infection of, 357–362
    inflammation of, 352–353, 357–362
        eosinophilic, 361
        lymphocytic (nonsuppurative), 360, 360f, 361f
        mixed cell, 360–361, 361f, 362f, 363f
        neutrophilic or suppurative, 352–353, 357–360, 359f, 360f
    leiomyosarcoma of, 373f
    in lipid storage disease, 347f
    lymphoma of, 368, 369f, 370f, 371f, 372f, 373f
    malignant histiocytosis of, 372f
    mast cell of, 340, 340f
        tumor of, 372f
    neoplasia of, 362–370, 365b, 365f, 366f
    nodular and regenerative hyperplasia of, 354–355, 355f
    normal cytology and artifacts of, 340–341, 340f, 341f, 342f
    nuclear inclusion of, 341–343, 343f, 344f, 345f
    pigments in, 348–352, 350t
    sampling from, 339
        contraindications to, 339, 339b
        indications for, 339, 339b
        technique of, 339–340
Lumbar cistern, cerebrospinal fluid collection from, 513–514
Lung lobe torsion, 268, 269f
Lung rupture, 269, 271f
Lungs, 204–237
    adenocarcinoma of, 25f
    bronchoalveolar lavage of, 205–206
    carcinoma of, 229f, 231f
    collection techniques for, 204–207
    cytology of, 209, 209f
    eosinophilic granulomatosis of, 212
    fine-needle aspiration of, 206
    hemorrhage in, 213–214, 214f
    hypersensitivity airway disorders, 214
    infectious causes of disease of
        Acanthamoeba spp. as, 224, 225f
        Aelurostrongylus abstrusus as, 224, 225f
        amebiasis, 224
        Angiostrongylus vasorum as, 227f, 228
        bacterial pneumonia, 212f
        Blastomyces dermatitidis as, 219–220, 221f

Lungs (Continued)
        Coccidioides immitis as, 220, 221f
        Crenosoma vulpis as, 226–228
        Eucoleus aerophila as, 225, 226t
        Filaroides hirthi as, 225–226, 226t, 227f
        fungal pneumonia, 219–222
        helminthic infestations, 224
        Histoplasma capsulatum as, 220, 221f
        lycoperdonosis, 222, 223f
        Mycobacteria, 217
        Neospora caninum as, 224
        Paragonimus kellicotti as, 224–225, 226f, 226t
        Pneumocystis carinii as, 220–221, 222f
        Sarcocystis neurona as, 224, 224f
        Sporothrix schenckii as, 221–222
        Toxoplasma gondii as, 222, 223f
        viral pneumonia, 215–216, 216f
        Yersinia pestis as, 219
    infectious inflammatory disorders of, 215–228
    inflammation of, 210–212
        chronic, 210, 213f
        eosinophilic, 211–212, 212f
        granulomatous, 211, 211f
        macrophagic and mixed, 211, 211f
        suppurative, 210–211, 210f, 211f, 213f
    metaplasia of, 213, 213f
    necrosis of, 213
    neoplasia of, 228–237
    nonrespiratory aspirate of, 209–210
    oropharyngeal contamination of, 209
    tissue injury in, 212–214
Lungworm, canine, 225–226, 227f
Lupus erythematosus cells, in immune-mediated disease of joints, 491, 492f
Lycoperdonosis, 222, 223f
Lymph nodes, 124–155
    biopsy of
        cytopathologic considerations, 124b, 126b
        indications for, 125, 126t
    collection and specimen preparation, 125–126, 126f
    cytopathologic biopsy considerations, 124, 124f
    endothelial venules of, 129
    hyperplastic, 127–131, 128f, 129f, 130f, 131f, 132f
    macrophages of, 124
    medullary cords of, 124
    metastasis to, 150–155, 151f, 152f, 153f, 154f, 155f, 156f
    Mott cells of, 129–131
    normal anatomy and histology, 124, 125f
    normal cytology and artifacts, 126–127, 126f, 127f, 128f
    plasma cells of, 124
    popliteal, 124b, 126t
    prescapular, 124b, 126t
    primary neoplasia of, 149–150
    reactive, 128f, 129f, 130f, 131f, 133f
    Russell bodies of, 129–131
    size of, 125
    specimen of, 13b
Lymphadenitis, 131–137
    eosinophilic, 132, 134f
    histiocytic or pyogranulomatous, 132–137, 133f, 134f, 135f, 136f, 137f, 138f
    neutrophilic, 132, 133f
Lymphadenomegaly, lymph node biopsy for, 125
Lymphangiosarcoma, 94–95

Lymphoblast, definition of, 138–139
Lymphoblastic lymphoma, 139
    B-cell, 143f, 144–145, 145f
    T-cell, 145, 145f, 146f
Lymphocyte-rich transudate, 267–268, 269f
Lymphocytes, 3f
    in body cavity fluid, 246
    in canine histiocytoma, 100f, 101f
    in cerebrospinal fluid, 515t
    in inflammation, 384–385
    in lymph nodes, 124
    in mycosis fungoides, 109–111, 113f
    in spleen, 158
Lymphocytic infiltration, 19, 19f
Lymphocytic lymphoma/leukemia, chronic, of B-cell origin, 143f
Lymphocytic portal hepatitis, hepatic inflammation in, 360f
Lymphocytosis
    neoplastic, 653
    peripheral, 654
    reactive, 653
Lymphoglandular bodies, 20–21, 21f, 139–140, 139f, 140f
Lymphoid cells, in body cavity fluid, 246, 246f
Lymphoid neoplasia, of spleen, 162–164
Lymphoid organ, cytopathology of, cytodiagnostic groups for, 124
Lymphoid precursors, splenic, 170
Lymphoid tissue, nasal-associated, 182, 185f
Lymphoma(s), 25, 137–149, 138f, 139f, 140f, 149b
    B-cell, 143f, 144–145, 145f
        mediastinal, 149, 150f
    bladder, 411, 411f
    of bone marrow, 510
    cell proliferation markers in, 141
    in central nervous system, 534, 537f, 538f
    chemotherapy for, hyperplastic spleen and, 159f
    classification of, 139t
    colonic, 317, 318f
    cutaneous, 109–113, 113b, 114f, 115f
    cytologic protocol for, 139b
    diagnosis of, PARR and, 658
    epitheliotropic, 109–111
    follicular, 143
    granular, metastatic, 155f
    hepatic, 368, 369f, 370f, 371f, 372f, 373f
    immunophenotyping for, 141, 654
    immunostaining in, 141
    of intestine, 314f
    laryngeal, 203, 203f
    of lung, 232–233, 234f, 235f
    lymphocytic, chronic, of B-cell origin, 143f
    lymphoglandular bodies in, 139–140, 139f
    lymphoplasmacytic, 141, 142f, 143f
    marginal zone, 143–144, 144f, 164, 166f
    monitoring and staging of, PARR and, 658
    nasal, 197–198, 198f
    neoplastic effusion from, 278–279, 278f, 279f, 280f
    versus reactive lymph nodes, 131
    renal, 405, 406f
    small lymphocytic, 141–143
    terms in evaluation of, 139b
    thymic, 173
    translocations and, 659
    T-zone, 141, 142f

Lymphomatoid granulomatosis, 236f
Lymphosarcoma, 138
Lymphosomes, 124f

M

Macronucleated medium-sized cell (MMC), 143–144
Macrophages
  alveolar, 210
  in body cavity fluids, 246, 246f
  in cerebrospinal fluid, 520–521, 520t
  foamy, in xanthomatosis, 42, 43f
  hemosiderin granules in, 19–20, 20f
  of lymph nodes, 124
  in spleen, 158, 161f
Macrophagic lesions, 17–18, 18f
Macrophagic splenitis, 161f
Magnesium ammonium phosphate crystals, 432f
Malassezia, 55, 56f
Mammary glands, 440–451
  adenocarcinomas of, canine, 446
  adenoma of, 446f
  anatomy of, normal, 440
  carcinoma of
    anaplastic, 447–448
    squamous cell, 449
  carcinosarcoma of, 446
  collection techniques for, 440
  cysts of, 441, 443f
  cytology of, normal, 440–441, 441f
  foam cells of, 440–441, 441f
  histology of, normal, 440, 441f
  histopathologic classification of, 442b
  hyperplasia of, 442–443, 443f
  infection of, 443–444
  inflammation of, 443–444
  lobules of, 441f
  neoplasia of, 445
    canine, 445–450, 447f, 448f, 449f
    cytologic examination of, 447f, 448f, 449f
    feline, 450–451, 450f
    stromal invasion in, 446
    treatment of, 451
  sarcoma of, 446
  specimens from, 440–451
Mannitol crystals, in urinary sediment, 438f
Marginal zone lymphoma, 143–144, 144f, 145f, 164, 166f
Mast cell(s)
  hepatic, 340, 340f
  in hyperplastic spleen, 158
  tumor of, 87f, 103–106, 105f, 106b, 106f, 107f, 108f, 109f, 110f
  eosinophilic lymphadenitis in, 132, 134f
  of liver, 372f
Mast cell tumor, 237
  C-Kit mutation PCR analysis for, 696–699t
  flow cytometry in, 655
Mastitis, 443–444, 444f
Mastocytoma, 166–168, 170f
Mastopathy, polycystic, 441
Matrix metalloproteinases (MMPs), in cerebrospinal fluid analysis, 518
May-Grunwald-Giemsa stain, 10–11
Mediastinal B-cell lymphoma, 149
Medullary cords, of lymph nodes, 124, 125f
Medulloblastoma, cerebrospinal fluid in, 536

Megaesophagus, thymoma and, 175–178
Megakaryocytes, splenic, 170
Meibomian adenoma, 74
Melan-A, 634
Melanocytes, 35
Melanocytic tumors, 95–98, 96f, 97f, 98b, 98f, 99f
Melanoma
  amelanotic, 97f
  lymph node metastasis in, 150–151
  nodular, 573–574
  oral, 291
  retrobulbar, 582f
Melanosis, nasal, 186
Membrane filtration technique, for cytologic preparation of cerebrospinal fluid, 518
MEN. see Multiple endocrine neoplasia
Meningeal cells, 542, 544f
Meningeal cysts, 533–534
Meninges, neoplasms of, 545–550
Meningiomas, 545–547, 545t, 546f, 547f, 548f, 549f
Meningoencephalitis
  bacterial, 525–526, 525f
  cerebrospinal fluid analysis for, 517
Merkel cell tumor, 115–116, 116f, 614
Mesenchymal nasal hamartoma, 193
Mesenchymal neoplasia/neoplasms, 23–25, 26f, 27b, 27f, 369–370, 373f
  of lung, 231–232
  nasal, 196–197, 197f
Mesenchymal tumors, 411, 411f
Mesocestoides infection, ascites with, 256
Mesothelial cells, 324
  in body cavity fluids, 245, 245f
  lining body cavities, 242
  in liver, 340–341, 342f
  in lung aspirate, 209f, 233f
  reactive, 245f
Mesothelioma, in neoplastic effusion, 274–278, 276f, 277f
Mesothelium, *versus* splenic imprint, 159f
Metabolic disease, genetic testing for, 696–699t
Metabolic lesions
  cytopathology report for, 691
  histopathology report for, 694
Metaplasia
  of lung, 213, 213f
  nasal, 185–186
Metastasis, to lymph nodes, 150–155, 151f, 152f, 153f, 154f, 155f, 156f
Metastatic neoplasia/neoplasms
  of bone, 503, 510f
  epithelial, 370, 373f, 374f, 375f
Metastatic osteosarcoma, 98
Metastatic tumor, immunochemical diagnosis of, 632–634
  cell line of differentiation, determination of, 634
  and cell-specific products, expression of, 634
    specific immunomarkers of, 634–635
  cytokeratin type, determination of, 634
  and vimentin, co-expression of, 634
Metritis, 460
Microabscess, Pautrier, 109–111
Microbial flora
  abnormal, in dry-mount fecal cytology, 381–383, 382f, 383b, 383f
  in dry-mount fecal cytology, 379

Microglia, 542, 544f
Microorganisms
  algae, 701–702, 703f
  bacteria, 701, 701–702f
  fungi, 701–702, 703f
  oomycetes, 701–702, 703f
  quick reference for morphologic features of, 706
  relative sizes of, 700f
  viruses, 700, 701f
Microscope basics, 665–669
  numerical aperture and resolution, 666–669
  optimizing usage, 665–666
  parts of, 665
Middle ear, 590–592, 590f, 591f, 592f, 593f
Mineralization, in pancreas, 324, 325f, 326f
Minimal residual disease, detection of, 658–659
Mitosis, 21–22, 24f, 686f
  abnormal, 687f
  in neoplasia, 24f
Mitotic figures, 685, 685–686f, 686f, 687f
  in canine histiocytoma, 98–100, 100f, 101f
  in mammary carcinoma, 447–448, 448f
Mitotic index, for lymphoma, 143f
Mixed cell inflammatory lesions, 18, 19f
MMC. see Macronucleated medium-sized cell
MODAL syndrome, 82–83, 83f
Monoclonal antibodies, in immunohistochemistry, 618
Monocyte/granulocyte lineage markers
  myeloperoxidase (MPO), 651
Monocytoid cells, in cerebrospinal fluid, 515t, 519t, 520–521
Mott cells, 129–131
Mucin, in myxoma, 86–87
Mucin clot test, 486–487, 487f
Mucinosis, 119–120
Mucins, 673
Mucoceles, 118–119
  laryngeal, 200
  salivary, 293–294, 298f
Mucoperiosteum, 590
Mucopurulent inflammation, 188f
Mucus, 21f
  of nasal cavity, 183
Multicellular parasites, 59, 702, 705f
Multinucleation, in neoplasia, 25f
Multiple endocrine neoplasia (MEN), 610
Multiple myeloma, bone lysis from, 505f, 506f, 507b, 507f, 508f, 510, 510f
Muscle, skeletal
  inflammatory cells in, 498
  normal, 16f
  tumors of, 498–499, 500f
Musculoskeletal system, 485–511
  synovial fluid in, 485–498
Myasthenia gravis, thymoma and, 175–178
Mycobacteriosis, 47–49, 48f, 49b, 49f
  cutaneous, 49
  lepromatous, 48
  in lung, 217
  tuberculous, 48
Mycoplasma infection, in lung, 219
Mycoplasmosis, conjunctival, 564f
Mycosis, nasal, 191
Mycosis fungoides, 109–111, 113f
Mycotic infection, 312f, 359f

Myelin, in cerebrospinal fluid, 532, 535f
Myelolipoma, 171, 173f
Myelomalacia, 532–533, 535f
Myopericytoma, canine, 87–91, 90f, 91b
Myositis, 498, 498f, 499f, 500f
Myxoma, 86–87, 87b, 87f
Myxosarcoma, 86–87, 87b, 88f

N

Nailbed cysts, 61–62, 62f
Naked nuclei
   versus lysed cell nuclei, 598f
   neoplasms, 26–28, 27b, 28b, 28f
Naked nuclei cytomorphology neoplasms, 237
NALT. *see* Nasal-associated lymphoid tissue
Nasal-associated lymphoid tissue (NALT), 182, 185f
Nasal cavity, 182–199
   adenocarcinoma of, 193–194, 195f
   anatomy of, 182
   biopsy of, fine-needle aspiration, 184
   brush cytology of, 184
   carcinoma of, 194f, 195f
      anaplastic, 193–194, 195f
      squamous cell, 193–194, 196f
      transitional, 196, 196f
   chondrosarcoma of, 196–197, 197f
   contamination of
      oropharyngeal, 184, 186f
      Simonsiella spp., 184, 186f
   dysplasia of, 185, 186f
   flush of, 183–184, 183f
   foreign bodies in, 186
   histology of, 182
   hyperplasia of, 185, 186f
   imprint cytology of, 184
   infection in, 187–193
      algal, 191
      Alternaria spp., 191
      Aspergillus spp., 189, 189t, 190f
      bacterial, 188–189, 188f
      Cryptococcus neoformans, 189t
      Cryptococcus spp., 189, 191f
      Eucoleus aerophilus, 225
      fungal, 189–191, 189t
      Histoplasma capsulatum, 189, 189t
      Linguatula serrata, 193
      parasitic, 193
      Penicillium spp., 189, 189t
      Pneumonyssoides caninum, 193
      protozoal, 189t, 193
      Rhinosporidium seeberi, 189t, 192–193, 192f
      viral, 187–188
   inflammatory disease of
      eosinophilic, 184
      noninfectious, 186–187
   lymphoid hyperplasia of, 197
   lymphoma of, 197–198, 198f
   metaplasia of, 185–186
   mucus of, 183
   neoplasia of, 193–199, 194t
      epithelial, 193–196
      mesenchymal, 196–197, 197f
   neuroendocrine tumors of, 198–199
   neuroepithelial tumors of, 198–199
   normal cytology of, 184, 185f
   oncocytoma of, 199

Nasal cavity *(Continued)*
   polyps in, 187f
   sample collection for, 182–184
   sample preparation from, 182–184
   swabs of, 183
   transmissible venereal tumor in, 198, 198f
Nasal flush, 183–184, 183f
Nasal swabs, 183
Nasolacrimal apparatus, 582, 583f
Nasopharyngeal polyps, 193, 194f
Necrosis, 21, 23f
   of lungs, 213
   pancreatic, 324, 325f, 326f
Necrotizing encephalitis, in small breed dogs, 528–529, 529f, 530f
Necrotizing vasculitis, 525
Needle, for specimen sampling, 1, 3f
Negative findings, in cytopathology report, 691
Neoplasia/neoplasms, 22–28, 27b
   anisokaryosis in, 25f
   basilar epithelial, 70–71, 70f, 71b, 71f
   of bile duct, 365–368, 366f, 367f
   of bone, 503–510, 510f
   of central nervous system, 534
   coarse chromatin in, 25f
   colonic, 317–318, 318f, 319f
   conjunctival, 565, 566f
   corneal, 571
   cytomorphologic categories of, 22–28, 24t, 26t
   epithelial, 228–231, 229f, 230f
   esophageal, 300–301, 301f
   of external ear and pinna, 587–589, 588f, 589f, 590f
   eyelid, 558, 560f
   gastric, 306–307, 306f
   general features of, 22
   hepatocellular, 362–370, 365b, 365f, 366f
   histopathologic description of, 692–693
   intestinal, 310–315, 314f, 315f
   of iris, 573–574, 574f, 575f
   laryngeal, 200–204
      mesenchymal, 201–203, 202f
   of lung, 228–237
      hemolymphatic, 232–237, 234f
      mesenchymal, 231–232, 233f
   mammary, 445, 446f, 447f, 448f, 449f
   of meninges, 545–550
   mesenchymal, 23–25, 26f, 27b, 27f
   mitotic figures in, 447–448, 448f
   multinucleation in, 25f
   multiple endocrine, 610
   naked nuclei, 26–28, 27b, 28b, 28f
   of nasal cavity, 193–199, 194t
      epithelial, 193–196
      mesenchymal, 196–197, 197f
   of nerve sheaths, 545–550
   of neuroepithelial cells, 550–553
   of nictitating membrane, 567, 568f
   nuclear molding in, 25f
   nuclear-to-cytoplasmic ratio in, 25f
   nucleoli in, prominent, 25f
   oral, 290–292, 291f, 292f, 293f, 294f, 295f, 296f, 297f
   of orbital cavity, 580–582
   ovarian, 454, 455f, 458f, 459f
      epithelial, 454–455, 455f
      germ cell, 456–458, 458f, 459f
      sex cord-stromal, 455–456, 456f, 457f

Neoplasia/neoplasms *(Continued)*
   of paranasal sinuses, 193–199
   pleomorphism in, 23f, 24t
   of prostate, 473–475, 474f, 475f
   renal, 402–406
   round cell, 25, 27b, 28b, 28f, 29t
   salivary, 294–296, 299f, 300f
   of spleen
      lymphoid, 160f, 162–166, 165f
      nonlymphoid, 166–170, 169f, 170f, 171f, 172f
   synovial, 495–498, 496f, 497f, 498b, 498f
   testicular, 478, 478f, 478t
   uterine, 461
   vaginal, 465–467, 466f, 467f, 468f, 470f
   vitreous body, 576
Neoplastic effusion, 244f, 272–279, 273f, 274f, 275f, 276f, 277f, 278f, 279f, 280f, 281f, 282f
   in lymphoma, 278–279, 278f, 279f, 280f
   mesothelioma in, 274–278, 276f, 277f
Neospora caninum infection
   in lungs, 224
   in respiratory tract, 189t
Neosporosis, 256f
Nephritis, mycobacterial, 402f
Nephroblastomas
   canine, 545t
   renal, 404–405, 405f
Nephron, 397
Nerve sheath tumors, 87, 88f, 89f, 90f
Nerve sheaths
   neoplasms of, 545–550
   tumors of
      benign, 550, 550f
      malignant, 551f
      peripheral, 545t, 548–550, 550f, 551f
Nervous system, 512–557
Neuroblastoma, 608
   metastatic, 156f
   olfactory, 198–199
Neuroendocrine carcinoma, 115–116, 116f
Neuroendocrine system, 596–617, 596b, 597t, 598f
Neuroendocrine tumor, nasal, 198–199
Neuroepithelial cells, neoplasms of, 550–553
Neuroepithelial tumor, nasal, 198–199
Neurons, 540–541, 541f, 542f
Neuron-specific enolase (NSE), 634
Neuropil, 540, 541f
Neutrophil(s), 10f
   in body cavity fluids, 246, 246f
   in cerebrospinal fluid, 515t, 519t, 520–521
      increased percentages of, 523
   degenerate, 17f
   fecal, in dry-mount fecal cytology, 383, 383f, 384f
   karyolysis of, 15, 17f
   karyorrhexis of, 15–17, 17f, 18f
   nondegenerate, 15, 17f
   pyknosis of, 15–17, 18f
   in suppurative inflammation of lungs, 207, 213f
   in uterine inflammation, 460
New methylene blue stain, 10, 10b, 11f
NGE. *see* Nodular granulomatous episcleritis
Nictitating membrane, 565–567
   cytology of, 565–566
   follicular conjunctivitis, 566, 567f
   neoplasia of, 567, 568f
   normal histology of, 565–566

Niemann-Pick disease, 347f
Nissl substance, 540
Nocardial/actinomycotic effusions, 265–266
Nocardiosis, 46–47, 47b, 47f
Nodular granulomatous episcleritis (NGE), 568f, 569f
Nodular hyperplasia, pancreatic, 325, 325b, 326f, 327f
Nodular panniculitis, 37–38, 38b, 41f
Nodular regenerative hyperplasia, of liver, 354–355, 355f
Nodules
　cutaneous, specimen of, 13b
　fibrohistiocytic, 158
　hyperplastic, 610–611
Nonchylous lymphocyte-rich transudate, 259, 259f
Noninfectious inflammation
　cytopathology report for, 691
　histopathology report for, 694
Noninfectious inflammatory disorders, 200
Nonlymphoid neoplasia, of spleen, 166–170, 169f, 170f, 171f, 172f
Non-neoplastic tumor, histopathologic description of, 693–694
Nonsuppurative joint disease, 491–493, 493f, 494f, 495f, 496f
Normal tissue, 15, 16f
NSE. see Neuron-specific enolase
Nuclear chromatin patterns, 685, 688f
Nuclear molding, in neoplasia, 25f
Nuclear streaming, 20–21, 21f
Nucleoli, in neoplasia, prominent, 25f
Numerical aperture, 666–669
Nurse cell, 173f

O

Oil red O stain, 673–674, 674f
Oligodendrocytes, 542, 543f
　tumors from, 550
Oligodendrogliomas, 550, 551f, 552f
Oncocytoma
　laryngeal, 203–204, 203t
　of nasal cavity, 199
Oomycete testing, 696–699t
Oomycetes, 57, 57b, 57f, 58f, 701–702, 703f
Oral cavity, 287–292
　epulis of, 291, 294f
　granular cell tumors of, 292, 296f
　hyperplasia of, 287
　inflammation of, 287–288, 288f, 289f, 290f, 291f
　melanoma of, 291, 295f
　neoplasia and, 291f
　　epithelial odontogenic, 294f
　normal cytology of, 287, 288f
　osteosarcoma of, 296f
　squamous cell carcinoma of, 300–301
Orbital cavity, 576–582
　inflammation of, 580, 580f
　neoplasia of, 580–582, 581f, 582f
Orchitis, 478
Oslerus osleri infection, 225–226, 226t, 227f
Osteoarthritis, 491–493
Osteoarthropathy, 491–493
Osteoblasts, 499–501, 502f, 503f
Osteoclast, 502f
　in degenerative joint disease, 491–493, 495f
Osteomyelitis, 501–503, 504f
　fungal, 503, 504f
Osteosarcoma, of bone, 503–505, 505f, 506f, 507b, 507f, 508f
Otic cytopathology, 582, 583f
Ovary(ies), 451–458
　anatomy of, normal, 451
　collection techniques for, 451
　cysts of, 453–454
　cytology of, normal, 452–453, 452f, 453f, 454f
　endometriosis, 454
　histology of, normal, 451, 451f
　inflammation of, 454
　neoplasia of, 454, 455f, 458f, 459f
　　epithelial, 454, 455f
　　germ cell, 456–458, 458f, 459f
　　sex cord-stromal, 455–456, 456f, 457f

P

Pacinian corpuscles, 322
Palisade pattern, 30, 30f
Pancreas, 322–338
　artifacts of, 324
　cystic lesions of, 324, 325f
　histology of, 322, 323f
　infectious inflammatory disorders of, 329–331
　neoplastic tumors of, 331–337
　nodular hyperplasia of, 16f, 325, 325b, 326f, 327f
　noninfectious inflammatory disorders of, 325–329
　normal anatomy of, 322, 323f
　normal cytology of, 324
　sample collection in, 322–324
　tissue injury of, 324, 325f, 326f
Pancreatic abscess, 329–330, 330f
Pancreatic adenoma, 331
Pancreatic carcinoma, 331–333, 331f, 332f, 333b, 333f
Pancreatic endocrine tumor (PET), 333f, 334f, 335b, 335f, 336b, 336f, 336t, 597t
Pancreatic flukes, 330, 330f
Pancreatic islets, 322
Pancreatic necrosis, 324, 325f, 326f
Pancreatic neoplasia, 337
Pancreatic nodular hyperplasia, 325, 325b, 326f, 327f
Pancreatic pseudocyst, 324, 325f
Pancreatic trematodiasis, 330f
Pancreatitis, 325–329
　acute, 327–329, 328f, 329b
　chronic, 329, 329b, 329f
　hepatic inflammation in, 358, 359f
Panel markers, in diagnostic immunohistochemistry, of tumors, 632t, 633f
Panniculitis, nodular, 37–38, 38b, 40f, 41f
Pannus, 569–570
Papanicolaou stain, 10
Papillary pattern, 30, 31f
Papilloma(s)
　choroid plexus, 552, 554f
　urothelial, 408, 409f
　viral, 64–67, 66f, 67f, 68f
Parabasal cells, of vagina, 461
Paraformaldehyde, as fixative, in electron microscopy, 636–637
Paraganglioma(s), 26–27, 28f, 605
　extra-adrenal, 605–606

Paragonimus kellicotti infection, 224–225, 226f, 226t
Paranasal sinuses, neoplasia of, 193
Paraneoplastic alopecia, 332–333
Parasites, in urinary sediment, 432
Parasitic infection, nasal, 193
Parathyroid gland, 597t, 604–605, 604t
　in dog and cat, 604t
　nonneoplastic, 604
　tumors of, 604–605, 605f
Parathyroiditis, lymphocytic, 604
Pathology reports, 691, 692f, 693f, 694f
　composing, 691
Patient safety checklist, 709, 710f
Pautrier microabscess, 109–111, 113f
Pavement pattern, 29, 29f
PCNA. see Proliferation cell nuclear antigen
PCR. see Polymerase chain reaction
PCR panel, 696–699t
Pearsonema plica, in urinary sediment, 432, 435f
Peculiar findings, 675
　based on cytopathologic characteristics, 677t
　basophilic materials, 677–679, 677t, 680f
　crystalline structures, 677, 677–678f, 677t
　eosinophilic materials, 679, 680f
　linear shapes, 677, 678–679f
　specimen acquisition and processing, 675–676, 675–676f, 676f
Pemphigus foliaceus, 42, 42b, 42f, 43f
Penicillium spp. infection, nasal, 189, 189t
Perianal gland adenoma, 76–78, 77f, 78b, 78f, 79f
Pericardial effusions, 269–272, 271f
　ancillary diagnostics of, 272
　canine, 269
　feline, 270
Pericardial fluid
　collection of, 242–243
　hematoidin crystals in, 20f
Pericardiocentesis, slide examination in, 9f
Perinuclear vacuolation, 67–68, 69f
Peripancreatic fat saponification, 324, 326f
Peripheral T-cell lymphoma, 141f, 147–149, 148f, 149f
Peritoneal effusions, 250–263
Peritoneal fluid, collection of, 242
Perivascular pattern, 31, 32f
Perivascular wall tumors, 87–91, 91b, 91f
Peroxidase, for immunohistochemistry, 624
PET. see Pancreatic endocrine tumor
Pet food toxicosis, 401f
Peyer's patch, 307–308, 309f
pH, of body cavity fluids, 283t
Phagocytosis, 32
Pheochromocytoma, 605, 608–610, 608f, 609f
Phlegmon, 329–330
Phycomycosis, gastric, 304
Physaloptera sp. infection, 303–304, 305f
Pigments, hepatic, 348–352, 350t
Pilomatricoma, 73, 74f, 75f
Pinna, 582–589
　inflammation of, 584–587, 584f, 585f, 586f, 587f
　neoplasia of, 587–589, 588f, 589f, 590f
　nonneoplastic tumors of, 587
　normal anatomy and histology of, 582–583, 583f, 584f
　normal cytology and artifacts of, 584, 584f
　response to tissue injury of, 587
　sample collection and preparation of, 583–584

Plan apochromat, 665
Plant material, in dry-mount fecal cytology, 380f
Plaque, eosinophilic, 39
Plasma cell(s)
　in hyperplastic spleen, 158, 168f
　of lymph nodes, 124
　tumors of
　　of bone marrow, 510
　　cerebrospinal fluid in, 536, 539f
Plasmacytic infiltration, 19, 19f
Plasmacytoma, 108–109, 109b, 110f, 111f, 112f
　colonic, 317, 319f
　laryngeal, 203
　of spleen, 165, 168f
Pleocytosis, 523–532
　eosinophilic, 526–527, 526f, 527f, 528f
　lymphocytic, 529f, 530f
　mixed cell, 532, 532f, 533f
　mononuclear, 527–532, 528f, 529f, 530f, 531f, 532f
　neutrophilic, 523–526, 523f, 524f, 525f
Pleomorphic fecal bacteria, in dry-mount fecal cytology, 389–390
Pleomorphism, in neoplasia, 23f
Pleural effusions, 264–269
Pleural fluid
　collection of, 242
　erythrophagocytosis and, 20f
Pneumocystis spp. infection, 189t
　in lung, 220–221, 222f
Pneumonia
　aspiration, 222
　bacterial, 212f, 216–219, 217f, 218f, 219f
　fungal, 219–222
　inhalation, 211
　lipid, 215, 215f
　mycotic, 219–222, 220f
　protozoal, 222–224
　viral, 215–216, 216f
Pneumonyssoides caninum infection, nasal, 193
PNL2, 634
Polarizing materials, 681, 681t, 682f, 683f, 684f
　basophilic, 677–679, 677t, 680f
　crystalline structures, 677, 677–678f, 677t
　eosinophilic, 679, 680f
　linear shapes, 677, 678–679f
　specimen acquisition and processing, 675–676, 675–676f, 676f
Pollen grains, in urinary sediment, 438f
Polyclonal antibodies, in immunohistochemistry, 618
Polymer methods, 624
Polymerase chain reaction (PCR), for antigen receptor rearrangements, 655–656, 656f
　clonality assays in cats and, 659
　methodology of, 656–658
　　data analysis in, 657–658
　　DNA amplification in, 657
　　sample collection in, 656
　sensitivity of, 658
　uses of
　　for clonal relationships between tumors, 658–659
　　for detection of minimal residual disease, 658–659
　　for diagnosis of lymphoma and leukemia, 658
　　for lymphoma, staging and monitoring of, 658

Polypoid cystitis, 407–408
Polyps, nasal, 187f
Postoperative exudates, 252, 252f
Potassium, in body cavity fluids, 283t
Primary bacterial peritonitis, 253–254, 253f
Proestrus, canine, 462, 463f, 464f
Proliferation cell nuclear antigen (PCNA), in lymphoma, 141
Proliferation markers, in veterinary oncology, 635
Proliferative lesions
　cytopathology report for, 691
　histopathology report for, 694
Prostate gland, 467–475
　anatomy of, normal, 469
　collection techniques for, 468–469
　cyst of, 16f, 470–471, 470f
　cytology of, normal, 469–470
　epithelial cells of, 469–470, 471f, 472f
　fine-needle aspiration of, 469
　histology of, normal, 469, 470f
　hyperplasia of, 16f, 471, 471f, 472f
　inflammation of, 471–473, 473f, 474f
　　fine-needle aspiration in, 468–469
　massage/wash of, 469
　neoplasia of, 473–475, 474f, 475f
　squamous epithelial cells of, 469
　squamous metaplasia of, 471, 472f
　transitional cells of, 469–470
　　carcinoma of, 474–475
　tubuloalveolar glands of, 469, 470f
Prostatitis, 473f, 474f
　acute, 473
　fine-needle aspiration in, 469
　septic, 473f
Protein
　in body cavity fluids, quantitation of, 243, 243b
　in cerebrospinal fluid, 515t, 516–517
　　abnormalities in, 523
Protein-cytologic dissociation, 523
Protein gene product (PGP) 9.5, 634
Proteinaceous debris, 20–21, 21f
Proteinosis, pulmonary alveolar, 214
Prototheca spp. infection, 316–317, 317f
　nasal, 191
Protothecosis, 57, 58f
　dry-mount fecal cytology in, 392f, 393f
　vitreocentesis, 579f
Protozoa, 702, 704f
Protozoal infection
　nasal, 193
　in respiratory tract, 189t
Protozoonosis, 266
Pseudocyst
　pancreatic, 324, 325f
　renal, 402, 402f
Pseudomycetoma, dermatophytic, 54–55, 55f
Purkinje cells, 540, 542f
Purulent lesions, 15
Pyelonephritis, 401–402
Pyknosis, 15–17, 18f
Pyoderma, 45–46, 45f, 46f
Pyogranulomatous inflammation, 18, 19f
Pyometra, 460
Pythiosis, 465, 466f
　gastric, 305f

R

Rabies infection, 531–532, 532f
Ragocytes, in immune-mediated disease, 491, 492f
"Rapid onsite evaluation" (ROSE), 707
Reactive lymphoid hyperplasia, of larynx, 200
Rectal cytopathology, 377–396
Rectum, 315–318
Red blood cells, in body cavity fluids, 244–245, 245b
Red cell cast, in urinary sediment, 423f
Reference laboratory, submitting cytology specimens to, 13f, 13–14, 14b
Reflux esophagitis, 297–298
Renal tubules
　cytology of, normal, 398–399, 399f
　normal, 397, 398f
Reproductive system, 440–484
　female, 440–467
　male, 467–482
Reproductive tract tears, 263, 263f
Resolution, 666–669
Respiratory system, 182–241
　nasal cavity in, 182–199
Retina, 574–575
　cytology of, 574, 576f, 577f
　normal histology of, 574, 576f, 577f
Retinal detachment, 578f
Rhabdomyoma, 498–499
　laryngeal, 201–203, 202f, 203t
Rhabdomyosarcoma, 95, 95f, 498–499, 500f, 501f, 502f
Rhinitis
　allergic, 186, 187f
　bacterial, 188–189, 188f
　cryptococcal, 190–191, 191f
　fungal, 189–191, 190f
　lymphoplasmacytic, 186–187
　parasitic, 193
　septic suppurative, 188f
Rhinosporidium seeberi infection, nasal, 189t, 192–193, 192f
Rhodococcal pleuropneumonia, 266, 266f
Rhodococcus equi, cellulitis from, 46
Romanowsky stains, 11f, 10–13
ROSE. *see* "Rapid onsite evaluation"
Round cell
　neoplasms, 25, 27b, 28b, 28f, 29t
　tumors, nasal, 197–198
Rubricytes, 170, 172f
Russell bodies, 129–131

S

Salivary gland, 292–296
　cytology of, normal, 292, 298f
　hyperplasia of, 292–293
　inflammation of, 293–294, 298f, 299f
　neoplasia of, 294–296, 299f, 300f, 580–582
　normal, 16f
Salmon fluke poisoning disease, 132–135, 136f
Sample, 706
Sample quality, of cytopathology report, 691
Sarcocystis neurona infection, of lungs, 224, 224f
Sarcoma(s), 9f
　anaplastic, with giant cells, 91–92, 92b, 92f
　histiocytic, 101, 101b, 102f, 103f
　of liver, 372f, 373f

Sarcoma(s) *(Continued)*
  nasal, 198, 236f
  of spleen, 168, 171f
  of mammary gland, 446
  renal, 405–406, 406b, 406f
  of synovial cell, 495–496, 497f, 498b, 498f
SCC. *see* Squamous cell carcinoma
Schizont, cytauxzoonosis, hepatic, 362f
Sclera, 567, 568f, 569f
Sebaceous adenoma, 73–74, 74b, 75f, 77f
Sebaceous carcinoma, 76, 76b, 77f
Sedimentation techniques, for cytologic preparation of cerebrospinal fluid, 518, 521f
Sedi-Stain, 417f
Semen
  abnormalities of, 481–482, 481f, 481t, 482f
  evaluation of, 468–469
Seminiferous tubules, 477f
Seminoma, 478–479, 479f
Seminoperitoneum, 263, 263f
Sepsis, bacterial, 17f
Seroma, 16f, 119, 120f
Serpulina spp, dry-mount fecal cytology in, 389–390, 389f
Sertoli cell tumor, 479, 479f, 480f
Sex cord-stromal tumors, ovarian, 455–456, 456f, 457f
Sézary syndrome, 109–111
Shandon Cytoblock Cell Block Preparation System, 689
Sialocele, 118–119, 120f, 293–294, 298f
Simonsiella spp., in oropharyngeal contamination, 184, 186f
Sinuses, paranasal, neoplasia of, 193
Sinusitis, chronic, 187, 187f
Skin
  cyst of
    apocrine, 63, 63b, 63f
    dermoid, 62–63, 63b
  inflammation of
    infectious, 45–59
    noninfectious, 35–45
  mycobacteriosis of, 47–49, 48f, 49f
  neoplasia of, 64–117
    epithelial, 64–83, 67b, 69f, 71f, 73f, 75f, 77f, 79f, 81f, 82f
    mesenchymal, 83–98, 83f, 85f, 87f, 91f, 92f, 93f, 94f, 95b, 97f
    naked nuclei, 114–117, 115f, 116f
    round or discrete cell, 98–114, 100f, 101f, 102f, 103f, 104f, 105f, 106b, 106f, 107f, 108f, 109f, 110f, 111f, 113f, 114f
  nodule of, specimen of, 13b
  non-neoplastic tumors, 61–64, 61b
  normal cytology and artifacts of, 35, 36f, 37f, 38f
  parasitic infestation of, 60f
  response of, to tissue injury, 117–121
  xanthoma of, 42–44, 43f, 44f
Smartphone telecytopathology basics, 669–670, 669f, 670f, 671f
  manual technique, 669
  over-the-eyepiece holders, 669–670, 671f
Sodium urate crystals, 426t, 427f
SOPs. *see* Standard operating procedures
Special objective adjustment rings, 667f
Specialized diagnostic testing sites, list of, 696, 696–699t

Specific gravity, of cerebrospinal fluid, 515t
Specimen(s), 1b, 706
  air-drying of, 623
  buffy coat technique, 9
  buffy-coat concentration technique for, 9f
  cerebrospinal fluid, handling of, 514
  collection of, 1–3
    diagnostic imaging-guided, 1–3, 3b
    equipment, 2, 3f
    techniques for, 1, 2, 2t, 3f
  compression (spread) preparation of, 4b, 4f
  compression (squash) preparation of, 3–5, 5b, 5f
  liver, 339
  mammary, 440–451
  management of, 1–14, 3–9, 6b
    fluids, 6–9, 9b, 7f, 9f, 10f
    sampling guidelines for, 1
    serum-coated slides for, 9b
    site-specific considerations
      for cutaneous nodule, 13b
      for lymph node, 13b
    staining of, 10–13, 12b, 13b
      abnormal, causes of, 12b
      with new methylene blue stain, 10, 10b, 11f
      with Papanicolaou stain, 10
      with Romanowsky stains, 11f, 10–13
      times of, 12
    touch imprint of, 5–6, 5f, 6f
Specimen overview, in cytopathology report, 691
Spherical aberration, 665
Spider bite reaction, 37, 40f
Spinal arachnoid cysts, 533–534
Spindle cells, in hemangiopericytoma, 87–91
Spiriliform bacteria, in dry-mount fecal cytology, 389f
Spirocerca lupi infection, 300
Spirocercosis, 270f
Spleen, 156–171
  anatomy and histology of, 156, 157f
  biopsy of
    artifacts on, 158f, 159f
    aspirate, 157, 157b, 158f, 161f, 162f
    indications for, 156–157
  ellipsoids of, 158, 158f
  extramedullary hematopoiesis of, 170–171, 172f, 173f
  granular lymphocytic leukemia of, 165, 167f
  hemangiosarcoma of, 166, 169f
  hyperplastic, 158, 159f
  inflammation of, 158–161
  lymphocytes in, 158
  macrophages in, 158, 161f
  mastocytoma of, 166–168, 170f
  myelolipoma of, 171, 173f
  neoplasia of
    lymphoid, 160f, 162–166, 165f
    nonlymphoid, 166–170, 169f, 170f, 171f, 172f
  plasmacytoma of, 165, 168f
  punctate vacuoles of, 166
  reactive, 158, 159f
  sarcoma of, histiocytic, 168, 171f
Splendore-Hoeppli reaction, 120–121, 120f
Splenitis, 158–161, 160f, 162f, 163f, 164f
  neutrophilic, 160f
Splenomegaly, splenic biopsy for, 156
Sporangia, 192–193, 192f

Sporothrix schenckii infection
  in lung, 221–222
  in respiratory tract, 189t
Sporotrichosis, 56–57, 56f, 57b
  nasal, 191
Squamous cell carcinoma (SCC), 67–69, 68b, 68f, 69b, 69f
  of bone, 510, 510f
  laryngeal, 200–201, 200f
  of lung, 230–231, 232f
  of mammary gland, 449
  nasal, 193–194, 196f
  of nictitating membrane, 567, 568f
  oral, 300–301
Staining, 10–13, 12b, 13b
  abnormal, causes of, 12b
  in immunodiagnosis
    background, 625–626, 626f, 627f, 628f, 629f, 630f, 631f
    false-negative, 625–626, 626f, 627f, 628f, 629f, 630f, 631f
    false-positive, 625–626, 626f, 627f, 628f, 629f, 630f, 631f
    lack of, 625
    weak, 625
  times for, 12
Stains
  histochemical, 639–642, 647f
    advantages of, 639–641
    disadvantages of, 641
    for intracellular and extracellular substances, 647f, 648t
    for microorganisms, 650t
    principles of, 641–642, 647f, 648t, 649f, 650t
    selected, and protocols, 672–674
      acid-alcohol, 672
      alkaline phosphatase, 672, 672f
      calcofluor white, 672, 673f
      Grimelius and Grocott-Gomori Methenamine Siver, 672, 673f
      immunocytochemistry, 674
      mucins and glycogen stains, 673
      oil red O, 673–674, 674f
Standard operating procedures (SOPs), 706, 707t
Starch granules, in urinary sediment, 437f
Steatitis, nodular, 37–38, 38b, 40f, 41f
Steatosis, 343–344
Sterile granulomatous dermatitis, 44
Steroid-responsive suppurative meningitis-arteritis, 525, 525f
Stomach, 301–307
  fundic glands of, 302f
  hyperplasia of, 303
  infection of
    Candida spp., 310
    Physaloptera sp., 303–304, 305f
  inflammation of, 303–306, 304f, 305f
  lymphocytic, 303f, 304f
  mucin granules of, 302f
  neoplasia of, 306–307, 306f
  neutrophilic gastritis, 304f
  normal cytology of, 301–303, 302f, 303f, 304f
  spiral-shaped bacteria of, 303f
Stomatitis
  eosinophilic, 289f
  neutrophilic, 289f
Storiform pattern, 30, 31f, 32f

Subarachnoid space, cerebrospinal fluid collection from, 513
Subcutis, 35, 36f
Subgross morphology
  of neoplasm, 692
  of non-neoplastic tumor, 693
Substage condenser, 666f
Sulfonamide crystals, 426t, 430f, 431f
Superficial cells, of vagina, 462
Suppurative joint disease, 488–491, 488f
Suppurative lesions, 15
Surface epithelium, in cerebrospinal fluid, 522
Sweat gland, tumors of, 80–82, 81f, 82b
Sweet spot, 3–4, 4f, 5b
Synovial fluid
  anatomy of, 485, 486f
  appearance of, 486–488
  cell and differential counts of, 488
  characteristics of, 486b
  classification of abnormal, 486t
  in degenerative joint disease, 491–493, 492f
  evaluation of, 485–498
  handling of, 485–486
  in hemarthrosis, 493–495, 496f
  hyaluronic acid in, 486
  in infectious arthritis, 489–491, 489f, 490b, 490f, 491b
  mucin clot test of, 486–487, 487f
  nondegenerate neutrophils in, 17f
  in noninfectious arthritis, 491, 491f, 492f
  production of, 485
  protein concentration in, 488
  sample collection of, 485–486
  in suppurative joint disease, 488–491, 488f
  viscosity of, 486–488, 487f
Synovium, neoplasia of, 495–496, 497f, 498b, 498f
Systemic mycoses, 254, 254f, 255f, 266
Systemic protozoonosis, 255, 256f
Systemic quantitative antigen EIA, 696–699t

T

T zone lymphoma, 654
Tape preparations, 6
Tarsocrural joint, sample collection from, 485–486
TCC. see Transitional cell carcinoma
Tears, 582
Telomerase, as marker, in veterinary oncology, 635
Tenosynovitis, bicipital, 491–493
Teratomas, ovarian, 456–457, 458f, 459f
Testes, 475–481
  anatomy of, normal, 476
  collection techniques for, 476
  cytology of, normal, 476–478, 477f
  fine-needle aspiration of, 475–476
  histology of, normal, 476, 477f
  inflammation of, 478
  neoplasia of, 478, 478f, 478t
  seminoma of, 478–479, 479f
  tumors of
    interstitial cell, 479–481, 480f
    Sertoli cell, 479, 479f, 480f
ThinPreps, for immunocytochemistry, 618–623
Thixotropy, 485–486
Thorax, removal of fluid from, 242
Thymic cyst, 175f
Thymic mass, 178f

Thymoma, 173–178, 176f, 177f, 178f, 179f
  detection of, by flow cytometry, 655f
Thymus, 171–178
  anatomy and histology of, 171–172, 174f
  biopsy of, 171–178
  Hassall's corpuscles of, 171–172, 174f
  non-neoplastic tumor, 173, 175f
Thyroid gland, 596–604, 597t, 598f
  naked nuclei neoplasm of, 114–115, 115f
  nonneoplastic diseases of, 596–599, 598f, 599t
    in cats, 599–604, 599f, 600f, 601f, 602f, 602t
    in dogs, 599–604, 599f, 600f, 601f, 602f, 602t
  normal, 598f
  tumors of, 26–27, 28f, 602t
    canine, 602–603
    feline, 603–604, 603f, 604b
Thyroid transcription factor-1 (TTF1), 634
Tick bite reaction, 37, 40f
Tissue injury, response to, 20f, 21f, 22f, 117–121
Total nucleated cell count, in body cavity fluids, 244–245, 245b
Touch imprint, 5–6, 5f, 6f
Toxoplasma gondii infection
  in lungs, 222, 223f
  mammary gland, 443–444
  in respiratory tract, 189t
Toxoplasma sp., in nervous system tissues, 544, 544f
Toxoplasmosis, 59, 59f, 256f
Trabecular pattern, 30, 31f
Trachea, 204–237
  anatomy of, 204
  collection techniques for, 204–207
  cytology of, 207–209, 207f, 207t, 208f
Tracheal wash, 204–205
Tracheitis
  bacterial, 216, 216f
  viral, 215
Tracheobronchial tract
  infectious causes of disease of, 212–213
  infectious inflammatory disorders of, 215–228
  inflammation of, 210–212
  metaplasia of, 213
  noninfectious inflammatory disorders of, 214–215
  normal cytology of, 207–209
Tracheobronchomalacia, 214
Transitional carcinoma, nasal, 196, 196f
Transitional cell carcinoma (TCC), 24f, 29f
  of prostate gland, 474–475, 476f
Transmissible venereal tumors (TVTs)
  canine, 113–114, 114b, 114f, 198, 198f
  vaginal, 466–467, 468f, 470f
Transthoracic fine-needle aspiration, 206–207
Transtracheal wash, 204b, 205f
Transudate, 246f, 247–248, 248f
Traumatic urethral catheterization, for bladder specimen, 407
Treponeme-like bacteria, in dry-mount fecal cytology, 389–390, 390f
Triaditis, 329
Trichoblastoma, 70, 71f, 72f
Trichoepithelioma, 72, 73f
Trichuris vulpis infection, 315–316
Triglycerides, in body cavity fluids, 283t
Trypomastigotes, 702
TTF1. see Thyroid transcription factor-1

Tumors
  common ultrastructural features of, 644–646t
  diagnosis of, organelle approach to, 643–644t
  diagnostic immunohistochemistry of, panel markers for, 631–632, 632t, 633f
  non-neoplastic, 193
TVTs. see Transmissible venereal tumors
Tympanokeratoma, 591–592
Tyrosine crystals, 424, 426t

U

Ultrasound, fine-needle aspiration biopsy guided by, 1–2, 3f
  of kidney, 397
Ultrasound gel, 3f
  as artifact, 158, 158f
Ureters, 406, 407f
  anatomy and histology of, normal, 397
Urethra
  anatomy and histology of, normal, 397, 406–407
  discharge from, 468
  inflammatory disorders of, 407–408, 408f
  normal cytology and artifacts of, 407, 407f
  specimen collection from, 407
Urinary sediment, 414–439
  artifacts, 437
  casts in, 421–423, 424b
    cellular, 422, 423f
    granular, 422, 424f
    hyaline, 421–422, 422f, 425f
    myoglobin, 423f
    red cell, 423f
    waxy, 423, 424f, 425f
  cellular components, 417–421
  collection, 414
  complete urinalysis, 414, 415b
  contaminated, 421f
  cotton fibers in, 437f
  crystals in, 423–428, 426t
    acid urine, 424–425, 431b
    alkaline urine, 425–428, 432f, 433f
    ammonium biurate, 426t, 433f
    amorphous urates, 426t, 427f
    bilirubin, 426t, 429f
    calcium carbonate, 426t, 434f
    calcium hydrogen phosphate dihydrate, 426t, 430f
    calcium oxalate dihydrate, 426t, 428f
    calcium oxalate monohydrate, 426t, 428f, 429f
    calcium phosphate, 426t, 430f
    cholesterol, 426t
    cystine, 426t, 430f
    magnesium ammonium phosphate, 432f
    radiopaque contrast dye, 437f
    sodium urate, 426t, 427f
    struvite, 432f
    sulfonamides, 426t, 430f, 431f
    tyrosine, 426t
    uric acid, 426t, 427f
  epithelial cells in, 417b, 418–421, 419f, 420f, 421f, 422f
  erythrocytes in, 417–418, 418b
  hyphal forms of fungi in, 435f
  infectious agents in, 428–434, 434b, 434f, 435f, 436f

Urinary sediment *(Continued)*
  leukocytes in, 418, 418b, 419f
  lipid droplets in, 416, 417f, 434, 437f
  mannitol crystals, 438f
  microscopic examination of, 415b
    recording of, 416–437
    Sedi-Stain in, 417f
  pollen grains in, 438f
  preparation of, 414–416
  specimen processing, 414–416
    dry-mount, 416
    wet-mount, 414–416, 416f, 417f
  spermatozoa, 434–437
  stained, 415–416
  starch granules in, 437f
  unstained, 415, 416f, 417f
  yeast in, 432, 436f
Urinary system, 397–413
Urine. *see* Urinary sediment
Urine BRAF mutation detection assay, for urothelial carcinoma, 696–699t
Uroabdomen, 261–263, 262f, 263f
Uroperitoneum effusion, 261–263, 262f, 263f
Uroplakin III, 634
Urothelial carcinoma
  renal, 404, 404f
  urine BRAF mutation detection assay for, 696–699t
Uterus, 458–461
  anatomy of, normal, 459
  collection techniques for, 459
  cystic endometrial hyperplasia-pyometra complex of, 460
  cytology of, normal, 460
  histology of, normal, 459, 459f
  neoplasia of, 461

Uvea
  anterior, 571
  posterior, retina, 574
Uveitis
  anterior, 572, 573f
  neutrophilic, 575f

V

Vacuolation, 347
Vagina, 461–467
  anatomy of, normal, 461
  basal cells of, 461
  collection techniques for, 461
  cytology of, normal, 461–462, 462f
  eosinophilic index of, 461
  in estrous cycle
    canine, 462–465, 463f, 463t, 464f
    feline, 465
    inflammation of, 465
  histology of, normal, 461
  intermediate cells of, 462
  leiomyoma of, 465–466, 466f
  neoplasia of, 465–467, 466f, 468f, 470f
  parabasal cells of, 461
  superficial cells of, 462
  transmissible venereal tumor of, 466–467, 468f, 470f
Vaginitis, 465, 465f, 466f
Venereal tumor, 25, 28f
  transmissible, canine, 113–114, 114b, 114f
Vernier scale usage, 669
Vestibular glands, 461
Veterinary diagnostic cytopathology services
  list of suggested content for, 707t
  quality management recommendations for, 706, 706f, 707t, 708f, 710f, 711b

Veterinary diagnostic cytopathology services *(Continued)*
  suggested quality metrics for, 711b
Vimentin, 634
Viral infections, nasal, 187–188
Viral papilloma, 64–67, 66f, 67f, 68f
Viruses, 700, 701f
  canine distemper, 531–532, 531f
  cerebrospinal fluid analysis for, 517
  feline leukemia, 131
Vitreocentesis, 575–576, 578f
Vitreous body, 575–576, 579f
  collection of, 575–576, 578f
  neoplasia of, 576
  normal cytology of, 575–576, 578f
Vomeronasal organ, 182

W

Whole slide imaging system validation, recommendations for, 711b
Windrowing, in synovial fluid, 487–488, 487f, 488f
Workflow path, 706, 706f

X

Xanthochromia, of cerebrospinal fluid, 516, 516f
Xanthomatosis, cutaneous, 42–44, 43f, 44b, 44f

Y

Yeast
  incidental, in dry-mount fecal cytology, 379f, 380f
  in urinary sediment, 432, 436f
Yersinia pestis infection, in respiratory tract, 219

bacteria (including *Mycoplasma* spp. and *Ureaplasma* spp.) into the prostate gland (Cunto et al., 2019). Hematogenous and local spread from other urogenital organs is also possible. *E. coli* is the most commonly isolated organism from both acute and chronic cases of prostatitis followed by *Staphylococcus aureus*, *Klebsiella* spp., *Proteus mirabilis*, *Mycoplasma canis*, *Pseudomonas aeruginosa*, *Enterobacter* spp., *Streptococcus* spp., *Pasteurella* spp., and *Haemophilus* spp. (Cunto et al., 2019). *Brucella canis* may infect the canine prostate, but it is more commonly associated with epididymal and testicular infection and clinical signs referable to those organs (Cunto et al., 2019). Anaerobic bacteria or fungal infections *(Blastomyces dermatitidis)* (Reed et al., 2010), *Cryptococcus neoformans*, and *Coccidioides* spp. also have been observed via hematogenous spread, urethral ascent, or penetration through the scrotum with descending prostate infection from a testicular source (Cunto et al., 2019). Infertility and chronic prostatitis caused by *Leishmania infantum* and *Bartonella* spp. infection have been rarely reported. Alteration of normal architecture by diseases such as prostatic hyperplasia, squamous metaplasia, and neoplasia can interfere with normal defense mechanisms or provide a medium (i.e., blood in cysts) for bacterial growth. Coalescing of focal areas of septic prostatitis or infection of prostatic cysts may result in prostatic abscesses.

Acute prostatitis is usually associated with systemic signs of illness (fever, anorexia, and lethargy); straining to urinate or defecate; hematuria; and edema of the scrotum, prepuce, and hind limb or pain on rectal palpation of the prostate gland. The dog may also experience locomotor problems because of caudal lumbar or abdominal pain. An inflammatory leukogram with or without a left shift is often present. Clinical signs in dogs with chronic prostatitis may be absent, or there may be recurrent urinary tract infection, poor semen quality with infertility, or occasionally decreased libido (Cunto et al., 2019). Intermittent or constant urethral discharge may also be noted. Prostatic abscesses may present with signs related to enlargement of the prostate (tenesmus, dysuria), constant or intermittent urethral discharge, and evidence of systemic illness related to endotoxemia or peritonitis. Treatment of prostatitis involves appropriate antibiotic therapy as determined by culture and sensitivity. In acute prostatitis, most antibiotics reach the site of infection because the prostate-lipid barrier is disrupted. Antibiotics for the treatment of chronic prostatitis should be selected for the ability to cross the lipid barrier, which is usually intact and for the ability to concentrate in the prostate. In addition to appropriate antibiotic therapy, prostatic abscesses can be treated surgically with marsupialization of the gland, placement of a drain, or prostatectomy. All of these surgical procedures are associated with significant complications. Castration should also be performed in dogs with prostatitis (Cunto et al., 2019).

Cytopathologic evaluation of samples from bacterial prostatitis contains large numbers of neutrophils, many of which exhibit degenerative changes of karyolysis and karyorrhexis (Figs. 13.64 and 13.65). Macrophages may also be present, especially in chronic prostatitis (Figs. 13.66 and 13.67). In the absence of previous antibiotic therapy, intracellular and extracellular organisms may be seen (Boland et al., 2003). Epithelial cells that are present may appear normal or hyperplastic as evidenced by increased cytoplasmic basophilia, increased N:C, and mild anisokaryosis (Fig. 13.68). Cellular atypia associated with prostatic epithelial cells in the presence of inflammation

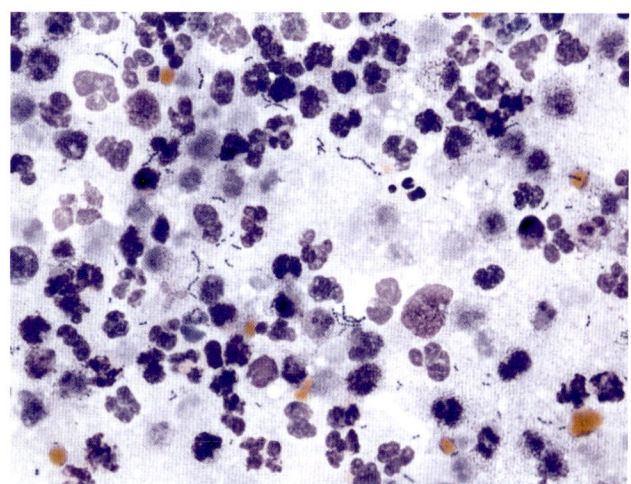

■ **FIGURE 13.64 Prostatic abscess. Prostate aspirate. Dog.** Many degenerate neutrophils, chains of bacterial cocci, and amorphous, basophilic debris (necrosis). Bacterial culture identified a pure growth of *Streptococcus canis* (group G). (Wright-Giemsa; HP oil.) (Courtesy Katie Boes, Virginia Polytechnic Institute and State University.)

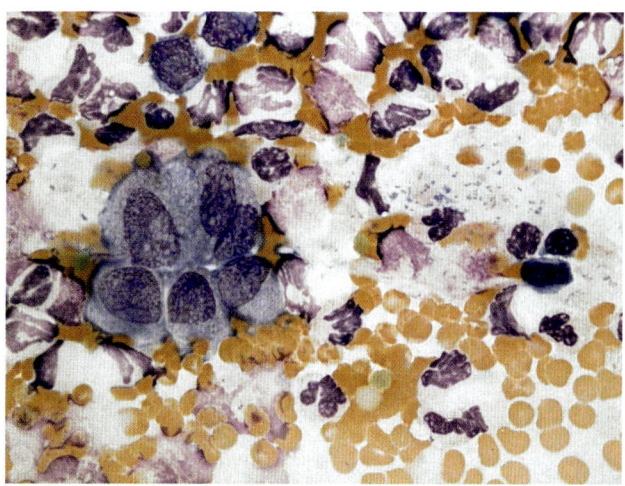

■ **FIGURE 13.65 Prostatic carcinoma with secondary bacterial prostatitis. Prostate aspirate. Dog.** A sheet of six neoplastic, round epithelial cells is surrounded by freely dispersed erythrocytes, degenerate and nondegenerate neutrophils, and extracellular bacteria. The bacteria are less than 1 μm in diameter, pleomorphic, and lightly basophilic, compatible with *Mycoplasma* spp. or *Ureaplasma* spp. (Wright-Giemsa; HP oil.) (Courtesy Katie Boes, Virginia Polytechnic Institute and State University.)

should be interpreted cautiously to avoid a false-positive diagnosis of neoplasia.

Prostatic Neoplasia

Malignant prostatic tumors are rare with a reported annual prevalence of 0.0% to 0.9%, with Shetland sheep dogs and Scottish terriers having an increased risk (Bryan et al., 2007). The same condition in cats is extremely rare (Foster, 2017b). Although prostatic cancers may occur in intact or castrated male dogs, castrated male dogs have an increased risk for urothelial (transitional cell) carcinoma, prostate adenocarcinoma, and

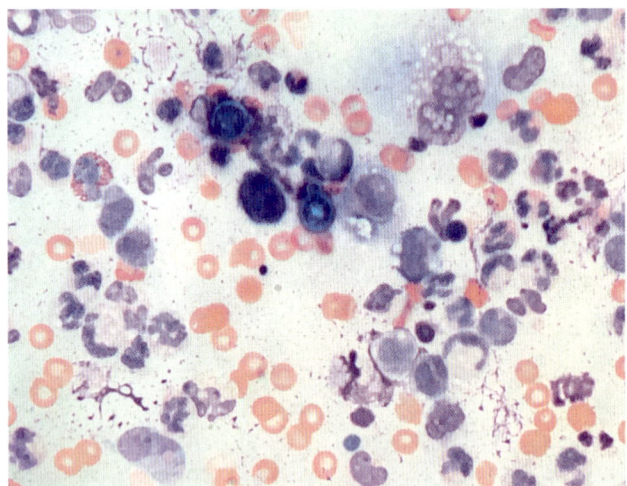

■ **FIGURE 13.66 Fungal prostatitis. Prostate aspirate. Dog.** This dog presented with a history of sudden inability to urinate; on rectal palpation, the prostate was markedly enlarged. Neutrophils, macrophages, and eosinophils were present along with two yeasts, one of which displays broad-based budding. The dog had been treated for dermal blastomycosis 4 months earlier. (Modified Wright; HP oil.) (Courtesy Rose Raskin, Purdue University.)

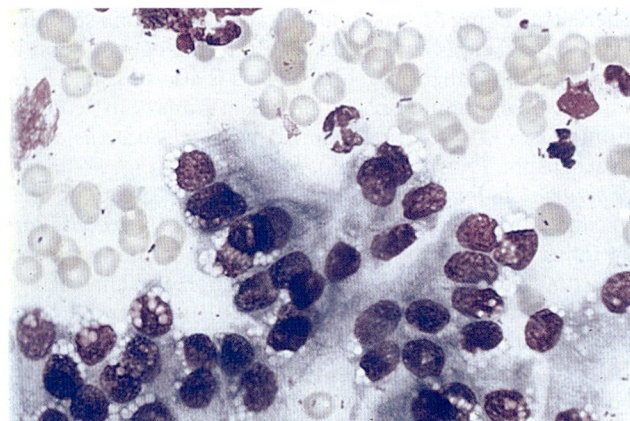

■ **FIGURE 13.68 Bacterial prostatitis. Prostate aspirate. Dog.** Prostatic epithelial cells and neutrophils are present in this example of acute septic prostatitis. Prostatic epithelial cells display increased cytoplasmic basophilia and cytoplasmic vacuolization compatible with hyperplasia. Neutrophils are degenerate as indicated by moderate karyolysis. Bacterial bacilli are present in the background and within the neutrophils. (Wright-Giemsa; HP oil.)

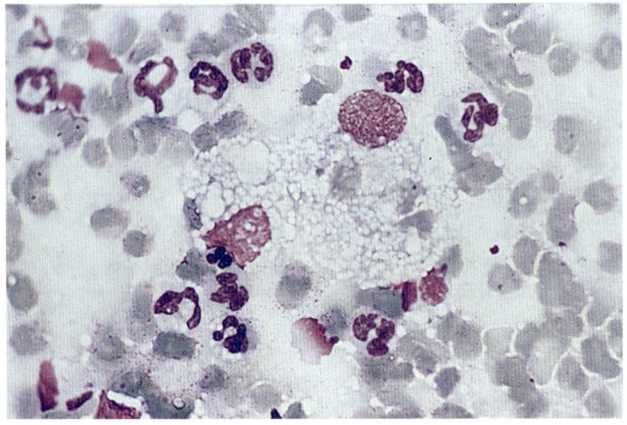

■ **FIGURE 13.67 Mixed-cell prostatitis. Prostate aspirate. Dog.** A mixed cell population is present in this case of chronic prostatitis. Increased numbers of neutrophils, the majority of which are nondegenerate, and two reactive macrophages are present. Infectious organisms were not seen in this sample. (Wright-Giemsa; HP oil.)

prostate carcinoma (Bryan et al., 2007). The mean age of diagnosis is 10 years (Cunto et al., 2019). Adenocarcinoma was the most commonly reported neoplasm of the prostate followed by urothelial (transitional cell) carcinoma arising from the prostatic urethra. However, other epithelial neoplasms have been described, such as undifferentiated carcinoma and SCC. Prostatic intraepithelial neoplasia, a precursor lesion of prostatic carcinoma, has been rarely reported in neoplastic prostate glands. Other malignant neoplasms have been rarely described such as lymphoma and malignant mesenchymal tumors, such as hemangiosarcoma and leiomyosarcoma, and prostatic sarcomatoid carcinoma (Pinto da Cunha et al., 2007; Agnew and MacLachlan, 2017). Canine prostatic carcinoma is an insidious disease, with many dogs showing no evidence of clinical abnormalities until late in the course of the malignancy. The most frequently detected abnormality during physical examination is prostatomegaly, which is identified in 52% of dogs with prostatic carcinoma. The enlargement is primarily asymmetrical (32%); however, sometimes symmetrical enlargement (6%) can be noted. Other physical abnormalities include depression, painful abdominal palpation, cachexia, pyrexia, dyspnea, dysuria, stranguria, hematuria, tenesmus, weight loss, gait abnormalities, and presence of an abdominal mass. Complete obstruction of urinary flow may result in hydroureter, hydronephrosis, and subsequent renal failure (Cunto et al., 2019).

Histologically, most canine prostatic carcinomas are of an intraalveolar pattern, but many also contain patterns similar to urothelial (transitional cell) carcinoma. Until further definition of a standardized immunohistochemical diagnostic panel, three general types of carcinoma of the prostate are histologically identified: (1) prostatic urothelial carcinoma (UC, transitional cell carcinoma), (2) prostatic adenocarcinoma, and (3) prostatic carcinoma with mixed urothelial and glandular phenotypes (i.e., when prostatic carcinoma shows mixed morphologic features within the same tissue section) (Palmieri et al., 2019a). Neoplastic canine prostate glands also frequently contain foci of prostatic hyperplasia, cystic glandular dilatation, and significant suppurative and lymphoplasmacytic inflammation. Interestingly, a significant increase in density of T and B lymphocytes in prostatic adenocarcinoma was found compared with normal prostate and in prostatic hyperplasia (Palmieri et al., 2019b).

Fine-needle aspiration is useful for the diagnosis of prostatic neoplasia, and there is good diagnostic agreement between cytopathology and histopathology for prostatic adenocarcinoma (Powe et al., 2004). Cytopathologic evaluation of FNA samples from prostatic adenocarcinoma usually reveals large numbers of deeply basophilic, frequently vacuolated epithelial cells arranged in variably sized clusters and sheets. N:C is often high, and anisokaryosis and anisocytosis can be moderate to marked. Nuclei are round to pleomorphic, and nucleoli are large, prominent, and often multiple. Binucleation may be noted. Prostatic adenocarcinoma (Fig. 13.69) and urothelial (transitional cell)